WRIGHT'S LIVER AND BILIARY DISEASE

WRIGHT'S LIVER AND BILIARY DISEASE

Pathophysiology, Diagnosis and Management

G.H. Millward-Sadler

BSc, MBChB, FRCPath, MHSM

Consultant Pathologist, Southampton University Hospitals;
Honorary Senior Lecturer, Faculty of Medicine, University of Southampton,
UK

R. Wright

MA, MD, DPhil, FRCP

Formerly Professor of Medicine, Faculty of Medicine, University of
Southampton, UK

M.J.P. Arthur

DM, MRCP

Professor of Medicine, Faculty of Medicine, University of Southampton;
Honorary Consultant Physician, Southampton University Hospitals, UK

THIRD EDITION
VOLUME ONE

W.B. SAUNDERS COMPANY LTD

London   Philadelphia   Toronto   Sydney   Tokyo

This book is printed on acid free paper

W.B. Saunders Company Ltd

24–28 Oval Road
London NW1 7DX

The Curtis Center
Independence Square West
Philadelphia, PA 19106–3399

55 Horner Avenue
Toronto, Ontario M8Z 4X6, Canada

Harcourt Brace Jovanovich (Australia) Pty Ltd,
30–52 Smidmore St
Marrickville, NSW 2204, Australia

Harcourt Brace Jovanovich Japan Inc.
Ichibancho Central Building, 22-1 Ichibancho
Chiyoda-ku, Tokyo 102, Japan

First published 1979
Second edition 1985
Third edition 1992

A catalogue record for this book is available from the British Library.

Volume 1   ISBN 0-7020-1655-1
Volume 2   ISBN 0-7020-1656-X
        Set   ISBN 0-7020-1392-7

Typeset by Photo-graphics, Honiton, Devon
Printed and bound in Great Britain by the University Press, Cambridge

Professor Ralph Wright

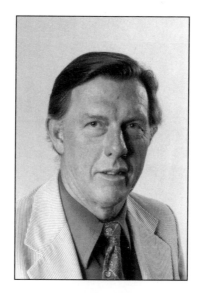

1930–1990

Ralph Wright, Professor of Medicine at the University of Southampton Medical School, graduated from Cape Town in 1954. Soon after specializing he spent a year as District Surgeon in a 300 bed hospital serving a large Zulu population. From there he went to the University of Natal Medical School where he led a team which pioneered a new treatment of tetanus neoatorum and halved its mortality. Throughout his life he had a strong love for the country and its peoples but an intense dislike of its political regime. He left South Africa in 1960 taking up a junior post in the Nuffield Department of Medicine at the Radcliffe Infirmary in Oxford from which he progressed to become May Reader in 1969. During this period in Oxford he published extensively with Dr Sidney Truelove on the immunopathology of diseases of the gut and whilst on a year's sabbatical with Dr Gerry Klatskin in Yale, described the association of the Australia antigen (HBsAg) with (acute and) chronic hepatitis. On his return he carried out a large survey on the association of halothane anaesthesia with acute liver disease.

In 1971 he was appointed Professor of Medicine in Southampton where he soon established a thriving department orientated towards gastrointestinal medicine and liver disease. From amongst the many papers and projects produced by his department he took an especial pride in the success of this international multi-author reference book on liver and biliary disease which he conceived and co-edited. He identified the need for an international reference book on liver disease that had a focused multidisciplinary approach. It was his reputation as a hepatologist that brought together from all parts of the world the large number of specialists whose contributions have made this book so successful.

Despite his international reputation as an expert in liver diseases, we will mostly remember him for his personal qualities. A keen sportsman he played in goal for the combined South African Universities football team in his student days, and in later life became an enthusiastic yachtsman. He was an open and approachable man of boundless energy who hated pomposity and pretentiousness and who believed firmly in the principles of equality in all aspects of his work and life. Above all else he was a man devoted to his family.

Working with him was a privilege. Knowing him was both a pleasure and an inspiration.

G.H. MILLWARD-SADLER
M.J.P. ARTHUR

Contents

VOLUME TWO

Contributors

Duncan Melville Ackery, MA, MB, MSc, FRCR
Consultant and Honorary Clinical Professor of Nuclear Medicine, Department of Nuclear Medicine, Southampton University Hospitals, Tremona Road, Southampton SO9 4XY, UK.
Radionuclide Imaging

K.G.M.M. Alberti, MA, DPhil, BM BCh, FRCP, FRCP(E), FRCPath
Professor of Medicine, Department of Medicine, The Medical School, Framlington Place, Newcastle upon Tyne NE2 4HH, UK.
Carbohydrate Metabolism, The Liver and the Endocrine System

Michael J.P. Arthur, DM, MCRP
Professor of Medicine, Faculty of Medicine, University of Southampton; Honorary Consultant Physician, Southampton University Hospitals, Tremona Road, Southampton SO9 4XY, UK.
Acute Viral Hepatitis, Liver Fibrosis and Cirrhosis

Irving S. Benjamin, BSc, MD, FRCS
Professor of Surgery and Director, Department of Surgery, King's College School of Medicine and Dentistry, Rayne Institute, 123 Coldharbour Lane, London SE5 9NU, UK.
Biliary Bypass and Reconstructive Surgery

D. Montgomery Bissell, MD
Professor of Medicine, San Francisco School of Medicine, University of California; Attending Physician, University of California Hospitals and San Francisco General Hospital Medical Center, San Francisco CA, USA.
Haem Metabolism

Richard M. Blaquière, BSc, MB ChB, FRCR
Consultant Radiologist, Wessex Bodyscanner Unit, Southampton University Hospitals, Tremona Road, Southampton SO9 4XY, UK.
Computed Tomography

T. Blanchard, BSc, MRCP
Research Fellow, London School of Hygiene and Tropical Medicine, Keppel Street, London WC1; Honorary Senior Registrar, Hospital for Tropical Diseases, London, UK.
The Liver in Infection

Leslie H. Blumgart, BDS, MD, FRCS
Direktor der Universitätsklinik für Viszerace und Transplantationschirurige, Inselspital, CH-3010, Berne, Switzerland;
Department of Surgery, Memorial Sloan-Kettering Cancer Center, 1275 York Avenue, NY 10021, USA.
Biliary Bypass and Reconstructive Surgery, Tumours of the Extrahepatic Biliary Tree and Pancreas

David J. Bouchier-Hayes, MCh, FRCSI, FRCS
Professor of Surgery, Department of Surgery, The Royal College of Surgeons in Ireland, Beaumont Hospital, Dublin 9, Republic of Ireland.
The Physiology of the Gallbladder

Nancy L.R. Bucher, MD
Research Professor of Pathology, Department of Pathology, Boston University School of Medicine, 80 East Concord Street, Boston, MA 02118, USA.
Regulatory Mechanisms in Hepatic Regeneration

F. Geoffrey Bull, BSc, DPhil
Senior Experimental Officer, Professorial Medical Unit, Southampton University Hositals, Tremona Road, Southampton SO9 4XY, UK.
Acute Viral Hepatitis

Sir Roy Y. Calne, MB BS, FRCS(Eng), MS, MA, FRCP, FRS
Professor of Surgery and Honorary Consultant Surgeon, Cambridge University Department of Surgery, Addenbrooke's Hospital, Hills Road, Cambridge CB2 2QQ, UK.
Surgical Aspects of Liver Transplantation

Joyce A. Carlson, MD, PhD
Assistant Chief of Staff, Department of Clinical Chemistry, University of Lund, Malmö General Hospital, S-214 O, Malmö, Sweden.
Apha-1-Antitrypsin Deficiency

Morag Chisholm, MB ChB, MD, FRCPath
Senior Lecturer in Haematology, Faculty of Medicine, University of Southampton; Consultant Haematologist, Southampton University Hospitals, Tremona Road, Southampton SO9 4XY, UK.
Haematological Disorders

Meinhard Classen, MD
Professor of Medicine, Head, 2nd Department of Medicine, Technical University of Munich, Klinikum rechts der Isar, Ismaninger Strasse 22, DW-8000 Munich 80, Germany.
Endoscopic Examination and Therapy

Russell E. Cowan, MD, MRCP
Consultant Physician, Essex County Hospital, Lexden Road, Colchester, Essex, UK.
Peritoneoscopy

Ara Darzi, FRCSI
Registrar in Surgery, The Central Middlesex Hospital, London, UK.
The Physiology of the Gallbladder

Mark Davenport, MC ChB, FRCS (Eng), FRCS (Glasg)
Lecturer in Paediatric Surgery, King's College Hospital and Medical School, Denmark Hill, London SE5 9RS, UK.
Paediatric Liver Disease: Surgical Aspects

J.L. Dawson, MS, FRCS
Consultant Surgeon, King's College Hospital and Medical School, Denmark Hill, London SE5 9RS, UK.
Normal Anatomy

Keith C. Dewbury, BSc, MB BS, FRCR
Consultant Radiologist, Southampton University Hospitals, Tremona Road, Southampton SO9 4XY; Honorary Clinical Senior Lecturer, Faculty of Medicine, University of Southampton, UK.
Ultrasound Imaging, Investigation of the Jaundiced Patient

Robert Dick, MB BS, FRACR, FRCR
Consultant Radiologist, Royal Free Hospital, London; Admissions Sub-Dean, Royal Free Hospital School of Medicine, Pond Street, London NW3 2QG, UK.
Angiography

David R. Fine, MB BS, MRCP, MD
Consultant Gastroenterologist, Southampton University Hospitals, Tremona Road, Southampton SO9 4XY, UK.
Calculous Disease and Cholecystitis

Josef E. Fischer, MD
Professor and Chairman, Department of Surgery, University of Cincinnati Medical Center, 231 Bethesda Avenue, Cincinnati, OH 45267-0558, USA.
Portal-Systemic Encephalopathy

Scott L. Friedman, MD
Assistant Professor of Medicine, University of California, San Francisco; Attending Gastroenterologist, San Francisco General Hospital, San Francisco, CA 94110, USA.
Liver Fibrosis and Cirrhosis

Peter J. Friend, MA, MB BChir, FRCS
University Lecturer and Honorary Consultant Surgeon, Addenbrooke's Hospital, Cambridge CB2 2QQ, UK.
Surgical Aspects of Liver Transplantation

Susan V. Gelding, MRCP
RD Lawrence Research Fellow, St Mary's Hospital Medical School, Paddington, London, UK.
The Liver and the Endocrine System

Charles F. George, BSc, MD, FRCP
Professor of Clinical Pharmacology, Faculty of Medicine, University of Southampton; Honorary Consultant Physician, Southampton University Hospitals, Tremona Road, Southampton SO9 4XY, UK.
The Liver and Response to Drugs

Richard H. George, MB ChB, FRCPath
Senior Clinical Lecturer, University of Birmingham; Consultant Microbiologist, Children's Hospital, Ladywood Middleway, Birmingham B16 8ET and Birmingham Maternity Hospital, Queen Elizabeth Medical Centre, Birmingham B15 2TG, UK.
The Liver and Response to Drugs

Norman Gitlin, MD, FRCP, FRCPE, FACP, FACG
Professor of Medicine, University of California, San Francisco; Chief of Gastroenterology, Veterans Administration Medical Center, Fresno, CA 93703, USA.
Liver Disease in Pregnancy

John L. Gollan, MD, PhD, FRACP, FRCP
Associate Professor of Medicine, Harvard Medical School, Boston; Consultant Physician, Children's Hospital Medical Center, Boston; Director, Gastroenterology Division, Brigham and Women's Hospital, 75 Francis Street, Boston MA 02115, USA.
Bilirubin Metabolism

Pierce A. Grace, MCh, FRCSI
Lecturer in Surgery, Department of Surgery, The Royal College of Surgeons in Ireland, Beaumont Hospital, Dublin 9, Republic of Ireland.
The Physiology of the Gallbladder

David S. Harry, PhD, BTech
Clinical Scientist, Honorary Lecturer, Department of Medicine, Royal Free Hospital, Pond Street, London NW3 2QG, UK.
Plasma Lipoproteins

Stephen Crane Hauser, MD
Assistant Professor of Medicine, Harvard Medical School, Boston; Director, Gastroenterology Clinics, Brigham and Women's Hospital, 75 Francis Street, Boston, MA 02115, USA.
Bilirubin Metabolism

Jay P. Heiken, MD
Associate Professor of Radiology, Co-Director, Computed Body Tomography, Mallinckrodt Institute of Radiology, Washington University School of Medicine, St Louis, Missouri, USA.
Magnetic Resonance Imaging

John Herbetko, MB BS, FRCR
Senior Registrar in Radiology, Southampton University Hospitals, Tremona Road, Southampton SO9 4XY, UK.
Ultrasound Imaging

R. Hickman, MB ChB, MD, CLM, FCS
Associate Professor, Department of Surgery, University of Cape Town; Deputy Director, MRC/UCT Liver Research Centre, Cape Town, South Africa.
Acute Liver Failure

R.J. Hift, MB ChB, FCP
Research Fellow, MRC/UCT Liver Research Centre, Department of Medicine, University of Cape Town and Groote Schuur Hospital, Cape Town, South Africa.
Acute Liver Failure

K.E.F. Hobbs, ChM, FRCS
Professor of Surgery, Royal Free Hospital School of Medicine; Honorary Consultant Surgeon, Royal Free Hospital Academic Department of Surgery, Royal Free Hospital, Pond Street, London NW3 2QG, UK.
The Surgery of Portal Hypertension

Alan F. Hofmann, MD, PhD, MD hon.causis
Professor of Medicine, Department of Medicine, T-013, University of California, San Diego, La Jolla, CA 92093, USA.
Bile Acids

G. Holdstock, DM, MRCP
Consultant Physician, Hillingdon Hospital, Pield Heath Road, Uxbridge UB8 3NN, UK.
Hepatic Changes in Systemic Disease, The Liver in Infection

Edward R. Howard, MS, FRCS
Consultant Surgeon and Honorary Senior Lecturer, King's College Hospital and Medical School, Denmark Hill, London SE5 9RS, UK.
Paediatric Liver Disease: Surgical Aspects

Colin W. Howden, MD, MRCP
Division of Digestive Diseases and Nutrition, University of South Carolina School of Medicine, 2 Richland Medical Park, Suite 506, Columbia, SC 29203, USA.
The Liver and Response to Drugs

Clement W. Imrie, BSc, MB ChB, FRCS
Honorary Senior Lecturer, University of Glasgow; Consultant Surgeon, Royal Infirmary, Glasgow G4 0SF, UK.
Tumours of the Extrahepatic Biliary Tree and Pancreas

J.P. Iredale, BM, MRCP
MRC Training Fellow, Professorial Medical Unit, Southampton University Hospitals, Tremona Road, Southampton SO9 4XY, UK.
Hepatic Changes in Systemic Disease

Kurt J. Isselbacher, MD
Professor of Medicine, Harvard Medical School; Chief, Gastrointestinal Unit, Massachusetts General Hospital, Boston, Massachusetts, USA.
Postoperative Jaundice

Shun Iwatsuki, MD
Associate Professor of Surgery, 5C Falk Clinic, 3601 Fifth Avenue, Pittsburgh, PA 15213, USA.
Portal-Systemic Shunting

Meron R. Jacyna, MD, MRCP
Consultant Physician and Gastroenterologist, Northwick Park Hospital, Harrow HA1 3UJ; Honorary Senior Lecturer, St Mary's Hospital Medical School, Paddington, London W2, UK.
Chronic Hepatitis

Neville Victor Jamieson, MA, MB BS, MD, FRCS
Honorary Consultant Surgeon and University Lecturer, Cambridge University Department of Surgery, Addenbrooke's Hospital, Hills Road, Cambridge CB2 2QQ, UK.
Surgical Aspects of Liver Transplantation

Anne-Marie Jezequel, MD
Professor of Pathology, University of Ancona School of Medicine, 60100 Ancona, Italy.
Normal Histology and Ultrastructure, Ultrastructural Pathology

C.D. Johnson, MChir, FRCS
Senior Lecturer and Honorary Consultant Surgeon, University Surgical Unit, Southampton University Hospitals, Tremona Road, Southampton SO9 4XY, UK.
Calculous Disease and Cholecystitis

Desmond G. Johnston, PhD, FRCP
Professor of Clinical Endocrinology, St Mary's Hospital Medical School, Norfolk Place, London W2 1PG, UK.
Carbohydrate Metabolism, The Liver and the Endocrine System

Peter S. Johnston, MB ChB, FRACS
University Lecturer and Honorary Consultant Surgeon, Addenbrooke's Hospital, Hills Road, Cambridge CB2 2QQ, UK.
Surgical Aspects of Liver Transplantation

D. Kahn, MB ChB, ChM, FCS
Senior Specialist and Senior Lecturer, MRC/UCT Liver Research Centre, Department of Surgery, University of Cape Town and Groote Schuur Hospital, Cape Town, South Africa.
Acute Liver Failure

Stephen Karran, MA, MChir, FRCS, FRCS(Ed)
Reader in Surgery, Faculty of Medicine, University of Southampton; Honorary Consultant Surgeon, Southampton University Hospitals, Tremona Road, Southampton SO9 4XY, UK.
Physical Aspects of Hepatic Regeneration, Investigation of the Jaundiced Patient, Calculous Disease and Cholecystitis

R.E. Kirsch, MB ChB, MD, MRCP, FCP(SA)
Professor of Medicine, University of Cape Town; Chief Specialist, Groote Schuur Hospital, Cape Town; Co-Director, MRC/UCT Liver Research Centre, Cape Town, South Africa.
Acute Liver Failure

J. Thomas LaMont, MD
Professor of Medicine, Chief of Gastroenterology and Hepatology, Boston University Medical Center, Boston, MA 02118, USA.
Postoperative Jaundice

R.H.S. Lane, MS, FRCS
Consultant Surgeon, Royal Hampshire County Hospital, Winchester, Hampshire SO22 5DG, UK.
Calculous Disease and Cholecystitis

Joel E. Lavine, MD, PhD
Assistant Professor of Pediatrics, Harvard Medical School; Assistant in Gastroenterology, The Children's Hospital, Boston, MA 02115, USA.
Acute Viral Hepatitis

Charles S. Lieber, MD
Professor of Medicine and Pathology, Mount Sinai School of Medicine (CUNY); Director, Section of Liver Disease and Nutrition, Alcohol Research and Treatment Center, GI Program, Bronx VA Medical Center, 120 West Kingsbridge Road, Bronx, NY 10468, USA.
Alcoholic Liver Disease

Padraic MacMathuna, MD, MRCPI
Honorary Lecturer, Liver Unit, King's College Hospital, Denmark Hill, London SE5 9PJ, UK.
Portal Hypertension

Arthur J. McCullough, MD
Associate Professor of Medicine, Case Western Reserve University School of Medicine; Director of Gastroenterology, Metro Health Medical Center, 3395 Scranton Road, Cleveland OH 44109, USA.
Protein Metabolism

William V. McDermott, Jr, FACS, AB, MD
Cheever Professor of Surgery, Emeritus, Harvard Medical School; Chairman (Ret.), Department of Surgery, New England Deaconess Hospital, USA.
Hepatic Resection

Neil McIntyre, BSc, MD, FRCP
Professor of Medicine and Chairman, University Department of Medicine, Royal Free Hospital School of Medicine, Pond Street, London NW3 2QG, UK.
Plasma Lipoproteins

Magnus I. McLaren, MB BS, MS, FRCS
Consultant Orthopaedic Surgeon, Queen Alexandra Hospital, Cosham, Portsmouth, UK.
Physical Aspects of Hepatic Regeneration

Hylton B. Meire, MB BS, FRCR
Consultant Radiologist, King's College Hospital, Denmark Hill, London SE5 9PJ UK.
Ultrasound Imaging

Giorgina Mieli-Vergani, MD, PhD
Senior Lecturer in Paediatric Hepatology and Consultant Paediatrician, King's College School of Medicine and Dentistry, London SE5 8RX, UK.
Paediatric Liver Disease: Medical Aspects

G.H. Millward-Sadler, BSc, MB ChB, FRCPath, MHSM
Consultant Pathologist, Southampton University Hospitals; Honorary Senior Lecturer, Faculty of Medicine, University of Southampton, Tremona Road, Southampton SO9 4XY, UK.
Normal Histology and Ultrastructure, Liver Biopsy, Acute Viral Hepatitis, Chronic Hepatitis, Liver Fibrosis and Cirrhosis, Hepatic Changes in Systemic Disease, The Liver in Infection, Hepatic Tumours, Alpha-1-Antitrypsin Deficiency

Kevin Moore, BSc, MB BS, MRCP
Senior Registrar, Department of Clinical Pharmacology, Hammersmith Hospital, Du Cane Road, London W12 0NN, UK.
Ascites and Renal Dysfunction

Marsha Y. Morgan, MB ChB, FRCP
Senior Lecturer in Medicine and Honorary Consultant Physician, University Department of Medicine, Royal Free Hospital and School of Medicine, Hampstead, London NW3 2QG, UK.
Nutrition and the Liver

Alex P. Mowat, MB ChB, FRCP, DCH, DObs, RCOG
Professor of Paediatric Hepatology and Consultant Paediatrician, King's College School of Medicine and Dentistry, King's College Hospital, London SE5 8RY, UK.
Paediatric Liver Disease: Medical Aspects

Horst Neuhaus, MD
2nd Department of Medicine, Technical University of Munich, Klinikum rechts der Isar, Ismaninger Strasse 22, DW-8000 Munich 80, Germany.
Endoscopic Examination and Therapy

G.B. Ong, PhD, FRCS, FRACS, FACS, FRCS(Ed)
Emeritus Professor, University of Hong Kong, Hong Kong.
Helminthic Diseases

Kendrick A. Porter, MD, DSc, FRCPath
Professor of Pathology, Department of Pathology, St Mary's Hospital Medical School, London W2 1PG, UK.
Portal-Systemic Shunting

L.W. Powell, MD, PhD, FRACP
Professor, Liver Unit, Department of Medicine, Royal Brisbane Hospital, Herston, Queensland 4029, Australia.
Haemochromatosis and Related Iron Storage Diseases

Rudolf Preisig, MD
Professor of Medicine and Clinical Pharmacology, Department of Clinical Pharmacology, University of Berne, Murtenstrasse 35, CH-3010 Berne, Switzerland.
Assessment of Liver Function

Christopher P. Price, MA, PhD, MCB, FRSC, FRCPath
Professor of Clinical Biochemistry, London Hospital Medical College, Turner Street, London E1 2AD, UK.
Assessment of Liver Function

Alan E. Read, CBE, MD, FRCP
Professor and Head of Professorial Medical Unit, University of Bristol; Honorary Consulting Physician, Bristol Royal Infirmary, Bristol BS2 8HW, UK.
The Liver and Drugs

Telfer B. Reynolds, MD
Clayton G. Loosli Professor of Medicine, USC School of Medicine, Division of Gastrointestinal and Liver Diseases, Department of Medicine (GNH7900), USC School of Medicine, 2025 Zonal Avenue, Los Angeles, CA 90033, USA.
Peritoneoscopy

Duncan A.F. Robertson, BSc, MD, MRCP
Consultant Physician, Royal United Hospital, Combe Park, Bath BA1 3NG, UK.
The Liver in Infection

S.C. Robson, MB ChB, MRCP, DCH, PhD
Specialist Physician and Lecturer, MRC/UCT Liver Research Centre, Department of Medicine, University of Cape Town and Groote Schuur Hospital, Cape Town, South Africa.
Acute Liver Failure

Mikko Salaspuro, MD
Professor of Alcohol Diseases, Research Unit of Alcohol Diseases, Helsinki University Central Hospital, 00290 Helsinki 29, Finland.
Alcoholic Liver Disease

S.J. Saunders, MD, FRCP, FCP
Vice Chancellor and Principal, University of Cape Town, South Africa.
Acute Liver Failure

Fenton Schaffner, MD
George Baehr Professor of Medicine and Chief, Mount Sinai School of Medicine, 1 Gustave L. Levy Place, New York, NY 10029-6574, USA.
Cholestasis

I. Herbert Scheinberg, MD
Professor of Medicine Emeritus and Head, Division of Genetic Medicine, Albert Einstein College of Medicine; Attending Physician, Bronx Municipal Hospital Center and Montefiore Hospital and Medical Center, Bronx, New York, USA.
Wilson's Disease

Sheila Sherlock, DBE, MD, FRCP
Professor of Medicine, Royal Free Hospital School of Medicine, (University of London), Pond Street, London NW3 2QG, UK.
Primary Biliary Cirrhosis

Thomas E. Starzl, MD, PhD
Professor of Surgery, 5C Falk Clinic, 3601 Fifth Avenue, Pittsburgh, PA 15213, USA.
Portal-Systemic Shunting

Irmin Sternlieb, MD
Professor of Medicine and Associate Director, Liver Research Center, Albert Einstein College of Medicine; Attending Physician, Bronx Municipal Hospital Center and Montefiore Hospital and Medical Center, Bronx, New York, USA.
Wilson's Disease

Alastair J. Strain, PhD
Senior Lecturer in Biochemistry, University of Birmingham; Scientific Director, Liver Research Laboratories, Liver Unit, Queen Elizabeth Hospital, Edgbaston, Birmingham B15 2TH, UK.
Regulatory Mechanisms in Hepatic Regeneration

Leo Strunin, MB BS, MD, FFARCS, FRCP(C)
BOC Professor of Anaesthesia, Hunterian Institute, The Royal College of Surgeons of England and The London Hospital Medical College, London, UK.
Anaesthetic Management of Patients

K.C. Tan, MB BS, FRCSE
Consultant Surgeon, King's College Hospital, Denmark Hill, London SE5 9RS, UK.
Normal Anatomy

Anthony S. Tavill, MD, FRCP
Professor of Medicine and Academic Director of Gastroenterology, Case Western Reserve University School of Medicine; Director of the Digestive and Liver Diseases Center, Mount Sinai Hospital Medical Center, 1 Mount Sinai Drive, Cleveland, OH 44106, USA.
Protein Metabolism

Irving Taylor, MD, ChM, FRCS
Professor of Surgery, University Surgical Unit, Faculty of Medicine, University of Southampton and Southampton University Hospitals, Tremona Road, Southampton SO9 4XY, UK.
Treatment of Liver Tumours

Roy Taylor, MB BS, MD, FRCP
Senior Lecturer and Honorary Consultant in Medicine, Department of Medicine, The Medical School, Framlington Place, Newcastle upon Tyne NE2 4HH, UK.
Carbohydrate Metabolism

J. Terblanche, MB ChB, ChM, FCS, FRCS, FRCPS, FACS
Professor and Head of Surgery, University of Cape Town and Groote Schuur Hospital, Cape Town; Co-Director MRC/UCT Liver Research Centre, Cape Town, South Africa.
Acute Liver Failure

H.C. Thomas, BSc, MB BS, PhD, FRCP, FRCPath
Professor and Chairman of Medicine, Department of Medicine, St Mary's Hospital Medical School; Consultant Hepatologist, St Mary's Hospital, London W2 1PG, UK.
Chronic Hepatitis

David R. Triger, MA, BM BCh, DPhil, FRCP
Professor of Postgraduate Medical Education, University of Sheffield Medical School, Beech Hill Road, Sheffield S10 2RX, UK.
Immunological Aspects, Alpha-1-Antitrypsin Deficiency

Niels Tygstrup,
Professor of Medicine, Rigshospitalet, Medical Department A, 9 Blegdamsvej, DK-2100 Copenhagen Ø, Denmark.
Assessment of Liver Function

Alan P. Venook, MD
Assistant Clinical Professor of Medicine, Cancer Research Institute, University of California, San Francisco, 400 Parnassus Avenue, San Francisco, CA 94143, USA.
Hepatic Tumours

M.D. Voigt, MB ChB, FCP
Specialist Physician and Lecturer, MRC/UCT Liver Research Centre, Department of Medicine, University of Cape Town and Groote Schuur Hospital, Cape Town, South Africa.
Acute Liver Failure

Alexander J. Walt, MB ChB, MS, FRCS, FRCS(C), FACS
Distinguished Professor of Surgery, Wayne State University Department of Surgery, University Health Center 6-B, 4201 St Antoine, Detroit, MI 48201; Surgeon, Harper Hospital, USA.
Liver Trauma

David Westaby, MA, FRCP
Consultant Physician and Honorary Senior Lecturer, Institute of Liver Studies, King's College Hospital and Medical School, London SE5 9PJ, UK.
Portal Hypertension

P.J. Whorwell, BSc, MD, FRCP
Department of Medicine, University Hospital of South Manchester, Manchester M20 8LR, UK.
Liver Biopsy

Stephen P. Wilkinson, BSc, MD, MRCP
Consultant Physician, Gloucestershire Royal Hospital, Gloucester GL1 3NN, UK.
Ascites and Renal Dysfunction

Roger Williams, MD, FRCP, FRCS, FRCPE, FRACS
Consultant Physician and Director, Institute of Liver Studies, King's College Hospital; Senior Lecturer, King's College School of Medicine and Dentistry, Denmark Hill, London SE5 9RS, UK.
Portal Hypertension, Ascites and Renal Dysfunction

Dennis H. Wright, BSc, MD, FRCPath
Professor of Pathology, Faculty of Medicine, University of Southampton; Honorary Consultant Pathologist, Southampton University Hospitals, Tremona Road, Southampton SO9 4XY, UK.
Immunological Aspects, Involvement of the Liver by Lympho-reticular Disease

R. Wright, MA, MD, DPhil, FRCP
Formerly Professor of Medicine, Faculty of Medicine, University of Southampton; Honorary Consultant Physician, Southampton University Hospitals, Tremona Road, Southampton SO9 4XY, UK.
Immunological Aspects, Investigation of the Jaundiced Patient, Hepatic Changes in Systemic Disease

Teresa Lyn Wright, BM, BS
Assistant Professor of Medicine, Veterans Administration Medical Center and the University of California, San Francisco, USA.
Hepatic Tumours, Medical Aspects of Liver Transplantation

Preface

The third edition of *Wright's Liver and Biliary Disease* incorporates major changes from the second edition in both personnel and content. Ralph Wright's tragic death in 1990 during the preparation of this edition was a huge loss and necessitated considerable reorganization. The most important problem was to replace Ralph's considerable expertise, knowledge and enthusiasm as editor: the solution—to invite Dr Michael J.P. Arthur to be editor—was simple. Dr Arthur is not only an active clinical hepatologist but has already established himself as a research worker of some authority both in the United Kingdom and abroad. He has recently been appointed to be the Professor of Medicine in the University of Southampton succeeding Ralph Wright, having prior to this been a Senior Lecturer in Ralph's Department. We separately include a tribute to Ralph Wright's life and achievements but would wish to record here our own personal indebtedness to the standards that he set and his vision of medicine in general and hepatology in particular, that we were able to share.

The easiest decision to take was to name the book after him: this was not only the unanimous desire of the current editors and publishers but also the request of many fellow hepatologists at home and abroad. We hope that it is a fitting dedication.

Prior to his death the decision had been taken to have only two editors for the third edition—reflecting the volume and burden borne in previous editions. We would like gratefully to acknowledge the quality of the contribution made by Professor George Alberti and Mr Stephen Karran and record with pleasure their continuing involvement with individual chapters in this edition.

Apart from changes at editorial level there have been changes to the format of the book which is now divided into two volumes for ease of handling. Colour photography has been incorporated into the text of the major clinical section of the book. We hope and believe that this considerably enhances the quality and attractiveness of the third edition.

Major changes have occurred within hepatology—which of course is the justification for this new edition. Fundamental advances in molecular biology have been applied to hepatology and have resulted in greater understanding of the basic pathophysiological mechanisms underlying many diseases of the liver. These advances are covered as an integral part of the relevant chapters but of particular note are those advances made in liver regeneration, the identification of hepatitis viruses, the role of viruses in the pathogenesis of hepatocellular carcinoma, matrix synthesis and degradation particularly in cirrhosis, and the genetics and processing of alpha-1-antitrypsin.

The range of investigative options has also increased and is recognised by incorporating a new chapter on magnetic resonance imaging. Percutaneous and biliary endoscopic diagnostic techniques are also considerably improved and these have been reviewed and illustrated in detail. The advances in endoscopy have not only enhanced diagnosis but have enabled new therapeutic techniques such as the stenting of tumours and endoscopic lithotripsy of gallstones to be developed. Other therapeutic modalities for treating diseases of the gallbladder and biliary tree—laparoscopic cholecystectomy, external lithotripsy of gallstones and the medical dissolution of gallstones, are now available. These have also been separately assessed so that the optimal choice of therapy for the individual patient with biliary disease can be made.

The major therapeutic advance has been the improvement in mortality and morbidity of patients undergoing liver transplantation. This is now a significant option in the treatment of many endstage liver diseases and has even been suggested as a primary treatment for some diseases. We have recognised the increasing importance of this by having two complementary chapters on medical and surgical aspects of liver transplantation.

It must be stated that the production of this book is a major effort requiring throughout the help, commitment and tolerance of many people. We wish formally and publicly to recognise their contribution, for without them we could not have produced this edition. Superb organizational and secretarial support has been provided by Mrs Gillian Clark and Mrs Barbara Thomas; no task was too difficult for them to attempt, no problem too difficult to tackle. As editors we have certainly tested them thoroughly. At W.B. Saunders Seán Duggan, Nicki Dennis and Carol Parr have all shown total commitment to the book, a willingness to help in any matter large or small and a patience that we must have considerably stretched—but never broken.

Most of all we would like to acknowledge the support, help and understanding of our wives, Hilary and Liz, and families. Their contribution to this text is immeasurable. Their encouragement and tenacity have been a source of inspiration and in the long hours of this book, their patience and devotion above and beyond that which could reasonably be expected. We love and thank them.

We also rest secure in the knowledge that they share our joy at completing this edition.

G.H. MILLWARD-SADLER
M.J.P. ARTHUR

PART 1

PATHOPHYSIOLOGY

CHAPTER 1

Anatomy of the Liver

J.L. Dawson & K.C. Tan

THE LIVER

Functionally the liver is a bilobed organ; each half has separate afferent and efferent blood vessels.[7,12] The contiguous surfaces of the two halves are closely applied and lie within a common capsule, so that there is no external evidence of this important division. The true division between right and left halves is also called the principal plane of the liver; it corresponds with a line which runs from the fundus of the gallbladder to the vena cava (Figure 1.1). The afferent vessels to the liver enter the organ at the hilum and branch in a recognizable pattern within the liver substance. They are accompanied by the branches of the bile ducts to make the portal triad.

The regular branching pattern of the portal triad within the hepatic parenchyma allows each half of the liver to be subdivided into four functional segments.[7] Knowledge of the intrahepatic segmental anatomy is especially important in the interpretation of selective angiograms and for the planning of hepatic resections.

The efferent vessels are the hepatic veins which run separately from the afferent vessels within the liver and drain directly into the inferior vena cava.

EXTERNAL APPEARANCE

The liver is the largest solid organ in the body and normally weighs between 1.2 and 1.8 kg. It is roughly wedge-shaped and the base of the wedge occupies the right side of the upper part of the peritoneal cavity. The right side of the liver is closely applied to the costal fibres and the central tendon of the right leaf of the diaphragm. The left liver (the apex of the wedge) reaches for a variable distance into the left upper part of the abdominal cavity, abutting the left leaf of the diaphragm. The posterior, upper and anterior surfaces of the liver are convex and the underside to the right of the midline is slightly concave.

Most of the liver substance is covered by peritoneum which, apart from a small area on the underside of the left liver, is related to the greater sac. The peritoneal attachments are asymmetrical and best understood by considering the development of the liver (see below).

SURFACE ANATOMY

In the healthy adult the upper border of the right liver reaches to the right fifth rib about 2 cm medial to the mid-clavicular line. This is usually 1 cm below the right nipple. The left liver reaches to the left sixth rib in the mid-clavicular line. This point is about 2 cm below the left nipple. The oblique inferior margin passes from the

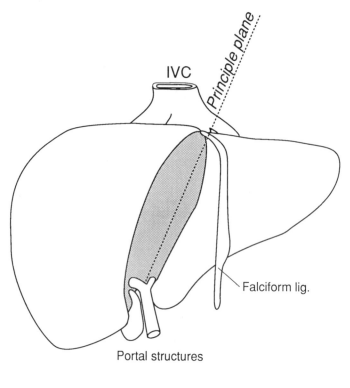

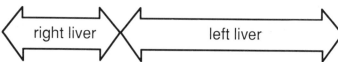

Figure 1.1 Diagram showing the two functional halves of the liver. The three hilar structures are represented by a single tube with left and right branches. The functional division into right and left halves by the principal plane corresponds with a line which runs from the fundus of the gallbladder to the left side of the inferior vena cava; it is not related to the attachment of the falciform ligament.

highest point on the left downwards to the right, passing through the fundus of the gallbladder. This latter point is where the transpyloric plane crosses the costal margin.

DEVELOPMENT

In the developing embryo the liver first appears as a hollow endodermal bud from the ventral aspect of the foregut. This bud grows ventrally and cranially into the ventral mesogastrium which has developed from the caudal part of the septum transversum. As it grows into the ventral mesogastrium it bifurcates and produces epithelial trabeculae called hepatic cylinders. These in turn branch and anastomose to form a close meshwork. These cells become the liver cells and the spaces between them become filled with blood sinusoids, which have developed from potentially angiogenic cells of the mesenchyme of the septum transversum,[18] giving the appearance of a vascular sponge. Thus, the hepatic cells in the adult come to lie in close contact with blood draining from the portal venous system.

The gallbladder and cystic duct develop as a separate bud (pars cystica) from the ventral–caudal surface of the main diverticulum. They are solid at first, but later in development they become canalized. As the mesoderm round the extrahepatic ducts begins to migrate into the liver along the main branches of the portal vein, the adjacent parenchymal cells develop into duct epithelium. This migration and transformation progresses from the hilum, peripherally, to the terminal branches of the portal vein. The hepatic artery and a branch of the vagus nerve also migrate into the liver with the mesoderm along the portal vein. Initially, the blood from the yolk sac is drained through the right and left vitelline veins, which also have numerous cross-channels. During development, complicated changes take place, with the disappearance of some segments and persistence of some communicating veins, until the normal adult arrangement of a single portal vein dividing into right and left branches at the hilum of the liver is achieved.

On the cephalic side of the liver, part of the vitelline venous system persists as the terminal segment of the inferior vena cava. During this time there are two umbilical veins, but the right soon disappears. The left runs in the free edge of the ventral mesogastrium and drains into the left branch of the portal vein. In the fetus there is a large venous channel within the sinusoidal system, the ductus venosum, which connects the left branch of the portal vein to the inferior vena cava. This channel allows oxygenated and nutritive blood from the placenta to bypass the liver and gain direct access to the inferior vena cava. The umbilical vein closes soon after birth and the adult remnant is known as the ligamentum teres. The ductus venosus closes and becomes the ligamentum venosum, which, in the adult, is found in the region of the attachment of the lesser omentum to the under surface of the liver (Figure 1.2).

As the development of the fetus proceeds, the viscera in the upper abdomen rotate and enormous growth of the liver occurs. Initially this increase in size is at a relatively greater rate than the body as a whole and the liver comes to occupy most of the space in the developing upper abdominal cavity and is approximately 10% of the body weight. Later this growth rate gradually diminishes and at birth the liver is only 5% of the body weight. This diminution affects the left lobe more than the right and the initial symmetry will be lost. The two leaves of the peritoneum which make up the ventral mesogastrium are taken up over the liver, almost completely covering it. In the adult, only the lesser omentum and falciform ligament remain as a double leaf of peritoneum, and the ligamentum teres notches the inferior border of the liver.

PERITONEAL ATTACHMENTS

In the adult, the falciform ligament stretches from the body wall to the liver. The line of its ventral attachment runs from the umbilicus along the posterior aspect of the anterior abdominal wall and the diaphragm in the midline

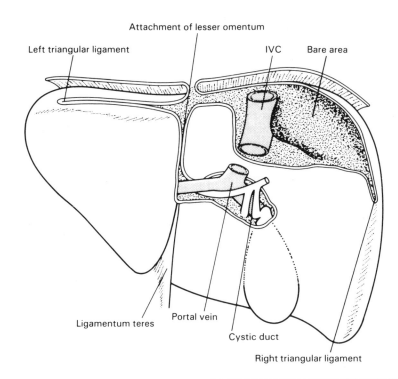

Left triangular ligament

Attachment of lesser omentum

IVC   Bare area

Ligamentum teres

Portal vein

Cystic duct

Right triangular ligament

Figure 1.2 Diagram of the posterior aspect of the liver to show the arrangement of the peritoneal attachments. Note the horizontal course of the left branch of the portal vein and the comparatively short course of the right branch.

as far back as the inferior vena cava opening just above the liver. Its attachment to the liver is to the right of the midline; thus, the falciform ligament lies in an oblique plane with its right surface facing anteriorly and its left surface facing posteriorly. The left leaf of the falciform ligament is continued laterally and to the left over the surface of the liver, where superiorly it becomes the left triangular ligament of the liver. This ligament consists of the two layers of peritoneum, from the anterior and posterior aspect of the left liver, which have been fused together and which suspend the lateral part of the left liver to the undersurface of the diaphragm. The left phrenic vessels run close to the diaphragmatic attachment of this ligament. Division of the left triangular ligament of the liver renders the lateral part of the left liver freely mobile. The medial end of the posterior aspect of the triangular ligament is continued into the two layers of the lesser omentum.

The lesser omentum is a double layer of peritoneum and represents that part of the ventral mesogastrium between the stomach and the liver; in its free lower margin run the three structures of the portal triad—the bile ducts anteriorly to the right, the hepatic artery anteriorly slightly to the left, and the portal vein immediately posterior to both structures. On the liver the right posterior leaf of the lesser omentum is reflected inferiorly over the front of the inferior vena cava and passes to the right. The two layers of the peritoneum are widely separated to encompass the bare area of the liver, except at the extreme right where they fuse to become the right triangular ligament of the liver (Figure 1.2). The upper reflection of the peritoneum is continued until it reaches the right lateral leaf of the falciform ligament. Division

of the right triangular ligament and the two diverging peritoneal reflections on the right liver, as far medially as the inferior vena cava, is required to mobilize the right liver and gain access to its posterior aspect.

THE LOBES OF THE LIVER

Before the bilateral nature of the liver was appreciated,[12] the liver was arbitrarily divided into two main lobes (right and left) and two accessory lobes (quadrate and caudate), according to peritoneal attachments and surface fissures. These divisions were purely descriptive and did not have much practical significance.

For the clinician the division of the liver into two functional halves called the right and left livers by the principal plane (Figure 1.1) is of considerable practical importance.[2,3,8,12,19] The principal plane passes from the middle of the gallbladder bed anteriorly to the left side of the inferior vena cava posteriorly. The branches of the portal triad are closely applied and arborize in a regular manner within the parenchyma.

The right and left halves of the liver are each further divided into two sectors by the right and left fissures, which correspond to the location of the right and left hepatic veins (Figure 1.3). The right fissure extends from the anterior border of the liver at a point midway between the right margin of the liver and the gallbladder fossa, to the confluence of the inferior vena cava and the right hepatic vein posteriorly. It divides the right half of the liver into an anterior and posterior sector. The left fissure is not well defined and extends from the left side of the inferior vena cava to a point between the dorsal one-third and ventral two-thirds of the left margin of the liver. It

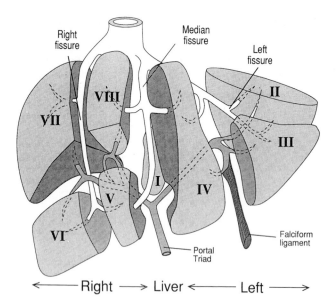

Figure 1.3 Diagram showing the liver subdivided into eight functional segments by the regular branching pattern of the portal triad according to Couinaud. Each segment has a precise afferent and efferent blood supply and biliary channels. The portal triad is represented by a single tube with divisions to the respective liver segments. The middle hepatic vein runs along the median fissure which corresponds to the principal plane and divides the liver into two functional halves. The right and left hepatic veins run along the right and left fissures; subdividing the right and left livers into two sectors each respectively.

also divides the left half of the liver into an anterior and posterior sector.

The regular branching pattern of the 'afferent structures' (i.e. the portal vein, hepatic artery and bile ducts) allows these sectors to be further subdivided into segments. Studies have shown that these segments have an independent vascular supply and biliary drainage.[2,8] The anterior and posterior sectors of the right half of the liver are subdivided into superior and inferior segments. In the left half of the liver, the anterior sector is subdivided by the umbilical fissure into medial and lateral segments. The posterior sector remains as a single segment. These are the eight segments described by Couinaud[2] and numbered clockwise from II to VIII; segment I denotes the caudate lobe (Figure 1.3). Each segment has a precise afferent and efferent blood supply and biliary channels. There is no collateral circulation between segments.

The caudate lobe (segment I) is best considered an autonomous part of the liver from a functional viewpoint. It is a pedunculated lobule in direct contact with the left side of the inferior vena cava and may extend posteriorly to it for a variable distance. It has a separate blood supply and bile drainage from the rest of the liver and its hepatic veins are independent and drain directly into the retrohepatic vena cava.

ARTERIAL BLOOD SUPPLY

The hepatic artery supplies arterial blood to the liver; it is responsible for approximately 25–30% of the total afferent blood flow but carries about 50% of the available oxygen. Hepatic artery obstruction in the intact liver is usually harmless but if it occurs in the transplanted liver, hepatic or biliary necrosis follows.

The common hepatic artery most commonly arises as a branch of the coeliac axis and passes forwards and to the right to gain access to the lesser omentum. As it does it raises a small fold of peritoneum, the right or inferior gastropancreatic fold, which lies at the lower margin of the inner aspect of the aditus to the lesser sac. Before it passes upwards to the hilum of the liver the hepatic artery gives off the right gastric and gastroduodenal arteries. It divides at the hilum of the liver into right and left branches and the intrahepatic course of these branches is shown. The division takes place at a variable level, sometimes it is high in the hilum, sometimes it is comparatively low down in the free edge of the lesser omentum. The right and left hepatic arteries usually lie on a plane posterior to the bile ducts at the hilum of the liver. The cystic artery, which supplies the gallbladder, is usually given off in the lesser omentum from the right branch of the hepatic artery and passes behind the bile ducts and cephalad to the cystic duct to reach the anterior surface of the gallbladder. Variations in the course of the cystic artery are not uncommon.

The blood supply to the supraduodenal part of the common bile duct is precarious. Elegant studies have shown that the blood supply to the human bile duct is mainly axial, the main contribution usually coming from below.[16] Small arteries both ascend and descend the length of the bile duct to form an arcade, the most important run along the lateral borders and are called the 3 o'clock and 9 o'clock arteries (Figure 1.4). Anteriorly the ascending vessels are mainly from the retroduodenal artery with the descending vessels from the right hepatic artery and cystic artery. Posteriorly most of the blood is supplied by the retroportal artery. This is a fairly consistent artery that may arise from the coeliac axis of the superior mesenteric artery, close to their origin. It runs behind the portal vein and terminates by joining either the right hepatic or retroduodenal artery. Throughout its course it contributes branches to the pericholedochal plexus. In human liver transplantation, the donor bile duct is more liable to become ischaemic than the recipient duct and this may be related to the length of the donor duct transplanted.[15]

Variations in the arrangement of the arterial supply to the liver are common and a completely normal arrangement is found in only 50% of subjects.[13] Part or all of the left liver may be supplied by an abnormal left hepatic artery which arises from the left gastric artery. All or part of the territory normally supplied by the right branch of the hepatic artery may come from a vessel which arises from the superior mesenteric artery. Such an abnormal

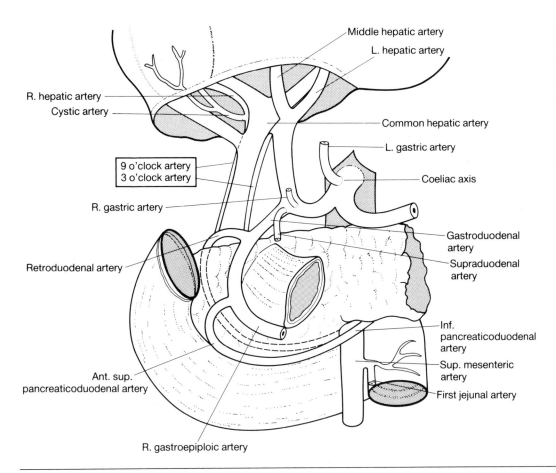

R. hepatic artery
Cystic artery

9 o'clock artery
3 o'clock artery

R. gastric artery

Retroduodenal artery

Ant. sup.
pancreaticoduodenal artery

R. gastroepiploic artery

Middle hepatic artery
L. hepatic artery

Common hepatic artery

L. gastric artery

Coeliac axis

Gastroduodenal artery

Supraduodenal artery

Inf. pancreaticoduodenal artery

Sup. mesenteric artery

First jejunal artery

Figure 1.4 Diagram showing the major arteries related to the supraduodenal part of the common bile duct. Small arteries both ascend and descend the length of the common bile duct to form an arcade, the most important run along the lateral borders and are called the 3 o'clock and 9 o'clock arteries. (Courtesy of the *British Journal of Surgery*, vol. 66, pp. 397–384 (1979)).

right hepatic artery passes up to the hilum of the liver, lying at first posterior to the portal vein, and often winds around its right margin in the lesser omentum. This arrangement may sometimes cause difficulty when the portal vein is being dissected free in the course of a portocaval shunt operation. Sometimes the superior mesenteric artery may share a common origin with the coeliac axis. All of these abnormal vessels are end-arteries, not accessory vessels, and their division results in lack of arterial supply to that part of the liver to which they are distributed. The branching of the hepatic artery within the liver is very similar to the pattern of the portal vein (Figures 1.5 and 1.6).

THE PORTAL VEIN

The valveless portal vein drains blood from the splanchnic area and carries approximately 75% of the total liver blood flow. It is formed behind the neck of the pancreas as an upward continuation of the superior mesenteric vein after this vessel has been joined by the splenic vein. It then lies posterior to the bile ducts and hepatic artery in the free edge of the lesser omentum. At the hilum of the liver the vein divides into right and left branches which run with the right and left hepatic arteries and the right and left hepatic ducts. Unlike the hepatic arterial supply anomalies are rare. There are always 2–3 consistent branches at its birfurcation supplying the porta hepatis

and the caudate lobe directly. The former are important during dissection of the porta hepatis as they can be a source of troublesome bleeding.

The portal vein shares a recognizable pattern of branching within the liver with the branches of the hepatic artery and bile duct. The three elements are enclosed in a fibrous sheath which enables all three components of the triad to be isolated and divided as one structure during surgery. The regular intrahepatic branching pattern allows the liver to be divided into seven segments as already described (see Figure 1.6).

The main right and left branches of the portal vein supply the right liver and left liver respectively. The right branch of the portal vein is usually less than 3 cm long and runs more vertically, hence its dissection is much more difficult than the left. It divides into anterior and posterior branches which supply the anterior and posterior parts of the right lobe. Each of these vessels divides again into superior and inferior branches (see Figures 1.6b and 1.3).

The left branch of the portal vein passes horizontally to the left to give branches which supply segments II and III. The vein is then joined by the obliterated umbilical vein as it turns medially. The terminal part of the vessel continues into segment IV which it supplies with ascending and descending branches (Figure 1.7). This arrangement of blood supply may lead to inadvertent devascularization of either the anterior or posterior sectors of the left half of the liver during liver resection.[3,17]

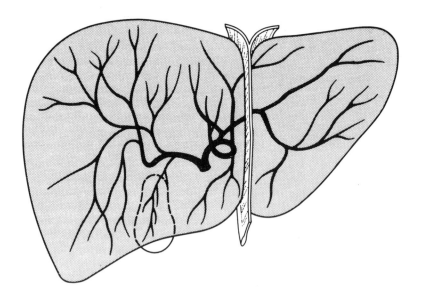

Figure 1.5 Diagram showing the intrahepatic distribution of the hepatic artery. Note the 'returning loop' of the left branch near the attachment of the falciform ligament. This is liable to injury here during resection of segments II and III.

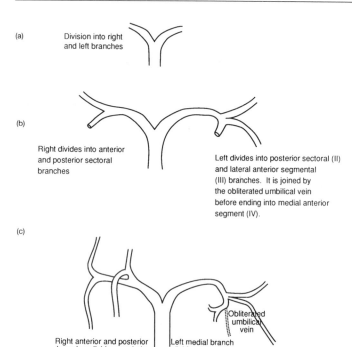

(a) Division into right and left branches

(b) Right divides into anterior and posterior sectoral branches

Left divides into posterior sectoral (II) and lateral anterior segmental (III) branches. It is joined by the obliterated umbilical vein before ending into medial anterior segment (IV).

(c) Right anterior and posterior branches divide superiorly and inferiorly

Left medial branch divides superiorly and inferiorly

Obliterated umbilical vein

Figure 1.6 Progressive branching of the intrahepatic portal vein and its distribution within the liver parenchyma. (a) Division into right and left branches. (b) Division of the right branch into anterior and posterior branches and of left branch into posterior and lateral anterior branches before ending as the medial anterior branch. (c) Four segments of the liver supplied by the right and three by the left branches; the caudate lobe (segment I) is supplied separately.

THE HEPATIC VEINS

All the hepatic veins drain into the inferior vena cava (Figure 1.8). There are three main hepatic veins, right, middle and left. They lie posterosuperiorly just below the diaphragm: a variable number of smaller ones (dorsal hepatic veins) drain from the posterior aspect of the right half of the liver and caudate lobe (segment I) directly into the retrohepatic vena cava which lies in a groove in the liver substance. The branches of the three main hepatic veins ramify in the hepatic parenchyma in a distribution that is quite separate from the portal triad structures.

The right hepatic vein drains most of the right half of the liver, namely segments V, VI and VII. The vein itself lies between the right anterior and posterior sectors, which is represented on the surface by the right fissure, which may be very obvious in occasional patients. More than a dozen branches join the vein on either side as it courses toward the right margin of the inferior vena cava into which it drains. Although it has a short extrahepatic course, in more than 60% of cases there are no branches in its last 1 cm, which facilitates ligation of the vein at its caval junction.

The middle hepatic vein lies in the principal plane between the right and left halves of the liver and drains mainly segments IV, V and VIII. Formed in the depths of the parenchyma near the fundus of the gallbladder, it passes in a dorsal direction to form a common trunk with the left hepatic vein in about 90% of cases before emptying into the inferior vena cava at the upper border of the liver posteriorly.[14] The left hepatic vein drains segments II and III.

The number of dorsal hepatic veins varies but may reach 15, and these pass from the right posterior sector of the liver directly into the inferior vena cava (not shown in Figure 1.8). They vary a great deal in size and are generally thin-walled. Great care should be taken during their dissection in a right hemihepatectomy.[11] The most caudal of these veins is the posteroinferior vein, which is consistent and usually large. Its size is in inverse proportion to the size of the right hepatic vein: the smaller the right hepatic vein the larger is the posteroinferior vein.

The right suprarenal gland may be firmly adherent to

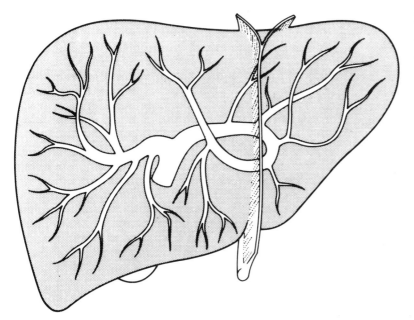

Figure 1.7 Diagram showing the intrahepatic distribution of the portal vein. Note that the left branch has a horizontal part which turns forwards towards the umbilical fissure. The branches to segments II and III come from the right side of this part of the vessel (the pars umbilicalis).

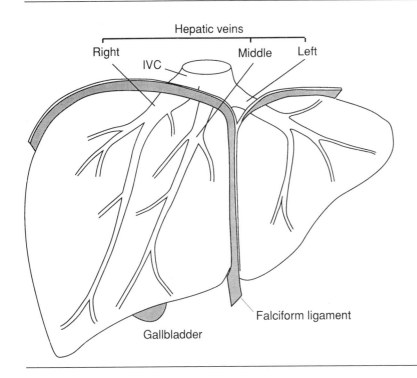

Hepatic veins

Right   IVC   Middle   Left

Gallbladder

Falciform ligament

Figure 1.8 Diagram showing the usual arrangement of the main hepatic veins (the small veins draining the posterior aspect of the right half of the liver and caudate lobe are not shown). The three hepatic veins run along the corresponding fissures, dividing the liver into four sectors (see Figure 1.3). The middle hepatic vein often forms a common trunk with the left hepatic vein before emptying into the inferior vena cava.

the liver or attached to it with some loose connective tissue. The right suprarenal vein is constant and large and usually drains directly into the infrahepatic vena cava above the right renal vein. Occasionally it may drain either into one of the dorsal hepatic veins, namely the posteroinferior vein, or into the junction with the right renal vein. It may be multiple in a small number of cases.[14]

The length of the inferior vena cava between the diaphragm and the upper margin of the hepatic veins is short and drains several large phrenic veins, especially on the right side.

LYMPH DRAINAGE

Lymph from the liver drains through superficial and deep channels. The convex surface drains into nodes along the falciform ligament, coeliac axis and oesophageal nodes. Some passes through the diaphragm into the xiphisternal nodes.

The under surface of the liver drains to nodes along the inferior vena cava and the common bile duct. The deep channels surround each branch of the portal vein and pass to the biliary and hepatic artery nodes. The nodes in these porta are arranged in an asymmetrical fashion and lie posterior to the portal vein and its left branch. On the right, nodes occur infrequently and are small. Nodal enlargement is an unlikely cause of obstruction to bile flow.[6]

NERVE SUPPLY

The nerve supply of the liver and biliary tree is derived from the hepatic plexus which is formed by sympathetic fibres from thoracic segments 7 to 10, parasympathetic fibres from both right and left vagi, and a few fibres from the right phrenic nerve.[1] The branches from the left vagus run in the upper part of the lesser omentum towards the hilum of the liver. Branches of the sympathetic and the right vagus travel with the hepatic arteries to reach the viscera. Afferent impulses from the liver and common duct travel in the sympathetic nerves.

THE BILIARY TREE

THE GALLBLADDER

The gallbladder is pear-shaped and lies on the under surface of the liver covered by peritoneum. It holds 50 to 75 ml of bile and is connected to the common hepatic duct by the cystic duct. The blind end, or fundus, usually projects beyond the lower edge of the liver and is the lowest point. About two-thirds of the circumference of the gallbladder is usually visible, the rest of the body is embedded in the liver tissue. Occasionally, the gallbladder may have a mesentery which potentially allows it to undergo torsion. In adult life a dilatation of the gallbladder at the point where the neck joins the cystic duct (Hartmann's pouch) is often seen at operation.

The cystic duct runs downwards with a sinuous course before joining the common hepatic duct to form the common bile duct. Its lumen contains a spiral valve of Heister and this 'concertina-ed' part of the cystic duct is surrounded by connective tissue and autonomic nerves. The cystic duct usually enters from the right side to form a T-junction, but the exact configuration of this junction varies greatly (Figure 1.9). For example, the cystic duct may run anterior or posterior to the bile duct, spiralling round it before joining it on its medial side. Sometimes the cystic duct joins the common bile duct and runs parallel with it for some distance before entering its lumen. From the outside there may be no obvious sulcus and the duct system is double-barrelled for a short distance. This arrangement may occasionally give rise to confusion during attempted exploration of the common bile duct. In addition, its inadvertent inclusion as part of the wall of the common bile duct during liver transplantation may result in an obstructing mucocoele.[9]

The gallbladder is supplied by the cystic artery, which is normally a branch of the right hepatic artery. The latter usually passes laterally behind the common hepatic duct before giving off the cystic artery, which reaches the gallbladder on the superior aspect of its neck. At this

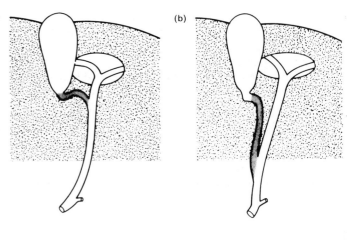

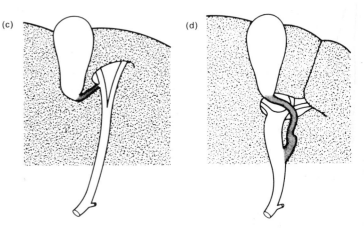

Figure 1.9 Diagram showing some of the common variations in the junction between the cystic duct and the common hepatic duct (CHD). (a) High union with the CHD. (b) Low union with the CHD. The ducts may be 'double-barrelled', i.e. they may share a common covering with no sulcus visible externally. (c) Union with the right hepatic duct. This is often associated with a low union of the right and left hepatic ducts. (d) Entry of the cystic duct low on the left side of the CHD. The cystic duct may cross either in front of or behind the CHD. After Grant (1947), *An Atlas of Anatomy*, Williams and Wilkins, Baltimore.

point the right hepatic artery turns cephalad to enter the liver. The cystic lymph node is closely related to the cystic artery on the wall of the gallbladder. These divide again so that four vessels runs towards the fundus, giving off tiny branches to produce a reticular pattern.[4] However, the origin and course of the cystic artery are variable. It may reach the gallbladder by passing caudal to the union of the cystic and common hepatic ducts. It may pass in front of the common hepatic duct and there may be two cystic arteries. The cystic artery pursues a straight course to the gallbladder and until it is divided at operation the cystic duct cannot be dissected free and 'straightened out'.

The veins draining the gallbladder show no constant pattern and drain directly into the liver; they also communicate with the meshwork of veins, the choledochal plexus, which surrounds and drains the bile ducts. This plexus communicates with the duodenal, pancreatic and gastric venous drainage.

The lymphatics of the gallbladder drain through the cystic and superior pancreatic and duodenal lymph nodes. The latter is constant and is sometimes known as the common duct node because it lies immediately to the right of the common bile duct at the junction of the first and second parts of the duodenum. It is a useful landmark during re-exploration of the common bile duct. As the cystic lymph node lies in close proximity to the cystic artery on the wall of the gallbladder, it is a useful landmark for the surgeon seeking the cystic artery.

THE BILE DUCTS

The bile ducts drain bile from the bile ductular and canalicular network of the acinus (see below). These ducts run with branches of the portal vein and hepatic artery in the portal tracts. The smallest interlobular ducts eventually join to form septal bile ducts and these finally form the right and left hepatic ducts. The left hepatic duct drains the three segments (II, III and IV) that constitute the left liver and the right hepatic duct drains segments V, VI, VII and VIII. The caudate lobe (segment I) is drained by one or several ducts joining the left and right hepatic ducts. The extrahepatic segment of the right duct is short, but the left duct has a much longer extrahepatic course. These ducts usually fuse at the hilum of the liver as they emerge from the capsule to form the common hepatic duct which runs caudally in the free edge of the lesser omentum. A normal biliary confluence of the right and left hepatic ducts is reported in only 56%.[10] Trifurcations are not uncommon, this usually involves either the right posterior or right anterior sectoral ducts joining the main bile duct separately. This anomaly is important because the first right branch may be mistaken for the cystic duct and tied off during cholecystectomy. In addition, during left hemihepatectomy the main duct may be mistaken for the left duct and be ligated just distal to the first right branch, thereby depriving half of the remaining right liver of biliary drainage.

The common hepatic duct is joined at a variable level by the cystic duct to form the common bile duct, normally about 2.5 cm above the duodenum. Variations in the anatomy of the biliary tree are common (Figure 1.9). The junction of right and left hepatic ducts may be low, e.g. 2–5 cm below the hilum of the liver. The cystic duct may join the right hepatic duct rather than the common hepatic duct. The common bile duct passes downwards behind the first part of the duodenum and the head of the pancreas. This part of the duct is often completely buried in the pancreas. The duct then inclines to the right to pass through the duodenal wall to open into the lumen about 10 cm from the pylorus. The lumen of the common duct is considerably reduced as it passes through the duodenal wall. A characteristic notch is seen on the operative cholangiogram which represents the upper border of the choledochal sphincter which surrounds the distal duct and extends upwards around the duct, reaching more proximally than the duodenal wall itself.[5] The pancreatic duct lies in close apposition to the narrow segment of bile duct and is also surrounded by the fibres of the choledochal sphincter. The common bile duct and pancreatic ducts have a common channel, from 2 to 7 mm long, which is usually called the ampulla of Vater, although there is in fact no dilatation or ampulla. The distal part of the duct is surrounded by the choledochal muscle and lies in the medial wall of the second part of the duodenum. The opening is recognized by a small elevation, the papilla, which can be seen and felt.

REFERENCES

1. Burnett, W., Cairns, F.W. & Bacsich, P. (1964) Innervation of the extrahepatic biliary system. *Annals of Surgery*, **123**, 8–26.
2. Couinaud, C. (1957) Le Foie. Les hepatectomies e'largies. In *Etudes Anatomiques et Chirugicales*, pp. 400–409. Paris: Masson & Cie.
3. Goldsmith, N.A. & Woodburne, R.T. (1957) The surgical anatomy pertaining to liver resection. *Surgery, Gynecology and Obstetrics*, **105**, 310–318.
4. Gordon, K.C.D. (1967) Cystic arterial patterns in diseased human gallbladders. *Gut*, **8**, 565–568.
5. Hand, B.H. (1973) Anatomy and function of the extrahepatic biliary system. *Clinics in Gastroenterology*, **2**, 3–29.
6. Hardy, K.J., Wheatley, I.C., Anderson, A.I.E. & Bond, R.J. (1976) The lymph nodes of the porta hepatis. *Surgery, Gynecology and Obstetrics*, **143**, 225–228.
7. Healey, J.E. (1954) Clinical anatomic aspects of radical hepatic surgery. *Journal of the International College of Surgeons*, **22**, 542.
8. Hjortjo, C.H. (1950) The topography of the intrahepatic duct system. *Acta Anatomica*, **11**, 599–615.
9. Koneru, B., Zajko, A.B., Linda, S., Marsh, J.W., Tzakis, A.G., Iwatsuki, S. & Starzl, T.E. (1989) Obstructing mucocoele of the cystic duct after transplantation of the liver. *Surgery, Gynecology and Obstetrics*, **168**, 394–396.
10. Kune, G.A. (1969) The anatomical basis of liver surgery. *Australian and New Zealand Journal of Surgery*, **39**, 117–126.
11. Longmire, W.P. & Cleveland, R.J. (1972) Surgical anatomy and blunt trauma of the liver. *Surgical Clinics of North America*, **52**, 587–589.
12. McIndoe, A.H. & Counseller, V.S. (1927) The bilaterality of the liver. *Archives of Surgery*, **15**, 589–611.
13. Michels, N.A. (1960) Newer anatomy of liver: variant blood supply and collateral circulation. *Journal of the American Medical Association*, **172**, 125.
14. Nakamura, S. & Tsuzuki, T. (1981) Surgical anatomy of the hepatic veins and inferior vena cava. *Surgery, Gynecology and Obstetrics*, **152**, 43–50.
15. Northover, J.M.A. & Terblanche, J. (1978) Bile duct blood supply: its importance in human liver transplantation. *Transplantation*, **26**, 67–69.
16. Northover, J.M.A. & Terblanche, J. (1979) A new look at the arterial supply of the bile duct in man and its surgical implications. *British Journal of Surgery*, **66**, 379–384.
17. Starzl, T.E., Bell, R.H., Beart, R.W. & Putnam, C.W. (1975) Hepatic trisegmentectomy and other liver resections. *Surgery, Gynecology and Obstetrics*, **141**, 429–437.
18. Streeter, G.L. (1942) Developmental horizons in human embryos. Descriptions of age group XII, 21–29 somites. *Contributions to Embryology*, **30**, 211–245.
19. Tung, T.T. (1979) *Les Re'sections Majeures et Mineures du Foie*. Paris: Masson.

CHAPTER 2

Normal Histology and Ultrastructure

G.H. Millward-Sadler & A-M. Jezequel

LIVER MICROANATOMY AND HISTOLOGY

The basic unit of the liver has classically been the lobule. This is identified from the microscopic anatomical features of the liver and is composed of a central efferent vein surrounded by parenchyma with portal tracts at the periphery. It does not correspond to the acinus, which is the functional unit of the liver.[164] The acinus is not well defined anatomically without injection studies but is formed from a central portal tract surrounded by parenchyma with the efferent veins now at the periphery and therefore no longer 'central'. Blood then drains from the acinus through several small efferent veins—the terminal hepatic veins. The lobule has the status of being the traditional established unit used to describe the architecture of the liver, but the acinus provides better understand-

ing of disease mechanisms. Even abnormal pathological features such as the stellate necrosis of ischaemic hepatitis are better appreciated using the acinus as the basic unit of architecture.

HEPATIC ARCHITECTURE

The acinus

The acinus is the functional unit of the liver and conceptually is a mass of parenchyma dependent on a unit blood supply provided through the portal tracts. Each acinus has a central portal tract of the smallest calibre—the terminal portal tract—which histologically is round on transverse section. Blood flows from the artery and portal vein of this terminal portal tract into the sinusoids, supplies the intervening parenchyma and then drains into

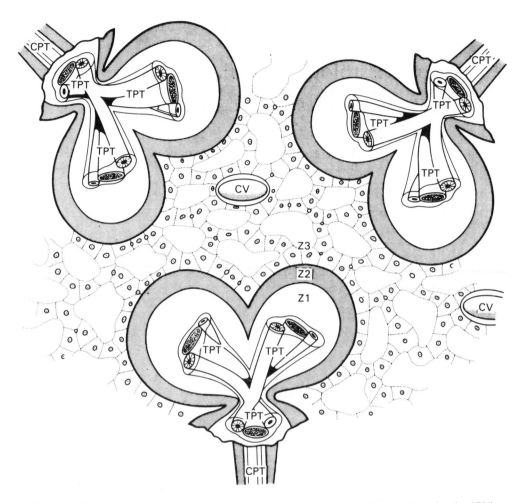

Figure 2.1 This is a diagrammatic representation of a lobule with the centrally positioned vein (CV) surrounded by parenchyma and with the portal tracts (TPT) at the periphery. Note that the portal tracts normally arise at differing heights and angles from the conducting tract and not, as represented here, by simultaneous division. Thus there may be as few as three or as many as six portal tracts seen around any one lobule.

Three conducting portal tracts (CPT) here each split into three terminal portal tracts (TPT). The parenchyma has been diagrammatically represented as three zones which do not have a morphologically visible counterpart in routine histology. Zone I (Z1) is immediately around the terminal portal tract. Zone 2 (Z2) surrounds zone 1, and zone 3 (Z3), drawn in as hepatocytes and sinusoids, fills in the spaces between the zone 2s down to the central efferent vein (CV).

Each terminal portal tract is surrounded by zoned parenchyma and constitutes an acinus. Each group of three acini with their conducting portal tract form a complex acinus. Nine potential acini are illustrated, of which six are more fully detailed to include zone 3 hepatocytes. No acinus is complete because each will drain to more than one central vein.

Note also that one lobule is formed from between three and six acini with approximately half of any one acinus contributing to the lobule.

the peripheral efferent veins—the central veins of the lobule. Each efferent vein, or terminal hepatic venule, receives blood from several acini.

The hepatocytes of each acinus are zoned by their position in relation to the portal tract, with those nearest the portal tract being in zone 1 and those furthest away being zone 3 (Figure 2.1). These zones cannot be identified by standard histological techniques but they do reflect the variation of function along the sinusoid.[114] This variation in function is coordinated so that the acinus acts as a physiological unit for any of several biochemical pro-

cesses.[73] A model for ammonia detoxification in the acinus has been proposed.[82] In this model there is a high-capacity, low-affinity system primarily located in the periportal zone which converts most of the ammonia in the portal blood to urea. A low-capacity but high-affinity system which converts ammonia and glutamic acid into glutamine is located in the perivenular zone and scavenges the efferent sinusoidal blood for residual ammonia.

Hepatocytes adjacent to the portal tract receive blood with the highest content of oxygen, insulin, glucagon and amino acids. This is believed to explain the higher metabolic activity of zone 1 hepatocytes and why the earliest signs of regeneration are found there. More direct morphological evidence has been produced. Autoradiography has demonstrated that protein synthesis[113] and uptake of galactose[69] occurs predominantly in zone 1 and the distribution of hepatocellular enzymes in the acinus also supports this concept.[184] Transaminases,[178] glutamyl transpeptidase,[138] alcohol dehydrogenase,[71] rhodamine B[21] and carbamylphosphate synthetase[57] are most easily demonstrated in periportal zone 1 while glutamine synthetase—specifically required for the conversion of ammonia and glutamic acid into glutamine,[60] the NADH ʊ.nd NADPH reductases and esterases—are predominantly in perivenular zone 3.[138]

The distribution of some of these functions is determined by the microenvironment of the hepatocytes. The periportal zone is the site of maximal oxygen consumption, gluconeogenesis and glycolysis. Experimentally this is instantly altered if the flow of blood through the acinus is reversed by retrograde perfusion of the liver and then the perivenular zone 3 becomes the site of maximal activity for these functions.[199] None the less, not all functions are changed by alteration in the microenvironment. Mixed-function oxidation remains predominantly located in perivenular hepatocytes even on retrograde perfusion of the liver[199] and glutamine synthetase remains confined to a small number of perivenular hepatocytes 1–2 layers thick,[60] suggesting that different control mechanisms, possibly genetically determined,[73,219] may operate.

Clearly the acinar zones will be inadequate to explain fully the physiological complexity of the acinus.[107] The challenge morphologically will be to correlate disordered structure and function at the microanatomical level in both acute and chronic liver disease.

Complex acinus

This is the term used for a group of three or more simple acini served by a common vascular bundle from a larger conducting portal tract.[164] The latter has a triangular outline on liver biopsy. Both the portal vein and the hepatic artery within this conducting portal tract subdivide into branches, each of which is terminal and supplies one acinus.

In addition to the simple acini, a complex acinus has a sheath of hepatocytes around the conducting portal tract which does not belong to any acinus but is supplied by a vascular twig arising directly from the vessels of the conducting tract. This sheath is a composite of small groups of hepatocytes and each group is called an acinulus. The perivenular zone 3 hepatocytes from the simple acini abut onto this acinular sleeve. Consequently, necrosis of zone 3 hepatocytes will appear not only to be perivenular but may also be found adjacent to some of the larger portal tracts, morphologically exaggerating the severity of the lesion. Such necrosis often has a stellate configuration and this is more readily explained using the concept of the acinus.

Acinar agglomerate

A further enlargement of the multi-acinar concept has also been described in which three or more of these complex acini are grouped together to form an acinar agglomerate. This also has a directly supplied sleeve of hepatocytes around its large vascular core. These complicated acinar agglomerates are not visualized in routine histological sections because their divisions branch to produce a three-dimensional network. Their complete demonstration requires vascular injection techniques with cleared thick sections of liver.

The biliary tree

Bile produced by the hepatocytes of an acinus flows through the canalicular network to the appropriate portal tract. The intrahepatic canaliculi do not run simply between hepatocytes in a straight line from efferent vein to portal tract but form a complicated three-dimensional network.[80,187] The anastomoses are so extensive that focal mechanical obstruction at simple or complex acinar level does not usually result in blockage of bile flow. At the portal tract interface the bile is excreted into the peripheral bile ductules—the cholangioles or ducts of Hering—and thence into the smallest of the interlobular bile ducts in the terminal portal tract. It is then excreted through the variously graded interlobular and septal bile ducts in the tracts of the supra-acinar complexes.

HISTOLOGY _____

Portal tracts

Stromal trabeculae in the liver are continuous with its capsule and extend from the porta hepatis into the liver by repeated branching. These trabeculae contain the various branches of the portal vein, hepatic artery and bile ducts as well as the lymphatics and nerve fibres. The stroma is a tightly woven meshwork of fibroblasts, types I and III collagen bundles and elastic fibres within a matrix of non-fibrillar collagens including types IV, V, and VI, fibronectin and laminin[74,77] (and see Chapter 32). Stroma around the bile ducts, especially those of septal calibre, is condensed into a concentrically orientated cuff of tissue. Basement membrane is found around the various arterial, portal venous and bile duct branches within the portal tract.

In biopsy specimens the majority of portal tracts will be terminal structures or their preterminal trunks. The former are visualized as round or oval tracts when cut in cross-section (Figure 2.2). The preterminal trunks are larger, and in cross-section are the smallest angular, frequently triangular, tracts. This appearance is created by the branching of the trunks into their terminal divisions. Consequently a longitudinal section of these trunks may show a bifurcating portal tract. All three branches are rarely identified in the plane of a single section in routine histological preparations.

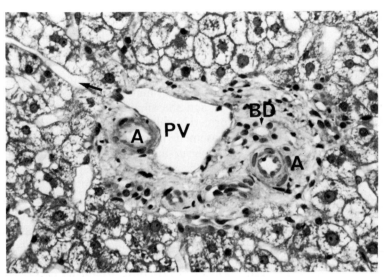

Figure 2.2 An oval cross-section of a terminal portal tract. The portal vein is the largest vascular space (PV) and a tributary has directly entered the sinusoid (arrow). Two arterioles are present (A). The endothelium and double layer of smooth muscle cells are clearly demonstrated in the arteriole on the right. A small interlobular bile duct (BD) is present just above this arteriole and small bile ductules are present along the lower margin of the tract.

The hepatic artery

Branches of the hepatic artery are intimately related to the corresponding branch of the portal vein. As well as branching, the artery spirals around the portal vein (Figure 2.3) and thus in a single histological section may appear as several unconnected arteries adjacent to a portal vein.

Arteries and arterioles that are commonly visualized in needle biopsy material have at most an intima, an internal elastic lamina and two or three layers of smooth muscle cells in the media (Figures 2.2 and 2.3). A cuff of adventitia surrounds the media and contains numerous unmyelinated nerve fibres. The terminal arterioles are much smaller, lack an internal elastic lamina and have an intima surrounded by a single layer of smooth muscle. They produce a leash of capillaries that encircles the accompanying interlobular bile duct and is termed the 'peribiliary plexus'.[128,198] This is believed to help regulate the composition of bile excreted by modifying the water and bicarbonate concentrations in a counter-current manner analogous to the loop of Henle in the kidney. Drainage of the plexus is both directly into the sinusoids[131] and into small branches of the portal veins.[198] A different leash of capillaries supplies the other portal tract structures and either drains directly into the sinusoidal network or may join the terminal portal venule immediately before it enters the network. A smooth muscle sphincter has been described around these latter capillaries which allows the volume and pressure of arterial blood to be controlled.[110,165]

The vascular supply to the rat liver has been studied by scanning electron microscopy using resin polymer corrosion casts of the appropriate vessel. These have supported earlier studies[135] and have also demonstrated that some arterioles terminate in zones 2 and 3 of the acinus.[102] The functional significance of such vessels has not been determined nor can their equivalent be recognized by standard light microscopic techniques.

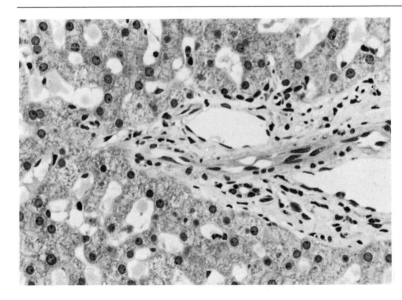

Figure 2.3 A terminal portal tract cut obliquely. The hepatic arteriole runs longitudinally from right to centre and, in spiralling around the portal vein, appears to separate it into the two branches. The limiting plate of hepatocytes is clearly defined along the lower margin of the portal tract as the layer of hepatocytes parallel to the edge of the tract and at right angles to the other plates of hepatocytes.

The portal vein

Branches of the portal vein are the largest blood-containing endothelial-lined space in the portal tract (Figures 2.2 and 2.3). The small veins only have a thin basement membrane surrounding the endothelium. Smooth muscle surrounds the endothelium in the largest veins but such branches are rarely identifiable within needle biopsy specimens. Both the 'conducting' and the 'axial distributing' veins, as described by Elias,[42] produce a large number of venules which empty into the periportal sinusoids. Many, if not all of these vessels as well as arising from terminals of the portal vein regulate the rate of flow of blood into the sinusoids.[102] As there are no muscle cells around the venules it has been suggested that this is only possible through the swelling and shrinking of reticuloendothelial cells at the junction of venule with sinusoid.[126] The mechanisms by which this postulated sphincter is controlled are not fully understood, but a response to vasodilators such as adenine nucleotide has been noted.[126] It has been postulated that adenosine regulates flow by controlling the hepatic arteriolar contribution, which is then varied in inverse proportion to the portal venous flow.[46,109] Increased arterial flow will also have the effect of lowering the adenosine concentration so that an autoregulatory mechanism becomes established. This autoregulatory 'adenosine washout' hypothesis identifies the arterial contribution as one that is responsive to portal blood flow rather than its primary regulator.

A second mechanism may also exist. McCuskey[126] has described different types of arterioportal anastomoses, one of which may be very effective in this respect. The arteriolar blood enters into the sinusoid just beyond the portal vein inlet but is directed against the flow of portal venous blood entering the sinusoid. Vasodilatation of these arterioles will therefore be a very effective method of reducing portal blood flow. These arteriovenous anastomoses have been confirmed by scanning electron microscopic examination of corrosion casts of the arterial tree but could not be demonstrated in the casts created from injection of the portal vein.[135] The mechanisms that control such a system are unknown as are any interrelationships with the adenosine washout hypothesis.

Bile ducts

The largest intrahepatic branches are the septal bile ducts (Figure 2.4), which, after repeated branching, diminish in calibre to interlobular ducts. The smallest interlobular bile duct is present in the terminal portal tract (Figure 2.2) and communicates through peripheral bile ductules with the canalicular network (Figure 2.3). All branches of the biliary tree down to the junction of the ductule with the hepatocytes have a basement membrane. This is a microscopically homogeneous layer of gel formed from mucopolysaccharides and glycoproteins—particularly laminin—and in contact with the duct epithelium on the one surface and closely associated with fine reticulin fibres of type IV collagen on the other surface. Because of its mucopolysaccharide component it can be well demonstrated by oxidation–aldehyde techniques such as periodic–acid Schiff (PAS) or methanamine–silver.[147] Bile duct basement membrane may be antigenically distinct from capillary basement membrane.[155]

Septal bile ducts are readily recognized by their large calibre, although the diameter may vary two- or threefold between the largest and the smallest. Characteristically the epithelium is formed by tall columnar mucus-secreting cells resting on a basement membrane. These cells have abundant clear cytoplasm and a small round or oval nucleus situated at the basal pole of the cell (Figure 2.4). The cytoplasm and apical border stain positively with the PAS technique and the acidic mucopolysaccharide carboxyl groups of the cytoplasm with alcian blue. Around these ducts is the basement membrane and then a concentric layering of stromal collagen containing the peribiliary arteriolar plexus.

The *interlobular bile ducts* are those found in the smaller portal tracts. They occupy a central position in the tract and are lined by a cuboidal epithelium resting on basement membrane. The cells have a small round nucleus and the cytoplasm is scanty and eosinophilic. Usually there is no PAS-positive staining of the cytoplasm or glycocalyx but on occasion a transition zone where a positively stained brush border occurs in cuboidal epithelium can be found. Staining with alcian blue is negative.

The smallest duct is formed from the amalgamation, rarely visualized, of bile ductules. These ductules are seen in the periphery of the tracts usually as an elongated double column of flattened cells (Figure 2.5). The nucleus is similar to those in other bile duct epithelium but the cytoplasm is even more scanty and has no special histochemical staining properties. The ductules link up directly with the hepatocytes and at this point the basement membrane ceases. This is the region sometimes referred to as the canal of Hering.

Other portal tract structures

These comprise the lymphatics and nerves. Lymphatics are present in all portal tracts and surround the artery and vein. They are also present in the walls of the larger branches of the portal and hepatic veins. Nerve bundles are identified only in the largest portal tracts of a wedge biopsy, but unmyelinated fibres can be demonstrated around arterioles by immunohistochemical techniques and electron microscopy.

Parenchyma

On standard light microscopy the cell plates are anastomosing Indian-file cords of polygonal hepatocytes which pass radially from portal tract to efferent hepatic vein. Around the portal tract is a concentric but discontinuous layer of hepatocytes from which these cords arise (Figure 2.3). This layer forms the limiting plate of the parenchyma on the portal tract interface and is a feature frequently altered in the many diseases affecting the liver. There is no morphological change in either the portal tract collagen

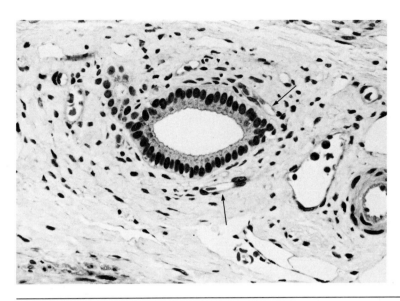

Figure 2.4 Septal bile duct lined by tall columnar epithelium with oval nuclei at the basal pole of the cells. The stroma immediately around the bile duct is more condensed and contains capillaries (arrows) which are part of the peribiliary plexus.

at its interface with the limiting plate or in the hepatocytes of the limiting plate when compared with their immediate neighbours. Communications between the portal vessels and the sinusoids breach the plate and so produce the discontinuity.

The Indian-file arrangement of hepatocytes between portal tracts and efferent veins is only a two-dimensional representation of the architecture, but the constancy of the arrangement in histological sections, whatever the plane in which they are examined, indicates a symmetrical meshwork of hepatocytes. This meshwork is formed by the series of fenestrated cell plates that are both anastomosing and continually curving (Figure 2.6). An analogy with the sponge can be made in which the air spaces represent intercommunicating sinusoids and the matrix the anastomosing cell plates (Figure 2.7).

In babies and small children, the cell plates are double and the adult single cell plate pattern is acquired slowly, usually by the age of 5 years. Above this age, twinning of cell plates is regarded as evidence of regeneration.

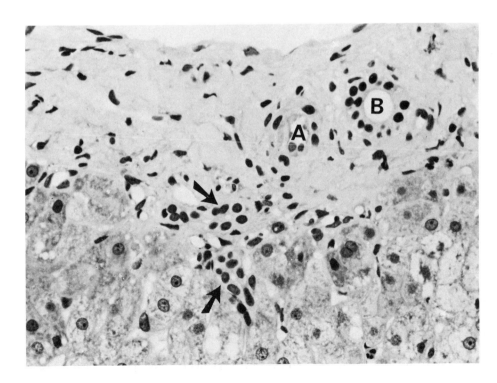

Figure 2.5 Bile ductules at the edge of a portal tract (arrows). It is an elongated double column of epithelial cells which have scanty cytoplasm. A tiny lumen can be seen. In the centre is an interlobular bile duct (B) with an hepatic arteriole (A).

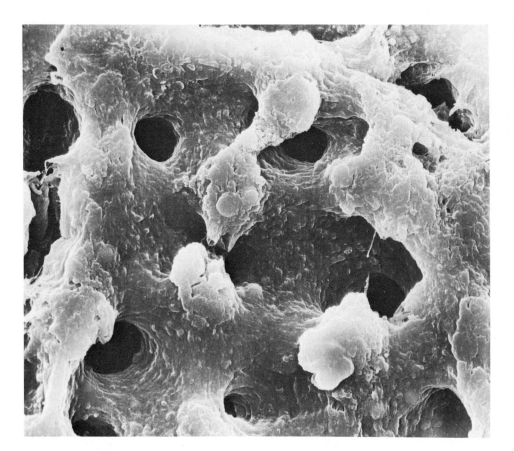

Figure 2.6 Scanning electron microscopy of human liver biopsy with a normal architecture. Note the continually curving nature of the cell plates.

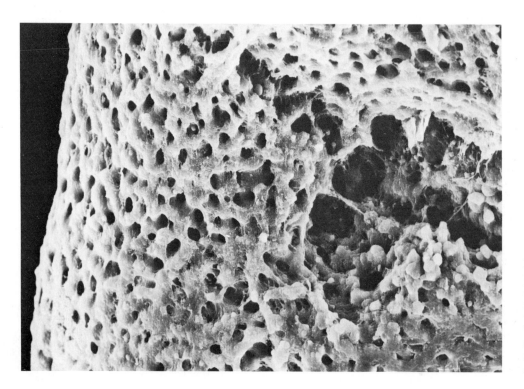

Figure 2.7 Scanning electron microscopy of normal human liver. The portal tract (right) is dividing into branches but the stroma has been torn out. The parenchyma shows a sponge-like arrangement of intercommunicating sinusoids and anastomosing cell plates.

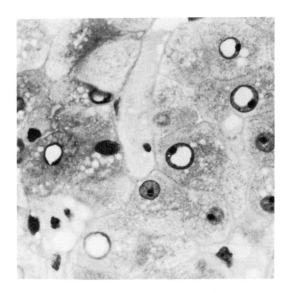

Figure 2.8 Periportal hepatocytes with vacuolated 'empty' nuclei. A membrane usually demarcates the vacuole which in the electron microscope can be identified as invagination of the nucleus by cytoplasm.

Hepatocytes

These are large polygonal cells 20–30 μm across which have a clearly defined cell margin and a prominent nucleus.

The nucleus is round, has finely dispersed chromatin condensed slightly around the nuclear envelope and contains a large nucleolus. Occasional hepatocytes are binucleate and the proportion increases with age or any stimulus to regeneration. Most cells also have diploid nuclei but again there are occasional tetraploid and polyploid nuclei to be found and these also increase in frequency with age and in response to regeneration. Polyploidy is represented morphologically by a larger, denser, more haematoxyphilic nucleus. The nucleus can be enlarged by intranuclear vacuoles which are cytoplasmic invaginations of the nuclear envelope (Figure 2.8). Such vacuoles are most frequent in periportal hepatocytes and often contain glycogen. Electron microscopy shows that these cytoplasmic invaginations are almost entirely composed of smooth endoplasmic reticulum with rosettes of glycogen between the membranes. Although described in association with diabetes mellitus and with Wilson's disease, these vacuoles are common in a wide variety of disorders and, for instance, are often present in patients with psoriasis without primary liver disease.

The abundant cytoplasm is eosinophilic but frequently shows a basophilic stippling due to the haematoxyphilia of the RNA in the rough endoplasmic reticulum. Sometimes the cytoplasm has distinct areas of eosinophilia and of basophilia which most commonly represent the light-microscopic equivalents of smooth and rough endoplasmic reticulum. The mitochondria can be seen as small round or elongated refractile eosinophilic bodies approximately 0.5–1.0 μm long but which can occasionally be up to 5 μm in maximum length. Plasma membranes are clearly defined and with care even the normal bile canaliculus can be identified between the opposing membranes of adjacent hepatocytes—most easily where the membranes of three hepatocytes converge. Perivenular hepatocytes frequently contain a granular brown lipofuscin pigment. This 'wear and tear' pigment must be differentiated from intrahepatic and canalicular bile which indicates cholestasis and is a pathological change. Lipofuscin granules are more uniform in size, refractile, and golden to dark brown in colour. They cluster around but are never present within the bile canaliculus. Although it is a normal wear and tear pigment, there are pathological conditions in which lipofuscin is present in excess (see Chapter 46).

By using histochemical, autoradiographic and immunological techniques a variety of other normal cell constituents can be demonstrated. These include glycogen, the bile canaliculus,[177,178] albumin,[49,66] and a wide variety of enzymes.[71,138,178,206]

The cytoskeleton of hepatocytes can also be visualized using immunohistochemical techniques.[48,145,172] From these studies the relative roles of microtubules, microfilaments and intermediate filaments are becoming more apparent (see below).

Microtubules are formed from tubulin and can be visualized using antibodies to this protein. They form a cytoplasmic network of strands which is present throughout the cytoplasm but is most dense in the region of the Golgi apparatus and along the sinusoidal plasma membrane.[125] Functionally they are involved in the secretion of locally synthesized proteins into the plasma.

Microfilaments are formed from myosin and actin and can be easily demonstrated immunocytochemically using anti-actin antibodies.[51] They are distributed along the internal face of the plasma membrane being particularly concentrated around the bile canaliculus. They are involved in bile secretion and with the functioning of the microvilli on the sinusoidal surface. Disruption of the microfilament network using cytochalasin B induces cholestasis.[152] In lymphocytes microfilaments are involved in the process of 'capping' and internalization of surface membrane antigens when the cells are exposed to the appropriate antibodies,[185] and it is possible that hepatocyte microfilaments are involved in similar responses in the course of immunologically mediated diseases of the liver.

Intermediate filaments are cytokeratins and can be seen extending from the plasma membrane to the perinuclear zone. Different cells have different cytokeratin subtypes. Hepatocytes normally have cytokeratins 8 and 18[145,172] but may develop other subtypes in response to chronic injury and in particular may acquire the subtypes 7 and 19 which are associated with bile duct epithelial cells.[90, 209] They form an irregular meshwork of fibrils which extends from the cytoplasmic faces of the plasma membrane to the perinuclear zone, where they are present in greatest concentration. Intermediate filaments are

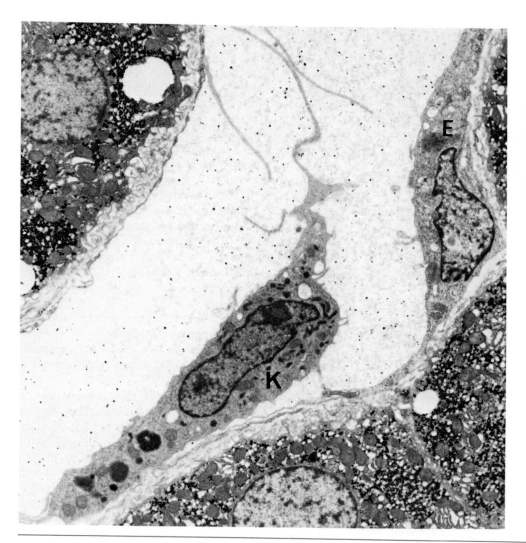

Figure 2.9 Transmission electron microscopy of human liver. A Kupffer cell (K) is demonstrated with elongated cytoplasmic processes extending into the sinusoid. Phagosomes are present as large dark intracytoplasmic bodies bottom left. Note the adjacent endothelial cell (E) with its attenuated cytoplasm extending between the Kupffer cell and subjacent hepatocyte.

responsible for the spatial organization and structural integrity of the hepatocyte.

Sinusoids

The sinusoids are wide vascular channels separating anastomosing plates of hepatocytes and lined by fenestrated endothelial cells (Figures 2.9 and 2.12). They contain highly mobile, tissue-specific macrophages—the Kupffer cells—and the recently described pit cells. The endothelial lining separates the vascular lumen of the sinusoid from the perisinusoidal space—the space of Disse—in which can be found a variety of matrix proteins, the fat-storing perisinusoidal (Ito) cells and the microvilli of the sinusoidal surface of the hepatocyte. These matrix proteins include fibrillar Type III collagen, which can be demonstrated by silver impregnation techniques (Figure 2.10) or by electron microscopy (Figure 2.26). Techniques for isolating and distinguishing sinusoidal cells have been established.[41,104,105]

Kupffer cells

These are sporadically distributed large stellate macrophages within the sinusoids (Figures 2.9 and 2.11). They are positioned at the junctions of sinusoids and are most frequent in periportal zones.[17] These macrophages are larger than endothelial cells with more cytoplasm and have cytoplasmic processes that extend into and sometimes across the sinusoid. Some of these processes anchor the cells to the wall of the sinusoid and have been seen both attached to the endothelial cell and also passing through the endothelial fenestrations into the space of Disse. The nucleus of the Kupffer cell is elongated with a plumper, slightly more irregular outline than the slimmer, smoother, elongated nucleus of the endothelial cell. Transitions between the two cell types do not occur.[215] Discrimination between the two is usually easy, especially if phagocytosis occurs. Otherwise it involves the histochemical or immunological demonstration in Kupffer cells of non-specific esterase, peroxidase, α_1-antitrypsin or muramidase (Figure 2.11), positive immunological staining using monoclonal antibodies,[121] or electron microscopy.

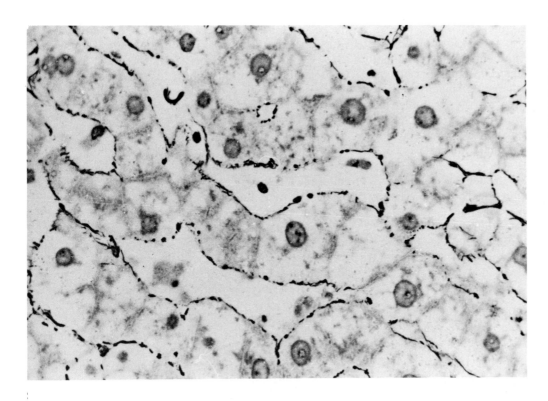

Figure 2.10 Reticulin architecture of liver. Wilder's reticulin on 2 μm methacrylate section of human liver to demonstrate the continuously intermittent deposit of silver along the sinusoidal surfaces of hepatocytes.

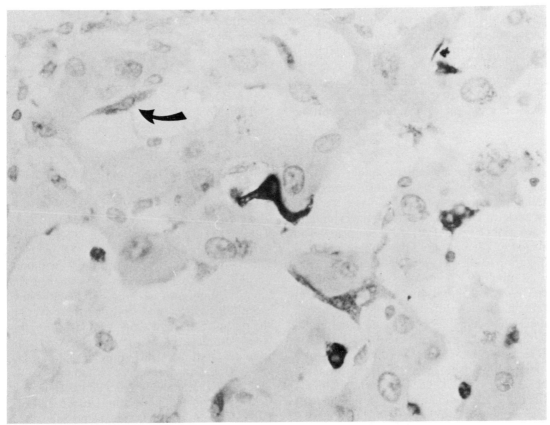

Figure 2.11 Demonstration of muramidase in a Kupffer cell using the peroxidase-antiperoxidase technique with primary antibody diluted at 1/1000. Note the negative endothelial cell (arrow).

The origin and kinetics of Kupffer cells are a controversial topic with both evidence for local maintenance and proliferation and for recruitment and replacement from bone marrow. It is probable that Kupffer cells are a stable, self-maintaining population of macrophages[17] capable of rapid proliferation but rapidly reinforced by recruitment from bone marrow when necessary.[16,39,61] Repopulation of the liver from the bone marrow following both bone marrow and liver transplantation has also been clearly demonstrated.[59,159,189]

Kupffer cells have a vital role in the defence mechanisms of the body[99,134,171] (see Chapter 9). They are actively pinocytosing and phagocytosing cells that have specific receptors enabling them to clear endotoxin and immune complexes.[22,134,171] There is also evidence that they are capable of directly causing hepatocellular damage and death.[50]

The pit cell

This cell can only be identified with confidence by electron microscopy (see below) and has only recently been identified in human liver.[19,100,106] Morphologically they are similar to large granular lymphocytes with 'natural killer' (NK) functions found in the spleen and other sites in the body but not lymph nodes. These NK cells antigenically carry the CD-56 and CD-57 markers as well as a CD-16 Fc receptor which distinguish them from activated cytotoxic T lymphocytes. Their role appears to be to eliminate tumour cells,[26,116] host cells that are antibody coated and host cells expressing viral markers.[24,26] They are present in very small numers elsewhere in the body so that their identification in the liver is of potential general immunological significance. Their role in the pathogenesis of chronic hepatitis remains to be clarified although one of the first reports identifying them in human liver was in a patient with autoimmune chronic active hepatitis.[101]

Endothelial cells

Endothelial cells of the liver sinusoid are unique amongst endothelial cells of the body.[218] On light microscopy they have thin attenuated inconspicuous cytoplasm with an elongated thin nucleus. Pores (fenestrae) in the cytoplasm of these cells are grouped together into 'sieve plates' and can only be clearly seen using the scanning electron microscope (Figure 2.13). Experimentally endothelial cells can be separated from other sinusoidal cells by centrifugal elutriation after enzymatic perfusion,[88,105] but their morphological staining characteristics are more variable. A major functional characteristic of liver sinusoidal endothelial cells is their capacity for endocytosis,[36,99,215] with endocytotic vesicles a correspondingly prominent feature on electron microscopy (see below). Factor 8-related antigen can be demonstrated in the sinusoidal endothelial cells of guinea pig liver,[166] but not in rat[88] or human liver and ulex lectin staining is also consistently negative.[150] Endothelial cells also can synthesize type IV collagen[88] and fibronectin,[166] while Fc receptors may be present on the cell membrane, at least in the rat.[203] Another way in which the liver sinusoidal endothelial cells are unusual is that they lack an electron-dense basement membrane. Consequently, very small particles can gain direct access to the space of Disse through the fenestrae of the sieve plates with the size of the particles in the microfiltrate being determined by the size of the fenestrae.

The space of Disse

The subendothelial space of Disse contains type III collagen fibrils and is rich in both the glycoprotein, fibronectin and the proteoglycan, heparan sulphate. It does not morphologically have a basement membrane. Although small deposits of basement membrane type IV collagen can be visualized by immunochemical staining, the presence of laminin, which elsewhere is a regular constituent of basement membranes, is more controversial. It has been claimed that laminin is not present in normal sinusoids and only appears in the space of Disse in pathological states.[67,76,122] Others have been able to demonstrate laminin in normal sinusoids albeit with much reduced intensity of staining by using high-titre, affinity-purified antibodies,[75,119,205] and laminin production by the perisinusoidal (Ito) cells has been demonstrated in culture.[35,55] In situ hybridization has also been used to localize laminin B1 chain-specific RNA transcripts to the perisinusoidal cells of the sinusoids.[127] More recently another matrix glycoprotein, tenascin, has been identified within the space of Disse but not within portal tracts.[205] Enhanced staining is seen at parenchymal–connective tissue interfaces in active liver disease, suggesting that tenascin has a transient role in early matrix organization.

There is increasing evidence that the matrix proteins are vital to the functional integrity of sinusoidal cells and hepatocytes. Considerable improvement in morphology and function of hepatocytes and perisinusoidal (Ito) cells occurs in tissue culture if a laminin-rich model basement membrane matrix is used.[11,56] The complex interplay of the proteins within the space of Disse and with the cells that secrete them that is more fully discussed in Chapter 32.

The perisinusoidal cell

This cell is situated within the space of Disse and has various names including the Ito cell,[89] the hepatic lipocyte and the fat-storing cell. It is a small stellate cell that may occupy the sinusoidal recess between the sinusoidal and lateral membranes of adjacent hepatocytes. Its major morphological feature, and one that gives it a name, is the presence of small droplets of fat within the cytoplasm. These droplets are rich in vitamin A, specifically retinyl esters,[13] and the cells are the major storage cell for the vitamin in the body. Vitamin A has a specific autofluorescence at 330 nm when examined in ultraviolet light so that the cells can be recognized with some confidence. A gold chloride technique can also be used for their morphological demonstration if liver biopsies are first prefixed in 0.05% chromic acid for up to 5 minutes at room temperature.[200,209] In rats the perisinusoidal cells can be stained immunochemically for desmin,[223] but it is difficult to demonstrate this protein, at least morphologically, in human perisinusoidal cells. This may simply reflect a lack of sensitivity in the techniques used to demonstrate desmin in the human liver. Techniques for the isolation, purification and culture of these cells have been established.[54] The perisinusoidal cell has been shown to secrete fibronectin, laminin, types I and III collagens, as well as collagenases. They probably have a major role in forming and maintaining the extracellular matrix in health and disease. This is considered in more detail in Chapter 32.

Hepatic veins and venules

The hepatic venous tree drains blood from the liver into the inferior vena cava. The smallest radicles are the terminal hepatic veins which drain the blood from the simple acinus. These efferent veins are little more than a dilated sinusoid without the fenestrations in the endothelial cells. The larger veins become surrounded by a fenestrated layer of collagen with smooth-muscle cells and lymphatics appearing in this wall.[158]

ULTRASTRUCTURE

The meaning of a 'normal' liver cell and the variety of selection criteria adopted in different studies have been extensively discussed[143] and the difficulties—practical and ethical—of selecting a reference population in human studies have been emphasized.

As visualized with the electron microscope, the one-cell-thick plates formed by the parenchymal cells are separated from the sinusoids by a thin endothelial lining. Bile canaliculi are seen as spaces between the hepatocytes and do not communicate with the subendothelial space (the space of Disse). This arrangement is evident in transmission (Figure 2.12) as well as in scanning electron microscopy (Figure 2.13).[23,40,47,138,169,177] The tridimensional aspects of liver ultrastructure have been well illustrated in a recent exhaustive review,[154] while some texts are especially concerned with the various facets of the relationships between liver cells, structure and function.[3]

THE HEPATOCYTE

Stereological studies show that hepatocytes account for about 78% of the liver volume in normal adult rats, with 6% for non-hepatocytes and 16% for intracellular spaces.[14] In man, the hepatocytes represent 80–88% of the parenchymal volume.[143,168]

The nucleus

The nucleus is separated from the cytoplasm by a double membrane and accounts for 7–8% of the parenchymal volume in animals and in man.[14,143,168] The space between the two leaflets of the nuclear membrane is considered to be part of the granular endoplasmic reticulum, although continuity is rarely found in thin sections. The outer membrane of the nucleus is studded with ribosomes and may extend into the cytoplasm as brief segments of rough endoplasmic reticulum. The inner membrane is smooth and lined with a polymeric protein or nuclear lamina. Recent work has demonstrated that the lamina is composed of intermediate-type filaments: the nuclear lamina would provide an architectural framework for the interphase nucleus and anchoring sites for interphase chromosomes.[63] Small clumps of heterochromatin are seen along the inner membrane and around the nucleolus. At intervals, the outer and inner membranes of the nucleus show close apposition to form the nuclear pores. These have been demonstrated in thin sections using negative staining, freeze etching, scanning electron microscopy in whole tissue, in isolated nuclei and in nuclear 'ghosts'.[81,103,173] The outer diameter of the nuclear 'pore complex' varies from 85 to 100 nm and the inner diameter measures from 25 to 40 nm, depending on the technique. A granule is sometimes evident in the centre of the pore complex, especially in nuclear ghosts sectioned parallel to the membrane surface. Besides the central granule, other structures or 'diaphragm material' such as fibres or tubules are seen inside the annulus but their significance has not been elucidated. No significant differences have been noted between the pore complexes from nuclei of normal rat liver or from hepatomas.[81]

The general and enzymatic composition of the nuclear envelope has been studied mainly on rat and bovine liver but this is difficult because of its close association with DNA, RNA and various proteins on the inner side and with cytoplasmic ribosomes and proteins on the outer side. Most, if not all, enzymes of the nuclear envelope are microsomal enzymes.[148] Some of them, such as nucleoside diphosphatase[140] or glucose-6-phosphatase,[68] have been demonstrated in situ by histochemical techniques.

In the nucleoplasm, most of the chromatin is present as euchromatin but the appearance varies with the mode of fixation. Clumps of heterochromatin are more evident when fixation with aldehydes (formaldehyde, acrolein or glutaraldehyde) precedes osmium tetroxide than when osmium is used alone. Next to the clumps of chromatin and separated from them by a clear halo are the perichromatin granules, which are about 40 nm in diameter (Figure 2.14). Enzymic digestion shows that they contain proteins and RNA fibrils, possibly a type of messenger RNA.[5] Clusters of small interchromatin granules, 20–25 nm in diameter, are dispersed in the nucleoplasm and are thought to be ribonucleoproteins.[5]

The nucleolus appears as a spongy network, roughly

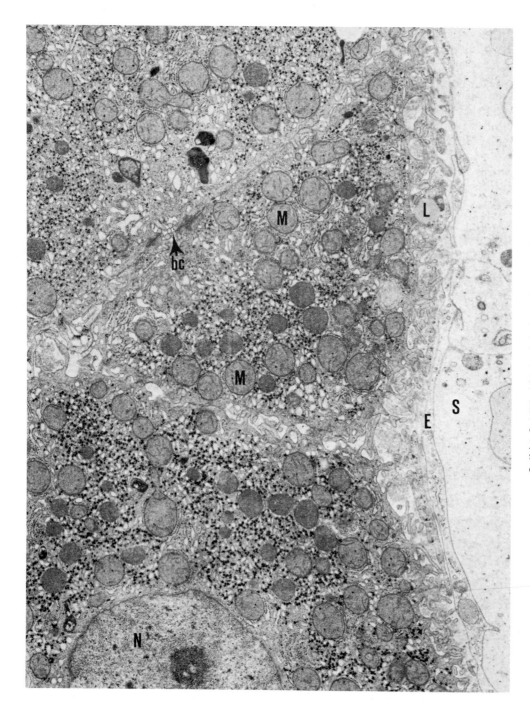

Figure 2.12 Low-power electron micrograph of normal human liver. Three hepatocytes are present in the field. They are separated from the sinusoidal lumen (S) by a thin layer of endothelium (E). A small lipid droplet (L), visible in the space of Disse, probably belongs to a lipocyte. The nucleus (N) and nucleolus of a hepatocyte are evident at the bottom of the photograph. In the cytoplasm, numerous mitochondria (M) and peroxisomes are present. The rough endoplasmic reticulum is preferentially located around the nucleus, the sinusoidal border and the mitochondria. The smooth endoplasmic reticulum is diffusely distributed throughout the cytoplasm. It shows a finely vesicular pattern and is associated with rosettes of glycogen. Some elements of the Golgi apparatus are present, together with lysosomes, next to a small bile canaliculus (bc). The junctional complexes on either side of the bile canaliculus are evident. × 9900.

circular in shape, not limited by a membrane (Figures 2.12 and 2.15). It is composed of 15 nm granules and 5–8 nm fibrils, both containing RNA, embedded in a protein matrix.[120] Transport of messenger RNA and other macromolecules to the cytoplasm is believed to be through the nuclear pores. There is also evidence that macromolecular complexes are transported from the cytoplasm to the nucleus. No visible transport of material across the nuclear membranes has yet been detected.

Nuclear inclusions are unusual in normal conditions, except for glycogen. The intranuclear glycogen is always in the form of isolated particles, about 30 nm in diameter, as opposed to the large rosette-like aggregates present in the cytoplasm (Figure 2.14). It occupies large areas, well circumscribed but without a limiting membrane, save for small dense deposits which are often encircled by a thick, finely fibrillar envelope. Although intranuclear glycogen is common in diabetes[40] and in various other conditions, including glycogen storage diseases,[8,169,179] it can also be an occasional finding in normal human liver.[118]

Small cytoplasmic areas, occasionally containing lipid droplets, may be entrapped in invaginations of the nuclear

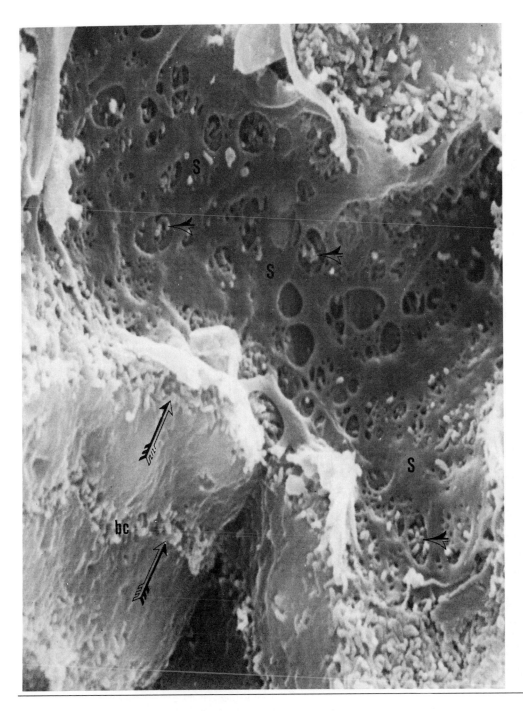

Figure 2.13 The sinusoidal endothelim (S), as seen with the scanning electron microscope, shows large and small fenestrations. The microvilli of an underlying hepatocyte are seen through these fenestrations (short arrows). The lower half of the picture shows a one-cell-thick liver cell plate with a bile canaliculus (bc) running through the central portion of the hepatocytes. Microvilli are seen along the bile canaliculus and along the sinusoidal surface of hepatocytes (long arrows). × 8500. Courtesy of Dr K. Miyai, Department of Pathology, University of California, San Diego.

membrane and, depending on the plane of section, may appear as intranuclear inclusions. These are more frequently observed in old animals and in some pathological situations.[2,138]

The cytoplasm

The cytoplasm of the hepatocytes contains a variety of organelles and membrane systems, which occupy roughly half of the cell volume.[14,84,143,168] The membranous system divides the cytoplasm into two compartments, cytoplasmic and intracisternal, and it also surrounds the various

organelles, isolating areas where specialized functions can be carried out.

Endoplasmic reticulum

The endoplasmic reticulum is made up of the rough endoplasmic reticulum, with membranes studded with ribosomes 15 nm in diameter, and the agranular or smooth endoplasmic reticulum, which lacks ribosomes (Figure 2.16). The total density of the endoplasmic reticulum is about 3.8 m/cm of parenchyma, with 62% and 38% respectively for the rough and smooth endoplasmic reticulum in adult rats.[14] In this species the two-cell layer

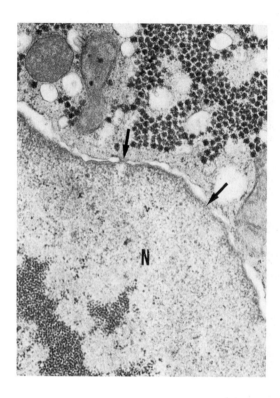

Figure 2.14 Part of a hepatocyte showing the perinuclear space interrupted by the nuclear pores (arrows). Some monoparticulate glycogen is present in the nucleus (N) whereas the intracytoplasmic glycogen has a rosette-like appearance. × 25 000.

adjacent to the central vein has approximately equal proportions of rough and smooth.[117] The relative proportion of the two aspects of the endoplasmic reticulum varies according to the species: in dogs, the rough and smooth endoplasmic reticulum represent respectively 40% and 60% of the total,[84] whereas in adult man the values are around 25% and 75%.[94,168] These species differences have not always been taken into account, especially in studies on humans, and numerous reports of 'hypertrophy' of the smooth endoplasmic reticulum in human hepatocytes should be interpreted with caution.

Rough endoplasmic reticulum This is arranged in flattened cisternae, often grouped around the nucleus and mitochondria, and along the sinusoidal border in the margin to areas of smooth endoplasmic reticulum and glycogen. This disposition is more evident in human liver, especially in the hepatocytes surrounding the central vein. Also, in human hepatocytes the cisternae of the rough endoplasmic reticulum appear more fragmented than in those of animals. Ribosomes are attached on the cytoplasmic side of the rough endoplasmic reticulum but can also be seen free in the cytoplasm, either isolated or arranged along a fine thread of messenger RNA in spirals or rosettes to constitute the polysomes, the functional unit of protein synthesis. Polysomes are also associated with the membrane of the endoplasmic reticulum but can be seen as such only in a tangential section of the membranous sheet. Synthesis of protein takes place at the

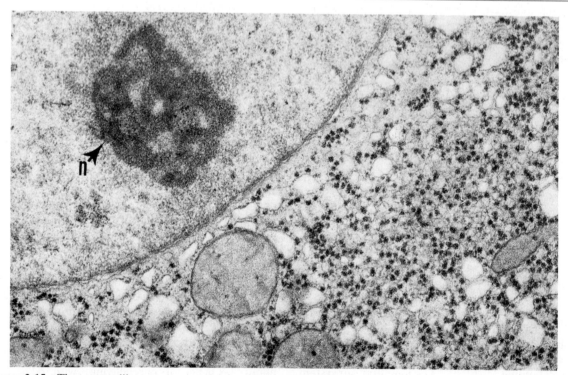

Figure 2.15 The sponge-like appearance of the nucleolus (n) is evident on this electron micrograph. The chromatin is slightly denser around the nucleolus and along the nuclear membrane than in the remaining nucleoplasm. × 25 000.

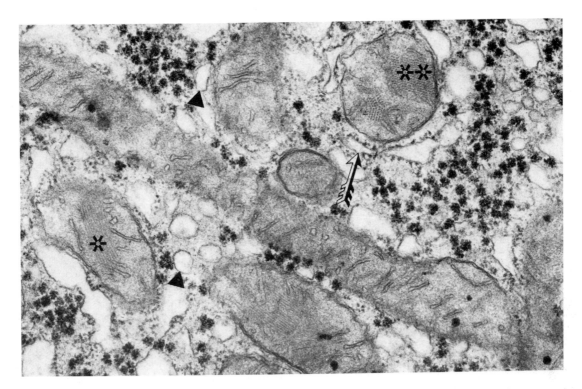

Figure 2.16 Part of the cytoplasm of a hepatocyte of a normal subject showing cisternae of rough (long arrow) and smooth (arrowheads) endoplasmic reticulum. Electron-dense rosettes of glycogen are dispersed throughout the cytoplasm. The mitochondria contain crystalline formations seen in longitudinal (single asterisk) or in cross-sections (double asterisk). × 37 500.

level of the rough endoplasmic reticulum. Morphological demonstration of albumin synthesis in the liver has been achieved by autoradiography[66] and by immune electron microscopy.[49] The heterogeneous distribution of the albumin in human liver has suggested that only a small number of hepatocytes are engaged in albumin synthesis. There is evidence that the immunocytochemical localization of proteins is dependent upon technical factors such as stirring during fixation, and addition of permeabilizing agents.[86,156] It is now accepted that every hepatocyte can engage in the synthesis of plasma proteins (prealbumin, albumin, fibrinogen, transferrin).

The membrane of the endoplasmic reticulum contains phospholipids and proteins arranged asymmetrically; the proteins are either buried (completely or partially) inside the phospholipid bilayer (integral proteins) or loosely bound to the polar surface of the membrane (peripheral proteins).[29,133]

Smooth endoplasmic reticulum and glycogen The smooth endoplasmic reticulum is distributed throughout the hepatocyte, mainly as small vesicles associated with glycogen. The glycogen has a stellate shape or a rosette-like appearance and is arranged in clusters of granules, each 10–20 nm in diameter (Figures 2.14 and 2.16). In man, the smooth endoplasmic reticulum is more diffusely distributed than in rat, dog or rabbit hepatocytes. Moreover, two types occur: the more common form, type 1,

has a finely vesicular honeycomb pattern and accounts for 77% of the smooth membranes, while the other, type 2, is made up of densely packed membranes without a cavitary system and accounts for 23% (Figure 2.17). Until now this dual configuration has been observed only in human liver. Its significance is suggested by the modifications which occur when there are changes in microsomal enzyme activity (see Chapters 15 and 20).

It is known that the smooth endoplasmic reticulum is mainly concerned with the synthesis of lipids, the accumulation of glycogen and the metabolism of drugs and steroids.[67,97] It contains enzymes for the synthesis of cholesterol and the formation of bile acids. Uridine diphosphate (UDP) glucuronyl transferase is also associated with the smooth endoplasmic reticulum.[182] Some enzymes of the endoplasmic reticulum have been demonstrated by ultrastructural histochemistry and include glucose-6-phosphatase,[68] nucleoside diphosphatase[140] and acetyl-CoA carboxylase.[222] Glucose-6-phosphatase is evenly distributed throughout the endoplasmic reticulum, including the nuclear envelope, but seems to develop asynchronously in the hepatocyte population.[115] Cytochrome P450 together with NADPH-cytochrome *c* reductase constitutes the microsomal monooxygenase system which plays a key role in the biotransformation of drugs and numerous endogenous compounds such as steroids. Multiple forms of P450 have been identified, and specific forms are inducible by various drugs,

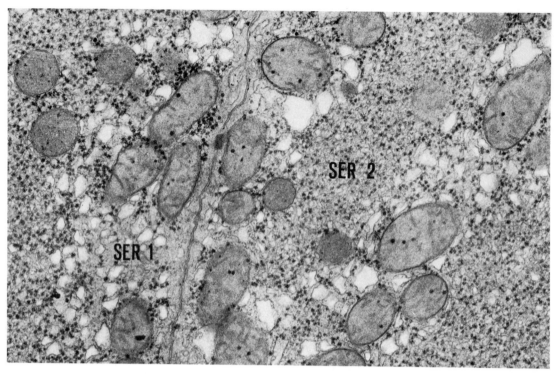

Figure 2.17 Part of two hepatocytes in human liver showing the variable pattern of distribution of the smooth endoplasmic reticulum. The SER type 1 (SER 1) has a grossly vesicular appearance, with vesicles varying in size and shape. The SER type 2 (SER 2) is formed of densely packed membranes concentrated in various areas of the cytoplasm and shows little or no evidence of a cavity system. × 21 000.

accompanied by a proliferation of smooth membranes (see Chapters 17 and 20).[144,180]

Studies in rats and mice on the endoplasmic reticulum during the perinatal period show that rough and smooth endoplasmic reticula are present at birth. Little variation in the rough endoplasmic reticulum is observed thereafter, but the smooth endoplasmic reticulum increases in association with the maturation of some microsomal enzymes.[29,30,31] The enzymes of the endoplasmic reticulum do not rise in parallel with the membranous compartment.[30,115] In rats the maximum increase in the smooth endoplasmic reticulum occurs 24–72 hours after birth but it continues to rise thereafter.[34,83,167,177] In human liver, a small amount of smooth endoplasmic reticulum has been found in young children up to 9 months of age, with an increase up to 18 years.[34,196] These data make it clear that the limits of 'normal' vary and that age should be carefully considered.

The Golgi apparatus

The Golgi apparatus is a specialized area of the smooth endoplasmic reticulum located in the vicinity of the bile canaliculi (Figure 2.18). It is arranged as a group of flattened saccules, vacuoles and small vesicles, which are sometimes seen budding off the extremities of the saccules. Multivesicular bodies and lysosomes are frequently associated with the Golgi areas. The cisternae usually appear empty, but in liver perfused with free fatty acids may be

filled with dense particles 30–100 nm in diameter. These have been identified as very low-density lipoproteins, later secreted in the space of Disse and the sinusoids.[79] The term GERL has been proposed to designate a specialized area of the endoplasmic reticulum which, together with the innermost elements of the Golgi apparatus, contributes to the formation of lysosomes. It is identified by acid phosphatase cytochemistry.[137] In normal animals, GERL is not conspicuous but it becomes enlarged and swollen in some experimental situations. The Golgi apparatus is a site for assembly and packaging of lipoproteins and glycoproteins which are then exported or incorporated into intracellular components. It has been shown to participate in the intracellular migration of albumin.[66] Experimental evidence would suggest that the Golgi apparatus is involved in the handling of some glutathione conjugates prior to their elimination in bile[96] but a specific role of the Golgi complex in the transport of biliary lipids seems to be excluded.[161] Much of the difficulty in fully understanding the role of the Golgi complex in the economy of the cell comes from the difficulties in isolating homogeneous and intact Golgi subfractions.

In adult rats the surface density of the Golgi membranes is 0.17 m^2/cm^3 of liver parenchyma, and these contribute 4% to the membranes of the endoplasmic reticulum in hepatocytes.[14] In adult man, the Golgi contributes about 6% to the membranes of the endoplasmic reticulum with a surface density of 0.23 $\mu m^2/\mu m^3$ of cytoplasm.[94,143] This

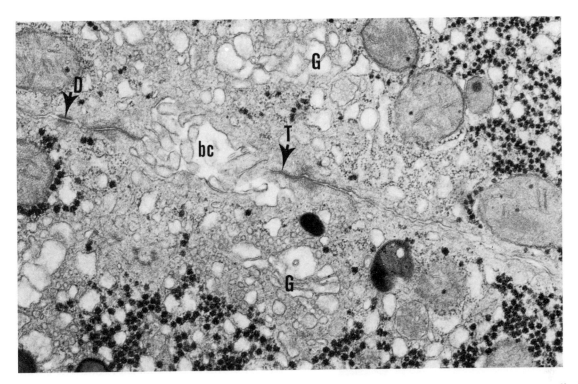

Figure 2.18 Part of two hepatocytes showing the specializations of the cell surface at the level of bile canaliculi. Microvilli of various sizes project into the lumen of the canaliculus (bc) and the Golgi apparatus (G) is evident in both hepatocytes at a short distance from the cell border. T = tight junctions; D = desmosomes. × 25 000.

appears to be higher in younger individuals.[34] In rats the maximum values are observed around 5 weeks of age[196] and a significant decrease in Golgi membranes occurs with ageing.[177]

Mitochondria

The mitochondria account for about 23% of the cytoplasmic volume in adult rat hepatocytes,[211] 24% in dogs[84] and 14–19% in adult man.[143,183] They measure 0.4–0.5 μm by 0.5–1 μm. Small intra-acinar differences have been observed, the mitochondria being longer, thinner and more numerous in perivenular areas than in periportal areas of rat liver;[117] the variation in mitochondrial number means that the mitochondrial volume density remains constant throughout the acinus.[4] The mitochondria are limited by a double membrane. The outer membrane is closely apposed to the rough endoplasmic reticulum and the inner membrane is folded in numerous invaginations to form the cristae (Figure 2.16). Negative staining reveals club-shaped particles associated with the inner membrane: the head, about 9 nm in diameter, is thought to represent the ATPase-coupling factor F1, while the stalk contains the components of the electron transfer system.[162] The matrix contains naked DNA, a small amount of RNA and ribosomes.[130] The dense granules, about 10–25 nm in diameter, often present in the matrix have been shown to bind various cations, especially calcium and phosphorus.[15,130] The mitochondria are involved in a variety of metabolic pathways, mainly the citric acid cycle,

fatty-acid activation and oxidation, steroid metabolism, respiration, nucleic acid and protein synthesis and haem biosynthesis. Ultrastructural cytochemistry has localized NADH$_2$–TNBT (tetranitro blue tetrazolium) reductase activity to the mitochondria in all hepatocytes, with a higher activity in portal areas.[118] The activity of cytochromes *c* and *b* has also been demonstrated in situ by various techniques.[118,139,201]

No major qualitative differences are evident in the structure of mitochondria in different species. The variety of profile shapes seen in thin sections is due to the morphological heterogeneity of mitochondria. Serial section analysis reveals V-shaped or club-shaped mitochondria, discs, cylinders or spheres.[4,190] Giant mitochondria, up to 5 μm, are occasionally observed in human hepatocytes and often contain bundles of filaments arranged in an orderly fashion (Figure 2.19). These were originally described as a pathological finding but are now well established as an occasional feature of normal human liver.[91,118,129,169,183,213] By optical diffraction, these inclusions are crystalline and made up of either phospholipid micelles or relatively large protein molecules.[193] A protein component in these crystals is also suggested by ultrastructural histochemistry.[175,176] Giant mitochondria seem to be frequently associated with steatosis. A light-microscopic study has shown that in normal or pathological liver tissue, giant mitochondria have a heterogeneous distribution and are found in clusters of a few hepatocytes,[149] which explains why they can be missed or overestimated

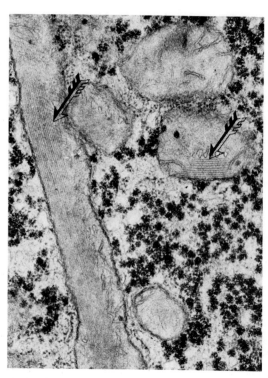

Figure 2.19 Group of mitochondria containing crystals shown in longitudinal section (arrows) in the hepatocytes of a normal subject. × 27 500.

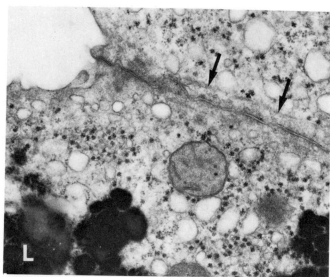

Figure 2.20 Part of two hepatocytes showing lipofuscin granules (L) in the lower left corner and a bundle of microfilaments (arrows) running parallel to the cell membrane. × 25 000.

in the electron microscope. Stacks of mitochondrial cristae are occasionally observed in human hepatocytes and have also been noted in livers of pathogen-free dogs.[65] In monkey liver, mitochondria show an intricate fibrillar pattern which in cross-section appears as groups of dots, sometimes arranged as annulets 65 nm in diameter.[170] The significance of these formations is still unknown.

The greatest pleomorphism and the greatest individual mitochondrial volume are found in the first 24 hours after birth.[168,190] In ageing rats and mice, the volume and shape of the average mitochondrion remain constant,[177,197] but the number of mitochondria and the surface density of mitochondrial cristae appear to decrease.[197]

Lysosomes

The heterogeneous class of organelles known as lysosomes actually represents residual bodies or secondary lysosomes, made up of particles limited by a single membrane, containing a variety of inclusions and showing acid phosphatase and β-glucuronidase activity.[118,136] These secondary lysosomes are a storage form, temporary or definitive, of degradation products of normal cell metabolism and auto or heterophagocytosis. In the hepatocytes, most residual bodies are preferentially located around the bile canaliculi (Figures 2.12 and 2.18). They include autophagic vacuoles, multivesicular bodies, ferritin-containing granules and lipofuscin granules (the most common residual body in human hepatocytes) (Figure 2.20). Lipofuscin granules are irregularly lobulated and show a complex

structure with electron-lucent regions, dense lipid-containing globules and ferritin-containing areas.[44,118] They have been considered as members of the lipolysosome (lipid-containing lysosomes) family, to which the electron-lucent lipid inclusions seen in golden hamsters also belong.[132] The volume occupied by the residual bodies in hepatocytes of adult rats varies from 0.3% to 0.9% of the cytoplasmic volume, without significant differences in volume density in various parts of the acinus.[118,211] The number of particles seems to be higher in perivenular areas.[114] In dog liver, the volume occupied by lysosomes is around 0.7% of the cytoplasmic volume,[84] whereas in man the values vary from 1.33[142] to 2% of the cytoplasmic volume.[168]

The maximal volume density of dense bodies in rats and mice is found at 24 hours after birth[167] in association with the formation of numerous autophagic vacuoles in the cytoplasm of hepatocytes.[93] The volume returns rapidly to adult values, which are reached by the third day post-partum.[167] Little difference in the relative volume of lysosomes seems to occur therafter, although a moderate but significant increase has been found in old virgin rats compared with old breeder rats.[177] Thus, except for the perinatal period, it appears that no gross changes in the volume density of residual bodies occur in normal individuals. This probably reflects the steady state in cell metabolism and turnover of the various cell components.

Peroxisomes

The peroxisomes (microbodies) are made up of granules about 0.25–1 μm in diameter, limited by a single membrane. The largest ones, up to 1.50 μm, are found in human liver.[141,194] They are occasionally arranged in clusters and are usually distributed in close proximity to the smooth endoplasmic reticulum and glycogen areas

(Figures 2.12 and 2.14). Slender communications between smooth endoplasmic reticulum and peroxisomes have been observed in rat and human liver. These suggest that hepatic peroxisomes may arise as dilatations of smooth endoplasmic reticulum cisternae,[141] but this is still a matter of controversy. The matrix of peroxisomes is homogeneous, of moderate electron density, and in some species contains a crystalline inclusion or core made up of the enzyme urate oxidase. This core is lacking in peroxisomes of human hepatocytes,[87,141,181] but marginal plates and a variety of matrical inclusions are irregularly observed.[194] Histochemical reactions based on the demonstration of catalase activity using 3',3'-diaminobenzidine[139,141] helped to characterize this group of organelles, and the term 'microperoxisomes' has been proposed for 'anucleoid' peroxisome-like structures in a variety of tissues.[141] In adult rats, the mean volume density of the peroxisomes represents about 1.5% of the cytoplasmic volume,[118,211] with higher values in perivenular areas.[118] The highest volume, 3.7%, is found in dog liver compared with 0.97–1.33% in man.[143,168] Adult values seem to be reached very rapidly following the sharp increase in volume density of peroxisomes noted in neonatal rats.[168]

The peroxisomes are involved in respiration, lipid metabolism, purine catabolism, alcohol metabolism and other reactions such as gluconeogenesis.[33,87,111] Peroxisomal respiration accounts for about 20% of the oxygen consumption by the liver and differs from mitochondrial respiration in that the energy produced is dissipated as heat rather than used in the formation of ATP. The respiratory pathway utilizes molecular oxygen, producing hydrogen peroxide (H_2O_2) which in turn is decomposed by peroxisomal catalase. Alcohol is one of the substrates undergoing peroxidation and about 10% of the clearance of ethanol could be mediated by this pathway.[146] The role of peroxisomes in fatty-acid metabolism has been demonstrated relatively recently:[111] long-chain fatty acids are the substrates for β-oxidation, the end-product being acetyl-CoA.[112] There is also evidence that peroxisomes are involved in side-chain oxidation of cholesterol and bile acid synthesis.[210] A number of pathological or experimental situations are known to be accompanied by alterations in the shape or number of peroxisomes (see Chapter 20).

The cytoskeleton

The cytoskeleton includes various types of cytoplasmic components: microfilaments, intermediate filaments and microtubules. The term should be applied only to the last two elements, since microfilaments are part of the contractile system of the cells.

Microfilaments are 4–7 nm in diameter and are composed of globular (G) actin molecules assembled to form the filamentous (F) actin. F actin microfilaments may associate into bundles of variable thickness. The meshwork extends throughout the cytoplasm, with higher concentrations in the peripheral cytoplasm (Figure 2.20),[52,151] especially the microvilli and around the bile canalic-

uli, and accounts for the polygonal staining pattern revealed by immunofluorescence.[9,37,85,142,221] The microfilaments are also the site of binding of smooth muscle autoantibody, identified as anti-actin antibody, present in patients with chronic liver disease.[52] The mode of association of actin filaments with cell membranes is still unclear. It is probable that microfilaments are involved in motile phenomena, and their association with bile canaliculi suggests that they play a role in bile secretion and the tone of the canalicular wall. Their dysfunction has been proposed as a mechanism for intrahepatic cholestasis.[43,151] Recently, the presence of hepatocyte myosin near the bile canaliculi in rabbit liver[202] and the colocalization of myosin and actin in rat liver[221] have been demonstrated by immunocytochemistry. This suggests that hepatocyte motility and especially normal bile flow are dependent upon an efficient actomyosin system.

The other two components of the cytoskeletal system are more diffusely distributed in the cytoplasm. Intermediate filaments are about 10 nm in diameter. They are especially evident in preparations of liver perfused with detergent solutions.[37,53] Intermediate filaments are heterogeneous in composition and indeed show a remarkable tissue-specific diversity.[172] This feature is used as a tool for a study of distribution of intermediate filament proteins in normal tissues[70] and tissue typing applied to tumour diagnosis.[145] In the liver, intermediate filaments of hepatocytes are of the cytokeratin type, specifically types 8 and 18,[145] while in cells of mesenchymal origin they contain vimentin. They are often closely associated with desmosomes. Bundles of intermediate filaments are occasionally present in the pericanalicular areas together with the microfilaments. Intermediate filaments are thought to play a role in the maintenance of cell shape, integration of cytoplasmic space and guidance of organelle movements.[37] Some pathological conditions have been related to alterations in this filamentous system (see Chapter 20).

Microtubules differ from the former two components in that they are hollow structures, with an outer diameter of about 25 nm, and extend for long distances in the cytoplasm.[37,191] They are composed of dimers of α- and β-tubulin and in the hepatocyte exist mainly as labile elements highly sensitive to the action of antitubulin drugs (see Chapter 20). They have been most extensively studied in cilia but are also a prominent component of the mitotic spindle. In a non-ciliated cell such as the hepatocyte there is still a prominent microtubular network even in interphase. They radiate out to the plasma membrane from focal condensations around the nucleus and around the Golgi apparatus. Their functions in the hepatocyte are uncertain: as in all cells they interact with the microfilament network and are considered to be involved in the maintenance of cell structure, but they are also probably concerned with intracytoplasmic transport of metabolites including some newly synthesized proteins.

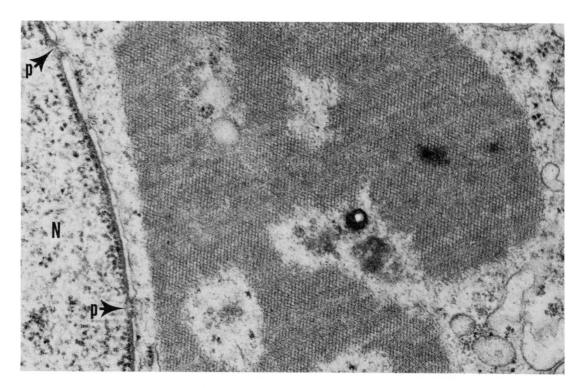

Figure 2.21 Large crystalline inclusion in the cytoplasm of a liver cell. The inclusion has no limiting membrane and is complex in shape with numerous cytoplasmic invaginations. The organization of the crystal shows a regular, honeycomb pattern in this plane or section. p = nuclear pore; N = nucleus. × 36 000.

Crystalline structures

The presence of crystalline formations in the cytoplasm of hepatocytes is irregularly observed. These formations occupy large areas of the hyaloplasm, often interspersed with rosettes of glycogen, and are not limited by a membrane (Figure 2.21). They measure 1–7 μm in length by 1–2.5 μm.[25,92,129,195] There is a variable internal arrangement: a regular honeycomb pattern is sometimes evident, with occasional cross-sections of filamentous components 6 nm thick with a spacing of 19 nm. The periodicity may also give a 'herring-bone' appearance in some sections.[25] The intracytoplasmic crystals are occasionally seen together with intramitochondrial crystals in the same cell, but the former are more rarely observed. Proteins are the most likely constituent of intracytoplasmic crystals as shown by optical diffraction analysis.[195]

Lipids

In normal conditions, the hepatocytes may also contain some lipid droplets. These account for 0.37% of the hepatocyte volume in normal rats,[14] 0.14% in dogs[84] and 0.3–2.1% in man.[143,168]

The plasma membrane

The hepatocyte is in contact with three compartments: the perisinusoidal space or space of Disse, the intercellular space, and the bile canaliculi. The membrane facing the perisinusoidal space forms numerous microvilli and represents 72% of the whole plasma membrane in rats.[14] In man, the membranes facing the sinusoidal and the intercellular spaces together represent 83.3% of the total plasma membrane.[143] There is histochemical and biochemical evidence that Na^+/K^+-ATPase activity (the Na^+ pump) is localized at the sinusoidal and lateral membranes, with little or no activity at the canalicular membrane.[12,108,160] Gamma-glutamyl transferase and glucagon-activated adenylate cyclase appear to be preferentially located in the sinusoidal domain.[45,214] Mg^{2+}-ATPase and alkaline phosphatase are localized predominantly at the canalicular surface.[12]

The microvilli which project into the space of Disse are occasionally in contact with the sinusoidal lumen through fenestrae in the endothelial cells. These are evident in transmission as well as in scanning electron microscopy (Figure 2.13). At the base of the microvilli, small regular invaginations of the cell membrane are often seen. Some of these invaginations are characterized by a specific protein (clathrin) coating specialized areas of the cell membrane and leading to the formation of a bristle coat on the cytoplasmic convex side, hence the name of 'coated pits'. These are 100–150 nm in diameter and are easily identified by their dense outline (Figure 2.22), evident even in unstained sections.[118,169] Eventually the coated pit is pinched off to form an intracytoplasmic coated vesicle. Coated pits and coated vesicles appear involved in receptor-mediated endocytosis and a shuttling mechanism for intracellular transfer of selected macromolecules.[186]

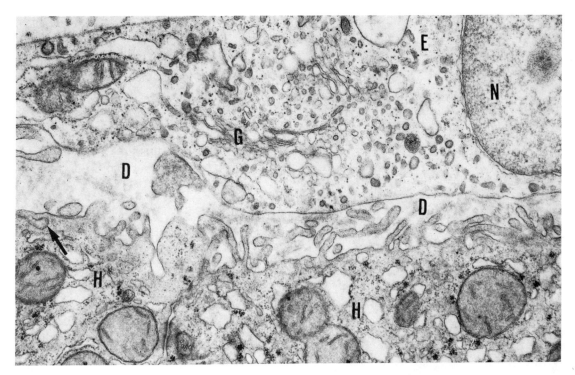

Figure 2.22 The space of Disse (D) is defined on one side by the hepatocytes (H) and on the other side by the sinusoidal lining cells. Part of an endothelial cell (E) is shown here with a large pale nucleus (N). The cytoplasm lacks phagocytic inclusions and shows some elements of the Golgi apparatus (G). Some pinocytic vesicles can be seen along the cell surface (arrow). × 21 000.

Along the lateral cell membranes, three classes of intercellular junctional complexes may be observed. *Tight junctions* (zonula occludentes) separate the intercellular spaces of perisinusoidal recesses from the canalicular lumen and control transepithelial flux between cells.[45,72] They are formed by the close apposition of strands of intermembranous particles present in the cell membranes and extend as a belt-like structure around the bile canaliculi.[156,208] Recent studies show that the permeability of tight junctions differs among various epithelia ('tight' or 'leaky'); those of the liver seem to be of an intermediate type. A tight junction (paracellular) pathway could be of importance for passage of water and electrolytes from the blood to the canaliculi. The relative importance of paracellular and transcellular fluid movements for the physiology of the bile secretion has been reviewed.[20]

Desmosomes are irregularly distributed along lateral cell membranes. They are formed by the close apposition of short, straight segments of the membranes of adjacent cells, separated by a space of about 25 nm, are filled with homogeneous electron-dense material, and are reinforced by a plaque on the cytoplasmic side of the membrane.[9] Microfilaments often originate from the desmosomes; they may be seen expanding fan-wise into the cytoplasm or running along the cell membranes and around the bile canaliculi as part of the microfilamentous network of the hepatocyte.

The third type, the gap junction, is made up of aggregates of intramembranous particles, associated in pairs across the intercellular space. These thus form a channel allowing direct exchange of ions and small molecules between cells.[45]

THE BILIARY TREE

The biliary tree includes the bile canaliculi (or bile capillaries), the ducts of Hering (preductules or intermediary portion), the bile ductules and the larger bile ducts located in the portal tracts.[187,188]

Canaliculi

The bile canaliculi are spaces formed by separation of adjacent cells (Figure 2.18). Numerous microvilli project into their lumen but extended areas may be deprived of microvilli even in normal conditions. The anastomosing network of bile canaliculi running between hepatocytes is well shown by scanning electron microscopy (Figure 2.13).[72] The four different types of canaliculi which have been distinguished in fetal and neonatal rat liver might represent various stages of maturation of the biliary pole of the liver cell, characterized by an increase in the surface/volume ratio of canaliculi.[38] In adult liver, the width and shape of the canaliculi are variable; altogether they represent 0.4% of the parenchymal volume.[14] The canaliculi of the perivenular zone seem to have fewer

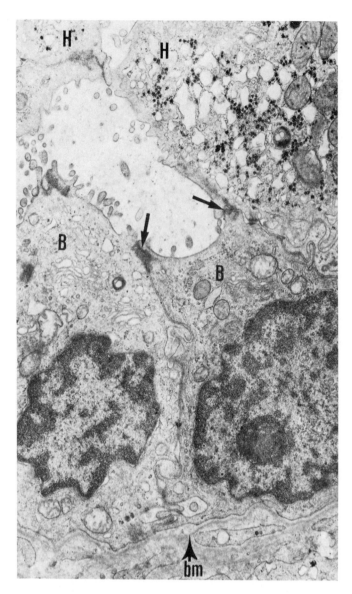

Figure 2.23 The lumen of a duct of Hering surrounded by both hepatocytes (H) and biliary epithelial cells (B). Tight junctions are evident around the lumen and between cells of different types (arrows). A basement membrane (bm) runs along the basal pole of the ductular cells. × 14 000.

microvilli and a narrower lumen than those in the periportal areas.[118] Both transmission electron microscopy[187] and scanning electron microscopy have failed to reveal any direct connection between the canaliculi and the perisinusoidal spaces.[72] A strong cohesion between hepatocytes is provided by tight junctions (zonula occludens); this resists mechanical disruption and permits isolation of intact segments of the bile canalicular network from the rest of the parenchyma.[153] Next to the tight junctions, the lateral cell membranes form the intermediate junction with an intercellular gap of about 20 nm. The staining of the bile canalicular membrane by phosphotungstic acid[187] or by ruthenium red[142] may be due to the presence of a

fuzzy coat on the cell surface. A high 5'-nucleotidase and Mg^{++}-ATPase activity is present at the canalicular level but in normal conditions the alkaline phosphatase activity is low.[118] On the cytoplasmic side, a zone of condensed cytoplasm or 'pericanalicular ectoplasm' reinforces the bile canalicular wall. It may be considered to be a differentiated area of the cytoplasm similar to the terminal web of intestinal columnar cells. Actin filaments are distributed around the canaliculi and extend into the microvilli, suggesting that the microfilaments are contractile, with a role in intracellular transport, bile flow and tone of the canalicular wall.

Ductules

The ducts of Hering or preductules are spaces limited by both hepatocytes and biliary epithelial cells without an intermediate cell type (Figure 2.23).[1,188] They can be found in both adult and newborn liver.[93,187] They represent a very short segment of the biliary tree which is in continuity at one end with the bile canaliculi and at the other end with the bile ductules. The latter are surrounded only by biliary epithelial cells or 'ductular cells'. The ductular cells are cuboidal, with cytoplasm lighter and more homogeneous than the cytoplasm of hepatocytes (Figure 2.24). Occasional 'dark' cells can be observed between the light ductular cells.[187] Whether at the level of the duct of Hering or at the ductular level, the biliary epithelium rests on a basement membrane (Figures 2.23, 2.24 and 2.25) which takes up phosphotungstic acid and appears more complex, with branching structures, in humans than in animals. The basement membrane can also be stained with periodic acid–silver methenamine in methacrylate-embedded material. This reaction has been attributed to a high glycoprotein content.[187] On the apical surface of the ductular cells, numerous microvilli project in the ductular lumen and occasional cilia have been observed.[192] The basal surface is straight and the lateral membranes may show complex interdigitations (Figure 2.24) or be separated from each other by wide gaps, especially towards the basal pole of the cells. Near the apical pole, strong cohesion is provided by junctional complexes, which are also seen at the point of contact between hepatocytes and ductular cells (Figures 2.23 and 2.24). The nucleus is located towards the basal pole of the cell, while the Golgi apparatus is located towards the luminal or the lateral surface (Figure 2.23). Small round or elongated mitochondria are dispersed in the cytoplasm. The endoplasmic reticulum is scarce and mainly of the smooth type. The cytoplasm also contains some lysosomes, a few lipid droplets and a rich network of filaments originating from the junctional complexes. These filaments probably represent a contractile system involved in intracellular transport.

Blood vessels and lymphatics are closely apposed to the ductules in the portal tracts and unmyelinated nerve fibres are sometimes seen next to the basement membrane of venules (Figure 2.25).[192]

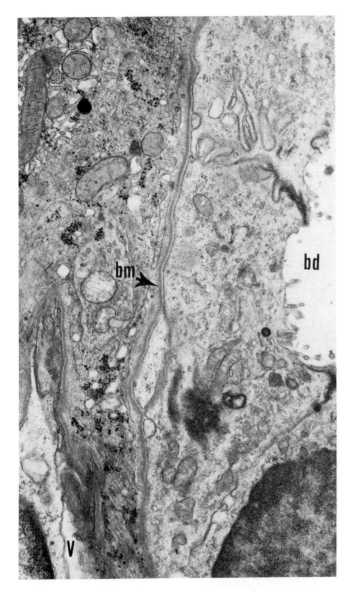

Figure 2.24 Part of a small portal tract showing the close apposition between the parenchymal cells and the bile ductule (bd). The ductular cells rest upon a thick basement membrane (bm) showing evidence of branching structure. Part of a venule (V) with an endothelial cell is also visible. × 10 500.

THE SINUSOID

The sinusoidal wall contains four types of cells: endothelial cells, Kupffer cells, perisinusoidal cells or Ito cells and pit cells. Kupffer cells and endothelial cells are littoral cells which are in contact with the lumen of the sinusoids, while the lipocytes are located in the space of Disse between the hepatocyte and the littoral cells.

Thin cytoplasmic extensions covering the microvilli of hepatocytes characterize the endothelial cells (Figures 2.22 and 2.26) while the Kupffer cells are voluminous with a prominent nucleus and numerous phagocytic inclusions.[215] Cytochemically, the cells may be distinguished by the lack of both peroxidase and phagocytic

activity in endothelial cells.[212,216] No transitional stages have been observed between the two types of cells.[215]

Endothelial cells

These form a "fenestrated" endothelium well demonstrated by scanning electron microscopy (Figure 2.13).[72] In rat liver, endothelial cells account for 2.8% of the parenchymal volume roughly equivalent to that of the Kupffer cells.[14] Their cytoplasm (Figure 2.22) contains small mitochondria which represent only 0.53% of the total mitochondrial volume of the hepatic parenchyma. The cisternae of the rough endoplasmic reticulum are connected with an anastomosing network of smooth membranes. The relative proportion is 60% of rough and 40% of smooth membranes. Together they represent only 3.3% of the total area of the endoplasmic reticulum of the parenchyma.[14] The Golgi apparatus represents 11.9% of the total Golgi membranes. Lysosomes are not prominent and constitute 7% of the cell volume.[14] Contrary to rat liver, human liver often shows large amounts of monoparticulate glycogen inside endothelial cells. A measure of the high process of pinocytosis in endothelial cells is given by the volume density of pinocytic vesicles, which is 2.51% of the cell volume.[14] The luminal surface of the endothelial cells, including the pinocytic vesicles, intracytoplasmic tubules and the mature face of the Golgi complex, stains with phosphotungstic acid, suggesting common physicochemical properties, perhaps related to a transfer process operating through membrane fusion between the cell surface and the inner cellular compartments.[32] Thus the endothelial lining can act as a filtration barrier, impeding the passage of particles larger than 10 nm (the size of intercellular pores), and also helps remove foreign material from the blood through uptake of macromolecules by endocytosis. The transport of particles and fluids into and out of the space of Disse is promoted by 'forced sieving' and 'endothelial massage' due to the interaction of blood cells and the fenestrated sinusoidal wall.[218]

Kupffer cells

The Kupffer cells constitute 2.1% of the parenchymal volume in adult rat liver[14] and appear more numerous in sinusoids around the portal tracts.[98] Their cytoplasm is more abundant than that of the endothelial cells. It contains numerous phagocytic inclusions, which represent 14% of the cell volume. The endoplasmic reticulum is scarce and is mainly found as rough endoplasmic reticulum.[14] Microtubules and microfilaments are commonly observed.[216] In rats, peroxidase activity is present in the perinuclear space, in endoplasmic reticulum and also in occasional annulate lamellae. This has been linked with the clearing of living microorganisms from the blood.[212,216] The surface of the Kupffer cells is sometimes indented to form peculiar wormlike structures about 140 nm in diameter with an irregular dense line in the

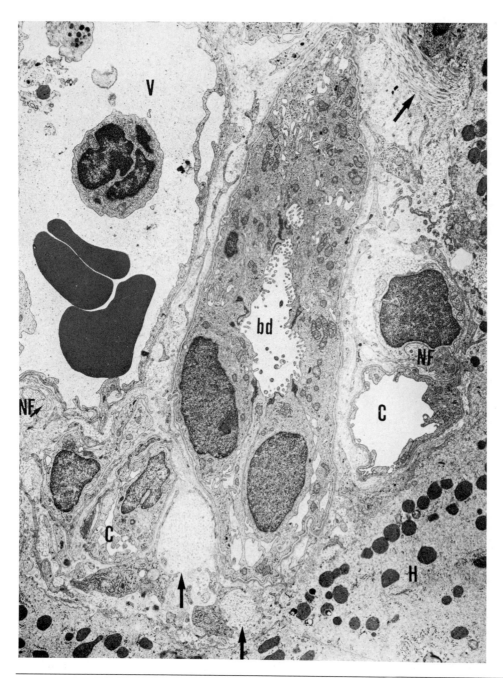

Figure 2.25 Low-power view of a small portal tract, showing the bile ductule (bd) surrounded by a basement membrane, venules (V) and capillaries (C). Bundles of collagen fibres are present (arrows) around the bile ductule and in close contact with hepatocytes (H). Small unmyelinated nerve fibres (NF) are seen close to the venule and a capillary. × 4000. From Sternlieb (1972),[192] with kind permission of the author and the publisher. © (1972) Williams and Wilkins Co., Baltimore.

centre. Together with a thick fuzzy coat on the cell surface and numerous 100 nm bristle-coated vesicles, the worm-like structures are evidence of the active pinocytosis of Kupffer cells.[124,212,216] The dense line present in the worm-like structures is produced by invagination of the cell surface and close apposition of the molecules of the fuzzy coat.[98]

Erythrocyte catabolism is one of the main functions of the Kupffer cell, but it appears to be limited to a specialized subpopulation (about 30%) of sinusoidal cells. This erythrophagocytic property may be directly related to the cellular content of microsomal haem oxygenase.[10]

Fat-storing cells

The perisinusoidal fat-storing cells or lipocytes in the perisinusoidal space are located beneath the endothelium, in close contact with hepatocytes, and sometimes project into perisinusoidal recesses between hepatocytes. Small bundles of collagen fibrils are often evident between the perisinusoidal cells and the hepatocytes (Figure 2.26). They appear to be present in the liver of all species, accounting for 1.40% of the parenchymal volume in normal adult rat liver[14] and 1.88% in man.[64,95] Their cytoplasm contains a few profiles of rough endoplasmic

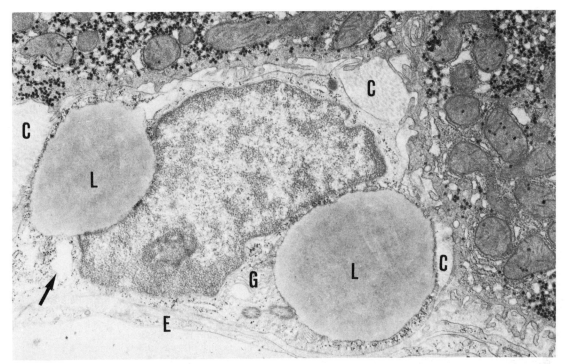

Figure 2.26 A lipocyte is located in the space between the endothelium (E) and the hepatocytes. Two large lipid droplets (L) occupy most of the cytoplasm of the lipocyte, and one of them is pressing against the nucleus. The cytoplasm contains little rough endoplasmic reticulum (arrow), and a small Golgi apparatus (G) next to two centrioles. Bundles of collagen fibres (C) are closely apposed to the lipocyte. × 14 000.

reticulum, monoparticulate glycogen isolated or in small clumps, and small mitochondria with a light matrix and short cristae. Centrioles are frequently observed. Perisinusoidal cells do not show evidence of phagocytosis, and pinocytic vesicles are rarely seen. The cytoplasm also contains a variable number of large round or star-shaped lipid droplets, which sometimes displace the nucleus. These droplets react strongly with gold chloride and exhibit intense vitamin A fluorescence.[209] Recent evidence supports the hypothesis that besides storage of vitamin A, perisinusoidal cells play a major role in fibrogenesis.[157] They contain collagen type I, III, IV and laminin in rough endoplasmic reticulum and nuclear envelope as shown by immunocytochemistry.[27,28,123] Extracellular matrix components may be also synthesized by perisinusoidal cells in primary cultures.[163,174] Spontaneous in vitro differentiation of perisinusoidal cells into myofibroblast-like cells is accompanied by an 11-fold increase in the secretion of collagen, especially of collagen type I, showing a similarity between in vitro and in vivo phenotypic alterations of these cells (see also Chapter 32).[62] No relationship between perisinusoidal cells and parenchymal steatosis has been found in adult human liver.[64,95] Although uncommon in normal liver, cells resembling mature fibroblasts are occasionally seen in the space of Disse. They are morphologically similar to perisinusoidal cells except for the absence of lipid droplets in their cytoplasm.

Pit cells

The 'pit' cell, has been described in the sinusoidal wall of rat liver. These cells are infrequent and have a dense nucleus and an electron-lucent cytoplasm. They are in contact with both the hepatocytes and the sinusoidal lumen and may replace the endothelium over a large area. They are also found in other locations in the body. Pit cells are characterized by the presence of intracytoplasmic granules, about 0.3 μm in diameter, which has suggested an endocrine function.[217] It is now proposed that pit cells represent large granular lymphocytes (LGL)[100] which correspond functionally to natural killer (NK) cells in various species. This hypothesis is supported by a study of LGL isolated from rat liver, showing morphological similarities between the two types of cells and suggesting that the pit cell should indeed be regarded as the tissue equivalent of LGL in rat[18] and in human liver.[19,106]

REFERENCES

1. Albot, G. & Jezequel, A.M. (1962) Le passage entre les canalicules biliaires trabéculaires et les canaux biliaires interlobulaires chez l'homme. *Presse Médicale*, **70**, 1485–1498.
2. Andrew, W. (1962) An electron microscope study of age changes in the liver of the mouse. *American Journal of Anatomy*, **110**, 1–18.
3. Arias, I.M., Jakoby, W.B., Popper, H. *et al.* (1988) *The Liver. Biology and Pathobiology*. New York: Raven Press.
4. Berger, E.R. (1973) Two morphologically different mitochondrial populations in the rat hepatocyte as determined by quantitative three-dimensional electron microscopy. *Journal of Ultrastructure Research*, **45**, 303–327.
5. Bernhard, W. (1971) Drug effects on the nucleus. In Clementi, F. & Ceccarelli, B. (eds) *Advances in Cell Pharmacology*, Vol. 1, pp. 49–67. New York: Raven Press.
6. Biagini, G. & Ballardini, G. (1989) Liver fibrosis and extracellular matrix. *Journal of Hepatology*, **8**, 115–124.
7. Bianchi, F.B., Biagini, G., Ballardini, G. *et al.* (1984) Basement membrane production by hepatocytes in chronic liver disease. *Hepatology*, **4**, 1167–1172.
8. Biava, C. (1963) Identification and structural forms of human particulate glycogen. *Laboratory Investigation*, **12**, 1179–1197.
9. Biava, C. (1964) Studies on cholestasis. A reevaluation of the fine structure of normal human bile canaliculi. *Laboratory Investigation*, **13**, 840–864.
10. Bissell, D.M., Hammaker, L. & Schmid, R. (1972) Liver sinusoidal cells. Identification of a sub-population for erythrocyte catabolism. *Journal of Cell Biology*, **54**, 107–119.
11. Bissell, D.M., Arenson, D.M., Maher, J.J. & Roll, F.J. (1987) Support of cultured hepatocytes by a laminin-rich gel. Evidence for a functionally significant subendothelial matrix in normal rat liver. *Journal of Clinical Investigation*, **79**, 801–812.
12. Blitzer, B.L. & Boyer, J.L. (1978) Cytochemical localization of Na^+/K^+ATPase in the rat hepatocyte. *Journal of Clinical Investigation*, **62**, 1104–1108.
13. Blomhoff, R., Holte, K., Naess, L. & Berg, T. (1984) Newly administered [3H] retinol is transferred from hepatocytes to stellate cells in liver for storage. *Experimental Cell Research*, **150**, 186–193.
14. Blouin, A., Bolender, R.P. & Weibel, E.R. (1977) Distribution of organelles and membranes between hepatocytes and non hepatocytes in the rat liver parenchyma. *Journal of Cell Biology*, **72**, 441–455.
15. Bonucci, E., Derenzini, M. & Marinozzi, V. (1973) The organic-inorganic relationship in calcified mitochondria. *Journal of Cell Biology*, **59**, 185–212.
16. Bouwens, L., Baekeland, M. & Wisse, E. (1984) Importance of local proliferation in the expanding Kupffer cell population of rat liver after zymosan stimulation and partial hepatectomy. *Hepatology*, **4**, 213–219.
17. Bouwens, L., Baekeland, M., de Zanger, R. & Wisse, E. (1986) Quantitation, tissue distribution and proliferation kinetics of Kupffer cells in normal rat liver. *Hepatology*, **6**, 718–722.
18. Bouwens, L., Remels, L., Baekeland, M. *et al.* (1987) Large granular lymphocytes of 'pit cells' from rat liver. Isolation, characterization and natural killer activity. *European Journal of Immunology*, **17**, 37–42.
19. Bouwens, L., Brouwer, A. & Wisse, E. (1989) Ultrastructure of human hepatic pit cells. In Wisse, E., Knook, D.L. & Decker, K. (eds) *Cells of the Hepatic Sinusoid*, Vol. 2, pp. 471–476. Rijswijk, The Netherlands: The Kupffer Cell Foundation.
20. Boyer, J.L. (1980) Newer concepts of hepatocytic bile formation. *Physiology Review*, **60**, 303–326.
21. Braakman, I., Groothuis, G.M.M. & Meijer, D.K.F. (1987) Acinar redistribution and heterogeneity in transport of the organic cation Rhodamine B in rat liver. *Hepatology*, **7**, 849–855.
22. Brouwer, A., Barelds, R.J., de Leeuw, A.M. *et al.* (1988) Isolation and culture of Kupffer cells from human liver. Ultrastructure, endocytosis and prostaglandin synthesis. *Journal of Hepatology*, **6**, 36–49.
23. Bruni, C. & Porter, K. (1965) The fine structure of the parenchymal cell of the normal rat liver. I. General observations. *American Journal of Pathology*, **46**, 691–755.
24. Bukowski, J.F., Woda, B.A., Habu, S. *et al.* (1983) Natural killer

cell depletion enhances virus synthesis and virus-induced hepatitis in vivo. *Journal of Immunology*, **131**, 1531–1538.
25. Burns, W.A., Vanderweide, G., Goldstein, L.I. & Chan, C.H. (1974) Cytoplasmic crystalline regions in hepatocytes of liver biopsy specimens. *Archives of Pathology*, **97**, 43–45.
26. Chin, T.W., Hollinger, F.B., Rich, R.R. *et al.* (1983) Cytotoxicity by NK-like cells from hepatitis-B immune patients to a human hepatoma cell line secreting HBsAg. *Journal of Immunology*, **130**, 173–178.
27. Clement, B., Rissel, M., Peyrol, S. *et al.* (1985) A procedure for light and electron microscopic intracellular immunolocalization of collagen and fibronectin in rat liver. *Journal of Histochemistry and Cytochemistry*, **33**, 407–415.
28. Clement, B., Grimaud, J., Campion, J. *et al.* (1986) Cell types involved in collagen and fibronectin production in normal and fibrotic human liver. *Hepatology*, **6**, 225–234.
29. Dallner, G. & Ericsson, J.L.E. (1976) Molecular structure and biological implication of the liver endoplasmic reticulum. In Popper, H. & Schaffner, F. (eds) *Progress in Liver Diseases*, Vol. 5, pp. 35–50. New York: Grune & Stratton.
30. Dallner, G., Siekevitz, P. & Palade, G.E. (1966) Biogenesis of endoplasmic reticulum membranes. I. Structural and chemical differentiation in developing rat hepatocyte. *Journal of Cell Biology*, **30**, 73–96.
31. Dallner, G., Siekevitz, P. & Palade, G.E. (1966) Biogenesis of endoplasmic reticulum membranes. II. Synthesis of constitutive microsomal enzymes in developing rat hepatocyte. *Journal of Cell Biology*, **30**, 97–118.
32. De Bruyn, P.P.H., Michelson, S. & Becker, R.P. (1977) Phosphotungstic acid as a marker for the endocytic-lysosomal system (vacuolar apparatus) including transfer tubules of the lining cells of the sinusoids in the bone marrow and liver. *Journal of Ultrastructure Research*, **58**, 87–95.
33. De Duve, C. (1966) Peroxisomes (microbodies) and related particles. *Physiological Reviews*, **46**, 323–357.
34. De La Iglesia, F.A., Sturgess, J.M., McGuire, E.J. & Feuer, G. (1976) Quantitative microscopic evaluation of the endoplasmic reticulum in developing human liver. *American Journal of Pathology*, **82**, 61–70.
35. de Leeuw, A.M., McCarthy, S.P., Geerts, A. & Knook, D. (1984) Purified rat liver fat-storing cells in culture divide and contain collagen. *Hepatology*, **4**, 392–403.
36. de Leeuw, A.M., Praaning-van Dalen, D.P., Brouwer, A. & Knook, D.L. (1989) Endocytosis in liver sinusoidal endothelial cells. In Wisse, E., Knook, D.L. & Decker, K. (eds) *Cells of the Hepatic Sinusoid*, Vol. 2, pp. 94–98. Rijswijk, The Netherlands: The Kupffer Cell Foundation.
37. Denk, H. & Franke, W.W. (1982) Cytoskeletal filaments. In Arias, I., Popper, H., Schachter, D. & Shafritz, D.A. (eds) *The Liver. Biology and Pathophysiology*, pp. 55–71. New York: Raven Press.
38. De Wolf-Peeters, C., De Vos, R., Desmet, V. *et al.* (1974) Electron microscopy and morphometry of canalicular differentiation in fetal and neonatal rat liver. *Experimental and Molecular Pathology*, **21**, 339–350.
39. Diesselhoff-Den Dulk, M.M.C., Crofton, R.W. & van Furth, R. (1979) Origin and kinetics of Kupffer cells during an acute inflammatory response. *Immunology*, **37**, 7–14.
40. Dominici, G. & Orlandi, F. (1961) Ultrastructural and microanalytical observations on human hepatic tissue removed by puncture biopsy in diabetic subjects. *Proceedings of the International Congress of Gastroenterology*, pp. 125–128. Amsterdam: Excerpta Medica.
41. Dooley, M., Bohman, R., Durstenfeld, A. & Cascarano, J. (1987) Identification and characterisation of liver non-parenchymal cells by flow cytometry. *Hepatology*, **7**, 696–703.
42. Elias, H. (1949) A re-examination of the structure of the mammalian liver. II. The hepatic lobule and its relations to the vascular and biliary system. *American Journal of Anatomy*, **85**, 379.
43. Erlinger, S. (1978) Cholestasis: pump failure, microvillous defect, or both? *Lancet*, **1**, 533–534.
44. Essner, E. & Novikoff, A.B. (1960) Human hepatocellular pigments and lysosomes. *Journal of Ultrastructure Research*, **3**, 374–391.
45. Evans, W.H. (1980) A biochemical dissection of the functional

polarity of the plasma membrane of the hepatocyte. *Biochimica et Biophysica Acta*, **604**, 27–64.

46. Ezzat, W.R. & Lautt, W.W. (1986) Hepatic arterial pressure-flow autoregulation is adenosine mediated. *American Journal of Physiology*, **252**, H836–H845.

47. Fawcett, D.W. (1955) Observations on cytology and electron microscopy of hepatic cells. *Journal of the National Cancer Institute*, **15**, 1475–1503.

48. Feldman, G. (1989) The cytoskeleton of the hepatocyte. Structure and functions. *Journal of Hepatology*, **8**, 380–386.

49. Feldmann, G., Penaud-Laurencin, J., Crassous, J. & Benhamou, J.P. (1972) Albumin synthesis by human liver cells. Its morphological demonstration. *Gastroenterology*, **63**, 1036–1048.

50. Ferluga, J. & Allison, A.C. (1978) Role of mononuclear infiltrating cells in the pathogenesis of hepatitis. *Lancet*, **2**, 610–611.

51. Franke, W.W., Schmid, W., Kartenbeck, J. *et al.* (1979) Characterisation of the intermediate-size filaments in liver cells by immunofluorescence and electron microscopy. *Biology of the Cell*, **34**, 99–110.

52. French, S.W. & Davies, P.L. (1975) Ulstrasture localization of actin-like filaments in rat hepatocytes. *Gastroenterology*, **68**, 765–774.

53. French, S.W., Kondo, I., Irie, T. *et al.* (1982) Morphologic study of intermediate filaments in rat hepatocytes. *Hepatology*, **2**, 29–38.

54. Friedman, S.L. & Roll, F.J. (1987) Isolation and culture of hepatic lipocytes, Kupffer cells, and sinusoidal endothelial cells by density gradient centrifugation with Stractan. *Analytical Biochemistry*, **161**, 207–218.

55. Friedman, S.L., Roll, F.J., Boyles, J. & Bissell, D.M. (1985) Hepatic lipocytes: the principal collagen-producing cells of normal rat liver. *Proceedings of the National Academy of Sciences of the USA*, **82**, 8681–8685.

56. Friedman, S.L., Roll, F.J., Boyles, J. *et al.* (1989) Maintenance of differentiated phenotype of cultured rat hepatic lipocytes by basement membrane matrix. *Journal of Biological Chemistry*, **264**, 10756–10762.

57. Gaasbeek Janzen, J.W., Lamers, W.H., Moorman, A.F.M. *et al.* (1985) Immunohistochemical localization of carbamylphosphate synthetase (ammonia) in adult rat liver: evidence for a heterogeneous distribution. *Journal of Histochemistry and Cytochemistry*, **33**, 1205–1211.

58. Gabbiani, G., Ryan, G.B., Lamelin, J.P. *et al.* (1973) Human smooth muscle auto-antibody. Its identification as antiactin antibody and a study of its binding to 'non-muscular' cells. *American Journal of Pathology*, **72**, 473–488.

59. Gale, R.P., Sparkes, R.S. & Golde, D.W. (1978) Bone marrow origin of hepatic macrophages [Kupffer cells] in humans. *Science*, **201**, 937–938.

60. Gebhardt, R. & Mecke, D. (1983) Heterogeneous distribution of glutamine synthetase among rat liver parenchymal cells in situ and in primary culture. *EMBO Journal*, **2**, 567–570.

61. Geerts, A., Schellinck, P., Bouwens, L. & Wisse, E. (1988) Cell population kinetics of Kupffer cells during the onset of fibrosis in rat liver by chronic carbon tetrachloride administration. *Journal of Hepatology*, **6**, 50–56.

62. Geerts, A., Vrijsen, R., Rauterberg, J. *et al.* (1989) In vitro differentiation of fat-storing cells parallels marked increase of collagen synthesis and secretion. *Journal of Hepatology*, **9**, 59–68.

63. Gerace, L. (1986) Nuclear lamina and organization of nuclear architecture. *Trends in Biochemical Science* (Nov.), 443–446.

64. Giampieri, M.P., Jezequel, A.M. & Orlandi, F. (1981) The lipocytes in normal human liver. A quantitative study. *Digestion*, **22**, 165–169.

65. Givan, K. & Jezequel, A.M. (1969) Infectious canine hepatitis. A virological and ultrastructural study. *Laboratory Investigation*, **20**, 36–45.

66. Glaumann, H. & Ericsson, J.L.E. (1970) Evidence for the participation of the Golgi apparatus in the intracellular transport of nascent albumin in the liver cell. *Journal of Cell Biology*, **47**, 555–567.

67. Goldblatt, P.J. (1969) The endoplasmic reticulum. In Lima de Faria, A. (ed.) *Handbook of Molecular Cytology*, pp. 1101–1129. New York: North-Holland.

68. Goldfischer, S., Essner, E. & Novikoff, A.B. (1964) The localization of phosphatase activity at the level of ultrastructure. *Journal of Histochemistry and Cytochemistry*, **12**, 72–95.

69. Goresky, C.A., Bach, G.G. & Nadeau, B.E. (1973) On the uptake of materials by the intact liver. The transport and net removal of galactose. *Journal of Clinical Investigation*, **52**, 991–1009.

70. Gown, A.M. & Vogel, A.M. (1984). Monoclonal antibodies to human intermediate filament proteins II. Distribution of filament proteins in normal human tissues. *American Journal of Pathology*, **114**, 309–315.

71. Greenberger, N.J., Cohen, R.B. & Isselbacher, K.J. (1965) The effect of chronic ethanol administration on liver alcohol dehydrogenase activity in the rat. *Laboratory Investigation*, **14**, 264–271.

72. Grisham, J.W., Nopanitaya, W. & Compagno, J. (1976) Scanning electron microscopy of the liver: a review of methods and results. In Popper, H. & Schaffner, F. (eds) *Progress in Liver Diseases*, Vol. 5, pp. 1–23. New York: Grune & Stratton.

73. Gumucio, J.J. (1989) Hepatocyte heterogeneity: the coming of age from the description of a biological curiosity to a partial understanding of its physiological meaning and regulation. *Hepatology*, **9**, 154–160.

74. Hahn, E.G. & Schuppan, D. (1983) Collagen metabolism in liver disease. In Bianchi, L., Gerok, W., Landmann, L. *et al.* (eds) *Liver in Metabolic Diseases* (Falk Symposium No. 35), pp. 309–323. Lancaster: MTP Press.

75. Hahn, E.G. & Schuppan, D. (1985) Ethanol and fibrogenesis in the liver. In Seitz H.K. & Kommerel, B. (eds). *Alcohol-related Diseases in Gastroenterology*, pp. 125–153. Berlin: Springer-Verlag.

76. Hahn, E., Wick, G., Pencev, D. & Timpl, R. (1980) Distribution of basement membrane proteins in normal and fibrotic human liver: Collagen Type IV, laminin, and fibronectin. *Gut*, **21**, 63–71.

77. Hahn, U., Schuppan, D. & Hahn, E.G. (1983) *Expression of new collagen types by portal fibroblasts in obstructive bile duct disease (OBDD)*. European Association for the Study of the Liver, Southampton. Abstract G17.

78. Ham, A.W. (1974) *Histology*, 7th edn. Philadelphia: J.B. Lippincott.

79. Hamilton, R.L., Regan, D.M., Gray, M.E. & Le Quire, V.S. (1967) Lipid transport in liver. I. Electron microscopic identification of very low density lipoproteins in perfused rat liver. *Laboratory Investigation*, **16**, 305–319.

80. Hanzon, V. (1952) Liver cell secretion under normal and pathologic conditions studied by fluorescence microscopy on living rats. *Acta Physiologica Scandinavica*, **28** (supplement 101), 1–268.

81. Harris, J.R., Price, M.R. & Willison, M. (1974) A comparative study on rat liver and hepatoma nuclear membranes. *Journal of Ultrastructure Research*, **48**, 17–32.

82. Haussinger, D., Sies, H. & Gerok, W. (1985) Functional hepatocyte heterogeneity in ammonia metabolism — the intercellular glutamine cycle. *Journal of Hepatology*, **1**, 3–14.

83. Herzfeld, A.M., Federman, M. & Greengard, O. (1973) Subcellular morphometric and biochemical analyses of developing rat hepatocytes. *Journal of Cell Biology*, **57**, 475–483.

84. Hess, F.A., Weibel, E.R. & Preisig, R. (1973) Morphometry of dog liver. Normal baseline data, *Virchows Archiv Abteilung B*, **12**, 303–317.

85. Holborow, E.J., Trenchev, P.S., Dorling, J. & Webb, J. (1975) Demonstration of smooth muscle contractile protein antigens in liver and epithelial cells. *Annals of the New York Academy of Sciences*, **254**, 489–504.

86. Horikawa, M., Chisaka, N., Yokoyama, S. & Onoe, T. (1976) Effect of stirring during fixation upon immunofluorescence results with distribution of albumin-producing cells in liver. *Journal of Histochemistry and Cytochemistry*, **24**, 926–932.

87. Hruban, Z. & Rechcigl, M.J. (1969) *Microbodies and Related Particles*, New York: Academic Press.

88. Irving, M.G., Roll, R.J., Huang, S. *et al* (1984) Characterisation and culture of sinusoidal endothelium from normal rat liver: lipoprotein uptake and collagen phenotype. *Gastroenterology*, **87**, 1233–1247.

89. Ito, T. & Nemoto, M. (1952) Ueber die Kupfferschen Sternzellen und die 'Fettspeicherungszellen' ('fat-storing cells') in der Blutkapillarenwand der menschlichen Leber. *Okajimas Folia Anatomica Japonica*, **24**, 243–258.

90. James, J., Lygidakis, N.J., van Eycken, P. *et al.* (1989) Application of keratin immunocytochemistry and Sirius Red staining in evaluating intrahepatic changes with acute extrahepatic cholestasis due to hepatic duct carcinoma. *Hepatogastroenterology*, **36**, 151–155.

91. Jezequel, A.M. (1959) Dégénérescence myélinique des mitochon-

dries de foie humain dans un épithélioma du cholédoque et un ictère viral. *Journal of Ultrastructure Research*, **3**, 210–215.

92. Jezequel, A.M. & Orlandi, F. (1972) Fine morphology of the liver as a tool in clinical pharmacology. In Jezequel, A.M. & Orlandi, F. (eds) *Liver and Drugs*, pp. 145–192. London: Academic Press.

93. Jezequel, A.M., Arakawa, K. & Steiner, J.W. (1965) The fine structure of the normal neonatal mouse liver. *Laboratory Investigation*, **14**, 1894–1930.

94. Jezequel, A.M., Koch, M. & Orlandi, F. (1974) A morphometric study of the endoplasmic reticulum in human hepatocytes. *Gut*, **15**, 737–747.

95. Jezequel, A.M., Koch, M.M. & Orlandi, F. (1980) Hepatic fibrosis. Role of perisinusoidal cells? *Italian Journal of Gastroenterology*, **12**, 37–40.

96. Jezequel, A.M., Bonazzi, P., Amabili, P. *et al.* (1982) Changes of the Golgi apparatus induced by diethylmaleate in rat hepatocytes. *Hepatology*, **2**, 856–862.

97. Jones, A.L. & Schmucker, D.L. (1977) Current concepts of liver structure as related to function. *Gastroenterology*, **73**, 833–851.

98. Jones, E.A. & Summerfield, J.A. (1982) Kupffer cells. In Arias, I., Popper, H., Schachter, D. & Shafritz, D.A. (eds) *The Liver, Biology and Pathophysiology*, pp. 507–523. New York: Raven Press.

99. Jones, E.A. & Summerfield, J.A. (1985) Functional aspects of hepatic sinusoidal cells. *Seminars in Liver Disease*, **5**, 157–174.

100. Kaneda, K., Dan, C. & Wake, K. (1983) Pit cells as natural killer cells. *Biomedical Research*, **4**, 567–576.

101. Kaneda, K., Kurioka, N., Seki, S. *et al.* (1984) Pit cell-hepatocyte contact in autoimmune hepatitis. *Hepatology*, **4**, 955–958.

102. Kardon, R.H. & Kessel, R.G. (1980) Three-dimensional organisation of the hepatic microcirculation in the rodent as observed by scanning electron microscopy of corrosion casts. *Gastroenterology*, **79**, 72–81.

103. Kirschner, R.H., Rusli, M. & Martin, T.E. (1977) Characterization of the nuclear envelope, pore complexes and dense lamina of mouse liver nuclei by high resolution scanning electron microscopy. *Journal of Cell Biology*, **72**, 118–132.

104. Knook, D.L. & Wisse, E. (ed.) (1982) *Sinusoidal Liver Cells*. Amsterdam: Elsevier Biomedical Press.

105. Knook, D.L., Blansjaar, N. & Sleyster, E.Ch. (1977) Isolation and characterisation of Kupffer and endothelial cells from the rat liver. *Experimental Cell Research*, **109**, 317–329.

106. Lafon, M.E., Boulard, A., Bioulac-Sage, P. *et al.* (1989) Isolation of pit cells from human liver: preliminary results. In Wisse, E., Knook, D.L. & Decker, K. (eds) *Cells of the Hepatic Sinusoid*, Vol. 2, pp. 488–489. Riswijk, The Netherlands: The Kupffer Cell Foundation.

107. Lamers, W.H., Hilberts, A., Furt, E. *et al.* (1989) Hepatic enzyme zonation: a re-evaluation of the concept of the liver acinus. *Hepatology*, **10**, 72–76.

108. Latham, P.S. & Kashgarian, M. (1979) The ultrastructural localization of transport ATPase in the rat liver at non-bile canalicular plasma membranes. *Gastroenterology*, **76**, 988–996.

109. Lautt, W.W. (1985) Mechanism and role of intrinsic regulation of hepatic arterial blood flow: the hepatic arterial buffer response. *American Journal of Physiology*, **249**, G549–G556.

110. Lautt, W.W. & Greenway, C.V. (1987) Conceptual review of the hepatic vascular bed. *Hepatology*, **5**, 952–963.

111. Lazarow, P.B. (1978) Rat liver peroxisomes catalyze the β oxidation of fatty acids. *Journal of Biological Chemistry*, **253**, 1522–1528.

112. Lazarow, P.B. (1982) Peroxisomes. In Arias, I., Popper, H., Schachter, D. & Shafritz, D.A. (eds) *The Liver. Biology and Pathophysiology*, pp. 27–39. New York: Raven Press.

113. LeBouton, A.V. (1968) Heterogeneity of protein metabolism between liver cells as studied by autoradiography. *Currents in Modern Biology*, **2**, 111–114.

114. LeBouton, A.V. (1969) Relations and extent of the zone of intensified protein metabolism in the liver acinus. *Currents in Modern Biology*, **3**, 4–8.

115. Leskes, A., Siekevitz, P. & Palade, G.E. (1971) Differentiation of endoplasmic reticulum in hepatocytes. I. Glucose-6-phosphatase distribution in situ. *Journal of Cell Biology*, **49**, 264–287.

116. Leu, R.W., Norton, T.R., Herriott, M.J. *et al.* (1985) Suppression of natural killer and lymphocyte functions associated with carcinogen-induced premalignant hyperplastic nodules in rat liver. *Cancer Research*, **45**, 3282–3287.

117. Loud, A.V. (1968) A quantitative stereological description of the ultrastructure of normal rat liver parenchymal cells. *Journal of Cell Biology*, **37**, 27–46.

118. Ma, M.H. & Biempica. L. (1971) The normal human liver cell. Cytochemical and ultrastructural studies. *American Journal of Pathology*, **62**, 353–390.

119. Maher, J.J., Friedman, S.L., Roll, F.J. & Bissell, D.M. (1988) Immunolocalisation of laminin in normal rat liver and biosynthesis of laminin by hepatic lipocytes in primary culture. *Gastroenterology*, **94**, 1053–1062.

120. Marinozzi, V. (1964) Cytochimie ultrastructurale du nucléole. RNA et proteines intranucléolaires. *Journal of Ultrastructure Research*, **10**, 433–456.

121. Martin, S.R., Moscicki, R.A., Ariniello, P.D. *et al.* (1989) Characterisation of rat Kupffer cells using monoclonal antibodies and flow cytometry. In Wisse, E. Knook, D.L. & Decker, K. (eds) *Cells of the Hepatic Sinusoid*, Vol. 2, pp. 439–442. Rijswijk, The Netherlands: The Kupffer Cell Foundation.

122. Martinez-Hernandez, A. (1984) The hepatic extracellular matrix. I. Electron immunohistochemical studies in normal rat liver. *Laboratory Investigation*, **51**, 57–74.

123. Martinez-Hernandez, A. (1985) The hepatic extracellular matrix. II: Electron immunohistochemical studies in rat CCl₄-induced cirrhosis. *Laboratory Investigation*, **53**, 166–186.

124. Matter, A., Orci, L., Forssmann, W.G. & Rouiller, C. (1968) The stereological analysis of the fine structure of the 'micropinocytosis vermiformis' in Kupffer cells of the rat. *Journal of Ultrastructure Research*, **23**, 272–279.

125. Maurice, M. & Feldmann, G. (1982) Quantitative, biochemical and ultrastructural studies of microtubules in rat liver during the acute inflammatory reaction. *Experimental Molecular Pathology*, **36**, 193–203.

126. McCuskey, R.A. (1966) A dynamic and static study of hepatic arterioles and hepatic sphincters. *American Journal of Anatomy*, **119**, 455–477.

127. Milani, S., Herbst, H., Schuppan, D. *et al.* (1989) Cellular localisation of laminin gene transcripts in normal and fibrotic human liver. *American Journal of Pathology*, **134**, 1175–1182.

128. Mitra, S.K. (1966) The terminal distribution of the hepatic artery with special references to arterio-portal anastomosis. *Journal of Anatomy*, **100**, 651–663.

129. Mugnaini, E. (1964) Filamentous inclusions in the matrix of mitochondria from human livers. *Journal of Ultrastructure Research*, **11**, 525–544.

130. Munn, E.A. (1974) *The Fine Structure of Mitochondria*. London: Academic Press.

131. Nakata, K. & Kanbe, A. (1966) The terminal distribution of the hepatic artery and its relationship to the development of focal liver necrosis following interruption of the portal blood supply. *Acta Pathologica Japonica*, **16**, 313–321.

132. Nehemiah, J.L. & Novikoff, A.B. (1974) Unusual lysosomes in hamster hepatocytes. *Experimental and Molecular Pathology*, **21**, 398–423.

133. Nilsson, O. & Dallner, G. (1977) Enzyme and phospholipid asymmetry in liver microsomal membranes. *Journal of Cell Biology*, **72**, 568–583.

134. Nishi, T., Bhan, A.K., Collins, A.B. & McCluskey, R.T. (1981) Effect of circulating immune complexes on Fc and C3 receptors of Kupffer cells in vivo. *Laboratory Investigation*, **44**, 442–448.

135. Nopanitayo, W., Grisham, J.W., Aghajanian, J.G. & Carson, J.L. (1978) Intrahepatic microcirculation: SEM study of the terminal distribution of the hepatic artery. *Scanning Electron Microscopy*, **11**, 837–842.

136. Novikoff, A.B. (1973) Lysosomes: a personal account. In Heis, H.G. & Van Hoof, F. (eds) *Lysosomes and Storage Diseases*, pp. 1–42. New York: Academic Press.

137. Novikoff, A.B. (1976) The endoplasmic reticulum. A cytochemist's view. A review. *Proceedings of the National Academy of Sciences of the USA*, **73**, 2781–2787.

138. Novikoff, A.B. & Essner, E. (1960) The liver cell: some new approaches to its study. *American Journal of Medicine*, **29**, 102–131.

139. Novikoff, A.B. & Goldfischer, S. (1969) Visualization of peroxisomes (microbodies) and mitochondria with diaminobenzidine. *Journal of Histochemistry and Cytochemistry*, **17**, 675–680.

140. Novikoff, A.B., Essner, E., Goldfischer, S. & Heus, M. (1962) Nucleoside phosphatase activities of cytomembranes. In Harris, R.J.C. (ed.) *The Interpretation of Ultrastructure*, pp. 149–192. New York: Academic Press.

141. Novikoff, P.M., Novkoff, A.B., Quintana, N. & Davis, C. (1973) Studies on microperoxisomes. III. Observations on human and rat hepatocytes. *Journal of Histochemistry and Cytochemistry*, **21**, 540–558.

142. Oda, M., Price, V.M., Fisher, M.M. & Phillips, M.J. (1974) Ultrastructure of bile canaliculi with special reference to the surface coat and the pericanalicular web. *Laboratory Investigation*, **31**, 314–323.

143. Orlandi, F. & Koch, M. (1976) The fine structure of liver cells. In Taylor, W. (ed.) *The Hepatobiliary System*, pp. 145–177. New York: Plenum Press.

144. Orrenius, S., Ericsson, J.L.E. & Ernster, L. (1965) Phenobarbital-induced synthesis of microsomal drug-metabolizing enzyme system and its relationship to the proliferation of endoplasmic membranes. *Journal of Cell Biology*, **25**, 627–639.

145. Osborn, M. & Weber, K. (1983) Biology of disease. Tumor diagnosis by intermediate filament typing: a novel tool for surgical pathology. *Laboratory Investigation*, **48**, 372–394.

146. Oshino, N., Jamieson, D., Sugano, T. & Chance, B. (1975) Optical measurement of catalase-hydrogen peroxide intermediate (compound I) in the liver of anesthetized rats and its implication for hydrogen peroxide production in situ. *Biochemical Journal*, **146**, 67–77.

147. Pearse, A.G.E. (1968) *Histochemistry; Theoretical and Applied*, 3rd edn, Vol. 1, pp. 294–380. London: J. & A. Churchill.

148. Pederson, T. (1975) Nuclei. In Altman, P.L. & Katz, D.D. (eds) *Cell Biology*, Vol. 1, pp. 363–400. Bethesda, Maryland: Federation of American Societies for Experimental Biology.

149. Perrin, C., Oudea, M.C., Lenne, Y. & Oudea, P. (1970) Les mitochondries géantes. Appreciation au microscope photonique de leur fréquence en pathologie humaine. *Pathologie Biologie*, **18**, 613–618.

150. Petrovic, L.M., Burroughs, A. & Scheuer, P.J. (1989) Hepatic sinusoidal endothelium: Ulex lectin binding. *Histopathology*, **14**, 233–244.

151. Phillips, M.J., Oda, M., Mak, E. & Fisher, M.M. (1975) Bile canalicular structure and function. In Goresky, C. & Fisher, M.M. (eds) *Jaundice*, pp. 367–382. New York: Plenum Press.

152. Phillips, M.J., Oda, M., Mak, E. *et al.* (1975) Microfilament dysfunction as a possible cause of intrahepatic cholestasis. *Gastroenterology*, **69**, 48–57.

153. Phillips, M.J., Oda, M., Mak, E. *et al.* (1976) The bile canalicular network in vitro. *Journal of Ultrastructure Research*, **57**, 163–167.

154. Phillips, M.J., Poucell, S., Patterson, J. & Valencia Mayoral, P. (1987) *The Liver: An Atlas and Text of Ultrastructural Pathology*. New York: Raven Press.

155. Pierce, G.B., Jr, Midgeley, A.R., Jr & SriRam, J. (1963) The histogenesis of basement membranes. *Journal of Experimental Medicine*, **117**, 339–348.

156. Pignal, F., Maurice, M. & Feldmann, G. (1982) Immunoperoxidase localization of albumin and fibrinogen in rat liver fixed by perfusion or immersion: effect of saponin on the intracellular penetration of labelled antibodies. *Journal of Histochemistry and Cytochemistry*, **30**, 1004–1014.

157. Popper, H. & Udenfriend, S. (1970) Hepatic fibrosis. *American Journal of Medicine*, **49**, 707–721.

158. Popper, H., Elias, H. & Petty, D.E. (1952) Vascular pattern of cirrhotic liver. *American Journal of Clinical Pathology*, **22**, 717–729.

159. Portmann, B., Schindler, A.-M., Murray-Lyon, I.M. & Williams, R. (1976) Histological sexing of a reticulum cell sarcoma arising after liver transplantation. *Gastroenterology*, **70**, 82–84.

160. Poupon, R.E. & Evans, W.H. (1979) Biochemical evidence that Na^+/K^+ATPase is located at the lateral region of the hepatocyte surface membrane. *FEBS Letters*, **108**, 374–378.

161. Prugh, M.F., Gregory, D.H., Vhlacevic, Z.R. & Swell, L. (1976) Role of the 'microtubular-Golgi' network in the hepatocellular transport of biliary lipids. *Gastroenterology*, **70**, A132/990.

162. Racker, E. & Horstman, L.L. (1967) Partial resolution of the enzymes catalyzing oxidative phosphorylation. XIII. Structure and function of submitochondrial particles completely resolved with respect to coupling factor. *Journal of Biological Chemistry*, **242**, 2547–2551.

163. Ramadori, G., Rieder, H., Knittel, T. *et al.* Fat-storing cells (FSC) of rat liver synthesize and secrete fibronectin. *Journal of Hepatology*, **4**, 190–197.

164. Rappaport, A.M. (1973) The microcirculatory hepatic unit. *Microvascular Research*, **6**, 212–228.

165. Rhodin, J.A.G. (1967) The ultrastructure of mammalian arterioles and precapillary sphincters. *Journal of Ultrastructure Research*, **18**, 181–223.

166. Rieder, H., Ramadori, G., Dienes, H.-P. & Meyer zum Buschenfelde, K.-H. (1987) Sinusoidal endothelial cells from guinea pig liver synthesize and secrete cellular fibronectin in vitro. *Hepatology*, **7**, 856–864.

167. Rohr, H.P., Wirz, A., Henning, L.G. *et al.* (1971) Morphometric analysis of the rat liver cell in the perinatal period. *Laboratory Investigation*, **24**, 128–139.

168. Rohr, H.P., Luthy, J., Gudat, F. *et al.* (1976) Stereology of liver biopsies from healthy volunteers. *Virchows Archiv Abteilung A*, **371**, 251–263.

169. Rouiller, C. & Jezequel, A.M. (1963) Electron microscopy of the liver. In Rouiller, C. (ed.) *The Liver*, pp. 195–264. New York: Academic Press.

170. Ruebner, B.H., Aguirre, J., Brayton, M.A. & Watanabe, K. (1971) Inclusions with helical substructure in hepatocytic mitochondria of Rhesus monkey. *Journal of Ultrastructure Research*, **35**, 499–507.

171. Ruiter, D.J., van der Menlen, J., Brouwer, A. *et al.* (1981) Uptake by liver cells of endotoxin following its intravenous injection. *Laboratory Investigation*, **45**, 38–45.

172. Rungger-Brandle, E. & Gabbiani, G. (1983) The role of cytoskeletal and cytocontractile elements in pathologic process. *American Journal of Pathology*, **110**, 360–390.

173. Sadowski, P. & Steiner, J.W. (1968) Electron microscopic and biochemical characteristics of nuclei and nucleoli isolated from rat liver. *Journal of Cell Biology*, **37**, 147–161.

174. Schafer, S., Zerbe, O. & Gressner, M. (1987) The synthesis of glycosaminoglycans in fat-storing cells of rat liver. *Hepatology*, **7**, 680–687.

175. Schaff, S., Lapis, K. & Andre, J. (1974) Study of the tridimensional structure of intramitochondrial crystalline inclusions. *Journal of Microscopy*, **20**, 259–264.

176. Schaff, S., Lapis, K. & Andre, J. (1974) Effect of proteolytic digestion on mitochondrial crystalline inclusions in Gilbert's syndrome. *Journal of Microscopy*, **20**, 265–270.

177. Schmucker, D.L. (1976) Age related change in hepatic fine structure: a quantitative analysis. *Journal of Gerontology*, **31**, 135–143.

178. Shank, R.E., Morrison, G., Cheng, C.H. *et al.* (1959) Cell heterogeneity within the hepatic lobule: quantitative histochemistry. *Journal of Histochemistry and Cytochemistry*, **7**, 237–239.

179. Sheldon, H., Silverberg, M. & Kerner, I. (1962) On the differing appearance of intranuclear and cytoplasmic glycogen in liver cells in glycogen storage disease. *Journal of Cell Biology*, **13**, 468–473.

180. Shiraki, H. & Guegenrich, F.P. (1984) Turnover of membrane proteins: kinetics of induction and degradation of seven forms of rat liver microsomal cytochrome P450, cytochrome P450 reductase and epoxide hydrolase. *Archives of Biochemistry and Biophysics*, **235**, 86–96.

181. Shnitka, T.K. (1966) Comparative ultrastructure of hepatic microbodies in some mammals and birds in relation to species differences. *Journal of Ultrastructure Research*, **16**, 598–625.

182. Siekevitz, P. (1976) Endoplasmic reticulum, microsomes, ribosomes and Golgi. In Altman, P.L. & Katz, D.D. (eds) *Cell Biology*, pp. 231–313. Bethesda, Maryland: Federation of American Societies for Experimental Biology.

183. Slabodsky-Brousse, N., Feldmann, G., Brousse, J. & Dreyfus, P. (1974) Étude stéréologique de la fréquence des mitochondries géantes hépatiques dans la maladie de Gilbert. Comparison avec le sujet normal. *Biologie et Gastroenterologie*, **7**, 179–186.

184. Sokal, E.M., Trivedi, P., Cheeseman, P. *et al.* (1989) The application of quantitative cytochemistry to study the acinar

distribution of enzymatic activities in human liver biopsy sections. *Journal of Hepatology*, **9**, 42–48.

185. Stackpole, C.W., Jacobsen, J.B. & Lardis, M.P. (1974) Two distinct types of capping of surface receptors on mouse lymphoid cells. *Nature*, **248**, 232–234.

186. Steer, C.J. & Klausner, R.D. (1982) Clathrin-coated pits and coated vesicles: functional and structural studies. *Hepatology*, **3**, 437–454.

187. Steiner, J.W. & Carruthers, J.S. (1961) Studies on the fine structure of the terminal branches of the biliary tree. *American Journal of Pathology*, **38**, 639–661.

188. Steiner, J.W., Jezequel, A.M., Phillips, M.J. *et al.* (1965) Some aspects of the ultrastructural pathology of the liver. In Popper, H., & Schaffner, F. (eds) *Progress in Liver Diseases*, Vol. 2, pp. 303–372. New York: Grune & Stratton.

189. Steinhoff, G., Behrend, M., Sorg, C. *et al.* (1989) Sequential analysis of macrophage tissue differentiation and Kupffer cell exchange after human liver transplantation. In Wisse, E., Knook, D.L. & Decker, K. (eds) *Cells of the Hepatic Sinusoid*, Vol. 2, pp. 406–409. Rijswijk, The Netherlands: The Kupffer Cell Foundation.

190. Stempak, J. & Laurencin, M. (1976) Mitochondrial forms in hepatic parenchymal cells in rats of several ages. *American Journal of Anatomy*, **145**, 261–281.

191. Sternlieb, I. (1965) Perinuclear filaments and microtubules in human hepatocytes and biliary epithelial cells. *Journal of Microscopy*, **4**, 551–558.

192. Sternlieb, I. (1972) Functional implication of human portal and bile ductular ultrastructure. *Gastroenterology*, **63**, 321–327.

193. Sternlieb, I. & Berger, J.E. (1969) Optical diffraction studies of crystalline structures in electron micrographs. *Journal of Cell Biology*, **43**, 448–455.

194. Sternlieb, I. & Quintana, N. (1977) The peroxisomes of human hepatocytes. *Laboratory Investigation*, **36**, 140–149.

195. Sternlieb, I., Berger, J.E., Biempica, L. *et al.* (1971) Cytoplasmic crystals in human hepatocytes. *Laboratory Investigation*, **25**, 503–508.

196. Sturgess, J.M. & De La Iglesia, F.A. (1972) Morphometry of the Golgi apparatus in developing liver. *Journal of Cell Biology*, **55**, 524–530.

197. Tate, E.L. & Herbener, G.H. (1976) A morphometric study of the density of mitochondrial cristae in heart and liver of ageing mice. *Journal of Gerontology*, **31**, 129–134.

198. Terada, T., Ishida, F. & Nakanuma, Y. (1989) Vascular plexus around intrahepatic bile ducts in normal liver and portal hypertension. *Journal of Hepatology*, **8**, 139–149.

199. Thurman, R.G. & Kauffman F.C. (1985) Sublobular compartmentation of pharmacological events (SCOPE): metabolic fluxes in periportal and pericentral regions of the liver lobule. *Hepatology*, **5**, 144–151.

200. Tosuka, S., Hasumura, Y. & Takeuchi, J. (1985) Histochemical characteristics of fat-storing cells in alcoholic liver disease: A study by the gold chloride method using needle biopsy specimens of the liver. *American Journal of Clinical Pathology*, **83**, 47–52.

201. Tsou, K.C., Mela, L., Gupta, P.D. & Lynn, D. (1976) Mitochondrial ultrastructure study with the new cytochrome *c* binding agent 4.4′diamino-2.2′-bipyridyl ferrous chelate. *Journal of Ultrastructure Research*, **54**, 235–242.

202. Ueno, T., Yasuura, S., Watanabe, S. *et al.* (1988) Immunocytochemical localization of myosin in the rabbit liver cell. *Journal of Histochemistry and Cytochemistry*, **36**, 803–806.

203. van der Laan-Klamer, S.M., Harms, G. & Hardouk, M.J. (1986) Immunohistochemical demonstration of Fc receptors in rat tissues using immune complexes as ligand. *Histochemistry*, **84**, 257–262.

204. van Eycken, P., Sciot, R. & Desmet, V.J. (1988) A cytokeratin immunohistochemical study of alcoholic liver disease: evidence that hepatocytes can express 'bile duct-type' cytokeratins. *Histopathology*, **13**, 605–617.

205. van Eyken, P., Sciot, R. & Desmet, V.J. (1990) Expression of the novel extracellular matrix component tenascin in normal and diseased human liver. *Journal of Hepatology*, **11**, 43–52.

206. Wachstein, M. (1959) Enzymic histochemistry of the liver. *Gastroenterology*, **37**, 525–537.

207. Wachstein, M. & Meisel, E. (1957) Histochemistry of hepatic phosphatases at a physiological pH with special reference to demonstration of bile canaliculi. *American Journal of Clinical Pathology*, **27**, 13–23.

208. Wade, J.B. & Karnovsky, M. (1974) The structure of the zonula occludens. A single fibril model based on freeze-fracture. *Journal of Cell Biology*, **60**, 168–180.

209. Wake, K. (1980) Perisinusoid stellate cells (fat-storing cells, interstitial cells, lipocytes), their related structure in and around liver sinusoids, and vitamin-A storing cells in extrahepatic organs. *International Review of Cytology*, **66**, 303–353.

210. Wanders, R.J.A., Schutgens, R.B.H. & Heymans, H.S.A. (1987) Deficient cholesterol side chain oxidation in patients without peroxisomes (Zellweger syndrome): evidence for the involvement of peroxisomes in bile acid synthesis in man. *Clinical Chimica Acta*, **162**, 295–301.

211. Weibel, E.R., Staubli, W., Gnagi, H.R. & Hess, F.A. (1969) Correlated morphometric and biochemical studies on the liver cell. *Journal of Cell Biology*, **42**, 68–91.

212. Widman, J.J., Cotran, R.S. & Fahimi, H.D. (1972) Mononuclear phagocytes (Kupffer cells) and endothelial cells. Identification of two functional cell types in rat liver sinusoids by endogenous peroxidase activity. *Journal of Cell Biology*, **52**, 159–170.

213. Wills, E.J. (1965) Crystalline structures in the mitochondria of normal human liver parenchymal cells. *Journal of Cell Biology*, **24**, 511–514.

214. Wisher, M.H. & Evans, W.H. (1975) Functional polarity of the rat hepatocyte surface membrane. Isolation and characterization of plasma-membrane subfractions from the blood-sinusoidal, bile canalicular and contiguous surfaces of the hepatocyte. *Biochemical Journal*, **146**, 375–388.

215. Wisse, E. (1972) An ultrastructural characterization of the endothelial cell in the rat liver sinusoid under normal and various experimental conditions, as a contribution to the distinction between endothelial and Kupffer cells. *Journal of Ultrastructure Research*, **38**, 528–562.

216. Wisse, E. (1974) Observation on the fine structure and peroxidase cytochemistry of normal rat liver Kupffer cells. *Journal of Ultrastructure Research*, **46**, 393–426.

217. Wisse, E., Van't Noordende, J.M., Van Dermeulen, J. & Daems, W. (1976) The pit cell: description of a new type of cell occurring in rat liver sinusoids and peripheral blood. *Cell and Tissue Research*, **173**, 423–435.

218. Wisse, E., de Zanger, R.B., Charels, K. *et al.* (1985) The liver sieve: Considerations concerning the structure and function of endothelial fenestrae, the sinusoidal wall and the space of Disse. *Hepatology*, **5**, 683–692.

219. Wojcik, E., Dvorak, C., Chianale, J. *et al.* (1988) Demonstration by in situ hybridisation of the zonal modulation of rat liver cytochrome P450b and P450e gene expression after phenobarbital. *Journal of Clinical Investigation*, **82**, 658–666.

220. Wood, R.L. (1961) Some structural features of the bile canaliculus in calf liver. *Anatomical Record*, **140**, 207–216.

221. Yasuura, S., Ueno, T., Watanabe, S. *et al.* (1989) Immunocytochemical localization of myosin in normal and phalloidin-treated rat hepatocytes. *Gastroenterology*, **97**, 982–989.

222. Yates, R.D., Higgins, J.A. & Barnett, R.J. (1969) Fine structural localization of acetylcoenzyme A carboxylase in rat liver hepatocytes. *Journal of Histochemistry and Cytochemistry*, **17**, 379–385.

223. Yokoi, Y., Namihisa, T., Kuroda, H. *et al.* (1984) Immunocytochemical detection of desmin in fat-storing cells (Ito cells). *Hepatology*, **4**, 709–714.

CHAPTER 3

Carbohydrate Metabolism in Liver Disease

K.G.M.M. Alberti, R. Taylor & D.G. Johnston

The liver is of prime importance in the regulation of carbohydrate metabolism.[13] It receives ingested carbohydrates via the portal circulation and plays a critical role in homeostasis by damping down sudden surges in the concentrations of fuels, thus preventing excessive fluctuations in systemic osmolality. Man is an intermittent feeder but uses glucose continuously and the liver is the major organ which prevents blood glucose levels falling during periods of fasting. Indeed, the blood glucose level in normal man shows surprisingly small fluctuations, little more than 10% of the mean level. Perhaps the most important role of the liver in metabolism is in preserving this constancy, thus ensuring a fixed, even and predictable supply of carbohydrate to extrahepatic tissues.

The metabolic functions of the liver are outlined in Table 3.1. It can be seen that many important reactions are virtually unique to the liver. In addition, many hormones exert regulatory roles in the liver, and the liver degrades several of these hormones, in certain cases being the only important site of their catabolism (see Chapter 7). Table 3.1 also shows that the main actions of the liver with regard to carbohydrate metabolism can be divided into glucose production, glucose storage, and metabolism of hexoses and sugars other than glucose, which are ingested but not utilized to any major extent elsewhere in the body.

In view of these critical roles of the liver in carbohydrate homeostasis it would be surprising if carbohydrate metabolism were not disturbed in liver disease. What *is* perhaps surprising is that the disturbance is not greater than that commonly found. This reflects the large reserve capacity of the liver parenchyma.

In this chapter we shall first review briefly the role of the normal liver in carbohydrate metabolism, with emphasis on the contrasts between the fed and starved states. The effects of different disorders of the liver on these processes will then be described. Most studies in man have concentrated on measurements of metabolites in blood, but where possible reference will be made to changes in intracellular enzymes and metabolites in

Table 3.1 Metabolic functions of the liver.

Substrate metabolism

Carbohydrates	Glucose storage as glycogen
	Glycogenolysis
	Gluconeogenesis[a]
	Glucose clearance
	Lactate clearance
	Non-glucose hexose metabolism[b]
Lipids	Triglyceride production (in part from glucose)
	VLDL production[b]
	Cholesterol synthesis
	NEFA synthesis and degradation
	Ketogenesis[b]
Proteins	Amino acid degradation
	Ureagenesis[b]
	Plasma protein synthesis[b]

Hormones

Major action on the liver	Insulin, glucagon, growth hormone, glucocorticoids, catecholamines, thyroxine
Catabolized by the liver	Insulin,[b] glucagon, growth hormone,[b] glucocorticoids,[b] thyroxine

Adapted from Alberti[4] and Alberti *et al.*[5]

[a] Takes place in liver and kidney.

[b] Primarily occurs in liver only.

diseased liver and relevant animal data will be discussed. Hormonal changes will be referred to only in so far as they impinge directly on regulatory processes in carbohydrate metabolism, as they are referred to in more detail in Chapter 7. Similarly the metabolism and acute effects of ethanol are described in detail elsewhere in this volume (Chapter 34) and will not be described here.

Several reviews provide further information on the general metabolic aspects of liver disease[1,5,31,47,69,74,129] and on the role of the liver in carbohydrate metabolism.[4,6,66,67,114,115,141,189]

THE REGULATION OF HEPATIC CARBOHYDRATE METABOLISM IN NORMAL MAN

THE FASTED STATE

In short-term starvation certain tissues have an obligatory requirement for glucose. These include the central nervous system, peripheral nerves, red blood corpuscles, white blood cells and fibroblasts, with a total requirement of some 160 g/day in normal man. Other tissues can use substrates such as fatty acids and ketone bodies, with the brain able to use the latter on adaptation to starvation. Only liver and, to a lesser extent, kidney contain the key enzyme glucose-6-phosphatase which allows glucose to be formed in the tissue and released into the circulation for use by other tissues. As ingested glucose disappears, so the liver releases glucose with the result that blood glucose concentration falls only slightly.

After an overnight fast approximately 75% of the released glucose is derived from glycogenolysis, with approximately 25% coming from gluconeogenesis. The liver contains only 70–80 g of glycogen after an overnight fast, so that the contribution of glycogenolysis to glucose production falls rapidly after the first 18 to 24 hours of fasting.[94] As starvation continues, the total body glucose requirement falls owing to the adaptation of the brain to ketone body utilization.[122] Thus after 5–6 weeks' fasting only 40 g glucose/day is required[123] and about half of this requirement is produced by the kidney.

The precursors for gluconeogenesis are lactate, pyruvate, glucogenic amino acids (mainly alanine) and glycerol. Lactate is quantitatively the most important, providing about half of non-glycogen glucose and approximately 20% of total glucose after an overnight fast. Total lactate turnover is some 140 g/day.[87] However, more than half this lactate is derived in turn from glucose metabolism (the Cori cycle) in extrahepatic tissues and from muscle glycogen, much of which is also derived originally from glucose released from the liver. This role of muscle glycogen as a glucose precursor has been elegantly demonstrated in the rat by Sugden, Sharples and Randle.[194] It can thus be considered that although lactate is a useful (albeit energetically wasteful) means whereby extrahepatic tissues can conserve glucose and divert fuels to other tissues via the liver, it is hardly, in the long term, a means for de novo glucose synthesis. This role must be reserved for amino acids, which are irreversibly converted to glucose and contribute 6–12% of total glucose production after an overnight fast but a much greater proportion with prolongation of the fast.

The importance of alanine as a gluconeogenic precursor was first formalized in 1970 by Felig et al.,[51] who had studied arteriovenous differences of amino acids across muscle during fasting. Alanine and glutamine accounted for more than 50% of the amino acids released. Alanine is then taken up in significant quantities by the splanchnic bed. Subsequently it has been shown that glutamine released by muscle is taken up mainly by gut and kidney while the alanine is taken up by the liver and converted to glucose (see review by Snell[183]).

Alanine is formed in peripheral tissues by transamination of pyruvate, the amino groups deriving from the other amino acids, particularly the branched-chain amino acids. It is immediately obvious that if, as was first postulated by Felig,[45] the carbon skeleton derived primarily from glucose then, again, no de novo glucose synthesis would be taking place. Garber, Karl and Kipnis[54] later showed that much of the carbon skeleton of alanine derives from the carbon skeleton of the other amino acids. The whole process can be considered as a molecular reorganization whereby many different amino acids reach the liver in the form of a single amino acid, which undoubtedly simplifies the regulatory processes required in the liver. Further amino groups in peripheral tissues will combine with glutamate to give glutamine, which will be disposed of in the gut and kidney. Much of this glutamine will then be converted to alanine and delivered to the liver. In the liver alanine is again transaminated, this time with oxaloacetate, forming pyruvate and aspartate. The latter participates in the urea cycle yielding urea while the pyruvate passes up the usual gluconeogenic pathway. The role of amino acids in gluconeogenesis is well reviewed by Pogson *et al.*[134]

It is worth pointing out the key regulatory steps in gluconeogenesis as these are most likely to be affected by disorders of the liver:

$$\text{Pyruvate} + CO_2 + \text{ATP} \xrightarrow{\text{pyruvate carboxylase}} \quad (1)$$
$$\text{oxaloacetate} + \text{ADP} + \text{Pi}$$

$$\text{Oxaloacetate} + \text{GTP} \xrightarrow{\text{PEP-carboxykinase}} \quad (2)$$
$$\text{phosphoenolpyruvate} + \text{GDP} + CO_2$$

$$\text{Fructose-1,6-bisphosphate} \xrightarrow{\text{fructose-1,6-bisphosphatase}} \quad (3)$$
$$\text{fructose-6-phosphate} + \text{Pi}$$

$$\text{Glucose-6-phosphate} + H_2O \xrightarrow{\text{glucose-6-phophatase}} \quad (4)$$
$$\text{glucose} + \text{orthophosphate}$$

The fine regulation of gluconeogenesis and its integration with the regulation of glycogenolysis are obviously important in the maintenance of constant blood glucose. Glucose, glucose precursors and hormones are all important in this regulation. The autoregulation of hepatic glucose production by glucose availability has been discussed since the classic early studies of Soskin and Levine.[186] In experimental studies several authors have shown that the liver no longer takes up glucose when portal vein levels fall below approximately 7 mmol/l (120 mg/dl).[27] Glucose enters the liver cell extremely rapidly and is converted by glucokinase to glucose-6-phosphate. This, together with glucose-6-phosphatase, forms a sensitive substrate cycle. Glucose-6-phosphate will influence glycogenesis while glucose itself has a direct inhibitory effect on liver phosphorylase.[189] These effects of glucose are more important in regulating glucose uptake (see below) than output by the liver.

Substrate availability appears to be important in determining the contribution of gluconeogenesis to glucose output. Both Dietze and his co-workers[40] and Lundholm and Schersten[97] have shown that gluconeogenesis in man increases with increasing precursor supply. Release of these precursors from the periphery will thus be all-important. A more detailed account of the regulation of gluconeogenesis can be found in Hue.[66]

In fasting man most of the changes in carbohydrate metabolism can be explained by changes in circulating hormone levels superimposed on these endogenous regulatory mechanisms. Thus, as blood glucose concentration falls, so insulin secretion will decrease and glucagon secretion will rise. There will also be a relative increase in the concentrations of glucocorticoids, growth hormone

and catecholamines when compared with insulin. The effect of insulin on amino acid transport and amino acid synthesis within peripheral tissues will be decreased and glucocorticoid effects will predominate. More amino acids, particularly alanine, will be released into the circulation. At the same time there will be increased extraction of alanine, due to increased glucagon, as well as enhanced extraction of other glucose precursors, by the liver. The normal constraints of insulin on gluconeogenesis will be lost and gluconeogenesis will increase. The importance of this hepatic extraction is shown by the observation that alanine levels in the circulation fall rather than rise on fasting.[135] Glycogenolysis will increase, owing partly to the lack of inhibition by both glucose and insulin. The liver is exquisitely sensitive to small increments in portal insulin concentration, with glycogenolysis being more sensitive than gluconeogenesis (see review by Cherrington[21]). Glycogenolysis will also be enhanced through activation of adenyl cyclase by glucagon and catecholamines. It is possible that other hormones, such as vasopressin and parathormone, also exert acute effects on hepatic glucose metabolism (see Hue[66] and Van de Werve and Jeanrenaud[202] for reviews of hormonal effects on gluconeogenesis).

In the longer term, lipolysis will increase, again owing to the relative lack of insulin. Increased non-esterified fatty acid (NEFA) supply to the liver in the presence of a relative increase in glucagon will result in enhanced ketogenesis. Ketone bodies thus become available as an alternative fuel. The brain then adapts to ketone body utilization, with a resultant fall in total body glucose requirement. This is synchronized with an inhibitory effect of ketone bodies on muscle amino acid release, thereby conserving protein.[177]

THE FED STATE

The main roles of the liver in the fed state are to prevent violent oscillations in peripheral substrate concentrations and to conserve, store and convert into suitable storage forms fuels which are ingested in excess of requirements at the time.

The main carbohydrates ingested by man: sucrose, which yields equimolar amounts of glucose and fructose; lactose, which yields glucose and galactose; and starch, which is broken down in the gut to glucose. Quantitatively glucose and fructose are the most important.

Glucose

Even after ingestion of large amounts of glucose there is relatively little fluctuation in blood glucose concentration. It can be calculated that if 100 g of glucose were infused and all remained in the circulation, blood glucose concentration would rise by 37 mmol/l (670 mg/dl), whereas the measured rise is rarely more than 4 mmol/l (72 mg/dl). Glucose must therefore be disposed of rapidly and in large quantities. The liver is obviously important in this disposal, a fact recognized by Bernard more than a hundred years ago, but arguments still rage as to the exact distribution of this ingested glucose between the liver and the periphery.

All ingested glucose passes through the liver before reaching the peripheral circulation. It has always been assumed that much of this glucose will be sequestered and metabolized by the liver and will not reach the peripheral circulation. There have been wide discrepancies in the estimates of the amount which actually passes through the liver between those using radioactive glucose turnover methods and those using catheterization techniques. Both methods are fraught with difficulties, the former because of recycling or exchange of the radioactive label, and the latter because of the inexact methods available for measuring hepatic blood flow and the stressful nature of the experiments.

The primary exponents of the catheterization technique have been Felig and his co-workers.[48,49] They showed that after oral ingestion of 100 g glucose only 40 g appeared in the hepatic vein over the next 180 minutes. At the same time, hepatic glucose production was decreased from the expected 25 g to near zero. They concluded that there was a net uptake of 85% or a real uptake of 60% of the glucose load.

More recently, Waldhausl et al.[206] have suggested that less than half a 75-g load is retained in the splanchnic bed, while Katz et al.[82] could only acount for 25–30% of the load being cleared by the liver. Overall, the consensus would be that 30–60% of an oral glucose load is taken up by the liver. In contrast, if glucose is slowly infused directly into the portal vein, no uptake can be demonstrated.[95] These observations are not inconsistent, in that oral ingestion of glucose is associated with stimulation of the enteroinsular axis[103,142] with a resulting surge of insulin secretion due to stimulation by both glucose and probably gastric inhibitory polypeptide (GIP).[42] The liver is very sensitive to small amounts of insulin in both man[48] and dog,[19] the effects being both direct and indirect through lowering the threshold for glucose autoregulation.[189] Bergman[12] has suggested that although autoregulation may be important for minute-to-minute adjustment of hepatic glucose metabolism, this effect is of short duration and insulin is required for the sustained uptake of glucose seen after oral glucose loading. Thus the effect of portal infusion of glucose will depend purely on the relatively insensitive autoregulatory process while oral glucose loading will be assisted by simultaneous insulin secretion into the portal vein.

The discrepancies between hepatic catheterization studies and turnover data have been more serious. Steele et al.[191], working with anaesthetized dogs, estimated that 72% of an oral [U[14]C]glucose load entered the peripheral circulation in the 3 hours following glucose ingestion. Hepatic glucose output decreased 42% while peripheral glucose utilization increased by 58%. It was estimated that about 16% of the glucose load was taken up on first passage through the liver. Since that time several thoughtful accounts of radioactive turnover methodology and its problems have appeared.[41,141,143] Radziuk et al.[145] have subsequently examined the problem of hepatic glucose uptake in normal man. They showed convincingly that on first passage of glucose through the liver a maximum of 8% is taken up directly, with 92% appearing in the peripheral circulation. By use of different labels they were able to show that only about 10% of the total glucose consumed was incorporated unchanged into glycogen.[140] Similar results have been shown in the rat[112] and dog.[34] Similar data have been obtained with intravenous glucose with an equivalent amount of glycogen coming from gluconeogenic precursors.[181] However, effects are more rapid with oral than with intravenous glucose, secondary to the higher insulin levels achieved.[142]

The low glucose uptake by the liver found with the tracer studies is not inconsistent with catheterization studies. The latter provide estimates of total hepatic glucose uptake while the radioactive studies indicate only that amount of glucose extracted on the first pass through the liver. In fact, extrapolation of these studies gives an estimate of total hepatic uptake of 40–50 g glucose of a 100 g load, and this is not dissimilar to the conclusions of Felig[46] and Waldhausl et al.[206] These data are also consistent with Mosora et al.,[108] who used a stable isotope method, and found that some 10% of an administered glucose load is oxidized within the first 3 hours of ingestion. It is important to realize that the importance of the liver in taking up an oral glucose load is not because of its anatomical location astride the portal vein but rather because of the sensitivity of the liver to insulin. The importance of oral rather than intravenous glucose feeding is due to the potentiation of insulin secretion by gut hormones, although recent data in the dog suggest that other, as yet unidentified, portal factors may be involved.[101]

The situation is further complicated by the fact that glycogen synthesis after a glucose load occurs not just from glucose but also from three carbon units such as lactate—the so called 'glucose paradox'.[81] Indeed, lactate may be quantitatively a more important precursor, with 60% of glycogen coming from lactate.[139] It is possible that a proportion of ingested glucose is converted to lactate in the small intestinal mucosa and this then passes to the liver for conversion into glycogen. This fits with recent data on zonation of liver parenchyma which identify marked differences between perivenous and peripheral hepatocytes, with some being predominantly glycogenic and others gluconeogenic (see Chapter 2).

It is evident that the liver is important in glucose disposal, although exact quantitation of both uptake and intracellular distribution remain to be determined. Both autoregulation by glucose and insulin effects are important, although the recent work of Sacca et al.,[160] using combined infusions of somatostatin, glucagon and variable amounts of insulin, suggests that the latter predominates. Similar studies by De Fronzo et al.[37] using euglycaemic and hyperinsulinaemic clamps demonstrated that at insulin concentrations of 10 mU/l (compared with increments of 3 mU/l used by Sacca *et al.*[160]) hepatic glucose output could be suppressed at supraphysiological glucose concentrations. Further experiments with oral glucose administration will be of interest in elucidating the nature of the elusive gut/portal factors.

The role of other hormones is less clear. Glucagon has been emphasized by Unger[201] and he has suggested that the ratio of glucagon to insulin is an important determinant of glucose metabolism. Glucagon has only short-term effects on glycogen breakdown but has a more sustained stimulatory effect on gluconeogenesis.[21] After glucose ingestion, glucagon levels fall and its effects are almost certainly overcome entirely by insulin plus glucose. The importance of glucagon in glucoregulation when insulin is present has been severely questioned.[179]

Other hormones such as glucocorticoids are probably more important than glucagon in counteracting the effects of insulin on glucose disposal in the liver. In the presence of excess amounts of glucocorticoids, glucose disposal is impaired, partly as a peripheral effect but also by a direct effect on the liver which is thought to be due to enhanced activity of the substrate cycle between glucose and glucose-6-phosphate[68] as well as to a direct stimulation of gluconeogenesis.

After rapid diffusion into the liver, glucose is phosphorylated to glucose-6-phosphate. At most a quarter will be stored as glycogen and a further 10% will pass down the glycolytic pathway.[168] Glucose will also be disposed of via the hexose monophosphate shunt. Both this and the glycolytic pathways will direct glucose towards glycerol and fatty acid synthesis for subsequent release as very low-density lipoprotein (VLDL)-triglyceride.

After glucose ingestion, changes in circulating concentrations of carbohydrate intermediates are found. These include a 50% rise in blood lactate and pyruvate concentration, which follows the rise in blood glucose concentration by 10–20 minutes.[172] The rise in lactate is not due to enhanced peripheral lactate production[71,91,142] and is unlikely to be due to enhanced hepatic glycolysis because of the relative inactivity of this pathway. It is most likely to be secondary to an insulin-induced inhibition of gluconeogenesis with a consequent decrease in hepatic uptake of gluconeogenic precursors. Blood citrate and 2-oxoglutarate concentrations also rise after oral glucose loading but the source and significance of these changes are unclear.

Most emphasis has been placed on the changes which occur after glucose feeding. Precise studies of hepatic carbohydrate metabolism after mixed feeding are more difficult to interpret. Obviously the hormonal milieu after a mixed meal is different from that following glucose alone, in that insulin secretion is likely to be enhanced while glucagon levels will tend to rise rather than fall. Using continuous in vivo glucose monitoring we have shown that blood glucose profiles were superimposable when 50 g glucose was taken alone or an equivalent amount of carbohydrate was taken in a mixed meal. It can be assumed that disposal of glucose will, in principle, be similar to that shown for pure glucose feeding, although with the former glucagon levels rise rather than fall.

Other hexoses

Quantitatively fructose forms an important source of calories in Western society. There is little doubt that the majority of ingested fructose is taken up by and metabolized in the liver. It is phosphorylated rapidly to fructose-1-phosphate and subsequently enters the glycolytic/gluconeogenic pathway.[53] In normal liver approximately 70% of a fructose load appears as lactate with the rest converted to glycogen. Fructose administration can also lead to a fall in hepatic ATP concentration and hyperuricaemia[208] but these changes are minor with oral ingestion of the normal dietary amounts of fructose.

Galactose and other rarer hexoses are also metabolized almost exclusively by the liver, being in the main converted to glucose or glycogen.

THE REGULATION OF HEPATIC CARBOHYDRATE METABOLISM IN PATIENTS WITH LIVER DISEASE

THE FASTED STATE _____

Blood glucose

Despite the importance of the liver in glucose production, fasting hypoglycaemia is surprisingly rare in liver disease.[161,212] There are two possible reasons for this. Firstly, the liver has a large reserve capacity and it has been suggested that normal glucose homeostasis can be maintained with as little as 20% of parenchymal cells functional. Secondly, the kidney is capable of gluconeogenesis and it is possible that this organ could take over a significant proportion of glucose production in chronic liver damage as it does in starvation. Owen *et al.*[124] could show little net renal glucose exchange after overnight or 3-day fasts in cirrhotic subjects, although there was marked variation within the cirrhotic group.

Hypoglycaemia when it occurs is generally found in acute fulminant hepatic disease (Table 3.2). Hypoglycaemia has been reported in acute viral hepatitis[50,96] although this has not been corroborated in our own studies (Table 3.3), where subjects were in a better nutritional state.[149] Hypoglycaemia has also been reported in association with toxic liver damage secondary to overdosage of agents such as chloroform and paracetamol. Ethanol-induced hypoglycaemia is regarded as a separate case because there is a specific biochemical reason for the hypoglycaemia and it occurs in normal as well as in diseased liver (see Chapter 34). Other causes of hepatogenous hypoglycaemia are shown in Table 3.2. It can be seen that most of these are acute disorders apart from rare instances of hypoglycaemia in cirrhosis and in association with primary hepatic

Table 3.2 Fasting hypoglycaemia in liver disease.

Cause	References
Acute viral hepatitis	Felig et al.,[50] Lindner[96]
Fulminant hepatitis	Moore et al.,[106] Samson et al.[162]
Primary hepatic carcinoma	Kronig and Bass,[88] McFadzean and Young[100]
Metastatic carcinoma	Keating and Wilder[83]
Cirrhosis	Samols and Holdsworth[161]
Cholangitis	Conn et al.,[29] Marks and Rose[99]
General hepatotoxins	
Chloroform	Stander[190]
Neoarsphenamine	Cross and Blackford[32]
Paracetamol	Record et al.[150]
Phosphorus	McIntosh[102]
Specific hepatotoxins	
Ethanol	See Chapter 34
Hypoglycin	Hassall and Reyle[60]

Based on Samols and Holdsworth.[161]

carcinoma. In this latter case the mechanism may be similar to that found in other large tumours such as mesenchymal tumours.[90] In other cases of chronic liver disease there is often mild hyperglycaemia after an overnight fast[6] (Table 3.2) and even after a 3-day fast Owen et al.[124] were unable to provoke hypoglycaemia in their cirrhotic subjects.

The possible causes of hepatogenic hypoglycaemia include: (a) impaired glycogen synthesis and breakdown, and (b) impaired gluconeogenesis. It should be pointed out that these processes may be impaired in hepatic disease even without overt hypoglycaemia occurring provided that the disturbance is mild or that compensatory mechanisms have come into play. These latter could include increased renal gluconeogenesis (see above) and provision of alternative substrates such as fatty acids, the levels of which are often increased in liver disease.[154]

Glycogen metabolism

A primary defect in many forms of liver disease may be a decreased capacity to store glycogen. Owen et al.,[124] with elegant catheterization studies, showed that after an overnight fast only about one-third of glucose production was derived from glycogen in cirrhotic subjects while 70–80% came from glycogen in normal subjects. The same conclusions can be drawn from studies where glucagon was administered. Felig et al.[50] showed a dimin-

Table 3.3 Fasting values for metabolites in liver disease. (Continued on facing page.)

Metabolite*	Cirrhosis		Hepatic coma	
	Patient	Control	Patient	Control
Glucose (mmol/l [mg/dl])	5.17 ± 0.33 (93 ± 6)	3.94 ± 0.33 (71 ± 6)[a]	5.83 ± 0.50 (105 ± 9)	5.44 ± 0.39 (98 ± 7)[d]
	4.59 ± 0.48 (83 ± 9)	4.58 ± 0.48 (82 ± 9)[b]		
	5.17 ± 0.17 (93 ± 3)	5.12 ± 0.11 (92 ± 2)[c]		
	5.44 ± 0.17 (98 ± 3)	5.44 ± 0.39 (98 ± 7)[d]		
Lactate (mmol/l)	0.88 ± 0.06	0.66 ± 0.05[c]	3.01 (1.03–15.4)‡	1.18 ± 0.05[i]
	1.02 ± 0.08	0.69 ± 0.06[e]		
Pyruvate (mmol/l)	0.086 ± 0.005	0.070 ± 0.005[c]	0.255 (0.120–0.350)	0.089 (0.045–0.160)[f]
	0.124 ± 0.040	0.118 ± 0.020[h]	0.305 ± 0.110	0.120 ± 0.010[j]
	0.112 (0.06–0.16)	0.089 (0.045–0.160)[f]	0.203 (0.054–0.643)‡	0.106 ± 0.004[i]
2-Oxoglutarate (mmol/l)	0.011 (0.010–0.013)	0.010 (0.006–0.021)[g]	0.040 (0.020–0.086)	0.012 (0.008–0.018)[f]
	0.009 ± 0.002§	0.004 ± 0.003[h]	0.020 ± 0.006	0.010 (0.006–0.021)[g]
	0.021 (0.018–0.030)	0.012 (0.008–0.018)		
Glycerol (mmol/l)	0.116 ± 0.011	0.058 ± 0.012[c]		
Alanine mmol/l	0.28 ± 0.02	0.29 ± 0.03[c]	1.036 ± 0.444†	0.412 (0.273–0.565)[k]
	0.33 ± 0.22	0.38 ± 0.02[s]	0.48 ± 0.10	0.38 ± 0.02[d]

Adapted from Johnston and Alberti.[74]
* Values are the median and range or the mean ± s.e. mean, and are given for whole blood except where otherwise stated.
† Values expressed as mmol/l plasma.
‡ Patients and controls had both received glucose; values are for arterial blood.
§ 38 patients with liver disease studied, 33 of whom had cirrhosis.

ished glycaemic response to glucagon in viral hepatitis patients and Yeung and Wang[211] obtained the same results in patients with postnecrotic cirrhosis, as did de Moura and Cruz[38] in a group of cirrhotic patients of varied aetiology. In Yeung and Wang's[211] series those subjects with the lowest glucose response had the most severe liver disease. There is also suggestive evidence of impaired glycogen metabolism in patients with acute hepatic failure secondary to paracetamol poisoning.[150] Against these positive reports are the negative findings of Strange *et al.*[193] and Van Itallie and Bentley[203], who could show no abnormality in the glucose response to glucagon in most patients with cirrhosis. These discrepancies may have been due to differing patient populations or to different nutritional states of the patients.

An impaired glucose response to glucagon could be explained in several ways. There may be decreased hepatic glycogen,[124] which could be due either to parenchymal damage per se, or to chronically increased glycogenolysis. The latter is a possibility as patients with liver disease have chronically elevated portal and peripheral glucagon levels with hyper-responsiveness to different physiological stimuli.[57,180] Alternatively, there may be tissue insensitivity to glucagon. Greco *et al.*[58] showed a diminished glycaemic response to glucagon in the presence of somatostatin despite higher glucagon levels in patients with hepatic cirrhosis. The report by Davies, Prudhoe and Douglas[33] of an increased plasma cyclic AMP response

to glucagon infusion in patients with cirrhosis, and extrahepatic and intrahepatic cholestasis, is of interest. It suggests that glucagon receptors are fully functional in these states, although the glucose response to glucagon was also normal in these patients. Davies and his colleagues also found that the cyclic AMP response was diminished in six of eight patients with portacaval shunts and that these patients had a somewhat lowered glucose response. This was also found by Sherwin *et al.*[180] and their patients had the highest glucagon values. It is worth pointing out that Sherwin's cirrhotic patients with normal hepatic blood flow had an exaggerated glucose response to glucagon infusion. Shunting is, therefore, important as a possible mechanism for diminishing delivery of appropriate stimuli to glycogen breakdown, and may result in an inaccurate picture of glycogen reserves.

Obviously, more direct studies of glycogenolysis and glycogenesis in man are required, particularly in view of the discrepant results obtained by different groups and the strikingly suggestive results of Owen *et al.* referred to above.[124]

Gluconeogenesis

Gluconeogenesis in patients with liver disease has been examined in four ways: indirectly by measurement of circulating gluconeogenic precursor concentrations and by measuring clearance of exogenous loads of these

Table 3.3 Continued

	Acute viral hepatitis		Untreated chronic active hepatitis		Paracetamol poisoning	
	Patient	Control	Patient	Control	Patient	Control
	3.31 ± 0.16 (60 ± 3)†	4.26 ± 0.06 (77 ± 1)[l] 3.84 ± 0.10 (69 ± 2)[m] 4.61 ± 0.39 (83 ± 7)[n]	4.22 ± 0.17 (76 ± 3)	3.67 ± 0.17 (66 ± 3)[p]	2.60 ± 0.20 (47 ± 4)	3.80 ± 0.10 (68 ± 2)[r]
	0.96 ± 0.13	0.72 ± 0.04[m]	0.76 ± 0.11	0.74 ± 0.05[p]	1.47 ± 0.24	0.72 ± 0.04[r]
	0.116 ± 0.016 0.078 ± 0.009 0.001 ± 0.026	0.120 ± 0.010[j] 0.072 ± 0.005[m] 0.073 ± 0.016[n]	0.064 ± 0.009	0.070 ± 0.006[p]	0.137 ± 0.026	0.072 ± 0.005[r]
	0.013 ± 0.002 0.024 ± 0.012	0.009 ± 0.001[m] 0.013 ± 0.002[a]	0.013 ± 0.001	0.011 ± 0.001[p]	0.015 ± 0.002	0.009 ± 0.001[r]
	0.087 ± 0.014	0.074 ± 0.005[m]	0.112 ± 0.013	0.077 ± 0.006[p]		
	0.322 ± 0.034	0.343 ± 0.021[l]	0.261 ± 0.016	0.309 ± 0.024[q]		

[a] Greco *et al.*[56]
[b] Amatuzio *et al.*[9]
[c] Johnston *et al.*[77]
[d] Sestoft and Rehfeld.[174]
[e] Klassen *et al.*[86]
[f] Summerskill *et al.*[195]
[g] Walshe[207]
[h] Dawson *et al.*[35]
[i] Record *et al.*[151]
[j] Amatuzio and Nesbitt.[8]
[k] Wu *et al.*[210]
[l] Felig *et al.*[50]
[m] Record *et al.*[149]
[n] Seligson *et al.*[173]
[p] Alberti *et al.*[6]
[q] Johnston *et al.*[75]
[r] Record *et al.*[150]
[s] Rosen *et al.*[157]

precursors; and directly by measuring transhepatic substrate balances or by using radioactive turnover techniques.

Precursor concentrations

The main gluconeogenic precursors are lactate, pyruvate, alanine and glycerol. Table 3.3 shows blood concentrations of these substrates after an overnight fast in a broad spectrum of hepatic disorders. Lactate concentrations are moderately elevated in acute viral hepatitis,[149] cirrhosis[3, 77,91,195] and paracetamol poisoning,[150] although values rarely exceed 2 mmol/l (18 mg/dl). In acute hepatic failure values may be higher.[151] Impaired hepatic clearance may be contributory but it should also be recognized that increased production may occur. This could be secondary to impaired pyruvate oxidation[146] due to the raised circulating fatty acid concentrations.[107] Pyruvate concentrations tend to parallel those of lactate.

Alanine concentrations are more variable. We could show no change in fasting whole blood concentrations in patients with cirrhosis, viral hepatitis or chronic active hepatitis, although Rosen *et al*.[157] showed a small decrease in cirrhotic subjects. In acute hepatic necrosis[157] or fulminant hepatic failure[152,210] alanine values were elevated, as were concentrations of the other glucogenic amino acids, glycine, glutamate and glutamine. The reason for the lack of abnormality of fasting alanine concentrations in all but the most severe forms of liver disease may be sought both in the peripheral tissues and in the liver. Systemic plasma insulin concentrations are raised in most forms of liver disease (see Chapter 7) and this will tend to drive alanine back into peripheral tissues, particularly muscle. Alternatively, glucagon levels are raised in liver disease and in normal man glucagon enhances hepatic alanine uptake,[22] although this mechanism may be impaired in viral hepatitis.[50]

Fasting concentrations of glycerol are also raised in approximately 50% of patients with liver disease.[4] Leg catheterization studies have shown that this is a consequence of lack of inhibition of adipose tissue lipolysis.[105]

Clearance studies

Interpretation of blood metabolite concentrations in terms of mechanisms and the role of individual tissues is difficult if not impossible. By infusing known amounts of precursors which are metabolized mainly in the liver, more information can be gained, although it will reveal more about maximal metabolic capacity than subtle alterations in regulatory processes.

Impaired hepatic lactate clearance in cirrhotic subjects was first demonstrated more than 50 years ago.[25,184] Although this has been confirmed more recently in the fed state,[30] hepatic lactate uptake was found to be normal in a hepatic vein catheterization study.[105]

Lactate has the disadvantage that it can be used by many different tissues, which may exhibit disturbed function in cirrhosis. We have instead used glycerol, which is particularly attractive as an experimental substrate

because more than 90% is metabolized by the liver. It is non-ionic, and therefore does not generate acid–base disturbances, and can be given safely in relatively high doses. Using a steady-state infusion technique we have estimated metabolic clearance and disappearance rates in normal and stable cirrhotic subjects.[78] Disappearance followed a double exponential curve with a fast first component and a much slower second component. The half-life of the first component was prolonged from 1.4 to 9.5 minutes in the cirrhotics, while the metabolic clearance rate was decreased from 37.5 to 24.5 ml/kg/min. We would suggest that the fast component, which represented 80–90% of total clearance, was the hepatic component, and the data give clear evidence of impaired hepatic handling of a relatively large load of gluconeogenic substrate.

In contrast to these clear-cut findings we were unable to show any alteration in alanine handling in cirrhotic subjects when using a continuous infusion protocol similar to that used for glycerol. This may have been due to the excessive glucagon response to alanine which is found in cirrhotic subjects[178] and which would tend to compensate any defect by stimulating hepatic alanine uptake.

Catheterization studies

All the results outlined so far give an indirect measure of hepatic gluconeogenetic capacity in liver disease. Direct measurement of hepatic gluconeogenic precursor uptake and glucose output is obviously preferable, but few data are available owing to the technical problems involved and ethical considerations.

In early studies, Myers[109] showed a 25% decrease in hepatic glucose production in cirrhotic subjects after an overnight fast. He did not establish the relative impairment of glycogenolysis and gluconeogenesis. More recently Feruglio *et al*.[52] have studied hepatosplanchnic glucose and lactate balances in normal and cirrhotic subjects. In the post-absorptive state there was no difference in glucose production between the two groups, and similarly splanchnic lactate balances were not different (uptake of 26.9 ± 18 mg/min [0.30 ± 0.20 mmol/min] in normals and 33.9 ± 47.2 mg/min [0.38 ± 0.52 mmol/min] in cirrhotics). On infusion of 1.5 mg glucagon over 30 minutes (a pharmacological dose) there was a twofold greater output of glucose from the liver in the normal subjects. In addition, lactate uptake doubled in normals but was unaltered in the cirrhotic patients. Too much weight should not be placed on these results as there was considerable between- and within-patient variation.

The best executed studies to date have been those of Owen *et al*.[124] and of Merli *et al*.[105] In both studies the patients were stable cirrhotics with normal arterial lactate, pyruvate, and glucose concentrations after an overnight fast. Hepatic glucose output was 40% and 50% lower than that of previously published control groups.[204] By contrast, their gluconeogenic precursor uptake was twice normal and accounted for two-thirds of glucose output, the deficit arising from decreased glycogenolysis. After a

3-day fast the entire glucose output could be accounted for by gluconeogenesis, compared with only two-thirds in normal subjects. Biopsy showed glycogen levels of only 1–3% net weight compared with 4–5% in round numbers.[117] Gluconeogenic enzyme contents were normal. There is a striking similarity, as pointed out by Owen, between the results found in cirrhotics and those reported by Nilssen, Furst and Hultman[118] for subjects receiving a carbohydrate-restricted diet, where liver glycogen content was decreased.

Providing that the nutritional status of the cirrhotic subjects is normal it can be concluded that in mild degrees of liver disease there is decreased hepatic glucose production but this is due to impaired glycogenolysis, not decreased gluconeogenesis. This appears to be true even in subjects with more severe cirrhosis.[124]

Glucose turnover studies

Few studies have examined glucose turnover in cirrhotic subjects. Perez *et al.*[130] were unable to demonstrate any abnormality in glucose output, uptake or metabolic clearance rate. At the time of study both peripheral plasma glucagon and insulin concentrations were twice normal. After injection of insulin, plasma glucose concentration showed a similar fall in both normal and cirrhotic subjects. There was a marked decrease in both glucose production and glucose uptake in response to hypoglycaemia in the cirrhotics. Insulin levels were similar in both groups but the glucagon response was markedly enhanced in the cirrhotics. This enhancement has also been found in cirrhotic dogs when similar tracer techniques have been used.[144] The authors suggest that the studies demonstrate both peripheral insulin resistance and hepatic glucagon insensitivity. Adlung *et al.*[1] using [^{14}C]glucose, have shown that glucose production starts when blood glucose concentration falls below 7 mmol/l (125 mg/dl) in normal subjects but only at 4.4 mmol/l (80 mg/dl) in patients with cirrhosis. This again could be due to hepatic insensitivity to glucagon, secondary perhaps to depleted glycogen stores.

More recently, Proietto, Alford and Dudley[137] have shown decreased basal hepatic glucose output (10.2 vs 13.6 μmol kg^{-1} min^{-1}) and a decreased metabolic clearance rate for glucose despite a twofold increase in peripheral insulin levels. The latter suggests peripheral resistance to insulin action. By contrast, hepatic glucose output responded normally to an insulin infusion. In our own studies[131] we have also found a diminished hepatic glucose output (8.1 vs 12.1 μmol kg^{-1} min^{-1}) and glucose clearance. Glucose recycling, a reflection of Cori cycle activity, was also diminished appropriately so that we could not confirm the relative increase in gluconeogenesis suggested by Owen *et al.*[124]

Animal studies

Animal models of liver disease have been used to determine more precisely the nature of the impairment in hepatic glucose production. Unfortunately there are major problems in relating animal models of alcoholic cirrhosis to the human condition. Studies have been performed in rats with diet-produced cirrhosis.[63] When livers from such rats were isolated and perfused there was a decrease in gluconeogenesis from both lactate and alanine. This was associated with a lower oxygen consumption and lower Krebs cycle activity. Fatty acids also failed to stimulate gluconeogenesis in the usual way, perhaps because of limited pyruvate carboxylase activity.

Administration of dimethylnitrosamine to rats over a 10-week period has been shown to produce a true cirrhotic process, rather than a chronic hepatitis.[72] This was found to be associated with increased insulin sensitivity in both muscle and adipose tissue, most likely as a direct consequence of co-existing malnourishment (body weight 237 ± 20 g vs 365 ± 13 g).[23] Future use of this promising model will demand careful attention to matching nutritional status to control animals. Galactosamine hepatitis has proved useful as a model for acute hepatitis.[85] Using this model we have shown increased blood lactate concentrations as in human hepatitis.[147] Perfused liver experiments revealed impaired gluconeogenic capacity from lactate, and direct measurement showed a marked decrease in activity of the key gluconeogenic enzyme, phosphoenolpyruvate carboxykinase, as well as of alanine aminotransferase.[148] In this model, as well as with carbon tetrachloride treatment, insulin binding to liver plasma membranes has been shown to be decreased.[10,163] Impaired gluconeogenesis has also been reported after bile duct ligation in the rat.[92,147] More work is required to validate these animal models as useful guides to human disease.

THE FED STATE _____

Normal feeding

Most studies of patients with liver disease have concentrated on the fasted state or on provocative tests such as glucose tolerance tests. Relatively little is known of circulating glucose and metabolic intermediates under normal conditions.

In an attempt to rectify this we have measured circulating hormones and metabolites over a 12-hour period in patients with differing degrees of alcoholic liver disease.[192] A reasonable nutritional state was ensured before testing. In normal subjects blood glucose concentration varied little through the 12 hours with increments of 1–2 mmol/l (18–36 mg/dl) after meals. These mealtime responses were exaggerated (a rise of 4–5 mmol/l (72 to 90 mg/dl)) in patients with mild alcoholic liver disease. In subjects with severe cirrhosis, glucose values rose from normal fasting levels to a mean of 11 mmol/l (198 mg/dl) with breakfast and remained there throughout the day. This hyperglycaemia was associated with marked fasting and postprandial peripheral hyperinsulinism (see Chapter 7), suggesting both insulin resistance and impaired degradation and/or increased secretion.

Diurnal patterns of gluconeogenic precursors were also distorted. Blood lactate concentrations showed exaggerated postprandial rises in mildly affected subjects. In patients with the more severe cirrhosis, fasting levels were already raised (Table 3.3) and after breakfast rose to more than 2 mmol/l (36 mg/dl) and remained elevated for the rest of the day. Surprisingly, the extent of hyperlactataemia in these cirrhotic patients showed a close correlation with two unrelated aspects of liver function, the rise in serum bilirubin and the fall in serum albumin. Pyruvate changed in a similar way to lactate although the lactate/pyruvate ratio was mildly increased, suggesting perhaps increased intrahepatic (free NADH/free NAD) ratio, although these ratios should be interpreted with caution. The increase in lactate is presumably due to inhibition of hepatic lactate uptake as in normal subjects (see above) with perhaps some contribution from hepatic fructose metabolism, derived from dietary sucrose. Hyperlactataemia after a glucose load has been shown to correlate with the insulin response in chronic active hepatitis and cirrhosis[3,30] but is not the result of increased peripheral glycolysis, at least as assessed using the forearm model in cirrhotic man.[91] In the cirrhotic subjects there is also defective lactate clearance[30] which will enhance the hyperlactataemia of the fed state. This point is of practical clinical importance in that lactic acidosis can be provoked relatively easily in patients with severe liver disease.

In contrast, diurnal levels of alanine were lowered in both mild and severe cirrhotic groups. This could be related to both the peripheral hyperinsulinism and to a selective increase in hepatic extraction secondary to the hyperglucagonaemia although the results of Felig *et al.*[51] make this hypothesis doubtful.

Glucose loading

Glucose intolerance in liver disease has been recognized since the first description of so-called 'hepatogenous diabetes' by Naunyn and Blanchs.[111] It occurs commonly in cirrhosis,[7,14,18,26,62,77,104,187] chronic active hepatitis,[6] acute viral hepatitis,[50,55,84,116,149] obstructive liver disease[185] and toxic hepatitis.[150] Many of these studies could be criticized in that patients were inadequately prepared in a nutritional sense; it is well known that malnutrition and fasting induce glucose intolerance and insulin resistance.[113] Adequate precautions were taken in many other studies and the incidence of oral glucose intolerance of 50–100% is impressive. One common finding is that more patients show intolerance to oral than to intravenous glucose.[31] This could be due partly to portasystemic shunting of glucose,[36] although, as shown by Radziuk *et al.*[145] only 8% of portal vein glucose is extracted at first pass. Thereafter all glucose, whether derived from the oral or the intravenous route, will reach the liver by the same routes. Alternatively, there could be defective gut hormone release.

Peripheral insulin levels have been measured in many

Table 3.4 Possible causes of glucose intolerance in hepatic disease.

General factors
  Poor nutritional state
  Potassium deficiency

Hepatic factors
  Decreased parenchymal mass
  Portosystemic shunting
  Decreased glycogen synthetic capacity
  Impaired insulin action
  Increased glucagon secretion
  Increased growth hormone secretion
  Haemosiderosis
  Hypoinsulinaemia

Extrahepatic factors
  Peripheral insulin resistance
  Increased NEFA levels
  Circulating antagonists

of the above studies. Hyperinsulinaemia after glucose loading appears to be associated particularly with hepatic cirrhosis and acute severe liver damage, while hypoinsulinaemia appears to be more characteristic of chronic active hepatitis and prolonged-course hepatitis. This is discussed in detail in Chapter 7, as is the problem of distinguishing hepatogenous diabetes from maturity-onset diabetes.

Intermediary metabolite changes after glucose loading

Measurements of lactate and pyruvate have been made during glucose tolerance tests in several different diseases of the liver. In alcoholic liver disease the lactate response to intravenous glucose is increased.[3,4] No consistent change was found in cases of viral hepatitis or paracetamol poisoning, while a consistently lowered response was found in patients with chronic active hepatitis.[6] In this latter group there was a close correlation with the initial insulin response to glucose. Similarly, after oral glucose loading there was a significant correlation between mean blood lactate and mean serum insulin ($r = 0.55$, $p < 0.05$).[77] The mechanism of these changes remains unclear, and it should be noted that overall there was no correlation between glucose tolerance and change in blood lactate concentration. Similarly, there were no consistent changes in 2-oxoglutarate, glycerol or the lipid metabolites, non-esterified fatty acids (NEFA) and ketone bodies.

Mechanism of glucose intolerance in liver disease (Table 3.4)

Although major advances in understanding have occurred in the last few years, it is still not possible to put forward a definitive explanation. There are several reasons why this is the case. Firstly, individual patients differ markedly in terms of nutrition, severity of cirrhosis, physical fitness, other disease processes and family history of non-insulin-dependent diabetes. All these factors will directly affect insulin sensitivity and the outcome of individual studies will be an effect of the characteristics represented in the study group. Secondly, it has proved difficult in man to establish the relative contribution of liver and extrahepatic tissues (mainly muscle) to the impaired glucose handling. Thirdly, it is highly likely that no one factor alone explains the glucose intolerance associated with cirrhosis, although insulin insensitivity must be a leading participant. Several relevant factors may be identified.

Insulin sensitivity in adipose tissue is decreased in alcoholic, primary biliary and cryptogenic cirrhosis[59,196] and lipolysis is relatively unrestrained in stable well-nourished cirrhotic subjects. This is reflected in raised plasma non-esterified fatty acids (NEFA) and glycerol.[44,105] Increased supply of NEFA to muscle (which comprises 35–40% of body weight) results in decreased muscle glucose metabolism by the glucose–fatty acid cycle. This is reflected in the data from indirect calorimetry, a respiratory quotient of 0.67 being observed,[156] and from ^{14}C-labelled fatty-acid infusions.[105,125] In the fasting state, when peripheral tissue glucose utilization and hepatic glucose output are balanced, decreased glucose utilization is associated with decreased hepatic glucose output as demonstrated by many groups.[124,131,137] After glucose ingestion, suppression of this low hepatic glucose output has much less effect than usual in modifying the rise in plasma glucose concentration. The switch to metabolism of glucose by peripheral tissues is not instantaneous and could account for the delay in fall of plasma glucose concentrations.

We have recently confirmed the possible importance of fatty acids in modifying peripheral glucose metabolism in cirrhosis. Patients had a twofold increase in basal NEFA levels, hyperinsulinaemia, glucose intolerance and impaired glucose clearance in response to insulin. When lipolysis was suppressed with acipimox, a nicotinic acid analogue, glucose intolerance and glucose clearance both improved although neither was normalized.

By measuring the amount of glucose required to keep plasma glucose constant during an insulin infusion (the hyperinsulinaemic, euglycaemic clamp technique), overall sensitivity to the stimulation of glucose metabolism by insulin may be determined. When either physiological (~50 mU/l) or supraphysiological (~1000 mU/l) insulin concentrations were employed, cirrhotic subjects required only about one-half the glucose required by controls.[20,70,196] The clamp technique is expected to reflect muscle tissue insulin sensitivity primarily, and this has been confirmed by studies on both forearm[17,61,91] and leg.[105] The mechanism of the lack of glucose uptake in response to insulin has been studied extensively. It is now clear that modest changes in insulin receptor numbers are unlikely to underlie such insulin insensitivity and that studies attempting to ascribe physiological relevance to measurement of blood cell insulin binding should be disregarded.[128,197] The transmission of the insulin signal into muscle has been shown to be grossly defective in non-insulin-dependent diabetes by measurement of the

activity of glycogen synthase before and during insulin infusion.[15,73] This approach is attractive because glycogen synthase is the rate-limiting enzyme for glucose storage as glycogen, and it has been applied in a study of seven subjects with alcoholic cirrhosis.[89] Although glycogen deposition was marginally lower, this study demonstrated a similar percentage response of expressed enzyme activity to insulin (cirrhotic, 13.9 ± 0.9 to 26.5 ± 1.1; control, 15.2 ± 1.1 to 30.9 ± 1.6). Hence, there is a difference in the insulin insensitivity of muscle in non-insulin-dependent diabetes and cirrhosis, there being no evident failure of insulin signalling in muscle of cirrhotic subjects. This implies perhaps that substrate competition is more important in inhibiting glucose uptake by muscle in cirrhosis.

Hepatic factors are also likely to be involved in the glucose intolerance. A decrease in parenchymal mass was the first postulated mechanism, but this is unlikely to be relevant in the majority of cirrhotic subjects.[127] Distortion of hepatic architecture is present in all subjects. It is now clear that cellular function differs in different parts of the liver acinus, periportal hepatocytes having higher capacity for gluconeogenesis, glycogen synthesis from lactate and glucose release from glycogen, and perivenous hepatocytes having higher capacity for glycolysis, glycogen synthesis from glucose and ketogenesis.[2,79] Disruption of functional zonation of hepatocytes and thickening of cell plates with increased diffusion distance for glucose and hormones may well contribute to glucose intolerance, but definitive information upon this is awaited. The effect of porto-systemic shunting upon glucose metabolism has been extensively studied. In a careful series of studies, Holdsworth and his colleagues[64,65] showed impaired glucose tolerance preoperatively which did not change after the operation, despite a further increase in peripheral insulin levels. Owen and his colleagues[16,126] demonstrated no change in the low hepatic glucose release and high ketone body output in the fasting state in the same patients before and 3–10 days after surgery. A similar lack of change in fasting hepatic glucose production has been documented 2 months[20] and 1 year[43,119] after surgical shunting. Furthermore, glucose metabolism was found to be the same in groups of patients with and without spontaneous portacaval shunts.[182] In contrast to this, data from normal conscious dogs suggest that some gut factor, perhaps not glucose, must be delivered by the portal system to achieve normal glucose tolerance.[95] Radziuk[145] has shown that only 8% of absorbed glucose is extracted by the liver at first pass and thus the reported lack of effect of porto-systemic shunting is not surprising. Finally, decreased activity of glucokinase has been reported in alcoholic cirrhosis, and as phosphorylation is the first step in cellular glucose metabolism this could explain subnormal rates of hepatic glucose uptake postprandially.[188]

Impaired insulin secretion may contribute to glucose intolerance in some liver diseases such as chronic active hepatitis,[6] although in most liver disorders hyperinsulinaemia is usually described. Undoubtedly, the reported insulin levels may be exaggerated by assay problems. Proinsulin levels are elevated twofold in cirrhosis and proinsulin cross-reacts approximately 50% in the insulin radioimmunoassay.[80] Split forms of proinsulin may also introduce a further overestimation.[198] Insulin secretion rates as assessed independently by C-peptide assay are sometimes increased[196] and portal vein insulin levels may be markedly increased,[57] although data in the literature are variable (see Chapter 7). Fractional hepatic extraction of insulin was found by one group to be decreased from 51% to 13% in alcoholic cirrhosis[120] and this will contribute to a decrease in insulin action at the liver as well as an increase in peripheral hyperinsulinaemia. It is difficult to implicate impaired insulin secretion as the cause of the glucose intolerance in most cases.

Anti-insulin hormones could also contribute to glucose intolerance by driving gluconeogenesis and/or glycogenolysis. Glucagon has already been discussed. Circulating concentrations of glucocorticoids are rarely raised, although their catabolism may be impaired.[4] Growth hormone could be more important, as it has been shown to produce peripheral tissue insulin resistance in normal and all other subjects.[155] Suppression of plasma growth hormone levels with somatostatin achieved a doubling of insulin-stimulated glucose disposal rates in four cirrhotic subjects,[175] but there is no relationship between plasma growth hormone levels and the degree of disturbance of carbohydrate metabolism.[153]

Among other postulated factors is potassium depletion, which has been suggested as a cause of impaired insulin secretion and glucose intolerance.[28,133] Improved glucose tolerance on potassium repletion is not found in all patients, and in any case it is unlikely that all patients with liver disease are potassium depleted. Circulating antagonists to insulin action or 'glucose intolerance factors' have been reported but never confirmed.[43,171]

In planning future studies of glucose intolerance in cirrhosis, several factors must be considered. The nutritional state, muscle mass and physical fitness should be matched with the control group. Severity of cirrhosis should be documented, as the prevalence of glucose intolerance has been shown to increase from just over 40% in Child's group A, to 52% in group B and 63% in group C.[14] Similarly, family history of diabetes should be matched since prevalence of glucose intolerance has been reported as 61% and 45% with and without family history.[14] Aetiology of the cirrhosis should be considered as a selection factor for studies since major differences in cellular function have been reported between adipocytes from subjects with alcoholic, primary biliary and cryptogenic cirrhosis.[196] Finally, further efforts are required to establish the relative importance of different tissues in the observed glucose handling.

Other carbohydrates

Less work has been done with other carbohydrates than with glucose, although it has been known for many years that galactose, for example, is cleared less readily in liver disease.[176] It is rational to consider that measurement of specific hexoses such as galactose could be used as tests of liver function since these are metabolized primarily in the liver. There has been only sporadic interest, owing no doubt to a combination of problems in measurement of these hexoses and the need for exogenous administration (see Chapter 17). Nakamura *et al.*[110] have reported the use of $[1\text{-}^{14}C]$D-galactose in the assessment of degree of intrahepatic shunting, while Tygstrup and Lundquist[200] have used galactose measurements in their investigations of the effect of ethanol on hepatic metabolism. Tengstrom[199] has published a thoughtful account of the use of the intravenous galactose tolerance test compared with other liver function tests, and it has no clear advantage over the more common tests. Royle *et al.*[158] have suggested the use of an intravenous galactose test as a measure of hepatic glucose output, but the clinical application of this has not yet been established.

More attention has been paid to fructose than to galactose because of its potentially injurious effects. Approximately 70% of fructose is converted rapidly to lactate in the liver. Normally this lactate would be metabolized rapidly but this does not occur with severe parenchymal damage. The amounts of fructose ingested normally as sucrose may contribute to the hyperlactataemia that we have noted in cirrhosis[192] but are probably not harmful. Problems arise when fructose is given intravenously as part of an intravenous feeding regimen. In this situation we have reported fatal lactic acidosis in patients with acute hepatic failure given fructose,[208] a problem which has been well reviewed by Cohen and Woods.[24] Sorbitol is also potentially hazardous, as it follows the same metabolic route as fructose. One interesting point is that fructose causes hepatic adenine nucleotide depletion.[98] This could well compromise hepatic regeneration after and during damage in that ATP and total adenine nucleotide levels are already low in the regenerating liver, at least in the experimental situation.[76]

There has also been some interest in the metabolism of xylose and xylulose in patients with liver disease, less from a pathophysiological viewpoint than in their use as liver function tests. The conversion of D-xylose to threitol, which normally occurs in liver and kidney, is diminished in patients with cirrhosis[132] but not to an extent sufficient to cause abnormal results in the oral D-xylose tolerance test. Similarly, there is diminished metabolism of xylulose after intravenous loading and fasting levels are raised in cirrhotic subjects.[121]

It is not surprising that metabolism of many non-glucose hexoses and pentoses is disturbed in hepatic disease. Specific information is still required on the exact nature of the lesions and the effect of different hepatic diseases on these processes. The metabolism of ethanol itself in liver disease is dealt with elsewhere in this volume (see Chapter 34).

Biopsy studies

Most of the work described above has been performed indirectly through studies in blood and urine. There is a paucity of direct information on the metabolism of liver in human liver disease owing to obvious technical and ethical problems. As stated above, more information is available using animal models but the absolute relevance of this remains to be proven. Some biopsy studies have been published. It should be remembered that if the disease process is not uniformly distributed through the liver there could be gross errors due to sampling problems. Thus a biopsy may contain a disproportionate amount of fat or fibrous tissue, as pointed out by Schmidt and Schmidt.[169] Kupffer cells may also show markedly different changes from biliary tract or parenchymal cells, as elegantly shown by Wootton, Neale and Moss.[209] Thus after experimental bile duct ligation 5'-nucleotidase activity increased in parenchymal cells but fell in Kupffer cells.

Schersten[165] has summarized many of the differences in metabolic activity between liver from patients with hepatitis and those with cholestasis. Among the earliest studies was that of Schmidt et al.[170] who showed decreased activity of glycerol-3-phosphate dehydrogenase, aldolase and glutamate dehydrogenase together with an increase in glucose-6-phosphate dehydrogenase in patients with viral hepatitis. This suggests increased pentose phosphate shunt activity. At the same time there may be decreased transport of NADH equivalents into the mitochondria because of the decreased glycerol-3-phosphate dehydrogenase activity. This would tend to increase intrahepatic lactate levels and may explain the accumulation of lactate in blood in such patients. Liver mitochondria from hepatitis patients may also be abnormal. Both a low oxygen uptake and uncoupled oxidative phosphorylation have been found.[167] Gross disturbances of endoplasmic reticulum function have also been described in hepatitis[165] but these have less relevance to carbohydrate metabolism.

In biopsies from patients with cholestatic jaundice there is similar evidence of decreased oxygen uptake by isolated mitochondria.[166,167] This may be due to a direct effect of bile acids and/or bilirubin.[93,136]

The problems of uneven biopsy in patients with hepatic cirrhosis are more severe. Diaz Gil et al.[39] found that cirrhotic livers appear to contain fewer mitochondria, together with decreased mitochondrial respiratory control and a marked fall in the levels of cytochrome-b_5 and cytochrome P450. Others have reported more variable changes in cytochrome-b_5 but a distinct fall in the level of cytochrome-aa_3 with a decreased $aa_3/c + c_1$ ratio.[164] These data are consistent with a change in respiratory control and may explain the earlier finding of Benga and Muresan[11] that cirrhotic livers had reduced ATP-synthesizing ability. By contrast, Owen et al.[124] found normal gluconeogenic enzyme activity in biopsies from cirrhotic livers, although glycogen content was decreased, as originally observed by Nilssen.[117] Sato et al.[164] also studied biopsies from patients with hepatocellular carcinoma where similar but more pronounced changes were found, and from patients with chronic hepatitis where the changes were extremely variable. More recently, low activity of glucose-6-phosphatase has been observed.[188] This could underlie low rates of release of glucose from liver glycogen stores but might merely reflect operation of other controlling factors.

The work reported to date has been somewhat disappointing, mainly owing to technical problems. Studies of substrate levels, as well as of enzyme activities, will be of interest. It is possible that techniques such as nuclear magnetic resonance (NMR) will be of use.

CONCLUSIONS

A great deal of factual information has now been obtained on carbohydrate metabolism in patients with liver disease and abnormalities have been described in fasting glucose and gluconeogenic precursor concentrations. Glucose intolerance is abnormal in the majority of cases, although there are still occasional difficulties in distinguishing liver disease associated with glucose intolerance from liver disease in patients who also have maturity-onset diabetes. Aberrations in circulating concentrations of lactate and other carbohydrate moieties are also found during glucose tolerance tests and in the fed state. Information on mechanisms as well as direct studies of metabolism in the diseased liver remain sparse. Emphasis in the future should be placed on turnover and catheterization techniques together with biopsy studies, particularly in conditions other than alcoholic cirrhosis.

REFERENCES

1. Adlung, J., Kelch, L., Peters, J. & Grazikowske, H. (1977) Leberglukosebildung und Insulinresistenz bei der Leberzirrhose. Untersuchungen mit ¹⁴C-glukose. *Zeitschrift für Gastroenterologie*, **15**, 553–564.
2. Agius, L., Peak M. & Alberti, K.G.M.M. (1990) Regulation of glycogen synthesis and gluconeogenic precursors by insulin in periportal and perivenous rat hepatocytes. *Biochemical Journal*, **266**, 91–102.
3. Alberti, K.G.M.M. (1972) Gluconeogenesis in liver disease. *Connecticut Medicine*, **36**, 568–671.

4. Alberti, K.G.M.M. (1974) Some metabolic aspects of liver disease. In Truelove, S.C. & Trowell, J. (eds.) *Topics of Gastroenterology*, pp. 341–359. Oxford: Blackwell.
5. Alberti, K.G.M.M., Johnston, D.G. & Sutton, G. (1979) Some aspects of carbohydrate metabolism in liver disease. In Crepaldi, G., Lefebvre, P.J. & Alberti, K.G.M.M. (eds.) *Diabetes, Hyperlipidaemia and Obesity*, pp. 29–39. London: Academic Press.
6. Alberti, K.G.M.M., Record, C.O., Williamson, D.H. & Wright, R. (1972) Metabolic changes in active chronic hepatitis. *Clinical Science*, **42**, 591–605.

7. Althausen, T.L., Gunther, L., Lagen, J.B. & Kerr, W.J. (1930) Modification of dextrose tolerance test as index of metabolic activity of liver. *Archives of Internal Medicine*, **46**, 482–493.

8. Amatuzio, D.S. & Nesbitt, S. (1950) A study of pyruvic acid in the blood and spinal fluid of patients with liver disease with and without hepatic coma. *Journal of Clinical Investigation*, **29**, 1486–1490.

9. Amatuzio, D.S., Schrifter, N., Stutzman, F.L. & Nesbitt, S. (1952) Blood pyruvic acid response to intravenous glucose or insulin in the normal and in patients with liver disease and with diabetes mellitus. *Journal of Clinical Investigation*, **31**, 751–755.

10. Bachmann, W., Haslbeck, M., Bottger, I. *et al.* (1979). Reduced insulin binding to hepatic plasma membranes in D-galactosamine-treated rats. *Diabetologia*, **17**, 101–109.

11. Benga, G. & Muresan, L. (1974) Human liver mitochondria. III. ATPase activity as an index of mitochondrial damage. *Medicine*, **10**, 131–139.

12. Bergman, R.N. (1977) Integrated control of hepatic glucose metabolism. *Federation Proceedings*, **36**, 265–270.

13. Bernard, C. (1876) Critique expérimentale sur la glycémie. Des conditions physiologiques à remplir pour constater la présence du sucre dans le sang. *Comptes Rendus Hebdomadaires des Séances de l'Academie des Science (Paris)*, **82**, 1405–1410.

14. Blancho, C.D.V., Gentile, S. & Marno, R. (1990) Alterations of glucose metabolism in chronic liver disease. *Diabetes Research and Clinical Practice*, **8**, 29–36.

15. Bogardus, C., Lillioja, S., Stone, K. *et al.* (1984) Correlation between muscle glycogen synthase activity and in vivo insulin action in man. *Journal of Clinical Investigation*, **73**, 1185–1190.

16. Bosch, J., Gomis, R., Kravetz, D. *et al.* (1984) Role of spontaneous portal-systemic shunting in hyperinsulinaemia of cirrhosis. *American Journal of Physiology*, **217**, G206–G212.

17. Butler, P., Record, C.O., Taylor, R. *et al.* (1991) Forearm glucose uptake in hepatic cirrhosis (submitted).

18. Campbell, J.A. & Tagnon, H.J. (1946) Intravenous glucose tolerance test in liver disease. *New England Journal of Medicine*, **234**, 216–221.

19. Camu, F. (1975) Hepatic balances of glucose and insulin in response to physiological increments of endogenous insulin during glucose infusions in dogs. *European Journal of Clinical Investigation*, **5**, 101–108.

20. Cavallo-Perin, P., Cassader, M. & Bozzo, C. (1985) Mechanism of insulin resistance in human liver cirrhosis. *Journal of Clinical Investigation*, **75**, 1659–1665.

21. Cherrington, A.D. (1981) Gluconeogenesis: its regulation by insulin and glucagon. In Brownlee, M. (ed.) *Diabetes Mellitus*, Vol. 3, pp. 49–117. New York: Garland STPM Press.

22. Chiasson, J.L., Liljenquist, J.E., Sinclair-Smith, B.C. & Lacy, W.W. (1975) Gluconeogenesis from alanine in normal postabsorptive man. Intrahepatic stimulatory effect of glucagon. *Diabetes*, **24**, 574–584.

23. Chowdhury, S.A. & Taylor, R. (1989) Insulin sensitivity in experimental cirrhosis. *Molecular and Cellular Biochemistry*, **89**, 69–72.

24. Cohen, R.D. & Woods, H.F. (1976) *Clinical and Metabolic Aspects of Lactic Acidosis*. Oxford: Blackwell Scientific.

25. Cohn, C. (1942) Sodium D-lactate tolerance as test of hepatic function. *Archives of Internal Medicine*, **70**, 829–835.

26. Coller, R.A. & Troost, F.L. (1929) Glucose tolerance and hepatic damage. *Annals of Surgery*, **90**, 781–793.

27. Coombes, B., Adams, R.H., Strickland, W. & Madison, L.L. (1961) The physiological significance of the secretion of endogenous insulin into the portal circulation. IV. Hepatic uptake of glucose during glucose infusion in non-diabetic dogs. *Journal of Clinical Investigation*, **40**, 1706–1718.

28. Conn, H.O. (1970) Cirrhosis and diabetes. IV. Effect of potassium chloride administration on glucose and insulin metabolism. *American Journal of Medical Science*, **259**, 394–404.

29. Conn, J.W., Newburgh, L.H., Johnston, M.W. & Sheldon, J.M. (1938) Study of deranged carbohydrate metabolism in chronic infectious hepatitis. *Archives of Internal Medicine*, **62**, 765–782.

30. Connor, H., Woods, H.F., Murray, J.D. & Ledingham, J.G.G. (1978) The kinetics of elimination of a sodium L-lactate load in man: the effect of liver disease. *Clinical Science and Molecular Medicine*, **54**, 33–34.

31. Creutzfeldt, W., Frerichs, H. & Sickinger, K. (1970) Liver diseases and diabetes mellitus. In Popper, H. & Schaffner, F. (eds) *Progress in Liver Diseases*, Vol. 3, pp. 371–407. London: Heinemann.

32. Cross, J.B. & Blackford, L.M. (1930) Fatal hepatogenic hypoglycemia following neoarsphenamine. *Journal of the American Medical Association*, **94**, 1739–1742.

33. Davies, T.F., Prudhoe, K. & Douglas, A.P. (1976) Plasma cyclic adenosine-3′,5′-monophosphate response to glucagon in patients with liver disease. *British Medical Journal*, **1**, 931–933.

34. Davis, M.A., Williams, P.E. & Cherrington, A.D. (1984) The effect of a mixed meal on hepatic lactate and gluconeogic precursor metabolism in the overnight fasted conscious dog. *American Journal of Physiology*, **10**, E362–E369.

35. Dawson, A.M., Rosenthal, W.S., deGroote, J. & Sherlock, S. (1957) Blood pyruvic acid and alphaketoglutaric-acid levels in liver disease and hepatic coma. *Lancet*, **1**, 392–396.

36. Debry, G. & Charles, J. (1965) Etude des perturbations du métabolisme des glucides chez les sujets atteints de cirrhose hepatique. *Diabète et Métabolisme*, **13**, 151–168.

37. DeFronzo, R.A., Simonson, D. & Ferrannini, E. (1982) Regulation of splanchnic and peripheral glucose uptake by insulin and hyperglycaemia in man. *Diabetes*, **32**, 35–45.

38. deMoura, M.C. & Cruz, A.G. (1968) Carbohydrate metabolism studies in cirrhosis of the liver. *American Journal of Digestive Diseases*, **13**, 891–906.

39. Diaz Gil, J., Rossi, I., Escartin, P. *et al.* (1977) Mitochondrial functions and content of microsomal and mitochondrial cytochromes in human cirrhosis. *Clinical Science and Molecular Medicine*, **52**, 599–606.

40. Dietze, G., Wicklmayr, M., Hepp, K.D. *et al.* (1976) On gluconeogenesis of human liver. Accelerated hepatic glucose formation induced by increased precursor supply. *Diabetologia*, **12**, 555–561.

41. Dunn, A., Chenoweth, M. & Bever, K. (1977) Use of ^{3}H and ^{14}C doubly labeled glucose and amino acids in the study of hormonal regulation of gluconeogenesis in rats. *Federation Proceedings*, **36**, 245–252.

42. Dupre, J., Ross, S.A., Watson, D. & Brown, J.C. (1973) Stimulation of insulin secretion by gastric inhibitory polypeptide in man. *Journal of Clinical Endocrinology and Metabolism*, **37**, 826–828.

43. Dzurikova, V., Cernacek, P., Niederland, T.R. & Dzurik, R. (1974) Isolation of an inhibitor responsible for abnormal glucose utilisation in liver disease. *Acta Diabetologica Latina*, **11**, 277–282.

44. Farrer, M., Fulcher, G. & Johnson, A.B. (1992) Operation of the glucose–fatty acid cycle in metabolism in patients with hepatic cirrhosis (submitted).

45. Felig, P. (1973) The glucose-alanine cycle. *Metabolism*, **22**, 179–207.

46. Felig, P. (1976) The liver in glucose homeostasis in normal man and in diabetes. In Vallance-Owen, J. (ed.) *Diabetes, its Physiological and Biochemical Basis*, pp. 93–123. Lancaster: MIT Press.

47. Felig, P. & Sherwin, R. (1976) Carbohydrate homeostasis, liver and diabetes. In Popper, H. & Schaffner, F. (eds) *Progress in Liver Diseases*, Vol. 5, pp. 149–171. New York: Grune & Stratton.

48. Felig, P. & Wahren, J. (1971) Influence of endogenous insulin secretion on splanchnic glucose and amino acid balance in man. *Journal of Clinical Investigation*, **50**, 1702–1911.

49. Felig, P., Wahren, J. & Hendler, R. (1975) Influence of oral glucose ingestion on splanchnic glucose and gluconeogenic substrate metabolism in man. *Diabetes*, **24**, 468–475.

50. Felig, P., Brown, W.V., Levine, R.A. & Klatskin, G. (1970) Glucose homeostasis in viral hepatitis. *New England Journal of Medicine*, **283**, 1436–1440.

51. Felig, P., Pozefsky, T., Marliss, E. & Cahill, G.F. (1970) Alanine: key role in gluconeogenesis. *Science*, **167**, 1003–1004.

52. Feruglio, F.S., Greco, F., Cesano, L. *et al.* (1966) The effects of glucagon on systemic and hepatosplanchnic haemodynamics and on net peripheral and hepatosplanchnic balance of glucose, lactic and pyruvic acids in normal subjects and cirrhotics. *Clinical Science*, **30**, 43–50.

53. Froesch, R. (1976) Disorders of fructose metabolism. *Clinics in Endocrinology and Metabolism*, **5**, 599–611.

54. Garber, A.J., Karl, I.E. & Kipnis, D.M. (1976) Alanine and glutamine synthesis and release from skeletal muscle. *Journal of Biological Chemistry*, **251**, 836–843.

55. Gioannini, I.P. & Scalise, G. (1971) Glucose tolerance in viral hepatitis. *Acta Diabetologica Latina*, **8**, 932–948.

56. Greco, A.V., Fedeli, G., Ghirlanda, G. *et al.* (1974) Behaviour of pancreatic glucagon, insulin and HGV in liver cirrhosis, after arginine and I.V. glucose. *Acta Diabetologica Latina*, **11**, 330–339.

57. Greco, A.V. Crucitti, F., Ghirlanda, G. *et al.* (1979) Insulin and glucagon concentrations in portal and peripheral veins in patients with hepatic cirrhosis. *Diabetologia*, **17**, 23–28.

58. Greco, A.V., Altomonte, L., Ghirlanda, G. *et al.* (1980) Somatostatin infusion in liver cirrhosis: glucagon control of glucose homeostasis. *Diabetologia*, **18**, 187–191.

59. Harewood, M.S., Proietto, J., Dudley, F. & Alford, F.P. (1982) Insulin action and cirrhosis: insulin binding and lipogenesis in isolated adipocytes. *Metabolism*, **31**, 1241–1246.

60. Hassall, C.H. & Reyle, K. (1955) Hypoglycin A and B, two biologically active peptides from *Blighia sapida*. *Biochemical Journal*, **60**, 334.

61. Hed, G., Lindblad, L.E., Nygren, A. & Sundblad, L. (1977) Forearm glucose uptake during glucose tolerance tests in chronic alcoholics. *Seandinavian Journal of Clinical and Laboratory Investigation*, **37**, 229–233.

62. Hed, R. (1958) Clinical studies in chronic alcoholism. II. Carbohydrate metabolism in chronic alcoholism with particular reference to glucose and insulin tolerances. *Acta Medica Scandinavica*, **162**, 195–202.

63. Henley, K.S., Laughrey, E.G. & Clancy, P.E. (1974) Gluconeogenesis in the fatty and cirrhotic liver of the rat. The effect of oleate and ethanol. In Lundquist, F. & Tygstrup, N. (eds) *Regulation of Hepatic Metabolism*, pp. 401–413. Copenhagen: Munksgaard.

64. Holdsworth, C.D. (1969) The gut and oral glucose tolerance. *Gut*, **10**, 422–427.

65. Holdsworth, C.D., Nye, L. & King, E. (1972) The effect of portacaval anastomosis on oral glucose tolerance and on plasma insulin levels. *Gut*, **13**, 58–63.

66. Hue, L. (1987) Gluconeogenesis and its regulation. *Diabetes/Metabolism Reviews*, **3**, 111–126.

67. Hue, L., Felieu, J.-E. & Van Schaftingen, E. (1981) Hormonal regulation of gluconeogenesis. In Hue, L. & Van de Werve, G. (eds) *Short-Term Regulation of Liver Metabolism*, pp. 141–158. Amsterdam: Elsevier/North Holland.

68. Issekutz, B. (1977) Studies on hepatic glucose cycles in normal and methyl prednisolone-treated dogs. *Metabolism*, **26**, 157–170.

69. Iversen, J. & Tygstrup, N. (1982) Carbohydrate metabolism in relation to liver physiology and disease. In Arias, I.M., Frenkel, M. & Wilson, J.P.H. (eds) *The Liver Annual 2*, pp. 1–15. Amsterdam: Excerpta Medica.

70. Iversen, J., Vilstrup, H. & Tygstrup, N. (1984) Kinetics of glucose metabolism in relation to insulin concentrations in patients with alcoholic cirrhosis and in healthy persons. *Gastroenterology*, **87**, 1138–1143.

71. Jackson, R.A., Advani, U., Perry, G. *et al.* (1973) Forearm glucose uptake during the oral glucose tolerance test in normal subjects. *Diabetes*, **22**, 442–458.

72. Jenkins, S.A., Grandison, A., Baxter, J.N. *et al.* (1985) A dimethylnitrosamine-induced model for cirrhosis and portal hypertension in the rat. *Journal of Hepatology*, **1**, 489–499.

73. Johnson, A.B., Argyraki, M., Thow, J.C. *et al.* (1990) Effects of intensive dietary treatment on insulin-stimulated skeletal muscle glycogen synthase activation and insulin secretion in newly presenting type 2 diabetic subjects. *Diabetic Medicine*, **7**, 420–428.

74. Johnston, D.G. & Alberti, K.G.M.M. (1976) Carbohydrate metabolism in liver disease. *Clinics in Endocrinology and Metabolism*, **5**, 675–702.

75. Johnston, D.G., Alberti, K.G.M.M. & Wright, R. (1984) Unpublished observations.

76. Johnston, D.G., Johnson, G.A. & Alberti, K.G.M.M. (1978) Hepatotrophic factors: implications for diabetes mellitus. In *Hepatotrophic Factors*, Ciba Symposium 55, pp. 357–373. Amsterdam: Elsevier.

77. Johnston, D.G., Alberti, K.G.M.M., Binder, C. *et al.* (1982) Hormonal and metabolic changes in hepatic cirrhosis. *Hormone and Metabolic Research*, **14**, 34–39.

78. Johnston, D.G., Alberti, K.G.M.M., Wright, R. & Blain, P.G. (1982) Glycerol clearance in alcoholic liver disease. *Gut*, **23**, 257–264.

79. Jungermann, K. (1987) Metabolic zonation of liver parenchyma: significance for the regulation of glycogen metabolism. *Diabetes/Metabolism Reviews*, **3**, 269–294.

80. Kasperska-Czyzykowa, T., Heding, L.G. & Czyzyk, A. (1983) Serum levels of true insulin, C-peptide and proinsulin in peripheral blood of patients with cirrhosis. *Diabetologia*, **25**, 506–509.

81. Katz, J. & McGarry, J. (1984) The Glucose Paradox. Is glucose a substrate for liver metabolism? *Journal of Clinical Investigation*, **74**, 1901–1909.

82. Katz, L.D., Glickman, M.G., Rapoport, S. *et al.* (1983) Splanchnic and peripheral disposal of oral glucose in man. *Diabetes*, **32**, 675–679.

83. Keating, F.R. & Wilder, J.M. (1941) Spontaneous hypoglycemia: report of cases. *Southern Medical Surgery*, **103**, 125–131.

84. Kelly, M., Walsh, H., Doyle, C. *et al.* (1972) Glucose homeostasis in viral hepatitis. *Digestion*, **6**, 286.

85. Keppler, D., Lesch, R., Reutter, W. & Decker, K. (1968) Experimental hepatitis induced by D-galactosamine. *Experimental and Molecular Pathology*, **9**, 279–290.

86. Klassen, G.A., Aronoff, A. & Karpati, G. (1969) Forearm metabolism in patients with chronic liver disease. *Clinical Science*, **37**, 455–470.

87. Kreisberg, R.A. (1972) Glucose-lactate interrelations in man. *New England Journal of Medicine*, **287**, 132–137.

88. Kronig, B. & Bass, E.U. (1973) Paraneoplastische Hypoglykämie bei Leberzellkarzinom. *Deutsche Medizinische Wochenschrift*, **98**, 322–325.

89. Krusynska, Y., Williams, N. & Perry, M. (1988) The relationship between insulin sensitivity and skeletal muscle enzyme activities in hepatic cirrhosis. *Hepatology*, **8**, 1615–1619.

90. Laurent, J., Debry, G. & Floquet, J. (1971) *Hypoglycaemic Tumours*. Amsterdam: Excerpta Medica.

91. Leatherdale, B.A., Chase, R.A., Rogers, J. *et al.* (1980) Forearm glucose uptake in cirrhosis and its relationship to glucose tolerance. *Clinical Science*, **59**, 191–198.

92. Lee, E., Ross, B.D. & Haines, J.R. (1972) The effect of experimental bile duct obstruction on critical biosynthetic functions of the liver. *British Journal of Surgery*, **59**, 564–568.

93. Lee, M.J. & Whitehouse, M.W. (1965) Inhibition of electron transport and coupled phosphorylation in liver mitochondria by cholanic (bile) acids and their conjugates. *Biochimica et Biophysica Acta*, **100**, 317–328.

94. Levenson, S.M. (1977) Starvation. In Richards, J.R. & Kinney, J.M. (eds) *Nutritional Aspects of Care of the Critically Ill*, pp. 3–94. Edinburgh: Churchill Livingstone.

95. Lickley, H.L.A., Chisholm, D.J., Rabinowitch, A. *et al.* (1975) Effects of portacaval anastomosis on glucose tolerance in the dog: evidence of an interaction between the gut and the liver in oral glucose disposal. *Metabolism*, **24**, 1157–1168.

96. Lindner, W. (1975) Hypoglykämie-Aglykämie bei Virushepatitis. *Münchener Medizinische Wochenschrift*, **117**, 855–860.

97. Lundholm, K. & Schersten, T. (1976) Gluconeogenesis in human liver tissue. An in vitro method for evaluation of gluconeogenesis in man. *Scandinavian Journal of Clinical and Laboratory Investigation*, **36**, 339–346.

98. Maenpaa, P.H., Raivio, K.O. & Kekomaki, M.P. (1968) Liver adenine nucleotides: fructose-induced depletion and its effect on protein synthesis. *Science*, **161**, 1253–1254.

99. Marks, V. & Rose, C.F. (1965) *Hypoglycaemia*, pp. 166–172. Oxford: Blackwell.

100. McFadzean, A.J.S. & Young, T.T. (1956) Hypoglycaemia in primary carcinoma of the liver. *Archives of Internal Medicine*, **98**, 720–731.

101. McGuiness, O.P., Steiner, K.E., Abumrad, N.N. (1987) Insulin action in vivo. In Alberti, K.G.M.M. & Krall, L.P. (eds) *Diabetes Annual*, Vol. 3, pp. 398–432. Amsterdam: Elsevier.

102. McIntosh, R. (1927) Acute phosphorus poisoning. Report of a case with recovery. *American Journal of Diseases of Children*, **34**, 595–602.

103. McIntyre, N., Holdsworth, C.D. & Turner, D.S. (1964) New interpretation of oral glucose tolerance. *Lancet*, **2**, 20–21.

104. Megyesi, C., Samols, E. & Marks, V. (1967) Glucose tolerance and diabetes in chronic liver disease. *Lancet*, **2**, 1051–1056.

105. Merli, M., Eriksson, L.S. & Hagenfeldt, L. (1986) Splanchnic and

leg exchange of free fatty acids in patients with liver cirrhosis. *Journal of Hepatology*, **3**, 348–355.

106. Moore, H., O'Farrell, W.R. & Heandon, M.F. (1934) Spontaneous hypoglycaemia associated with hepatitis. *British Medical Journal*, **1**, 225–226.

107. Mortiaux, A. & Dawson, A.M. (1961) Plasma free fatty acid in liver disease. *Gut*, **2**, 204–209.

108. Mosora, F., Lefebvre, P., Pirnay, F. *et al.* (1976) Quantitative evaluation of the oxidation of exogenous glucose load using naturally labeled C-glucose. *Metabolism*, **25**, 1575–1582.

109. Myers, J.D. (1950) Net splanchnic glucose production in normal man and in various disease states. *Journal of Clinical Investigation*, **29**, 1421–1429.

110. Nakamura, S., Sasaki, K., Takezawa, Y. *et al.* (1974) Physiological measurement of intrahepatic shunted blood flow by method of continuous infusion of D-galactose-1-C^{14}. *Angiology*, **25**, 484–489.

111. Naunyn, B. (1906) Der diabetes Mellitus. In Holder, A. (ed.) *Nothnagels Handbuch*, Vol. 7.2. Vienna.

112. Newgard, C.B., Hirsch, L.J., Foster, D.W. & McGarry, J.D. (1983) Studies on the mechanism by which exogenous glucose is converted into glycogen in the rat. *Journal of Biological Chemistry*, **258**, 8046–8052.

113. Newman, W.P. & Brodows, R.G. (1983) Insulin action during acute starvation: evidence for selective insulin resistance in normal man. *Metabolism*, **32**, 590–596.

114. Newsholme, E.A. (1976) Role of the liver in integration of fat and carbohydrate metabolism and clinical implications in patients with liver disease. In Popper, H. & Schaffner, F. (eds) *Progress in Liver Diseases*, Vol. 5, pp. 125–135. New York: Grune & Stratton.

115. Newsholme, E.A. & Leech, A.R. (1983) Carbohydrate metabolism in the liver. In *Biochemistry for the Medical Sciences*, pp. 442–480. Chichester: Wiley.

116. Nieschlag, E., Kremer, G.J. & Mussgnug, U. (1970) Insulin, Glucosetoleranz und freie Fettsäuren während und nach akuter Hepatitis. *Klinische Wochenschrift*, **48**, 381–383.

117. Nilssen, L.H. (1973) Liver glycogen content in man in the post-absorptive state. *Scandinavian Journal of Clinical and Laboratory Investigation*, **32**, 317–323.

118. Nilssen, L.H., Furst, P. & Hultman, E. (1973) Carbohydrate metabolism of the liver in normal man under varying dietary conditions. *Scandinavian Journal of Clinical and Laboratory Investigation*, **32**, 331–337.

119. Nosadini, R., Avogaro, A., Mollo, F. *et al.* (1984) Carbohydrate and lipid metabolism in cirrhosis. Evidence that hepatic uptake of gluconeogenic precursors and of fatty acids depends upon effective hepatic blood flow. *Journal of Endocrinology and Metabolism*, **58**, 1125–1132.

120. Nygren, A., Adner, N., Sundblad, L. & Wiechel, K.C. (1985) Insulin uptake by the human alcoholic cirrhotic liver. *Metabolism*, **34**, 48–52.

121. Oka, H., Suzuki, S., Suzuki, H. & Oda, T. (1976) Increased urinary excretion of L-xylulose in patients with liver cirrhosis. *Clinica Chimica Acta*, **67**, 131–136.

122. Owen, O.E., Morgan, A.P., Kemp, H.G.. *et al.* (1967) Brain metabolism during fasting. *Journal of Clinical Investigation*, **46**, 1589–1595.

123. Owen, O.E., Felig, P., Morgan, A.P. *et al.* (1969) Liver and kidney metabolism during prolonged fasting. *Journal of Clinical Investigation*, **48**, 574–583.

124. Owen, O.E., Reichle, A., Mozzoli, A. *et al.* (1981) Hepatic and renal substrate flux rates in patients with hepatic cirrhosis. *Journal of Clinical Investigation*, **68**, 240–252.

125. Owen, O.E., Trapp, V.E., Reichard, G.A. *et al.* (1983) Nature and quantity of fuels consumed in patients with alcoholic cirrhosis. *Journal of Clinical Investigation*, **72**, 1821–1832.

126. Owen, O.E., Mozzoli, M.A., Reichle, F.A. *et al.* (1985) Hepatic and renal metabolism before and after portosystemic shunts in patients with cirrhosis. *Journal of Clinical Investigation*, **76**, 1209–1217.

127. Pachmann, D.J. (1940) Oral and intravenous dextrose tolerance tests in cases of acute (catarrhal) hepatitis. *American Journal of Diseases of Children*, **60**, 1277–1288.

128. Pedersen, O. (1983) Insulin receptor assays used in human studies: Merits and limitations. *Diabetes Care*, **6**, 301–309.

129. Petrides, A.S. & De Fronzo, R.A. (1989) Glucose metabolism in cirrhosis: A review with some perspectives for the future. *Diabetes/Metabolism Reviews*, **5**, 691–709.

130. Perez, G., Trimarco, B., Ungaro, B. *et al.* (1978) Glucoregulatory response to insulin-induced hypoglycemia in Laennec's cirrhosis. *Journal of Clinical Endocrinology and Metabolism*, **46**, 778–783.

131. Piniewska, D.M., McCulloch, A.J., Bramble, M.G. *et al.* (1986) Glucose turnover in compensated hepatic cirrhosis. *Hormone Metabolic Research*, **18**, 834–837.

132. Pitkanen, H. (1977) The conversion of D-xylose into D-theitol in patients with portal liver cirrhosis. *Clinica Chimica Acta*, **80**, 49–54.

133. Podolsky, S., Zimmerman, H.J., Burrows, B.A. *et al.* (1973) Potassium depletion in hepatic cirrhosis. *New England Journal of Medicine*, **288**, 644–648.

134. Pogson, C.I., Munoz-Clares, R.A., Elliott, K.R.F. *et al.* (1981) Interactions of amino acids with gluconeogenesis. In Hue, L. & Van de Werve, G. (eds) *Short-term Regulation of Liver Metabolism*, pp. 339–357. Amsterdam: Elsevier/North Holland.

135. Pozefsky, T., Tancredi, R.G., Moxley, R.T. *et al.* (1976) Effects of brief starvation on muscle amino acid metabolism in non-obese man. *Journal of Clinical Investigation*, **57**, 444–449.

136. Pressman, B.C. & Lardy, H.A. (1956) Effect of surface active agents on the latent ATPase of mitochondria. *Biochimica et Biophysica Acta*, **100**, 317–328.

137. Proietto, J., Alford, F.B. & Dudley, F.J. (1980) The mechanism of the carbohydrate intolerance of cirrhosis. *Journal of Clinical Endocrinology and Metabolism*, **51**, 1030–1036.

138. Proietto, J., Dudley, F.J., Aitken, P. *et al.* (1984) Hyperinsulinaemia and insulin resistance of cirrhosis: The importance of insulin hypersecretion. *Clinical Endocrinology*, **21**, 657–665.

139. Radziuk, J. (1982) Carbon transfer in the measurement of glycogen synthesis from precursors during absorption of an ingested glucose load. *Federation Proceedings*, **41**, 88–90.

140. Radziuk, J. (1982) Sources of carbon in hepatic glycogen synthesis during absorption of an oral glucose load in humans. *Federation Proceedings*, **41**, 110–116.

141. Radziuk, J. (1987) Tracer methods and the metabolic disposal of a carbohydrate load in man. *Diabetes/Metabolism Reviews*, **3**, 231–268.

142. Radziuk, J. & Inculet, R. (1983) The effects of ingested and intravenous glucose on forearm uptake of glucose and glucogenic substrate in normal man. *Diabetes*, **32**, 977–981.

143. Radziuk, J. & Vranic, M. (1977) Estimating rapid changes in the rates of glucose production from glycogenolysis and recycling through lactate. *Federation Proceedings*, **36**, 236–238.

144. Radziuk, J., Dupre, J., McDonald, T.J. *et al.* (1977) Decreased sensitivity of glucose turnover in hepatic cirrhosis in dogs. *Clinical Research*, **25**, 397.

145. Radziuk, J., McDonald, T.J., Rubenstein, D. & Dupre, J. (1978) Initial splanchnic extraction of ingested glucose in normal man. *Metabolism*, **27**, 657–669.

146. Randle, P.J., Garland, P.B., Hales, C.N. & Newsholme, E.A. (1963) The glucose and fatty acid cycle. Its role in insulin sensitivity and the metabolic disturbance of diabetes mellitus. *Lancet*, **2**, 785–789.

147. Record, C.O. & Alberti, K.G.M.M. (1973) Glucose tolerance and blood metabolite changes in galactosamine hepatitis and obstructive jaundice in the rat. *European Journal of Clinical Investigation*, **3**, 130–135.

148. Record, C.O., Alberti, K.G.M.M. & Williamson, D.H. (1972) Metabolic studies in experimental liver disease resulting from D(+)-galactosamine administration. *Biochemical Journal*, **130**, 37–44.

149. Record, C.O., Alberti, K.G.M.M., Williamson, D.H. & Wright, R. (1973) Glucose tolerance and metabolic changes in human viral hepatitis. *Clinical Science and Molecular Medicine*, **45**, 677–690.

150. Record, C.O., Chase, R.A., Alberti, K.G.M.M. & Williams, R. (1975) Disturbances in glucose metabolism in patients with liver damage due to paracetamol overdose. *Clinical Science and Molecular Medicine*, **49**, 473–479.

151. Record, C.O., Iles, R.A., Cohen, R.D. & Williams, R. (1975) Acid–base and metabolic disturbances in fulminant hepatic failure. *Gut*, **16**, 144–149.

152. Record, C.O., Buxton, B., Chase, R.A. *et al.* (1976) Plasma and

brain amino acids in fulminant hepatic encephalopathy. *European Journal of Clinical Investigation*, **6**, 387–394.

153. Riggio, O., Merli, M., Cangiano, C. *et al.* (1982) Glucose intolerance in liver cirrhosis. *Metabolism*, **31**, 627–634.

154. Riggio, O., Merli, M., Cantafora, A. *et al.* (1984) Total and individual free fatty acid concentrations in liver cirrhosis. *Metabolism*, **33**, 646–651.

155. Rizza, R.A., Mandarino, L.J. & Gerich, J.E. (1982) Effects of growth hormone on insulin action in man. Mechanisms of insulin resistance, impaired suppression of glucose production and impaired stimulation of glucose utilisation. *Diabetes*, **31**, 663–669.

156. Rornijn, J.A., Jansen, P.L.M., Chamuleau, R.A.F.M. *et al.* (1989) Glucose/fatty acid metabolism in cirrhosis during short-term starvation. *Hepatology*, **10**, 709.

157. Rosen, H.M., Yoshimura, N., Hodgman, J.M. & Fischer, J.E. (1977) Plasma amino acid patterns in hepatic encephalopathy of differing etiology. *Gastroenterology*, **72**, 483–487.

158. Royle, G., Kettlewell, M.G.W., Ilic, V. & Williamson, D.H. (1978) The metabolic response to galactose as a measure of hepatic glucose release in man. *Clinical Science and Molecular Medicine*, **54**, 107–109.

159. Rubin, E. & Lieber, C.S. (1968) Hepatic microsomal enzymes in man and rat. Induction and inhibition by ethanol. *Science*, **162**, 690–691.

160. Sacca, L., Cicala, M., Trimarco, B. *et al.* (1982) Differential effects of insulin on splanchnic and peripheral glucose disposal after an IV glucose load in man. *Journal of Clinical Investigation*, **70**, 117–126.

161. Samols, E. & Holdsworth, D. (1968) Disturbances in carbohydrate metabolism: liver disease. In Dickens, F., Randle, P.J. & Whelan, W.J. (eds) *Carbohydrate Metabolism and its Disorders*, Vol. 2, pp. 289–336. London: Academic Press.

162. Samson, R.I., Trey, C., Timme, A.H. & Saunders, S.J. (1967) Fulminating hepatitis with recurrent hypoglycemia and haemorrhage. *Gastroenterology*, **53**, 291–300.

163. Sasaki, S., Masaki, N., Yashiro, H. & Takebe, K. (1983) Defect in insulin binding to receptor on liver plasma membrane in liver injury rat. *Hormone and Metabolic Research*, **15**, 19–23.

164. Sato, N., Kamada, T., Abe, H. *et al.* (1977) Simultaneous measurement of mitochondrial and microsomal cytochrome levels in human liver biopsy. *Clinica Chimica Acta*, **80**, 243–251.

165. Schersten, T. (1972) Metabolic differences between hepatitis and cholestasis in human liver. In Popper, H. & Schaffner, F. (eds) *Progress in Liver Diseases*, Vol. 4, pp. 133–150. New York: Grune & Stratton.

166. Schersten, T., Bjorkerud, S., Jakoi, L. & Bjorntorp, P. (1966) Oxidation and phosphorylation reactions in isolated liver mitochondria in normal and icteric conditions. *Scandinavian Journal of Gastroenterology*, **1**, 284–291.

167. Schersten, T., Bjorntorp, P., Bjorkerud, S. *et al.* (1970) Liver cell function in infectious hepatitis in man. *Acta Hepato-Splenologica*, **17**, 375–392.

168. Schimassek, H., Walli, A.K., Langhans, W. & Mayer, P. (1974) Glycolysis and gluconeogenesis in the rat liver. In Lundquist, F. & Tygstrup, N. (eds) *Regulation of Hepatic Metabolism*, pp. 92–104. Copenhagen: Munksgaard.

169. Schmidt, E. & Schmidt, F.W. (1962–1963) Die Auswirkungen verschiedener Extraktions-Arten auf Enzym-Aktivitäts-Bestimmungen in Lebergewebe. *Enzymologia Biologica et Clinica*, **2**, 223–232.

170. Schmidt, E., Schmidt, F.W. & Wildhirt, E. (1958) Aktivitäts-Bestimmungen von Enzymen des energieliefernden Stoffwechsels in der menchlichen Leber bei der akuten Hepatitis und ihren Ausheilungszustanden. *Klinische Wochenschrift*, **36**, 227–233.

171. Schwartz, K. & Mertz, W. (1957) A glucose tolerance factor and its differentiation from factor 3. *Archives of Biochemistry and Biophysics*, **72**, 515–518.

172. Selam, J.-L., Noy, G. & Alberti, K.G.M.M. (1984) Unpublished observations.

173. Seligson, D., McCormick, G.J. & Sborov, V. (1952) Blood ketoglutarate and pyruvate in liver disease. *Journal of Clinical Investigation*, **31**, 661 (abstract).

174. Sestoft, L. & Rehfeld, J.F. (1970) Insulin and glucose metabolism

in liver cirrhosis and in liver failure. *Scandinavian Journal of Gastroenterology (Supplement)*, **7**, 133–136.

175. Shankar, T.P., Solomon, S.S. & Duckworth, W.C. (1988) Growth hormone and carbohydrate intolerance in cirrhosis. *Hormone and Metabolism Research*, **20**, 579–583.

176. Shay, H., Schloss, E.M. & Bell, M.A. (1931) Metabolism of galactose: considerations underlying use of galactose in tests of function of liver. *Archives of Internal Medicine*, **47**, 391–402.

177. Sherwin, R.S., Hendler, R.G. & Felig, P. (1975) Effect of ketone infusions on amino acid and nitrogen metabolism in man. *Journal of Clinical Investigation*, **55**, 1382–1390.

178. Sherwin, R.S., Joshi, P., Hendler, R. *et al.* (1974) Hyperglucagonaemia in Laennec's cirrhosis, the role of portal-systemic shunting. *New England Journal of Medicine*, **290**, 239–242.

179. Sherwin, R.S., Fisher, M., Hendler, R. & Felig, P. (1976) Hyperglucagonaemia and blood glucose regulation in normal, obese and diabetic subjects. *New England Journal of Medicine*, **294**, 455–461.

180. Sherwin, R.S., Fisher, M., Bessoff, J. *et al.* (1978) Hyperglucagonaemia in cirrhosis: altered secretion and sensitivity to glucagon. *Gastroenterology*, **74**, 1224–1228.

181. Shikima, H. & Ui, M. (1978) Glucose load diverts hepatic gluconeogenic product from glucose to glycogen in vivo. *American Journal of Physiology*, **235**, E354–360.

182. Smith-Laing, G., Sherlock, S. & Faber, O.K. (1979) Effects of spontaneous portal-systemic shunting on insulin metabolism. *Gastroenterology*, **76**, 685–690.

183. Snell, K. (1980) Muscle alanine synthesis and hepatic gluconeogenesis. *Biochemical Society Transactions*, **8**, 205–213.

184. Soffer, L.J., Dantes, D.A., Newburger, R. & Sobotka, J. (1937) Metabolism of sodium D-lactate by patients with acute diffuse parenchymal injury of liver. *Archives of Internal Medicine*, **60**, 822–886.

185. Soler, N.G., Exon, P.D. & Paton, A. (1974) Carbohydrate tolerance and insulin responses in obstructive jaundice. *British Medical Journal*, **4**, 447–451.

186. Soskin, S. & Levine, R. (1946) *Carbohydrate Metabolism*. Chicago: University of Chicago Press.

187. Soskins, S. & Mirsky, I.A. (1935) Influence of progressive toxemic liver damage upon dextrose tolerance curve. *American Journal of Physiology*, **112**, 649–656.

188. Soteniemi, E.A., Keinanen, K. & Lahtela, J.T. (1985) Carbohydrate intolerance associated with reduced hepatic glucose phosphorylating and releasing enzyme activities and peripheral insulin resistance in alcoholics with liver cirrhosis. *Journal of Hepatology*, **1**, 277–290.

189. Stalmans, W. (1976) The role of the liver in the homeostasis of blood glucose. *Current Topics in Cellular Regulations*, **11**, 51–97.

190. Stander, H.J. (1924) A chemical study of a case of chloroform poisoning. *Johns Hopkins Medical Bulletin*, **35**, 46–49.

191. Steele, R., Bjerknes, C., Rathgeb, I. & Altzuler, N. (1968) Glucose uptake and production during the oral glucose tolerance test. *Diabetes*, **17**, 415–421.

192. Stewart, A., Johnston, D.G., Alberti, K.G.M.M. *et al.* (1983) Hormonal and metabolic profiles in alcoholic liver disease. *European Journal of Clinical Investigation*, **13**, 397–403.

193. Strange, R.C., Mjos, O.D., Hendon, T. & Jynge, P. (1977) The effect on plasma cyclic AMP and glucose concentrations in patients with alcoholic cirrhosis. *Acta Medica Scandinavica*, **202**, 87–88.

194. Sugden, M.C., Sharples, C. & Randle, P.J. (1976) Carcass glycogen as a potential source of glucose during short-term starvation. *Biochemical Journal*, **160**, 817–819.

195. Summerskill, W.H.J., Wolfe, S.J. & Davidson, C.S. (1957) The metabolism of ammonia and aketo-acids in liver disease and hepatic coma. *Journal of Clinical Investigation*, **36**, 361–372.

196. Taylor, R., Heine, R.J., Collins, J. *et al.* (1985) Insulin action in hepatic cirrhosis: in vivo and in vitro studies. *Hepatology*, **5**, 64–71.

197. Taylor, R. (1986) Insulin receptors and the clinician. *British Medical Journal*, **292**, 919–922.

198. Temple, R.C., Carrington, C.A., Luzio, S.D. *et al.* (1989) Insulin deficiency in non-insulin dependent diabetes. *Lancet*, **1**, 293–295.

199. Tengstrom, B. (1966) An intravenous galactose tolerance test with an enzymatic determination of galactose. A comparison with other

diagnostic aids in hepatobiliary disease. *Scandinavian Journal of Clinical and Laboratory Investigation*, **18** (*Supplement* 92), 132–142.

200. Tygstrup, N. & Lundquist, F. (1962) The effect of ethanol on galactose elimination in man. *Journal of Laboratory and Clinical Medicine*, **59**, 637–644.
201. Unger, R.H. (1971) Glucagon and the insulin:glucagon ratio in diabetes and other catabolic illnesses. *Diabetes*, **20**, 834–838.
202. Van de Werve, G. & Jeanrenaud, B. (1987) Liver glycogen metabolism: An overview. *Diabetes/Metabolism Reviews*, **3**, 47–48.
203. Van Itallie, T.B. & Bentley, W.B.A. (1955) Glucagon-induced hyperglycemia as an index of liver function. *Journal of Clinical Investigation*, **34**, 1730–1737.
204. Wahren, J., Felig, P., Cerasi, E. & Luft, R. (1972) Splanchnic and peripheral glucose and amino acid metabolism in diabetes mellitus. *Journal of Clinical Investigation*, **51**, 1870–1878.
205. Wahren, J., Sato, Y., Osman, J. *et al*. (1984) Turnover and splanchnic metabolism of free fatty acids and ketones in insulin dependent diabetics at rest and in response to exercise. *Journal of Clinical Investigation*, **73**, 1367–1376.
206. Waldhausl, W.K., Gasic, S., Bratusch-Marrain, P. & Nowotny, P. (1983) The 75-g oral glucose tolerance test: effect on splanchnic metabolism of substrates and pancreatic hormone release in healthy man. *Diabetologia*, **25**, 489–495.
207. Walshe, J.M. (1955) Glutamic acid in hepatic coma. *Lancet*, **1**, 1235–1239
208. Woods, H.F. & Alberti, K.G.M.M. (1972) Dangers of intravenous fructose. *Lancet*, **2**, 1354–1357.
209. Wootton, A.M., Neale, G. & Moss, D.W. (1977) Enzyme activities of cells of different types isolated from livers of normal and cholestatic rats. *Clinical Science and Molecular Medicine*, **52**, 585–590.
210. Wu, C., Bollman, J.L. & Butt, H.R. (1955) Changes in free amino acids in the plasma during hepatic coma. *Journal of Clinical Investigation*, **34**, 845–849.
211. Yeung, R.T.T. & Wang, C.C.L. (1974) A study of carbohydrate metabolism in postnecrotic cirrhosis of liver. *Gut*, **15**, 907–912.
212. Zimmerman, H.J., Thomas, L.J. & Scherr, E.H. (1953) Fasting blood sugar in hepatic disease with reference to infrequency of hypoglycemia. *Archives of Internal Medicine*, **91**, 577–584.

CHAPTER 4

Plasma Lipoproteins and the Liver

David S. Harry & Neil McIntyre

The major lipids of plasma are cholesterol and cholesteryl esters, phospholipids and triglycerides. Cholesterol is present in all mammalian plasma membranes and is a precursor of bile acids and steroid hormones. Apart from the hydroxyl group at C-3 and the double bond between C-5 and C-6, it is a fully saturated hydrocarbon. It is chemically unreactive and virtually insoluble in water, and is thus suited to its structural role in membranes. The cholesterol of membranes and of bile is free sterol, but in plasma and tissues cholesteryl esters are also present; the 3β-OH group of cholesterol is esterified with the carboxyl group of a long-chain fatty acid. Cholesteryl esters are even less soluble in water than cholesterol; their function can be regarded as the storage and transport of cholesterol molecules.

There are several types of phospholipid. They are major constituents of membranes and take part in many important biochemical reactions, including intracellular signalling via breakdown of phosphoinositides. They contain one or more phosphoric acid groups and all except phosphatidic acid have another polar group—a nitrogenous base such as choline, ethanolamine or sphingosine, the amino acid serine, or the polyalcohol inositol. In phosphoglycerides, one or two long-chain fatty acids are attached to the glycerol backbone.

In triglycerides the three hydroxyl groups of glycerol are esterified with a variety of fatty acids. Triglyceride is the major form in which fat is stored (in adipose tissue) or transported in plasma (as chylomicrons and very low-density lipoproteins, see below).

Cell surface membranes

The plasma membrane of mammalian cells is made up of two layers of phospholipid and cholesterol with which various proteins are associated. In each layer the polar groups of the phospholipids and the hydroxyl group of cholesterol face outwards, making contact with the water of either the extracellular space or the intracellular fluid. The interior of the membrane is made up of the hydrocarbon parts of the cholesterol molecules and the fatty acyl chains of phospholipids; both are aligned perpendicularly to the plane of the membrane. The components of the two sides of the bilayer meet, end to end, in the middle of the membrane and form a hydrophobic domain in which lipid-soluble substances can

Table 4.1 Characteristics of the major plasma lipoproteins

Characteristic	Chylomicrons	VLDL	LDL$_1$	LDL$_2$	HDL$_2$	HDL$_3$
Electrophoretic mobility[a]	Origin	Pre-beta	Beta	Beta	Alpha	Alpha
Density[b] (g/ml)	0.95	1.006	1.006–1.019	1.019–1.063	1.063–1.125	1.125–1.210
Diameter (nm)	75	30–80	20–40	20–22	7–10	5–7
Concentration in fasting plasma (mg/dl)	None	20–300	10–20	200–400	40–100[c] 60–150[d]	120–300[c] 200–350[d]
Composition (per cent by weight)						
Protein	1–2	8–12	18–20	21–23	40–45	50–55
Cholesterol (free)	2–3	7–10	9–11	8–10	3–6	3–5
Cholesteryl ester	2–6	10–14	15–18	36–40	14–18	10–12
Phospholipid	5–8	15–20	16–20	21–23	25–30	20–23
Triglyceride	80–90	50–60	30–34	8–10	3–6	3–6

[a] On paper, agarose, or cellulose acetate.
[b] Solvent density.
[c] Males.
[d] Females.

dissolve. The various phospholipids are distributed asymmetrically in the membrane. On the outside, sphingomyelin, and often lecithin, predominate; on the inside, the major phospholipids are phosphatidylethanolamine, phosphatidylserine and phosphatidylinositol.

LIPOPROTEINS

In plasma the water-insoluble lipids are associated with specific proteins. Some relatively polar lipids are bound to albumin (unesterified fatty acids and lysolecithin) or to specific binding proteins (such as retinol). The major plasma lipids are carried in large macromolecular complexes—the lipoproteins. Several classes are recognized; these can be separated on the basis of their hydrated density (by ultracentrifugation), size (by gel filtration), net charge (by electrophoresis) or other surface properties (precipitation techniques), or by their apoprotein composition (by immunoaffinity chromatography). Their physicochemical characteristics and compositions are given in Table 4.1.

The lipoproteins of normal plasma are roughly spherical particles with a hydrophobic core. They are covered by a single layer of amphipathic molecules (phospholipid, cholesterol and one or more specific polypeptides, termed apolipoproteins, or apoproteins for convenience); small amounts of non-polar lipids are also present. Non-covalent, mainly hydrophobic, forces stabilize the lipoprotein structure, but exchange and transfer of their constituent lipids and apolipoproteins occurs during metabolism.

Chylomicrons are very large particles that float on standing; on electrophoresis they remain at the origin. *Very low-density lipoproteins* (VLDL) float at a density of 1.006 g/ml (the density of protein-free plasma) and migrate to a pre-β position on paper electrophoresis.

Low-density lipoproteins (LDL) were originally defined as the lipoproteins having a density range of 1.006–1.063 g/ml. This fraction, however, contains at least two types of particle: intermediate density lipoproteins (IDL or LDL$_1$; density 1.006–1.019 g/ml) and the major component (classical LDL or LDL$_2$; density 1.019–1.063 g/ml). IDL, unlike LDL$_2$, contains apoproteins other than apo-B—principally apo-E and apo-C apoproteins. In chylomicrons and VLDL, the core consists mainly of triglyceride, whilst LDL, the major carrier of plasma cholesterol, has a core consisting primarily of cholesteryl ester.

High-density lipoproteins (HDL) float at a density of 1.063–1.21 g/ml and migrate farthest on electrophoresis to the α position. HDL are heterogeneous: HDL$_1$, HDL$_2$ and HDL$_3$ can be identified by analytical ultracentrifugation; some HDL particles contain apoA-I and apoA-II, some only apoA-I; apoA-I-rich HDL may migrate in the pre-β band on electrophoresis. The minor subclass, HDL$_1$, which is rich in apo-E may also be present in the density range 1.063–1.125 g/ml. HDL have the highest protein-to-lipid ratio and their surface is largely occupied by helical regions of apoproteins interdigitating with lecithin and sphingomyelin molecules.

There are few reports on the nature and appearance of lipoproteins in the extravascular space. Chylomicrons and very large VLDL particles may be excluded from interstitial tissue fluid, but studies on synovial fluid, peripheral and pericardial lymph, ascitic fluid and pleural effusions have shown substantial amounts of the other lipoproteins.[140] Differences in composition and morphology have been noted between the lipoproteins of interstitial tissue fluid and the corresponding class in plasma. This suggests that lipoproteins may be modified in transit between these spaces; this may have important consequences for their metabolic fate.

Table 4.2 Apoproteins of plasma lipoproteins

Apoprotein	Molecular weight	Major component	Minor component	Function
A-I	28 300	HDL	CM	LCAT activator
A-II	17 400[a]	HDL	CM	LCAT inhibitor?
B-100	549 000	LDL, VLDL		High-affinity receptor binding
B-48	263 500	CM	VLDL	
C-I	6 600	VLDL, CM	HDL	LPL inhibitor
C-II	9 100	VLDL, CM	HDL	LPL activator
C-III	8 800	VLDL, CM	HDL	Unknown
D (A-III)	32 500		CM, VLDL, HDL	High-affinity receptor binding
E	34 000			
A-IV	46 000		CM, VLDL, HDL	Unknown

[a] Dimeric form.
CM, chylomicrons; LCAT, lecithin–cholesterol acyltransferase; LPL, lipoprotein lipase.

Apoproteins[83]

The plasma lipoproteins are the polypeptide chains found in the various plasma lipoprotein subfractions. They appear to be structural components of lipoprotein particles, and several have other important functions. In 1966 Gustafson et al.[63] proposed the existence of three major groups of apoproteins: apoA in HDL, apoB in LDL and apoC in VLDL. This is now considered an oversimplification. The ABC nomenclature has survived, however, although there have been additions to it. The main apoprotein groups are described by capital letters, nonidentical polypeptides by roman numerals, and polymorphic forms by arabic numbers. All lipoprotein fractions, with the possible exception of normal LDL, contain more than one type of apoprotein (Table 4.2).

ApoA The major HDL proteins are apoA-I and apoA-II; both have a C-terminal glutamine residue. Plasma apoA-I is a single polypeptide chain of 243 amino acids of known sequence; its gene is on chromosome 11 close to those for apoC-III and apoA-IV. ApoA-I is synthesized by liver and intestine. It has a lipid binding domain and is the chief activator of lecithin-cholesterol acyltransferase (LCAT).

Plasma apoA-II is a protein of 154 amino acids, made up of two identical polypeptide chains linked by a single disulphide bond at position 6 of their sequences. The gene is on chromosome 1. ApoA-II activates hepatic triglyceride lipase.

ApoB-100 and apoB-48 Plasma apoB-100 and apoB-48 are two apoproteins, sharing a number of features, that are found in plasma lipoproteins. ApoB-100, which is produced in the liver, is one of several apoproteins present in VLDL and IDL. In LDL_2 it is the only protein found. These lipoproteins contain only one apoB molecule per particle. The molecular weight of ApoB-48 is 48% that of B-100 and the polypeptide chain is the N-terminal end of the B-100 molecule. It is produced in the intestine and is found in plasma chylomicrons and chylomicron remnants.[74]

There is only one gene for apoB, which is found on chromosome 2. In the liver it codes for apoB-100 (a polypeptide of 4536 amino acids, molecular weight 549 000 daltons); it is the largest monomeric protein yet identified, and the most hydrophobic of the apoproteins and thus difficult to study. In the intestine the same gene codes for apoB-48, which has 2152 amino acid residues. The production of these two different polypeptides from the same gene appears to be due to a novel mechanism. A stop codon (UAA) is introduced into the intestinal mRNA instead of the CAA which normally encodes Gln-2153 in apoB-100; this change is not dictated by the gene sequence at that point but involves a post-transcriptional modification of the mRNA. ApoB-100 binds to the LDL receptor; apoB-48 does not because the section of apoB-100 responsible for binding is not present in apoB-48.

ApoC There are at least three different types of apoC: C-I, C-II and C-III. They are the major apoproteins of VLDL and chylomicrons. The genes for apoC-I and apoC-II are on chromosome 19; the gene for apoC-III on chromosome 11. ApoC-I is a peptide of 57 amino acids which, like apoA-I, is an activator of LCAT. Mature apoC-II is a polypeptide chain of 73 amino acids which activates lipoprotein lipase. ApoC-III contains 79 amino acid residues; a carbohydrate chain is attached to the threonine at position 74. The oligosaccharide chain contains one residue each of galactose and galactosamine and 0–2 residues of sialic acid. ApoC-III occurs in three forms in plasma, each having the same polypeptide chain but a different content of sialic acid; they can be separated on polyacrylamide gel electrophoresis, giving bands which are designated as $apoC-III_0$, $apoC-III_1$ and $apoC-III_2$.

ApoE ApoE is found in plasma chylomicrons, VLDL and HDL. Its gene is on chromosome 19, and encodes for a single polypeptide chain of 299 amino acids which is subsequently glycosylated. There are three common alleles of apoE—E2, E3 and E4—of which E3 is the most common. ApoE4 differs from apoE3 because there is an arginine instead of cysteine at residue 112, while in apoE2 cysteine replaces the arginine-158 of apoE3. The latter substitution affects the ability of apoE2 to bind to the LDL and chylomicron remnant receptors; a number of other apoE variants have been described. There are six common genotypes E2/E2, E3/E3, E4/E4, E2/E3, E2/E4 and E3/E4.

ApoE is synthesized primarily in the liver but also in a number of other tissues including spleen, kidney, adrenals, gonads, brain and macrophages.

Other apoproteins

Lp(a) A lipoprotein fraction, called Lp(a), with a lipid composition like that of LDL_2, is present in human plasma but its concentration is variable. It migrates between the normal β and pre-β bands. Lp(a) results from covalent binding of a carbohydrate-rich apoprotein, apo(a), to apoB-100 via disulphide bridges. There are at least six molecular weight isoforms of apo(a) resulting from different alleles at the same locus. The type of isoform present seems to determine the level of Lp(a) present in plasma. Sequencing of apo(a) has revealed considerable homology with plasminogen.

The function of Lp(a) has not been established. Variation in plasma levels within individuals suggests that it behaves like an acute-phase reactant. The presence of large amounts of Lp(a) appears to increase the risk of coronary artery disease.[30] Its present role in atherogenesis remains uncertain; however, some elements in its structure suggest an affinity for binding to other macromolecules, and it may be involved in the activation/inhibition of the thrombogenic cascade and of platelet adhesion. Removal of apo(a) from Lp(a) particles (with retention of the apoB-100) greatly enhances the affinity of the LDL for LDL receptors.

There are a number of other apoproteins in plasma. ApoD, a minor constituent of HDL and VLDL, has been implicated in the activation of LCAT, although this is now disputed. Several 'trace' apoproteins have been described, including apoA-IV, apoF, α-glycoprotein, two threonine-poor apoproteins and the amyloid protein.

Synthesis and secretion of lipoproteins

Most studies of lipoprotein synthesis and secretion have been done in the rat and other experimental animals, but the mechanisms are probably similar in the human.[159]

Only the intestine and liver appear to synthesize and secrete plasma lipoproteins. Chylomicrons are made in the mucosal cells of the small intestine during dietary fat absorption. VLDL are produced in the liver and intestine. HDL are made in the liver and intestine, and within the plasma. LDL are produced mainly, in man perhaps entirely, within the plasma as a result of the catabolism of VLDL (see below). Newly synthesized gut and liver HDL ('nascent HDL') are disc-like particles consisting of bilayers of free cholesterol and phospholipid and small amounts of apoproteins. Similar particles may be produced from the redundant cholesterol and phospholipid released from the surface of chylomicrons and VLDL during triglyceride hydrolysis. Intestinal HDL is rich in apoA; hepatic HDL is rich in apoE.

Studies on the subcellular aspects of synthesis and secretion have been confined largely to VLDL and chylomicrons. Apoproteins are synthesized on the ribosomes and linked to lipid in the smooth endoplasmic reticulum where the enzymes for lipogenesis are found. Particles which look like VLDL and chylomicrons can be seen in vesicles of the smooth endoplasmic reticulum. They are transferred to the Golgi organelles, where carbohydrate is added by the enzyme glycoprotein glycosyl transferase;[84] they accumulate in secretory vesicles, derived from the Golgi, which migrate to the lateral cell membrane and fuse with the lateral plasmalemma. In the small intestine, particles are discharged into the intercellular space; in the liver, they are discharged into the space of Disse.[129]

The VLDL found in the Golgi organelles of rat liver and intestine have a similar composition to circulating VLDL, but contain less apoC and more phospholipid.[68, 89] When they are incubated with plasma or HDL their composition becomes closer to that of circulating VLDL, which suggests transfer of protein and lipid between VLDL and HDL (see below).

We have some understanding of the factors controlling the production of chylomicrons and VLDL. Chylomicron production depends on the amount of dietary fat presented for absorption. With large fat loads, individual particles also tend to be larger, presumably to reduce the amount of surface material (especially apoproteins) that mucosal cells have to synthesize. The size of intestinal VLDL particles may vary with the type of fatty acid absorbed. VLDL production by the liver is increased when the liver is presented with a large energy load, either as preformed fatty acids or as carbohydrates which are converted to fatty acids and then incorporated into triglycerides.

There is no evidence that chylomicron and VLDL production is driven by the production of apoproteins, and there is little change in the apoB synthesis rate with change in the lipoprotein production rate. However, if apoprotein synthesis is blocked, the synthesis and secretion of lipoproteins may be impaired. This can be brought about experimentally.[54] In the rare inherited disorder abetalipoproteinaemia more messenger for apoB is present than in normal subjects, and apoB is present intracellularly, but there is an impairment of secretion of apoB-containing lipoproteins; neither chylomicrons nor VLDL are released and small intestinal enterocytes become engorged with fat droplets.

A lipoprotein with α mobility has been isolated from

the Golgi apparatus of rat liver which reacts with immunological identity to the major apoprotein of HDL.[88] The composition of HDL before secretion is unknown, but 'nascent' HDL, isolated from the perfusate of an isolated rat liver system, are markedly different from circulating HDL.[64] Nascent HDL are small discs, 20 nm in diameter and 4 nm thick, which are made up of a single lipid bilayer. They are composed almost exclusively of polar lipids and protein and are particularly rich in apoE.[42] These discs assume the composition and spherical shape of 'normal' HDL when incubated with plasma containing LCAT.[58]

Little is known about the factors regulating the production of HDL. HDL levels are higher in premenopausal women than in men and are increased by oestrogens and reduced by androgens. They are decreased with high-carbohydrate diets but increased by alcohol.[73] An inverse relationship exists between the amount of VLDL-triglyceride and plasma HDL levels.

Metabolism of plasma lipoproteins

Lipoprotein metabolism is complex; it involves the activity of three enzymes—lipoprotein lipase, hepatic lipase and lecithin–cholesterol acyltransferase (LCAT)—and the transfer of constituent lipids and lipoproteins between the various lipoprotein classes, either by specific transfer proteins or by 'equilibration'.

Lipoprotein lipase (LPL) (EC 3.1.1.34) is synthesized within cells but the active form is present on the luminal surface of capillary endothelial cells, where it is bound to a heparin-like glycosaminoglycan. It is displaced from this site by heparin which remains bound to the enzyme; an association with either heparin or the glycosaminoglycan seems essential for lipolytic activity. LPL also has binding sites for lipid and for apoC-II (which activates LPL), and a separate site is responsible for triglyceride hydrolysis. The natural substrate for LPL is the triglyceride in the core of chylomicrons and VLDL. ApoC-II is required as a cofactor for maximal activity.

The gene for lipoprotein lipase is on chromosome 8. It codes for a protein of 448 amino acids which shows similarities to hepatic triglyceride lipase and to pancreatic lipase.[86] LPL activity is found in many tissues including adipose tissue, skeletal muscle, myocardium, mammary gland, placenta, brain and lung, and it is synthesized by different cell types and tissues including macrophages, Kupffer cells, adipocyte and muscle cells. It is not clear whether this results from products of a single gene. The LPL in different tissues appear to be different proteins and to show different substrate affinities. Rat heart LPL, for example, has a much higher affinity than adipose tissue LPL; it therefore seems likely that the heart would be able to obtain energy from circulating triglyceride (TG) even during fasting, when TG levels are low; at this time the adipose tissue would hydrolyse little circulating TG, although it would hydrolyse its own fat stores thus releasing free fatty acids (FFA) into the bloodstream.

After fat feeding, or during carbohydrate-induced hypertriglyceridaemia, adipose tissue LPL would hydrolyse more circulating TG and store the released fatty acids; the high-affinity LPLs would already be saturated and would play little part in disposing of the excess TG. The LPL in different tissues also respond differently to various hormonal stimuli. The LPL activity of adipose tissue rises with fat or carbohydrate feeding and falls with fasting, probably in response to circulating levels of insulin and other hormones; breast LPL is responsive to prolactin and rises markedly during lactation.

Hepatic triglyceride lipase is an enzyme which is synthesized and secreted by hepatocytes and then bound to the endothelial cells of the liver. The gene is on chromosome 15. Like lipoprotein lipase it is released from its binding site by heparin and then its plasma activity can be measured. In animal studies it appears to play a role in the intraplasmatic metabolism of VLDL and IDL but its precise role in man has not yet been established. Hepatic lipase requires apoA-II as a cofactor. Hepatic lipase hydrolyses triglycerides in vitro but its main physiological action may be hydrolysis of phospholipid on the surface of lipoproteins to promote interconversion of HDL_2 to HDL_3 and possibly VLDL catabolism to LDL.

Lipoprotein lipase and hepatic lipase are barely detectable in normal human plasma, but both are released into the circulation following the intravenous injection of heparin, allowing their measurement as 'post-heparin lipolytic activity'.

Lecithin–cholesterol acyltransferase

Lecithin–cholesterol acyltransferase (EC 2.3.1.43) or 'LCAT' is secreted from the liver into plasma, where it catalyses the transfer of a fatty acid from the 2-position of lecithin to the 3β-OH group of free cholesterol to produce cholesteryl ester and lysolecithin. It plays a major role in the turnover of plasma cholesterol and lecithin. The reaction, which is activated by apoA-I and possibly apoC-I, appears to take place on the surface of HDL particles. LCAT plays an important role in the metabolism of the HDL subclasses.

The amino acid sequence of mature LCAT is known.[94, 151] It has 416 amino acids including several stretches of hydrophobic residues and four potential sites for glycosylation; plasma LCAT is a heavily glycosylated protein, carbohydrate making up about 25% of its mass. The gene is on chromosome 16. The 1550-base LCAT mRNA has been detected in liver, testes and brain[94,142] and in HepG2 cells but not in small intestine, spleen, pancreas, placenta or adrenal tissue. LCAT activity increases linearly in the perfusate from an isolated rat liver system[106,138] and LCAT appears in the medium of cultured rat hepatocytes.[101] In rats, plasma cholesteryl ester fell following hepatectomy[47] and evisceration lowered in vitro plasma cholesterol-esterifying activity.[15] Rats given carbon tetrachloride[147] or ethionine,[85] or subjected to partial hepatectomy,[43] showed reduced plasma LCAT activity.

Triglyceride transport

Rapid changes occur in the surface components of newly synthesized, triglyceride-rich lipoproteins (chylomicrons and VLDL) when they enter the extracellular space. In lymph and plasma, they lose phospholipid and intestinal apoA-IV to HDL particles and receive cholesterol and E and C apoproteins (including apoC-II, the cofactor for lipoprotein lipase). These surface changes promote inter-action with lipoprotein lipase which hydrolyses the core triglyceride into free fatty acids for uptake by peripheral tissues. As triglyceride is removed, the chylomicrons and VLDL shrink and redundant surface components (cholesterol, phospholipid and C apoproteins) are lost to HDL. The remaining particles are termed 'remnants'. During triglyceride hydrolysis, cholesteryl ester, made by LCAT, is transferred from HDL to VLDL remnants via the cholesteryl ester transfer protein (or triglyceride transfer protein)—a hydrophobic glycoprotein with a molecular weight between 63 000 and 69 000 daltons. It is probably reduced by the liver and its gene is on chromosome 16. Its major function appears to be the transfer of cholesteryl ester from HDL to VLDL and IDL, and thus to LDL, but it may also transport triglycer-ide from VLDL to the other lipoprotein fractions.[124]

In the rat and rabbit, chylomicron and VLDL remnants are rapidly cleared by the liver through binding of their apoE by a specific receptor on the hepatocyte surface. In man, VLDL remnants (IDL) are converted to LDL through further hydrolysis of triglycerides and this path-way appears to be the major source of LDL. Each VLDL remnant retains its apoB during the transformation to LDL; the other apoproteins are transferred to other lipoprotein particles, and the lipid composition changes owing to further lipid transfer and the action of hepatic lipase.

Human chylomicron remnants are not converted to LDL; they are removed and rapidly catabolized by the liver. The difference in fate between the two remnant particles may be related to differences in apolipoprotein composition, particularly the amount of apoE relative to the amount of apoC, and the type of apoB present in the remnant. The apolipoprotein-B of chylomicrons (designated apoB-48), unlike the apoB of VLDL (apoB-100), does not bind to the apoB receptor of the liver; this may influence remnant catabolism. Further details of the complex relationship between lipoproteins during the metabolism of chylomicrons and VLDL may be found in a recent review.[9]

Cholesterol transport

The cholesterol nucleus is not degraded in man; choles-terol losses from the body (to balance the input from the diet and by synthesis) occur by shedding of cholesterol in the skin and intestinal epithelia and by faecal excretion (the major pathway) of biliary and dietary cholesterol, bile salts and metabolites of unabsorbed cholesterol. Clearly, net movement of cholesterol in the exchangeable pool, including that in most extrahepatic cells and on the surface of lipoproteins, must be towards the liver if excessive accumulation is to be prevented.

Cholesterol delivery to peripheral tissues

Although most cells can synthesize cholesterol, many obtain cholesterol by uptake and degradation of LDL. Uptake of LDL cholesterol by extrahepatic cells would not help to remove cholesterol from the body as they cannot degrade it (except to steroid hormones in the adrenals, etc.), but it would enable cells to conserve the energy required for *de novo* cholesterol synthesis.

LDL are produced in plasma as a consequence of the intravascular catabolism of VLDL but some LDL may be secreted directly by the liver and intestine. Direct hepatic secretion may occur in homozygous familial hypercholes-terolaemia.[143] Dolphin[37] isolated LDL-like particles from the secretory vesicles of rat hepatocyte and an LDL, presumed to be of intestinal origin, has been isolated from human chyle.[4] Nakaya and colleagues[99] reported that pig liver can remove LDL from the plasma and return it to the circulation together with newly synthesized LDL. Whether this is true of other species is not known.

Many peripheral cells (and hepatocytes) have high-affinity receptors on their surface membrane which bind with either apoB-100 or apoE (the 'B,E' receptors or LDL_r). These receptors are located in clathrin-coated pits which seal off into vesicles and migrate into the cell, carrying LDL and/or apoE-rich lipoprotein as well as ligands attached to other receptors. Following ingestion, the lipoprotein particles are transported to lysosomes where their apoprotein is degraded and their cholesteryl ester is hydrolysed. The resulting increase in free choles-terol enhances acyl CoA-cholesterol acyltransferase (ACAT) activity so that excess cholesterol is stored as newly synthesized cholesteryl ester; cholesterol synthesis is inhibited, and production of LDL_r is switched off to limit further entry of lipoprotein into the cell.[60] The LDL_r is responsible for uptake of LDL (which is rich in apoB-100) and will also bind with lipoprotein particles rich in apoE (such as chylomicron and VLDL remnants, and HDL_1—a minor subclass of HDL which increases with cholesterol feeding—and HDL from many patients with liver disease; see below). ApoE-rich particles appear to be removed by specific apoE receptors which are present in hepatocyte membranes. It therefore seems likely that apoE-rich particles are removed primarily by the liver.

The LDL_r appear to be responsible for the removal of about 80% of LDL from plasma in normal subjects. The rest is removed by non-specific endocytosis and via the 'scavenger' pathway; the latter mechanism involves phagocytic cells of the reticulo-endothelial system which clear LDL that has been chemically modified, e.g. by oxidation, methylation, or by complexating with other molecules. Patients with homozygous type II hypercholesterolaemia have a defective LDL_r mechanism; they have very high levels of plasma LDL which is removed largely through non-receptor mechanisms.

Many years ago it was assumed that LDL was degraded exclusively in the liver. However, the discovery of the LDL-receptor pathway in cultured cells[60] suggested that the liver might be relatively unimportant in LDL degradation; LDL is cleared rapidly by hepatectomized pigs and little catabolism of LDL apoB takes place in perfused rat liver. More recently the in vivo uptake of LDL by various tissues has been estimated using LDL covalently labelled with radioactive sucrose (which does not affect binding by the LDL_r of cultured cells). When this modified LDL is engulfed by the cells, apoprotein degradation products escape; the radioactive sucrose is trapped, allowing the rate and sites of uptake to be estimated. Studies in rats, rabbits and pigs indicate that from one-half to two-thirds of total body LDL degradation occurs in the liver. The role of the receptor-dependent and receptor-independent pathways in clearing LDL from the circulation and the contribution of the liver to this clearance therefore remains unresolved in normal man.[16,17]

THE EFFECTS OF LIVER DISEASE ON PLASMA LIPIDS AND LIPOPROTEINS

In 1862 Austin Flint[44] found a high *blood* cholesterol level in three jaundiced patients (probably with parenchymal liver disease) and attributed it to failure of the diseased liver to remove cholesterol from the blood. Fifty years later Widal *et al.*[163] showed that hypercholesterolaemia in obstructive jaundice was due to elevation of free cholesterol. This was confirmed by Epstein[41] who noted that ester cholesterol could be high, normal or low in obstructive jaundice. In severe parenchymal liver disease a low cholesteryl ester was found and was attributed to liver damage.

Triglyceride and phospholipid changes in liver disease have received less attention. Triglyceride (originally measured as 'neutral fat'), although normal in most patients with liver disease, is occasionally elevated in obstructive jaundice and in infectious hepatitis, but the plasma is not turbid.[90,116] Lipid phosphorus is high in obstructive jaundice and shows a good correlation with cholesterol levels, because of a virtually linear relationship between lecithin and free cholesterol. Normal total plasma phospholipid levels are found in parenchymal liver disease, but lecithin is often increased.[116] Lysolecithin falls in jaundiced patients when liver damage is severe, and is often low in obstructive jaundice when lecithin is markedly elevated.[52]

The lipid composition of whole plasma provides an incomplete picture of the plasma lipid changes occurring with liver disease. Unfortunately, methods for separating the individual lipoprotein fractions were, and still are, costly and time consuming, and for many years progress was slow.

Gofman *et al.*[59] pioneered the ultracentrifugal separation of plasma lipoproteins, and studied the striking hyperlipidaemia sometimes seen with obstructive jaundice. This emphasis on the study of obstructive jaundice has persisted to the present day; by comparison the lipoprotein changes of parenchymal liver disease have been neglected.

Lecithin—cholesterol acyltransferase and triglyceride lipase activity

The fall in plasma cholesteryl ester levels after hepatectomy in animals[47] and the demonstration of a cholesterol-esterifying system in liver homogenates[96] seemed originally to support the idea that the reduced plasma cholesteryl ester level in liver disease was due to decreased production by the damaged liver.

In 1935, however, Sperry[144] showed that plasma esterifies free cholesterol in vitro, and this activity was found to be reduced in many patients with liver disease.[24,158] The significance of these observations became clear after demonstration of the quantitative importance of the plasma enzyme LCAT in the formation of plasma cholesteryl ester,[55,56] and the discovery of familial LCAT deficiency, a rare disorder in which plasma cholesteryl esters are extremely low.[102]

Plasma LCAT is secreted by the liver and several reports indicate that plasma LCAT activity is reduced in human liver disease, and that this reduction correlates well with the amount of plasma cholesterol present as ester.[22,52,139,150] The low activity appears to be due to reduced plasma enzyme and not to inhibitors, absence of activators, or lack of suitable substrate lipoproteins.[24,139] The low LCAT activity may be due to defective synthesis or impaired release of the enzyme from the damaged liver.

Plasma triglycerides are normally cleared by peripheral and hepatic triglyceride lipases. Hypertriglyceridaemia may occur in acute and chronic hepatitis and in cholestasis[98,115] and is associated with abnormal TG-rich LDL particles.[1,98] Muller *et al.*[98] and Bolzano *et al.*[14] demonstrated normal peripheral lipase activity in patients with liver disease in whom hepatic lipase activity was strikingly reduced. They suggested, probably erroneously, that the high triglyceride in LDL is due to decreased hepatic lipase (see below).

The lipoproteins of obstructive jaundice

In primary biliary cirrhosis, cholesterol and phospholipid levels may be far higher than in extrahepatic biliary obstruction. The increase in total β-globulin is disproportionately large when compared with the increase of protein in this fraction.[80] In chronic biliary obstruction there is massive LDL elevation and a marked reduction in HDL.[59] Moreover, the LDL composition in obstructive jaundice is abnormal:[39] a Cohn fraction normally containing HDL contains LDL rich in free cholesterol, with a low cholesterol-to-phospholipid ratio, and a low protein content. This fraction does not react to antisera against normal LDL.[128] Several abnormal LDL are thought to be present and heterogeneity of LDL in obstructive jaundice has been postulated.[49]

Lipoprotein-X (LP-X)

Antibodies have been used to remove 'normal' LDL from the LDL fraction of patients with primary biliary cirrhosis.[148] The lipoprotein remaining is rich in phospholipid and free cholesterol; triglyceride and cholesteryl esters are virtually absent. The small amount of protein present has an amino acid composition like that of VLDL, and an antiserum to it reacts with VLDL but not with normal LDL or HDL.

These findings have been confirmed and extended by other groups.[134,136] The abnormal lipoprotein has been called lipoprotein-X or LP-X, because it was thought to contain a specific apolipoprotein, apo-X, but after delipidation apo-X appears identical with apo-C, the group of peptides associated with VLDL.

On electron microscopy sera containing LP-X show coin-shaped or disc-shaped particles (40–60 nm across and about 10 nm thick) tending to form rouleaux.[65] They appear as partially flattened vesicles surrounded by a continuous lipid bilayer (Figure 4.1). These sera may contain larger structures—stacked layers or lamellar whorls—which may be continuous with the rouleaux.[122] Free cholesterol and lecithin are present in LP-X in an approximately 1 : 1 molar ratio.

LP-X is present in 99% of patients with histological cholestasis, and absent in 97% of those without cholestasis,[95,135] but this observation is of little diagnostic value as 'cholestasis' may be found in parenchymal liver disease such as hepatitis and cirrhosis. Furthermore, LP-X may be undetectable in patients with surgical or other forms of obstruction to the biliary tree.[38,87,126,127,135,161] This limits the value of LP-X even for screening.

The direction of change in LP-X concentration in plasma has also been examined,[87,126] but the distinction between 'extrahepatic' and 'intrahepatic' obstruction can not be made on the basis of plasma LP-X levels, nor on the measurement of trends. We believe that the LP-X test is of little clinical value in the management of jaundice in adults.

In children the test may be useful. In a study of 14 children with extrahepatic biliary obstruction, all had LP-X in their serum and the level rose after 2 weeks of cholestyramine.[119] In comparison, six with neonatal hepatitis had no LP-X before or after cholestyramine, while seven with intrahepatic cholestasis showed a fall in LP-X or no change (one patient).

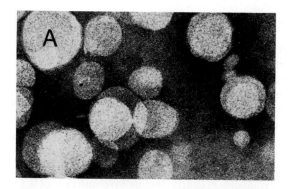
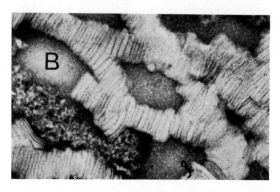
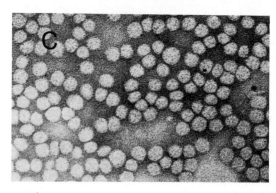

Figure 4.1 A, Large triglyceride-rich LDL (× 182 000). B, Lipoprotein-X (LP-X) (× 182 000). C, Normal-sized LDL (× 182 000). In obstructive jaundice and parenchymal liver disease this is triglyceride rich when plasma LCAT activity is low.

Other lipoprotein changes in obstructive jaundice

LDL In obstructive jaundice there is excess lipid in the LDL fraction but the composition depends on plasma LCAT activity. With high LCAT activity, LDL is virtually normal and on electron microscopy looks like LDL of normal subjects.

With low LCAT activity the picture is complex. LP-X appears, and accounts for most of the striking increase in free cholesterol and phospholipid in LDL. A large (30–70 nm) triglyceride-rich particle is present when the plasma triglyceride is high[1,79,98] (Figure 4.1); it contains B and C apoproteins. It may result from reduced hepatic lipase activity,[98] but a similar particle is present in patients with familial LCAT deficiency who have normal hepatic and peripheral lipase activity.

The excess plasma triglyceride found in obstructive jaundice is not accounted for by increased VLDL. Some is present in large LDL particles; the rest is in normal-sized (20 nm) LDL particles. When LCAT is high, the composition of normal-sized particles is normal, but as LCAT activity falls their triglyceride increases and their cholesteryl ester falls. Triglyceride and cholesteryl ester are non-polar lipids and form the core of the spherical LDL particle; if the particle size is constant then an increase in one must be accompanied by a decrease in the other. Lipoprotein lipase removes triglyceride from VLDL during its conversion to LDL. Cholesteryl ester, produced by LCAT, seems to be incorporated first into VLDL and thus into LDL. LDL with a high triglyceride-to-cholesteryl ester ratio might result if the B apoprotein carried more triglyceride than usual from VLDL (perhaps because lipase activity was reduced). A low plasma LCAT activity would have the same effect on the ratio if, as a result, less cholesteryl ester was transferred to the B apoprotein. The normal-sized LDL of familial LCAT deficiency is also triglyceride-rich; in these patients hepatic and peripheral lipase activity is normal. This suggests that in obstructive jaundice the primary cause of triglyceride-rich, normal-sized LDL is reduced LCAT activity, a hypothesis supported by the correlation which exists between the cholesteryl ester-to-triglyceride ratio of these particles and plasma LCAT activity.

VLDL When plasma LCAT activity is high in obstructive jaundice, the lipoprotein pattern on paper or agarose electrophoresis is normal. A pre-B band is seen and VLDL has a normal composition. When LCAT activity falls, only a broad, densely staining B band is seen. Although a pre-B band is absent VLDL can be isolated by preparative ultracentrifugation. Its electrophoretic mobility is abnormal; it runs in the broad B band,[136] probably because it has an altered apoprotein composition.[122] When LCAT activity is low, VLDL composition is abnormal; it has a high protein, phospholipid and free cholesterol content, and a low cholesteryl ester and triglyceride content.

HDL Gofman *et al.*[59] emphasized the 'wipe out' of HDL in chronic biliary obstruction. Alpha-lipoprotein is often absent on plasma electrophoresis and this appears related to low plasma LCAT activity; when it is high, a prominent α-band is visible. Even when LCAT activity is low, HDL can be isolated by ultracentrifugation; its concentration is low and uptake of electrophoretic stains is further impaired by its low content of cholesteryl ester.

The composition and physicochemical characteristics of HDL particles in obstructive jaundice are poorly documented. This reflects, in part, the heterogeneity of normal plasma HDL.

It has been shown, using agarose column chromatography, that HDL in obstructive jaundice could contain at

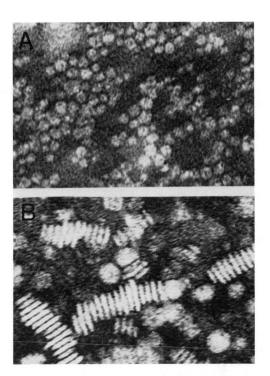

Figure 4.2 A, Normal HDL (× 220 000). B, Abnormal 'nascent' HDL, found in obstructive jaundice and parenchymal liver disease when plasma LCAT activity is low (× 220 000).

least three distinct particles.[1] When LCAT was high or normal, high levels of virtually normal HDL were present; only one peak was seen on chromatography, which was normal on electron microscopy (Figure 4.2). With low LCAT levels there were two major peaks; one looked like normal HDL, but it had a high TG and free cholesterol and a low cholesteryl ester (CE) and phospholipid. The other peak was rich in free cholesterol and phospholipid and had a low CE and protein; this fraction contained 'stacked discs' (4 nm thick and 15–20 nm in diameter; Figure 4.2) resembling those found in familial LCAT deficiency[103] and in the 'nascent' HDL secreted by perfused rat liver when LCAT activity is inhibited.[66] In some patients with low LCAT, small amounts of tiny, spherical particles were found in a third HDL peak which were rich in TG and phospholipid; they are also seen in familial LCAT deficiency and are thought to be of intestinal origin.

Reduced serum apoA-I and apoA-II levels are found in cholestasis, with a disproportionate reduction of apoA-II; because HDL_3 has a lower apoA-I : apoA-II ratio than HDL_2, Fujii *et al.*[48] suggested not only decreased total HDL but a more profound decrease in HDL_3. This preferential reduction in HDL_3 levels has been confirmed using sequential,[5,72] zonal[78] or density gradient ultracentrifugation[162] and gradient gel electrophoresis.[96] Because conversion of HDL_3 to HDL_2 is catalysed by LCAT, whereas the transformation of HDL_2 to HDL_3 requires hepatic lipase, it is proposed that the observed elevation of the HDL_2 : HDL_3 ratio in obstructive jaundice reflects a combination of low hepatic lipase activity with normal or intermediate LCAT activity.[132] Reduced LCAT activity is considered a sensitive indicator of hepatic dysfunction,[34,137] and it is therefore unclear how hepatic lipase activity can be low without a corresponding decrement in LCAT secretion. One explanation may be the recent finding that a heat-labile plasma inhibitor of hepatic lipase is present in patients with primary biliary cirrhosis,[72] but confirmation of this factor and its identification await further studies. In severe advanced liver disease HDL concentrations are very low, because LCAT activity is markedly reduced, and the increased $HDL_2 : HDL_3$ ratio is less apparent.[72]

The most striking HDL apoprotein abnormality in obstructive jaundice is an elevation in apoE.[26,31,45,78,110] Very high apoE levels correlate with a slow moving α-lipoprotein band on electrophoresis which tends to appear in the HDL_1 position by zonal ultracentrifugation.[78] ApoE-rich HDL particles can be isolated by heparin–sepharose chromatography,[149] and immunoaffinity chromatography suggests there may be two subclasses, one containing apoE as its sole constituent and another in which apoA-I is also present.[31] In extrahepatic biliary obstruction a discoidal HDL fraction has been found, rich in free cholesterol and phospholipid and containing almost entirely apoE as its protein; presumably these particles represent nascent HDL of hepatic origin.

The hyperlipidaemia of obstructive jaundice[93]

Hyperlipidaemia can occur in obstructive jaundice even when the individual lipoprotein fractions appear to have a normal composition.[1] This may be due to the regurgitation of biliary lipids into plasma. When bile ducts are occluded, canaliculi become distended and may rupture.[8,40] Epstein[41] therefore argued that entry of bile, rich in free cholesterol, into the bloodstream caused hypercholesterolaemia. However, in rats cholesterol from bile would account for only one-third of the excess cholesterol found in plasma 24 hours after biliary obstruction. Cholesterol synthesis increases in rat liver after bile duct ligation,[46] but plasma free cholesterol still rises markedly even if increased cholesterol synthesis is prevented by cycloheximide.[68] Plasma phospholipid also rises with biliary obstruction but there is no agreement that phospholipid synthesis increases following biliary obstruction.[62,145]

How does cholesterol enter plasma in such large amounts? Being insoluble in water, it presumably needs to be transferred in a lipoprotein or as a complex with phospholipid, as in biliary micelles or in LP-X. There are no data to suggest that more cholesterol is secreted in normal lipoproteins, and early electron-microscopic studies[28,146] of the liver in obstructive jaundice did not show LP-X awaiting secretion. Particles resembling LP-X have subsequently been found in canaliculi, in cytoplasmic vacuoles, in spaces between hepatocytes, and in the space of Disse on electron microscopy of liver from rats following bile duct ligation.[42] It was suggested that phospholipid-rich particles were formed within the canaliculi and transported to the space of Disse in pinocytotic vesicles.

The discovery of familial LCAT deficiency suggested another factor contributing to the hypercholesterolaemia of liver disease, one which accounted for other lipid and lipoprotein changes. Patients with this rare condition show a hyperlipidaemic pattern similar to that found with obstructive jaundice and with almost identical lipoprotein changes.[103] They even have target erythrocytes in the blood, a common finding in obstructive jaundice and one which appears to be secondary to the lipoprotein abnormalities.[29]

Low values for activity were found in early studies on obstructive jaundice,[22,51] suggesting that reduced LCAT activity might be implicated in the production of the plasma lipid and lipoprotein abnormalities. However, it was recognized from the beginning that reduced LCAT activity alone could not account for all the changes.[92] With obstructive jaundice and low LCAT activity, free cholesterol is often far higher than with familial absence of the enzyme. Secondly, plasma cholesteryl ester levels may be low, normal or even elevated with obstructive jaundice; they are invariably low in familiar LCAT deficiency. This variation in plasma cholesteryl ester levels seems to be related to variable LCAT activity, which may be low, normal or markedly elevated in obstructive jaundice,[75] and there is a good correlation between the two variables.

Reduced LCAT activity may contribute to increased plasma lipid levels of obstructive jaundice as the mean total plasma lipid is higher in patients with low LCAT than in obstructed patients with normal or high LCAT activity.[1] The difference is not striking and both groups of patients have a far higher mean plasma lipid than normal subjects (8.8 mmol/l). Clearly, a factor other than LCAT activity is operating in these patients.

The hyperlipidaemia of obstructive jaundice seems to be best explained by regurgitation of lecithin from the obstructed biliary tree into the blood. A biliary factor has been implicated because plasma cholesterol rises when the bile duct of the rat is anastomosed to the inferior vena cava.[18] Initially bile salts were incriminated but subsequently it was found that infusion of phospholipid (brain lecithin) alone gave plasma cholesterol-to-phospholipid ratios almost identical to those found in rats following bile duct ligation.[19]

These studies were supported by observations in bile duct obstructed, cholecystectomized dogs.[123] Free cholesterol and lecithin rose in plasma as their concentrations fell in the stagnant bile: the regurgitation of phospholipid normally excreted in the bile accounted for the phospholipid accumulating in plasma. When purified egg lecithin was infused into the biliary tree, almost all of it appeared in plasma, and as the plasma lecithin increased so did the plasma cholesterol.

But where does the extra cholesterol come from? Hypercholesterolaemia occurs even if phospholipid is infused into hepatectomized animals.[20,21] These studies suggest that the cholesterol accumulating in blood is derived partly from the partitioning of pre-existing tissue cholesterol into the excess phospholipid in the plasma, and that the rest is derived from an increase in cholesterol synthesis—in the liver and possibly in other tissues as well.

It seems likely that some of the cholesterol does come from the liver as a significant increase in hepatic cholesterol synthesis is observed following phospholipid infusion;[121] this does not occur if an equimolar amount of cholesterol is given with lecithin. Presumably lecithin removes cholesterol from the liver and cholesterol synthesis increases as a compensatory mechanism. This observation is of particular interest as it offers a partial explanation for the increased cholesterol synthesis found with biliary ligation.[27]

Studies of cholesterol synthesis in humans with obstructive jaundice have concluded that total cholesterol and bile acid synthesis are low in patients with chronic cholestatic liver disease, as both biliary and faecal steroid outputs are only half of those seen in controls.[76] Hepatic HMG-CoA reductase activity (the rate limiting enzyme of cholesterol biosynthesis) is reduced in biopsies from patients with extrahepatic biliary obstruction,[100] but an increased rate of cholesterol synthesis (measured as incorporation of acetate into digitonin-precipitable steroids) has also been reported in several patients with obstructive jaundice.[105] This area deserves further study.

The regurgitation of phospholipid and secondary accumulation of free cholesterol can obviously account for the appearance in plasma of LP-X in which these two compounds are present in a 1 : 1 molar ratio. Why should phospholipid regurgitation increase the concentration of apparently normal lipoproteins (as in obstructed patients with high LCAT levels)? The reason is not known. Intravenous infusions of phospholipid into human volunteers with normal plasma lipids (and presumably with normal LCAT) have demonstrated an increase in cholesteryl ester and LDL.[156] This suggests that normal lipoproteins might accumulate if the patient has enough plasma LCAT to cope with the extra substrate. These studies also demonstrated a transient accumulation of phospholipid, suggesting that LCAT might have been temporarily overloaded. High rates of regurgitation from the biliary tree might similarly exceed the esterification capacity in obstructed patients with normal or high LCAT levels, and this could explain why LP-X is found in some of these patients.[12] Such results fit with a study in rats[23] when, following acute bile duct ligation, there was a marked rise in plasma free cholesterol and phospholipid (which was presumably in LP-X). An increase in LCAT activity and in plasma cholesteryl ester also occurred which was subsequently found to be present in the LDL fraction.

With severe and prolonged obstruction, liver function becomes impaired; LCAT levels fall and are inversely related to the level of plasma bilirubin. Free cholesterol, lecithin and LP-X should then accumulate in plasma as they do in LCAT deficiency. However, the amount present would not depend only on LCAT activity. If there was a large amount of regurgitation from bile, plasma lecithin and free cholesterol would be able to reach the very high levels found in some patients with chronic obstruction. If the liver cells fail, bile flow and presumably regurgitation would fall, and this might account for the drop in plasma lecithin and cholesterol seen with end-stage biliary obstruction.

The lipoproteins of parenchymal liver disease

The plasma lipid changes in parenchymal liver disease were described earlier in this chapter. Relatively few detailed studies have been done on the corresponding lipoprotein abnormalities. Studies of plasma LDL concentration in cirrhosis have demonstrated either minor changes[117] or significant elevations[118] (100–400 Svedberg units).

In early acute hepatitis, lipoprotein fractions are abnormal;[39] the ratio of cholesteryl ester to free cholesterol is low with an abnormal electrophoretic mobility. The lipoproteins return to normal with recovery from acute liver disease.

More recent studies with agarose gel electrophoresis have shown that the α- and pre-β bands disappear early in acute viral hepatitis and reappear with recovery.[53,113,114,135] Early in the attack the β band is broader, stains more densely, and migrates slightly faster than normal. In patients with viral hepatitis α-lipoprotein is usually absent in the early stages of mild or moderate cases, but gradually reappears with recovery.[152] In severe cases it is absent for longer periods and does not reappear in those who eventually die.[152]

In our own studies on parenchymal liver disease, such changes appear to relate to LCAT activity.[33] When LCAT is normal or high, the lipoprotein electrophoretic pattern is normal; with moderate reduction of LCAT activity there is loss of the pre-β band, and with severe reduction both the pre-β and the α bands disappear.

Patients with parenchymal and obstructive liver disease demonstrate similar changes.[136] Despite the absence of pre-β and α bands, both VLDL and HDL can be obtained with ultracentrifugation. The concentration of VLDL is normal (see Muller *et al.*[98]) and it has a normal composition, lipid : protein ratio and particle size; the abnormal electrophoretic mobility can be attributed to the absence of apoA. HDL in these patients has an increased protein : lipid ratio; this and its abnormal mobility are attributed to an impaired ability of apoA to bind lipid, although apoA is thought to be present in normal amounts (but see below).

Plasma lipid and lipoproteins have been studied serially in 11 cases of acute viral hepatitis.[115] High plasma triglyceride is found not in VLDL, but in LDL which contains less cholesteryl ester than usual. With recovery the cholesteryl ester content of the LDL rises and the triglyceride falls reciprocally. HDL are present in reduced amounts and on analytical ultracentrifugation there are at least two HDL components.

As in obstructive liver disease, hypertriglyceridaemia is found in patients with parenchymal liver disease[98] and this is associated with the appearance of large (30–70 nm) triglyceride-rich particles in the LDL fraction, which are called B-2 lipoprotein. This may explain the increased LDL triglyceride previously reported by other workers.[77,115]

In patients with acute alcoholic liver disease (characterized by massive fatty liver, alcoholic hepatitis and intrahepatic cholestasis), striking abnormalities of plasma lipoproteins are found and are associated with a marked decrease in plasma LCAT activity.[131] The predominant lipoprotein is the triglyceride-rich LDL described by Muller et al.[98] LP-X is also present as a minor component of LDL. Most of the HDL consists of long chains of bilamellar discs. A similar picture is observed with galactosamine-induced hepatic injury in the rat.[130]

In many of the above studies patients demonstrated features of cholestasis and it is difficult to distinguish the effects of parenchymal disease from those of intrahepatic biliary obstruction. We studied plasma lipoproteins in patients with parenchymal liver disease of varying severity and with a wide range of plasma LCAT activity.[33] None had obvious evidence of intra- or extrahepatic cholestasis. Patients with normal or high LCAT activity have lipoproteins of normal structure, electrophoretic mobility and composition. Patients with low LCAT activity show a number of abnormalities. Their HDL are decreased in amount, are of abnormal composition and consist largely of stacked discs on electron microscopy, similar to those found in low-LCAT obstructive jaundice and in familial LCAT deficiency. The similarity of these HDL changes in obstructive and parenchymal liver disease suggests that they are due to LCAT deficiency per se, presumably because the enzyme is not available to act on 'nascent' HDL. The percentage protein content of the HDL is reduced and our findings, together with others,[11,115] do not support the suggestion of Seidel et al.[136] that lipid binding by the apoA of HDL is decreased in liver disease.

There have been a number of studies on HDL apoproteins in liver disease. A low serum apoA-1 has been found in patients with several types of liver disease.[164] In parenchymal liver disease, but not with extrahepatic obstruction, there is a good correlation with LCAT activity. Although there is a poor negative correlation with plasma LP-X, a possible relationship between these two indices has been emphasized. Subsequently a reduction of both apoA-I and apoA-II in patients with liver disease has been reported;[78,164] in acute hepatitis, decompensated cirrhosis and hepatoma, and more strikingly with extrahepatic and intrahepatic obstruction, there is a disproportionate reduction in apoA-II. As HDL$_3$ has a higher proportion of apoA-II than HDL$_2$, it is suggested that HDL$_3$ levels might be more affected in liver disease. This idea is supported by the observation that there is no difference in total HDL between cirrhotics and normal subjects, but a striking reduction in HDL$_3$ cholesterol.[104] Koga et al.[78] also found that the low total HDL in parenchymal liver disease is due solely to low HDL$_3$

levels, with no change in HDL$_2$. The levels of HDL$_3$ cholesterol correlate with those of other plasma proteins secreted by the liver and suggest that HDL$_3$ synthesis by the liver is reduced. In patients with acute alcoholic hepatitis 'light' HDL (HDL$_2$) reappears in plasma before 'heavy' HDL (HDL$_3$).[162] As many of these patients have cholestatic features, the reappearance of HDL$_2$ before HDL$_3$ may be due to the action of LCAT on LP-X like particles, or on 'nascent' HDL-like material. Studies on 'pure' parenchymal patients would resolve these questions.

The HDL fraction is apoE rich in parenchymal liver disease,[149,162] as in cholestatic liver disease, and the apoE-containing particles may be devoid of apoA-II.[91] This apoE-rich HDL appears to influence cellular metabolism in a number of ways (see below).

The LDL fraction, in contrast to patients with obstructive jaundice, shows only one peak on gel filtration, regardless of plasma LCAT activity; when LCAT activity is low, the particles in this peak, which are of the same size and shape as normal LDL, have an abnormal composition.[33] Like the 'normal-sized' LDL particles often found in low-LCAT obstructive jaundice and in familial LCAT deficiency, they are deficient in cholesteryl ester and rich in triglyceride. The appearance in plasma of triglyceride-rich LDL in all these low-LCAT states suggests that it is a direct consequence of LCAT deficiency, perhaps because less cholesteryl ester is produced to take the place of triglyceride in the core of particles during the catabolism of VLDL to LDL. Our findings[33] also show that an increased triglyceride content of LDL in parenchymal liver disease is not necessarily due to the presence of B-2 lipoprotein as suggested by Muller et al.[98]

Patients with 'low-LCAT' parenchymal liver disease have low total plasma lipids, and it is therefore surprising that the plasma concentration of LDL is normal. The markedly reduced levels of its precursor, VLDL, suggests that LDL catabolism must also be reduced, but this hypothesis needs to be tested by LDL turnover studies.

THE CLINICAL IMPLICATIONS OF THE PLASMA LIPOPROTEIN ABNORMALITIES OF LIVER DISEASE

Xanthomatosis

There are few overt clinical consequences of the plasma lipoprotein abnormalities found with liver disease. When plasma lipid levels are very high, as in chronic obstructive jaundice, cutaneous xanthomata may appear.[3] These may be scanty or widespread, with a characteristic distribution in the palmar creases, on the palms and soles, around the eyes, and over the elbows, buttocks and knees. Areas subject to pressure or trauma are also involved. When palmar and plantar xanthomatosis is severe, there may be skin tenderness due to mild sensory neuropathy associated with xanthomatous deposits in the peripheral nerves.[154]

There are few good descriptions of the histology of the xanthomata of biliary obstruction and we are not aware of any electron-microscopic observations. The chemical composition of these deposits has received little attention, but in one report all the cholesterol was present in the form of ester.[153] We have analysed several and found a large proportion of ester, although free cholesterol was also present.

We believe, on the basis of in vitro studies, that cholesterol accumulates in these tissues because of unrestricted 'diffusion' from the free-cholesterol-rich lipoproteins present in the plasma of these patients. Esterification within the cells not only leads to storage of cholesteryl ester, but maintains a concentration gradient for continued transfer of the free cholesterol.

Ischaemic heart disease
Aortic atheroma in hyperlipidaemic patients with primary biliary cirrhosis has been studied.[2] Paradoxically the extent of atheroma seemed inversely related to plasma lipid levels. Four patients with marked cutaneous xanthomatosis had minimal atheroma, but three prexanthomatous patients had arterial lesions which were disproportionately severe in relation to the age and sex of the patients. Despite these observations it is generally accepted that ischaemic heart disease is uncommon in patients with primary biliary cirrhosis; in three series ischaemic heart disease was found in only a small number of patients, but in another series of over 50 patients, 4 had suffered a myocardial infarct and 2 had severe angina.[133] This problem deserves further study.

Treatment of hypercholesterolaemia
Many workers have treated the elevated plasma cholesterol levels in patients with chronic obstruction. There is little to suggest that dietary measures are of value and steroids confer no obvious benefit.[133] Cholestyramine given for pruritus lowers serum cholesterol and there may be some clearing of xanthomas.[32,160]

In patients treated with clofibrate there was a paradoxical increase in the cholesterol or in the size of xanthomas.[133] In bile duct-ligated rats treated with clofibrate the free cholesterol and phospholipid increase is much greater than in animals subjected to bile duct ligation alone, whereas ester cholesterol and triglyceride concentrations are lower.[120] These results are difficult to explain. Hypercholesterolaemia may be a consequence of regurgitation of biliary phospholipid from damaged ductules; in the rat clofibrate may enhance biliary lecithin output but this effect is not consistently found in man.[67] Further studies of this phenomenon are indicated.

Mechanical methods have been used to reduce cholesterol levels in two patients with severe xanthomatous neuropathy.[157] In one, plasmapheresis was used; the other patient was treated with plasma exchange. In both there was a striking fall in plasma cholesterol, symptoms improved, and xanthomas regressed. These methods are time consuming and inconvenient for the patient, but they are effective for severe neuropathic symptoms and for disfiguring xanthomas.

One of our patients with primary biliary cirrhosis has been successfully treated with a combination of plasma exchange and mevinolin—an experimental drug which inhibits cholesterol biosynthesis.[155]

Effects on laboratory tests
Obstructive hypercholesterolaemia affects some laboratory tests. Lipoprotein electrophoresis is used to type hyperlipidaemias. Because a broad, densely staining β band is found in association with high cholesterol and increased triglyceride in obstructive jaundice, a diagnosis of type IIa or type III hyperlipoproteinaemia is often made,[10] and dietary and other advice may be given on this basis. It is inappropriate as the lipoprotein abnormalities of liver disease are quite different from those of conventional hyperlipoproteinaemias.

Sera from patients with liver disease inhibit the haemolytic effect of streptolysin O, and antistreptolysin O titres are falsely high. The effect is due to an increased serum free cholesterol.[6] A true measure of antistreptolysin O is possible with pretreatment of the serum with isoamyl alcohol.[6] Automated white cell counts may be falsely elevated in some patients with extreme hypercholesterolaemia secondary to liver disease because saponin, a compound used to prepare samples, fails to haemolyse red cells completely.[25] This may occur because of formation of a stable complex between saponin and plasma free cholesterol that prevents lysis of red cells.

Effects on cell membranes
The surface components of lipoproteins are altered in severe liver disease. Free cholesterol increases relative to total phospholipid (i.e. the cholesterol-to-phospholipid ratio is high), the proportion of lecithin increases relative to other phospholipids, the ratio of polyunsaturated to saturated and monounsaturated fatty acids in phospholipids is reduced, and there are abnormalities in the apoprotein composition of lipoprotein subfractions. Surface lipids of lipoproteins exchange and equilibrate with those in the surface membranes of cells and it is not surprising that similar lipid abnormalities are found in the red cells and platelets in liver disease. These may affect membrane function by changing membrane fluidity, by altering binding of charged substances to specific phospholipid head groups, by affecting interaction of hydrophobic substances with the interior of the membrane, by changing the state of water at the surface and in the interior of the membrane, and by reducing the concentration of arachidonic acid, which is a precursor of prostaglandins and thromboxanes.

Increase in the cholesterol to phospholipid (C : P) ratio of cell membranes, and reduction in the proportion of polyunsaturated fatty acids in membrane phospholipids, will reduce membrane fluidity; increase in the lecithin-to-sphingomyelin ratio will increase it. Changes in membrane fluidity affect many membrane properties and functions, including permeability. Alterations in the activity of membrane proteins which act as receptors, transport proteins and/or enzymes have been found when membrane fluidity and membrane lipid composition are changed. Membrane fluidity is decreased in erythrocytes from patients with liver disease and this is due mainly to an increase in the C : P ratio of the membrane.[109] In severe liver disease a reduction in the ouabain-insensitive sodium efflux of red cells has been demonstrated and this correlates with the increase in C : P ratio.[107] Reduction in red cell sodium efflux in liver disease is due to inhibition of frusemide-sensitive sodium transport, although impairment of Na^+K^+-ATPase-mediated sodium transport (the sodium pump) can be inhibited in vitro if red cell membranes are further enriched with cholesterol.[69–71] Anion exchange, i.e. pyruvate influx with chloride or hydroxyl efflux, is also reduced and the sensitivity of this process to frusemide is almost identical to that of sodium transport.[69–71] It seems likely that both processes are mediated via the band AE-I intramembrane protein. It appears to be the maximal velocity of anion exchange which is reduced and not the affinity of binding sites for anions.

When normal platelets are enriched with cholesterol they have an increased sensitivity to the aggregating agents ADP and adrenaline. Platelets from patients with liver disease are cholesterol-rich but their aggregability is diminished. Impairment of platelet aggregation was associated with an increase in the lecithin-to-sphingomyelin ratio and with a reduction in the amount of arachidonic acid present in whole platelets and in platelet phospholipids.[108] Arachidonic acid is a precursor of thromboxane A_2, a key component in platelet aggregation; our suggestion that a reduction in arachidonic acid might result in diminished production of the proaggregatory thromboxane A_2 has been confirmed.[81,82]

It seems likely that the membranes of other tissues are affected by the lipoprotein abnormalities found in liver disease. Renal failure occurs in some patients with familial LCAT deficiency. Large amounts of cholesterol and phospholipid accumulate in the renal cortex and there is histological evidence of lipid deposition in glomeruli. Progressive renal failure and similar histological changes have been seen in patients with advanced liver disease and low plasma LCAT activity.[50] The sensitivity to noradrenaline of renal and other blood vessels is increased in liver disease and in jaundiced animals; the sensitivity of isolated kidneys and arteries to noradrenaline is also increased when they are perfused or incubated with the lipoproteins of jaundiced plasma.[13] These observations suggest that lipoprotein abnormalities may underlie some of the renal abnormalities seen in patients with liver disease.

Effects on cellular metabolism

Changes in the apoprotein composition of the lipoproteins may also be expected to have important functional effects. The HDL of patients with severe liver disease are rich in apoE, which competes with the apoB of LDL for binding to the B,E receptor present on the surface of many cells. This receptor controls the cellular intake of LDL particles, the major carriers of plasma cholesterol. The HDL of liver disease does indeed interfere with LDL uptake by cells:[110] this may explain the relatively normal levels of LDL found in patients with severe parenchymal liver disease,[33] despite a profound reduction in the plasma levels of VLDL, normally the precursor particle of LDL. Reduction of cellular uptake of LDL may have important implications for intracellular cholesterol metabolism, even though the abnormal HDL particles, with their cholesterol, are ingested following binding. The clinical significance of these phenomena, if any, is at present a matter for speculation.

The abnormal HDL of liver disease have a number of other biological effects. HDL isolated from patients with cirrhosis inhibits ADP-induced platelet aggregation.[35] This anti-aggregatory effect of cirrhotic HDL appears to be related to its high apoE content, as apoE-enriched HDL_1 from normal plasma also impairs the reactivity of platelets to a variety of agonists, apparently by binding to saturable sites on the cell surface.[36] ApoE-rich HDL from jaundiced patients also inhibits mitogen-induced lymphocyte transformation[112] and this may account, in part, for the increased susceptibility to infection in liver disease.

Red cell shape in liver disease

In many patients with liver disease the red cell membrane contains more cholesterol, or more cholesterol and phospholipid, than normal erythrocytes. This causes expansion of the surface area without a corresponding change in volume; as a result there is a change in shape. In wet preparations these erythrocytes are seen as 'bowl' shaped but drying prior to staining distorts them and in conventional blood films they appear as 'target' cells.[7] Target cells may result from impaired handling of free cholesterol and lecithin, itself a consequence of low LCAT activity, and this explanation would also account for their appearance in familial LCAT deficiency.[57]

In rare cases, bizarrely shaped cells, similar to the acanthocytes seen in abetalipoproteinaemia, may be seen in the peripheral blood of cirrhotic patients. Overt haemolysis is seen in these subjects and the syndrome is called 'spur-cell' anaemia.[141] It has been suggested that this disorder is due to marked elevation of the C : P ratio. This seems unlikely as the ratio may be just as high in familial LCAT deficiency, in which target cells are seen, but not acanthocytes.[29] It was also suggested[29] that acanthocytes are produced in vivo by modification of more regularly spiculated cells called echinocytes; several groups have shown that echinocytes are produced in vitro by incubating normal red cells in sera from patients with spur cell anaemia. Echinocytes are rarely reported in dried stained smears from patients with liver disease but they are evident in wet film preparations from many patients with cirrhosis.[61,111] We have found that HDL from patients whose blood contains echinocytes transforms normal red cells into echinocytes within seconds, and there is a close correlation between the number of echinocytes found in the blood of an individual patient and the ability of that patient's HDL to transform normal red cells.[111] The transformation to echinocytes is not accompanied by transfer of cholesterol or phospholipid to the cell, as suggested by Cooper.[29] The change in shape produced in vitro could be reversed by adding normal HDL or albumin to the cells; the echinocytes seen in liver disease also revert towards normal when these materials are added and the improvement in shape is not accompanied by a reduction in red cell cholesterol.

The biological significance of these red cell shape changes is unknown, except in the overt haemolytic anaemia which is found when acanthocytes are present. It is not clear whether the presence of echinocytes may contribute to the reduced red cell life which has been reported in liver disease. It is possible that factors which distort the red cell membrane may affect the membranes of other cells in some way, and so contribute, together with changes in membrane lipids, to the general metabolic changes seen in severe liver disease.

Because lipoprotein research, using adequate methods, is relatively difficult and time-consuming, few groups have studied the lipoproteins of liver disease in any depth. Even smaller numbers of workers have shown interest in the cellular changes which may result from the lipoprotein abnormalities found. This neglect has been unfortunate. It seems likely that many of the metabolic disturbances seen in patients with liver disease may be secondary to changes in the composition and function of cell membranes. The area clearly deserves further study as it may be possible to reverse many of the lipoprotein abnormalities, at least on a temporary basis; this may help in the management of severe hepatitis and in the preparation of jaundiced patients for surgery.

REFERENCES _____

1. Agorastos, J., Fox, D., Harry, D.S. & McIntyre, N. (1978) Lecithin: cholesterol acyltransferase and the lipoprotein abnormalities of obstructive jaundice. *Clinical Science and Molecular Medicine*, **54**, 369–379.
2. Ahrens, E.H. (1950) The lipid disturbance in biliary obstruction and its relationship to the genesis of arteriosclerosis. *Bulletin of the New York Academy of Medicine*, **26**, 151–162.
3. Ahrens, E.H., Jr & Kunkel, H.G. (1949) The relationship between serum lipids and skin xanthomata in eighteen patients with primary biliary cirrhosis. *Journal of Clinical Investigation*, **28**, 1565–1574.
4. Alaupovic, P., Furman, R.H., Falor, W.H. *et al.* (1968) Isolation and characterization of human chyle chylomicrons and lipoproteins. *Annals of the New York Academy of Sciences*, **149**, 791–807.
5. Aly, A., Carlson, K., Johansson, C. *et al.* (1984) Lipoprotein abnormalities in patients with primary biliary cirrhosis. *European Journal of Clinical Investigation*, **14**, 155–162.
6. Badin, J. & Barillee, A. (1969) Dosage spécifique de l'antistreptolysine O sérique après élimination des lipoprotéines per l'alcool isoamylique. *Annales de Biologie Clinique*, **27**, 395–402.
7. Barrett, A.M. (1938) A special form of erythrocyte possessing increased resistance to hypotonic saline. *Journal of Pathology and Bacteriology*, **46**, 603–618.
8. Barron, E.S.G. & Bumstead, J.H. (1928) The pathogenesis of early obstructive jaundice. *Journal of Experimental Medicine*, **47**, 999–1012.
9. Barter, J.P., Hopkins, G.J. & Calvert, G.D. (1982) Transfers and exchanges of esterified cholesterol between plasma lipo-proteins. *Biochemical Journal*, **208**, 1–7.
10. Beaumont, J.L., Carlson, L.A. & Cooper, G.R. *et al.* (1970) Classification of hyperlipidaemias and hyperlipoproteinaemias. *Bulletin of the World Health Organisation*, **43**, 891–915.
11. Blomhoff, J.P. (1974) High density lipoproteins in cholestasis. *Scandinavian Journal of Gastroenterology*, **9**, 591–596.
12. Blomhoff, J.P., Skrede, S. & Ritland, S. (1974) Lecithin cholesterol acyltransferase and plasma proteins in liver disease. *Clinica Chimica Acta*, **53**, 197–207.
13. Bloom, D., McAlden, T.A. & Rosendorff, C. (1975) Effects of jaundiced plasma on vascular sensitivity to noradrenaline. *Kidney International*, **8**, 149–157.
14. Bolzano, K., Krempler, F. & Sandhofer, R. (1975) Hepatic and extrahepatic triglyceride lipase activity in post-heparin plasma of normals and patients with cirrhosis of the liver. *Hormone and Metabolic Research*, **7**, 238–241.
15. Brot, N., Lossow, W.J. & Chaikoff, I.L. (1962) In vitro esterification of cholesterol by plasma: the effect of evisceration. *Journal of Lipid Research*, **3**, 413–415.

16. Brown, M.S. & Goldstein, J.L. (1983) Lipoprotein receptors in the liver. Control signals for plasma cholesterol traffic. *Journal of Clinical Investigation*, **72**, 743–747.
17. Brown, M.S. & Goldstein, J.L. (1983) Lipoprotein metabolism in the macrophage. Implications of cholesterol deposition in atherosclerosis. *Annual Review of Biochemistry*, **52**, 223–261.
18. Byers, S.O. & Friedman, M. (1962) The relation of biliary retention of cholesterol, distention of the biliary tract, the shunting of bile to the vena cava, and the removal of the gastro-intestinal tract to the hypercholesterolemia consequent on biliary obstruction. *Journal of Experimental Medicine*, **95**, 19–24.
19. Byers, S.O. & Friedman, M. (1957) Cholesterol and phospholipid concentration in hepatic lymph and bile during phosphatide-induced hypercholesterolemia. *Proceedings of the Society for Experimental Biology and Medicine*, **96**, 702–705.
20. Byers, S.O. & Friedman, M. (1969) Probable sources of plasma cholesterol during phosphatide-induced hypercholesterolemia. *Lipids*, **4**, 123–128.
21. Byers, S.O., Friedman, M. & Sugiyama, T. (1962) Mechanism underlying phosphatide-induced hypercholesterolemia. *Journal of Biological Chemistry*, **237**, 3375–3380.
22. Calandra, S., Martin, M.J. & McIntyre, N. (1971) Plasma lecithin-cholesterol transferase activity in liver disease. *European Journal of Clinical Investigation*, **1**, 352–360.
23. Calandra, S., Martin, M.J., O'Shea, M.J. & McIntyre, N. (1972) The effect of experimental biliary obstruction on the structure and lipid content of rat erythrocytes. *Biochimica et Biophysica Acta*, **260**, 424–432.
24. Castro Mendoza, H. & Diaz, C.J. (1949) The cholesterase of the serum (Sperry's enzyme) under normal and pathological conditions. *Bulletin of the Institute of Medical Research (Madrid)*, **2**, 81–93.
25. Charache, S. & Margolis, S. (1969) Effect of plasma from patients with liver disease on resistance of red blood cells to lysis by saponin. *Journal of Laboratory and Clinical Medicine*, **73**, 951–955.
26. Coulhoun, M.P., Tallet, F., Younger, J. *et al.* (1985) Changes in human high density lipoproteins in patients with extrahepatic biliary obstruction. *Clinica Chimica Acta*, **145**, 163–172.
27. Cooper, A.D. & Ockner, R.K. (1974) Studies of hepatic cholesterol synthesis in experimental acute biliary obstruction. *Gastroenterology*, **66**, 586–595.
28. Cooper, A.D., Jones, A.L., Koldinger, R.E. & Ockner, R.K. (1974) Selective biliary obstruction: a model for the study of lipid metabolism in cholestasis. *Gastroenterology*, **66**, 584–585.
29. Cooper, R.A. (1970) Lipids in human red cell membrane; normal composition and variability in disease. *Seminars in Hematology*, **7**, 296–322.

30. Dahlen, G., Berg, K. & Frick, M.H. (1976) Lp(a) lipoprotein/pre B lipoprotein serum lipids and atherosclerotic disease. *Clinical Genetics*, **9**, 558–566.

31. Danielsson, B., Ekman, R., Johansson, B.G. *et al.* (1978) Lipoproteins in plasma from patients with low LCAT activity due to biliary obstruction. *Scandinavian Journal of Clinical and Laboratory Investigation*, **38** (Supplement 150), 214–217.

32. Datta, D.V. & Sherlock, S. (1963) Treatment of pruritus of obstructive jaundice with cholestyramine. *British Medical Journal*, **1**, 216–219.

33. Day, R.C., Harry, D.S., Owen, J.S. & McIntyre, N. (1979) Plasma lecithin: cholesterol acyltransferase and the lipoprotein abnormalities of parenchymal liver disease. *Clinical Science and Molecular Medicine*, **56**, 575–583.

34. De Martiis, M., Barlattini, A., Parenzi, A. & Sebastiani, F. (1983) Pattern of lecithin-cholesterol acyltransferase activity in the course of liver cirrhosis. *Journal of International Medical Research*, **11**, 232–238.

35. Desai, K., Mistry, P., Bagget, C. *et al.* (1989) Inhibition of platelet aggregation by abnormal high density lipoprotein particles in plasma from patients with cirrhosis. *Lancet*, **1**, 693–695.

36. Desai, K., Bruckdorfer, K.R., Hutton, R.A. & Owen, J.S. (1989) Binding of apoE rich high density lipoprotein particles by saturable sites on human blood platelets inhibits agonist-induced platelet aggregation. *Journal of Lipid Research*, **30**, 831–840.

37. Dolphin, P.J. (1982) Serum and hepatic nascent lipoproteins in normal and hypercholesterolemic rats. *Journal of Lipid Research*, **22**, 971–989.

38. Eder, G., Wiess, W., Neumayr, A. *et al.* (1977) Conclusions of LP-X determinations in more than 2500 patients. In Peeters, H. (ed.) *Proteides of Biological Fluids*, Vol. 25, pp. 341–347. Oxford: Pergamon Press.

39. Eder, H.A., Russ, E.M., Rees Pritchett, R.A. *et al.* (1955) Protein-lipid relationship in human plasma; in biliary cirrhosis, obstructive jaundice and acute hepatitis. *Journal of Clinical Investigation*, **34**, 1147–1162.

40. Eppinger, H. (1902) Beiträge zur normalen und pathol Histologie der menschilichen Gallencapillaren mit bes. Berücksichtigung der Pathogenese des Ikterus. *Beiträge zur Pathologischen Anatomie*, **31**, 230–295.

41. Epstein, E.Z. (1932) Cholesterol of the blood plasma in hepatic and biliary disease. *Archives of Internal Medicine*, **50**, 203–222.

42. Felker, T.E., Fainara, M., Hamilton, R.L. & Havel, R.J. (1977) Secretion of the arginine-rich and A-I apolipoproteins by the isolated perfused rat liver. *Journal of Lipid Research*, **18**, 465–473.

43. Fex, G. & Wallinder, L. (1973) Liver and plasma cholesteryl ester metabolism after partial hepatectomy in the rat. *Biochimica et Biophysica Acta*, **316**, 91–97.

44. Flint, A., Jr (1862) Experimental researches into an excretory function of the liver; consisting in the removal of cholesterine from the blood, and its discharging from the body in the form of stercorine. *American Journal of Medical Science*, **44**, 305–365.

45. Floren, C.-H., Gustafson, A. (1985) Apolipoproteins A-I, A-II and E in cholestatic liver disease. *Journal of Laboratory and Clinical Investigation*, **45**, 103–108.

46. Fredrickson, D.S., Loud, A.V., Hinkelman, B.T. *et al.* (1954) The effect of ligation of the common bile duct on cholesterol synthesis in the rat. *Journal of Experimental Medicine*, **99**, 43–53.

47. Friedman, M. & Byers, S.O. (1955) Observations concerning the production and excretion of cholesterol in mammals. XVI The relationship of the liver to the content and control of plasma cholesterol ester. *Journal of Clinical Investigation*, **34**, 1369–1374.

48. Fujii, S., Koga, S., Shono, T. *et al.* (1981) Serum apoprotein A-I and A-II levels in liver disease and cholestasis. *Clinical Chimica Acta*, **115**, 321–329.

49. Furman, R.H. & Conrad, L.L. (1957) Ultracentrifugal characterisation of the lipoprotein spectrum in obstructive jaundice: studies of serum lipid relationships in intra and extrahepatic biliary obstruction. *Journal of Clinical Investigation*, **36**, 713–722.

50. Gjone, E. (1981) Familial lecithin: cholesterol acyltransferase deficiency—a new metabolic disease with renal involvement. *Advances in Nephrology*, **10**, 167–185.

51. Gjone, E. & Blomhoff, J.P. (1970) Plasma lecithin-cholesterol acyltransferase in obstructive jaundice. *Scandinavian Journal of Gastroenterology*, **5**, 305–308.

52. Gjone, E. & Orning, O.M. (1966) Plasma phospholipids in patients with liver disease. *Scandinavian Journal of Clinical and Laboratory Investigation*, **18**, 209–261.

53. Gjone, E., Blomoff, J.P. & Wiencke, I. (1971) Plasma lecithin: cholesterol acyltransferase activity in acute hepatitis. *Scandinavian Journal of Gastroenterology*, **6**, 161–168.

54. Glickman, R.M. & Kirsch, K. (1973) Lymph chylomicron formation during the inhibition of protein synthesis. *Journal of Clinical Investigation*, **52**, 2910–2920.

55. Glomset, J.A. (1962) The mechanism of the plasma cholesterol esterification reaction: plasma fatty acid transferase. *Biochimica et Biophysica Acta*, **65**, 128–135.

56. Glomset, J.A. (1968) The plasma lecithin: cholesterol acyltransferase reaction. *Journal of Lipid Research*, **9**, 155–167.

57. Glomset, J.A., Norum, K.R. & Gjone, E. (1983) Familial lecithin: cholesterol acyltransferase deficiency. In Stanbury, J.B., Wyngaarden, J.B., Fredrickson, D.S. *et al.* (eds) *The Metabolic Basis of Inherited Disease*, 5th edn., Chap. 31, pp. 643–654. New York: McGraw-Hill.

58. Glomset, J.A., Norum, K.R., Nichols, A.V. *et al.* (1975) Plasma lipoproteins in familial lecithin : cholesterol acyltransferase deficiency: effects of dietary manipulation. *Scandinavian Journal of Clinical and Laboratory Investigation*, **35** (Supplement 142), 1–55.

59. Gofman, J.W., Da Lalla, O., Glazier, F. *et al.* (1954) The serum lipoprotein transport system in health, metabolic disorders, atherosclerosis and coronary heart disease. *Plasma*, **2**, 413–484.

60. Goldstein, J.L. & Brown, M.S. (1977) Atherosclerosis: the low density lipoprotein receptor hypothesis. *Metabolism*, **26**, 1256–1275.

61. Grahn, E.P., Dietz, A.A., Stefani, S.S. & Donnelly, W.J. (1968) Burr cells, haemolytic anaemia and cirrhosis. *American Journal of Medicine*, **45**, 78–87.

62. Gregory, P.B. & Beck, R. (1973) Lecithin metabolism during experimental cholestasis in the rat. *Gastroenterology*, **65**, 543 (abstract).

63. Gustafson, A., Alaupovic, P. & Furman, R.H. (1966) Studies of the composition and structure of serum lipoproteins. Separation and characterization of phospholipid-protein residues obtained by partial delipidization of very low density lipoproteins of human serum. *Biochemistry*, **5**, 632–646.

64. Hamilton, R.L. (1972) Synthesis and secretion of plasma lipoproteins. *Advances in Experimental Biology and Medicine*, **26**, 7–24.

65. Hamilton, R.L., Havel, R.J., Kane, J.P. *et al.* (1971) Cholestasis: lamellar structure of the abnormal human serum lipo-protein. *Science*, **172**, 475–478.

66. Hamilton, R.L., Williams, M.C., Fielding, C.J. & Havel, R.J. (1976) Discoidal bilayer structure of nascent high density lipoproteins from perfused rat liver. *Journal of Clinical Investigation*, **58**, 667–680.

67. Hanson, K.C., Deal, J., Schmidt, G. & Brunworth, D. (1974) Effect of clofibrate on hepatic, biliary and serum lipids in the rat. *Gastroenterology*, **64**, 740 (abstract).

68. Harry, D.S., Dini, M. & McIntyre, N. (1973) Effect of cholesterol feeding and biliary obstruction on hepatic cholesterol biosynthesis in the rat. *Biochimica et Biophysica Acta*, **296**, 209–220.

69. Jackson, P. & Morgan, D.B. (1982) The relation between membrane cholesterol and phospholipid and sodium efflux in erythrocytes from healthy subjects and patients with chronic cholestasis. *Clinical Science*, **62**, 101–107.

70. Jackson, P. & Morgan, D.B. (1982) The relation between membrane cholesterol content and anion exchange in the erythrocytes of patients with cholestasis. *Biochimica et Biophysica Acta*, **693**, 99–104.

71. Jackson, P. & Morgan, D.B. (1983) Cholesterol and facilitated transport systems of the erythrocyte membrane. *Clinical Chemistry Abstracts*, p. 32.

72. Jahn, C.E., Schaefer, E.J., Taam, L.A. *et al.* (1985) Lipoprotein abnormalities in primary biliary cirrhosis: association with hepatic lipase inhibition as well as altered cholesterol esterification. *Gastroenterology*, **89**, 1266–1278.

73. Johansson, B.G. & Medhus, A. (1974) Increase in plasma α-lipoproteins in chronic alcoholics after acute abuse. *Acta Medica Scandinavica*, **195**, 273–277.

74. Kane, P.J., Hardman, D.A. & Paulus, H.E. (1980) Heterogeneity of apolipoprotein B: isolation of a new species from human chylomicrons. *Proceedings of the National Academy of Sciences of the USA*, **770**, 2465–2469.

75. Kepkay, D.L., Poon, R. & Simon, J.B. (1973) Lecithin : cholesterol acyltransferase and serum cholesterol esterification in obstructive jaundice. *Journal of Laboratory and Clinical Medicine*, **81**, 172–181.

76. Kesaniemi, A.Y., Salaspuro, M.P., Vuoristo, M. & Miettinen, T.A. (1982) Biliary lipid secretion in chronic cholestasis liver disease. *Gut*, **23**, 931–938.

77. Klor, U., Ditschuneit, H.H., Rakow, D. & Ditschuneit, H. (1972) Further characterisation of dyslipoproteinaemia in hepatic disease. *European Journal of Clinical Investigation*, **2**, 291 (abstract).

78. Koga, S., Shono, T., Inoue, M. & Ibayashi, H. (1983) Quantitative determinations of HDL_2 and HDL_3 in patients with liver disease. *Gastroenterologica Japonica*, **18**, 32–40.

79. Kostner, G.M., Laggner, P., Prexl, H.J. & Holasek, A. (1976) Investigation of the abnormal low-density lipoproteins occurring in patients with obstructive jaundice. *Biochemical Journal*, **157**, 401–407.

80. Kunkel, H.G. & Ahrens, E.H., Jr (1949) The relationship between serum lipids and the electrophoretic pattern with particular reference to patients with primary biliary cirrhosis. *Journal of Clinical Investigation*, **28**, 1575–1579.

81. Laffi, G., La Villa, G., Pinzani, M. *et al.* (1986) Altered renal and platelet arachidonic metabolism in cirrhosis. *Gastroenterology*, **90**, 274–282.

82. Laffi, G., Cominelli, F., Ruggiero, M. *et al.* (1988) Altered platelet function in cirrhosis of the liver: impairment of inositol lipid and arachidonic acid metabolism in response to agonists. *Hepatology*, **8**, 1620–1626.

83. Li, W.-H., Tanimura, M., Luo, C.-C. *et al.* (1988) The apolipoprotein multigene family: biosynthesis, structure, structure-function relationships and evolution. *Journal of Lipid Research*, **29**, 245–271.

84. Lo, C.-H. & Marsh, J.B. (1970) Biosynthesis of plasma lipoproteins. Incorporation of C-glucosamine by cells and sub-cellular fractions of rat liver. *Journal of Biological Chemistry*, **245**, 5001–5006.

85. Lossow, W.J., Shah, S.N., Brot, N. & Chaikoff, I.L. (1983) Effect of ethionine treatment on esterification in vitro of free (4-C) cholesterol by rat plasma. *Biochimica et Biophysica Acta*, **70**, 593–595.

86. Lusis, A.J. (1988) Genetic factors affecting blood lipoproteins: the candidate gene approach. *Journal of Lipid Research*, **29**, 347–429.

87. Magnani, R.H. & Alaupovic, P. (1976) Utilisation of the quantitive assay of lipoprotein-X in the differential diagnosis of extrahepatic and intrahepatic diseases. *Gastroenterology*, **71**, 87–93.

88. Mahley, R.H., Bersot, T.P. & Lequire, V.S. (1970) Identity of very low density lipoprotein apoproteins of plasma and liver Golgi apparatus. *Science*, **168**, 380–382.

89. Mahley, R.W., Bennett, B.D., Morre, D.J. *et al.* (1971) Lipoproteins associated with the Golgi apparatus isolated from epithelial cells of rat small intestine. *Laboratory Investigation*, **25**, 435–444.

90. Man, E.B., Kartin, B.L., Durlacher, S.H. & Peters, J.B. (1945) The lipids of serum and liver in patients with hepatic diseases. *Journal of Clinical Investigation*, **24**, 623–643.

91. Marcell, Y.L., Vezina, C., Emond, D. & Suzue, G. (1980) Heterogeneity of human high density lipoproteins with and without apoE and their roles as substrates for the lecithin-cholesterol acyltransferase reaction. *Proceedings of the National Academy of Sciences*, **77**, 2969–2973.

92. McIntyre, N., Calandra, S. & Pearson, A.J.G. (1974) Lipid and lipoprotein abnormalities in liver disease: the possible role of lecithin : cholesterol acyltransferase deficiency. *Scandinavian Journal of Clinical and Laboratory Investigation*, **33** (Supplement 137), 115–120.

93. McIntyre, N., Harry, D.S. & Pearson, A.J.G. (1975) The hypercholesterolaemia of obstructive jaundice. *Gut*, **16**, 379–391.

94. McLean, J., Wion, K., Drayna, D. *et al.* (1986) Human lecithin : cholesterol acyltransferase gene, complete sequence and sites of expression. *Nucleic Acids Research*, **14**, 9387–9406.

95. Milewski, B. & Palynyczko, Z. (1975) Evaluation of the usefulness of serum lipoprotein-X (LP-X) detection test for the diagnosis of cholestasis in chronic liver diseases. *Polish Archives of Medicine*, **53**, 445–452.

96. Miyata, Y., Innoui, M., Masumoto, A. *et al.* (1984) A study on the disorders of lipoproteins and apolipoproteins in patients with primary biliary cirrhosis. *Acta Hepatologica Japonica*, **25**, 54–61.

97. Mukherjee, S., Kunitake, G. & Alfin-Slater, R.B. (1958) The esterification of cholesterol with palmitic acid by rat liver homogenates. *Journal of Biological Chemistry*, **23**, 91–96.

98. Muller, P., Fellin, R., Lambrecht, J. *et al.* (1974) Hypertriglyceridemia secondary to liver disease. *European Journal of Clinical Investigation*, **4**, 419–428.

99. Nakaya, N., Chung, B.H., Patsch, J.R. & Taunton, D.D. (1977) Synthesis and release of low density lipoprotein by the isolated perfused pig liver. *Journal of Biological Chemistry*, **252**, 7530–7532.

100. Nicolau, G., Shefer, S., Salen, G. & Mosbach, E.H. (1974) Regulation of cholesterol and bile acid synthesis in patients with gallstones and biliary obstruction. *Hepatologie*, **5**, 231 (abstract).

101. Nordby, G., Berg, T., Nilsson, M. & Norum, K.R. (1976) Secretion of lecithin : cholesterol acyltransferase from isolated rat hepatocytes. *Biochimica et Biophysica Acta*, **450**, 68–77.

102. Norum, K.R. & Gjone, E. (1967) Familial plasma lecithin cholesterol acyltransferase deficiency. Biochemical study of a new inborn error of metabolism. *Scandinavian Journal of Clinical and Laboratory Investigation*, **20**, 231–243.

103. Norum, K.R., Glomset, J.A., Nichols, A.V. & Forte, T. (1971) Plasma lipoproteins in familial lecithin : cholesterol acyltransferase deficiency: physical and chemical studies of low and high density lipoproteins. *Journal of Clinical Investigation*, **50**, 1131–1140.

104. Okazaki, M., Hara, I., Tanaka, A. *et al.* (1981) Decreased serum HDL_3 cholesterol levels in cirrhosis of the liver. *New England Journal of Medicine*, **304**, 1608.

105. Orlandi, F. (1975) Personal communication.

106. Osuga, T. & Portman, O.W. (1971) Origin and disappearance of plasma lecithin : cholesterol acyltransferase. *American Journal of Physiology*, **220**, 735–741.

107. Owen, J.S. & McIntyre, N. (1978) Erythrocyte lipid composition and sodium transport in human liver disease. *Biochimica et Biophysica Acta*, **510**, 168–176.

108. Owen, J.S., Hutton, R.A., Day, R.C. *et al.* (1981) Platelet lipid composition and platelet aggregation in human liver disease. *Journal of Lipid Research*, **22**, 423–430.

109. Owen, J.S., Bruckdorfer, K.R., Day, R.C. & McIntyre, N. (1982) Decreased erythrocyte membrane fluidity and altered lipid composition in human liver disease. *Journal of Lipid Research*, **23**, 124–132.

110. Owen, J.S., Goodall, H., Mistry, P. *et al.* (1984) Abnormal high density lipoproteins from patients with liver disease regulate cholesterol metabolism in cultured skin fibroblasts. *Journal of Lipid Research*, **25**, 919–931.

111. Owen, J.S., Brown, D.J.C., Harry, D.S. *et al.* (1985) Erythrocyte echinocytosis in liver disease. Role of abnormal plasma high density lipoproteins. *Journal of Clinical Investigation*, **76**, 2275–2285.

112. Owen, J.S., Brown, D.J.C., Chu, P. *et al.* (1985) The effect of high density lipoproteins from patients with liver disease on erythrocyte morphology and lymphocyte transformation. *Gastroenterology*, **79**, 1119.

113. Paradopoulos, N.M. & Charles, M.A. (1970) Serum lipoprotein patterns in liver disease. *Proceedings of the Society for Experimental Biology and Medicine*, **134**, 797–799.

114. Pearson, A.J.G. (1972) Triglyceride in obstructive liver disease. *Abstracts of the 5th Meeting of the International Association for the Study of the Liver*, Versailles, p. VI.

115. Pearson, A.J.G., Pyrovolakis, J. & McIntyre, N. (1974) Plasma lipids and lipoprotein changes in acute viral hepatitis. *Digestion*, **10**, 322 (abstract).

116. Phillips, G.B. (1960) The lipid composition of serum in patients with liver disease. *Journal of Clinical Investigation*, **39**, 1639–1650.

117. Pierce, F.T. & Gofman, J.W. (1951) Lipoproteins, liver disease and atherosclerosis. *Circulation*, **4**, 25–28.

118. Pierce, F.T., Kimmel, J.R. & Burns, T.W. (1954) Lipoproteins in infectious and serum hepatitis. *Metabolism*, **3**, 228–239.

119. Poley, J.R., Alaupovic, P., Magnani, H.N. *et al.* (1974) Quantitive serum lipoprotein-X (LP-X) before and after cholestyramine (CSM) in the diagnosis of extrahepatic biliary atresia (EBA). *Gastroenterology*, **66**, 761 (abstract).

120. Pyrovolakis, J., Pearson, A.J.G., Harry, D.S. *et al.* (1975) Elev-

ation of plasma cholesterol by clofibrate in rats with biliary obstruction. In Gerok, W. & Sickinger, K. (eds) *Drugs and the Liver*, pp. 381–386. Stuttgart: Schattauer Verlag.

121. Quarfordt, S.H. & Jakoi, L. (1973) Alterations of hepatic cholesterol synthesis in rats by lecithin and lecithin : cholesterol mesophase infusions. *Gastroenterology*, **65**, 566 (abstract).

122. Quarfordt, S.H., Oelschlaeger, H. & Krigbaum, W.R. (1972) Liquid crystalline lipid in the plasma of humans with biliary obstruction. *Journal of Clinical Investigation*, **51**, 1979–1988.

123. Quarfordt, S.H., Oelschlaeger, H., Krigbaum, W.R. *et al.* (1973) Effect of biliary obstruction on canine plasma and biliary lipids. *Lipids*, **8**, 522–530.

124. Quinn, D., Shirai, K. & Jackson, R.L. (1983) Lipoprotein lipase: mechanism of action and role in lipoprotein metabolism. *Progress in Lipid Research*, **22**, 35–78.

125. Ritland, S. (1975) Quantitive determination of the abnormal lipoprotein of cholestasis, LP-X, in liver disease. *Scandinavian Journal of Gastroenterology*, **10**, 5–15.

126. Ritland, S., Blomhoff, J.P. & Gjone, E. (1973) Lecithin : cholesterol acyltransferase and lipoprotein-X in liver disease. *Clinica Chimica Acta*, **49**, 251–259.

127. Ross, A., Murphy, G.M., Wilkinson, P.A. *et al.* (1970) Occurrence of an abnormal lipoprotein in patients with liver disease. *Gut*, **11**, 1035–1037.

128. Russ, E.M., Raymunt, J. & Barr, D.P. (1956) Lipoproteins in primary biliary cirrhosis. *Journal of Clinical Investigation*, **35**, 133–144.

129. Sabesin, S.M. & Frase, S. (1977) Electron microscopic studies of the assembly, intracellular transport and secretion of chylomicrons by rat intestine. *Journal of Lipid Research*, **18**, 496–511.

130. Sabesin, S.M., Kuiken, L.B. & Ragland, J.B. (1975) Lipoprotein and lecithin : cholesterol acyltransferase in galactosamine-induced rat liver injury. *Science*, **190**, 1302–1304.

131. Sabesin, S.M., Hawkins, H.L., Kuiken, L. & Ragland, J.B. (1977) Abnormal plasma lipoproteins and lecithin : cholesterol acyltransferase deficiency in alcoholic liver disease. *Gastroenterology*, **72**, 510–518.

132. Sabesin, S.M. & Weidman, S.W. (1985) Lipoprotein abnormalities in primary biliary cirrhosis: information concerning control of plasma high density lipoprotein levels. *Gastroenterology*, **89**, 1426–1429.

133. Schaffner, F. (1969) Paradoxical elevation of serum cholesterol by clofibrate in patients with primary biliary cirrhosis. *Gastroenterology*, **57**, 253–255.

134. Seidel, D., Alaupovic, P. & Furman, R.H. (1969) A lipoprotein characterizing obstructive jaundice. I Method for quantitative separation and identification of lipoproteins in jaundiced subjects. *Journal of Clinical Investigation*, **48**, 1211–1223.

135. Seidel, D., Gretz, H. & Ruppert, C. (1973) Significance of the LP-X test in differential diagnosis of jaundice. *Clinical Chemistry*, **19**, 86–91.

136. Seidel, D., Greten, H., Greisen, H.P. *et al.* (1972) Further aspects on the characterisation of high and very low density lipoproteins in patients with liver disease. *European Journal of Clinical Investigation*, **2**, 359–364.

137. Simko, V., Kelley, R.E. & Dinscoy, H.P. (1965) Predicting severity of liver disease: twelve laboratory tests evaluated by multiple regression. *Journal of International Medical Research*, **13**, 249–254.

138. Simon, J.B. & Boyer, J.L. (1971) Production of lecithin : cholesterol acyltransferase by the isolated perfused rat liver. *Biochimica et Biophysica Acta*, **218**, 549–551.

139. Simon, J.B. & Schieg, R. (1970) Serum cholesterol esterification in liver disease: importance of lecithin : cholesterol acyltransferase. *New England Journal of Medicine*, **283**, 841–846.

140. Sloop, C.H., Dory, L. & Roheim, P.S. (1987) Interstitial fluid lipoproteins. *Journal of Lipid Research*, **28**, 225–237.

141. Smith, J.A., Lonergan, E.T. & Sterling, K. (1964) Spur-cell anaemia: haemolytic anaemia with red cells resembling acanthocytes. *New England Journal of Medicine*, **271**, 396–398.

142. Smith, K.M., Lawn, R.M. & Wilcox, J.N. (1990) Cellular localization of apolipoprotein D and lecithin-cholesterol transferase mRNA in Rhesus monkey tissues by in situ hybridization. *Journal of Lipid Research*, **31**, 995–1004.

143. Soutar, A.K., Myant, N.B. & Thompson, G.R. (1977) Simultaneous measurements of apolipoprotein B turnover in very low and low density lipoproteins in familial hypercholesterolaemia. *Atherosclerosis*, **28**, 247–256.

144. Sperry, W.M. (1935) Cholesterol esterase in blood. *Journal of Biological Chemistry*, **111**, 467–478.

145. Stakeberg, H., Lundborg, H. & Schersten, T. (1974) Rate of in vitro incorporation of precursors into hepatic lipids and proteins in patients with extrahepatic cholestasis. *European Journal of Clinical Investigation*, **4**, 399–403.

146. Stein, O., Alkan, M. & Stein, Y. (1973) Obstructive jaundice lipoprotein particles studied in ultrathin sections of livers of bile duct-ligated mice. *Laboratory Investigation*, **29**, 166–172.

147. Sugano, M., Hori, K. & Wada, M. (1969) Hepatotoxicity and plasma cholesterol esterification by rats. *Archives of Biochemistry*, **129**, 588–596.

148. Switzer, S. (1967) Plasma lipoproteins in liver disease: 1 Immunologically distinct low-density lipoproteins in patients with biliary obstruction. *Journal of Clinical Investigation*, **46**, 1855–1866.

149. Tada, N., Nestel, P.J., Fidge, N. & Campbell, G. (1981) Abnormal apoprotein composition in alcoholic hepatitis. *Biochimica et Biophysica Acta*, **64**, 207–220.

150. Takahashi, Z. & Muto, Y. (1968) The importance of lecithin: cholesterol acyltransferase in diseases of the liver and biliary tree (in Japanese). *Japanese Journal of Gastroenterology*, **65**, 1139–1142.

151. Tata, F., Chavez, E., Markham, A.F. *et al.* (1987) The isolation and characterization of cDNA and genetic clones for human lecithin–cholesterol acyltransferase. *Biochimica et Biophysica Acta*, **910**, 142–148.

152. Thalassinos, N., Hatzioannou, J., Scliros, Ph. *et al.* (1975) Plasma a-lipoprotein pattern in acute viral hepatitis. *American Journal of Digestive Diseases*, **20**, 148–155.

153. Thannhauser, S.J. & Magendantz, H. (1938) The different clinical groups of xanthomatous diseases: a clinical physiological study of 22 cases. *Annals of Internal Medicine*, **11**, 148–155.

154. Thomas, P.K. & Walker, J.G. (1965) Xanthomatous neuropathy in primary biliary cirrhosis. *Brain*, **88**, 1079–1088.

155. Thompson, G.R. (1983) Plasma exchange and affinity chromotrographic therapy for hyperlipidaemia: a review. *Apheresis Bulletin*, **1**, 26–31.

156. Thompson, G.R., Jadhav, A., Nava, M. & Gotto, A.M., Jr (1976) Effects of intravenous phospholipid on low-density lipoprotein turnover in man. *European Journal of Clinical Investigation*, **6**, 241–248.

157. Turnberg, L.A., Mahoney, M.P., Gleeson, M.H. *et al.* (1972) Plasmaphoresis and plasma exchange in the treatment of hyperlipaemia and xanthomatous neuropathy in patients with primary biliary cirrhosis. *Gut*, **13**, 976–981.

158. Turner, K.B., McCormack, G.H. & Richards, A. (1953) The cholesterol-esterifying enzymes of human serum. I. In liver disease. *Journal of Clinical Investigation*, **32**, 801–806.

159. Tytgat, G.N., Rubin, C. & Saunders, D.R. (1971) Synthesis and transport of lipoprotein particles by intestinal absorptive cells in man. *Journal of Clinical Investigation*, **50**, 2056–2078.

160. Van Itallie, T.B., Hashim, S.A., Crampton, R.S. & Tennent, D.M. (1961) The treatment of pruritus and hypercholesterolaemia of primary biliary cirrhosis with cholestyramine. *New England Journal of Medicine*, **265**, 469–474.

161. Vergani, C., Pietrogrande, M. & Grondona, M.C. (1973) Study of the abnormal lipoprotein-X in obstructive and non-obstructive jaundice. *Clinica Chimica Acta*, **48**, 243–248.

162. Weidman, S.W., Ragland, J.B. & Sabesin, S.M. (1982) Plasma lipoprotein composition in alcoholic hepatitis: accumulation of apolipoprotein E-rich high density lipoprotein and preferential reappearance of 'light'-HDL during partial recovery. *Journal of Lipid Research*, **23**, 556–569.

163. Widal, F., Weil, A. & Laudat, M. (1912) La lipemie des Brightiques: rapports de la retinite des Brightiques avec l'azotemie et la cholesterolemie. *Semaine Medicale*, **32**, 529–531.

164. Yamamoto, K., Koga, S. & Ibayashi, H. (1978) Apoprotein A-I in cholestatic liver disease. *Clinica Chimica Acta*, **87**, 85–92.

CHAPTER 5

Protein Metabolism and the Liver

Anthony S. Tavill & Arthur J. McCullough

The liver plays a major role in the metabolism of amino acids and proteins. It processes the nutritional supply of amino acids delivered by portal venous inflow both for its own needs and for the requirements of peripheral tissue, predominantly the muscles. In addition, it is the recipient of amino acids (mainly alanine and glutamine) from the muscles, which play a vital role within the liver in gluconeogenesis and transamination reactions. Furthermore, ammonia derived intrahepatically by deamination of alanine and other amino acids, and ammonia generated extrahepatically by nucleotide metabolism or by bacterial degradation of intestinal protein and urea, is efficiently eliminated as urea by the hepatic enzymes of the Krebs–Henseleit urea cycle. The liver is the exclusive or major site of synthesis of virtually all the plasma proteins, and is an important route of degradation of many of these proteins and hormones. Recent information also suggests that certain proteins may be excreted into bile after uptake and endocytosis by the hepatocyte. Finally, there is evidence that the liver may modulate overall body protein metabolism by virtue of its role in the metabolism of those hormones which have significant effects on the fate of amino acids in peripheral tissues.

In both acute and chronic liver disease, control of both

amino acid and protein metabolism may be disturbed by the combined effects of reduction in functional hepatocyte mass and portal systemic shunting. It is becoming increasingly apparent that alterations in muscle protein metabolism may occur concomitantly with liver disease as a result of associated nutritional and hormonal disturbances. These abnormalities have considerable relevance to the pathogenesis and management of portal systemic encephalopathy and to the rational nutritional support of these frequently malnourished patients.

This chapter will attempt to describe the qualitative and quantitative role of the liver in protein metabolism in the context of dietary nitrogen supply, and will review important carbohydrate–protein interactions. Also, recent data on associated body protein turnover and amino acid oxidation will be critically reviewed and their relevance to nutritional therapy in liver disease will be discussed. The specific functions of the liver in the synthesis and secretion of certain specialized plasma proteins will be described, and attention will be given to the effects of alcohol and liver disease on these functions. Finally, the role of the liver in the metabolism of iron storage and transport proteins will be discussed in the context of hepatic iron overload diseases.

QUANTITATIVE ASPECTS OF HEPATIC PROTEIN METABOLISM

HEPATIC PROTEIN TURNOVER

The term 'protein turnover' is used to convey the concept of continuing synthesis and degradation. In the case of both the constituent and secretory proteins of the liver, turnover is a random process which occurs without regard to the longevity of individual protein molecules.[329] On a fractional basis the liver is one of the most active organs in protein turnover, surpassed only by the intestinal mucosa and pancreas, but muscle protein by virtue of its larger mass makes a much more important contribution to overall body protein turnover. Total body protein in an average 70 kg adult is approximately 12 kg, turning over at a rate of between 200 and 300 g/day.[107,358,380] Muscle protein synthesis and degradation constitute about 53% of total turnover. In absolute terms muscle protein turnover of about 130 g/day makes the single largest contribution to the free amino acid pool of the body. As such, the ability of the body to modulate the balance between the synthesis and degradation of muscle protein provides a means for the supply of amino acids when dietary protein is limited. Such a labile source of amino acids is required for essential functions of the liver, e.g. gluconeogenesis, during relative deprivation of dietary protein and carbohydrate. A normal dietary protein intake of 90 g/day may be reduced to about 45 g/day before negative nitrogen balance is reached.[360] At that point net degradation of muscle protein provides the principal means for the continuous supply of amino acids for

gluconeogenesis and the priority synthesis of other essential proteins.

Hepatic protein synthesis constitutes about 20% of total body protein turnover, viz. approximately 48 g/day in a 70-kg adult. This is divided roughly equally between the synthesis of constituent and export proteins,[359] with albumin comprising the single most important secretory protein.[368] The average synthesis of albumin of 12 g/day (120–200 mg kg^{-1} day^{-1})[279,295] constitutes about 25% of total hepatic protein synthesis and about 50% of total hepatic export protein synthesis.

TOTAL NITROGEN ECONOMY

The total body amino acid pool receives contributions from the degradation of body protein and from dietary protein which is completely hydrolysed to amino acids in the process of digestion and intestinal absorption. Although the total flux in this system is derived from about 250 g of body protein and about 90 g of dietary protein, there is compartmentation of amino acid flow through the portal system. In this system dietary protein mixes with the endogenous proteins derived from exfoliation of intestinal cells (about 50 g), secreted enzyme proteins from the salivary glands, stomach, intestine and pancreas (about 16 g) and a small amount of plasma protein lost by exudation into the intestinal lumen (1–2 g).[75] In the absorptive period following a meal about 23% of the incoming portal venous nitrogen is passed on to the peripheral tissues.[69] The remainder is processed in the liver to urea (57%) or for hepatic protein synthesis (20%). Between meals there is a fall in the total flux of nitrogen in the portal vein. Only that derived from digestion of endogenous protein continues, and as a consequence the rate of ureagenesis falls to about one-third of the level in the absorptive period. There is no net transport of amino acids to the periphery, and in fact there is net hepatic uptake of nitrogen, largely as alanine released from muscle protein degradation. Hepatic tissue protein also goes into a catabolic phase and together with the amino acids released from muscle makes a contribution to ureagenesis and gluconeogenesis. Plasma protein synthesis seems to be relatively well buffered from these short-term changes in amino acid supply and continues at a normal rate with little circadian variation.[69,246]

HEPATIC AMINO ACID FLUXES

Following a meal containing protein there are large changes in amino acid concentration in the portal venous blood[58] which are not mirrored by those occurring in the peripheral blood. Not only does the liver pass on only 23% of the incoming amino acid nitrogen to the periphery, but it also selectively modifies the profile of the individual amino acids reaching the systemic blood. For example, there is a relative hepatic barrier to the branched-chain amino acids (BCAA). These amino acids, valine, leucine and isoleucine, account for more than 60% of the total amino acids appearing in systemic blood, although they constitute only about 20% of the amino acids in dietary protein. Rather, there is a predominance of hepatic metabolism of the aromatic amino acids (AAA), phenylalanine, and tyrosine, and also methionine, while the BCAA are relayed peripherally to be metabolized predominantly by muscle.[349]

The events related to the variations in protein intake are mediated by a variety of enzymes in liver and muscle which take part in intermediary amino acid metabolism.[139] These are concerned with gluconeogenesis, ureagenesis, transamination and synthesis of non-essential amino acids. For example, the synthesis of the first four of the enzymes of the urea cycle in the liver, carbamyl phosphate synthetase, ornithine transcarbamylase, arginino-succinate synthetase and arginino-succinase, is induced by increasing dietary protein, while the fifth enzyme, arginase is increased in concentration by reduction in its degradation.[292,293] At the same time there is decreased activity of BCAA transaminase in muscle,[202] which is responsible for a reduction in BCAA degradation during periods of exogenous protein supply.

Branched-chain amino acids play a vital role in both muscle and hepatic protein metabolism.[79] BCAA undergo degradation as a source of energy for muscle, for the provision of both the carbon skeletons for pyruvate and the nitrogen required for their transamination to alanine and glutamine (Figure 5.1). During an overnight fast there is net release of these two amino acids from the protein reservoir in muscles. The net flux of alanine is largely mopped up by the liver, where its carbon skeleton becomes a source of glucose and its nitrogen undergoes transamination or ureagenesis. In contrast, glutamine is largely taken up by the kidney as a source of ammonia and by the gut as an energy source. After dietary protein–calorie ingestion the BCAA play a unique role in reversing the negative nitrogen balance induced by fasting. Being largely excluded from hepatic uptake, they constitute the main source of amino acid supply to muscle.[349] Because they comprise only 20% of the amino acid residues in muscle protein, incoming BCAA are available for oxidation as an important energy source as well as for anabolic incorporation into protein. The keto acid derivatives of the BCAA are a vital source of the pyruvate which is oxidized for energy or which undergoes transamination to alanine and glutamine.

The concept of cyclical anabolism–catabolism of muscle protein and the associated fluxes of alanine are based on the observations of Felig et al.[78,80] The proposed glucose–alanine cycle (Figure 5.1) consists of a compartment in muscle in which incoming glucose is a source of pyruvate which is transaminated to alanine. Alanine in turn is transported to the liver compartment where it is the major amino acid source for gluconeogenesis and ureagenesis. During fasting, the net formation of glucose in the liver is derived from alanine released by degradation of muscle protein. After appropriate feeding, this catabolic phase is reversed by net synthesis of muscle protein, with

an accompanying sharp reduction in net flux of alanine to the liver. The anabolic–catabolic phases of the cycle are under the intrinsic control of the hormones insulin and glucagon. Insulin secretion, which is maximal after feeding, limits the uptake of alanine by the liver and thereby restricts this source of gluconeogenesis and the associated catabolism of BCAA in muscle. Glucagon secretion, which is maximal in the fasted state, promotes muscle protein[56] and BCAA degradation, stimulates alanine synthesis and uptake by liver, and leads to enhanced gluconeogenesis and ureagenesis. The normal relationships between insulin and glucagon secretion are critical for the maintenance of a compensated cycle of muscle protein anabolism and catabolism. In liver disease these relationships may be disturbed, with profound consequences for the maintenance of the normal nutritional state of the patient, and for the maintenance of normal BCAA metabolism.

ALTERATIONS IN AMINO ACID AND PROTEIN METABOLISM IN LIVER DISEASE

ROLE OF PROTEIN–CALORIE MALNUTRITION (see also Chapter 6)

Most of the data on the prevalence of protein–calorie malnutrition (PCM) have been derived from patients with alcoholic liver disease, although to some degree PCM is manifested in other forms of longstanding liver disease, particularly in the late stages of primary biliary cirrhosis and post-hepatitic cirrhosis. In a recent review of 362 patients reported in eight separate studies, 60% had evidence of significant weight loss. Although dietary intake of protein and calories tends to be restricted in alcoholics prior to the onset of liver disease, it is unusual for PCM to become overt until significant liver disease has developed. McCullough and co-workers have compared the data on the frequency of PCM in alcoholics with and without liver disease in a series of prospective studies,[187] and report that, although methods of nutritional assessment vary among studies, there was usually significant malnutrition in the presence of liver disease. The largest and most detailed data are derived from 363 patients in the Veteran Administration Cooperative Study,[193] which reported 100% prevalence of PCM in alcoholic liver disease, the extent of which correlated with the biochemical extent of liver dysfunction but not with the severity of liver disease as judged by the presence of cirrhosis. In this study ingested alcohol constituted the single largest source of calories (47.4%), while dietary protein was the smallest source of total calorie intake (7.6%). All the markers of malnutrition increased with the severity of liver dysfunction; these included lean body mass, fat stores, immune function, nitrogen balance and visceral protein status reflected by serum albumin and transferrin concentrations. The major impact of malnutrition in alcoholic liver disease is conveyed in a subsequent

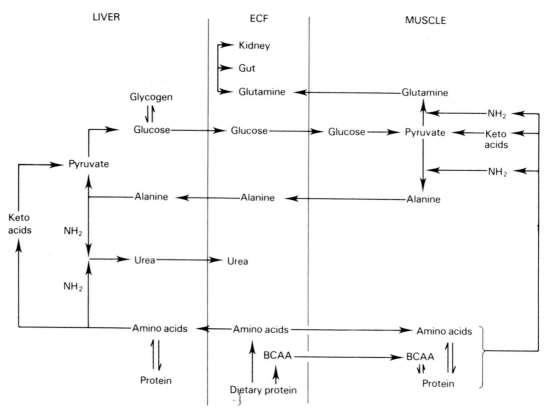

Figure 5.1 Carbohydrate–protein exchange between muscle and liver in normal humans (based upon data presented by Felig et al.[78,80]) After an overnight fast there is net release of amino acids by muscle predominantly as alanine and glutamine. These are derived by transamination of pyruvate, the carbon skeletons being provided by both degraded amino acids and glucose. Branched chain amino acids (BCAA) are particularly important in the provision of nitrogen for alanine synthesis, and also possibly the carbon skeletons. Alanine is utilized for gluconeogenesis by the liver and urea is formed as a by-product. The kidney and the gut are the main sites of uptake of glutamine, where it is used for ammonia production and as a possible source of energy respectively. Following dietary protein ingestion, muscle goes into an anabolic phase; there is selective hepatic escape and muscle uptake of dietary BCAA, reduced muscle output of alanine and glutamine, and a reduced rate of hepatic gluconeogenesis. Hepatic tissue protein also goes into an anabolic phase following protein ingestion. Although about 14% of dietary amino acids are used for hepatic protein synthesis, up to 50–60% may be deaminated to urea and keto-acid analogues.

report from the V.A. Cooperative Study which demonstrated a clear negative correlation between PCM and survival.[194]

Although a variety of metabolic factors including maldigestion, malabsorption and decreased hepatic storage have been implicated[196] in the PCM of chronic liver disease, poor dietary intake of nutrients is by far the most important factor.[196,197,207] Having stated this there is growing evidence for intrinsic defects in energy and protein metabolism which cannot be explained solely by inadequate supply of exogenous calories and protein.[186]

DISTURBANCES IN AMINO ACID AND PROTEIN METABOLISM

The spectrum of disordered nitrogen metabolism in chronic liver disease is wide. Characteristics include abnormal patterns of plasma amino acids and skeletal muscle wasting. First, the characteristic pattern of plasma amino acids has been described in established cirrhosis; namely,

low levels of the BCAA leucine, isoleucine and valine and elevated levels of the AAA tyrosine and phenylalanine, as well as methionine.[73,206,209,289,387] This pattern may be observed in the presence or absence of portal systemic encephalopathy and protein intolerance, and its presence does not appear to be related to the severity or activity of liver disease,[185] or to the ability to maintain positive nitrogen balance.[361]

Second, objective evidence for the associated changes in muscle protein metabolism in chronic liver disease is very limited. Studies have been confined to the measurement of urinary excretion of 3-methylhistidine (3MH) or to the fluxes of labelled amino acid precursors as indicants of protein turnover. 3MH is a uniquely modified amino acid residue in myofibrillar proteins which is excreted quantitatively after the degradation of muscle proteins. Based on measurements in cirrhotics with and without muscle wasting, increased fractional rates of myofibrillar protein turnover have been calculated.[388] Independent support for this observation have been provided by radioisotopic studies using ^{14}C-labelled tyrosine.[233,234] Increased amino acid flux in patients with cirrhosis or fulminant hepatic failure apparently reflected increased endogenous protein degradation without increased amino acid oxidation. Major reservations have been expressed with regard to some of the fundamental assumptions of the methodology employed in the foregoing studies.[186] More recent studies using [1-^{13}C]leucine as a tracer or [^{15}N]glycine incorporation into urinary nitrogenous end-products indicate that protein turnover in stable cirrhosis is not increased in the fasting state.[81,201,217,305,326] In response to feeding, the data are conflicting. Labelled leucine studies revealed no increase in protein turnover[201] while labelled glycine studies suggest that cirrhotics have enhanced protein turnover in response to feeding.[326] In the light of these conflicting data, more definitive studies which undertake both evaluation of the mechanisms of the reduced plasma concentrations of the BCAA and measurement of BCAA turnover and muscle protein metabolism are awaited.

There has been a great deal of speculation on the mechanism of depression of plasma levels of BCAA in patients with advanced liver disease. Both direct and indirect data suggest strongly that the phenomenon is multifactorial in origin. As reviewed by Shaw and Lieber,[307] there may be synergistic roles for alcohol, nutrition and liver disease in patients with alcoholic hepatitis and cirrhosis. Although dietary protein deficiency may contribute to the reduction, it was felt that liver disease and in particular the degree of associated portal systemic shunting were far more important in its pathogenesis.[178,308] Chronic liver disease and shunting is accompanied by hyperinsulinaemia and hyperglucagonaemia, the former probably due to both increased pancreatic β-cell secretion and decreased hepatic degradation, the latter primarily due to increased α-cell secretion.[306,309] These hormonal disturbances have been postulated to contribute to increased catabolism of BCAA by muscle and possibly also by adipose tissue.[125,173,308,314] Direct evidence for the role of insulin in the reduced BCAA concentrations has been sought by studies in normal volunteers[290] and in cirrhotics.[175] Insulin infusions were followed by a fall in BCAA and branched-chain keto acid (BCKA) levels in normals, even after return to normoglycaemia. However, the rate of fall in BCAA was lower in cirrhotics subjected to euglycaemic insulin infusions than controls, indicating that factors in addition to hyperinsulinism are probably responsible for the low BCAA levels. Furthermore, following a protein meal, cirrhotics show an exaggerated increase in BCAA which parallels the degree of glucose intolerance, the evidence pointing to a defect in substrate response to insulin in peripheral tissues.[176]

The absolute increase in plasma concentrations of other amino acids compared to BCAA in cirrhosis is evidence of decreased intrinsic ability of the diseased liver to clear the non-BCAA efficiently.[346] Although there is evidence that the urea cycle is operating at only 60% of capacity under normal circumstances,[114] the enzymes of the cycle are induced by feeding a high-protein diet.[292] In liver disease this adaptive ability may be severely limited by reduced activity of the enzymes of the urea cycle,[142,171] resulting in a reduction in the maximal rate of urea synthesis,[283] elevation in plasma amino acids (particularly the AAA) and hyperammonaemia.[304] Finally, it has been noted using indirect calorimetry and tracer analysis of [^{14}C]palmitate that patients with alcoholic cirrhosis after an overnight fast derived 69% of their calories from fat (cf. normals 40%), a situation which only develops in normal subjects after 2–3 days of total starvation.[239] This disturbed pattern of fuel homeostasis was suggested as a contributory factor to the cachexia observed in certain patients with alcoholic cirrhosis. The synergistic roles of dietary deficiency, loss of functioning hepatocyte mass, portal systemic shunting and associated hormonal imbalance may serve to explain the wasting of fat and protein which is almost invariable in decompensated cirrhosis. Nevertheless, much work remains to be done to document accurately the precise mechanism of wasting of skeletal muscle. Analogy with other diseases which result in muscle protein wasting suggests that depression of muscle protein synthesis is the final common pathway for all the pathogenetic factors operating in chronic liver disease.[212,263]

THERAPEUTIC USE OF BRANCHED-CHAIN AMINO ACIDS AND KETO ACIDS

The association of low plasma branched-chain amino acids and muscle protein wasting in patients with liver disease has been offered as a rationale for the use of oral or intravenous nutritional supplementation with BCAA-enriched amino acids. Although such solutions were initially proposed as specific therapy for patients with hepatic encephalopathy and protein intolerance,[83] attention has turned to their use for the improvement of the nutritional status of cirrhotics with or without encephalopathy. In particular, it has been suggested that BCAA may have a particular therapeutic value in reversing the abnormal plasma amino acid pattern and promoting an anabolic trend in muscle metabolism. In uncontrolled studies of patients with hepatic encephalopathy and protein intolerance there was a positive correlation between the amount of intravenous or enteral BCAA administered and improved nitrogen balance,[86,140] while in six cirrhotics without encephalopathy or muscle wasting, anticatabolic effects were observed in the form of reduced 3-methylhistidine excretion.[174] Since it has been shown that patients with alcoholic liver disease may well be able to tolerate standard amino acid solutions, and may show improved biochemical function, histopathology and survival following such treatment,[3,4,35,62,228,312] it is unclear whether BCAA are a superior source of nitrogen to standard amino acid mixtures. Data from these earlier studies suggested that BCAA may serve a specific role in reducing degradation of myofibrillar protein in cirrhotic patients. Several studies compared BCAA-enriched mixtures with standard mixtures administered orally (two studies) or intravenously (three studies) with discrepant results.[137, 177,227,235,269] A detailed evaluation of some of these studies[187,334] concluded that standard amino acid solutions achieved better nitrogen balance than BCAA-enriched mixtures although other workers have suggested that BCAA were superior in long-term use.[43,177,189,200,376] Differences other than BCAA/AAA composition exist in these modified formulations, making interpretation of specific metabolic effects difficult, and prompting caution in their use, given the limited capacity of the diseased liver to clear relatively heavy loads of certain amino acids.[347] In summary, although the use of BCAA in the therapy of hepatic encephalopathy shows promise based on published data,[72,229] there remains no general agreement regarding their efficacy and cost-effectiveness in the overall nutritional management of chronic liver disease.[208] There is consensus in the view that routine protein restriction in cirrhotic patients is not justified and may be harmful. Rather, supplementation in the form of intravenous or enteral tube feeding in the acute hospital setting, and long-term amino acid administration, may improve survival and nutritional status. Even such simple manoeuvres such as altering the timing of protein supplementation may prove efficacious in patients with liver disease.[329] Accordingly, although BCAA-enriched solutions offer potential advantages in the nutritional support of patients with chronic liver disease, it is premature to advocate their wholesale use until more precise evaluation of their efficacy in humans is available, and until guidelines for patient selection and end-points of therapy have been defined.

The first step in the metabolism of BCAA in the periphery is their reversible transamination to the α-keto analogues, α-ketoisovalerate (from valine), α-ketoisocaproate (from leucine) and α-keto-β-methylvalerate (from isoleucine). The next step is the irreversible oxidative decarboxylation of the BCKA by BCKA dehydrogenase. Theoretically, it is therefore possible for BCKA to substitute for BCAA as essential dietary constituents. Leucine promotes protein synthesis and decreases protein degradation in skeletal muscle and this effect is mediated by its keto analogue α-ketoisocaproate.[337] Furthermore, the efficient uptake of BCKA by muscle is accompanied by formation of the corresponding BCAA, and a reduction in alanine release.[353] Although there is little transamination of BCAA in the liver, there is a hepatic capability for the oxidation of BCKA and for the acceptance of nitrogen by BCKA from glutamine.[353] Also, since leucine and BCKA stimulate hepatic protein synthesis and suppress degradation,[145,299] BCKA offer a potential means for promoting overall anabolism both in the periphery (predominantly muscle) and in the liver (reviewed by Walser[354]). In obese fasting subjects, daily intravenous infusions of BCKA had a nitrogen-sparing effect[288] and in cirrhotics, intravenous administration of α-keto-isocaproate reduced the muscle output of alanine without an increase in the output of leucine or other amino acids.[73]

Additionally in this study, hepatic ureagenesis fell by 50%. Since about 33% of the infused α-keto-isocaproate is taken up by muscle, it is important to know the relative rates of transamination and oxidative decarboxylation of the BCKA within muscle tissue. Based on stable isotopic data, in the postabsorptive state in man, the ratio of these two pathways of leucine metabolism was about 10 : 1, falling to 4 : 1 in the fed state.[181] These observations indicate the potential of BCKA to promote net nitrogen retention in vivo possibly by inhibiting protein degradation in muscle rather than by stimulating protein synthesis, as has been observed for the parent BCAA, leucine.[100] At this time it is not possible to extrapolate these results for α-ketoisocaproic acid to other BCKA. For example, it has recently been suggested that the overall capacity for α-ketoisovaleric acid decarboxylation is greater than the capacity for valine transamination.[291]

To date, studies of the response to BCKA therapy in patients with chronic liver disease have concentrated on their anticipated beneficial effects on hepatic encephalopathy with only limited evaluation of their potential nutritional value. The most encouraging results have been observed with the ornithine salts of BCKA, which were observed to be superior to BCAA in improving encephalopathy and reducing hyperammonaemia.[116] In contrast, the administration of calcium salts of BCKA has produced inconsistent results. Little benefit has been noted by some workers[350] while others have noted some improvement in plasma amino acid patterns[33,116,170] or nitrogen balance and muscle composition. In summary, the therapeutic uses of branched-chain keto acids have not been established. As with BCAA there is a need for more quantitative data, and in particular for those markers of metabolic improvement which provide evidence of net protein anabolism. Although commercial preparations are not available, specific formulations for use in liver disease are being prepared and investigated.

THE ROLE OF THE LIVER IN PROTEIN SYNTHESIS AND DEGRADATION

OVERVIEW OF MECHANISMS OF TURNOVER

The concepts of turnover of hepatic proteins have been reviewed in detail elsewhere.[329,331,333] The term 'turnover' implies a continuous process of synthesis and degradation; modulation of turnover may be influenced by primary changes in either of these metabolic processes. Homeostasis is primarily geared to restoration of steady-state conditions, namely a reattainment of the balance between synthesis and degradation. In a teleological sense the apparent energy-wasting mechanisms of degradation provide a means of adaptation to environmental changes which primarily affect synthesis.[294] Likewise, the synthetic process is endowed with the potential for dynamic responses to pathological alterations in degradation.

In the last two decades there have been major advances

in the understanding of the cellular biology of the hepatocyte. The hepatocyte synthesizes both constituent proteins and secretory proteins. It therefore possesses a relatively segregated synthetic machinery; constituent proteins are synthesized predominantly on free polyribosomes, whereas secretory proteins begin their translational process on polyribosomes bound to the rough endoplasmic reticulum.[118,260] Proteins destined for export are subsequently channelled into the transport pathway through the smooth endoplasmic reticulum (SER) and Golgi apparatus and microtubular apparatus, where they may undergo post-translational modifications prior to secretion.

The liver also plays a major role in the degradation of both constituent and secretory proteins. There are both lysosomal and non-lysosomal pathways for the degradation of endogenous and exogenous proteins and these may be controlled by different mechanisms. The hepatocyte is equipped with a selection of specific receptors which recognize and bind certain glycoproteins, with subsequent uptake within endocytotic vesicles which are directed towards either lysosomal or non-lysosomal routes of degradation. Finally, it is apparent that some of these uptake mechanisms are linked to specific ligands which may be released within the hepatocyte or in certain instances may be excreted intact into the biliary canaliculus. The carrier protein may be degraded within the cell or may be excreted without undergoing degradation by exocytosis into the plasma (a process called 'diacytosis') or into the bile by a vesicular transport mechanism.

Regulatory mechanisms in protein turnover which are responsive to dietary energy or protein supply and to hormonal influences may be relatively non-specific, affecting both constituent and secretory proteins in a general way. Other regulatory mechanisms of synthesis and degradation are more specific to individual proteins and show unique responses to substrates, drugs, prosthetic groups and ligands. The general and specific aspects of protein turnover will be discussed separately. The specific aspects will be considered for the specialized proteins (usually secretory) of hepatic origin. In addition to the physiological regulation of these processes, recent information on disturbances in regulation resulting from malnutrition, alcohol and liver disease will be discussed.

PROTEIN SYNTHESIS AND SECRETION _____

In the traditional schema of protein synthesis all forms of cellular RNA are transcribed from chromosomal DNA and are transported from the nucleus to constitute the three cytoplasmic forms of RNA, ribosomal (rRNA), transfer (tRNA) and messenger RNA (mRNA). The nucleotide sequence of the mRNA provides the information governing the specific sequence of amino acids in a particular protein. The tRNA, which binds the activated amino acid is then called in by a series of initiation factors to bind to the ribosome on the 5′ end of the mRNA. During the subsequent translation of the messenger, the polypeptide is propagated in a sequence controlled by the specific sequence of triple nucleotide frames. Translation proceeds from the 5′ end to the 3′ end of the mRNA and the completed polypeptide is released. Transcriptional control of protein synthesis is exerted by the amount of mRNA which has been formed from the genome, while translational control is governed by the efficiency of the protein-synthesizing machinery. The most efficient synthetic unit is a strand of mRNA fully loaded with ribosomes which are being translocated along the message at a maximum rate. Indeed, hepatocytes which have been stimulated to synthesize protein at a maximum rate show a preponderance of so-called aggregated polyribosomes, i.e. mRNA associated with a full complement of ribosomes and nascent polypeptide chains being propagated from the N-terminal end of the molecule.

At a transcriptional level, control of protein synthesis may be mediated by regulation of the activities of DNA and RNA polymerases and ribonucleases. At a translational level the activity of polyribosomes may be regulated by factors influencing initiation, elongation and release of the polypeptide chain and the supply of high-energy phosphates, ATP and GTP, and Mg^{2+} ions. For those proteins which enter the secretory pathway, a variety of post-translational factors may also play a role in governing the rate at which they appear in the circulation. The secretory apparatus itself is subject to a degree of control. For example, albumin takes about 1–2 minutes for the polyribosome to translate the complete polypeptide chain, which then traverses the smooth endoplasmic reticulum (SER) to reach the Golgi apparatus in 15–20 minutes. Although the liver does not store large quantities of secretory proteins, there is evidence that the Golgi bodies vary in volume in proportion to the rate of synthesis.[95,247] Recent studies have demonstrated by biochemical and autoradiographic techniques that the Golgi apparatus is the site of maximum glycosylation of both secretory and membrane glycoproteins.[24,37,38] Although the major site of action of colchicine is more distal in the secretory pathway, viz. at the level of the microtubules, the drug also induces structural and functional changes in the stacked cisternal membranes of the Golgi.[12] In general, there is a correlation between the rate of glycosylation and the rate of protein secretion,[11] although in certain circumstances glycosylation is not essential for secretion.[127]

Vesicles derived from the Golgi apparatus encapsulate the protein and are guided to the exterior of the cell by the activity of the cytoskeletal components, microfilaments and microtubules. These terminal events in the secretory pathway may be separately controlled or damaged by factors which have minimal effects on the earlier events in protein synthesis. Microtubules are cylindrical cytoplasmic organelles which have been implicated in the movement of ribosomes and secretory and lysosomal vesicles during protein synthesis, secretion and degradation. The structural protein of microtubules is tubulin, a dimer composed of two polypeptides (M_r about 55 000).

The assembly of microtubules is based on the polymerization of tubulin subunits and their subsequent organization into protofilaments.[285] Microtubules play a role in the secretion of a variety of proteins by the hepatocyte by promoting migration of secretory vesicles from the Golgi complex towards the plasma membrane of the hepatocyte.[157,158,184,259] Colchicine is thought to exert its inhibitory effect on protein secretion primarily by inhibiting polymerization of tubulin,[77,236,261] while adenosine triphosphate (ATP) promotes microtubule assembly by specifically binding to tubulin.[382]

Finally, it is apparent from both biochemical and immunocytochemical studies that there may be intra-acinar functional heterogeneity of hepatocytes in protein synthesis and secretion. For example, although only 10–35% of parenchymal cells contain albumin at any point of time,[76,110] all parenchymal cells are capable of the synthesis and secretion of export proteins.[313] It is possible that hepatocytes rotate their synthetic and secretory efforts and lie fallow for some time after a burst of activity. In spite of the overwhelming evidence for the totipotentiality of parenchymal cells in protein synthesis and secretion, it has been shown recently that different secretory proteins migrate from the RER to the Golgi at their own characteristic rates.[153,166] Therefore, regulation of transport of individual proteins in the region of the RER where vesicles bud en route to the Golgi is another possible site of control, even though subsequent packaging of secretory proteins on the distal side of the Golgi apparatus is probably a shared process.[375]

Effects of amino acid supply on protein synthesis

Measurement of the rates of incorporation of [¹⁴C]leucine into liver proteins indicates that the entire protein mass of the liver turns over completely each day.[192] It is not surprising, therefore, that quite rapid changes in hepatic protein mass and rate of protein synthesis and secretion can be induced by changing amino acid supply to the liver. In vivo, limitation of dietary protein intake produces an early decrease in hepatic albumin synthesis.[48,94,120,126] This is followed by a compensatory fall in degradation. On refeeding a diet replete in protein, these effects can be reversed. Synthesis is initially stimulated to supranormal levels, to be followed by a gradual increase in degradation.[144] Rapid reversal of the synthetic defect was shown by refeeding in vivo, or by supplying the perfused liver with a high concentration of amino acids.[129,141,205,276] A quantitative relationship between the level of amino acid supply and the rate of total protein and albumin synthesis has been shown in the isolated perfused rat liver. There was a linear increase in protein synthesis with increase in amino acid supply up to five times normal plasma levels of total amino acids.[84] Total synthesis could be stimulated almost twofold by this manoeuvre. Interestingly, it was shown that amino acids released from endogenous protein degradation can sustain protein synthesis when exogenous supply is limited, confirming earlier data on the important role of degradation of constituent proteins in sustaining intracellular amino acid pools.[89]

The effects of repletion with amino acids differ depending on whether protein deprivation has been short-term or long-term. For example, low albumin and transferrin synthesis resulting from long-term deprivation of dietary protein in the rat may not be reversible by supplying amino acids to the isolated perfused rat liver at high concentrations.[330] In these circumstances short-term translational effects operating at the level of the polyribosome are probably reinforced by long-term and less rapidly reversible effects occurring at a transcriptional level. Indeed, the supply of ribosomal, messenger and transfer RNA may be rate-limiting in these circumstances[50,70,143,224] and longer periods of repletion are required for reversal of the effects of their deficiency. Another mechanism which has recently been described for the short-term control of protein synthesis by amino acid supply depends on the subcellular compartmentation of mRNA. Under normal circumstances 75–80% of the polyribosomes within the hepatocyte are associated with the RER. In response to protein deprivation there may be a shift of membrane-bound mRNA and associated ribosomes into the free cytosolic pool where the mRNA becomes untranslatable for export protein synthesis. This shift is reversible with protein feeding, and the balance between the two pools may provide a means for rapid modulation of protein synthesis in response to amino acid supply or other regulatory factors.[303,371]

Among essential amino acids, tryptophan has been shown to play a special role in regulating protein synthesis.[222,277,310,311] During starvation or protein deprivation the amount of tryptophan tRNA may be rate-limiting for the translation of mRNA. This may be because tryptophan is the least abundant amino acid in constituent protein, and, as indicated above, recycling of endogenous amino acids from degraded tissue protein becomes a means for sustaining protein synthesis in these circumstances. In addition to its unique effects on polypeptide translation, tryptophan also plays a role in the rate of synthesis of both mRNA and rRNA.[115,345] It has been shown recently that transcriptional control by tryptophan may be mediated by two important enzymes which regulate the translocation of RNA from the nucleus to the cytoplasm, protein phosphokinase and phosphoprotein phosphohydrolase. Tryptophan was shown to stimulate rapidly and specifically the activity of these two enzymes after a period of fasting.[226] Although it would be very unusual to find a unique deficiency of tryptophan in the context of protein malnutrition in man, rare situations have been described in which tryptophan has been diverted into unique metabolic pathways, resulting in protein wasting and hypoproteinaemia.[325]

Hormonal effects on protein synthesis

Hormonal influences on hepatic protein metabolism are closely integrated with nutritional effects, and their summation represents the combined effects on synthesis and degradation. It should be emphasized that conclusions drawn from in vitro studies of isolated organs, cells or cell-free systems do not take into account complex hormonal and nutritional interactions which occur as an integrated response to endocrine disturbances in vivo. However, it is useful to be aware of the predominant metabolic effects of the major hormones.

Insulin is an anabolic hormone for the synthesis of both constituent and secretory proteins. It is necessary for the maximal synthesis of albumin in isolated hepatocytes[60, 130] and in the isolated perfused rat liver.[134] It stimulates the synthesis of both soluble and secretory proteins in isolated hepatocytes[46] and it has translational effects on polyribosome structure and function.[240] It also plays a role in DNA synthesis during hepatic regeneration,[318] RNA synthesis[121a] and in the transcription of mRNA in the liver of rats with spontaneous, insulin-dependent diabetes.[131] In addition, it has an anticatabolic effect on the degradation of tissue proteins.[203,213] A fall in the insulin : glucagon ratio is observed in a number of clinical hypercatabolic/hypoanabolic states.[341,342] In these circumstances the effects of relative insulin deficiency may be reinforced by glucagon-induced degradation of protein and promotion of gluconeogenesis and ureagenesis.[103,198,199]

Corticosteroids have a stimulatory effect on hepatic protein synthesis at both transcriptional and translational levels.[52,65,71,128,134] Administration or excess secretion of corticosteroids in man is associated with increased synthesis and degradation of albumin.[36,271,272,321]

Physiological concentrations of thyroid hormones may have selective effects in stimulating the synthesis of certain liver-produced proteins.[117] In long-standing experimental hypothyroidism, the synthesis of both export and constituent proteins is depressed in a non-selective manner.[243] In vivo, triiodothyronine (T3) regulates a variety of mRNA species but several of these may be mediated by an indirect effect on the pituitary output of growth hormone. In certain cases, the combined action of T3 and growth hormone is required for maintenance of normal levels of mRNA, suggesting a complex multifactorial regulation of hepatic mRNAs.[159]

In summary, it is apparent that hormonal control of protein metabolism is complex, and in vivo other factors may complicate the outcome of endocrine disturbances, such as changes in nutrition and amino acid supply, and fluid distribution, as well as interaction between the rates of secretion of individual endocrine glands. In liver disease there may be abnormal synthesis or defective degradation of hormones or hormone-binding proteins, with the appearance in the circulation of a variety of abnormal desialylated binding glycoproteins.[179,180] Little is known about the role of these abnormal proteins

in regulating the effects of their hormone ligands on target organs.

Effects of alcohol on protein synthesis and secretion

The role of alcohol and its metabolites, and the interaction of alcohol with amino acid supply in influencing hepatic protein synthesis and secretion is complex. A number of recent reviews have helped to delineate the various controversies.[19,160,280,281,315,340] Unfortunately, the field remains confusing and contradictory and reviewers present their individual viewpoints of the controversial issues.

This section will attempt to synthesize the available information and to reconcile somewhat opposing views. All the original references from the various groups of workers will not be cited since they can be found in their respective reviews (see Chapter 34).

Four major areas of controversy have arisen in the course of the last two decades of research in this field. First, it is apparent that the effects of alcohol on protein metabolism are influenced by the type of experimental model used, namely whether alcohol is administered in vivo or in vitro to isolated organs or cells; and whether it is administered acutely or chronically before the measurement of protein synthesis and secretion. Second, there are the important issues of whether alcohol influences primarily synthesis or secretion, and the relative extent to which constituent or secretory proteins are affected. Third, there is a need to evaluate the evidence favouring mediation of the alcohol effect by alcohol itself or by its various metabolic products. Finally, newer areas of controversy concerning the mechanism of secretory defects are developing. In particular, recent biochemical and biophysical data on the interaction of alcohol and acetaldehyde with intracellular macromolecules offer exciting new insights into pathogenetic mechanisms.

Alcohol administered acutely in vitro to the isolated perfused liver, isolated hepatocytes and cell-free systems is associated with a fall in the synthesis of constituent and secretory proteins. This is due in part to the disaggregation of polyribosomes, and can be reversed or prevented by high concentrations of amino acids, in particular tryptophan and arginine, and by polyamines.[280] In regard to albumin synthesis and polyribosome disaggregation, there are many similarities between the effects of alcohol and that of a short-term fast.[281] Although 10 mmol/l concentrations of the aforementioned amino acids are capable of reversing the acute effects of either fasting or ethanol, they are not effective in preventing or reversing the effects of a combination of the two stresses, e.g. the acute administration of ethanol to the perfused liver from a fasted donor rabbit. It is probable that the inhibitory effect of ethanol can be accounted for by inhibition of specific amino-acyl tRNA synthetases, which leads to blockage of polypeptide chain elongation.[57] In contrast, the acute administration of alcohol in vivo results in inhibition of the appearance of secretory proteins, but no change in the synthesis of total hepatic constituent proteins.[160]

The chronic effects of alcohol are perhaps more relevant to alcoholic liver disease in man. Long-term administration of a diet containing at least 36% of the caloric intake as alcohol does not inhibit synthesis of either constituent or export proteins. On the contrary, total liver protein and intrahepatic albumin may be increased as a result of enhanced synthesis.[160] Molecular hybridization techniques provide supportive data for these observations, showing a significant increase in protein synthesis per unit weight of RNA, particularly in membrane-bound polyribosomes from chronically treated rats.[385] Associated with this increase in synthesis there is a defect in vivo in the secretory process, leading to retention of those proteins destined for export from the hepatocyte.[18] Although other workers have not been able to reproduce the secretory defect by exposing hepatocytes acutely to 100 mmol/l alcohol,[211] there is a great deal of accumulated evidence to show that glycoproteins, which form a major fraction of secreted proteins, are predominantly retained within the microsomal fraction of liver from rats acutely or chronically exposed to 10 mmol/l alcohol.[315,316,339] By means of fucose labelling of the carbohydrate moiety of glycoproteins, it has been shown that alcohol administration interferes with the final stages of secretion following incorporation of the terminal sugars in the Golgi complex.[316,348] The secretory defect has been used to explain the swelling of the hepatocyte due to accumulation of protein and water. While earlier reports suggest that alcohol inhibits lipoprotein synthesis and the incorporation of labelled glucosamine into the carbohydrate moiety of lipoproteins,[204] others have shown enhanced lipoprotein synthesis and secretion after both acute and chronic alcohol consumption, offering this as a partial explanation for the hyperlipaemia of the chronic alcoholic.[15,16]

The third question of the mediation of alcohol's effects on protein synthesis and secretion has been addressed by several groups of workers. Acetaldehyde at concentrations encountered in blood in vivo inhibits the synthesis of constituent proteins, and the glycosylation and secretion of exported glycoproteins.[160,280,281,315] Furthermore, the inhibition of alcohol oxidation to acetaldehyde by 4-methylpyrazole, an inhibitor of alcohol dehydrogenase, protects against the effects of alcohol, suggesting that acetaldehyde is an important mediator of the defects in protein synthesis in vitro and in vivo.[348] It should be noted that a protective effect can also be acquired by the use of agents which correct for alcohol-induced alterations in the redox state of the liver.

Finally, the pharmacological mechanism of alcohol-induced inhibition of secretion is a question of major importance. Chronic ethanol feeding has been reported to reduce cellular polymerized tubulin, leading to defective microtubular structure and function.[17,182] Other workers have been unable to find any alterations in the polymerization of tubulin in vitro by alcohol, while acetaldehyde caused impairment of polymerization only at high concen-

trations.[132] Quantitative morphometry has also failed to reveal any change in the number or structure of hepatic microtubules after chronic ethanol feeding,[26] raising questions about the functional relevance of changes in tubulin polymerization to the observed secretory defects produced by alcohol.

An alternative mechanism of injury which is currently being explored is the binding of alcohol metabolites to cellular macromolecules. Recent research has led to the development of a hypothesis for the role of acetaldehyde in the pathogenesis of liver injury. This hypothesis proposes that 'during ethanol oxidation in the liver, acetaldehyde forms stable adducts via binding to reactive lysine residue of preferential target proteins, resulting in selective functional impairment of these proteins, ultimately leading to liver cell injury'.[132] In vitro evidence supports the concept of differential susceptibility for the formation of stable adducts based on the reactivity of lysine residues in various intracellular proteins. In this regard it is interesting to note that the α-chain of tubulin is the preferential site of stable adduct formation, suggesting that in tubulin reactivity to acetaldehyde the α-chain may contain very selective target lysine residues. Other direct evidence for the formation of acetaldehyde–protein adducts in vivo has been provided by immunotransblot detection of an altered 37-kD cytosolic protein in the livers of alcohol-fed rats.[163,164] Functionally, the formation of stable adducts may explain alterations in a variety of cell trafficking phenomena, such as membrane assembly, protein secretion, and receptor-mediated endocytosis, in addition to long-term inhibition of important enzyme systems responsible for intermediary metabolism and xenobiotic degradation. Changes in cellular biosynthesis coupled with defects in protein degradation[63] (see below) and the possible damaging autoimmunological reactivity of neoantigens produced by the humoral response to acetaldehyde adducts formed in vivo[231] may play a role in initiating and perpetuating alcoholic liver injury. In spite of much accumulated evidence it is still premature to conclude that the formation of stable acetaldehyde adducts are the direct precursor of irreversible liver injury. To prove this hypothesis it will be necessary to demonstrate a clear-cut correlation between adduct formation and the specific function of the altered protein.

In summary, a perspective on the role of alcohol on hepatic protein metabolism reveals areas of consensus and areas of continued controversy. It is agreed that alcohol may have effects on diverse sites in the schema of protein synthesis and secretion, that derangements result from its metabolism or its metabolic products, and that protection may be offered by specific inhibitors of its metabolism or by nutritional means. Uncertainties remain with regard to its precise effects on secretion, to the mechanism of the secretory defects and to the pathogenesis of the architectural disorganization of the hepatocyte which may accompany the metabolic protein disturbances in alcohol-induced liver injury.

PROTEIN DEGRADATION _____

The liver, as befits an organ with a high rate of protein turnover, is equipped with a variety of efficient mechanisms for the degradation of both constituent and secreted proteins. First, the hepatocyte possesses several proteolytic mechanisms for the degradation of endogenous proteins, which make a major contribution to the supply of amino acids for other essential metabolic purposes in the postabsorptive intervals between meals. As will be discussed below, some of these are responsive to physiological regulators while others are not. Second, there are specific carbohydrate receptors on the hepatocyte plasma membrane which are potentially involved in the degradation of endogenous and exogenous glycoproteins. Third, Kupffer cells make a significant contribution to the overall degradative capacity of the liver. In addition to their propensity for phagocytosis of relatively large circulating particles, these macrophages are capable of intense proteolysis, lipolysis and carbohydrate breakdown of membrane constituents.[96] Fourth, export proteins may undergo proteolysis before completion of the secretory process. In some specialized examples (see below), this degradative step is only partial and is an obligatory prerequisite for the extracellular appearance of a secreted protein from a longer intracellular precursor molecule. In other situations, the secretory protein is completely destroyed within minutes of being synthesized.[28] In particular, when secretion is halted by microtubular inhibitors, retention of secretory products is followed by degradation.[97] This event is associated with fusion of lysosomes with secretory vesicles, a process termed 'crinophagy'. In physiological secretory proteolysis, limited degradation may take place in the trans-Golgi elements in a region called GERL (Golgi-endoplasmic reticulum-lysosome), where certain proteases are known to be located. Finally, there is considerable evidence for a mechanism of hepatic protein degradation which involves biliary secretion of protein. This mechanism has been postulated to consist of two hepatocytic pathways of biliary protein secretion: (i) a direct pathway of uptake, transport and secretion of intact protein into bile via endocytotic vesicles; and (ii) an indirect pathway involving fusion of vesicles with lysosomes of the GERL which may be responsible for sequestering and degrading macromolecules prior to secretion.[265] The following section will limit further discussion to the role of the liver in the degradation of endogenous proteins, and the receptor-mediated pathway of degradation of modified glycoproteins and the biliary secretion of proteins.

Degradation of endogenous proteins

More than 99% of constituent proteins of the liver are degraded by lysosomal proteases. These proteins have variable half-lives which are responsive to physiological regulators of proteolysis such as insulin, glucagon and amino acids. About 0.2% of hepatic proteins have ultrashort half-lives which are not susceptible to physiological

regulation. These are degraded by non-lysosomal mechanisms, possibly as a result of structural modifications which render them susceptible to proteolysis within the cytosol of the cell.[215]

On the basis of experiments in the rat, the liver rapidly loses a considerable fraction of its constituent protein in response to caloric deprivation. The high degree of sensitivity of the liver to gluconeogenic requirements enables it to precede muscle protein degradation in taking on responsibility for the liberation of amino acids during the postabsorptive period. This proteolysis can be inhibited by physiological portal venous concentrations of a selective group of amino acids comprising leucine, phenylalanine, tyrosine, tryptophan and glutamine. At three- to four-fold plasma concentrations these amino acids are also capable of blocking the catabolic action of glucagon.[251] Considerable evidence has been accumulated in recent years to indicate that the bulk of intracellular membrane and soluble cytosolic protein is degraded by a lysosomal pathway. Mortimore[215] has reviewed the evidence that hepatocytes can sequester and digest portions of their cytoplasm. Experimentally, this process of autophagy has been induced by nutritional and hormonal factors, e.g. starvation and glucagon, and can be inhibited by a number of lysosomotropic agents. Either these agents raise the lysosomal pH to a level which inhibits acid hydrolase activity (e.g. chloroquine or amines), or they are direct inhibitors of thiol or carboxyl proteinases (e.g. leupeptin or pepstatin). In either mechanism, their influence on protein turnover provides strong evidence that lysosomal autophagy plays a major role in accelerated rates of degradation. Correlation between the rate of release of valine from fixed protein and the aggregate volume of autophagic vacuoles is strongly indicative that the latter are the site of protein turnover.[296] This is reinforced by the finding that the size of sequestered intralysosomal protein pools is related directly to rates of protein degradation in basal and accelerated states.[214] Nevertheless, controversy does exist with regard to the mechanism of *basal* protein turnover. The wide range of rates of turnover of individual proteins can be explained by a flexible process of microautophagy in which variations in the size and binding activity of these small primary vesicles could yield diverse rates of degradation, depending on the spectrum of cytoplasmic and membrane-associated proteins entrapped by this process.[5] It is possible that basal proteolysis is composed of both a neutral and a complementary acidic lysosomal mechanism, which explains why lysosomotropic agents do not invariably influence basal turnover. In contrast, the inducible autophagic mechanism is recruited by nutritional and hormonal factors and plays a role in a number of hypercatabolic, pathological states.[10]

Receptor-mediated degradation of glycoproteins

The term 'receptor-mediated endocytosis' is used to describe the process of specific binding and internalization of macromolecules and/or associated ligands. For the liver in protein degradation, particular interest lies in the carbohydrate recognition system for receptor-mediated endocytosis of glycoproteins, as reviewed by Neufeld and Ashwell,[230] McFarlane,[188] Stockert and Morell,[323] Wileman et al.,[365] Stahl and Schwartz[317] and Steer and Ashwell.[319] Following removal of the terminal sialic acid and exposure of the penultimate galactose residues, plasma glycoproteins are rapidly endocytosed by the liver with subsequent lysosomal degradation. Hepatocytes possess saturable receptors specific for asialoglycoproteins (ASGP), which are internalized with bound protein, deliver the proteins to their lysosomal degradation site, and recycle intact to the plasma membrane of the cell. Additionally, there are other receptors which are particularly avid for ligand-binding glycoproteins which are transported in endocytotic vesicles to the biliary canaliculus for excretion in bile, or recycle as an intact glycoprotein–receptor complex to the sinusoidal surface of the cell after delivering the ligand to its site of utilization, a process termed diacytosis (see below). Both of these vesicular transport mechanisms effectively bypass lysosomal degradation. Finally, since the initial discovery of the galactose recognition system, a total of four carbohydrate recognition systems have been described in the liver. Galactose and fucose receptors appear to be confined to parenchymal cells, while receptors for N-acetylglucosamine and mannose have been identified in Kupffer cells. Although there is a large mass of information on all these processes we still lack insights into the physiological role of the ASGP-receptor pathway of degradation. For example, it is not known how and where glycoproteins are desialylated in vivo.

The current view of the sequence of events involved in the uptake and degradation of ASGPs has recently been summarized by Stockert and Morell;[323] additional references will be provided in this summary. Analysis of the receptor protein from rat hepatocytes has revealed it to be a glycoprotein composed of two non-identical subunits of M_r 48 000 and 42 000 and coded for by at least two genes.[66] Immune electron microscopic studies show that the highest surface density of receptors is on the sinusoidal face of the hepatocyte.[183] After initial binding of the ASGP to the receptor there is migration of the complex to clathrin 'coated pits' of the sinusoidal plasma membrane (Figure 5.2). Internalization ensues as the coated pits are pinched off to become coated vesicles. The site of dissociation of the receptor–ligand complex is thought to be in prelysosomal vesicles termed CURL (compartment of uncoupling of receptor and ligand)[34,93,111] by a mechanism involving a fall in pH. There is much evidence for recycling of the receptor to the plasma membrane and delivery of the ligand to the lysosomal compartment, as well as recent data to show that the receptor–ligand complex may recycle intact prior to dissociation on the internal surface of the hepatocyte.[363] At least two major pathways of fusion of the coated endocytotic vesicle with primary lysosomes lead to degra-

dation of the desialylated glycoprotein to carbohydrates and amino acid constituents.[47] However, a failure of acidification of the migrating endosome leads to trapping of the protein ligand in a prelysosomal compartment and inhibition of ASGP degradation.[112,366]

While receptor-mediated endocytosis undoubtedly exists as a specific catabolic pathway within hepatocytes for this special class of modified proteins, the physiological substrate and the function of the hepatic receptor remain unknown. It is intriguing that in patients with liver disease there may be abnormal levels of a heterogeneous group of circulating ASGPs[179,180] in association with an increase in the plasma concentration of polymeric IgA, which is a powerful competitive inhibitor of binding of ASGPs to the hepatic receptor protein.

Biliary excretion of proteins

In contradistinction to the degradative fate of the majority of desialylated glycoproteins which enter the intracellular pathway by the above route, a small component effectively bypasses the lysosomes and appears as intact protein in bile. A variety of specific vesicular active transport mechanisms exist which are responsible for the biliary excretion of both intact and degraded macromolecules. Quantitative autoradiography showed two pathways of vesicular transport in the hepatocyte.[264,265] In the first the endocytotic vesicle is transported directly to the canalicular membrane, while in the second vesicles containing labelled macromolecules are directed to the Golgi region and its associated system of lysosomes and endoplasmic reticulum (GERL) before fusing with the canalicular membrane (Figure 5.2). The appearance of labelled degradation products in bile is evidence that the second pathway may be responsible for sequestering and degrading macromolecules prior to biliary secretion or return to the circulation.[82,264,265,270] In effect, the first pathway is also a route of degradation for protein macromolecules as their appearance in the intestinal lumen leads to digestion by exocrine proteases in most instances.

The complexity of the biliary excretory pathway has been compounded as more individual proteins or protein degradation products have been discovered in bile. With current knowledge these can be divided into three groups.[221,267] First, there are plasma proteins which appear in bile at very low concentrations relative to their plasma levels. Their rate of transport from plasma to bile shows a direct relationship to their molecular weight.[335] It has been proposed that they reach the canaliculus by a non-receptor-mediated pathway involving a paracellular route from the peribiliary capillaries. Second, there are proteins which are present in bile at much higher concentrations relative to plasma. These utilize the specific receptor-mediated transcellular pathway described above. The best-studied examples of this group of proteins are polymeric and secretory IgA[121,218,265] in which the principal specific membrane receptor is secretory component,[220] and the haptoglobin–haemoglobin complex

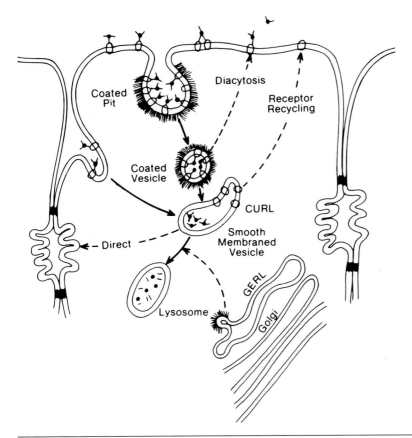

Figure 5.2 The stages and pathways of receptor-mediated endocytosis of asialoglycoproteins proposed by biochemical and morphological studies. Receptor (O) recognizes the ligand ⅄ at the plasma membrane, resulting in internalization of the receptor–ligand complex. This process occurs predominantly at the sinusoidal surface in coated regions, and occasionally at the lateral surface of the hepatocyte. The majority of the complex dissociates in prelysosomal vesicles (CURL) by a change to an acid pH, and the receptor recycles to the plasma membrane while the ligand enters the lysosomal compartment to be degraded. A small fraction of the ligand is excreted intact into bile (direct route) or returns, still bound to receptor, to the cell surface by *diacytosis*. (From Stockert and Morell[323] with kind permission of the authors and the American Association for the Study of Liver Diseases.)

(Hp.Hb)[119] for which a specific receptor has been isolated from the hepatocyte plasma membrane.[168] Other proteins, of relatively high molecular size, also show consistently higher concentration in bile relative to plasma concentrations. In addition to secretory IgA and hapto-globin–haemoglobin complexes, these include IgM, ceruloplasmin and β_2-glycoprotein-1. The accumulation of polymeric IgA in plasma in hepatobiliary disease has been explained by a combination of increased local production and decreased excretion by the biliary route.[44,64,149,156,266] Third, direct evidence has been provided for a lysosome-to-bile hepatic excretory pathway which may function as a route for the elimination of degradation products of endogenous and exogenous macromolecules.[151,152] Both this route and the specific transport pathway may be influenced profoundly by the administration of microtubule-modulating agents.[219,302] Paradoxically, colchicine may increase the biliary output of those proteins, which normally appear in bile in very low concentrations.[14,99] It has been suggested that disruption of the microtubular system at the sinusoidal face of the hepatocyte leads to the accumulation of secretory vesicles which are discharged spuriously into the biliary canaliculus under these circumstances. Finally, it should be noted that there are non-plasma proteins which may enter bile by the detergent action of bile salts on the membranes of the canalicular surface of the hepatocyte. The enzymes alkaline phosphodiesterase and 5′-nucleotidase are examples of such proteins.

In addition to the transcellular and paracellular routes for hepatic biliary protein secretion postulated above, a third route has been suggested by Sternlieb and Quintana[322] on the basis of ultrastructural and kinetic studies. The close anatomical association between peribiliary capillaries and bile ductular cells provides a means for efficient selective transport of macromolecules in the direction of the duct lumen.[374] So far this pathway has been demonstrated only for anterograde flow (plasma → ductular or ductal cell → bile). Attempts to induce retrograde trafficking through this pathway have failed, at least for sIgA.[135]

PATHOPHYSIOLOGY OF SPECIFIC LIVER-PRODUCED PROTEINS

This section will review aspects of metabolism of individual proteins of hepatic origin. These aspects include the control of gene expression; specific features of synthesis, secretion and degradation; and in certain instances the exploitation of disturbances in the above processes for the diagnosis and management of patients with liver disease. Wherever possible, references to comprehensive review articles are provided, with more recent original publications as additional source material. The reader is referred to the reviews for detailed earlier references.

ALBUMIN _____

Human plasma albumin is the most abundant circulating protein. It exists as a single polypeptide chain of 575 amino acid residues devoid of a significant carbohydrate component.[244,245] It is quantitatively the most important mediator of the plasma colloid osmotic pressure, and it also functions as the principal plasma transport protein for certain organic anions, cations, hormones, fatty acids and tryptophan. Evidence derived from experiments in hepatectomized animals, and from the isolated perfused liver, indicate that the liver is the exclusive site of biosynthesis of albumin. Rothschild et al.[279] have reviewed comprehensively the data on normal albumin metabolism in humans. A normal adult synthesizes and secretes about 120 mg kg^{-1} day^{-1} into a total exchangeable pool of 3.5–5.0 g/kg body weight, of which 38–45% is located intravascularly. The plasma albumin concentration varies between 35 and 45 g/l. Therefore, in a normal 70-kg male adult the liver synthesizes about 12 g of albumin into a total exchangeable pool of 300 g (120 g located intravascularly, 180 g extravascularly). In a steady metabolic state this synthesis is balanced by degradation of an equal amount of albumin at a multiplicity of sites (see below).

Two aspects of the molecular biology of albumin synthesis are worthy of special discussion. The first pertains to the role of a free or uncommitted pool of mRNA in the regulation of albumin synthesis. Such a pool may constitute a significant component of total designated RNA within the hepatocyte. This pool may be called on in times of need to promote increased protein synthesis. Although molecular hybridization techniques have shown that 98% of specific albumin mRNA is located in membrane-bound polyribosomes,[371] under conditions of starvation or protein deprivation there is a shift from the rough endoplasmic reticulum (RER) into the free cytosolic pool.[303,372] On refeeding or protein repletion there is a return of these albumin mRNA sequences to the RER, with an associated marked translational response. It is thought that modulation of this balance may provide a means for responding rapidly to a variety of nutritional and other regulatory factors.

The second important concept is so-called 'signal sequence' regulation, which is particularly well illustrated by the process of translation of albumin. The albumin molecule which is translated in the RER has 24 extra amino acids at the N-terminal end of the poypeptide. This is called preproalbumin, in which 18 of the 24 amino acids constitute the *signal* or *leader* sequence. This sequence is necessary for the vectorial transfer of nascent protein across the membrane of the RER. More precisely, a signal-recognition protein (SRP) acts as a messenger permitting the RER to recognize the signal sequence and thereby promote attachment of the ribosome to a 'docking' protein in the membrane.[195,355] The signal sequence is cleaved as the polypeptide chain is completed on the ribosome, leaving proalbumin to migrate from the RER to the Golgi, where the propeptide is removed. The intracellular precursor proalbumin has been identified by chromatographic techniques, and has been shown to have an N-terminal extension of five or six amino acids.[136,257,284,343] The conversion of proalbumin to plasma albumin probably takes place in the trans-Golgi elements of the GERL where the putative cleavage protease, cathepsin B, may be located.[232] The released free hexapeptide has been identified within the hepatocyte, and has been shown to exert a regulatory role in the rate of synthesis and release of albumin.[362] Regulation of the translation of plasma albumin can therefore potentially take place at many sites, but in particular the signal sequence site and the rate of cleavage of both the pre- and propeptides are feasible sites of control.

Although albumin is subjected to most of the non-specific regulatory mechanisms in protein synthesis and degradation which affect other secretory and constituent proteins, there are some factors which are thought to influence albumin metabolism disproportionately. For example, ornithine, an amino acid intermediate of the urea cycle, is not incorporated into protein but has a marked stimulatory effect on albumin synthesis by the isolated perfused liver. Ornithine is the immediate precursor of polyamines, substances which have been shown to exert protection against inhibition of albumin synthesis by alcohol and carbon tetrachloride. Oratz and co-workers[237] have provided evidence to show that ornithine stimulates albumin synthesis by promoting polyamine synthesis. Second, the liver responds to reduction in extracellular colloid osmotic pressure by increasing its rate of synthesis and secretion of albumin.[61,275] It is probable that the osmotic environment is modulated by relatively small changes in the concentration of osmotically active macromolecules in the restricted interstitial space of the liver.[272,273,274] These may in turn influence the rate of appearance of albumin at some point in the biosynthetic or secretory pathway.

Although the precise tissue sites of degradation of albumin are uncertain, analysis of kinetic data in man and experimental animals has suggested that catabolism takes place in close proximity to the circulating plasma pool. Recent more direct data using [^{14}C]sucrose labelled albumin, which allows the products of degradation to be retained at the site of catabolism, indicate that on a whole-organ basis the liver itself, muscle and kidney are the largest individual contributors, accounting for 7–10% each of total degradation.[373] Degraded albumin was found in all tissues, supporting the notion that all cells possess the capability to degrade proteins. Nevertheless, the highest rates occur in those organs with a partially discontinuous or fenestrated capillary endothelium which allows easy access to their cells.

Many patients with liver disease and hypoalbuminaemia have low rates of turnover of plasma albumin, even though the total exchangeable pool is not invariably reduced.[27,68,320,328,367] In these circumstances, it is thought that a reduction in the rate of hepatic albumin synthesis is the primary effect of the disease process, with a reduction in the fractional rate of degradation following secondarily.[328] Additionally, in patients with ascites there is an abnormal intravascular : extravascular distribution, with a greater proportion of the total albumin located in the extravascular compartment. In cirrhotics, newly synthesized albumin may not be released normally into plasma but may be lost at source directly into lymph and ascites.[386] In certain patients with ascites, albumin synthesis may be normal or elevated.[278] Hypoalbuminaemia in these patients probably reflects dilution by abnormal salt and water retention. Finally, if the experimental data reviewed above, pertaining to the effects of alcohol on the liver, are applicable to the patient with alcoholic liver disease, then it is possible that part of the defect in albumin appearance in the plasma reflects a primary defect in secretion rather than biosynthesis. It should be noted that in patients with non-alcoholic liver disease, e.g. chronic active hepatitis, hypoalbuminaemia may be associated with very low rates of albumin synthesis.[36] Although albumin synthesis could be selectively stimulated in these patients by appropriate corticosteroid therapy, there was little effect on plasma albumin concentration or intravascular pool size, attesting to the role of prednisone in simultaneously promoting protein degradation.

ALPHA-1-FETOPROTEIN[1,8] _____

The presence of circulating α-1-fetoprotein (AFP) is a manifestation of carcinofetal reversion, in which proliferating malignant cells recapitulate some of the phenotypic characteristics of developing fetal tissues. The molecular basis of this phenomenon is thought to be a derepression of fetal genomes which are normally repressed as differentiation occurs. AFP is a single-chain glycoprotein with M_r approximately 70 000 daltons containing about 4% carbohydrate. Based on the recently reported nucleotide sequence of human AFP mRNA, the complete sequence of the 590 amino acids in AFP has been deduced.[210] There is a 39% overall sequence homology with human albumin, but because of differences in the number of disulphide bridges there are differences in the secondary structures of the two proteins. Nevertheless, there are important developmental, genetic, structural and functional similarities, which reflect the likelihood that the genes for albumin and AFP have remained linked throughout their approximate 500 million years of evolution.[98, 148] Their relationship is based on previous and current work demonstrating in addition to sequence homology, similarities in their chemical and physical properties, in particular with regard to binding of bilirubin, fatty acids and other organic anions.[25,124]

AFP is synthesized predominantly by embryonic mammalian yolk sac and liver. Although there is a coordinated reciprocal relationship between the plasma levels of AFP and albumin in pre- and postnatal development, this does not appear to be based on a reciprocal expression of the two genes.[336] Therefore, although the AFP and albumin genes arose in evolution as a consequence of duplication of an ancestral gene, they are apparently modulated independently in committed cells. Similarly, there is no evidence for a reciprocal relationship between hepatic AFP mRNA and albumin mRNA during liver regeneration or carcinogenesis.[242,248,255,301] Interestingly, a human hepatocellular carcinoma derived from a male patient whose serum was HB_sAg and AFP positive, has been used to establish a cell line in culture since 1973. AFP was not expressed during cell culture in vitro, but when transplanted into athymic (nude) mice the xenograft expressed AFP production.[20] Furthermore, in this experimental situation, phenotypic expression was directly related to the rate of DNA replication and tumour mass.

About 80–90% of human hepatocellular carcinomas synthesize AFP, but the range of associated plasma AFP concentrations varies widely. The quantitative variation has necessitated the use of highly sensitive techniques for detection. The concentration of AFP is a function of factors in addition to the size of the tumour (see also Chapter 40). The nature of the carcinogen, the degree of differentiation of the tumour and the age of the patient all influence the level. Abnormal concentrations have been observed following acute hepatic injury of viral or toxic origin. It has been suggested that these reflect the regenerative response, but this may not occur after partial hepatectomy, indicating that a distinctive form of injury and regeneration is required to evoke derepression of the AFP genome.[9]

ALPHA-1-ANTITRYPSIN (α_1AT) (see Chapter 43) __

Genetic deficiency of the serine protease inhibitor, α_1AT is accompanied by the early onset of degenerative lung disease and in some cases by liver disease. α_1AT deficiency due to the homozygous PiZZ phenotype is associated with neonatal hepatitis, chronic active hepatitis, juvenile cirrhosis and primary hepatocellular carcinoma (PHC). Liver disease is usually evident only in phenotypes in which there is less than 15% of normal protease inhibitory activity in the plasma and exclusively in those genetic variants in which inclusion bodies are found within hepatocytes (see below).

α_1AT inhibits a variety of serine proteases by forming an inactive complex on a mole : mole basis with the enzyme. It is composed of a single polypeptide chain and three carbohydrates side chains (M_r 50 000). As with other secreted proteins, α_1AT is synthesized with an N-terminal signal peptide[39,105,106] which is cleaved during polypeptide propagation. Cotranslational glycosylation of the polypeptide backbone occurs in a stepwise fashion during intracellular transport.[344] The deficiency state which occurs in the homozygous PiZZ phenotype is associated with the production of the Z protein, in which glutamic acid is substituted for lysine in the 342 position. Since this mutation possesses normal protease-binding activity, an explanation has been sought for the low plasma α_1AT concentration in the PiZZ phenotype.

Increased degradation of the circulating Z protein has been excluded, so that either a decreased rate of synthesis or faulty processing are the two alternative explanations. No evidence has been found for a transcriptional defect in mRNA synthesis, and the Z mRNA is translated at a normal rate at least as far as the stage of core glycosylation.[21,74] In all likelihood the amino acid substitution at position 342 of the normal M protein causes a partial blockage in the processing or intracellular transport of the Z protein, subsequent to core glycosylation. This leads to deficient secretion of a functionally normal protein, with an anomalous primary sequence and lacking the full complement of terminal carbohydrate residues. As a consequence there is retention within the hepatocyte of the non-secretable protein. Ultrastructural studies of the liver in patients with α_1AT deficiency have correlated PAS positive granules with amorphous, proteinaceous material within dilated vesicles of the RER. Although these deposits are antigenically identical to α_1AT, they differ in carbohydrate content and amino acid sequence. It has been suggested that the failure to negotiate the normal secretory pathway leads to aggregation of the protein within the RER. It has been further speculated that the liver disease of α_1AT deficiency may be related to retention of α_1AT in the hepatocyte rather than to the associated plasma deficiency, because it occurs only in variants that produce inclusions and has not been reported in those, such as the S variant or PiNull variant, which give an isolated plasma deficiency without hepatic inclusions.[91]

Recently, data on the human α_1AT transgenic mouse model have been presented by two laboratories.[40,92] Both have succeeded in injecting genomic clones containing the Z mutation into mouse embryos, with subsequent expression of the mutant α_1AT mRNA. In those transgenic mice with a critical number of mutant genomic copies it was possible to demonstrate hepatocytes filled with PAS-positive globules of α_1AT antibody-reactive material. Geller and coworkers[92] showed a polymorphonuclear leucocyte response to the accumulated α_1AT, and they were also able to demonstrate perisinusoidal fibrosis and dysplastic changes in groups of hepatocytes in older transgenic animals. Carlson and coworkers[40] reported the association of the abnormal α_1AT-containing hepatocytes and inflammation with the presence of normal amounts of mouse α_1AT in the sera of their animals, supporting the view that liver damage is the result of the accumulation of the abnormal protein rather than the absence of a circulating protease inhibitor.

There is considerable evidence to show that α_1AT plays an important role in inhibiting natural tissue proteases.[41] The protein is a relatively small and polar molecule with ready access to interstitial fluids. The single reactive site of the molecule which is responsible for protease binding is situated around methionine 358. This reactive centre functions as a bait for the protease by mimicking the site of attack on a natural substrate (e.g. leucocyte elastase → elastin). While the methionine 358 is susceptible to attack by other cytotoxic mechanisms (e.g. free radical

oxidation) it can also be regenerated by met-O-peptide reductase activity in the tissues.[2] A rare mutant has been described in which substitution of arginine for methionine 358 converts α_1AT to antithrombin III.[238] The young boy possessing this mutant protein reacted normally to acute phase stimuli by increasing α_1AT synthesis. Unfortunately, the phenotypic response was a major increase in antithrombin activity, with resultant severe episodic bleeding. This illustrates the specificity of the reactive centre; methionine is the preferred cleavage site for leucocyte elastase, and arginine is the preferred cleavage site for thrombin, the target enzyme of antithrombin. α_1AT is therefore an ideally constructed molecule for the protection of tissues against naturally occurring proteases, and its deficiency may lead to uncontrolled enzymic attack particularly in the context of other inflammatory stimuli.

For this reason therapeutic strategies in α_1AT deficiency have been aimed primarily at restoring normal protease binding activity in the circulation. Encouraging results have been obtained by stimulating α_1AT synthesis with danazol, an impeded androgen, in heterozygotes with intermediate deficiency.[101] No apparent injurious effects were observed, which may in theory have been possible due to increased hepatic retention of non-secretable α_1AT. In homozygotes with severe deficiency, concentrations up to only 50 mg/dl were achieved. Since levels in excess of 80 mg/dl (normal 200 mg/dl) are needed to maintain normal protease–antiprotease homeostasis within the lung, it has not encouraged investigators to use this treatment for the prevention of lung disease. To date, only liver transplantation has succeeded in restoring normal plasma antiprotease activity, and in converting the recipient to the normal phenotype of the donor.[256]

COAGULATION FACTORS[262,324] (see Chapter 8)

The liver plays an integral role in haemostasis as both an organ of synthesis and one of degradation. It is responsible for the synthesis of most of the coagulation proteins, fibrinogen (factor I), prothrombin (factor II) and factors V, VII, IX and X. All except fibrinogen require vitamin K for synthesis and secretion in an activated form. The liver is also responsible for the synthesis and degradation of fibrinolytic factors, and for the clearance of activated clotting factors from the circulation. Recent data have confirmed that the liver synthesizes factor XII (Hageman factor).[287] Severe liver disease is associated with prolongation of the one-stage prothrombin time, which is a marker of the depressed synthesis of factors II, V, VII and X. It is unusual for fibrinogen levels to be significantly reduced unless the liver disease is complicated by disseminated intravascular coagulation.

Fibrinogen is a large dimeric protein, M_r approximately 340 000 composed of three non-identical polypeptide chains, Aα, Bβ and γ chains. Molecular cloning techniques have provided evidence for coordinated regulation of the three genes controlling the synthesis of the respective mRNAs for these chains.[53,54,138] Consequently, translation can proceed in parallel in response to a stimulus to fibrinogen synthesis providing that the hormonal milieu is optimal.[104,250,381] The stimulation of fibrinogen synthesis by defibrination or acute inflammation has led to the search for a putative humoral factor which acts as an intermediary messenger to the liver. As a result of inflammation the plasminolytic product of fibrinogen, fragment D, is greatly increased in the circulation, and this has been shown to be a transferable factor capable of stimulating the liver to synthesize fibrinogen.[23,85,146] Specific plasminolytic fragments of fibrinogen do not interact directly with the hepatocyte to stimulate fibrinogen synthesis, but rather they stimulate leucocytes in vivo in a dose-dependent manner to produce a potent hepatocyte-stimulating factor (HSF), which in turn acts on hepatocytes to increase the synthesis of fibrinogen and several other plasma proteins, including haptoglobin.[88,268]

Prothrombin is the protease precursor of thrombin, and is synthesized in the liver as a glycoprotein of M_r 72 000 consisting of a single polypeptide chain. As a secretory protein, prothrombin is characteristically synthesized as a hepatic precursor with an N-terminal extension or signal peptide. Both glycosylation and cleavage of the signal peptide probably occur as cotranslational events prior to release of the polypeptide chain from the ribosome. The biosynthesis of functionally active prothrombin requires a post-translational modification of ten glutamyl residues in the N-terminal domain of the molecule. This modification consists of carboxylation on the γ carbon to yield γ-carboxyglutamyl residues, which confer both metal-binding properties and coagulant activity.[161] The reaction requires vitamin K, molecular O_2 and CO_2, and an intact hepatic microsomal carboxylase system. Additional rate-limiting reactions which are essential to γ-carboxylation are reduction of vitamin K to vitamin K hydroquinone and its subsequent conversion to vitamin K 2,3-epoxide. These preliminary reactions are coupled to each other and to the final activation step of carboxylation.[150,351,352] The mechanism of regulation of prothrombin synthesis under vitamin K-replete conditions is not known with certainty. Fragments of prothrombin containing γ-carboxyglutamate residues produce a dose-dependent induction of prothrombin synthesis,[102] suggesting that synthesis may be regulated in vivo by products of degradation released during the coagulation process.

In contrast to fibrinogen, prothrombin and other coagulation proteins, the role of the liver in the synthesis of plasminogen has been uncertain until recently. Plasminogen is the precursor of the proteolytic enzyme plasmin, which is responsible for the dissolution of intravascular fibrin deposits. The decreased titre of plasma plasminogen in many patients with advanced cirrhosis suggests that the liver may be a major site of production. This has been confirmed in humans undergoing hepatic transplantation[258] and in hepatocyte cultures and the isolated perfused liver from experimental animals.[30,286]

In addition to the quantitative deficiency in the synthesis of coagulation and plasminolytic factors, patients with advanced liver disease may also manifest qualitative disturbances in the synthesis of fibrinogen and prothrombin which may contribute to a bleeding diathesis. For example, low-molecular-weight forms of fibrinogen may be found in the plasma which may represent partial degradation products of native fibrinogen.[165] In addition, functionally abnormal fibrinogens may be found which have a reduced clotting ability based on a defect in fibrin monomer polymerization.[241] These may be synthesized by the diseased liver or may be formed as a result of post-translational modifications after synthesis. How these modifications arise is unknown, but they may aggravate the clotting abnormalities of liver disease. Finally, while it is recognized that an abnormality of prothrombin biosynthesis contributes to the prolongation of the prothrombin time in acute and chronic liver disease, it is not always known to what extent this is due to impaired protein synthesis or to impaired γ-carboxylation. Certain patients with cirrhosis or hepatitis have impaired vitamin K-dependent carboxylation of prothrombin. Regardless of the prothrombin time, up to 90% of patients with liver disease may have detectable under-carboxylated prothrombin in their plasma, which is unresponsive to vitamin K.[29,51] As evidenced by the lack of correlation with prothrombin time, the inadequacy of vitamin K carboxylation appears to be unrelated to the severity of the liver disease. In contrast, the degree of aberrant protein synthesis has been shown to reach much higher levels in patients with primary hepatocellular carcinoma (PHC). Des-γ-carboxyprothrombin, an abnormal prothrombin, was detected in 91% of patients with biopsy-proven PHC at mean levels of 900 ng/ml, compared to levels of 10 ng/ml in patients with chronic active hepatitis.[162] There is clearly potential for the exploitation of this marker for the early detection of transition of chronic liver disease to PHC.[87,338]

IRON TRANSPORT AND STORAGE PROTEINS[6,7,108,113,223,225,332,369] (see Chapter 36) _____

The liver plays a major role in the maintenance of whole-body iron homeostasis by serving as the major storage organ for iron and as the principal site of synthesis of the plasma iron-transport protein, transferrin. Increases in hepatic storage iron content are brought about by sequestration of iron in a non-toxic form as ferritin. As requirements for iron for the synthesis of haem are increased at extrahepatic sites of haem synthesis, iron is released from ferritin to the free binding sites on plasma transferrin. In addition to transferrin-bound iron, the liver is also capable of uptake of iron in the form of haem–haemopexin, haemoglobin–haptoglobin and circulating ferritin. The complex interactions of hepatic and extrahepatic iron have been reviewed.[13]

The liver is the principal but not the exclusive site of transferrin synthesis. The elevated concentrations of plasma transferrin seen in iron deficiency reflect an increased rate of hepatic transferrin synthesis. An inverse correlation between levels of intrahepatic ferritin iron and hepatic transferrin synthesis suggests that the ambient storage iron exerts a negative feedback control on transferrin synthesis at a molecular level.[190,191,216] In other circumstances it has been shown that transferrin synthesis can be modulated without inducing significant changes in ferritin storage iron[90] and that an increase in storage iron to a level of iron overload does not alter transferrin synthesis, although secretion is inhibited.[59] It remains to be shown how other regulatory factors, e.g. oxygen supply, may influence a metabolically active subcompartment of hepatic iron such as the postulated iron transit pool, which is distinct from ferritin or other storage forms of iron. Although synthesis probably plays the predominant role in the regulation of transferrin concentrations in plasma, there are other situations, such as toxic or inflammatory disease, where enhanced degradation seems to be responsible for the observed reduction in plasma iron-binding capacity.

Transferrin-bound iron is the major physiological source of hepatic iron. Iron uptake from this source can take place by two mechanisms:[13] first by non-specific, non-saturable binding followed by fluid-phase endocytosis, and second by specific, saturable, receptor-mediated binding of ferric transferrin.[31] At high levels of plasma transferrin saturation associated with plentiful iron supply, the non-saturable pathway is operative, whereas at normal levels of transferrin saturation the receptor-mediated pathway is dominant. It has been estimated that each hepatocyte possesses between 37 000 and 66 000 specific receptors with a high affinity for diferric transferrin, that is transferrin with both its binding sites occupied by Fe^{3+}.[49,377,378,379] Interest has been expressed in the possible role of the hepatic transferrin receptor in hereditary haemochromatosis. Using a specific monoclonal antibody for the human transferrin receptor it has been shown that expression of the receptor on the surface of the hepatocyte is completely absent.[297] With adequate treatment of iron overload by phlebotomy, others have shown that the receptor is re-expressed.[167] This and other experimental evidence[298] suggests that there is a reciprocal relationship between transferrin receptor expression and the level of iron supply. The precise mediator of this physiological control is not known, nor can the effect of the down-regulation of the specific transferrin receptor on the other mechanisms of hepatic iron uptake be judged.

Following binding to the receptor, the evidence points to the uptake of the transferrin–iron–receptor complex into the interior of the hepatocyte by a process of endocytosis via clathrin-coated pits and vesicles.[31] A non-lysosomal endocytotic vesicle is formed and iron is released from transferrin when the pH is reduced below 5.5. Undegraded transferrin is quickly recycled to the exterior of the cell with its receptor by diacytosis. At the neutral pH of the cell surface the apotransferrin is released from the receptor to be reutilized for iron uptake at sites of iron absorption or other storage sites. The acidic endosome cycle provides a feasible explanation for the dissociation between iron donation and transferrin degradation, but remains to be demonstrated in its entirety for the normal hepatocyte.

Iron which is available to the hepatocyte in excess of requirements for utilization for haem synthesis or for the synthesis of iron-containing proteins is stored primarily as ferritin. In pathological iron overload, haemosiderin progressively becomes the predominant storage form of iron. Ferritin is a water-soluble macromolecule composed of 24 subunits with a total molecular weight of the protein moiety of 450 000 daltons. The microheterogeneity of tissue ferritins is based on varying proportions of heavy (H) and light (L) subunits. Each ferritin molecule can accommodate up to 4500 atoms of iron, with an average under physiological circumstances of about 2500–3000 atoms per molecule. Apoferritin synthesis occurs predominantly on free polyribosomes. Iron stimulates apoferritin biosynthesis,[67] with preferential promotion of the synthesis of L subunits, favouring the assembly of L-rich apoferritin protein shells.[32,249,364] Unassembled subunits are inhibitory to mRNA translation. Iron, by promoting assembly, removes this inhibition and allows mRNA to be efficiently translated,[356,357,383,384] probably through a specific iron-responsive element located in the 5′ untranslated portion of the ferritin messenger RNA.[42,154,155,282] Furthermore, iron produces an increase in the absolute and relative content of L-rich isoferritins, not only by stimulating protein synthesis but also by enhancing degradation of H-rich isoferritins and preferentially retarding the degradation of iron-rich L-rich isoferritins.[32,147]

Catabolism of hepatic ferritin occurs by two routes, a lysosomal route which predominates in Kupffer cells, and by non-lysosomal cytosolic proteolysis which predominates in normal hepatocytes. In iron overload the lysosomal pathway becomes operative in parenchymal cells, and within membrane-bound lysosomes the protein component of ferritin is digested by hydrolytic enzymes, leaving the stable ferric hydroxide core and denatured protein. The resulting conglomerate, haemosiderin, is an insoluble, amorphous deposit containing protein without a defined composition, and ferric hydroxide polymers which may undergo specific structural changes with various forms of iron overloading.[172] Changes in the structure of ferritin as it ages and fills with iron may be the trigger for its uptake by lysosomes.[122,123] In conditions of hepatic iron overload there is evidence that the haemosiderin content of the liver is increased to a greater extent than the ferritin content, suggesting that the lysosomal pathway of degradation is induced at critical levels of intracellular ferritin.[22,300]

In comparison with tissue ferritin, circulating serum ferritin is present in minute concentrations and contains relatively little iron. This suggests that the protein does not reach the plasma in normal circumstances by leakage from damaged cells. Rather, it is possible that it is synthesized on membrane-bound polyribosomes, and may be subjected to some degree of regulation by iron supply even though iron is not incorporated into the protein. Serum ferritin has been used as a diagnostic screening procedure for iron overload syndromes in many laboratories[253] and it has shown excellent correlation with hepatic iron stores measured by other means. States other than iron overload can cause an elevated serum ferritin level. For example, hepatocellular necrosis, inflammation, malignant neoplasms and lymphomas may lead to excess secretion or release of ferritin into the circulation. As evidenced by studies of experimentally induced hepatic necrosis, the serum ferritin in these circumstances contains higher iron concentrations and probably reflects leakage from damaged cells.[389] Although correction for the degree of necrosis in liver disease does yield a better correlation between serum ferritin and liver iron stores,[254] in patients with primary haemochromatosis and excess alcohol ingestion serum ferritin is a reliable indicator of liver iron stores only in the absence of active liver disease.[45]

Serum and tissue isoferritin patterns change with iron status in patients with primary haemochromatosis and these are reversible by effective phlebotomy therapy.[109, 252] Marked differences exist in turnover of the various circulating isoferritins. Labelled human serum ferritin has a slow rate of clearance, with a plasma half-life of between 27 and 30 hours,[370] whereas spleen ferritin disappears from the circulation within minutes.[55] It has been suggested that the difference in turnover may reflect the relative content of H and L subunits, the degree of iron accretion in the central core of the apoferritin shell, or the extent of glycosylation of the protein subunits (normal serum ferritin has a higher carbohydrate content). In some way these may play a role in regulating the uptake of circulating ferritin at sites of degradation. Indeed, the identification of a specific ferritin receptor on hepatocytes may provide an explanation for the rapid removal of tissue ferritin from the circulation.[169]

SUMMARY

The liver plays a central role in body protein metabolism. As a major processor of amino acids derived from dietary protein and from the degradation of endogenous proteins, it has a vital role in regulating the flux of amino acids amongst tissues and in overall nitrogen balance. Both constituent and secretory proteins are in a state of dynamic equilibrium with the free amino acid pool of the body, and their turnover is subject to influences by nutritional and hormonal factors, some of which may be severely disturbed in patients with liver disease. Based on newer insights into abnormalities of amino acid and protein metabolism, innovative strategies are being devised for the correction or prevention of protein wasting in liver disease. A wealth of new information has been acquired on the regulation of protein turnover at a cellular level. The role of amino acid supply in hepatic protein synthesis and degradation has been defined with greater precision, while the effects of alcohol on protein secretion in particular have been further elucidated. Exciting new data have been reviewed on the role of the lysosome in the degradation of both exogenous and endogenous proteins, while the elucidation of the receptor-mediated pathways for uptake and degradation of modified glycoproteins offers promise for better understanding of the role of the liver in the regulation of protein degradation in general. Finally, the study of specific secretory proteins has pointed to the role of molecular modifications in the regulation of synthesis, secretion and degradation. Knowledge of specific molecular features of certain proteins which have been altered by abnormal gene control, disease, drugs and alcohol has offered insights into pathogenesis, diagnosis or treatment of various congenital or acquired liver diseases.

Acknowledgements

This work was supported in part by Grants DK 31505 and DK 39527 from the National Institutes of Health. We would like to express our appreciation to Jane Shantery and Joyce McCrory for expert secretarial assistance.

REFERENCES

1. Abelev, G.I. (1989) Alpha-fetoprotein: 25 years of study (Review). *Tumour Biology*, **10**, 63–74.
2. Abrams, W.R., Weinbaum, G., Weissbach, L. *et al.* (1981) Enzymatic reduction of oxidized α-1-proteinase inhibitor restores biological activity. *Proceedings of the National Academy of Sciences of the USA*, **78**, 7483–7486.
3. Achord, J.L. (1987) Malnutrition and the role of nutritional support in alcoholic liver disease. *American Journal of Gastroenterology*, **82**, 1–7.
4. Achord, J.L. (1987) A prospective clinical trial of peripheral amino acid-glucose supplementation in acute alcoholic hepatitis. *American Journal of Gastroenterology*, **82**, 871–875.
5. Ahlberg, J., Marzella, L. & Glaumann, H. (1982) Uptake and degradation of proteins by isolated rat liver lysosomes. Suggestions of a microautophagic pathway of proteolysis. *Laboratory Investigation*, **47**, 523–532.
6. Aisen, P. & Brown, E.G. (1977) The iron-binding function of transferrin in iron metabolism. *Seminars in Hematology*, **14**, 31–53.
7. Aisen, P. & Listowsky, I. (1980) Iron transport and storage proteins. *Annual Review of Biochemistry*, **49**, 357–393.
8. Alpert, E. (1976) Human alpha-1-fetoprotein. In Popper, H. & Schaffner, F. (eds) *Progress in Liver Diseases*, Vol. 5, pp. 337–349. New York: Grune & Stratton.
9. Alpert, E. & Feller, E.R. (1978) α-Fetoprotein (AFP) in benign liver disease. Evidence that normal liver regeneration does not induce AFP synthesis. *Gastroenterology*, **74**, 856–858.
10. Amenta, J.S. & Brocher, S.C. (1981) Minireview: Mechanisms of turnover in cultured cells. *Life Sciences*, **28**, 1195–1208.
11. Andus, T., Gross, V., Tran-Thi, T.A. *et al.* (1983) The biosynthesis of acute-phase proteins in primary cultures of rat hepatocytes. *European Journal of Biochemistry*, **133**, 561–571.
12. Azhar, S., Hwang, S.F. & Reaven, E.P. (1983) Effect of antimicro-

tubule agents on terminal glycosyltranferases and other enzymes associated with rat liver subcellular fractions. _Biochemical Journal_, **212**, 721–731.

13. Bacon, B.R. & Tavill, A.S. (1984) The role of the liver in normal iron metabolism. _Seminars in Liver Disease_, **4**, 181–192.

14. Barnwell, S.G. & Coleman, R. (1983) Abnormal secretion of proteins into bile from colchicine-treated isolated perfused rat livers. _Biochemical Journal_, **216**, 409–414.

15. Baroana, E. & Lieber, C.S. (1970) Effects of chronic ethanol feeding on serum lipoprotein metabolism in the rat. _Journal of Clinical Investigation_, **49**, 769–778.

16. Baroana, E., Pirola, R.C. & Lieber, C.S. (1973) Pathogenesis of postprandial hyperlipemia in rats fed ethanol-containing diets. _Journal of Clinical Investigation_, **52**, 296–303.

17. Baroana, E., Leo, M.A., Borowsky, S.A. & Leiber, D.S. (1977) Pathogenesis of alcohol-induced accumulation of protein in the liver. _Journal of Clinical Investigation_, **60**, 546–554.

18. Baroana, E., Pikkarainen, P., Salaspuro, M. _et al._ (1980) Acute effects of ethanol on hepatic protein synthesis and secretion in the rat. _Gastroenterology_, **79**, 104–111.

19. Baroana, E. & Lieber, C.S. (1982) Effects of alcohol on hepatic transport of proteins. _Annual Review of Medicine_, **33**, 281–292.

20. Bassendine, M.F., Wright, N.A., Thomas, H.C. & Sherlock, S. (1983) Growth characteristic of α-foetoprotein-secretory human hepatocellular carcinoma in athymic (nude mice). _Clinical Science_, **64**, 643–648.

21. Bathurst, I.C., Stenflo, J., Errington, D.M. & Carrell, R.W. (1983) Translation and processing of normal (PiMM) and abnormal (PiZZ) human α₁-antitrypsin. _FEBS Letters_, **153**, 270–274.

22. Beaumont, C., Simon, M., Smith, P.M. & Worwood, M. (1980) Hepatic and serum ferritin concentrations in patients with idiopathic hemochromatosis. _Gastroenterology_, **79**, 877–883.

23. Bell, W.R., Kessler, C.M. & Townsend, R.R. (1983) Stimulation of fibrinogen biosynthesis by fibrinogen fragments D and E. _British Journal of Haematology_, **53**, 599–610.

24. Bennett, G. & O'Shaughnessy, D. (1981) The site of incorporation of sialic acid residues into glycoproteins and the subsequent fates of these molecules in various rat and mouse cell types as shown by radioautography after injection of [³H]_N_-acetylmannosamine. _Journal of Cell Biology_, **88**, 1–15.

25. Berde, C.B., Nagai, M. & Deutsch, H.F. (1979) Human α-fetoprotein: fluorescent studies on binding and proximity relationships for fatty acids and bilirubin. _Journal of Biological Chemistry_, **254**, 12609–12614.

26. Berman, W.J., Gil, J., Jennett, R.B. _et al._ (1983) Ethanol, hepatocellular organelles, and microtubules. A morphometric study in vivo and in vitro. _Laboratory Investigation_, **48**, 760–767.

27. Berson, S.A. & Yalow, R.S. (1954) The distribution of I¹³¹-labelled human serum albumin introduced into ascitic fluid: analysis of the kinetics of a three compartment quaternary transfer system in man and speculation on possible sites of degradation. _Journal of Clinical Investigation_, **33**, 377–387.

28. Bienkowski, R.S. (1983) Review article: Intracellular degradation of newly synthesized secretory proteins. _Biochemical Journal_, **214**, 1–10.

29. Blanchard, R.A., Furie, B.C., Jorgensen, J. _et al._ (1981) Acquired vitamin K-dependent carboxylation deficiency in liver disease. _New England Journal of Medicine_, **305**, 242–248.

30. Bohmfalk, J.F. & Fuller, G.M. (1980) Plasminogen is synthesized by primary cultures of rat hepatocytes. _Science_, **209**, 408–410.

31. Bomford, A.B. & Munro, H.N. (1985) Transferrin and its receptor: their roles in cell function. _Hepatology_, **5**, 870–875.

32. Bomford, A., Conlon-Hollingshead, C. & Munro, H.N. (1981) Adaptive responses of rat tissue isoferritins to iron administration. Changes in subunit synthesis, isoferritin abundance and capacity for iron storage. _Journal of Biological Chemistry_, **256**, 948–955.

33. Borghi, L., Novarini, A., Ghinelli, F. _et al._ (1982) Preliminary report on nutritional effects of α-ketoacids in chronic hepatic and renal failure. _Journal of Parenteral and Enteral Nutrition_, **6**, 328.

34. Breitfield, P.P., Simmons, C.F., Jr. & Strous, G.J.A.M. (1985) Cell biology of the asialoglycoprotein receptor system: a model of receptor-mediated endocytosis. _International Review of Cytology_, **97**, 47.

35. Cabre, E., Gonzalez-Huix, F., Abad-Lacruz, A. _et al._ (1990) Effect of total enteral nutrition on the short-term outcome of severely malnourished cirrhotics. A randomized controlled trial. _Gastroenterology_, **98**, 715–720.

36. Cain, G.D., Mayer, G. & Jones, E.A. (1970) Augmentation of albumin but not fibrinogen synthesis by corticosteroids in patients with hepatocellular disease. _Journal of Clinical Investigation_, **49**, 2198–2204.

37. Carey, D.J. & Hirschberg, C.B. (1981) Kinetics of glycosylation and intracellular transport of sialoglycoproteins in mouse liver. _Journal of Biological Chemistry_, **255**, 4348–4354.

38. Carey, D.J. & Hirschberg, C.B. (1981) Topography of sialoglycoproteins and sialyltransferases in mouse and rat liver Golgi. _Journal of Biological Chemistry_, **256**, 989–993.

39. Carlson, J. & Stenflo, J. (1982) The biosynthesis of rat α₁-antitrypsin. _Journal of Biological Chemistry_, **257**, 12987–12994.

40. Carlson, J.A., Rogers, B.B., Sifers, R.N. _et al._ (1989) Accumulation of PiZ α-1-antitrypsin causes liver damage in transgenic mice. _Journal of Clinical Investigation_, **83**, 1183–1190.

41. Carrell, R.W., Jeppsson, J.O., Laurell, C.B. _et al._ (1982) Structure and variation of human α₁-antitrypsin. _Nature_, **298**, 329–334.

42. Casey, J.L., Hentze, M.W., Koeller, D.M. _et al._ (1988) Iron-responsive elements: regulatory RNA sequences that control mRNA levels and translation. _Science_, **240**, 924–928.

43. Cerra, F.B., McMillen, M., Angelico, R. _et al._ (1983) Cirrhosis, encephalopathy, and improved results with metabolic support. _Surgery_, **94**, 612–619.

44. Chandy, K.G., Hubscher, S.G., Elias, E. _et al._ (1983) Dual role of the liver in regulating circulating polymeric IgA in man: studies on patients with liver diseases. _Clinical and Experimental Immunology_, **52**, 207–218.

45. Chapman, R.W., Morgan, M.Y., Laulicht, M. _et al._ (1982) Hepatic iron stores and markers of iron overload in alcoholics and patients with idiopathic hemochromatosis. _Digestive Diseases and Sciences_, **27**, 909–916.

46. Clark, R.L. & Hansen, R.J. (1980) Insulin stimulates synthesis of soluble proteins in isolated rat hepatocytes. _Biochemical Journal_, **190**, 615–619.

47. Clarke, B.L., Oka, J.A. & Weigel, P.H. (1987) Degradation of asialoglycoproteins mediated by the galactosyl receptor system in isolated hepatocytes: Evidence for two parallel pathways. _Journal of Biological Chemistry_, **262**, 17284.

48. Cohen, S. & Hansen, J.D.L. (1962) Metabolism of albumin and γ-globulin in kwashiorkor. _Clinical Science_, **23**, 351–359.

49. Cole, E.S. & Glass, J. (1983) Transferrin binding and iron uptake in mouse hepatocytes. _Biochimica et Biophysica Acta_, **762**, 102–110.

50. Conde, R.D. & Franze-Fernandez, M.T. (1980) Increased transcription and decreased degradation control the recovery of liver ribosomes after a period of protein starvation. _Biochemical Journal_, **192**, 935–940.

51. Corrigan, J.J., Monette, J. & Earnest, D.L. (1982) Prothrombin antigen and coagulant activity in patients with liver disease. _Journal of the American Medical Association_, **248**, 1736–1739.

52. Cox, R.F. & Matthias, A.P. (1969) Cytoplasmic effects of cortisol in liver. _Biochemical Journal_, **115**, 777–787.

53. Crabtree, G.R. & Kant, J.A. (1981) Molecular cloning of cDNA for the α, β and γ chains of rat fibrinogen. A family of coordinately regulated genes. _Journal of Biological Chemistry_, **256**, 9718–9723.

54. Crabtree, G.R. & Kant, J.A. (1982) Coordinate accumulation of the mRNA's for the α, β and γ chains of rat fibrinogen following defibrination. _Journal of Biological Chemistry_, **257**, 7277–7279.

55. Cragg, S.J., Corell, A.M., Burch, A. _et al._ (1983) Turnover of ¹³¹I-human spleen ferritin in plasma. _British Journal of Haematology_, **55**, 83–92.

56. Daniel, P.M., Pratt, O.E. & Spargo, E. (1977) The metabolic homeostatic role of muscle and its function as a store of protein. _Lancet_, **2**, 446–448.

57. David, E.T., Fischer, I. & Moldave, K. (1983) Studies on the effect of ethanol on eukaryotic protein synthesis in vitro. _Journal of Biological Chemistry_, **258**, 7702–7706.

58. Denton, A.E. & Elvehjem, C.A. (1954) Amino acid concentration in the portal vein after ingestion of amino acids. _Journal of Biological Chemistry_, **206**, 455–460.

59. Desverne, B., Baffet, G., Loyer, P. _et al._ (1989) Chronic iron overload inhibits protein secretion by adult rat hepatocytes main-

tained in long-term primary culture. *European Journal of Cell Biology*, **49**, 162–170.

60. Dich, J. & Gluud, C.N. (1975) Effect of insulin on albumin production and incorporation of [¹⁴C]leucine into proteins in isolated parenchymal liver cells from normal rats. *Acta Physiologica Scandinavica*, **94**, 236–243.

61. Dich, J., Hansen, S.E. & Thieden, H.D. (1973) Effect of albumin concentration and colloid osmotic pressure on albumin synthesis in the perfused rat liver. *Acta Physiologica Scandinavica*, **89**, 352–358.

62. Diehl, A.M., Boitnott, J.K., Herlong, H.F. *et al.* (1983) Effect of parenteral amino acid supplementation in alcoholic hepatitis. *Hepatology*, **5**, 216–220.

63. Donohue, T.M. Jr, Zetterman, R.K. & Tuma, D.H. (1989) Effect of chronic ethanol administration on protein catabolism in rat liver. *Alcoholism (NY)*, **13**, 498–57.

64. Dooley, J.S., Potter, B.J., Thomas, H.C. & Sherlock, S. (1982) A comparative study of the biliary secretion of human dimeric and monomeric IgA in the rat and man. *Hepatology*, **2**, 323–327.

65. Drews, J. & Braverman, G. (1976) Alterations in the nature of ribonucleic acid synthesized in rat liver during regeneration and after cortisol administration. *Journal of Biological Chemistry*, **242**, 801–808.

66. Drickamer, K., Mamon, J.F., Binns, G. & Leung, J.O. (1984) Primary structure of the rat liver asialoglycoprotein receptor. Structural evidence for multiple polypeptide species. *Journal of Biological Chemistry*, **259**, 770–778.

67. Drysdale, J.W. & Shafritz, D.A. (1975) In vitro stimulation of apoferritin synthesis by iron. *Biochemica et Biophysica Acta*, **383**, 97–105.

68. Dykes, P.W. (1968) The rates of distribution and catabolism of albumin in normal subjects and in patients with cirrhosis of the liver. *Clinical Science*, **34**, 161–183.

69. Elwyn, D.H. (1970) The role of the liver in regulation of amino acid and protein metabolism. In Munro, H.M. (ed.) *Mammalian Protein Metabolism*, Vol. IV, pp. 523–558. New York: Academic Press.

70. Enwonwu, C.O. & Munro, H.N. (1970) Rate of RNA turnover in rat liver in relation to intake of protein. *Archives of Biochemistry and Biophysics*, **138**, 532–539.

71. Enwonwu, C.O. & Munro, H.N. (1971) Changes in liver polyribosome patterns following administration of hydrocortisone and actinomycin. *Biochemica et Biophysica Acta*, **238**, 264–276.

72. Eriksson, L.S. & Conn, H.O. (1989) Branched-chain amino acids in the management of hepatic encephalopathy: An analysis of variants (Special article). *Hepatology*, **10**, 228–246.

73. Ericksson, L.S., Hagenfeldt, L. & Wahren, J. (1982) Intravenous infusion of α-oxoisocaproate: influence on amino acid and nitrogen metabolism in patients with liver cirrhosis. *Clinical Science*, **62**, 285–293.

74. Errington, D.M., Bathurst, I.C., Janus, E.D. & Carrell, R.W. (1982) In vitro synthesis of M and Z forms of human α1-antitrypsin. *FEBS Letters*, **148**, 83–86.

75. Fauconneau, G. & Michel, M.C. (1970) The role of gastrointestinal tract in the regulation of protein metabolism. In Munro, H.N. (ed.) *Mammalian Protein Metabolism*, Vol. IV, pp. 481–522. New York: Academic Press.

76. Feldmann, G., Penaud-Laurencin, J., Grassous, J. & Benhamou, J.P. (1972) Albumin synthesis by human liver cells: its morphological demonstration. *Gastroenterology*, **63**, 1036–1048.

77. Feldmann, G., Maurice, M., Sapin, C. & Benhamou, J.P. (1975) Inhibition by colchicine of fibrinogen translocation in hepatocytes. *Journal of Cell Biology*, **67**, 237–243.

78. Felig, P. (1973) The glucose-alanine cycle. *Metabolism*, **22**, 179–207.

79. Felig, P. (1975) Amino acid metabolism in man. *Annual Review of Biochemistry*, **44**, 933–955.

80. Felig, P., Wahren, J., Sherwin, R. & Palaiologos, G. (1977) Amino acid and protein metabolism in diabetes mellitus. *Archives of Internal Medicine*, **137**, 507–513.

81. Fern, E.B., Garlick, P.J., McNurlan, M.A. *et al.* (1981) The excretion of isotope in urea and ammonia for estimating protein turnover in men with [¹⁵N]glycine. *Clinical Science*, **61**, 217–228.

82. Finck, M.H., Reichen, J., Vierling, J.M. *et al.* (1985) Hepatic uptake and disposition of human polymeric IgA, in perfused rat liver: evidence for incomplete biliary excretion and intrahepatic degradation. *American Journal of Physiology*, **148**, G450–G455.

83. Fischer, J.E., Rosen, H.M., Ebeid, A.M. *et al.* (1976) The effect of normalization of plasma amino acids on hepatic encephalopathy in man. *Surgery*, **80**, 77–91.

84. Flaim, K.E., Peavy, D.E., Everson, W.V. & Jefferson, L.S. (1982) The role of amino acids in the regulation of protein synthesis in perfused rat liver. I. Reduction in rates of synthesis resulting from amino acid deprivation and recovery during flow-through perfusion. *Journal of Biological Chemistry*, **257**, 2939–2938.

85. Franks, J.J., Kirsch, R.E., Frith, L.O'C. *et al.* (1981) Effect of fibrinogenolytic products D and E on fibrinogen and albumin synthesis in the rat. *Journal of Clinical Investigation*, **67**, 575–580.

86. Freund, H., Dienstag, J., Lehrich, J. *et al.* (1982) Infusion of branched chain enriched acid solution in patients with hepatic encephalopathy. *Annals of Surgery*, **196**, 109–220.

87. Friedman, P.A. (1984) Editorial: Vitamin K-dependent proteins. *New England Journal of Medicine*, **310**, 1458–1460.

88. Fuller, G.M., Otto, J.M., Woloski, B.M. *et al.* (1985) The effects of hepatocyte simulating factor on fibrinogen synthesis in hepatocyte monolayers. *Journal of Cell Biology*, **101**, 1481.

89. Gan, J.C. & Jeffay, H. (1967) Origins and metabolisms of the intracellular amino acid pools in rat liver and muscle. *Biochimica et Biophysica Acta*, **148**, 448–459.

90. Gardiner, M.E. & Morgan, E.H. (1981) Effect of reduced atmospheric pressure and fasting on transferrin synthesis in the rat. *Life Sciences*, **29**, 1641–1648.

91. Garver, R.I., Jr, Nornex, J.-F., Nukiwa, T. *et al.* (1986) Alpha-1-antitrypsin deficiency and emphysema caused by homozygous inheritance of non-expressing alpha-1-antitrypsin genes. *New England Journal of Medicine*, **314**, 762–766.

92. Geller, S.A., Nichols, W.S., Dycaico, M.J. *et al.* (1990) Histopathology of α-antitrypsin liver disease in a transgenic mouse model. *Hepatology*, **12**, 40–47.

93. Geuze, H.J., Slot, J.W., Strous, G.J.A.M. *et al.* (1983) Intracellular site of asialoglycoprotein receptor-ligand uncoupling: double-label immunoelectron microscopy during receptor-mediated endocytosis. *Cell*, **32**, 277–287.

94. Gersovitz, M., Munro, H.N., Udall, J. & Young, V.R. (1980) Albumin synthesis in young and elderly subjects using a new stable isotope methodology: Response to level of protein uptake. *Metabolism*, **29**, 1075–1086.

95. Glaumann, H. & Ericsson, J.L.E. (1970) Evidence for the participation of the Golgi apparatus in the intracellular transport of nascent albumin in the liver cell. *Journal of Cell Biology*, **47**, 555–567.

96. Glaumann, H. & Marzella, L. (1981) Degradation of membrane components by Kupffer cell lysosomes. *Laboratory Investigation*, **45**, 479–490.

97. Glaumann, H., Sandberg, P.O. & Marzella, L. (1982) Degradation of secretory content in Golgi-enriched fractions from rat liver after vinblastine administration. *Experimental Cell Research*, **140**, 201–213.

98. Godbout, R., Ingram, R. & Tilghman, S.M. (1986) Multiple regulatory elements in the intergenic region between the α-fetoprotein and albumin genes. *Molecular Cell Biology*, **6**, 477.

99. Godfrey, P.P., Lembra, L. & Coleman, R. (1982) Effects of colchicine and vinblastine on output of proteins into bile. *Biochemical Journal*, **208**, 153–157.

100. Goldberg, A.L. & Tischler, M.E. (1981) Regulatory effects of leucine on carbohydrate and protein metabolism. In Walser, M. & Williamson, J.R. (eds) *Metabolism and Clinical Implications of Branched-chain Amino and Keto Acids*, p. 205. New York: Elsevier.

101. Gradek, J.E., Fulmer, J.D., Gelfand, J.A. *et al.* (1980) Danazol-induced augmentation of serum α1-antitrypsin levels in individuals with marked deficiency of this antiprotease. *Journal of Clinical Investigation*, **66**, 82–87.

102. Graves, C.B., Munns, T.W., Carlisle, T.L. *et al.* (1981) Induction of prothrombin synthesis by prothrombin fragments. *Proceedings of National Academy of Sciences of the USA*, **78**, 4772–4776.

103. Green, M. & Miller, L.L. (1960) Protein catabolism and protein synthesis in perfused livers of normal and alloxan-diabetic rats. *Journal of Biological Chemistry*, **235**, 3202–3208.

104. Grieninger, G., Oddoux, C., Diamond, L. *et al.* (1989) Regulation of fibrinogen synthesis and secretion by the chicken hepatocyte. *Annals of the New York Academy of Sciences*, **557**, 15707.

105. Gross, V., Geiger, T., Tran-Thi, T.A. *et al.* (1982) Biosynthesis and secretion of α1-antitrypsin in primary cultures of rat hepatocytes. *European Journal of Biochemistry*, **129**, 317–323.

106. Gross, V., Kaiser, C., Tran-Thi, T.A. *et al.* (1983) N-terminal amino acid sequences of precursor and mature forms of α-1-antitrypsin. *FEBS Letters*, **151**, 201–205.

107. Halliday, D. & McKeran, R.O. (1975) Measurement of muscle protein synthetic rate from serial muscle biopsies and total body protein turnover in man by continuous intravenous infusion of L-[^{15}N]lysine. *Clinical Science and Molecular Medicine*, **49**, 581–590.

108. Halliday, J.W. & Powell, L.W. (1988) Ferritin and cellular iron metabolism. *Annals of the New York Academy of Sciences*, **526**, 101–112.

109. Halliday, J.W., McKeering, L.V., Tweedale, R. & Powell, L.W. (1977) Serum ferritin in haemochromatosis: changes in the isoferritin composition during venesection therapy. *British Journal of Haematology*, **36**, 395–404.

110. Hamashima, Y., Harter, J.G. & Coons, A.H. (1964) The localization of albumin and fibrinogen in human liver cells. *Journal of Cell Biology*, **20**, 271–279.

111. Harford, J., Bridges, K., Ashwell, G. & Klausner, R.D. (1983) Intracellular dissociation of receptor-bound asialoglycoproteins in cultured hepatocytes. A pH-mediated nonlysosomal event. *Journal of Biological Chemistry*, **258**, 3191–3197.

112. Harford, J., Klausner, R.D. & Ashwell, G. (1984) Inhibition of the endocytic pathway for asialoglycoprotein catabolism. *Biology of the Cell*, **52**, 173.

113. Harrison, P.M. (1977) Ferritin: an iron storage molecule. *Seminars in Haematology*, **14**, 55–70.

114. Hems, R., Ross, B.D., Berry, M.N. & Krebs, H.A. (1966) Gluconeogenesis in the perfused rat liver. *Biochemical Journal*, **101**, 284–292.

115. Henderson, A.R. (1970) The effect of feeding with a tryptophan-free amino acid mixture on rat liver magnesium ion-activated deoxyribonucleic acid polymerase. *Biochemical Journal*, **120**, 205–214.

116. Herlong, H.F., Maddrey, W.C. & Walser, M. (1980) The use of ornithine salts of branched-chain keto acids in portal-systemic encephalopathy. *Annals of Internal Medicine*, **93**, 545–550.

117. Hertzberg, K.M., Pindyck, J., Mosesson, M.W. & Grieninger, G. (1981) Thyroid hormone stimulation of plasma protein synthesis in cultured hepatocytes. *Journal of Biological Chemistry*, **256**, 563–566.

118. Hicks, S.J., Drysdale, J.W. & Munro, H.N. (1969) Preferential synthesis of ferritin and albumin by different populations of liver polysomes. *Science*, **164**, 584–585.

119. Hinton, R.H., Dobrota, M. & Mullock, B.M. (1980) Haptoglobin transfer of haemoglobin from serum into bile. *FEBS Letters*, **112**, 247–250.

120. Hoffenberg, R., Black, E. & Brock, J.F. (1966) Albumin and γ-globulin tracer studies in protein depletion states. *Journal of Clinical Investigation*, **45**, 143–152.

121. Hoppe, C.A., Connolly, T.P. & Hubbard, A.L. (1985) Transcellular transport of polymeric IgA in the rat hepatocyte: Biochemical and morphological characterization of the transport pathway. *Journal of Cell Biology*, **191**, 2113–2123.

121a. Horvat, A. (1980) Stimulation of RNA synthesis in isolated nuclei by an insulin-induced factor in liver. *Nature*, **286**, 906.

122. Hoy, T.G. & Jacobs, A. (1981) Ferritin polymers and the formation of haemosiderin. *British Journal of Haematology*, **49**, 593–602.

123. Hoy, T.G. & Jacobs, A. (1981) Changes in the characteristics and distribution of ferritin in iron loaded cell cultures. *Biochemical Journal*, **193**, 87–92.

124. Hsia, J.C., Er, S.S., Tan, C.T. *et al.* (1980) α-Fetoprotein specificity for arachidonate, bilirubin, decosahexaenoate and palmitate. *Journal of Biological Chemistry*, **255**, 4224–4227.

125. Iwasaki, Y., Sato, H., Ohkubo, A. *et al.* (1980) Effect of spontaneous portal-systemic shunting on plasma insulin and amino acid concentrations. *Gastroenterology*, **78**, 677–683.

126. James, W.P.T. & Hay, A.M. (1968) Albumin metabolism: effect of the nutritional state and dietary protein intake. *Journal of Clinical Investigation*, **47**, 1958–1972.

127. Jansen, R.G. & Tamaoki, T. (1983) Secretion and glycosylation of α-fetoprotein by the mouse yolk sac. *Biochemical Journal*, **212**, 313–320.

128. Jeejeebhoy, K.N., Bruce-Robertson, A., Sodtke, U. & Foley, M. (1970) The effect of growth hormone on fibrinogen synthesis. *Biochemical Journal*, **119**, 243–249.

129. Jeejeebhoy, K.N., Bruce-Robertson, A., Ho, J. & Sodtke, U. (1975) The effect of ethanol on albumin and fibrinogen synthesis in vivo and in hepatocyte suspension. In Rothschild, M.A., Oratz, M. & Schreiber, S.S. (eds) *Alcohol and Abnormal Protein Biosynthesis: Biochemical and Clinical*, p. 373. New York: Pergamon Press.

130. Jeejeebhoy, K.N., Phillips, M.J., Bruce-Robertson, A. *et al.* (1975) Albumin, fibrinogen and transferrin synthesis in isolated rat hepatocyte suspensions. *Biochemical Journal*, **146**, 141–155.

131. Jefferson, L.S., Liao, W.S.C., Peavy, D.E. *et al.* (1983) Diabetes induced alterations in liver protein synthesis. Changes in relative abundance of mRNAs for albumin and other plasma proteins. *Journal of Biological Chemistry*, **258**, 1369–1375.

132. Jennett, R.B., Tuma, D.H. & Sorrell, M.F. (1990) Effects of acetaldehyde on hepatic proteins. *Progress in Liver Diseases*, **9**, 325–333.

133. Jennett, R.B., Tuma, D.J. & Sorrell, M.F. (1980) The effect of ethanol and its metabolites on microtubule formation. *Pharmacology*, **21**, 363–368.

134. John, D.W. & Miller, L.L. (1969) Regulation of net biosynthesis of serum albumin and acute phase plasma proteins. *Journal of Biological Chemistry*, **244**, 6134–6142.

135. Jones, A.L., Hradek, G.T., Schmucker, D.L. & Underdown, B.J. (1984) The fate of polymeric and secretory immunoglobulin A after retrograde infusion into the common bile duct of rats. *Hepatology*, **4**, 1173.

136. Judah, J.D., Gamble, M. & Steadman, J.H. (1973) Biosynthesis of serum albumin in rat liver. Evidence for the existence of 'proalbumin'. *Biochemical Journal*, **134**, 1083–1091.

137. Kanematsu, T., Koyenagi, N., Matsumata, T. *et al.* (1988) Lack of preventive effect of branched-chain amino acid solution on post-operative hepatic encephalopathy in patients with cirrhosis. A randomized, prospective trial. *Surgery*, **104**, 482–488.

138. Kant, J.A. & Crabtree, G.R. (1983) The rat fibrinogen genes. Linkage of the Aα and γ chain genes. *Journal of Biological Chemistry*, **258**, 4666–4667.

139. Kaplan, J.H. & Pitot, H.C. (1970) The regulation of intermediary amino acid metabolism in animal tissues. In Munro, H.N. (ed.) *Mammalian Protein Metabolism*, Vol. IV, pp. 388–443. New York: Academic Press.

140. Keohane, P.P., Attrill, H., Grimble, G. *et al.* (1983) Enteral nutrition in malnourished patients with hepatic cirrhosis and acute encephalopathy. *Journal of Parenteral and Enteral Nutrition*, **7**, 346–350.

141. Kelman, L., Saunders, S.J., Wicht, S. *et al.* (1972) The effect of amino acids on albumin synthesis by the isolated perfused rat liver. *Biochemical Journal*, **129**, 805–809.

142. Khatra, B.S., Smith, R.B., Millikan, W.J. *et al.* (1974) Activities of Krebs-Henseleit enzymes in normal and cirrhotic human liver. *Journal of Laboratory and Clinical Medicine*, **84**, 708–715.

143. Kido, H., Shimazu, Y., Ueki, M. & Ogata, K. (1973) Effects of protein deficiency on serum albumin synthesizing activity with special reference to the presence of transcriptional controls. *Journal of Biochemistry (Tokyo)*, **74**, 747–756.

144. Kirsch, R., Frith, L., Black, E. & Hoffenberg, R. (1968) Regulation of albumin synthesis and catabolism by alteration of dietary protein. *Nature*, **217**, 578–579.

145. Kirsch, R.E., Frith, L.O'C & Saunders, S.J. (1976) Stimulation of albumin synthesis by keto analogues of amino acids. *Biochimica et Biophysica Acta*, **442**, 437–441.

146. Kirsch, R.E. & Franks, J.J. (1982) Fibrinogen synthesis in the isolated perfused rat liver: stimulation by a humoral factor associated with trauma. *Hepatology*, **2**, 205–208.

147. Kohgo, Y., Yokota, M. & Drysdale, J.W. (1980) Differential turnover of rat liver isoferritins. *Journal of Biological Chemistry*, **255**, 5195–5200.

148. Krumlauf, R., Hammer, R.E., Tilghman, S.M. & Brinster, R.L. (1985) Development regulation of α-fetoprotein genes in transgenic mice. *Molecular and Cellular Biology*, **5**, 1639.

149. Kutteh, W.H., Prince, S.J., Phillips, J.O. *et al.* (1982) Properties of immunoglobulin A in serum of individuals with liver diseases and in hepatic bile. *Gastroenterology*, **82**, 184–193.

150. Larson, A.E., Friedman, P.A. and Suttie, J.W. (1981) Vitamin K-dependent carboxylation: Stoichiometry of carboxylation and vitamin K 2,3-epoxide formation. *Journal of Biological Chemistry*, **256**, 11032–11035.

151. LaRusso, N.F. & Fowler, S. (1979) Coordinate secretion of acid hydrolases in rat bile. Hepatic exocytosis of lysosomal protein. *Journal of Clinical Investigation*, **64**, 948–954.

152. LaRusso, N.F., Kost, L.J., Carter, J.A. & Barham, S.S. (1982) Triton WR 1339, a lysosomotropic compound, is excreted into bile and alters the biliary excretion of lysosomal enzymes and lipids. *Hepatology*, **2**, 209–215.

153. Ledford, B.E. & Davis, D.F. (1983) Kinetics of serum protein secretion by hepatoma cells. Evidence for multiple secretory pathways. *Journal of Biological Chemistry*, **258**, 3304–3308.

154. Leibold, E.A. & Munro, H.N. (1988) Cytoplasmic protein binds in vitro to a highly conserved region of ferritin heavy-and-light-subunit mRNAs. *Proceedings of the National Academy of Sciences of the USA* **85**, 2171–2175.

155. Leibold, E.A., Laudano, A. & Yu, Y. (1990) Structural requirements of iron-responsive elements for binding of the protein involved in both transferrin receptor and ferritin mRNA post-trancriptional regulation. *Nucleic Acids Research*, **18**, 1819–1824.

156. LeMaitre-Coelho, I., Jackson, G.D.F. & Vaerman, J.P. (1978) High levels of secretory IgA and free secretory component in the serum of rats with bile duct obstruction. *Journal of Experimental Medicine*, **147**, 934–939.

157. LeMarchand, Y., Singh, A., Assimacopoulos-Jeannet, F. *et al.* (1973) A role for the microtubular system in the release of very low density lipoproteins by perfused mouse livers. *Journal of Biological Chemistry*, **248**, 6862–6870.

158. LeMarchand, Y., Patzelt, C., Assimacopoulos-Jeannet, F. *et al.* (1974) Evidence for a role of the microtubular system in the secretion of newly synthesized albumin and other proteins by the liver. *Journal of Clinical Investigation*, **53**, 1512–1517.

159. Liaw, C., Seelig, S., Mariash, C.N. *et al.* (1983) Interactions of thyroid hormone, growth hormone, and a high carbohydrate, fat-free diet in regulating several rat liver messenger ribonucleic acid species. *Biochemistry*, **22**, 213–221.

160. Lieber, C.S. (1980) Alcohol, protein metabolism and liver injury. *Gastroenterology*, **79**, 373–390.

161. Liebman, H.A., Furie, B.C. & Furie, B. (1982) Hepatic vitamin K-dependent carboxylation of blood clotting proteins. *Hepatology*, **2**, 488–494.

162. Liebman, H.A., Furie, B.C., Tong, M.J. *et al.* (1984) Des-γ-carboxy (abnormal) prothrombin as a serum marker of primary hepatocellular carcinoma. *New England Journal of Medicine*, **310**, 1427–1431.

163. Lin, R.C., Fillenworth, M.J., Minter, R. & Lumeng, L. (1990) Formation of the 37-kD protein acetaldehyde adduct in primary cultured hepatocytes exposed to alcohol. *Hepatology*, **11**, 401–407.

164. Lin, R.C. & Lumeng, L. (1989) Further studies on the 37-kD liver protein acetaldehyde adduct that forms in vivo during chronic alcohol ingestion. *Hepatology*, **10**, 807–814.

165. Lipinski, B., Lipinska, I., Nowak, A. & Gurewich, V. (1977) Abnormal fibrinogen heterogeneity and fibrinolytic activity in advanced liver disease. *Journal of Laboratory and Clinical Medicine*, **90**, 187–194.

166. Lodish, H.F., Kong, N., Snider, M. & Strous, G.J.A.M. (1983) Hepatoma secretory proteins migrate from rough endoplasmic reticulum to Golgi at characteristic rates. *Nature*, **304**, 80–83.

167. Lombard, M., Bomford, A., Hynes, M. *et al.* (1989) Regulation of the hepatic transferrin receptor in hereditary hemochromatosis. *Hepatology*, **9**, 1–5.

168. Lowe, M.E. & Ashwell, G. (1982) Solubilization and assay of an hepatic receptor for the haptoglobin-hemoglobin complex. *Archives of Biochemistry and Biophysics*, **216**, 704–710.

169. Mack, U., Powell, L.W. & Halliday, J.W. (1983) Detection and isolation of a hepatic membrane receptor for ferritin. *Journal of Biological Chemistry*, **258**, 4672–4675.

170. Maddrey, W.C., Chura, C., Coulter, A.W. *et al.* (1976) Effects of keto-analogues of essential amino acids in portal-systemic encephalopathy. *Gastroenterology*, **71**, 190–195.

171. Maier, K.P., Volk, B., Hoppe-Seyler, G. & Gerok, W. (1974) Urea cycle enzymes in normal liver and in patients with alcoholic hepatitis. *European Journal of Clinical Investigation*, **4**, 193–195.

172. Mann, S., Wade, V.J., Dickson, D.P. *et al.* (1988) Structural specificity of haemosiderin iron cores in iron-overload diseases. *FEBS Letters*, **234**, 69–72.

173. Marchesini, G., Zoli, M., Angiolini, A. *et al.* (1981) Muscle protein breakdown in liver cirrhosis and the role of altered carbohydrate metabolism. *Hepatology*, **1**, 294–299.

174. Marchesini, G., Zoli, M., Dondi, C. *et al.* (1982) Anticatabolic effect of branched-chain amino acid enriched solutions in patients with liver cirrhosis. *Hepatology*, **2**, 420–425.

175. Marchesini, G., Forlani, G., Zoli, M. *et al.* (1983) Effect of euglycemic insulin infusion on plasma levels of branched-chain amino acids in cirrhosis. *Hepatology*, **3**, 184–187.

176. Marchesini, G., Bianchi, G., Zoli, M. *et al.* (1983) Plasma amino acid response to protein ingestion in patients with cirrhosis. *Gastroenterology*, **85**, 283–290.

177. Marchesini, G., Dioguardi, F.S., Bianchi, G.P., *et al.* (1990) Long-term oral branched-chain amino acid treatment in chronic hepatic encephalopathy. A randomized double-blind case controlled trial. *Journal of Hepatology*, **11**, 92–101.

178. Marco, J., Diego, J., Villaneuva, M.L. *et al.* (1973) Elevated plasma glucagon levels in cirrhosis of the liver. *New England Journal of Medicine*, **289**, 1107–1111.

179. Marshall, J.S., Green, A.M., Pensky, J. *et al.* (1974) Measurement of circulating desialylated glycoproteins and correlation with hepatocellular damage. *Journal of Clinical Investigation*, **54**, 555–562.

180. Marshall, J.S., Williams, S., Jones, P. & Hepner, G.W. (1978) Serum desialylated glycoproteins in patients with hepatobiliary dysfunction. *Journal of Laboratory and Clinical Medicine*, **92**, 30–37.

181. Matthews, D.E., Bier, D.M., Rennie, M.J. *et al.* (1981) Regulation of leucine metabolism in man: a stable isotope study. *Science*, **214**, 1129–1131.

182. Matsuda, Y., Baroana, E., Salaspuro, M. & Lieber, C.S. (1979) Effects of ethanol on liver microtubules and Golgi apparatus. *Laboratory Investigation*, **41**, 455–463.

183. Matsuura, S., Nakada, H., Sawamura, T. & Tashiro, Y. (1982) Distribution of an asialoglycoprotein receptor on rat hepatocyte cell surface. *Journal of Cell Biology*, **95**, 864–875.

184. Maurice, M. & Feldmann, G. (1982) Quantitative biochemical and ultrastructural studies of microtubules in rat liver during the acute inflammatory reaction. *Experimental Molecular Pathology*, **36**, 193–203.

185. McCullough, A.J., Czaja, A.J., Jones, J.D. & Go, W.L.W. (1981) The nature and prognostic significance of serial amino acid determinations in severe chronic active liver disease. *Gastroenterology*, **81**, 645–652.

186. McCullough, A.J., Mullen, K.D. & Tavill, A.S. (1983) Branched-chain amino acids as nutritional therapy in liver disease: Dearth or surfeit. *Hepatology*, **3**, 269–271.

187. McCullough, A.J., Mullen, K.D., Smanik, E.J. *et al.* (1989) Nutritional therapy and liver disease. *Gastroenterology Clinics of North America*, **18**, 619–643.

188. McFarlane, I.G. (1983) Editorial review: Hepatic clearance of serum glycoproteins. *Clinical Science*, **64**, 127–135.

189. McGhee, A., Henderson, J.M., Millikan, W.J. *et al.* (1983) Comparison of the effects of Hepatic-Aid and a casein modular diet on encephalopathy, plasma amino acids, and nitrogen balance in cirrhotic patients. *Annals of Surgery*, **197**, 288–293.

190. McKnight, G.S., Lee, D.C., Hemmaplardh, D. *et al.* (1980) Transferrin gene expression: effects of nutritional iron deficiency. *Journal of Biological Chemistry*, **255**, 144–147.

191. McKnight, G.S., Lee, D.C. & Palmiter, R.D. (1980) Transferrin gene expression: regulation of mRNA transcription in chicken liver by steroid hormones and iron deficiency. *Journal of Biological Chemistry*, **255**, 148–153.

192. McNurlan, M.A. & Garlick, P.J. (1980) Contribution of rat liver

and gastrointestinal tract to whole-body protein synthesis on the rat. *Biochemical Journal,* **186**, 381–383.

193. Mendenhall, C.L., Anderson, S., Weesner, R.E. *et al.* (1984) Protein-calorie malnutrition associated with alcoholic hepatitis. *American Journal of Medicine,* **76**, 211–222.

194. Mendenhall, C.L., Tosch, T., Weesner, R.E. *et al.* (1986) VA cooperative study on alcoholic hepatitis II. Prognostic significance of protein-calorie malnutrition. *American Journal of Clinical Nutrition,* **43**, 213–218.

195. Meyer, D.I., Krause, E. & Dobberstein, B. (1982) Secretory protein translocation across membranes — a role of the "docking protein". *Nature,* **297**, 647–650.

196. Mezey, E. (1978) Liver disease and nutrition. *Gastroenterology,* **4**, 770–783.

197. Mezey, E. (1978) Liver disease and protein needs. *Annual Review of Nutrition,* **2**, 21–50.

198. Miller, L.L. (1960) Glucagon: a protein catabolic hormone in the isolated perfused rat liver. *Nature,* **185**, 248.

199. Miller, L.L. (1961) Some direct actions of insulin glucagon and hydrocortisone on the isolated perfused rat liver. *Recent Progress in Hormone Research,* **17**, 539–568.

200. Millikan, W.J., Henderson, J.M., Warren, W.E. *et al.* (1983) Total parenteral nutrition with F080^R in cirrhotics with subclinical encephalopathy. *Annals of Surgery,* **197**, 294–304.

201. Millikan, W.H., Henderson, J.M., Galloway, J.R. *et al.* (1985) In vivo measurements of leucine metabolism with stable isotopes in normal subjects and in those with cirrhosis fed conventional and branched-chain amino acid enriched diets. *Surgery,* **98**, 405–412.

202. Mimura, T., Yamada, C. & Swenseid, M.E. (1968) Influence of dietary protein levels and hydrocortisone administration on the branched chain transaminase activity in rat tissues. *Journal of Nutrition,* **95**, 493–498.

203. Mondon, C.E. & Mortimore, G.E. (1967) Effects of insulin on amino acid release and urea formation in perfused rat liver. *American Journal of Physiology,* **212**, 173–178.

204. Mookerjea, Y. & Chow, A. (1969) Impairment of glycoprotein synthesis in acute ethanol intoxication in rats. *Biochimica et Biophysica Acta,* **184**, 83–92.

205. Morgan, E.H. & Peters, T. (1971) The biosynthesis of rat serum albumin. V. Effect of protein depletion and refeeding on albumin and transferrin synthesis. *Journal of Biological Chemistry,* **246**, 3500–3507.

206. Morgan, M.Y., Marshall, A.W., Milsom, J.P. & Sherlock, S. (1982) Plasma amino acid patterns in liver disease. *Gut,* **23**, 362–370.

207. Morgan, M.Y. (1982) Alcohol and nutrition. *British Medical Bulletin,* **38**, 21–29.

208. Morgan, M.Y. (1990) Branched-chain amino acids in the management of chronic liver disease. Facts and fantasies (Leader). *Journal of Hepatology,* **11**, 133–141.

209. Morgan, M.Y., Milsom, J.P. & Sherlock, S. (1978) Plasma ratio of valine, leucine and isoleucine to phenylalanine and tyrosine in liver disease. *Gut,* **19**, 1068–1073.

210. Morinaga, T., Saga, M., Wegmann, T.G. & Tamaoki, T. (1983) The primary structures of human α-fetoprotein and its mRNA. *Proceedings of the National Academy of Sciences of the USA,* **80**, 4604–4608.

211. Morland, J., Rothschild, M.A., Oratz, M. *et al.* (1981) Protein secretion in suspensions of isolated rat hepatocytes: no influence of acute ethanol administration. *Gastroenterology,* **80**, 159–165.

212. Morrison, W.L., Bouchier, I.A.D., Gibson, J.N.A. & Rennie, M.J. (1990) Skeletal muscle and whole-body protein turnover in cirrhosis. *Clinical Science,* **78**, 613–619.

213. Mortimore, G.E. & Mondon, C.E. (1970) Inhibition by insulin of valine turnover in liver. *Journal of Biological Chemistry,* **245**, 2375–2383.

214. Mortimore, G.E. & Ward, W.F. (1981) Internalization of cytoplasmic protein by hepatic lysosomes in basal and deprivation-induced proteolytic states. *Journal of Biological Chemistry,* **256**, 7659–7665.

215. Mortimore, G.E. (1982) Mechanisms of cellular protein catabolism. *Nutrition Reviews,* **40**, 1–12.

216. Morton, A.G. & Tavill, A.S. (1977) The role of iron in the regulation of hepatic transferrin synthesis. *British Journal of Haematology,* **36**, 383–394.

217. Mullen, K.D., Denne, S.C., McCullough, A.J. *et al.* (1986) Leucine metabolism in stable cirrhosis. *Hepatology,* **6**, 622–630.

218. Mullock, B.M., Hinton, R.H., Dobrota, M., Peppard, J. & Orlans, E. (1979) Endocytic vesicles in liver carry polymeric IgA from serum into bile. *Biochimica et Biophysica Acta,* **587**, 381–391.

219. Mullock, B.M., Hinton, R.H., Dobrota, M., Peppard, J. & Orlans, E. (1980) Distribution of secretory component in hepatocytes and its mode of transfer into bile. *Biochemical Journal,* **190**, 819–826.

220. Mullock, B.M., Jones, R.S., Peppard, J. & Hinton, R.H. (1980) Effect of colchicine on the transfer of IgA across hepatocytes into bile in isolated perfused rat livers. *FEBS Letters,* **120**, 278–282.

221. Mullock, B.M., Shaw, L.J., Fitzharris, B. *et al.* (1985) Sources of proteins in human bile. *Gut,* **26**, 500–509.

222. Munro, H.M. (1968) Role of amino acid supply in regulating ribosome function. *Federation Proceedings,* **27**, 1231–1237.

223. Munro, H.N. & Linder, M.C. (1978) Ferritin: Structure, biosynthesis and role in iron metabolism. *Physiological Reviews,* **58**, 317–396.

224. Munro, H.N., Hubert, C. & Baliga, B.S. (1975) Regulation of protein synthesis in relation to amino acid supply — a review. In Rothschild, M.A., Oratz, M. & Schreiber, S.S. (eds) *Alcohol and Abnormal Protein Synthesis, Biochemical and Clinical,* pp. 33–66. New York: Pergamon Press.

225. Munro, H.N., Aziz, N., Leibold, E.A. *et al.* (1988) The ferritin genes: structure, expression, and regulation. *Annals of the New York Academy of Science,* **526**, 113–123.

226. Murty, C.N., Hornseth, R., Verney, E. & Sidranksy, H. (1983) Effect of tryptophan on enzymes and proteins of hepatic nuclear envelopes of rats. *Laboratory Investigation,* **48**, 256–262.

227. Muto, Y. & Yoshida, T. (1983) Effect of oral supplementation with branched-chain amino acid granules on improvement in decompensated liver cirrhosis: a cross-over controlled trial. In Ogoshi, S. & Okada, A. (eds) *Parenteral and Enteral Hyperalimentation,* pp. 280–292 New York. Elsevier. 1983.

228. Nasrallah, S.M. & Galambos, J.T. (1980) Amino acid therapy of alcoholic hepatitis. *Lancet,* **2**, 1276–1277.

229. Naylor, C.D., O'Rourke, K., Detsky, A.S. & Baker, J.P. (1989) Parenteral nutrition with branched-chain amino acids in hepatic encephalopathy. A meta-analysis. *Gastroenterology,* **97**, 1022–1042.

230. Neufeld, E.F. & Ashwell, G. (1980) Carbohydrate recognition systems for receptor-mediated pinocytosis. In Lennarz, W.J. (ed.) *The Biochemistry of Glycoproteins and Proteoglycans,* pp. 241–266. New York: Plenum Press.

231. Niemala, O., Klajner, F., Orrego, H. *et al.* (1987) Antibodies against acetaldehyde-modified protein epitopes in human alcoholics. *Hepatology,* **7**, 1210–1214.

232. Oda, K. & Ikehara, Y. (1981) Monensin inhibits the conversion of proalbumin to serum albumin in cultured rat hepatocytes. *Biochemical and Biophysical Research Communications,* **105**, 766–772.

233. O'Keefe, S.J.D., Abraham, R.R., Davis, M. & Williams., R. (1980) Protein turnover in acute and chronic liver disease. *Acta Chirurgica Scandinavica,* **507**, (Supplement), 91–101.

234. O'Keefe, S.J.D., Abraham, R.R., El-Zayadi, A. *et al.* (1981) Increased plasma tyrosine concentrations with cirrhosis and fulminant hepatic failure associated with increased plasma tyrosine flux and reduced hepatic oxidation capacity. *Gastroenterology,* **81**, 1017–1024.

235. Okuno, M., Nagayama, M., Tallai, T. *et al.* (1985) Post-operative total parenteral nutrition in patients with liver disorders. *Journal of Surgical Research,* **39**, 93–102.

236. Olmsted, J.B. & Borisy, G.G. (1973) Microtubules. *Annual Review of Biochemistry,* **42**, 507–540.

237. Oratz, M., Rothschild, M.A., Schreiber, S.S. *et al.* (1983) The role of the urea cycle and polyamines in albumin synthesis. *Hepatology,* **3**, 567–571.

238. Owen, M.C., Brennan, S.O., Lewis, J.H. & Carrell, R.W. (1983) Mutation of antitrypsin to antithrombin: α₁-antitrypsin Pittsburgh (358 Met→Arg), a fatal bleeding disorder. *New England Journal of Medicine,* **309**, 694–698.

239. Owen, O.E., Trapp, V.E., Reichard, G.A., Jr *et al.* (1983) Nature and quantity of fuels consumed in patients with alcoholic cirrhosis. *Journal of Clinical Investigation,* **72**, 1821–1831.

240. Pain, V.M., Lanoix, J., Bergeron, J.J.M. & Clemens, M.J. (1974)

Effects of diabetes on the ultrastructure of the hepatocyte and on the distribution and activity of ribosomes in the free and membrane-bound populations. *Biochimica et Biophysica Acta*, **353**, 487–498.

241. Palascak, J.E. & Martinez, J. (1977) Dysfibrinogenemia associated with liver disease. *Journal of Clinical Investigation*, **60**, 89–95.

242. Panduro, A., Shalasky, F., Weiner, F.R. *et al.* (1986) Transcriptional switch from albumin to α-fetoprotein and changes in transcription of other genes during carbon tetrachloride induced liver regeneration. *Biochemistry*, **25**, 1414.

243. Peavy, D.E., Taylor, J.M. & Jefferson, L.S. (1981) Protein synthesis in perfused rat liver following thyroidectomy and hormone treatment. *American Journal of Physiology*, **240**, E19–E23.

244. Peters, T. Jr (1970) Serum albumin. *Advances in Clinical Chemistry*, **13**, 37–41.

245. Peters, T.J. Jr (1985) Serum albumin. In Anfinsen, C.B., Edsall, J.T. & Richards, F.M. (eds) *Advances in Protein Chemistry*, Vol. 37, p. 161. New York: Academic Press.

246. Peters, T. & Peters, J.C. (1972) The biosynthesis of rat serum albumin. VI. Intracellular transport of albumin and rates of albumin and liver protein synthesis in vivo under various physiological conditions. *Journal of Biological Chemistry*, **247**, 3858–3863.

247. Peters, T. Jr, Fleischer, B. & Fleischer, S. (1971) The biosynthesis of rat serum albumin. IV. Apparent passage of albumin through the Golgi apparatus during secretion. *Journal of Biological Chemistry*, **246**, 240–244.

248. Petropoulos, C., Andrews, C., Tamaoki, T. & Fausto, N. (1983) α-Fetoprotein and albumin mRNA levels in liver regeneration and carcinogenesis. *Journal of Biological Chemistry*, **258**, 4901–4906.

249. Pietrangelo, A., Rocchi, E., Schiaffonati, L. *et al.* (1990) Liver gene expression during chronic dietary iron overload in rats. *Hepatology*, **11**, 798–804.

250. Plant, P.W. & Grieninger, G. (1986) Noncoordinate synthesis of the fibrinogen subunits in hepatocytes cultured under hormone-deficient conditions. *Journal of Biological Chemistry*, **261**, 2331.

251. Poso, A.R., Wert, J.J. & Mortimore, G.E. (1982) Multifunction control by amino acids of deprivation-induced proteolysis in liver. *Journal of Biological Chemistry*, **257**, 12114–12120.

252. Powell, L.W., Alpert, E., Isselbacher, K.J. & Drysdale, J.W. (1974) Abnormality in tissue isoferritin distribution in idiopathic haemochromatosis. *Nature*, **250**, 333–335.

253. Powell, L.W., Bassett, M.L. & Halliday, J.W. (1980) Hemochromatosis: 1980 Update. Gastroenterology, **78**, 374–381.

254. Prieto, J., Barry, M. & Sherlock, S. (1975) Serum ferritin in patients with iron overload and with acute and chronic liver diseases. *Gastroenterology*, **68**, 525–533.

255. Princen, H.M.G., Selten, G.C.M., Selten-Verteegen, A.M.E. *et al.* (1982) Distribution of mRNA's of fibrinogen polypeptides and albumin in free and membrane-bound polyribosomes and induction of α-foetoprotein mRNA synthesis during liver regeneration after partial hepatectomy. *Biochimica Biophysica Acta*, **699**, 121–130.

256. Putnam, C.W., Porter, K., Peters, R.L. *et al.* (1977) Liver replacement for alpha₁-antitrypsin deficiency. *Surgery*, **81**, 258–261.

257. Quinn, P.S., Gamble, M. & Judah, J.D. (1975) Biosynthesis of serum albumin in rat liver. Isolation and probable structure of 'proalbumin' from rat liver. *Biochemical Journal*, **146**, 389–393.

258. Raum, D., Marcus, D., Alper, C.A. *et al.* (1980) Synthesis of human plasminogen by the liver. *Science*, **208**, 1036–1037.

259. Reaven, E.P. & Reaven, G.M. (1980) Evidence that microtubules play a permissive role in hepatocyte very low density lipoprotein secretion. *Journal of Cell Biology*, **84**, 28–39.

260. Redman, C.M. (1969) Biosynthesis of serum proteins and ferritin by free and attached ribosomes of rat liver. *Journal of Biological Chemistry*, **244**, 4308–4315.

261. Redman, C.M., Bannerjee, D., Howell, K. & Palade, G.E. (1975) Colchicine inhibition of plasma protein release from rat hepatocytes. *Journal of Cell Biology*, **66**, 42–59.

262. Regoeczi, E. (1974) Fibrinogen. In Allison, A.C. (ed.) *Structure and Function of Plasma Proteins*, Vol. 1, pp. 133–167. London: Plenum Press.

263. Rennie, M.J., Edwards, R.H.T., Emery, P.W. *et al.* (1983) Hypothesis: Depressed protein synthesis is the dominant characteristic of muscle wasting and cachexia. *Clinical Physiology*, **3**, 387–398.

264. Renston, R.H., Jones, A.L., Christiansen, W.D. *et al.* (1980) Evidence for a vesicular transport mechanism in hepatocytes for biliary secretion of immunoglobulin A. *Science*, **208**, 1276–1278.

265. Renston, R.H., Maloney, D.G., Jones, A.L. *et al.* (1980) Biliary secretory apparatus: evidence for a vesicular transport mechanism for proteins in the rat, using horseradish peroxidase and [¹²⁵I]insulin. *Gastroenterology*, **78**, 1373–1388.

266. Renston, R.H., Zsigmond, G., Bernhoff, R.A. *et al.* (1983) Vesicular transport of horseradish peroxidase during chronic bile duct obstruction in the rat. *Hepatology*, **31**, 673–680.

267. Reuben, A. (1984) Biliary proteins. *Hepatoplogy*, **4**, 465–505.

268. Ritchie, D.G., Levy, B.A., Adams, M.A. & Fuller, G.M. (1982) Regulation of fibrinogen synthesis by plasmin-derived fragments of fibrinogen and fibrin: an indirect feedback pathway. *Proceedings of the National Academy of Sciences of the USA*, **79**, 1530–1534.

269. Rocchi, E., Casaanelli, M., Gilbertini, P. *et al.* (1981) Standard or branched-chain amino acid infusions as short-term nutritional support in liver cirrhosis? *Journal of Parenteral and Enteral Nutrition*, **9**, 447–451.

270. Rosenblum, J.D., Raab, B.K. & Alpers, D.H. (1982) Hepatobiliary and pancreatic clearance of circulating pancreatic amylase. *American Journal of Physiology*, **243**, G21–G27.

271. Rothschild, M.A., Schreiber, S.S., Oratz, M. & McGee, H.L. (1958) The effects of adrenocortical hormones on albumin metabolism studied with ¹³¹I-albumin. *Journal of Clinical Investigation*, **37**, 1229–1235.

272. Rothschild, M.A., Oratz, M., Wimer, E. & Schreiber, S.S. (1961) Studies on albumin synthesis. Effects of dextran and cortisone on albumin metabolism in rabbits studied with ¹³¹I-albumin. *Journal of Clinical Investigation*, **40**, 545–554.

273. Rothschild, M.A., Oratz, M., Franklin, E.C. & Schreiber, S.S. (1962) The effect of hyperglobulinemia on albumin metabolism in hyperimmunized rabbits studied with ¹³¹I-albumin. *Journal of Clinical Investigation*, **41**, 1564–1571.

274. Rothschild, M.A., Oratz, M., Evans, C. & Schreiber, S.S. (1964) Alterations in albumin metabolism after serum and albumin infusions. *Journal of Clinical Investigation*, **43**, 1874–1880.

275. Rothschild, M.A., Oratz, M., Evans, C.E. & Schreiber, S.S. (1966) Role of hepatic interstitial albumin in regulating albumin synthesis. *American Journal of Physiology*, **210**, 57–62.

276. Rothschild, M.A., Oratz, M., Mongelli, J. & Schreiber, S.S. (1968) Effects of a short term fast on albumin synthesis studied in vivo in the perfused liver and on amino acid incorporation by hepatic microsomes. *Journal of Clinical Investigation*, **47**, 2591–2599.

277. Rothschild, M.A., Oratz, M., Mongelli, J. *et al.* (1969) Amino acid regulation of albumin synthesis. *Journal of Nutrition*, **98**, 395–403.

278. Rothschild, M.A., Oratz, M., Zimmon, D.S. *et al.* (1969) Albumin synthesis in chronic subjects studied with [¹⁴C]carbonate. *Journal of Clinical Investigation*, **48**, 344–350.

279. Rothschild, M.A., Oratz, M. & Schreiber, S.S. (1972) Albumin synthesis. *New England Journal of Medicine*, **286**, 748–757, 816–821.

280. Rothschild, M.A., Oratz, M., Morland, J. *et al.* (1980) Effects of ethanol on protein synthesis and secretion. *Pharmacology Biochemical Behaviour*, **13** (Supplement 1), 31–36.

281. Rothschild, M.A., Oratz, M. & Schreiber, S.S. (1983) Effects of nutrition and alcohol on albumin synthesis. *Alcoholism: Clinical and Experimental Research*, **7**, 28–30.

282. Rouault, T.A., Hentze, M.W., Caughman, S.W. *et al.* (1988) Binding of a cytosolic protein to the iron-responsive element of human ferritin messenger RNA. *Science*, **241**, 1207–1210.

283. Rudman, D., Difulco, T.J., Galambos, J.T. *et al.* (1973) Maximal rates of excretion and synthesis of urea in normal and cirrhotic subjects. *Journal of Clinical Investigation*, **52**, 2241–2249.

284. Russell, J.H. & Geller, D.M. (1973) Rat serum albumin biosynthesis: evidence for a precursor. *Biochemical and Biophysical Research Communications*, **55**, 239–245.

285. Sabesin, S.M. (1981) Editorial: Microtubules-biological machines at the molecular level. *Gastroenterology*, **81**, 810–813.

286. Saito, H., Hamilton, S.M., Tavill, A.S. *et al.* (1980) Production and release of plasminogen by isolated perfused rat liver. *Proceedings of the National Academy of Sciences of the USA*, **77**, 6837–6840.

287. Saito, H., Hamilton, S.M., Tavill, A.S. *et al.* (1983) Synthesis and

release of Hageman factor (factor XII) by the isolated perfused rat liver. *Journal of Clinical Investigation*, **72**, 948–954.

288. Sapir, D.G. & Walser, M. (1977) Nitrogen sparing induced early in starvation by infusion of branched-chain keto acids. *Metabolism*, **26**, 301–308.

289. Sato, Y., Eriksson, S., Hagenfeldt, L. & Wahren, J. (1981) Influence of branched chain amino acid infusion on arterial concentrations and brain exchange of amino acids and patients with hepatic cirrhosis. *Clinical Physiology*, **1**, 151–165.

290. Schauder, P., Schroder, K., Matthaei, D. *et al.* (1983) Influence of insulin on blood levels of branched keto and amino acids in man. *Metabolism*, **32**, 323–327.

291. Schauder, P., Schroder, K., Herbertz, L. *et al.* (1984) Oral administration of α-ketoisovaleric acid or valine in humans: Blood kinetics and biochemical effects. *Journal of Laboratory and Clinical Medicine*, **103**, 597–605.

292. Schimke, R.T. (1963) Studies on factors affecting the levels of urea cycle enzymes in rat liver. *Journal of Biological Chemistry*, **238**, 1012–1018.

293. Schimke, R.T. (1964) The importance of both synthesis and degradation in the control of arginase levels in rat liver. *Journal of Biological Chemistry*, **239**, 3808–3817.

294. Schimke, R.T. (1970) Regulation of protein degradation in mammalian tissues. In Munro, H.N. (ed.) *Mammalian Protein Metabolism*, Vol. IV, pp. 178–228. New York: Academic Press.

295. Schultze, H.E. & Heremans, J.F. (1966) *Molecular Biology of Human Proteins*, Vol. I, p. 475. Amsterdam: Elsevier.

296. Schworer, C.M., Schiffer, K.A. & Mortimore, G.E. (1981) Quantitative relationship between autophagy and proteolysis during graded amino acid deprivation in perfused rat liver. *Journal of Biological Chemistry*, **256**, 7652–7658.

297. Sciot, R., Paterson, A.C., Van den Oord, J.J. & Desmet, V.J. (1987) Lack of hepatic transferrin receptor expression in hemochromatosis. *Hepatology*, **7**, 831–837.

298. Sciot, R., Verhoeven, G., Van Eyken, P. *et al.* (1990) Transferrin receptor expression in rat liver: Immunohistochemical and biochemical analysis of the effects of age and iron storage. *Hepatology*, **11**, 416–427.

299. Seglen, P.O. (1978) Effects of amino acids, ammonia and leupeptin on protein synthesis and degradation in isolated rat hepatocytes. *Biochemical Journal*, **174**, 469–474.

300. Selden, C., Owen, M., Hopkins, J.M.P. & Peters, T.J. (1980) Studies on the concentration and intracellular localization of iron proteins in liver biopsy specimens from patients with iron overload with special reference to their role in lysosomal disruption. *British Journal of Haematology*, **44**, 593–603.

301. Selten, G.C.M., Princen, H.M.G., Selten-Verteegen, A.M.E. *et al.* (1982) Sequence content of α-fetoprotein, albumin and fibrinogen polypeptide mRNAs in different organs, developing tissues, and in liver during carcinogenesis in rats. *Biochimica Biophysica Acta*, **699**, 131–137.

302. Sewell, R.B., Barham, S.S., Zinmeister, A.R. & LaRusso, N.F. (1984) Microtubule modulation of biliary excretion of endogenous and exogenous hepatic lysosomal constituents. *American Journal of Physiology*, **246**, G8–G15.

303. Shafritz, D.A. (1979) Molecular hybridization probes for research in liver disease: Studies with albumin cDNA. *Gastroenterology*, **77**, 1335–1348.

304. Shambaugh, G.E. (1978) Urea biosynthesis. II. Normal and abnormal regulation. *American Journal of Clinical Nutrition*, **31**, 126–133.

305. Shanbhogue, R.L.K., Bistrian, B.R., Lakshman, K. *et al.* (1987) Whole body leucine, phenylalanine, and tyrosine kinetics in end-stage liver disease before and after hepatic transplantation. *Metabolism*, **36**, 1047–1053.

306. Shankar, T.P., Solomon, S.S., Duckworth, W.C. *et al.* (1983) Studies of glucose intolerance in cirrhosis of the liver. *Journal of Laboratory and Clinical Medicine*, **102**, 459–469.

307. Shaw, S. & Lieber, C.S. (1983) Plasma amino acids in the alcoholic: Nutritional aspects. *Alcoholism: Clinical and Experimental Research*, **7**, 22–27.

308. Sherwin, R., Joshi, P., Hendler, R. *et al.* (1974) Hyperglucagonemia in Laennec's cirrhosis. *New England Journal of Medicine*, **290**, 239–242.

309. Sherwin, R.S., Fisher, M., Bessoff, J. *et al.* (1978) Hyperglucagonemia of cirrhosis: altered secretion and sensitivity to glucagon. *Gastroenterology*, **74**, 1224–1228.

310. Sidransky, H., Verney, E. & Sarma, D.S.R. (1971) Effect of tryptophan on polyribosomes and protein synthesis in liver. *American Journal of Clinical Nutrition*, **24**, 779–785.

311. Sidransky, H., Sarma, D.S.R., Bongiorno, M. & Verney, E. (1968) Effect of dietary tryptophan on hepatic polyribosomes and protein synthesis in fasted mice. *Journal of Biological Chemistry*, **243**, 1123–1132.

312. Simon, D. & Galambos, J.T. (1988) A randomized controlled trial of peripheral parenteral nutrition in moderate and severe alcoholic hepatitis. *Journal of Hepatology*, **7**, 200–207.

313. Smith-Kielland, A., Bengtsson, G., Svendsen, L. & Morland, J. (1982) Protein synthesis in different populations of rat hepatocytes separated according to density. *Journal of Cell Physiology*, **110**, 262–266.

314. Soeters, P.B. & Fischer, J.E. (1976) Insulin, glucagon, amino acid imbalance and hepatic encephalopathy. *Lancet*, **2**, 880–882.

315. Sorrell, M.F. & Tuma, D.J. (1979) Effects of alcohol on hepatic metabolism: selected aspects. *Clinical Science*, **57**, 481–489.

316. Sorrell, M.F., Nauss, J.M., Donohue, T.M. & Tuma, D.J. (1983) Effects of chronic ethanol administration on hepatic glycoprotein secretion in the rat. *Gastroenterology*, **84**, 580–586.

317. Stahl, P. & Schwartz, A.L. (1986) Perspectives: receptor-mediated endocytosis. *Journal of Clinical Investigation*, **77**, 657.

318. Starzl, T.E., Porter, K.A., Watanabe, K. & Putnam, C.W. (1976) Effects of insulin, glucagon, and insulin/glucagon infusions on liver morphology and cell division after complete portacaval shunt in dogs. *Lancet*, **1**, 821–825.

319. Steer, C.J. & Ashwell, G. (1990) Receptor-mediated endocytosis: mechanisms, biologic function and molecular properties. In Zakim D. & Boyer, T.D. (eds) *Hepatology: A Textbook of Liver Disease*, pp. 137–182. Philadelphia: W.B. Saunders.

320. Sterling, K. (1951) Serum albumin turnover in Laennec's cirrhosis as measured by ^{131}I-tagged albumin. *Journal of Clinical Investigation*, **30**, 1238–1242.

321. Sterling, K. (1960) The effect of Cushing's syndrome upon serum albumin metabolism. *Journal of Clinical Investigation*, **39**, 1900–1908.

322. Sternlieb, I. & Quintana, N. (1985) Special article: Biliary proteins and ductular ultrastructure. *Hepatology*, **5**, 129–143.

323. Stockert, R.J. & Morell, A.G. (1983) Hepatic binding protein: The galactose-specific receptor of mammalian hepatocytes. *Hepatology*, **3**, 750–757.

324. Suttie, J.W. & Jackson, C.M. (1977) Prothrombin structure, activation and biosynthesis. *Physiological Reviews*, **57**, 1–70.

325. Swain, C.P., Tavill, A.S. & Neale, G. (1976) Studies of tryptophan and albumin metabolism in a patient with carcinoid syndrome, pellagra and hypoproteinemia. *Gastroenterology*, **71**, 484–489.

326. Swart, G.R., Van Den Berg, J.W.O., Wahimera, J.L.D. *et al.* (1988) Elevated protein requirements in cirrhosis of the liver investigated by whole body protein turnover studies. *Clinical Science*, **75**, 101–107.

327. Swart, G.R., Zillikens, M.C., Van Vuure, J.K. & Van den Berg, J.W.O. (1989) Effect of a late evening meal on nitrogen balance in patients with cirrhosis of the liver. *British Medical Journal*, **299**, 1202–1203.

328. Tavill, A.S., Craigie, A. & Rosenoer, V.M. (1968) The measurement of the synthetic rate of albumin in man. *Clinical Science*, **34**, 1–28.

329. Tavill, A.S. (1972) The synthesis and degradation of liver produced proteins. *Gut*, **13**, 225–241.

330. Tavill, A.S., East, A.G., Black, E.G. *et al.* (1973) Regulatory factors in the synthesis of plasma proteins by the isolated perfused rat liver. *Ciba Foundation Symposium*, **9** (New Series), 155–180.

331. Tavill, A.S. & Hoffenberg, R. (1976) Turnover of plasma proteins. In Allison, A.C. (ed.) *Structure and Function of Plasma Proteins*, Vol. 2, pp. 107–144. New York: Plenum Press.

332. Tavill, A.S. & Morton, A.G. (1978) Transferrin metabolism and the liver. In Powell, L.W. (ed.) *Metals in the Liver*, pp. 93–130. New York: Marcel Dekker.

333. Tavill, A.S. & Swain, C.P. (1979) The protein secretory activities of the liver. In Duthie, H.L. & Wormsley, K.G. (eds) *Scientific*

334. Tavill, A.S. (1985) Hepatic protein metabolism: Basic and applied biochemical and clinical aspects. In Arias, I.M., Frenkel, M. & Wilson, J.H.P. (eds) *Liver Annual 4*. Amsterdam: Elsevier, pp. 53–96.

Basis of Gastroenterology, pp. 249–287. Edinburgh: Churchill-Livingstone.

335. Thomas, P., Toth, C.A. & Zamcheck, N. (1982) The mechanism of biliary excretion of α_1-acid glycoprotein in the rat: Evidence for a molecular weight, nonreceptor-mediated pathway. *Hepatology*, **2**, 800–803.

336. Tilghman, S.M. & Belayew, A. (1982) Transcriptional control of the murine albumin/α-fetoprotein locus during development. *Proceedings of the National Academy of Sciences of the USA*, **79**, 5254–5257.

337. Tischler, M.E., Desautels, M. & Goldberg, A.L. (1982) Does leucine, leucyl-tRNA, or some metabolite of leucine regulate protein synthesis and degradation in skeletal and cardiac muscle? *Journal of Biological Chemistry*, **257**, 1613–1621.

338. Tsai, S.L., Huang, G.T., Yang, P.M. *et al.* (1990) Plasma des-gamma-carboxyprothrombin in the early stage of hepatocellular carcinoma. *Hepatology*, **11**, 481–488.

339. Tuma, D.J. & Sorrell, M.F. (1981) Effects of ethanol on the secretion of glycoproteins by rat liver slices. *Gastroenterology*, **80**, 273–278.

340. Tuma, D.J. & Sorrell, M.F. (1988) Effects of ethanol on protein trafficking in the liver. *Seminars in Liver Disease*, **8**, 69–80.

341. Unger, R.H. (1971) Glucagon physiology and pathophysiology. *New England Journal of Medicine*, **285**, 443–449.

342. Unger, R.H. (1972) Insulin/glucagon rates. *Israel Journal of Medical Sciences*, **8**, 252–257.

343. Urban, J., Inglis, A.S., Edwards, K. & Schreiber, G. (1974) Chemical evidence for the difference between albumins from microsomes and serum and a possible precursor-product relationship. *Biochemical and Biophysical Research Communications*, **61**, 494–501.

344. Verbanac, K.M. & Heath, E.C. (1983) Biosynthesis and processing of rat α 1-antitrypsin. *Archives of Biochemistry and Biophysics*, **223**, 149–157.

345. Veseley, J. & Cihak, A. (1970) Enhanced DNA-dependent RNA polymerase and RNA synthesis in rat liver nuclei after administration of L-tryptophan. *Biochimica et Biophysica Acta*, **204**, 614–616.

346. Vilstrup, H., Bucher, D., Krog, B. & Damgard, S.E. (1982) Elimination of infused amino acids from plasma of control subjects and of patients with cirrhosis of the liver. *European Journal of Clinical Investigation*, **12**, 197–202.

347. Vilstrup, H., Bucher, D. & Krog, B. (1982) Elimination of infused amino acids from plasma of control subjects and patients with cirrhosis of the liver. *European Journal of Clinical Investigation*, **12**, 197–202.

348. Volentine, G.D., Tuma, D.J. & Sorrell, M.F. (1984) Acute effects of ethanol on hepatic glycoprotein secretion in the rat in vivo. *Gastroenterology*, **86**, 225–229.

349. Wahren, J., Felig, P. & Hagenfeldt, J. (1976) Effect of protein ingestion on splanchnic and leg metabolism in normal man and in patients with diabetes mellitus. *Journal of Clinical Investigation*, **57**, 987–999.

350. Walker, S., Gotz, R., Czygan, P. *et al.* (1982) Oral keto analogs of branched-chain amino acids in hyperammonemia in patients with cirrhosis of the liver. A double-blind crossover study. *Digestion*, **24**, 105–111.

351. Wallin, R. & Hutson, S. (1982) Vitamin K dependent carboxylation: evidence that at least two microsomal dehydrogenases reduce vitamin K to support carboxylation. *Journal of Biological Chemistry*, **257**, 1583–1586.

352. Wallin, R. & Suttie, J.W. (1982) Vitamin K-dependent carboxylase: evidence for cofractionation of carboxylase and epoxidase activities and for carboxylation of a high-molecular weight microsomal protein. *Archives of Biochemistry and Biophysics*, **214**, 155–163.

353. Walser, M., Lund, P., Ruderman, N.B. & Coulter, A.W. (1973) Synthesis of essential amino acids from their α-keto-analogues by perfused rat liver and muscle. *Journal of Clinical Investigation*, **52**, 2865–2877.

354. Walser, M. (1984) Therapeutic aspects of branched-chain amino and keto acids. *Clinical Science*, **66**, 1–15.

355. Walter, P. & Blobel, G. (1982) Signal recognition particle contains a 7S RNA essential for protein translocation across the endoplasmic reticulum. *Nature*, **299**, 691–698.

356. Watanabe, N. & Drysdale, J.W. (1981) Natural enrichment of ferritin mRNA in mRNP particles. *Biochemical Biophysical Research Communications*, **103**, 207–212.

357. Watanabe, N. & Drysdale, J.W. (1981) Evidence for distinct mRNA's for ferritin subunits. *Biochemical Biophysical Research Communications*, **98**, 507–511.

358. Waterlow, J.C. (1967) Lysine turnover in man measured by intravenous infusion of L[U-^{14}C] lysine. *Clinical Science*, **33**, 507–515.

359. Waterlow, J.C. & Stephen, J.M.L. (1968) The effect of low protein diets on the turnover rates of serum, liver and muscle proteins in the rat measured by continuous infusion of L-[U-^{14}C]lysine. *Clinical Science*, **35**, 287–305.

360. Waterlow, J.C. & Payne, P.R. (1975) The protein gap. *Nature*, **258**, 113–117.

361. Weber, F.L. & Reiser, B.J. (1982) Relationship of plasma amino acids to nitrogen balance and portal systemic encephalopathy in alcoholic liver disease. *Digestive Diseases and Sciences*, **27**, 103–110.

362. Weigand, K., Schmid, M., Villringer, A. *et al.* (1982) Hexa- and pentapeptide extension of proalbumin: feedback inhibition of albumin synthesis by its propeptide in isolated hepatocytes and in the cell-free system. *Biochemistry*, **21**, 6053–6059.

363. Weigel, P.H. & Oka, J.A. (1984) Recycling of the hepatic asialoglycoprotein receptor in isolated rat hepatocytes. *Journal of Biological Chemistry*, **259**, 1150–1154.

364. White, K. & Munro, H.N. (1988) Induction of ferritin subunit synthesis by iron is regulated at both the transcriptional and translational levels. *Journal of Biological Chemistry*, **263**, 8938–8942.

365. Wileman, T., Harding, C. & Stahl, P. (1985) Review article: receptor-mediated endocytosis. *Biochemical Journal*, **232**, 1–14.

366. Wileman, T., Boshens, R.L. & Schlesinger, P. (1984) Monensin inhibits recycling of macrophage mannose-glycoprotein receptors and ligand delivery to lysosomes. *Biochemical Journal*, **220**, 665–675.

367. Wilkinson, P. & Mendenhall, C.L. (1963) Serum albumin turnover in normal subjects and patients with cirrhosis measured by ^{131}I-labelled human albumin. *Clinical Science*, **25**, 281–292.

368. Wilson, S.H. & Hill, N.Z. & Hoagland, M.D. (1967) Physiology of rat-liver polysomes. Protein synthesis by stable polysomes. *Biochemical Journal*, **103**, 567–572.

369. Wixom, R.L., Prutkin, L. & Munro, H.N. (1980) Hemosiderin: nature, formation and significance. *International Review of Experimental Pathology*, **22**, 193–225.

370. Worwood, M., Cragg, S.J., Williams, A.M. *et al.* (1982) The clearance of ^{131}I-human plasma ferritin in man. *Blood*, **60**, 827–833.

371. Yap, S.H., Strair, S.K. & Shafritz, D.A. (1977) Distribution of rat liver albumin mRNA membrane-bound and free in polyribosomes as determined by molecular hybridization. *Proceedings of the National Academy of Sciences of the USA*, **74**, 5397–5401.

372. Yap, S.H., Strair, R.K. & Shafritz, D.A. (1978) Effect of a short term fast on the distribution of cytoplasmic albumin messenger ribonucleic acid in rat liver. Evidence for formation of free albumin messenger ribonucleoprotein particles. *Journal of Biological Chemistry*, **253**, 4944–4950.

373. Yedgar, S., Carew, T.E., Pittman, P.C. *et al.* (1983) Tissue sites of catabolism of albumin in rabbits. *American Journal of Physiology*, **244**, E101–E107.

374. Yokota, S. (1984) Immunocytochemical evidence for a vesicular transport of albumin across the epithelium in the rat interlobular bile duct. *Biochemical Research*, **5**, 303–310.

375. Yokota, S. & Fahimi, H.D. (1981) Immunocytochemical localization of albumin in the secretory apparatus of rat liver parenchymal cells. *Proceedings of the National Academy of Sciences of the USA*, **78**, 4970–4974.

376. Yoshida, T., Muto, Y., Moriwaki, H. & Yamato, M. (1989) Effect of long-term oral supplementation with branched-chain amino acid granules in the prognosis of liver cirrhosis. *Gastroenterologica Japonica*, **24**, 692–698.

377. Young, S.P. & Aisen, P. (1980) The interaction of transferrin with isolated hepatocytes. *Biochimica et Biophysica Acta*, **633**, 145–153.
378. Young, S.P. & Aisen, P. (1981) Transferrin receptors and the uptake and release of iron by isolated hepatocyte. *Hepatology*, **1**, 114–119.
379. Young, S.P., Bomford, A. & Williams, R. (1983) Dual pathways for the uptake of rat asialotransferrin by rat hepatocytes. *Journal of Biological Chemistry*, **258**, 4972–4976.
380. Young, V.R., Steffee, W.P., Pencharz, P.B. *et al.* (1975) Total human body protein synthesis in relation to protein requirements at various ages. *Nature*, **253**, 192–194.
381. Yu, S., Sher, B., Kudryk, B. & Redman, C.M. (1984) Fibrinogen precursors: order of assembly of fibrinogen chains. *Journal of Biological Chemistry*, **259**, 105–174.
382. Zabrecky, J.R. & Cole, R.D. (1982) Binding of ATP to tubulin. *Nature*, **296**, 757–759.
383. Zahringer, J., Konijn, A.M., Baliga, B.S. & Munro, H.N. (1975) Mechanism of iron induction of ferritin synthesis. *Biochemical, Biophysical Research Communications*, **65**, 583–590.
384. Zahringer, J., Baliga, B.S. & Munro, H.N. (1976) Novel mechanism for translational control in regulation of ferritin synthesis by iron. *Proceedings of the National Academy of Sciences of the USA*, **73**, 857–861.
385. Zern, M.A., Chakraborty, P.R., Ruiz-Opazo, N. *et al.* (1983) Development and use of a rat albumin cDNA clone to evaluate the effect of chronic ethanol administration on hepatic protein synthesis. *Hepatology*, **3**, 317–322.
386. Zimmon, D.S., Oratz, M., Kessler, R. *et al.* (1969) Albumin to ascites: demonstration of a direct pathway bypassing the systemic circulation. *Journal of Clinical Investigation*, **48**, 2074–2078.
387. Zinneman, H.H., Seal, U.S. & Doe, R.P. (1969) Plasma and urinary amino acids in Laennec's cirrhosis. *American Journal Digestive Disease*, **14**, 118–126.
388. Zoli, M., Marchesini, G., Dondi, C. *et al.* (1982) Myofibrillar protein catabolic rates in cirrhotic patients with and without muscle wasting. *Clinical Science*, **62**, 683–686.
389. Zuyderhout, F.M.J., Jorning, G.G.A., Dehaan, J.G. *et al.* (1980) Rat liver storage iron and plasma ferritin during D-galactosamine-HCL-induced hepatitis. *Clinical Science*, **58**, 321–325.

CHAPTER 6

Nutrition and the Liver

Marsha Y. Morgan

The liver plays a central role in the metabolism of the nutrients essential for well-being and for life. Nutrient metabolism may be disturbed, with detrimental consequences, in individuals with hepatobiliary disease. Conversely, liver damage may result from dietary inadequacies, dietary excesses and dietary contaminants, or as a result of various nutritional manoeuvres or therapies. The nutritional status of all patients with hepatobiliary disease should be assessed carefully and monitored regularly. Dietary manipulation and specific nutrient therapy play an important role in the management of these individuals.

In this chapter the nutritional role of the liver and the effects of hepatobiliary disease on nutrient metabolism will be discussed. The damaging effects of dietary inadequacies and excesses, and of certain dietary contaminants on liver structure and function will be considered. Finally, the nutritional management of patients with liver and biliary disease will be detailed.

THE NUTRITIONAL ROLE OF THE LIVER AND THE EFFECTS OF HEPATOBILIARY DAMAGE

Food may be broadly defined as any ingested substance that can be assimilated and utilized for supporting growth, maintaining bodily function, repairing or maintaining cells and tissues and satisfying energy requirements. The diet is the source of some 40 to 50 nutrients which are classically divided into six categories: carbohydrate, fat, protein, vitamins, minerals and water. The caloric requirements of the body can be met by the three bulk dietary components, carbohydrate, fat and protein; of these only protein is indispensable. A number of other nutrients including certain amino acids, fatty acids, minerals and the vitamins are termed essential because they cannot be synthesized de novo. The minimum daily requirement of these essential nutrients is the smallest quantity needed to maintain normal mass, composition, morphology and physiological function of the various organs and tissues of the body, to prevent clinical and biochemical signs of the corresponding deficiency state and, in children, to maintain normal growth. Requirements differ from one individual to another and the requirements of a given individual may change with alterations in the composition and nature of the diet as a whole. For these reasons dietary allowances are recommended which incorporate a margin of safety sufficient to meet the needs of 90–95% of the population, and which take account of differences in requirements according to age, sex, levels of physical activity, pregnancy and lactation.[152,206] Nutritional requirements and tolerances may change in patients with hepatobiliary disease.

ENERGY

Energy requirements are determined, in a given individual, by body size and composition, by age and by the level of physical activity. Healthy adults require 0.13–0.15 MJ (30–35 kcal)/kg or 8–15 MJ (2000 to 3600 kcal)/24 h.[152,206] Dietary carbohydrate should provide 50–55% of total daily energy requirements, fat 30–35%, and protein 10–20%.

The liver plays a central role in energy balance and fuel homeostasis, so that changes in these variables might be expected in individuals with acute and chronic liver disease. To date only one study has been undertaken in patients with acute hepatitis[542] and this is open to criticism. Thus, although the authors report that there were no appreciable changes in energy metabolism in these patients, apart from a decrease in the protein oxidation rate, few patient details are provided and the dietary intakes of the patients and control subjects in the period prior to study are likely to have differed significantly. Further studies are warranted. Several studies have been undertaken in patients with chronic liver disease[183,398,439,460,501,542] but these are generally unsatisfactory; the study populations are heterogeneous and poorly characterized, particularly with regard to the severity of the liver injury, and control populations are small and imperfectly matched, particularly with regard to age. In addition, results are often expressed inappropriately with little regard to the effects of body composition on metabolic variables. In consequence, although most workers agree that the resting respiratory quotient (RQ) is reduced in these patients, indicating use, in the fasting state, of a fat-enriched metabolic mixture, there is little consensus

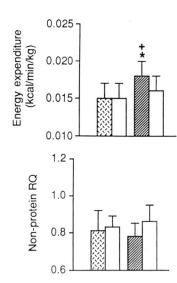

Figure 6.1 Mean ± SD resting energy expenditure and non-protein respiratory quotients (RQ) in 32 patients with cirrhosis and in 32 healthy matched healthy volunteers. Stippled, compensated cirrhosis (n=20); hatched, decompensated cirrhosis (n=12); open, healthy volunteers. Values significantly difference between patients with decompensated cirrhosis and healthy volunteers, *, $p < 0.001$. Values significantly different between patients with compensated and decompensated cirrhosis, +, $p < 0.001$. (Levine et al.[346])

as to the effects of chronic liver disease on resting energy expenditure.

The results of a recent study, conducted by Levine and coworkers,[346] have helped clarify this situation. These workers measured calorimetric variables in a large group of patients with cirrhosis of carefully defined aetiology and severity, exercising controls for drinking behaviour and disturbances of body composition secondary to fluid retention. Reference data were obtained from a population of healthy individuals carefully matched to the study population, on an individual basis, for age, sex, ethnicity and for important anthropometric and dietary variables.

The mean, resting energy expenditure in the cirrhotic patients was significantly increased, compared with control values, whether expressed in absolute terms or in relation to body composition. This increase in resting energy expenditure was independent of the sex of the patient and the aetiology of the liver injury but was related to its severity. Thus, the mean resting energy expenditure in patients with compensated disease was comparable to that in their pair-matched controls, whereas the mean resting energy expenditure in patients with decompensated disease was significantly increased compared to the pair-matched control value (Figure 6.1). However, the difference in mean resting energy expenditure between patients with compensated and decompensated cirrhosis was only significant when related to body weight, and only relatively weak, though significant, correlations were observed between resting energy expenditure and serum bilirubin concentrations and prothrombin times. These workers also found that the mean, resting non-protein RQ was lower in cirrhotic patients than in control subjects (Figure 6.1).

The changes observed in energy expenditure and fuel utilization in patients with cirrhosis can be attributed, at least in part, to the changes occurring in carbohydrate and fat metabolism. In healthy individuals, the net splanchnic glucose production rate, after an overnight fast, averages 8.6 mmol/min/1.73 m^2.[627] Approximately 80% of glucose release is attributed to glycogenolysis while the remainder is attributed to gluconeogenesis from lactate, pyruvate, amino acids and glycerol. The liver glycogen content in healthy individuals, after an overnight fast, averages only 44 mg/g, so that the contribution of glycogenolysis to glucose production falls rapidly after 18–24 hours without feeding.

In patients with liver disease the capacity to store glycogen is decreased because of spatial limitations secondary to fibrosis and/or because of parenchymal damage per se.[450,461] It might, therefore, be expected that, in patients with liver disease, net splanchnic glucose production rates and the contribution of glycogenolysis to glucose production, after an overnight fast, would be reduced. In addition, as circulating concentrations of gluconeogenic precursors[146] and of glucagon[379] are increased in patients with liver disease, and as gluconeogenesis increases with increasing precursor supply[162] and in response to glucagon, the contribution made to glucose production by gluconeogenesis might be expected to increase in these patients. Gluconeogenesis, unlike glycogenolysis, is an energy-requiring process.[203] Thus, if in patients with liver disease a significant increase occurs in the contribution of gluconeogenesis to splanchnic glucose production, after an overnight fast, then hepatic oxygen consumption might increase and this would be reflected in an increase in resting energy expenditure.

The findings of Owen and colleagues[461] support this hypothesis. In an elegant catheterization study these workers showed that, after an overnight fast, the net splanchnic glucose production rate in cirrhotic patients averaged 5.3 mmol/min/1.73 m^2, which is only 62% of the glucose release rate documented in healthy volunteers by Wahren and colleagues.[627] The total net splanchnic extraction rate of gluconeogenic precursors in the cirrhotic patients was about 2-fold greater than that reported in healthy volunteers. As glucagon levels were uniformly raised in the cirrhotic patients, it is likely that the majority of gluconeogenic precursors were quantitatively converted to, and released as glucose to account for, on average, 3.58 mmol/min/1.73 m^2 of the splanchnic glucose production rate. Thus, after an overnight fast, gluconeogenesis accounted for 67% of hepatic glucose release in these cirrhotic patients. Owen and colleagues[461] also showed that the activities of key gluconeogenic enzymes in cirrhotic patients, in vitro, were similar to those in healthy subjects and that the activities appeared more than sufficient to sustain the rates of hepatic gluconeogenesis observed in vivo.

If glucose production rates are reduced in patients with cirrhosis, then fuel homeostasis can only be maintained if compensatory changes occur in the metabolism of other major fuels, and this has been shown to happen. Owen and colleagues,[460] measured plasma free fatty acid concentrations in 8 patients with cirrhosis and 10 healthy volunteers after an overnight fast and determined fatty acid oxidation and turnover rates, using [^{14}C]palmitate. Plasma free fatty acid concentrations were 2-fold greater in cirrhotic patients as a result of increased lipolysis, and an increase of similar magnitude was observed in the free fatty acid oxidation rate which, in the cirrhotic patients, was equivalent to a mean ($\pm$ SEM) of 0.71 $\pm$ 0.07 kcal/min or to 67 $\pm$ 5% of total energy requirements. Thus, the primary mechanism for maintaining fuel homeostasis in cirrhotic patients, in the fasting state, appears to be augmented lipolysis and free fatty acid oxidation, which contribute about two-thirds of total energy requirements and almost 80% of non-protein calorie requirements. Utilization of this fat-enriched 'metabolic mixture', in the fasting state, will be reflected by a reduction in non-protein RQ values.

Thus, patients with chronic liver disease have increased total caloric requirements and their ability to store glycogen is impaired. These findings have nutritional implications.

CARBOHYDRATE

Ingested carbohydrate is absorbed as monosaccharides of which glucose and fructose are quantitatively the most important. Glucose plays a central metabolic role as it is the optimal fuel for many tissues, and is an obligatory fuel for erythrocytes, fibroblasts, the renal medulla and the brain, except during starvation. The phosphorylated forms of fructose are important intracellular intermediates in the metabolism of glucose.

The most important dietary sources of carbohydrate are bread, potatoes, cereals, cakes, biscuits, milk and the sugar added as a sweetener to foods and drinks. Sixty per cent of carbohydrate is ingested in the form of starch and 25% as sucrose. Carbohydrate should provide approximately half of the total daily energy requirements, with a high percentage from unrefined sources to ensure an adequate intake of dietary fibre.

The liver is of prime importance in the regulation of carbohydrate metabolism as it receives absorbed monosaccharides from the portal vein and provides an even and predictable supply of glucose to extrahepatic tissue, when required. The liver removes 25–50% of ingested glucose, although probably less than 10% is taken up on first passage.[486] Glucose diffuses rapidly into the liver where it is used for energy, stored as glycogen or converted to fat. The remaining 50–75% enters peripheral tissues where it is oxidized or stored as glycogen. As circulating concentrations of glucose fall, so more is released from the liver. After an overnight fast, 75% of released glucose is derived from glycogenolysis; the remainder is formed by gluconeogenesis using lactate, pyruvate, alanine and glycerol as precursors. Glucose, glucose precursors and hormones are all important in the regulation of gluco-genesis, gluconeogenesis and glycogenolysis. The major portion of fructose in the portal vein is removed by the liver on first pass. Approximately one-third is metabolized immediately to pyruvate and lactate; the remainder is rapidly phosphorylated.

Carbohydrate metabolism is disturbed in patients with liver disease, although the abnormalities are not as striking as might be anticipated. Hypoglycaemia is common in patients with fulminant hepatic failure, presumably because of impairment of glycogen synthesis and break-down, and of gluconeogenesis. Hypoglycaemia, however, is rare in patients with chronic liver disease unless provoked by oral hypoglycaemic agents. Patients with cirrhosis commonly show fasting hyperglycaemia and glucose intolerance. Glucose intolerance is also frequently observed in patients with acute viral hepatitis, hepatic steatosis, toxic liver damage and autoimmune chronic active hepatitis. More patients show intolerance to oral than to intravenous glucose[135] which can only partly be explained by portal–systemic shunting of blood.[271,486] The mechanism of glucose intolerance in patients with liver disease is largely unknown, but there is much evidence to suggest that relative insensitivity of tissues to insulin may be a major factor; the exact nature of the insulin resistance observed in these patients remains to be eluci-dated. Patients with cirrhosis may show higher serum fructose concentrations after an oral load,[385] most likely as a consequence of portal–systemic shunting of blood;[569] this is of no significant consequence.

FAT

Fat is a metabolic fuel and a major source of the fat-soluble vitamins and essential fatty acids.

Dietary fat is mainly triglyceride and is provided from such 'visible' sources as butter, margarine, cooking fat, vegetable oils and meat fat, and from 'invisible' sources such as nuts, egg yolk and lean meat. Cakes, biscuits, gravies and sauces, because of their content of butter, cooking fat, milk or eggs, are additional rich sources of dietary lipid.

Naturally occurring fat contains both saturated and unsaturated fatty acids. The most important are the long-chain fatty acids which have carbon chain lengths of 16 or more. They include the common saturated fatty acids (palmitic (C_{16}) and stearic (C_{18})), the mono-unsaturated oleic ($C_{18}\Delta 9$), where Δ signifies the position of the double bond or bonds and the polyunsaturated fatty acids (linoleic ($C_{18}\Delta 9, 12$), linolenic ($C_{18}\Delta 9, 12, 15$) and arachidonic ($C_{20}\Delta 5, 8, 11, 14$)). Medium-chain triglycerides contain fatty acids with chain lengths shorter than C_{16}.

No recommendations have been made for either the total caloric intake of lipid or for the relative amounts of contained saturated and unsaturated fatty acids. However, a daily minimum of 40 g of dietary fat is required for palatability and fat should provide 30–35% of total daily energy requirements. Fat-soluble vitamin requirements are easily met with a palatable diet; the essential fatty acid requirement can be met by daily ingestion of 11 mmol (3 g) of linoleic acid.

Following ingestion, dietary fat is emulsified by bile salts. Pancreatic lipase splits the ester linkages of the long-chain triglycerides at positions 1 and 3 of the glycerol backbone to produce two fatty acids and a 2-monoglycer-ide. These associate with bile acids and phosphatidyl-choline to form micelles which incorporate cholesterol and fat-soluble vitamins into their core. These micelles come into contact with the small intestinal microvilli and their fatty acids, monoglyceride, cholesterol and fat-soluble vitamins are taken up by the enterocytes. The monoglyceride and fatty acids are synthesized to triglycer-ide within the enterocyte which is then, together with cholesterol, cholesterol esters, phospholipids, apoproteins and fat-soluble vitamins, packaged into chylomicrons to leave the gut in intestinal lymph. Medium-chain triglycer-ides do not require bile salts or pancreatic lipase for their digestion; they pass directly through the mucosal cells into the portal blood and are bound to albumin for transport in unesterified form.

The major lipids of plasma are: (i) cholesterol, which is an important constituent of all mammalian plasma membranes and a precursor of bile acids and steroid hormones; (ii) cholesterol esters, which store and trans-port cholesterol molecules; (iii) phospholipids, which are major constituents of membranes and take part in many important biochemical reactions, including intracellular signalling via breakdown of phosphoinositides; and (iv) triglyceride, which is the major form in which fat is transported in plasma and stored in adipose tissue.

Plasma lipids are associated with proteins. Unesterified fats and the phospholipid lysolecithin are bound to albu-min or to specific proteins such as retinol-binding protein. However, the majority of plasma lipids are carried by lipoproteins; these are large macromolecular complexes which are manufactured in the liver or intestine and which contain cholesterol, phospholipid, one or more specific polypeptides termed apoproteins and small quantities of non-polar lipids. The lipoproteins are classified, on the basis of certain physicochemical properties, as chylo-microns, very low-density lipoproteins (VLDL), low-density lipoproteins (LDL) and high-density lipoproteins (HDL). Triglycerides are mainly transported in chylomi-crons and in VLDL, while cholesterol is transported mainly in LDL.

The lipoproteins are subsequently broken down by peripheral and hepatic lipases and by lecithin–cholesterol acyltransferase (LCAT). Once triglyceride has been released from chylomicrons and VLDL it is hydrolysed by lipoprotein lipase to free fatty acids which are available for uptake in the periphery. Fatty acids, particularly the polyunsaturated fatty acids, may be incorporated into cell structures and play an important role in membrane interchange, thus influencing the activity of some key enzymes and receptors. In addition, polyunsaturated fatty acids with 20 carbon atoms are precursors of prostaglandins and related eicosanoids. The cholesterol released from LDL is not degraded in man; cholesterol losses from the body occur by shedding of cholesterol in skin cells and intestinal epithelia, and by faecal excretion of biliary and dietary cholesterol, bile salts and metabolites of unabsorbed cholesterol.

In patients with parenchymal liver disease or chronic cholestasis, the flow of bile salts is usually reduced and this interferes with fat emulsification and triglyceride hydrolysis by pancreatic lipase. Some hydrolysis of triglyceride still occurs and free fatty acids and monoglyceride continue to be absorbed in relatively large amounts. Thus, steatorrhoea is usually modest; its severity is roughly proportional to the degree of hepatocellular damage or biliary obstruction. When luminal concentrations of bile salts are low, micelle formation is seriously disrupted and this will impair the absorption of fat-soluble vitamins and cholesterol, as these depend on micellar solubility for their uptake.

A number of changes are observed in circulating lipid, lipoprotein and fatty acid concentrations in individuals with both parenchymal liver disease and chronic cholestasis. Circulating cholesterol and triglyceride concentrations may increase as a result of regurgitation of biliary lipids into plasma and because of a reduction in plasma LCAT activity secondary to impaired hepatic synthesis or defective enzyme release from the damaged liver.[8] Changes may also occur in the structure, electrophoretic mobility and composition of the lipoprotein fractions, predominantly in patients in whom plasma LCAT activity is reduced.[147] Total plasma fatty acid concentrations may be increased in patients with chronic liver disease,[396,460] and absolute and relative increases may be observed in the plasma concentrations of individual fatty acids.[603] The constituent fatty acids of triglyceride, phospholipids and cholesterol esters may show increased saturation and a concomitant decrease in polyunsaturated fatty acids, probably as a result of impaired hepatic essential fatty acid metabolism.[463] Recently, Cabré and colleagues,[88,90] reported a reduction in total plasma concentrations of saturated fatty acids, linoleate and polyunsaturated fatty acids in patients with alcoholic cirrhosis; the reduction in polyunsaturated fatty acids and linoleate was proportionally greater than the reduction in saturated and monoenoic fatty acids. The reductions observed in polyunsaturated fatty acids were greatest in those patients with the most severe liver disease, those most nutritionally compromised and those actively abusing alcohol.

Xanthelasma may develop in patients with chronic liver disease who have very high serum lipid concentrations; these typically appear around the eyes, on the palms and soles and over bony prominences.[9] Rarely a xanthomatous peripheral neuropathy may develop.[610] Changes may be observed in the cholesterol and/or phospholipid content of erythrocyte membranes in patients with long-standing liver disease which result in changes in red-cell shape and

possibly survival. Similarly, the changes observed in plasma lipoproteins in these patients may induce alterations in the membrane fluidity of a variety of cells. Deficiency of polyunsaturated fatty acids may result in impaired synthesis of prostaglandins and related compounds.

PROTEIN

Protein is an energy source and provides the body with amino acids for endogenous protein synthesis. The amino acids threonine, valine, methionine, leucine, isoleucine, phenylalanine, lysine and tryptophan are 'essential' in both children and adults, while arginine and histidine are additionally essential during childhood.

Dietary protein is derived from animal sources such as meat, fish, eggs, milk and cheese and from vegetable sources such as peas, beans, lentils, other pulses, cereals, bread and flour. Approximately one-third of dietary protein ingested in the United Kingdom is of animal origin. Daily protein requirements are influenced by the caloric intake and by the biological value of the proteins ingested. The biological value of a protein is defined as the proportion which is retained following absorption, and depends primarily on its content of essential amino acids. In general, animal proteins have higher biological values than vegetable proteins. If calories are deficient, then the daily protein requirement is inversely proportional to the energy intake. A diet which provides less than 10% of total food energy as protein is likely to be unpalatable and may be deficient in other nutrients such as easily absorbable iron, vitamin B_{12}, riboflavin, nicotinic acid and trace elements such as zinc. A daily dietary protein intake of 0.5 g/kg body weight will maintain bodily function in a healthy adult; daily intakes of 0.65 g/kg in adult women and of 0.70 g/kg in adult males are considered 'safe'. Daily requirements for the eight essential amino acids vary from 250 to 1100 mg. About 30 g of non-essential amino acids is also required for protein synthesis. However, it has recently been suggested, on the basis of studies with stable isotopes, that the recommended intakes for amino acids may significantly underestimate actual needs.[653]

Dietary protein is completely hydrolysed during the process of digestion and intestinal absorption and the amino acids released enter the portal vein. There they mix with amino acids derived from the digestion and absorption of exfoliated cellular protein, secreted enzyme protein and a small amount of exuded plasma protein.

Hepatocyte uptake of amino acids is governed by transport mechanisms which are stereospecific, saturable for certain amino acids, and may exhibit cross-inhibition.[465] In consequence, there are selective differences in hepatic amino acid uptake and metabolism. Alanine uptake, for example, exceeds that of all other amino acids, while the branched-chain amino acids leucine, isoleucine and valine are poorly extracted by the liver; their main site of metabolism is skeletal muscle.[409]

In healthy individuals, plasma amino acid concentrations vary with age, sex and dietary intake[417] and with the amount of exercise taken.[20] After an overnight fast, women have lower plasma concentrations of several amino acids than men, although these differences disappear postprandially.[417] With a dietary intake of 1 g/kg body weight, which would be considered normal for a British population, no significant diurnal variation is found in the plasma amino acid concentrations; if protein intake is increased to 1.5 g/kg, then significant variations are seen, throughout the day, in the plasma concentrations of proline, half-cysteine, methionine and the three branched-chain amino acids.[417]

The liver plays a central role in protein and amino acid metabolism. It processes dietary amino acids and reprocesses amino acids released from muscle protein degradation. It regulates the supply of amino acids to peripheral tissues such as muscle, and converts excess amino acids into urea for excretion in the urine. Ammonia derived from the intrahepatic deamination of amino acids and generated extrahepatically from the metabolism of nucleotides, from the metabolism of glutamine in the gut wall and as a result of bacterial degradation of intestinal protein and urea, is efficiently eliminated, as urea, by the hepatic urea-cycle enzymes. The liver utilizes amino acids, particularly alanine and glutamine, for gluconeogenesis and for protein synthesis. It is the exclusive or major site of synthesis for virtually all the plasma proteins and is an important site for degradation of many of these proteins and of the hormones. The liver may modulate overall body protein metabolism because of its role in the metabolism of hormones which regulate peripheral amino acid metabolism.

Daily protein requirements are increased in patients with cirrhosis.[213,601] Their minimal daily protein requirement has been calculated as 0.75 g/kg and their daily safe level of protein intake as 58 g or 1.2 g/kg.[601] Diets may be suboptimal because of anorexia, nausea, abdominal distension and/or ascites or else dietary restriction may have been enforced for the management of hepatic encephalopathy and fluid retention. In consequence, these patients are often in negative nitrogen balance[195] and show reduced lean body mass and muscle wasting.[435]

It has been suggested that the increased protein requirement arises because these patients cannot store glycogen[450,461] and in consequence show a reduction in the contribution of glycogenolysis to hepatic glucose release and a compensatory increase in gluconeogenesis.[461] This results in additional loss of amino acids and depletion of tissue protein stores; extra dietary protein is then required to help replenish the deficit.

This hypothesis is supported by evidence from two groups of workers that whole-body protein synthesis and breakdown rates are increased in patients with cirrhosis.[455,602] However, other workers have found the rate of protein synthesis in cirrhotic patients to be unchanged[410,439] or else decreased.[435] Obviously further studies are needed to clarify this situation.

In patients with acute and chronic liver disease, synthesis of plasma proteins, for example albumin and prothrombin, may be reduced. Additionally, in patients with severe liver disease, qualitative changes may occur in certain proteins, for example fibrinogen, which alter or attenuate their function.

Blood urea concentrations may be low in patients with chronic liver disease, reflecting a reduction in urea synthesis rates.[553] Conversely, blood ammonia concentrations may be elevated secondary to impaired hepatic function and portal–systemic shunting of blood. The increase in circulating ammonia concentrations has been implicated in the genesis of hepatic encephalopathy.

Significant changes occur in plasma amino acid concentrations in patients with liver disease which appear to relate to the severity of the liver disease, its activity and its aetiology.[432] In patients with fulminant hepatic failure, plasma concentrations of all the amino acids are high except those of the branched-chain amino acids, which are normal or low.[491] These changes reflect release of amino acids into the plasma from peripheral tissues and from the necrosing liver, and failure of hepatic amino acid uptake. The branched-chain amino acids are predominantly metabolized by muscle, so that their plasma concentrations are largely unaffected. In patients with chronic liver disease, plasma concentrations of the branched-chain amino acids are reduced, while concentrations of one or both of the aromatic amino acids phenylalanine and tyrosine are increased, together with methionine.[424,432, 474] These changes reflect impaired hepatic function, portal–systemic shunting of blood, hyperinsulinaemia and hyperglucagonaemia, and have been implicated in the genesis of hepatic encephalopathy.

In patients with minimal, potentially reversible liver damage, for example alcoholic fatty liver or acute viral hepatitis, plasma concentrations of the branched-chain amino acids and proline are reduced.[432] These changes are not readily explained but indicate that amino acid metabolism is disturbed even in the presence of minor liver injury.

FAT-SOLUBLE VITAMINS[380] _____

Vitamin A[229,230]

Vitamin A originates in the diet as retinol, which is found in the tissues of animals and saltwater fish mainly as the ester, retinyl palmitate, and as 3,4-dehydroretinol, which is found mainly in freshwater fish. Plant carotenoids, such as β-carotene, can be hydrolysed in the small-intestinal epithelial cells to retinaldehyde and then reduced to retinol. Fish liver oils are the richest source of vitamin A, but substantial amounts are present in mammalian liver, kidney, dairy produce and eggs. β-Carotene is found in dark green leafy vegetables such as parsley and spinach, and in carrots; approximately 50% of dietary vitamin A is provided in this form. In healthy adults the recommended daily intake is 4000–5000 IU (1.2–1.5 mg) of vitamin A or 800–1000 retinol equivalents (1 retinol equivalent = 1 μg of retinol, 6 μg of β-carotene or 3.33 IU of vitamin A activity).[152,206]

Retinol is present in the diet mainly in esterified form. Most of the retinyl esters are hydrolysed in the intestinal lumen and brush border before absorption. Although retinol is lipophilic, and its absorption is linked to that of lipid and is enhanced by bile, its uptake by intestinal cells is governed by a carrier-mediated process and is facilitated by the presence of a cytosolic protein, cellular retinol-binding protein. The retinol is largely re-esterified in enterocytes before leaving the gut, and enters the liver in chylomicron remnants. Appreciable quantities of retinol are absorbed directly into the circulation. Retinol and retinyl esters are stored primarily in the liver. β-Carotene is less well absorbed; its uptake is, therefore, more affected by disorders of fat absorption and micelle formation. A proportion of β-carotene is converted to retinol in the intestinal wall; this is then esterified and transported in the lymph. Some β-carotene is absorbed unchanged and circulates in association with lipoproteins. β-Carotene is stored primarily in the liver but also in body fat.

The concentration of retinyl esters in the liver is approximately 100–300 μg/g compared with a concentration of 1 μg/g in tissues such as kidney, lung or intraperitoneal fat; the retinal pigment epithelium contains approximately 10 μg/g. Before release into the circulation, hepatic retinyl esters are hydrolysed and 90–95% of the retinol formed is bound to an α_1-globulin, retinol-binding protein, which circulates in the blood complexed with transthyretin, a thyroxine-binding prealbumin. The formation of this complex prevents metabolism and excretion of the retinol–retinol-binding protein moiety. Retinyl esters comprise less than 5% of total retinoids in the blood; they are associated with lipoproteins. Plasma concentrations of retinol are maintained at the expense of hepatic reserves. Thus, plasma retinol concentrations do not provide an accurate assessment of overall vitamin A status, although low plasma retinol concentrations indicate a significant reduction in hepatic vitamin A stores. Retinol is conjugated with β-glucuronide, which is excreted in bile and can be reabsorbed. It is also oxidized to retinal and retinoic acid which, together with other water-soluble metabolites, are excreted in the urine and faeces.

Vitamin A plays an essential role in the function of the retina. It is necessary for the growth and differentiation of epithelial tissues and is required for bone growth, reproduction and embryonic development. Vitamin A, together with certain carotenoids, appears to enhance the function of the immune system, to reduce the consequences of some infectious diseases, and to protect against the development of certain malignancies. Retinol also appears to have a specific biochemical function in the synthesis of mannose- and galactose-containing glycoproteins and glycolipids.

In the retina, vitamin A forms a series of carotenoid proteins that provide the molecular basis for visual excitation. In order to be photochemically active, retinol must be converted to its aldehyde, retinal, which requires the zinc-dependent enzyme retinal dehydrogenase.[576] Vitamin E may be necessary to prevent peroxidation of vitamin A in the retina.[506] Vitamin A, as retinal, also plays an important role in spermatogenesis; in vitro it acts synergistically with insulin, follicle-stimulating hormone and testosterone to stimulate production of androgen-binding protein by Sertoli cells.[302]

Symptoms and signs of vitamin A deficiency appear when plasma concentrations fall below 0.35–0.70 μmol/l (10–20 μg/100 ml) or when the hepatic concentrations of retinoids are less than 5–20 μg/g. The most recognizable manifestation of vitamin A deficiency is impaired dark adaptation, possibly leading to night blindness. In addition, adults may develop follicular hyperkeratosis and children xerophthalmia. Deficiency in adults should be treated with oral vitamin A, 50 000 IU (15 mg) daily. In children, a single intramuscular injection of 30 mg of retinol as the water-miscible palmitate has been advocated, followed by intermittent oral treatment with vitamin A in oil.

Vitamin A metabolism is disturbed in patients with chronic hepatobiliary disease. Absorption of the vitamin may be impaired whenever bile secretion is reduced. Hepatic synthesis and release of retinol-binding protein may be reduced in patients with parenchymal liver damage,[268,300,368,568] resulting in impaired release of vitamin A from hepatic stores. In addition, hepatic synthesis of transthyretin may be significantly impaired, resulting in urinary loss of the retinol–retinol-binding protein complex. In individuals chronically abusing alcohol, the microsomal cytochrome P450 enzyme system is induced, resulting in enhanced hepatic vitamin A metabolism and a reduction in retinoid stores.[344] In addition, the dehydrogenase required to convert retinol to retinal has an affinity for ethanol 50 times greater than for retinol; therefore ethanol in the circulation could act as a competitive enzyme inhibitor.[333] Ethanol also increases urinary zinc excretion and this might further impair the function of vitamin A.[298] Hepatic vitamin A stores are reduced in individuals with non-alcoholic liver disease[38,541] and in individuals chronically abusing alcohol, whether or not they have significant liver injury.[38,290,344] Both groups of individuals may, therefore, develop vitamin A deficiency.

Vitamin A deficiency is relatively common in patients with primary biliary cirrhosis; the lowest plasma values are found in the most severely cholestatic patients.[440] Deficiency is usually manifest as impaired dark adaptation; overt night blindness is rarely encountered.[261,434] As individuals may be unaware of even severe impairment of dark adaptation, visual function should be checked routinely in all patients with chronic cholestasis. Regular monthly intramuscular injections of 10 000 IU (3 mg) of vitamin A should be given to patients with primary biliary cirrhosis who are jaundiced. However, as the disease progresses it would seem advisable to give oral supplements of 25 000 IU (7.5 mg) daily.[629] At present there is insufficient evidence to support the use of regular zinc supplementation.

Children with chronic cholestasis may show electrical abnormalities of the retina that could be attributed to lack of vitamin A, vitamin E, or both.[13] Studies in animals indicate that a combined deficiency accelerates the loss of photoreceptor cells.[506] Supplementation with both vitamins is, therefore, recommended.

Individuals chronically abusing alcohol may develop hypogonadism and impaired dark adaptation, possibly as a result of vitamin A deficiency.[368] Management involves abstinence from alcohol, the institution of a nutritionally sound diet and oral vitamin A, 30 000 IU (9 mg) daily for 3–5 days. There is no evidence that the hypogonadism responds to vitamin A supplementation alone.

Chronic ingestion of high doses of vitamin A, over a prolonged period, can result in the development of liver injury.[251,527]

Vitamin D[253,272,494]

Many forms of vitamin D exist but only two are of nutritional or biological significance: vitamin D_2 (ergocalciferol) is synthesized in the skin by ultraviolet irradiation of ergosterol, which is derived from yeasts and fungi, while vitamin D_3 (cholecalciferol) is synthesized in the skin by ultraviolet irradiation of 7-dehydrocholesterol, which is derived from animal sources. The only structural difference between D_2 and D_3 is in the side-chain; in the absence of a subscript, the term vitamin D refers to either compound.

Vitamin D is unique among vitamins in that, with adequate sunlight, no dietary intake is needed, as the entire bodily requirements can be met by skin photolysis reactions. Only when skin irradiation is limited or insignificant is there a real need for dietary supplementation. The richest sources of dietary vitamin D are fish liver oils, animal liver and dairy produce; crystalline vitamin D is added to a variety of foods including milk, milk products, margarine and cereals. The daily requirements for vitamin D in adults have not been established; daily intakes in the region of 200–400 IU (5–10 μg) of cholecalciferol have been recommended for adults, and of 400 IU (10 μg) for children.[152,206]

Ingested vitamin D is absorbed from the small intestine in association with dietary fat and requires micellar solubilization for its uptake. Newly absorbed vitamin D leaves the gut in lymphatics, primarily as a lipoprotein complex in the chylomicron fraction. Subsequently, the vitamin is either stored unchanged in the liver, skeletal muscle or adipose tissue or else is converted into one of its biologically active, hydroxylated, forms which circulate in plasma bound to a specific α_1-globulin designated vitamin D-binding protein.

The vitamin D formed by skin photolysis diffuses into the circulation via cutaneous blood and lymph capillaries. It associates with vitamin D-binding protein in plasma and is only gradually taken up by the liver.

Vitamin D is hydroxylated in the liver to 25-hydroxy-cholecalciferol (25-(OH)D), or calcifediol, which is the major circulating form of the vitamin. In healthy individuals there is marked seasonal variation in serum 25-(OH)D concentrations, which are maximal in autumn and minimal at the end of winter. Further hydroxylation of 25-(OH)D occurs in the kidney, with formation of 1,25-dihydroxycholecalciferol (1,25-(OH)$_2$D), or calcitriol, which is now believed to be the active form of the vitamin. When supplies of calcium and phosphorus are adequate, 24,25-dihydroxycholecalciferol (24,25-(OH)$_2$D) is the major metabolite of 25-(OH)D rather than 1,25-(OH)$_2$D. Some vitamin D may be 1-α-hydroxylated to form 1-α-vitamin D [1α-(OH)D] before 25-hydroxylation occurs. Vitamin D is inactivated by microsomal drug-metabolizing enzymes or else is excreted unchanged in the bile to undergo enterohepatic recirculation.

The active forms of vitamin D, together with para-thyroid hormone and calcitonin, play an important role in regulating calcium and phosphorus homeostasis, in particular the maintenance of plasma calcium and phosphorus concentrations. Vitamin D promotes calcium and phosphorus absorption from the small intestine, mobilizes calcium and phosphorus from bone and increases calcium retention by the kidney. 1,25-(OH)$_2$D also affects maturation and differentiation of mononuclear cells and influences lymphokine production.[15] It also inhibits proliferation and induces differentiation of malignant cells.[71,252] Vitamin D deficiency results in defective mineralization of bone, with development of rickets in children and osteomalacia in adults; it is treated with oral cholecalciferol, 500–5000 IU (12.5–125 μg) daily. 1α-(OH)D and 1α-25-(OH)$_2$D should be used to treat vitamin D deficiency in patients with renal disease.

Patients with long-standing cholestasis or severe parenchymal liver disease may have low circulating serum 25-(OH)D concentrations.[126,137,260,440] A small percentage of these patients will develop osteomalacia which is characterized by bone pain and fractures.[23,157] The aetiology of the vitamin D deficiency is multifactorial, but poor diet, reduced exposure to sunlight, malabsorption and increased urinary losses of water-soluble metabolites all play a role. It might be expected that in the presence of severe liver disease hydroxylation of vitamin D would be impaired, but there is little evidence that this occurs.[325,477] Both vitamin D and its metabolites have been used to treat osteomalacia in patients with long-standing cholestasis and severe parenchymal liver disease.[127,128,360,493] Patients with primary biliary cirrhosis and those with long-standing biliary obstruction should receive prophylactic intramuscular vitamin D, 10 000 IU (0.25 mg) monthly.

Low serum 25-(OH)D concentrations are also found in individuals chronically abusing alcohol, irrespective of whether they have associated liver disease;[154,156,264,423,477] the aetiology is multifactorial and includes poor dietary intake, malabsorption and possibly increased urinary losses of water-soluble metabolites. Many such individuals have osteopenia, but the percentage with osteomalacia is probably very small. The bone lesion responds to vitamin D and its metabolites once the individual has stopped drinking and liver function has improved.[423,477]

Prolonged ingestion of vitamin D supplements is associated with the development of hypercalcaemia with metastatic tissue calcification.[253]

Vitamin E[47,380,573]

Vitamin E activity is found in naturally occurring tocopherols; α-tocopherol is the most abundant and has the greatest biological activity. The main sources of vitamin E in the diet are polyunsaturated vegetable oils, cereal products and eggs. Daily intakes of 8 mg (12 IU) of d-α-tocopherol for women and of 10 mg (15 IU) of d-α-tocopherol for men are recommended.[152,206] The activity of 1 mg of d-α-tocopherol is equal to 1 α-tocopherol equivalent. The vitamin is prescribed as d-α-tocopherol acetate, which has a potency of 1.36 IU/mg; d-α-tocopherol succinate, which has a potency of 1.21 IU/mg, is also available.

Esterified tocopherols are hydrolysed in the intestinal lumen and micellar solubilization is necessary for maximal absorption. Aqueous dispersions, which are more readily absorbed, are available for use when natural absorption is impaired. Free tocopherol is transported from the intestine in chylomicrons and is taken up by the liver in chylomicron remnants. It is then secreted in VLDL and subsequently becomes associated with plasma β-lipoproteins. There does not appear to be a specific plasma transport protein. Circulating tocopherol is taken up slowly by tissues and stored in fat, skeletal muscle and liver; tissue concentrations vary widely. Vitamin E is metabolized in the liver and its metabolites are excreted in bile and urine.

Vitamin E inhibits oxidation of unsaturated fatty acids and other oxygen-sensitive compounds by interacting with selenium and ascorbate. Its ability to prevent lipid peroxidation is of fundamental importance to all cells. It also has free radical scavenging properties and may have a cardioprotective effect by favouring redistribution of cholesterol into the HDL fraction.[262]

Vitamin E deficiency is associated with the development of increased red cell fragility and haemolytic anaemia.[658] While these changes may reflect alterations in lipid peroxidation, they may also indicate a role for the vitamin in normal haematopoiesis.[165,177] A neurological syndrome has been described in association with vitamin E deficiency; its features include peripheral neuropathy, cerebellar degeneration and abnormal eye movements.[47,177,238,247,509,573] In both male and female rats, deficiency of vitamin E results in infertility; its role in human fertility is unknown.

Children with chronic cholestasis develop a neurological syndrome which has been attributed to vitamin E deficiency[177,509] and which responds, at least in part, to treatment with α-tocopherol.[238] They also develop retinal degeneration which has been attributed to deficiency of

vitamin E, vitamin A, or both.[13] Established deficiency can be treated with oral d-α-tocopherol acetate in a daily dose of 50–200 IU (37–147 mg)/kg body weight. If oral supplementation is unsuccessful, then dl-α-tocopherol may be given intravenously in a dose of 1–2 IU (1–2 mg)/kg daily. In adults with chronic cholestasis or with parenchymal liver damage, vitamin E deficiency, if present, tends to be mild and subclinical.[290,403,413,440,606] Although red-cell survival is shortened in these patients, its aetiology is multifactorial and lack of vitamin E is of only minor importance. The polyunsaturated fatty acid content of erythrocyte membranes is reduced in jaundiced patients and this may attenuate the effects of vitamin E deficiency.

Vitamin K[295,380,598]

Vitamin K activity is associated with at least two distinct natural substances; vitamin K_1 (phytonadione), which is present in most edible vegetables, particularly spinach, cabbage, cauliflower, peas and cereals, and vitamin K_2 (a series of menaquinones), which is produced in the mammalian intestine by Gram-positive bacteria. All other compounds which possess vitamin K-like activity are structurally related to the simpler compound, menadione. Daily intakes of the order of 45–80 μg or of 1 μg/kg body weight are recommended for adults.

Vitamins K_1 and K_2 are dependent for their absorption on micellar solubilization, whereas menadione and its water-soluble derivatives are absorbed, even in the absence of bile. Vitamin K_1 is absorbed by an active process in the proximal small intestine, while vitamin K_2 and the menadiones are absorbed by passive diffusion in the distal small intestine and colon. Following absorption, vitamins K_1 and K_2 leave the gut by way of the lymph, while menadione and its water-soluble derivatives enter the bloodstream directly. Vitamin K_1 is rapidly metabolized in the liver and its metabolites are excreted in bile and urine. Body stores of vitamin K are small but take several weeks to deplete.

Vitamin K is essential for the hepatic synthesis of the procoagulant Factors II (prothrombin), VII, IX and X. It is also necessary for the hepatic synthesis of γ-carboxyglutamic acid (Gla), a metal-binding amino acid which is required for the functional activity of vitamin K-dependent coagulation proteins and certain other proteins in cortical bone, renal tissue, lung, spleen, pancreas and placenta. Vitamin K is also required for production of protein C and protein S. Protein C, a serine protease, is synthesized in the liver and, in its activated form, functions as an anticoagulant by inactivating Factors V and VII; it also facilitates clot lysis.[125] Protein S, a glycoprotein, is synthesized mainly in the liver and its free form acts as a cofactor in the inactivation of Factors V and VII by protein C.

Deficiency of vitamin K is associated with a marked decrease in the activities of Factors II, VII, IX and X; this may be associated with a bleeding tendency. The prothrombin produced by the liver in the presence of vitamin K deficiency contains a considerably reduced number of Gla residues so that it is unable to bind calcium and to function normally. Similar abnormalities may occur in the other proteins which require vitamin K for post-translational modification. Vitamin K deficiency is treated with parenteral vitamin K_1 in daily doses of 1–10 mg.

In patients with both acute and chronic liver disease, circulating concentrations of the blood clotting proteins may be reduced and the prothrombin time prolonged. Several factors are responsible, including vitamin K deficiency due to poor dietary intake, malabsorption and cholestasis, diminished hepatic protein synthesis and increased consumption of clotting factor following bleeding and fibrinolysis. In a percentage of patients there are low but detectable concentrations of an abnormal prothrombin in the plasma.[52] Improvement may occur in the prothrombin time in patients with parenchymal liver disease following parenteral vitamin K_1, but in general coagulation remains prolonged until liver function improves. Paradoxically, the administration of large doses of vitamin K_1 or its analogues to patients with severe parenchymal liver disease may result in further depression of the prothrombin concentration; the mechanism is unknown. Patients with obstructive jaundice absorb vitamin K poorly; defects in their clotting time can be corrected by parenteral administration of vitamin K_1. Patients with primary biliary cirrhosis and those with long-standing biliary obstruction should be given prophylactic intramuscular vitamin K_1, 10 mg monthly; cutaneous hypersensitivity to injected vitamin K_1 may develop.[198]

WATER-SOLUBLE VITAMINS[142,381]

Thiamine[142,381]

Thiamine is synthesized by a variety of plants and micro-organisms, but not by animal tissues. It is widely distributed in food and the richest sources in the United Kingdom are bread, flour, potatoes and meat; eggs, fruit, nuts, vegetables, whole-grain cereals and fortified breakfast cereals are rich additional sources. A limited amount of thiamine may be synthesized by intestinal bacteria. A large portion of the vitamin in vegetable products is in the form of thiamine itself, whereas in animal tissues it is mainly present as phosphate esters. Daily thiamine intakes of 1.0 mg for women and 1.5 mg for men or of 120 μg/MJ (0.5 mg/1000 kcal) of total energy intake are recommended.[152,206] Requirements increase in proportion to increases in metabolic rate and are greatest when carbohydrate is the main source of dietary energy. Fresh fish, shrimps, clams, mussels and some raw animal tissues contain thiaminases which inactivate thiamine, while betel nuts and tea leaves contain a thiamine antagonist. Excessive ingestion of these foods will substantially increase thiamine requirements.

At low, or physiological, concentrations thiamine is absorbed from the small intestine by a sodium-dependent, active transport process. At high or pharmacological concentrations, transport across the intestine may also occur by passive diffusion. Thiamine passes to the liver, where it is phosphorylated to thiamine pyrophosphate. The body of a healthy adult contains about 25 mg of thiamine. It is stored in a variety of tissues, principally as the pyrophosphate. Heart muscle contains 2–3 μg/g; brain, liver and kidney about 1 μg/g and skeletal muscle 0.5 μg/g. Thiamine circulates in free form in the plasma and as the pyrophosphate in erythrocytes and leucocytes. It is catabolized to a number of metabolites, some of which are excreted in urine, together with unchanged thiamine.

Thiamine pyrophosphate, the physiologically active form of thiamine, functions in carbohydrate metabolism as a coenzyme in the decarboxylation of α-keto acids, for example pyruvate and α-ketoglutarate, and as a cofactor for transketolase in the hexose–monophosphate shunt. In recent years it has been suggested that thiamine may have a specific role in neuromuscular transmission, independent of its function as a coenzyme in general metabolism.[132, 544]

Thiamine deficiency leads to disorders of the cardiovascular (wet beri-beri) and nervous systems (dry beri-beri and the Wernicke–Korsakoff syndrome). Beri-beri heart disease may develop acutely or chronically and usually results in high-output cardiac failure. Parenteral administration of thiamine rapidly restores peripheral vascular resistance but, as improvement of the myocardial abnormality is often delayed, treatment may be complicated by the development of low-output cardiac failure. Wernicke's encephalopathy is characterized by a confusional state, variable degrees of ophthalmoplegia and ataxia. The central feature of Korsakoff psychosis is a memory defect specifically involving short-term memory; confabulation may be present. Wernicke's encephalopathy and Korsakoff's psychosis are not separate clinical entities but represent successive stages of a single disease process; hence the term the Wernicke–Korsakoff syndrome. Treatment with oral or intramuscular thiamine hydrochloride, in doses of up to 600 mg daily, results in improvement in the features of the Wernicke's encephalopathy but the Korsakoff's psychosis improves in only 50% of patients. Dry beri-beri manifests as a symmetrical, bilateral sensorimotor peripheral neuropathy; it is non-specific and cannot be distinguished from other 'nutritional' neuropathies; it responds reasonably well to thiamine supplementation given in a dose of 40 mg daily.

The factors which determine the manifestations of thiamine deficiency in individual patients are poorly understood. Several factors are, however, known to be important, including the duration and severity of the thiamine deficiency, the amount of physical activity undertaken and the daily caloric intake. A moderate degree of chronic thiamine deficiency coupled with a high carbohydrate intake and severe physical exertion favours the development of cardiovascular disease. An equal deficiency coupled with caloric restriction and relative

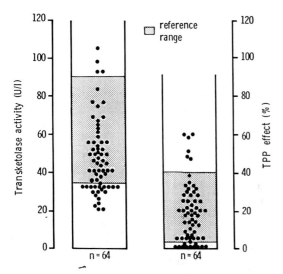

Figure 6.2 Erythrocyte transketolase activity in 64 individuals with alcohol-related liver disease of varying severity both before and after stimulation in vitro with the coenzyme thiamine pyrophosphate (TPP effect). (Camilo et al.[94])

inactivity favours the development of peripheral neuropathy. Genetic factors might also be important. Blass and Gibson,[53] for example, showed that the transketolase in fibroblasts cultured from four patients with Wernicke–Korsakoff's syndrome bound thiamine pyrophosphate only one-tenth as avidly as fibroblasts from healthy volunteers. More studies are needed to confirm this finding.[540]

Thiamine deficiency has been reported in between 9% and 80% of individuals chronically abusing alcohol, irrespective of the presence of significant liver disease.[94, 141,191,234,338,340,517,578,648] In the majority of patients, however, biochemical evidence of thiamine deficiency is not accompanied by symptoms or signs of hypovitaminosis. The widely varying incidence of thiamine deficiency in the various reported series may be explained partly by the diversity of methods used to assess thiamine deficiency and partly by differences in patient populations.

Several factors contribute to the development of thiamine deficiency in individuals chronically abusing alcohol, including reduced dietary intake, increased metabolic demands and impaired intestinal absorption;[73] additional factors play a role in patients with alcohol-related liver disease, including deficiency of the thiamine pyrophosphate apoenzyme,[189] impaired conversion of the vitamin to its active form and a reduction in hepatic storage capacity. Camilo and coworkers,[94] found low erythrocyte transketolase activity in 19 (30%) of 64 normally nourished alcohol abusers with well-compensated liver disease (Figure 6.2). In 6 of the 19, addition of thiamine pyrophosphate in vitro (TPP effect) stimulated transketolase activity, indicating depleted thiamine stores. In the remaining 13 patients, the TPP effect was normal or low, suggesting a deficiency or an inability to use the transketolase apoenzyme, as a result either of long-

standing thiamine deficiency or of the presence of liver disease. A further 8 patients (13%) had normal transketolase activity but a low TPP effect, perhaps reflecting failure of the coenzyme TPP to recombine with the transketolase apoenzyme in the presence of normal thiamine stores. In the majority of alcohol abusers, subclinical thiamine deficiency can be corrected by use of oral thiamine hydrochloride, 10–100 mg daily, in divided doses. In patients with overt deficiency, high dose parenteral preparations should be used.

Subclinical thiamine deficiency has been described in patients with fulminant hepatic failure;[328] biochemical abnormalities correct following thiamine supplementation. Opinions vary as to the incidence of thiamine deficiency in patients with chronic non-alcoholic liver disease. Morgan and coworkers,[426] found evidence of biochemical thiamine deficiency in only one (3%) of 31 patients with cryptogenic cirrhosis or chronic active hepatitis, whereas Rossouw and colleagues,[517] found evidence of thiamine deficiency in 6 (43%) of 14 patients with chronic non-alcoholic liver disease; the patients in the latter study were, however, severely ill and showed evidence of hepatic decompensation.

Riboflavin[142,381,504]

Riboflavin is widely distributed in plants and animals but not in large amounts. The richest dietary sources are brewer's yeast, milk, cheese, green vegetables, offal, whole-grain and enriched cereals and bread. Requirements for riboflavin seem to relate to resting metabolic rate; daily intakes of 1.4 mg for women and of 1.6 mg for men or, for both sexes, of 0.16 mg/MJ (0.6 mg/1000 kcal) have been recommended.[152,206]

Riboflavin is absorbed from the upper small intestine by a specific, active transport mechanism. A percentage of the absorbed riboflavin is phosphorylated to flavin mononucleotide (FMN) in the intestinal mucosa. Both free and phosphorylated riboflavin enter the portal vein, where they bind to albumin and other plasma proteins. Riboflavin and FMN may undergo further phosphorylation, in the liver, to flavin adenine dinucleotide (FAD). The main storage sites are liver and kidney but the stores are not extensive and so are easily depleted. A small amount of riboflavin appears to be excreted in the bile and hence undergoes enterohepatic recirculation. However, the vitamin is mainly excreted in the urine, predominantly in free form.

FMN and FAD are the physiologically active forms of riboflavin. They serve a vital role in metabolism as coenzymes for a wide variety of respiratory flavoproteins; they are, for example, essential for oxidative phosphorylation, dehydrogenation of fatty acids, the conversion of folic acid to 5-N-methyltetrahydrofolic acid, the conversion of pyridoxine to its 5' phosphate and for the activity of the flavin-dependent purine enzyme xanthine oxidase. In addition, covalently attached flavins are essential to the structure of enzymes such as succinate dehydrogenase and monoamine oxidase.

In man, riboflavin deficiency results in the development of cheilosis, angular stomatitis, glossitis, scrotal skin changes, seborrhoeic dermatitis of the face, a generalized dermatitis, a normochromic, normocytic anaemia associated with pure red-cell hypoplasia and a neuropathy. In some individuals the cornea becomes vascularized and cataracts form. All these features can be rapidly reversed with oral riboflavin, 5–10 mg daily. Deficiency of this vitamin rarely occurs in isolation and certain features of the riboflavin deficiency syndrome, such as cheilosis and glossitis, occur with deficiencies of the other B vitamins.

Riboflavin deficiency has been reported in between 15% and 50% of individuals abusing alcohol, with or without liver disease.[25,33,61,77,255,340,511] Several factors contribute to the deficiency, including poor dietary intake and reduced availability secondary to a direct effect of ethanol on the enzymes responsible for FMN and FAD hydrolysis.[472] Despite the fact that biochemical riboflavin deficiency is common in alcohol abusers, clinical symptoms of hypovitaminosis are rare.[340,511]

Very little information is available on riboflavin status in patients with non-alcoholic liver disease; the incidence of biochemical riboflavin deficiency in patients with non-alcoholic cirrhosis varies from 4% to 6%.[118,338,426]

Niacin[142,258,381]

Niacin is the generic term for both nicotinic acid and nicotinamide. It is found in liver, meat, fish, whole-grain and enriched breads and cereals, nuts, and also in coffee and tea; fruit, most vegetables, milk and eggs are poor sources. Many foods, especially cereals, contain bound forms of niacin from which the vitamin is not nutritionally available. Niacin is not a vitamin, in the true sense, in that it can be formed from the essential amino acid, tryptophan. One niacin equivalent is equal to 1 mg of niacin or 60 mg of dietary tryptophan: only 1.5% of dietary tryptophan is converted to niacin under normal circumstances, although this percentage may increase in the absence of dietary niacin. In women, daily intakes of 15 niacin equivalents and in men of 18 niacin equivalents or, for both sexes, of 2.7 niacin equivalents/MJ (11.3 niacin equivalents/1000 kcal) are recommended.[152, 206]

Both nicotinic acid and nicotinamide are readily absorbed throughout the intestinal tract and the vitamin is distributed to all tissues. The principal route of metabolism is to N'-methylnicotinamide and its derivatives, which are in turn metabolized further. Otherwise, little is known about the absorption, fate and excretion of this vitamin.[258]

Niacin is an essential component of nicotinamide adenine dinucleotide (NAD) and nicotinamide adenine dinucleotide phosphate (NADP), coenzymes for a multitude of important oxidation–reduction reactions essential for tissue respiration. NAD also participates as a substrate

in the transfer of adenosine diphosphate (ADP)–ribosyl moieties to proteins.[223] Nicotinic acid will depress blood lipids and can prevent the rise in plasma triglycerides, phospholipids and free fatty acids observed after acute alcohol ingestion.[296] This latter effect has been attributed to inhibition of peripheral free fatty acid release and to inhibition of liver alcohol dehydrogenase and hence the shift in redox state. However, if nicotinic acid is given to rats chronically fed ethanol then the development of hepatic steatosis is potentiated.[580]

Niacin deficiency is one of the major factors in the development of pellagra. The clinical features of this condition include dermatitis, inflammation of mucous membranes, diarrhoea and psychiatric disturbances. Skin changes, especially on the hands, may be useful in detecting early deficiency. The condition is treated with nicotinamide, 500 mg orally or 75 mg intravenously, daily, in divided doses.

Pellagra is now rare in industrialized countries but when diagnosed it is often associated with chronic alcohol abuse.[164,282,583,588,619] Biochemical evidence of niacin deficiency has been found in a percentage of individuals abusing alcohol in some series[144,190] but not in others.[311,448,516] Hepatic niacin concentrations are reduced in individuals abusing alcohol and the percentage reduction increases with increasing severity of liver injury.[28,208,340] Potential mechanisms for niacin deficiency in individuals chronically abusing alcohol include poor dietary intake, decreased conversion to active coenzyme forms, decreased hepatic storage and increased requirements. It has also been suggested that, in individuals chronically abusing alcohol, zinc deficiency may potentiate the development of pellagra, probably through an effect on pyridoxine metabolism.[619,620]

In patients with fulminant liver failure, blood levels of niacin are variable.[516] Biochemical niacin deficiency is rarely encountered in patients with non-alcoholic chronic liver disease.[426]

Vitamin B_6[142,279,341,381]

The biological activity of the vitamin B_6 group is displayed by pyridoxine, pyridoxal and pyridoxamine and their 5′-phosphate esters. The vitamin is widely and uniformly distributed in all foods but substantial losses occur during cooking; lean meat, liver, vegetables and whole-grain breads and cereals are among the richest sources. Daily intakes for healthy women of 1.6 mg and of 2 mg for healthy men are recommended, but requirements may increase if dietary protein intake is high.[152,206]

Vitamin B_6 is absorbed from the jejunum and ileum by passive diffusion and is then converted, predominantly in the liver but also in skeletal muscle and kidney, to the active coenzyme form, pyridoxal-5′-phosphate. The coenzyme is transported in plasma bound to albumin. The major circulating forms of the vitamin are pyridoxal-5′-phosphate, together with pyridoxal and 4-pyridoxic acid.[122,364] Circulating pyridoxal can enter cells and is reutilized to synthesize pyridoxal-5'-phosphate. Ultimately most pyridoxal-5'-phosphate is metabolized to 4-pyridoxic acid.

Pyridoxal-5'-phosphate acts as a cofactor for a large number of enzymes involved in amino acid metabolism, including transaminases, decarboxylases, synthetases and hydroxylases. It is of particular importance, in man, in the metabolism of tryptophan, glycine, serine, glutamate, and the sulphur-containing amino acids. Pyridoxal-5'-phosphate is also required for the synthesis of the haem precursor 6-aminolaevulinic acid, for breakdown of glycogen and for syringomyelin biosynthesis. A large percentage of body pyridoxine is found in muscle phosphorylase, where it probably acts as an enzyme stabilizer. It also plays an important, although ill-understood role, in neuronal excitability, and modulates the actions of steroid hormones by interacting with steroid receptor complexes.

Clinical symptoms of vitamin B_6 deficiency include neuromuscular irritability, peripheral neuropathy, dermatitis, cheilosis, stomatitis, anaemia and impaired immunity. The vitamin is widely present in food, thus dietary pyridoxine deficiency has never been recognized in human adults, although it can occur in infants fed highly processed formula feeds. Pyridoxine deficiency can arise in adults either during treatment with drugs such as isoniazid, cycloserine, hydralazine and D-penicillamine, which act as pyridoxine antagonists, or as a result of genetically determined abnormalities in vitamin B_6 metabolism.[207] Pyridoxine, in an oral dose of 30 mg daily, will correct the deficiency in patients taking isoniazid, while doses of up to 100 mg daily may be required in subjects taking D-penicillamine or in the presence of a one of the genetically determined clinical states of 'pyridoxine dependency'. Vitamin B_6 should be given prophylactically to patients receiving pyridoxine antagonists, in a dose of 25 mg daily.

Low circulating levels of pyridoxal-5'-phosphate have been reported in between 30% and 50% of alcohol abusers with minimal liver damage and in between 80% and 100% of those with cirrhosis,[60,160,257,267,329,338,340,363,421,452,581] mainly as a result of an increase in pyridoxal-5'-phosphate degradation.[329,421] The factors responsible for this accelerated degradation are largely unknown, although acetaldehyde can produce this effect.[363] Ethanol itself interferes with the conversion of pyridoxine to pyridoxal-5'-phosphate[266] and this may contribute to the reduction in circulating pyridoxal-5'-phosphate concentrations. In individuals with alcohol-related cirrhosis, circulating pyridoxal concentrations have been reported as both increased[257] and decreased.[452] Similarly 24-hour urinary excretion of 4-pyridoxic acid has been reported as both increased[452] or unchanged.[257] Deficiency is corrected with oral pyridoxine hydrochloride, 50–150 mg daily in divided doses. However, the plasma pyridoxal-5'-phosphate response to administered pyridoxine may be impaired in patients with cirrhosis.[257,581] These individuals have raised serum alkaline phosphatase activity which may dephosphorylate the circulating pyridoxal-5'-phosphate to pyridoxal.[17,257,399,645]

Plasma pyridoxal-5'-phosphate concentrations are within the reference range in patients with acute viral hepatitis[421] but the concentrations are more variable in patients with fulminant hepatic failure.[516] Low plasma pyridoxal-5'-phosphate concentrations may also be found in patients with non-alcoholic chronic liver disease;[329,452,655] increased pyridoxal-5'-phosphate degradation is the major aetiological factor, although reduced plasma albumin concentrations may be of additional importance. In these individuals, however, plasma pyridoxal concentrations and urinary excretion of 4-pyridoxic acid are normal, so that the plasma pyridoxal-5'-phosphate concentration may be an unreliable indicator of overall vitamin B_6 status.[452] It has been suggested that in these individuals the excess pyridoxal generated by dephosphorylation of pyridoxal-5'-phosphate, possibly under the influence of circulating alkaline phosphatase, may be taken up by tissues rather than being excreted. In consequence, although plasma pyridoxal-5'-phosphate concentrations are reduced in patients with non-alcoholic liver disease, tissue levels of pyridoxal-5'-phosphate remain normal.[257,365,452]

Folic acid[142,265]

Folic acid is the common name for pteroylmonoglutamic acid. It is synthesized by many different plants and bacteria. Offal, green leafy vegetables, pulses, oranges, nuts, bananas and bread are the richest sources. However, some forms of dietary folic acid are labile and may be destroyed by cooking. Thus, fruit and raw vegetables probably constitute the primary dietary sources of the vitamin. Daily intakes of 200 µg of folate are recommended for healthy adults.[152,206]

Food folates are present mainly as reduced polyglutamates and require deconjugation in the gut lumen to mono- and diglutamates before absorption in the proximal jejunum. A percentage of the formed glutamates undergoes reduction and methylation by mucosal cells to the active form, 5-methyltetrahydrofolate (5-methyl THFA), which then enters the portal circulation; the remainder of the absorbed folate is transported unchanged. Folates circulate in the plasma in free form, or else loosely bound to plasma proteins or firmly bound to high-affinity carriers. Folates appear to be taken up by tissues, including the liver, by a carrier-mediated transport mechanism. 5-Methyl THFA is excreted in the bile and undergoes reabsorption by the gut. This enterohepatic circulation may provide as much as 200 µg or more of folate each day for recycling to body tissues. The total body content of folic acid is normally 5–10 mg, about half of which is present in the liver, mainly as the polyglutamate form of 5-methyl THFA.

In the form of its tetrahydro derivatives, such as 5-formimino THFA and 5,10-methylene THFA, folate functions as a participant in one-carbon transfer reactions; thus, it is involved in the synthesis of purine and pyrimidine nucleotides, in a number of amino acid interconversions and in the generation of formate for the 'formate pool'.

Folic acid deficiency results in reduced replication of rapidly dividing cells, especially those in the bone marrow and the gastrointestinal tract. A macrocytic, megaloblastic anaemia may develop and is the major haematological manifestation of deficiency. The gastrointestinal manifestations include glossitis, cheilosis and diarrhoea. Neurological abnormalities occur only rarely. Folic acid deficiency may arise during treatment with drugs which interfere with its absorption and conversion to 5-methyl THFA, such as, phenytoin, phenobarbitone and the oral contraceptives, or during treatment with drugs which inhibit dihydrofolate reductase, such as methotrexate, pyrimethamine and triamterene. Deficiency is treated with oral folic acid, 10–20 mg daily, for 2 weeks; a maintenance dose of 5–10 mg daily may be required.

Individuals chronically abusing alcohol may develop folate deficiency though they are rarely symptomatic; the incidence of low serum or red-cell folate concentrations varies from 6% to 87% in reported series and is independent of the degree of liver damage.[100,224,243,259,285,314,322,433,612,649,652] Several factors are of aetiological importance, including dietary inadequacy, intestinal malabsorption, impaired delivery of circulating folate to tissues, decreased hepatic retention, increased urinary excretion and possibly altered enterohepatic recycling.[242,528,637] Cessation of alcohol abuse and oral folic acid supplements, 5–15 mg daily, will correct the deficiency.

The excretion of urinary folate is increased in patients with acute viral hepatitis,[495,604] presumably because stored folate is released from the liver and the plasma binding capacity is overwhelmed. Serum and red-cell folate values are low in less than a quarter of patients with chronic non-alcoholic liver disease.[314,322,426,433,652]

Vitamin B$_{12}$[142,265]

Vitamin B$_{12}$ is a complex organometallic compound which is present in animal tissue but not in plant tissue; it can be synthesized by a number of microorganisms, including a proportion of those normally present in the human intestine. The chief dietary sources are liver, meat, fish, eggs, cheese and milk. Daily intakes of about 2.0 µg are recommended for healthy adults.[152,206]

Vitamin B$_{12}$ is attached, in coenzyme form, to protein in food. During ingestion, proteolysis occurs and the released vitamin B$_{12}$ forms a stable complex with R binder, which is one of a group of closely related glycoproteins found in intestinal secretions such as, saliva, gastric juice and bile, and also in granulocytes and plasma. The binding protein is removed in the presence of gastric acid and pancreatic proteases, releasing the vitamin, which then binds to intrinsic factor, a glycoprotein produced by the parietal cells of the stomach. The vitamin B$_{12}$-intrinsic factor complex is resistant to proteolytic digestion and travels to the distal ileum where it binds to specific receptors on the mucosal brush border. The vitamin B$_{12}$

is then transferred from the ileal receptor across the mucosa to the capillary circulation where it binds, initially, to a β-globulin, transcobalamin II.

The vitamin B$_{12}$-transcobalamin II complex is rapidly taken up by the liver, bone marrow and other proliferating cells. Although transcobalamin II is the transport protein for newly absorbed vitamin B$_{12}$, most vitamin B$_{12}$ circulates bound to transcobalamin I, a glycoprotein closely resembling gastric R binder. This situation arises because the vitamin B$_{12}$ bound to transcobalamin II is rapidly cleared from the blood while clearance of the vitamin B$_{12}$ bound to transcobalamin I requires many days. The liver contains from 50% to 90% of total body stores of vitamin B$_{12}$ which range from 1 to 10 mg; the vitamin is stored as its coenzyme, 5-deoxyadenosylcobalamin. Vitamin B$_{12}$ is not catabolized and loss occurs by excretion, largely in the bile. Approximately 0.5–5.0 µg of vitamin B$_{12}$ is excreted in bile daily, 65–75% of which is reabsorbed. Normally less than 0.25 µg of vitamin B$_{12}$ is lost in the urine each day.

Vitamin B$_{12}$ is converted, in the liver, to its active coenzyme forms, methylcobalamine and 5-deoxyadenosylcobalamin. The coenzymes are involved in many metabolic processes and, as they are necessary for nucleic acid synthesis, are important for maintaining growth, haematopoiesis, epithelial cell function and possibly myelin integrity. Methylcobalamin is required for the transmethylation of homocysteine to methionine and its derivative, S-adenosylmethionine. 5-Deoxyadenosylcobalamin is also a cofactor for the enzyme methylmalonyl-CoA mutase in the oxidation of odd-numbered fatty acids.

Deficiency of vitamin B$_{12}$ leads to haematological, gastrointestinal and neurological abnormalities. The main haematological manifestation is a macrocytic, megaloblastic anaemia; thrombocytopenia also may occur. The gastrointestinal manifestations are usually mild and include glossitis, cheilosis and diarrhoea; malabsorption may lead to moderate weight loss. The neurological manifestations include a peripheral neuropathy, subacute combined degeneration of the spinal cord, a cerebellar syndrome and disturbances of mentation that vary from mild irritability to severe dementia or frank psychosis. The haematological and gastrointestinal manifestations respond well to parenteral vitamin B$_{12}$, but remission of the neurological features may be incomplete.

Plasma vitamin B$_{12}$ concentrations are usually within the reference range in individuals abusing alcohol, irrespective of the degree of any associated liver disease,[100,224,433] but hepatic vitamin B$_{12}$ concentrations may be reduced.[28,208] Ethanol has been shown to interfere with binding of the vitamin B$_{12}$-intrinsic factor complex, and may reduce in vivo uptake of vitamin B$_{12}$: neither of these factors appears to be of clinical significance.

Plasma vitamin B$_{12}$ concentrations are low in only a very small percentage of patients with chronic, non-alcoholic liver disease;[338,426] the aetiology of the vitamin B$_{12}$ deficiency in these patients is unclear as both absorption and transport of the vitamin are normal.[510]

High circulating vitamin B_{12} concentrations have been reported in patients with viral hepatitis, hepatic steatosis, alcoholic hepatitis, cholangitis, liver abscess, metastatic carcinoma and cirrhosis, most likely because of release from injured hepatocytes.[27,356,485] Patients with pernicious anaemia may indeed undergo 'spontaneous remission' if they develop hepatitis, suggesting that under normal circumstances not all the hepatic stores of vitamin B_{12} are available for haematopoiesis.

Changes may also occur in the plasma binding of vitamin B_{12} in patients with liver disease. Patients with acute hepatitis, for example, have low plasma levels of vitamin B_{12} binding capacity, possibly secondary to hyperbilirubinaemia, and, in consequence, have high levels of free plasma vitamin B_{12}, whereas in patients with chronic liver disease, concentrations of the bound form increase.[294]

Pantothenic acid[142,381,475]

Pantothenic acid is widely distributed in natural foods and is probably an essential nutrient; offal, beef and egg yolk are rich sources. Diets containing 4–8 mg of pantothenic acid daily are considered adequate.[152,206]

Pantothenic acid is readily absorbed from the small intestine by simple diffusion. It is present in tissues, probably in the bound form of coenzyme A, in concentrations ranging from 2 to 45 $\mu g/g$; the concentration in liver exceeds that in all other tissues. Pantothenic acid is not metabolized within the body to any great extent and is largely excreted in urine.

The vitamin is transformed within the body to 4'-phosphopantetheine which is then incorporated into the functional forms of the vitamin, coenzyme A and acyl carrier protein. Coenzyme A is a cofactor for a variety of enzyme-catalysed reactions involving transfer of two-carbon groups. Such reactions are important in the oxidative metabolism of carbohydrates, gluconeogenesis, degradation of fatty acids and the synthesis of sterols, steroid hormones and porphyrins. Pantothenate also participates in the post-translational modification of proteins, including N-terminal acetylation, acetylation of internal amino acids and fatty acid acetylation. Such modifications influence the intracellular localization, stability and activity of proteins.

Pantothenic acid deficiency has not been recognized in humans consuming a normal diet, presumably because of its ubiquitous presence in food. Experimental pantothenic acid deficiency results in the development of paraesthesia in the extremities, muscle cramps, impaired coordination, fatigue, headache, abdominal cramp and vomiting.[212] The burning or electric foot syndrome which developed in prisoners in World War II responded to administered pantothenic acid and probably represents a specific feature of deficiency.[151]

Plasma pantothenic acid concentrations are variable in individuals chronically abusing alcohol;[28,61,338,339] the lowest values are observed in individuals with decompensated liver disease.[338,340] Hepatic pantothenic acid concentrations are reduced in individuals with alcohol-related liver injury.[28] The mechanisms responsible for the reduced vitamin levels have not been elucidated. No information is available on pantothenic acid status in patients with non-alcoholic liver disease.

Biotin[142,370,381]

Biotin is widely distributed in natural foods, although in small amounts; brewer's yeast, offal, egg yolk, milk, fish and nuts are the richest sources. The daily requirements of biotin are unknown, but diets providing a daily intake of 30–100 μg are considered adequate.[206] Part of the biotin synthesized by intestinal bacteria is also available for absorption.

Ingested biotin is rapidly absorbed from the gastrointestinal tract and is readily excreted in the urine, predominantly in the form of intact biotin, and in lesser amounts as the metabolites bis-norbiotin and biotin sulphoxide.

Biotin is a cofactor for the enzymatic carboxylation of pyruvate, acetyl coenzyme-A, proprionyl coenzyme-A and β-methylcrotonyl coenzyme-A, and as such plays an important role in carbon dioxide fixation in both carbohydrate and fat metabolism.

There is no evidence that spontaneous biotin deficiency can occur in man except in individuals who consume large quantities of raw egg white, as this contains avidin, a glycoprotein which possess a strong affinity for biotin and binds to it, preventing its absorption. The symptoms and signs of biotin deficiency, as observed in these individuals, include dermatitis, atrophic glossitis, hyperaesthesia, muscle pain, lassitude, anorexia, nausea, mild anaemia and non-specific changes in the electrocardiograph. Symptomatic biotin deficiency has been reported in children and in adults receiving long-term total parenteral nutrition, and manifests as severe exfoliative dermatitis and alopecia.[222,605,642]

Low plasma and liver biotin concentrations have been found in individuals chronically abusing alcohol,[28,190,340] but no clinical symptoms of deficiency have been recorded; the mechanism of the deficiency is unknown. No information is available on the biotin status of patients with non-alcoholic liver disease.

Vitamin C[347,381]

Vitamin C is widely distributed in a variety of fruits and vegetables; citrus fruits, blackcurrants and rosehips are particularly rich sources. Most green leafy vegetables and fruits contain reasonably large amounts of the vitamin, although apples are generally a poor source. Root vegetables, such as potatoes, are a useful source because of the amounts eaten. Storage of unprocessed fruits and vegetables for prolonged periods leads to loss of the vitamin; processed fruits and vegetables retain 50% or more of their vitamin C content. Daily intakes of 30–60 mg are recommended for healthy adults.[152,206]

Vitamin C is readily absorbed from the intestinal tract and is distributed in all body tissues. The highest concentrations are found in glandular tissues, the lowest in muscle and storage fat. The vitamin is partly metabolized and partly excreted unchanged in the urine. A major route of metabolism involves conversion to urinary oxalate.

Vitamin C functions as a cofactor in a number of hydroxylation and amidation reactions. It is required for, or facilitates, the conversion of certain proline and lysine residues in procollagen to hydroxyproline and hydroxylysine in the course of collagen synthesis; it is a cofactor in the conversion of folic to folinic acid and the hydroxylation of dopamine to form noradrenaline; it plays an important role in microsomal drug metabolism. It also promotes the activity of an amidating enzyme thought to be involved in the processing of certain peptide hormones such as oxytocin, antidiuretic hormone and cholecystokinin; it directly stimulates collagen peptide synthesis, promotes intestinal absorption of iron by reducing non-haem ferrous iron to its ferric state, and plays an ill-defined role in adrenal steroidogenesis.

Deficiency of vitamin C leads to scurvy. The main symptoms of this disorder arise from pathological lesions in the blood vessels and connective-tissue matrix and include perifollicular hyperkeratosis and haemorrhage, purpura, haemorrhages into muscles and joints, swollen, friable and bleeding gums in patients with teeth, poor wound healing and anaemia. In infancy and childhood haemorrhage may occur into the periosteum of long bones, causing painful swellings and occasionally epiphysial separation.

Treatment with oral vitamin C, 500 mg daily in divided doses, will reverse these changes.

Individuals chronically abusing alcohol often have low leucocyte vitamin C concentrations, probably as a result of dietary deficiency.[36,154,169,340,413] Low leucocyte vitamin C levels have also been found in patients with viral hepatitis, cryptogenic cirrhosis, chronic aggressive hepatitis, primary biliary cirrhosis and hepatocellular carcinoma.[36,169,426] Poor dietary intake may be important in explaining these low vitamin levels, but daily intakes of vitamin C were acceptable in the patients with primary biliary cirrhosis studied by Beattie and Sherlock.[36] These patients were, however, taking cholestyramine and it was suggested that this drug might interfere with vitamin C absorption. These authors also showed that vitamin C deficiency interfered with antipyrine metabolism and speculated that such deficiency might affect the microsomal oxidation of other drugs.

MINERALS

Iron[265]

Iron is present in many foods; the richest sources are offal, brewer's yeast, wheatgerm, egg yolks, oysters, certain dried beans and fruit; most lean meat, poultry, fish, green vegetables and cereals contain moderate amounts. The main sources of dietary iron in the United Kingdom are meat, bread, flour, potatoes and other vegetables. Daily iron intakes of 0.5–1.0 mg are recommended for healthy men and non-menstruating women, and of 1.0–2.0 mg for women who menstruate.[152,206] In healthy individuals only 10% of food iron is absorbed; thus, daily intakes should exceed dietary requirements by a factor of ten. The average diet provides 1.4 mg/MJ (6 mg/1000 kcal) of iron or about 10–20 mg/24 h; as such it may not provide enough iron for women who are menstruating. Absorption may be more efficient when iron requirements are increased.

The rate of iron absorption is of prime importance in determining body iron status, but the nature of the absorptive system is poorly understood;[111] a carrier-mediated process is proposed.[565,591] After acidification and partial digestion in the stomach, food iron is presented to the intestinal mucosa of the duodenum and proximal jejunum and is taken up by the absorptive cells; it is then transported directly into the plasma or stored as mucosal ferritin. Absorption is regulated by the relative activities of these two pathways, which are in some way determined by the internal state of iron metabolism. Iron derived from haemoglobin and other haem proteins of animal origin is absorbed as the intact haem molecule. Most other forms of iron are more easily absorbed in the ferrous form. Phytates and phosphates in food form complexes with iron and reduce its absorption; achlorhydria and the administration of antacids also decrease iron absorption. Reducing agents such as ascorbic acid facilitate iron absorption by converting ferric to ferrous iron; meat facilitates iron absorption by stimulating gastric acid production. Absorption is also increased when iron intake is deficient, when iron stores are depleted or when erythropoiesis is enhanced; even under these circumstances absorption is limited to between 3 and 4 mg of dietary iron daily.

Absorbed iron is transported bound to transferrin, a β_1-glycoprotein synthesized in the liver. Iron is delivered from transferrin to intracellular sites by means of a specific transferrin receptor in the plasma membrane. A major portion of circulating iron is transported to the bone marrow for haemoglobin synthesis and to other sites for the manufacture of other essential iron-containing compounds, including myoglobin and a variety of iron-dependent enzymes. The remaining iron is stored either in the reticuloendothelial system or in the liver and muscle. Approximately one-third of total storage iron is found in the liver as ferritin, either in the form of individual molecules or aggregated as haemosiderin; over 95% of hepatic iron is located in hepatocytes. The remaining two-thirds of storage iron is equally divided between muscle and the reticuloendothelial cells of the spleen and bone marrow. The body of a healthy man contains approximately 50 mg/kg body weight of iron, while that of a healthy woman contains 35 mg/kg. About two-thirds of body iron circulates in haemoglobin, while only 3 mg circulates as transferrin. A very small proportion of total body iron, perhaps 150 mg, is present in myoglobin and in the haem enzymes concerned with electron transfer. The remaining 1000 mg in men and 100–400 mg in women is stored in the liver, spleen, bone marrow and muscle, complexed to protein, as ferritin and haemosiderin.

Daily iron losses average less than 1 mg in men and 2 mg in women who menstruate. The main loss occurs from desquamation of epithelial cells from the skin and the gastrointestinal tract. In women, menstrual iron loss is highly variable but averages 17 mg monthly. The net loss of iron during a normal pregnancy is about 700 mg.

Iron is essential for normal haematopoiesis and for the integrity of epithelial tissues. Most individuals with iron deficiency are asymptomatic; symptoms develop in proportion to the degree of anaemia and the constitution of the patient, and relate to the cause of the deficiency. In general, the clinical manifestations are those common to all chronic anaemias and include fatigue, headache, tachycardia, exertional dyspnoea, ankle oedema and pallor. In occasional patients, abnormalities of epithelial tissues may occur, including glossitis, angular stomatitis, spooning of the nails and dysphagia. Oral iron, for example ferrous sulphate 600 mg daily, in divided doses, will correct the abnormalities, but the cause of the deficiency must be sought and ameliorated if possible.

Abnormalities of iron metabolism are common in chronic alcohol abusers. Iron deficiency, with or without anaemia, is found in up to 25% of such individuals[130,280,314] and its presence is generally attributed to gastrointestinal bleeding and/or inadequate dietary intake. Conversely, individuals abusing alcohol may have increased serum iron concentrations and increased saturation of their total iron binding capacity.[107,109,354,595] The mechanisms responsible for these findings are unclear, but as the abnormalities occur independently of the severity of any liver disease they probably reflect a direct effect of alcohol on iron metabolism.[130,354] Additionally, liver iron concentrations are mildly to moderately increased in approximately one-third of alcohol abusers independently of the presence, or the degree, of alcohol-related liver injury.[31,109]

Several explanations have been suggested for these findings, none of them entirely satisfactory. Originally it was supposed that the hepatic siderosis reflected the iron content of the beverages consumed. However, it has been clearly shown that there is no relationship between the degree of hepatic siderosis and either the amount of alcohol or the amount of iron ingested in alcoholic beverages (Figure 6.3).[109,283,419] Equally, it has been suggested that the high serum iron concentrations and increased transferrin saturations observed in these patients might enhance liver iron uptake.[641] However, although the uptake of transferrin-bound ^{52}Fe is increased in individuals abusing alcohol, independently of the degree of liver damage, it is also increased in patients with non-alcoholic liver disease (Figure 6.4).[107] It has also been

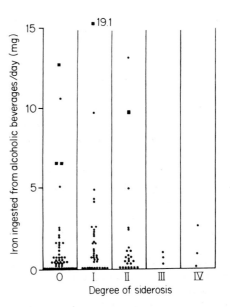

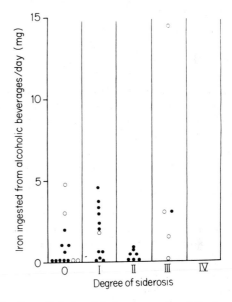

Figure 6.3 *Top*: Relationship between the daily ingestion of beverage iron and the degree of hepatic siderosis in men chronically abusing alcohol (■, men drinking wine exclusively). *Bottom*: Relationship between the daily ingestion of beverage iron and the degree of hepatic siderosis in women chronically abusing alcohol (○, premenopausal women). (Jakobovits *et al.*[283])

suggested that iron absorption might be increased in individuals chronically abusing alcohol, but this does not appear to be the case (Figure 6.5).[108] While increased iron absorption may not be observed in response to chronic alcohol ingestion, intermittent increases in iron absorption may occur in relation to high circulating concentrations of ethanol (Figures 6.6 and 6.7).[108] This finding may explain, at least in part, the increased iron stores in some individuals chronically abusing alcohol. It is also possible that the hepatic siderosis might reflect

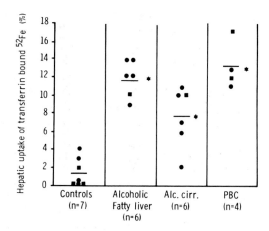

Figure 6.4 Hepatic uptake of transferrin-bound ^{52}Fe in healthy volunteers and in patients with alcoholic fatty liver, alcoholic cirrhosis and primary biliary cirrhosis (PBC); ——, group mean value; ●, men; ■, women. Significance of the difference between mean values in the patient groups and in the control subjects, *, $p < 0.01$. (Chapman *et al.*[107])

defective release of transferrin-bound or non-transferrin bound iron from tissue stores, perhaps as a direct effect of alcohol.

Serum iron[526] and serum ferritin[483] concentrations are often raised in individuals with acute viral hepatitis. The mechanism is not clear, but release of transferrin from damaged cells, diminished haemoglobin synthesis and impaired iron storage may all play a role.

Evidence of iron deficiency, with or without anaemia, occurs in approximately 25% of patients with cryptogenic cirrhosis and chronic active hepatitis;[426] its presence is attributed to either poor dietary intake or occult gastrointestinal blood loss. Iron deficiency is uncommon in patients with non-alcoholic chronic liver disease in the absence of malabsorption, gastrointestinal haemorrhage or a bleeding diathesis.

Hepatic iron overload, as observed in idiopathic haemochromatosis, nutritional iron overload or as a complication of certain haematological disorders, can lead to the development of liver damage.

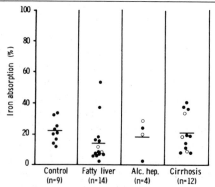

Figure 6.5 ^{59}Fe absorption in healthy volunteers and in alcohol abusers with liver disease of varying severity; ——, group mean value; ●, men; ○, women. (Chapman *et al.*[108])

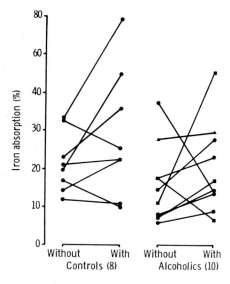

Figure 6.6 ^{59}Fe absorption in healthy volunteers and in alcohol abusers with liver disease of varying severity. Absorption was measured from a test meal with or without added alcohol in a dose of 0.5 g/kg body weight; ●, fatty liver; ▲, alcoholic hepatitis; ■, cirrhosis. (Chapman *et al.*[108])

Calcium[253]

The most important dietary sources of calcium are dairy products, mainly milk and cheese, and bread. Varying quantities of calcium are present in domestic water supplies. The average diet in the United Kingdom provides 600–800 mg of calcium daily, while the average diet in the United States provides 200–2500 mg; considerably less than half the calcium ingested is absorbed. The

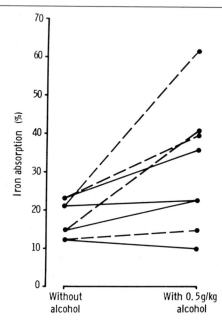

Figure 6.7 The effects of acute alcohol administration on ^{59}Fe absorption in four healthy volunteers. Alcohol was given in a dose of 0.5 g/kg body weight both orally (——) and intravenously (– – –) (Chapman *et al.*[108])

recommended daily allowance for healthy adults is 500 mg in the United Kingdom and 800–1200 mg in the United States.[152,206]

Calcium from food and from intestinal secretions is absorbed in soluble, ionized form from the proximal small intestine; intestinal absorption is thought to be mediated either by calcium-specific channels or by a carrier, but the mechanism is not completely understood. Intestinal absorption is enhanced by vitamin D and parathyroid hormone; intake of a calcium-deficient diet results in an increase in fractional absorption. Phosphates, phytates and oxalates in food form complexes or insoluble salts with calcium and decrease its absorption; absorption may also be impaired in the presence of steatorrhoea, while diarrhoea may be associated with increased faecal loss. Alcohol appears to depress duodenal calcium absorption, at least in experimental animals.[324]

Following absorption, calcium enters the plasma, where it circulates either as free ions or bound to plasma proteins or, to a small extent, as diffusible complexes. The concentration of free calcium ions is of critical importance for a variety of functions and is subjected to precise hormonal control, largely via parathyroid hormone; circulating calcium concentrations are kept remarkably constant. Calcium enters the plasma via absorption from the intestinal tract and following reabsorption from bone mineral. Calcium leaves the extracellular fluid via secretion into the gastrointestinal tract, urinary excretion and deposition in bone mineral. The body of a healthy adult contains 1–2 kg of calcium, over 98% of which is in the skeleton. Bone resorption and formation are usually tightly coupled, with approximately 500 mg of calcium entering and leaving the skeleton daily.

Calcium is essential for the functional integrity of the nervous and muscular systems; it has a major influence on the excitability of nerves and muscles and on the release of neurotransmitters. Calcium is also necessary for normal cardiac function and is an important factor in maintenance of the integrity of membranes and coagulation of the blood. In addition, it mediates the intracellular action of many hormones. Decrease in the concentration of free calcium ions secondary to, for example, reduced dietary intake of calcium and vitamin D, malabsorption of calcium and vitamin D or hypoparathyroidism, is accompanied by increased neuromuscular irritability and the syndrome of tetany. Hypomagnesaemia and alkalosis lower the threshold for tetany, whereas hypokalaemia and acidosis raise the threshold. Hypercalcaemia secondary to, for example, hyperparathyroidism, vitamin D excess, sarcoidosis or neoplasia, is accompanied by anorexia, nausea, vomiting, constipation, polyuria and polydypsia, hypotonia and depression and, when of long-standing, by metastatic tissue calcification.

Bone density may be decreased in individuals chronically abusing alcohol,[449] as a result of a decrease in the mineral rather than the organic phase of bone.[291] Several explanations have been suggested, including disturbances of calcium metabolism secondary to poor dietary intake and fat malabsorption, and increased urinary losses of calcium and magnesium.[298] There is evidence that alcohol directly affects osteoblastic function, resulting in diminished bone formation and reduced bone mineralization.[156, 330] These changes in bone mass may contribute to the increased incidence of bone fractures reported in individuals abusing alcohol and to their tendency to develop osteonecrosis of the femoral head. Withdrawal of alcohol is probably the most important therapeutic manoeuvre.

Patients with non-alcohol-related chronic liver disease and patients with long-standing biliary obstruction may develop osteoporosis.[375] Several factors are of importance in its development, including calcium deficiency secondary to poor dietary intake and fat malabsorption.[308] It is not easily treated, but the provision of a nutritious diet, high in protein, together with calcium supplementation, may lead to improvement. There is evidence to suggest that calcium provided in the form of hydroxyapatite might be more beneficial than calcium provided as a simple salt.[179] Medium-chain triglycerides may be given to these patients not only as a fat source but also to promote calcium uptake. No information is available on the efficacy and safety of biphosphate, oestrogen, fluoride or calcitonin in the treatment of osteoporosis associated with chronic liver disease.

A small number of patients with primary biliary cirrhosis experience severe bone pain despite provision of adequate amounts of vitamin D and calcium. The cause of the bone pain is uncertain but it may respond to intravenous infusions of calcium.[10]

Zinc[184,481,586]

Zinc is widely distributed in food, particularly in meat, shellfish, liver, gelatin, bread, cereals, lentils, peas, beans and rice. However, phytates in the diet will tightly bind zinc, thereby limiting its absorption; thus, the zinc from vegetable sources is generally unavailable. The recommended daily intake for a healthy adult is 15 mg.[152,206]

Zinc is absorbed, in competition with copper, in the duodenum and jejunum. The mechanism of zinc absorption is not clear but seems to be related to the zinc content of the intestinal mucosa and to be regulated by metallothionein.[134] Following absorption, zinc is transported from the intestine in the portal vein. After oral or parenteral administration, appreciable amounts of zinc accumulate in the liver bound to thioneins, which are low-molecular-weight proteins synthesized in the presence of zinc. The body of a healthy adult contains 1.6–2.9 g of zinc, 98% of which is intracellular. Skin, bone, muscle, prostate and visceral organs are relatively rich in zinc; the liver contains about 3% of total body stores. In plasma, 60% of circulating zinc is loosely bound to albumin, 30–40% to a specific α_2-macroglobulin and a small percentage to transferrin and γ-globulin; approximately 1% is associated with amino acids such as histidine and cysteine.[68] The major route of zinc excretion is in faeces;

faecal zinc is largely derived from pancreatic juice with a small contribution from bile.[335] In addition, approximately 0.66 mg of zinc is excreted daily in the urine, and sweat contains 10 mg/100 ml.

Zinc is a component of many metalloenzymes such as alkaline phosphatase, alcohol dehydrogenase, carbonic anhydrase, thymidine kinase, DNA and RNA polymerases, collagenase, carboxypeptidase and superoxide dismutase. It is also a component of a number of metal–protein complexes, in particular metallothionein. It is important for microtubular and microfilament production, and for stabilization of microsomal and lysosomal membranes.[45] It is also important for epithelial differentiation, immune responses, DNA and RNA synthesis and repair, prostaglandin metabolism, fatty acid metabolism, sensory functions, cerebral function and platelet aggregation. It plays a role in the storage and secretion of insulin. It is important for bone development, wound healing, growth and sexual maturation, for the conversion of retinol to retinal and for hepatic secretion of retinol-binding protein.

Hypogonadal dwarfism, sometimes complicated by hepatosplenomegaly, has been described in rural Iranian and Egyptian boys who subsist on diets of mainly bread and beans and very little animal protein. These youths have decreased zinc concentrations in plasma, erythrocytes and hair and decreased serum concentrations of the zinc-dependent enzyme alkaline phosphatase. Growth and sexual maturation improve following a nutritionally adequate diet but the effect is enhanced by addition of zinc. Acrodermatitis enteropathica is an autosomal recessive disorder which manifests as severe chronic diarrhoea, wasting, alopecia and roughened, thickened and ulcerated skin around body orifices. Serum and hair zinc concentrations are extremely low and leucocyte chemotaxis is impaired. The condition responds promptly to administered zinc, although the exact mechanism of the zinc deficiency is not known. Acrodermatitis enteropathica has also been observed in patients on long-term parenteral nutrition who are inadequately zinc supplemented; the condition reverses quickly when zinc supplements are given. Wound healing is delayed in patients who are zinc deficient and is quickly restored following oral zinc supplementation. Zinc may also play a role in the maintenance of normal taste; patients with decreased taste acuity may improve following oral zinc sulphate, 660 mg daily, in divided doses.

The assessment of zinc status in man is difficult. Serum concentrations can be affected by a variety of factors[482] and, even within individuals, zinc concentrations, in a given tissue, may vary substantially.[546] Thus, although marked changes occur in the zinc content of tissues, blood and urine in many human diseases, the relationship of such alterations to the underlying condition is, for the most part, poorly understood.

Circulating concentrations of zinc are reduced and urinary zinc excretion is increased in individuals chronically abusing alcohol, irrespective of the presence or degree of any associated alcoholic liver disease.[57,228,244,297,306,366,503,617] In patients with cirrhosis, zinc concentrations in plasma may be low because of a reduction in the fraction bound to albumin; the amount bound to α_2-macroglobulin is normal[68] or else increased.[539] Leucocyte zinc concentrations may be reduced in these patients[228,305] but erythrocyte zinc concentrations are usually normal.[228] Hepatic zinc concentrations are reduced in individuals with alcoholic liver disease, irrespective of its severity.[57,69,313,412,416,503,617]

Decreased circulating zinc concentrations have also been observed in patients with a variety of non-alcoholic liver diseases, including acute viral hepatitis,[297] fulminant hepatic failure,[96] chronic persistent and chronic active hepatitis,[57,228,306] primary biliary cirrhosis,[228] cirrhosis,[575] haemochromatosis,[75] Indian childhood cirrhosis,[420] and schistosomiasis.[408] Reduced hepatic zinc concentrations have also been observed in patients with a variety of non-alcoholic liver diseases.[46,57,313,416]

The mechanisms responsible for these changes in blood and tissue zinc concentrations in patients with liver disease are not entirely clear. Dietary zinc intake may be reduced if the diet is inadequate or the patient is anorexic. Zinc absorption may be impaired,[163,545,575] although it has also been reported to be increased.[412,415] The presence of portal–systemic shunting of blood and of decreased hepatocyte function might explain the low hepatic zinc concentrations observed in these individuals, but hepatic zinc extraction has been reported to be normal or high in patients with liver disease.[307] Finally, ethanol enhances urinary zinc excretion,[298] as will the use of thiazide diuretics.

A number of abnormalities have been reported in patients with liver disease which might reflect the presence of zinc deficiency.[83,184,481] For example, patients with long-standing cholestasis and patients with parenchymal liver disease may develop impaired dark adaptation as a result of vitamin A deficiency.[13,261] Zinc plays an important role in vitamin A metabolism as it is necessary for conversion of retinol to retinal and for the hepatic secretion of retinol-binding protein. While most patients with liver disease and impaired dark adaptation respond to vitamin A alone, others require additional supplementation with zinc.[261,434] Indeed, it has been suggested that patients with chronic liver disease and low leucocyte concentrations may show photoreceptor dysfunction regardless of their vitamin A status.[306]

Patients with liver disease may display abnormalities of taste and smell, which have been treated, with varying degrees of success, with zinc supplementation.[592,638] Patients with cirrhosis and hypogonadism tend to have low serum zinc concentrations,[3] but do not benefit, in this regard, from zinc supplementation.[226] It has been postulated that zinc deficiency may play a role in the pathogenesis of hepatic encephalopathy as serum zinc concentrations are reduced in patients with this syndrome and correlate inversely with blood ammonia concentrations;[236,492] use of zinc supplements is associated with improvement in neuropsychiatric status.[492] Zinc deficiency has also been implicated in the pathogenesis of alcohol-related liver injury, particularly the development of fibrosis;[367,437,464] no information is available currently on the potential benefits of zinc supplementation in individuals chronically abusing alcohol in relation to the development of liver injury. Finally, patients with cirrhosis show abnormal handling of sulphur-containing amino acids and decreased conversion of ornithine to citrulline; both abnormalities might reflect zinc deficiency.

Thus, there is circumstantial evidence that patients with liver disease may become zinc deficient. Further studies are obviously needed to define the role of zinc supplementation in these individuals.

Magnesium[204,524]

Magnesium is widely distributed in ordinary foods. The richest sources are cocoa, nuts, barley, oats, oatmeal, wholemeal flour, soya flour and lima beans. The average diet provides 250–500 mg a day, of which less than half is absorbed. The recommended daily intake for healthy adults is 300–400 mg.[152,206]

Magnesium is absorbed from the small intestine by an active transport system which is vitamin D dependent; it then enters the circulation. The body of a 70-kg adult contains 2.5 g of magnesium, of which approximately one-half is found in bone, mainly in the mineral lattice. The remainder is located in skeletal and cardiac muscle, liver, kidney, brain and interstitial fluid; the amount in extracellular fluid is extremely small. About two-thirds of the magnesium in plasma is in free form, while the rest is bound to proteins. Plasma magnesium concentrations are maintained within narrow limits, but little information is available on the factors responsible for retaining this homeostasis. Plasma magnesium concentrations correlate best with those of the exchangeable magnesium of bone; a good correlation exists between plasma and intracellular magnesium concentrations. Magnesium is excreted mainly by the kidney but over 90% of the filtered cation is reabsorbed from the proximal renal tubule. Magnesium acts as a cofactor for many enzymatic reactions, particularly those involved in high-energy phosphate metabolism. It is also involved in the reversible association of intracellular particles and in the binding of macromolecules to subcellular organelles. Body mechanisms for preserving magnesium are extremely efficient; thus, spontaneous magnesium deficiency is rarely encountered. Volunteers fed magnesium-deficient regimens develop hypomagnesaemia which is inconsistently accompanied by hypokalaemia and hypocalcaemia. These individuals may develop neuromuscular disorders akin to those observed with hypocalcaemia.

The incidence and implications of magnesium deficiency in patients with liver disease have received little attention, although magnesium has been incriminated in the fibrotic response of rat liver to carbon tetrachloride and alcohol[490] and in the neurological response of cirrhotic patients to ammonia.[205] Magnesium deficiency has been documented in individuals chronically abusing alcohol, with or without liver disease, and may be accompanied by clinical signs of deficiency. Alcohol increases urinary magnesium excretion,[298] but other factors must also be important. Hypomagnesaemia has been reported in patients with cirrhosis[593] but it is rarely accompanied by clinical evidence of deficiency. However, Lim and Jacob,[353] studied a group of cirrhotic patients with anorexia, muscle weakness and cramps, and found that while plasma and bone magnesium concentrations were normal, muscle magnesium values were low; their symptoms resolved following magnesium supplementation over a period of 6 weeks. The mechanism of magnesium deficiency in patients with liver disease, when it occurs, is unknown, although urinary magnesium concentrations may increase in patients with secondary hyperaldosteronism and in those taking diuretics.

Selenium

Selenium is present in a wide variety of foods. Cereal products, meat, poultry and fish are the richest sources; milk, vegetables and fruit contain only small amounts. Intakes may vary significantly between populations, largely because of differences in the selenium content of soils and other soil–plant factors. Selenium in food is available in a number of forms, although information is incomplete. Thus, 40% of the selenium in wheat is present as protein-bound selenomethionine but the chemical nature and quantitative distribution of the remainder is unknown; it may include selenate and selenocysteic acid. In animal tissues, selenium is present as selenocysteine, selenomethionine, selenosulphide, selenopersulphides and metal selenides. Not all forms of dietary selenium are equally available, although information on bioavailability is incomplete. Dietary intakes of 50–200 mg of selenium daily are considered adequate and safe.[206]

Selenium is absorbed in the distal ileum. It is transported in plasma bound to a specific protein, probably produced in the liver.[436] It is stored in the liver, spleen, heart and nails. Newly absorbed selenium is rapidly excreted in the urine; it may also be excreted in sweat and bile.

Selenium is an essential component of a number of enzymes, most importantly glutathione peroxidase, which catalyses the breakdown of lipid peroxides and other organic peroxides generated during cellular metabolism. This enzyme is an antioxidant and, together with vitamin E, superoxide dismutase and glutathione, serves to protect lipid membranes from oxidative stress and lipid peroxidation. Populations with low serum selenium concentrations may show reduced glutathione peroxidase activity but this is of no obvious clinical consequence. However, in areas of China where the soil selenium is particularly low, children may develop a cardiomyopathy which is thought to be a feature of deficiency. This so-called Kershan's disease can be prevented by use of sodium selenite supplementation.

Serum, plasma and erythrocyte selenium concentrations are reduced in individuals abusing alcohol, irrespective of the presence of liver disease.[1,102,172,173,175,290,323,606,616] Deficiency may arise because of poor dietary intake or because of reduced hepatic production of the transport protein. Hepatic selenium concentrations are reduced in patients with alcoholic cirrhosis.[174,416,503] No changes have been observed in serum, plasma or blood glutathione peroxidase activity in individuals abusing alcohol,[606] although platelet glutathione peroxidase activity is reduced in patients with alcoholic cirrhosis.[290] Increased lipid peroxidation is thought to be a major pathogenic factor in the development of alcohol-related liver injury. Selenium deficiency is associated with reduced glutathione peroxidase activity and hence reduced antioxidant activity and enhanced lipid peroxidation. Selenium deficiency has, therefore, been implicated in the pathogenesis of alcohol-related liver injury.[174]

Very little information is available on the selenium status of patients with non-alcoholic liver disease. Both reduced serum[2,594] and hepatic[416] selenium concentrations have been reported.

DIET AND OTHER NUTRITIONAL FACTORS IN THE PRODUCTION OF HEPATIC DAMAGE

Liver damage may result from dietary inadequacies, dietary excesses and dietary contaminants, or else as a result of various nutritional manoeuvres or therapies.

MALNUTRITION AND UNDERNUTRITION[484]

Animals fed diets deficient in choline, protein and/or vitamins develop fatty liver and cirrhosis.[249] As a result, the concept of nutritional liver injury arose and, for some considerable time, malnutrition was nominated as a factor in human cirrhosis, particularly in the tropics. In countries where malnutrition is endemic, however, environmental hygiene tends to be poor and large reservoirs of potentially hepatotoxic viruses, parasites and food-borne contaminants are present. Thus, it is now considered unlikely that cirrhosis is related to malnutrition per se and 'nutritional' cirrhosis is a term of doubtful significance.[145,608] Nevertheless, liver injury, short of cirrhosis, can accompany both malnutrition and undernutrition.

The term protein–calorie malnutrition is used to encompass the various clinical forms of malnutrition which result from an inadequate intake of calories, or protein, or both.[625,632] These disorders are particularly common in the Third World where the food supply is often limited, but may also occur in the Western world, as a consequence either of disease or of unusual dietary habits or food fads.[113,566] In its most extreme forms protein–calorie malnutrition manifests as one of two clinical syndromes, kwashiorkor and marasmus.

Kwashiorkor, first described in malnourished African children several decades ago, but still widely prevalent in tropical and subtropical regions, results from consumption of a diet severely restricted in protein but adequate in calories from carbohydrate and fat sources.[414] The syndrome classically develops when a child is weaned from breast milk, which provides a balanced intake of nutrients, to a diet composed mainly of starch in the form of maize. Kwashiorkor is characterized by growth failure, hair and skin changes and peripheral oedema. Lean muscle mass and body fat stores are preserved, at least initially, but visceral protein production is seriously disturbed. The liver is often grossly enlarged, containing 30–50% fat by weight,[317] predominantly in the form of neutral fat or triglyceride.[115] The intrahepatic accumulation of fat results from the combined effects of excess delivery of fatty acids to the liver and/or enhanced lipogenesis, combined with impaired lipid transport from the liver secondary to apoprotein deficiency. Although the liver may be markedly enlarged, serum enzyme concentrations may be normal or at most minimally abnormal,[489] although coagulation defects have been described.[250]

All the features of kwashiorkor improve dramatically when protein is supplied; fat clears from the liver within a short period of time. Hepatic fibrosis may develop if the disorder is severe and of long standing, but it is never marked and does not evolve to cirrhosis.[131,488]

Marasmus affects children in tropical and subtropical regions and arises when the diet is deficient in both protein and energy. It is characterized by stunted growth, loss of fat stores, generalized loss of lean body mass but maintenance of visceral protein production, at least initially. The liver in children with marasmus is not usually palpable and the changes that occur in liver histology are non-specific; neither fibrosis nor cirrhosis develop. Grossly undernourished adults show no signs of liver disease and no important histological changes in the liver.[556] Institution of a normal diet results in the reversal of any clinical or histological abnormalities.

Most children and adults with protein–calorie malnutrition, both in the Third World and in the Western world, present with mixed features of kwashiorkor and marasmus, or more commonly still, with chronic mild to moderate malnutrition, which in children is manifest by retardation in height and weight and delayed psychomotor and mental development, but which in adults may be essentially asymptomatic.

DIETARY EXCESSES

Alcohol abuse is a well-recognized cause of liver disease; excessive energy intake, resulting, as it does, in the development of obesity, may also cause liver injury. Liver damage may also develop in individuals consuming excessive amounts of vitamins A and possibly in individuals consuming excessive dietary iron.

Alcohol[6,281,422,430]

Alcohol is not an essential nutrient but is a 'normal' constituent of the diet of many individuals. It is a metabolic fuel, which in Western diets, supplies 4–6% of total daily energy requirements.

Alcohol is the most important cause of liver disease in the Western world today[405,428] (see Chapter 34). The majority of alcoholics will develop hepatic steatosis at some stage of their drinking career, but only 20–30% will develop cirrhosis.[337,342] An individual's susceptibility to developing significant alcohol-related liver injury is probably determined by a number of genetic,[56,155,636] constitutional,[210,383,451] and environmental factors.[105,349]

In susceptible individuals, liver damage results from the prolonged daily ingestion of 60 g or more of alcohol, although intakes of 20–40 g may be sufficient in women.[121,451] Significant liver disease may not appear for 20 years but in some individuals may develop in as little as 5 years. Alcoholic liver injury appears to progress from fatty liver through alcoholic hepatitis to cirrhosis.[348]

Fatty change is the most common liver lesion seen, but although fat accumulation represents a profound metabolic disturbance of the liver, it is not necessarily harmful. Certainly cirrhosis may develop in an alcoholic who has never had fatty change and isolated fatty change has not been shown to proceed directly to cirrhosis, in man.

Alcoholic hepatitis develops in only a proportion of drinkers, even after decades of abuse, and is assumed to be a precirrhotic lesion, although its natural history is not well understood.[343] Thus, in approximately 50% of individuals with alcoholic hepatitis the liver lesion may persist for several years, while in 10% the lesion may heal despite continued alcohol abuse.[215] It has, therefore, been suggested that although alcoholic hepatitis may contribute, when present, to the evolution to cirrhosis, it is not a *sine qua non* of such progression. A number of alternative precursor lesions of cirrhosis have been suggested, including, perisinusoidal fibrosis,[446] occlusive lesions in the terminal hepatic venules,[231] and perivenular fibrosis.[444,621,650]

Cirrhosis is generally considered to be an irreversible lesion. Once established it may remain asymptomatic for many years, but decompensation tends to develop at a rate of 10% per annum;[139] hepatocellular carcinoma develops in approximately 20% of individuals with alcoholic cirrhosis, almost invariably in those who have remained abstinent from alcohol.[334]

The relative importance of alcohol toxicity and malnutrition in the pathogenesis of liver injury in individuals abusing alcohol has been debated for years; both factors are probably important. Alcohol has been shown to be directly hepatotoxic, independently of dietary intake, in both chronic alcohol abusers[351] and healthy volunteers.[523] In these early experiments, ethanol was substituted isocalorically for carbohydrate in diets that contained either normal or increased amounts of protein. Liver biopsies were obtained a maximum of 3 weeks later and the presence of fatty change was taken to indicate hepatotoxicity. However, the fatty change observed might simply have reflected an adaptive response to obligatory ethanol metabolism. It might also be argued that a diet which is adequate under normal circumstances might not be adequate when alcohol is substituted for carbohydrate to comprise 50% of total daily energy intake. Such a sharp decrease in carbohydrate intake would limit glycogen reserves and gluconeogenesis,[19] and might lead to loss of the protein-sparing effect of carbohydrate. Additionally, the high fat-to-carbohydrate ratio of the diets might interfere with ethanol oxidation[639] and fat metabolism.[293,350] Despite these reservations about the original studies, ample evidence has accrued to support the view that alcohol directly damages liver cells; the exact mechanism of damage remains in debate.[281]

Although alcohol is believed to be directly hepatotoxic, it is of interest that in individuals with established alcoholic liver disease, alcohol in amounts up to 300 g daily does not impede recovery.[466,499,596,626] Indeed, provided that patients are adequately nourished, improvement occurs despite continued alcohol abuse. Patek and Post[466] allowed a group of patients with decompensated alcoholic cirrhosis and severe malnutrition to stabilize in hospital on a nutritious, high-protein diet. Alcohol was then reintroduced and quantities equivalent to one-third to one-half of a bottle of spirits daily were given for up to 18 months. Improvement continued in both clinical signs and laboratory test results. Erenoglu and coworkers[180] randomized patients recovering from liver failure to treatment with either high- or low-protein diets; all received approximately 160 g of alcohol daily. The majority of patients taking the high-protein diet showed clinical, biochemical and histological improvements, while patients taking the low-protein diet either remained stable or deteriorated slightly. These findings suggest that the patients' nutritional status might play an important role in limiting or repairing alcohol-related liver damage.

Alcohol provides 30 kJ (7.1 kcal)/g, so that a bottle of spirits provides 6300 kJ (1500 kcal), or one-half of recommended daily energy requirements for a healthy individual. Alcohol does not, however, provide equivalent caloric food value when compared, for example, with carbohydrate. In addition, alcoholic beverages contain only small amounts of nutrients, which are inadequate to meet daily requirements (Table 6.1). Many individuals chronically abusing alcohol maintain food intake (Figure 6.8), so that their total daily calorie intakes equal or exceed those of healthy non-drinkers.[393,427,448] However, their body weights are invariably lower.[562] This suggests that the calories derived from alcohol have little or no value in terms of maintaining body weight and hence nutritional reserves. Support for this suggestion is gained from a number of studies in which patients were fed alcohol under carefully controlled conditions. Mezey and Faillace[404] fed a diet which provided 2600 kcal daily to 56 individuals with a history of alcohol abuse, and noted

Table 6.1 Alcohol, energy and nutrient content of various beverages

Constituent (per 100 ml)	Beer	Wine	Fortified wine (sherry, vermouth)	Spirits (70% proof)
Alcohol (g)	2.2–4.3	8.7–10.2	13.0–15.9	31.5
Energy (kcal)	25–39	66–94	116–157	222
Carbohydrate (g)	1.5–4.2	0.3–5.9	1.4–15.9	Trace
Protein (g)	0.2–0.3	0.1–0.3	Trace	Trace–0.3
Thiamine (mg)	Trace	Trace	Trace	–
Riboflavin (mg)	0.02–0.04	0.01	Trace–0.01	–
Nicotinic acid (mg)	0.30–0.51	0.06–0.09	0.04–0.10	–
Pyridoxine (mg)	0.012–0.023	0.012–0.023	0.004–0.010	–
Folic acid (μg)	4.0–8.8	0.1–0.2	Trace–0.1	–
Vitamin B_{12} (μg)	0.11–0.17	Trace	Trace	–
Iron (mg)	Trace–0.05	0.5–1.2	0.34–0.53	Trace
Calcium (mg)	4–11	3–14	4–9	Trace
Magnesium (mg)	6–10	6–11	4–13	Trace

Data from Paul and Southgate.[468]

that they all gained weight. Seventeen of these patients were provided with an extra 1800 kcal daily in the form of spirits, but no additional weight gain was observed. Pirola and Lieber[473] showed that if alcohol was substituted isocalorically for up to 50% of dietary carbohydrate, weight loss occurred. They also showed that addition of 2000 kcal daily as alcohol to the diet had no consistent effect on body weight, whereas addition of 2000 kcal daily as chocolate resulted in consistent weight gain (Figure 6.9).

The calories provided by alcohol are, therefore, inefficiently utilized, probably because oxidation is not coupled by phosphorylation to produce adenosine

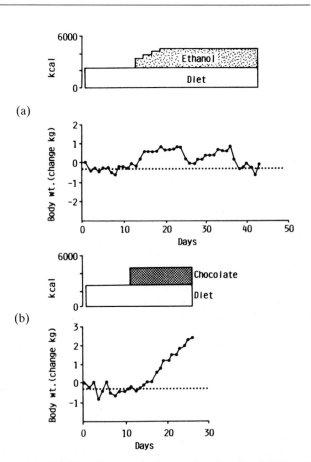

Figure 6.9 (a) The effect on body weight of adding 2000 kcal/day as ethanol to the diet of one subject. The dotted line represents the mean weight change during the control period. (b) The effect on body weight of adding 2000 kcal/day as chocolate to the diet of the same subject. The dotted line represents the mean change during the control period. (Pirola and Lieber.[473])

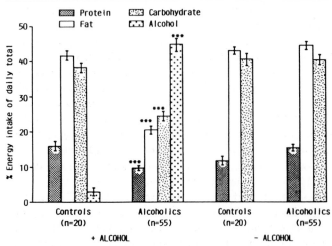

Figure 6.8 Mean (±SEM) percentage contributions made by protein, fat and carbohydrate to total daily energy intake in control subjects and alcohol abusers both with and without the energy contribution from alcohol.
***Values significantly different from values in control subjects, $p < 0.01$. (Morgan.[427])

triphosphate (ATP). Thus, although alcohol generates large amounts of reduced nicotinamide adenine dinucleotides (NADH), much is wasted in shifting redox state. In addition, chronic alcohol intake causes mitochondrial dysfunction, with the result that NADH reoxidation, electron transport and phosphorylation processes may be impaired. Finally, chronic alcohol ingestion induces the activity of the hepatic microsomal ethanol-oxidizing system, thereby increasing its contribution to alcohol metabolism. Utilization of this process for metabolizing alcohol is energy-wasting because it is not coupled with oxidative phosphorylation and so generates heat instead of conserving chemical energy. Induction of this energy-wasteful pathway for alcohol metabolism may explain, at least in part, the increase in energy expenditure observed in individuals chronically abusing alcohol.[431] Alcohol is, therefore, an inefficient metabolic fuel.

Individuals chronically abusing alcohol may be malnourished not only because alcohol is a nutrient-poor, inefficient caloric fuel but also because of its effects on nutrient absorption, metabolism, storage and requirements. However, the relationship between malnutrition and the liver injury seen in individuals chronically abusing alcohol needs further clarification. While malnutrition may not initiate liver injury, it is undoubtedly important in limiting and repairing damage.

The mainstay of nutritional therapy in individuals with alcoholic liver disease is discontinuation of alcohol and provision of a well-balanced diet; specific deficiencies, for example of vitamins or trace metals, should be corrected.

Calories[14,24,42,120,185,309]

The basal energy expenditure of any given individual, in good health, is reasonably constant and can be met with a basal caloric intake of 5.4–8.3 MJ (1300–2000 kcal)/24 h. If body mass is to remain constant, then the caloric intake must match the energy expenditure. Calories ingested surplus to requirements are stored as triglyceride in adipose tissue. Body weight will increase if excess calories are consumed over time; the weight gain is proportional to the total excess energy consumed; approximately 30% of the excess weight is lean body mass. Obesity is defined as a body mass index (weight (kg)/height (m^2)) in excess of 25. It is associated with the development, both in adults and in children, of parenchymal liver damage and the formation of gallstones.

The most common histological lesion observed in obese individuals is fatty change;[167,239,318,520,630,640,657] the fat comprises triglyceride, fatty acids and mono- and diglycerides.[390] The amount of fat deposited in the liver does not relate to the degree of obesity. Mild to moderate degrees of hepatic inflammation and fibrosis are also commonly observed; the fibrosis is more severe and more extensive in individuals with morbid obesity of long standing who have severe fatty change.[630] A small proportion of obese individuals develop steatohepatitis which histologically mimics alcoholic hepatitis.[7,159,318,336,362,425,479] There is no relationship between the development of non-alcoholic steatohepatitis and the degree of obesity. However, in individual patients the development of this liver lesion may be preceded by a period of rapid weight loss.[479] Non-alcoholic steatonecrosis may progress to cirrhosis in a small number of patients but generally it is a clinically mild, slowly progressive lesion.[336,479] There is little correlation between the structural and functional abnormalities of the liver observed in obese individuals.[166,167,217,239,443,640]

The mechanism of the fatty change in obese individuals is not clear. These individuals tend to take diets low in protein but high in fat and carbohydrate, so that dietary imbalance may play a role.[167] Additionally, 50% of obese subjects, or more, show carbohydrate intolerance[640,657] which may be a contributory factor, although no relationship exists between the degree of hepatic abnormality and the disturbance of carbohydrate metabolism.[640] It is of interest that the hepatic lipid stores in obese individuals can be mobilized in the absence of exogenous calories and protein.

Transient increases are observed in serum bilirubin and enzyme concentrations and in bromsulphophthalein retention in obese subjects who lose weight acutely through fasting or semistarvation; these abnormalities subside when normal dietary intake is resumed.[520] Gradual weight loss, to within 15% of ideal body weight, is associated with improvement in liver function test results.[640] Fatty infiltration of the liver decreases, to a degree, after moderate weight loss,[640] while after repeated short periods of fasting, fatty change diminishes but fibrosis may become more prominent.[520] More extensive and rapid weight loss results in a progressive reduction in the degree of fatty infiltration, and occasionally in a diminution of periportal fibrosis.[167] Near-normal liver histology is observed in obese subjects who achieve and maintain substantial weight reduction.[167]

The presence of obesity increases the risk of gallstone formation, particularly stones of cholesterol or mixed type. In the general population the frequency of gallstones in individuals aged 18 years or older is approximately 11%.[30,211] In contrast, the frequency in obese subjects is 23%, and in the morbidly obese 30–35%.[30,185] Several factors are of importance in the genesis of gallstones in the obese, including increased bile saturation,[496,497] impaired gallbladder motility,[202,387] and the ingestion of high-fat, high-carbohydrate diets.[550]

Weight loss may be associated with an increased risk of gallstone formation if the saturation index of bile remains unchanged or increases. This can be prevented by prophylactic use of ursodeoxycholic acid in a dose of 10–15 mg/kg.[76] Both chenodeoxycholic acid and ursodeoxycholic acid, in daily doses of 15 mg/kg, have been used successfully to dissolve gallstones in obese adolescents.[476] The effectiveness of treatment may improve if weight is lost simultaneously.[496,633]

Other nutrients

Excess intake or absorption of vitamin A,[39,380] and of iron[232,265,607] may result in liver injury.

An intake of retinoids greatly in excess of requirements results in development of a toxic syndrome known as hypervitaminosis A.[39,187,251,527] Toxicity in children usually results from overenthusiastic vitamin therapy and can arise with intakes as small as 1500 IU/kg (7.5–15 mg) daily for 30 days. Toxicity in adults results from extended vitamin supplementation, food fads or the use of high-dose retinoids for treatment of certain skin complaints; it is uncommon in adults consuming less than 100 000 IU (30 mg) of vitamin A daily, although mild symptoms of chronic intoxication have been detected in individuals whose intakes have averaged 33 000 IU (10 mg) daily for 6 months.[39] Individuals chronically abusing alcohol are more susceptible to the hepatotoxic effects of vitamin A and may develop liver damage when taking only moderate amounts of supplements.[345]

The syndrome is characterized by skin and hair changes, pain and tenderness of bones and joints, hyperostosis, anorexia, fatigue, weight loss, benign intracranial hypertension, hypoprothrombinaemia and hepatosplenomegaly. The changes within the liver include hypertrophy of fat-storing cells, fibrosis, sclerosis of central veins and cirrhosis. Increased concentrations of the vitamin are found in the serum, mainly in the form of retinyl esters; concentrations of retinol in plasma in excess of 3.5 μmol/l (100 μg/100 ml) are usually diagnostic. The concentration of retinol-binding protein is normal and the excess retinol circulates in association with lipoproteins. Symptoms improve when the vitamin is withdrawn. Birth defects have been identified in the offsprings of women consuming approximately 25 000–40 000 IU (7.5–12 mg) of vitamin A daily during the first trimester of pregnancy.

It has been suggested that the mandatory fortification of food with iron might lead to an increase in the incidence of iron-storage disease.[136] However, it is uncertain whether prolonged iron intake can result in excess iron accumulation in healthy individuals. In Ethiopia the daily ingestion of up to 200 mg of iron, as dirt iron, causes only modest increases in reticuloendothelial iron stores.[270] Equally, intakes of medicinal iron totalling 1000 g over many years only rarely results in significant iron overload.[292] Massive iron overload is nevertheless seen in South African negroes who use iron pots for cooking and fermenting beer and, as a result, ingest up to 200 mg of iron daily.[63] Many of these subjects show evidence of ascorbic acid deficiency,[551] and this may have profound effects on iron metabolism.[64,110] Thus, excess dietary iron may not be the only factor important in the development of so-called Bantu haemochromatosis. The excess iron can be removed by venesection, but dietary iron intake should also be reduced.

It is possible that as individuals in the Western world become more health conscious, other, as yet unrecognized syndromes of 'dietary excess' or 'dietary imbalance' may arise as a result of self-administered dietary supplements.

INTESTINAL BYPASS SURGERY[24,185]

Surgical bypass of the small intestine has been used for the treatment and control of severe obesity since the early 1960s. The procedure is undoubtedly efficacious, but is almost invariably complicated by increased fat deposition in the liver.[79,166,167,216,239,273,530,571] Fatty change may regress within 1–2 years of surgery, but in many patients it persists for considerably longer.[166,216,239] A minority of patients develop steatonecrosis, fibrosis and frank cirrhosis;[216,239] the morphology and pathological sequence of these changes are indistinguishable from those observed in individuals chronically abusing alcohol.[159,216,469] The development of cirrhosis is usually insidious and unheralded by any major changes in liver function;[166,167,239] death may occur from hepatic failure.[70,78,245,278,374,376,391,582]

The majority of the 31 obese individuals studied by Haines and colleagues,[239] showed varying degrees of fatty infiltration and portal fibrosis in their presurgery liver biopsy; mild perivenular fibrosis was noted in 7 patients (26%) and developing cirrhosis in 1 (4%). Following the surgical procedure, hepatic steatosis increased in all patients, reaching maximum severity in 3–6 months and then gradually regressing; portal fibrosis increased in severity in 25 patients (93%) while perivenular fibrosis persisted in the 7 individuals in whom it was present preoperatively and developed de novo in a further 9. More significant lesions, such as steatonecrosis, central hyaline necrosis and/or cirrhosis developed in 7 patients (23%) as early as 3 months and as late as 24 months post-surgery. The patients who developed steatonecrosis and/or cirrhosis were older, had invariably shown perivenular fibrosis on the initial liver biopsy and, 3 months post-surgery, had lost significantly more weight and had significantly higher serum aspartate transaminase values than the subjects who showed steatosis only. These authors suggest that the presence of perivenular fibrosis preoperatively identified patients at greater risk of developing significant liver disease following surgery.[239] Similar conclusions were drawn by Clain and Lefkowich.[120]

Arrest, improvement and at least partial recovery of the liver injury have been achieved by restoration of intestinal continuity, by enteral and parenteral hyperalimentation and by use of metronidazole.[78,166,216,239,278,316]

The mechanism of the liver injury following bypass surgery remains speculative. Most observers believe that the liver injury results from complex nutritional deficiencies which arise during the period of rapid weight loss immediately following surgery.[16,216,254,358,369,438] Others favour a hepatotoxic insult, directly or indirectly related to bacterial overgrowth of the bypassed intestinal segment.[143,166,316,457]

The hepatic changes observed in these patients are similar to those of protein–calorie malnutrition and, indeed, following bypass surgery patients tend to favour low-protein diets high in carbohydrate and fat. The plasma amino acid patterns observed following bypass surgery[438] and in Kwashiorkor[533] are very similar and the hepatic lesions in both conditions have been shown to reverse with nutritional therapy.[16,358,369] In protein-deficient patients the liver is more susceptible to the toxic effects of various agents and impairment of the local immune response in the intestine facilitates penetration by potentially hepatotoxic substances. Protein repletion may facilitate reversal of the liver lesion by improving host defence mechanisms. It could also be argued that, while the steatosis observed following bypass surgery is morphologically similar to that observed with protein–calorie malnutrition, it develops at a time when patients show no clinical or laboratory evidence of protein depletion and still have ample energy reserves. Also, while nutritional therapy may have a favourable effect on the hepatic lesion, liver injury may progress despite provision of essential nutrients.[78] Although the role of malnutrition in the genesis of hepatic steatosis following intestinal bypass surgery needs to be clarified, protein depletion is likely to be a permissive or potentiating factor.

The relationship between the development of liver injury and the presence of bacterial overgrowth in the bypassed segment is also debated. Colonic bacteria have been identified in the excluded small intestine[133] and nonspecific inflammatory changes develop in the mucosa of the bypassed segment.[168] Moreover, the hepatic steatosis has been shown to reverse with use of metronidazole.[166] However, significant bacterial overgrowth may not occur[216] and circulating bacterial endotoxin has not been found in these patients. Additionally, hepatic injury resembling alcoholic hepatitis may develop in obese subjects following gastroplasty in which the stomach is not bypassed but is merely partitioned.[91,246]

Gallstones are prevalent in obese individuals and their incidence probably increases in those whose obesity is treated with an intestinal bypass procedure, irrespective of the surgical technique employed.[14,24,149,186,609,633] Several pathogenic mechanisms have been proposed, including mobilization of cholesterol as a result of marked postoperative weight loss,[407,536] increase in the saturation index of bile due to increased faecal bile acid loss and reduction in the bile acid pool,[32,186,579] and reduction in biliary cholesterol solubilization secondary to changes in bile acid concentrations.[480] It is thought that the mechanism of gallstone formation after gastric operations for obesity might relate more directly to the weight loss.

Ursodeoxycholic acid may be absorbed in patients who have undergone ileal surgery[332] and appears to be well-tolerated by patients with long-standing jejunoileostomies. It could be used prophylactically in patients undergoing jejunoileal bypass or gastric surgery for obesity to prevent gallstone formation. Some difficulty might be encountered in patients who have undergone gastric restrictive surgery because of the large size of the medication.

In view of the potentially serious hepatobiliary consequences associated with intestinal bypass surgery, great caution should be exercised in using this method for treating and controlling obesity.

PARENTERAL NUTRITION[26,29,201,286,321,534]

Total parenteral nutrition is an effective method for supplying energy and nutrients to support life, when oral or enteral feeding is impossible or contraindicated. Most total parenteral nutritional regimens supply energy in the form of carbohydrate, fat and amino acids, with supplements of vitamins, minerals and trace metals as required; glucose is the most commonly used carbohydrate and fat is usually supplied as the soybean emulsion Intralipid.

Individuals receiving total parenteral nutrition may develop hepatobiliary abnormalities for a number of reasons; they may, for example, be malnourished; they may have small-bowel disease or have undergone small intestinal resection, or they may be septicaemic and/or suffer failure or dysfunction of multiple organ systems. There is clear evidence that the use of total parenteral nutrition, per se, may be associated with abnormalities of hepatobiliary function which may result in significant morbidity and possibly even death; the spectrum of abnormalities includes asymptomatic biochemical changes, hepatic steatosis with progression to steatohepatitis, fibrosis and cirrhosis, acalculous cholecystitis, cholelithiasis and intrahepatic cholestasis.

Overall, the complications of total parenteral nutrition are more severe in infants than in adults. The most frequent and predictable hepatobiliary complication associated with use of total parenteral nutrition is the development of cholestasis in infants, especially those born prematurely. The other common complications of this form of nutritional support, such as the development of fatty change or the accumulation of biliary sludge and stones, may occur in individuals of any age.

Many individuals receiving total parenteral nutrition develop abnormal biochemical test results, but it is often difficult to establish a cause and effect relationship because of the possible contribution of the patient's underlying disease process. Equally, it is difficult to assess the relevance of such changes in terms of hepatic morphology because liver biopsies are only infrequently taken.

Lindor and colleagues[355] retrospectively reviewed the liver function tests of 48 patients who had received total parenteral nutrition for between 2 and 4 weeks, and found significant increases in serum concentrations of bilirubin in 10 (21%), alkaline phosphatase in 26 (54%) and aspartate transaminase in 32 (67%); maximal values were observed between the ninth and twelfth days. Liver biopsies were undertaken in 4 patients and showed periportal steatosis.

Bengoa and coworkers[40] examined liver function test results in 92 adults with inflammatory bowel disease during total parenteral nutrition. Twenty (22%) had abnormal liver function test results from the outset. Within 2 weeks serum alkaline phosphatase and aspartate transaminase activities had increased, in the majority of patients, and increased serum bilirubin concentrations were observed in 23 (25%). Liver biopsies were performed in the 4 patients with the highest serum aspartate trans-aminase concentrations, and showed only minor, non-specific changes. Discontinuation of total parenteral nutrition was associated with a prompt return of the biochemical abnormalities to baseline values.

Finally, Robertson and colleagues[505] retrospectively assessed liver function test results in 127 general surgical patients who had received a course of intravenous nutrition. Test results were abnormal in 101 patients (80%) at the outset. Serum concentrations of γ-glutamyl transferase increased in all patients by the fourth week of treatment but the changes were usually transient; the changes in serum alkaline phosphatase activity were more persistent. The incidence of biochemical abnormalities was significantly greater in individuals with major sepsis and in those who were malnourished; significant increases in serum bilirubin concentrations were only observed in individuals transfused more than 8 units of blood.

The alterations in liver function test results in patients receiving total parenteral nutrition may simply reflect 'infusate imbalance'. The use of high-calorie infusions in dextrose-based regimens is associated with a greater incidence of abnormalities than use of regimens in which 30–50% of the calories are provided as lipid emulsion.[101, 392] However, use of regimens in which lipid provides in excess of 60% of non-protein calories is associated with the development of cholestasis.[11]

Fatty change is the most common liver lesion to develop in association with total parenteral nutrition; the accumulated lipid is almost entirely triglyceride.[299] The clinical significance of the hepatic fat accumulation is not known. Thus, although it undoubtedly reflects abnormal liver cell metabolism, its presence does not predict pro-gressive liver cell dysfunction or damage. Several mechan-isms may be responsible for this change, reflecting meta-bolic alterations associated with the patients' nutritional status, their disease state and the use of this form of nutritional support per se.

Calorie overload in excess of basal energy expenditure is thought to be a major factor associated with the development of hepatic steatosis in patients receiving total parenteral nutrition.[355,361,647] Infusion of large amounts of glucose is thought to be the most likely contributor. At infusion rates as low as 4 mg/kg /min, less than half of the infused glucose is oxidized; higher rates of glucose infusion result in lipid and glycogen deposition in the liver and may also affect fatty acid oxidation, thereby contributing to the steatosis.[535,585,647] Provision of a proportion of non-protein calories as fat blunts the increase in hepatic lipids,[86] but administration of large amounts of lipid may also cause hepatic fat accumu-lation.[58,386] It has, therefore, been recommended that the non-protein calorie intake, during total parenteral nutrition, be reduced to provide a calorie-to-nitrogen ratio of 150 kcal to 1 g of nitrogen and that 30–50% of the non-protein calories be provided as lipid emulsion.

Carnitine is essential for long-chain fatty acid oxidation; carnitine deficiency is associated with the development of hepatic steatosis.[303] The fluids used for total parenteral nutrition do not contain carnitine but it can be synthesized endogenously from methionine and lysine. Nevertheless, low circulating and hepatic carnitine concentrations have been documented in patients receiving total parenteral nutrition.[67] Carnitine supplementation is associated with restoration of carnitine concentrations in the blood and liver but has little effect on liver structure or on the liver fat content.[65]

Choline is essential for the integrity of all membranes, for the transport of lipids and for neural function; choline deficiency is possibly associated with the development of hepatic steatosis.[116] The fluids used for parenteral nutrition do not contain choline but it can be synthesized de novo provided there is a supply of methionine. Plasma choline concentrations are low in individuals on un-supplemented enteral and parenteral feeding regimens, [116] but the relationship between choline deficiency and the development of hepatic steatosis in patients receiving total parenteral nutrition is unknown.

The prolonged use of total parenteral nutrition is associated with the development of progressive liver injury including steatohepatitis, progressive cholestasis, fibrosis and cirrhosis; patients may be asymptomatic or may develop symptoms and signs of progressive liver dysfunc-tion and failure.[66] The prevalence of this complication is unknown but it is thought to occur uncommonly.[66,275] Equally, the contribution of total parenteral nutrition per se to the development of the liver injury is undocu-mented.[584]

Acalculous cholecystitis and cholelithiasis may develop both in adults,[18,401,470,512] and in children.[41,150,315,644] In a prospective evaluation of 21 children requiring total parenteral nutrition for a minimum of 3 months, 9 (43%) were found to have developed gallstones.[513] In a prospective ultrasonographic study, gallbladder sludge was shown to develop in 18 (44%) of 41 neonates receiving total parenteral nutrition after a mean period of 10 days.[389] Evolution of sludge into 'sludge balls' was observed in 5 infants and 2 developed uncomplicated gallstones. Messing and coworkers[401] also used ultrasonography to assess the prevalence of gallbladder sludge and lithiasis in 23 adults receiving total parenteral nutrition who were free of hepatobiliary disease at the outset of treatment. The incidence of sludge formation during the first 3 weeks of treatment was 6%, increasing to 50% between the fourth and sixth weeks and reaching 100% with treatment periods in excess of 6 weeks. Gallstones were found, together with sludge, in 6 patients, 3 of whom required cholecystectomy after a mean of 43 days of treatment.

The bile in patients receiving total parenteral nutrition is thick and dark and may contain cholesterol crystals with microlithiasis and calcium bilirubinate precipitates.[12, 97] The gallstones are pigmented and contain large amounts of calcium bilirubinate.[577]

The biliary complications of total parenteral nutrition

arise secondary to biliary stasis; it is unclear whether this develops as a result of increased bile lithogenicity with cholesterol crystal formation or from altered gallbladder function.[98,388]

If total parenteral nutrition is to continue for more than just a few weeks, then gallbladder contraction should be stimulated by intermittent enteral feeding, if possible,[170,567] or else by use of intravenous cholecystokinin or cerulin.[548]

Use of total parenteral nutrition may also be complicated by the development of intrahepatic cholestasis both in adults,[99,462] and in children, particularly pre-term infants.[34,44,276,487,507,611] The histological changes in infants receiving total parenteral nutrition are non-specific and highly variable. The major component is intrahepatic cholestasis alone or in conjunction with bile duct proliferation and occasionally periportal inflammation.[123,276,487,507,656] Fibrosis and even cirrhosis may develop in infants undergoing prolonged total parenteral nutrition.[123,487,507] In adults, the histological picture is of a mixed portal and periportal inflammatory infiltrate, periportal canalicular bile plugs and bile duct proliferation.[11,531,555]

The cholestasis which develops during total parenteral nutrition results from failure of bile secretion, or excretion, rather than from primary hepatocellular failure. Nevertheless, the mechanisms responsible for its development remain unclear.[400,521,643] In infants, the incidence of intrahepatic cholestasis during total parenteral nutrition correlates inversely with gestational age and body weight, suggesting that immaturity of hepatic excretory mechanisms must play a role. Equally, the requirements for certain essential nutrients such as taurine,[138,219] and essential fatty acids[500] may not be met, and immaturity of various biosynthetic enzyme systems might lead to deficiencies of nutrients such as carnitine and choline which are not usually considered essential; deficiencies of molybdenum, vitamin E and selenium have also been proposed.

The basic components of the infusate have also been blamed for the development of the intrahepatic cholestasis but the evidence is not convincing.[188,478] Other infusate components may cause liver injury; aluminium, for example, can accumulate in the liver and is hepatotoxic.[319,320]

Cholestasis has been observed in sick infants and adults after fasting and this led to the suggestion that lack of enteral nutrition with suppression or lack of hormone stimulation of the hepatobiliary system might be of aetiological importance in the development of intrahepatic cholestasis in relation to total parenteral nutrition.[276,487] Finally, the possibility that the cholestasis might in some way relate to intestinal overgrowth with anaerobic bacteria must also been considered;[99,462] these individuals may be predisposed to intestinal bacterial overgrowth because of bowel inactivity.

The intrahepatic cholestasis observed in individuals receiving prolonged total parenteral nutrition regresses when treatment is discontinued. It can be ameliorated during treatment by stimulating bile flow with small lipid and protein meals or with cholecystokinin; a trial of metronidazole may be warranted.[99,326,331]

In general, total parenteral nutrition should be used for the shortest possible time; excess calories should be avoided and 30–50% of non-protein calories should be provided as fat. Patients should be very carefully monitored throughout.

INBORN ERRORS OF METABOLISM _____

Tyrosinaemia, galactosaemia and fructose intolerance (see Chapter 44)

Children with hereditary tyrosinaemia,[227] galactosaemia[552] and hereditary fructose intolerance[225] may develop liver damage in response to normal dietary constituents. They present soon after birth and successful management depends on early diagnosis and exclusion of the offending substance from the diet. The mechanism of the liver injury in these conditions is not understood but it is assumed to relate to the accumulation of toxic metabolites of tyrosine, galactose or fructose.

Wilson's disease (hepatolenticular/hepatocerebral degeneration)[570,586] (see Chapter 35)

Wilson's disease is an autosomal, recessively inherited disorder of copper metabolism in which hepatic lysosomes fail to excrete copper into the bile. The excess intracellular copper inhibits the formation of caeruloplasmin from apocaeruloplasmin and copper, hence circulating concentrations of this glycoprotein are characteristically low. The capacity of hepatocytes to store copper is eventually exceeded; copper is released into the circulation and accumulates in the brain, kidney and cornea. Toxicity occurs as a result of binding of the excess copper to various cellular proteins. The gene for Wilson's disease is located on chromosome 13.

Clinical manifestations of copper excess are rare before the age of 6 years; most patients present in adolescence, although an occasional patient may remain in good health until their sixth decade. The hepatic manifestations tend to occur earlier than the neurological manifestations; nevertheless, fewer than 50% of patients present with evidence of liver involvement. The clinical picture of hepatic Wilson's disease varies from an acute, often fulminant hepatitis, to an asymptomatic inactive cirrhosis. Neurological and psychiatric abnormalities may coexist; Kayser–Fleischer rings are almost invariably present; sunflower cataracts, haematological, endocrine and skeletal abnormalities may also be present.

Abnormal fat and glycogen deposits are the earliest abnormalities observed in the liver biopsy on light microscopy. Mitochondrial abnormalities, said to be specific for this disorder, are seen on electron microscopy. At a later stage, necrosis, inflammation, fibrosis, bile duct proliferation and cirrhosis develop. The rate and mode of progression from steatosis, through fibrosis to cirrhosis, are variable.

The diagnosis of hepatic Wilson's disease is generally based on finding Kayser–Fleischer rings, a serum caeruloplasmin concentration below 13 μmol/l (200 mg/100 ml), urinary copper excretion in excess of 1.5 μmol (100 μg)/24 h, a hepatic copper concentration of 4–47 μmol (25–3000 μg)/g dry weight and compatible histological changes in the liver. Screening of all first-degree relatives should be undertaken; if, in these individuals, serum caeruloplasmin concentrations are less than 13 μmol/l (200 mg/100 ml), and there is evidence of copper deposition in the cornea, or elevated serum aspartate transaminase activity, then liver biopsy should be undertaken. Hepatic copper concentrations in excess of 4 μmol (250 μg)/g dry weight and compatible histological change will confirm the diagnosis.

Wilson's disease is fatal if untreated. Treatment consists of removing excess copper by use of a chelating agent. D-Penicillamine is the drug of choice and life-long therapy is required. Dietary copper intake should be kept as low as possible; patients should be advised to avoid shellfish, dried fruit, nuts, broccoli, chocolate, mushrooms and liver, and to restrict the amount of salt and pepper they use for flavouring. If local water supplies contain copper in excess of 1.6 μmol/l (0.1 mg/100 ml), demineralized water should be used. Domestic water softeners should not be used, as they may substantially increase the copper content of the water.

Copper and zinc compete with one another for absorption from the small intestine;[194] zinc supplementation could, therefore, be used to reduce copper absorption. Negative or neutral copper balance can be achieved in patients with Wilson's disease who received no treatment other than oral zinc, although not consistently.[74,590] However, while zinc therapy may have a place in the management of patients intolerant of chelating agents, it is unnecessary in patients who are able to take D-penicillamine.

As D-penicillamine is a pyridoxine antagonist, patients receiving this drug should be given prophylactic pyridoxine, 25 mg daily.

Genetic haemochromatosis[232,607] (see Chapter 36)

Genetic haemochromatosis is an autosomal, recessively inherited disorder of iron metabolism in which excess iron gradually accumulates in various body tissues. The gene for haemochromatosis susceptibility is located on the short arm of chromosome 6 in proximity to the HLA-A3 locus. The most common haplotypes associated with this disorder are A3,B14, and A3,B7. Although the control of iron absorption is known to be defective in this disease, the underlying metabolic defect has not been defined. After absorption, the excess iron is deposited in the parenchymal cells of the liver, pancreas, heart and pituitary in the form of haemosiderin. The rate of accretion of absorbed iron is both slow and variable; an excess of 20 g of storage iron is needed to produce tissue damage. The precise

cytopathological mechanisms by which excess iron causes cellular injury are unknown. Several possible mechanisms have been proposed, including intracellular disruption of iron-laden lysosomes, increased lipid peroxidation and stimulation of collagen biosynthesis.

Clinically overt disease is much more common in men; the low incidence in women relates to iron loss during menstruation and pregnancy. Men with haemochromatosis usually present between the ages of 40 and 60 years with symptoms and signs of hepatic and cardiac impairment, diabetes and hypogonadism. Over 90% show skin pigmentation which is largely due to melanin deposition. An arthropathy develops in 20–50% of individuals, although its pathogenesis is unknown. Women tend to present some 10 years later than men. Individuals diagnosed by means of pedigree analysis show a much lower incidence of hepatic, cardiac, and endocrine abnormalities but a similar incidence of arthropathy.

Haemosiderin deposits in the liver appear first in the periportal parenchyma; iron is deposited more extensively over time and a characteristic 'holly leaf' pattern of fibrosis emerges. Cirrhosis develops comparatively late in the disease. Hepatocellular carcinoma develops in about 35% of patients; it is the most common cause of death in treated individuals.

Patients with haemochromatosis have increased saturation of their transferrin iron, high serum ferritin concentrations and, most importantly, excess hepatic iron stores. Its genetic origin is determined by the absence of causes of secondary iron overload, the presence of an appropriate HLA haplotype and a family history of iron overload or the subsequent discovery of iron overload in asymptomatic relatives. Screening of all first-degree relatives should be undertaken; in men a transferrin saturation in excess of 62% and in women in excess of 50% is highly suggestive; the diagnosis is confirmed by assessing tissue iron stores. HLA-typing can be used to assess the risk to unaffected relatives; the risk in individuals sharing neither haplotype with the proband is virtually zero, whereas the risk in individuals sharing both haplotypes is very high.

Hepatic iron concentrations are increased in 30% of individuals abusing alcohol, irrespective of the severity of their liver disease.[109] As approximately 25% of patients with genetic haemochromatosis abuse alcohol, difficulty might arise in interpreting hepatic siderosis in alcohol abusers. However, liver iron concentrations in excess of 1 g/100 g dry weight are only observed in patients with the genetic disorder.[109]

Excess iron is effectively removed from the body by repeated venesection, following which the liver and spleen decrease in size, liver function tests return to normal and hepatic fibrosis may decrease. Based on weekly or biweekly removal of one unit of blood (250 mg of iron), it may take 2–3 years to remove the excess tissue iron stores; maintenance phlebotomy will be required, perhaps 3–6 times a year, thereafter, to maintain the transferrin saturation at about 50%. Iron depletion does not protect against the development of hepatocellular carcinoma once cirrhosis is present. While there is no need to restrict dietary iron intake, patients should be warned about the dangers of alcohol excess, not only because alcohol may increase iron absorption[108,112] but because of its own hepatotoxic potential.

Secondary haemochromatosis arises in relation to a variety of dyserythropoietic anaemias;[537,564] it is observed in both the sporadic and familial forms of porphyria cutanea tarda,[37,327] and in idiopathic neonatal iron storage disease.[560]

TOXIC FOODS AND DIETARY CONTAMINANTS[522] —

Liver damage can be caused by the accidental ingestion of toxic agents. The fungus *Amanita phalloides* contains a potent hepatotoxin; liver damage occurs in proportion to the amount ingested. Following small amounts of amanitotoxin the liver shows perivenular necrosis with ceroid pigment in Kupffer cells around necrotic areas; if large amounts are ingested, severe steatosis and extensive or massive necrosis develop. No antitoxin is available; treatment is supportive.

Plants of the genera *Senecio*, *Crotalaria* and *Heliotropium* contaminate grain, and subsequently bread, and are used to make herbal teas. The pyrrolizidine alkaloids they contain have been linked to the development of veno-occlusive disease in which both small and medium-sized hepatic veins become blocked. Veno-occlusive disease has been described in South Africa, Jamaica, Afghanistan, India and America.

Aflatoxins are derived from species of *Aspergillus* and are known to contaminate stored foods and groundnuts. A significant correlation has been found between aflatoxin ingestion and the incidence of hepatocellular carcinoma in several areas of Africa and Asia.[618,646] Danish workers exposed to aflatoxin via the respiratory route while handling contaminated crops imported for animal feed production show an increased risk of developing hepatocellular carcinoma, the magnitude of which increases over time exposed.[459] In areas of the world such as Taiwan and China, where hepatitis B virus infection is the major aetiological agent for hepatocellular carcinoma, there is no association between aflatoxin ingestion and development of this tumour.[95]

NUTRITIONAL MANAGEMENT OF PATIENTS WITH HEPATOBILIARY DISEASE

Nutritional deficiencies may arise in individuals with hepatobiliary disease and may adversely affect hepatic function, perpetuate liver injury and ultimately affect prognosis.[92,195,241,395] Children with chronic liver disease may be particularly compromised because they develop resistance to the growth-promoting, diabetogenic and lipolytic effects of growth hormone.[80] In consequence, they show growth failure, short stature and, if the onset of the disease is within the first few years of life, intellectual impairment.[587]

These individuals, therefore, require dietary advice and nutritional support. Specific dietary modifications may be necessary in patients with chronic parenchymal liver disease or chronic cholestasis, and specific dietary restrictions may be necessary in individuals with complications of chronic liver disease, such as fluid retention and hepatic encephalopathy. Vigorous nutritional support may be necessary for patients with fulminant hepatic failure, severe alcoholic hepatitis and end-stage liver disease, particularly if they are candidates for liver transplantation.[158,233,304,558] Aggressive nutritional support, beginning at the time of diagnosis, might help to offset the delays in growth and intellectual development in children with chronic liver disease;[587] selective use of somatomedin might help promote growth in these children.[301]

In order to provide a rational basis for dietary advice and therapy, nutritional status should be assessed initially and then again at suitable intervals. Careful and continuous attention to diet is mandatory, as in many instances nutrient deficiencies arise as the result of inadequate or ill-conceived dietary advice.

RECOGNITION OF NUTRIENT DEFICIENCIES[557] ____

Various techniques have been used to assess nutritional status, although no one method provides all the necessary information. In the past too much reliance has been placed on the use of weight alone or on the weight-to-height ratio as a routine measure of metabolic status. Weight is only a useful indicator of nutritional status when lean body mass has decreased; in the presence of fluid retention its measurement is misleading. Equally, deficiencies of individual nutrients, for example vitamins or trace metals, while important in themselves, say little about the patients' general state of nutrition and health.

In practice, nutritional status is best assessed by combining the results of the nutritional history, physical examination, anthropometric measurements and selected laboratory analyses (Table 6.2). Although the methods of assessment are not unduly time-consuming or complicated to perform, the extent to which they can be employed will depend on the staff and facilities available. Thus, while it should be possible to undertake a full assessment in hospitalized patients, it may not be possible to do so in individuals attending as outpatients, unless they are reliable enough to collect urine samples and are willing to document their dietary intake accurately.

The nutritional history serves to identify individuals with liver disease 'at risk' of developing malnutrition. It also provides information on the possible role of dietary inadequacies in the genesis of malnutrition. The nutritional history is a composite of information derived from the clinical history, from the dietary history and from measurements of changes in body weight, food intake and excretory losses.

The dietary history provides information on food intake,

Table 6.2 Overview of the nutritional assessment

Variable	Content	How recorded	Staff
History	Clinical data, gross nutritional state, brief clinical history, denture wearer	Pre-printed form	Any—with minimal training
	Food intake, food consumption patterns	Interview plus computer analysis	Dietitian
	Daily weight, food intake, food received extra, altered behaviour, excreta	Pre-printed form	Nurse
Physical examination	Physical examination from a nutritional perspective	Clinical history	Clinician
Anthropometry	Weight/height, body mass index, skinfold thicknesses, mid-arm circumference, elbow breadth, grip strength	Pre-printed form	Any—with some training
Laboratory	Various—albumin, electrolytes, vitamins, minerals, others	Pre-printed form	Technical staff

eating habits and meal consumption patterns and is best undertaken by use of a modified research dietary interview technique,[84] concentrating on the average nutrient intake in the week prior to review. Careful prompting, together with the use of food models, helps overcome inaccuracies.[382] An estimate of the number of grams of individual foods consumed daily can be made and the approximate intakes of total calories, fat, carbohydrate, protein, vitamins and minerals assessed by reference to food composition tables.[468] This process is greatly facilitated by use of a computer program. The calculated dietary intakes can then be compared with recommended daily intakes.[152, 206] These data are of limited usefulness because very little information is available on the requirements for nutrients in individuals with liver disease or in individuals who take up to 50% of their total calories as alcohol. However, they provide an invaluable baseline for therapy.

Body weight, food intakes and excretory losses are measured daily by nursing staff. Food intake is assessed by inspecting food trays and estimating the percentage of food actually eaten. Care should be taken to document food brought in from outside as, in many instances, this might equal or exceed in amount the intake of hospital food. Fluid balance and stool charts enable excretory losses to be documented.

A detailed clinical examination provides an impression of overall nutritional status and evidence of malnutrition such as muscle wasting, peripheral neuropathy, glossitis, and hair, skin and nail changes (Table 6.3).[85]

An anthropometric assessment will provide information on the three major tissues available to meet energy requirements, namely skeletal muscle, fat and visceral protein (Table 6.4). Anthropometric indices are simply and easily obtained and their values, when compared against standards compiled for healthy males and females,[50,72,171,287,288,402,624] provide estimates of fat stores and lean body mass (Table 6.5). The creatinine/height index is not thought to be a reliable measure of lean body mass in individuals with liver disease.

Great care must be taken when using anthropometric indices to assess nutritional status in children with chronic liver disease. Assessments using weight/height percentiles are misleading as the weight of the enlarged liver and spleen may contribute substantially to total body weight, thereby producing erroneously high values and hence underestimates of the degree of malnutrition. As chronic malnutrition may lead to stunting, that is a deficit in height for age, the normative data used for comparison should be based on height age rather than on chronological age. Measurements of triceps skinfold thickness and mean arm circumference afford better estimates of nutritional status in children and should be used in preference to other indices.[574]

Measurement of serum albumin and transferrin concentrations provides an estimate of visceral protein status, but these findings should be interpreted with caution in patients with liver disease, particularly if the liver disease is alcohol-related. Plasma protein synthesis may be impaired in patients with liver disease per se independently of their nutritional status.[359,397] In addition, alcohol directly inhibits protein synthesis;[518,519] thus, in individuals actively abusing alcohol, circulating albumin and transferrin concentrations may be low but will return towards reference values with abstinence from alcohol.[413]

Total lymphocyte counts and delayed skin hypersensitivity tests are usually performed as part of the nutritional assessment, as an indirect measure of nutritional status. These data should also be interpreted with caution in individuals with liver disease, particularly if alcohol-related. Skin anergy is commonly observed in patients with cirrhosis;[43,413] total lymphocyte counts are often significantly reduced in individuals who are actively abusing alcohol but return promptly towards reference values within a few days of alcohol withdrawal (Figure 6.10).[413]

Deficiencies of specific nutrients, such as vitamins and

Table 6.3 Clinical findings and the nutritional assessment

Clinical finding	Consider deficiency	Comment
Hair, nails		
Hair easily pluckable, sparse, straight, depigmented, dull;	Protein	
Spoon-shaped brittle, ridged or lined nails	Iron	
Skin		
Petechiae, purpura, corkscrew hairs	Ascorbic acid	
Pigmentation, desquamation	Niacin (pellagra)	Sun-exposed areas: symmetrical
Follicular hyperkeratosis	Vitamin A	Keratin plugs in follicles
Dry, scaling	Non-specific	
Subcutaneous fat loss	Calories	Minimal fat reserves if triceps skinfold 6 mm ($\frac{1}{4}$ inch) between fingers
Eyes		
Dull, dry conjunctiva	Vitamin A	
Blepharitis	B-complex	
Ophthalmoplegia	Thiamine	Wernicke's syndrome: prompt treatment necessary
Perioral		
Angular fissures, scars	B-complex, iron, protein	Also seen with ill-fitting dentures
Cheilosis	Pyridoxine, niacin, riboflavin, protein	
Oral		
Ageusia, disgeusia	Zinc	Also associated with altered sense of smell
Glossitis, depapillation	Niacin, riboflavin, B_{12}, folate, iron	
Swollen, bleeding gums	Ascorbic acid	
Glands		
Parotid enlargement	Protein	
Heart		
Enlargement, tachycardia, high-output failure	Thiamine	'Wet beriberi'
Musculoskeletal		
Muscle wasting evident in temporal area, dorsum of hand between thumb and index finger, calf muscles	Protein–calorie	
Pain in calves, weak thighs	Thiamine	
Oedema	Protein, thiamine	
Bone pain, osteomalacia	Vitamin D, calcium, protein	Poor calcium intake, no sun, steatorrhoea
Neurological		
Ophthalmoplegia, footdrop	Thiamine	Wernicke's encephalopathy
Confabulation, disorientation	Thiamine	Korsakoff's psychosis
Decreased position and vibration sense, ataxia	B_{12}	Subacute combined cord degeneration
Weakness, paresthesia in legs	Thiamine, pyridoxine, pantothenic acid, B_{12}	Nutritional polyneuropathy
Other		
Delayed healing and tissue repair	Vitamin C, zinc, protein, calories	

minerals, may be detected using a variety of laboratory procedures (Table 6.6). Again, care must be taken in the interpretation of test results. Thus, many individuals who are abusing alcohol will show subnormal circulating concentrations of vitamins and minerals on admission to hospital, but values may return towards reference values following short-term abstinence from alcohol, without specific supplementation.[77,413]

The results from these various examinations must then be combined to provide an overall assessment of nutritional status. At present these relatively simple techniques for nutritional assessment have not been validated in patients with liver disease against more objective data which reflect metabolism more closely. In recent years a number of techniques have been devised to monitor whole-body metabolism, muscle protein turnover

Table 6.4 Anthropometric variables used to assess lean body mass, body fat and visceral protein stores

Measure	Body compartments assessed	Method of assessment
Weight (kg)/height (cm), (wt/ht)	Overall nutritional status	Direct measurements
Body mass index, (wt/ht^2)	Overall nutritional status	Derived measurement
Mid-arm circumference (cm), (MAC)	Overall nutritional status	Direct measurement
Triceps skinfold thickness (mm), (TSF)	Fat stores	Direct measurement
Mid-arm muscle circumference (cm), (MAMC)	Lean body mass	Derived measurement MAMC = MAC−(π × TSF)
Creatinine (mg/24 h)/height (cm) (cr/ht)	Lean body mass	24 h urinary creatinine excretion (mg) estimated on 2 consecutive days
Serum albumin (g/l)	Visceral protein	Direct measurement
Serum transferrin (g/l)	Visceral protein	Direct measurement

Table 6.5 Measures used for anthropometric assessment

Procedure	Apparatus	Method
Height determination	Vertical wall measure	Foam slippers, feet together, stand erect, head-Frankfort horizontal plane
Weight	Beam or lever balance	Light clothing, consistent, standard time
Weight if bed-ridden	Bed balance scale	Light clothing, consistent, standard time
Skinfolds	Harpenden or Lange callipers	Triceps—halfway between olecranon and acromion on belly of muscle
		Biceps—same position but on belly of biceps
		Subscapular—1 cm below inferior angle scapula
		Suprailiac—1 cm above iliac crest: side of body specified.
Mid-arm circumference (MAC)	Tape measure	Same position as for triceps skinfold (TSF).
Mid-arm muscle circumference (MAMC)		MAMC (cm) = MAC (cm) − [π × TSF (mm)]
Hand grip strength	Standard sphygmomanometer cuff manometer	Inflate sphygmomanometer to 30 mmHg, subject squeezes bag; pressure recorded on manometer

and fuel utilization, which should provide more objective data. Doubly-labelled water, $D_2{}^{18}O$, has been used to determine energy expenditure in free-living subjects[352, 543] and the results utilizing this technique compare very favourably with those obtained using confining procedures which restrict daily activity. A number of stable isotopic methods are now available for studying muscle protein turnover which provide information previously unavailable.[178,193,651,654] Total body conductivity and biological impedance can be used to determine total body water, sodium and fat. Dual-photon absorptiometry can be used to measure the density of bone and, by extrapolation, total body bone mineral. These techniques are all minimally invasive, and, when fully validated, may provide information on body composition that is now only available using expensive and technically demanding procedures such as total body neutron activation, whole-body counting and radioisotopic dilution.[124] None of these techniques has been used to study the effects of liver disease or of obligatory ethanol metabolism on nutrient handling.

INCIDENCE OF MALNUTRITION

Although it is now well recognized that individuals with liver disease are at risk for developing malnutrition, surprisingly little information is available on the prevalence of nutritional deficiencies in these populations, and the data available are often of questionable quality.

A number of difficulties arise in trying to evaluate the data on the prevalence of malnutrition in patients with alcohol-related liver disease. It is widely assumed that the majority of individuals who abuse alcohol are malnourished, but the studies on which these observations are based generally tend to focus on unrepresentative populations of derelict, often physically ill individuals,[458,467] or else deduce information on overall nutritional status from single nutrient deficiencies.[208, 418] There is evidence to suggest that frank deficiency disease is uncommon in individuals with alcohol-related liver injury[35,94,197] and that, when present, malnutrition

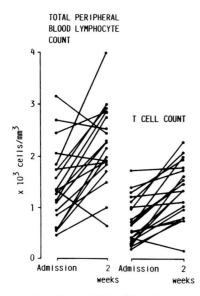

TOTAL PERIPHERAL
BLOOD LYMPHOCYTE
COUNT

T CELL COUNT

$\times 10^3$ cells/mm^3

Admission 2 weeks Admission 2 weeks

Figure 6.10 Total peripheral blood lymphocyte and T lymphocyte counts in individuals chronically abusing alcohol on admission to hospital and after 2 weeks hospitalization. (Mills *et al.*[413])

is only mild to moderate in degree.[81,413,427,448] However, these findings have been largely ignored.

Surprisingly little information is available on the overall nutritional status of individuals with alcoholic liver disease. Very few studies have focused specifically on these patients,[81,93,393,413,427,454,562] and those that are available are often incomplete; some additional data are available from nutritional surveys undertaken in hospitalized patients, a proportion of whom were chronically abusing alcohol.[49,59]

Data are available from some of these studies on the proportion of patients showing anthropometric abnormalities, and these can usefully be compared (Table 6.7). The results of these studies show that, in general, individuals with alcoholic liver disease maintain body weight, although they tend to lose weight during periods of active drinking.[649] In the majority of studies, 30% or more of the individuals surveyed showed a reduction of lean body mass, whilst 50% or more showed reduced fat stores. However, the findings of two studies stand in contrast to the others.[81,413] Mills and coworkers[413] assessed 30 men chronically abusing alcohol, 19 of whom (63%) had alcoholic hepatitis or cirrhosis on liver biopsy. The mean

Table 6.6 Method available for measurement of various nutrients with indications of deficient, low and acceptable values

Nutrient	Test employed (units)	Deficient levels	Low levels	Acceptable levels
Protein	Serum albumin (g/l)	<30	30–35	>35
	Serum transferrin (g/l)			1.2–2.0
Vitamin A	Plasma retinol (μmol/l)	<0.5	0.5–0.7	0.7–1.7
Vitamin D	Serum 25-hydroxycholecalciferol (μmol/l)	<3.5	3.5–9.0	9–44
Vitamin E	Plasma vitamin E (mg/1α-tocopherol)	<3.0	3–5	5–10
Vitamin K	Plasma prothrombin time (s)	>3 s prolonged corrected by IM vitamin K_1		Comparable to control
Thiamine	Erythrocyte transketolase activity (U/l)	<34	34–90	
	Stimulation with TPP^a (%)	>40		3.5–40
Riboflavin	EGR activity coefficient^b	>1.4	1.2–1.4	1.2
Nicotinamide	*N*-Methylnicotinamide excretion (mg/g creatinine)	<0.5	0.5–1.6	1.6
Pyridoxine	EGPT activity coefficient^c	>1.25		<1.25
	EGOT activity coefficient^c	<2.00		>2.00
	Plasma pyridoxal-5′-phosphate (μg/l)			10.0–20.0
Folic acid	Serum folic acid (μg/l)	<3.0		3.0–20.0
	Erythrocyte folic acid (μg/l)	<160		160–640
Vitamin B_{12}	Serum vitamin B_{12} (ng/l)	<120	120–160	160–925
Vitamin C	Leucocyte ascorbic acid (μg/10^9 WBC)	<20		23–51
Iron	Serum iron (μmol/l)	<10		11–36
	Plasma total iron binding capacity (μmol/l)	>90		53–85
Calcium	Serum calcium (mmol/l)	<1.9	1.9–2.1	2.1–2.6
	24-h urinary calcium (mmol/l)	<1.5	1.5–2.5	2.5–7.5
Phosphorus	Serum inorganic phosphate (mmol/l)	<0.5	0.5–0.7	0.7–1.25
	24-h urinary phosphate (mmol)	<10	10–15	15–20
Zinc	Plasma zinc (μmol/l)	<8	8–12	12–17
	24-h urinary zinc (μmol)	<3	3–6	6–9
Magnesium	Serum magnesium (mmol/l)	<0.5	0.5–0.7	0.7–1.0
	24-h urinary magnesium (mmol)	<1.5	1.5–3.0	3.0–5.0

^{a} TPP, thiamine pyrophosphate.
^{b} EGR activity coefficient, erythrocyte glutathione reductase activity with and without added coenzyme flavine adenine dinucleotide.
^{c} EGPT (EGOT) activity coefficient, erythrocyte aminotransferase activity with and without added coenzyme pyridoxal phosphate.

Table 6.7 Incidence of anthropometric abnormalities in individuals abusing alcohol

First author, date, and reference number	Patients (n)	Liver disease	Weight/height	Ideal body weight	Triceps skinfold thickness	MAC[a]	MAMC[b]	Creatinine/height	Serum albumin
					(% abnormal)				
Bollet 1973[59]	29	?	–	24	–	–	–	–	56
Bistrian 1976[51]	52	?	31	–	75	–	50	–	–
O'Keefe 1980[454]	32	?	6	–	55	–	–	–	66
Morgan 1981[427]	55	33% cirrhosis	7	–	51	33	29	40	18
Camilo 1982[93]	103	70% cirrhosis	41	–	64	–	55	–	59
Mill 1983[413]	30	63% cirrhosis	–	3	10	–	13	–	59
Mendenhall 1984[393]	284	100% hepatitis ± cirrhosis	63	–	86	–	52	85	71

[a] MAC, mean arm circumference.
[b] MAMC, mean arm muscle circumference.

body weight on admission was 108% of standard with 7 patients (23%) weighing more than 120% of standard. No indications were given as to whether these patients were retaining fluid or whether allowance was made for this in the calculations. The mean triceps skinfold thickness was 107% of standard, with only very few patients showing depletion of fat stores. The mean mid-arm circumference was reduced to 90% of standard, although very few patients showed more than moderate depletion of lean body mass. Bunout and coworkers[81] assessed nutritional and anthropometric variables in 84 chronic alcohol abusers admitted to a treatment facility, 12 (14%) of whom had acute alcoholic hepatitis and/or cirrhosis. Mean anthropometric variables were within 80–100% of commonly used standards. Of particular interest was the fact that the patients with significant liver disease were, if anything, overnourished, with significantly increased anthropometric indices.

It is difficult to reconcile the findings of these two studies with those of Morgan[427] and Mendenhall and coworkers.[393] The patients were of similar age, probably of similar socioeconomic class and consumed similar amounts of alcohol. Nevertheless, the discrepancies in these findings serve as a reminder of the heterogeneous nature of populations of alcohol abusers and of the importance of clearly delineating the demography of such patient groups. Overall, the incidence of anthropometric abnormalities in individuals abusing alcohol, as represented by the studies detailed, is no greater than in general medical and surgical patients, 44–50% of whom show anthropometric abnormalities.[48,49,51]

In a number of studies, sufficient details of the patient populations were given to enable the relationship between nutritional status, judged clinically and anthropometrically, and the severity of alcohol-related liver injury to be explored. In patients with well-compensated liver disease,[413,427] the incidence of malnutrition was independent of the presence of cirrhosis (Figure 6.11). However, in patients with decompensated liver disease,[93,393] the incidence of malnutrition increased with increasing severity of liver injury (Figure 6.12).

Much more information is available on the incidence of vitamin and mineral deficiencies in alcohol abusers, but problems also arise in the interpretation of these data. Thus, the patient populations studied often vary considerably both in terms of their social circumstances and in terms of their physical status. In the majority of studies, very little information is provided on recent drinking behaviour and no attempt has been made to standardize the timing of sample collection. The methods available for assessing vitamin status are often indirect and several different assay procedures have been used. Values designated 'low' or 'deficient' are often arbitrarily defined and the 'cut-off' points tend to vary from series to series. Finally, while it is generally believed that subnormal vitamin and mineral values may be deleterious, there is rarely evidence to support this contention. Indeed, the incidence of frank deficiency disease in individuals chronically abusing alcohol is generally low,[197,340] although the incidence of low circulating concentrations of vitamins and minerals is generally high.

Very little information is available on the nutritional status of unselected populations of patients with non-alcoholic liver injury.[359,427,574] Rather more information

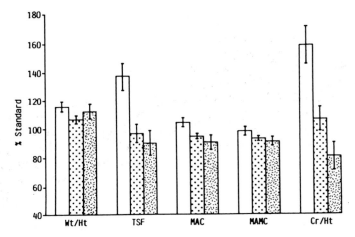

Figure 6.11 Mean (± SEM) anthropometric measures, expressed as percentage of standard, in alcohol abusers in relation to the severity of their liver disease. Open, healthy volunteers (*n* = 20); dotted, alcohol abuser with minimal liver damage (*n* = 37); stippled, alcohol abuser with cirrhosis (*n* = 18). Wt/Ht, weight (kg)/height (cm); TSF, triceps skinfold thickness (mm); MAC, mean arm circumference (cm); MAMC, mean arm muscle circumference (cm); Cr/Ht, creatinine (mg/24 h)/height (cm). > 90% standard, not depleted; 80–90% standard, mildly depleted; 60–80% standard, moderately depleted; < 60% standard, severely depleted. (Morgan[427])

is available on the nutritional status of candidates for hepatic transplantation, the majority of whom have non-alcoholic liver disease.[158] However, these patients, by their very nature, tend to be malnourished and so cannot be considered representative.

Loguercio and colleagues[359] undertook a carefully controlled assessment of 108 patients with liver disease, 69 (64%) of whom had non-alcoholic cirrhosis. They found a high incidence of malnutrition, overall, with fat stores more severely compromised than lean body mass. There was no relationship between the prevalence or degree of malnutrition and the aetiology of the liver injury, but a clear relationship with the severity of the liver injury. Thus, the triceps skinfold thickness was significantly reduced in 12 (19%) of the 63 patients with compensated

cirrhosis but in 22 (49%) of the 45 with decompensated disease.

Morgan[427] surveyed 92 patients with liver disease, of whom 37 (40%) had either primary biliary cirrhosis or autoimmune chronic active hepatitis. The prevalence of malnutrition, overall, was relatively high. However, the patients with primary biliary cirrhosis showed depletion of both lean body mass and fat stores, whereas lean body mass was generally preserved in the other patient groups.

The relationship between the aetiology of liver injury and the severity of malnutrition has been observed by other workers. DiCecco and coworkers,[158] for example, surveyed 74 liver transplant candidates and commented on the extreme muscle and fat wasting observed in patients with primary biliary cirrhosis; in their series the patients with acute hepatitis were the most severely malnourished. Sokol and Stall[574] undertook anthropometric evaluations in 56 children, aged 1 month to 10 years, with stable chronic liver disease not requiring hepatic transplantation. Wasting and stunting were frequently observed, but there was definite variation in the prevalence of malnutrition, within subgroups of patients, in relation to the aetiology of their liver injury; patients with arteriohepatic dysplasia were the most compromised.

Very limited information is available on the prevalence of vitamin and mineral deficiencies in patients with non-alcoholic liver disease. It is generally believed, and there is some evidence to support the contention, that patients with acute liver disease show deficiencies of the B vitamins[381] and that patients with chronic cholestasis are deficient in fat-soluble vitamins.[380] Many of the comments made earlier in relation to the interpretation of the data on specific deficiencies in patients with alcoholic liver disease, pertain here also.

NUTRITIONAL THERAPY IN LIVER DISEASE: GENERAL CONSIDERATIONS[54,371] _____

Patients with liver disease are often given dietary advice that is of doubtful value and which may even prove harmful. High-calorie, low-protein diets are frequently prescribed for patients with uncomplicated hepatitis, but

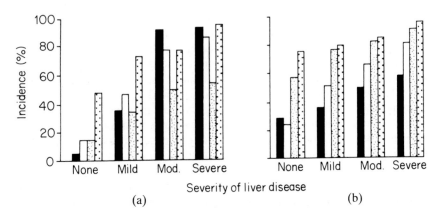

(a)   (b)

Figure 6.12 Percentage of chronic alcohol abusers showing abnormalities of measured variables in relation to the presence and severity of their liver disease. (a) Kwashiorkor-like: solid, plasma albumin; open, plasma transferrin; stippled, lymphocyte count; dotted, skin anergy. (b) Marasmus: solid, mean arm muscle circumference; open, % ideal body weight; stippled, creatinine/height index; dotted, triceps skin fold thickness. (Mendenhall *et al.*[393])

these diets may cause serious undernutrition with loss of lean body mass. Jaundiced patients are often advised to take low-fat or fat-free diets even if they are fat tolerant; such diets are unpalatable, they often provide inadequate calories and, if continued for long periods, may lead to deficiencies of essential fatty acids and fat-soluble vitamins. Patients with liver disease are generally advised to abstain from alcohol, irrespective of the aetiology of their liver damage; while this advice is essential for patients with alcohol-related liver injury, there is no contraindication to modest alcohol intake by others.

In general, patients with liver disease should take a diet which provides adequate intakes of calories, protein, vitamins and minerals. However, it is likely that a diet which is adequate for a healthy individual may not be adequate in the presence of liver disease. For these reasons, dietary intake must be carefully monitored and adjusted in order to achieve positive nitrogen balance and correction of any nutritional deficiencies.

Many patients with liver disease are anorexic or suffer from nausea or abdominal distension. Maintenance of an adequate oral intake may prove difficult under these circumstances. Patients should be encouraged to eat and should be offered small amounts of attractively prepared food, at frequent intervals, since large meals often provoke nausea. If a reasonable dietary intake can be achieved and body weight is maintained, nothing further is required.

It is often difficult to sustain an adequate oral intake in patients with persistent anorexia and nausea or to increase oral intake beyond a certain limit in malnourished patients. Diets can be homogenized and taken in liquid form, in small quantities and at frequent intervals. It is preferable, where possible, to continue oral food intake. Where there are marginal nutrient deficits, proprietary formulated feeds can be used for supplementation. Where nutrient deficits are greater, feeds can be specially prepared using a number of proprietary constituents; carbohydrate is supplied as a glucose polymer (Maxijul: Scientific Hospital Supplies (SHS)), fat as double cream, long-chain triglycerides (Calogen: SHS), or medium-chain triglycerides (Portagen: Mead Johnson), and nitrogen as whey protein isolate (Maxipro: SHS). Approximately 0.8 MJ (200 kcal) should be provided for each gram of nitrogen, 40% from fat and 60% from carbohydrate. Vitamins of the B group should be added (Abidec: Parke-Davis & Co.) and attempts made to enhance the taste of the supplement by use of fruit juice or milk-shake flavourings.

If oral feeding proves impossible, due to anorexia, food intolerance or vomiting, a fine-bore, nasogastric tube can be passed and liquid feed given slowly, preferably at night. If abdominal distension and vomiting continue, the nasogastric tube can be endoscopically repositioned in the jejunum. Patients should still be encouraged to eat whatever food they can. Difficulties may still be experienced with enteral feeding and the volume of feed needed to supply daily requirements may be excessive for those who are fluid intolerant. In these circumstances, par-

enteral feeding may be necessary. If some oral or enteral intake is possible, then an estimate should be made of that intake and the deficit given parenterally. Difficulty might arise in balancing the diet if there is significant malabsorption, in which case the amount of nutrition given parenterally will have to be determined by trial and error.

Dietary requirements for certain nutrients differ when given parenterally. More than 90% of ingested carbohydrate, fat, sodium, potassium and chloride are absorbed, so that recommended daily allowances apply whether nutrients are given enterally or parenterally. Other nutrients, in particular the essential minerals, are much less well absorbed, so that parenteral requirements are substantially less than enteral requirements. It is also likely that enteral and parenteral requirements for certain amino acids will differ. The timing of parenteral supply is also important. For example, if protein synthesis is to be supported, all the essential amino acids must be supplied simultaneously; if even one essential amino acid is administered at a different time from the other essential and non-essential amino acids, protein assimilation is curtailed. Similarly, if amino acids, lipids, glucose and minerals are infused at differing times, several nutrients may not be assimilated. For these reasons the parenteral requirements of many essential nutrients remain uncertain.

Several additional problems arise when providing parenteral nutrition for individuals with liver disease. They may be fluid intolerant, so that the volume infused may need to be restricted to 1 litre or less. It may also be necessary to modify the amino acid solutions used. Cysteine and tyrosine are synthesized in the liver from methionine and phenylalanine. These amino acids are virtually insoluble in water and their concentrations in commercially available amino acid mixtures are extremely low. In patients with cirrhosis, synthesis of cysteine and tyrosine may be impaired and deficiencies may arise during parenteral feeding.[411,525] The sulphur-containing amino acid cysteine is non-essential, since under normal circumstances it is readily synthesized from methionine. Cirrhotic patients may acquire a defect in the hepatic transulphation pathway so that if they are given methionine-containing but cysteine-free amino acid preparations, hypocysteinaemia may develop.[117] Under these circumstances cysteine becomes an essential nutrient and without it protein synthesis may become seriously impeded. Similar remarks can be made about choline[116] and carnitine.[554] In addition, many formulations used in patients with liver disease are nutritionally incomplete or else contain quantities of amino acids, such as glycine, proline, lysine, threonine and arginine, which may not be adequately cleared when ureagenic capacity is limited.[622]

For many years the presence of liver disease was considered a contraindication to the use of intravenous lipid solutions, even by the manufacturers.[240] Very little explanation was available other than that use of these preparations might lead to the accumulation of 'fat pigment' in liver cells, and early experiences with cotton-seed emulsions called for caution in their use in patients with liver disease. Even so, several early reports showed that lipid solutions could be used safely in patients with liver disease,[310,547] and this has been confirmed in more recent studies.[441,442,515] Thus, if patients with liver disease require parenteral nutrition there is no contraindication to the careful use of intravenous glucose, amino acids and Intralipid.

Several drugs prescribed for patients with liver disease cause malabsorption, impaired utilization or urinary hyperexcretion of nutrients. Use of neomycin and cholestyramine may lead to malabsorption of several nutrients, including fat, vitamins and minerals. D-Penicillamine impairs the utilization of pyridoxine and increases the urinary excretion of zinc, pyridoxine and copper. Diuretics increase the urinary excretion of several minerals. Careful note must therefore be made of all drugs prescribed.

Subclinical vitamin deficiencies may occur in patients with liver disease, more especially in individuals abusing alcohol. These are difficult to identify and their measurement is often complex and expensive. Multivitamin therapy is cheap and is assumed harmless if recommended doses are not exceeded. Thus, the common practice of giving vitamin supplements to these patients has a reasonable therapeutic basis. If deficiencies are clinically overt, then more specific therapy is required.

NUTRITIONAL MANAGEMENT OF INDIVIDUAL DISORDERS

Viral or drug-related hepatitis

Patients with few symptoms should be encouraged to eat a normal diet. Even patients with anorexia, nausea and vomiting can usually take some food by mouth and enough fluid to prevent dehydration. Patients tend to prefer small meals and these should be given frequently throughout the day. During the acute illness, requirements for protein and energy are similar to those of any moderately hypercatabolic illness; daily protein requirements increase to 120 g and energy requirements to 8–12 MJ (2000–3000 kcal). Although early studies suggested that patients with hepatitis might benefit from taking high-protein, high-calorie feeds,[106,269] such diets should not be forced. Fat should not be restricted; low-fat diets are bulky, generally unappetizing and may aggravate anorexia. If anorexia and vomiting persist it may be necessary to feed the patient enterally or even parenterally. As patients with severe hepatitis may not be able to excrete a water load, very careful monitoring of fluid balance is necessary.

Patients with hepatitis are usually advised to abstain from alcohol during the acute illness and for 6 months afterwards. There is no good evidence that alcohol in moderation has a deleterious effect on the liver either during the acute illness or during convalescence. Nevertheless, excessive amounts of alcohol are hepatotoxic in their

own right and relapse of hepatitis following alcohol abuse has been reported.[140]

Fulminant hepatic failure

Patients with fulminant hepatic failure may develop profound, recurrent hypoglycaemia because their glycogen stores are reduced and glycogenolysis and gluconeogenesis are impaired. They may also become rapidly malnourished because of marked loss of nitrogen which occurs secondary to the endocrine response to massive hepatic necrosis. Additional nitrogen losses occur when artificial liver-support systems, such as charcoal haemoperfusion or polyacrylonitrile membrane haemodialysis, are employed.[114]

These patients, therefore, need a constant supply of glucose, which should be given intravenously as 10–20% glucose solutions in a volume sufficient to provide 150–200 g over 24 hours. They should, in addition, receive nutritional support designed to suppress protein catabolism, increase protein anabolism and so optimize conditions for hepatic regeneration. O'Keefe and colleagues[453] showed that amino acid/glucose solutions, infused intravenously to provide 3 g of amino acid and 5 g of glucose hourly, were well-tolerated by patients with fulminant hepatic failure and that their use was associated with decreased protein catabolism, improved plasma amino acid profiles and increased circulating insulin concentrations.

No formal trials of the use of parenteral nutrition in patients with fulminant hepatic failure have been published to date.

Acute alcoholic hepatitis[5]

Patients with acute alcoholic hepatitis usually have a long history of alcohol abuse and may have neglected their diet in the weeks or months before admission. Quite marked deterioration may occur in their clinical state, once hospitalized, and this is generally attributed to loss of the calorie intake from alcohol.[248,256,357,384,529] Nutritional support should, therefore, be provided in the form of a high-protein, high-calorie diet from the time of admission. Patients should be encouraged to eat, and their intake should be recorded. Supplemental drinks should be provided as soon as it becomes obvious that their dietary intake is insufficient. Enteral and parenteral feeding may be necessary. High-dose vitamins should be given parenterally.

Very little information is available regarding the precise nutritional requirements of patients with alcoholic hepatitis. In one of the few studies available,[634] seven patients with acute alcoholic hepatitis were investigated under metabolic ward conditions. Nitrogen balance became positive in three of five patients receiving 1 g protein/kg body weight daily and remained positive in the other two. The remaining two patients received 0.5 g protein/kg daily and attained positive nitrogen balance within 2 weeks.

The improvements in nitrogen balance resulted from a fall in urinary nitrogen excretion, probably because of a fall in the excretion of urinary urea. Thus, in patients with alcoholic hepatitis, daily protein intakes of 30 g are associated with negative nitrogen balance, while daily intakes in the region of 70–100 g ensure positive nitrogen balance.

Improving the nutritional status of patients with alcoholic hepatitis should, in theory, aid recovery. Although a number of controlled trials of hyperalimentation have been undertaken in these patients, it is still unclear whether nutritional therapy influences the course of the disease. The studies that have been undertaken to date can be criticized for several reasons; first, the number of patients treated is generally small; second, the dietary intake in control patients is almost invariably suboptimal; third, the monitoring procedures are generally inadequate; and fourth, the only outcome variable consistently recorded is death.

The first controlled trial of nutritional supplementation in patients with alcoholic hepatitis was reported in 1980 by Nasrallah and Galambos.[445] In this trial, 35 patients with alcoholic hepatitis were studied, one-third of whom had cirrhosis. All patients were given a diet providing 100 g of protein and 3000 kcal daily. The 17 patients allocated to the treatment group received, in addition, approximately 40 g daily of an intravenous balanced amino acid mixture for 3 days followed by 80 g daily for an additional 25 days. No placebo infusion was used. Dietary intakes were comparable in both control and treatment groups, but represented only a proportion of the food they received. During the trial period significant improvements were seen in plasma bilirubin and albumin concentrations in the supplemented patients. Four (22%) of the 18 control patients died, whilst all 17 of the treated patients survived; this difference is statistically significant. These results must be interpreted with caution because the mortality from alcoholic hepatitis tends to be higher in women,[532] and in this study there were proportionally more women in the control group. Anthropometric variables and nitrogen balance were not assessed.

Diehl and coworkers[161] studied 15 patients with biopsy-proven alcoholic hepatitis who showed evidence of moderate malnutrition. All patients were allowed ad libitum consumption of a hospital diet. Five patients received an amino acid–glucose infusion for a month, whilst the remaining 10 patients received intravenous glucose alone, for the same period. Total daily calorie intakes were similar in both groups, but the mean daily protein intake in the amino acid–glucose group was 138.6 g compared with an intake of 97.5 g in the group receiving glucose alone. Clinical and biochemical abnormalities improved significantly in both groups. A greater improvement was seen in nitrogen balance in the patients receiving amino acids, but no changes were observed in the various anthropometric measures. Fatty infiltration resolved more quickly in the treated patients, but otherwise treatment had little effect on hepatic histology. These authors found

significant correlations between certain clinical, laboratory and histological abnormalities and the quantity of alcohol consumed before admission, and appear to suggest that the outcome of the trial was more influenced by the severity of the initial illness than by the use of parenteral amino acid supplements.

In a more detailed study, Calvey and coworkers[92] gave a daily diet containing 40–80 g of protein, 1800–2400 kcal and 22 mmol of sodium to 64 patients with severe alcoholic hepatitis, with or without cirrhosis. Twenty-one patients received an additional 65 g of protein and 2000 non-protein kcal daily, whilst a further 21 patients received 45 g of protein, 20 g of branched-chain amino acids and 2000 non-protein kcal daily. The supplements were given orally, enterally, or, if necessary, parenterally, for approximately 3 weeks. Twenty-three patients (36%) died during the trial but there was no significant difference in mortality between the three treatment groups. Nitrogen balance studies were undertaken in 49 patients with adequate renal function and it is of interest that the mortality rate was only 3.3% in patients who achieved positive nitrogen balance but 57.9% in the patients who did not. There was no evidence of benefit, in this respect, from supplementation, nor was there evidence of benefit in the subgroup receiving parenteral supplementation. These findings confirm those of Fiaccadori and coworkers,[195] who observed a marked decrease in survival in cirrhotic patients who were unable to maintain nitrogen equilibrium.

Achord[4] undertook a prospective, randomized trial of parenteral amino acid–glucose supplementation in 40 patients with a clinical or histological diagnosis of alcoholic hepatitis, approximately 60% of whom had established cirrhosis. The patients were randomized to receive a standard hospital diet, providing 2674 kcal and 100 g of protein daily, or a standard hospital diet together with a daily intravenous infusion of an amino acid–glucose solution which provided an additional 860 kcal and 42 g of protein. The study lasted for 21 days. Fourteen (67%) of the 21 patients randomized to diet alone and 14 (74%) of the 19 patients randomized to diet with intravenous supplementation completed the study. Oral intake varied considerably in the patients in both groups, but most were taking a minimum of 1200 kcal daily by the second week of the study.

At the end of the study significant improvements were observed in the mean serum bilirubin and aspartate transaminase concentrations in patients receiving the standard hospital diet, and in the mean serum bilirubin, aspartate transaminase and albumin concentrations in patients receiving the standard diet with intravenous supplementation. Alcoholic hyaline was observed in 6 of 8 initial liver biopsies in each group; at the end of the study, hyaline was observed in 5 (82%) of 6 liver biopsies from patients receiving the standard hospital diet but in only one (17%) of six biopsies from patients receiving diet with intravenous supplementation. These numbers are too small for statistical analysis. None of the patients receiving the standard hospital treatment died during the study period, although 3 died within 10 days of its completion. One patient receiving diet with intravenous supplementation died of liver failure, but when this death occurred is not stated. Anthropometric variables and nitrogen balance were not assessed.

Few conclusions can be drawn from this study because the feeding regimens were neither isocaloric nor isonitrogenous. Thus, although the author implies that the use of intravenous supplementation might benefit patients with alcoholic hepatitis, this conclusion is not supported by the data.

Simon and Galambos[563] undertook a prospective, randomized trial of parenteral amino acid, glucose and lipid supplementation in 34 patients with alcoholic hepatitis, biopsy-proven in 56%, who were classified, on the basis of clinical and laboratory variables, as having moderate or severe disease. Within these groups patients were randomized to receive either a daily diet providing 2400 kcal and 100 g of protein, together with a liquid supplement providing unspecified amounts of calories and protein, or to receive the same oral regimen supplemented with an intravenous infusion of 2 litres of an amino acid–glucose solution and 500 ml of Intralipid providing, between them, an additional 70 g of conventional amino acids and approximately 2000 kcal daily; the study lasted for 28 days.

Ten of the 12 patients with moderate alcoholic hepatitis completed the study; there were no deaths in this group and parenteral supplementation conferred no benefit either clinically or biochemically. In the patients with severe alcoholic hepatitis, intravenous supplementation was associated with significant improvement in serum bilirubin and transferrin concentrations but had no effect on mortality. Thus, the mortality rates in the patients treated conventionally were 16.7% during the study and 25% during the hospitalization, compared with rates of 30% and 40% respectively in the patients receiving the intravenous supplement.

No information is provided on the actual dietary intakes in these patients, but obviously the two regimens were neither isocaloric nor isonitrogenous. Similarly, anthropometric variables and nitrogen balance were not assessed. It is, therefore, difficult to comment on the overall effect of this type of supplementation on morbidity, and the number of patients studied is too small to allow comment on the effect on mortality. However, it is important to note that the addition of 70 g of conventional amino acids and 2.5 litres of fluid to the dietary regimen of these patients had no deleterious effect on their mental state or fluid balance.

Mendenhall and coworkers[394] studied the changes in nutritional status of 57 patients with moderate to severe alcoholic hepatitis over a 30-day period. Thirty-four patients received a routine hospital diet which provided 2500 kcal daily, with the protein and sodium contents adjusted to suit individual needs. The remaining 23 patients were given a minimum of 1000 kcal daily as hospital food together with a liquid supplement providing 2000 kcal from carbohydrate and 220 kcal from an amino acid mixture rich in branched-chain amino acids (Hepatic-Aid). Five (22%) of the 23 patients given the nutritional supplement withdrew from treatment, largely because of problems with the enteral feed. In the patients who found the nutritional supplement acceptable, more significant improvements were observed in nutritional variables than in the non-supplemented group. Mortality rates were 16.7% in the supplemented and 20.6% in the non-supplemented patients.

The two regimens used in this study were not comparable in that they were neither isocaloric nor isonitrogenous. Thus, it is not possible to conclude that enteral feeding confers benefit in this situation or that it has advantages over a diet adequate in protein and calories consumed ad libitum. The trial does show that it is possible to feed these patients enterally and that enteral feeds are relatively well tolerated. Similar conclusions were also reached by other workers.[572]

In only one of these studies in patients with acute alcoholic hepatitis did protein and calorie supplementation influence mortality.[445] In others there was evidence of a beneficial effect on morbidity in terms of liver function test results, but as the monitoring of nutritional status and nitrogen balance was, in the majority of studies, suboptimal, no firm conclusions can be made. Thus, at present, no confident recommendation can be made regarding the usefulness of nutritional supplements in patients with alcoholic hepatitis. In view of the observation that the inability to attain positive nitrogen balance is associated with a significant mortality,[92] every attempt should be made to ensure that these patients receive adequate amounts of calories and protein.

Cirrhosis[430]

Patients with cirrhosis have increased protein requirements[214,601] and increased total calorie requirements.[346] They should, therefore, take a well-balanced diet providing a daily intake of 60–80 g of protein and between 8 and 12 MJ (2000–3000 kcal) depending on their level of physical activity. These patients are also unable to store hepatic glycogen adequately[450,461] and so might benefit from dietary regimens which provide a constant supply of carbohydrate throughout the 24-hour period. This could be achieved by feeding frequent carbohydrate-rich meals throughout the waking hours, together with a late night meal or carbohydrate load, or else by use of agents such as acarbose which delay carbohydrate absorption, resulting in its sustained release.[600]

Patients with decompensated cirrhosis may be protein depleted and yet at the same time protein intolerant. As excess dietary protein may precipitate hepatic encephalopathy in these patients,[372,471,549] daily protein intakes are often reduced to 40 or 50 g and this leads to further depletion of body protein stores. Attempts have, therefore, been made to find a nitrogen source which is better tolerated than dietary protein.

Branched-chain amino acids have an anticatabolic effect in patients with liver disease, probably because of their ability to serve as an energy substrate for muscle and because of their effects on muscle protein synthesis and degradation. It has been shown, for example, that muscle catabolism decreases in cirrhotic patients, over 3 days, following daily infusion of 40 g of a branched-chain-enriched amino acid mixture.[377]

Branched-chain amino acid mixtures are well tolerated by patients who are otherwise clearly protein intolerant.[103,394] It has, therefore, been suggested that branched-chain amino acids might provide a useful nutritional supplement for patients with chronic liver disease.

A number of uncontrolled studies have been undertaken in which branched-chain amino acid-enriched mixtures have been used as dietary supplements in cirrhotic patients, the majority of whom had abused alcohol. In two early studies it was shown that cirrhotic patients who were intolerant of standard amino acid solutions could tolerate up to 125 g of a branched-chain-enriched amino acid solution infused over 24 hours, and could achieve positive nitrogen balance.[200,209] In a further study involving 74 cirrhotic patients in negative nitrogen balance, use of an oral or intravenous branched-chain-enriched amino acid mixture resulted in reversal of the nitrogen balance usually within 1 week.[195] As these trials are anecdotal, no comment can be made as to whether branched-chain amino acid mixtures provide a superior nitrogen source to either dietary protein or a balanced amino acid mixture given by the same route.

However, a total of 13 controlled studies have now been undertaken which provide data on the efficacy and safety of this form of nutritional support in patients with cirrhosis (Table 6.8). Seven of these studies were specifically designed to address these questions;[62,82,89,119,456,508,631] the remaining six trials were designed to assess the efficacy and safety of these supplements in patients with chronic hepatic encephalopathy but provide some nutritional data in addition.[176,237,373,377,561,599]

All the patients studied had cirrhosis, but the aetiology of the liver lesion varied from study to study (Table 6.8). Many of the patients were protein depleted but the exact numbers in any given study are poorly documented. In six studies, the patient numbers exceeded 30 but in the remainder the number were generally much smaller. In only three studies were patients treated beyond 30 days. In all studies patients were randomized to receive either a control or an experimental regimen, except in the study undertaken by Okita and colleagues,[456] in which patients served as their own controls and received both the control and experimental regimens in set order. Six studies included a cross-over phase in their design.

In seven studies the control and experimental regimens were isonitrogenous, if not isocaloric, whereas in the remaining six studies the experimental regimen invariably provided more energy and protein than the control regimen (Table 6.8). A proportion of the nitrogen in all the experimental regimens was provided in the form of branched-chain amino acids.

The results of these studies are difficult to interpret for a number of reasons. First, the variation in population size, trial duration, trial regimens and control regimens make comparisons difficult, if not impossible. Second, outcome variables are poorly defined: in the majority of studies the main outcome variable is morbidity, usually in relation to some aspect of the nutritional assessment. In some studies the effects on morbidity are assessed in relation to dietary regimens which are clearly incomparable in their provision of energy and protein. In others morbidity is assessed in relation to regimens which are comparable in their provision of energy and nitrogen, at least in theory, but in which the nitrogen sources differ. In a minority of studies mortality is the main outcome variable. Finally, outcomes are not stratified by the nutritional status of the patient.

A number of conclusions can, nevertheless, be drawn. First, patients with cirrhosis will tolerate high-protein, high-calorie diets; second, high-protein, high-calorie intakes are accompanied by improvements in nitrogen balance and 'nutritional indices' in the majority of patients with cirrhosis; and third, improvements in nutritional status can be achieved, whatever the nitrogen source, provided that the amount given exceeds 9.6 g daily ($\equiv$ 60 g of protein). At present there is little evidence to show that branched-chain amino acid supplementation is superior to supplementation with other nitrogen sources.

Cholestasis

The severity of the nutritional disturbances associated with acute cholestasis depends on the degree of biliary obstruction and its reversibility. Steatorrhoea may occur but it is rarely gross, as large amounts of fat can be absorbed from the intestine even when luminal concentrations of bile salts are low and the micellar phase is reduced; severe reduction in micelle formation will, however, affect the absorption of fat-soluble vitamins. When the obstruction is easily remediable there is little indication for special dietary advice. Vitamin K_1, 10 mg daily, should be given preoperatively and dehydration and other obvious metabolic disturbances should be corrected, as far as possible.

In patients with chronic cholestasis associated with, for example, primary or secondary biliary cirrhosis, sclerosing cholangitis, or biliary atresia, specific dietary advice is needed. If patients are fat intolerant, dietary fat should be reduced and carbohydrate intake increased to balance the calorie loss. However, fat intake should not be restricted too rigorously as this will reduce the palatability of the diet. Medium-chain triglycerides may be given, preferably in the form of an emulsion which can be made into milkshakes. Fat-soluble vitamins should be supplemented monthly in the form of intramuscular injections of 10 mg vitamin K_1, 10 000 IU (10 mg) of vitamin

Table 6.8 Controlled trials of 'nutritional therapy' in patients with chronic liver disease

First author, date, and reference number	Trial design	Patients (n)	Aetiology of cirrhosis	Trial duration (days)	Trial regimen (daily)	Alternative regimen (daily)	Outcome
Swart 1981[599]	Single-centre Randomized Cross-over	8	Chronic active hepatitis 50%	30 alternating 5 day regimens	Diet containing BCAA[a]-rich protein (35% BCAA) 40, 60, 80 g at 10-day intervals	Diet containing mixed protein (20% BCAA) 40, 60, 80 g at 10-day intervals	Nitrogen balance positive on intakes of 60 g and 80 g Minimal protein requirements averaged 48 g/day on both regimens
Bory 1982[62]	Single-centre Randomized	74	Alcoholic 63%	15	BCAA–enriched enteral feed	Standard hospital diet	24-Hour creatinine excretion, 'nutritional indices', serum albumin and prothrombin time improved on enteral feed
McGhee 1983[373]	Single-centre Randomized Double-blind Cross-over	4	Mixed	11 on each regimen	30 g Hepatic-Aid[b] 20 g Casein + 260 g CHO[c] 80 g fat } 2000 kcal	50 g Casein + 260 g CHO 80 g fat } 2000 kcal	Nitrogen balance maintained on each regimen
Simko 1983[561]	Single-centre Randomized Single-blind	15	Alcoholic	90	Usual diet + 20-60 g Hepatic-Aid	Usual diet + placebo powder	4 BCAA and 1 placebo patient dropped out Calorie intake, fat stores and serum transferrin concentrations increased significantly on BCAA
Watanabe 1983[631]	Single-centre Randomized Cross-over	2	Mixed	? 14 on each regimen	1600 kcal 40 g protein + 600 kcal 37 g protein } as BCAA supplement	2072 kcal 74 g protein	Nitrogen balance positive on BCAA
Guanieri 1984[237]	Single-centre Randomized	8	Mixed	100–120	Calorie-reduced basal diet + 20 g Hepatic-Aid CHO Fat } 1120 kcal	Calorie-reduced basal diet + CHO Fat } 1120 kcal	Fat stores Plasma proteins Cr/Ht index Nitrogen balance Muscle RNA/DNA } Increased with BCAA
Christie 1985[119]	Single-centre Randomized Double-blind Cross-over	8	Alcoholic 75%	9 on each regimen	Diet containing 40 g protein + BCAA supplement 20 g increments × 3	Diet containing 40 g protein + Casein supplement 20 g increments × 3	Significant increase in nitrogen balance on both regimens
Egberts 1985[176]	Single-centre Randomized Double-blind Cross-over	22	Alcoholic 87%	7 on each regimen	Diet containing 1 g protein/kg 35 kcal/kg + BCAA 0.25 g/kg	Diet containing 1 g protein/kg 35 kcal/kg + Casein 0.25g/kg	Significant increase in nitrogen balance on both regimens
Okita 1985[456]	Single-centre Cross-over	10	Alcoholic 70%	14 control; 14 trial; 14 control, in order	Oral diet 40 g protein 1500 kcal + 40 g protein 630 kcal } supplement rich in BCAA	Oral diet 80 g protein 2100 kcal	Improved nitrogen balance and serum prealbumin concentrations on supplemented regimen
Rocchi 1985[508]	Singel-centre Randomized	36	Alcoholic 50%	5	_A_ Oral diet + IV BCAA 0.5 g/kg _B_ Oral diet + IV BCAA 1.0 g/kg	_C_ Oral diet + IV BCAA-enriched 0.8 g/kg _D_ Oral diet + IV balanced AA 0.5 g/kg	Improved nitrogen balance in groups B, C and D
Bunout 1989[82]	Single-centre Randomized	36	Alcoholic	15–30	Diet containing BCAA-rich protein 1.5 g/kg, energy 50 kcal/kg	Standard diet, protein 0.8 g/kg energy 35 kcal/kg	No difference in nutritional status between groups
Cabré 1990[89]	Single-centre Randomized	35	Alcoholic 66%	18–30	BCAA-enriched, energy-dense enteral feed, 2115 kcal/day 40 mmol sodium/day	Standard low-sodium hospital diet, 2200 kcal/day	Actual intake in control group 1370 kcal/day Enteral feed withdrawn in two patients Significant increase in serum albumin in enteral group
Marchesini 1990[377]	Multicentre Randomized Double-blind Partial cross-over	64	Alcoholic 56%	90 on each regimen	Usual diet + 2.4 g BCAA/10 kg	Usual diet + 1.8 g casein/10 kg	Significant increase in nitrogen balance on both regimens after 6 months

[a] BCAA, branched-chain amino acids. [b] Hepatic-Aid, commercial branched-chain-enriched amino acid supplement. [c] CHO, carbohydrate.

A and 10 000 IU (0.25 mg) of vitamin D. Children with chronic cholestasis might benefit from supplementation with parenteral vitamin E given in a dose of 1.4–2.8 IU (1–2 mg)/kg at intervals determined by the plasma concentrations. Calcium supplements may be required by both children and adults. There is some evidence that calcium provided in the form of hydroxyapatite might be more beneficial than calcium provided as a simple salt.[179] Medium-chain triglycerides promote calcium uptake.

A sample high-protein, high-energy, low-fat diet suitable for patients with steatorrhoea and a sample low-fat diet with added medium-chain triglycerides suitable for patients with chronic cholestasis are given in the Appendix.

DIETARY MANAGEMENT OF THE COMPLICATIONS OF LIVER DISEASE

Fluid retention

Patients with both subacute and chronic liver disease may develop significant fluid retention which manifests as ascites and peripheral oedema. In general, the development of ascites is associated with a poor prognosis.[22] Fluid retention may develop gradually and spontaneously or its appearance may be precipitated by events such as gastrointestinal bleeding which further impair hepatic function. Spontaneous bacterial peritonitis may develop in patients with ascites; it is often subclinical and its development carries a high mortality.

The pathogenesis of ascites formation is complex and multifactorial (see Chapter 51). However, as these patients retain both salt and water, manipulation of dietary salt and water intake may be of therapeutic benefit.

The degree of renal functional disturbance may be assessed arbitrarily from the ability of the kidney to excrete salt and to clear free water.[21] Patients with fluid retention who pass relatively large amounts of urinary sodium and are able to generate free water may respond to sodium restriction alone without the need for diuretics. A 'no added salt' diet together with avoidance of salty foods will reduce the daily sodium intake to 50 mmol (50 mEq). It may be necessary to reduce intake further, for a short period of time, by complete avoidance of salt in the cooking and the use of special salt-free bread, cakes and biscuits; care should be taken to avoid salt-containing medications such as antacids and certain antibiotics; in this way the daily sodium intake can be reduced to 20 mmol (20 mEq). In patients with low urinary sodium excretion but an ability to generate free water, diuretics are usually needed in addition to dietary sodium restriction. Major problems arise in patients who have low urinary sodium excretion and cannot generate free water; these patients are usually hyponatraemic and require daily fluid restriction to around 1 litre, in addition to sodium restriction and diuretics; their prognosis is particularly poor.

Reynolds and coworkers[498] examined the advantages of treating ascites without sodium restriction. Diets were more palatable and uraemia and hyperuricaemia, which often complicate more vigorous regimens, were observed only infrequently. Hyponatraemia developed in a number of patients but this could have been avoided if dietary fluid intake had been restricted. Patients were, however, concerned about their appearance, and the time taken to achieve fluid loss was sometimes unacceptable.

The apparent advantages of treating ascites without sodium restriction, observed by Reynolds and colleagues,[498] were not confirmed by two other groups of workers.[153, 220] Gauthier and colleagues[220] studied the effects of sodium restriction in 140 patients with alcoholic cirrhosis and moderately severe ascites. All patients were initially treated with bed rest and with dietary sodium restriction to 21 mmol daily and fluid restriction to 1 litre daily. After 4–7 days, patients were randomly allocated either to remain on the sodium restricted diet or to take an unrestricted diet which provided 51–68 mmol of sodium daily. Diuretics were prescribed as necessary. After 14 days of treatment, body weight and abdominal girth were significantly reduced in the patients on the sodium restricted diet; serum sodium concentrations were significantly lower in these patients at this time, but the decrease was transient and was not accompanied by an increase in blood urea concentration. There were no significant differences between the two groups at 3 months.

Once the fluid retention has been treated successfully, it may be necessary to continue sodium restriction to prevent fluid reaccumulation. Care must be taken not to restrict sodium too rigorously for too long a period. Patients should be monitored frequently and the dietary sodium restriction reviewed and modified as indicated.

Patients with cirrhosis may develop refractory ascites and this has deleterious effects on their nutritional status. Blendis and coworkers[55] have shown that successful insertion of a peritoneovenous shunt is associated, over time, with significant improvements in nitrogen balance, total body potassium and total body nitrogen.

Sample low-sodium diets are given in the Appendix.

Hepatic encephalopathy[430]

Treatment of hepatic encephalopathy depends upon measures designed to reduce the circulating levels of toxins. This is usually achieved by decreasing the gut protein load, altering the intestinal flora, reducing the rate of absorption of protein and protein fragments, decreasing intestinal transit time and bowel cleansing.

Dietary protein restriction has been the mainstay of treatment for hepatic encephalopathy for many years and there is little doubt that it is effective.[372,597,613] However, protein requirements are significantly increased in patients with cirrhosis, with the majority requiring a daily minimum of 35–50 g,[214] or 0.75 g/kg body weight[601] to maintain nitrogen balance. Institution of a protein-restricted diet may, therefore, compromise the nutritional status of the patient. Thus, while it might be necessary, and reasonable, to restrict dietary protein intake in the short term, long-term restriction should be avoided. During an acute episode of hepatic encephalopathy, protein intake should be reduced initially to 20 g daily. Thereafter, protein intake should be increased by increments of 10 g every third day until the maximum tolerated, which should be of the order of 60 g or 1 g/kg body weight daily, whichever is greater. Dietary protein should be distributed fairly evenly throughout the day.

The type of protein ingested is also thought to be important, as patients with cirrhosis show variations in their tolerance to dietary protein, depending on its source.[613] Thus, dairy protein is better tolerated than protein from mixed sources[192] and vegetable protein is better tolerated than meat protein.[148,235,312,614] Vegetable protein diets contain significantly more dietary fibre than isonitrogenous meat protein diets; the enhanced tolerance to vegetable protein is thought to reflect the effects of dietary fibre on colonic function, namely decreased transit time, reduced intraluminal pH and increased faecal ammonia excretion.[218,263,635] Alternatively, consumption of a purely vegetable diet may result in alteration of the bowel flora with beneficial effect. In addition, plasma arginine and ornithine concentrations tend to be higher in patients on vegetable protein diets[148] and this may additionally facilitate ammonia removal via the Krebs–Henseleit cycle.

The acceptability of vegetable protein diets varies widely from population to population. In developed countries, where the dietary fibre content of the staple diet is low, diets containing more than 50 g of vegetable protein are considered bulky and often produce early satiety, abdominal distension, flatulence and diarrhoea. In underdeveloped countries, where the staple diet contains significant amounts of fibre, these diets tend to be better accepted. In general, patients should be encouraged to take as high a percentage of vegetable protein as they can, and provided that they are not also salt restricted, which makes the diet unpalatable, daily intakes of 30–40 g of vegetable protein can usually be achieved.

The aromatic amino acids serve as precursors for the physiological neurotransmitters noradrenaline and dopamine. The free brain concentrations of these amino acids are determined, in part, by their plasma concentrations but also by the concentrations of the other neutral amino acids, including the branched-chain amino acids, with which they compete for passage across the blood–brain barrier. In 1971, Fischer and Baldesarini[199] hypothesized that in patients with liver disease, in whom plasma concentrations of the aromatic amino acids are high and concentrations of the branched-chain amino acids are low, passage of neurotransmitter precursors into the brain might be augmented. Phenylalanine in high concentration might compete with tyrosine, within the brain, as a substrate for tyrosine hydroxylase, the key enzyme in catecholamine synthesis, resulting in decreased conversion of tyrosine to dopamine and noradrenaline.

In addition, the excess amounts of phenylalanine and tyrosine might be decarboxylated to β-phenylethanol-amine and octopamine, which, although structurally similar to the physiological neurotransmitters, possess only one-hundredth of their neurotransmitter potency. These weak neurotransmitters might then compete with the true neurotransmitters for receptor sites, resulting in impairment of cerebral function. Later, this original 'false neurotransmitter' hypothesis was modified to implicate ammonia, via the formation of glutamine, as a promoter of amino acid transport across the blood–brain barrier[284] (see Chapter 47).

It therefore follows that if the abnormal plasma amino acid pattern observed in patients with chronic liver disease is important in the pathogenesis of hepatic encephalopathy, then correcting the plasma amino acid profile, by use of intravenous or oral mixtures with low concentration of aromatic and high concentrations of branched-chain amino acids, might benefit patients with this condition.

The results of several early studies in which intravenous branched-chain amino acid-enriched solutions were used to treat episodes of hepatic encephalopathy in patients with cirrhosis were encouraging, but, as they were generally uncontrolled, no firm conclusions could be made about the efficacy and safety of this form of treatment. Subsequently, a number of randomized, controlled clinical trials have been published[87,104,196,277,406,514,589,623,628] but they are not easily compared as the trial designs are not standardized to any great degree (Table 6.9). For example, there is wide variation in the aetiology and severity of the liver injury, in the cause and severity of the precoma/coma, and in its duration before the trial. Equally, although in all nine studies the treatment groups received an infusion of a branched-chain amino acid mixture and hypertonic glucose, the nature of the amino acid solution varies from trial to trial. There is, in addition, little consensus on the nature of the control regimen or on the need for adjuvant therapy with lactulose and/or neomycin in the treatment group. The duration of treatment varies from trial to trial, though in most it was continued for 48 h after 'wake-up'. End-points for determining treatment outcome are not clearly defined, but in most the time to 'wake-up', generally to Grade 0 or I, is noted and the percentage survival is recorded.

It is extremely difficult to interpret the results of these studies in view of the non-standardized way in which they were conducted. In six of the nine studies, infusion of branched-chain amino acid mixtures had no significant effect on recovery or survival in comparison to the chosen control regimen.[87,277,406,514,623,628] In one study the use of branched-chain amino acids had a significant effect on recovery from precoma but not on mortality,[104] while in another treatment with branched-chain amino acids was associated with an accelerated recovery from precoma.[589] In one study, treatment with branched-chain amino acids and/or lactulose was found to be more effective than treatment with lactulose alone.[196]

These trials have recently been subjected to extensive

Table 6.9 Randomized, controlled trials of intravenous branched-chain amino acids (BCAA) in the treatment of acute hepatic encephalopathy in patients with cirrhosis

First author, date, and reference number	Trial design	Patients (n)	Episodes treated (n)	Aetiology of cirrhosis (% alcoholic)	Coma grade (% III/IV)	Trial duration (days)	Treatment regimen (daily)	Control regimen (daily)	Oral intake (daily)	Response to treatment (No.(%) improved) BCAA	Control	Combined	Study mortality (No.(%) deaths) BCAA	Control	Combined	Comments	Conclusion
Rossi-Fanelli 1982[514]	Multi-centre	34	34	32	100	2–4	BCAA-rich (BS692) + 20% glucose	Lactulose + 20% glucose	Nil	12/17 (71)	8/17 (47)	3/7 (43)	3/17 (18)	4/17 (24)	4/7 (57)	Patients failing to respond after 4 days given BCAA *and* lactulose	No significant effect of BCAA on recovery or mortality
Wahren 1983[628]	Multi-centre Double-blind	50	50	76	96	<5	BCAA (KabiVitrum) + 50% glucose 20% lipid	5% glucose + 50% glucose 20% lipid	Nil	14/25 (56)	12/25 (48)	—	10/25 (40)	5/25 (20)	—	Eight patients also received lactulose ± neomycin	No significant effect of BCAA on recovery or mortality
Cerra 1985[104]	Multi-centre Double-blind	75	75	92	?	14	BCAA-rich (F080) + 25% glucose	Neomycin + 25% glucose	Nil until symptom free	16/30 (53)	5/29 (17)	—	12/40 (30)	13/35 (37)	—	20% dropped out; 15% crossed to other regimen on day 4. Results selectively analysed	Significant effect of BCAA on recovery but not on mortality
Fiaccadori 1985[196]	Multi-centre	48	48	52	50	7	BCAA-rich (BS666) + 30% glucose ± lactulose	Lactulose + 30% glucose	?	15/16 (94)	10/16 (63)	16/16 (100)	0	0	0	—	Treatment with BCAA ± lactulose significantly better than treatment with lactulose alone
Michel 1985[406]	Multi-centre Double-blind	70	70	81	64	5	BCAA-rich + 30% glucose 20% lipid	Conventional AA mixture + 30% glucose 20% lipid	Nil	12/36 (33)	10/34 (29)	—	7/36 (19)	7/34 (21)	—	—	No significant effect of BCAA on recovery or mortality
Vilstrup 1985[623]	Multi-centre Double-blind	65	65	91	69	<16	BCAA-rich (Pf 8) + Lactulose + 50% glucose	Lactulose + 50% glucose	?	17/32 (53)	17/33 (52)	—	11/32 (30)	10/33 (34)	—	—	No significant effect of BCAA on recovery or mortality
Strauss 1986[589]	Two-centre	29	32	91	34	?5	BCAA-rich (F080) + hypertonic glucose	Neomycin	Low-protein when grade I/II	14/16 (88)	14/16 (88)	—	2/16 (13)	2/16 (13)	—	—	No significant effect of BCAA on recovery or mortality. Speed of recovery faster with BCAA
Caballería Rovira 1987[87]	Single-centre	20	20	?	35	<5	BCAA-rich (F080)	Neomycin + lactulose	Protein-free diet?	6/10 (60)	6/10 (60)	—	2/10 (20)	2/10 (20)	—	—	No significant effect of BCAA on recovery or mortality
Hwang 1988[277]	Single-centre	55[a]	60[a]	15 (8/52)	89[a]	<5	BCAA-rich (Aminoleban) + neomycin + lactulose + 10% dextrose	Neomycin + lactulose + 10% dextrose	Nil days 0–3 <20 g protein days 3–5	19/27[a] (70)	15/28[a] (54)	—	10/27[a] (37)	14/28[a] (50)	—	—	No significant effect of BCAA on recovery or mortality

[a] Included 3 patients with fulminant hepatic failure.

review and reanalysis by two groups of workers, who unfortunately came to different conclusions. Eriksson and Conn[181] reviewed seven of the nine studies and undertook an extensive reanalysis of one. They concluded that 'BCAA therapy, whether pure or combined with other amino acids, irrespective of the amount administered does not affect significantly the outcome of patients with acute hepatic encephalopathy.' Naylor and coworkers[447] applied meta-analytical methods to review the results of seven of the nine studies, though unfortunately they seem to have used preliminary data, published earlier than the definitive studies, in three cases. They concluded that pooled analysis of five of the studies showed that treatment with branched-chain amino acids was associated with a highly significant improvement in mental recovery from severe encephalopathy over follow-up times varying from 5 to 14 days. The case fatality data could not be pooled, although the most conservative interpretation of data from three of the studies showed that treatment with branched-chain amino acids was associated with a significant reduction in mortality. However, the authors caution that although the study results to date are promising, they 'do not permit an unqualified conclusion in favour of use of BCAA solutions and hypertonic glucose as a nutritional support regimen for cirrhotic patients with high-grade HE'. They stipulate that confirmatory randomized, controlled trials, with longer follow-up periods, are warranted.

Early studies showed that the use of oral branched-chain-enriched amino acid supplements might be efficacious in treating persistent hepatic encephalopathy or in preventing recurrence of episodic encephalopathy in patients with chronic liver disease. The number of patients treated was small and the observations were uncontrolled. However, in recent years a number of randomized, controlled clinical trials of this form of treatment have been undertaken.[176,182,237,274,373,378,502,538,559,561,599]

Many of the criticisms of the intravenous studies in acute hepatic encephalopathy can also be made of these studies. Thus, with few exceptions, the numbers of patients treated in the various studies is small and the treatment periods are short (Table 6.10). Wide variation is observed in the degree of encephalopathy on entry into the study and in the trial and control regimens employed. In only one study was a branched-chain amino acid mixture used as an alternative to treatment with lactulose,[502] while in the others it was used either as an adjunct or as an alternative in individual patients, depending on whether lactulose was given simultaneously. In several studies, the 'comagenic' potential of branched-chain amino acid mixtures was compared with that of isonitrogenous amounts of dietary protein or casein, although in only one study was lactulose discontinued. In 6 of the 11 studies a cross-over design was employed but, in general, wash-out periods between treatments were not allowed and the correct statistical analyses to allow separation of the effects of the two regimens were not employed. Overall, the end-points of treatment are not clearly defined, although in most trials patients were monitored, throughout, by clinical examination, psychometric assessment and measurements of blood ammonia concentrations and electroencephalogram mean cycle frequencies.

In 8 of the 11 studies, no improvement was noted in mental state, psychometric test performance or in electroencephalogram mean cycle frequencies in patients given branched-chain amino acid mixtures. Horst and colleagues[274] found that the incidence of encephalopathy was less in patients treated with the amino acid supplement than in patients treated with isonitrogenous amounts of dietary protein, while Egberts and colleagues[176] recorded significantly better psychometric performance in patients given the amino acid rather than a casein supplement. Marchesini and coworkers[378] reported significant improvements in mental state, psychometric test results and/or electroencephalogram mean cycle frequencies in patients given branched-chain amino acids but not in patients given casein. As such, this is the only truly positive study and so deserves separate consideration.

These workers undertook a randomized, double-blind study of branched-chain amino acids against equinitrogenous amounts of casein in 64 patients with grade I to II hepatic encephalopathy over one 3-month period. The patients were carefully monitored during the treatment period using the Portal–Systemic Encephalopathy (PSE) Index[129] and the end-points of the trial were clearly delineated, with improvement in encephalopathy being defined as a change of at least one grade in the score of two or more of the five variables of the PSE Index. Patients remained on their usual dietary protein intake of 45–65 g daily and received lactulose in a dose of 20–40 g to ensure daily passage of two semi-soft stools. Thus, treatment with the branched-chain amino acids was tested not as an alternative but as an adjunct to conventional therapy.

During the treatment period, improvement in encephalopathy was demonstrated in 24 (80%) of the 30 patients given branched-chain amino acids but in only 12 (35%) of the 34 patients given casein. This difference is statistically significant both on an intention-to-treat basis, which included the three patients who dropped out, and on the basis of treatment given. The patient groups were well matched and the results of this parallel comparison of agents is very convincing.

At the end of the 3 months of parallel comparison the authors continued with an unconventionally designed, single-blind, partial cross-over study. Patients who had improved on either the branched-chain amino acid or the casein supplements continued treatment with the same agent for a further 3 months, but those who had not improved were crossed over, after a 2 week wash-out period, to 3 months of supplementation with the alternative agent. Twenty of the 24 patients who had improved with branched-chain amino acids were followed for a further 3 months and improvement was maintained in 19. Nine of the 12 patients who improved with casein were monitored beyond 3 months and improvement was

Table 6.10 Randomized, controlled trials of oral branched-chain amino acids (BCAA) in patients with chronic hepatic encephalopathy

First author, date, and reference number	Trial design	Patients (n)	Mental state (grade)	Pretrial regimen	Trial period (days)	Trial regimen (daily)	Alternative/control regimen (daily)	Comment	Findings
Schäfer 1981[538]	Single-centre Double-blind Cross-over	8	I–II	Protein restriction 8/8 Lactulose 5/8	30–60 on each regimen	Usual diet + 45 g protein (34% BCAA)	(a) Usual diet + 45 g milk protein (20% BCAA) (b) Usual diet + 125 g CHO[a]	Lactulose 5/8 BCAA-enriched protein well tolerated; milk protein poorly tolerated	No significant effect of BCAA on NCT[b] results or EEG[c] mcf
Swart 1981[599]	Single-centre Cross-over	8	0	Protein restriction 8/8 Lactulose 8/8	30 alternating 5 days regimens	Diet containing BCAA-rich protein (35% BCAA) 40,60,80 g at 10-day intervals	Diet containing mixed protein (20% BCAA) 40,60,80 g at 10-day intervals	Lactulose 8/8	No significant effect of BCAA on mental state, NCT results or EEG mcf
Eriksson 1982[182]	Single-centre Double-blind Cross-over	7	I–II	Protein restriction 4/7 Lactulose	14 on each regimen	Usual diet + 30 g BCAA 5 g sucrose	Usual diet + 34 g maltodextrine 11 g sucrose	Lactulose 4/7 BCAA well tolerated	No significant effect of BCAA on mental state, psychometric test results or EEG mcf
McGhee 1983[373]	Single-centre Double-blind Cross-over	4	0	Protein restriction 4/4	11 on each regimen	30 g Hepatic-Aid[d] 20 g casein + 260 g CHO } 2000 kcal	50 g Casein + 260 g CHO } 2000 kcal	Both regimens well tolerated	No significant effect of BCAA on psychometric test results or EEG mcf
Siez 1983[559]	Single-centre Double-blind Cross-over	14	0–I	Protein restriction 14/14 Lactulose 14/14	90 on each regimen	Usual diet + 44 g protein (30% BCAA) 80 g CHO	Usual diet + 125 g CHO	Lactulose 14/14 BCAA well tolerated	No significant effect of BCAA on NCT results or EEG mcf
Simko 1983[561]	Single-centre Single-blind	15	0–I	Lactulose/neomycin ?/15	90	Usual diet + 20–60 g Hepatic-Aid	Usual diet + placebo powder	Lactulose/neomycin ?/15 4 BCAA; 1 placebo dropped out	No adverse effects of BCAA on mental state or NCT results

Study	Design	No. of patients	Grade of encephalopathy	Entry / compliance	Duration (days)	BCAA regimen	Control regimen	Co-treatment / tolerability	Outcome
Guarnieri 1984[237]	Single-centre	8	< II	Protein restriction 8/8 Lactulose/ neomycin ?/8	100–120	Calorie-reduced basal diet + 29 g Hepatic-Aid CHO } 1120 Fat } kcal	Calorie-reduced basal diet + CHO } 1120 Fat } kcal	Lactulose/neomycin ?/8 All patients malnourished; supplement well-tolerated	No significant effect of BCAA on mental state or EEG mcf
Horst 1984[274]	Multicentre Double-blind	26	0–II	Protein restriction 26/26 Lactulose ± neomycin 25/26	30	Diet containing 20 g protein + Hepatic-Aid 20 g BCAA added at weekly intervals	Diet containing 20 g protein + 20 g dietary protein added at weekly intervals	Lactulose 2/26 BCAA well tolerated	Incidence of encephalopathy significantly less with BCAA
Riggio 1984[502]	Single-centre	28	0–II	Protein restriction 28/28 Lactulose 28/28	90	Diet containing 0.5 g/kg protein days 0–60 0.8 g/kg protein days 60–90 + 0.3 g/kg BCAA days 0–90	Diet containing 0.5 g/kg protein days 0–60 0.8 g/kg protein days 60–90 + Lactulose days 0–90	5/14 BCAA dropped out ? cause	One patient in each group developed grade II hepatic encephalopathy
Egberts 1985[176]	Single-centre Double-blind Cross-over	22	0	Lactulose 14/22	7 on each regimen	Diet containing 1 g protein/kg 35 kcal/kg + BCAA 0.25 g/kg	Diet containing 1 g protein/kg 35 kcal/kg + casein 0.25 g/kg	Lactulose 14/22	Psychometric test results significantly better on BCAA
Marchesini 1990[373]	Multicentre Double-blind Partial cross-over	64	I–II	Protein restriction 64/64 Lactulose 64/64	90	Usual diet + 2.4 g BCAA/10 kg	Usual diet + 1.8 g casein/10 kg	Lactulose 64/64	Significant improvements in mental state, NCT results and EEG mcf on BCAA

[a] CHO, carbohydrate.
[b] NCT, Number Connection Test.
[c] EEG, electroencephalogram.
[d] Hepatic-Aid, commercial branched-chain-enriched amino acid supplement.
mcf, mean cycle frequency.

sustained in four. Of the 20 patients eligible to cross over from casein to branched-chain amino acids, only 10 did so and in 8 the PSE Index improved. However, of the 5 patients eligible to cross over from branched-chain amino acids to casein, only 2 did so, and improvement in encephalopathy was observed in one. It is difficult to understand why these authors did not undertake a conventional cross-over study from the outset. The design of the second phase of the study is unconventional and its description is so complex that the results of the initial parallel comparison become 'watered-down' in the reading of the text. Nevertheless, the results of the parallel comparison stand.

It is unclear why the results of this study[378] differ from the majority of the other studies in this field. These workers did carefully preselect their patient population, excluding individuals who were abusing alcohol, were malnourished or who had had a recent gastrointestinal bleed, and this may have had some bearing on the results. No information is provided on the numbers of patients excluded, but five centres participated in the study yet only 64 patients were recruited over a 2-year period, indicating that perhaps the majority of patients seen were not eligible for inclusion. The results of the study are, nevertheless, encouraging, although it would be premature, on the basis of one study, to recommend use of oral branched-chain amino acid supplements to treat chronic hepatic encephalopathy.

Marchesini and colleagues[378] treated a highly selected population of patients and it may be that treatment should be confined to such highly motivated, relatively well individuals. Studies in more disadvantaged patient populations are obviously needed before the characteristics of patients suitable for treatment can be defined. Even if suitable patient groups can be identified, compliance with treatment might well be poor. Thus, although Marchesini and colleagues[378] excluded patients known to be poorly compliant with diet and drug treatment, 14 (22%) of the 64 patients admitted to their study were non-compliant with the treatment regimen. The rate of non-compliance increased, as might be expected, with increasing length of treatment.

It is apparent that further randomized, controlled studies are required to define the efficacy of branched-chain amino acids in the management of chronic hepatic encephalopathy. Any future studies should give prime consideration to the cost and cost-effectiveness of treatment.

Sample low-protein and vegetable protein diets are given in the Appendix.

Carbohydrate intolerance

Glucose intolerance is commonly observed in patients with a variety of liver diseases. Individuals with chronic liver disease and mild glucose intolerance may benefit from dietary manipulation. They should be encouraged to take 45–55% of their total energy intake as carbo-

hydrate and approximately one-third as fat. Complex carbohydrates which have low glycaemic indices and which are rich in soluble fibre, such as pulses, pasta and cereals, are recommended;[289] sucrose intake should be limited to 30 g daily and its use as a sweetener in drinks should be avoided; most of the dietary fat should be unsaturated. Provided that the postprandial blood glucose levels are not persistently elevated and that the immediate preprandial blood sugar concentrations do not exceed 6.0 mmol/l, no further measures are needed.

Patients with severe parenchymal liver disease complicated by hepatic encephalopathy and glucose intolerance have been shown to benefit from institution of a vegetable protein diet supplemented with dietary fibre.[615]

A sample diet suitable for a patient with chronic parenchymal liver disease and mild to moderate glucose intolerance is given in the Appendix.

APPENDIX

Miss Angela Madden, Senior Dietitian at the Royal Free Hospital, kindly assisted in the compilation of this appendix.

High-protein, high-energy, low-fat diet

Approximately 80 g protein, 35 g fat, and 10.8 MJ (2400 kcal).

DAILY	570 ml (1 pint) skimmed milk (extra skimmed milk powder may be added to increase protein content)
BREAKFAST	Fruit or fruit juice
	Cereal or porridge with sugar and skimmed milk
	1 egg, lean grilled bacon, lean ham or fish
	Bread and scrape of low-fat spread, for example, Gold, Delight, Outline
	Marmalade, honey or jam
	Tea or coffee with skimmed milk
MID-MORNING	Skimmed-milk shake (skimmed milk, skimmed milk powder and flavouring such as Nesquik or Crusha)
LUNCH	Average portion lean meat, no visible fat, or large portion white fish or chicken
	Potatoes, rice or spaghetti
	Vegetables or salad, no oil
	Skimmed milk pudding, fruit or jelly
	Stewed or tinned fruit
TEA	Tea with skimmed milk
	Plain biscuits
SUPPER	As lunch
BED-TIME	Skimmed-milk shake

Energy intake may be increased by fruit drinks plus

glucose, or a glucose polymer. The use of high-carbo-hydrate foods such as potatoes, rice or spaghetti should be encouraged. Build Up (Nestlé) is a useful low-fat calorie and protein supplement that is palatable when made up with skimmed milk.

Low-fat diet with added medium-chain triglyceride

Long-chain fat should be restricted to reduce steatorrhoea, and medium-chain triglycerides (MCT) added to the diet to increase the energy content. These should be introduced slowly into the diet over several days, as they may cause gastrointestinal disturbance if administered rapidly. MCT are available as oil, an emulsion (Liquigen) or powdered milk (Portagen or MCT Formula 1). Adults will find the first two more useful, while infants and children will also require MCT milk. All three are available on prescription in the United Kingdom and patients will benefit most from individual practical advice from a dietition on how to use them. The oil should never be taken undiluted but always mixed with at least an equal quantity of fluid or food.

DAILY	570 ml (1 pint) skimmed milk plus 60 ml (4 tablespoons) Liquigen and up to 50 ml MCT oil for cooking, baking or adding to foods
BREAKFAST	Fruit or fruit juice Cereal, supplemental milk and sugar Bread and scrape of low-fat spread Marmalade or honey Tea or coffee with supplemental milk and sugar as desired
MID-MORNING	Coffee or tea, supplemental milk Plain biscuits
LUNCH	Lean meat, no visible fat, or white fish Potatoes mashed with MCT or fried with MCT, or bread with scrape of low-fat spread Custard or milk pudding made with supplemented milk Tinned or stewed fruit, jelly or jam
TEA	Tea or coffee with supplemental milk
SUPPER	As lunch
BED-TIME	Supplemental milk drink

Diets restricted in sodium

DAILY	300 ml (approximately 0.5 pint) milk for tea and cereal
BREAKFAST	Fruit or fruit juice, if desired Shredded Wheat, Puffed Wheat or porridge made without salt 1 egg, tomatoes, mushrooms 2 slices ordinary bread Salt-free butter
	Jam, marmalade or honey Milk from allowance on cereal and in tea
MID-MORNING	Tea or coffee, milk from allowance
LUNCH	Meat or fish—home prepared without salt Potatoes, rice or pasta, or salt-free bread Vegetables or salad Fruit, jelly, unsalted pastry
TEA	Tea with milk from allowance Salt-free cake or biscuit—home prepared using appropriate recipe
SUPPER	As lunch
BED-TIME	Remainder of milk in tea or coffee Salt-free bread, salt-free butter and jam or salt-free cake or biscuit

This regimen provides approximately 40 mmol (40 mEq) of sodium daily. Salt should not be used in cooking or added at table, and foods forbidden and allowed are given below.

Foods allowed freely
Fruit, fresh, canned or frozen; dates
Fresh or frozen vegetables
Salt-free bread, matzos, salt-free crispbread
Puffed Wheat, Shredded Wheat, Sugar Puffs, unsalted porridge
Plain rice, dried pasta, semolina, sago, tapioca
Sugar, glucose, honey, marmalade, jam
Boiled sweets, peppermints, chewing gum, dark chocolate
Pepper, herbs, spices, vinegar, powdered mustard
Meat, fish, eggs
Milk in limited quantities only
Tea, coffee, fresh fruit juice
Mineral waters, except Vichy water, Badoit, Ferrarelle
Salt substitutes (based on potassium chloride) may be used if serum potassium is normal or low, for example Ruthmol
Unsalted butter, all cooking oils, double cream

Foods not allowed
Ordinary biscuits, cakes
Ordinary bread above daily allowance
Self-raising flour, baking powder
Rice Krispies, Cornflakes, All-Bran and all other cereals except those on the 'allowed freely' list
Cheese, ice-cream
Yoghurt—unless taken in place of milk
Evaporated or condensed milk
Sausages, beefburgers
Ham, bacon, tinned meats, meat paste
Tinned fish, smoked fish, fish paste, fish fingers, fish in sauce
All commercial ready meals
Meat extract, yeast extract

Tinned vegetables, including baked beans
Tinned or packet soups, instant mashed potato
Ketchup, pickles, ready-made mustard, soy sauce, all
  other bottled sauces
Milk chocolate, toffees, fudge, fruit gums, fruit pastilles
Lucozade, soda water, Vichy water, Badoit, Ferrarelle
Tomato juice
Sultanas, raisins
Potato crisps, salted nuts and other savoury snacks

Diets restricted in protein

DAILY	200 ml milk for tea, cereal, etc.
BREAKFAST	Fruit or fruit juice One egg—cooked any way 1 slice ordinary bread, butter and marmalade Small serving of cereal with milk from allowance Tea or coffee, sugar and milk from allowance
MID-MORNING	Tea or coffee, sugar and milk from allowance Plain biscuit
LUNCH	Fruit juice or clear vegetable soup A 25-g portion of cooked meat, fish or cheese or one egg Vegetables or salad Potatoes, rice or pasta Tinned fruit, sugar and double cream
TEA	Tea or coffee, sugar and milk from allowance Piece of cake or 1 slice bread, butter and jam
SUPPER	As lunch
BED-TIME	As mid-morning

This regimen provides approximately 40 g of protein
daily. The diet can be increased to provide 60 g of protein
daily by increasing the meat, fish or cheese portion to
75 g at both lunch and supper.

It is essential with all restricted protein diets to provide
an adequate energy intake to ensure optimal protein
utilization. The energy content of the diet can be increased
by ensuring the inclusion of non-protein fat and carbohydrate foods. Glucose polymers taken, for example, in
fruit juice, provide a concentrated source of energy for
patients with small appetites.

Foods allowed freely on all diets restricted in protein

Butter, margarine, lard, oil, double cream
Sugar, glucose, marmalade, jam, honey
Low-protein bread, biscuits and pasta (available on
  prescription in the United Kingdom)
Boiled sweets, fruit juice, squash, fizzy drinks

Vegetable protein diet

Approximately 80 g protein, 11.7 MJ (2600 kcal) and
60 mmol (60 mEq) sodium. No salt to be added at table.

BREAKFAST	200 ml orange juice Porridge and sugar 2 slices wholemeal toast Butter, jam
MID-MORNING	50 g peanuts 200 ml orange juice
LUNCH	100 mg soya-protein meat Baked potato Grilled tomatoes Wholemeal bread with butter Peaches with double cream
SUPPER	150 g boiled rice Onions fried in butter 50 g kidney beans Tinned pineapple with double cream

Low-sodium, vegetable protein diet

Approximately 65 g protein, 11.7 MJ (2600 kcal) and
40 mmol (40 mEq) sodium. No salt to be added in cooking
or at table.

BREAKFAST	200 ml orange juice Porridge and sugar 2 slices wholemeal toast Salt-free butter and jam
MID-MORNING	50 g peanuts 200 ml orange juice
LUNCH	Fried mushrooms 200 g baked potato Grilled tomatoes French beans 1 slice of wholemeal bread Salt-free butter Peaches and syrup Double cream
SUPPER	150 g boiled rice Onions fried in salt-free butter 50 g kidney beans Tinned pineapple and double cream

Diet suitable for individuals with mild carbohydrate intolerance

Approximately 100 g protein, 73 g fat (two-thirds polyunsaturated fatty acids), 283 g carbohydrate, 46 g fibre, 9.5 MJ
(2100 kcal). Approximately 52% of total energy is supplied by carbohydrate and 30% by fat.

DAILY	570 ml (1 pint) skimmed milk 45 g (1.5 oz) polyunsaturated margarine
BREAKFAST	Large bowl of high-fibre cereal 2 slices of wholemeal bread Margarine from allowance ± Marmite

	spread if desired Tea/coffee with skimmed milk
MID-MORNING	Tea/coffee with skimmed milk or low calorie drink Piece of fresh fruit
LUNCH	Average portion lean meat, chicken or fish with no visible fat Large jacket potato Vegetables or salad, no oil Stewed or tinned fruit, unsweetened Low-fat natural yoghurt or custard made from skimmed milk and artificial sweeteners
TEA	Tea with skimmed milk

| SUPPER | Average portion lean meat, chicken or fish with no visible fat
4 slices of wholemeal bread
Margarine from allowance
Salad with up to 10 ml polyunsaturated oil as dressing
Fresh fruit, or baked apple, no sugar added |
| BED-TIME | Tea/coffee with skimmed milk
1 digestive or wholemeal biscuit |

Saccharine or aspartame tablets, for example Sweetex, Hermesetas or Canderel, may be used for sweetening.

REFERENCES

1. Aaseth, J., Thomassen, Y., Alexander, J. & Norheim, G. (1980) Decreased serum selenium in alcoholic cirrhosis. *New England Journal of Medicine*, **303**, 944–945 (letter).
2. Aaseth, J., Alexander, J., Thomassen, Y. *et al.* (1982) Serum selenium levels in liver diseases. *Clinical Biochemistry*, **15**, 281–283.
3. Abdu-Gusau, K., Elegbede, J.A. & Akanya, H.O. (1989) Serum zinc, retinol and retinol-binding protein levels in cirrhotics with hypogonadism. *European Journal of Clinical Nutrition*, **43**, 53–57.
4. Achord, J.L. (1987) A prospective randomized clinical trial of peripheral amino acid-glucose supplementation in acute alcoholic hepatitis. *American Journal of Gastroenterology*, **82**, 871–875.
5. Achord, J.L. (1987) Malnutrition and the role of nutritional support in alcoholic liver disease. *American Journal of Gastroenterology*, **82**, 1–7.
6. Achord, J.L. (1988) 1987 Henry Baker lecture. Nutrition, alcohol and the liver. *American Journal of Gastroenterology*, **83**, 244–248.
7. Adler, M. & Schaffner, F. (1979) Fatty liver hepatitis and cirrhosis in obese patients. *American Journal of Medicine*, **67**, 811–816.
8. Agorastos, J., Fox, C., Harry, D.S. & McIntyre, N. (1978) Lecithin-cholesterol acyltransferase and the lipoprotein abnormalities of obstructive jaundice. *Clinical Science and Molecular Medicine*, **54**, 369–379.
9. Ahrens, E.H. Jr. & Kunkel, H.G. (1949) The relationship between serum lipids and skin xanthomata in eighteen patients with primary biliary cirrhosis. *Journal of Clinical Investigation*, **28**, 1565–1574.
10. Ajdukiewicz, A.B., Agnew, J.E., Byers, P.D. *et al.* (1974) The relief of bone pain in primary biliary cirrhosis with calcium infusions. *Gut*, **15**, 788–793.
11. Allardyce, D.B. (1982) Cholestasis caused by lipid emulsions. *Surgery, Gynecology and Obstetrics,* **154**, 641–647.
12. Allen, B., Bernhoft, R., Blanckaert, N. *et al.* (1981) Sludge is calcium bilirubinate associated with bile stasis. *American Journal of Surgery*, **141**, 51–56.
13. Alvarez, F., Landrieu, P., Laget, P. *et al.* (1983) Nervous and occular disorders in children with cholestasis and vitamin A and E deficiencies. *Hepatology*, **3**, 410–414.
14. Amaral, J.F. & Thompson, W.R. (1988) Gallbladder disease in morbidly obese patients. *American Journal of Surgery*, **149**, 547–557.
15. Amento, E.P. (1987) Vitamin D and the immune system. *Steroids*, **49**, 55–72.
16. Ames, F.C., Copeland, E.M., Leeb, D.C. *et al.* (1976) Liver dysfunction following small-bowel bypass for obesity: non-operative treatment of fatty metamorphosis with parenteral hyperalimentation. *Journal of the American Medical Association*, **235**, 1249–1252.
17. Anderson, B.B., O'Brien, H., Griffen, G.E. & Mollin, D.L. (1980) Hydrolysis of pyridoxal-5′-phosphate in plasma in conditions with raised alkaline phosphatase. *Gut*, **21**, 192–194.
18. Anderson, J.L. (1972) Acalculous cholecystitis—a possible compli-

cation of parenteral hyperalimentation. Report of a case. *Medical Annals of the District of Columbia*, **41**, 438–450.
19. Arky, R.A. (1971) The effect of alcohol on carbohydrate metabolism: carbohydrate metabolism in alcoholics. In Kissin, B. & Begleiter, H. (eds) *The Biology of Alcoholism*, vol. 1 *Biochemistry*, pp. 197–227. New York: Plenum Press.
20. Armstrong, M.D. & Stave, U. (1973) A study of plasma free amino acid levels. I. Study of factors affecting validity of amino acid analyses. *Metabolism*, **22**, 549–560.
21. Arroyo, V. & Rodés, J. (1975) A rational approach to the treatment of ascites. *Postgraduate Medical Journal*, **51**, 558–562.
22. Arroyo, V., Ginés, P., Planas, R. *et al.* (1986) Management of patients with cirrhosis and ascites. *Seminars in Liver Disease*, **6**, 353–369.
23. Atkinson, M., Nordin, B.E.C. & Sherlock, S. (1956) Malabsorption and bone disease in prolonged obstructive jaundice. *Quarterly Journal of Medicine*, **25**, 299–312.
24. Ayub, A. & Faloon, W.W. (1979) Gallstones, obesity and jejunoileostomy. *Surgical Clinics of North America*, **59**, 1095–1101.
25. Baines, M. (1978) Detection and incidence of B and C vitamin deficiency in alcohol-related illness. *Annals of Clinical Biochemistry*, **15**, 307–312.
26. Baker, A.L. & Rosenberg, I.H. (1987) Hepatic complications of total parenteral nutrition. *American Journal of Medicine*, **82**, 489–497.
27. Baker, H., Frank, O. & DeAngelis, B. (1987) Plasma vitamin B_{12} titres as indicators of disease severity and mortality of patients with alcoholic hepatitis. *Alcohol and Alcoholism*, **22**, 1–5.
28. Baker, H., Frank, O., Ziffer, H. *et al.* (1964) Effect of hepatic disease on liver B-complex vitamin titers. *American Journal of Clinical Nutrition*, **14**, 1–6.
29. Balistreri, W.F. & Bove, K.E. (1990) Hepatobiliary consequences of parenteral alimentation. In Popper, H. & Schaffner, F. (eds) *Progress in Liver Diseases*, vol. IX, pp. 567–601. Philadelphia: W.B. Saunders.
30. Barbara, L., Sama, C., Morselli Labate, A.M. *et al.* (1987) A population study on the prevalence of gallstone disease: the Sirmione Study. *Hepatology*, **7**, 913–917.
31. Barry, M. (1974) Progress report: iron and the liver. *Gut*, **15**; 324–334.
32. Barry, R.E., Barisch, J., Bray, G.A. *et al.* (1977) Intestinal adaptation after jejunoileal bypass in man. *American Journal of Clinical Nutrition*, **30**, 32–42.
33. Bayoumi, R.A. & Rosalki, S.B. (1976) Evaluation of methods of coenzyme activation of erythrocyte enzymes for detection of vitamins B_1, B_2, and B_6. *Clinical Chemistry*, **22**, 327–335.
34. Beale, E.F., Nelson, R.M., Bucciarelli, R.L. *et al.* (1979) Intrahepatic cholestasis associated with parenteral nutrition in premature infants. *Pediatrics*, **64**, 342–347.

35. Bean, W.B., Vitter, R.W. & Blankenhorn, M.A. (1949) Incidence of pellagra. *Journal of the American Medical Association*, **140**, 872–873.

36. Beattie, A.D. & Sherlock, S. (1976) Ascorbic acid deficiency in liver disease. *Gut*, **17**, 571–575.

37. Beaumont, C., Fauchet, R., Phung, L.N. *et al.* (1987) Porphyria cutanea tarda and HLA-linked hemochromatosis. Evidence against a systematic association. *Gastroenterology*, **92**, 1833–1838.

38. Bell, H., Nilsson, A., Norum, K.R. *et al.* (1989) Retinol and retinyl esters in patients with alcoholic liver disease. *Journal of Hepatology*, **8**, 26–31.

39. Bendich, A. & Langseth, L. (1989) Safety of vitamin A. *American Journal of Clinical Nutrition*, **49**, 358–371.

40. Bengoa, J.M., Hanauer, S.B., Sitrin, M.D. *et al.* (1985) Pattern and prognosis of liver function test abnormalities during parenteral nutrition in inflammatory bowel disease. *Hepatology*, **5**, 79–84.

41. Benjamin, D.R. (1982) Cholelithiasis in infants: the role of total parenteral nutrition and gastrointestinal dysfunction. *Journal of Pediatric Surgery*, **17**, 386–389.

42. Bennion, L.J. & Grundy, S.M. (1978) Risk factors for the development of cholelithiasis in man. *New England Journal of Medicine*, **299**, 1161–1167.

43. Berenyi, M.R., Straus, B. & Cruz, D. (1974) In vitro and in vivo studies of cellular immunity in alcoholic cirrhosis. *American Journal of Digestive Diseases*, **19**, 199–205.

44. Bernstein, J., Chang, C.H., Brough, A.J. & Heidelberger, K.P. (1977) Conjugated hyperbilirubinemia in infancy associated with parenteral alimentation. *Journal of Pediatrics*, **90**, 361–367.

45. Bettger, W.J. & O'Dell, B.L. (1981) A critical physiological role of zinc in the structure and function of biomembranes. *Life Sciences*, **28**, 1425–1438.

46. Bhandari, B., Sharda, B. & Mehta, R. (1981) Study of zinc and copper in Indian childhood cirrhosis. *Journal of the Association of Physicians of India*, **29**, 641–644.

47. Bieri, J.G., Corash, L. & Hubbard, V.S. (1983) Medical uses of vitamin E. *New England Journal of Medicine*, **308**, 1063–1071.

48. Bistrian, B.R., Blackburn, G.L., Hallowell, E. & Heddle, R. (1974) Protein status of general surgical patients. *Journal of the American Medical Association*, **230**, 858–860.

49. Bistrian, B.R., Blackburn, G.L., Vitale, J. *et al.* (1976) Prevalence of malnutrition in general medical patients. *Journal of the American Medical Association*, **235**, 1567–1570.

50. Blackburn, G.L., Bistrian, B.R. & Maini, B.S. (1976) *Manual for Nutritional/Metabolic Assessment of the Hospitalised Patient*. Chicago: American College of Surgeons.

51. Blackburn, G.L., Bistrian, B.R., Maini, B.S. *et al.* (1977) Nutritional and metabolic assessment of the hospitalized patient. *Journal of Parenteral and Enteral Nutrition*, **1**, 11–22.

52. Blanchard, R.A., Furie, B.C., Jorgensen, M. *et al.* (1981) Acquired vitamin K-dependent carboxylation deficiency in liver disease. *New England Journal of Medicine*, **305**, 242–248.

53. Blass, J.P. & Gibson, G.E. (1977) Abnormality of a thiamine-requiring enzyme in patients with Wernicke–Korsakoff syndrome. *New England Journal of Medicine*, **297**, 1367–1370.

54. Blendis, L.M. (1989) Nutritional management of patients with chronic liver disease. *Baillière's Clinical Gastroenterology*, **3**, 91–108.

55. Blendis, L.M., Harrison, J.E., Russell, D.M. *et al.* (1986) Effects of peritoneovenous shunting on body composition. *Gastroenterology*, **90**, 127–134.

56. Blum, K., Noble, E.P., Sheridan, P.J. *et al.* (1990) Allelic association of human dopamine D_2 receptor gene in alcoholism. *Journal of the American Medical Association*, **263**, 2055–2060.

57. Bode, J.C., Hanisch, P., Henning, H. *et al.* (1988) Hepatic zinc content in patients with various stages of alcoholic liver disease and in patients with chronic active and chronic persistent hepatitis. *Hepatology*, **8**, 1605–1609.

58. Boelhouwer, R.U., King, W.W., Kingsnorth, A.N. *et al.* (1983) Fat-based (Intralipid 20%) versus carbohydrate-based total parenteral nutrition: effects on hepatic structure and function in rats. *Journal of Parenteral and Enteral Nutrition*, **7**, 530–533.

59. Bollet, A.J. & Owens, S. (1973) Evaluation of nutritional status of selected hospitalized patients. *American Journal of Clinical Nutrition*, **26**, 931–938.

60. Bonjour, J.P. (1980) Vitamins and alcoholism. III. Vitamin B_6. *International Journal for Vitamin and Nutrition Research*, **50**, 215–230.

61. Bonjour, J.P. (1980) Vitamins and alcoholism. V. Riboflavin, VI. Niacin, VII. Pantothenic acid, and VIII. Biotin. *International Journal for Vitamin and Nutrition Research*, **50**, 425–440.

62. Bory, F., Kravetz, D., Bruguera, M. *et al.* (1982) Estudio controlada sobre el efecto nutricional de una nueva dieta enteral en la cirrosis hepática. *Gastroenterologia y Hepatologia*, **5**, 371–377.

63. Bothwell, T.H., Seftel, H., Jacobs, P. *et al.* (1964) Iron overload in Bantu subjects: studies on the availability of iron in Bantu beer. *American Journal of Clinical Nutrition*, **14**, 47–51.

64. Bothwell, T.H., Bradlow, B.A., Jacobs, P. *et al.* (1964) Iron metabolism in scurvy with special reference to erythropoiesis. *British Journal of Haematology*, **10**, 50–58.

65. Bowyer, B.A., Miles, J.M., Haymond, M.W. & Fleming, C.R. (1988) L-Carnitine therapy in home parenteral nutrition patients with abnormal liver tests and low plasma carnitine concentrations. *Gastroenterology*, **94**, 434–438.

66. Bowyer, B.A., Fleming, C.R., Ludwig, J. *et al.* (1985) Does long-term home parenteral nutrition in adult patients cause chronic liver disease? *Journal of Parenteral and Enteral Nutrition*, **9**, 11–17.

67. Bowyer, B.A., Fleming, C.R, Ilstrup, D. *et al.* (1986) Plasma carnitine levels in patients receiving home parenteral nutrition. *American Journal of Clinical Nutrition*, **43**, 85–91.

68. Boyett, J.D. & Sullivan, J.F. (1970) Distribution of protein-bound zinc in normal and cirrhotic serum. *Metabolism*, **19**, 148–157.

69. Boyett, J.D. & Sullivan, J.F. (1970) Zinc and collagen content of cirrhotic liver. *American Journal of Digestive Diseases*, **15**, 797–802.

70. Braddeley, R.M. (1976) Results of jejuno-ileostomy for gross refractory obesity. *British Journal of Surgery*, **63**, 801–806.

71. Braidman, I.P. & Anderson, D.C. (1985) Extra-endocrine functions of vitamin D. *Clinical Endocrinology*, **23**, 445–460.

72. Bray, G.A. (1979) Nomogram for body mass index. In *Obesity in America*. US Department of Health, Education and Welfare, Publication No. (NIH) 79-359, p.6. Washington D.C.: US Department of Health, Education and Welfare.

73. Breen, K.J., Buttigieg, R., Iossifidis, S. *et al.* (1985) Jejunal uptake of thiamin hydrochloride in man: influence of alcoholism and alcohol. *American Journal of Clinical Nutrition*, **42**, 121–126.

74. Brewer, G.J., Hill, G.M., Prasad, A.S. *et al.* (1983) Oral zinc therapy for Wilson's disease. *Annals of Internal Medicine*, **99**, 314–320.

75. Brissot, P., Le Treut, A., Dien, G. *et al.* (1978) Hypovitaminemia A in idiopathic hemochromatosis and hepatic cirrhosis. Role of retinol-binding protein and zinc. *Digestion*, **17**, 469–478.

76. Broomfield, P., Chopra, R., Sheinbaum, R. *et al.* (1987) Formation and prevention of lithogenic bile and gallstones during weight loss. *Gastroenterology*, **92**, 1721 (abstract).

77. Brown, L.M., Rowe, A.E., Ryle, P.R. *et al.* (1983) Efficacy of vitamin supplementation in chronic alcoholics undergoing detoxification. *Alcohol and Alcoholism*, **18**, 157–166.

78. Brown, R.G., O'Leary, J.P. & Woodward, E.R. (1974) Hepatic effects of jejunoileal bypass for morbid obesity. *American Journal of Surgery*, **127**, 53–58.

79. Buchwald, H., Lober, P.H. & Varco, R.I. (1974) Liver biopsy findings in seventy-seven consecutive patients undergoing jejuno-ileal bypass for morbid obesity. *American Journal of Surgery*, **127**, 48–52.

80. Bucuvalas, J.C., Cutfield, W., Horn, J. *et al.* (1990) Resistance to the growth-promoting and metabolic effects of growth hormone in children with chronic liver disease. *Journal of Pediatrics*, **117**, 397–402.

81. Bunout, D., Gattas, V., Iturriaga, H. *et al.* (1983) Nutritional status of alcoholic patients: its possible relationship to alcoholic liver damage. *American Journal of Clinical Nutrition*, **38**, 469–473.

82. Bunout, D., Aicardi, V., Hirsch, S. *et al.* (1989) Nutritional support in hospitalized patients with alcoholic liver disease. *European Journal of Clinical Nutrition*, **43**, 615–621.

83. Burch, R.E., Hahn, H.K.J. & Sullivan, J.F. (1978) Other metals and the liver, with particular reference to zinc. In Powell, L. (ed.), *Metals and the Liver*, pp. 333–361. New York: Dekker.

84. Burke, B.S. (1947) Dietary history as a tool in research. *Journal of the American Dietetic Association*, **23**, 1041–1046.

85. Butterworth, C.E., Jr. & Weinsier, R.L. (1978) Malnutrition in hospital patients: assessment and treatment. In Goodhart, R.S. & Shils, M.E. (eds), *Modern Nutrition in Health and Disease*, 6th edn, pp. 667–684. Philadelphia: Lea and Febiger.

86. Buzby, G.P., Mullen, J.L., Stein, T.P. & Rosato, E.F. (1981) Manipulation of TPN caloric substrate and fatty infiltration of liver. *Journal of Surgical Research*, **31**, 46–54.

87. Caballería Rovira, E., Arogo López, J.V., Masso Ubeda, R.M. et al. (1987) Tratamiento de la encefalopatía hepática con aminoácidos de cadena ramificada (BCAA) por vía oral: 1. Encefalopatía hepática aguda. *Revista Española de los Enfermedades del Aparato Digestive*, **72**, 116–122.

88. Cabré, E., Periago, J.L., Abad-Lacruz, A. et al. (1988) Polyunsaturated fatty acid deficiency in liver cirrhosis: its relation to associated protein-energy malnutrition (preliminary report). *American Journal of Gastroenterology*, **83**, 712–717.

89. Cabré, E., Gonzalez-Huix, F., Abad-Lacruz, A. et al. (1990) Effect of total enteral nutrition on the short-term outcome of severely malnourished cirrhotics. A randomized controlled trial. *Gastroenterology*, **98**, 715–720.

90. Cabré, E., Periago, J.L., Abad-Lacruz, A. et al. (1990) Plasma fatty acid profile in advanced cirrhosis: unsaturation deficit of lipid fractions. *American Journal of Gastroenterology*, **85**, 1597–1604.

91. Cairns, S.R., Kark, A.E. & Peters, T.J. (1986) Raised hepatic free fatty acids in a patient with acute fatty liver after gastric surgery for morbid obesity. *Journal of Clinical Pathology*, **39**, 647–649.

92. Calvey, H., Davis, M. & Williams, R. (1985) Controlled trial of nutritional supplementation, with and without branched chain amino acid enrichment, in treatment of acute alcoholic hepatitis. *Journal of Hepatology*, **1**, 141–151.

93. Camilo, M.E. & Pinto Correia, J. (1982) Estvido da nutriçao na doença hepática alcoólica. *Revista Portuguesa de Clínica e Terapêutica*, **7**, 43–48.

94. Camilo, M.E., Morgan, M.Y. & Sherlock, S. (1981) Red blood cell transketolase activity in alcoholic liver disease. *Scandinavian Journal of Gastroenterology*, **16**, 273–279.

95. Campbell, T.C., Chen, J.S., Liv, C.B. et al. (1990) Nonassociation of aflatoxin with primary liver cancer in a cross-sectional ecological survey in the People's Republic of China. *Cancer Research*, **50**, 6882–6893.

96. Canalese, J., Sewell, R.B., Poston, L. & Williams, R. (1985) Zinc abnormalities in fulminant hepatic failure. *Australian and New Zealand Journal of Medicine*, **15**, 7–9.

97. Cano, N. & Gerolami, A. (1983) Intrahepatic cholestasis during total parenteral nutrition. *Lancet*, **1**, 985 (letter).

98. Cano, N., Cicero, F., Ranieri, F. et al. (1986) Ultrasonographic study of gallbladder motility during total parenteral nutrition. *Gastroenterology*, **91**, 313–317.

99. Capron, J.-P., Ginston, J.-L., Herve, M.-A. & Braillon, A. (1983) Metronidazole in prevention of cholestasis associated with total parenteral nutrition. *Lancet*, **1**, 446–447.

100. Carney, M.W.P. & Sheffield, B. (1978) Serum folate and B_{12} and haematological status of in-patient alcoholics. *British Journal of Addiction*, **73**, 3–8.

101. Carpentier, Y.A. & Van Brandt, M. (1981) Effect of total parenteral nutrition on liver function. *Acta Chirurgia Belgica*, **80**, 141–144.

102. Casaril, M., Stanzial, A.M., Gabrielli, G.B. et al. (1989) Serum selenium in liver cirrhosis: correlation with markers of fibrosis. *Clinica Chimica Acta*, **182**, 221–227.

103. Cerra, F.B., McMillen, M., Angelico, R. et al. (1983) Cirrhosis, encephalopathy, and improved results with metabolic support. *Surgery*, **94**, 612–619.

104. Cerra, F.B., Cheung, N.K., Fischer, J.E. et al. (1985) Disease-specific amino acid infusion (F080) in hepatic encephalopathy: a prospective, randomised, double-blind, controlled trial. *Journal of Parenteral and Enteral Nutrition*, **9**, 288–295.

105. Chalmers, T.C. (1972) Potential contributors of multiple risk factors in the etiology of cirrhosis. In Lee, D.H.K. & Loten, P. (eds), *Multiple Factors in the Causation of Environmentally-Induced Disease*, pp. 29–42. New York: Academic Press.

106. Chalmers, T.C., Eckhardt, R.D., Reynolds, W.E. et al. (1955) The treatment of acute infectious hepatitis. Controlled studies of the effects of diet, rest, and physical reconditioning on the acute course of the disease and on the incidence of relapses and residual abnormalities. *Journal of Clinical Investigation*, **34**, 1163–1235.

107. Chapman, R.W., Morgan, M.Y., Bell, R. & Sherlock, S. (1983) Hepatic iron uptake in alcoholic liver disease. *Gastroenterology*, **84**, 143–147.

108. Chapman, R.W., Morgan, M.Y., Boss, A.M. & Sherlock, S. (1983) Acute and chronic effects of alcohol on iron absorption. *Digestive Diseases and Sciences*, **28**, 321–327.

109. Chapman, R.W., Morgan, M.Y., Laulicht, M. et al. (1982) Hepatic iron stores and markers of iron overload in alcoholics and patients with idiopathic hemochromatosis. *Digestive Diseases and Sciences*, **27**, 909–916.

110. Chapman, R.W.G., Hussain, M.A.M., Gorman, A. et al. (1982) Effect of ascorbic acid deficiency on serum ferritin concentration in patients with β-thalassaemia major and iron overload. *Journal of Clinical Pathology*, **35**, 487–491.

111. Charlton, R.W. & Bothwell, T.H. (1983) Iron absorption. *Annual Review of Medicine*, **34**, 55–68.

112. Charlton, R.W., Jacobs, P., Seftel, H. & Bothwell, T.H. (1964) Effect of alcohol on iron absorption. *British Medical Journal*, **2**, 1427–1429.

113. Chase, H.P., Kumar, V., Caldwell, R.T. & O'Brien, D. (1980) Kwashiorkor in the United States. *Pediatrics*, **66**, 972–976.

114. Chase, R.A., Davies, M., Trewby, P.N. et al. (1978) Plasma amino acid profiles in patients with fulminant hepatic failure treated by repeated polyacrylonitrile membrane hemodialysis. *Gastroenterology*, **75**, 1033–1040.

115. Chaudhuri, A.D., Bhattacharyya, A.K. & Mukherjee, A.M. (1972) The liver in pre-kwashiorkor and kwashiorkor-marasmus syndromes. *Transactions of the Royal Society of Tropical Medicine and Hygiene*, **66**, 258–262.

116. Chawla, R.K., Wolf, D.C., Kutner, M.H. & Bonkovsky, H.L. (1989) Choline may be an essential nutrient in malnourished patients with cirrhosis. *Gastroenterology*, **97**, 1514–1520.

117. Chawla, R.K., Lewis, F.W., Kutner, M.H. et al. (1984) Plasma cysteine, cystine, and glutathione in cirrhosis. *Gastroenterology*, **87**, 770–776.

118. Chen, C. & Liao, T. (1960) Histochemical study on riboflavin. *Journal of Vitaminology*, **6**, 171–195.

119. Christie, M.L., Sack, D.M., Pomposelli, J. & Horst, D. (1985) Enriched branched-chain amino acid formula versus a casein-based supplement in the treatment of cirrhosis. *Journal of Parenteral and Enteral Nutrition*, **9**, 671–678.

120. Clain, D.J. & Lefkowitch, J.H. (1987) Fatty liver disease in morbid obesity. *Gastroenterology Clinics of North America*, **16**, 239–252.

121. Coates, R.A., Halliday, M.L., Rankin, J.G. et al. (1986) Risk of fatty infiltration or cirrhosis of the liver in relation to ethanol consumption: a case-control study. *Clinical and Investigative Medicine*, **9**, 26–32.

122. Coburn, S.P. & Mahuren, J.D. (1983) A versatile cation-exchange procedure for measuring the seven major forms of vitamin B_6 in biological samples. *Analytical Biochemistry*, **129**, 310–317.

123. Cohen, C. & Olsen, M.M. (1981) Pediatric total parenteral nutrition: liver histopathology. *Archives of Pathology and Laboratory Medicine*, **105**, 152–156.

124. Cohn, S.H. (1987) New concepts of body composition. In Ellis, K.J., Yasumura, S. & Morgan, W.D. (eds), *In Vivo Body Composition Studies*, pp. 1–14. London: Institute of Physical Sciences in Medicine.

125. Comp, P.C., Jacocks, R.M., Ferrell, G.L. & Esmon, C.T. (1982) Activation of protein C in vivo. *Journal of Clinical Investigation*, **70**, 127–134.

126. Compston, J.E. (1986) Hepatic osteodystrophy: vitamin D metabolism in patients with liver disease. *Gut*, **27**, 1073–1090.

127. Compston, J.E., Crowe, J.P. & Horton, L.W.L. (1979) Treatment of osteomalacia associated with primary biliary cirrhosis with oral 1-alpha-hydroxy vitamin D_3. *British Medical Journal*, **2**, 309.

128. Compston, J.E., Horton, L.W.L. & Thompson, R.P.H. (1979) Treatment of osteomalacia associated with primary biliary cirrhosis with parenteral vitamin D_2 or oral 25-hydroxyvitamin D_3. *Gut*, **20**, 133–136.

129. Conn, H.O., Leevy, C.M., Vlahcevic, Z.R. et al. (1977) Comparison of lactulose and neomycin in the treatment of chronic portal-

systemic encephalopathy. A double blind controlled trial. *Gastroenterology*, **72**, 573–583.

130. Conrad, M.E. & Barton, J.C. (1980) Anemia and iron kinetics in alcoholism. *Seminars in Hematology*, **17**, 149–163.

131. Cook, G.C. & Hutt, M.S.R. (1967) The liver after kwashiorkor. *British Medical Journal*, **3**, 454–457.

132. Cooper, J.R. & Pincus, J.H. (1979) The role of thiamine in nervous tissue. *Neurochemical Research*, **4**, 223–229.

133. Corrodi, P., Wideman, P.A., Sutter, V.L. *et al.* (1978) Bacterial flora of the small bowel before and after bypass procedure for morbid obesity. *Journal of Infectious Diseases*, **137**, 1–6.

134. Cousins, R.J. (1979) Regulatory aspects of zinc metabolism in liver and intestine. *Nutrition Reviews*, **37**, 97–103.

135. Creutzfeldt, W., Frerichs, H. & Sickinger, K. (1970) Liver diseases and diabetes mellitus. In Popper, H. & Schaffner, F. (eds), *Progress in Liver Diseases*, vol. III, pp. 371–407. London: Heinemann.

136. Crosby, W.H. (1977) Current concepts in nutrition: who needs iron? *New England Journal of Medicine*, **297**, 543–545.

137. Cuthbert, J.A., Pak, C.Y., Zerwekh, J.E. *et al.* (1984) Bone disease in primary biliary cirrhosis: increased bone resorption and turnover in the absence of osteoporosis or osteomalacia. *Hepatology*, **4**, 1–8.

138. Dahlstrom, K.A., Ament, M.E., Laidlaw, S.A. & Kopple, J.D. (1988) Plasma amino acid concentrations in children receiving long-term parenteral nutrition. *Journal of Pediatric Gastroenterology and Nutrition*, **7**, 748–754.

139. D'Amico, G., Morabito, A., Pagliaro, L. & Marubini, E. (1986) Survival and prognostic indicators in compensated and decompensated cirrhosis. *Digestive Diseases and Sciences*, **31**, 468–475.

140. Damodaran, K. & Hartfall, S.J. (1944) Infective hepatitis in the garrison of Malta. *British Medical Journal*, **2**, 587–590.

141. Dancy, M., Evans, G., Gaitonde, M.K. & Maxwell, J.D. (1984) Blood thiamine and thiamine phosphate ester concentrations in alcoholic and non-alcoholic liver diseases. *British Medical Journal*, **289**, 79–82.

142. Danford, D.E. & Munro, H.N. (1988) Liver in relation to B vitamins. In Arias, I.M., Jakoby, W.B., Popper, H., Schachter, D. & Shafritz, D.A. (eds) *The Liver: Biology and Pathology,* 2nd edn, pp. 505–523. New York: Raven Press.

143. Danö, P., Nielson, O.V., Petri, M. & Jörgensen, B. (1975) Liver morphology and liver function before and after intestinal shunt operation for obesity. *Scandinavian Journal of Gastroenterology*, **10**, 409–416.

144. Dastur, D.K., Santhadevi, N., Quadros, E.V. *et al.* (1976) The B-vitamins in malnutrition with alcoholism: a model of intervention relationships. *British Journal of Nutrition*, **36**, 143–159.

145. Davidson, C.S. (1970) Nutrition, geography, and liver diseases. *American Journal of Clinical Nutrition*, **23**, 427–436.

146. Dawson, A.M., de Groote, J., Rosenthal, W.S. & Sherlock, S. (1957) Blood pyruvic-acid and alpha-ketoglutaric-acid levels in liver disease and hepatic coma. *Lancet*, **1**, 392–396.

147. Day, R.C., Harry, D.S., Owen, J.S. *et al.* (1979) Lecithin-cholesterol acyltransferase and the lipoprotein abnormalities of parenchymal liver disease. *Clinical Science*, **56**, 575–583.

148. De Bruijn, K.M., Blendis, L.M., Zilm, D.H. *et al.* (1983) Effect of dietary protein manipulations in subclinical portal-systemic encephalopathy. *Gut*, **24**, 53–60.

149. Deitel, M. & Petrov, I. (1987) Incidence of symptomatic gallstones after bariatric operations. *Surgery, Gynecology and Obstetrics*, **164**, 549–552.

150. Demarquez, J.L., Cadier, L., Billeaud, C. *et al.* (1980) Surveillance de la nutrition parentérale chez l'enfant: intérêt de l'échographie de la vésicule et dos voies biliaires. *Agressologie*, **21**, 137–141.

151. Denny-Brown, D. (1947) Neurological conditions resulting from prolonged and severe dietary restriction. *Medicine*, **26**, 41–113.

152. Department of Health and Social Security. (1979) *Recommended Daily Intakes of Energy and Nutrients for Groups of People in the United Kingdom. Report by the Committee on Medical Aspects of Food Policy.* Report on Health and Social Subjects, No. 15. London: HMSO.

153. Descos, L., Gauthier, A., Levy, V.G. *et al.* (1983) Comparison of six treatments of ascites in patients with liver cirrhosis. A clinical trial. *Hepatogastroenterology*, **30**, 15–20.

154. Devgun, M.S., Fiabane, A., Paterson, C.R. *et al.* (1981) Vitamin and mineral nutrition in chronic alcoholics including patients with Korsakoff's psychosis. *British Journal of Nutrition*, **45**, 469–472.

155. Devor, E.J. & Colinger, C.R. (1989) Genetics of alcoholism. *Annual Review of Genetics*, **23**, 19–36.

156. Diamond, T., Stiel, D., Lunzer, M. *et al.* (1989) Ethanol reduces bone formation and may cause osteoporosis. *American Journal of Medicine*, **86**, 282–288.

157. Dibble, J.B., Sheridan, P., Hampshire, R. *et al.* (1982) Osteomalacia, vitamin D deficiency and cholestasis in chronic liver disease. *Quarterly Journal of Medicine*, **51**, 89–103.

158. DiCecco, S.R., Wieners, E.J., Wiesner, R.H. *et al.* (1989) Assessment of nutritional status of patients with end-stage liver disease undergoing liver transplantation. *Mayo Clinic Proceedings*, **64**, 95–102.

159. Diehl, A.M., Goodman, Z. & Ishak, K.G. (1988) Alcohollike liver disease in nonalcoholics. A clinical and histologic comparison with alcohol-induced liver injury. *Gastroenterology*, **95**, 1056–1062.

160. Diehl, A.M., Potter, J., Boitnott, J. *et al.* (1984) Relationship between pyridoxal 5'-phosphate deficiency and aminotransferase levels in alcoholic hepatitis. *Gastroenterology*, **86**, 632–636.

161. Diehl, A.M., Boitnott, J.K., Herlong, H.F. *et al.* (1985) Effect of parenteral amino acid supplementation in alcoholic hepatitis. *Hepatology*, **5**, 57–63.

162. Dietze, G., Wicklmayr, M., Hepp, K.D. *et al.* (1976) On gluconeogenesis of human liver. Accelerated hepatic glucose formation induced by increased precursor supply. *Diabetologia*, **12**, 555–561.

163. Dinsmore, W., Callender, M.E., McMaster, D. *et al.* (1985) Zinc absorption in alcoholics using zinc-65. *Digestion*, **32**, 238–242.

164. Dogliotti, M., Liebowiez, M., Downing, D.T. & Strauss, J.S. (1977) Nutritional influences of pellagra on sebum composition. *British Journal of Dermatology*, **97**, 25–28.

165. Drake, J.R. & Fitch, C.D. (1980) Status of vitamin E as an erythropoietic factor. *American Journal of Clinical Nutrition*, **33**, 2386–2393.

166. Drenick, E.J., Fisher, J. & Johnson, D. (1982) Hepatic steatosis after intestinal bypass—prevention and reversal by metronidazole, irrespective of protein–calorie malnutrition. *Gastroenterology*, **82**, 535–548.

167. Drenick, E.J., Simmons, F. & Murphy, J.F. (1970) Effect on hepatic morphology of treatment of obesity by fasting, reducing diets and small-bowel bypass. *New England Journal of Medicine*, **282**, 829–834.

168. Drenick, E.J., Ament, M.E., Finegold, S.M. & Passaro, E., Jr. (1977) Bypass enterology: an inflammatory process in the excluded segment with systemic complications. *American Journal of Clinical Nutrition*, **30**, 76–89.

169. Dubey, S.S., Palodhi, G.R. & Jain, A.K. (1987) Ascorbic acid, dehydroascorbic acid and glutathione in liver disease. *Indian Journal of Physiology and Pharmacology*, **31**, 279–283.

170. Dunn, L., Hulman, S., Weiner, J. & Kliegman, R. (1988) Beneficial effects of early hypocaloric enteral feeding on neonatal gastrointestinal function: preliminary report of a randomized trial. *Journal of Pediatrics*, **112**, 622–629.

171. Durnin, J.V.G.A. & Rahaman, M.M. (1967) The assessment of the amount of fat in the human body from measurement of skin fold thickness. *British Journal of Nutrition*, **21**, 681–689.

172. Dutta, S.K., Miller, P.A., Greenberg, L.B. & Levander, O.A. (1983) Selenium and acute alcoholism. *American Journal of Clinical Nutrition*, **38**, 713–718.

173. Dworkin, B.M., Rosenthal, W.S., Gordon, G.G. & Jankowski, R.H. (1984) Diminished blood selenium levels in alcoholics. *Alcoholism: Clinical and Experimental Research*, **8**, 535–538.

174. Dworkin, B.M., Rosenthal, W.S., Stahl, R.E. & Panesar, N.K. (1988) Decreased hepatic selenium content in alcoholic cirrhosis. *Digestive Diseases and Sciences*, **33**, 1213–1217.

175. Dworkin, B., Rosenthal, W.S., Jankowski, R.H. *et al.* (1985) Low blood selenium levels in alcoholics with and without advanced liver disease. Correlations with clinical and nutritional status. *Digestive Diseases and Sciences*, **30**, 838–844.

176. Egberts, E.-H., Schomerus, H., Hamster, W. & Jürgens, P. (1985) Branched chain amino acids in the treatment of latent portosystemic encephalopathy. A double-blind placebo-controlled crossover study. *Gastroenterology*, **88**, 887–895.

177. Elias, E., Muller, D.P.R. & Scott, J. (1981) Association of

spinocerebellar disorders with cystic fibrosis or chronic childhood cholestasis and a very low serum vitamin E. *Lancet*, **2**, 1319–1321.

178. Emery, P.W., Edwards, R.H.T., Rennie, M.J. *et al.* (1984) Protein synthesis in muscle measured in vivo in cachectic patients with cancer. *British Medical Journal*, **289**, 584–586.

179. Epstein, O., Kato, Y., Dick, R. & Sherlock, S. (1982) Vitamin D, hydroxyapatite, and calcium gluconate in treatment of cortical bone thinning in post-menopausal women with primary biliary cirrhosis. *American Journal of Clinical Nutrition*, **36**, 426–430.

180. Erenoglu, E., Edreira, J.G. & Patek, A.J. Jr. (1964) Observations on patients with Laennec's cirrhosis receiving alcohol while on controlled diets. *Annals of Internal Medicine*, **60**, 814–823.

181. Eriksson, L.S. & Conn, H.O. (1989) Branched-chain amino acids in the management of hepatic encephalopathy: an analysis of variants. *Hepatology*, **10**, 228–246.

182. Eriksson, L.S., Persson, A. & Wahren, J. (1982) Branched-chain amino acids in the treatment of chronic hepatic encephalopathy. *Gut*, **23**, 801–806.

183. Eriksson, L.S., Thorne, A. & Wahren, J. (1989) Diet-induced thermogenesis in patients with liver cirrhosis. *Clinical Physiology*, **9**, 131–141.

184. Evans, G.W. (1986) Zinc and its deficiency diseases. *Clinical Physiology and Biochemistry*, **4**, 94–98.

185. Faloon, W.W. (1988) Hepatobiliary effects of obesity and weight-reducing surgery. *Seminars in Liver Disease*, **8**, 229–236.

186. Faloon, W.W., Rubulis, A., Knipp, J. *et al.* (1977) Fecal fat, bile acid and sterol excretion and biliary lipid changes in jejuno-ileostomy patients. *American Journal of Clinical Nutrition*, **30**, 21–31.

187. Farrell, G.C., Bhathal, P.S. & Powell, L.W. (1977) Abnormal liver function in chronic hypervitaminosis A. *American Journal of Digestive Diseases*, **22**, 724–728.

188. Farrell, M.K., Balistreri, W.F. & Suchy, F.J. (1982) Serum-sulfated lithocholate as an indicator of cholestasis during parenteral nutrition in infants and children. *Journal of Parenteral and Enteral Nutrition*, **6**, 30–33.

189. Fennelly, J., Baker, H., Frank, O. & Leevy, C.M. (1963) Deficiency of thiamine pyrophosphate apoenzyme in liver disease. *Clinical Research*, **11**, 182 (abstract).

190. Fennelly, J., Frank, O., Baker, H. & Leevy, C.M. (1964) Peripheral neuropathy of the alcoholic: 1, aetiological role of aneurin and other B-complex vitamins. *British Medical Journal*, **2**, 1290–1292.

191. Fennelly, J., Frank, O., Baker, H. & Leevy, C.M. (1967) Red blood cell-transketolase activity in malnourished alcoholics with cirrhosis. *American Journal of Clinical Nutrition*, **20**, 946–949.

192. Fenton, J.C.B., Knight, E.J. & Humpherson, P.L. (1966) Milk-and-cheese diet in portal-systemic encephalopathy. *Lancet*, **1**, 164–165.

193. Fern, E.B., Garlick, P.J. & Waterlow, J.C. (1985) Apparent compartmentation of body nitrogen in one human subject: its consequences in measuring the rate of whole-body protein synthesis with ^{15}N. *Clinical Science*, **68**, 271–282.

194. Festa, M.D., Anderson, H.L., Dowdy, R.P. & Ellersieck, M.R. (1985) Effect of zinc intake on copper excretion and retention in men. *American Journal of Clinical Nutrition*, **41**, 285–292.

195. Fiaccadori, F., Ghinelli, F., Pedretti, G. *et al.* (1984) Different nutritional approaches in liver cirrhosis. Effects on nitrogen balance. Preliminary report. In Gentilini, P. & Dianzani, M.U. (eds) *Frontiers of Gastrointestinal Research*, vol. 8. *Liver Cirrhosis*, pp. 254–265. Basel: Karger.

196. Fiaccadori, F., Ghinelli, F., Pedretti, G. *et al.* (1985) Branched-chain enriched amino acid solutions in the treatment of hepatic encephalopathy: a controlled trial. *Italian Journal of Gastroenterology*, **17**, 5–10.

197. Figueroa, W.G. (1953) Lack of avitaminosis among alcoholics: its relation to fortification of cereal products and general nutritional status of the population. *Journal of Clinical Nutrition*, **1**, 179–199.

198. Finkelstein, H., Champion, M.C. & Adam, J.E. (1987) Cutaneous hypersensitivity to vitamin K$_1$ injection. *Journal of the American Academy of Dermatology*, **16**, 540–545.

199. Fischer, J.E. & Baldessarini, R.J. (1971) False neurotransmitters and hepatic failure. *Lancet*, **2**, 75–80.

200. Fischer, J.E., Rosen, H.M., Ebeid, A.M. *et al.* (1976) The effect of normalisation of plasma amino acids on hepatic encephalopathy in man. *Surgery*, **80**, 77–91.

201. Fisher, R.L. (1989) Hepatobiliary abnormalities associated with total parenteral nutrition. *Gastroenterology Clinics of North America*, **18**, 645–666.

202. Fisher, R.S., Stelzer, F., Rock, E. & Malmud, L.S. (1982) Abnormal gallbladder emptying in patients with gallstones. *Digestive Diseases and Sciences*, **27**, 1019–1024.

203. Flatt, J.P. (1972) On the maximal possible rate of ketogenesis. *Diabetes*, **21**, 50–53.

204. Flink, E.B. (1981) Magnesium deficiency. Etiology and clinical spectrum. *Acta Medica Scandinavica Supplementum*, **647**, 125–137.

205. Flink, E.B., Konig, T.J. & Brown, J.L. (1955) The association of low serum magnesium concentrations and deleterious effects of ammonia in hepatic cirrhosis. *Journal of Laboratory and Clinical Medicine*, **46**, 814–815.

206. Food and Nutrition Board, National Research Council. (1989) *Recommended Daily Allowances*, 10th edn. Washington D.C.: National Academy of Sciences.

207. Fowler, B. (1985) Recent advances in the mechanism of pyridoxine-responsive disorders. *Journal of Inherited Metabolic Disease, Supplement*, **8**(1), 76–83.

208. Frank, O., Luisada-Opper, A., Sorrell, M.F. *et al.* (1971) Vitamin deficits in severe alcoholic fatty liver of man calculated from multiple reference units. *Experimental and Molecular Pathology*, **15**, 191–197.

209. Freund, H., Dienstag, J., Lehrich, J. *et al.* (1982) Infusion of branched-chain enriched amino acid solution in patients with hepatic encephalopathy. *Annals of Surgery*, **196**, 209–220.

210. Frezza, M., di Padova, C., Pozzato, G. *et al.* (1990) High blood alcohol levels in women: the role of decreased gastric alcohol dehydrogenase activity and first-pass metabolism. *New England Journal of Medicine*, **322**, 95–99.

211. Friedman, G.D., Kannel, W.B. & Dawber, T.R. (1966) The epidemiology of gallbladder disease: observations in the Framingham Study. *Journal of Chronic Diseases*, **19**, 273–292.

212. Fry, P.C., Fox, H.M. & Tao, H.G. (1976) Metabolic response to a pantothenic acid deficient diet in humans. *Journal of Nutritional Science and Vitaminology*, **22**, 339–346.

213. Gabuzda, G.J., Jr. & Davidson, C.S. (1954) Protein metabolism in patients with cirrhosis of the liver. *Annals of the New York Academy of Sciences*, **57**, 776–785.

214. Gabuzda, G.J. & Shear, L. (1970) Metabolism of dietary protein in hepatic cirrhosis. Nutritional and clinical considerations. *American Journal of Clinical Nutrition*, **23**, 479–487.

215. Galambos, J.T. (1972) Natural history of alcoholic hepatitis. III. Histological change. *Gastroenterology*, **63**, 1026–1035.

216. Galambos, J.T. (1976) Jejunoileal bypass and nutritional liver injury. *Archives of Pathology and Laboratory Medicine*, **100**, 229–231.

217. Galambos, J.T. & Wills, C.E. (1978) Relationship between 505 paired liver tests and biopsies in 242 obese patients. *Gastroenterology*, **74**, 1191–1195.

218. García-Compean, D., Uribe, M., Rico, N. *et al.* (1987) Fiber content rather than protein determines tolerance to nitrogen load in chronic portal systemic encephalopathy: a randomised trial. *Hepatology*, **7**, 1034 (abstract).

219. Gaull, G.E. (1986) Taurine as a conditionally essential nutrient in man. *Journal of the American College of Nutrition*, **5**, 121–125.

220. Gauthier, A., Levy, V.G., Quinton, A. *et al.* (1986) Salt or no salt in the treatment of cirrhotic ascites: a randomised study. *Gut*, **27**, 705–709.

221. Gerber, M.A. & Popper, H. (1972) Relation between central canals and portal tracts in alcoholic hepatitis. A contribution to the pathogenesis of cirrhosis in alcoholics. *Human Pathology*, **3**, 199–207.

222. Gillis, J., Murphy, F.R., Boxall, L.B. & Pencharz, P.B. (1982) Biotin deficiency in a child on long-term TPN. *Journal of Parenteral and Enteral Nutrition*, **6**, 308–310.

223. Gilman, A.G. (1987) G proteins: transducers of receptor-generated signals. *Annual Review of Biochemistry*, **56**, 615–649.

224. Gimsing, P., Melgaard, B., Andersen, K. *et al.* (1989) Vitamin B-12 and folate function in chronic alcoholic men with peripheral

neuropathy and encephalopathy. _Journal of Nutrition_, **119**, 416–424.

225. Gitzelmann, R., Steinmann, B. & Van den Berghe, G. (1989) Disorders of fructose metabolism. In Scriver, C.R., Beaudet, A.L., Sly, W.S. & Valle, D. (eds) _The Metabolic Basis of Inherited Diseases_, 6th edn, pp. 399–424. New York: McGraw-Hill.

226. Goldiner, W.H., Hamilton, B.P., Hyman, P.D. & Russell, R.M. (1983) Effect of the administration of zinc sulfate on hypogonadism and impotence in patients with chronic stable hepatic cirrhosis. _Journal of the American College of Nutrition_, **2**, 157–162.

227. Goldsmith, L.A. & Laberge, C. (1989) Tyrosinemia and related disorders. In Scriver, C.R., Beaudet, A.L., Sly, W.S. & Valle, D. (eds) _The Metabolic Basis of Inherited Diseases_, 6th edn, pp. 547–562. New York: McGraw-Hill.

228. Goode, H.F., Kelleher, J. & Walker, B.E. (1990) Relation between zinc status and hepatic functional reserve in patients with liver disease. _Gut_, **31**, 694–697.

229. Goodman, D.S. (1984) Vitamin A and retinoids in health and disease. _New England Journal of Medicine_, **310**, 1023–1031.

230. Goodman, D.S. (1988) Vitamin A metabolism and the liver. In Arias, I.M., Jakoby, W.B., Popper, H., Schachter, D. & Shafritz, D.A. (eds) _The Liver: Biology and Pathobiology_, 2nd edn, pp. 467–474. New York: Raven Press.

231. Goodman, Z.D. & Ishak, K.G. (1982) Occlusive venous lesions in alcoholic liver disease. A study of 200 cases. _Gastroenterology_, **83**, 786–796.

232. Gordenk, V.R., Bacon, B.R. & Brittenham, G.M. (1987) Iron overload: causes and consequences. _Annual Review of Nutrition_, **7**, 485–508.

233. Goulet, O.J., de Ville de Goyet, J., Otte, J.B. & Ricour, C. (1987). Preoperative nutritional evaluation and support for liver transplantation in children. _Transplantation Proceedings_, **19**, 3249–3255.

234. Graudal, N., Torp-Pedersen, K., Bonde, J. _et al._ (1987) The influence of hepatic insufficiency due to alcoholic cirrhosis on the erythrocyte transketolase activity (ETKA). _Liver_, **7**, 91–95.

235. Greenberger, N.J., Carley, J., Schenker, S. _et al._ (1977) Effect of vegetable and animal protein diets in chronic hepatic encephalopathy. _American Journal of Digestive Diseases_, **22**, 845–855.

236. Grungreiff, K., Abicht, K., Kluge, M. _et al._ (1988) Clinical studies on zinc in chronic liver diseases. _Zeitschrift für Gastroenterologie_, **26**, 409–415.

237. Guarnieri, G.F., Toigo, G., Situlin, R. _et al._ (1984) Muscle biopsy studies on malnutrition in patients with liver cirrhosis: preliminary results of long-term treatment with a branched-chain amino acid enriched diet. In Capocaccia, L., Fischer, J.E. & Rossi-Fanelli, F. (eds) _Hepatic Encephalopathy in Chronic Liver Failure_, pp. 193–208. New York: Plenum Press.

238. Guggenheim, M.A., Ringel, S.P., Silverman, A. & Grabert, B.E. (1982) Progressive neuromuscular disease in children with chronic cholestasis and vitamin E deficiency: diagnosis and treatment with alpha tocopherol. _Journal of Pediatrics_, **100**, 51–58.

239. Haines, N.W., Baker, A.L., Boyer, J.L. _et al._ (1981) Prognostic indicators of hepatic injury following jejunoileal bypass performed for refractory obesity: a prospective study. _Hepatology_, **1**, 161–167.

240. Hallberg, D., Holm, I., Obel, A.L. _et al._ (1967) Fat emulsions for complete intravenous nutrition. _Postgraduate Medical Journal_, **43**, 307–316.

241. Halliday, A.W., Benjamin, I.S. & Blumgart, L.H. (1988) Nutritional risk factors in major hepatobiliary surgery. _Journal of Parenteral and Enteral Nutrition_, **12**, 43–48.

242. Halstead, C.H. (1980) Folate deficiency in alcoholism. _American Journal of Clinical Nutrition_, **33**, 2736–2740.

243. Halstead, C.H. & Tamura, T. (1979) Folate deficiency in liver disease. In Davidson, C.S. (ed.) _Problems in Liver Disease_, pp. 91–100. New York: Grune and Stratton.

244. Halstead, J.A., Hackley, B., Rudzki, C. & Smith, J.C., Jr. (1968) Plasma zinc concentration in liver diseases. Comparison with normal controls and certain other chronic diseases. _Gastroenterology_, **54**, 1098–1105.

245. Halverson, J.D., Wise, L., Wazna, M.F. & Ballinger, W.F. (1978) Jejunoileal bypass for morbid obesity: a critical appraisal. _American Journal of Medicine_, **64**, 461–475.

246. Hamilton, D.L., Vest, T.K., Brown, B.S. _et al._ (1983) Liver injury with alcoholiclike hyalin after gastroplasty for morbid obesity. _Gastroenterology_, **85**, 722–726.

247. Harding, A.E., Muller, D.P.R., Thomas, P.K. & Willison, H.J. (1982) Spinocerebellar degeneration secondary to chronic intestinal malabsorption: a vitamin E deficiency syndrome. _Annals of Neurology_, **12**, 419–424.

248. Hardison, W.G. & Lee, F.I. (1966) Prognosis in acute liver disease of the alcoholic patient. _New England Journal of Medicine_, **275**, 61–66.

249. Hartcroft, W.S. (1961) Experimental reproduction of human hepatic disease. In Popper, H. & Schaffner, F. (eds) _Progress in Liver Diseases_, vol. I, pp. 68–85. New York: Grune and Stratton.

250. Hassanein, E.A. & Tankovsky, I. (1973) Disturbances of coagulation mechanism in protein-calorie malnutrition. _Tropical and Geographical Medicine_, **25**, 158–162.

251. Hathcock, J.N., Hattan, D.G., Jenkins, M.Y. _et al._ (1990) Evaluation of vitamin A toxicity. _American Journal of Clinical Nutrition_, **52**, 183–202.

252. Haussler, M.R. (1986) Vitamin D receptors: nature and function. _Annual Review of Nutrition_, **6**, 527–562.

253. Haynes, R.C. Jr. (1990) Agents affecting calcification: calcium, parathyroid hormone, calcitonin, vitamin D, and other compounds. In Gilman, A.G., Rall, T.W., Nies, A.S. & Taylor, P. (eds) _Goodman and Gilman's The Pharmacological Basis of Therapeutics_, 8th edn, pp. 1497–1522. New York: Pergamon Press.

254. Heimberger, S.L., Steiger, E., LoGerfo, P. _et al._ (1975) Reversal of severe fatty hepatic infiltration after intestinal bypass for morbid obesity by calorie-free amino acid infusion. _American Journal of Surgery_, **129**, 229–235.

255. Hell, D. & Six, P. (1977) Thiamin-, riboflavin- und pyridoxin-versorgung bei chronischem alkoholismus. _Deutsche Medizinische Wochenschrift_, **102**, 962–966.

256. Helman, R.A., Temko, M.H., Nye, S.W. & Fallon, H.J. (1971) Alcoholic hepatitis. Natural history and evaluation of prednisolone therapy. _Annals of Internal Medicine_, **74**, 311–321.

257. Henderson, J.M., Codner, M.A., Hollins, B. _et al._ (1986) The fasting B_6 vitamin profile and response to a pyridoxine load in normal and cirrhotic subjects. _Hepatology_, **6**, 464–471.

258. Henderson, L.M. (1984) Niacin. _Annual Review of Nutrition_, **3**, 289–307.

259. Herbert, V., Zalusky, R. & Davidson, C.S. (1963) Correlation of folate deficiency with alcoholism and associated macrocytosis, anemia and liver disease. _Annals of Internal Medicine_, **58**, 977–988.

260. Herlong, H.F., Recker, R.R. & Maddrey, W.C. (1982) Bone disease in primary biliary cirrhosis: histologic features and response to 25-hydroxyvitamin D. _Gastroenterology_, **83**, 103–108.

261. Herlong, H.F., Russell, R.M. & Maddrey, W.C. (1981) Vitamin A and zinc therapy in primary biliary cirrhosis. _Hepatology_, **1**, 348–351.

262. Hermann, W.J., Jr., Ward, K. & Faucett, J. (1979) The effect of tocopherol on high-density lipoprotein cholesterol: a clinical observation. _American Journal of Clinical Pathology_, **72**, 848–852.

263. Herrman, R., Shakoor, T. & Weber, F.L., Jr. (1987) Beneficial effects of pectin in chronic hepatic encephalopathy. _Gastroenterology_, **92**, 1795 (abstract).

264. Hickish, T., Colston, K.W., Bland, J.M. & Maxwell, J.D. (1989) Vitamin D deficiency and muscle strength in male alcoholics. _Clinical Science_, **77**, 171–176.

265. Hillman, R.S. (1990) Hematopoietic agents: growth factors, minerals and vitamins. In Gilman, A.G., Rall, T.W., Nies, A.S. & Taylor, P. (eds), _Goodman and Gilman's The Pharmacological Basis of Therapeutics_, 8th edn, pp. 1277–1310. New York: Pergamon Press.

266. Hines, J.D. (1975) Hematologic abnormalities involving vitamin B_6 and folate metabolism in alcoholic subjects. _Annals of the New York Academy of Sciences_, **252**, 316–327.

267. Hines, J.D. & Cowan, D.H. (1970) Studies on the pathogenesis of alcohol-induced sideroblastic bone-marrow abnormalities. _New England Journal of Medicine_, **283**, 441–446.

268. Hirosowa, K. & Yamada, E. (1973) The localisation of the vitamin A in the mouse liver as revealed by electron microscope radioautography. _Journal of Electron Microscopy_, **22**, 337–346.

269. Hoagland, C.L., Labby, D.H., Kunkel, H.G. & Shank, R.E. (1946) An analysis of the effect of fat in the diet on recovery

in infectious hepatitis. *American Journal of Public Health*, **36**, 1287–1292.

270. Hofvander, Y. (1968) Hematological investigations in Ethiopia with special reference to a high iron intake. *Acta Medica Scandinavica Supplementum*, **494**, 11–74.

271. Holdsworth, C.D., Nye, L. & King, E. (1972) The effect of portacaval anastomosis on oral carbohydrate tolerance and on plasma insulin levels. *Gut*, **13**, 58–63.

272. Holick, M.F. (1988) Vitamin D: photobiology, metabolism, and clinical application. In Arias, I.M., Jakoby, W.B., Popper, H., Schachter, D. & Shafritz, D.A. (eds) *The Liver: Biology and Pathobiology*, 2nd edn, pp. 475–493. New York: Raven Press.

273. Holzbach, R.T., Wieland, R.G., Lieber, C.S. *et al.* (1974) Hepatic lipid in morbid obesity: assessment at and subsequent to jejunoileal bypass. *New England Journal of Medicine*, **290**, 296–299.

274. Horst, D., Grace, N.D., Conn, H.O. *et al.* (1984) Comparison of dietary protein with an oral branched chain-enriched amino acid supplement in chronic portal-systemic encephalopathy: a randomized controlled trial. *Hepatology*, **4**, 279–287.

275. Howard, L., Heaphey, L.L. & Timchalk, M. (1986) A review of the current national status of home parenteral and enteral nutrition from the provider and consumer perspective. *Journal of Parenteral and Enteral Nutrition*, **10**, 416–424.

276. Hughes, C.A., Talbot, I.C., Ducker, D.A. & Harran, M.J. (1983) Total parenteral nutrition in infancy: effect on the liver and suggested pathogenesis. *Gut*, **24**, 241–248.

277. Hwang, S.-J., Chan, C.-Y., Wu, J.-C. *et al.* (1988) A randomized controlled trial for the evaluation of the efficacy of branched chain amino acid-enriched amino acid solution in the treatment of patients with hepatic encephalopathy. *Chinese Journal of Gastroenterology*, **5**, 185–192.

278. Iber, F.L. & Cooper, M. (1977) Jejunoileal bypass for the treatment of massive obesity. Prevalence, morbidity and short- and long-term consequences. *American Journal of Clinical Nutrition*, **30**, 4–14.

279. Ink, S.L. & Henderson, L.M. (1984) Vitamin B₆ metabolism. *Annual Review of Nutrition*, **4**, 445–470.

280. Isa, L., Jean, G., Silvani, A. *et al.* (1988) Evaluation of iron stores in patients with alcoholic liver disease: role of red cell ferritin. *Acta Haematologica*, **80**, 85–88.

281. Ishak, K.G., Zimmerman, H.J. & Ray, M.B. (1991) Alcoholic liver disease: pathologic, pathogenetic and clinical aspects. *Alcoholism: Clinical and Experimental Research*, **15**, 45–66.

282. Ishii, N. & Nishihara, Y. (1981) Pellagra among chronic alcoholics: clinical and pathological study of 20 necropsy cases. *Journal of Neurology, Neurosurgery and Psychiatry*, **44**, 209–215.

283. Jacobovits, A.W., Morgan, M.Y. & Sherlock, S. (1979) Hepatic siderosis in alcoholics. *American Journal of Digestive Diseases*, **24**, 305–310.

284. James, J.H., Ziparo, V., Jeppsson, B. & Fischer, J.E. (1979) Hyperammonaemia, plasma aminoacid imbalance, and blood-brain aminoacid transport: a unified theory of portal-systemic encephalopathy. *Lancet*, **2**, 772–775.

285. Jandl, J.H. & Lear, A.A. (1956) The metabolism of folic acid in cirrhosis. *Annals of Internal Medicine*, **45**, 1027–1044.

286. Jeejeebhoy, K.N. (1988) Hepatic complications of total parenteral nutrition. Need for prospective investigations. *Hepatology*, **8**, 428–429.

287. Jelliffe, D.B. (1966) The assessment of the nutritional status of the community. *WHO Monograph 53*. Geneva: World Health Organization.

288. Jelliffe, D.B. & Jelliffe, E.F.P. (1971) Age-dependent anthropometry. *American Journal of Clinical Nutrition*, **24**, 1377–1379.

289. Jenkins, D.J., Shapira, N., Greenberg, G. *et al.* (1989) Low glycemic index foods and reduced glucose, amino acid, and endocrine responses in cirrhosis. *American Journal of Gastroenterology*, **84**, 732–739.

290. Johansson, U., Johnsson, F., Joelsson *et al.* (1986) Selenium status in patients with liver cirrhosis and alcoholism. *British Journal of Nutrition*, **55**, 227–233.

291. Johnell, O., Nilsson, B.E. & Wiklund, P.E. (1982) Bone morphometry in alcoholics. *Clinical Orthopaedics and Related Research*, **165**, 253–258.

292. Johnson, B.F. (1968) Hemochromatosis resulting from prolonged oral iron therapy. *New England Journal of Medicine*, **278**, 1100–1101.

293. Jones, D.P. & Greene, E.A. (1966) Influences of dietary fat on alcoholic fatty liver. *American Journal of Clinical Nutrition*, **18**, 350–357.

294. Jones, P.N., Mills, E.H. & Capps, R.B. (1957) The effect of liver on serum vitamin B₁₂ concentrations. *Journal of Laboratory and Clinical Medicine*, **49**, 910–922.

295. Jorgensen, M.J., Furie, B.C. & Furie, B. (1988) Vitamin K-dependent blood coagulation proteins. In Arias, I.M., Jakoby, W.B., Popper, H., Schachter, D. & Shafritz, D.A. (eds) *The Liver: Biology and Pathobiology*, 2nd edn, pp. 495–503. New York: Raven Press.

296. Kaffarnik, H., Schneider, J., Schubotz, R. *et al.* (1978) Plasma lipids, triglyceride/fatty acid patterns, and plasma insulin in fasted healthy volunteers during continuous ingestion of ethanol. Influence of lipolysis inhibited by nicotinic acid. *Atherosclerosis*, **29**, 1–7.

297. Kahn, A.M., Helwig, H.L., Redeker, A.G. & Reynolds, T.B. (1965) Urine and serum zinc abnormalities in disease of the liver. *American Journal of Clinical Pathology*, **44**, 426–435.

298. Kalbfleisch, J.H., Lindeman, R.D., Ginn, H.E. & Smith, W.O. (1963) Effects of ethanol administration on urinary excretion of magnesium and other electrolytes in alcoholic and normal subjects. *Journal of Clinical Investigation*, **42**, 1471–1475.

299. Kaminski, D.L., Adams, A. & Jellinek, M. (1980) The effect of hyperalimentation on hepatic lipid content and lipogenic enzyme activity in rats and man. *Surgery*, **88**, 93–100.

300. Kanai, M., Raz, A. & Goodman, DeW.S. (1968) Retinol-binding protein: the transit protein for vitamin A in human plasma. *Journal of Clinical Investigation*, **47**, 2025–2044.

301. Kappy, M.S. (1987) Regulation of growth in children with chronic illness. Therapeutic implications for the year 2000. *American Journal of Diseases of Children*, **141**, 489–493.

302. Karl, A.F. & Griswold, M.D. (1980) Actions of insulin and vitamin A on Sertoli cells. *Biochemical Journal*, **186**, 1001–1003.

303. Karpati, G., Carpenter, S., Engel, A.G. *et al.* (1975) The syndrome of systemic carnitine deficiency. Clinical, morphologic, biochemical, and pathophysiologic features. *Neurology*, **25**, 16–24.

304. Kaufman, S.S., Scrivner, D.J. & Guest, J.E. (1989) Preoperative evaluation, preparation, and timing of orthotopic liver transplantation in the child. *Seminars in Liver Disease*, **9**, 176–183.

305. Keeling, P.W.N., Jones, R.B., Hillon, P.J. & Thompson, R.P.H. (1980) Reduced leucocyte zinc in liver disease. *Gut*, **21**, 561–564.

306. Keeling, P.W.N., O'Day, J., Ruse, W. & Thompson, R.P.H. (1982) Zinc deficiency and photoreceptor dysfunction in chronic liver disease. *Clinical Science*, **62**, 109–111.

307. Keeling, P.W.N., Ruse, W., Bull, J. *et al.* (1981) Direct measurement of the hepatointestinal extraction of zinc in cirrhosis and hepatitis. *Clinical Science*, **61**, 441–444.

308. Kehayoglou, A.K., Holdsworth, C.D., Agnew, J.E., Whelton, M.J. & Sherlock, S. (1968) Bone disease and calcium absorption in primary biliary cirrhosis with special reference to vitamin-D therapy. *Lancet*, **1**, 715–718.

309. Kern, F. (1983) Epidemiology and natural history of gall-stones. *Seminars in Liver Disease*, **3**, 87–96.

310. Kern, F., Jr., Jackson, R.G., Martin, T.E. & Mueller, J.F. (1957) Some effects of multiple intravenous infusions of a cottonseed oil emulsion in patients with Laennec's cirrhosis of the liver. *Metabolism*, **6**, 743–757.

311. Kershaw, P.W. (1967) Blood thiamin and nicotinic acid levels in alcoholism and confusional states. *British Journal of Psychiatry*, **113**, 387–393.

312. Keshavarzian, A., Meek, J., Sutton, C. *et al.* (1984) Dietary protein supplementation from vegetable sources in the management of chronic portal systemic encephalopathy. *American Journal of Gastroenterology*, **79**, 945–949.

313. Kiilerich, S., Dietrichson, O., Loud, F.B. *et al.* (1980) Zinc depletion in alcoholic liver diseases. *Scandinavian Journal of Gastroenterology*, **15**, 363–367.

314. Kimber, C., Deller, D.J., Ibbotson, R.N. & Lander, H. (1965) The mechanism of anaemia in chronic liver disease. *Quarterly Journal of Medicine*, **34**, 33–64.

315. King, D.R. Ginn Pease, M.E., Lloyd, T.V. *et al.* (1987) Parenteral

nutrition with associated cholelithiasis: another iatrogenic disease of infants and children. *Journal of Pediatric Surgery*, **22**, 593–596.

316. Kirkpatrick, J.R. (1987) Jejunoileal bypass. A legacy of late complications. *Archives of Surgery*, **122**, 610–614.

317. Kirsch, R.E. & Saunders, S.J. (1972) Nutrition and the liver. *South African Medical Journal*, **46**, 2072–2078.

318. Klain, J., Fraser, D., Goldstein, J. *et al.* (1989) Liver histology abnormalities in the morbidly obese. *Hepatology*, **10**, 873–876.

319. Klein, G.L. (1989) Aluminium in parenteral products: medical perspective on large and small volume parenterals. *Journal of Parenteral Science and Technology*, **43**, 120–124.

320. Klein, G.L., Heyman, M.B., Lee, T.C. *et al.* (1988) Aluminium-associated hepatobiliary dysfunction in rats: relationships to dosage and duration of exposure. *Pediatric Research*, **23**, 275–278.

321. Klein, S. & Nealon, W.H. (1988) Hepatobiliary abnormalities associated with total parenteral nutrition. *Seminars in Liver Disease*, **8**, 237–246.

322. Klipstein, F.A. & Lindenbaum, J. (1965) Folate deficiency in chronic liver disease. *Blood*, **25**, 443–456.

323. Korpela, H., Kumpulainen, J., Luoma, P.V. *et al.* (1985) Decreased serum selenium in alcoholics as related to liver structure and function. *American Journal of Clinical Nutrition*, **42**, 147–151.

324. Krawitt, E.L. (1975) Effect of ethanol ingestion on duodenal calcium transport. *Journal of Laboratory and Clinical Medicine*, **85**, 665–671.

325. Krawitt, E.L., Grundman, M.J. & Mawer, E.B. (1977) Absorption, hydroxylation and excretion of vitamin D_3 in primary biliary cirrhosis. *Lancet*, **2**, 1246–1249.

326. Kubota, A., Okada, A., Imura, K. *et al.* (1990) The effect of metronidazole on TPN-associated liver dysfunction in neonates. *Journal of Pediatric Surgery*, **25**, 618–621.

327. Kushner, J.P., Edwards, C.Q., Dadone, M.M. & Skolnick, M.H. (1985) Heterozygosity for HLA-linked hemochromatosis as a likely cause of the hepatic siderosis associated with sporadic porphyria cutanea tarda. *Gastroenterology*, **88**, 1232–1238.

328. Labadarios, D., Rossouw, J.E., McConnell, J.B. *et al.* (1977) Thiamine deficiency in fulminant hepatic failure and effects of supplementation. *International Journal for Vitamin and Nutrition Research*, **47**, 17–22.

329. Labadarios, D., Rossouw, J.E., McConnell, J.B. *et al.* (1977) Vitamin B_6 deficiency in chronic liver disease—evidence for increased degradation of pyridoxal 5'-phosphate. *Gut*, **18**, 23–27.

330. Labib, M., Abdel-Kader, M., Ranganath, L. *et al.* (1989) Bone disease in chronic alcoholism: the value of plasma osteocalcin measurement. *Alcohol and Alcoholism*, **24**, 141–144.

331. Lambert, J.R. & Thomas, S.M. (1985) Metronidazole prevention of serum liver enzyme abnormalities during total parenteral nutrition. *Journal of Parenteral and Enteral Nutrition*, **9**, 501–503.

332. LaRusso, N.F. & Thistle, J.L. (1981) Ursodeoxycholic acid ingestion after ileal resection. Effect on biliary bile acid and lipid composition. *Digestive Diseases and Sciences*, **26**, 705–709.

333. Leathen, J.H. (1970) Nutrition. In Johnson, A.D., Gomes, W.R. & Vandemark, N.L. (eds) *The Testis*, vol. 3, pp. 188–190. New York: Academic Press.

334. Lee, F.I. (1966) Cirrhosis and hepatoma in alcoholics. *Gut*, **7**, 77–85.

335. Lee, H.H., Hill, G.M., Sikha, V.K.N.M. *et al.* (1990) Pancreatico-biliary secretion of zinc and copper in normal persons and patients with Wilson's disease. *Journal of Laboratory and Clinical Medicine*, **116**, 283–288.

336. Lee, R.G. (1989) Nonalcoholic steatohepatitis: a study of 49 patients. *Human Pathology*, **20**, 594–598.

337. Leevy, C.M. (1968) Cirrhosis in alcoholics. *Medical Clinics of North America*, **52**, 1445–1455.

338. Leevy, C.M., Thompson, A. & Baker, H. (1970) Vitamins and liver injury. *American Journal of Clinical Nutrition*, **23**, 493–499.

339. Leevy, C.M., George, W.S., Ziffer, H. & Baker, H. (1960) Pantothenic acid, fatty liver and alcoholism. *Journal of Clinical Investigation*, **39**, 1005 (abstract).

340. Leevy, C.M., Baker, H., tenHove, W. *et al.* (1965) B-Complex vitamins in liver disease of the alcoholic. *American Journal of Clinical Nutrition*, **16**, 339–346.

341. Leklem, J.E. (1988) Vitamin B_6 metabolism and function in humans. In Leklem, J.E. & Reynolds, R.D. (eds) *Clinical and Physiological Applications of Vitamin B_6*, pp. 3–28. New York: Alan R. Liss.

342. Lelbach, W.K. (1966) Leberschäden bei chronischm alkoholismus I–III. *Acta Heptosplenologica*, **13**, 321–349.

343. Lelbach, W.K. (1975) Cirrhosis in the alcoholic and its relation to the volume of alcohol abuse. *Annals of the New York Academy of Sciences*, **252**, 85–105.

344. Leo, M.A. & Lieber, C.S. (1982) Hepatic vitamin A depletion in alcoholic liver injury. *New England Journal of Medicine*, **307**, 597–601.

345. Leo, M.A. & Lieber, C.S. (1983) Hepatic fibrosis after long-term administration of ethanol and moderate vitamin A supplementation in the rat. *Hepatology*, **3**, 1–11.

346. Levine, J.A. Stanger, L.C. & Morgan, M.Y. (1991) Resting and postprandial energy expenditure and fuel utilisation in patients with cirrhosis. *Hepatology* (in press).

347. Levine, M. (1986) New concepts in the biology and biochemistry of ascorbic acid. *New England Journal of Medicine*, **314**, 892–899.

348. Lieber, C.S. (1975) Liver disease and alcohol: fatty liver, alcoholic hepatitis, cirrhosis and their interrelationships. *Annals of the New York Academy of Sciences*, **252**, 63–84.

349. Lieber, C.S. (1985) Alcohol and the liver: metabolism of ethanol, metabolic effects and the pathogenesis of injury. *Acta Medica Scandinavica Supplementum*, **703**, 11–55.

350. Lieber, C.S. & DeCarli, L.M. (1970) Quantitative relationship between amount of dietary fat and severity of alcoholic fatty liver. *American Journal of Clinical Nutrition*, **23**, 474–478.

351. Lieber, C.S., Jones, D.P. & DeCarli, L.M. (1965) Effects of prolonged ethanol intake: production of fatty liver despite adequate diets. *Journal of Clinical Investigation*, **44**, 1009–1021.

352. Lifson, N., Gordon, G.B. & McClintock, R. (1955) Measurement of total carbon dioxide production by means of $D_2^{18}O$. *Journal of Applied Physiology*, **7**, 704–710.

353. Lim, P. & Jacob, E. (1972) Magnesium deficiency in liver cirrhosis. *Quarterly Journal of Medicine*, **41**, 291–300.

354. Lindenbaum, J. & Lieber, C.S. (1969) Hematologic effects of alcohol in man in the absence of nutritional deficiency. *New England Journal of Medicine*, **281**, 333–338.

355. Lindor, K.D., Fleming, C.R., Abrams, A. & Hirschkorn, M.A. (1979) Liver function values in adults receiving parenteral nutrition. *Journal of the American Medical Association*, **241**, 2398–2400.

356. Linnell, J. (1975) The fate of cobalamins *in vivo*. In Babior, B.M. (ed.) *Cobalamin: Biochemistry and Pathophysiology*, pp. 287–333. New York: John Wiley.

357. Lischner, M.W., Alexander, J.F. & Galambos, J.T. (1971) Natural history of alcoholic hepatitis. I. The acute disease. *American Journal of Digestive Diseases*, **16**, 481–494.

358. Lockwood, D.H., Amatruda, J.M., Moxley, R.T. *et al.* (1977) Effect of oral amino acid supplementation on liver disease after jejunoileal bypass for morbid obesity. *American Journal of Clinical Nutrition*, **30**, 58–63.

359. Loguercio, C., Sava, E., Marmo, R. *et al.* (1990) Malnutrition in cirrhotic patients: anthropometric measurements as a method of assessing nutritional status. *British Journal of Clinical Practice*, **44**, 98–101.

360. Long, R.G., Varghese, Z., Meinhard, E.A., Skinner, R.K., Wills, M.R., & Sherlock, S. (1978) Parenteral 1,25-dihydroxycholecalciferol in hepatic osteomalacia. *British Medical Journal*, **1**, 75–77.

361. Lowry, S.F. & Brennan, M.F. (1979) Abnormal liver function during parenteral nutrition: relation to infusion excess. *Journal of Surgical Research*, **26**, 300–307.

362. Ludwig, J., Viggiano, T.R., McGill, D.B. & Ott, B.J. (1980) Non-alcoholic steatohepatitis: Mayo Clinic experience with a hitherto unnamed disease. *Mayo Clinic Proceedings*, **55**, 434–438.

363. Lumeng, L. & Li, T.K. (1974) Vitamin B_6 metabolism in chronic alcohol abuse. Pyridoxal phosphate levels in plasma and the effects of acetaldehyde on pyridoxal phosphate synthesis and degradation in human erythrocytes. *Journal of Clinical Investigation*, **53**, 693–704.

364. Lumeng, L., Lui, A. & Li, T.-K. (1980) Plasma content of B_6 vitamers and its relationship to hepatic vitamin B_6 metabolism. *Journal of Clinical Investigation*, **66**, 688–695.

365. Lumeng, L., Schenker, S., Li, T.K., Brashear, R.E. & Compton, M.C. (1984) Clearance and metabolism of plasma pyridoxal 5'-

phosphate in the dog. *Journal of Laboratory and Clinical Medicine*, **103**, 59–69.

366. McClain, C.J. & Su, L.C. (1983) Zinc deficiency in the alcoholic: a review. *Alcoholism: Clinical and Experimental Research*, **7**, 5–10.

367. McClain, C.J., Antonow, D.R., Cohen, D.A. & Shedlofsky, S.I. (1986) Zinc metabolism in alcoholic liver disease. *Alcoholism: Clinical and Experimental Research*, **10**, 582–589.

368. McClain, C.J., Van Thiel, D.H., Parker, S. *et al.* (1979) Alterations in zinc, vitamin A, and retinol-binding protein in chronic alcoholics: a possible mechanism for night blindness and hypogonadism. *Alcoholism: Clinical and Experimental Research*, **3**, 135–141.

369. McClelland, R.N., DeShazo, C.V., Heimbach, D.M. *et al.* (1970) Prevention of hepatic injury after jejunoileal bypass by supplemental jejunostomy feedings. *Surgical Forum*, **21**, 368–370.

370. McCormick, D.B. & Olson, R.E. (1984) Biotin. In Olson, R.E., Broquist, H.P., Chichester, C.O., Darby, W.J., Kolbye, A.C. & Stalvey, R.M. (eds) *Present Knowledge in Nutrition*, 5th edn, pp. 365–376. Washington DC: Nutrition Foundation.

371. McCullough, A.J., Mullen, K.D., Smanik, E.J. *et al.* (1989) Nutritional therapy and liver disease. *Gastroenterology Clinics of North America*, **18**, 619–643.

372. McDermott, W.V. Jr. & Adams, R.D. (1954) Episodic stupor associated with an Eck fistula in the human with particular reference to the metabolism of ammonia. *Journal of Clinical Investigation*, **33**, 1–7.

373. McGhee, A., Henderson, M., Millikan, W.J. *et al.* (1983) Comparison of the effects of Hepatic-Aid and a casein modular diet on encephalopathy, plasma amino acids and nitrogen balance in cirrhotic patients. *Annals of Surgery*, **197**, 288–293.

374. McGill, D.B., Humphreys, S.R., Baggenstoss, A.H. & Dickson, E.R. (1972) Cirrhosis and death after jejunoileal shunt. *Gastroenterology*, **63**, 872–877.

375. Maddrey, W.C. (1990) Bone disease in patients with primary biliary cirrhosis. In Popper, H. & Schaffner, F. (eds) *Progress in Liver Diseases*, vol. IX, pp. 537–554. Philadelphia: W.B. Saunders.

376. Mangla, J.C., Hoy, W., Kim, Y. & Chopek, M. (1974) Cirrhosis and death after jejunoileal shunt for obesity. *American Journal of Digestive Diseases*, **19**, 759–765.

377. Marchesini, G., Zoli, M., Dondi, C. *et al.* (1982) Anticatabolic effect of branched-chain amino acid-enriched solutions in patients with liver cirrhosis. *Hepatology*, **2**, 420–425.

378. Marchesini, G., Dioguardi, F.S., Bianchi, G.P. *et al.* (1990) Long-term oral branched-chain amino acid treatment in chronic hepatic encephalopathy: a randomized double-blind casein-controlled trial. *Journal of Hepatology*, **11**, 92–101.

379. Marco, J., Diego, J., Villanueva, M.L. *et al.* (1973) Elevated plasma glucagon levels in cirrhosis of the liver. *New England Journal of Medicine*, **289**, 1107–1111.

380. Marcus, R. & Coulston, A.M. (1990) Fat-soluble vitamins: vitamins A, K and E. In Gilman, A.G., Rall, T.W., Nies, A.S. & Taylor, P. (eds) *Goodman and Gilman's The Pharmacological Basis of Therapeutics*, 8th edn, pp. 1553–1571. New York: Pergamon Press.

381. Marcus, R. & Coulston, A.M. (1990) Water-soluble vitamins: the vitamin B complex and ascorbic acid. In Gilman, A.G., Rall, T.W., Nies, A.S. & Taylor, P. (eds) *Goodman and Gilman's The Pharmacological Basis of Therapeutics*, 8th edn, pp. 1530–1552. New York: Pergamon Press.

382. Marr, J.W. (1971) Individuals dietary surveys: purposes and methods. *World Review of Nutrition and Dietetics*, **13**, 105–164.

383. Marshall, A.W., Kingstone, D., Boss, A.M. & Morgan, M.Y. (1983) Ethanol elimination in males and females: relationship to menstrual cycle and body composition. *Hepatology*, **3**, 701–706.

384. Marshall, J.B., Burnett, D.A., Zetterman, R.K. & Sorrell, M.F. (1983) Clinical and biochemical course of alcoholic liver disease following sudden discontinuation of alcoholic consumption. *Alcoholism: Clinical and Experimental Research*, **7**, 312–315.

385. Martin, L.W. & Bryant, L.R. (1962) The use of fructose to determine the patency of portal-systemic shunts. *Archives of Surgery*, **85**, 783–791.

386. Martins, F.M., Weinberg, A., Meurling, S. *et al.* (1984) Serum lipids and fatty acids composition of tissues in rats on total parenteral nutrition (TPN). *Lipids*, **19**, 728–737.

387. Marzio, L., Capone, F., Neri, M. *et al.* (1988) Gallbladder kinetics in obese patients: effect of a regular meal and low-calorie meal. *Digestive Diseases and Sciences*, **33**, 4–9.

388. Mashako, M.N., Bernard, C., Cezard, J.P. *et al.* (1987) Effect of total parenteral nutrition, constant rate enteral nutrition and discontinuous oral feeding on plasma cholecystokinin immunoreactivity in children. *Journal of Pediatric Gastroenterology and Nutrition*, **6**, 948–952.

389. Matos, C., Avni, E.F., van Gansbeke, D., Pardov, A. & Struyven, J. (1987) Total parenteral nutrition (TPN) and gallbladder diseases in neonates. Sonographic assessment. *Journal of Ultrasound in Medicine*, **6**, 243–248.

390. Mavrelis, P.G., Ammon, H.V., Gleysteen, J.J. *et al.* (1983) Hepatic free fatty acids in alcoholic liver disease and morbid obesity. *Hepatology*, **3**, 226–231.

391. Maxwell, J.D., Sanderson, I., Butler, W.H. *et al.* (1977) Hepatic structure and function after modified jejunoileal bypass surgery for obesity. *British Medical Journal*, **2**, 726–729.

392. Meguid, M.M., Akahoshi, M.P., Jeffers, S. *et al.* (1984) Amelioration of metabolic complications of conventional total parenteral nutrition: a prospective randomized study. *Archives of Surgery*, **119**, 1294–1298.

393. Mendenhall, C.L., Anderson, S., Weesner, R.E. *et al.* (1984) Protein-calorie malnutrition associated with alcoholic hepatitis. Veterans Administration Cooperative Study Group on Alcoholic Hepatitis. *American Journal of Medicine*, **76**, 211–222.

394. Mendenhall, C., Bongiovanni, G., Goldberg, S. *et al.* (1985) VA Cooperative Study on Alcoholic Hepatitis. III: Changes in protein-calorie malnutrition associated with 30 days of hospitalization with and without enteral nutritional therapy. *Journal of Parenteral and Enteral Nutrition*, **9**, 590–596.

395. Mendenhall, C.L., Tosch, T., Weesner, R.E. *et al.* (1986) VA cooperative study on alcoholic hepatitis II: prognostic significance of protein-calorie malnutrition. *American Journal of Clinical Nutrition*, **43**, 213–218.

396. Merli, M., Eriksson, L.S., Hagenfeldt, L. & Wahren, J. (1986) Splanchnic and leg exchange of free fatty acids in patients with liver cirrhosis. *Journal of Hepatology*, **3**, 348–355.

397. Merli, M., Romiti, A., Riggio, O. & Capocaccia, L. (1987) Optimal nutritional indexes in chronic liver disease. *Journal of Parenteral and Enteral Nutrition, Supplement*, **11**(5), 130S–134S.

398. Merli, M., Riggio, O., Romiti, A. *et al.* (1990) Basal energy production rate and substrate use in stable cirrhotic patients. *Hepatology*, **12**, 106–112.

399. Merrill, A.H. Jr., Henderson, J.M., Wang, E. *et al.* (1986) Activities of the hepatic enzymes of vitamin B_6 metabolism for patients with cirrhosis. *American Journal of Clinical Nutrition*, **44**, 461–467.

400. Merritt, R.J. (1986) Cholestasis associated with total parenteral nutrition. *Journal of Pediatric Gastroenterology and Nutrition*, **5**, 9–22.

401. Messing, B., Bories, C., Kunstlinger, F. & Bernier, J.-J. (1983) Does total parenteral nutrition induce gall bladder sludge formation and lithiasis? *Gastroenterology*, **84**, 1012–1019.

402. Metropolitan Life Insurance Company (1960) Desirable weights for men and women according to height and frame. Ages 25 and over. *Metropolitan Life Insurance Company Statistical Bulletin*, **41**, Feb. p. 6, March p. 1.

403. Mezes, M., Par, A., Nemeth, P. & Javor, T. (1986) Studies of the blood lipid peroxide status and vitamin E levels in patients with chronic active hepatitis and alcoholic liver disease. *International Journal of Clinical Pharmacology Research*, **6**, 333–338.

404. Mezey, E. & Faillace, L.A. (1971) Metabolic impairment and recovery time in acute ethanol intoxication. *Journal of Nervous and Mental Disease*, **153**, 445–452.

405. Mezey, E., Kolman, C.J., Diehl, A.M. *et al.* (1988) Alcohol and dietary intake in the development of chronic pancreatitis and liver disease in alcoholism. *American Journal of Clinical Nutrition*, **48**, 148–151.

406. Michel, H., Bories, P., Aubin, J.P. *et al.* (1985) Treatment of acute hepatic encephalopathy in cirrhotics with branched-chain amino acids enriched versus a conventional amino acids mixture. A controlled study of 70 patients. *Liver*, **5**, 282–289.

407. Miettinen, T.A. (1968) Fecal steroid excretion during weight

reduction in obese patients with hyperlipidemia. _Clinica Chimica Acta_, **19**, 341–344.

408. Mikhail, M.M. & Mansour, M.M. (1982) Complications of human schistosomiasis and their effect on levels of plasma copper, zinc and serum vitamin A. _Human Nutrition: Clinical Nutrition_, **36**, 289–296.

409. Miller, L.L. (1961) The role of the liver and the non-hepatic tissues in the regulation of free amino acid levels in the blood. In Holden, J.T. (ed.) _Amino Acid Pools_, pp. 708–721. Amsterdam: Elsevier.

410. Millikan, W.J., Jr., Henderson, J.M., Galloway, J.R. _et al._ (1985) In vivo measurement of leucine metabolism with stable isotopes in normal subjects and in those with cirrhosis fed conventional and branched-chain amino acid-enriched diets. _Surgery_, **98**, 405–413.

411. Millikan, W.J. Jr., Henderson, J.M., Warren, W.D. _et al._ (1983) Total parenteral nutrition with FO80^R in cirrhotics with subclinical encephalopathy. _Annals of Surgery_, **197**, 294–304.

412. Mills, P.R., Fell, G.S., Bessent, R.G. _et al._ (1983) A study of zinc metabolism in alcoholic cirrhosis. _Clinical Science_, **64**, 527–535.

413. Mills, P.R., Shenkin, A., Anthony, R.S. _et al._ (1983) A study of zinc metabolism in alcoholic cirrhosis. _Clinical Science_, **64**, 527–535.

413. Mills, P.R., Shenkin, A., Anthony, R.S. _et al._ (1983) Assessment of nutritional status and in vivo immune responses in alcoholic liver disease. _American Journal of Clinical Nutrition_, **38**, 849–859.

414. Millward, D.J. (1979) Protein deficiency, starvation and protein metabolism. _Proceedings of the Nutrition Society_, **38**, 77–88.

415. Milman, N., Hvid-Jacobsen, K., Hegnhoj, J. & Sorensen, S.S. (1983) Zinc absorption in patients with compensated alcoholic cirrhosis. _Scandinavian Journal of Gastroenterology_, **18**, 871–875.

416. Milman, N., Laursen, J., Podenphat, J. & Asnaes, S. (1986) Trace elements in normal and cirrhotic human liver tissue. I. Iron, copper, zinc. _Archives of Internal Medicine_, **135**, 1053–1057.

417. Milsom, J.P., Morgan, M.Y. & Sherlock, S. (1979) Factors affecting plasma amino acid concentrations in control subjects. _Metabolism_, **28**, 313–319.

418. Minot, G.R., Strauss, M.B. & Cobb, S. (1933) "Alcoholic" polyneuritis, dietary deficiency as a factor in its production. _New England Journal of Medicine_, **208**, 1244–1249.

419. Miralles Garcia, J.M. & de Castro del Pozo, S. (1976) Iron deposits in chronic alcoholics. Special studies in relation to the iron content of red wine. _Acta Hepato-Gastroenterologica_, **23**, 10–19.

420. Misra, P.K., Srivastava, K.L. & Chawla, A.C. (1989) Serum and hair zinc in Indian childhood cirrhosis. _Indian Pediatrics_, **26**, 22–25.

421. Mitchell, D., Wagner, C., Stone, W.J. _et al._ (1976) Abnormal regulation of plasma pyridoxal 5′-phosphate in patients with liver disease. _Gastroenterology_, **70**, 988 (abstract).

422. Mitchell, M.C. & Herlong, H.F. (1986) Alcohol and nutrition: caloric value, bioenergetics, and relationship to liver damage. _Annual Review of Nutrition_, **6**, 457–474.

423. Mobarhan, S.A., Russell, R.M., Recker, R.R. _et al._ (1984) Metabolic bone disease in alcoholic cirrhosis: a comparison of the effect of vitamin D_2, 25-hydroxyvitamin D, or supportive treatment. _Hepatology_, **4**, 266–273.

424. Montanari, A., Simoni, I., Vallisa, D. _et al._ (1988) Free amino acids in plasma and skeletal muscle of patients with liver cirrhosis. _Hepatology_, **8**, 1034–1039.

425. Moran, J.R., Ghishan, F.K., Halter, S.A. & Greene, H.L. (1983) Steatohepatitis in obese children: a cause of chronic liver dysfunction. _American Journal of Gastroenterology_, **78**, 374–377.

426. Morgan, A.G., Kelleher, J., Walker, B.E. & Losowsky, M.S. (1976) Nutrition in cryptogenic cirrhosis and chronic aggressive hepatitis. _Gut_, **17**, 113–118.

427. Morgan, M.Y. (1981) Enteral nutrition in chronic liver disease. _Acta Chirurgica Scandinavica Supplementum_, **507**, 81–90.

428. Morgan, M.Y. (1985) The epidemiology of alcohol related liver disease in the United Kingdom. In Hall, P. (ed.) _Alcoholic Liver Disease: Pathology, Epidemiology and Clinical Aspects_, pp. 193–229. London: Edward Arnold.

429. Morgan, M.Y. (1990) Branched chain amino acids in the management of chronic liver disease: facts and fantasies. _Journal of Hepatology_, **11**, 133–141.

430. Morgan, M.Y. & Levine, J.A. (1988) Alcohol and nutrition. _Proceedings of the Nutrition Society_, **47**, 85–98.

431. Morgan, M.Y., Stanger, L.C. & Levine, J.A. (1989) Resting and post-prandial energy expenditure in alcoholic patients and control subjects. _Clinical Nutrition, Supplement_, **8**, 114 (abstract).

432. Morgan, M.Y., Marshall, A.W., Milsom, J.P. & Sherlock, S. (1982) Plasma amino acid patterns in liver disease. _Gut_, **23**, 362–370.

433. Morgan, M.Y., Camilo, M.E., Luck, W. _et al._ (1981) Macrocytosis in alcohol related liver disease: its value for screening. _Clinical and Laboratory Haematology_, **3**, 35–44.

434. Morrison, S.A., Russell, R.M., Carney, E.A. & Oaks, E.V. (1978) Zinc deficiency: a cause of abnormal dark adaptation in cirrhotics. _American Journal of Clinical Nutrition_, **31**, 276–281.

435. Morrison, W.L., Bouchier, I.A.D., Gibson, J.N.A. & Rennie, M.J. (1990) Skeletal muscle and whole-body protein turnover in cirrhosis. _Clinical Science_, **78**, 613–619.

436. Motsenbocker, M.A. & Tappel, A.L. (1982) A selenocysteine-containing selenium-transport protein in rat plasma. _Biochimica et Biophysica Acta_, **719**, 147–153.

437. Moussavian, S.N., Bozian, R.C., Hamilton, F.N. _et al._ (1981) Fatty liver induced by zinc deficiency in the rat. _Hepatology_, **1**, 533 (abstract).

438. Moxley, R.T., III, Pozefsky, T. & Lockwood, D.H. (1974) Protein nutrition and liver disease after jejunoileal bypass for morbid obesity. _New England Journal of Medicine_, **290**, 921–926.

439. Mullen, K.D., Denne, S.C., McCullough, A.J. _et al._ (1986) Leucine metabolism in stable cirrhosis. _Hepatology_, **6**, 622–630.

440. Munoz, S.J., Heubi, J.E., Balistreri, W.F. & Maddrey, W.C. (1989) Vitamin E deficiency in primary biliary cirrhosis: gastrointestinal malabsorption, frequency and relationship to other lipid-soluble vitamins. _Hepatology_, **9**, 525–531.

441. Muscaritoli, M., Cangiano, C., Cascino, A. _et al._ (1986) Exogenous lipid clearance in compensated liver cirrhosis. _Journal of Parenteral and Enteral Nutrition_, **10**, 599–603.

442. Nagayama, M., Takai, T., Okuno, M. & Umeyama, K. (1989) Fat emulsion in surgical patients with liver disorders. _Journal of Surgical Research_, **47**, 59–64.

443. Nakamura, S., Takezawa, Y., Nakajima, Y. & Maeda, T. (1980) Elevation of glutamic pyruvic transaminase and gamma-glutamyl transpeptidase in obesity. _Tohoku Journal of Experimental Medicine_, **132**, 473–478.

444. Nakano, M., Worner, T.M. & Lieber, C.S. (1982) Perivenular fibrosis in alcoholic liver injury: ultrastructure and histologic progression. _Gastroenterology_, **83**, 777–785.

445. Nasrallah, S.M. & Galambos, J.T. (1980) Amino acid therapy of alcoholic hepatitis. _Lancet_, **2**, 1276–1277.

446. Nasrallah, S.M., Nassar, V.H. & Galambos, J.T. (1980) Importance of terminal hepatic venule thickening. _Archives of Pathology and Laboratory Medicine_, **104**, 84–86.

447. Naylor, C.D., O'Rourke, K., Detsky, A.S. & Baker, J.P. (1989) Parenteral nutrition with branched-chain amino acids in hepatic encephalopathy. A meta-analysis. _Gastroenterology_, **97**, 1033–1042.

448. Neville, J.N., Eagles, J.A., Samson, G. & Olson, R.E. (1968) Nutritional status of alcoholics. _American Journal of Clinical Nutrition_, **21**, 1329–1340.

449. Nilsson, B.E. & Westlin, N.E. (1973) Changes in bone mass in alcoholics. _Clinical Orthopaedics and Related Research_, **90**, 229–232.

450. Nilsson, L.H. (1973) Liver glycogen content in man in the postabsorptive state. _Scandinavian Journal of Clinical and Laboratory Investigation_, **32**, 317–323.

451. Norton, R., Batey, R., Dwyer, T. & MacMahon, S. (1987) Alcohol consumption and the risk of alcohol related cirrhosis in women. _British Medical Journal_, **295**, 80–82.

452. Ohgi, N. & Hirayama, C. (1988) Vitamin B_6 status in cirrhotic patients in relation to apoenzyme of serum alanine aminotransferase. _Clinical Biochemistry_, **21**, 367–370.

453. O'Keefe, S.J.D., Abraham, R.R., Davis, M. & Williams, R. (1981) Protein turnover in acute and chronic liver disease. _Acta Chirurgica Scandinavica Supplementum_, **507**, 91–101.

454. O'Keefe, S.J., El-Zayadi, A.R., Carraher, T.E. _et al._ (1980) Malnutrition and immuno-incompetence in patients with liver disease. _Lancet_, **2**, 615–617.

455. O'Keefe, S.J., Abraham, R., El-Zayadi, A. _et al._ (1981) Increased plasma tyrosine concentrations in patients with cirrhosis and fulminant hepatic failure associated with increased tyrosine flux

and reduced hepatic oxidation capacity. *Gastroenterology*, **81**, 1017–1024.

456. Okita, M., Watanabe, A. & Nagashima, H. (1985) Nutritional treatment of liver cirrhosis by branched-chain amino acid-enriched nutrient mixture. *Journal of Nutritional Science and Vitaminology*, **31**, 291–303.

457. O'Leary, J.P., Hollenbeck, J.I. & Woodward, E.R. (1974) Pathogenesis of hepatic failure after obesity bypass. *Surgical Forum*, **25**, 356–359.

458. Olsen, A.Y. (1950) The study of dietary factors, alcoholic consumption and laboratory findings in 100 patients with hepatic cirrhosis and 200 non-cirrhotic controls. *American Journal of the Medical Sciences*, **220**, 477–484.

459. Olsen, J.H., Dragsted, L. & Autrup, H. (1988) Cancer risk and occupational exposure to aflatoxins in Denmark. *British Journal of Cancer*, **58**, 392–396.

460. Owen, O.E., Trapp, V.E., Reichard, G.R. Jr. *et al.* (1983) Nature of quantity of fuels consumed in patients with alcoholic cirrhosis. *Journal of Clinical Investigation*, **72**, 1821–1832.

461. Owen, O.E., Reichle, F.A., Mozzoli, M.A. *et al.* (1981) Hepatic, gut, and renal substrate flux rates in patients with hepatic cirrhosis. *Journal of Clinical Investigation*, **68**, 240–252.

462. Pallares, R., Sitges-Serra, A., Fuentes, J. *et al.* (1983) Cholestasis associated with total parenteral nutrition. *Lancet*, **1**, 758–759.

463. Palombo, J.D., Lopes, S.M., Zeisel, S.H. *et al.* (1987) Effectiveness of orthotopic liver transplantation on the restoration of cholesterol metabolism in patients with end-stage liver disease. *Gastroenterology*, **93**, 1170–1177.

464. Panés, J., Parés, A., Torra, M. *et al.* (1985) Evidence that zinc depletion may favour hepatic fibrogenesis in alcoholic liver disease. *Journal of Hepatology, Supplement*, **1**(2), S300 (abstract).

465. Pardridge, W.M. & Jefferson, L.S. (1975) Liver uptake of amino acids and carbohydrates during a single circulatory passage. *American Journal of Physiology*, **228**, 1155–1161.

466. Patek, A.J. Jr. & Post, J. (1941) Treatment of cirrhosis of the liver by a nutritious diet and supplements rich in vitamin B complex. *Journal of Clinical Investigation*, **20**, 481–505.

467. Patek, A.J. Jr., Toth, I.G., Saunders, M.G. *et al.* (1975) Alcohol and dietary factors in cirrhosis. *Archives of Internal Medicine*, **135**, 1053–1057.

468. Paul, A.A. & Southgate, D.A.T. (ed.) (1978) *McCance and Widdowson's The Composition of Foods*, 4th edn. London: HMSO.

469. Peters, R.L., Gay, T. & Reynolds, T.B. (1975) Post-jejunoileal-bypass hepatic disease: its similarity to alcoholic hepatic disease. *American Journal of Clinical Pathology*, **63**, 318–331.

470. Petersen, S.R. & Sheldon, G.F. (1979) Acute acalculous cholecystitis: A complication of hyperalimentation. *American Journal of Surgery*, **138**, 814–817.

471. Phillips, G.B. & Davidson, C.S. (1954) Acute hepatic insufficiency of the chronic alcoholic. *Archives of Internal Medicine*, **94**, 585–603.

472. Pinto, J., Huang, Y. & Rivlin, R. (1984) Selective effects of ethanol and acetaldehyde upon intestinal enzymes metabolizing riboflavin: mechanism of reduced flavin bioavailability due to ethanol. *American Journal of Clinical Nutrition*, **39**, 685 (abstract).

473. Pirola, R.C. & Lieber, C.S. (1972) The energy cost of the metabolism of drugs, including ethanol. *Pharmacology*, **7**, 185–196.

474. Plauth, M., Egberts, E.H., Abele, R. *et al.* (1990) Characteristic pattern of free amino acids in plasma and skeletal muscle in stable hepatic cirrhosis. *Hepato-Gastroenterology*, **37**, 135–139.

475. Plesofsky-Vig, N. & Brambl, R. (1988) Pantothenic acid and coenzyme A in cellular modifications of proteins. *Annual Review of Nutrition*, **8**, 461–482.

476. Podda, M., Zuin, M., Dioguardi, M.L. & Festorazzi, S. (1982) Successful treatment of gallstones with bile acids in obese adolescents. *Archives of Disease in Childhood*, **57**, 956–958.

477. Posner, D.B., Russell, R.M., Absood, S. *et al.* (1978) Effective 25-hydroxylation of vitamin D_2 in alcoholic cirrhosis. *Gastroenterology*, **74**, 866–870.

478. Postuma, R. & Trevenen, C.L. (1979) Liver disease in infants receiving total parenteral nutrition. *Pediatrics*, **63**, 110–115.

479. Powell, E.E., Cooksley, W.G.E., Hanson, R. *et al.* (1990) The natural history of nonalcoholic steatohepatitis: a follow-up study of forty-two patients for up to 21 years. *Hepatology*, **11**, 74–80.

480. Prakash, G., Drenick, E.J., Wexler, H. *et al.* (1987) Microbial flora in the bypassed jejunum of patients with biliopancreatic bypass for obesity. *American Journal of Clinical Nutrition*, **46**, 273–276.

481. Prasad, A.S. (1985) Clinical manifestation of zinc deficiency. *Annual Review of Nutrition*, **5**, 341–363.

482. Prasad, A.S. (1985) Laboratory diagnosis of zinc deficiency. *Journal of the American College of Nutrition*, **4**, 591–598.

483. Prieto, J., Barry, M. & Sherlock, S. (1975) Serum ferritin in patients with iron overload and with acute and chronic liver disease. *Gastroenterology*, **68**, 525–533.

484. Quigley, E.M.M. & Zetterman, R.K. (1988) Hepatobiliary complications of malabsorption and malnutrition. *Seminars in Liver Disease*, **8**, 218–228.

485. Rachmilewitz, M., Moshkowitz, B., Rachmilewitz, B. *et al.* (1972) Serum vitamin B_{12} binding proteins in viral hepatitis. *European Journal of Clinical Investigation*, **2**, 239–242.

486. Radziuk, J., McDonald, T.J., Rubenstein, D. & Dupre, J. (1978) Initial splanchnic extraction of ingested glucose in normal man. *Metabolism*, **27**, 657–669.

487. Rager, R. & Finegold, M.J. (1975) Cholestasis in immature newborn infants: is parenteral alimentation responsible? *Journal of Pediatrics*, **86**, 264–269.

488. Ramalingaswami, V. (1964) Perspectives in protein malnutrition. *Nature*, **201**, 546–551.

489. Rao, A., Cherian, A., Onvora, C.V. & Suvarnabai, P.C. (1985) Serum aminotransferases and gamma-glutamyl transferase in protein energy malnutrition. *Tropical and Geographical Medicine*, **37**, 11–14.

490. Rayssiguier, Y. & Durlach, J. (1981) Déficit magnésique marginal et lésions hépatiques expérimentales du rat. *Médecine et Chirurgie Digestives*, **10**, 313–315.

491. Record, C.O., Buxton, B., Chase, R.A. *et al.* (1976) Plasma and brain amino acids in fulminant hepatic failure and their relationship to hepatic encephalopathy. *European Journal of Clinical Investigation*, **6**, 387–394.

492. Reding, P., Duchateau, J. & Bataille, C. (1984) Oral zinc supplementation improves hepatic encephalopathy. Results of a randomised controlled trial. *Lancet*, **2**, 493–495.

493. Reed, J.S., Meredith, S.C., Nemchausky, B.A. *et al.* (1980) Bone disease in primary biliary cirrhosis: reversal of osteomalacia with oral 25-hydroxyvitamin D. *Gastroenterology*, **78**, 512–517.

494. Reichel, H., Koeffler, H.P. & Norman, A.W. (1989) The role of the vitamin D endocrine system in health and disease. *New England Journal of Medicine*, **320**, 980–991.

495. Retief, F.P. & Huskison, Y.J. (1969) Serum and urinary folate in liver disease. *British Medical Journal*, **2**, 150–153.

496. Reuben, A., Maton, P.N., Murphy, G.M. & Dowling, R.H. (1985) Bile lipid secretion in obese and non-obese individuals with and without gallstones. *Clinical Science*, **69**, 71–79.

497. Reuben, A., Qureshi, Y., Murphy, G.M. & Dowling, R.H. (1985) Effect of obesity and weight reduction on biliary cholesterol saturation and the response to chenodeoxycholic acid. *European Journal of Clinical Investigation*, **16**, 133–142.

498. Reynolds, T.B., Lieberman, F.L. & Goodman, A.R. (1978) Advantages of treatment of ascites without sodium restriction and without complete removal of excess fluid. *Gut*, **19**, 549–553.

499. Reynolds, T.B., Redeker, A.G. & Kuzma, O.T. (1965) Role of alcohol in pathogenesis of alcoholic cirrhosis. In McIntyre, N. & Sherlock, S. (eds) *Therapeutic Agents and the Liver*, pp. 131–142. Oxford: Blackwell.

500. Richardson, T.J. & Sgoutas, D. (1975) Essential fatty acid deficiency in four adult patients during total parenteral nutrition. *American Journal of Clinical Nutrition*, **28**, 258–263.

501. Riggio, O., Romiti, A., Merli, M. *et al.* (1989) Post-prandial energy expenditure and substrate utilisation in cirrhotic patients after a mixed meal. *Clinical Nutrition Supplement*, **8**, 108 (abstract).

502. Riggio, O., Cangiano, C., Cascino, A. (1984) Long term dietary supplement with branched chain amino acids: a new approach in the prevention of hepatic encephalopathy: results of a controlled study in cirrhotics with porto-caval anastomosis. In Capocaccia, L., Fischer, J.E. & Rossi-Fanelli, F. (eds) *Hepatic Encephalopathy in Chronic Liver Failure*, pp. 183–192. New York: Plenum Press.

503. Ritland, S. & Aaseth, J. (1987) Trace elements and the liver. *Journal of Hepatology*, **5**, 118–122.

504. Rivlin, R.S. (1984) Riboflavin. In Olson, R.E., Broquist, H.P., Chichester, C.O. *et al.* (eds) *Present Knowledge in Nutrition*, 5th edn, pp. 285–302. Washington DC: Nutrition Foundation.

505. Robertson, J.F., Garden, O.J. & Shenkin, A. (1986) Intravenous nutrition and hepatic dysfunction. *Journal of Parenteral and Enteral Nutrition*, **10**, 172–176.

506. Robison, W.G. Jr., Kuwabara, T. & Bieri, J.G. (1980) Deficiencies of vitamins E and A in the rat. Retinal damage and lipofuscin accumulation. *Investigative Ophthalmology and Visual Sciences*, **19**, 1030–1037.

507. Rodgers, B.M., Hollenbeck, J.I., Donnelly, W.H. & Talbert, J.L. (1976) Intrahepatic cholestasis with parenteral alimentation. *American Journal of Surgery*, **131**, 149–155.

508. Rocchi, E., Cassanelli, M., Gibertini, P., *et al.* (1985) Standard or branched-chain amino acid infusions as short-term nutritional support in liver cirrhosis? *Journal of Parenteral and Enteral Nutrition*, **9**, 447–451.

509. Rosenblum, J.L., Keating, J.P., Prensky, A.L. & Nelson, J.S. (1981) A progressive neurological syndrome in children with chronic liver disease. *New England Journal of Medicine*, **304**, 503–508.

510. Rosenthal, W.S. & Glass, G.B.J. (1970) Vitamin B₁₂ and the liver. In Popper, H. & Schaffner, F. (eds) *Progress in Liver Diseases*, vol. III, pp. 118–146. London: Heinemann.

511. Rosenthal, W.S., Adham, N.F., Lopez, R. & Cooperman, J.M. (1973) Riboflavin deficiency in complicated chronic alcoholism. *American Journal of Clinical Nutrition*, **26**, 858–860.

512. Roslyn, J.J., Pitt, H.A., Mann, L.L. *et al.* (1983) Gallbladder disease in patients on long-term parenteral nutrition. *Gastroenterology*, **84**, 148–154.

513. Roslyn, J.J., Berquist, W.E., Pitt, H.A. *et al.* (1983) Increased risk of gallstones in children receiving total parenteral nutrition. *Pediatrics*, **71**, 784–789.

514. Rossi-Fanelli, F., Riggio, O., Cangiano, C. *et al.* (1982) Branched-chain amino acids vs lactulose in the treatment of hepatic coma. A controlled study. *Digestive Diseases and Sciences*, **27**, 929–935.

515. Rössner, S., Johansson, C., Walldius, G. & Aly, A. (1979) Intralipid clearance and lipoprotein pattern in men with advanced alcoholic liver cirrhosis. *American Journal of Clinical Nutrition*, **32**, 2022–2026.

516. Rossouw, J.E., Labadarios, D., Davis, M. & Williams, R. (1978) Water-soluble vitamins in severe liver disease. *South African Medical Journal*, **54**, 183–186.

517. Rossouw, J.E., Labadarios, D., Krasner, N. *et al.* (1978) Red blood cell transketolase activity and the effect of thiamine supplementation in patients with chronic liver disease. *Scandinavian Journal of Gastroenterology*, **13**, 133–138.

518. Rothschild, M.A., Oratz, M. & Schreiber, S.S. (1974) Alcohol, amino acids, and albumin synthesis. *Gastroenterology*, **67**, 1200–1213.

519. Rothschild, M.A., Oratz, M., Zimmon, D. *et al.* (1969) Albumin synthesis in cirrhotic subjects with ascites studied with carbonate-¹⁴C. *Journal of Clinical Investigation*, **48**, 344–350.

520. Rozental, P., Biava, C., Spencer, H. & Zimmerman, H. (1967) Liver morphology and function tests in obesity and during total starvation. *American Journal of Digestive Diseases*, **12**, 198–208.

521. Roy, C.C. & Belli, D.C. (1985) Hepatobiliary complications associated with TPN: an enigma. *Journal of the American College of Nutrition*, **4**, 651–660.

522. Rubin, E. & Farber, J.L. (1990) Environmental diseases of the digestive system. *Medical Clinics of North America*, **74**, 413–424.

523. Rubin, E. & Lieber, C.S. (1968) Alcohol-induced hepatic injury in nonalcoholic volunteers. *New England Journal of Medicine*, **278**, 869–876.

524. Rude, R.K. & Singer, F.R. (1981) Magnesium deficiency and excess. *Annual Review of Medicine*, **32**, 245–259.

525. Rudman, D., Kunter, M., Ansley, J.D. *et al.* (1981) Hypotyrosinemia and failure to retain nitrogen during total parenteral nutrition of cirrhotic patients. *Gastroenterology*, **81**, 1025–1035.

526. Rumball, J.M., Stone, C.M. & Hasset, C. (1959) The behaviour of serum iron in acute hepatitis. *Gastroenterology*, **36**, 219–223.

527. Russell, R.M., Boyer, J.L., Bagheri, S.A. & Hruban, Z. (1974) Hepatic injury from chronic hypervitaminosis A resulting in portal hypertension and ascites. *New England Journal of Medicine*, **291**, 435–440.

528. Russell, R.M., Rosenberg, I.H., Wilson, P.D. *et al.* (1983) Increased urinary excretion and prolonged turnover time of folic acid during ethanol ingestion. *American Journal of Clinical Nutrition*, **38**, 64–70.

529. Sabesin, S.M. (1978) Clinical conference: alcoholic hepatitis. *Gastroenterology*, **74**, 276–286.

530. Salmon, P.A. & Reedyk, L. (1975) Fatty metamorphosis in patients with jejunoileal bypass. *Surgery, Gynecology and Obstetrics*, **141**, 75–84.

531. Salvian, A.J. & Allardyce, D.B. (1980) Impaired bilirubin secretion during total parenteral nutrition. *Journal of Surgical Research*, **28**, 547–555.

532. Saunders, J.B., Davis, M. & Williams, R. (1981) Do women develop alcoholic liver disease more readily than men? *British Medical Journal*, **282**, 1140–1143.

533. Saunders, S.J., Truswell, A.S., Barbezat, G.O. *et al.* (1967) Plasma free aminoacid pattern in protein-calorie malnutrition: reappraisal of its diagnostic value. *Lancet*, **2**, 795–797.

534. Sax, H.C. & Bower, R.H. (1988) Hepatic complications of total parenteral nutrition. *Journal of Parenteral and Enteral Nutrition*, **12**, 615–618.

535. Sax, H.C., Talamini, M.A., Brackett, K. & Fischer, J.E. (1986) Hepatic steatosis in total parenteral nutrition: failure of fatty infiltration to correlate with abnormal serum hepatic enzyme levels. *Surgery*, **100**, 697–704.

536. Schaefer, E.J., Woo, R., Kibata, M. *et al.* (1983) Mobilization of triglyceride but not cholesterol or tocopherol from human adipocytes during weight reduction. *American Journal of Clinical Nutrition*, **37**, 749–754.

537. Schafer, A.I., Cheron, R.G., Dluhy, R. *et al.* (1981) Clinical consequences of acquired transfusional iron overload in adults. *New England Journal of Medicine*, **304**, 319–324.

538. Schäfer, Von K., Winther, M.B., Ukida, M. *et al.* (1981) Influence of an orally administered protein mixture enriched in branched chain amino acids on the chronic hepatic encephalopathy (CHE) of patients with liver cirrhosis. *Zeitschrift für Gastroenterologie*, **19**, 356–362.

539. Schechter, P.J., Giroux, E.L., Schlienger, J.L. *et al.* (1976) Distribution of serum zinc between albumin and α₂-macroglobulin in patients with decompensated hepatic cirrhosis. *European Journal of Clinical Investigation*, **6**, 147–150.

540. Schenker, S., Henderson, G.I., Hoyumpa, A.M. Jr. & McCandless, D.W. (1980) Hepatic and Wernicke's encephalopathy: current concepts of pathogenesis. *American Journal of Clinical Nutrition*, **33**, 2719–2726.

541. Schindler, R., Friedrich, D.H., Kramer, M. *et al.* (1988) Size and composition of liver vitamin A reserves of human beings who died of various causes. *International Journal for Vitamin and Nutrition Research*, **58**, 146–154.

542. Schneeweiss, B., Graninger, W., Ferenci, P. *et al.* (1990) Energy metabolism in patients with acute and chronic liver disease. *Hepatology*, **11**, 387–393.

543. Schoeller, D.A., van Santen, E., Peterson, D.W. *et al.* (1980) Total body water measurement in humans with ¹⁸O and ²H labeled water. *American Journal of Clinical Nutrition*, **33**, 2686–2693.

544. Schoffeniels, E. (1983) Thiamine phosphorylated derivatives and bioelectrogenesis. *Archives Internationales de Physiologie et de Biochimie*, **91**, 233–242.

545. Schölmerich, J., Krauss, E., Wietholtz, H. *et al.* (1987) Bioavailability of zinc from zinc-histidine complexes. II. Studies on patients with liver cirrhosis and the influence of the time of application. *American Journal of Clinical Nutrition*, **45**, 1487–1491.

546. Schölmerich, J., Wietholtz, H., Buchsel, R. *et al.* (1984) Zinc and vitamin A deficiency in gastrointestinal diseases. *Leber, Magen, Darm*, **14**, 288–295.

547. Schuberth, O. (1963) Clinical results of intravenous fat emulsions. *Bibliotheca Nutritio et Dieta*, **5**, 387–402.

548. Schwartz, J.B., Merritt, R.J., Rosenthal, P. *et al.* (1988) Ceruletide to treat neonatal cholestasis. *Lancet*, **1**, 1219–1220 (letter).

549. Schwartz, R., Phillips, G.B., Seegmiller, J.E. *et al.* (1954) Dietary protein in the genesis of hepatic coma. *New England Journal of Medicine*, **251**, 685–689.

550. Scragg, R.K., McMichael, A.J. & Baghurst, P.A. (1984) Diet, alcohol, and relative weight in gall stone disease: a case-controlled study. *British Medical Journal*, **288**, 1113–1119.

551. Seftel, H.C., Malkin, C., Schmaman, A. *et al.* (1966) Osteoporosis, scurvy, and siderosis in Johannesburg Bantu. *British Medical Journal*, **1**, 642–646.

552. Segel, S. (1989) Disorders of galactose metabolism. In Scriver, C.R., Beaudet, A.L., Sly, W.S. & Valle, D. (eds) *The Metabolic Basis of Inherited Diseases*, 6th edn, pp. 453–480. New York: McGraw Hill.

553. Shambaugh, G.E. (1978) Urea biosynthesis II. Normal and abnormal regulation. *American Journal of Clinical Nutrition*, **31**, 126–133.

554. Shapira, G., Chawla, R.K., Berry, C.J. *et al.* (1986) Cysteine, tyrosine, choline, and carnitine supplementation of patients on total parenteral nutrition. *Nutrition International*, **2**, 334–339.

555. Sheldon, G.F., Peterson, S.R. & Sanders, R. (1978) Hepatic dysfunction during hyperalimentation. *Archives of Surgery*, **113**, 504–508.

556. Sherlock, S. & Walsh, V.M. (1951) Hepatic structure and function. In *Studies of Undernutrition, Wuppertal 1946–1949*. Medical Research Council Special Report Series No. 275, pp. 111–134. London: Medical Research Council.

557. Shronts, E.P. (1988) Nutritional assessment of adults with end-stage hepatic failure. *Nutrition in Clinical Practice*, **3**, 113–119.

558. Shronts, E.P., Teasley, K.M., Thoele, S.L. & Cerra, F.B. (1987) Nutritional support of the adult liver transplant candidate. *Journal of the American Dietetic Association*, **87**, 441–451.

559. Siez, A., Walker, S., Czygan, P. *et al.* (1983) Branched-chain amino acid-enriched elemental diet in patients with cirrhosis of the liver. A double blind crossover trial. *Zeitschrift für Gastroenterologie*, **21**, 644–650.

560. Silver, M.M., Beverley, D.W., Valberg, L.S. *et al.* (1987) Perinatal hemochromatosis. Clinical, morphologic and quantitative iron studies. *American Journal of Pathology*, **128**, 538–554.

561. Simko, V. (1983) Long-term tolerance of a special amino acid oral formula in patients with advanced liver disease. *Nutrition Reports International*, **27**, 765–773.

562. Simko, V., Connell, A.M. & Banks, B. (1982) Nutritional status in alcoholics with and without liver disease. *American Journal of Clinical Nutrition*, **35**, 197–203.

563. Simon, D. & Galambos, J.T. (1988) A randomized controlled study of peripheral parenteral nutrition in moderate and severe alcoholic hepatitis. *Journal of Hepatology*, **7**, 200–207.

564. Simon, M., Beaumont, C., Briere, J. *et al.* (1985) Is the HLA-linked haemochromatosis allele implicated in idiopathic refractory sideroblastic anaemia? *British Journal of Haematology*, **60**, 75–80.

565. Simpson, R.J. & Peters, T. (1987) Iron-binding lipids of rabbit duodenal brush-border membrane. *Biochemica et Biophysica Acta*, **898**, 181–186.

566. Sinatra, F.R. & Merritt, R.J. (1981) Iatrogenic kwashiorkor in infants. *American Journal of Diseases of Children*, **135**, 21–23.

567. Slagle, T.A. & Gross, S.J. (1988) Effect of early low-volume enteral substrate on subsequent feeding tolerance in very low birth weight infants. *Journal of Pediatrics*, **113**, 526–531.

568. Smith, J.C. Jr, Brown, E.D., White, S.C. & Finkelstein, J.D. (1975) Plasma vitamin A and zinc concentration in patients with alcoholic cirrhosis. *Lancet*, **1**, 1251–1252 (letter).

569. Smith, L.H. Jr, Ettinger, R.H. & Seligson, D. (1953) A comparison of the metabolism of fructose and glucose in hepatic disease and diabetes mellitus. *Journal of Clinical Investigation*, **32**, 273–282.

570. Smithgall, J.M. (1985) The copper-controlled diet: recurrent aspects of dietary copper restriction in management of copper metabolism disorders. *Journal of the American Dietetics Association*, **85**, 609–610.

571. Snodgrass, P.J. (1970) Obesity, small-bowel bypass and liver disease. *New England Journal of Medicine*, **282**, 870–871.

572. Soberon, S., Pauley, M.P., Duplantier, R. *et al.* (1987) Metabolic effects of enteral formula feeding in alcoholic hepatitis. *Hepatology*, **7**, 1204–1209.

573. Sokol, R.J. (1988) Vitamin E deficiency and neurologic disease. *Annual Review of Nutrition*, **8**, 351–373.

574. Sokol, R.J. & Stall, C. (1990) Anthropometric evaluation of children with chronic liver disease. *American Journal of Clinical Nutrition*, **52**, 203–208.

575. Solis-Herruzo, J., De Cuenca, B. & Munoz-Rivero, M.C. (1989) Intestinal zinc absorption in cirrhotic patients. *Zeitschrift für Gastroenterologie*, **27**, 335–338.

576. Solomans, N.W. & Russell, R.M. (1980) The interaction of vitamin A and zinc: implications for human nutrition. *American Journal of Clinical Nutrition*, **33**, 2031–2040.

577. Soloway, R.D., Trotman, B.W., Maddrey, W.C. & Nakayama, F. (1986) Pigment gallstone composition in patients with hemolysis or infection/stasis. *Digestive Diseases and Sciences*, **31**, 454–460.

578. Somogyi, J.C. (1976) Early signs of thiamine deficiency. *Bibliotheca Nutritio et Dieta*, **23**, 78–85.

579. Sorensen, T.I.A., Bruusgaard, A., Pedersen, L.R. & Krag, E. (1977) Lithogenic index of bile after jejunoileal bypass operation for obesity. *Scandinavian Journal of Gastroenterology*, **12**, 449–451.

580. Sorrell, M.F., Baker, H., Tuma, D.J. *et al.* (1976) Potentiation of ethanol fatty liver in rats by chronic administration of nicotinic acid. *Biochimica et Biophysica Acta*, **450**, 231–238.

581. Spannuth, C.L., Mitchell, D., Stone, W.J. *et al.* (1978) Vitamin B_6 nutriture in patients with uremia and with liver disease. In National Research Council (ed.) *Human Vitamin B_6 Requirements*, pp. 180–192. Washington DC: National Academy of Science.

582. Spin, F.P. & Weismann, R.E. (1975) Death from hepatic failure after jejunoileal anastomosis. *American Journal of Surgery*, **130**, 88–91.

583. Spivak, J.L. & Jackson, D.L. (1977) Pellagra: an analysis of 18 patients and a review of the literature. *John Hopkins Medical Journal*, **140**, 295–309.

584. Stanko, R.T., Nathan, G., Mendelow, H. & Adibi, S.A. (1987) Development of hepatic cholestasis and fibrosis in patients with massive loss of intestine supported by prolonged parenteral nutrition. *Gastroenterology*, **92**, 197–202.

585. Stein, T.P. & Mullen, J.L. (1985) Hepatic fat accumulation in man with excess parenteral glucose. *Nutrition Research*, **5**, 1347–1351.

586. Sternlieb, I. (1988) Copper and zinc. In Arias, I.M., Jakoby, W.B., Popper, H. *et al.* (eds) *The Liver: Biology and Pathobiology*, 2nd edn, pp. 525–533. New York: Raven Press.

587. Stewart, S.M., Uauy, R., Kennard, B.D. *et al.* (1988) Mental development and growth in children with chronic liver disease of early and late onset. *Pediatrics*, **82**, 167–172.

588. Stratiagos, J.D. & Katsambas, A. (1977) Pellagra: a still existing disease. *British Journal of Dermatology*, **96**, 99–106.

589. Strauss, E., dos Santos, W.R., da Silva, E.C. *et al.* (1986) Treatment of hepatic encephalopathy: a randomized clinical trial comparing a branched chain enriched amino acid solution to oral neomycin. *Nutritional Support Services*, **6**, 18–21.

590. Stremmel, W. & Strohmeyer, G. (1988) Oral zinc therapy is not always effective for treatment of Wilson's disease. *Hepatology*, **8**, 1335 (abstract).

591. Stremmel, W., Lotz, G., Nierderau, C. *et al.* (1987) Iron uptake by rat duodenal microvillous membrane vesicles: evidence for a carrier mediated transport system. *European Journal of Clinical Investigation*, **17**, 136–145.

592. Sturniolo, G.C., Parisi, G., Martin, A. *et al.* (1985) Taste and smell alterations in liver cirrhosis: a double blind crossover trial of oral zinc treatment. *Journal of Hepatology, Supplement*, **1**(1), S136 (abstract).

593. Stutzman, F.L. & Amatuzio, D.S. (1953) Blood serum magnesium in portal cirrhosis and diabetes mellitus. *Journal of Laboratory and Clinical Medicine*, **41**, 215–219.

594. Sullivan, J.F., Blotcky, A.J., Jetton, M.M. *et al.* (1979) Serum levels of selenium, calcium, copper, magnesium, manganese and zinc in various human diseases. *Journal of Nutrition*, **109**, 1432–1437.

595. Sullivan, L.W. & Herbert, V. (1964) Suppression of hematopoiesis by ethanol. *Journal of Clinical Investigation*, **43**, 2048–2062.

596. Summerskill, W.H.J., Wolfe, S.J. & Davidson, C.S. (1957) Response to alcohol in chronic alcoholics with liver disease: clinical, pathological and metabolic changes. *Lancet*, **1**, 335–340.

597. Summerskill, W.H.J., Wolfe, S.J. & Davidson, C.S. (1957) The management of hepatic coma in relation to protein withdrawal and certain specific measures. *American Journal of Medicine*, **23**, 59–76.

598. Suttie, J.W. (1987) Recent advances in hepatic vitamin K metabolism and function. *Hepatology*, **7**, 367–376.

599. Swart, G.R., Frenkel, M. & van den Berg, J.W.O. (1981) Minimum

protein requirements in advanced liver disease; a metabolic ward study of the effects of oral branched chain amino acids. In Walser, M. & Williamson, J.R. (eds) *Metabolism and Clinical Implications of Branched Chain Amino and Ketoacids*, pp. 427–432. New York: Elsevier/North Holland.

600. Swart, G.R., Zillikens, M.C., van Vuure, J.K. & van den Berg, J.W.O. (1989) Effect of a late evening meal on nitrogen balance on patients with cirrhosis of the liver. *British Medical Journal*, **299**, 1202–1203.

601. Swart, G.R., van den Berg, J.W.O., van Vuure, J.K. *et al.* (1989) Minimum protein-requirements in liver cirrhosis determined by nitrogen-balance measurements at three levels of protein intake. *Clinical Nutrition*, **8**, 329–336.

602. Swart, G.R., van den Berg, J.W., Wattimena, J.L. *et al.* (1988) Elevated protein requirements in cirrhosis of the liver investigated by whole body protein turnover studies. *Clinical Science*, **75**, 101–107.

603. Szebeni, J., Eskelson, C., Sampliner, R. *et al.* (1986) Plasma fatty acid pattern including diene-conjugated linoleic acid in ethanol users and patients with ethanol-related liver disease. *Alcoholism: Clinical and Experimental Research*, **10**, 647–650.

604. Tamura, T. & Stokstad, E.L.R. (1977) Increased folate excretion in acute hepatitis. *American Journal of Clinical Nutrition*, **30**, 1378–1379.

605. Tanaka, K. (1981) New light on biotin deficiency. *New England Journal of Medicine*, **304**, 839–840.

606. Tanner, A.R., Bantock, I., Hinks, L. *et al.* (1986) Depressed selenium and vitamin E levels in an alcoholic population. Possible relationship to hepatic injury through increased lipid peroxidation. *Digestive Diseases and Sciences*, **31**, 1307–1312.

607. Tavill, A.S., Sharma, B.K. & Bacon, B.R. (1990) Iron and the liver: genetic hemochromatosis and other hepatic iron overload disorders. In Popper, H. & Schaffner, F. (eds) *Progress in Liver Diseases*, vol. IX, pp. 281–305. Philadelphia: W.B. Saunders.

608. Thaler, H. (1975) Relation of steatosis to cirrhosis. *Clinics in Gastroenterology*, **4**, 273–280.

609. Thiet, M.D., Mitrelstaedt, C.A., Herbst, C.A. & Buckwalter, J.A. (1984) Cholelithiasis in morbid obesity. *Southern Medical Journal*, **77**, 415–417.

610. Thomas, P.K. & Walker, J.G. (1965) Xanthomatous neuropathy in primary biliary cirrhosis. *Brain*, **88**, 1079–1088.

611. Touloukian, R.J. & Downing, S.E. (1973) Cholestasis associated with long-term parenteral hyperalimentation. *Archives of Surgery*, **106**, 58–62.

612. Unger, K.W. & Johnson, D., Jr. (1974) Red blood cell mean corpuscular volume: a potential indicator of alcohol usage in a working population. *American Journal of the Medical Sciences*, **267**, 281–289.

613. Uribe, M. (1985) Dietary management of portal-systemic encephalopathy. In Conn, H.O. & Bircher, J. (eds) *Hepatic Encephalopathy: Management with Lactulose and Related Carbohydrates*, pp. 95–112. East Lancing, Michigan: Medi-Ed Press.

614. Uribe, M., Márquez, M.A., Ramos, G.G. *et al.* (1982) Treatment of chronic portal-systemic encephalopathy with vegetable and animal protein diets: a controlled crossover study. *Digestive Diseases and Sciences*, **27**, 1109–1116.

615. Uribe, M., Dibildox, M., Malpica, S. *et al.* (1985) Beneficial effect of vegetable protein diet supplemented with psyllium plantago in patients with hepatic encephalopathy and diabetes mellitus. *Gastroenterology*, **88**, 901–907.

616. Valimäki, M.J., Harju, K.J. & Ylikahri, R.H. (1983) Decreased serum selenium in alcoholics—a consequence of liver dysfunction. *Clinica Chimica Acta*, **130**, 291–296.

617. Vallee, B.L., Wackner, W.E.C., Bartholomay, A.F. & Robin, E.D. (1956) Zinc metabolism in hepatic dysfunction. I. Serum zinc concentrations in Laënnec's cirrhosis and their validation by sequential analysis. *New England Journal of Medicine*, **255**, 403–408.

618. Van Rensburg, S.J., Cook-Mozaffari, P., Van Schalkwyk, D.J. *et al.* (1985) Hepatocellular carcinoma and dietary aflatoxin in Mozambique and Transkei. *British Journal of Cancer*, **51**, 713–726.

619. Vannucchi, H. & Moreno, F.S. (1989) Interaction of niacin and zinc metabolism in patients with alcoholic pellagra. *American Journal of Clinical Nutrition*, **50**, 364–369.

620. Vannucchi, H., Kutnink, M.D., Sauberlich, M. & Howede, E. (1986) Interaction among niacin, vitamin B_6 and zinc in rats receiving ethanol. *International Journal for Vitamin and Nutrition Research*, **56**, 355–362.

621. Van Waes, L. & Lieber, C.S. (1977) Early perivenular sclerosis in alcoholic fatty liver: an index of progressive liver injury. *Gastroenterology*, **73**, 646–650.

622. Vilstrup, H., Bucher, D., Krog, B. & Damgard, S.E. (1982) Elimination of infused amino acids from plasma of control subjects and of patients with cirrhosis of the liver. *European Journal of Clinical Investigation*, **12**, 197–202.

623. Vilstrup, H., Gluud, C., Hardt, F. *et al.* (1985) Branched chain enriched amino acid nutrition does not change the outcome of hepatic coma in patients with cirrhosis of the liver. *Journal of Hepatology, Supplement*, **1**(2), S347 (abstract).

624. Vital Health Statistics Data. (1966) Average weight for men and women by age and height. United States 1960–1962. *Weight by Height and Age of Adults*, US National Health Service, Publication No. 1000, Series 11, No. 14, Washington DC: US National Health Service.

625. Viteri, F.E. & Torun, B. (1980) Protein-calorie malnutrition. In Goodhart, R.S. & Shils, M.E. (eds) *Modern Nutrition in Health and Disease*, 6th edn, pp. 697–720. Philadelphia: Lea & Febiger.

626. Volwiler, W., Jones, C.M. & Mallory, T.B. (1948) Criteria for the measurement of results of treatment in fatty cirrhosis. *Gastroenterology*, **11**, 164–182.

627. Wahren, J., Felig, P., Cerasi, E. & Luft, R. (1972) Splanchnic and peripheral glucose and amino acid metabolism in diabetes mellitus. *Journal of Clinical Investigation*, **51**, 1870–1878.

628. Wahren, J., Denis, J., Desurmont, P. *et al.* (1983) Is intravenous administration of branched chain amino acids effective in the treatment of hepatic encephalopathy? A multicenter study. *Hepatology*, **3**, 475–480.

629. Walt, R.P., Kemp, C.M., Lyness, L. *et al.* (1984) Vitamin A therapy for night blindness in primary biliary cirrhosis. *British Medical Journal*, **288**, 1030–1031.

630. Watanabe, A., Kobayashi, M., Yoshitomi, S. & Nagashima, H. (1989) Liver fibrosis in obese patients with fatty livers. *Journal of Medicine*, **20**, 357–362.

631. Watanabe, A., Shiota, T., Okia, M. & Nagashima, H. (1983) Effect of a branched chain amino acid-enriched nutritional product on the pathophysiology of the liver and nutritional state of patients with liver cirrhosis. *Acta Medica Okayama*, **37**, 321–333.

632. Waterlow, J.C. (1979) Childhood malnutrition—the global problem. *Proceedings of the Nutrition Society*, **38**, 1–9.

633. Wattchow, D.A., Hall, J.C., Whiting, M.J. *et al.* (1983) Prevalence and treatment of gall stones after gastric bypass surgery for morbid obesity. *British Medical Journal*, **286**, 763.

634. Weber, F.L. Jr. & Reiser, B.J. (1982) Relationship of plasma amino acids to nitrogen balance and portal-systemic encephalopathy in alcoholic liver disease. *Digestive Diseases and Sciences*, **27**, 103–110.

635. Weber, F.L. Jr., Minco, D., Fresard, K.M. & Banwell, J.G. (1985) Effects of vegetable diets on nitrogen metabolism in cirrhotic subjects. *Gastroenterology*, **89**, 538–544.

636. Weiner, F.R., Eskreis, D.S., Compton, K.V. *et al.* (1988) Haplotype analysis of a type I collagen gene and its association with alcoholic cirrhosis in man. *Molecular Aspects of Medicine*, **10**, 159–168.

637. Weir, D.G., McGing, P.G. & Scott, J.M. (1985) Folate metabolism, the enterohepatic circulation and alcohol. *Biochemical Pharmacology*, **34**, 1–7.

638. Weismann, K., Christensen, E. & Dreyer, V. (1979) Zinc supplementation in alcoholic cirrhosis. A double-blind clinical trial. *Acta Medica Scandinavica*, **205**, 361–366.

639. Westerfeld, W.W. & Schulman, M.P. (1959) Metabolism and caloric value of alcohol. *Journal of the American Medical Association*, **170**, 197–203.

640. Westwater, J.O. & Fainer, D. (1958) Liver impairment in the obese. *Gastroenterology*, **34**, 686–693.

641. Wheby, M.S. & Umpiere, G. (1964) Effect of transferrin saturation on iron absorption in man. *New England Journal of Medicine*, **271**, 1391–1395.

642. Whitehead, C.C. (1981) The assessment of biotin status in man and animals. *Proceedings of the Nutrition Society*, **40**, 165–172.

643. Whitington, P.F. (1985) Cholestasis associated with total parenteral nutrition in infants. *Hepatology*, **5**, 693–696.

644. Whitington, P.F. & Black, D.D. (1980) Cholelithiasis in premature infants treated with parenteral nutrition and furosemide. *Journal of Pediatrics*, **97**, 647–649.

645. Whyte, M.P., Mahuren, J.D., Vrabel, L.A. & Coburn, S.P. (1985) Markedly increased circulating pyridoxal-5′-phosphate levels in hypophosphatasia. Alkaline phosphatase acts in vitamin B_6 metabolism. *Journal of Clinical Investigation*, **76**, 752–756.

646. Wogan, G.N. (1989) Dietary risk factors for primary hepatocellular carcinoma. *Cancer Detection and Prevention*, **14**, 209–213.

647. Wolfe, R.R., O'Donnell, T.F. Jr., Stone, M.D. *et al.* (1980) Investigation of factors determining the optimal glucose infusion rate in total parenteral nutrition. *Metabolism*, **29**, 892–900.

648. World, M.J., Ryle, P.R. & Thomson, A.D. (1985) Alcoholic malnutrition and the small intestine. *Alcohol and Alcoholism*, **20**, 89–124.

649. World, M.J., Ryle, P.R., Jones, D. *et al.* (1984) Differential effect of chronic alcohol intake and poor nutrition on body weight and fat stores. *Alcohol and Alcoholism*, **19**, 281–290.

650. Worner, T.M. & Lieber, C.S. (1985) Perivenular fibrosis as precursor lesion of cirrhosis. *Journal of the American Medical Association*, **254**, 627–630.

651. Wrong, O.M., Vince, A.J. & Waterlow, J.C. (1985) The contribution of endogenous urea to faecal ammonia in man, determined by ^{15}N labelling of plasma urea. *Clinical Science*, **68**, 193–199.

652. Wu, A., Chanarin, I. & Levi, A.J. (1974) Macrocytosis of chronic alcoholism. *Lancet*, **1**, 829–831.

653. Young, V.R. (1987) 1987 McCollum award lecture. Kinetics of human amino acid metabolism: nutritional implications and some lessons. *American Journal of Clinical Nutrition*, **46**, 709–725.

654. Yudkoff, M., Nissim, I., Glassman, M. & Segal, S. (1984) Whole body nitrogen kinetics in man: determination from plasma [*guanidino*-^{15}N]arginine. *Clinical Science*, **66**, 337–342.

655. Zaman, S.N., Tredger, J.M., Johnson, P.J. & Williams, R. (1986) Vitamin B_6 concentrations in patients with chronic liver disease and hepatocellular carcinoma. *British Medical Journal*, **293**, 175.

656. Zarif, M.A., Pildes, R.S., Szanto, P.B. & Vidyasagar, D. (1976) Cholestasis associated with administration of L-amino acids and dextrose solutions. *Biology of the Neonate*, **29**, 66–76.

657. Zelman, S. (1952) The liver in obesity. *Archives of Internal Medicine*, **90**, 141–156.

658. Zipursky, A., Brown, E.J., Watts, J. *et al.* (1987) Oral vitamin E supplementation for the prevention of anemia in premature infants: a controlled trial. *Pediatrics*, **79**, 61–68.

CHAPTER 7

The Liver and the Endocrine System

S.V. Gelding, K.G.M.M. Alberti & D.G. Johnston

The liver is of key importance in the functioning of much of the endocrine system. It has a major role in the metabolic degradation of many hormones (see Table 7.1) and it is to be expected therefore that abnormalities of circulating hormone concentrations will be found in subjects with liver disease. This is of clinical importance in the interpretation of blood concentrations of individual hormones. The liver is also the prime target organ for the action of many hormones, and hepatic disease may be associated with diminished or altered hormone effects despite an apparently normal circulating concentration. In addition, the liver may be necessary for production of a 'secondary messenger' essential for the full effects of a particular hormone to be manifested, e.g. the somatomed-ins and growth hormone. These and other mechanisms of endocrine abnormality in liver disease are outlined in Table 7.2.

The endocrine abnormalities associated with liver disease are often similar in hepatic disease of varied aetiology but in certain conditions, such as haemochromatosis, endocrine changes are either specific or occur with such frequency that they are considered separately. In view of the importance of alcohol in the pathogenesis or progression of much of the liver disease seen in Western societies, a separate discussion of the endocrine effects of alcohol is included. Finally, we will discuss the hepatic disorders observed in patients with primary disease of the endocrine system.

Table 7.1 Hormones catabolized by liver.

Catabolism primarily by liver
  Insulin
  Glucagon (3500-dalton)
  Growth hormone
  Glucocorticoids
  Oestrogens
  Progesterone
  Parathyroid hormone
  Some gut hormones

Catabolism by liver and other tissues
  Thyroid hormones
  Luteinizing hormone
  Antidiuretic hormone
  Testosterone
  Aldosterone
  Oxytocin
  Adrenocorticotrophic hormone
  Thyroid-stimulating hormone
  Thyrotrophin-releasing hormone

ENDOCRINE CHANGES IN LIVER DISEASE

INSULIN

Normal physiology

The liver is a major organ in the regulation of carbohydrate, protein and lipid metabolism and as such is an important target tissue for insulin action. It is also important in insulin degradation.

Insulin is secreted directly into the portal venous system, the rate of secretion being influenced by many factors other than blood glucose concentration; these include amino acids, gut hormones and stress. The liver is sensitive to small changes in insulin secretion; thus a twofold rise in portal venous insulin concentration in overnight-fasted man is sufficient to inhibit hepatic glucose production completely.[118] This fine control of hepatic metabolism may be aided by the fact that the liver is exposed to much

Table 7.2 Mechanisms of endocrine abnormality in liver disease.

- Impaired metabolism of hormones by the diseased liver
- Increased hormone secretion by endocrine organs
- Decreased hormone secretion by endocrine organs
- Abnormal control mechanisms for hormone secretion by endocrine organs
- Decreased hormone production or activation by the diseased liver or by non-endocrine tissues
- Production of a variant hormone where heterogeneous molecular forms exist
- Alterations in target tissue response
- Abnormalities induced through nutritional alterations or therapeutic agents

higher insulin concentrations than are peripheral tissues, as a result of direct secretion into the portal venous system.[36] A further factor increasing the portal–peripheral venous difference is hepatic degradation of insulin. Most evidence available from animals and man suggests that approximately 50% of the insulin secreted by the pancreas is degraded in the first passage through the liver.[40,52,60a,173,189,190,232,261,275,280,328] Hepatic extraction of insulin is not saturated over a fivefold range of insulin levels in normal man.[40]

Insulin in liver disease

It is to be expected that liver disease will be associated with abnormalities of insulin metabolism. Hepatic cirrhosis is consistently associated with elevated peripheral venous immunoreactive insulin concentrations (Table 7.3). Hyperinsulinaemia is observed in the fasting state and in response to normal meals, oral or intravenous glucose, amino acids and tolbutamide.[77,82,149,183,186,205,247,275,307,369] Similar findings have been demonstrated, although less consistently, in liver failure[338,362,414] and in acute viral hepatitis.[119,245,272,313] Liver damage with paracetamol (acetaminophen) overdose is associated with normal fasting insulin concentrations but an exaggerated insulin response to intravenous glucose.[314] Chronic active hepatitis, on the other hand, may be associated with hypoinsulinaemia and a delayed insulin response to intravenous glucose,[7] although basal and stimulated hyperinsulinaemia have also been reported.[27,49]

Mechanisms of hyperinsulinaemia

Peripheral hyperinsulinaemia is therefore the rule for most forms of liver disease unless pancreatic damage is also present.[11] The hyperinsulinaemia may result from either hypersecretion or diminished degradation. The bulk of evidence suggests that the latter is more important.[57,58,170,181,184,186,220,340] In the pancreatic B cell, proinsulin is cleaved to insulin and the connecting peptide, C-peptide, plus some basic amino acids. C-peptide and insulin are released in equimolar quantities[169] but evidence so far suggests that C-peptide is degraded by the kidney and not significantly by the liver.[191,373] If renal function is normal, peripheral C-peptide levels are unlikely to be influenced by liver disease and will provide a better indication of insulin secretion than measurement of peripheral insulin levels alone. Studies have shown that fasting C-peptide concentrations are normal in hyperinsulinaemic cirrhotics, suggesting that, despite high peripheral insulin concentrations, insulin secretion is not increased. In addition, after oral glucose, cirrhotics with a high peripheral insulin response have similar C-peptide values to those with normal peripheral insulin values.[175] It therefore appears that hyperinsulinaemia both in fasting and after oral glucose results from diminished degradation rather than hypersecretion of insulin, at least in cirrhotic subjects. Support for this hypothesis comes from studies involving direct measurements of portal and peripheral venous insulin levels.[150] However, some investigators using either insulin-infusion studies[74,364] or C-peptide and insulin measurements[11] have concluded that hypersecretion of insulin was more important in production of the hyperinsulinaemia, while other studies have suggested that both diminished insulin degradation and increased secretion of insulin were present.[57,58,192,311,334] Insulin-infusion techniques are less reliable in that when insulin is given through a peripheral vein, relatively more of this insulin is likely to be cleared by non-hepatic tissues and a substantial defect in hepatic insulin clearance may go undetected. To overcome this problem, combined peripheral and portal infusion studies have been performed and demonstrate that insulin uptake is markedly reduced in cirrhosis.[275] Results from studies with simultaneous insulin and C-peptide measurement will be influenced by the presence of fasting hyperglycaemia and the resultant increased stimulus to insulin secretion in these patients. In most, but not all, studies where the fasting blood glucose was normal, hyperinsulinaemia was considered to reflect diminished insulin degradation.

Abnormalities in the regulation of insulin secretion have also been postulated as contributing to the hyperinsulinaemia of cirrhosis[58] in those with insulin hypersecretion. Impaired suppression of insulin release by insulin itself, reduced first-phase secretion in response to glucose and reduced pancreatic content of insulin have all been demonstrated.[233,271,341]

The hyperinsulinaemia of liver disease is associated with insulin resistance, as is observed in other hyperinsulinaemic conditions. Whatever the cause of the hyperinsulinaemia in liver disease, insulin resistance must coexist if hypoglycaemia is not to be the result.

The interpretation of insulin immunoassay results is complicated by the interference of precursor proinsulin molecules which are present in excess in cirrhosis and cross-react with insulin in the radioimmunoassay but have a low insulin-like biological activity. The recent development of a specific two-site immunoradiometric assay that can distinguish intact and split proinsulin from insulin[381] may help to elucidate the aetiology of documented peripheral hyperinsulinaemia in liver disease.

Table 7.3 Basal values for hormones in liver disease.

	Cirrhosis		Acute viral hepatitis		Chronic active hepatitis	
	Patient	Control	Patient	Control	Patient	Control
Insulin (mU/l)	17 ± 2.4^a	8.9 ± 2.1	23.0 ± 9.3^f	9 ± 4	8.1 ± 0.9^i	6.4 ± 0.7
	28 ± 7^b	11 ± 3	10.3 ± 2.1^g	6.4 ± 0.5		
	16.3^c	3.8	8.7 ± 1^h	$12.2 \pm 1.3\dagger$		
	12 ± 5^d	12 ± 2				
	22 ± 2^e	8 ± 1				
Glucagon (ng/l)	342 ± 28^b	105 ± 12				
	239 ± 32^e	146 ± 10				
	243 ± 41^j	89 ± 16				
	320 ± 15^{bb}	90 ± 12				
Growth hormone (μg/l)	6.9 ± 0.9^b	2.8 ± 0.7	8.6 ± 2.1^g	6.4 ± 0.5	3.8 ± 1^i	6.7 ± 2.1
	9.4 ± 7.1^k	2.5 ± 0.9	3.9 ± 1.7^l	$0.3–5$		
	10.7 ± 4.6^l	$0.3–5$				
	8.4 ± 1.4^m	2.5 ± 0.9				
Thyroxine (T$_4$) (nmol/l)	97 ± 5^n	108 ± 3	147 ± 19^p	111 ± 4	102 ± 6^{bb}	$46–150$
	94 ± 6°	84 ± 3		$74\ (42–120)$	97 ± 6^{cc}	94 ± 3
	104 ± 8^p	111 ± 4	$154\ (112–222)^{dd}$		136 ± 13^{ee}	108 ± 4
	86 ± 5^{cc}	94 ± 3				
Triiodothyronine (T$_3$) (nmol/l)	0.51 ± 0.05^n	1.94 ± 0.05	2.29 ± 0.32^p	1.94 ± 0.06	1.85 ± 0.10^{bb}	$1.5–3$
	1.31 ± 0.12^p	1.94 ± 0.06		$1.9\ (1.2–3.0)$	2.0 ± 0.1^{cc}	2.2 ± 0.1
	1.2 ± 0.1^{cc}	2.2 ± 0.1	$2.4\ (1.4–5.2)^{dd}$		3.1 ± 0.3^{ee}	2.8 ± 0.2
Free thyroxine (pmol/l)	15.3 ± 0.6^{cc}	12.7 ± 0.4			15.3 ± 1.0^{cc}	12.7 ± 0.4
	50.2 ± 2.2^n	36.0 ± 1.3				
Free triiodothyronine (pmol/l)	4.5 ± 0.2^{cc}	6.5 ± 0.2			5.5 ± 0.3^{cc}	6.5 ± 0.2
	2.5 ± 0.2^n	5.8 ± 0.3				
Thyroid stimulating hormone (TSH) (mU/l)	8 ± 1^n	4.6 ± 0.3	5.5 ± 0.4^p	3.1 ± 0.1	10.4 ± 0.8^{bb}	$8–18.7$
	5 ± 0.4^o	3.6 ± 0.2			2.7 ± 0.2^{cc}	2.4 ± 0.1
	7.1 ± 0.6^p	3.1 ± 0.1	$1.1\ (0.2–3.2)^{dd}$	$1.1\ (0.2–4.2)$	3.4 ± 1.2^{ee}	3.1 ± 0.2
	3.1 ± 0.2^{cc}	2.4 ± 0.1				

Role of portosystemic anastomoses

Diminished insulin degradation in liver cirrhosis may result from parenchymal damage, portosystemic shunting or both. Considerable intrahepatic portosystemic shunting may occur in patients who have no demonstrable large-vessel anastomoses. Animal experiments with diversion of portal or pancreatic venous blood into the systemic circulation have produced conflicting results: some workers have demonstrated a hyperinsulinaemic effect,[218,337,363] while others have not.[73,353,412] Human studies have shown a rise in basal and stimulated peripheral insulin concentrations in cirrhotic subjects after surgical portacaval anastomosis.[115,167,247,329,351] This would suggest that portal bypass is an important factor in diminished insulin metabolism, but the possibility remains that the bypass procedure itself may produce further liver damage. Evidence against a major role for portal bypass is provided by studies in subjects with long-standing portal venous block who had extensive natural or surgically created portosystemic anastomoses. These subjects had ostensibly normal liver function and normal liver biopsy histology on light microscopy.[185,361] Fasting hyperinsulinaemia did not occur and fasting C-peptide concentrations were normal. Only at high rates of insulin secretion was a defect in insulin degradation observed. Thus, significant liver damage is necessary for hyperinsulinaemia to occur and parenchymal damage is likely to be more important than portosystemic anastomosis alone in the hyperinsulinaemia of cirrhosis.

Table 7.3 Continued

	Cirrhosis		Acute viral hepatitis		Chronic active hepatitis	
	Patient	Control	Patient	Control	Patient	Control
Testosterone* (nmol/l)	7.6 (3.8–19.1)[q]	22.6 (16.7–27.4)			17.3 ± 3.4[u]	26.4 ± 1.1
	17.0 ± 3.1[r]	26.4 ± 2.4			6.9 ± 1.9[v]	8.0 ± 1.1†
	8.1 ± 1.7[s]	19.7 ± 1.8				
	10.5 ± 0.8[t]	20.8 ± 3.2				
	11.6 ± 1.7[u]	26.4 ± 1.1				
	10.8 ± 2.3[v]	8 ± 1.1‡				
Oestradiol* (pmol/l)	109 ± 8[w]	86 ± 7			93 ± 11[u]	70 ± 4
	115 ± 7[u]	70 ± 4			89 ± 30[v]	85 ± 15
	159 ± 24[x]	84 ± 11				
	174 ± 19[s]	100 ± 7				
	117 ± 16[r]	112 ± 5				
Luteinizing hormone* (LH) (U/l)	24.1 ± 2.5[s]	12.1 ± 1.1			18 ± 2[u]	12 ± 1
	19.5 ± 5.5[y]	11.8 ± 2.5			3.2 ± 0.4[v]	2.4 ± 0.2
	4 ± 0.4[z]	0.8–13.3				
	18 ± 1[u]	12 ± 1				
	19.1 ± 3.4[aa]	8.8 ± 1.4				
Follicle stimulating hormone* (FSH)(U/l)	12.8 ± 2.3[s]	8.4 ± 2				
	10.1 ± 1.7[y]	5.6 ± 1.7				
	3.1 ± 0.4[z]	0.2–8.3				
	20.7 ± 5.1[aa]	11.5 ± 2.9				
Prolactin (mU/l)	1135 ± 178[ff]	270 ± 20				
	315 ± 53[gg]	203 ± 35§				

Values for plasma or serum samples, mean ± standard error of the mean, or range.
* Values are for male subjects.
† Values are for a group of hypoglycaemic subjects.
‡ Testosterone measured as 17-β-hydroxy androgen, μg/l.
§ 13 out of 16 patients had cirrhosis.

Values are adapted from the following papers:
[a] Johnston *et al.*[186]
[b] Greco *et al.*[149]
[c] West *et al.*[419]
[d] Sestoft and Rehfeld[338]
[e] Marco *et al.*[234]
[f] Nieschlag *et al.*[272]
[g] Record *et al.*[313]
[h] Felig *et al.*[119]
[i] Alberti *et al.*[7]
[j] Sherwin *et al.*[347]
[k] Conn and Daughaday[77]
[l] Hernandez *et al.*[164]
[m] Zanoboni and Zanoboni-Muciaccia[433]
[n] Chopra *et al.*[66]
[o] Cuttelod *et al.*[84]
[p] Nomura *et al.*[273]
[q] Coppage and Cooner[79]
[r] Distiller *et al.*[98]
[s] Chopra *et al.*[65]
[t] Gordon *et al.*[146]
[u] Kley *et al.*[200]
[v] Galvao-Teles *et al.*[137]
[w] Pentikäinen *et al.*[292]
[x] Korenman *et al.*[206]
[y] Schalch *et al.*[331]
[z] Mowat *et al.*[262]
[aa] Van Thiel *et al.*[401]
[bb] Sheridan *et al.*[344]
[cc] Borzio *et al.*[38]
[dd] Hegedüs *et al.*[161]
[ee] Schussler *et al.*[335]
[ff] Van Thiel *et al.*[404]
[gg] Panerai *et al.*[287]

GLUCAGON _____

Normal physiology

In normal man, the importance of the liver in the metabolism of glucagon is uncertain. Many of the difficulties in determining its role are attributable to the heterogeneity of total plasma immunoreactive glucagon (IRG). Total plasma IRG is composed of multiple fractions: the 3500-dalton component is the biologically active form of the hormone and the 9000-dalton moiety may be a precursor of the 3500-dalton form but is itself biologically inactive; the significance of other forms such as the 2000-dalton and 160 000-dalton fractions is uncertain. Thus, although the 3500-dalton moiety is the biologically active one, total plasma IRG may measure all components, depending on the antibody used, and significant changes in 3500-dalton glucagon may occur without a measurable change in total IRG.

Some studies using total plasma IRG measurement have suggested that the kidneys are of major importance in glucagon metabolism, with the liver assuming a minor role,[120,123,127,319] whereas others have suggested that the liver is the major site of glucagon metabolism.[45,213,423] The importance of gel filtration and measurement of each particular fraction of IRG is illustrated by the study of Jaspan and colleagues.[177] Thus, in the rat, the liver selectively metabolizes 3500-dalton glucagon with an extraction in fasted animals of 81% ± 5% while extracting only minimal quantities of 9000-dalton and > 40 000-dalton glucagon. If these results can be extrapolated to man, hepatic glucagon metabolism may therefore be of major physiological importance.

Studies using radiolabelled glucagon in the dog _in vivo_ and _in vitro_[158] have identified a peptide product of glucagon metabolism by the liver. This metabolic product, glucagon (4–29), is also present in human plasma. The fragment lacks the terminal three residues of the hormone and is biologically inactive but is detected in the carboxy-terminal glucagon radioimmunoassay. It represents approximately 25% of the immunoreactive glucagon detected. Thus, the true hepatic clearance of glucagon may have been further underestimated in past studies.

Glucagon in liver disease

All of the earlier studies in human liver disease give information only about total IRG concentrations. Marco and colleagues[234] found mean fasting plasma glucagon levels of 455 ± 63 pg/ml in cirrhotic patients with a portacaval shunt, 217 ± 23 pg/ml in patients with liver disease but no evidence of portosystemic anastomoses, and 146 ± 10 pg/ml in control subjects. Sherwin _et al._[347] found elevated plasma IRG concentrations only if portosystemic shunting was present. The importance of portal bypass is further suggested by experiments in normal dogs in which progressive hyperglucagonaemia occurred after surgical portacaval anastomosis.[363] Elevated plasma glucagon concentrations are also found in human subjects with chronic portal venous block and extensive natural or surgically created portosystemic anastomoses, despite normal liver function on routine biochemistry and normal liver biopsy to light microscopy. In chemically induced liver injury in rats without portosystemic shunts, circulating IRG levels have been reported as normal[10] or increased.[170] Decreased extraction of glucagon by the isolated perfused rat liver has been documented in carbon tetrachloride-induced liver damage.[170]

The importance of portal venous bypass in the production of hyperglucagonaemia suggests that diminished hepatic breakdown, rather than hypersecretion of glucagon, may be the major factor, a situation analogous to that for insulin. This may not be solely the case. Sherwin and colleagues,[348] measuring specifically 3500-dalton glucagon, found a two- to sixfold increase in basal plasma levels in cirrhotics with demonstrable portosystemic anastomoses, but values were normal in cirrhotics without portal venous bypass. Metabolic clearance rate of 3500-dalton glucagon was normal in all subjects, suggesting that the elevated plasma concentrations observed in cirrhotics with portosystemic anastomoses were the result of hypersecretion of glucagon. In addition, in experimentally produced portal hypertension in rats,[353] glucagon hypersecretion was proposed on the basis of increased arterial and portal IRG levels. Pancreatic islet glucagon concentration is also increased after portocaval anastomosis in rats.[271] By contrast, Alford and colleagues,[8] measuring total plasma immunoreactive glucagon, observed a decrease in the metabolic clearance rate in human cirrhotics after portacaval anastomosis compared with the values obtained before surgery in the same patients. Glucagon clearance was normal before surgical bypass. These authors concluded that hyperglucagonaemia before shunting reflected A-cell hypersecretion, whereas after portal bypass both hypersecretion and diminished degradation contributed to the elevated fasting glucagon levels. Regional blood-flow studies revealed that the raised plasma glucagon levels in portocaval-shunted rats were directly related to an increase in cardiac output and portal venous inflow.[207] These circulatory changes are unlikely to be causative in the hyperglucagonaemia but rather the reverse, as glucagon itself has been implicated in producing the increased blood flow.

Metabolic consequences of hyperglucagonaemia

The pathophysiological importance of hyperglucagonaemia in liver disease is uncertain because glucagon concentrations bear no relation to the degree of glucose intolerance or other metabolic disturbances.[114,186] The elevated plasma concentrations observed do not fall normally in response to glucose and show abnormal increases after alanine or arginine stimulation.[149,150] Similar abnormalities of glucagon regulation have been observed in most[170,271] but not all[10] *in vitro* studies on isolated islets. The liver in man is the major organ on which glucagon exerts its glycogenolytic and gluconeogenic actions, but portal bypass or hepatic parenchymal damage may serve to decrease the metabolic effect. A diminished blood glucose response to exogenous glucagon has been observed in viral hepatitis,[119] in post-necrotic cirrhosis[430] and in cirrhosis of varied aetiology.[91] Against these positive reports are other studies in which no abnormality in the blood glucose response to glucagon could be demonstrated in the majority of patients with cirrhosis.[340,374,396] These discrepancies may have been due to differing patient populations or to differences in the nutritional states of the patients.

An impaired glucose response to glucagon can be explained in several ways. There may be decreased hepatic glycogen due to parenchymal damage, inadequate nutrition or to increased glycogenolysis for some other reason. Alternatively, there may be damage to glucagon receptors. The report by Davies *et al.*[88] of an increased plasma cyclic AMP response to glucagon infusion in patients with cirrhosis and extrahepatic and intrahepatic cholestasis is of interest. It suggests that glucagon receptors are fully functional in these states; the normal glucose response to glucagon in the same patients suggested that no other major post-receptor block to glucagon action was present. These authors also found that the cyclic AMP response was diminished in six out of eight patients with portacaval shunts and that shunted patients had a significantly lowered glucose response. This was observed also by Sherwin's group[348] and their patients with shunts had the highest glucagon levels. In the latter study, patients with normal hepatic blood flow had an exaggerated glucose response to glucagon infusion. Shunting is therefore important as a major mechanism for diminished delivery of glucagon to the liver and consequent decrease in both glucagon degradation and in glucagon-stimulated glycogenolysis.

It is also possible that glucagon-induced hyperglycaemia occurs by a different mechanism in certain patients with liver disease. The glycaemic response in normal subjects to intravenous alanine, a potent stimulus of glucagon release, occurs within 10–20 minutes and probably reflects glycogenolysis. In cirrhotic subjects the maximal increase in glucose is similar but may be delayed to 30–60 minutes.[347] This corresponds to the time required for glucagon to stimulate glucose synthesis from [14C]alanine. The hyperglycaemic effect of glucagon in liver disease may therefore be due more to a stimulating effect on gluconeogenesis rather than on glycogenolysis.

GROWTH HORMONE _____

Normal physiology

Turnover of growth hormone in plasma is rapid, with a half-disappearance time of 19 minutes.[283] Secretion is pulsatile and its control is complex; the effects of stress, non-esterified fatty acids, amino acids, glucose depri-vation, adrenergic stimulation and deep sleep have been reviewed.[96,187,265,321] There is also evidence of negative feedback by somatomedins or by the growth hormone molecule itself.[1,157] The liver and kidneys are the major sites of growth hormone degradation. Growth hormone release from the pituitary is determined by the hypothalamus. The hypothalamus produces a stimulatory factor or factors (growth hormone-releasing hormone, GHRH) and an inhibitory factor (somatostatin).

Growth hormone in liver disease

Basal growth hormone levels may be elevated in various forms of liver disease, particularly cirrhosis (see Table 7.3) with the highest levels frequently observed in those patients with the most severe disease.[209,369] The rise in growth hormone has been attributed to a decrease in metabolic clearance. Thus, Owens and coworkers,[283] using a constant infusion technique to achieve a variety of serum growth hormone levels, showed a decrease in metabolic clearance of unlabelled human growth hormone in 10 out of 17 patients with hepatic cirrhosis. Cameron *et al.*,[51] using radiolabelled human growth hormone, obtained similar results. Taylor and colleagues[380] showed that the liver was responsible for 90% of the metabolic clearance of human growth hormone but found normal values in patients with liver disease. In addition, Pimstone *et al.*[299] showed normal clearance of endogenous growth hormone during infusion of somatostatin in four patients with severe liver disease who had elevated basal growth hormone values.

Thus, evidence for delayed growth hormone clearance is inconclusive and, although in some subjects it may contribute to the elevation in basal values, it does not explain the paradoxical rise in growth hormone after oral glucose in some patients with liver disease or the exaggerated growth hormone response to insulin-induced hypoglycaemia and arginine in others.[27,187,209,264,327,341] In liver disease, glucose fails to inhibit the growth hormone-releasing hormone (GHRH) stimulated growth hormone (GH) release, perhaps through a failure to stimulate hypothalamic somatostatin secretion. It should be noted that the elevated fasting and post-prandial somatostatin levels in the peripheral circulation in cirrhosis[341] reflect increased somatostatin production in the gastrointestinal tract, and the small amount of circulating somatostatin has probably very little effect on growth hormone secretion.[411] Altered hypothalamic-pituitary control of growth hormone secretion is also suggested by the growth hormone response to intravenous thyrotrophin-releasing hormone, which is not observed in normal subjects.[209,287,433] Altered dopaminergic control of growth hormone secretion also requires investigation, particularly in patients with hepatic failure in whom a defect in dopaminergic neurotransmission has been postulated.[126,209]

Other factors which are known to influence growth hormone secretion, including circulating oestrogen concentrations, recent alcohol ingestion and nutritional status, cannot explain the abnormal growth hormone regulation observed in liver disease.

Somatomedins

Many of the actions of growth hormone are secondary to the production of a group of small peptides, the somatomedins. Present evidence suggests that somatomedins are produced in part by the liver. Somatomedin activity falls after partial hepatectomy in rats and rises as the liver regenerates.[394] Isolated rat liver perfusion experiments have demonstrated an increase in somatomedin activity in the perfusate when growth hormone was added to the perfusion medium.[242,243] In similar experiments, livers from hypophysectomized rats released less somatomedin activity than livers from intact animals, and activity could be increased by the addition of growth hormone to the perfusate.[298] Other hormones, such as insulin and the thyroid hormones, and nutritional status also influence hepatic somatomedin production.[256] Studies on partially hepatectomized rats on a controlled food intake following surgery have demonstrated transient reductions in somatomedin activity measured in a bioassay using costal cartilage. Activity was increased above that observed in control rats during the subsequent 7 days of hepatic regeneration. This suggests either that somatomedin production increased or that production of a somatomedin inhibitor decreased as the liver regenerated. In hypophysectomized animals somatomedin activity remained persistently low after partial hepatectomy and these rats exhibited reduced liver regeneration. Thus, pituitary factors are involved both in hepatic regeneration and in the enhanced somatomedin activity associated with liver regeneration.[393]

Wu and colleagues[426] studied serum somatomedin activity in a group of patients with chronic liver disease, in whom activity was assessed by ^{35}S uptake into chick embryo pelvic rudiments. Nine out of ten cirrhotics showed low activity which correlated with the degree of liver damage. Elevated basal growth hormone levels were found in seven patients, all of whom had decreased somatomedin activity. Similar findings have been obtained using a somatomedin radioreceptor assay.[378] In catheterization studies, the expected gradient of somatomedin activity across the liver is absent in cirrhosis, suggesting a decrease in hepatic production.[332,333] Agner[5] found increased basal growth hormone levels in alcoholics, but levels were higher in those with cirrhosis than in those with fatty change or normal liver histology. The cirrhotics also had a greater growth hormone response to thyrotropin-releasing hormone (TRH) than those patients with less severe liver disease. Since there was no associated effect of liver disease on TRH stimulation of thyroid-stimulating hormone or prolactin, the enhanced growth hormone stimulation may reflect reduced negative feedback as a consequence of the reduced somatomedin levels rather than a defect in the hypothalamo–pituitary axis.[5,341]

Abnormal oestrogen metabolism in cirrhotic subjects may contribute, as oestrogen administration decreases the somatomedin response to growth hormone both in animals[297] and man,[421,422] but no relationship has been evident between somatomedin levels and oestrogen concentrations. Similarly, no relationship with nutritional status is evident in cirrhotic patients, although inadequate nutrition might potentially decrease somatostatin production.

Metabolic effects

The metabolic effects of a chronic elevation in growth hormone concentration in subjects with liver disease are probably diminished by the decreased somatomedin response. Patients may have raised growth hormone levels for years but not develop acromegaly. Growth hormone may play some role in the abnormal carbohydrate metabolism observed (see Chapter 3) but levels do not correlate with any index of glucose tolerance.

CORTISOL

Normal physiology

Cortisol is the major glucocorticoid hormone and its secretion is influenced by the diurnal rhythm, negative feedback by the cortisol molecule and stress, of which stress is the most potent stimulus. In the basal state, circulating cortisol is 95% bound to protein, largely cortisol-binding globulin and, to a lesser extent, albumin. It is degraded primarily in the liver and its metabolites are excreted mainly conjugated in the glucuronate or sulphate form.

Plasma cortisol levels in liver disease

Clinical evidence of cortisol excess, such as striae, obesity, facial mooning and acne, may be seen in some patients with liver disease, in particular those with chronic active hepatitis. Studies of plasma cortisol levels have shown different results. Peterson[295] and most other workers have shown normal values, although Sholiton et al.[350] showed lower values throughout the day. A loss of the normal diurnal variation has also been described[369,390] but in the most detailed study the normal cortisol diurnal rhythm was preserved, although the secretory peaks were decreased in number and duration.[323] Absent cortisol responses to insulin hypoglycaemia and pseudo-Cushing's syndrome, both described in alcoholics (see below), are more likely to result from alcohol ingestion than associated liver disease.

The significance of total plasma cortisol measurements is uncertain in view of the decrease in serum albumin and, particularly, cortisol-binding globulin in subjects with liver disease.[221,323] Studies which take protein binding into account have clarified this. McCann and Fulton[241] showed a small but significant decrease in total 11-hydroxycorticosteroid concentrations throughout the day in a group of patients with a variety of liver diseases. Free hormone levels were normal in the morning and slightly higher than for controls at 23:00 h. Kley *et al.*[199] found normal total levels and free hormone concentrations in subjects with liver disease. The nature of the liver disease may be of relevance. Orbach demonstrated raised levels of cortisol-binding globulin, and increased serum cortisol binding as measured by charcoal uptake of ^{125}I cortisol, in patients with chronic active hepatitis but not in cirrhotics. The increase in protein binding could delay hormone clearance and account for reports of elevated serum cortisol concentrations in patients with chronic hepatitis.[281]

Cortisol metabolism in liver disease

The liver is the major organ of catabolism of adrenal corticosteroids and it is to be expected that abnormalities of clearance will be found in liver disease. Radioactive cortisol is cleared more slowly in cirrhotic subjects, and after cortisol or ACTH infusion, plasma 17-hydroxycorticosteroids remain elevated longer than normal.[43,108,295] Impairment of A-ring reduction has been demonstrated, as has impairment of 6-β-hydroxylase and of the conjugation mechanism.[317,434] Normal or near normal plasma cortisol levels in the presence of diminished clearance implies a decrease in cortisol production rate but two studies have failed to demonstrate such a decreased rate in cirrhotic subjects[241,434] and this requires further clarification. Twenty-four-hour urinary free cortisol excretion is diminished[241] as is 17-hydroxysteroid and 17-ketosteroid excretion.[342] This does not necessarily imply diminished adrenal steroid production as urinary excretion may be modified by alterations in glomerular filtration known to occur in cirrhotic patients. The possibility of an increase in extrahepatic hormone metabolism has not been investigated.

Metabolic effects

There is as yet no evidence to suggest that alterations in the amount or action of glucocorticoids are important in the production of the metabolic changes observed in subjects with liver disease. The roles of cortisol deficiency in the pathogenesis of alcoholic hypoglycaemia and of cortisol excess in the pathogenesis of alcoholic ketosis are discussed below.

THYROID HORMONES

Normal physiology

In normal subjects, the thyroid produces 100 nmol/24 h (78 μg/24 h) of thyroxine (T_4). Of this, 20 nmol/24 h (16 μg/24 h) is conjugated, excreted in bile or undergoes oxidative deamination.[56,136] The remainder is de-iodin-ated to either triiodothyronine (T_3) (35 nmol/24 h; 23 μg/24 h)[41,304,377] or reverse triiodothyronine (rT_3) (45 nmol/24 h; 29 μg/24 h).[62,139] The same enzyme (iodothyronine deiodinase) is involved in T_3 production and rT_3 clearance but rT_3 is the preferred substrate and is catalysed 400 times more efficiently than T_4.[411a] Reverse T_3 may be considered biologically inactive at pathophysiological concentrations[303] but T_3 is several times more potent than T_4 on a molar basis.[44] Peripheral conversion of T_4 to T_3 may therefore be considered to be a form of hormone activation. Only 5 nmol/24 h (3 μg/24 h) of T_3 is secreted directly by the thyroid.[56,63]

Hepatectomy in dogs severely impairs production of T_3 but not of rT_3 from exogenously administered T_4.[129] This suggests that the liver is a major organ of T_4 to T_3 conversion, and that production of rT_3 occurs in extrahepatic tissues. Thus, the liver has a major role in thyroid hormone metabolism, being involved in conjugation, biliary excretion and oxidative deamination of thyroxine and peripheral de-iodination of thyroxine to triiodothyronine. Abnormalities of thyroid hormone metabolism are therefore to be expected in subjects with liver disease. In addition to the major thyroid hormones (T_4, T_3 and rT_3) other iodothyronines and their derivatives have been identified in human serum.[64] These include three diiodothyronines, two monoiodothyronines, thyronine, and acetic acid analogues of T_4 and T_3. Mono- and diiodotyrosine have also been isolated. As with T_3 and rT_3, production of the iodothyronines and iodotyrosines occurs predominantly outside the thyroid.[64,140,358]

Thyroid hormones in liver disease

The majority of patients with liver disease are clinically euthyroid; this view is supported by indirect measures of thyroid hormone action such as Achilles tendon reflex time and indices of myocardial contractility.[66] However, many standard laboratory techniques may give misleading results suggesting hyper- or hypothyroidism.

^{131}Iodine uptake

Patients with acute alcohol related liver disease may have elevated thyroid uptake and clearance of radioactive iodine (^{131}I).[349] This has been attributed to iodine deficiency secondary to malnutrition, although evidence for this is not conclusive. The elevated ^{131}I uptake returns to normal if the patients are admitted to hospital and it can be suppressed with T_3. Accelerated ^{131}I uptake may also be found in hepatobiliary giardiasis.[215] Uptake of ^{131}I has been found to be decreased in acute infective hepatitis, particularly in patients with severe disease.[92,397] Chronic liver disease, particularly alcoholic cirrhosis, may be associated with increased ^{131}I uptake by a mechanism similar to that of acute alcoholic damage.[263,349] Uptake may be low in chronic active hepatitis.[344]

Thyroid hormone levels

The daily production rate of T_4 in liver disease is mildly decreased.[62] Serum total and free T_4 levels are normal, slightly increased or slightly decreased in most studies of subjects with a variety of liver diseases[38,54,66,171,273,335,344,413] (see Table 7.3). In occasional patients, the total T_4 may be considerably increased or decreased in association with an altered level of thyroxine-binding proteins.[171,344] Some insight into a possible mechanism for the biochemical changes in acute liver disease has been provided by the studies of Hegedüs *et al.*[162] This group observed raised total T_4 and thyroxine-binding globulin (TBG) in patients with acute viral hepatitis and the volume of the thyroid gland (measured by ultrasound) was increased by approximately 50%. There was a significant correlation between the TBG levels and aspartate transaminase concentrations. All of these changes reverted to normal after recovery from the hepatitis. It was suggested that the rise in TBG, possibly released from damaged hepatocytes, resulted in thyroid hypertrophy in an attempt to meet the demand for increased thyroxine production.

The combination of a low total T_4 with an elevated free T_4 is frequently observed in patients with severe decompensated liver disease, and reflects a decrease in thyroid hormone-binding proteins.[64] Patients with severe liver disease may also possess a circulating inhibitor which prevents thyroid hormones binding to serum proteins. Estimation of the free thyroxine index, calculated from serum thyroxine and thyroid hormone binding level, usually reveals a normal result in liver disease.[344]

Total and free T_3 levels may be diminished, sometimes profoundly, and they correlate negatively with the degree of liver damage as indicated by clinical criteria and liver function tests.[28,54,66,163,174] Nomura and colleagues[273] have shown T_4 to T_3 conversion in four cirrhotic patients to be decreased to less than half that seen in normal subjects (15.6% compared with 35.7%). In addition, two patients convalescing from alcoholic hepatitis showed a progressive return of serum T_3 levels to normal as liver function improved. Diminished T_4 to T_3 conversion appears the likely mechanism for the low serum T_3 levels observed in liver disease, although decreased serum binding also contributes. The direct thyroid secretion of T_3 is normal,[66] as is the metabolic clearance rate of T_3. The reduction in serum T_3 concentration in those who are ill with acute and chronic liver disease is similar to, but more marked than, that observed in subjects with a variety of other acute and chronic illnesses.[48,54]

Hepatic cirrhosis is associated with an increase in both total and dialysable rT_3.[66] Again, this is not specific for liver disease, similar changes being observed in acute febrile illness and in patients with disseminated carcinoma.[48] It is also a feature of chronic malnutrition, as whenever serum albumin falls below 35 g/l in patients with a variety of conditions, the low T_3 is associated with a rise in rT_3.[294] In malnutrition the elevated rT_3 levels result from a decrease in the metabolic clearance rate of rT_3, while the production of rT_3 is similar to that observed in normal controls. When viewed in the context of the decreased T_4 production rate, the proportion of T_4 converted to rT_3 is either normal or increased and T_3 production is clearly diminished.[62,68] A reciprocal relationship between serum T_3 and rT_3 is observed in patients with chronic liver disease.[55]

The effect of alcohol on thyroid function may not only be determined by the resulting hepatic pathology. Agner reported a reduction in serum T_3 and rT_3 in alcoholics with cirrhosis, fatty change or normal liver on histology but only those with cirrhosis had raised TBG levels. Regardless of the pathology, alcohol has a predominant effect on T_3 levels, possibly by causing increased T_4 metabolism via routes other than to T_3 or rT_3. Binding protein levels are determined more by the extent of the liver disease. There is no evidence for a major defect in hypothalamic-pituitary control of TSH release in chronic alcoholism.[5] Minor abnormalities have been observed. Röjdmark *et al.* investigated the effect of TRH stimulation in chronic alcoholics, 24 hours after alcohol withdrawal. A reduced TSH response was observed and could be normalized by pretreatment with metoclopramide, a dopamine-receptor blocking agent. Increased dopaminergic inhibition of TSH release by the pituitary may therefore be implicated in the reduced response of TSH to its releasing hormone in chronic alcoholism.[320]

Circulating concentrations of the diiodothyronines ($3,3'$-T_2; $3'5'$-T_2; $3,5$-T_2) and monoiodothyronine ($3'$-T_1) have also been investigated in liver disease. Serum $3,3'$-T_2 and $3,5$-T_2 concentrations are decreased and follow the direction of T_3 levels, while serum $3'5'$-T_2 and $3'$-T_1 levels are raised, paralleling the changes in rT_3. Information is now available on the kinetics of these metabolites in liver disease[67,111–113] but their biological significance remains unclear.

Thus, biochemical assessment of thyroid function will usually yield results appropriate to the clinical status if free thyroxine index is measured, but T_3 concentrations may be low and rT_3 levels high. In view of the metabolic potency of T_3, this may suggest hypothyroidism in these subjects, although clinical criteria are against this.

Thyroid-stimulating hormone concentration

Estimation of serum thyroid-stimulating hormone (TSH) concentration is the most sensitive index of thyroid hypofunction available at present if hypothalamic and pituitary function is normal. In several reports, TSH levels have been elevated to twice normal in chronic liver disease,[66,84,161,273] suggesting mild hypothyroidism. TSH levels increase with increasing severity of cirrhosis,[28] but there is no correlation between thyroid hormone levels and TSH.[272] In addition, peak TSH response to thyrotrophin-releasing hormone (TRH), which is exaggerated in primary hypothyroidism, is normal or decreased in liver disease.[5,38,66,305] Van Thiel *et al.* reported raised basal TSH levels, and TSH responses to TRH were exaggerated in this study in chronic liver disease patients, with restoration of TSH values towards normal after liver transplantation.[409] A delay in TSH clearance may be the mechanism for the elevated basal circulating levels.

Evidence for hypothyroidism in liver disease is therefore inconclusive and there is no indication for thyroid replacement therapy in those subjects with low circulating T_3 levels if clinical criteria suggest they are euthyroid.

Thyroid hormones in chronic active hepatitis

Chronic active hepatitis should be considered separately from other forms of liver disturbance in that the incidence of autoimmune thyroid disease is much increased.[100,344] Thyroid function may be normal, increased or decreased.[281,312,384] Primary biliary cirrhosis is also associated with an increased incidence of autoimmune thyroiditis[101,345] (see Chapter 33).

CALCIUM METABOLISM _____

Bone changes in liver disease

Bone thinning and spontaneous fractures occur in patients with chronic cholestatic[17] and alcoholic[225] liver disease, and this hepatic osteodystrophy may result from osteomalacia, osteoporosis or both. Symptomatic bone disease is rare in non-alcoholic, chronic hepatocellular disease,[290] but common in cholestatic disease. In a series of 36 patients with chronic cholestatic liver disease, 42% reported symptoms and had histological evidence of osteoporosis.[368] Osteoporosis has been considered the most common abnormality, but osteomalacia also occurs and early abnormalities of mineralization can be detected in primary biliary cirrhosis at presentation.[257] Between 42% and 75% of patients with established primary biliary cirrhosis have histological evidence of osteomalacia.[95,225] Alcoholic and other forms of liver disease, particularly if associated with chronic cholestasis, may also be associated with osteomalacia as well as with osteoporosis.

The incidence of osteomalacia may have been overestimated in the past owing to inadequate diagnostic methods. Radiological techniques such as bone densitometry do not distinguish between osteoporosis and osteomalacia and nor does measurement of circulating calcium, phosphate and alkaline phosphatase concentrations.[225] Bone histology on non-decalcified sections is necessary with measurement of osteoid tissue and of calcification fronts by double tetracycline labelling.

Pathogenesis of bone pathology

Parathyroid hormone

The aetiology of bone changes is multifactorial. The liver appears to be an important organ for the metabolism of parathyroid hormone,[116] at least in the isolated perfused rat liver. Intact 1–84 amino acid PTH and the NH_2 terminal 1–34 immunoreactive PTH are cleared at the same rate but the mid-molecule and COOH terminal 39–84 PTH are cleared more slowly. This selective hepatic clearance may in part account for the predominance of COOH terminal PTH fragments in plasma.[87] Two-thirds of the intact PTH is extracted via a saturable calcium-independent process by Kupffer cells, and one-third of intact PTH with all 1–34 PTH is extracted by a separate process involving specific hepatocyte receptors and sinusoidal lining cells. This second mechanism can also be saturated and is decreased in hypocalcaemia.[85] The importance of these different processes *in vivo* in man is uncertain, as are the consequences of liver disease for parathyroid hormone metabolism. Kupffer cell dysfunction has been implicated in the development of osteoporosis as these cells are responsible for cleaving intact PTH to the carboxyl fragment. Patients with primary biliary cirrhosis have raised intact PTH levels and reduced carboxyl PTH values, which could be attributed to impaired Kupffer cell function; the consequent increased concentration of intact PTH could contribute to osteoporosis.[160] Hypophosphataemia is a frequent finding in hepatic disease and there have been reports of hypercalcaemia in patients with chronic liver disease awaiting transplantation.[141] Immunoassayable parathyroid hormone levels in such patients are generally normal and radiological osteitis fibrosa has not been reported. Occasional patients with osteomalacia have raised circulating parathyroid hormone levels, suggesting secondary hyperparathyroidism.[86]

Fonseca *et al.* have demonstrated elevated PTH concentrations in patients with primary biliary cirrhosis despite normal or slightly elevated serum calcium and vitamin D levels. This may indicate autonomous PTH secretion and it is possible that vitamin D deficiency and consequent secondary hyperparathyroidism are very early features of the disease.[130] There has also been a report of parathyroid adenomas in patients with cirrhosis followed up after portacaval anastomosis,[282] perhaps reflecting tertiary hyperparathyroidism. It should be noted that not all studies have found evidence of any form of PTH excess in patients with chronic liver disease and bone disease.[225]

Calcium and vitamin D

Many alcoholics have diets low in protein, calcium and most vitamins,[212] and patients with cryptogenic cirrhosis and chronic active hepatitis may be deficient in vitamins A and E and carotene.[260] In addition, calcium malabsorption has been demonstrated in primary biliary cirrhosis and hepatocellular disease.[2,193,257,420] An increase in non-absorbed gut fat, secondary to diminished bile salt secretion, may allow formation of insoluble calcium soaps in the gut lumen.[420] Calcium absorption may be further decreased by malabsorption of fat-soluble vitamin D (D_3); absorption of the latter correlates negatively with faecal fat excretion.[86] Vitamin D given parenterally will correct the defect in calcium absorption but large doses may be necessary, suggesting some resistance to its action. In order to exert its physiological effects, D_3 is hydroxylated in the liver to $25\text{-}(OH)D_3$ and subsequently in the kidney to $1,25\text{-}(OH)_2D_3$.[134,309] Blood concentrations of $25\text{-}(OH)D_3$ are decreased in 40–50% of patients with a variety of liver diseases.[86,95,224,308] It is possible theoretically that resistance to vitamin D action, even when given parenterally, may result from impaired hydroxylation by the diseased liver.[188] Studies in patients with primary biliary cirrhosis and with alcoholic cirrhosis suggest that any defect in 25-hydroxylation is mild and insufficient in itself to explain the low plasma $25\text{-}(OH)D_3$ levels found.[86,226,240,308] A complicating factor is that in liver disease total $25\text{-}(OH)D_3$ levels may be misleading owing to reduced levels of vitamin D-binding globulin. When free $25\text{-}(OH)D_3$ and $1,25\text{-}(OH)_2D_3$ concentrations are measured, they are often normal.[34,35]

A further influence on calcium homeostasis may be interference with the enterohepatic circulation of $25\text{-}(OH)D_3$; in normal subjects one-third of an intravenous dose of $25\text{-}(OH)D_3$ appears in the duodenum over a 24-hour period and, of this, one-quarter is subsequently reabsorbed in the terminal ileum.[15] Malabsorption of enterically secreted $25\text{-}(OH)D_3$[75] may contribute to the lowering of plasma levels in liver disease but most of the vitamin D excreted in bile is in a polar inactive form, malabsorption of which would not be sufficient to account for vitamin D deficiency.[160] Increased urinary losses of vitamin D metabolites in primary biliary cirrhosis, though positively related to serum bilirubin concentration, are probably not quantitatively significant.[240] In this condition the main causes of vitamin D deficiency are inadequate dietary intake and lack of ultraviolet light. The major lesion resides in the hepatobiliary tree and hepatocellular function in primary biliary cirrhosis is spared until late in the disease. In contrast, in alcoholic liver disease, hepatic dysfunction is an early feature: Mawer *et al.* demonstrated that vitamin D hydroxylation was impaired and that it correlated negatively with the bilirubin level and pro-thrombin time.[240]

Osteocalcin

Serum osteocalcin (bone Gla-protein) measurement by radioimmunoassay has been proposed to provide a non-invasive assessment of bone turnover. Osteocalcin is a 49-amino-acid peptide which is synthesized by osteoblasts and is activated by a vitamin K-dependent carboxylation. Decreased serum osteocalcin levels have been reported in primary biliary cirrhosis with a relative excess of the inactive non-carboxylated fraction and a reduction in the active carboxylated form. This may be due to vitamin K deficiency.[130] Combined with bone histology, serum osteocalcin levels have provided further evidence of reduced bone formation as the major cause of osteodystrophy in primary biliary cirrhosis.[166] Diamond *et al.* demonstrated lower bone turnover rates and serum osteocalcin levels in patients with alcoholic liver disease, haemochromatosis and chronic cholestasis than were observed in patients with chronic active hepatitis, although values

in chronic active hepatitis were still lower than in a normal population. These measurements were most abnormal in patients with the most severe hepatic dysfunction.[93] Other investigators have been unable to demonstrate a relationship between bone density and the nature or degree of liver disease. The relative contribution of factors such as immobility and menopausal state remains to be evaluated.[9]

Treatment of bone pathology

Studies in subjects with primary biliary cirrhosis and established bone pathology suggest that vitamin D given parenterally in large doses (100 000 units monthly for 6–72 months) may produce circulating $25\text{-}(OH)D_3$ concentrations in the normal range;[357] it can also be administered prophylactically. Histological osteomalacia may be reversed by such treatment.[76] In view of such results, expensive synthetic vitamin D analogues such as $1\text{-}(OH)D_3$ and $25\text{-}(OH)D_3$ may not be necessary in those patients requiring treatment. These potent analogues may be of value in patients taking cholestyramine, which interferes with the enterohepatic circulation of $25\text{-}(OH)D_3$ or in patients taking hepatic microsomal enzyme inducers, e.g. phenobarbitone or spironolactone, which increase vitamin D degradation to inactive products.[75,318] It seems reasonable, in addition, to provide extra dietary calcium by oral supplements. Corticosteroid therapy aggravates the bone pathology.[160,368]

SEX HORMONES _____

Male patients with cirrhosis of varied aetiology become feminized and females become masculinized, but the changes in male cirrhotics have been more extensively studied.

Normal physiology

Testosterone is the principal androgen secreted by testicular Leydig cells in normal man and it requires conversion to a more potent metabolite, dihydrotestosterone, for full effect. Dihydrotestosterone formation can occur both in the circulation and in peripheral target tissues. Testosterone has a high affinity for a carrier protein in blood, sex hormone-binding globulin (SHBG), and androgenic activity is believed to be related only to the unbound (free) testosterone concentration, although the evidence for this is not strong. Testosterone is degraded particularly in the liver and it is conjugated as sulphates or glucuronides before excretion in the urine as 17-oxosteroids. Testosterone production is stimulated by luteinizing hormone (LH), and testosterone exerts negative feedback on LH secretion. Other less potent androgens include androstenedione, which is secreted by both the testes and the adrenals, and dehydroepiandrosterone, which is primarily an adrenal hormone.

The other principal function of the testis is spermatogenesis, and spermatogenic activity is closely related to plasma follicle-stimulating hormone (FSH) concentration. The seminiferous tubules secrete a hormone, inhibin, which is responsible for negative feedback control of FSH secretion. Testosterone is also necessary for normal spermatogenesis and it is likely that the close apposition of the Leydig cells to the tubules may allow high concentrations of androgens to reach the developing spermatogonia.

Primary testicular disease producing androgen deficiency is associated with elevated plasma LH concentrations and, if spermatogenesis is decreased, plasma FSH levels are raised. In hypothalamic–pituitary disease, plasma gonadotrophin levels are low. The response to intravenous luteinizing hormone-releasing hormone (LRH) administration is exaggerated in primary testicular disease and diminished, or peak LH or FSH levels are delayed, in disease of the pituitary or hypothalamus.

The principal biologically active, naturally occurring oestrogen is oestradiol, with oestrone and oestriol relatively much less potent. Small amounts of oestrogens are produced by the testes and, to a lesser extent, the adrenals in normal man, but the major proportion is derived from peripheral conversion of testosterone and androstenedione to oestradiol and oestrone, respectively. Control of oestrogen secretion and of androgen–oestrogen interconversion in normal man is poorly understood. Oestradiol in blood is bound to SHBG, but its affinity for SHBG is much lower than that of testosterone. SHBG production is increased markedly by oestrogens. Oestrogens are metabolized largely by the liver, conjugated with glucuronic or sulphuric acid, and excreted in bile and urine.

Sex hormones in liver disease

Clinical features
The association of cirrhosis with gynaecomastia was first described in 1834[203] and documented by Corda[80] and Silvestrini,[354] who added testicular atrophy to the pathological complex. Most (80%) of cirrhotic males are impotent[20] and seminal fluid is grossly abnormal in the remainder.[262,401] More than 50% have clinical[20,223,310] and histological[29] evidence of testicular atrophy, in particular atrophy of the germinal epithelium with interstitial fibrosis and thickening of the tubular lamina propria. Testicular atrophy is said to be more common in alcoholic than in other forms of cirrhosis,[20,310] although this is disputed.[398] Secondary sexual characteristics are also diminished, with decreased body[20,109] and facial[401] hair. Benign prostatic hypertrophy occurs less frequently and is delayed in cirrhotic subjects.[29,375]

Gynaecomastia occurs in 40% of cirrhotic men,[20,137,223,310,376] and also in young men with chronic active hepatitis. It may be unilateral or bilateral and results from true glandular hyperplasia. It is said to occur more commonly in alcoholic cirrhosis than in other forms of liver disease,[20,137,376] although not all studies have found this.[262,310] In alcoholism, Gavaler has distinguished hypo-

gonadism (characterized by reduced fertility and testicular atrophy, loss of libido, impotence, lack of prostatic hypertrophy with age and reduced plasma testosterone level) from the syndrome of feminization (in which gynaecomastia occurs, and plasma oestrogen levels are raised). Hypogonadism is a consequence of alcohol abuse and may occur in the absence of cirrhosis, whereas feminization is a later feature and develops only once cirrhosis is established.[138]

Vascular spider naevi are often considered a consequence of feminization as they occur in normal women with increased frequency in the second to fifth month of pregnancy. They also frequently occur in normal subjects, especially children, and occasionally in rheumatoid disease. In addition, they are not commonly observed in male patients with prostatic carcinoma given high therapeutic doses of oestrogen. In subjects with liver disease, vascular spider naevi appear and regress with no clinical or biochemical evidence of other endocrine change.[20] It is unlikely, therefore, that the pathogenesis of vascular naevi in liver disease is related solely to abnormal sex hormone metabolism.

Testosterone
Total plasma testosterone concentration is decreased in cirrhotic subjects compared with normal controls in most, but not all, studies; the values are lowest in those with the most severe disease.[20,65,79,144,196,199,200] The production rate of testosterone is one-quarter of that found in normal subjects.[146,168] In addition, 15% of the circulating testosterone in cirrhotic men is derived not from the testes but from peripheral conversion of androstenedione of adrenal origin compared with 1% in normal males.[146] Testosterone output by the testes of cirrhotic patients is therefore markedly decreased. SHBG concentration is increased in cirrhosis[142,155,201,322,324,410] and, as testosterone has a high affinity for SHBG, free testosterone levels are decreased more than would be suggested by total plasma testosterone measurement. The rise in SHBG also leads to a decrease in testosterone clearance.[20,146] Hepatic vein catheterization studies suggest that hepatic uptake of sex steroids accounts for 50% of their total clearance and the exact proportion is determined by liver function and by the degree of binding to SHBG. Metabolism in peripheral tissues accounts for the remainder. There is some evidence that in severe decompensated liver disease, reduced protein synthesis results in a return of SHBG levels to normal.[89]

Oestrogens
Oestradiol is the most active of the biologically occurring oestrogens. There is little agreement between different studies on total plasma oestradiol concentrations in cirrhotic patients. They have been reported as normal[137,152,398,401] mildly raised[20,206,292] or markedly increased.[59,65,155,279] Oestradiol, like testosterone, is bound in plasma to SHBG, but similarly disparate results have been found when measuring unbound plasma oestradiol as with the

total hormone measurements.[20,65,137,152] There is evidence that free oestradiol concentrations may be raised only in those patients with the most severe liver disease,[199] perhaps accounting for the variable results in other studies. The metabolic clearance rate of oestradiol is normal in cirrhotic subjects and the production rate may be normal[20] or increased.[279]

Oestrone is a biological precursor of oestradiol but has only one-twelfth the feminizing potency.[165] Plasma levels are raised in cirrhotic patients[59,152,279,292] as is the oestrone production rate.[104] Metabolic clearance of oestrone is normal. Oestriol, which also has low biological activity, is present in raised concentrations in the plasma in cirrhotic patients.[152,292]

The low feminizing potency of oestrone and oestriol makes the pathophysiological significance of these findings doubtful. Oestradiol, which is biologically the most active, is certainly metabolized by the liver[3,4] but the Edmonson hypothesis[105] that feminization in liver disease results from diminished oestrogen metabolism is now untenable as the sole mechanism. Increased peripheral conversion of testosterone to oestradiol and of androstenedione to oestrone occurs in liver disease[20,279,365,399] but, as plasma testosterone and testosterone production rate are decreased, the quantitative importance of this is unclear. If oestrogens are of prime importance in feminization, target tissue factors may be operative. Increased local oestrogen synthesis in the breast may occur from androgens that have escaped hepatic metabolism as a consequence of portal systemic shunts.[406] Alcohol feeding in the rat increases hepatic oestrogen receptors[103] and it is possible that this occurs also in tissues other than the liver. Finally, hepatic metabolism of oestrogens is abnormal in liver disease[42] and metabolites of oestradiol such as 16-α-hydroxyoestrone, which may have marked oestrogenic activity, are increased in cirrhosis.[128] The biochemical processing of sex hormones by the diseased liver warrants further study.

Since the metabolic clearance of oestrogens is normal in cirrhosis but that of testosterone is decreased, it has been postulated that these hormones bind to different isoforms of SHBG, rather than to a single competitive binding site. Terasaki *et al.*, using the techniques of isoelectric focusing and chromatography, have demonstrated differences in the biochemical characteristics of oestradiol-binding SHBG and testosterone-binding SHBG.[382]

The pathogenesis of feminization must therefore remain uncertain. The possibility that masculinization/feminization is related more to the androgen-to-oestrogen ratio than the absolute concentration of either hormone group has also received attention. In this context, the free hormone levels may be important. Testosterone binds more avidly to SHBG than does oestradiol, so that a rise in SHBG will decrease free testosterone more than free oestradiol. Idiopathic haemochromatosis is associated with testicular atrophy and low testosterone levels, but gynaecomastia is unusual. SHBG levels are not elevated

in haemochromatosis and this may minimize the effect of testicular deficiency and relative oestrogen excess. Trials of testosterone administration for the feminization of liver disease have been disappointing. Although plasma androgen : oestrogen ratio is increased by such treatment, liver function impairment and portal systemic shunting enable the testosterone to bypass hepatic clearance, and later increased peripheral conversion results in raised oestrogen concentrations.[142] Data on SHBG, free testosterone and free oestradiol levels during treatment are lacking. No real symptomatic benefit has been demonstrated, although objective assessment is difficult.[138,143]

Some workers have demonstrated lower testosterone : oestrogen ratios in patients with cirrhosis and hepatocellular carcinoma than in patients with cirrhosis alone[156,269] and have suggested that this ratio may predict the development of carcinoma.

It is worth adding that, in some cirrhotics, therapy with spironolactone may be a cause of gynaecomastia,[71] as indeed it is in patients with normal liver function.

The liver is not just important as a site for the metabolism of sex hormones but it is also a target tissue for some of their actions. Hepatic production of hormone-binding proteins and hepatic levels of certain steroid-metabolizing enzymes are critically dependent on sex hormone exposure. The consequences of liver disease on these aspects of sex hormone action are unknown. The liver contains both androgen and oestrogen receptors, but animal studies have shown that after partial hepatectomy hepatic sex hormone receptors develop increased responsiveness to oestrogens.[133] Alterations in hepatic oestrogen receptor number and response have also been associated with benign hepatic neoplasms and hyperplasia.[306]

Sex hormone changes in women in liver disease

There have been a limited number of studies on sex hormones in liver disease in women; testosterone levels may be normal or raised, oestradiol and oestrone levels are normal[53,110] or raised[21] and SHBG may also be unchanged or elevated. In primary biliary cirrhosis, the SHBG level is related to the degree of liver dysfunction.[110] The concentration of the adrenal androgen dehydroepiandrosterone sulphate tends to be reduced, and it correlates with the degree of liver disease. Androstenedione levels may be raised, as in men, or they may be decreased.

Gonadotrophins

Studies of urinary gonadotrophin excretion determined by bioassay in male cirrhotic subjects have shown low,[99,300] normal[223] or elevated values.[325] Radioimmunoassay of plasma gonadotrophins has shown equally variable results.[20,65,137,196,262,401] A large multicentre study[20] showed normal plasma LH levels in 64–73% of 117 male subjects, elevated levels in 16–32% and decreased levels in 4–11%. FSH levels were normal in 82%, elevated in

9–10% and decreased in 8–9%. Almost all subjects with low LH and FSH levels were severely ill with liver failure or alcoholic hepatitis. Thus, in compensated liver cirrhosis, the majority of patients have normal basal gonadotrophin levels.

Decreased plasma testosterone levels, despite normal plasma LH concentrations, suggest primary testicular failure; Baker *et al.*[20] showed an inverse correlation between plasma LH and testosterone levels. LH response to luteinizing hormone-releasing hormone (LRH) is exaggerated in primary testicular failure, and in cirrhotic subjects with compensated disease the LH response to LRH has been reported as normal or exaggerated.[20,98,262] Interpretation is hampered by delayed clearance of LH in liver disease. Testosterone responses to small doses of exogenous human chorionic gonadotrophin, which has predominant LH activity, are diminished.[20] This also favours the presence of a primary testicular defect, although the rise in testosterone after higher doses of chorionic gonadotrophin is normal.[365,401]

In the presence of a normal hypothalamus and pituitary, primary testicular failure in other conditions is associated with elevated LH concentrations. Therefore, normal LH levels in liver disease suggest a hypothalamic–pituitary defect. Against this are the LH response obtained to LRH, which should be diminished, or the peak LH value should be delayed, in hypothalamic–pituitary disease, and the finding of a normal LH response to clomiphene in patients with compensated cirrhosis. Only in patients with uncompensated disease are LH and FSH levels low and the response to LRH and clomiphene diminished.[20,401]

As well as abnormalities in basal and stimulated LH concentrations, there may also be a disturbance in the nature of the LH secretion in liver disease. LH is normally secreted in a series of pulses; Bannister *et al.* have demonstrated attenuated release and loss of this pulsatility in alcoholic cirrhotics with hypogonadism and normal basal LH levels, but normal LH pulsatility in those cirrhotics without hypogonadism and raised basal LH concentrations.[22]

Thus, evidence for a primary testicular defect in testosterone secretion is strong but there is probably, in addition, a defect in hypothalamic–pituitary control of gonadotrophin secretion, particularly in severely ill patients.

Prolactin

The role of prolactin secretion in the production of hypogonadism is uncertain. Hyperplasia and hypertrophy of prolactin-secreting cells have been described postmortem in the anterior pituitary of patients with hepatic cirrhosis.[106] In both alcoholic and non-alcoholic cirrhotics, basal serum prolactin levels have been reported as normal,[151,201,274,287,379,427,432] or increased,[398,402,418] while decreased values have been reported in alcoholic fatty liver.[404] The serum prolactin response to intravenous TRH has also been reported as normal[151] or increased,[287,432] although occasional patients with basal hyperprolactinaemia fail to respond to TRH.[403] A generally normal response to insulin-induced hypoglycaemia has been observed in a variety of liver diseases.[258] An extensive study of 150 patients with liver diseases of varied aetiology showed 12% to have serum prolactin levels above the reference range.[258,259] Prolactin levels did not correlate with severity of the liver disease, or the presence of gynaecomastia, confirming the findings of some[391,418,432] but not all,[89,404] other investigators. The aetiology of the liver disease also bore no relation to prolactin levels, although Wenze and Schmitz[418] found hyperprolactinaemia in more than 50% of patients with cirrhosis of alcoholic origin compared with 11% in non-alcoholic cirrhotics.

The mechanism of hyperprolactinaemia in subjects with liver disease is uncertain. Prolactin levels do rise in response to an increase in circulating oestrogen concentrations[429] but no relationship between prolactin and oestrogen levels has been observed in liver disease.[258,404] A positive relationship between serum prolactin and plasma tryptophan levels has been observed[287] and is of interest, as tryptophan is a precursor of the prolactin secretagogue, serotonin. Alcohol may have a direct effect on prolactin secretion,[398] although this is disputed.[388] Irrespective of the mechanism, the lack of correlation with hypogonadism in male subjects and the absence of galactorrhoea in cirrhotics strongly suggest that prolactin is not of major importance.

In summary, there are multiple abnormalities of sex hormones in liver disease, particularly cirrhosis, but there is still much disagreement on the extent, nature and aetiology of these changes. Similarly, there is no clear explanation for the clinically common feminization syndrome.

HAEMOCHROMATOSIS

Haemochromatosis is considered separately because endocrine abnormalities occur so frequently.

Diabetes mellitus

Incidence

Diabetes mellitus occurs in 40–50% of subjects with idiopathic haemochromatosis, depending on criteria for diagnosis of both diabetes and haemochromatosis.[26,102,246,276,343,372] Of these 70% ultimately require insulin.[276] Some cases of idiopathic haemochromatosis go undetected amongst patients attending diabetic clinics. One study recorded a prevalence rate of previously unrecognized haemochromatosis of 1 in 100 compared to 1 in 250 in the general population.[296]

Aetiology

Pancreatic iron content is increased 50–100-fold in idiopathic haemochromatosis.[124] Generalized pancreatic fibrosis occurs and the characteristic islet abnormalities are pigmentation, decrease in number or absence, and fibrosis.[343] Pigmentation affects only B cells, A cells being normal.[244]

It is uncertain whether diabetes is the direct result of excessive iron deposition, but the occasional improvement of the diabetes with venesection favours this idea. Genetic factors are certainly important; diabetes was found in first-degree relatives of 25% of patients with idiopathic haemochromatosis and diabetes but in first-degree relatives of only 4% of subjects with haemochromatosis without diabetes.[102]

Thus, in addition to the presence of raised serum iron levels or frank haemochromatosis in close relatives, the predisposition to diabetes appears to be genetically determined. Diabetes is also infrequent in patients with haemochromatosis without frank cirrhosis,[372] although this may only reflect the severity of the disease at the time of study. Cirrhosis itself may contribute to the glucose intolerance observed but is unlikely to be a major factor in the production of fasting hyperglycaemia and the full syndrome of diabetes mellitus (see Chapter 3).

Insulin secretion and action

The cause of diabetes in idiopathic haemochromatosis is deficient insulin secretion. After intravenous glucose, insulin is promptly released but release is not sustained.[372] The average insulin requirement of insulin-dependent subjects is 50 units/day[276] but some patients exhibit remarkable resistance to exogenous insulin, with daily requirements of up to 4640 units of bovine insulin.[102] The mechanism of this resistance is uncertain. Basal glucagon levels are increased in diabetes with haemochromatosis, as is the glucagon response to intravenous arginine,[288] but glucagon levels are similar to those found in other forms of insulin-dependent diabetes (IDDM).

The effect of venesection on glucose tolerance is variable and is probably dependent on the severity and reversibility of pancreatic damage at the time of treatment. In one major study,[102] 20 out of 49 patients showed a decrease in insulin requirements and four subjects were able to stop taking exogenous insulin completely. Other studies have shown results that are much less impressive.

Complications of diabetes

Complications of diabetes occur with the same frequency as in subjects with other forms of IDDM. These complications are not seen in patients with haemochromatosis if diabetes is absent. Of 72 patients with haemochromatosis and diabetes, 22% had evidence of nephropathy, neuropathy or peripheral vascular disease.[102] The incidence of retinopathy is also similar to that in other patients with IDDM.[289]

Fat atrophy with bovine insulin injections occurs more commonly in patients with haemochromatosis than in IDDM without haemochromatosis, particularly in male subjects,[102] but the mechanism is obscure.

Hypothalamic–pituitary function

Hypogonadism

Since the early descriptions of the disease, hypogonadism has been recognized as a feature and subsequent reports suggest that it occurs in 50–80% of subjects.[246,255,355,370,371] The incidence of hypogonadism is lower in women, presumably owing to the protective effects of iron loss from menstruation, pregnancy and lactation on the liver disease. Sexual function in males is decreased in association with testicular atrophy and a reduction in body hair, and plasma testosterone levels are decreased. Unlike with other causes of chronic liver disease, men with idiopathic haemochromatosis rarely develop gynaecomastia. Kley *et al.* compared sex hormone concentrations and metabolism in men with idiopathic haemochromatosis with men with alcoholic cirrhosis. The former had normal oestrogen levels and SHBG levels and normal peripheral androgen metabolism, suggesting that oestrogenic activity was normal. In contrast, all parameters of oestrogen activity were increased in the alcoholic cirrhotics.[201]

Despite earlier reports,[124] symptoms and signs of hypogonadism correlate poorly with the severity of liver disease. Plasma testosterone levels tend to be lower, and SHBG levels higher, in patients with cirrhosis such that free testosterone concentrations may be markedly decreased.[83] Excessive iron deposition occurs in the pituitary,[31,194,230,343] but the testes, though often atrophic, rarely contain excess iron. Even then the deposition of iron is limited to the vessel walls and spares the interstitial Leydig cells and the germinal epithelium. Hypogonadism has been postulated to result from decreased gonadotrophin secretion but studies so far have produced conflicting results. Stocks and Powell[371] found that 14 out of 32 patients showed decreased plasma LH levels, and Walsh and colleagues[415] found a decreased LH and FSH response to LRH in 2 out of 12 patients who also had low plasma testosterone levels. Similarly, decreased basal and stimulated gonadotrophin values have been found by other workers,[61,94,195,246,389,416] but Simon and colleagues[355] found that basal gonadotrophin levels were normal or elevated in 23 out of 29 patients and concluded that there was a primary testicular defect. This is supported by the decreased testosterone response to exogenous human chorionic gonadotrophin which has been observed in some,[246] but not all studies.[83] On the other hand, a positive correlation has been noted between serum LH and free testosterone, suggesting that hypoandrogenism is the result of selective gonadotrophin deficiency at least in some patients.[83] Other aspects of hypothalamic–pituitary function may be abnormal, such as an impaired decline in serum prolactin following administration of levodopa,[228] but the significance of these abnormalities is uncertain at present.

It is likely that hypogonadism in haemochromatosis is multifactorial in origin. Some patients have deficient secretion of other pituitary hormones in addition to gonadotrophins, and hypothalamic–pituitary disease is likely to be of importance. In subjects with raised gonadotrophin levels, primary testicular disease seems likely. The severity of iron overload and its distribution in particular tissues may be important. Feller et al.[121] found little evidence of sex hormone dysfunction in patients in the pre-cirrhotic stage of haemochromatosis. Other influences may be the severity of the cirrhosis, alcohol intake and autonomic neuropathy secondary to diabetes mellitus. Cundy et al. in a study of 30 men with idiopathic haemochromatosis found that diabetic neuropathy contributed significantly to sexual dysfunction. The diabetes had no effect on the biochemical findings of hypogonadism.[83] Symptomatic and biochemical improvement in hypogonadal men following venesection has been reported; Kelly and colleagues reported restoration of sexual function and sex hormone concentrations in one patient with haemochromatosis and evidence of hypothalamic–pituitary dysfunction and in one patient with evidence of primary testicular failure.[194] These patients, however, had only minimal disturbance of sex hormone levels. Siemons and Mahler demonstrated recovery of reproductive function, biochemistry and testicular histology in a man with haemochromatosis and hypogonadism due to hypothalamic–pituitary disease.[352] In a larger series of patients, Lufkin et al. were unable to detect any improvement in endocrine function after 2 years of venesection to produce iron depletion.[228] This group suggested that endocrine parenchymal damage in haemochromatosis was not solely a function of iron deposition.

O'Hare and Rolla observed that adequate erythropoiesis during phlebotomy required normal androgen levels, so that testosterone replacement was necessary in patients with hypogonadism and haemochromatosis.[277] Testosterone deficiency has also been associated with an increased incidence of osteoporosis. Hypogonadal men with haemochromatosis had lower 25-(OH) vitamin D and lower albumin levels than eugonadal patients. Venesection may have a role in the prevention of reduced bone density by increasing osteoblastic function.[94]

Other aspects of hypothalamic–pituitary function
Other aspects of hypothalamic–pituitary function may be abnormal. A decreased growth hormone response to insulin hypoglycaemia and arginine infusion has been shown in occasional patients.[228,370,371] A diminished cortisol response to insulin hypoglycaemia and TSH response to TRH have also been described. Basal prolactin levels may be normal, increased or decreased and patients frequently demonstrate a subnormal prolactin response to intravenous TRH.[30,216,228,246,415,416]

Other endocrine glands
Haemosiderin deposits are found in other endocrine glands, such as the adrenals, thyroid and parathyroids.[302] Occasional patients with primary hypothyroidism have been described, although it is uncertain whether autoimmune thyroiditis was also present.

ENDOCRINE EFFECTS OF ALCOHOL

Alcohol ingestion is of such importance in many subjects with liver disease that it is worthy of separate comment. The endocrine effects of alcohol are multiple and the subject has been extensively reviewed.[39,145,182,408,424,425] Only those effects that are of clinical importance will be discussed.

In assessment of clinical studies of endocrine effects of alcohol, it is important to note the exact experimental conditions and type of subject studied. Thus, effects of acute alcohol administration differ considerably from those seen with chronic ingestion: endocrine changes in the habituated may be very different from those seen in alcohol-naive subjects; the effects of alcohol in chronic alcohol abusers must be separated from the less-specific effects of liver damage.

Adrenocortical function
Alcohol consumed in moderate doses by normal subjects has little effect on cortisol secretion.[178] Only in the presence of intoxication and usually with blood ethanol levels in excess of 217 mmol/l (100 mg/dl) is a rise in plasma cortisol observed.[249,254] This is probably a non-specific stress effect mediated via the hypothalamic–pituitary–adrenal axis.[178] Alcoholic subjects with tolerance to the intoxicating effects of alcohol may not show a rise in adrenocortical secretion despite blood alcohol levels in excess of 217 mmol/l (100 mg/dl).[254]

Many of the clinical features of chronic alcohol abuse resemble those of Cushing's syndrome, e.g. body habitus, florid complexion and thin skin.[97,254] Chronic alcoholics have higher morning cortisol levels than normal,[253] but this is abolished by alcohol or barbiturate administration or long-term abstinence,[250] and may be related to alcohol withdrawal symptoms. Occasional alcoholic patients present with the clinical and biochemical features of advanced Cushing's syndrome.[132,291,316,359,360] Plasma cortisol levels are raised and may not suppress adequately with dexamethasone[360] (non-suppressibility of serum cortisol by dexamethasone may be observed in alcoholics even in the absence of physical stigmata of hypercortisolism).[197] If alcohol is withdrawn, the biochemical features return to normal during the next 2–3 weeks. The mechanism for alcohol-induced pseudo-Cushing's syndrome is unknown but elevated or normal ACTH levels suggest that the defect is mediated at a hypothalamic–pituitary rather than adrenal level.[197] It does not appear to be related to the severity of the liver damage, as most of the subjects described had only mild liver disturbance.

Adrenocortical insufficiency is more common than alcohol-induced pseudo-Cushing's syndrome. The cortisol response to insulin hypoglycaemia is either absent or severely attenuated in more than 25% of chronic alcoholic subjects, whether still drinking or recently abstinent.[60,154,176,236,238] In none of the subjects studied did plasma cortisol rise by more than 137 nmol/l (5 μg/dl) despite adequate hypoglycaemia. The adrenal glands themselves are functionally normal with adequate fasting plasma cortisol levels,[239] cortisol secretion rate[235] and response to ACTH or tetracosactrin,[252] suggesting that the abnormality lies in the hypothalamic–pituitary–adrenal axis. The impairment was reversible in one patient who was studied after 6 months' abstinence from alcohol. The importance of the deficiency may lie in its role in the pathogenesis of alcoholic hypoglycaemia. A possible mechanism has been provided from experiments in chronically alcohol-fed rats. Hypothalamic CRF content was decreased in these animals and the pulse frequency of CRF secretion was increased. It has been postulated that this may down-regulate pituitary CRF receptors and lead to deficient ACTH release in response to stressful stimuli such as hypoglycaemia.[315] Similar impairments in growth hormone and prolactin secretion in response to insulin hypoglycaemia have been reported.[60]

Sex hormones

Alcohol has effects on hypothalamic–pituitary and testicular function independent of liver disease. The effects may be different in habitual drinkers from those in non-drinkers. Short-term feeding of large doses of alcohol (220 g/day) to healthy volunteers is associated with dampening of the normal pattern of episodic bursts in testosterone secretion[147] and the mean plasma testosterone concentration falls after 5 days. The effect of alcohol to decrease testosterone production by the testes has been postulated as secondary to an increase in the testicular NADH to NAD$^+$ ratio resulting in decreased activity of NAD-dependent enzyme systems involved in steroidogenesis.[107,148,398] Other effects on testicular steroid synthesis independent of NAD may coexist.[69,266] There may also be competitive inhibition of the alcohol dehydrogenase-dependent conversion of retinol to retinal, the latter being essential for normal spermatogenesis.[400] Loss of germ cells in seminiferous tubules results, with testicular atrophy. Alcohol itself and its metabolites, acetaldehyde and acetate, all decrease testosterone output from the rat testis,[408] with acetaldehyde having the most potent action.[18,70] A similar effect of acetaldehyde is observed in the canine testis.[39] Finally, ethanol may decrease testicular gonadotrophin receptor number, an effect which has been observed after ethanol feeding in the rat.[33]

A decrease in testosterone production rate is evident after 24 hours of alcohol feeding in man.[145] Alcohol may also increase the metabolic clearance of testosterone, but in short-term experiments in normal subjects it has no effect on the peripheral conversion of testosterone to oestradiol or of androstenedione to oestrone. Despite alterations in testosterone secretion, no consistent changes in plasma LH or FSH are observed in normal subjects over several weeks of alcohol ingestion,[147] although other investigators have demonstrated a short-term rise in LH.[222,251,431] The absence of a rise in LH despite decreased plasma testosterone levels after several weeks

of excessive alcohol consumption in normal subjects suggests an impairment of hypothalamic–pituitary function. A similar alcohol-induced impairment of LH release has been observed in the rat,[405] but not in the dog.[286]

In chronic alcoholics, alcohol ingestion is also associated with a decrease in plasma testosterone levels,[219,248] with a possible rebound in the post-drinking period. Wright and colleagues[425] found basal plasma LH values to be raised in 6 out of 13 actively drinking male alcoholics and these patients showed an exaggerated LH response to LRH. Plasma total 17-hydroxyandrogens were normal in these subjects and showed no relationship with LH values.

Thus, the effects of alcohol on sex hormone metabolism are complex and dependent on previous ethanol ingestion. In patients with alcoholic cirrhosis, the relative roles of alcohol ingestion and liver disease *per se* in production of the sex hormone abnormalities remain uncertain. In one study, circulating testosterone levels were significantly lower and LH and oestrone levels were higher in alcoholics with cirrhosis than in those without, suggesting that liver disease was of major importance.[395] By contrast, circulating testosterone levels, spermatozoa counts and seminal fluid volume were lower in a group of alcoholic men than in a group of haemophiliac patients matched for the degree of liver dysfunction.[407] The latter authors concluded that factors other than liver disease were more important. In addition there is evidence that in men with alcoholic liver disease, testosterone levels are significantly lower and oestrogen levels are higher than in men with non-alcoholic liver disease. Disturbances in sex hormones occur due to liver disease alone, but in certain studies these abnormalities have been more severe when alcohol was the underlying cause.[23]

Alcohol-related fasting hypoglycaemia

Hypoglycaemia may occur in severe liver disease, particularly fulminant hepatic failure (see Chapter 3), but it may also occur in association with alcohol use and abuse in the presence of a normal liver or relatively mild liver dysfunction. Such patients usually present with a blood glucose concentration of 1.5 mmol/l (27 mg/dl) or less.[237] Patients may be children, but are typically chronic alcoholics with a history of ingestion of moderate to large amounts of alcohol 6–36 hours before admission, and are usually malnourished.[231] They may be stuporose or comatose, usually smell of alcohol, and are often hypothermic. Diagnosis is established on the clinical findings, hypoglycaemia and the blood alcohol level (usually less than 21.7 mmol/l (100 mg/l). Lactic acidosis and ketoacidosis are common. Treatment consists of administration of intravenous glucose, with or without hydrocortisone[238] but a mortality of 10–20% in spite of glucose therapy has been reported.[231] It is possible that hypoglycaemia may be a cause of the unexplained sudden deaths known to occur in alcoholics.[210]

The mechanism is probably multifactorial. A major factor is likely to be inhibition of gluconeogenesis by alcohol.[122,135,208] Oxidation by alcohol dehydrogenase results in an increase in the NAD/NAD$^+$ ratio, which reduces pyruvate concentrations and its conversion to phosphoenolpyruvate, a rate-limiting step in gluconeogenesis. Glycogen stores are usually depleted. Plasma insulin levels are low and glucagon levels high,[180,285,385] although a report with measurement of plasma insulin and C-peptide concentrations[181] suggests that insulin secretion may still be inappropriately high for the blood glucose levels in certain patients. Growth hormone and cortisol levels are raised, but less than might be anticipated in view of the severity of the hypoglycaemia.[14,180] The importance of an abnormality in the hypothalamic–pituitary–adrenal axis in more than 25% of chronic alcoholics (see above) is suggested by evidence that adrenocortical insufficiency predisposes to development of alcohol-induced hypoglycaemia in experimental situations.[14] A defect in growth hormone secretion during insulin hypoglycaemia[12,60] may also play a role in certain patients.

Alcohol may also be important in the potentiation of drug-induced hypoglycaemia, particularly that secondary to insulin.[237] Growth hormone, cortisol and glucagon responses to insulin-induced hypoglycaemia are reduced in normal subjects during acute ethanol infusion, but recovery from hypoglycaemia is accelerated.[204] Alcohol may induce reactive hypoglycaemia when given with glucose[278] and there is slender evidence that chronic alcoholics may demonstrate reactive hypoglycaemia more than controls.[72,117,237,386,387]

Alcoholic ketoacidosis

This uncommon condition occurs in non-diabetic alcoholic patients who almost always have abnormal liver function tests.[78,179,217,284] Females are affected more than males, and there is a history of heavy chronic alcohol intake preceding a drinking 'binge' 2–3 days before presentation. There is a history of abdominal pain, vomiting and lack of solid food; on examination, patients are conscious but tachypnoeic, not grossly salt- and water-depleted, and usually have diffuse epigastric tenderness. Blood glucose estimation is normal and, in one series of six subjects,[78] mean arterial pH was 7.25 with an anion gap of 18. Plasma phosphate level may be low and accompanied by red-cell haemolysis.[383] Blood ketone body and non-esterified fatty-acid concentrations are high, but testing plasma or urine with a standard nitroprusside reagent (Acetest or Ketostix) may reveal mild ketosis only, as 3-hydroxybutyrate, which is not measured by this method, is elevated considerably more than acetoacetate and acetone. The principal differential diagnosis is from lactic acidosis, which also occurs in alcoholic liver disease (see Chapter 3) and direct measurement of blood ketone body and lactate concentrations is necessary. Treatment with intravenous glucose, saline and small amounts of sodium bicarbonate leads to prompt recovery.

The mechanism of production of alcoholic ketoacidosis is uncertain; altered mitochondrial function has been proposed. Serum insulin concentrations are low, cortisol markedly increased, and growth hormone levels mildly raised.[78] A ketogenic effect of cortisol in insulin-deficient man has been demonstrated[6,330] and this, combined with increased catecholamine release, may be of importance. It is also possible that there may be direct conversion of alcohol to ketone bodies through acetate, as acetate infusion causes a rise in circulating ketone body levels. The absolute contribution of this route remains to be established. Finally, ketosis develops despite the fact that fatty-acid oxidation may be decreased secondary to the increase in the NADH to NAD$^+$ ratio as a result of alcohol oxidation.[125]

HEPATIC DISTURBANCE IN ENDOCRINE DISEASE

Diabetes mellitus

Hepatotrophic effects of insulin

There is considerable experimental evidence that insulin and other hormones are necessary for maintenance of normal hepatic architecture and for regeneration after injury.

The so-called hepatotrophic effects of substances in the portal blood have been noted, under several experimental conditions, to include hypertrophy, hyperplasia, glycogen storage and increase of several other synthetic functions. *In vitro* work has suggested that insulin may have an important role in the maintenance of hepatocyte integrity.[214] Extensive work *in vivo* in dogs by Starzl and colleagues[367] has elaborated on these findings. Experiments in which portal blood was directed at one part of the liver and systemic blood at another have shown the importance of the portal blood in the maintenance of normal liver architecture and in the normal regenerative response to injury. The more recent studies by these workers suggest that insulin is a major factor, although glucagon secretion and the insulin : glucagon ratio may also be of importance.[46,47] The role of other pancreatic hormones and the numerous gut hormones is at present uncertain (see also Chapter 11).

The liver in diabetes mellitus

The liver in normal man is exposed to much higher insulin concentrations in the portal blood than are found in the systemic circulation.[36] If this is important in maintaining liver structure, it is to be expected that insulin-treated diabetic subjects would show a high incidence of hepatic abnormality in that insulin is given systemically rather than portally. Perisinusoidal fibrosis is a frequent feature in the liver in insulin-dependent diabetes;[270] studies in a rat model suggest that the lesion is related to the genetic predisposition to diabetes rather than to the hyperglycaemia.[32] Structural abnormalities may even be expected in non-insulin-dependent diabetes (NIDDM), in which insulin and glucagon are still secreted, as there is a change in their relative proportions, with glucagon preponderant.[392]

Fatty liver

Many pathological changes have been reported in diabetic livers but most are acutely reversible phenomena such as the hepatic enlargement seen in ketoacidosis. Excessive glycogen deposition has been reported,[37] but the most consistent change is that of fatty infiltration.

Creutzfeldt *et al.*[82] in their classic review of 1759 biopsies from different centres, reported fatty changes in from 21% to 78% of diabetics. The incidence is lower in insulin-dependent diabetes (25%) than in NIDDM (63%).[159] This difference probably results from the increased number of obese patients in the NIDDM series. Patients selected for biopsy may also not be representative of diabetics as a whole, as biopsy was performed for a clinical reason such as hepatomegaly or abnormality of liver function. Autopsy studies are also unrepresentative as patients have died from diverse causes and the metabolic status is uncertain, but such studies have shown the incidence of fatty liver to be lower, at 20–30% compared with 15–25% in the non-diabetic population. In an unselected series using bright liver ultrasound, Foster *et al.*[131] suggested a 23% prevalence of fatty infiltration.

Fatty change is not specific to diabetes. Progression is slow over many years and it may remain static for long periods.[211] In a comparison of fatty change due to alcoholic hepatitis with that due to non-insulin-dependent diabetes, there was marked similarity, but periportal rather than perivenular lesions and nuclear vacuolation were more common in diabetes.[270] In addition, the frequency of fatty infiltration was lowest in insulin-dependent diabetes, suggesting that insulin lack may not be a major factor in its pathogenesis.

Hepatic cirrhosis

Intolerance to oral or intravenous glucose is a common finding in subjects with liver disease.[180] This differs from diabetes in that it is usually mild and is not generally associated with fasting hyperglycaemia. Peripheral insulin concentrations are raised. It is therefore vital to distinguish between the glucose intolerance of cirrhosis and the occurrence of cirrhosis in subjects with essential diabetes. Many previous studies have failed to make this distinction.

Standard liver function tests in well-controlled diabetics reveal little difference from the normal population,[131] but in a review of published autopsy reports the frequency of cirrhosis in diabetics ranged from 5.7% to 21.4% compared with 2.3–13.4% in non-diabetics. In two of the series reported, figures were the same in diabetics and non-diabetics, while in four there was a clear preponderance of cirrhosis in diabetic subjects. In the two best clinical studies[81,267] in the literature, a higher incidence of cirrhosis was found in diabetics (3.7% and 9.2% in diabetics compared with 1.2% and 1.8% in normals). Even in these studies, criteria for distinction between the glucose intolerance of cirrhosis and diabetes are questionable and in only 40% of the subjects with both diabetes and cirrhosis was the diabetes diagnosed first.

Evidence for an increased overall incidence of cirrhosis in diabetes is therefore tenuous. There is, nevertheless, a high incidence of post-necrotic cirrhosis in diabetic subjects,[229] presumably due to the higher incidence of viral hepatitis (type B). Seige and Thierbach[336] have shown that cirrhosis follows viral hepatitis more frequently in diabetics than in non-diabetics. Normal pancreatic secretion may therefore be of importance in the response to viral infection or other liver injury, but there is little evidence in man that pancreatic hyposecretion in diabetes leads to a serious loss of hepatic structural integrity in the absence of a further liver insult.

Hyperthyroidism

Histological changes

Many changes in liver histology have been reported in hyperthyroidism, e.g. decreased glycogen content, fatty change, focal necrosis, diffuse or perivenular necrosis, simple atrophy, nodule formation and cirrhosis with lymphoid infiltration,[25,50,301,339,417] but most of these findings probably result from cardiac failure or severe weight loss and are not specific to hyperthyroidism. In other studies of patients with milder disease diagnosed at an earlier stage, histological changes have been unimpressive; in particular, severe perivenular necrosis and cirrhosis are not seen.[16,293]

Changes in hepatic ultrastructure have been reported in experimental hyperthyroidism; in particular, increased size and number of mitochondria with increased cristae formation per mitochondrion were seen.[202] These changes are not specific and are also seen after administration of ethanol and other substances.

Chronic active hepatitis[384] and sclerosing cholangitis[24,198] occur more frequently in thyroid disease than would be expected by chance.

Liver function

Despite an increase in cardiac output, hepatic blood flow is not increased in hyperthyroidism.[268] Hepatic oxygen consumption is, however, increased, so that hepatocytes extract more oxygen, and this may contribute to the perivenular necrosis found occasionally in severely hyperthyroid subjects. In experimental hyperthyroidism, increased glycogen synthase activity mediated via synthase phosphatase has been demonstrated.[37a] There is no correlation between hepatic histology and standard tests of liver function. In a series of 570 patients, increased bromosulphthalein retention was found in only 8% and elevation of aspartate aminotransferase, bilirubin and alkaline phosphatase occurred less frequently.[16] In a smaller series, the bromosulphthalein retention was found to be inversely related to a reduced hepatic glutathione level, and it improved after antithyroid drug therapy which also increased hepatic glutathione.[356] Clinical jaundice is found in hyperthyroidism usually only in the presence of a complication, e.g. infection or cardiac failure, as is seen in 20–25% of patients with a thyroid crisis.[172] Intrahepatic cholestatic jaundice in hyperthyroidism has been reported,[428] but in general, jaundice in a subject with uncomplicated mild hyperthyroidism should arouse suspicion of coexistent liver disease; thyrotoxicosis may aggravate an underlying defect in bilirubin metabolism such as Gilbert's disease.[153]

Hypothyroidism

Jaundice may be found in neonatal thyroid deficiency, and, although symptoms or signs of disturbed liver function are not usually encountered in adult hypothyroidism, jaundice in adult primary hypothyroidism has also been

reported.[13] Defective canalicular bile production has been postulated due to decreased ATP activity. Serum levels of aspartate aminotransferase, lactate dehydrogenase and creatine phosphokinase may be elevated; these return to normal after 2–4 weeks' replacement therapy. These abnormalities are thought to represent altered metabolism of the enzymes rather than liver damage.[90]

Exudative ascites and effusions in other body cavities may occur in hypothyroidism, unrelated to liver or cardiac pathology,[326] although perivenular congestion and fibrosis have been reported on liver biopsy.[19]

Acromegaly

The liver is enlarged in acromegaly as part of the generalized organomegaly. Standard liver function tests are normal, but bromosulphthalein excretion time may be increased.[346]

REFERENCES

1. Abrams, R.L., Crumbach, M.M. & Kaplan, S.L. (1971) The effect of intravenous administration of human growth hormone on the plasma growth hormone, cortisol, glucose and free fatty acid response to insulin: evidence for growth hormone autoregulation in man. *Journal of Clinical Investigation*, **50**, 940–950.
2. Adjukiewicz, A.B., Agnew, J.E., Byers, P.D. *et al.* (1974) The relief of bone pain in primary biliary cirrhosis with calcium infusions. *Gut*, **15**, 788–793.
3. Aldercreutz, H. (1970) Oestrogen metabolism in liver disease. *Journal of Endocrinology*, **46**, 129–163.
4. Aldercreutz, H. (1974) Hepatic metabolism of oestrogens in health and disease. *New England Journal of Medicine*, **290**, 1081–1083.
5. Agner, T., Hagen, C., Bent, N.A. and Hegedüs, L. (1986) Pituitary–thyroid function and thyrotropin, prolactin and growth hormone responses to TRH in patients with chronic alcoholism. *Acta Medica Scandinavica*, **220**, 57–62.
6. Alberti, K.G.M.M. & Johnston, D.G. (1977) Cortisol and catabolism: a new perspective. *Clinical Science and Molecular Medicine*, **52**, 333–336.
7. Alberti, K.G.M.M., Record, C.O., Williamson, D.H. & Wright, R. (1972) Metabolic changes in active chronic hepatitis. *Clinical Science*, **42**, 591–605.
8. Alford, F.P., Dudley, F.J., Chisholm, D.J. & Findlay, D.M. (1979) Glucagon metabolism in normal subjects and in cirrhotic patients before and after portasystemic venous shunt surgery. *Clinical Endocrinology*, **11**, 413–424.
9. Almdal, T., Schaadt, O., Vesterdal Jorgensen, J. *et al.* (1989) Vitamin D, parathyroid hormone, and bone mineral content of lumbar spine and femur in primary biliary cirrhosis. *Journal of Internal Medicine*, **225**, 207–213.
10. Alwmark, A., Mamlock, V., Greeley, G.H. *et al.* (1987) Insulin and glucagon production in experimental cirrhosis. *Annals of Surgery*, **205**(1), 9–12.
11. Anderson, B.N., Hagen, C., Faber, O.K. *et al.* (1983) Glucose tolerance and B cell function in chronic alcoholism: its relation to hepatic histology and exocrine pancreatic function. *Metabolism*, **32**, 1029–1032.
12. Andreani, D., Tamburrano, G. & Javicoli, M. (1976) Alcohol hypoglycaemia: hormonal changes. In Andreani, D., Lefebvre, P.J. & Marks, V. (eds) *Hypoglycaemia*, Proceedings of the European Symposium, Rome, pp. 95–105. Stuttgart: Thieme.
13. Ariza, C.R., Frati, A.C. & Sierra, I. (1984) Hypothyroidism-associated cholestasis. *Journal of the American Medical Association*, **252**, 2392.
14. Arky, R.A. & Freinkel, N. (1966) Alcohol hypoglycaemia. V. Alcohol infusion to test gluconeogenesis in starvation, with specific reference to obesity. *New England Journal of Medicine*, **274**, 426–433.
15. Arnauld, S.B., Goldsmith, R.S. & Lambert, P.W. (1975) 25-Hydroxy-vitamin D₃: evidence of an enterohepatic circulation in man. *Proceedings of the Society for Experimental Biology and Medicine*, **149**, 570–572.
16. Ashkar, F.S., Miller, R., Smoak, W.M. & Gilson, A.J. (1971) Liver disease in hyperthyroidism. *Southern Medical Journal*, **64**, 462–465.
17. Atkinson, M., Nordin, B.E.C. & Sherlock, S. (1956) Malabsorption and bone disease in prolonged obstructive jaundice. *Quarterly Journal of Medicine*, **25**, 299–313.
18. Badr, F.M., Bartke, A., Dalterio, S. & Bulger, W. (1977) Suppression of testosterone production by ethyl alcohol. Possible mode of action. *Steroids*, **30**, 647–655.
19. Baker, A., Kaplan, M. & Wolfe, H. (1972) Central congestive fibrosis of the liver in myxoedema ascites. *Annals of Internal Medicine*, **77**, 927–929.
20. Baker, H.W.G., Burger, H.G., de Kretser, D.M. *et al.* (1976) A study of the endocrine manifestations of hepatic cirrhosis. *Quarterly Journal of Medicine*, **45**, 145–178.
21. Bannister, P., Sheridan, P. & Losowsky, M.S. (1985) Plasma concentrations of sex hormones in postmenopausal women in non-alcoholic cirrhosis. *Clinical Endocrinology*, **23**, 335–340.
22. Bannister, P., Handley, T., Chapman, C. & Losowsky, M.S. (1986) Hypogonadism in chronic liver disease: impaired release of luteinising hormone. *British Medical Journal*, **293**, 1191–1193.
23. Bannister, P., Oakes, J., Sheridan, P. & Losowsky, M.S. (1987) Sex hormone changes in chronic liver disease: a matched study of alcoholic versus non-alcoholic liver disease. *Quarterly Journal of Medicine*, **63**, No. 240: 305–313.
24. Bartholomew, L.G., Cain, J.C., Woolner, L.B. *et al.* (1963) Sclerosing cholangitis: its possible association with Riedel's struma and fibrous retroperitonitis. Report of two cases. *New England Journal of Medicine*, **269**, 8–12.
25. Beaver, D.C. & Pemberton, J. de J. (1933) The pathologic anatomy of the liver in exophthalmic goitre. *Annals of Internal Medicine*, **7**, 687–708.
26. Becker, D.R. & Miller, M. (1960) Presence of diabetic glomerulosclerosis in patients with hemochromatosis. *New England Journal of Medicine*, **263**, 367–373.
27. Becker, M.D., Cook, G.C. & Wright, A.D. (1969) Paradoxical elevation of growth hormone in active chronic hepatitis. *Lancet*, **2**, 1035–1039.
28. Becker, U., Gluud, C. & Bennett, P. (1988) Thyroid hormones and thyroxine-binding globulin in relation to liver function and serum testosterone in men with alcoholic cirrhosis. *Acta Medica Scandinavica*, **224**, 367–373.
29. Bennett, H.S., Baggenstoss, A.H. & Butt, H.R. (1950) The testis,

breast and prostate of men who die of cirrhosis of the liver. *American Journal of Clinical Pathology*, 20, 814–828.

30. Bercovici, J.P., Darragon, T., Caroff, J. & Le Roy, J. (1979) L'exporation hypophysaire des haemochromatoses idiopathic. *Semaine des Hôpitaux de Paris*, 55, 1606–1612.

31. Bergeron, C. & Kovacs, K. (1978) Pituitary sclerosis; a histologic immunocytologic and ultrastructural study. *American Journal of Pathology*, 93, 295–306.

32. Bernuau, D., Guillot, R., Durand-Schneider, A. *et al.* (1985) Liver perisinusoidal fibrosis in BB rats with or without overt diabetes. *American Journal of Pathology*, 120, 38–45.

33. Bhalla, V.K., Chen, C.J.H. & Gnanaprakasam, M.S. (1979) Effects of in vivo administration of human chorionic gonadotrophin and ethanol on the processes of testicular receptor depletion and replenishment. *Life Sciences*, 24, 1315–1324.

34. Bikle, D.D., Gee, E., Halloran, B. & Haddad, J.G. (1984) Free 1,25-dihydroxyvitamin D levels in serum from normal subjects, pregnant subjects, and subjects with liver disease. *Journal of Clinical Investigation*, 74, 1966–1971.

35. Bikle, D.D., Halloran, B., Gee, E. *et al.* (1986) Free 25-hydroxyvitamin D levels are normal in subjects with liver disease and reduced total 25-hydroxyvitamin D levels. *Journal of Clinical Investigation*, 78, 748–752.

36. Blackard, W.G. & Nelson, N.C. (1970) Portal and peripheral vein immunoreactive insulin concentrations before and after glucose infusion. *Diabetes*, 19, 302–306.

37. Bogoch, A., Casselman, W.G.B., Kaplan, A. & Bockus, H.L. (1955) Studies of hepatic function in diabetes mellitus, portal cirrhosis and other liver diseases; correlation of clinical, biochemical and liver needle biopsy findings. *American Journal of Medicine*, 18, 354–384.

37a.Bollen, M. & Stalmans, W. (1988) The effects of the thyroid status on the activation of glycogen synthase in liver cells. *Endocrinology*, 122, 2915–2919.

38. Borzio, M., Caldara, R., Borzio, F. *et al.* (1983) Thyroid function tests in chronic liver disease: evidence for multiple abnormalities despite clinical euthyroidism. *Gut*, 24, 631–636.

39. Boyden, T.W. & Pamenter, R.W. (1983) Effects of ethanol on the male hypothalamic–pituitary–gonadal axis. *Endocrine Reviews*, 4, 389–395.

40. Bratusch-Marrain, P.R., Waldhausl, W.K., Gasic, S. & Holfer, A. (1984) Hepatic disposal of biosynthetic human insulin and porcine C-peptide in humans. *Metabolism*, 33, 151–157.

41. Braverman, L.E., Vagenakis, A., Downs, P. *et al.* (1973) Effects of replacement doses of sodium L-thyroxine on the peripheral metabolism of thyroxine and triiodothyronine in man. *Journal of Clinical Investigation*, 52, 1010–1017.

42. Breuer, H. & Höller, M. (1982) Hepatic metabolism of steroids. In Langer, M., Chiandussi, L., Chopra, I.J. & Martini, L. (eds) *The Endocrines and The Liver*, pp. 77–92. Serono Symposium No. 51. London: Academic Press.

43. Brown, H., Willardson, D.G., Samuels, L.T. & Tyler, F.H. (1954) 17-Hydroxycorticosteroid metabolism in liver disease. *Journal of Clinical Investigation*, 33, 1524–1532.

44. Brown, J., Chopra, J.J., Cornell, J.S. *et al.* (1974) Thyroid physiology in health and disease. *Annals of Internal Medicine*, 81, 68–81.

45. Buchanan, K., Solomon, S., Vance, J. *et al.* (1968) Glucagon clearance by the isolated perfused rat liver. *Proceedings of the Society for Experimental Biology and Medicine*, 128, 620–623.

46. Bucher, N.L.R. & Swaffield, M.N. (1975) Regulation of hepatic regeneration in rats by synergistic action of insulin and glucagon. *Proceedings of the National Academy of Sciences of the USA*, 72, 1157–1160.

47. Bucher, N.L.R. & Weir, G.C. (1976) Insulin, glucagon, liver regeneration, and DNA synthesis. *Metabolism*, 25 (supplement 1), 1423–1425.

48. Burger, A., Nicod, P., Suter, P. *et al.* (1976) Reduced active thyroid hormone levels in acute illness. *Lancet*, 1, 653–655.

49. Buzzeli, G., Bonora, E., Coscelli, C. *et al.* (1982) Glucagon intolerance in chronic active hepatitis. In Langer, M., Chiandussi, L., Chopra, I.J. & Martini, L., *The Endocrines and The Liver*, pp. 355–370. Serono Symposium No. 51. London: Academic Press.

50. Cameron, G.R. & Karunaratne, W. (1935) Liver changes in exophthalmic goitre. *Journal of Pathology*, 41, 267–282.

51. Cameron, D.P., Burger, H.G., Catt, K.J. *et al.* (1972) Metabolic clearance of human growth hormone in patients with hepatic and renal failure and in the isolated perfused pig liver. *Metabolism*, 21, 895–904.

52. Camu, F. (1975) Hepatic balances of glucose and insulin in response to physiological increments of endogenous insulin during glucose infusions in dogs. *European Journal of Clinical Investigation*, 5, 101–108.

53. Carlström, K., Eriksson, S. & Rannevik, G. (1986) Sex steroids and steroid binding proteins in female alcoholic liver disease. *Acta Endocrinologica*, 111, 75–79.

54. Carter, J.N., Eastman, C.J., Corcoran, J.M. & Lazarus, L. (1974) Effect of severe chronic illness on thyroid function. *Lancet*, 2, 971–974.

55. Cavalieri, R.R. (1980) In Oppenheimer, J.H. (ed.) *Thyroid Today*, vol. 3, no. 7. Deerfield, Illinois: Flint Laboratories.

56. Cavalieri, R.R. & Rapoport, B. (1977) Impaired peripheral conversion of thyroxine to triiodothyronine. *Annual Review of Medicine*, 28, 57–65.

57. Cavallo-Perin, P., Cassader, M., Bozzo, A. *et al.* (1985) Mechanism of insulin resistance in human liver cirrhosis. Evidence of a combined receptor and postreceptor defect. *Journal of Clinical Investigation*, 75, 1659–1665.

58. Cavallo-Perin, P., Bruno, A., Nuccio, P. *et al.* (1986) Feedback inhibition of insulin secretion is altered in cirrhosis. *Journal of Clinical Endocrinology and Metabolism*, 63, 1023–1027.

59. Cedard, L., Mosse, A. & Klotz, H.P. (1970) Les oestrogenes plasmatiques dans les gynecomasties et les hepatopathies. *Annales d'Endocrinologie*, 31, 453–458.

60. Chalmers, R.J., Bennie, E.H., Johnson, R.H. & Masterton, G. (1978) Growth hormone, prolactin and corticosteroid responses to insulin hypoglycaemia in alcoholics. *British Medical Journal*, 1, 745–748.

60a.Chap, Z., Ishida, T., Chou, J. *et al.* (1987) First-pass hepatic extraction and metabolic effects of insulin and insulin analogues. *American Journal of Physiology*, 252, E209–217.

61. Charbonnel, B., Chupin, M., LeGrand, A. & Guillon, J. (1981) Pituitary function in idiopathic haemochromatosis: hormonal study in 36 male patients. *Acta Endocrinologica*, 98, 178–183.

62. Chopra, I.J. (1976) An assessment of daily turnover and significance of thyroidal secretion of 3,3′,5′-triiodothyronine (reverse T_3) in man. *Journal of Clinical Investigation*, 58, 32–40.

63. Chopra, I.J. (1978) Nature, source and biological significance of thyroid hormones in blood. In Werner, S.C. & Ingbar, S.H. (eds) *The Thyroid: A Fundamental and Clinical Text*. New York: Harper & Row.

64. Chopra, I.J. (1982) Thyroid hormone metabolism in chronic liver disease. In Langer, M., Chiandussi, L., Chopra, I.J. & Martini, L. (eds) *The Endocrines and The Liver*, pp. 185–193. Serono Symposium No. 51. London: Academic Press.

65. Chopra, I.J., Tulchinsky, D. & Greenway, F.L. (1973) Estrogen–androgen imbalance in hepatic cirrhosis. *Annals of Internal Medicine*, 79, 198–203.

66. Chopra, I.J., Solomon, D.H., Chopra, U. *et al.* (1974) Alterations in circulating thyroid hormones and thyrotropin in hepatic cirrhosis: evidence of euthyroidism despite subnormal serum triiodothyronine. *Journal of Clinical Endocrinology and Metabolism*, 39, 501–511.

67. Chopra, I.J., Geola, F., Solomon, D.H. & Maciel, R.M.B. (1978) 3′,5′-Diiodothyronine in health and disease: studies by a radioimmunoassay. *Journal of Clinical Endocrinology and Metabolism*, 47, 1198–1207.

68. Chopra, I.J., Solomon, D.H., Hepner, G.W. & Morgenstein, A. (1979) Misleadingly low free thyroxine index and usefulness of reverse triiodothyronine measurement in non-thyroidal illnesses. *Annals of Internal Medicine*, 90, 905–912.

69. Cicero, T.J. & Bell, R.D. (1980) Effects of ethanol and acetaldehyde on the biosynthesis of testosterone in the rodent testis. *Biochemical and Biophysical Research Communications*, 94, 814–819.

70. Cicero, T.J., Bell, R.D., Meyer, E.R. & Badger, T.M. (1980) Ethanol and acetaldehyde directly inhibit testicular steroidogenesis. *Journal of Pharmacology and Experimental Therapeutics*, 213, 228–233.

71. Clark, E. (1965) Spironolactone therapy and gynecomastia. *Journal of the American Medical Association*, 193, 163–164.

72. Cohen, S. (1976) A review of hypoglycemia and alcoholism with or without liver disease. *Annals of the New York Academy of Sciences*, **273**, 338–342.

73. Collin, J., Taylor, R.M.R. & Johnston, I.D.A. (1977) Carbohydrate tolerance with portal and systemic venous drainage of the pancreas. *British Journal of Surgery*, **64**, 180–182.

74. Collins, J.R., Lacy, W.W., Stiel, J.N. & Crofford, O.B. (1970) Glucose intolerance and insulin resistance in patients with liver disease. II. A study of etiological factors and evaluation of insulin actions. *Archives of Internal Medicine*, **126**, 608–614.

75. Compston, J.E. & Thompson, R.P.H. (1977) Intestinal absorption of 25-hydroxyvitamin D and osteomalacia in primary biliary cirrhosis. *Lancet*, **1**, 721–724.

76. Compston, J.E., Horton, L.W.L. & Thompson, R.P.H. (1979) Treatment of osteomalacia with primary biliary cirrhosis with parenteral vitamin D2 or oral 25-hydroxyvitamin D3. *Gut*, **20**, 133–136.

77. Conn, H.O. & Daughaday, W.H. (1970) Cirrhosis and diabetes v serum growth hormone levels in Laennec's cirrhosis. *Journal of Laboratory and Clinical Medicine*, **76**, 678–688.

78. Cooperman, M.T., Davidoff, F., Spark, R. & Pallota, J. (1974) Clinical studies of alcoholic ketoacidosis. *Diabetes*, **23**, 433–439.

79. Coppage, W.S. & Cooner, A.E. (1965) Testosterone in human plasma. *New England Journal of Medicine*, **273**, 902–907.

80. Corda, L. (1925) Sulla c.d. reviviscenza della mamella maschile viella cirrosi epatica. *Minerva Medica*, **5**, 1067–1069.

81. Creutzfeldt, W. (1959) Morphologische Befunde an der Leber von Diabetikern nach langfristiger Sulphonylharnstoff behandlung und an verschiedenen Organen nach Synthalin und DBI-Vergiftung beim Tier. In *Diabetes Mellitus*. Proceedings of 3rd Congresse Internationale Diabetes Federation, p. 267. Stuttgart: Thieme.

82. Creutzfeldt, W., Frerichs, H. & Sickinger, K. (1970). Liver diseases and diabetes mellitus. In Popper, H. & Schaffner, F. (eds) *Progress in Liver Disease*, vol. 3, pp. 380–407. New York: Grune & Stratton.

83. Cundy, T., Bomford, A., Butler, J. *et al.* (1989) Hypogonadism and sexual dysfunction in hemochromatosis: the effects of cirrhosis and diabetes. *Journal of Clinical Endocrinology and Metabolism*, **69**, 110–116.

84. Cuttelod, S., LeMarchand-Beraud, T., Magnenat, P. *et al.* (1974) Effect of age and role of kidneys and liver on thyrotropin turnover in man. *Metabolism*, **23**, 101–113.

85. D'Amour, P. & Huet, P. (1989) Ca^{2+} concentration influences the hepatic extraction of bioactive human PTH-(1–34) in rats. *American Journal of Physiology*, **256** (1, pt 1), E87–92.

86. Danielsson, A., Lorentzon, R. & Larsson, S.E. (1982) Intestinal absorption and 25-hydroxylation of vitamin D in patients with primary biliary cirrhosis. *Scandinavian Journal of Gastroenterology*, **17**, 349–355.

87. Daugaard, H., Egfjord, M. & Olgaard, K. (1988) Metabolism of intact parathyroid hormone in isolated perfused rat liver and kidney. *American Journal of Physiology*, **254** (6, pt 1), E740–748.

88. Davies, T.F., Prudhoe, K. & Douglas, A.P. (1976) Plasma cyclic adenosine-3′,5′-monophosphate response to glucagon in patients with liver disease. *British Medical Journal*, **1**, 931–933.

89. De Besi, L., Zucchetta, P., Zotti, S. & Mastrogiacomo, I. (1989) Sex hormones and sex hormone binding globulin in males with compensated and decompensated cirrhosis of the liver. *Acta Endocrinologica*, **120**, 271–276.

90. De Groot, L.J. & Stanbury, J.B. (1975) Adult hypothyroid states and myxoedema. In *The Thyroid and its Diseases*, pp. 405–471. New York: Wiley.

91. De Moura, M.C. & Cruz, A.G. (1968) Carbohydrate metabolism studies in cirrhosis of the liver. *American Journal of Digestive Diseases*, **13**, 891–896.

92. Desai, K.B., Ganatra, R.D. & Sharma, S.M. (1971) Thyroid uptake studies in infectious hepatitis. *Journal of Nuclear Medicine*, **2** (supplement 5), 828–833.

93. Diamond, T.H., Stiel, D., Lunzer, M. *et al.* (1989) Hepatic osteodystrophy. Static and dynamic bone histomorphometry and serum Gla-protein in 80 patients with chronic liver disease. *Gastroenterology*, **96**, 213–221.

94. Diamond, T., Stiel, D. & Posen, S. (1989) Osteoporosis in hemochromatosis: iron excess, gonadal deficiency, or other factors? *Annals of Internal Medicine*, **110**, 430–436.

95. Dibble, J.B., Sheridan, P., Hampshire, R. *et al.* (1982) Osteomalacia, vitamin D deficiency and cholestasis in chronic liver disease. *Quarterly Journal of Medicine*, **201**, 89–103.

96. Dieguez, C., Page, M.D. & Scanlon, M.F. (1988) Growth hormone, neuroregulation and its alterations in disease states. *Clinical Endocrinology*, **28**, 109–143.

97. Dillon, R.S. (1973) *Handbook of Endocrinology*. Philadelphia: Lea & Febiger.

98. Distiller, L.A., Sagel, J., Dubowitz, B. *et al.* (1976) Pituitary–gonadal function in men with alcoholic cirrhosis of the liver. *Hormone and Metabolic Research*, **8**, 461–465.

99. Dohan, F.C., Richardson, E.M., Bluemle, L.W. & Gyorgy, P. (1952) Hormone excretion in liver disease. *Journal of Clinical Investigation*, **31**, 481–498.

100. Doniach, D., Roitt, I.M., Walker, J. G. & Sherlock, S. (1966) Tissue antibodies in primary biliary cirrhosis, active chronic (lupoid) hepatitis, cryptogenic cirrhosis and other liver diseases and their clinical implications. *Clinical and Experimental Immunology*, **1**, 237–262.

101. Doniach, D., Walker, J.G., Roitt, I.M. & Berg, P.A. (1970) Current concepts: autoallergic hepatitis. *New England Journal of Medicine*, **282**, 86–89.

102. Dymock, I.W., Cassar, J., Pyke, D.A. *et al.* (1972) Observations on the pathogenesis, complications and treatment of diabetes in 115 cases of hemochromatosis. *American Journal of Medicine*, **52**, 203–210.

103. Eagon, P.K., Zdunck, J.R., van Thiel, D.H. *et al.* (1981) Alcohol-induced changes in hepatic estrogen binding proteins: a mechanism explaining feminisation in alcoholics. *Archives of Biochemistry and Biophysics*, **211**, 48–54.

104. Edman, C.D., MacDonald, P.C. & Combes, B. (1975) Extra-glandular production of oestrogen in subjects with liver disease. *Gastroenterology*, **69**, A–19/819.

105. Edmonson, H.A., Glass, S.J. & Soll, S.N. (1939) Gynecomastia associated with cirrhosis of the liver. *Proceedings of the Society for Experimental Biology and Medicine*, **42**, 97–99.

106. El Etreby, M.F. & Gunzel, P. (1974) Sex hormones—effects on prolactin cells in the rat, dog, monkey and man. *Acta Endocrinologica, Supplementum*, **189**, 3–15.

107. Ellingboe, J. & Varanelli, C.C. (1979) Ethanol inhibits testosterone biosynthesis by direct action on Leydig cells. *Research Communications in Chemical Pathology and Pharmacology*, **24**, 87–102.

108. Englert, E. Jr., Brown, H., Wallach, S. & Simons, J. (1957) Metabolism of free and conjugated 17-hydroxycorticosteroids in subjects with liver disease. *Journal of Clinical Endocrinology*, **17**, 1395–1406.

109. Eppinger, H. (1925) *cited in* The Vienna Convention. Diseases of metabolism and of the digestive tract (letter). *Journal of the American Medical Association*, **85**, 1572–1574.

110. Eriksson, S., Carlström, K. & Rannevik, G. (1989) Sex steroids and steroid binding proteins in primary biliary cirrhosis. *Journal of Steroid Biochemistry*, **32**, 427–431.

111. Faber, J., Kirkegaard, C., Lumholtz, B. *et al.* (1979). Measurements of serum 3′,5′-diiodothyronine and 3,3′-diiodothyronine concentrations in normal subjects and in patients with thyroid and non-thyroid disease: studies of 3′,5′-diiodothyronine metabolism. *Journal of Clinical Endocrinology and Metabolism*, **48**, 611–617.

112. Faber, J., Thomsen, H.F., Lumholtz, I.B. *et al.* (1981). Kinetic studies of thyroxine, 3,5,3′-triiodothyronine, 3,3′5′-triiodothyronine, 3′,5′-diiodothyronine, 3,3′-diiodothyronine and 3′-monoiodothyronine in patients with liver cirrhosis. *Journal of Clinical Endocrinology and Metabolism*, **53**, 978–984.

113. Faber, J., Kirkegaard, C., Thomsen, H.F. *et al.* (1983) The extrathyroidal conversion of 3,5,3′-triiodothyronine to 3,5-diiodothyronine in patients with liver cirrhosis. *Journal of Clinical Endocrinology and Metabolism*, **57**, 428–431.

114. Falluca, F., Ziparo, V., Giangrande, L. *et al.* (1981) Exaggerated glucagon secretion in diabetic and non-diabetic subjects with surgical portocaval anastomosis. *Hormone and Metabolic Research*, **13**, 545–547.

115. Falluca, F., Giangrande, L., Del Balzo, P. *et al.* (1982) The function of islet alpha- and beta-cells in cirrhotic patients with portocaval shunts. In Langer, M., Chiandussi, L., Chopra, I.J. &

Martini, L. (eds) *The Endocrines and The Liver*, pp. 371–380. Serono Symposium No. 51. London: Academic Press.

116. Fang, V.S. & Tashjian, A.H., Jr (1972) Studies on the role of the liver in the metabolism of parathyroid hormone effects of partial hepatectomy and incubation of the hormone with tissue homogenates. *Endocrinology*, **90**, 1177–1184.

117. Farmer, R.W., Farrell, G., Pellizzari, E.D. & Fabre, L.F. (1971) Serum insulin levels during oral glucose tolerance tests in chronic alcoholics. *Federation Proceedings*, **30**, 250 (abstract).

118. Felig, P. & Wahren, J. (1971) Influence of endogenous insulin secretion on splanchnic glucose and amino acid balance in man. *Journal of Clinical Investigation*, **50**, 1702–1711.

119. Felig, P., Brown, W.V., Levine, R.A. & Klatskin, G. (1970) Glucose homeostasis in viral hepatitis. *New England Journal of Medicine*, **283**, 1436–1440.

120. Felig, P., Gusberg, R., Hendler, R. *et al.* (1974) Concentrations of glucagon and the insulin : glucagon ratio in the portal and peripheral circulation. *Proceedings of the Society for Experimental Biology and Medicine*, **147**, 88–90.

121. Feller, E.R., Pont, A. & Wands, J.R. (1977) Familial hemochromatosis physiological studies in the pre-cirrhotic stage of the disease. *New England Journal of Medicine*, **296**, 1422–1426.

122. Field, J.B., Williams, H.E. & Mortimer, G.E. (1963). Studies on the mechanism of ethanol-induced hypoglycemia. *Journal of Clinical Investigation*, **42**, 497–506.

123. Field, J.B., Bloom, G., Petruska, M. *et al.* (1976) Effects of stimulation of insulin and glucagon secretion on hepatic glucose production, insulin/glucagon ratio and hepatic extraction of insulin and glucagon. *Clinical Research*, **24**, 485A.

124. Finch, S.C. & Finch, C.A. (1955) Idiopathic hemochromatosis and iron storage disease. *Medicine*, **34**, 381–430.

125. Fink, R. & Rosalki, S.B. (1978) Clinical biochemistry of alcoholism. *Clinics in Endocrinology and Metabolism*, **7**, 297–319.

126. Fischer, J.E. & Baldessarini, R.J. (1971) False neurotransmitters and hepatic failure. *Lancet*, **2**, 75–79.

127. Fischer, M., Sherwin, R.S., Hendler, R. & Felig, P. (1976) Kinetics of glucagon in man: effects of starvation. *Proceedings of the National Academy of Sciences of the USA*, **73**, 1735–1739.

128. Fishman, J. & Martucci, C. (1980) Biological properties of 16-hydroxyestrone. Implications in estrogen physiology and the pathophysiology of cirrhosis and systemic lupus erythematosis. *Journal of Clinical Endocrinology and Metabolism*, **51**, 611–615.

129. Flock, E.V., Bollman, J.L., Grindlay, J.H. & Stobie, G.H. (1961) Partial deiodination of L-thyroxine. *Endocrinology*, **69**, 626–637.

130. Fonseca, V., Epstein, O., Gill, D.S. *et al.* (1987) Hyperparathyroidism and low serum osteocalcin despite vitamin D replacement in primary biliary cirrhosis. *Journal of Clinical Endocrinology and Metabolism*, **64**, 873–877.

131. Foster, K.J., Griffith, A.H., Dewbury, K. *et al.* (1980) Liver disease in patients with diabetes mellitus. *Postgraduate Medical Journal*, **56**, 767–772.

132. Frajra, R. & Angeli, A. (1977) Alcohol-induced pseudo-Cushing's syndrome. *Lancet*, **1**, 1050–1051.

133. Francavilla, A., Eagon, P.K., DiLeo, A. *et al.* (1986) Sex hormone-related functions in regenerating male rat liver. *Gastroenterology*, **91**, 1263–1270.

134. Fraser, D.R. & Kodicek, E. (1970) Unique biosynthesis by kidney of a biological active vitamin D metabolite. *Nature*, **228**, 764–766.

135. Freinkel, N., Singer, D.L., Arky, R.A. *et al.* (1963) Alcohol hypoglycaemia. I. Carbohydrate metabolism of patients with clinical alcohol hypoglycaemia and the experimental reproduction of the syndrome with pure ethanol. *Journal of Clinical Investigation*, **42**, 1112–1133.

136. Galton, V.A. & Nisula, B.C. (1972) The enterohepatic circulation of thyroxine. *Journal of Endocrinology*, **54**, 187–193.

137. Galvao-Teles, A., Anderson, D.C., Burke, C.W. *et al.* (1973) Biologically active androgens and oestradiol in men with chronic liver disease. *Lancet*, **1**, 173–177.

138. Gavaler, J.S. & Van Thiel, D.H. (1988) Gonadal dysfunction and inadequate sexual performance in alcoholic cirrhotic men. *Gastroenterology*, **95**, 1680–1683.

139. Gavin, L., Castle, J., McMahon, F. *et al.* (1976) Metabolic clearance and production rates of 3,5,3'-triiodothyronine (T3) and 3,3'5'-T3 (reverse T3) in man. *Clinical Research*, **24**, 427A.

140. Geola, F., Chopra, I.J., Solomon, D.H. & Maciel, R.M.B. (1979) Metabolic clearance and production of 3',5'-diiodothyronine and 3,3'-diiodothyronine in man. *Journal of Clinical Endocrinology and Metabolism*, **48**, 297–301.

141. Gerhardt, A., Greenberg, A., Reilly, J.J. Jr & Van Thiel, D.H. (1987) Hypercalcaemia. A complication of advanced chronic liver disease. *Archives of Internal Medicine*, **147**, 274–277.

142. Gluud, C., Dejgaard, A., Bennett, P. & Svenstrup, B. (1987) Androgens and oestrogens before and following oral testosterone administration in male patients with and without alcoholic cirrhosis. *Acta Endocrinologica*, **115**, 385–391.

143. Gluud, C., Wantzin, P., Eriksen, J. & the Copenhagen Study Group for Liver Diseases (1988) No effect of oral testosterone treatment on sexual dysfunction in alcoholic cirrhotic men. *Gastroenterology*, **95**, 1582–1587.

144. Gluud, C. & the Copenhagen Study Group for Liver Diseases (1987) Serum testosterone concentrations in men with alcoholic cirrhosis: background for variation. *Metabolism*, **36**, 373–378.

145. Gordon, G.G. & Southren, A.L. (1977) Metabolic effects of alcohol on the endocrine system. In Lieber, C.S. (ed.) *Metabolic Aspects of Alcohol*. Lancaster: MTP Press.

146. Gordon, G.G., Olivo, J., Rafii, F. & Southren, A.L. (1975) Conversion of androgens to estrogens in cirrhosis of the liver. *Journal of Clinical Endocrinology and Metabolism*, **40**, 1018–1026.

147. Gordon, G.G., Altman, K., Southren, A.L. *et al.* (1976) Effect of alcohol administration on sex hormone metabolism in normal men. *New England Journal of Medicine*, **295**, 793–797.

148. Gordon, G.G., Vittek, J., Southren, A.L. *et al.* (1980) Effect of chronic alcohol ingestion on the biosynthesis of steroids in rat testicular homogenate in vitro. *Endocrinology*, **106**, 1880–1885.

149. Greco, A.V., Fedeli, G., Ghirlanda, G. *et al.* (1974) Behaviour of pancreatic glucagon, insulin and HGH in liver cirrhosis after arginine and i.v. glucose. *Acta Diabetologica Latina*, **11**, 330–339.

150. Greco, A.V., Crucitti, F., Ghirlanda, G. *et al.* (1978) Insulin and glucagon concentrations in portal and peripheral veins in patients with cirrhosis. *Diabetologia*, **17**, 23–28.

151. Green, J.R.B. (1977) Mechanism of hypogonadism in cirrhotic males. *Gut*, **18**, 843–853.

152. Green, J.R.B., Mowat, N.A.G., Fisher, R.A. & Anderson, D.C. (1976) Plasma oestrogens in men with chronic liver disease. *Gut*, **17**, 426–430.

153. Greenberger, N.J., Milligan, F.D., De Groot, L.J. & Isselbacher, K.J. (1964) Jaundice and thyrotoxicosis in the absence of congestive heart failure. *American Journal of Medicine*, **36**, 840.

154. Greenwood, F.C., Landon, J. & Stamp, T.C. (1966) The plasma sugar, free fatty acid, cortisol, and growth hormone response to insulin. *Journal of Clinical Investigation*, **45**, 429–436.

155. Guechot, J., Vaubourdolle, M., Ballet, F. *et al.* (1987) Hepatic uptake of sex steroids in men with alcoholic cirrhosis. *Gastroenterology*, **92**, 203–207.

156. Guechot, J., Peigney, N., Ballet, F. *et al.* (1988) Sex hormone imbalance in male alcoholic cirrhotic patients with and without hepatocellular carcinoma. *Cancer*, **62**, 760–762.

157. Hagen, T.C., Lawrence, A.M. & Kirsteins, L. (1972) Autoregulation of growth hormone secretion in normal subjects. *Metabolism*, **21**, 603–610.

158. Hagopian, W.A. & Tager, H.S. (1987) Hepatic glucagon metabolism. *Journal of Clinical Investigation*, **79**, 409–417.

159. Hanefield, M., Naumann, H.J. & Haller, H. (1967) Statistische Untersuchungen über den Einfluss des Diabetes typs und der Therapieform auf die Ausprägung und Frequenz der Leberverfettung bei Diabetes Mellitus. *Deutsche Zeitschrift für Verdauungs- und Stoffwechselkrankheiten*, **27**, 13–19.

160. Heaf, J.G. (1985) Hepatic osteodystrophy. *Scandinavian Journal of Gastroenterology*, **20**, 1035–1040.

161. Hegedüs, L., Kastrup, J., Feldt-Rasmussen, U. & Hyltoft Petersen, P. (1983) Serum thyroglobulin in acute and chronic liver disease. *Clinical Endocrinology*, **19**, 231–237.

162. Hegedüs, L. (1986) Thyroid gland volume and thyroid function during and after acute hepatitis infection. *Metabolism*, **35**, 495–498.

163. Hepner, G.W. & Chopra, I.J. (1979) Serum thyroid hormone levels in patients with liver disease. *Archives of Internal Medicine*, **139**, 1117–1120.

164. Hernandez, A., Zorilla, E. & Gershberg, H. (1969) Decreased

insulin production, elevated growth hormone levels, and glucose intolerance in liver disease. *Journal of Laboratory and Clinical Medicine*, **73**, 25–33.

165. Hisaw, F.L. (1959) Comparative effectiveness of estrogens on fluid inhibition and growth of the rat's uterus. *Endocrinology*, **64**, 276–289.

166. Hodgson, S.F., Rolland Dickson, E., Wahner, H.W. *et al.* (1985) Bone loss and reduced osteoblast function in primary biliary cirrhosis. *Annals of Internal Medicine*, **103**, 855–860.

167. Holdsworth, C.D., Nye, L. & King, E. (1972) The effect of portacaval anastomosis on oral carbohydrate tolerance and on plasma insulin levels. *Gut*, **13**, 58–63.

168. Horton, R. & Tait, J.F. (1966) Androstenedione production and interconversion rates measured in peripheral blood and studies on the possible site of its conversion to testosterone. *Journal of Clinical Investigation*, **45**, 301–313.

169. Horwitz, D.L., Starr, J.L., Mako, M.E. *et al.* (1975) Proinsulin, insulin and C-peptide concentrations in human portal and peripheral blood. *Journal of Clinical Investigation*, **55**, 1278–1283.

170. Ikeda, T., Takeuchi, T., Ito, Y. *et al.* (1986) Secretion and degradation of insulin and glucagon in carbon tetrachloride-induced liver injury rats. *American Journal of Physiology*, **251** (6, Pt 1) E660–663.

171. Inada, M. & Sterling, K. (1967) Thyroxine turnover and transport in Laennec's cirrhosis of the liver. *Journal of Clinical Investigation*, **46**, 1275–1282.

172. Ingbar, S.H. (1978) Thyroid storm or crisis. In Werner, S.C. & Ingbar, S.H. (eds) *The Thyroid: A Fundamental and Clinical Text*, pp. 800–804. London: Harper & Row.

173. Ishida, T., Lewis, R.M., Hartley, C.J. *et al.* (1983) Comparison of hepatic extraction of insulin and glucagon in conscious and anesthetized dogs. *Endocrinology*, **112**, 1098–1109.

174. Israel, Y., Walfish, P.G., Orrego, H. *et al.* (1979) Thyroid hormones in alcoholic liver disease. Effect of treatment with 6-n-propylthiouracil. *Gastroenterology*, **76**, 116–122.

175. Iwasaki, Y., Ohkubo, A., Kajinuma, H. *et al.* (1978) Degradation and secretion of insulin in hepatic cirrhosis. *Journal of Clinical Endocrinology and Metabolism*, **47**, 774–779.

176. Jacobs, H.S. & Nabarro, J.D. (1969) Tests of hypothalamic–pituitary–adrenal function in man. *Quarterly Journal of Medicine*, **38**, 475–493.

177. Jaspan, J.B., Huen, A.H.J., Morely, C.G. *et al.* (1977) The role of the liver in glucagon metabolism. *Journal of Clinical Investigation*, **60**, 421–428.

178. Jenkins, J.S. & Connolly, J. (1968) Adrenocortical response to ethanol in man. *British Medical Journal*, **2**, 804–805.

179. Jenkins, D.W., Eckel, R.E. & Craig, J.W. (1971) Alcoholic ketoacidosis. *Journal of the American Medical Association*, **217**, 177–183.

180. Joffe, B.I., Seftel, H.C. & Van As. M. (1975) Hormonal response in ethanol-induced hypoglycemia. *Journal of Studies on Alcohol*, **36**, 550–554.

181. Joffe, B.I., Shires, R., Seftel, H.C. & Heding, L.G. (1977) Plasma insulin, C-peptide and glucagon levels in acute phase of ethanol-induced hypoglycaemia. *British Medical Journal*, **2**, 678–679.

182. Johnson, P.J. (1984) Sex hormones and the liver. *Clinical Science*, **66**, 369–376.

183. Johnston, D.G. & Alberti, K.G.M.M. (1976) Carbohydrate metabolism in liver disease. *Clinics in Endocrinology and Metabolism*, **5**, 675–702.

184. Johnston, D.G., Alberti, K.G.M.M., Faber, O.K. *et al.* (1977) Hyperinsulinism of hepatic cirrhosis: diminished degradation or hypersecretion? *Lancet*, **1**, 10–13.

185. Johnston, D.G., Alberti, K.G.M.M., Wright, R. *et al.* (1978) C-peptide and insulin in liver disease. *Diabetes*, **27**(supplement), 201–206.

186. Johnston, D.G., Alberti, K.G.M.M., Binder, C. *et al.* (1982) Hormonal and metabolic changes in hepatic cirrhosis. *Hormone and Metabolic Research*, **14**, 34–39.

187. Johnston, D.G., Davies, R.R. & Prescott, R.W.G. (1985) Regulation of growth hormone secretion in man: a review. *Journal of the Royal Society of Medicine*, **78**, 319–327.

188. Jung, R.T., Davie, M., Hunter, J.O. *et al.* (1978) Abnormal vitamin D metabolism in cirrhosis. *Gut*, **19**, 290–293.

189. Kaden, M., Harding, P. & Field, J.B. (1973) Effect of intraduodenal glucose administration on hepatic extraction of insulin in the anaesthetised dog. *Journal of Clinical Investigation*, **52**, 2016–2028.

190. Kanazawa, Y., Kuzuya, T., Ide, T. & Kosaka, K. (1966) Plasma insulin response to glucose in femoral hepatic and pancreatic veins in dogs. *American Journal of Physiology*, **211**, 442–448.

191. Katz, A.I. & Rubenstein, A.H. (1973) Metabolism of proinsulin, insulin and C-peptide in the rat. *Journal of Clinical Investigation*, **52**, 1113–1121.

192. Kawai, K., Hayakawa, H., Yoshika, K. *et al.* (1977) Plasma insulin and C-peptide levels in cirrhotic and uremic patients. *Diabete et Metabolisme*, **3**, 7–10.

193. Kehayoglou, A.K., Agnew, J.E., Holdsworth, C.D. *et al.* (1968) Bone disease and calcium absorption in primary biliary cirrhosis. *Lancet*, **1**, 715–719.

194. Kelly, T.M., Edwards, C.Q., Meikle, A.W. & Kushner, J.P. (1984) Hypogonadism in hemochromatosis: reversal with iron depletion. *Annals of Internal Medicine*, **101**, 629–632.

195. Kent, J.R., Aronow, W. & Meister, L. (1969) Hypogonadotrophic hypogonadism in hemochromatosis. *California Medicine*, **111**, 450–452.

196. Kent, J.R., Scaramuzzi, R.J., Lauwers, W. *et al.* (1973) Plasma testosterone, estradiol and gonadotrophins in hepatic insufficiency. *Gastroenterology*, **64**, 111–115.

197. Kirkman, S. & Nelson, D.H. (1988) Alcohol-induced pseudo-Cushing's disease: a study of prevalence with review of the literature. *Metabolism*, **37**, 390–394.

198. Kittridge, R.D. & Nash, A.D. (1974) The many facets of sclerosing fibrosis. *American Journal of Roentgenology*, **122**, 288–298.

199. Kley, H.K., Strohmeyer, G. & Kruskemper, H.L. (1979) Effect of testosterone application on hormone concentrations of androgens and estrogens in male patients with cirrhosis of the liver. *Gastroenterology*, **76**, 235–241.

200. Kley, H.K., Nieschlag, E., Wiegelmann, W. *et al.* (1975) Steroid hormones and their binding in plasma of male patients with fatty liver, chronic hepatitis and liver cirrhosis. *Acta Endocrinologica*, **79**, 275–285.

201. Kley, H.K., Niederau, C., Stremmel, W. *et al.* (1985) Conversion of androgens to estrogens in idiopathic hemochromatosis: comparison with alcoholic liver cirrhosis. *Journal of Clinical Endocrinology and Metabolism*, **61**, 1–6.

202. Klion, F., Segal, R. & Schaffner, R. (1971) The effect of altered thyroid function on the ultrastructure of human liver. *American Journal of Medicine*, **50**, 317–324.

203. Koechling, D., cited in Berzoni, M. (1934) Gynäkomastie und Lebercirrhose. *Virchows Archiv für Pathologie*, **293**, 679–723.

204. Kolaczynski, J.W. Ylikahri, R., Härkonen, M. & Koivisto, V.A. (1988) The acute effect of ethanol on counterregulatory response and recovery from insulin-induced hypoglycaemia. *Journal of Clinical Endocrinology and Metabolism*, **67**, 384–388.

205. Kopetz, K. & Wehrmann, P. (1970) Stoffwechselveränderungen nach Glucose und tolbutamid-belastung bei Lebercirrhosen und ihre Rolle in der Pathogenese des hepatogenen diabetes mellitus. *Klinische Wochenschrift*, **48**, 1265–1276.

206. Korenman, S.G., Perrin, L.E. & McCallum, T. (1969) Estradiol in human plasma: demonstration of elevated levels in gynaecomastia and in cirrhosis. *Journal of Clinical Investigation*, **48**, 45a (abstract).

207. Kravetz, D., Arderiu, M., Bosch, J. *et al.* Casamitjana, R. and Rodes, J. (1987) Hyperglucagonaemia and hyperkinetic circulation after portocaval shunt in the rat. *American Journal of Physiology*, **252** (2, Pt 1): G257–261.

208. Krebs, H.A., Freedland, R.A., Hems, R. & Stubbs, M. (1969) Inhibition of hepatic gluconeogenesis by alcohol. *Biochemical Journal*, **112**, 117–124.

209. Langer, M., Masala, A., Rassu, S. *et al.* (1982) Growth hormone secretion in chronic liver disease. In Langer, M., Chiandussi, L., Chopra, I.J. & Martini, L. (eds) *The Endocrines and the Liver*, pp. 278–287. Serono Symposium No. 51. London: Academic Press.

210. Lavric, W. (1971) Alcohol as a cause of sudden unexpected death. *Medical Journal of Australia*, **1**, 1224–1227.

211. Leevy, C.M. (1952) Fatty liver: a study of 270 patients with biopsy proven fatty liver and a review of the literature. *Medicine*, **41**, 249–278.

212. Leevy, C.M., Thomson, P. & Baker, H. (1970) Vitamins and liver injury. *American Journal of Clinical Nutrition*, **23**, 493–498.

213. LeFebvre, P. & Luyckx, A. (1970) Modification par le foie isole et perfuse de l'effet exerce par le glucagon sur la graisee epididymaire du rat. *Société Belge d'Endocrinologie*, **26**, 369–374.

214. Leffert, H.L. (1974) Growth control of differentiated foetal rat hepatocytes in primary monolayer culture. VII. Hormonal control of DNA synthesis and its possible significance to the problem of liver regeneration. *Journal of Cell Biology*, **62**, 792–801.

215. Lepyavko, A.G. (1970) Functional state of the thyroid gland in patients with lambliasis with predominant involvement of the hepatobiliary system. *Klinicheskaia Meditsina*, **48**, 83–86.

216. Levy, C.L. & Carlson, H.E. (1978) Decreased prolactin reserve in hemochromatosis. *Journal of Clinical Endocrinology and Metabolism*, **47**, 444–446.

217. Levy, L.J., Duga, J., Girgis, M. & Gordon, E.E. (1973) Ketoacidosis associated with alcoholism in non-diabetic subjects. *Annals of Internal Medicine*, **78**, 213–219.

218. Lickley, H.L.A., Chisholm, D.J., Rabinowitch, A. *et al.* (1975) Effects of portacaval anastomosis on glucose tolerance in the dog: evidence of an interaction between the gut and the liver in oral glucose disposal. *Metabolism*, **24**, 1157–1168.

219. Liegel, J., Fabre, L.F., Howard, P.Y. & Farmer, R.W. (1972) Plasma testosterone and sex hormone binding globulin (SBG) in alcoholic subjects. *Physiologist*, **15**, 918 (abstract).

220. Limberg, B. & Kommerell, B. (1984) Correction of altered plasma amino acid pattern in cirrhosis of the liver by somatostatin. *Gut*, **25**, 1291–1295.

221. Lindholm, J. (1982) Steroid-binding proteins and the liver. In Langer, M., Chiandussi, L., Chopra, I.J. & Martini, L. (eds) *The Endocrines and The Liver*, pp. 93–100. London: Academic Press.

222. Linnoila, M., Prinz, P.N., Wonsowicz, C.J. & Lepaluoto, J. (1980) Effect of moderate doses of ethanol and phenobarbital on pituitary and thyroid hormones and testosterone. *British Journal of Addiction*, **75**, 207–212.

223. Lloyd, C.W. & Williams, R.H. (1948) Endocrine changes associated with Laennec's cirrhosis of the liver. *American Journal of Medicine*, **4**, 315–330.

224. Long, R.G., Wills, M.R., Skinner, R.K. & Sherlock, S. (1976) Serum-25-hydroxy-vitamin-D in untreated parenchymal and cholestatic liver disease. *Lancet*, **2**, 650–652.

225. Long, R.G., Meinhard, E., Skinner, R.K. *et al.* (1978) Clinical biochemical and histological studies of osteomalacia, osteoporosis and parathyroid function in chronic liver disease. *Gut*, **19**, 85–90.

226. Long, R.G., Skinner, R.K., Wills, M.R. & Sherlock, S. (1978) Formation of vitamin D metabolites from ^{3}H- and ^{14}C-radiolabelled vitamin D-3 in chronic liver diseases. *Clinica Chimica Acta*, **85**, 311–317.

227. Long, R.G., Varghese, Z., Wills, M.R. & Sherlock, S. (1978) Plasma calcium and magnesium fractions in liver disease. *Clinica Chimica Acta*, **84**, 239–245.

228. Lufkin, E.G., Baldus, W.P., Bergstralh, E.J. & Kao, P.C. (1987) Influence of phlebotomy treatment on abnormal hypothalamic–pituitary function in genetic hemochromatosis. *Mayo Clinic Proceedings*, **62**, 473–479.

229. MacDonald, R.A. & Mallory, G.K. (1958) The natural history of post-necrotic cirrhosis. *American Journal of Medicine*, **24**, 334–357.

230. MacDonald, R.A. & Mallory, G.K. (1960) Hemochromatosis and hemosiderosis. *Archives of Internal Medicine*, **105**, 686–700.

231. Madison, L.L. (1968) Ethanol-induced hypoglycaemia. *Advances in Metabolic Disorders*, **3**, 85–108.

232. Madison, L.L., Combes, B., Unger, R.H. & Kaplan, N. (1959) The relationship between the mechanism of action of the sulphonylureas and the secretion of insulin into the portal circulation. *Annals of the New York Academy of Sciences*, **74**, 548–556.

233. Magnusson, I. & Tranberg, K.G. (1987) Impaired early insulin response to intravenous glucose in alcoholic liver cirrhosis. *Scandinavian Journal of Gastroenterology*, **22**, 301–307.

234. Marco, J., Diego, J., Villaneuva, M.L. *et al.* (1973) Elevated plasma glucagon levels in cirrhosis of the liver. *New England Journal of Medicine*, **289**, 1107–1111.

235. Margraf, H.W., Moyer, C.A., Ashford, L.E. & Lavelle, L.W. (1967) Adrenocortical function in alcoholics. *Journal of Surgical Research*, **7**, 55–62.

236. Marks, V. (1975) Alcohol and changes in body constituents: glucose and hormones. *Proceedings of the Royal Society of Medicine*, **68**, 377–380.

237. Marks, V. (1978) Alcohol and carbohydrate metabolism. *Clinics in Endocrinology and Metabolism*, **7**, 333–349.

238. Marks, V. & Rose, F.C. (1981) *Hypoglycaemia*. Oxford: Blackwell.

239. Marks, V. & Wright, J. (1977) Endocrinological and metabolic effects of alcohol. *Proceedings of the Royal Society of Medicine*, **70**, 337–344.

240. Mawer, E.B., Klass, H.J., Warnes, T.W. & Berry, J.L. (1985) Metabolism of vitamin D in patients with primary biliary cirrhosis and alcoholic liver disease. *Clinical Science*, **69**, 561–570.

241. McCann, V.J. & Fulton, T.T. (1975) Cortisol metabolism in chronic liver disease. *Journal of Clinical Endocrinology and Metabolism*, **40**, 1038–1044.

242. McConaghey, P. (1972) The production of 'sulphation factor' by rat liver. *Journal of Endocrinology*, **52**, 1–9.

243. McConaghey, P. & Sledge, C.B. (1970) Production of 'sulphation factor' by perfused liver. *Nature*, **225**, 1249–1250.

244. McGavran, M.H. & Hartroft, W.S. (1956) The pre-dilection of pancreatic beta cells for pigment deposition in hemochromatosis and hemosiderosis. *American Journal of Clinical Pathology*, **32**, 631.

245. McIlroy, M., Walsh, C.H., Doyle, C. *et al.* (1976) Glucose tolerance in viral hepatitis. *Irish Journal of Medical Science*, **145**, 3–6.

246. McNeil, L.W., McKee, L.C., Lorber, D. & Rabin, D. (1983) The endocrine manifestations of hemochromatosis. *American Journal of the Medical Sciences*, **285**, 7–13.

247. Megyesi, C., Samols, E. & Marks, V. (1967) Glucose tolerance and diabetes in chronic liver disease. *Lancet*, **2**, 1051–1056.

248. Mendelson, J.H. & Mello, N.K. (1976) Behavioural and biochemical interrelations in alcoholism. *Annual Review of Medicine*, **27**, 321–323.

249. Mendelson, J.H. & Stein, S. (1966) Serum cortisol levels in alcoholic and non-alcoholic subjects during experimentally induced ethanol intoxication. *Psychosomatic Medicine*, **28**, 616–626.

250. Mendelson, J., Ogata, M. & Mello, N.K. (1971) Adrenal function and alcoholism. I. Serum cortisol. *Psychosomatic Medicine*, **33**, 145–157.

251. Mendelson, J.H., Mello, N.K. & Ellingboe, J. (1977) Effects of acute alcohol intake on pituitary–gonadal hormones in normal human males. *Journal of Pharmacology and Experimental Therapeutics*, **202**, 676–682.

252. Merry, J. & Marks, V. (1969) Plasma hydrocortisone response to ethanol in chronic alcoholics. *Lancet*, **1**, 921–923.

253. Merry, J. & Marks, V. (1972) The effect of alcohol, barbiturate and diazepam on hypothalamic–pituitary–adrenal function in chronic alcoholics. *Lancet*, **2**, 990–992.

254. Merry, J. & Marks, V. (1973) Hypothalamic–pituitary–adrenal function in chronic alcoholics. In Cross, M.M. (ed.) *Alcoholic Intoxication and Withdrawal: Experimental Studies*, p. 167. Advances in Experimental Biology and Medicine. New York: Plenum Press.

255. Milder, M.S., Cook, J.D., Stray, S. & Finch, C.A. (1980) Idiopathic hemochromatosis an interim report. *Medicine*, **59**, 34–49.

256. Miller, L.L., Schalch, D.S. & Draznin, B. (1981) Role of liver in regulating somatomedin activity: effects of streptozotocin diabetes and starvation on the synthesis and release of insulin-like growth factor and its carrier protein by the isolated perfused rat liver. *Endocrinology*, **108**, 1265–1270.

257. Mitchison, H.C., Malcolm, A.J., Bassendine, M.F. & James, O.F.W. (1988) Metabolic bone disease in primary biliary cirrhosis at presentation. *Gastroenterology*, **94**, 463–470.

258. Morgan, M.Y. (1982) Basal and dynamic prolactin secretion in liver disease. In Langer, M., Chiandussi, L., Chopra, I.J. & Martini, L. (eds) *The Endocrines and the Liver*, pp. 303–320. Serono Symposium No. 51. London: Academic Press.

259. Morgan, M.Y. & Sherlock, S. (1978) Serum prolactin in liver disease and its relationship to gynaecomastia. *Gut*, **19**, 170–174.

260. Morgan, A.G., Kelleher, J., Walker, B.E. & Losowsky, M.S. (1976) Nutrition in cryptogenic cirrhosis and chronic active hepatitis. *Gut*, **17**, 113–118.

261. Mortimer, G.E. & Tietze, F. (1959) Studies on the mechanism of capture and degradation of insulin I-131 by the cyclically perfused rat liver. *Annals of the New York Academy of Sciences*, **82**, 329–337.

262. Mowat, N.A.G., Edwards, C.R.W., Fisher, R. *et al.* (1976) Hypothalamic–pituitary–gonadal function in men with cirrhosis of the liver. *Gut*, **17**, 345–350.

263. Mueller, R., Brausch, C.C., Hirsch, E.Z. *et al.* (1954) Thyroid I-131 uptake in liver disease. *Journal of Clinical Endocrinology and Metabolism*, **14**, 1287–1299.

264. Muggeo, M., Tiengo, A., Fedele, D. & Crepaldi, G. (1979) Altered control of growth hormone secretion in patients with cirrhosis of the liver. *Archives of Internal Medicine*, **139**, 1157–1160.

265. Müller, E.E. (1974) Growth hormone and the regulation of metabolism. In McCann, S.M. (ed.) *MTP International Review of Science, Physiology, Series One*, vol. 5. Endocrine Physiology. London: Butterworth.

266. Murono, E.P., Lin, T., Osterman, J. & Nankin, H.R. (1980) Direct inhibition of testosterone synthesis in rat testis interstitial cells by ethanol: possible sites of action. *Steroids*, **36**, 619–631.

267. Müting, D., Lackas, N., Reikowski, H. & Richmond, S. (1966) Leberzirrhose und Diabetes mellitus. *Deutsche Medicinische Wochenschrift*, **91**, 1433–1438.

268. Myers, J.D., Brannon, E.S. & Holland, B.C. (1950) A correlative study of the cardiac output and the hepatic circulation in hyperthyroidism. *Journal of Clinical Investigation*, **29**, 1069–1077.

269. Nagasue, N., Ogawa, Y., Yukaya, H. *et al.* (1985) Serum levels of estrogens and testosterone in cirrhotic men with and without hepatocellular carcinoma. *Gastroenterology*, **88**, 768–772.

270. Nagore, N. & Scheuer, P.J. (1988) The pathology of diabetic hepatitis. *Journal of Pathology*, **156**, 155–160.

271. Nakamura, T., Otsuki, M., Tani, S. *et al.* (1988) Pancreatic endocrine function in cirrhotic rats. *Metabolism*, **37**, 892–899.

272. Nieschlag, E., Kremer, G.J. & Mussgnug, J. (1970) Insulin. Glucose-toleranz und freie Fettsauren Während und nach akuter Hepatitis. *Klinische Wochenschrift*, **48**, 381–385.

273. Nomura, S., Pittman, C.S., Chambers, J.B. *et al.* (1975) Reduced peripheral conversion of thyroxine to triiodothyronine in patients with hepatic cirrhosis. *Journal of Clinical Investigation*, **56**, 643–652.

274. Nunziata, V., Ceparano, G., Mazzacca, G. *et al.* (1978) Prolactin secretion in non-alcoholic liver cirrhosis. *Digestion*, **18**, 157–161.

275. Nygren, A., Adner, N., Sundblad, L. & Wiechel, K. (1985) Insulin uptake by the human alcoholic cirrhotic liver. *Metabolism*, **34**, 48–52.

276. Oakley, W.G. (1968) Pancreatic diabetes and haemochromatosis. In Oakley, W.G., Pyke, D.A. & Taylor, K.W. (eds) *Clinical Diabetes and its Biochemical Basis*, pp. 663–680. Oxford: Blackwell.

277. O'Hare, J. & Rolla, A.P. (1985) Hemochromatosis, hypogonadism, testosterone, and erythropoiesis. *Annals of Internal Medicine*, **102**, 871–872.

278. O'Keefe, S.J.D. & Marks, V. (1977) Lunchtime gin and tonic a cause of reactive hypoglycaemia. *Lancet*, **1**, 1286–1288.

279. Olivo, J., Gordon, G.G., Rafii, F. & Southren, A.L. (1975) Estrogen metabolism in hyperthyroidism and cirrhosis of the liver. *Steroids*, **26**, 47–56.

280. Ooms, H.A. (1973) *Emploi des Insulines Radioiodees comme Traceurs en Biologie*. Bruxelles: Arscia Editions.

281. Orbach, O. & Schussler, G.C. (1989) Increased serum cortisol binding in chronic active hepatitis. *American Journal of Medicine*, **86**, 39–42.

282. Orloff, M.J. (1987) Hyperparathyroidism, cirrhosis, and portocaval shunt. A new clinical syndrome. *American Journal of Surgery*, **155**, 76–81.

283. Owens, D., Srivastava, M.C., Tompkins, C.V. *et al.* (1973) Studies on the metabolic clearance rate, apparent distribution space and plasma half disappearance time of unlabelled human growth hormone in normal subjects and in patients with liver disease, renal disease, thyroid disease and diabetes mellitus. *European Journal of Clinical Investigation*, **3**, 284–294.

284. Palmer, J.P. (1983) Alcoholic ketoacidosis: clinical and laboratory presentation, pathophysiology and treatment. *Clinics in Endocrinology and Metabolism*, **12**, 381–389.

285. Palmer, J.P. & Ensinck, J.W. (1975) Stimulation of glucagon secretion by ethanol induced hypoglycaemia in man. *Diabetes*, **24**, 295–300.

286. Pamenter, R.W., Boyden, T.W. & Silvert, M.A. (1981) Chronic ethanol ingestion enhances Gn RH stimulated LH responses of castrated male dogs. *Journal of Reproduction and Fertility*, **63**, 91–94.

287. Panerai, A.E., Salerno, F., Manneschi, M. *et al.* (1977) Growth hormone and prolactin responses to thyrotrophin-releasing hormone in patients with severe liver disease. *Journal of Clinical Endocrinology and Metabolism*, **45**, 134–140.

288. Passa, P., Luyckx, A.S., Carpentier, J.L. *et al.* (1977) Glucagon secretion in diabetic patients with haemochromatosis. *Diabetologia*, **13**, 509–513.

289. Passa, P., Rosselie, F., Ganville, C. & Canivet, J. (1977) Retinopathy and plasma growth hormone levels in idiopathic hemochromatosis with diabetes. *Diabetes*, **26**, 113–120.

290. Paterson, C.R. & Losowsky, M.S. (1967) The bones in chronic liver disease. *Scandinavian Journal of Gastroenterology*, **2**, 293–300.

291. Paton, A. (1976) Alcohol-induced Cushingoid syndrome (letter) *British Medical Journal*, **25**, 1504.

292. Pentikäinen, P.J., Pentikäinen, L.A., Azarnoff, D.L. & Dujoune, C.A. (1975) Plasma levels and excretion of oestrogens in urine in chronic liver disease. *Gastroenterology*, **69**, 20–27.

293. Perin, E. & Sode, J. (1970) The liver in Graves' disease. *Medical Annual*, **39**, 563–570.

294. Persson, H. Bennegard, K., Lundberg, P. *et al.* (1985) Thyroid hormones in conditions of chronic malnutrition. *Annals of Surgery*, **201**, 45–52.

295. Peterson, R.E. (1960) Adrenocortical steroid metabolism and adrenal cortical function in liver disease. *Journal of Clinical Investigation*, **39**, 320–331.

296. Phelps, G., Chapman, I., Hall, P. *et al.* (1989) Prevalence of genetic haemochromatosis among diabetic patients. *Lancet*, **2**, 233–234.

297. Phillips, L.S., Herington, A.C. & Daughaday, W.H. (1975) Steroid hormone effects on somatomedin. I. Somatomedin action in vivo. *Endocrinology*, **97**, 780–786.

298. Phillips, L.S., Herington, A.C., Karl, I.E. & Daughaday, W.H. (1976) Comparison of somatomedin activity in perfusates of normal and hypophysectomised rat livers with and without added growth hormone. *Endocrinology*, **98**, 606–614.

299. Pimstone, B.L., Le Roith, D., Epstein, S. & Kronheim, S. (1975) Disappearance rates of plasma growth hormone after intravenous somatostatin in renal and liver disease. *Journal of Clinical Endocrinology and Metabolism*, **41**, 392–395.

300. Pincus, I.J., Rakoff, A.E., Cohn, E.M. & Tumen, H.J. (1951). Hormonal studies in patients with chronic liver disease. *Gastroenterology*, **19**, 735–754.

301. Pipher, J. & Poulsen, E. (1947) Liver biopsy in thyrotoxicosis. *Acta Medica Scandinavica*, **127**, 439.

302. Pirart, J. & Gatez, P. (1958) L'etiologie de l'hemochromatose non transfusionelle: revue de la question: étude de l'heredité dans 21 familles. *Semaine des Hôpitaux de Paris*, **34**, 1044–1051.

303. Pittman, C.S. & Pittman, J.A. (1974) Relation of chemical structure to the action and metabolism of thyroactive substances. *Handbook of Physiology*, **3**, 233–253.

304. Pittman, C.S., Chambers, J.B. & Read, V.H. (1971). The extrathyroidal conversion rate of thyroxine to triiodothyronine in normal man. *Journal of Clinical Investigation*, **50**, 1187–1196.

305. Pokroy, N., Epstein, S., Hendricks, S. & Pimstone, B. (1974) Thyrotrophin response to intravenous thyrotrophin-releasing hormone in patients with hepatic and renal disease. *Hormone and Metabolic Research*, **6**, 132–136.

306. Porter, L., Elm, M.S., Van Thiel, D.H. & Eagon, P.K. (1987) Hepatic estrogen receptor in human liver disease. *Gastroenterology*, **92**, 735–745.

307. Portugal-Alvarez, J., de Clamagirand, C.P., Souto, J.M. *et al.* (1974) Relationship between growth hormone, insulin and urinary oestrogens in hepatic cirrhosis. *Acta Diabetologica Latina*, **11**, 1–8.

308. Posner, D.B., Russell, R.M., Absood, S. *et al.* (1978). Effective 25-hydroxylation of vitamin D_2 in alcoholic cirrhosis. *Gastroenterology*, **74**, 866–870.

309. Pouchon, G., Kennan, A.L. & De Luca, H.F. (1969) Activation

of vitamin D by the liver. *Journal of Clinical Investigation*, **48**, 2032–2037.

310. Powell, L.W., Mortimer, R. & Harris, O.D. (1971) Cirrhosis of the liver—a comparative study of the four major aetiological groups. *Medical Journal of Australia*, **1**, 941–950.

311. Proietto, J., Dudley, F.J., Aitken, P. & Alford, F.P. (1984) Hyperinsulinaemia and insulin resistance of cirrhosis: the importance of insulin hypersecretion. *Clinical Endocrinology*, **21**, 657–665.

312. Read, A.E., Harrison, C.V. & Sherlock, S. (1963) 'Juvenile cirrhosis' part of a system disease. The effect of corticosteroid therapy. *Gut*, **4**, 378–384.

313. Record, C.O., Alberti, K.G.M.M., Williamson, D.H. & Wright, R. (1973) Glucose tolerance and metabolic changes in human viral hepatitis. *Clinical Science and Molecular Medicine*, **45**, 677–690.

314. Record, C.O., Chase, R.A., Alberti, K.G.M.M. & Williams, R. (1975) Disturbances in glucose metabolism in patients with liver damage due to paracetamol overdose. *Clinical Science and Molecular Medicine*, **49**, 473–479.

315. Redei, E., Branch, B.J., Gholami, S. *et al.* (1988) Effects of ethanol on CRF release in vitro. *Endocrinology*, **123**, 2736–2743.

316. Rees, L.H., Besser, G.M., Jeffcoate, W.J. *et al.* (1977) Alcohol induced pseudo-Cushing's syndrome. *Lancet*, **1**, 726–728.

317. Renner, E., Horber, F.F., Jost, G. *et al.* (1986) Effect of liver function on the metabolism of prednisone and prednisolone in humans. *Gastroenterology*, **90**, 819–828.

318. Richens, A. (1976) In Richens, A. & Woodford, F.P. (eds) *Anticonvulsant Drugs and Enzyme Induction*, p. 3. Amsterdam: Elsevier, Excerpta Medica.

319. Röjdmark, S., Bloom, G., Chou, M.C.Y. & Field, J.B. (1978) Hepatic extraction of exogenous insulin and glucagon in the dog. *Endocrinology*, **102**, 806–813.

320. Röjdmark, S., Adner, N., Andersson, E.H. *et al.* (1984) Prolactin and Thyrotropin responses to thyrotropin-releasing hormone and metoclopramide in men with chronic alcoholism. *Journal of Clinical Endocrinology and Metabolism*, **59**, 595–600.

321. Root, A.W. (1976) Clinical studies of human growth hormone. *Pharmacology and Therapeutics*, **1**, 19–43.

322. Rosenbaum, W., Christy, N.P. & Kelly, W.G. (1966) Electrophoretic evidence for the presence of an estrogen-binding β-globulin in human plasma. *Journal of Clinical Endocrinology and Metabolism*, **26**, 1399–1403.

323. Rosman, P.M., Farag, A., Benn, R. *et al.* (1982) Modulation of pituitary–adrenocortical function: decreased secretory episodes and blunted circadian rhythmicity in patients with alcoholic liver disease. *Journal of Clinical Endocrinology and Metabolism*, **55**, 709–717.

324. Rosner, W. (1972) A simplified method for the quantitative determination of testosterone-estradiol-binding globulin activity in human plasma. *Journal of Clinical Endocrinology and Metabolism*, **34**, 983–988.

325. Rupp, J., Cantarow, A., Rakoff, A.E. & Paschkis, K.E. (1951) Hormone excretion in liver disease and in gynecomastia. *Journal of Clinical Endocrinology*, **11**, 688–699.

326. Sachdev, Y. & Hall, R. (1975) Effusions into body cavities in hypothyroidism. *Lancet*, **1**, 564–566.

327. Samaan, N.A., Stone, D.B. & Eckhardt, R.D. (1969) Serum glucose insulin and growth hormone in chronic hepatic cirrhosis. *Archives of Internal Medicine*, **124**, 149–152.

328. Samols, E. & Ryder, J.A. (1961) Studies on tissue uptake of insulin in man using a differential immunoassay for endogenous and exogenous insulin. *Journal of Clinical Investigation*, **40**, 2092–2102.

329. Samols, E. & Turner, M.D. (1968) Disturbances in carbohydrate metabolism liver disease. In Dickens, F., Randle, P.J. & Whelan, W.J. (eds) *Carbohydrate Metabolism and its Disorders*, p. 298. London: Academic Press.

330. Schade, D.S., Eaton, R.P. & Standefer, J. (1977) Glucocorticoid regulation of plasma ketone body concentration in insulin-deficient man. *Journal of Clinical Endocrinology and Metabolism*, **44**, 1069–1079.

331. Schalch, D.S., Gonzalez-Barcena, D., Kastin, A.J. *et al.* (1975) Plasma gonadotrophins after administration of LH-releasing hormone in patients with renal or hepatic failure. *Journal of Clinical Endocrinology and Metabolism*, **41**, 921–925.

332. Schimpff, R.M., Lebrec, D. & Donnadieu, M. (1977) Somatomedin

production in normal adults and cirrhotic patients. *Acta Endocrinologica*, **86**, 355–362.

333. Schimpff, R.M., Lebrec, D. & Donnadieu, M. (1978) Serum somatomedin activity measured as sulphation factor in peripheral hepatic and renal veins of patients with alcoholic cirrhosis. *Acta Endocrinologica*, **88**, 729–736.

334. Schlienger, J.L., Blickle, F., Demangeat, C. *et al.* (1978) Analyse de l'insulinosecretion par le dosage du peptide C au cours des hepatopathies alcoholiques. *Nouvelle Presse Medicale*, **7**, 4011–4014.

335. Schussler, G.C., Schaffner, F. & Korn, F. (1978) Increased serum thyroid hormone binding and decreased free hormone in chronic active liver disease. *New England Journal of Medicine*, **299**, 510–515.

336. Seige, K. & Thierbach, V. (1959) Posthepatitische Schäden bei Diabetes mellitus. *Verhandlungen der Deutschen Gesellschaft für Innere Medizin*, **65**, 705–709.

337. Sells, R.A., Calne, R.H., Hadjiyanakis, V. & Marshall, V.C. (1972) Glucose and insulin metabolism after pancreatic transplantation. *British Medical Journal*, **3**, 678–681.

338. Sestoft, L. & Rehfeld, J.F. (1970) Insulin and glucose metabolism in liver cirrhosis and in liver failure. *Scandinavian Journal of Gastroenterology, Supplement*, **7**, 133–136.

339. Shaffer, J.M. (1940) Disease of the liver in hyperthyroidism. *Archives of Pathology*, **29**, 20–30.

340. Shankar, T.P., Drake, S. & Solomon, S.S. (1987) Insulin resistance and delayed clearance of peptide hormones in cirrhotic rat liver. *American Journal of Physiology*, **252** (6, Pt 1): E772–777.

341. Shankar, T.P., Fredi, J.L., Himmelstein, S. *et al.* (1986) Elevated growth hormone levels and insulin resistance in patients with cirrhosis of the liver. *American Journal of Medical Sciences*, **291**, 248–254.

342. Shedl, H.P. (1965) Steroid hormone metabolism in liver disease. In Popper, H. & Schaffner, F. (eds) *Progress in Liver Diseases*. New York: Grune & Stratton.

343. Sheldon, J.H. (1935) *Haemochromatosis*. Oxford University Press.

344. Sheridan, P., Chapman, C. & Losowsky, M.S. (1978) Interpretation of laboratory tests of thyroid function in chronic active hepatitis. *Clinica Chimica Acta*, **86**, 73–80.

345. Sherlock, S. (1989) Primary biliary cirrhosis. In *Diseases of the Liver and Biliary System*, pp. 273–288. Oxford: Blackwell.

346. Sherlock, S. (1989) Nutritional and metabolic liver diseases. In *Diseases of the Liver and Biliary System*, pp. 470–500. Oxford: Blackwell.

347. Sherwin, R.S., Joshi, P., Hendler, R. *et al.* (1974) Hyperglucagonemia in Laennec's cirrhosis, the role of portal-systemic shunting. *New England Journal of Medicine*, **290**, 239–242.

348. Sherwin, R.S., Fisher, M., Bessoff, J. *et al.* (1978) Hyperglucagonemia in cirrhosis: altered secretion and sensitivity to glucagon. *Gastroenterology*, **74**, 1224–1228.

349. Shipley, R.A. & Chudzik, E.B. (1957) Thyroidal uptake and plasma clearance of ^{131}I and [127]I in cirrhosis of the liver. *Journal of Clinical Endocrinology and Metabolism*, **17**, 1229–1236.

350. Sholiton, L.J., Werk, E.E. Jr & Marnell, R.T. (1961) Diurnal variation of adrenocortical function in non-endocrine disease states. *Metabolism*, **10**, 632–646.

351. Shurberg, J.L., Resnick, R.H., Koff, R.S. *et al.* (1977) Serum lipids, insulin and glucagon after portacaval shunt in cirrhosis. *Gastroenterology*, **72**, 301–304.

352. Siemons, L.J. & Mahler, C.H. (1987) Hypogonadotrophic hypogonadism in hemochromatosis: recovery of reproductive function after iron depletion. *Journal of Clinical Endocrinology and Metabolism*, **65**, 585–587.

353. Sikuler, E., Polio, J., Groszmann, R.J. & Hendler, R. (1987) Glucagon and insulin metabolism in a portal-hypertensive rat model. *American Journal of Physiology*, **253** (2, Pt 1): G110–115.

354. Silvestrini, R. (1926) La reviviscenza mammaria nell uomo affeto da cirrosi del Laennec. *Reforma Medica*, **42**, 701–704.

355. Simon, M., Franchimont, P., Murie, N. *et al.* (1972) Study of somatotropic and gonadotrophin pituitary function in idiopathic haemochromatosis (31 cases). *European Journal of Clinical Investigation*, **2**, 384–389.

356. Sir, T., Wolff, C., Soto, J.R. *et al.* (1987) Relationship between

hepatic levels of glutathione and sulphobromophthalein retention in hyperthyroidism. *Clinical Science*, **73**, 235–237.

357. Skinner, R.K., Long, R.G., Sherlock, S. & Wills, M.R. (1977) 25-Hydroxylation of Vitamin D in primary biliary cirrhosis. *Lancet*, **1**, 720–721.

358. Smallridge, R.C., Wartofsky, L., Green, B.J. *et al.* (1979) 3'-L-monoidiothyronine: development of a radioimmunoassay and demonstration of in vivo conversion from 3',5'-diiodothyronine. *Journal of Clinical Endocrinology and Metabolism*, **48**, 32–36.

359. Smals, A., Kloppenborg, P., Njo, K.T. *et al.* (1976) Alcohol-induced Cushingoid syndrome. *British Medical Journal*, **2**, 1298.

360. Smals, A.G.H., Njo, K.T., Knoben, J.M. *et al.* (1977) Alcohol-induced Cushingoid syndrome. *Journal of the Royal College of Physicians*, **12**, 36–41.

361. Smith-Laing, G., Sherlock, S. & Faber, O.K. (1979) Effects of spontaneous portal-systemic shunting on insulin metabolism. *Gastroenterology*, **76**, 685–690.

362. Soeters, P.B. & Fischer, J.E. (1976) Insulin, glucagon, amino acid imbalance, and hepatic encephalopathy. *Lancet*, **2**, 880–881.

363. Soeters, P., Weir, G., Ebeid, A.M. & Fischer, J.E. (1977) Insulin, glucagon, portal systemic shunting and hepatic failure in the dog. *Journal of Surgical Research*, **23**, 183–188.

364. Sönksen, P.H., Jones, R.H., Tompkins, C.V. *et al.* (1976) The metabolism of insulin in vivo. *Excerpta Medica International Congress Series*, **413**, 204–210.

365. Southren, A.L., Gordon, G.G., Olico, J. *et al.* (1973) Androgen metabolism in cirrhosis of the liver. *Metabolism*, **22**, 695–702.

366. Starzl, T.E., Porter, K.A., Francavilla, J.A. *et al.* (1978) A hundred years of the hepatotrophic controversy. In *Hepatotrophic Factors*. Ciba Foundation Symposium 55 (new series). Amsterdam: North-Holland & Elsevier, Excerpta Medica.

367. Starzl, T.E., Porter, K.A., Hayashida, N. *et al.* (1980) Further studies on hepatic stimulatory substance (SS) after partial hepatectomy. *Journal of Surgical Research*, **29**, 471–474.

368. Stellon, A.J. Davies, A., Compston, J. & Williams, R. (1985) Osteoporosis in chronic cholestatic liver disease. *Quarterly Journal of Medicine*, **57**, 783–790.

369. Stewart, A., Johnston, D.G., Alberti, K.G.M.M. *et al.* (1983) Hormone and metabolic profiles in alcoholic liver disease. *European Journal of Clinical Investigation*, **13**, 397–403.

370. Stocks, A.E. & Martin, F.I.R. (1968) Pituitary function in hemochromatosis. *American Journal of Medicine*, **45**, 839–845.

371. Stocks, A.E. & Powell, L.W. (1972) Pituitary function in idiopathic haemochromatosis and cirrhosis of the liver. *Lancet*, **2**, 298–300.

372. Stocks, A.E. & Powell, L.W. (1973) Carbohydrate intolerance in idiopathic haemochromatosis and cirrhosis of the liver. *Quarterly Journal of Medicine*, **42**, 733–749.

373. Stoll, R.W., Touber, J.L., Menathan, L.H. & Williams, R.H. (1970) Clearance of porcine insulin, proinsulin and connecting peptide by the isolated rat liver. *Proceedings of the Society for Experimental Biology and Medicine*, **133**, 894–896.

374. Strange, R.C., Mjos, O.D., Hendon, T. & Jynge, P. (1977) The effect of glucagon on plasma cyclic AMP and glucose concentrations in patients with alcoholic cirrhosis. *Acta Medica Scandinavia*, **202**, 87–88.

375. Stumpf, H.H. & Wilens, S.L. (1953) Inhibitory effects of portal cirrhosis of liver on prostatic enlargement. *Archives of Internal Medicine*, **91**, 304–309.

376. Summerskill, W.H.J., Davidson, C.S., Dible, J.H. *et al.* (1960) Cirrhosis of the liver: a study of alcoholic and non-alcoholic patients in Boston and London. *New England Journal of Medicine*, **262**, 1–9.

377. Surks, M.I., Schadlow, A.R., Stock, J.M. & Oppenheimer, J.R. (1973) Determination of iodothyronine absorption and conversion of L-thyroxine (T4) to L-triiodothyronine (T3) using turnover rate techniques. *Journal of Clinical Investigation*, **52**, 805–811.

378. Takano, K., Hizuka, N., Shizume, K. *et al.* (1977) Serum somatomedin peptides measured by somatomedin A radio receptor assay in chronic liver disease. *Journal of Clinical Endocrinology and Metabolism*, **45**, 828–832.

379. Tarquini, B., Gheri, R., Anichini, P. *et al.* (1977) Circadian study of immunoreactive prolactin in patients with cirrhosis of the liver. *Gastroenterology*, **73**, 116–119.

380. Taylor, A.L., Upman, R.L., Salam, A. & Mintz, D.H. (1972) Hepatic clearance of human growth hormone. *Journal of Clinical Endocrinology*, **34**, 395–399.

381. Temple, R.C., Carrington, C.A., Luzio, S.D. *et al.* (1989) Insulin deficiency in non-insulin dependent diabetes mellitus. *Lancet*, **i**, 293–295.

382. Terasaki, T., Nowlin, D.M. & Pardridge, W.M. (1988) Differential binding of testosterone and estradiol to isoforms of sex hormone-binding globulin: selective alteration of estradiol binding in cirrhosis. *Journal of Clinical Endocrinology and Metabolism*, **67**, 639–643.

383. Territo, M.C. & Tanaka, K.R. (1974) Hypophosphatemia in chronic alcoholism. *Archives of Internal Medicine*, **134**, 445–447.

384. Thompson, W.G. & Hart, I.R. (1973) Chronic active hepatitis and Graves' disease. *American Journal of Digestive Diseases*, **18**, 111–119.

385. Tiengo, A., Fedele, D., Dolzani, L. *et al.* (1976) Hormonal counterregulation in ethanol-induced hypoglycaemia-glucagon and cortisol secretion in pigs. In Andreani, D., Lefebvre, P.J. & Marks, W. (eds) *Hypoglycaemia*. Proceedings of the European Symposium. Rome, pp. 105–111. Stuttgart: Thieme.

386. Tintera, J.W. (1966) Stabilising homeostasis in the recovered alcoholic through endocrine therapy: evaluation of the hypoglycaemia factor. *Journal of the American Geriatrics Society*, **14**, 126–150.

387. Tintera, J.W. & Lovell, H.W. (1949) Endocrine treatment of alcoholism. *Geriatrics*, **4**, 274–280.

388. Toro, G., Kolodny, R.C., Jacobs, L.S. *et al.* (1973) Failure of alcohol to alter pituitary and target organ hormone levels. *Clinical Research*, **21**, 205.

389. Tourniare, J., Fevre, M., Mazenod, B. & Ponsin, G. (1974) Effects of clomiphene citrate and synthetic LHRH on serum luteinizing hormone (LH) in men with idiopathic hemochromatosis. *Journal of Clinical Endocrinology and Metabolism*, **38**, 1122–1124.

390. Tucci, J.R., Albacete, R.A. & Martin, M.M. (1966) Effect of liver disease upon steroid circadian rhythms in man. *Gastroenterology*, **50**, 637–644.

391. Turkington, R.W. (1972) Serum prolactin levels in patients with gynecomastia. *Journal of Clinical Endocrinology and Metabolism*, **34**, 62–66.

392. Unger, R.H. (1976) Diabetes and the alpha cell. *Diabetes*, **25**, 136–151.

393. Unterman, T.G. & Phillips, L.S. (1986) Circulating somatomedin activity during hepatic regeneration. *Endocrinology*, **119**, 185–192.

394. Uthne, K. & Uthne, T. (1972) Influence of liver resection and regeneration on somatomedin (sulfation factor) activity in sera from normal and hypophysectomised rats. *Acta Endocrinologica*, **71**, 255–264.

395. Valimaki, M., Salaspuro, M., Harkonen, M. & Ylikahri, R. (1982) Liver damage and sex hormones in chronic male alcoholics. *Clinical Endocrinology*, **17**, 469–477.

396. Van Itallie, T.B. & Bentley, W.B.A. (1955) Glucagon-induced hyperglycemia as an index of liver function. *Journal of Clinical Investigation*, **34**, 1730–1737.

397. Vanotti, A. & Beraud, T. (1959) Functional relationships between liver, thyroxine-binding protein of serum and the thyroid. *Journal of Clinical Endocrinology and Metabolism*, **19**, 466–477.

398. Van Thiel, D.H. & Lester, R. (1976) Alcoholism: its effect on hypothalamic–pituitary–gonadal function. *Gastroenterology*, **71**, 318–327.

399. Van Thiel, D.H. & Loriaux, D.L. (1979) Evidence for an adrenal origin of plasma estrogens in alcoholic men. *Metabolism*, **28**, 536–541.

400. Van Thiel, D.H., Gavaler, J. & Lester, R. (1974) Ethanol inhibition of vitamin A metabolism in the testes: possible mechanism for sterility in alcoholics. *Science*, **186**, 941–942.

401. Van Thiel, D.H., Lester, R. & Sherins, R.J. (1974) Hypogonadism alcoholic liver disease: evidence for a double defect. *Gastroenterology*, **67**, 1188–1199.

402. Van Thiel, D.H., Gavaler, J.S., Lester, R. *et al.* (1975) Plasma estrone, prolactin, neurophysin and sex steroid-binding globulin in chronic alcoholic men. *Metabolism*, **24**, 1015–1019.

403. Van Thiel, D.H., McClain, C.J., Elson, M.K. *et al.* (1978) Hyperprolactinemia and thyrotropin-releasing factor (TRH) responses in men with alcoholic liver disease. *Alcoholism: Clinical and Experimental Research*, **2**, 344–348.

404. Van Thiel, D.H., McClain, C.J., Elson, M.K. *et al.* (1978) Evidence for autonomous secretion of prolactin in some alcoholic men with cirrhosis and gynecomastia. *Metabolism. Clinical and Experimental*, **27**, 1778–1784.

405. Van Thiel, D.H., Gavaler, J.S., Cobb, C.F. *et al.* (1979) Alcohol-induced testicular atrophy in the adult male rat. *Endocrinology*, **105**, 888–895.

406. Van Thiel, D.H., Gavaler, J.S., Slone, F.S. *et al.* (1980) Feminisation in alcoholic man due in part to portal hypertension: a rat model. *Gastroenterology*, **78**, 81–91.

407. Van Thiel, D.H., Gavaler, J.S., Spero, J.A. *et al.* (1981) Patterns of hypothalamic–pituitary–gonadal dysfunction in man with liver disease due to differing etiologies. *Hepatology*, **1**, 39–46.

408. Van Thiel, D.H., Gavaler, J.S., Cobb, C.F. & Chiao, Y.-B. (1982) Effects of ethanol upon the hypothalamic–pituitary–gonadal axis. In Langer, M., Chiandussi, L., Chopra, I.J. & Martini, L. (eds) *The Endocrines and The Liver*, pp. 117–134. London: Academic Press.

409. Van Thiel, D.H., Gavaler, Judith, S., Tarter, R. *et al.* (1985) Pituitary and thyroid hormone levels before and after orthotopic hepatic transplantation and their responses to thyrotropin-releasing hormone. *Journal of Clinical Endocrinology and Metabolism*, **60**, 569–574.

410. Vermeulen, A., Verdonck, L., Van der Straeton, M. & Orie, N. (1969) Capacity of the testosterone binding globulin in human plasma and influence of specific binding of testosterone on its metabolic clearance rate. *Journal of Clinical Endocrinology and Metabolism*, **29**, 1470–1480.

411. Verillo, A., de Teresa, A., Martino, C. *et al.* (1986) Circulating somatostatin concentrations in healthy and cirrhotic subjects. *Metabolism*, **35**, 130–135.

411a.Visser, T.J., Kaptein, E., Terpstra, O.T. & Krenning, E.P. (1988) Deiodination of thyroid hormone by human liver. *Journal of Clinical Endocrinology and Metabolism*, **67**, 17–24.

412. Waddell, W.R. & Sussman, K.E. (1967) Plasma insulin after diversion of portal and pancreatic venous blood to vena cava. *Journal of Applied Physiology*, **22**, 808–812.

413. Walfish, P.G., Orrego, H., Israel, Y. *et al.* (1979) Serum triiodothyronine and other clinical and laboratory indices of alcoholic liver disease. *Annals of Internal Medicine*, **91**, 13–16.

414. Walker, C., Peterson, W. & Unger, R. (1974) Blood ammonia levels in advanced cirrhosis during therapeutic elevation of the insulin : glucagon ratio. *New England Journal of Medicine*, **211**, 168–171.

415. Walsh, C.H., Wright, A.D., Williams, J.W. & Holder, G. (1976) A study of pituitary function in patients with idiopathic haemochromatosis. *Journal of Clinical Endocrinology and Metabolism*, **43**, 866–872.

416. Walton, C., Kelly, W.F., Laing, I. & Bu'Lock, D.E. (1983) Endocrine abnormalities in idiopathic haemochromatosis. *Quarterly Journal of Medicine*, **205**, 99–110.

417. Weller, C.V. (1930) Hepatic lesions associated with exophthalmic goitre. *Transactions of the Association of American Physicians*, **45**, 71–85.

418. Wernze, H. & Schmitz, E. (1977) Plasma prolactin and prolactin release in liver cirrhosis. *Acta Hepato Gastroenterologica*, **24**, 97–101.

419. West, T.E.T., Owens, D., Sönksen, P.H. *et al.* (1975) Metabolic responses to monocomponent human insulin infusions in normal subjects and patients with liver and endocrine disease. *Clinical Endocrinology*, **4**, 573–584.

420. Whelton, M.J., Kehayoglou, A.K., Agnew, J.E. *et al.* (1971) Calcium absorption in parenchymatous and biliary disease. *Gut*, **12**, 978–983.

421. Wiedemann, E. & Schwartz, E. (1972) Suppression of growth hormone-dependent human serum sulfation factor by estrogen. *Journal of Clinical Endocrinology and Metabolism*, **34**, 51–58.

422. Wiedemann, E., Schwartz, E. & Frantz, A.G. (1976) Acute and chronic estrogen effects upon serum somatomedin activity, growth hormone and prolactin in man. *Journal of Clinical Endocrinology*, **42**, 942–952.

423. Williams, R.M., Hay, J.S. & Tjaden, M. (1959) Degradation of insulin ^{131}I and glucagon ^{131}I and factors influencing it. *Annals of the New York Academy of Sciences*, **74**, 13–21.

424. Wright, J. (1978) Endocrine effects of alcohol. *Clinics in Endocrinology and Metabolism*, **7**, 351–367.

425. Wright, J.W., Merry, J., Fry, D. & Marks, V. (1976) Pituitary function in chronic alcoholism. In Cross, M.M. (ed.) *Alcohol Intoxication and Withdrawal, Advances in Experimental Medicine and Biology*, p. 253. New York: Plenum Press.

426. Wu, A., Grant, D.B., Hambley, J. & Levi, A.J. (1974) Reduced serum somatomedin activity in patients with chronic liver disease. *Clinical Science and Molecular Medicine*, **47**, 359–366.

427. Yamaguchi, K., Fukushima, H. & Uzawa, H. (1979) Response of human growth hormone, prolactin and thyrotrophin releasing hormones in liver cirrhosis and diabetes mellitus. *Endocrinologica Japonica*, **26**, 81–88.

428. Yao, J.D.C., Gross, J.B., Jr, Ludwig, J. & Purnell, D.C. (1989) Cholestatic jaundice in hyperthyroidism. *American Journal of Medicine*, **86**, 619–620.

429. Yen, S.S.C., Ehara, Y. & Siler, T.M. (1974) Augmentation of prolactin secretion by estrogen in hypogonad women. *Journal of Clinical Investigation*, **53**, 652–655.

430. Yeung, R.T.T. & Wang, C.C.L. (1974) A study of carbohydrate metabolism in postnecrotic cirrhosis of the liver. *Gut*, **15**, 907–912.

431. Ylikahri, R.H., Huttunen, M.O., Harkonen, M. *et al.* (1978) Acute effects of alcohol on anterior pituitary secretion of the tropic hormones. *Journal of Clinical Endocrinology and Metabolism*, **46**, 175–720.

432. Zanoboni, A. & Zanoboni-Muciaccia, W. (1975) Gynaecomastia in alcoholic cirrhosis (letter). *Lancet*, **2**, 876.

433. Zanoboni, A. & Zanoboni-Muciaccia, W. (1977) Elevated basal growth hormone levels and growth hormone response to TRH in alcoholic patients with cirrhosis. *Journal of Clinical Endocrinology and Metabolism*, **45**, 576–578.

434. Zumoff, B., Bradlow, H.L., Gallagher, T.F. & Hellman, L. (1967) Cortisol metabolism in cirrhosis. *Journal of Clinical Investigation*, **46**, 1735–1743.

CHAPTER 8

Haematological Disorders in Liver Disease

Morag Chisholm

THE PHYSIOLOGICAL ROLE OF THE LIVER IN HAEMOPOIESIS AND HAEMOSTASIS

The liver is the primary site of erythropoiesis in the fetus from the ninth to the twenty-fourth week of gestation, but thereafter the bone marrow becomes the major source of red blood cells. Granulocytes and platelets are produced in the liver from the early weeks of fetal life, but the production of these cells is taken over by the bone marrow as the fetus develops. The potential for haemopoiesis is retained into adult life and in conditions where bone marrow function fails, as for example in myelofibrosis, the liver may again become an active site of haemopoiesis.

The major functions of the liver in relation to the blood are shown in Table 8.1. The major haematinics essential for haemopoiesis are iron, vitamin B$_{12}$ and folate. The liver's role in relation to these will be summarized briefly.

Red cell destruction and breakdown

Destruction and breakdown of the red cells take place in the liver and other parts of the reticuloendothelial (RE) system. A detailed description is given in Chapter 14. In summary, when the red cell is destroyed, iron and globin are split off and the residual haem is broken down in Kupffer and other RE cells to bilirubin, which is then carried in the plasma to the liver, bound to albumin. The bilirubin then enters the hepatic cells and undergoes conjugation to glucuronic acid, to form a water-soluble compound which passes via the bile duct to the intestine.

Table 8.1 Physiological role of the liver in haemopoiesis and haemostasis

Production of blood cells in utero
Reticuloendothelial function
    Red cell destruction and breakdown
    Transferrin production
    Clearance and breakdown of activated coagulation factors
Bilirubin metabolism and excretion
Storage organ for vitamin B_{12}, folate and iron
Production of coagulation factors

Urobilinogen is formed which is partly excreted and partly reabsorbed, and is finally excreted both in the urine and the faeces.

Iron metabolism

Transferrin, the major carrier protein for iron, is synthesized in the liver and other reticuloendothelial tissues. To a limited extent the liver acts as a storage organ for iron. The average iron content of a healthy male is about 70 mmol (4 g) and most of this is in the circulating haemoglobin. A small amount (approximately 5.5 mmol [0.3 g]) is stored in the liver either as ferritin, a water-soluble protein iron complex, or in the Kupffer cells as haemosiderin, an insoluble compound easily visible on light microscopy using special stains such as Prussian blue.

Vitamin B_{12} and folate metabolism

A large part of the body stores of vitamin B_{12} are present in the liver, the normal content ranging from 0.6 to 1.5 μg vitamin B_{12}/g wet weight. Folic acid is also stored in the liver, with a mean normal level of 7.1 μg/g.[36] The hepatic contents of vitamin B_{12} and folate correlate well with blood levels. There would appear to be few haemopoietic consequences of altered metabolism of these essential vitamins by liver disease per se. The changes described result mainly from associated abnormalities such as alcoholism and poor nutrition.

Coagulation factors

The current hypothesis of blood coagulation proposes that a series of reactions, which begins either with activation of factor XII by contact with exposed subendothelial collagen (intrinsic pathway) or with activation of factor VII by tissue substances known as thromboplastins (extrinsic pathway), leads to the formation of a thrombus consisting of closely interwoven fibrin and platelets. The coagulation factors are present in the plasma mostly in trace amounts as proenzymes or precursor proteins (zymogens), but during the process of clotting become activated and interact with each other sequentially as shown in Figure 8.1.

The following factors are produced in the liver: fibrinogen, the vitamin K dependent factors II, VII, IX and X, the soluble components of the protein C system,[72] the labile factors V and VIII, the contact factors XI and XII, and factor XIII, the fibrin stabilizing factor.[262] Most are produced exclusively in the liver, have a short half-life ranging from a few hours to a few days, and are reduced in hepatocellular failure. This latter observation was for a long time the main evidence to support the hypothesis that the liver was the site of production of the coagulation proteins. More recently, with the establishment in culture of hepatoma and other liver cell lines, it has been possible to characterize many of the coagulation factors in the culture fluid by direct assay, immunocytochemistry, and by the detection of specific RNAs. cDNAs encoding for several coagulation factors and inhibitors including protein C and antithrombin III have been isolated from human liver libraries and the structure of the hepatic genes for some of the coagulation factors is now known.[134] This is an exciting new field with discoveries to come.

Vitamin K-dependent factors

The synthesis of factors II, VII, IX and X is dependent both on normal liver function and on an adequate supply of vitamin K. Natural vitamin K is fat soluble and its absorption from the gut is facilitated by bile salts. It is obtained from the diet and from the synthetic activity of intestinal bacteria. Conditions such as malabsorption, obstructive jaundice and antibiotic therapy, and antagonists such as warfarin will lead to vitamin K deficiency. The role of vitamin K in the production of factors II, VII, IX and X has been defined.[239] The basic precursor proteins are produced in the liver, but are non-functional and are unable to participate in the clotting cascade. Vitamin K is essential for the next step and directs the insertion of a second carboxyl group into the γ-carbon of glutamic acid residues. This results in a unique amino acid, γ-carboxyglutamic acid, which confers coagulant activity on the precursor proteins,[234] enabling them to bind to phospholipid surfaces in the presence of calcium and to actively promote coagulation. In vitamin K deficiency the protein precursors known as PIVKA (i.e. protein induced by vitamin K absence or antagonists) accumulate in the plasma and can be detected by coagulation tests in vitro[109] and by immunological techniques.[92] The abnormal protein, des-γ-carboxy prothrombin, detectable by radioimmunoassay, has been shown to be useful as a marker of early vitamin K deficiency in serum and plasma.[160]

Other coagulation factors

Fibrinogen is synthesized almost exclusively by the liver, where it is produced by the parenchymal cells.[80] Unlike most of the other clotting factors, fibrinogen is present in measurable amounts in the plasma (6–12 μmol/l [2–4 g/l]) and has a relatively long half-life of 5 days. Both fibrinogen and factor VIII are acute-phase reactant

EXTRINSIC SYSTEM   INTRINSIC SYSTEM

Figure 8.1 The coagulation cascade. Dotted arrows indicate conversion to the activated form (a). PF3 = platelet factor 3 (phospholipid).

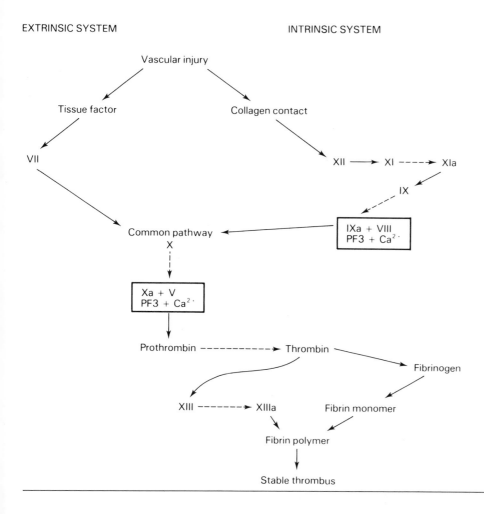

Fibrinolytic and inhibiting factors

proteins and are often raised in liver disease. Experimental work has shown that factor VIII is produced by the liver, spleen and other reticuloendothelial cells, and immunological techniques have demonstrated the production of the protein, factor VIII-related antigen now known as von Willebrand Factor (VWF), in vascular endothelial cells.[19] Factor VIII coagulant activity is labile, and its demonstration in tissue therefore difficult. Using an immunohistological technique for the assay of factor VIII clotting antigen (C Ag), Exner and colleagues[70] have demonstrated high factor VIII C Ag concentrations in lymph nodes, lungs and in normal sinusoidal endothelial cells; these were not noted in haemophilic tissues.[233] On the other hand, immunoradiometric assay (IRMA) has demonstrated higher factor VIII C Ag concentrations in hepatocytes and other cells than in endothelial cells,[135] suggesting that the liver is a major site of factor VIII production and that factor VIII C Ag is rapidly exported from the liver following its synthesis. Differences of technique may explain these contrasting results.

Factor XIII, the fibrin stabilizing factor, is probably synthesized in the liver[262] as well as in the megakaryocytes.[213]

A summary of the factors involved in fibrinolysis, the means whereby thrombi are broken down, is shown in Figure 8.2.

Plasminogen is synthesized by the liver[232] and is the inactive precursor of plasmin. Plasminogen activators are present in the plasma and blood cells (intrinsic activators) and in most tissues and body fluids (tissue-type plasminogen activators: tPA). The binding of tPA to fibrin greatly enhances its affinity for plasminogen and increases its conversion to plasmin. tPA is present in the vascular endothelium and as a result of genetic engineering is available for clinical use.

Plasmin is a potent proteolytic enzyme which is able to break down fibrin, and other coagulation factors including fibrinogen if not held in check. Plasmin breaks down fibrin into a number of small peptides known as fibrin degradation products (FDP). At a later stage cross-linked D-dimers (XDP) are produced. The measurement of FDPs and XDPs is useful as a marker of fibrin/fibrinogen breakdown in the circulation.

The action of plasmin in breaking down fibrin is limited by a number of circulating antiplasmins and plasminogen

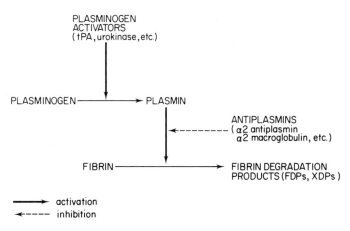

activation
inhibition

Figure 8.2 The fibrinolytic system.

activator inhibitors. The fast-acting plasminogen activator inhibitor (PAI) is synthesized by endothelial cells; low levels promote fibrinolysis and increased levels are associated with thrombosis. Of the antiplasmins shown in Figure 8.2, alpha-2-antiplasmin, synthesized in the liver, is physiologically important, deficiency being associated with a lifelong bleeding disorder due to excessive fibrinolysis.[143]

The liver plays an important role in the removal of activated factors and inhibitor–coagulation factor complexes from the circulation and in the production of fibrinolytic promoters and inhibitors. Plasma contains at least six inhibitors: the most important of these is antithrombin III (ATIII), which is synthesized in the liver[71] and endothelial cells. It is a major inhibitor of thrombin, and activated factors IXA, XA, XIA and XIIA and plasmin. Heparin markedly potentiates the inactivation of thrombin by ATIII, which is also known as heparin cofactor I. Low ATIII levels occur in liver disease, disseminated intravascular coagulation (DIC), and following thrombosis and heparin therapy. Congenital deficiency of ATIII is associated with a thrombotic tendency.[65,148] Other inhibitors, which include heparin cofactor II, have various substrates and are of less physiological importance, and deficiency is rarely associated with clinical problems in haemostasis.

ABNORMALITIES OF HAEMOPOIESIS

Liver disease may result in abnormalities of haemopoiesis ranging from morphological changes of the red cell to severe anaemia. White cell abnormalities occur but are less striking. Disturbed haemostasis is common due to thrombocytopenia and impaired synthesis of the coagulation factors or their excessive consumption and loss. Although there is some overlap, it will be convenient to discuss the effects of liver disease on haemopoiesis and haemostasis separately.

Red cell abnormalities

The normal mature red cell is a biconcave disc and, using the international terminology proposed by Bessis and colleagues,[13] is referred to as a discocyte. Red cell shape is maintained by a number of factors, including the ratio of the red cell membrane surface area to its volume. The membrane is basically a lipid bilayer; cholesterol and phospholipids comprise approximately 90% of the total membrane lipid.[27] The ratio of cholesterol to phospholipid (CP ratio) in the membrane is an important factor determining normal red cell shape. The membrane lipids may undergo a change in composition because of an alteration in plasma lipids, as has been shown in vitro by incubating red cells in sera with different lipid constituents.[53] In liver disease the cholesterol and phospholipid content of the plasma may rise, leading to an increased erythrocyte content of both, with possibly an altered ratio[49] (see Chapter 4). As a result of this and other factors as yet poorly understood, certain morphological changes occur in liver disease.

Macrocytosis

The macrocytosis associated with liver disease, particularly cirrhosis and obstructive jaundice, has excited much attention. The frequency varies, but approximately 60–65% of patients with liver disease will have macrocytic blood films.[14,15,233] The erythrocytes have been described as 'thin' macrocytes or leptocytes because they have a diminished thickness but an increased diameter. Early studies showed that thin macrocytosis was associated with a macronormoblastic marrow and was noted in just over one-third of patients with various liver diseases, including acute hepatitis and established obstructive jaundice, provided hepatocellular damage was present.[14,15] The survival of these cells is shortened but there is no clear association with anaemia.[104] This type of macrocytosis resolves after improvement in liver function rather than after treatment with vitamin B_{12} or folate.

True or 'thick' macrocytosis is seen in less than 10% and is noted only in patients with cirrhosis, mainly alcoholic. Megaloblastic erythropoiesis is common in this group and is almost certainly due to nutritional deficiency of folate.

Thus the underlying pathogenesis of macrocytosis in liver disease varies. Increased membrane cholesterol has been demonstrated in the leptocytes of liver disease[188,263] and an increased CP ratio in the red cell membrane could cause the broadening and flattening of the red cell. Reticulocytosis in response to haemolysis or blood loss may be a contributory factor[138] and the erythroid hyperplasia and macronormoblastic maturation associated with the bone marrow response to haemolysis also plays a part. In addition, it is likely that alcohol has a direct effect on erythropoiesis resulting in macrocytosis. Finally, in a small number of patients, macrocytosis will be due to folate deficiency.

Target cell formation

Target cells ('codocytes' according to the international classification) are bell shaped on scanning electron microscopy, but on dried films assume a characteristic target shape. Altered red cell membrane-to-volume ratio, either due to an absolute increase in membrane content, as in liver disease, or because of a decrease in intracellular haemoglobin content, as in iron deficiency, will result in target cell formation. Target cells in liver disease have an increased content of cholesterol and phospholipid but, because of a proportionately greater rise in the membrane lecithin, the CP ratio is not as raised as in acanthocytosis, another red cell abnormality seen in liver disease.[49]

Target cells are also thin macrocytes and were noted in one-third of patients with liver disease in Bingham's study.[14,15] They are commonly noted in the blood of patients with obstructive jaundice or hepatitis with associated obstruction,[53] but the reasons for the development of the defect are not clear. No consistent correlation between the plasma lipids and those of the red cell membrane has been observed.[53,188] It has been suggested that excess bile salts found in obstructive liver disease may inhibit the enzyme lecithin cholesterol acyltransferase (necessary for the esterification of cholesterol to lysolecithin), leading to raised plasma cholesterol and an associated increase in red cell membrane cholesterol. It is obvious that other factors must also be important since hypercholesterolaemia due to other diseases does not cause increased membrane cholesterol (see Chapter 4).[189]

Stomatocytosis

Stomatocytes are cup-shaped red cells in which the central circular area is replaced by a 'mouth-like' unstained area due to a dimple on one side. Stomatocytosis, or 'key hole' abnormality, has been defined as more than 4% stomatocytes in the peripheral blood, and has been described in chronic liver disease, particularly alcoholic. Agents that have been shown to induce stomatocytosis[13] include cationic drugs and a low pH, and in hereditary stomatocytosis an elevated membrane lecithin as well as abnormalities in red cell enzyme content have been reported.[205] Douglass and Twomey[62] described stomatocytosis in patients with alcoholic liver disease, but there was no clear correlation between the degree of stomatocytosis, red cell survival and anaemia. The mechanism underlying the phenomenon is not understood.

Spiculated red cells

Normal red cells (discocytes) may become crenated or spiculated under the influence of extrinsic and intrinsic factors and on changing their shape may be transformed into echinocytes or acanthocytes. An echinocyte is a spiculated cell with 10–30 spicules regularly distributed over the surface of the cell, while an acanthocyte is a spheroidal cell with 2–20 spicules of variable length irregularly distributed over its surface.[12]

Echinocytosis is usually an in vitro phenomenon brought about by contact with glass, fatty acids, lysolecithin, anionic drugs, a raised pH and other factors. The abnormality is usually reversible, and care must be taken in making blood films. Conditions in which true echinocytosis exists include uraemia, neonatal hepatitis and heparin therapy. Echinocytes are frequently found in the blood in liver disease (see Chapter 4) but require a wet film or scanning electron microscopy for their demonstration, neither of which is routinely used in haematology laboratories.[198] Echinocyte formation can be induced by incubating normal red cells with normal low-density lipoproteins, probably as a result of binding of apolipoprotein B to the cell membrane.[121] Normal high-density lipoproteins (HDL) do not induce echinocytosis but the abnormal HDL from patients with liver disease may do so.[198] The phenomenon is of unproven clinical significance.

Acanthocytosis is rare in liver disease but has received considerable attention. A markedly increased CP ratio has been noted in acanthocytes associated with liver disease. This is due to increased membrane cholesterol, the total phospholipid content remaining normal. As a result there is increased membrane rigidity of the red cell, which is thus less deformable and has a shortened survival. The defect does not lie in the red cell; normal red cells become abnormal on being transfused into patients with acanthocytosis.[48] The shortened red cell survival may or may not be associated with haemolytic anaemia and is found in established liver disease, usually alcoholic in origin. The spleen has an important role in contributing to the acanthocytosis, shortened survival and haemolytic anaemia.[51] Passage of red cells with a rigid membrane through the filtering system of the spleen leads in time to the development of spiculation and finally destruction by the spleen. Acanthocytosis is irreversible since affected red cells taken from a patient with liver disease continue to have a shortened survival when transfused into normal subjects.[50,227]

White cell abnormalities

Several leucocyte alterations have been described in patients with cirrhosis of the liver,[9] ranging from neutrophilia to neutropenia and lymphopenia. The white count is usually normal but neutropenia is not uncommon. Hypersplenism is one obvious contributing factor, but the degree of splenomegaly and neutropenia do not necessarily correlate. Impaired production has been suggested as a reason, but a review of the bone marrow appearance in cirrhosis does not support this.

Leucocytosis as a response to infection, blood loss, haemolysis and malignant infiltration may occur when these complications arise in patients with liver disease. The specific changes associated with acute viral hepatitis and alcoholic liver disease will be described later in this chapter.

Platelet abnormalities

Moderate thrombocytopenia is a common accompaniment of established liver disease.[61,75] Severe thrombocytopenia is unusual in uncomplicated cirrhosis, the platelet count usually being above the level associated with spontaneous bleeding (more than $30 \times 10^9/l$). There are many reasons for thrombocytopenia in patients with liver disease, but commonly it is secondary to splenomegaly and portal hypertension.[4] Under normal conditions approximately one-third of the circulating platelets are within the spleen, and splenomegaly, whatever its aetiology, can result in thrombocytopenia, although the total platelet mass may not be reduced.[4] The platelet half-life is moderately shortened in patients with chronic liver disease, usually alcoholic in aetiology.[247]

The degree of thrombocytopenia does not appear to correlate with the life span, splenic platelet pool or spleen size.[247] Megakaryocytes are present in normal numbers in the bone marrow[9] and it is not clear why increased platelet production cannot achieve normal blood levels. It is possible that because the *total* circulating platelet mass is maintained there is no increased stimulus to thrombocytopoiesis. Portacaval shunt[101] and splenectomy[171,236] will improve the thrombocytopenia in a proportion of patients.

Alcohol is another important cause of thrombocytopenia in liver disease and is associated with impaired megakaryocyte response and shortened platelet survival.[55] Other causes include acute severe blood loss, especially when treated by massive blood transfusion with stored blood, and increased consumption secondary to disseminated intravascular coagulation. Rarer causes of thrombocytopenia are acute viral hepatitis[133] and folate deficiency, when an associated megaloblastic anaemia and leucopenia may be present. In primary biliary cirrhosis, raised platelet-associated IgG was noted in patients with thrombocytopenia, suggesting immune-mediated platelet destruction.[6]

Abnormal platelet function may occur in liver disease and is characterized by impaired platelet aggregation associated with the presence of fibrinogen degradation products (FDPs) or fibrin monomer complexes and other evidence of intravascular coagulation.[5,243] Platelet membrane glycoprotein I is reduced.[193] Abnormal platelet aggregation is common in alcoholics even when liver function is normal. Defective production of thromboxane, a potent platelet aggregant has been demonstrated in patients with fatty infiltration of the liver.[114]

The bleeding time (BT), a useful test of platelet function, may be prolonged in patients with cirrhosis. The mechanism is not clear; thrombocytopenia is common in cirrhosis but there is no direct correlation with the platelet count. The synthetic vasopressin derivative desmopressin (DDAVP) which corrects the BT in von Willebrands disease and other disorders of platelet function,[142] shortens the long BT in patients with cirrhosis.[30,176] The mechanism is not known; baseline factor VIII-related

activities and their response to DDAVP are normal in cirrhotic patients. DDAVP shortens the long activated partial thromboplastin time but not the prothrombin time and the clinical benefit of DDAVP in liver disease needs to be assessed in controlled studies.

Anaemia in liver disease

While inevitably there will be case selection, surveys of the frequency of anaemia in chronic liver disease indicate that just over one-third of patients with biopsy-documented disease will be anaemic.[60,126,141,146] The anaemia is commonly normochromic, normocytic or macrocytic; a microcytic picture would suggest associated blood loss and resultant iron deficiency or, rarely, a sideroblastic anaemia. Under certain circumstances such as blood loss, acute haemolysis and folic acid deficiency, the anaemia may be marked but it is usually of moderate severity and does not correlate with the degree of hepatocellular failure.

Table 8.2 Anaemia in liver disease

Macrocytic
Normoblastic or macronormoblastic
Megaloblastic
Haemolytic
Anaemia due to altered iron metabolism
Iron deficiency
Sideroblastic
Impaired iron utilization
Dilutional anaemia and hypersplenism

Table 8.2 lists the various types of anaemia found in liver disease whatever the underlying pathology. Rarely, aplastic anaemia occurs in acute viral hepatitis but is not found in chronic liver disease.

Macrocytic anaemia

Macrocytosis is reported in up to 65% of patients with various types of liver disease but, in the majority, erythropoiesis is macronormoblastic and the haemoglobin is maintained. The macrocytosis of cirrhosis and obstructive jaundice is not corrected by folic acid or vitamin B_{12}, but may resolve with improved liver function. Disturbances of folate metabolism causing a true megaloblastic anaemia are much less common and are usually due to alcohol excess and associated nutritional deficiency; vitamin B_{12} deficiency is very rarely a factor in the anaemia of liver disease.

Abnormalities of folic acid and vitamin B_{12} metabolism Complex disturbances of folate metabolism are described in liver disease associated with alcohol (see Chapter 34). There is little evidence that these are important in liver disease due to other causes. Poor dietary intake can lead to low serum folate levels within 3–4 weeks[110] and must always be considered as a factor

Table 8.3 Incidence of megaloblastic anaemia in liver disease

Reference	Number of patients studied	Megaloblastic anaemia	
Jarrold and Vilter[126]	30	20	
Krasnow et al.[146]	350	22	
Klipstein and Lindenbaum[141]	40	4	11.8%
Deller et al.[60]	46	9	

Table 8.4 Haemolytic syndromes in liver disease

Acute viral hepatitis
  Autoimmune
Chronic liver disease
  Hyperlipidaemia
  Hypersplenism
  'Spur cell' anaemia
  Autoimmune

contributing to anaemia in patients with systemic illness, whatever its cause. Low serum folate levels have been reported in approximately 50% of patients with liver disease but mostly in the alcoholic.[60,111,141] However, the serum folate is a very sensitive index of folate deficiency; low red cell folate levels, which have also been reported, [120] are a better index of significant deficiency. Hepatic folate has been measured in a variety of disorders, including alcoholism, where it is commonly reduced and correlates well with the serum folate level.[155]

Disturbances of vitamin B_{12} metabolism are usually of a minor nature. Reduced liver stores are found in patients with a variety of liver disorders,[129] but serum levels are usually normal or even raised, particularly in patients with hepatocellular damage.[60,141,212] Presumably this is associated with depletion of hepatic stores. In an acute self-limiting disease, such as viral hepatitis, a rapid return to normal serum vitamin B_{12} levels occurs with recovery.[195]

Clinical features Anaemia is a late development in cirrhosis and is not uncommon; true megaloblastic anaemia is rare (Table 8.3). In one prospective study of 350 patients with cirrhosis, the bone marrow was examined in 96 patients with moderately severe anaemia and was megaloblastic in only seven (2% of the total).[146] The erythroid hyperplasia and macronormoblastic picture commonly seen[190] is found in the absence of bleeding and is related to the shortened red cell life. Chronic alcoholism and dietary deficiency are the major causes of folate deficiency, and folic acid is the haematinic of choice for megaloblastic anaemia in these patients. Treatment with vitamin B_{12} is not indicated. The diet of alcoholics who develop megaloblastic anaemia may not be obviously different from the diet of those who do not,[125] and other factors, such as an increased requirement for folic acid because of haemolysis, must be important.

Haemolytic anaemias

Many of the features of haemolysis, e.g. raised serum bilirubin, reduced or absent haptoglobins and shortened red cell survival, are found in liver disease per se without associated anaemia, and their significance in the presence of anaemia may be difficult to evaluate.

Laboratory findings A moderate reticulocytosis is a common finding in patients with chronic liver disease.[126] Macrocytes, target cells and acanthocytes due to the altered membrane lipids may be noted, but in most patients these findings will not be associated with overt haemolytic anaemia. Spherocytosis and a leucoerythroblastic picture have been described when florid haemolytic anaemia develops.[273]

The bone marrow will show increased cellularity and normoblastic or macronormoblastic maturation, indicating that increased haemopoiesis is required to maintain the haemoglobin concentration at near normal levels.[273]

Increased osmotic resistance to saline is a feature of red cells with an increased surface area such as target cells. A mild to moderate shortening of red cell survival is often present in patients with liver disease because of increased membrane lipid and rigidity of the red cell.[203, 235] Increased red cell destruction has been demonstrated using radioactive chromium, and increased splenic radioactivity suggests that the spleen is the site of destruction.[235] The degree to which this occurs is in part related to the spleen size[124,139] and the role of the spleen in potentiating red cell destruction has been emphasized.[51] However, variable splenic uptake of radioisotopes and the failure of splenectomy to improve the condition indicates that other factors are involved and reticuloendothelial hyperplasia elsewhere has been suggested.

Clinical features Low-grade haemolysis is frequently present in acute and chronic liver disease but anaemia is not common because of increased, compensatory erythropoiesis. It is difficult to estimate the frequency of anaemia in patients with liver disease from available reports because of case selection. Factors such as the severity and chronicity of the liver disease, its underlying aetiology, alcohol intake, hyperlipaemia and the degree of splenic enlargement may all play some part in determining the severity of anaemia.

There would appear to be several distinct haemolytic syndromes associated with chronic liver disease (Table 8.4). Self-limiting haemolysis accompanied by hyperlipidaemia and low-grade fever, usually precipitated by alcoholic excess, is known as Zieve's syndrome.[272] The patients are not acutely ill, hepatomegaly is due to fatty infiltration and spontaneous recovery usually occurs. Zieve[273] distinguished this syndrome from the condition in which patients had a significantly enlarged spleen, a much longer history of illness, and advanced liver disease and severe cirrhosis on biopsy. Haematologically there was little difference between the two groups except that haemolysis was characteristically brief in the hyperlipidaemic patients, and a low platelet and white count were seen in the patients with hypersplenism. No evidence of an autoimmune process was found in either group.

The mechanisms underlying Zieve's syndrome may be related to alcohol-induced vitamin E deficiency.[91] This, together with altered membrane lipid composition, leads to pyruvate kinase instability resulting in acute haemolysis. Such a mechanism would be similar to that described in favism, where exposure to fava beans precipitates haemolysis in patients with glucose-6-phosphate dehydrogenase deficiency, an inherited metabolic error, and fits with the reports of acute viral hepatitis precipitating haemolysis in patients with this defect.[39,41] Vitamin E deficiency has also been associated with a mild chronic haemolytic anaemia and increased red cell sensitivity to hydrogen peroxide lysis in a group of children with severe chronic liver disease.[74] The red cell membrane phospholipid content and the cholesterol phospholipid ratio were similar in replete and deficient children and the underlying mechanism of the vitamin E-associated abnormality is not known.

'Spur cell' anaemia, an acute haemolytic anaemia associated with acanthocytosis, is usually found in patients with advanced alcoholic cirrhosis and a poor prognosis, although there have been a few reports in non-alcoholic liver disease.[162] The evidence suggests that the defect is due to the large amount of cholesterol in the red cell membrane and is acquired by normal red cells on contact with the plasma of patients with acanthocytosis. The shortened survival of the acanthocytes persists after transfusion into normal recipients.[48,227]

Cooper and colleagues showed that absence of the spleen allows normal red cell survival[51] and it was suggested that the production of 'spur cell' anaemia took place in two stages. Within 12–24 h of contact and acquisition of cholesterol the red cell developed irregular spicules. Subsequently over a period of days, in the presence of an intact spleen, there was a progressive loss of red cell membrane and the deformity increased, the red cell being finally destroyed in the spleen. Splenectomy may be helpful in patients with severe haemolysis, but clearly the indications for this must be critically assessed as these patients will often have established liver disease.

A Coombs-positive autoimmune haemolytic anaemia is occasionally described in chronic liver disease, particularly in chronic active hepatitis.[201] The antibody, when it has been characterized, has usually been of the IgG type with Rh specificity, but other specificities have been reported.[161]

As is apparent from the above discussion, there is considerable overlap between the haemolytic syndromes described in liver disease. Indeed, the concept that these are distinct from each other with specific pathogenic mechanisms has been challenged.[162] The practical point of making such a distinction would appear to lie in assessing the prognostic implication of the haemolytic episodes. Treatment has little to offer in this situation;

alcohol withdrawal and general measures directed at improving the underlying liver disease will obviously be attempted. The rare autoimmune haemolytic anaemia may respond to corticosteroids and a short course at a high dose (60 mg prednisolone for an initial period of two weeks) is worth trying.

Anaemia due to altered iron metabolism

Many of the abnormalities of iron metabolism associated with liver disease are secondary to other factors such as associated blood loss or alcoholism. In established liver disease uncomplicated by blood loss, the serum iron is usually normal or raised,[37] the iron-binding capacity (transferrin) normal or low, and the transferrin saturation increased. In acute liver damage the serum iron and ferritin levels are raised,[206] possibly because of release from liver cells.

Increased iron absorption is documented in patients with cirrhosis.[46,267] The mechanism is poorly understood. Several possibilities have been suggested, including chronic pancreatitis, a direct effect of alcohol on iron absorption and iron overloading as a consequence of defective erythropoiesis or haemolysis.

Iron-deficiency anaemia   The frequency with which signs of iron deficiency (hypochromic anaemia, low serum iron and ferritin, high transferrin and reduced saturation) are seen in patients with chronic liver disease varies. In chronic liver disease uncomplicated by gastrointestinal haemorrhage or bleeding diathesis, iron deficiency is not common. The presence of an iron-deficiency anaemia should alert the physician to the likelihood of chronic blood loss, which is frequent in advanced liver disease.[139, 225]

Sideroblastic anaemia   Sideroblastic anaemia is an uncommon complication of liver disease and is usually due to alcohol. Severe dietary deficiency may alter the picture, but impaired iron utilization is evident with a rise in serum iron, transferrin saturation and increased iron in the bone marrow erythroblasts and reticuloendothelial cells.[66,117]

The basic defect which leads to the development of sideroblasts would appear to be in haem synthesis. An interference in the production of pyridoxal phosphate, a cofactor of δ-aminolaevulinic acid synthetase, a mitochondrial enzyme essential for haem production, has been implicated in some cases. As a result of the failure to produce haem, iron accumulates in the red cell where it may lie randomly in the cytoplasm, forming a pathological sideroblast, or in the mitochondria encircling the nucleus, forming a 'ring' sideroblast. On electron microscopy the mitochondria in alcohol-induced sideroblasts are swollen and deformed.[119] Large numbers of ring sideroblasts are found in the bone marrow of chronic alcoholics, but the defect may be reversed by abstinence from alcohol or intravenous administration of pyridoxal phosphate.[118]

The association of iron overload and alcoholism has led

to controversy regarding the role of alcohol in the aetiology of haemochromatosis.[170] This complex problem is discussed in Chapter 36.

Anaemia due to chronic disease

Chronic disorders such as chronic infection and collagen disease can result in 'the anaemia of chronic disease' and this may also be a cause of anaemia in chronic liver disease. The blood picture is usually of a normochromic normocytic moderate anaemia but it may be hypochromic microcytic and difficult to distinguish from iron deficiency. The serum iron is low but, unlike the situation in iron deficiency, the ferritin is normal and transferrin levels are reduced. Bone marrow examination shows some degree of failure. The defining feature is increased reticuloendothelial iron and reduced iron in the developing red cells, the so-called 'RE block' of chronic disease,[167] which is probably due to the defective release of iron from cells, particularly macrophages. Two possible mechanisms for this have been suggested: liberation of lactoferrin and induction of apoferritin synthesis.[153]

The anaemia is usually moderate and the clinical picture is dominated by the underlying disease process. The treatment is control of the underlying disease. Iron therapy should not be given and blood transfusion is not indicated in most cases since there is no evidence that patients benefit from a higher haemoglobin concentration.

Dilutional anaemia and hypersplenism

The anaemia of chronic liver failure is often complicated by portal hypertension and hypersplenism, and the increased plasma volume associated with splenomegaly may give a false impression of the degree of anaemia present. In a study of patients with chronic liver disease, true anaemia, as defined by a fall in the circulating red cell mass, was present in 40% but an apparent anaemia, as defined by a fall in the venous haematocrit, was noted in an additional 30%.[225] Lieberman and Reynolds[159] showed that an increase in the plasma volume was an important factor contributing to the low haemoglobin in a large number of patients with cirrhosis. Thus, as in the anaemia of pregnancy, haemodilution contributes to the anaemia of cirrhosis. The pathogenesis of the increased plasma volume is not clear but it must be partly due to portal hypertension.

The shortened red cell survival in this condition correlates with the splenomegaly. When the red cell shape is abnormal, prolonged trapping in the spleen may cause significant anaemia.

The leucopenia associated with hypersplenism is mainly due to neutropenia, which may be quite severe.[251] While there is some correlation between splenic size and resultant pancytopenia, this is not necessarily predictable and the degree of neutropenia and thrombocytopenia is not always related to the spleen size.

Correction of the portal hypertension by portacaval shunt may reduce the increased plasma volume but it does not usually return to normal.[159] The haematological

abnormalities show some improvement in approximately one-third of cases.[171] Splenectomy may succeed in correcting severe pancytopenia and could be combined with a portacaval shunt under certain circumstances.

THE HAEMATOLOGY OF SPECIFIC LIVER DISORDERS

The features associated with particular liver disorders are listed in Table 8.5.

Table 8.5 Liver disorders with specific haematological features

Acute viral hepatitis
Alcoholic liver disease
Non-alcoholic cirrhosis
Hepatocellular carcinoma
Hepatic vein thrombosis
Liver transplantation

Acute viral hepatitis

Significant anaemia is a rare complication of acute viral hepatitis; leucocyte and platelet abnormalities are noted much more frequently. Mild transient anaemia is not uncommon,[47,76] but occasionally the anaemia is severe and is usually either haemolytic or hypoplastic.[140]

Abnormalities in the peripheral blood are common. Macrocytosis is often present by the time jaundice is clinically evident and persists until recovery. Leucopenia develops before the onset of jaundice,[107] but by the seventh to fourteenth day the white count returns to normal. Initially there is both a lymphopenia and neutropenia, but by the second week there is often a lymphocytosis.[47] Atypical mononuclear cells seen during the first week are of the type commonly seen in viral infections. Features of these cells, referred to as 'virocytes', include cytoplasmic vacuolation, basophilic cytoplasm and large irregular nucleus occasionally containing nucleoli.[168] The platelet count is usually normal or even raised, but transient thrombocytopenia has been reported. The erythrocyte sedimentation rate (ESR) is variable in the early stages of infective hepatitis,[185,253] but by the time the disease is well established the ESR will be moderately elevated in the majority of patients, particularly in HBsAg-negative infections.[253] Raised serum levels of vitamin B_{12} have been reported.[208]

Haemolytic anaemia is an uncommon complication of acute viral hepatitis and the frequency is difficult to estimate.[57] Most reports are of small numbers but in one large series of 1200 patients 2% developed this complication.[79] The Coombs direct antiglobulin test is positive in some cases, and red cell antibodies may be demonstrated. A moderate shortening of the red cell survival is reported but the fragility is normal and a mild reticulocytosis occurs.[47] It usually presents a few weeks after the onset of viral hepatitis, is self-limiting and rarely of clinical significance. Patients with glucose-6-phosphate dehydrogenase deficiency run an increased risk of developing this complication.[39] No treatment is necessary, although the use of steroids may be considered if the anaemia is severe. The pathogenesis is unknown, but extrinsic factors such as lytic enzymes released from damaged liver cells, a direct haemolytic effect of the causative virus, incomplete cold agglutinins, and other autoimmune reactions have all been considered.

Prolonged hyperbilirubinaemia following acute viral hepatitis is described and was thought to be in part caused by haemolysis. There is no real evidence to support this and it is possible that impaired hepatocellular function or slow resolution of the hepatitis is the cause.[45]

Aplastic anaemia is a rare and serious complication of viral hepatitis and is associated with a high mortality. Four in a series of over 5000 Greek children hospitalized for viral hepatitis had aplastic anaemia, giving an incidence of 0.07%.[202] The incidence is higher in hepatitis-prevalent countries such as Taiwan where there is a high annual incidence of aplastic anaemia (10 per million children) one quarter of which are thought to be post-hepatitic.[158]

Serologic studies of hepatitis-associated aplastic anaemia have failed to identify the causative agent and it has been presumed that the hepatitis C virus (HCV) is a significant cause. An overall prevalence of anti-HCV positivity of 10.2% was found in a recent French study of 118 patients with severe aplastic anaemia. However, there was no significant difference in the HCV antibody rate in the hepatitis-associated cases (15.8%) and the rest where the aetiology was either known (7.9%) or unknown (9.8%).[204] This could reflect the presence of subclinical hepatitis in the 'non-hepatitic' cases and further study is needed to establish the role of the HCV in post-hepatitic aplastic anaemia.

The underlying mechanisms are poorly understood; in many reported cases the hepatitis was improving or had resolved when striking pancytopenia developed.[103] Failure of the liver to detoxicate intermediary metabolites or drugs, direct viral-induced bone marrow damage, virally initiated autoimmune mechanisms, and individual susceptibility have all been considered. Lymphopaenia and altered helper (CD4) and suppressor (CD8) lymphocyte percentages and ratios have been reported in post-hepatitic aplastic anaemia.[144] These changes were not seen in non-A non-B hepatitis without aplasia and so may be of pathogenetic relevance. The leucopenia which is an early feature in the course of hepatitis suggests that temporary bone marrow depression can occur and transient pancytopenia must be more common than the full-blown aplasia. Transient red cell aplasia has also been reported.[222]

In a review of 195 patients with aplastic anaemia following viral hepatitis,[103] a slightly higher incidence in males was noted and females had a worse prognosis; only 8.5% survived compared with an overall survival for the group of approximately 15%. No other factor of prognostic significance was determined. Eighteen per cent of the patients had been exposed to chloramphenicol. The mean interval between the onset of hepatitis and pancytopenia was 9.3 weeks and the survival time after pancytopenia was 11.3 weeks. The longest interval between the onset of hepatitis and death was 78 weeks.

Bone marrow transplantation for aplastic anaemia associated with viral hepatitis has been performed;[245] with improving techniques this measure would appear to offer the best chance of cure in this frequently fatal condition.

Alcoholic liver disease

Excessive intake of alcohol will have a direct toxic effect on blood and bone marrow and will result in metabolic disturbances and consequent haemopoietic abnormalities (Table 8.6). Several reviews describe these in detail.[36,164] Red cell, white cell and platelet production may all be affected. Provided caloric and vitamin intake is maintained, the haematological sequelae of alcoholism are usually not marked,[166] the major effect being mediated through associated factors such as impaired nutrition, vitamin deficiency and altered liver function.

Metabolic disturbances.

The extent to which the haemopoietic abnormalities reported in alcoholic liver disease are due to direct toxicity of alcohol or to associated nutritional deficiency is debatable. Both mechanisms appear to operate; in addition to poor diet and increased requirements for folate, alcoholism leads to folate deficiency by interfering with folate metabolism and intestinal absorption. Megaloblastic anaemia is rare in well-nourished alcoholics taking a reasonable diet, and there is a clear correlation between decreased dietary folate and megaloblastic anaemia. The folate content of alcohol is another important

Table 8.6 Blood findings in alcoholism

Peripheral blood
Red cells
   Macrocytosis
   Stomatocytosis
   Target cells
   Acanthocytosis
White cells
   Neutropenia
   Altered granulocyte function
Platelets
   Thrombocytopenia
   Altered platelet function

Bone marrow
Vacuolation of precursors
Variable cellularity
Secondary changes due to
   Folate deficiency
   Haemolysis
   Iron overload with sideroblastosis.
   Iron deficiency
Impaired megakaryocytopoiesis

factor: megaloblastic anaemia is seen more commonly in drinkers of spirits and wine, which have little or no folate, compared with drinkers of beer, which has a higher folate content.[164]

A direct effect of alcohol on haemopoiesis and folate metabolism was shown in a carefully executed study by Sullivan and Herbert[237] in three subjects with megaloblastic anaemia taking alcohol and maintained on a folate-deficient diet. Removal of alcohol was associated with reticulocytosis, a fall in serum iron and a return to normoblastic erythropoiesis; resumption of alcohol had the opposite effect. A greater dose of folate than is usual was needed to correct the megaloblastic anaemia as long as alcohol intake continued; erythropoiesis and white cell and platelet production were all depressed. Malabsorption due to a direct effect of ethanol on the gut mucosa may be important. In one study[105] ten days of heavy alcohol intake caused decreased absorption of labelled folic acid, and continued alcohol consumption led to steatorrhoea in 60%, impaired D-xylose excretion in 76% and abnormal vitamin B_{12} absorption in 53% of patients. Folate deficiency per se can cause impairment of small-bowel function and it is likely that alcohol excess and folate deficiency act synergistically to depress this further.[164] Increased loss of folate in the urine and faeces[241] is another significant factor leading to folate deficiency in chronic alcoholism. This evidence suggests that alcohol only interferes with folate absorption when folate deficiency is already present.

The metabolic block induced by alcohol is complex and is dealt with in detail in Chapter 34. There have been several reviews[112,116,261] and alcohol has been reported to affect folate metabolism in many ways. Inhibition of the liver enzyme tetrahydrofolate formylase, thus preventing incorporation of ^{14}C-labelled formate into DNA, by large doses of alcohol has been reported.[11] In addition, alcohol may block the release of N-5-methyltetrahydrofolic acid from storage pools, causing deficiency in the bone marrow.[150] An enterohepatic folate circulation which is influenced by body serum and hepatic folate levels may be important but the means whereby alcohol affects this process is still not clear. Weir and colleagues believe that current evidence does not support the claim that alcohol blocks excretion of hepatic folate into bile to a significant extent.[261]

Alcohol is known to result in significant abnormalities of iron-metabolism (see Chapter 36). Severe blood loss or, rarely, dietary deficiency may alter the picture but usually there is an increase in reticuloendothelial iron stores and ring sideroblasts in the bone marrow, a raised serum iron, and an increased transferrin saturation. Withdrawal of alcohol rapidly reverses these abnormalities and this suggests that alcohol has a direct toxic effect. A metabolic block in the conversion of pyridoxine to pyridoxal phosphate[118] is suggested by low pyridoxine phosphate serum levels and reversal of the sideroblastic changes by pyridoxal phosphate, whereas intravenous pyridoxine did not have the same effect. The picture is obviously complex; pyridoxine supplements as well as an adequate diet can prevent the sideroblastic change[166] and altered folate metabolism may be a necessary prerequisite.[66]

Laboratory findings

Macrocytosis is the commonest morphological change seen in the peripheral blood of patients with alcoholic liver disease, being reported in 70–90% of chronic alcoholics.[187,269] It is suggested that macrocytosis should alert the clinician to the possibility of alcohol abuse,[268] particularly mean corpuscular volume (MCV) values greater than 100 fl. There is usually no associated anaemia or neutrophil hypersegmentation. The MCV is moderately raised with Coulter 'S' values of 97–105 fl. Most patients have normal folate levels[269] and the macrocytosis disappears slowly in alcohol withdrawal, taking 1–4 months;[164] folate supplementation will not correct the macrocytosis if alcohol abuse continues. The pathogenesis is not clearly established, but a direct toxic effect and red cell membrane changes resulting from altered phospholipid fatty acid composition[42] are both implicated.

Macrocytosis is also a feature of aplastic and other dyserythropoietic anaemias; it is thus likely that the macrocytosis of alcoholism could be due in part to the toxic effect of alcohol on erythropoiesis.

The bone marrow changes noted in acute alcoholism are quite striking and occur frequently.[179] The overall cellularity of the marrow may be reduced, although the bone marrow usually shows normal or increased cellularity with the development of cirrhosis.[139] There is vacuolation of the erythroid precursors and, to a lesser extent, myeloid precursors, which rapidly disappears after alcohol withdrawal. The chemical nature of the vacuoles has not been elucidated by cytochemical techniques[166] and under the electron microscope they are seen to be formed by a process of red cell membrane invagination,[270] suggesting a direct toxic effect of alcohol on the cells. This is confirmed by the observation that both alcohol and its metabolite acetaldehyde inhibit the proliferation of haemopoietic progenitor cells in a reversible fashion, with erythroid precursors being particularly sensitive even at low concentrations.[182]

Eichner and Hillman[66] studied 65 patients with chronic alcoholism and concluded that the bone marrow changes and development of anaemia takes place in a predictable fashion. Initially, reduced dietary intake and excessive alcohol leads to a negative vitamin balance characterized by a marked drop in the serum folate level, a finding noted in 80% of alcoholics with cirrhosis. After 1–3 weeks of continued folate deficiency,[111] the red cell folate falls and erythropoiesis becomes megaloblastic; soon after this, sideroblastic changes occur.[166] This effect may be prevented by small doses of pyridoxine. Adequate iron stores are essential for the development of this picture. Recovery rapidly takes place with a normal diet or abstinence from alcohol and erythropoiesis will become normoblastic, vacuolation will disappear and marrow iron stores will decrease. Five to ten days after stopping alcohol the bone marrow will show erythroid hyperplasia and the reticulocyte count will be high. The picture at this stage is indistinguishable from a haemolytic anaemia and if lipaemia is noted an erroneous diagnosis of Zieve's syndrome may be made. Folic acid is the haematinic of choice and will correct the megaloblastic picture.

Haemolytic anaemia and the distinct haemolytic syndromes, i.e. Zieve's syndrome, 'spur cell' anaemia and chronic haemolytic anaemia, have been discussed previously.

Stomatocytosis is a transient phenomenon associated with acute alcoholism in approximately one-quarter of patients in one study.[62] This is occasionally associated with haemolysis but there is no direct correlation between the degree of stomatocytosis and the occurrence of haemolysis.[162] Target cells are not usually described in alcoholism, their presence suggesting obstructive jaundice and established cirrhosis. Acanthocytosis may be present when acute haemolytic anaemia complicates alcoholic liver disease. While there is good evidence that increased cholesterol and altered membrane lipids are important in the development of these abnormalities, the exact pathogenesis of these changes is not understood.

Other causes of anaemia such as iron deficiency due to gastrointestinal blood loss, hypersplenism and dilutional anaemia have all been described in patients with chronic alcoholic liver disease.[162]

The effect of alcohol on the white cell series is less well described. Vacuolation of the white cell precursors in the bone marrow and of the mature cells in the peripheral blood[127] and neutropenia,[169] together with an impaired leucocyte response to infections,[180] have been reported. Patients with alcoholic liver disease may have increased susceptibility to infection and, although simple depression of the cough reflex by alcoholic intoxication may explain the frequency of pneumonia,[8] an impaired granulocyte response to acute bacterial infection has been demonstrated.[38,180] The reason for this is not clear; neutropenia is uncommon and, if present, is usually mild,[67,169] and other factors such as defective reticuloendothelial clearance of organisms,[249] a direct toxic effect of alcohol on granulocyte mobilization[28] and defective cellular immunity[7] have all been suggested. Lymphocyte abnormalities described include a reduced count that usually accompanies the neutropenia and recovers on alcohol withdrawal, a reduction in T cell number, and impaired lymphocyte transformation.[36]

A direct toxic effect on the marrow has also been suggested as a cause of the thrombocytopenia noted in acute alcoholism. Heavy alcohol intake for only 6 days will impair megakaryocytopoiesis and the accelerated platelet production usually seen after induced thrombocytopenia.[238] Long-standing alcohol intake will cause thrombocytopenia in most patients, counts between 50 and 100 × 10⁹/l being common,[56] and indeed Cowan and Hines[56] have suggested that alcoholism is the commonest cause of thrombocytopenia in the United States. Reduced

platelet survival may be a contributory factor. On resuming a normal diet with alcohol abstinence, the platelet count rises within 2–3 days, daily increases being of the order of 20 to 30 × 10⁹/l. Failure of the thrombocytopenia to respond within a week of alcohol withdrawal should suggest some other underlying mechanism. Rebound thrombocytosis is well described.[165] Impaired platelet aggregation is a common finding in alcoholics and, when associated with fatty infiltration of the liver, the bleeding time is prolonged and blood thromboxane capacity is diminished.[114] These findings do not correlate directly with ethanol ingestion.

The anaemia associated with long-standing alcoholism and cirrhosis is multifactorial; alcohol withdrawal, treatment with folic acid, control of the associated coagulation abnormalities and bleeding problems are obvious therapeutic measures which may result in haematological improvement and amelioration of the patient's general condition. The final factor determining the outcome will be the degree of hepatocellular failure.

Non-alcoholic cirrhosis

Most clinical and experimental studies of anaemia in patients with chronic liver disease have included a large number of alcoholic patients. While the pathogenesis of the haematological abnormalities in alcoholic and non-alcoholic cirrhosis must be similar to some extent, since haemolysis, hypersplenism, blood loss and the disturbances associated with chronic disease are present in both conditions, there are differences, although none are specific. Nevertheless, application of a quadratic multiple discriminant analysis of 25 commonly ordered laboratory tests resulted in the differentiation of alcoholic from non-alcoholic liver disease with 100% accuracy.[217] Standard liver tests did not materially affect this discrimination. The haematological parameters used were the haemoglobin, the haematocrit, white blood cell and red blood cell counts, the mean corpuscular haemoglobin concentration, the mean corpuscular haemoglobin, and the mean corpuscular volume, the latter being clearly abnormal (mean of 102.6 fl) in alcoholic liver disease.

The metabolic and nutritional consequences of alcoholism are lacking, and folic acid deficiency and megaloblastic anaemia are rarely seen in non-alcoholic liver disease.[140,141] The striking sideroblastic change noted in chronic alcoholics is similarly much less evident in non-alcoholic cirrhosis, although it has been described.[119]

Although target cells are described in alcoholic patients, they are usually associated with cholestasis and characteristically are most striking in obstructive jaundice. As mentioned previously, target cells have an increased osmotic resistance but a normal survival, and, provided liver function is normal, are not associated with anaemia.[52] Their significance lies in drawing attention to the possibility of liver disease. Another interesting feature noted in about one-third of a small group of patients with chronic active hepatitis was a moderate eosinophilia.[266]

Increased plasma cells have been reported in the bone marrow of patients with cirrhosis and were proportional to the hypergammaglobulinaemia, a common finding in chronic liver disease.[126]

Autoimmune haemolytic anaemia is a rare complication in patients with chronic active hepatitis or primary biliary cirrhosis (PBC)[122,201] and excites interest because of the association of diseases of an autoimmune nature. Typically, the antibody is IgG in type and shows Rh specificity. Treatment with steroids may be successful in reducing haemolysis of this type. In non-immune haemolytic anaemia associated with PBC, the degree of liver dysfunction is an important factor in the production of the anaemia.[122]

Hepatocellular carcinoma

Erythrocytosis is a rare complication of hepatocellular carcinoma, although well recognized,[130,181,250] the frequency being between 5 and 10%. Most hepatocellular carcinomas are superimposed on pre-existing cirrhosis and, because there is often an increased plasma volume in this condition, the frequency of an absolute increase in red cell mass may be higher. It has been suggested that at haematocrit levels as low as 48% an increased red cell mass would invariably be present.[130] The clinical features of hepatocellular carcinoma are described in Chapter 42.

Splenomegaly, leucocytosis and thrombocytosis, features usually suggesting the diagnosis of polycythaemia vera, do not have the same significance in this situation. Splenomegaly may be present because of the pre-existing cirrhosis. Leucocytosis is reported in one-third of cases of hepatocellular carcinoma and is usually mild,[69] although a leukaemoid reaction has been described. An increased platelet count is unusual in the erythrocytosis complicating hepatocellular carcinoma. The oxygen saturation and blood pressure were normal in a small group of patients with this condition and raised plasma erythropoietin levels were noted in about half. Attempts to show that increased amounts of erythropoietin are generated by the liver tumour are not convincing[246] and although experimental studies in nephrectomized rats have suggested that the liver is an extrarenal source of erythropoietin, this is not proven.[84] Increased production by rapidly growing liver tissue of a substrate which is converted by an enzymatic renal factor to active erythropoietin has been proposed as one mechanism whereby erythrocytosis develops.[94] No substance with direct erythropoietin activity has been isolated from normal or neoplastic liver tissue.

The abnormal protein des-γ-carboxy prothrombin seems to be a useful marker of primary hepatocellular carcinoma.[160] Levels were high in 67% of 76 patients with this diagnosis and were low in patients with metastatic carcinoma and chronic active hepatitis. Taken together with alpha-fetoprotein levels, 84% of patients with hepatocellular carcinoma could be identified. The abnormal prothrombin was not corrected by vitamin K and disappeared with tumour resection, so it seems likely that it is

synthesized by tumour cells. Abnormal fibrinogen function (DF) has been described in association with hepatocellular carcinoma;[95] while not specific, it may also be of value in distinguishing primary from metastatic carcinoma of the liver.

Hepatic vein thrombosis

In most cases of hepatic vein thrombosis (Budd–Chiari syndrome) the aetiology is unknown. Reports of this disorder[254] and thrombosis of the portal vein[255] and other abdominal vessels complicating the myeloproliferative disorders have strongly supported their association. In 147 well-documented cases of hepatic vein thrombosis reviewed by Valla and colleagues,[254] overt polycythaemia was present in 61 patients. The incidence is not high in patients known to have a myeloproliferative disorder. In a study of 500 such patients 10% of patients with polycythaemia rubra vera, 13% with essential thrombocythaemia, 1% with idiopathic myelofibrosis and none of over 200 patients with chronic myeloid leukaemia developed hepatic vein thrombosis.[2] A causal relationship between a thrombotic event and haematological and coagulation abnormalities at the time of diagnosis was not established.[2] The condition is fatal in about one-third of cases and the majority of survivors will have late sequelae including liver cirrhosis.[254]

Recent advances in the diagnosis of myeloproliferative disorders suggest that evidence of the disorder at an early stage can be found in most patients developing hepatic vein thrombosis.[25] Findings include chromosomal abnormalities and altered bone marrow colony culture growth patterns.[199,254] Similar abnormalities have been found in patients with portal vein thrombosis.[255] The mechanism underlying the thrombosis remains unclear; vasculitis, complement-induced platelet activation, and paroxysmal nocturnal haemoglobinuria-like abnormalities have been described[25] but a direct role has not been established.

As the cause of hepatic vein thrombosis in the myeloproliferative disorders is not known, therapy and prophylaxis are empirical. Control of overt disease is clearly required and long-term anticoagulation for recurrent thrombosis is indicated. The management of patients with evidence of occult myeloproliferative disorders will depend on the clinical situation. Because of the risk of recurrent thrombosis, prophylactic anticoagulation in patients with the Budd–Chiari syndrome who have had a liver transplant seems advisable.[32]

Liver transplantation

Massive blood loss is a problem in orthotopic liver transplantation (OTL) despite advances in surgical technique and supportive measures. It carries with it a significant mortality and in 1218 liver transplants carried out in 32 European centres, 14% died of haemorrhage.[16] In a report from Pittsburgh of 70 first transplants,[22] three times as much blood was given to eight patients who died compared with the survivors and the use of FFP and platelets was also greater. In an attempt to define the patients likely to have haemorrhagic complications, a pre-operative coagulation abnormality score (CAS) based on the prothrombin time (PT), activated partial thromboplastin time (APTT), thrombin time, fibrinogen, platelet count, antithrombin III (ATIII), fibrinogen split products and euglobulin clot lysis time was devised. This correlated with intra-operative red cell usage and mortality and was most abnormal in patients with post-necrotic cirrhosis. Even with the exclusion of operative deaths there was a strong negative correlation between the CAS and survival at 6 months.[22] Other pre-transplantation parameters predictive of increased blood loss include a history of ascites, reduced urinary sodium and reduced plasma ATIII levels.[102] Portal hypertension was not thought to be a significant factor in this study as cholestasis did not affect blood loss, but contrary results have been reported.[31]

Three stages of OTL are described: stage 1 the pre-anhepatic phase when dissection and removal of the diseased liver is taking place; stage 2 the anhepatic stage; and stage 3 the post-anhepatic phase when the new liver is inserted and the restoration of portal blood flow occurs. The coagulation abnormalities in the three stages have been closely studied.[157,197,207]

Serious abnormalities in the coagulation and fibrinolytic systems are not usually present in the pre-anhepatic stage. The nature of the underlying liver disease is an important factor; post-necrotic cirrhosis, fulminant hepatic failure and alpha-1-antitrypsin deficiency are associated with significant reduction of coagulation factors.[207] In severe liver failure, marked derangement of the clotting factors occurs and is of prognostic importance; a PT of greater than 100 s[191] and a factor V level below 20% in comatose patients[10] being indications for liver transplantation.

In the anhepatic phase, early studies reported DIC and hyperfibrinolysis but modern carefully monitored support with blood and blood products prevents significant derangement of clotting factors in most cases.[207] Nevertheless, increased fibrinolytic activity and increased plasma tissue type plasminogen activator (tPA) have been demonstrated at the end of this stage and are associated with high intra-operative blood loss.[64,200] The lack of hepatic clearance of activated clotting factors is a likely major contributing factor to the coagulation disturbances at this stage.

The quality of the donor liver is important in restoring the haemostatic balance and improvements in graft preservation have reduced the bleeding complications in stage 3. The coagulation factors and platelets which had been falling steadily through the operation reached their nadir at this point. Activation of fibrinolysis in late stage 2 leads to destruction of coagulation factors in stage 3.[157] Minimal evidence of DIC was noted in the study and the ATIII levels did not change much throughout OTL. Factor VIII levels fell rapidly in the third stage, particularly when blood usage was high, presumably owing to inadequate replacement since blood and FFP are poor sources of factor VIII. A global test of coagulation and fibrinolysis, the thromboelastograph (TEG), correlated positively with the coagulation profile and was shown to be a rapid and reliable monitoring system in patients undergoing OTL.[131,197]

Once the operation is complete, the PT and APTT normalize rapidly and in 41 patients followed for the first 10 postoperative days the mean activities of all procoagulant factors were normal on day 1 except for factors V and VII, which normalized by day 3.[230] Supernormal levels of factor VIII were noted with peak values on day 5. In contrast, the anticoagulant proteins, ATIII, protein C and protein S, were reduced in many patients and thrombin/antithrombin complexes were elevated, denoting in vivo activation of coagulation. This imbalance between the forces driving and those inhibiting coagulation are consistent with a hypercoagulable stage.[106,230] Thrombotic complications such as hepatic artery thrombosis, although uncommon, are catastrophic and low-dose heparin infusion was used successfully in an uncontrolled study to prevent this occurring.[230] It was less successful in 3 of 14 children following OTL when the combination of heparin and ATIII infusions did not prevent portal vessel thrombosis. Here too a hypercoagulable state was present, reduced protein C, raised thrombin/antithrombin complexes and raised plasminogen activator inhibitor (PAI) levels being noted.[106] Protein C replacement could be useful in preventing these thrombotic complications.

In conclusion, although evidence of defective haemostasis is found in patients during OTL and in the postoperative period, in the majority this is not associated with a haemorrhagic or thrombotic tendency. Surgical difficulties, more likely following previous abdominal surgery, may be a significant factor leading to massive intra-operative blood loss. It is clearly important to define the small percentage of patients who may have life-threatening haemostatic complications but preoperative coagulation screening does not always allow an accurate prediction of subsequent blood usage.[214] There is no general agreement as to the value of a wide range of tests over and above the standard conventional tests, PT, APTT and platelet count. Currently such data are being pooled and the results may provide a firmer base for intra-operative monitoring and management.[21]

Red cells, FFP and platelet concentrates will be given as required to correct abnormalities and control bleeding. Cryoprecipitate is a good source of fibrinogen and factor VIII and may be useful in persistent haemostatic failure. The role of specific factor replacement, such as ATIII and protein C has not been defined but may have a place in severe haemostatic failure. Increased fibrinolysis is a consistent abnormality and has prompted the empirical use of fibrinolytic inhibitors such as ε-aminocaproic acid (EACA) and aprotinin (Trasylol).[274] The effect of EACA in vitro was assessed by the TEG[197]; in patients with increased fibrinolysis, low-dose EACA therapy corrected the severe fibrinolysis and was not associated with thrombotic complications.[132] The clinical significance of this is uncertain and controlled studies of fibrinolytic inhibitors, including aprotinin, which may prove to be a better drug, are necessary to determine their role in OTL.

The first successful liver transplantation carried out in 1985 in a haemophiliac with chronic active hepatitis cured his severe factor VIII deficiency.[156] Subsequent reports have confirmed the clinical cure of both haemophilia A[23] and haemophilia B (factor IX deficiency)[184] by liver transplantation.

COAGULATION DISTURBANCES ASSOCIATED WITH LIVER DISEASE

Effect on coagulation factors

Table 8.7 summarizes the coagulation abnormalities noted in liver disease.

Vitamin K-dependent factors

Deficiency of the vitamin K-dependent factors II, VII, IX and X causes abnormalities in both the extrinsic and intrinsic pathways, resulting in prolongation of the prothrombin time (PT) and the cephalin or activated partial thromboplastin time (APTT), respectively. Failure to synthesize these factors is an early consequence of liver disease; prolongation of the PT and APTT may be noted while other biochemical tests of liver function are still normal. Two additional tests which are sensitive to deficiency of these factors are: (a) the thrombotest, sensitive to the anticoagulant effect of precursor proteins induced by vitamin K absence (PIVKA); and (b) the normotest, which is not affected by PIVKA. These two tests may be used to try to distinguish between hepatocellular failure and vitamin K deficiency but in practice these tests are probably no more helpful than the PT alone.[257] The PT is considered the best screening test for coagulation defects in liver disease.[99,145] The APTT is usually also prolonged in liver disease; it occasionally may be abnormal when the PT is within the normal range.[61,154]

Assay of the individual factors has been carried out to see whether this is helpful in assessing the degree of liver damage, particularly in acute situations such as paracetamol (acetaminophen) poisoning and fulminant hepatitis. Factor VII has the shortest half-life (approximately 6 hours) and severe reduction (below 9%) was shown to carry a poor prognosis in a small group of patients with acute hepatic failure.[63] Significantly lower factor VII levels were noted in patients with decompensated liver cirrhosis who died within the next 6 weeks when compared with survivors; no difference was detected when factor VII was studied 2–4 months before death.[54]

The vitamin K-dependent factors may be reduced in patients with liver disease because of failed synthesis, but will also fall in obstructive jaundice because of impaired absorption of the fat-soluble vitamin K. Treatment with vitamin K can be used to distinguish the underlying

mechanism of a coagulation defect in patients with liver disease since this will not correct the coagulation abnormality of hepatocellular failure.[220,229] Not uncommonly, however, there may be a degree of obstruction superimposed on underlying hepatocellular failure and some improvement of the coagulation defect may result from vitamin K therapy. In addition, poor nutrition associated with severe liver disease may lead to vitamin K deficiency and here too response to vitamin K therapy may be observed.[73]

Activated protein C with its cofactor protein S is a major inhibitor of coagulation. Congenital deficiency leads to thromboembolic disease[100] with protean manifestations including portal vein thrombosis.[194] Reduced levels, roughly proportional to the degree of liver decompensation are reported in chronic liver disease,[174] acute hepatitis,[258] and fulminant hepatic failure.[151] The biologically active free protein S is also moderately reduced in liver disease.[58] The role of deficiency of these proteins in the haemorrhagic tendency in liver disease has not been established.

The abnormal prothrombin described by Liebman et al.[160] in vitamin K-deficient subjects and patients with hepatocellular carcinoma was noted in low concentration in the majority of patients with acute hepatitis and alcoholic cirrhosis. Small amounts of γ-carboxyglutamic acid-incomplete protein C in liver disease and high levels in hepatocellular carinoma have been reported.[271]

Fibrinogen

Significant fibrinogen deficiency will prolong the thrombin time, a useful screening test which is also sensitive to the presence of fibrin degradation products (FDPs) and an abnormal fibrinogen molecule. The reptilase time[86] is also prolonged in hypofibrinogenaemia and may be more sensitive to a qualitative abnormality of fibrinogen than the thrombin time. Quantitative methods such as that of Ratnoff and Menzie[211] are most accurate but are time consuming. Semiquantitative methods such as fibrin clot weight and fibrinogen titre are clinically useful, but are also sensitive to FDPs and fibrinolysis.[224] Most modern automated coagulometers estimate the fibrinogen concentration as part of the PT assessment. The results are accurate and useful in the investigation of patients with liver disease and DIC.

Fibrinogen is an 'acute-phase' reactive protein and is raised in response to a variety of stimuli, including infection, obstruction and neoplasms. Raised levels have been reported in obstructive jaundice[260] and following extensive liver resection. In mild to moderate liver disease, fibrinogen levels are normal.[61,252] Reduced fibrinogen levels have been described in fulminant hepatic failure[40] and following liver transplantation.[78] Increased fibrinogen turnover, as evidenced by a shortened ^{125}I-labelled fibrinogen half-life and corrected by an infusion of ATIII,[221] suggests that intravascular coagulation plays a role in these disturbances.

An abnormal fibrinogen molecule has been described

Table 8.7 A summary of the coagulation abnormalities in liver disease

Coagulation defect and laboratory diagnosis		Clinical significance
Vitamin K Dependent Factors		
(i) Reduction due to failure of hepatic synthesis	Prothrombin time prolonged; corrects in vitro with normal plasma. APTT less affected	An early sign of liver decompensation[98,145] Gross prolongation (ratio > 4.8,[63] PT > 100 s[191]) indicative of poor prognosis in fulminant hepatic failure Complete correction of PT by vitamin K noted in obstructive jaundice[220,229]
	Factors VII, IX, XI and II reduced	Marked reduction of factor VII a poor prognostic sign[54,63]
	Protein C[174,258,151] and protein S[58]	Role in bleeding and thrombosis not established
(ii) Qualitative abnormality	Abnormal prothrombin (PIVKA) detected by RIA, ELISA, etc.	Increased in liver cirrhosis Marked increase noted in hepatocellular carcinoma[160]
Fibrinogen		
(i) Quantitative abnormality	Usually within normal range (2–4 g/l) in mild/moderately severe liver disease[61,252]	(i) Increased (acute phase reactant protein) in infection, neoplasm, obstruction, jaundice[260] (ii) Low in fulminant hepatic failure[40] liver transplantation[78]
(ii) Qualitative abnormality	Dysfibrinogenaemia diagnosed by long thrombin time and reptilase time[86] and abnormal fibrin polymerization	Uncertain significance; noted in cirrhosis but not in obstructive jaundice, may be associated with bleeding[99]
Factor VIII	Raised level on functional and immunological assay (Normal range 50–150 iu/dl)	Levels raised in acute viral hepatitis,[183] cirrhosis[96,196] and fulminant hepatic failure[152] Higher antigen levels noted in obstructive jaundice[137]
Other factors		
Factor V – not Vitamin K dependent	Usually normal but may be reduced	Levels < 20% associated with poor prognosis in fulminant hepatic failure[10]
Contact factors (XI and XII)	May be reduced[210]	Not clinically significant
Factor XIII	Does not affect PT and APTT; diagnosed by screening test	Reduced in cirrhosis[173] but not in obstructive jaundice,[260] not clinically significant
Antithrombin III	May be reduced (normal range 80–120 iu/dl)	Low levels found in chronic liver disease and fulminant hepatic failure,[87] significance in thrombosis and bleeding uncertain
Fibrinolysis		
(i) Increased fibrinolytic activity	Short ECLT (normal 60–350 min) Low plasminogen[244] Increased tPA activity[113] Decreased tPA inhibitor activity[113] Reduced alpha-2-antiplasmin[178]	Increased in cirrhosis[77,83,147,209] after surgical resection of the liver,[259] liver transplantation[207,230] Contribution to bleeding diathesis not established; may be important in liver transplantation
(ii) Decreased fibrinolytic activity	Long ECLT > 350 min	Noted in acute hepatic failure,[40] obstructive jaundice[128]
Disseminated intravascular coagulation		
	Routine diagnostic criteria: Long PT, APTT, reduced fibrinogen low platelets, raised FDPs (> 100 ng/l) XDPs (> 6000 ng/l)	Laboratory evidence of DIC commonly found in liver disease[18] Clinically significant DIC rare[115]
	Research techniques: Increased fibrinogen breakdown[44,252] Increased fibrinopeptide A[43,186] Raised thrombin-antithrombin complexes[240] and alpha-2-antiplasmin complexes[240]	

in liver disease.[99,227] A simple colorimetric method using reptilase[99] demonstrated abnormalities of fibrin polymerization in 50% of patients with advanced liver disease. The part played by the dysfibrinogenaemia (DF) in the bleeding diathesis associated with severe liver disease is uncertain. In the patients studied by Green and colleagues[99] it appeared to be of prognostic significance; in 13 patients bleeding from oesophageal varices, most of those who died had an abnormal fibrinogen, whereas it was not detected in those who survived. Fibrin polymerization was normal in their patients with obstructive jaundice, suggesting that this test might help to differentiate obstructive jaundice from severe parenchymal liver disease. The nature of the abnormality is unknown; indeed, it has not yet been established that the defective fibrin monomer polymerization is due to a biochemically abnormal fibrinogen molecule. No molecular or structural defect in fibrinogen or derivative polypeptide chains was shown on examination of isolated fibrins on polyacrylamide gel electrophoresis.[149] Decreased D-galactose content of fibrinogen and an increase in sialic acid content[228] have been reported, and release from damaged liver cells of a precursor of fibrinogen has been suggested.[29] Comparison of the hepatocellular carcinoma-associated dysfibrinogen with the fibrinogen found in fetal plasma shows striking similarities[95] and both have been shown to have increased sialic acid content in the fibrinogen molecule. Reduction of the sialic acid content restored normal function to the tumour-associated fibrinogen, suggesting that these findings are related. Sialyl transferase, an enzyme capable of transferring sialic acid to a variety of asialo proteins and present in the liver, is increased in patients with liver disease and DF,[81] but also occurs in other conditions not associated with DF.[215] Experimental work in rats[82] suggests that DF in liver disease may be a manifestation of liver cell regeneration rather than liver cell damage. Further work, including serial studies in patients with acute liver injury, are needed to clarify this controversy.

Factor VIII

Factor VIII assays are of little help in clinically evaluating the coagulation defect in liver disease. Raised levels of both factor VIII and von Willebrand Factor (VWF) have been described in a variety of liver disorders, including acute viral hepatitis[183] (even in a haemophiliac[90]), alcoholic cirrhosis[96] and non-alcoholic cirrhosis.[196] Antigenic concentrations of the VIII and VWF were reported to be much higher than the biological activities of these factors and were highest in patients with cholestatic liver disease.[137] Parenteral vitamin K induced a fall in the factor VIII levels in patients who were vitamin K deficient[136] but not in those who were replete, suggesting a link with protein C deficiency. The protein C levels were at the lower end of the normal range but did not change with therapy. It is possible that an abnormal protein C molecule induced by vitamin K deficiency[271] could be functionally inactive, leading to reduced inactivation of factor VIII

and resultant higher levels. The observation that the factor VIII activity was significantly higher than the VWF antigen in patients with fulminant hepatic failure,[152] a condition associated with marked reduction of protein C levels,[151] supports this hypothesis. Further study assessing antigenic and functional protein C and factor VIII activities is needed to resolve this interesting problem.

Other reasons for the raised factor VIII levels in liver disease have been suggested. In acute hepatitis the rise in factor VIII may be due to release from the hepatocytes, a mechanism thought to account for the raised serum vitamin B_{12} levels in this condition. Increased production of factor VIII, a reactive protein, by the RE system in response to the disease process or impaired denaturation and clearance of the factor VIII molecule by the damaged liver are possible. Factor VIII levels rise significantly during normal pregnancy and the underlying mechanism here may be compensated low-grade intravascular coagulation;[6a] low-grade intravascular coagulation in liver disease might similarly result in raised factor VIII levels.

Factor V

Factor V is synthesized by the liver and, as it is not vitamin K dependent, low levels should theoretically help distinguish hepatocellular failure from obstructive jaundice. In practice, factor V assay does not appear to be a useful test for this purpose.[257] This is partly due to the fact that factor V may be raised in patients with acute infections or could be reduced because of disseminated intravascular coagulation. Very low levels have been reported in fulminant hepatic failure,[10] and a value of <20% is associated with a poor prognosis.

Other factors

Assay of the contact factors XI and XII has shown that reduced levels are present in patients with hepatic disease.[210] Clinically it is unlikely that this observation is significant; even severe congenital deficiency of these factors gives rise to surprisingly few bleeding problems.

Factor XIII is easily assessed by a simple screening test (clot solubility in 5 mol/l urea or 2% monochloracetic acid). Reduced levels of factor XIII have been reported in hepatocellular disease[173] but not in obstructive jaundice.[260] Low-grade intravascular coagulation might also explain this finding.

Abnormal platelet function has been described in patients with liver disease. Clinically this may be suggested by a prolonged bleeding time. In fulminant hepatic failure, impaired aggregation to adenosine diphosphate (ADP) and collagen and structural abnormalities on electron microscopy were demonstrated.[216] Defective aggregation to ristocetin[35] and to ADP and thrombin[243] in cirrhosis may be due to the inhibitory effect of FDPs and fibrin monomers.[242]

Fibrinolytic activity in liver disease

The basic reactions activating and controlling fibrinolysis are shown in Figure 8.2 and have been described on pp 205–206. The development of highly specific antibodies and chromogenic substrates has advanced the assessment of the fibrinolytic system and immunological and functional assays are now established for its major components. These include plasminogen and plasmin, plasminogen activators and inhibitors, circulating antiplasmins (alpha-2-antiplasmin, alpha-2-macroglobulin and ATIII) and fibrin/fibrinogen breakdown products (FDPs, XDPs and fibrinopeptide A (FPA)).[59] Techniques such as the euglobulin clot lysis time (ECLT) and whole-blood clot lysis time measure variations in fibrinolytic activity and are useful screening tests for hyperfibrinolysis. Additional research methods are being used in this expanding field.

Although there is conflicting evidence,[20] increased fibrinolytic activity has frequently been noted in cirrhosis of the liver,[77,93,147,209] following surgical resection of the liver[259] and liver transplantation.[207,231] Decreased fibrinolytic activity has been reported in acute hepatic failure[40] and in obstructive jaundice,[128] where it was associated with raised triglyceride levels.

The underlying mechanism leading to changes in the fibrinolytic system is complex. Increased fibrinolysis can result from primary activation of the fibrinolysis or could be secondary to underlying disseminated intravascular coagulation (DIC). Primary activation may be due to increased conversion of plasminogen to plasmin or to defects of the antiplasmins and other inhibiting factors (see Figure 8.2). Low plasminogen levels reported in liver disease[244] could be a consequence of this or of hepatic synthetic failure. Increased tissue type plasminogen activators (tPA),[16,20,113] and impaired clearance of circulating plasminogen activators[77] are described in cirrhosis; both could result in increased fibrinolysis. In a study of 30 cirrhotic patients, increased tPA activity but not tPA antigen levels correlated with fibrinolytic activity, as measured by whole-blood lysis. An equally significant correlation with decreased tPA inhibitor levels was also noted,[113] suggesting that the capacity of plasma inhibitors to limit tPA may be a critical factor in the development of accelerated fibrinolysis.

The major inhibitor of plasmin, alpha-2-antiplasmin, is reduced in cirrhotic patients[178] with increased fibrinolysis.[113] Congenital deficiency of this antiplasmin is associated with a severe haemorrhagic tendency[3] and could have significant clinical consequences for patients with cirrhosis.[20,83] Other coagulation defects are present in such patients and the specific contribution of accelerated fibrinolysis to bleeding complications is not established.

Disseminated intravascular coagulation

The abnormalities of fibrinolysis described in the preceding section could all be secondary to underlying DIC. The occurrence of DIC is well documented in liver disease, although pathological evidence of it was only found at autopsy in 4 out of 184 cases dying with liver disease.[192] The definitive event in DIC is activation of thrombin, leading to the conversion of fibrinogen to fibrin and formation of fibrin and platelet thrombi with consumption of coagulation factors and platelets. Fibrinolytic mechanisms are activated and plasmin is formed, leading to the digestion of fibrin, fibrinogen and other clotting factors and their consequent depletion. Fibrinogen breakdown products accumulate, fibrin polymerization is impaired and bleeding may ensue. Clearly, in liver disease the combination of release of thromboplastic substances from the diseased liver, impaired production of coagulation factors and inhibitors and defective hepatic clearance of activated coagulation factors could lead to systemic coagulation.

Established criteria for the diagnosis of significant DIC are prolongation of the PT, APTT and thrombin time, reduced fibrinogen and platelets and elevated FDPs.[34] More sophisticated sensitive tests to detect intravascular coagulation have been applied to the study of patients with liver disease, with conflicting results.

Increased fibrinogen breakdown which corrected with heparin has been reported in cirrhosis.[44,252] A later study confirmed these findings[232] in advanced cirrhosis and in addition showed increased catabolism of plasminogen and platelets; there was no increase in fibrinogen-related antigens, however, suggesting that intravascular coagulation was not the underlying mechanism.

Elevated FDPs which measure both fibrinogen and fibrin-related material are reported in uncomplicated liver disease but not at levels which are diagnostic of DIC.[115,256] Cross-linked D-dimer degradation products (XDPs) resulting from factor XIII action on fibrin are more specific for fibrin degradation, are similarly raised in liver disease, but are still well below the DIC range.[240] Immunoblotting demonstrated a spectrum of plasmin degradation products including XDPs in only 7 of 35 patients, with liver disease and in all 7, other illnesses known to be associated with DIC were present.[256]

Raised levels of fibrinopeptide A (FPA) formed by thrombin activation of fibrin, a sensitive but non-specific index of DIC, is reported in cirrhosis.[43,186] In one study[178] they were associated with reduced levels of alpha-2-antiplasmin but normal fibrinogen and FDP levels and an absence of bleeding and thus no convincing evidence of DIC. Thrombin–antithrombin and plasmin–alpha-2-antiplasmin complexes are raised in liver disease, suggesting actual generation of thrombin and plasmin, but clearance of these products has not been evaluated.[240]

Deficiency of the main inhibitor of thrombin, ATIII, occurs in a variety of liver disorders including chronic liver disease and fulminant hepatic failure.[87] Hereditary deficiency of ATIII predisposes to thrombosis[177] and it is suggested that low levels in liver disease may lead to thrombosis,[106] intravascular coagulation and a bleeding tendency.[87] ATIII concentrates were unable to maintain plasma ATIII levels in 7 of 12 patients with fulminant hepatic failure who died; gross haemostatic failure with thrombocytopenia and extensive bleeding was present and it is not clear how fundamental the low ATIII levels were to the fatal outcome. Another antithrombin, heparin cofactor II (HCII), is reduced in DIC and hepatic failure, in parallel with ATIII levels in most patients. A significant correlation between decreased HCII levels and a low serum albumin suggested failure of hepatic synthesis.[248]

The foregoing account has provided much evidence that coagulation and fibrinolytic abnormalities associated with DIC occur in liver disease. Nevertheless, clinically significant DIC is rare in uncomplicated cirrhosis of the liver[115] and other trigger factors such as infection,[34] release of endotoxin from the gut,[210] surgery, shock, infusions of prothrombin complex concentrates may be required to produce the full syndrome.[33]

Clinical significance of the coagulation abnormalities

Patients with established liver disease may bleed for many reasons. Commonly haemorrhage is due to local causes such as oesophageal varices, gastritis or peptic ulceration. Impaired production of the coagulation factors, especially factors II, VII, IX and X, is common, and thrombocytopenia and abnormal platelet function may be present. Intravascular coagulation and consumption coagulopathy may contribute to the bleeding problem. Massive transfusion by stored bank blood, low in coagulation factors and platelets, can aggravate or even induce a coagulation defect.

Use of coagulation tests to assess function and prognosis

The prothrombin time (PT) and activated partial thromboplastin time (APTT) are used routinely to screen patients with liver disease and may be considered as liver function tests, occasionally being abnormal when other biochemical tests are within normal limits. With any degree of cellular damage the PT and APTT will be abnormal, but bleeding complications will not necessarily be present.[229] In general there is good correlation between coagulation abnormalities and the degree of liver failure; for example, bleeding was noted in three-quarters of patients with acute liver failure[40] and in some was the direct cause of death. Failed synthesis of the clotting factors and disseminated intravascular coagulation are the main reasons for bleeding in such patients, and serial coagulation tests have been used to assess progress and prognosis. In one study of acute liver failure, clotting tests rapidly became abnormal and hepatic coma occurred in patients whose PT ratio rose above 2.2.[40] Another group showed that the PT ratio was excessively prolonged (greater than 4.8) in all who died.[63] Gross prolongation of the PT (> 100 s) in fulminant hepatic failure is taken as an indication for liver transplantation.[191] Similarly, the thrombotest levels are related to prognosis in acute hepatic failure.[115] Of specific factor assays, factor VII appears to be the most significant, levels below 9% being associated with a fatal outcome.[63]

Factor V levels are also thought to be important, a level below 20% in comatose patients being used as an indication for transplantation.[10] In chronic liver disease the factor VII level and the PT correlate well and are equally useful in assessing hepatocellular function. The differential diagnosis of obstructive jaundice and hepatocellular failure is not helped by detailed coagulation factor analysis. A therapeutic test of vitamin K_1 by parenteral injection (10 mg daily for three days) is helpful: persistent abnormalities indicate functional impairment of the hepatic cells.

Tests such as the PT and APTT are screening tests and may be normal even when specific coagulation factors are as low as 25–30% of normal; reductions of this order would be unlikely to lead to bleeding complications. Isolated factor deficiencies have been reported and the association of amyloidosis and factor X deficiency is well recognized.[88]

The clinical significance of laboratory evidence of a coagulation defect is difficult to assess. Many patients with gross abnormalities have little or no spontaneous bleeding. When complications such as oesophageal varices or gastric erosions arise, however, the coagulation defect may prevent normal haemostasis. The greater the coagulation defect, the more likely it is that bleeding will occur, but the picture is complex. Bleeding as a result of thrombocytopenia is also a variable phenomenon. As a general rule patients with a platelet count greater than $30 \times 10^9/l$ will not bleed spontaneously, but abnormal platelet function may be present. Platelet counts as low as $10 \times 10^9/l$ are rare in patients with liver disease unless there are other complications such as DIC or blood loss; at this level thrombocytopenic bleeding is common, but is not necessarily present.

Management of the coagulation defect

Non-bleeding patients

In patients about to undergo surgery or liver biopsy, correction of the coagulation defect is necessary. If this cannot be achieved, the decision to proceed with operation or biopsy will depend on its clinical indication.

Vitamin K_1 by intravenous injection 10 mg daily is given for three days, although maximal correction of the PT is usually achieved within 24 h. Abnormality persisting beyond this period indicates hepatocellular dysfunction. The use of fresh frozen plasma (FFP) and prothrombin complex concentrates (PCC) may temporarily correct the defect, the haemostatic effect lasting for a few hours and being sufficient to enable liver biopsy to be carried out safely. In patients undergoing liver biopsy, the PT should not be more than 3 s beyond the control time (INR of 1.4 or less).[226] Plugged biopsy techniques should be considered (see Chapter 19). Invasive procedures other than liver biopsy may be carried out safely in patients with a moderately prolonged PT of 15–29 s without prophylactic FFP; bleeding complications were rare in a series of 71 invasive procedures[85] managed in this way.

The decision to use PCC or FFP will depend on the circumstances. FFP must be given in large amounts with the attendant problems of fluid overload and would not be the therapy of choice in patients undergoing surgery. PCC is made up in a small volume of diluent and patients with congenital factor IX deficiency requiring surgery are treated successfully with these preparations. Multiple deficiencies associated with liver disease are more difficult to correct and complications are more likely to occur. Early users of PCC in patients with liver disease reported intravascular coagulation which occasionally proved fatal[17,89] and it was subsequently shown that the concentrates contained activated products. Improved fractionation techniques and exclusion of factor VII has reduced this risk and several of the available products contain only factors II, IX and X. With improved in vitro testing for spontaneous thrombin generation,[218] concentrates are now considered safe in patients with liver disease even when factor VII is not excluded.[97,175] The current NHS factor IX product (type 9A) contains factors II, X and IX and is heat-treated at 68°C for 72 h. It contains heparin in low concentration (not more than 5000 units/l) but it is still considered advisable to limit the use of these concentrates in patients with an increased risk of thrombosis.[264] Such a hypercoagulable state would be suggested by a history of a previous thrombotic episode or coagulation abnormalities such as low levels of antithrombin III.

With the introduction in 1985 of heat treatment of clotting concentrates, post-transfusion hepatitis and HIV transmission by this means have been virtually eliminated. Prior to this, most haemophiliac patients, following exposure to factor VIII concentrates, developed abnormal liver function and in approximately 20%[108] chronic liver disease, mainly due to hepatitis C, developed.[172] The risk was always much less with PCC. FFP is not heat-treated and a small risk of viral transmission remains; one in 75 000 UK donors are HIV seropositive and six in every thousand donors are HCV antibody positive.[26]

Thus the new PCC which is heat treated and has added heparin should be a safer product than FFP but no data on the efficacy and risk of thrombosis following the use of these new concentrates in liver disease is available. A study carried out in 1976 showed that a combination of FFP (8 ml/kg body weight) and a four-factor concentrate (12 u/kg body weight) best corrected the defect in patients being prepared for liver biopsy.[175] A single dose of FFP (12 mg/kg) was not effective nor was concentrate that lacked factor VII. Maximal correction was achieved within 5 min of administration and a second dose could be given with some further improvement. In practice patients are usually given an initial dose of 2–4 u FFP, the PT is checked again and if it is still prolonged a further dose of 2–4 u is given. Biopsy is usually abandoned or deferred if the PT correction is not adequate.

Associated thrombocytopenia is an obvious hazard in patients undergoing liver biopsy but moderate thrombocytopenia is not a contraindication. Liver biopsy was per-

formed without complication in 74 patients whose platelet count was greater than $60 \times 10^9/l$. Three of 13 patients with lower counts bled.[223] The bleeding time is a simple practical manoeuvre which should be performed in any doubtful case; significant prolongation would be considered an absolute contraindication to elective liver biopsy or surgery. Prophylactic platelet concentrates may be used; the formula that 1 unit of platelets/m² body surface area will raise the count by $12 \times 10^9/l$ is a useful guideline as to how much should be given to raise the count to a 'safe' level, which is generally thought to be above $100 \times 10^9/l$.

Bleeding patients

Extensive haemorrhage from gastrointestinal lesions such as oesophageal varices and gastric erosions may give rise to a life-threatening situation. Local measures to stem the blood loss such as the use of Sengstaken–Blakemore tubes are discussed in Chapter 48. Any associated coagulation defect will be treated vigorously with the measures described above. The benefit is usually temporary, and repeated administration of FFP and or PCC is often necessary to maintain haemostasis. When massive haemorrhage occurs, rapid replacement with stored bank blood may aggravate the coagulation defect and it is recommended that approximately 10% of the blood given should be fresh (i.e. less than 24 h old). If this is not possible, comparable infusions of FFP and platelet concentrates should be given. Marked thrombocytopenia will be temporarily corrected by platelet transfusion, but it may be difficult to achieve a sustained rise in the platelet count. It is difficult to correlate the platelet count and a bleeding tendency since many patients do not bleed even with counts below $30 \times 10^9/l$. The mean platelet volume (MPV) as measured by electronic counters may be a useful predictor of a haemorrhagic state; thrombocytopenic patients with a MPV less than 6.4 fl were more likely to bleed.[68] Defects of platelet function are difficult to correct, but transfusion with platelet concentrates is worth trying.

Correction of the long bleeding time in some patients with liver disease by DDAVP,[1,30,176] is interesting but its role in the management of bleeding patients needs to be assessed in clinical trials. Treatment with ATIII concentrates in cirrhosis,[221] fulminant hepatic failure[87] and during liver transplantation[106] will correct low ATIII levels but here too their role in correcting haemorrhage and preventing thrombosis is not yet established.

The treatment of DIC

The treatment of DIC is unsatisfactory and is difficult. Fortunately most patients with liver disease and DIC do not bleed.[89,115] The main problem is to assess to what extent the intravascular coagulation is contributing to the bleeding problem. Management of DIC may be summarized as follows:

1. Treatment or remove the underlying cause.
2. Replace the missing factors.

3. Take measures to stop continuing thrombosis if necessary.

Trigger factors such as infection, shock, dehydration and vascular stasis must obviously be treated by appropriate methods, and measures which achieve this may be sufficient to control the condition. Serial laboratory assessment will be important to gauge the progress and control of the disease.

No obvious trigger factors may be present and the decision to treat the coagulation defect will depend on the condition of the patient and laboratory evidence of a deteriorating situation.

The bleeding patient with evidence of severe consumption coagulopathy will need to be given replacement therapy. This approach has been questioned on the basis that the bleeding diathesis is due in part to the presence of breakdown products of fibrin and other activated products and their replacement may 'add fuel to the fire'. Such a theory is difficult to prove and if a patient has a severe coagulation defect and is bleeding, specific therapy should be given. If fresh blood, which contains platelets, red cells and coagulation factors, is not available, packed red cells and fresh frozen plasma should be given instead. Prothrombin and other concentrates should not be used in DIC. Severe hypofibrinogenaemia may be treated by cryoprecipitate, a rich source of fibrinogen and factor VIII.

If the situation is deteriorating clinically in spite of these measures and there is laboratory evidence of continuing DIC, treatment with heparin should be considered. Since liver disease is often complicated by varices or other gastrointestinal lesions which may bleed, the use of anticoagulants must be viewed with extreme caution.

Results of heparin therapy are variable but its value has not yet been proved by any controlled prospective trial. An uncontrolled study of 20 patients with acute hepatic necrosis treated with heparin and fresh frozen plasma suggested that it might be beneficial,[40] but a later study in paracetamol-induced hepatic necrosis showed no significant difference when FFP was compared with FFP and heparin.[89]

Increased survival of ^{125}I-labelled fibrinogen was noted in a small group of patients with cirrhosis treated with low-dose heparin[44] and this might be a safer alternative to full-dosage heparin since its prophylactic use in surgical patients is not followed by significant bleeding.[123] In the absence of convincing evidence that heparin administration leads to significant improvement in DIC[18] the present recommendation would be to reserve this for cases where therapy as outlined previously has failed to reverse life-threatening haemorrhage or thrombosis.

The use of fibrinolytic inhibitors such as ϵ-aminocaproic acid and tranexamic acid (Cyklokapron) has been considered for patients where excess fibrinolysis is a major component of the coagulopathy.[205] Such drugs will interfere with protective physiological mechanisms and have theoretical dangers in their use, but could be considered, possibly with heparin. Aprotinin may be a useful alternative.[274]

When other measures have failed, the use of plasma exchange to replace defective plasma, possibly containing circulating fibrin complexes and FDPs, without the attendant problems of circulatory overload might be considered. Such measures would have only a temporary effect but could tide the patient over a life-threatening episode of haemostatic failure, allowing time for recovery of liver function.

REFERENCES _____

1. Agnell, G., Berrettini, M., De Cunto, M. & Nenci, G.G. (1983). Desmopressin-induced improvement of abnormal coagulation in chronic liver disease. Lancet, 1, 645.
2. Anger, B.R., Seifried, E., Scheppach, J. & Heimpèl, H. (1989) Budd–Chiari syndrome and thrombosis of other abdominal vessels in chronic myeloproliferative diseases. Klinische Wochenschrift, 67, 818–825.
3. Aoki, N., Saito, H., Kamiya, T. et al. (1979) Congenital deficiency of α_2 plasmin inhibitor associated with severe haemorrhagic tendency. Journal of Clinical Investigation, 63, 877–884.
4. Aster, R.H. (1966) Pooling of platelets in the spleen: role in the pathogenesis of hypersplenic thrombocytopenia. Journal of Clinical Investigation, 45, 645–657.
5. Ballard, H.S. & Marcus, A.J. (1976) Platelet aggregation in portal cirrhosis. Archives of Internal Medicine, 136, 316–319.
6. Bassendine, M.F., Collins, J.D., Stephenson, J. et al. (1985) Platelet associated immunoglobulins in primary biliary cirrhosis: A cause of thrombocytopenia? Gut, 26, 1047–1079.
6a. Bennett, B. & Ratnoff, O.D. (1972) Changes in antihaemophilic factor (AHF factor VIII) procoagulant activity and AHF-like antigen in normal pregnancy and following exercise and pneumoencephalography. Journal of Laboratory and Clinical Medicine, 80, 256–263.
7. Berenyi, M.R., Straus, B. & Cruz, D. (1974) In vitro and in vivo studies of cellular immunity in alcoholic cirrhosis. American Journal of Digestive Diseases, 19, 199–205.
8. Berkowitz, H., Reichel, J. & Shim, C. (1973) The effect of ethanol

on the cough reflex. Clinical Science and Molecular Medicine, 45, 527–531.
9. Berman, L., Axelrod, A.R., Horan, T.N. et al. (1949) The blood and bone marrow in patients with cirrhosis of the liver. Blood, 4, 511–533.
10. Bernuau, J., Bourliere, M., Rueff, B. & Benhamou, J.P. (1990) Transplantation for fulminant hepatic failure. Lancet, 335, 407.
11. Bertino, J.R., Ward, J., Sartorelli, A.C. & Silber, R. (1965) An effect of ethanol on folate metabolism. Journal of Clinical Investigation, 44, 1028.
12. Bessis, M. (1977) Blood Smears Reinterpreted. p. 64. New York: Springer International.
13. Bessis, M., Weed, R. & Le Blond, P. (1973) Red Cell Shape: Physiology, Pathology, Ultrastructure. New York: Springer-Verlag.
14. Bingham, J. (1959) The macrocytosis of hepatic disease. I. Thin macrocytosis. Blood, 14, 244–254.
15. Bingham, J. (1960) The macrocytosis of hepatic disease. II. Thick macrocytosis. Blood, 15, 694–707.
16. Bismuth, H., Castaing, D., Ericzon, B.G. et al. (1987) Hepatic transplantation in Europe: First report of the European Liver Transplant Registry. Lancet, 2, 674–676.
17. Blatt, P.M., Lundblad, R.L., Kingdon, M.S. et al. (1974) Thrombogenic materials in prothrombin complex concentrates. Annals of Internal Medicine, 81, 766–770.
18. Bloom, A.L. (1975) Annotation: intravascular coagulation and the liver. British Journal of Haematology, 30, 1–7.

19. Bloom, A.L., Giddings, J.C. & Wilks, C.J. (1973) Factor VIII on the vascular intima: possible importance in haemostasis and thrombosis. *Nature: New Biology*, **241**, 217–219.
20. Boks, A.L., Brommer, E.J.P., Schalm, S.W. & Van Vliet, H.H.D.M. (1986) Hemostasis and fibrinolysis in severe liver failure and their relation to haemorrhage. *Hepatology*, **6**, 79–86.
21. Bontempo, F.A. (1987) Monitoring of coagulation during liver transplantation—how much is enough? *Mayo Clinic Proceedings*, **62**, 848–849.
22. Bontempo, F.A., Lewis, J.H., Van Thiel, D.H. *et al.* (1985) The relation of pre-operative coagulation findings to diagnosis, blood usage and survival in adult liver transplantation. *Transplantation*, **39**, 532–536.
23. Bontempo, F.A., Lewis, J.H., Gorenc, T.J. *et al.* (1987) Liver transplantation in hemophilia A. *Blood*, **69**, 1721–1724.
24. Booth, N.A., Anderson, J.A. & Bennett, B. (1984) Plasminogen activators in alcoholic cirrhosis: demonstration of increased tissue type and urokinase type activator. *Journal of Clinical Pathology*, **37**, 772–777.
25. Boughton, B.J. (1990) Hepatic and portal vein thrombosis. *British Medical Journal*, **302**, 192–193.
26. Boulton, F. (1991) Director, Wessex Regional Transfusion Service. Personal Communication.
27. Brain, M.C. (1977) Red cell membrane structure and function. In Hoffbrand, A.V., Brain, M.C. & Hirsh, J. (eds) *Recent Advances in Haematology*, pp. 27–41. Edinburgh, London and New York: Churchill Livingstone.
28. Brayton, R.G., Stokes, P.E., Schwartz, M.S. & Louria, D.B. (1970) Effect of alcohol and various diseases on leukocyte mobilization, phagocytosis and intracellular bacterial killing. *New England Journal of Medicine*, **282**, 123–128.
29. Brodsky, I., Siegel, M.H., Kahn, S.B. *et al.* (1970) Simultaneous fibrinogen and platelet survival with (^{75}Se) selenomethionine in man. *British Journal of Haematology*, **18**, 341–355.
30. Burroughs, A.K., Matthews, K., Qadiri, M. *et al.* (1985) Desmopressin and bleeding time in patients with cirrhosis. *British Medical Journal*, **291**, 1377–1381.
31. Butler, P., Israel, L., Nusbacher, A. *et al.* (1985) Blood transfusion in liver transplantation. *Transfusion*, **25**, 120–123.
32. Campbell, D.A., Rolles, K., Jamieson, N. *et al.* (1988) Hepatic transplantation with peri-operative and long term anticoagulation as treatment for Budd–Chiari syndrome. *Surgery, Gynaecology and Obstetrics*, **166**, 511–518.
33. Carr, J.M. (1989) Disseminated intravascular coagulation in cirrhosis. *Hepatology*, **10**, 103–110.
34. Cash, J.D. (1977) Disseminated intravascular coagulation. In Poller, L. (ed.) *Recent Advances in Blood Coagulation*, pp. 293–311. Edinburgh, London and New York: Churchill Livingstone.
35. Castillo, R., Maragall, S., Rodés, J. *et al.* (1977) Increased factor VIII complex and defective ristocetin induced platelet aggregation in liver disease. *Thrombosis Research*, **11**, 899–906.
36. Chanarin, I. (1982) Haemopoiesis and alcohol. *British Medical Bulletin*, **38**, 81–86.
37. Chiandussi, L., Bianco, A., Massaro, A. *et al.* (1964) The quantitative determination of iron kinetics and haemoglobin synthesis in anaemia of cirrhosis studies with ^{59}Fe. *Blut*, **10**, 120.
38. Chomet, B. & Gach, B.M. (1967) Lobar pneumonia and alcoholism: an analysis of thirty seven cases. *American Journal of Medical Science*, **253**, 300–304.
39. Choremis, C., Kattamis, Ch. A., Kyriazakou, M. & Gavrillidou, E. (1966) Viral hepatitis in G6PD deficiency. *Lancet*, **1**, 269–270.
40. Clark, R., Rake, M.O., Flute, P.T. & Williams, R. (1973) Coagulation abnormalities in acute liver failure. *Scandinavian Journal of Gastroenterology*. **19** (Supplement 8), 63–70.
41. Clearfield, H.R., Brody, J.I. & Tumen, H.J. (1969) Acute viral hepatitis, glucose-6-phosphate dehydrogenase deficiency and hemolytic anaemia. *Archives of Internal Medicine*, **123**, 689–691.
42. Clemens, M.R., Kessler, W., Schied, H.W. *et al.* (1986) Plasma and red cell lipids in alcoholics with macrocytosis. *Clinica Chemica Acta*, **156**, 321–328.
43. Coccheri, S., Mannucci, P.M., Palareti, G. *et al.* (1982) Significance of plasma fibrino peptide A and high molecular weight fibrinogen in patients with liver cirrhosis. *British Journal of Haematology*, **52**, 503–509.
44. Coleman, M., Finlayson, N., Bettigole, R.E. *et al.* (1975) Fibrinogen survival in cirrhosis: improvement by low dose heparin. *Annals of Internal Medicine*, **83**, 79–81.
45. Conrad, M.E. (1969) Persistent haemolysis after infectious hepatitis. *Gut*, **10**, 516–521.
46. Conrad, M.E., Berman, A. & Crosby, W.H. (1962) Iron kinetics in Laennec's cirrhosis. *Gastroenterology*, **43**, 385–390.
47. Conrad, M.E., Schwartz, F.D. & Young, A.A. (1964) Infectious hepatitis—a generalised disease. *American Journal of Medicine*, **37**, 789–801.
48. Cooper, R.A. (1969) Anaemia with spur cells: a red cell defect acquired in serum and modified in the circulation. *Journal of Clinical Investigation*, **48**, 1820–1831.
49. Cooper, R.A. (1970) Lipids of human red cell membrane: normal composition and variability in disease. *Seminars in Hematology*, **7**, 296–322.
50. Cooper, R.A. & Jandl, J.H. (1968) Bile salts and cholesterol in the pathogenesis of target cells in obstructive jaundice. *Journal of Clinical Investigation*, **47**, 809–822.
51. Cooper, R.A., Kimball, D.B. & Durocher, J.R. (1974) Role of the spleen in membrane conditioning and hemolysis of spur cells of liver disease. *New England Journal of Medicine*, **290**, 1279–1284.
52. Cooper, R.A., Diloy-Puray, M., Lando, P. & Greenberg, M.S. (1972) An analysis of lipoproteins, bile acids and red cell membranes associated with target cells and spur cells in patients with liver disease. *Journal of Clinical Investigation*, **51**, 3182–3192.
53. Cooper, R.A., Arner, E.C., Wiley, J.S. & Shattil, S.J. (1975) Modification of red cell membrane structure by cholesterol-rich lipid dispersions. A model for the primary spur cell defect. *Journal of Clinical Investigation*, **55**, 115–126.
54. Cordova, C., Violi, F., Alessandri, C. *et al.* (1986) Prekallikrein and factor VII as prognostic indexes of liver failure. *American Journal of Clinical Pathology*, **85**, 579–582.
55. Cowan, D.H. (1973) Thrombokinetic studies in alcohol related thrombocytopenia. *Journal of Laboratory and Clinical Medicine*, **81**, 64–76.
56. Cowan, D.H. & Hines, J.D. (1971) Thrombocytopenia of severe alcoholism. *Annals of Internal Medicine*, **74**, 37–43.
57. Dacie, J.V. (1967) *The Haemolytic Anaemias, Part III—Secondary or Symptomatic Anaemias.* pp. 826–837. London: J. & A. Churchill.
58. D'Angelo, A., D'Angelo, S.V., Esmon, C.T. & Comp, P.C. (1988). Acquired deficiencies of protein S. *Journal of Clinical Investigation*, **81**, 1445–1454.
59. Davidson, J.F. & Walker, I.D. (1987) Assessment of the fibrinolytic system. In *Haemostasis and Thrombosis*, 2nd edn., pp. 953–965. Edinburgh: Churchill Livingstone.
60. Deller, D.J., Kimber, C.L. & Ibbotson, R.N. (1965) Folic acid deficiency in cirrhosis of the liver. *American Journal of Digestive Diseases*, **10**, 35–42.
61. Donaldson, G.W.K., Davies, S.H., Darg, A. & Richmond, J. (1969) Coagulation factors in chronic liver disease. *Journal of Clinical Pathology*, **22**, 199–204.
62. Douglass, C.C. & Twomey, J.J. (1970) Transient stomatocytosis with haemolysis: a previously unrecognised complication of alcoholism. *Annals of Internal Medicine*, **72**, 159–164.
63. Dymock, I.W., Tucker, J.S., Woolf, I.L. *et al.* (1975) Coagulation studies as a prognostic index in acute liver failure. *British Journal of Haematology*, **29**, 385–395.
64. Dzik, W.H., Arkin, C.F., Jenkins, R.L. & Stump, D.C. (1988) Fibrinolysis during liver transplantation in humans. Role of tissue-type plasminogen activator. *Blood*, **71**, 1090–1095.
65. Egeberg, O. (1965) Inherited antithrombin deficiency causing thrombophilia. *Thrombosis et Diathesis Haemorrhagica*, **13**, 516–530.
66. Eichner, E.R. & Hillman, R.S. (1971) The evolution of anemia in alcoholic patients. *American Journal of Medicine*, **50**, 218–232.
67. Eichner, E.R., Buchanan, B., Smith, J.W. & Hillman, R.S. (1972) Variations in the hematologic and medical status of alcoholics. *American Journal of Medicine*, **263**, 35–42.
68. Eldor, A., Avitzour, M., Or, R. *et al.* (1982) Prediction of haemorrhagic diathesis in thrombocytopenia by mean platelet volume. *British Medicial Journal*, **285**, 397–400.
69. Eppstein, S. (1964) Primary carcinoma of the liver. *American Journal of the Medical Sciences*, **247**, 137.
70. Exner, T., Joshua, D.E., Rickard, K.A. & Kronenberg, H. (1982)

Detection of antihaemophilic factor by immunoradiometric assays in lymph node and lung extracts. In *Proceedings of the VIIIth International Congress on Thrombosis and Haemostasis.* p. 167. Stuttgart: Schattauer.

71. Fair, D.S. & Bahnak, B.R. (1984) Human hepatoma cells secrete single chain factor X, prothrombin and antithrombin III. *Blood*, **64**, 194.

72. Fair, D.S. & Marlar, R.A. (1986) Biosynthesis and secretion of factor VII, protein C, protein S and the protein C inhibitor from a human hepatoma cell line. *Blood*, **67**, 64–70.

73. Feldshon, S.D., Earnest, D.L. & Corrigan, J.J. (1983) Impaired coagulant factor synthesis is more important than impaired carboxylation in the coagulopathy of liver disease. *Hepatology*, **3**, 858.

74. Fernandez-Zamorano, A., Arnalich, F., Codoceo, R. *et al.* (1988) Hemolytic anaemia and susceptibility to hydrogen peroxide hemolysis in children with vitamin E deficiency and chronic liver disease. *Journal of Medicine*, **19**, 317–334.

75. Finkbiner, R.B., McGovern, J.J. Goldstein, R. & Bunker, J.P. (1959) Coagulation defects in liver disease and response to transfusion during surgery. *American Journal of Medicine*, **26**, 199–213.

76. Finks, R.M. & Blumberg, R.W. (1945) Epidemic hepatitis with and without jaundice: some clinical studies on two hundred and twenty five patients among troops in a combat zone. *Archives of Internal Medicine*, **76**, 102.

77. Fletcher, A.P., Biederman, D., Moore, D. *et al.* (1964) Abnormal plasminogen–plasmin system activity (fibrinolysis) in patients with hepatic cirrhosis. *Journal of Clinical Investigation*, **43**, 681–695.

78. Flute, P.T., Rake, M.O., Williams, R. *et al.* (1969) Liver transplantation in man. IV. Haemorrhage and thrombosis. *British Medical Journal*, **3**, 20–23.

79. Fodor, O. & Tanasescu, R. (1962) Anemiile hemolitice immunologice posthepatice. *Medicina Interna (Bucuresti)*, **14**, 1469–1476.

80. Forman, W.B. & Barnhart, M.I. (1964) Cellular site for fibrinogen synthesis. *Journal of the American Medical Association*, **187**, 128–132.

81. Francis, J.L. & Armstrong, D.J. (1983) Acquired dysfibrinogenaemia. *Medical Laboratory Sciences*, **40**, 165–175.

82. Francis, J.L., Simmonds, V.J. & Armstrong, D.J. (1983) The effect of phenobarbitone administration on sialyltransferase activity and fibrinogen bound sialic acid in rats. *Thrombosis Research*, **31**, 507–512.

83. Francis, R.P. & Feinstein, D.I. (1984) Clinical significance of accelerated fibrinolysis in liver disease. *Haemostasis*, **14**, 460.

84. Fried, W. (1972) The liver as a source of extrarenal erythropoietin production. *Blood*, **40**, 671–677.

85. Friedman, E.W. & Sussman, I.I. (1989) Safety of invasive procedures in patients with the coagulopathy of liver disease. *Clinical and Laboratory Haematology*, **11**, 199–204.

86. Funk, C., Gmur, J., Herold, R. & Straub, P.W. (1971) Reptilase-R. A new reagent in blood coagulation. *British Journal of Haematology*, **21**, 43–52.

87. Fujiwara, K., Okita, K., Akamatsu, K. *et al.* (1988) Antithrombin III concentrate in the treatment of fulminant hepatic failure. *Gastroenterology Japan*, **23**, 423–427.

88. Galbraith, P.A., Sharma, N., Parker, W.L. & Kilgour, J.M. (1974) Acquired factor X deficiency: altered plasma antithrombin activity and association with amyloidosis. *Journal of the American Medical Association*, **230**, 1658–1660.

89. Gazzard, B.G., Lewis, M.L., Ash, G. *et al.* (1974) Coagulation factor concentrates in the treatment of the haemorrhagic diathesis of fulminant hepatic failure. *Gut*, **15**, 993–998.

90. Gazzard, B.G., Clark, R., Flute, P.J. & Williams, R. (1975) Factor VIII levels during the course of acute hepatitis in a haemophiliac. *Journal of Clinical Pathology*, **28**, 972–974.

91. Goebel, K.M., Goebel, F.D., Schubotz, R. & Schneider, J. (1977) Red cell metabolic and membrane features in haemolytic anaemia of alcoholic liver disease (Zieve's syndrome). *British Journal of Haematology*, **35**, 573–585.

92. Goodnight, S.H., Jr, Feinstein, D.I., Østerad, B. & Rapaport, S.I. (1971) Factor VII antibody neutralizing material in hereditary and acquired factor VII deficiency. *Blood*, **38**, 1–8.

93. Goodpasture, E.W. (1914) Fibrinolysis in chronic hepatic insufficiency. *Bulletin of the Johns Hopkins Hospital*, **25**, 330.

94. Gordon, A.S., Zanjani, E.D. & Zalusky, R. (1970). A possible mechanism for the erythrocytosis associated with hepatocellular carcinoma in man. *Blood*, **35**, 151–157.

95. Gralnick, H.R., Givelber, H. & Abrams, E. (1978) Dysfibrinogenemia associated with hepatoma: increased carbohydrate content of the fibrinogen molecule. *New England Journal of Medicine*, **299**, 221–226.

96. Green, A.J. & Ratnoff, O.D. (1974) Elevated antihaemophiliac factor (AHF factor VIII) procoagulant activity and AHF-like antigen in alcoholic cirrhosis of the liver. *Journal of Laboratory and Clinical Medicine*, **83**, 189–197.

97. Green, G., Dymock, I.W., Poller, L. & Thomson, J.M. (1975) The use of a factor VII rich prothrombin complex concentrate in liver disease. *Lancet*, **1**, 1311–1314.

98. Green, G., Poller, L., Thomson, J.M. & Dymock, I.W. (1976) Factor VII as a marker of hepatocellular synthetic function in liver disease. *Journal of Clinical Pathology*, **29**, 971–975.

99. Green, G., Thomson, J.M., Dymock, I.W. & Poller, L. (1976) Abnormal fibrin polymerization in liver disease. *British Journal of Haematology*, **34**, 427–439.

100. Griffin, J.H., Evatt, B., Zimmerman, T.S. *et al.* (1981) Deficiency of protein C in congenital thrombotic disease. *Journal of Clinical Investigation*, **68**, 1370–1373.

101. Grossi, C.E., Rousselot, L.M. & Parke, W.F. (1964) Control of fibrinolysis during portocaval shunts. *Journal of the American Medical Association*, **187**, 1005–1008.

102. Haagsma, E.B., Gips, C.H., Wesenhagen, H. *et al.* (1985) Liver disease and its effect on haemostasis during liver transplantation. *Liver*, **5**, 123–128.

103. Hagler, L., Pastore, R.A., Bergin, J.J. & Wrensch, M.R. (1975) Aplastic anaemia following viral hepatitis. *Medicine*, **54**, 139–164.

104. Hall, C.A. (1960) Erythrocyte dynamics in liver disease. *American Journal of Medicine*, **28**, 541–549.

105. Halsted, C.H., Robles, E.A. & Mezey, E. (1973) Intestinal malabsorption in folate deficient alcoholics. *Gastroenterology*, **64**, 526–532.

106. Harper, P.L., Luddington, R.J., Carrell, R.W. *et al.* (1988) Protein C deficiency and portal thrombosis in liver transplantation in children. *Lancet*, **2**, 924–927.

107. Havens, W.P. & Marck, R.E. (1946) The leukocytic response of patients with experimentally induced infectious hepatitis. *American Journal of the Medical Sciences*, **212**, 129.

108. Hay, C.R.M., Preston, F.E., Triger, D.R. & Underwood, J.C.E. (1985) Progressive liver disease in haemophilia: An understated problem? *Lancet*, **1**, 1495–1498.

109. Hemker, H.C., Veltkamp, J.J., Hensen, A. & Leoliger, E.A. (1963) Nature of prothrombin biosynthesis: preprothrombinaemia in vitamin K deficiency. *Nature*, **200**, 589–590.

110. Herbert, V. (1962) Experimental nutritional folate deficiency in man. *Transactions of the Association of American Physicians*, **75**, 307.

111. Herbert, V., Zalusky, R. & Davidson, C.S. (1963) Correlation of folate deficiency with alcoholism and associated macrocytosis, anaemia and liver disease. *Annals of Internal Medicine*, **58**, 977–988.

112. Herbert, V. (1980) Hematologic complications of alcoholism. *Seminars in Hematology*, **XVII**, 83–176.

113. Hersch, S.L., Kunelis, T. & Francis, R.B. (1987) The pathogenesis of accelerated fibrinolysis in liver cirrhosis: A critical role for tissue plasminogen activator inhibitor. *Blood*, **69**, 1315–1319.

114. Hillbom, M., Muuronen, A. & Neiman, J. (1987) Liver disease and platelet function in alcoholics. *British Medical Journal*, **295**, 581.

115. Hillenbrand, P., Parbhoo, S.B., Jedrychowski, A. & Sherlock, S. (1974) Significance of intravascular coagulation and fibrinolysis in acute hepatic failure. *Gut*, **15**, 83–88.

116. Hillman, R.S. & Steinberg, S.E. (1982) The effects of alcohol on folate metabolism. *Annual Review of Medicine*, **33**, 345–354.

117. Hines, J.D. (1969) Reversible megaloblastic and sideroblastic marrow abnormalities in alcoholic patients. *British Journal of Haematology*, **16**, 87–101.

118. Hines, J.D. & Cowan, D.H. (1970) Studies on the pathogenesis of alcohol-induced sideroblastic bone marrow abnormalities. *New England Journal of Medicine*, **283**, 441–446.

119. Hines, J.D. & Grasso, J.A. (1970) The sideroblastic anaemias. *Seminars in Hematology*, **7**, 86–106.

120. Hoffbrand, A.V. (1972) The red cell folate assay. MD Thesis, University of Oxford.
121. Hui, D.Y. & Harmony, J.A.K. (1979) Interaction of plasma lipoproteins with erythrocytes. I. Alteration of erythrocyte morphology. *Biochimica et Biophysica Acta*, **550**, 407–424.
122. Hume, R., Williamson, J.M. & Whitelaw, J.W. (1970) Red cell survival in biliary cirrhosis. *Journal of Clinical Pathology*, **23**, 397–401.
123. International Multicentre Trial (1975) Prevention of fatal postoperative pulmonary embolism by low doses of heparin. *Lancet*, **2**, 45–51.
124. Jandl, J.H. (1955) The anaemia of liver disease: observations on its mechanism. *Journal of Clinical Investigation*, **34**, 390–404.
125. Jandl, J.H. & Lear, A.A. (1956) The metabolism of folic acid in cirrhosis. *Annals of Internal Medicine*, **45**, 1027–1044.
126. Jarrold, T. & Vilter, R.W. (1949) Haematologic observations in patients with chronic hepatic insufficiency. *Journal of Clinical Investigation*, **28**, 286–292.
127. Jarrold, T., Will, J.J. & Davies, A.R. (1967) Bone marrow erythroid morphology in alcoholic patients. *American Journal of Clinical Nutrition*, **20**, 716–722.
128. Jedrychowski, A., Hillenbrand, P., Ajdukiewicz, A.B. *et al.* (1973) Fibrinolysis in cholestatic jaundice. *British Medical Journal*, **1**, 640–642.
129. Joske, R.A. (1963) The vitamin B_{12} content of human liver tissue obtained by aspiration biopsy. *Gut*, **4**, 231–235.
130. Kan, Y.W., McFadzean, A.J.S., Todd, D. & Tso, S.C. (1961) Further observations on polycythaemia in hepatocellular carcinoma. *Blood*, **18**, 592–598.
131. Kang, Y.G., Martin, D.J., Marquez, J. *et al.* (1985) Intra-operative changes in blood coagulation and thrombelastographic monitoring in liver transplantation. *Anesthesia and Analgesia*, **64**, 888–896.
132. Kang, Y.G., Lewis, J.H., Navalgund, A. *et al.* (1987) Epsilon-aminocaproic acid for treatment of fibrinolysis during liver transplantation. *Anesthesiology*, **66**, 766–773.
133. Karpatkin, S., Strick, N., Karpatkin, M.B. & Siskind, G.W. (1972) Cumulative experience in the detection of antiplatelet antibody in 234 patients with idiopathic thrombocytopenic purpura, systemic lupus erythematosus and other clinical disorders. *American Journal of Medicine*, **52**, 776–785.
134. Kelly, D.A. & Summerfield, J.A. (1987) Hemostasis in liver disease. *Seminars in Liver Disease*, **7**, 182–191.
135. Kelly, D.A., Summerfield, J.A. & Tuddenham, E.G.D. (1984) Localisation of factor VIII C antigen in guinea-pig tissues and isolated liver cell fractions. *British Journal of Haematology*, **56**, 535–543.
136. Kelly, D.A., Mikami, S., Tuddenham, E.G.D. & Summerfield, J.A. (1984) Unexpected effect of vitamin K on factor VIII in liver disease. *Gut*, **25**, A543–544.
137. Kelly, D.A., O'Brien, F.J., Hutton, R.A. *et al.* (1985) The effect of liver disease on factors V, VIII and protein C. *British Journal of Haematology*, **61**, 541–548.
138. Kilbridge, T.M. & Heller, P. (1969) Determinants of erythrocyte size in chronic liver disease. *Blood*, **34**, 739–746.
139. Kimber, C., Deller, D.J., Ibbotson, R.H. & Lander, H. (1965) The mechanism of anaemia in chronic liver disease. *Quarterly Journal of Medicine*, **34**, 33–64.
140. Kivel, R.M. (1961) Haematologic aspects of acute viral hepatitis. *American Journal of Digestive Diseases*, **6**, 1017–1031.
141. Klipstein, F.A. & Lindenbaum, J. (1965) Folate deficiency in chronic liver disease. *Blood*, **25**, 443–456.
142. Kobrinsky, N.L., Israels, E.D., Gerrard, J.M. *et al.* (1984) Shortening of bleeding time by 1-deamino-8-D-arginine vasopressin in various bleeding disorders. *Lancet*, **1**, 1145–1148.
143. Koie, K., Kamiya, T., Ogata, K. & Takamatsu, J. (1978) α_2 Plasmin-inhibitor deficiency (Miyasato disease). *Lancet*, **2**, 1334–1336.
144. Kojima, S., Matsuyama, K., Kodera, Y. & Okada, J. (1989) Circulating activated suppressor T lymphocytes in hepatitis associated aplastic anaemia. *British Journal of Haematology*, **71**, 147–151.
145. Koller, F. (1973) Theory and experience behind the use of coagulation tests in diagnosis and prognosis of liver disease. *Scandinavian Journal of Gastroenterology*, **19** (Supplement 8) 59–61.
146. Krasnow, S.E., Walsh, J.R., Zimmerman, H.J. & Heller, P. (1957) Megaloblastic anaemia in 'alcoholic' cirrhosis. *Archives of Internal Medicine*, **100**, 870–880.
147. Kwaan, H.C., McFadzean, A.J.S. & Cook, J. (1956) Plasma fibrinolytic activity in cirrhosis of the liver. *Lancet*, **1**, 132–136.
148. *Lancet* (1983) Familial antithrombin III deficiency. *Lancet*, **1**, 1021–1022.
149. Lane, D.A., Scully, M.F., Thomas, D.P. *et al.* (1977) Acquired dysfibrinogenaemia in acute and chronic liver disease. *British Journal of Haematology*, **35**, 301–307.
150. Lane, F., Goff, P., McGuffin, R. & Hillman, R. (1973) The influence of ethanol on folate metabolism. *Blood*, **42**, 998.
151. Langley, P.G. & Williams, R. (1988) The effect of fulminant hepatic failure on protein C antigen and activity. *Thrombosis and Haemostasis*, **59**, 316–318.
152. Langley, P.G., Hughes, R.D. & Williams, R. (1985) Increased factor VIII complex in fulminant hepatic failure. *Thrombosis and Haemostasis*, **54**, 693–696.
153. Lee, G.R. (1983) The anaemia of chronic disease. *Seminars in Hematology*, **XX**, 61–80.
154. Lee, S., Yip, M. & Sachs, H.J. (1972) Factor IX deficiency in liver disease. *Journal of the American Medical Association*, **221**, 1410–1412.
155. Leevy, C.M., Baker, H., Tenhove, W.W. *et al.* (1965) B-complex vitamins in liver disease of the alcoholic. *American Journal of Clinical Nutrition*, **16**, 339–346.
156. Lewis, J.H., Bontempo, F.A., Spero, J.A. *et al.* (1985) Liver transplantation in a hemophiliac. *New England Journal of Medicine*, **312**, 1189.
157. Lewis, J.H., Bontempo, F.A., Awad, S.A. *et al.* (1989) Liver transplantation: intra-operative changes in coagulation factors in 100 first transplants. *Hepatology*, **9**, 710–714.
158. Liang, D.C., Lin, K.H., Lin, D.T. *et al.* (1990) Post hepatic aplastic anaemia in children in Taiwan, a hepatitis prevalent area. *British Journal of Haematology*, **74**, 487–491.
159. Lieberman, F.L. & Reynolds, T.B. (1967) Plasma volume in cirrhosis of the liver. *Journal of Clinical Investigation*, **46**, 1297–1308.
160. Liebman, H.A., Furie, B.C., Tong, M.J. *et al.* (1984) Des-γ-carboxy (abnormal) prothrombin as a serum marker of primary hepatocellular carcinoma. *New England Journal of Medicine*, **310**, 1427–1431.
161. Lightwood, A.M. & Scott, G.L. (1973) Auto-immune haemolytic anaemia due to red cell antibodies of different specificities in a patient with chronic hepatitis. *Vox Sanguinis*, **24**, 331–336.
162. Lindenbaum, J. (1977) Metabolic effects of alcohol on the blood and bone marrow. In Lieber, C.S. (ed.) *Metabolic Aspects of Alcoholism*, pp. 215–247. Baltimore: University Park Press.
163. Lindenbaum, J. (1980) Folate and vitamin B_{12} deficiencies in alcoholism. *Seminars in Hematology*, **17**, 119–129.
164. Lindenbaum, J. (1986) Hematologic complications of alcohol abuse. *Seminars in Liver Disease*, **7**, 169–181.
165. Lindenbaum, J. & Hargrove, R.L. (1968) Thrombocytopenia in alcoholics. *Annals of Internal Medicine*, **68**, 526–532.
166. Lindenbaum, J. & Lieber, C.S. (1969) Hematologic effects of alcohol in man in the absence of nutritional deficiency. *New England Journal of Medicine*, **281**, 333–338.
167. Lipschitz, D.A., Cook, J.D. & Finch, C.A. (1974) A clinical evaluation of serum ferritin as an index of iron stores. *New England Journal of Medicine*, **290**, 1213–1216.
168. Litwins, J. & Liebowitz, S. (1951) Abnormal lymphocytes ('virocytes') in virus diseases other than infectious mononucleosis. *Acta Haematologica*, **5**, 223.
169. Liu, Y.K. (1973) Leukopenia in alcoholics. *American Journal of Medicine*, **54**, 605–610.
170. MacDonald, R.A. (1963) Idiopathic haemochromatosis: genetic or acquired? *Archives of Internal Medicine*, **112**, 184–190.
171. MacPherson, A.I.S. & Innes, J. (1953) Peripheral blood picture after operation for portal hypertension. *Lancet*, **1**, 1120–1123.
172. Makris, M., Preston, F.E., Triger, D.R. *et al.* (1990) Hepatitis C antibody and chronic liver disease in haemophilia. *Lancet*, **335**, 1117–1119.
173. Mandel, E.E. & Gerhold, W.M. (1969) Plasma fibrin stabilizing factor: acquired deficiency in various disorders. *American Journal of Clinical Pathology*, **52**, 547–556.

174. Mannucci, P.M. & Vigano, S. (1982) Deficiencies of protein C, an inhibitor of blood coagulation. *Lancet*, **2**, 463–466.

175. Mannucci, P.M., Franchi, F. & Dioguardi, N. (1976) Correction of abnormal coagulation in chronic liver disease by combined use of fresh frozen plasma and prothrombin. *Lancet*, **2**, 542–545.

176. Mannucci, P.M., Vicente, V., Vianello, L. *et al.* (1986) Controlled trial of desmopressin in liver cirrhosis and other conditions associated with a prolonged bleeding time. *Blood*, **67**, 1148–1153.

177. Marciniak, E., Farley, C.H. & de Simone, P.A. (1974) Familial thrombosis due to antithrombin III deficiency. *Blood*, **43**, 219–231.

178. Marongiu, F., Mamusa, A.M., Mameli, G. *et al.* (1985) Alpha-2-antiplasmin and disseminated intravascular coagulation in liver cirrhosis. *Thrombosis Research*, **37**, 287–294.

179. McCurdy, P.R., Pierce, L.E. & Rath, C.E. (1962) Abnormal bone marrow morphology in acute alcoholism. *New England Journal of Medicine*, **266**, 505–507.

180. McFarland, W. & Leibre, E.P. (1963) Abnormal leukocyte response in alcoholism. *Annals of Internal Medicine*, **59**, 865–877.

181. McFadzean, A.J.S., Todd, D. & Tsang, K.C. (1958) Polycythaemia in primary carcinoma of the liver. *Blood*, **13**, 427–435.

182. Meagher, R.C., Sieber, F. & Spivak, J.L. (1982) Suppression of hematopoietic-progenitor cell proliferation by ethanol and acetaldehyde. *New England Journal of Medicine*, **307**, 845–849.

183. Meili, E.O. & Straub, P.W. (1970) Elevation of factor VIII in acute fatal liver necrosis. *Thrombosis et Diathesis Haemorrhagica*, **24**, 161–174.

184. Merion, R.M., Delius, R.E., Campbell, D.A. & Turcotte, J.G. (1988) Orthotopic liver transplantation totally corrects factor IX deficiency in hemophilia B. *Surgery*, **104**, 929–931.

185. Miles, J.A.R. (1945) The erythrocyte sedimentation rate in infective hepatitis. *British Medical Journal*, **1**, 767–769.

186. Mombelli, G., Monotti, R., Haeberli, A. & Straub, P.W. (1987) Relationship between fibrino peptide A and fibrinogen/fibrin fragment E in thromboembolism, DIC and various non-thromboembolic diseases. *Thrombosis and Haemostasis*, **58**, 758–763.

187. Morgan, M.Y., Camilo, M.E., Luck, W. *et al.* (1981) Macrocytosis in alcohol-related liver disease: its value for screening. *Clinical and Laboratory Haematology*, **3**, 35–44.

188. Neerhout, R.C. (1968) Abnormalities of erythrocyte stromal lipids in hepatic disease. *Journal of Laboratory and Clinical Medicine*, **71**, 438–477.

189. Neehout, R.C. (1968) Erythrocyte stromal lipids in hyperlipemic states. *Journal of Laboratory and Clinical Medicine*, **71**, 448–454.

190. Nunnally, R.M. & Levine, I. (1961) Macronormoblastic hyperplasia of the bone marrow in hepatic cirrhosis. *American Journal of Medicine*, **30**, 972–975.

191. O'Grady, J.G., Alexander, G.J.M., Hayllar, K.M. & Williams, R. (1989) Early indicators of prognosis in fulminant hepatic failure. *Gastroenterology*, **97**, 439–445.

192. Oka, K. & Tanaka, K. (1979) Intravascular coagulation in autopsy cases with liver disease. *Thrombosis and Haemostasis*, **42**, 564.

193. Ordinas, A., Maragatt, S., Castillo, R. & Nurden, A.T. (1979) A glycoprotein I defect in the platelets of three patients with severe cirrhosis of the liver. *Thrombosis Research*, **13**, 297–302.

194. Orozco, H., Guraieb, E., Takahashi, T. *et al.* (1988) Deficiency of protein C in patients with portal vein thrombosis. *Hepatology*, **8**, 1110–1111.

195. Østergaard Kristensen, H.P. (1959) The blood vitamin B_{12} level in liver disease. *Acta Medica Scandinavica*, **163**, 515–523.

196. Outryve, M., van Baele, G., Weerdi, G.A. de & Barbier, F. (1973) Antihaemophilic factor A (FVIII) and serum fibrin-fibrinogen degradation products in hepatic cirrhosis. *Scandinavian Journal of Haematology*, **11**, 148–152.

197. Owen, C.A., Rettke, S.R., Bowie, E.J.W. *et al.* (1987) Hemostatic evaluation of patients undergoing liver transplantation. *Mayo Clinic Proceedings*, **62**, 761–772.

198. Owen, J.S., Brown, D.J.C., Harry, D.S. *et al.* (1985) Erythrocyte echinocytosis in liver disease: the role of abnormal plasma high-density lipoproteins. *Journal of Clinical Investigation*, **76**, 2275–2285.

199. Pagliuca, A., Mufti, G.J., Tahernia, J.M. *et al.* (1990) In vitro colony culture and chromosomal studies in hepatic and portal vein thrombosis—possible evidence of an occult myeloproliferative state. *Quarterly Journal of Medicine*, **76**, 981–989.

200. Palareti, G., De Rosa, V., Fortunato, G. *et al.* (1988) Control of hemostasis during orthotopic liver transplantation. *Fibrinolysis*, **2** (Supplement 3), 61–66.

201. Pengelly, C.D.R. & Jennings, R.C. (1971) Active chronic hepatitis and haemolytic anaemia associated with Rh-specific antibodies. *Postgraduate Medical Journal*, **47**, 683–686.

202. Pikis, A., Kavaliotis, J. & Manios, S. (1988) Incidence of aplastic anaemia in viral hepatitis in children. *Scandinavian Journal of Infectious Diseases*, **20**, 109–110.

203. Pitcher, C.S. & Williams, R. (1963) Reduced red cell survival in jaundice and its relation to abnormal glutathione metabolism. *Clinical Science*, **24**, 239–252.

204. Pol, S., Driss, F., Devergie, A. *et al.* (1990). Is hepatitis C virus involved in hepatitis-associated aplastic anaemia? *Annals of Internal Medicine*, **113**, 435–437.

205. Poller, L. (1977) Coagulation abnormalities in liver disease. In Poller, L. (ed.) *Recent Advances in Blood Coagulation*, pp. 266–292. Edinburgh: Churchill Livingstone.

206. Prieto, J., Barry, M. & Sherlock, S. (1975) Serum ferritin in patients with iron overload and with acute and chronic liver diseases. *Gastroenterology*, **68**, 525–533.

207. Porte, R.J., Knot, E.A.R. & Bontempo, F.A. (1989) Hemostasis in liver transplantation. *Gastroenterology*, **97**, 488–501.

208. Rachmilewitz, M., Aronovitch, J. & Grossowicz, N. (1956) Serum concentrates of Vitamin B_{12} in acute and chronic liver disease. *Journal of Laboratory and Clinical Medicine*, **48**, 339.

209. Ratnoff, O.D. (1949) Studies on a proteolytic enzyme in human plasma. *Bulletin of the Johns Hopkins Hospital*, **84**, 29.

210. Ratnoff, O.D. (1977) The haemostatic defects of liver disease. In Ogston, D. & Bennett, B. (eds) *Haemostasis: Biochemistry, Physiology and Pathology*, pp. 446–466. New York: Wiley.

211. Ratnoff, O.D. & Menzie, C. (1951) A new method for the determination of fibrinogen in small samples of plasma. *Journal of Laboratory and Clinical Medicine*, **37**, 316–320.

212. Retief, F.P., VandenPlas, L. & Visser, H. (1969) Vitamin B_{12} binding proteins in liver disease. *British Journal of Haematology*, **16**, 231–240.

213. Rider, D.M., McDonagh, R.P. & McDonagh, J. (1978) A possible contributory role of the platelet in the formation of plasma factor XIII. *British Journal of Haematology*, **39**, 579–588.

214. Ritter, D.M., Owen, C.A., Bowie, E.J.W. *et al.* (1989) Evaluation of preoperative hematology–coagulation screening in liver transplantation. *Mayo Clinic Proceedings*, **64**, 216–223.

215. Ronquist, G., Rimsten, A., Westman, M. & Cerven, E. (1980) Serum sialyltransferase activity in benign and malignant diseases. *Acta Chirurgica Scandinavica*, **146**, 247–252.

216. Rubin, M.H., Weston, M.J., Bullock, G. *et al.* (1977) Abnormal platelet function and ultrastructure in fulminant hepatic failure. *Quarterly Journal of Medicine*, **183**, 339–352.

217. Ryback, R.S., Eckardt, M.J., Felsher, B. & Rawlings, R.R. (1982) Biochemical and hematologic correlates of alcoholism and liver disease. *Journal of the American Medical Association*, **248**, 2261–2265.

218. Sas, G., Owens, R.E., Smith, J.K. *et al.* (1975) In vitro spontaneous thrombin generation in human factor IX concentrates. *British Journal of Haematology*, **31**, 25–35.

219. Savage, D. & Lindenbaum, J. (1986) Anemia in alcoholics. *Medicine*, **65**, 322–338.

220. Scanlon, G.H., Brinkhouse, K.M., Warnerm, E.D. *et al.* (1939) Plasma prothrombin and the bleeding tendency with special reference to jaundiced patients and vitamin K therapy. *Journal of the American Medical Association*, **112**, 1898–1901.

221. Schipper, H.G. & ten Cate, J.W. (1982) Antithrombin III transfusion in patients with hepatic cirrhosis. *British Journal of Haematology*, **52**, 25–33.

222. Sears, D.A., George, J.N. & Gold, M.S. (1975) Transient red blood cell aplasia in association with viral hepatitis. Occurrence four years apart in siblings. *Archives of Internal Medicine*, **135**, 1585–1589.

223. Sharma, P., McDonald, G.B. & Banaji, M. (1982) The risk of bleeding after percutaneous liver biopsy: Relation to platelet count. *Journal of Clinical Gastroenterology*, **4**, 451–453.

224. Sharp, A.A., Howie, B., Biggs, R. & Methuen, D.T. (1958) Defibrination syndrome in pregnancy: value of various diagnostic tests. *Lancet*, **2**, 1309–1312.

225. Sheehy, T.W. & Berman, A. (1960) The anaemia of cirrhosis. *Journal of Laboratory and Clinical Medicine*, **56**, 72–82.
226. Sherlock, S., Dick, B. & Van Leewen, D. (1985) Liver biopsy today. *Journal of Hepatology*, **1**, 75–85.
227. Smith, J.A., Lonergan, E.T. & Sterling, K. (1964) Spur cell anemia. Hemolytic anemia with red cells resembling acanthocytosis in alcoholic cirrhosis. *New England Journal of Medicine*, **271**, 396–398.
228. Soria, J., Coupier, J., Samama, M. *et al.* (1970) Dysfibrinogenaemia without bleeding tendency with abnormal polymerization of fibrin monomers in a case of severe hepatitis. *XII Congress of the International Society of Haematology, New York. Abstracts.* p. 180.
229. Spector, I. & Corn, M. (1967) Laboratory tests of haemostasis. The relation to haemorrhage in liver disease. *Archives of Internal Medicine*, **119**, 577–582.
230. Stahl, R.L., Duncan, A., Hooks, M.A. *et al.* (1990) A hypercoagulable state follows orthotopic liver transplantation. *Hepatology*, **12**, 553–558.
231. Starzl, T.E., Marchioro, T.L., Von Kaulla, K.N. *et al.* (1963) Homotransplantation of the liver in humans. *Surgery, Gynecology and Obstetrics*, **117**, 659–676.
232. Stein, S.F. & Harker, L.A. (1982) Kinetic and functional studies of platelets, fibrinogen and plasminogen in patients with hepatic cirrhosis. *Journal of Laboratory and Clinical Medicine*, **99**, 217–230.
233. Stel, H.V., Vander, K., Wast, H. & Veerman, E.C.I. (1983) Detection of Factor VIII coagulant antigen in human liver tissue. *Nature*, **303**, 530–532.
234. Stenflo, J. (1974) Vitamin K and the biosynthesis of prothrombin. IV. Isolation of peptides containing prosthetic groups from normal prothrombin and corresponding peptides from dicoumarol-induced prothrombin. *Journal of Biological Chemistry*, **249**, 5527–5535.
235. Subhiyah, B.W. & Al-Hindawi, A.Y. (1967) Red cell survival and splenic accumulation of radio-chromium in liver cirrhosis with splenomegaly. *British Journal of Haematology*, **13**, 773–778.
236. Sullivan, B.H., Jr, & Tumen, H.J. (1961) The effect of portacaval shunt on thrombocytopenia associated with portal hypertension. *Annals of Internal Medicine*, **55**, 598–603.
237. Sullivan, L.W. & Herbert, V. (1964) Suppression of haematopoiesis by ethanol. *Journal of Clinical Investigation*, **43**, 2048–2062.
238. Sullivan, L.W., Adams, W.H. & Liu, Y.K. (1977) Induction of thrombocytopenia by thrombopheresis in man: patterns of recovery in normal subjects during ethanol ingestion and abstinence. *Blood*, **49**, 197–207.
239. Suttie, J.W. (1974) Metabolism and properties of a liver precursor to prothrombin. *Vitamins and Hormones*, **32**, 463–481.
240. Takahashi, H., Tatewaki, W., Wada, K. *et al.* (1989) Thrombin and plasmin generation in patients with liver disease. *American Journal of Haematology*, **32**, 30–35.
241. Tamura, T. & Halsted, C.H. (1983) Folate turnover in chronically alcoholic monkeys. *Journal of Laboratory and Clinical Medicine*, **101**, 623.
242. Thomas, D.P. (1972) Abnormalities of platelet aggregation in patients with alcoholic cirrhosis. *Annals of the New York Academy of Sciences*, **201**, 243–250.
243. Thomas, D.P., Ream, V.J. & Stuart, R.K. (1967) Platelet aggregation in patients with Laënnec's cirrhosis of the liver. *New England Journal of Medicine*, **276**, 1344–1348.
244. Thomas, D.P., Niewiarowski, S., Myers, A.R. *et al.* (1970) A comparative study of four methods for detecting fibrinogen degradation products in patients with various diseases. *New England Journal of Medicine*, **283**, 663–668.
245. Thomas, E.D., Buckner, C.D., Clift, R.A. *et al.* (1977) Current status of marrow transplantation for leukaemia or aplastic anaemia. In Hoffbrand, A.V., Brain, M.C. & Hirsh, J. (eds), *Recent Advances in Haematology*, pp. 111–125. Edinburgh: Churchill Livingstone.
246. Thorling, E.B. (1972) Paraneoplastic erythrocytosis and inappropriate erythropoietin production. *Scandinavian Journal of Haematology*, **1** (Supplement 17), 1–166.
247. Toghill, P.J. & Green, S. (1983) Platelet dynamics in chronic liver disease using the [III]indium oxine label. *Gut*, **24**, 49–52.
248. Tollefsen, D.M. & Pestka, C.A. (1985) Heparin cofactor II activity in patients with disseminated intravascular coagulation and hepatic failure. *Blood*, **66**, 769–774.

249. Triger, D.R., Alp, M.H. & Wright, R. (1972) Bacterial and dietary antibodies in liver disease. *Lancet*, **1**, 60–63.
250. Tso, S.C. & Hua, A.S.P. (1974) Erythrocytosis in hepatocellular carcinoma—a compensatory phenomenon. *British Journal of Haematology*, **28**, 497–503.
251. Tumen, H.J. (1970) Hypersplenism and portal hypertension. *Annals of the New York Academy of Sciences*, **170**, 332–344.
252. Tytgat, G.M., Collen, D. & Verstraete, M. (1971) Metabolism of fibrinogen in cirrhosis of the liver. *Journal of Clinical Investigation*, **50**, 1690–1701.
253. Vahrman, J. (1971) Viral hepatitis and the ESR. *British Medical Journal*, **2**, 466–467.
254. Valla, D., Casadevall, N., Lacombe, C. *et al.* (1985) Primary myeloproliferative disorder and hepatic vein thrombosis. A prospective study of erythroid colony formation in vitro in 20 patients with Budd–Chiari syndrome. *Annals of Internal Medicine*, **103**, 329–334.
255. Valla, D., Casadevall, N., Huisse, M.G. *et al.* (1988) Etiology of portal vein thrombosis in adults. *Gastroenterology*, **94**, 1063–1069.
256. Van de Water, L., Carr, J.M., Aronson, D. & McDonagh, J. (1986) Analysis of elevated fibrin(ogen) degradation product levels in patients with liver disease. *Blood*, **67**, 1468–1473.
257. Veltkamp, J.J. & Kreuning, J. (1973) Diagnostic value of coagulation studies in chronic liver disease. *Scandinavian Journal of Gastroenterology*, **19** (Supplement 8), 93–95.
258. Vigano, S., Mannucci, P.M., D'Angelo, A. *et al.* (1986) The significance of protein C antigen in acute and chronic liver biliary disease. *American Journal of Clinical Pathology*, **84**, 454–458.
259. Von Kaulla, K.N., Kaye, H., Von Kaulla, E. *et al.* (1966) Changes in blood coagulation before and after hepatectomy or transplantation in dogs and man. *Archives of Surgery*, **92**, 71–79.
260. Walls, W.D. & Losowsky, M.J. (1971) The hemostatic defect of liver disease. *Gastroenterology*, **60**, 108–119.
261. Weir, D.G., McGing, P.G. & Scott, J.M. (1985) Folate metabolism, the enterohepatic circulation and alcohol. *Biochemical Pharmacology*, **34**, 1–7.
262. Weisberg, L.J., Shiu, D.T., Conkling, P.R. & Shuman, M.A. (1987) Identification of normal human peripheral blood monocytes and liver as sites of synthesis of coagulation factor XIII α-chain. *Blood*, **70**, 579–582.
263. Werre, J.M., Helleman, P.W., Verloop, M.C. & Degier, J. (1970) Causes of macroplasia of erythrocytes in diseases of the liver and biliary tract with special reference to leptocytosis. *British Journal of Haematology*, **19**, 223–235.
264. White, G.C., Roberts, H.R., Kingdon, H.S. & Lundblad, R.L. (1977) Prothrombin complex, concentrates: potentially thrombogenic materials and clues to the mechanisms of thrombosis in vivo. *Blood*, **49**, 159–170.
265. Wiley, J.S., Ellory, J.C., Shuman, M.A. *et al.* (1975) Characteristics of the membrane defect in the hereditary stomatocytosis syndrome. *Blood*, **46**, 337–356.
266. Willcox, R.G. & Isselbacher, K.J. (1961) Chronic liver disease in young people. *American Journal of Medicine*, **30**, 185.
267. Williams, R., Williams, H.S., Scheuer, P.J. *et al.* (1967) Iron absorption and siderosis in chronic liver disease. *Quarterly Journal of Medicine*, **36**, 151–165.
268. Wright, S.G. & Ree, G.H. (1978) Blood in the alcohol stream. *Lancet*, **1**, 49–50.
269. Wu, A., Chanarin, I. & Levi, A.J. (1974) Macrocytosis of chronic alcoholism. *Lancet*, **1**, 829.
270. Yeung, K.Y., Klug, P.P., Brower, M. & Lessin, L.S. (1973) Mechanism of alcohol induced vacuolization in human bone marrow cells. *Blood*, **42**, 998.
271. Yoshikawa, Y., Sakata, Y., Toda, G. & Oka, H. (1988) The acquired vitamin K-dependent γ-carboxylation deficiency in hepatocellular carcinoma involves not only prothrombin but also protein C. *Hepatology*, **8**, 524–530.
272. Zieve, L. (1958) Jaundice, hyperlipemia, hemolytic anemia: a heretofore unrecognized syndrome associated with alcoholic fatty liver and cirrhosis. *Annals of Internal Medicine*, **48**, 471–496.
273. Zieve, L. (1966) Hemolytic anemia in liver disease. *Medicine*, **45**, 497–505.
274. Neuhaus, P., Bechstein, W.O., Lefebre, B., Blumhardt, G. and Slama, K. (1989) Effect of aprotinin on intraoperative bleeding and fibrinolysis in liver transplantation. *Lancet*, **2**, 924–925.

CHAPTER 9

Immunological Aspects of Liver Disease

D.R. Triger & Ralph Wright

Diseases affecting the liver are notable for the frequency with which immunological phenomena are detectable. Since the liver is a major component of the reticuloendothelial system, such disturbances might be expected, although the mechanism behind many of these abnormalities is poorly understood. The lack of knowledge concerning the aetiology and pathogenesis of liver diseases has prompted investigators to search for an immunological explanation for both the initiation and the perpetuation of many of these disorders. This chapter considers the current status of the liver as a part of the immune system and also reviews the immunological phenomena associated with damage to the liver. The specific immune responses to the hepatitis viruses are dealt with in Chapters 30 and 31.

EXPERIMENTAL EVIDENCE FOR THE IMMUNOLOGICAL ROLE OF THE INTACT LIVER

The liver occupies a strategic anatomical position between the gastrointestinal tract and the systemic circulation. Studies in germ-free mice indicate that the intestinal microorganisms provide the major stimulus to γ-globulin production, presumably by the absorption of intact bacteria or their antigenic components into both the lymphatic and portal venous systems.[92]

Supporting experimental evidence has been provided by the ability to demonstrate the presence of radiolabelled type-specific *E. coli* antigen in the liver of coliform-free rabbits following oral feeding.[88] Warshaw *et al.*[115] have studied the absorption of bovine serum albumin (BSA) by the rat small intestine using cannulation of the mesenteric lymphatic duct and portal vein. Following instillation of tritium-labelled BSA into the duodenum, they were able to demonstrate the uptake of [³H]BSA into both lymph and blood and prove that the absorbed BSA was immunologically identical to the instilled protein.

Antigens in the portal venous blood must pass through the hepatic sinusoids before reaching the systemic circulation, and particulate antigens, such as sheep erythrocytes[109] or *Salmonella adelaide*,[100] have been shown to be trapped there in significant quantities. Although the liver is the largest organ in the reticuloendothelial system and is capable of trapping and phagocytosing more antigen than any other component, it may handle antigens differ-

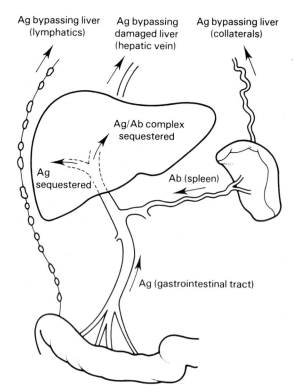

Ag bypassing liver (lymphatics)

Ag bypassing damaged liver (hepatic vein)

Ag bypassing liver (collaterals)

Ag/Ab complex sequestered

Ag sequestered

Ab (spleen)

Ag (gastrointestinal tract)

Figure 9.1   The sequestration of exogenous antigen by the liver.

ently. Whereas the spleen is able to phagocytose antigens and process them for antibody production, the liver appears to process and degrade antigens much more rapidly and completely without the production of antibody.[47] This may be due to the absence of significant numbers of lymphoid cells in the normal liver, in contrast to other organs in the reticuloendothelial system.

These experimental studies suggest that the liver may act as a filter of exogenous antigens absorbed from the gastrointestinal tract by sequestering part or all of those present in the portal venous system and thereby reducing the amount of antigen available to the antibody-producing components elsewhere (Figure 9.1). The possibility that this might be a significant in vivo function of the liver was first suggested by Cantor and Dumont.[19] They found that the circulating antibody response in dogs immunized with intramuscular dinitrochlorobenzene (DNCB) was significantly reduced if the animals were fed the hapten prior to the injections, and that this reduction was abolished if the animals were subjected to portacaval shunting before the start of the experiment. They suggested that the liver might help prevent sensitization to antigen absorbed from the gastrointestinal tract into the portal venous system. Subsequent work has emphasized this role of the liver by showing that repeated injection of small amounts of sheep erythrocytes into the portal venous system of rats results in a significantly lower antibody production compared with similar immunization via the inferior vena cava.[109] Supporting evidence has been provided by studies of circulating antibody after the

effective phagocytic hepatic function has been altered in various ways, including reticuloendothelial blockade with colloidal carbon,[96] carbon tetrachloride-induced necrosis,[105] portacaval anastomosis[54] and portacaval transposition.[10] All these procedures result in increases in both total and specific antibody production.

Central to this argument is the functional capability of the liver macrophage or Kupffer cell. The cells lining the liver sinusoids are divided into endothelial cells, perisinusoidal (Ito) cells, pit cells and Kupffer cells. These groups are morphologically distinct and now that they can be clearly separated and studied using elutriation, their functions are being characterized (see Chapter 2). At any given time, only about 30% of cells are phagocytic. Little is known about the kinetics of the macrophages, except that they are sessile under normal conditions and may have a very slow turnover. They are not uniformly distributed throughout the liver, being concentrated in the vicinity of the portal triads and less frequent in the perivenular zones.[95] They are probably derived from cells within the bone marrow, spleen and peripheral blood and are recruited from these sites following liver damage. These cells rarely divide within the liver under normal conditions, although division can be induced experimentally by agents such as zymosan. The macrophages of the reticuloendothelial system have many varied and important immunological functions related chiefly to handling of antigen and participation in T and B cell interaction, as well as playing a vital role in the repair of tissue damage.

Extrapolating these experimental observations to clinical medicine, a disturbance of phagocytic function of the liver may be implicated in the mechanism of the hyperglobulinaemia which frequently accompanies liver disease and which is considered later in this chapter. Kupffer cells possess several distinct immunological functions. Most human Kupffer cells express major histocompatibility (MHC) class II antigens[46] which are required for the activation of helper/inducer T lymphocytes. They also play an important role in the clearing of microorganisms and immune complexes, possibly by enhancement of free radical production which induces cell killing.[6]

IMMUNOLOGICAL MECHANISMS ASSOCIATED WITH LIVER DISEASE

A wide variety of immunological disturbances have been reported in both acute and chronic liver disease. Disturbances in immunity can be broadly divided into two groups: those involving alterations in B cell function or humoral antibody production, and those in which cellular immunity (T cell function) is affected. The discovery of interleukins has greatly improved our understanding of the mechanisms whereby antigens are recognized by specific lymphocytes. A detailed description of these cytokines may be found elsewhere.[80,81]

DISTURBANCES IN B CELL FUNCTION _____

Early studies of serum proteins in chronic liver disease recognized a reversal in albumin to globulin ratio together with an absolute increase in serum globulin. More specifically, it has been shown that this is mainly due to an increase in serum immunoglobulins,[28] with elevations in IgG being most striking in chronic active hepatitis, IgA in alcoholic liver disease and IgM in primary biliary cirrhosis, although there is a considerable overlap. Havens et al.[40] showed that the raised serum globulin was due to increased synthesis, and this was supported by observations that patients with hepatic cirrhosis had an enhanced capacity to produce circulating antibodies to administered antigens, such as diphtheria toxoid and tetanus antitoxin.[39] Subsequent reports failed to confirm this increased antibody production,[16] but interest in the mechanism of hyperglobulinaemia revived following the demonstration of increased anti-salmonella agglutinins in patients with chronic active hepatitis.[86] This was followed by the report of increased antibody titres to intestinal tract organisms (E. coli and bacteroides) and dietary proteins in patients with cirrhosis and chronic active hepatitis.[107] Increases in E. coli antibody titres were also observed in patients with acute viral hepatitis, these titres returning to normal following resolution of the hepatitis. In contrast, antibody titres to Haemophilus influenzae (a non-intestinal tract organism) were normal throughout the acute hepatitis and were not elevated in chronic liver disease, which argues against a non-specific immune response. Simultaneously, Bjørneboe et al.[15] confirmed high E. coli antibody titres in alcoholic cirrhosis and also observed an increase in E. coli antibody titres in patients following portacaval shunt. These observations suggested that Kupffer cells may fail to sequester antigen absorbed from the gut, either because of functional impairment or as a result of shunting of portal blood, an idea which was well supported by the experimental studies cited earlier.

This explanation fails to account for the grossly elevated antibody titres to certain viruses, notably measles, rubella and cytomegalovirus (CMV), which have been reported in patients with chronic active hepatitis.[110] Although elevated titres to CMV are also found in alcoholic cirrhosis, the raised measles and rubella antibody levels seem to occur only in chronic active hepatitis associated with autoantibodies. Cross-reactivity with these autoantibodies was ruled out by absorption experiments.

These apparently unrelated phenomena led us to suggest a number of different mechanisms to account for the hypergammaglobulinaemia of liver disease[106] (Table 9.1). There is evidence of increased antibody production in patients with liver disease. The spleen and lymph nodes, which are commonly enlarged in patients with chronic liver disease, are the sites of increased concentrations of antibody, demonstrated by immunofluorescence. Immunoglobulins are not normally detectable in the intact liver, although it is capable of synthesizing all other serum proteins. Increased stimulus to antibody production may be provided by the presence of antigens responsible for the liver disease, e.g. the hepatitis virus. Non-specific antigenic stimuli, such as E. coli, may also contribute for reasons discussed earlier. Some of the antibody production may be accounted for by the presence of autoantibodies, which will be considered in greater detail in the next section.

None of these stimuli is likely to be considerable, but other mechanisms may enhance their ability to induce antibody production. The liver may be unable to sequester antigens because of a functional loss of Kupffer cells, either due to a quantitative loss in the Kupffer cell population or because the cells themselves are committed to other functions, such as handling the products of liver cell breakdown that occurs in acute liver cell necrosis. Alternatively, the antigens may fail to reach the liver because of alterations in liver blood flow which often accompany hepatic disorders, or because of shunting of portal blood past the hepatic sinusoids. Prytz et al.,[87] when noting a further increase in serum γ-globulin and E. coli antibody titres in patients following portacaval anastomosis, suggested that extrahepatic shunting may play an important role in producing high serum globulin levels, especially of IgG. This has not been confirmed by Simjee et al.,[93] who favour defective Kupffer cell function or intrahepatic shunting to explain the high bacterial antibody titres. The finding of normal humoral immunity in patients with extrahepatic portal vein thrombosis[117] is further evidence against hyperglobulinaemia being largely due to extrahepatic shunting. Endotoxin is found in higher concentration in the portal compared with the peripheral venous system, and also in higher concentrations in the plasma of cirrhotic than non-cirrhotic subjects. This E. coli lipopolysaccharide is produced in the gastrointestinal tract and is believed to bypass the damaged liver. There is good experimental evidence to show that endotoxin also induces the release of numerous enzymes by Kupffer cells such as interleukins, leukotrienes and superoxides which are likely to affect immune function.[78] Evidence that such mechanisms play a significant role in man is comparatively sparse at present.[103]

The high viral antibody titres in chronic active hepatitis might be related to release of viral antigens sequestered in the liver, analogous to the measles infection which accompanies subacute sclerosing panencephalitis and which leads to comparably high antibody titres, but to measles virus alone. Evidence in support of persistent measles infection is provided by the finding that many patients with chronic active hepatitis have measles virus genome detectable in their peripheral blood mononuclear cells using a 50-base oligonucleotide probe.[90]

T cell function is commonly suppressed in liver disorders and it has been postulated that a disturbance in T/B cell regulation might lead to excessive immunoglobulin production. Mononuclear cells from cirrhotic patients produce increased amounts of IgG compared with those from normal subjects.[12] Although there is an inverse correlation between the suppressor cell activity and serum

Table 9.1 Hyperglobulinaemia in liver disease

	Hepatic	Extrahepatic
Stimulus to production	Infective agent, e.g. virus ?Autoantigens	?Autoantigens Antigenic stimuli not related to pathogenesis
Mechanism of production	Intrahepatic shunting Loss of Kupffer cells Saturation of Kupffer cell phagocytic function	Collateral circulation Reduced liver blood flow Decreased immune surveillance (T/B interaction)
	Release of antigens sequestered in liver Adjuvant effect of liver tissue Loss of normal immunosuppressive effect of liver	Mitogenic stimulus of endotoxin Alterations in T cell subpopulations

IgG,[82] there appear to be serum factors which are capable of stimulating increased immunoglobulin production. Interleukin-6 (IL-6) is a probable example of this, as high serum IL-6 levels have been shown to correlate with serum IgA in alcoholic liver disease and this interleukin is produced in increased amounts by leucocytes.[22] As will be described later, T cell function can now be defined in terms of the relative activity of different population subsets and evidence is accumulating to suggest that the regulatory balance between these may be disturbed in chronic liver disease.

There is considerable evidence to suggest that sequential liver transplantation prolongs the survival of renal and other allografts in experimental animals.[50,94] Although the mechanism is not clearly understood, it may relate to the absorption or neutralization of preformed antibodies by the donor liver. Fung *et al.*[30] have recently reported a series of patients with preformed lymphocytotoxic antibodies undergoing combined liver/kidney transplantation in whom successful grafting was accompanied by a significant reduction or even disappearance of these circulating antibodies.

It seems likely that no single mechanism can account for the elevation in globulins seen in acute and chronic liver disease and their relative importance awaits further elucidation.

Autoantibodies

Gajdusek[31] reported complement-fixing antibodies in the serum of patients with liver disease against an extract of normal human liver, an observation which stimulated much research into the incidence of tissue autoantibodies in hepatic and other disorders. Although most of these have been shown to be neither organ- nor species-specific, many have proved to be useful clinical markers in the investigation of hepatic disease. Details of the occurrence and importance of some of these antibodies are shown in Table 9.2.

Antinuclear antibody

Haserick *et al.*[38] were the first to demonstrate a specific factor in the γ-globulin fraction of patients with systemic lupus erythematosus (SLE) which was responsible for the so-called LE cell phenomenon. This antinuclear factor, subsequently renamed 'antinuclear antibody', can be demonstrated by a variety of immunological techniques, including indirect immunofluorescence, complement fixation, latex precipitation and tanned red cell agglutination. The antibodies are directed against several nuclear constituents, notably deoxyribonucleoprotein, ribonucleic acid and nucleohistones, and they belong to all three major immunoglobulin classes. Because of the heterogeneous nature of the antigen against which they are directed, different immunofluorescent patterns may be produced by antinuclear antibodies: these have been classified as nuclear dots, fine speckled, homogeneous, nucleolar, or centromere.[13] Most of these patterns appear to be non-specific, although reports of associations with primary biliary cirrhosis will be discussed later. The immunoglobulin class and titre of the antibodies are of some diagnostic value, as will be discussed later.

Although most commonly found in the sera of patients with SLE, antinuclear antibodies are also found in most connective-tissue disorders and occasionally in otherwise healthy individuals. An increased frequency is observed in chronic active hepatitis, primary biliary cirrhosis and some drug-associated hepatitis, in contrast to other forms of liver disease.[23] Reports on the frequency of this antibody in the normal population and in certain forms of liver disease (see Table 9.2) are very variable, much of the conflict arising from the difficulty in defining positivity. Low antibody titres of 1 : 10 or less are accepted by most authorities as unimportant, while titres equal to or greater than 1 : 80 are universally considered to be significant. IgG class antibodies are more commonly associated with pathological processes than IgM antibodies.

Table 9.2 Autoantibodies associated with liver disease

Autoantibody	Disease	Frequency (%)	Comments
Antinuclear antibody	Chronic active hepatitis	20–50	High-titre IgG
	Primary biliary cirrhosis	15–40	
	Drug-associated chronic active hepatitis	10–30	
Anti-DNA antibody	All types of liver disease	30–60	
Anti-smooth muscle antibody	Chronic active hepatitis	20–60	High-titre IgG
	Primary biliary cirrhosis	10–30	
	Viral hepatitis	50–80	Low-titre IgM, transient
	Alcoholic liver disease	10–15	Low-titre IgM
Antimitochondrial antibody	Primary biliary cirrhosis	80–95	
	Chronic active hepatitis	10–25	
Bile canalicular antibody	Chronic active hepatitis/primary biliary cirrhosis	20–40	
Liver membrane antibody	HBsAg-negative		
	Acute hepatitis	15	
	Chronic active hepatitis	40	
	Cirrhosis	60	

Anti-DNA antibodies

More specific characterization of the antinuclear antibodies, combined with increasingly sophisticated immunological techniques, led to the development of a radioimmunoassay for double-stranded (native) DNA and the demonstration that it appeared to be specific for SLE.[45] These dsDNA antibodies are also frequently found in patients with autoimmune chronic active hepatitis and they occur in such a wide range of liver disorders as to be of little diagnostic value.[56]

It is of interest that Fournié et al.[29] have shown the induction of anti-DNA antibodies in animals following the injection of bacterial lipopolysaccharides, raising the possibility that the mechanism of anti-DNA antibody production might be related to the elevated *E. coli* antibody titres considered earlier. Alternatively, hepatic- or viral-specific DNA might act as an antigenic stimulus.

Smooth-muscle antibody

Although first described by Johnson et al.[48] in patients with chronic active hepatitis, this autoantibody has been reported in many disorders, both hepatic and non-hepatic. Indirect immunofluorescence remains the sole means of detection and by this technique smooth-muscle antibody may stain the smooth muscle of bile canaliculi, renal glomeruli and thyroid epithelial cells. This antibody reacts with actin and other components of the cytoskeleton.[62] The highest antibody titres are usually found in chronic active hepatitis, are usually of IgG class, and when present may be of diagnostic value. However, lower antibody titres, mainly IgM, are found transiently in viral infections such as viral hepatitis and infectious mononucleosis. We have observed similar reactions in patients with alcoholic

liver disease; such antibodies may also be found in association with malignant disease without any apparent hepatic involvement.

Mitochondrial antibody

This autoantibody is of considerable clinical importance because of its frequent occurrence in primary biliary cirrhosis and rarity in other disorders (see Chapter 32). It is found in over 85% of patients with this disorder, and although some authors report its presence in 10–20% of patients with chronic active hepatitis, this probably reflects a clinical overlap between these two disorders.

There appears to be an increased incidence of antimitochondrial antibody in patients with connective-tissue disorders[108] as well as in the relatives of patients with primary biliary cirrhosis.[32] Although such patients frequently have minor histological abnormalities in the liver, there is no evidence that they invariably progress to develop primary biliary cirrhosis and it is thought that the autoantibody may represent a marker of potential autoimmune disease. On the other hand, the antimitochondrial antibody titre usually falls or even disappears following successful orthotopic liver transplantation,[36] suggesting that elimination or effective immunosuppression of the disease can be achieved. The antimitochondrial antibody in many subjects with no evidence of liver disease is indistinguishable from that found in patients with primary biliary cirrhosis both by titre and immunoglobulin subclass[108] although these have yet to be examined by the most sensitive techniques available (see below).

The autoantibody is predominantly of IgG_3 subclass.[88a] Indirect immunofluorescence is the most widely used technique, but many other methods have been successfully

Table 9.3 Clinical and laboratory characteristics of the antimitochondrial antibodies and antigens

Autoantibody	Immunofluorescent characteristics	Mitochondrial antigen	Clinical association
M1	Diffuse staining of rat kidney and liver Weak staining of human gastric parietal cell	Inner mitochondrial membrane	Cardiolipin antibody
M2	Granular staining of rat kidney and liver Strong staining of human parietal cells	Inner mitochondrial membrane Sucrose density gradient 1.19–1.28 Trypsin sensitive Antigens of M.W. 70, 45 and 39 kD	'Classical' PBC antibody
M3	Similar to M2 but more coarsely granular	Outer mitochondrial membrane not detectable by Western blot	Drug-induced pseudo-lupus syndromes
M4	Similar to M2 Complement fixing	Outer mitochondrial membrane Sucrose density gradient 1.08–1.12 Trypsin insensitive	Chronic active hepatitis/PBC hybrid Associated with M2
M5	Coarse granular or diffuse staining of rat kidney and liver	Outer mitochondrial membrane 61 and 57 kD antigenic determinants	Connective-tissue disorders
M6	Granular fluorescence of kidney proximal tubules	Not visualized by Western blot	Iproniazid hepatitis
M7	Specific to heart mitochondria Not complement fixing	Inner mitochondrial membrane Antigens M.W. 90 and 64 kD	Myocarditis: cardiomyopathies
M8	Complement fixing	Outer mitochondrial membrane Sucrose density gradient 1.14–1.24 Trypsin sensitive	Progressive PBC Only in association with M2
M9	Detected by ELISA using protein-treated sonicated mitochondrial particles from rat liver	Organ specific Outer membrane of liver mitochondria Trypsin insensitive Antigens of M.W. 98 and 59 kD	Early PBC Often in absence of M2

used, including immunoblotting which is the latest and most sensitive to be employed. There have been considerable advances in our knowledge of the antimitochondrial antibody and antigen. The antigens recognized by mitochondrial antibodies are heterogeneous and neither organ nor species specific. Berg and colleagues[11] have reported antibodies to no fewer than nine separate antigens, which they have classified on the basis of their immunofluorescent and biochemical properties (Table 9.3). While many are found in a variety of non-hepatic disorders, antibodies to M2, M4, M8 and M9 appear to be specific for PBC and the German workers have claimed that prognosis of the liver disease may be predicted by the antibody pattern.[11,58] Thus, in a follow-up period of between 6 and 16 years they noted that none out of 4 patients with M9 antibody alone had died compared with 9 out of 23 in whom M2 and M4 and/or M8 were present. An intermediate mortality of 3 out of 32 was observed in patients with M9 and/or M2 antibodies. If confirmed, this would be a unique example of an autoantibody pattern being shown to have a prognostic significance.

Using immunoblotting techniques, sera from over 90% of patients with PBC have been shown to react with three major M2 peptides of 70, 45, and 39 kD molecular weight (Figure 9.2). From a rat liver cDNA library, a 1370-base pair insert has been cloned, sequenced and demonstrated by use of expression vectors to code for a polypeptide that reacts specifically with sera from PBC patients and corresponds to the 70-kD mitochondrial autoantigen.[33] This has also been shown to have sequence homology with the purified E_2 sub-unit of pyruvate dehydrogenase enzyme complex in *E. coli*.[119] More recently it has been shown that PBC-specific mitochondrial antigens with molecular weights of 70 and 50 kD are recognized by antisera against a number of mutants of a range of bacteria.[97] This finding supports the hypothesis of a possible bacterial aetiology for primary biliary cirrhosis. Since this autoantigen would appear to be homologous with the subunit of a critical and ubiquitous enzyme pathway, its role and relevance to the disease is uncertain. Advances in molecular biological techniques should help determine whether these antibodies reflect cross-reactivity

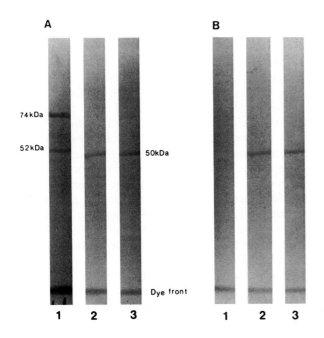

Figure 9.2 Reactivity of two different sera (A and B) from patients with PBC with components of the mitochondrial 2-oxo-acid dehydrogenase complexes. Proteins subjected to SDS-PAGE, transferred to nitrocellulose, and incubated with sera at a dilution of 1 : 1000. *Lane 1*: E_2 and protein X components of pyruvate dehydrogenase complex. *Lane 2*: E_2 component of branched chain 2-oxo-acid dehydrogenase complex. *Lane 3*: E_2 component of 2-oxoglutarate dehydrogenase complex. (Reproduced by kind permission of Dr M.F. Bassendine, University of Newcastle-upon-Tyne, England.)

with biliary epithelial or bacterial products, or whether they represent a more fundamental process relating to the pathogenesis of PBC.

Soluble liver antibody

Manns and co-workers have reported[69] a group of patients with HBsAg-negative chronic active hepatitis whose serum contained autoantibodies directed against a soluble liver antigen. Many of these patients have no other detectable autoantibodies in their serum. Clinically they were indistinguishable from autoimmune chronic active hepatitis and they responded well to immunosuppressive therapy. Soluble liver antigen is distinct from liver-specific lipoprotein (see below). Further studies concerning its nature are required.

Liver–kidney microsomal antibody

Rizzetto and colleagues were the first to describe circulating antibodies reacting with microsomes in kidney and liver in a group of patients with 'idiopathic' chronic active hepatitis.[89] In a large study from France,[42] LKM-positive patients tended to be young females with particularly aggressive liver damage in whom other autoantibodies were usually absent. Nevertheless, they generally responded to immunosuppressive therapy and behaved

like other patients with autoimmune chronic active hepatitis. This antibody appears to be a 50-kD polypeptide, although more recently an additional 66-kD polypeptide antigen has been recognized which may be part of the monooxygenase complex.[20]

The antibody found in chronic active hepatitis (LKM-1) should be distinguished from a similar autoantibody reported in association with tienilic acid-induced hepatitis (LKM-2). Both antibodies are directed against the cytochrome P450 complex in the endoplasmic reticulum but react with different isoenzymes.[3,9]

Bile canalicular antibody

This liver-specific antibody has been reported in the serum of some patients with chronic active hepatitis and primary biliary cirrhosis, but it has not proved useful as a diagnostic tool. Since immunofluorescent staining of bile canaliculi can be seen with sera containing strongly positive antibodies to smooth muscle, and this can be absorbed with purified actin,[60] it seems likely that the bile canalicular antibody is identical to smooth-muscle antibody.

"Liver-specific protein antibody" (LSP)

Meyer zum Büschenfelde and colleagues[72] have purified and characterized two proteins from supernatants of liver cell homogenates (LP1 and LP2) with which they were able to induce, by prolonged immunization in rabbits, a chronic hepatitis resembling human chronic active hepatitis. Further studies on LP1, which has since become known as liver-specific protein (LSP), have shown that it is closely associated with the plasma membrane of hepatocytes.[44] An autoantibody to this liver cell membrane antigen can be detected by immunofluorescence using isolated rabbit hepatocytes and the same group[99] have shown that it is specific for liver disorders. They reported its presence in 38% of patients with chronic active hepatitis, 16% with acute viral hepatitis and 61% with cirrhosis, while others have found it in acute hepatitis A and B, but rarely in non-A non-B hepatitis or in paracetamol (acetaminophen)-induced hepatic necrosis.[70] It is also found in active alcoholic liver disease, where it appears to correlate closely with the presence of a lymphocyte infiltrate on liver biopsy.[84] There was no correlation with the presence of other autoantibodies in any liver disorders. While there are many pointers to the possible role of LSP as an autoantigen in chronic liver disease, further investigation shows that its structure is highly complex, with both liver specific and organ cross-reacting components. Detailed studies of the individual specific antigens are required before any firm conclusions about its pathogenetic significance can be drawn.

Other liver-specific proteins may also exist. Sugamara and Smith[98] have purified and characterized a human liver protein of molecular weight between 40 000 and 80 000 daltons which has been termed F-antigen. Arakawa *et al.*[5] have induced the antigen by giving rabbits carbon tetrachloride and have shown it to be liver-specific. These workers have also detected it in patients with active liver disease but in only a small minority. It is immunologically distinct from LP-2, but its place in the pathogenesis of chronic liver disease has yet to be established.

Other autoantibodies

Anti-γ-globulin antibodies (rheumatoid factors) may be frequently found in all forms of chronic liver disease. Autoantibodies to thyroid and gastric parietal cells are found with increased frequency in patients with chronic active hepatitis, but the incidence in other types of liver disease is unremarkable.

Using immunofluorescent techniques, complement and immunoglobulins can sometimes be detected in the reticuloendothelial system. As mentioned earlier, immunoglobulins are not normally found in the intact liver, but in certain types of liver disease they are readily detectable. It is not known whether they are synthesized within the liver or merely deposited there from elsewhere. The type or nature of the immunoglobulin deposition does not appear to correlate with any clinical or histological parameters of liver disease.

DISTURBANCES IN T CELL FUNCTION _____

Studies of cellular immunity in liver disease have shown almost uniform depression in this arm of the immune response. Several tests are currently available for the assessment of T cell function.

In vivo response to skin test antigens

Using a variety of such antigens, depressed cell-mediated immunity has been demonstrated in all forms of chronic liver disease and even in patients with extrahepatic portal venous obstruction and apparently normal liver function.[117] On the other hand, the results in patients with acute hepatitis have been conflicting.

In vitro tests of mononuclear cell function

Function may be studied either in response to non-specific mitogens such as phytohaemagglutininin (PHA) or to specific antigens (e.g. LSP, hepatitis B virus). Lymphocyte transformation or leucocyte migration inhibition (LMI) are the standard techniques used for this test. Using lymphocyte transformation in response to phytohaemagglutinin, there is general agreement that cellular immunity is impaired in all forms of acute and chronic liver disease. Interpretation of these results, however, is problematical. The finding is non-specific since impairment of PHA transformation may be observed in many non-hepatic inflammatory disorders. Recent experimental studies suggest that PHA may stimulate both T and B cells, so its value as an index of T cell function must be questioned. Furthermore, several groups have demonstrated that a serum factor is involved in the impaired lymphocyte transformation, once more raising doubts as to the specificity of the test. The nature of this serum factor is unknown, but soluble immune complexes have been implicated.

Analysis of T cell subpopulations

The total circulating T cell population is significantly reduced in acute and chronic liver disease,[21,101] but the development of monoclonal antibodies as markers of T lymphocyte subpopulations now permits more precise characterization. The results of such studies in chronic liver disease have been conflicting and, although the CD4/CD8 (helper/suppressor T cell) ratio is usually reduced, attempts to correlate these changes with clinical activity or disease progression have been unsuccessful.

Studies based entirely on circulating blood cell population may be criticized because they reflect the activity of cells in transit to the liver rather than at the site of the inflammation. Examination of liver tissue for T cell subsets has shown that CD8-positive cytotoxic cells predominate in areas of local damage irrespective of the underlying cause of the chronic liver disease.[71]

Critical evaluation of the information provided by monoclonal antibodies is difficult for a number of reasons. Correlation between the number of cells of a particular subset and their function is poor; for example, the CD8 population is increased in acute hepatitis while suppressor cell function in this condition is generally recognized as being reduced. A major limitation of current monoclonal antibodies is the inability to separate suppressor and cytotoxic cells, and until this is possible conclusions on the helper/suppressor cell ratio as an index of immune regulation will be limited. While the antibodies appear to be specific for given antigenic receptors, it is recognized that individual cells may possess more than one type of receptor. To date, these studies have done little to advance the knowledge of cellular immunity in liver disease.

OTHER IMMUNOLOGICAL MECHANISMS _____

Immune complex disorders

Serum complement levels are often low in both acute and chronic liver disease and, while impaired synthesis by the liver may be a factor, there is good evidence to suggest that the low serum level is partly due to the complement consumption which occurs during the formation of antigen–antibody complexes. Experimentally induced complexes are usually cleared from the circulation by the liver and in cirrhotic animals this property is severely impaired.[100]

In situations where the antigen can be defined and quantified (such as hepatitis B surface antigen), good correlation can often be found between the extrahepatic complications of the infection, such as glomerulonephritis or arthritis and the presence of complexes (see Chapter 31). Problems arise when the antigen is unknown. Numerous tests exist for the detection of immune complexes in the serum but they measure complexes of different sizes. It is increasingly recognized that circulating immune complexes may arise in response to any form of inflammation.

It remains uncertain whether or not any of these complexes play a role in initiating or potentiating chronic inflammatory liver disease. Examples of the possible role of immune complexes in various liver disorders will be discussed later.

Cytotoxicity

The in-vitro demonstration of cytotoxicity has formed the basis of much research into the immune mechanisms of liver cell damage. Several types of cell killing are described. Cytotoxic T cell receptors recognize specific antigens on the surface of target cells, providing both target cell and T cell express the same MHC class I antigen. This is believed to be particularly important in the destruction of virus antigen, although data concerning hepatitis B infection are conflicting. Killer (K) cell cytotoxicity depends upon the presence of a specific IgG antibody on a target cell which is attached by a high-affinity but non-specific Fc receptor on the K cell. This phenomenon, known as antibody-dependent cell-mediated cytotoxicity (ADCC), is believed to be responsible for the liver damage produced by reactions against LSP antigens.[66] A third type of cytotoxic mechanism involves cells which do not elicit ADCC and which kill independently of prior sensitization, the so-called natural killer (NK) cells. Morphologically, the NK cells are identical to the pit cells which are a normal component of the liver sinusoid and there is evidence suggesting that pit cells are functionally similar to NK cells (see Chapter 2). Their role in relation to liver disease is not clear, although they are thought to be important as a first-line defence against viral infection and tumour cells. A cytotoxic assay which has been frequently employed is the autologous cytotoxic assay, in which peripheral mononuclear cells are cultured with hepatocytes isolated from the patient's own liver biopsy.[73] The relevance of this technique to clinical disease remains uncertain: it seems likely that additional factors are implicated, including possible immunosuppressor serum factors released by the liver itself.[25]

Interferon

Interferons are a class of proteins produced by cells in response to viruses and other inducers and which have potent antiviral activity. These properties are of particular relevance to chronic hepatitis B and C infection, in which their efficacy has already been established (see Chapter 31). In addition they are known to possess powerful immunoregulatory properties, which include modulating antibody production, affecting cell-mediated immune response, enhancing the expression of MHC antigens on mononuclear cells and enhancing NK cell activity. A detailed review of these effects in chronic viral hepatitis has recently been published.[24]

IMMUNOLOGICAL PHENOMENA ASSOCIATED WITH LIVER DISEASES

CHRONIC ACTIVE HEPATITIS (see also Chapter 31) _____

Much confusion exists in the literature concerning the immunological phenomena associated with chronic active hepatitis, in part at least owing to a failure to distinguish between subgroups of the disease. All have the histological picture of mononuclear cell infiltration, erosion of the limiting plate and piecemeal necrosis regardless of the aetiology.

It is now recognized that the histological features of chronic active hepatitis may be seen as a response to a wide range of stimuli, including hepatitis B, hepatitis C, Wilson's disease, alpha-1-antitrypsin deficiency, alcohol and drugs. In addition, a group of patients (mainly young and middle-aged females) are recognized in whom no aetiology is currently discernible and who are described as having 'autoimmune' or lupoid hepatitis. These patients commonly show striking abnormalities in B-cell parameters. The hyperglobulinaemia associated with this condition is often much higher than is found in any other liver disorder and is largely associated with IgG elevation. Autoantibodies are often found in this group of patients, particularly high-titre IgG class antinuclear and anti-smooth-muscle antibodies. Some of these patients, both clinically and histologically, resemble patients with primary biliary cirrhosis; this is reflected by the increased incidence of positive antimitochondrial antibodies. There is a strong association with the histocompatibility antigens A1, B8 and DR3.[55] This probably indicates that there is a susceptibility gene within the HLA region which interacts with other factors (possibly genetic and environmental), resulting in the clinical disease of auto-immune CAH. Such an HLA association has not been described with chronic active hepatitis due to other aetiologies. Inherited defects in C4 serum levels have been reported in association with autoimmune chronic active hepatitis.[112] Since this component of complement is essential for virus neutralization, the observation supports the hypothesis that viral persistence could be an important aetiological factor in the disorder. Extrahepatic manifestations, such as ulcerative colitis, pleurisy, renal tubular acidosis and endocrine disturbances, are also unusually common in autoimmune chronic active hepatitis. In contrast, polyarteritis nodosa, arthritis and glomerulonephritis are well recognized in association with HBsAg-positive chronic active hepatitis, and are thought to be related to the deposition of HBsAg-related antigen–antibody complexes in the tissues.

The mechanism behind the systemic manifestations in the non-hepatitis B group is unknown. Immune complex formation and deposition is possible, but cannot be established without prior identification of the antigen. Cross-reacting antigens, released after damage to hepatocytes, might elicit an immune response on selected target organs, such as the kidney tubule, as has been postulated to account for the accompanying renal tubular acidosis.[111]

To date there has been no satisfactory explanation for why certain individuals develop chronic active hepatitis in response to stimuli such as alcohol or drugs. Similarly, the initiating factors responsible for autoimmune chronic active hepatitis remain unknown.

PRIMARY BILIARY CIRRHOSIS
(see also Chapter 33)

The most striking serological abnormality associated with this condition is the presence of the antimitochondrial antibody, which is a valuable aid to clinical diagnosis. Although found occasionally in other disorders, the autoantibody has proved valuable in distinguishing this condition from extrahepatic biliary obstruction. The presence and titre of the antibody is in no way related to either the clinical or histological features of the disease and it is unaffected by treatment with immunosuppressive drugs and only transiently by liver transplantation. Antinuclear and anti-smooth-muscle antibodies are found in approximately 20% of patients with primary biliary cirrhosis.[102] The multiple nuclear dot pattern appears to correlate with the sicca syndrome,[61] while the presence of anti-centromere antibodies is related to sclerodactyly.[13] In addition, several other antibodies have been reported in PBC, including those directed against histones,[83] acetylcholine[63] and cardiolipin.[113]

The earliest histological lesion involves damage to the bile ducts, with IgM-staining plasma cells and CD8-positive T lymphocytes evident in this vicinity. There is also an aberrant expression of HLA-DR antigens on bile duct epithelium[7] and this may amplify T cell cytotoxic responses.

All three major immunoglobulins may be raised in this condition, although IgM is the most consistently elevated. At least part of this may be due to an exaggerated secondary IgM response to repeated antigenic exposure.[116] This suggests an in vivo abnormality in immunoglobulin class switching and is consistent with the defective helper/suppressor cell ratio noted in PBC. The abnormality may be genetically determined since there is a high incidence of IgM elevation in first-degree relatives of PBC patients.[104] Nevertheless, attempts to demonstrate an HLA association in PBC have been largely unsuccessful, apart from one report of DR8 in the condition.[35] Elevated levels of serum IgG_3 also occurs commonly; lymphocytes from patients with PBC have been shown in culture to secrete spontaneously high levels of this immunoglobulin.[14] Although modest elevations in total serum globulins are usually found, they are not nearly as high as those seen in lupoid hepatitis. The impairment in cell-mediated immunity seen in both skin and in vitro tests seems to be more marked in primary biliary cirrhosis. This condition is frequently characterized by the presence of granulomas within the liver and occasionally in other tissues, thus raising the possibility of its association with Crohn's disease or sarcoidosis, which may also be associated with anergic phenomena. The in vitro tests, however, are known to be non-specific in nature and more specific discriminants of these disorders have, to date, failed to reveal a common aetiology.

Although increased levels of circulating immune complexes have been reported in PBC, their significance and validity has been questioned.[34] Much of the controversy surrounding their presence as well as the observed abnormalities of complement may relate to the abnormal properties of IgM in this disease.[65]

Epstein and colleagues[26] have drawn attention to similarities between primary biliary cirrhosis and chronic graft-versus-host disease. They have suggested that the histological lesion of primary biliary cirrhosis might reflect a lymphocyte-mediated attack on host bile duct epithelium. This interesting idea has important implications with regard to therapy, but at present lacks any substantial proof.

ALCOHOLIC LIVER DISEASE
(see also Chapter 34)

Autoantibody production is not a noted feature in alcoholic liver disease, although low-titre smooth-muscle antibodies are occasionally found. Serum immunoglobulin levels are frequently elevated, particularly IgG and IgA. The IgG levels often reflect the general disease activity, but raised IgA levels, which are more often the most striking abnormality, occur independently of disease activity or severity. Once again, the reason for this selective elevation is unknown. In both normal and alcoholic sera, monomeric 7SIgA predominates, although polymeric IgA is the major form synthesized in vitro in both groups.[49] The elevated *E. coli* antibody titres noted in alcoholic liver disease are of IgM and not IgA class,[93] and, although immune complexes in the glomeruli of patients with alcoholic cirrhosis are rich in IgA,[18] this may well be secondary to the high serum levels. This may result from an increased antigenic load, either because alcohol alters the gut bacterial flora or because it facilitates uptake across the bowel mucosa. Alternatively, alcohol may suppress hepatic reticuloendothelial function, thereby preventing hepatic sequestration of antigens. As mentioned earlier, the non-specific in vitro tests of cellular immunity have generally shown impaired T cell function.

Immune mechanisms have been proposed and an attempt to explain the wide differences in individual susceptibility to harmful effects on the liver. It is recognized that, whereas fatty liver alone rarely predisposes to cirrhosis, alcoholic hepatitis is usually although not invariably a pre-cirrhotic disorder. It seems unlikely that alcohol itself induces immunological responses, but several of its metabolites have been implicated. Alcoholic hyalin, when added to lymphocytes from patients with alcoholic hepatitis, causes a significant increase in the stimulation index and production of migration-inhibition factor.[64]

Circulating antibodies to alcoholic hyalin can also be detected in the serum of patients with alcoholic liver disease.[51] Acetaldehyde, a major metabolite of alcohol oxidation, has also been suggested as an immunogen, possibly by forming adducts on the plasma membrane which stimulate liver damage.[8] Furthermore, alcohol itself may act by damaging liver cell components, against which serum antibodies undoubtedly develop,[76] but the relation to the liver damage is uncertain.

Antinuclear and anti-smooth-muscle antibodies are found infrequently in alcoholic liver disease, but they appear to be much commoner in women than in men.[59] Since it is widely believed that females are more susceptible to the effects of alcohol-related liver damage than males, this has been cited as evidence in support of the role of immune mechanisms in potentiating alcoholic liver disease. Data on histocompatibility antigens in alcoholic liver disease are conflicting. Although it has been suggested that patients with HLA-B8 are more prone to develop alcoholic cirrhosis,[91] this has not been confirmed by others.

VIRAL HEPATITIS _____

The specific immunological phenomena related to the hepatitis viruses are discussed in Chapters 30 and 31. There are, in addition, non-specific immunological disturbances in acute hepatitis. Serum IgG levels are slightly elevated in both, but IgM levels are said to be higher in HBsAg-negative patients than in hepatitis B,[85] although this has been disputed by other workers. Serum complement is usually low in the early stages of the illness, rising to normal or above later. Anti-smooth-muscle antibodies can frequently be detected in serum at some stage of the disease, but they are usually of low titre and transient. Antinuclear and antimitochondrial antibodies are only rarely found in acute viral hepatitis and then usually only in low titre. Non-specific elevation of antibody titres to gut-associated bacteria such as *E. coli* may occur transiently during hepatitis. Impairment of T cell function may be demonstrated by in vitro tests during acute hepatitis, with restoration to normal activity on recovery from the hepatitis. To date, however, none of the tests has proved to be of value in predicting which patients will recover uneventfully and which will progress to chronic liver disease.

As in acute hepatitis, low-titre anti-smooth-muscle antibodies are commonly detected in chronic hepatitis but they are of no diagnostic or prognostic significance. Two recent studies in chronic non-A non-B (mainly C) hepatitis have shown that the serum IgG levels correlate well with the histological severity of the liver lesion, with normal immunoglobulins being found in CPH, the highest levels in established cirrhosis, and intermediate levels in CAH.[41, 43] No such association has yet been described in chronic hepatitis B infection.

DRUG-ASSOCIATED HEPATITIS
(see also Chapters 30 and 46) _____

Many drugs may produce hepatic damage, either as a toxic reaction or on the basis of a hypersensitivity phenomenon. Distinction between the two mechanisms may often be difficult, but certain features tend to support the concept of a hypersensitivity reaction:

1. The liver damage produced by the drug is not dose dependent.
2. Withdrawal of the drug leads to an improvement in liver function, which deteriorates when the patient is subjected to further challenge with small doses of the drug.
3. Extrahepatic manifestations suggestive of an allergic reaction (e.g. rash, arthralgia, eosinophilia) may accompany the liver reaction. The absence of one or more of these phenomena does not exclude the possibility of a hypersensitivity reaction.

Dose-independent reactions may occur either as a result of metabolism of the drug through a minor metabolic pathway or as a consequence of an immune-mediated reaction. Indeed, both mechanisms may operate, and as our knowledge of biochemical pathways increases so more and more immunological phenomena are likely to be explicable at a molecular level.

It is now recognized that almost every type of acute and chronic hepatic lesion can be mimicked by a drug, although usually only one particular lesion is related to any given drug. The importance of drug-associated hepatic damage is that recognition of the condition and appropriate treatment, which is usually simple withdrawal of the precipitating agent, may prevent progressive liver disease and more serious and even fatal further reactions can be avoided if appropriate advice on the hazards of reintroducing such drugs is given. A few of the drug-related hepatic disorders have been selected for further discussion.

Chlorpromazine

This is recognized as causing a pure cholestatic reaction, with no evidence of a hepatitis-like picture. It is probably the commonest drug-associated liver lesion, occurring in up to 2% of all individuals receiving chlorpromazine. Cholestasis has been reported to occur after a single tablet, and jaundice and pruritis may continue for many months, when it may be mistaken for extrahepatic obstruction. Challenge with repeat administration will usually reproduce the clinical features, but is mostly avoided because of the possibility of inducing prolonged symptoms. Despite the deep and prolonged icterus that may develop, this condition is benign and usually resolves without any residual damage, although progressive damage may ensue.[68] Eosinophilia is an occasional but unremarkable finding. Immunological tests are generally unrewarding. Disturbances in serum immunoglobulins are rare and although serum autoantibodies are sometimes present these are non-specific.[42] Lymphocyte transformation using chlorpromazine as a mitogen is sometimes positive, but it is not sufficiently reliable to be of diagnostic value.

α-Methyldopa

α-Methyldopa is associated with both acute and chronic liver disease. Many cases present with acute hepatitis developing within a few months of starting therapy and which resolves on stopping the drug. In others, the progression of liver disease is insidious and diagnosis may not be made until cirrhosis and its complications have occurred. This is increasingly the mode of presentation today: relatively few patients are commenced on this drug for the treatment of hypertension, so that newly presenting cases are usually the result of many years of therapy. The serological and immunoglobulin abnormalities, when present, are identical to those seen in autoimmune chronic active hepatitis. It is impossible to distinguish between the two conditions but in all suspected cases the drug should be discontinued and an alternative preparation prescribed if indicated. A Coombs' positive haemolytic anaemia may be present, but this is found in 30% of all patients taking α-methyldopa and occurs independently of liver damage. Exposure both in vivo and in vitro of normal human lymphocytes to therapeutic concentrations of the drug leads to reduction in concanavalin-A-induced suppressor cell activity.[57] The authors have suggested that this might lead to unregulated autoantibody production by B cells in affected patients, but why the liver should be the target organ for damage is not clear.

Tienilic acid

The association of acute hepatitis with tienilic acid has been particularly well described in France,[42] where this diuretic has been available for many years. The hepatitis is often severe but it usually resolves following withdrawal of the drug. Patients in whom such improvement does not occur respond rapidly to immunosuppressive therapy. It is characterized by the presence of an anti-liver–kidney microsome antibody (anti-LKM2) whose immunofluorescence pattern differs from the anti-LKM1 seen in juvenile chronic active hepatitis. This antibody appears to occur exclusively in patients with tienilic acid-induced hepatitis since it is absent from the serum of patients with normal liver function tests who take the drug. The responsible antigen has been identified as a cytochrome P450 isoenzyme which metabolizes tienilic acid.[9] Association with other immunological abnormalities is uncommon.

Halothane (see also Chapter 53)

Despite much controversy during the past 25 years, it is now generally recognized that a small but significant number of patients develop abnormalities in liver function following repeated administration of halothane.[118] These abnormalities are generally minor, but occasionally a true hepatitis-like picture, which may even be fulminant, may appear. Repeated exposure using minute quantities of

halothane can produce hepatic disturbances, suggesting the sensitivity phenomenon is not dose related. Although the lesion produced is usually an acute hepatitis, repeated exposure may in some cases lead to a chronic active hepatitis with cirrhosis. Unexplained pyrexia is a common finding, and skin rashes and eosinophilia occur occasionally. Cross-sensitization with other halogenated anaesthetics occurs infrequently if at all. Serum immunoglobulin disturbances in this condition are minimal and anti-nuclear and anti-smooth-muscle antibodies are produced only occasionally and in low titre. It has been possible to demonstrate circulating antibodies which react with an antigen present on the hepatocytes from halothane pre-treated rabbits.[52] Although these appear to be specific to halothane-associated hepatitis, they are only present in 75% of sera from such patients and it is not clear whether they are involved in the pathogenesis of liver damage. The same group have identified three polypeptide antigens of molecular weight 100, 76 and 57 kD against which such antibodies might be directed. It appears that these antibodies recognize epitopes consisting of the trifluoroacetyl group together with associated structural features of protein carriers.[53] The notion that halothane-associated liver damage is due to metabolism of the drug via the reductive pathway is supported by animal studies, and since halothane hepatitis occurs particularly frequently in elderly obese subjects this has been cited as evidence to support similar metabolism in humans. The animal model differs in several important aspects from the human and there is at present little evidence to support the idea of excessive reductive halothane metabolism in halothane hepatitis.[77]

Even if a metabolic basis for halothane hepatitis can be demonstrated, there remains the question of why only a small proportion of patients exposed to repeated halothane suffer liver damage. Farrell and colleagues[27] have reported that lymphocytes from patients and some of their relatives are susceptible to electrophilic metabolites of phenytoin which are generated by rat liver microsomes in the presence of an epoxide hydrolase inhibitor. If this mechanism has any relevance to the pathogenesis of halothane hepatitis, it would support the concept of an abnormal lymphocyte response in susceptible individuals. It also points to a genetic predisposition, but to date familial cases of halothane hepatitis have only seldom been reported.[37]

Isoniazid

The hepatitis-like pattern associated with the antituberculous drug isoniazid provides a good example of the problems of ascribing hypersensitivity phenomena to a drug.[17] The onset of liver damage is variable and often prolonged following exposure to the drug, although re-challenge with isoniazid may produce the clinical and biochemical effects usually associated with drug hypersensitivity reactions. Anti-nuclear antibodies commonly appear in the serum of patients receiving isoniazid, but their presence does not relate to liver damage or other systemic disturbance. In contrast to most drug-associated hepatitis in which autoantibodies are produced, isoniazid reactions have been reported more commonly in males than females. Fever, chills, skin rashes and eosinophilia are notably uncommon in association with isoniazid-associated liver damage. Lymphocyte transformation in the presence of isoniazid has produced conflicting results. There is evidence to suggest that genetically determined rapid acetylation of isoniazid might be related to the frequency with which liver damage occurs, raising the possibility that a metabolite of isoniazid may be the provoking substance.[17] The exact nature of the biochemical disturbance still awaits elucidation.

CONCEPTS OF IMMUNOLOGICAL INJURY

Current theories are based on the assumption that the immune-mediated damage is initiated by antigens expressed on the surface of the hepatocytes. While the liver-specific protein is too crude and heterogeneous, McFarlane and Eddleston[67] have provided evidence to suggest that the asialoglycoprotein receptor may be a candidate for this role. Nevertheless, it seems probable that this is likely to be only one of a number of similar receptors.

Although the concept of autoimmunity or autoreactivity in liver disease has by no means been abandoned, increasing interest is being directed to identifying specific antigens responsible for inducing immune reactions in the liver. Most progress has been made with respect to drug-associated hepatic damage, where the active metabolites of implicated drugs together with specific biochemical pathways are being increasingly identified. Several examples have been described earlier in this chapter. Advances concerning specific viral and microbial antigens have been less dramatic; even here the work involving the mitochondrial antigens in PBC and the measles virus genome in chronic active hepatitis offer promise for the future. It seems probable that the increasing use of molecular biological techniques such as amplification by polymerase chain reaction will prove valuable tools in this direction.

Defective T cell function undoubtedly plays a role in the perpetuation of hepatic inflammation and in the development of chronic liver disease, but the precise mechanism is uncertain and may be multifactorial. Interaction between T and B lymphocytes, T lymphocytes and Kupffer cells, as well as imbalance between suppressor and helper T cell subpopulations, are all likely candidates (Fig. 9.3) and each may be important in specific immune-mediated processes. Interleukin-2 is likely to play a crucial role, and quantitative differences in both serum IL-2[4] and IL-2R[1,75] have been demonstrated in chronic liver disease of various aetiologies. T cell-independent mechanisms also contribute to immunologically mediated damage. Natural killer (NK) cell and antibody-dependent cellular

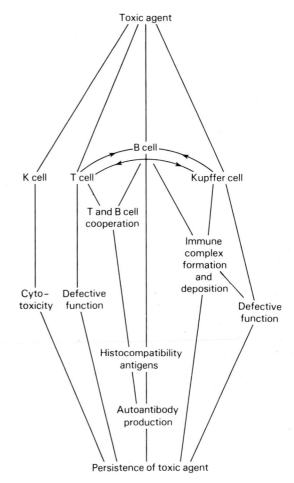

Figure 9.3 Some possible mechanisms involved in the immunological response to liver injury.

cytotoxicity have both been shown to be significant factors in certain situations.

The ability of the Kupffer cell to eliminate viral and other potential toxins and antigens merits further study. Defects in Kupffer cell function in man, due either to an intrinsic defect, competitive blockade, or vascular shunting, may lead to a persistence of the provoking agent which could result in chronic liver damage. Alternatively, this process might induce an inappropriate immune response which would itself be the cause of further damage.

Genetic factors are also likely to play a role in modulating immune responses. The association of A1 B8 DR3 with auto-immune chronic active hepatitis is the only consistent report of an HLA marker in chronic liver disease. Evidence in support of an MHC antigen association with defective immune function is provided by a recent study showing that homozygotes for HLA B8 SCO3 DR3 had a significantly subnormal response to hepatitis B vaccine.[2] HLA-independent factors may also contribute. Krawitt and colleagues,[60] in a family study of first-degree relatives of patients with autoimmune chronic active hepatitis have shown defects in suppressor cell function which are independent of circulating autoantibodies as well as gene segregation for HLA or immunoglobulin allotypes. The demonstration of sensitization to LSP in 24% of first-degree relatives and 27% of spouses of patients with autoimmune chronic active hepatitis suggests the possibility that an environmental factor may influence immune responsiveness.[79]

In conclusion, present knowledge suggests that many distinct but possibly interrelated immunological mechanisms are involved in both the initiation and perpetuation of many liver disorders. It remains impossible to decide whether most of these abnormalities occur as a consequence of the liver damage or whether they are instrumental in producing the destruction. Modern tools of molecular biology now offer hope that individual and specific antigens will become identifiable and such advances will permit greater understanding of the immunological processes involved.

REFERENCES

1. Alberti, A., Chemello, I., Fattovich, G. *et al.* (1989) Serum levels of soluble interleukin-2 receptors in acute and chronic viral hepatitis. *Digestive Diseases and Sciences,* **34,** 1559–1563.
2. Alner, C.A., Kruskall, M.S., Marcus-Bagley, D. *et al.* (1989) Genetic prediction of non response to hepatitis B vaccine. *New England Journal of Medicine,* **321,** 708–712.
3. Alvarez, F., Bernard, D., Homberg, J.C. & Kreibich, G. (1985) Anti-liver-kidney microsome antibody recognises a 50,000 molecular weight protein of the endoplasmic reticulum. *Journal of Experimental Medicine,* **161,** 1231–1236.
4. Anastassakos, Ch., Alexander, G.J.M., Wolstencroft, R.A. *et al.* (1988) Interleukin-1 and interleukin-2 activity in chronic hepatitis B virus infection.*Gastroenterology,* **94,** 999–1005.
5. Arakawa, Y., Bull, D.M., Schott, C.F. & Davidson, C.S. (1976) F-antigen: nature, liver specificity and release in experimental liver injury. *Gastroenterology,* **17,** 118–122.
6. Arthur, M.J.P., Kowalski-Saunders, P. & Wright, R. (1986). Corynebacterium parvum elicited hepatic machrophages demonstrate enhanced respiratory burst activity compared with resident Kupffer cells in the rat. *Gastroenterology,* **91,** 174–181.
7. Ballardini, G., Mirakian, R., Bianchi, F.B. *et al.* (1984) Aberrant expression of HLA-DR antigens on bile duct epithelium in primary biliary cirrhosis: relevance to pathogenesis. *Lancet,* **2,** 1009–1013.
8. Barry, R.E. & McGivan, J.H.D. (1985) Acetaldehyde alone may initiate hepatocellular damage in acute alcoholic liver disease. *Gut,* **26,** 1065–1069.
9. Beaune, P., Dansette, P.M., Mansuy, D. *et al.* (1987) Human anti-endoplasmic reticulum auto-antibodies appearing in a drug-induced hepatitis are directed against a human liver cytochrome P-450 that hydroxylates the drug. *Proceedings of the National Academy of Sciences of the USA,* **84,** 551–555.
10. Benjamin, I.S., Ryan, C.J., McLay, A.L.C. *et al.* (1976) The effects of portacaval shunting and portacaval transposition on serum IgG levels in the rat. *Gastroenterology,* **70,** 661–664.
11. Berg, P.A. & Klein, R. (1987) Immunology of primary biliary cirrhosis. *Baillières Clinical Gastroenterology,* **1,** 675–706.
12. Berger, S.R., Helms, R.A. & Bull, D.M. (1979) Cirrhotic hyperglobulinaemia. Increased rates of immunoglobulin synthesis by circulating lymphoid cells. *Digestive Diseases and Sciences,* **24,** 741–745.
13. Bernstein, R.M., Neuberger, J.M., Bunn, C.G. *et al.* (1984) Diversity of auto-antibodies in primary biliary cirrhosis and chronic active hepatitis. *Clinical and Experimental Immunology,* **55,** 553–560.
14. Bird, P., Calvert, J.F., Mitchison, H. *et al.* (1988) Lymphocytes from patients with primary biliary cirrhosis spontaneously secrete high levels of IgG$_3$ in culture. *Clinical and Experimental Immunology,* **71,** 475–480.
15. Bjørneboe, M., Prytz, H. & Ørskov, F. (1972) Antibodies to intestinal microbes in serum of patients with cirrhosis of the liver. *Lancet,* **1,** 58–60.
16. Bjørneboe, M., Jensen, K.B., Scheibel, I. *et al.* (1970) Tetanus antitoxin production and gamma globulin level in patients with cirrhosis of the liver. *Acta Medica Scandinavica,* **188,** 541–546.
17. Black, M., Mitchell, J.R., Zimmerman, H.J. *et al.* (1975) Isoniazid-associated hepatitis in 114 patients. *Gastroenterology,* **69,** 289–302.
18. Callard, P., Feldmann, G., Prandi, D. *et al.* (1975) Immune complex type glomerulonephritis in cirrhosis of the liver. *American Journal of Pathology,* **80,** 329–340.
19. Cantor, H.M. & Dumont, A.E. (1967) Hepatic suppression of sensitisation to antigen absorbed into the portal system. *Nature,* **215,** 744–745.
20. Codoner-Franch, P., Paradis, K., Guegen, M. *et al.* (1989) A new antigen recognised by anti-liver-kidney microsome antibody (LKMA). *Clinical and Experimental Immunology,* **75,** 354–358.
21. DeHoratius, R.J., Strickland, R.G. & Williams, R.C., Jr. (1974) T and B lymphocytes in acute and chronic hepatitis. *Clinical Immunology and Immunopathology,* **2,** 353–360.
22. Deviere, J., Content, J., Denys, C. *et al.* (1989) High interleukin-6 serum levels and increased production by leucocytes in alcoholic liver cirrhosis. Correlation with IgA serum levels and lymphokines production. *Clinical and Experimental Immunology,* **77,** 221–225.
23. Doniach, D., Roitt, I.M., Walker, J.G. & Sherlock, S. (1966) Tissue antibodies in primary biliary cirrhosis, active chronic hepatitis, cryptogenic cirrhosis and other liver diseases and their clinical implications. *Clinical and Experimental Immunology,* **1,** 237–262.
24. Eddleston, A.L.W.F. & Dixon, B. (1990) Interferons in the treatment of chronic virus infection of the liver. Macclesfield: Pennine Press.
25. Edgington, T.S. (1983) Immune responses and liver disease, perhaps. But what about target organ defenses? *Hepatology,* **3,** 767–768.
26. Epstein, O., Thomas, H.C. & Sherlock, S. (1980) Primary biliary cirrhosis is a dry gland disease with features of chronic graft versus host disease. *Lancet,* **1,** 1166–1168.
27. Farrell, G., Prendergast, D. & Murray, M. (1985) Halothane hepatitis. Detection of a constitutional susceptibility factor. *New England Journal of Medicine,* **313,** 1310–1314.
28. Feizi, T. (1968) Serum immunoglobulins in liver disease. *Gut,* **9,** 193–198.
29. Fournié, G.J., Lambert, P.H. & Miescher, P.A. (1974) Release of DNA in circulating blood and induction of anti-DNA antibodies after injection of bacterial lipopolysaccharides. *Journal of Experimental Medicine,* **140,** 1189–1206.
30. Fung, J., Makowka, L., Tzakis, A. *et al.* (1988) Combined liver-kidney transplantation: Analysis of patients with pre-formed lymphocytotoxic antibodies. *Transplantation Proceedings,* **20,** Supplement 1, 88–91.
31. Gajdusek, D.C. (1957) An 'auto-immune' reaction against human tissue antigens in certain chronic diseases. *Nature,* **179,** 666–668.
32. Galbraith, R.M., Smith, M., Mackenzie, R.M. *et al.* (1974) High prevalence of seroimmunological abnormalities in relatives of patients with CAH and PBC. *New England Journal of Medicine,* **290,** 63–69.
33. Gershwin, M.E., MacKay, I.R., Sturgess, A. & Coppel, R.I. (1987) Identification and specificity of a cDNA encoding the 70Kd mitochondrial antigen recognized in primary biliary cirrhosis. *Journal of Immunology,* **138,** 3525–3531.
34. Goldberg, H., Kaplan, M.M., Mitamuri, T. *et al.* (1982) Evidence against an immune complex pathogenesis of primary biliary cirrhosis. *Gastroenterology,* **83,** 677–683.
35. Gores, G.J., Moore, S.B., Fisher, L.D. *et al.* (1987) Primary biliary cirrhosis: associations with class II major histocompatibility complex antigens. *Hepatology,* **7,** 889–892.
36. Haagsma, E.B., Manns, M., Klein, R. *et al.* (1987) Sub-types of antimitochondrial antibodies in Primary Biliary Cirrhosis before and after orthotopic liver transplantation. *Hepatology,* **7,** 129–133.
37. Haft, R.H., Bunker, J.F., Goodman, M.H. & Gregory, P.B. (1981)

Halothane hepatitis in three pairs of closely related women. *New England Journal of Medicine*, **304**, 1023–1024.

38. Haserick, J.R., Lewis, L.A. & Bortz, D.W. (1950) Blood factor in acute disseminated lupus erythematosus. 1. Determination of gamma globulin as specific plasma fraction. *American Journal of Medical Sciences*, **219**, 660–663.

39. Havens, W.P., Meyerson, R.M. & Klatchko, J. (1957) Production of tetanus antitoxin by patients with hepatic cirrhosis. *New England Journal of Medicine*, **257**, 637–643.

40. Havens, W.P., Dickensheets, J., Bierly, J.N. & Eberhard, T.P. (1954) The half-life of I^{131} labelled normal human gamma globulin in patients with hepatic cirrhosis. *Journal of Immunology*, **73**, 256–258.

41. Hay, C.R.M., Preston, F.F., Triger, D.R. *et al.* (1987) Predictive markers of chronic liver disease in haemophilia. *Blood*, **69**, 1595–1599.

42. Homberg, J.C., Abuaf, N., Bernard, O. *et al.* (1987) Chronic active hepatitis associated with anti-liver/kidney microsome antibody type I: a second type of "auto-immune" hepatitis. *Hepatology*, **7**, 1333–1339.

43. Hopf, U., Moller, B., Kuther, D. *et al.* (1990) Long-term follow-up of post-transfusion and sporadic non-A, non-B hepatitis and frequency of circulating antibodies to hepatitis C virus (HCV). *Journal of Hepatology*, **10**, 69–76.

44. Hopf, U. & Meyer zum Büschenfelde, K.H. (1974) Studies on the pathogenesis of experimental chronic active hepatitis in rabbits. II Demonstration of immunoglobulin on isolated hepatocytes. *British Journal of Experimental Pathology*, **55**, 509–513.

45. Hughes, G.V.R. (1971) Significance of anti-DNA antibodies in systemic lupus erythematosus. *Lancet*, **2**, 861–863.

46. Hume, D.A., Allan, W., Hogan, P.G. & Doe, W.F. (1987) Immunohistochemical characterisation of macrophages in liver and gastrointestinal tract. Expression of CD4, HLA-DR, OKM1 and the mature marker 25F9 in normal and diseased tissue. *Journal of Leukocyte Biology*, **42**, 474–484.

47. Inchley, C.J. (1969) The activity of mouse Kupffer cells following intravenous injection of T4, bacteriophage. *Clinical and Experimental Immunology*, **5**, 173–187.

48. Johnson, G.D., Holborow, E.J. & Glynn, L.E. (1965) Antibody to smooth muscle in patients with liver disease. *Lancet*, **2**, 878–879.

49. Kalsi, J., Delacroix, D. & Hodgson, H.J.F. (1982) High serum IgA levels in alcoholic cirrhosis do not reflect impaired clearance of polymeric IgA by the liver. *Gut*, **23**, A460–461.

50. Kamada, N. (1985) The immunology of experimental liver transplantation in the rat. *Immunology*, **55**, 369–389.

51. Kanagasundaram, N., Kakumu, S., Chen, I. & Leevy, C.M. (1977) Alcoholic hyalin antigen (AHAg) and antibody (AHAb) in alcoholic hepatitis. *Gastroenterology*, **73**, 1368–1373.

52. Kenna, J.G., Neuberger, J. & Williams, R. (1984) An enzyme linked immunosorbent assay for detection of antibodies against halothane altered hepatocyte antigens. *Journal of Immunological Methods*, **75**, 3–14.

53. Kenna, J.G., Satoh, H., Christ, D.D. & Pohl, L.R. (1988) Metabolic basis for a drug hypersensitivity: antibodies in sera from patients with halothane hepatitis recognise liver neoantigens that contain the trifluoroacetyl group derived from halothane. *Journal of Pharmacology and Experimental Therapeutics*, **245**, 1103–1109.

54. Keraan, M., Meyers, O.L., Engelbrecht, G.H.C. *et al.* (1974) Increased serum immunoglobulin levels following portacaval shunt in the rat. *Gut*, **15**, 468–472.

55. Kilby, A.E., Albertini, R.J. & Krawitt, E.L. (1986) HLA typing and autoantibodies in hepatitis B surface antigen-negative chronic active hepatitis. *Tissue Antigens*, **28**, 214–217.

56. Kingham, J.G.C., Rassam, S., Ganguly, N.K. *et al.* (1978) DNA-binding antibodies and hepatitis B markers in acute and chronic liver disease. *Clinical and Experimental Immunology*, **33**, 204–210.

57. Kirtland, H., Daniel, M.D., Mohler, M.D. & Horwitz, D.A. (1980) Methyldopa inhibition of suppressor lymphocyte function. *New England Journal of Medicine*, **302**, 825–831.

58. Klein, R., Kloppel, G., Fischer, R. *et al.* (1988) The antimitochondrial antibody M-9. A marker for the diagnosis of early primary biliary cirrhosis. *Journal of Hepatology*, **6**, 299–306.

59. Krasner, N., Davis, M., Portmann, B. & Williams, R. (1977) Changing pattern of alcoholic liver disease in Great Britain: relation to sex and signs of auto-immunity. *British Medical Journal*, **1**, 1497–1500.

60. Krawitt, E.L., Kilby, A.F., Albertini, R.J. *et al.* (1988) An immunogenetic study of suppressor cell activity to autoimmune chronic active hepatitis. *Clinical Immunology and Immunopathology*, **46**, 249–257.

61. Kurki, P., Gripenberg, M., Teppu, A.M. & Salaspuro, M. (1984) Profile of anti-nuclear antibodies in chronic active hepatitis, primary biliary cirrhosis and alcoholic liver disease. *Liver*, **4**, 134–138.

62. Kurki, P., Miettinen, A., Salaspuro, M. *et al.* (1983) Cytoskeleton antibodies in chronic active hepatitis, primary biliary cirrhosis and alcoholic liver disease. *Hepatology*, **3**, 297–302.

63. Kyriatsoulis, A., Manns, M., Gerken, G. *et al.* (1988) Immunochemical characterization of anti-acetylcholine receptor antibodies in primary biliary cirrhosis. *Journal of Immunology*, **6**, 283–290.

64. Leevy, C.M., Chen, T. & Zetterman, R. (1975) Alcoholic hepatitis, cirrhosis and immunologic reactivity. *Annals of the New York Academy of Sciences*, **252**, 106–115.

65. Lindgren, S. & Eriksson, S. (1982) IgM in primary biliary cirrhosis: Physiochemical and complement activating properties. *Journal of Laboratory and Clinical Medicine*, **99**, 636–645.

66. McFarlane, I.G. & Williams, R. (1985) Review: liver membrane antibodies. *Journal of Hepatology*, **1**, 313–319.

67. McFarlane, I.G. & Eddleston, A.L.W.F. (1989) Chronic active hepatitis. In Targan, S.R. & Shanahan, F. (eds) *Immunology and Immunopathology of the Liver and Gastrointestinal Tract*, pp. 281–304. New York: Igaku-Shin.

68. Maddrey, W.C. & Boitnott, J.K. (1977) Drug-induced chronic liver disease. *Gastroenterology*, **77**, 1348–1353.

69. Manns, M., Gerken, G., Kyriatsoulis, A. *et al.* (1987) Characterization of a new subgroup of autoimmune chronic active hepatitis by autoantibodies against a soluble liver antigen. *Lancet*, **1**, 292–294.

70. Meliconi, R., Perperas, A., Jensen, D. *et al.* (1982) Anti-LSP antibodies in acute liver disease. *Gut*, **23**, 603–607.

71. Meyer, S.C., Moebius, U., Manns, M.M. *et al.* (1988) Clonal analysis of human T lymphocytes infiltrating the liver in chronic active hepatitis B and primary biliary cirrhosis. *European Journal of Immunology*, **18**, 1447–1452.

72. Meyer zum Büschenfelde, K.H., Kössling, F.K. & Miescher, P.A. (1972) Experimental chronic active hepatitis in rabbits following immunisation with human liver proteins. *Clinical and Experimental Immunology*, **11**, 99–108.

73. Mondelli, M., Mieli-Vergani, G., Alberti, A. *et al.* (1982) Specificity of T-lymphocyte cytotoxicity to autologous hepatocytes in chronic hepatitis B Virus infection: evidence that T cells are directed against HBV core antigen expressed on hepatocytes. *Journal of Immunology*, **129**, 2773–2778.

74. Moult, P.J.A., Adjukiewicz, A.B., Gaylarde, P.M. *et al.* (1975) Lymphocyte transformation in halothane-related hepatitis. *British Medical Journal*, **2**, 69–70.

75. Muller, C., Knoflach, P. & Zielinski, C.C. (1989) Soluble interleukin-2 receptor in acute viral hepatitis and chronic liver disease. *Hepatology*, **10**, 928–932.

76. Neuberger, J., Crossley, I.R., Saunders, J.B. *et al.* (1984) Antibodies to alcohol altered liver cell determinants in patients with alcoholic liver disease. *Gut*, **25**, 300–304.

77. Neuberger, J. & Kenna, J.G. (1987) Halothane hepatitis: a model of immune mediated drug hepatoxicity. *Clinical Science*, **72**, 263–270.

78. Nolan, J.P. (1989) Intestinal endotoxins as mediators of hepatic injury. *Hepatology*, **10**, 887–891.

79. O'Brien, C.J., Vento, S., Donaldson, P.T. *et al.* (1986) Cell mediated immunity and suppressor-T-cell defects to liver derived antigens in families of patients with autoimmune chronic active hepatitis. *Lancet*, **1**, 350–353.

80. O'Garra, A. (1989) Interleukins and the immune system 1. *Lancet*, **1**, 943–947.

81. O'Garra, A. (1989) Interleukins and the immune system 2. *Lancet*, **1**, 1003–1005.

82. Pan Bo Rong, Kalsi, J. & Hodgson, H.J.F. (1983) Hyper-globulinaemia correlates with decreased suppressor cell activity in chronic liver disease. *Clinical Science and Molecular Medicine*, **64**, 41P.

83. Penner, E., Muller, S., Zimmermann, D. & Van Regenmortel, M.H.V. (1987) High prevalence of antibodies to histones among

patients wih primary biliary cirrhosis. *Clinical and Experimental Immunology*, **70**, 47–52.

84. Perperas, A., Tsantoulas, D., Portmann, A. *et al.* (1981) Autoimmunity to a liver membrane lipoprotein and liver damage in alcoholic liver disease. *Gut*, **22**, 149–152.

85. Peters, C.J. & Johnson, K.M. (1972) Serum immunoglobulin levels in Australia antigen positive and Australia antigen negative hepatitis. *Clinical and Experimental Immunology*, **11**, 381–391.

86. Protell, R.L., Soloway, R.D., Martin, W.J. *et al.* (1971) Antisalmonella agglutinins in chronic active liver disease. *Lancet*, **ii**, 330–332.

87. Prytz, H., Bjørneboe, M., Johansen, T.S. & Ørskov, F. (1974) The influence of portosystemic shunt operation on immunoglobulins and *Escherichia coli* antibodies in patients with cirrhosis of the liver. *Acta Medica Scandinavica*, **196**, 109–112.

88. Ravin, H.A., Rowley, D., Jenkins, C. & Fine, J. (1960) On the absorption of bacterial endotoxin from the gastro-intestinal tract of the normal and shocked animal. *Journal of Experimental Medicine*, **112**, 783–792.

88a. Riggione, O., Stokes, R.P. & Thompson, R.A. (1983) Predominance of IgG3 subclass in primary biliary cirrhosis. *British Medical Journal*, **286**, 1015–1016.

89. Rizzetto, M., Swana, G. & Doniach, D. (1973) Microsomal antibodies in active chronic hepatitis and other disorders. *Clinical and Experimental Immunology*, **15**, 331–344.

90. Robertson, D.A.F., Zhang, S.I., Guy, E.C. & Wright, R. (1987) Persistent measles virus genome in autoimmune chronic active hepatitis. *Lancet*, **1**, 9–11.

91. Saunders, J.B., Wodak, A.D., Haines, A. *et al.* (1982) Accelerated development of alcoholic cirrhosis in patients with HLA B8. *Lancet*, **1**, 1381–1384.

92. Sell, S. & Fahey, J.L. (1967) Relationship between gamma-globulin metabolism and low serum gamma-globulin in germ-free mice. *Journal of Immunology*, **93**, 81–87.

93. Simjee, A.E., Hamilton-Miller, J.M.T., Thomas, H.C. *et al.* (1975) Antibodies to *Escherichia coli* in chronic liver diseases. *Gut*, **16**, 871–875.

94. Simpson, K.M., Bunch, D.I., Amemiva, H. *et al.* (1970) Humoral antibodies and coagulation mechanisms in the accelerated or hyperacute rejection of renal homografts in sensitized canine recipients. *Surgery*, **68**, 77–85.

95. Sleyster, E.C. & Knook, D.L. (1982) Relation between localization and function of rat liver Kupffer cells. *Laboratory Investigation*, **47**, 484–490.

96. Souhami, R.L. (1972) The effect of colloidal carbon on the organ distribution of sheep red cells and the immune response. *Immunology*, **22**, 685–694.

97. Stemerowicz, R., Hopf, U., Moller, B. *et al.* (1988) Are antimitochondrial antibodies in primary biliary cirrhosis induced by R (rough)-mutants of enterobacteriaceae. *Lancet*, **2**, 1166–1170.

98. Sugamara, K. & Smith, J.B. (1976) Purification and characterisation of human liver specific F antigen. *Clinical and Experimental Immunology*, **26**, 28–34.

99. Tage-Jensen, U., Arnold, W., Dietrichson, O. *et al.* (1977) Liver-cell-membrane autoantibody specific for inflammatory liver diseases. *British Medical Journal*, **1**, 206–208.

100. Thomas, H.C., MacSween, R.N.M. & White, R.G. (1973) Role of the liver in controlling the immunogenicity of commensal bacteria in the gut. *Lancet*, **1**, 1288–1291.

101. Thomas, H.C., Freni, M., Sanchez-Tapias, J. *et al.* (1976) Peripheral blood lymphocyte populations in chronic liver disease. *Clinical and Experimental Immunology*, **26**, 222–227.

102. Triger, D.R. (1990) Primary biliary cirrhosis. *Medicine International*, **84**, 3470–3472.

103. Triger, D.R. (1991) Endotoxaemia in liver disease—time for reappraisal? *Journal of Hepatology*, **12**, 136–138.

104. Triger, D.R. Muggleton, R.J. & Carter, N.D. (1989) IgM abnormalities in the families of patients with primary biliary cirrhosis. *Journal of Gastroenterology and Hepatology*, **4**, Supplement 1, 58–59.

105. Triger, D.R. & Wright, R. (1973) Studies on the hepatic uptake of antigen. II. The effect of hepatotoxins on the immune response. *Immunology*, **25**, 951–956.

106. Triger, D.R. & Wright, R. (1973) Hyperglobulinaemia in liver disease. *Lancet*, **1**, 1494–1496.

107. Triger, D.R., Alp, M.H. & Wright, R. (1972) Bacterial and dietary antibodies in liver disease. *Lancet*, **1**, 60–63.

108. Triger, D.R., Charlton, C.A.C. & Ward, A.M. (1982) What does the antimitochondrial antibody mean? *Gut*, **23**, 814–818.

109. Triger, D.R., Cynamon, M.H. & Wright, R. (1973) Studies on the hepatic uptake of antigen. I. Comparison of inferior vena cava and portal vein routes of immunization. *Immunology*, **25**, 941–950.

110. Triger, D.R., Kurtz, J.B. & Wright, R. (1974) Viral antibodies and auto-antibodies in chronic liver disease. *Gut*, **15**, 94–98.

111. Tsantoulas, D.C., McFarlane, I.G., Portmann, B. *et al.* (1974) Cell-mediated immunity to human Tamm–Horsfall glycoprotein in autoimmune liver disease with renal tubular acidosis. *British Medical Journal*, **4**, 491–494.

112. Vergani, D., Wells, L., Larcher, V.F. *et al.* (1985) Genetically determined low C4: a predisposing factor to autoimmune chronic active hepatitis. *Lancet*, **2**, 294–298.

113. Verrier Jones, J., Mosher, D.P., Jones, E. *et al.* (1989) Antibodies to cardiolipin in patients with primary biliary cirrhosis. *Canadian Journal of Gastroenterology*, **3**, 98–102.

114. Walton, B., Simpson, B.R., Strunin, L. *et al.* (1976) Unexplained hepatitis following halothane. *British Medical Journal*, **i**, 1171–1176.

115. Warshaw, A.L., Walker, W.A. & Isselbacher, K.J. (1974) Protein uptake by the intestine: evidence for absorption of intact macromolecules. *Gastroenterology*, **66**, 987–992.

116. Watmough, D., French, M.A. & Triger, D.R. (1987) Antibody responses to tetanus toxoid in patients with primary biliary cirrhosis. *Journal of Pathology*, **70**, 683–686.

117. Webb, L.J., Ross, M., Markham, R.L. *et al.* (1980) Immune function in patients with extrahepatic portal vein obstruction and the effect of splenectomy. *Gastroenterology*, **79**, 99–105.

118. Wright, R., Eade, O.E., Chisholm, K. *et al.* (1975) Controlled prospective study of the effect on liver function of multiple exposures to halothane. *Lancet*, **1**, 817–820.

119. Yeaman, S.J., Fussey, S.P., Danner, D.J. *et al.* (1988) Primary biliary cirrhosis identification of two major M2 mitochondrial autoantigens. *Lancet*, **1**, 1067–1070.

CHAPTER 10

Physical Aspects of Hepatic Regeneration

Stephen Karran and Magnus McLaren

Extensive resection of normal liver is compatible with survival and return to full health because of the capacity of the remnant to regenerate. Recovery has been reported following 80–90% resection (see Chapter 54). Not only is there rapid increase in the size of the liver cells (hypertrophy) but there is also active cell division and multiplication (hyperplasia), with the peak of mitotic activity occurring some 24–36 h after hepatectomy in parenchymal cells and later in sinusoidal and Kupffer cells[20] (Figure 10.1). In both animals and man there is thus an early increase in the mass and number of cells so that the liver tissue is restored with remarkable rapidity. In addition, repeated hepatectomy is feasible in the same animal following recovery.[42] Liver function also recovers quickly following the restoration of tissue,[7] provided no prior liver damage existed and that complications such as infection or anoxia are avoided. The severity of metabolic abnormality resulting from hepatectomy is directly related to the extent of the resection.[49] The restoration of mass, cell population and function constitutes 'regeneration', which may be contrasted with normal developmental growth and the additive forms of growth seen in pregnancy, lactation and hyperplasia.

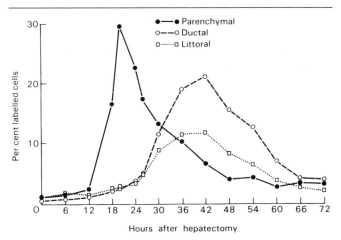

Figure 10.1 Mitotic activity in parenchymal, littoral and Kupffer cells following partial hepatectomy in the rat. (From ref. 10, with kind permission of the authors and the publisher, Little, Brown.)

RATE OF REGENERATION

Regeneration of the liver occurs in many species. Man, rodents, dogs, pigs, frogs and birds all exhibit a similar ability to restore lost or damaged tissue. The rate at which the remnant grows varies from species to species. In the rat, for example, following 67% hepatectomy,[22] normal mass and volume are restored within 7–10 days[25] (Figure 10.2). In dogs the process is slower. In children and young adults there is evidence that considerable restoration is detectable within the first 10 days following

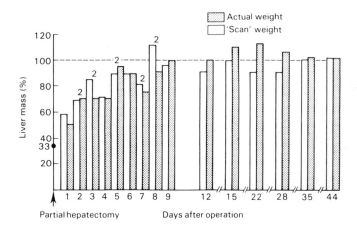

Figure 10.2 Histogram of liver growth in the rat following 67% hepatectomy assessed by in vivo imaging and sacrificial weight measurements. Liver mass is given as a percentage of the calculated prehepatectomy weight. (From ref. 25, with kind permission of the authors and the editor of the *Journal of Nuclear Medicine*.)

hemihepatectomy and this progresses considerably within the first few weeks[7] (Figure 10.3). Full restoration of mass has been recognized within 6 months,[2,18] but the process is probably more rapid than this in previously fit young patients. The radioisotope image in Figure 10.4 was obtained in a 9-year-old girl 3 weeks after splenectomy and right hemihepatectomy had been performed following a road traffic accident. It can be seen that not only has the remnant grown to the right to fill most of the space previously occupied by the right lobe of the liver, but also towards the left to occupy the splenic space. Similar conclusions can be made from observations on three patients who died from head and chest injuries at 1, 6 and 10 days after right hemihepatectomy (Figure 10.5). There was a rapid increase in the mass of the residual liver, so that in the patient who died 10 days after

resection the normal liver weight had been very nearly regained in this short space of time.

From these imaging studies and weight calculations it therefore appears that the growth of the remnant commences very rapidly after operation, provided complications such as anoxia and sepsis are avoided. Within a few weeks this process is well advanced and liver function returns rapidly to normal.[49] Previous estimates that suggest that 4–6 months are necessary before full restoration of mass is achieved are therefore almost certainly conservative in fit young patients.[30,31,36]

As the remnant grows, its shape is largely determined by external pressure. No new lobes develop, although the new liver that is formed is microscopically normal. The residual lobes grow until they are equal in size and volume to the original liver; a small amount of 'overshoot' may be seen. The remnant adapts itself to the available space as it grows. For example, following right hemihepatectomy in man the remnant grows in a globular fashion until it becomes moulded within the confines of the diaphragm and abdominal wall (Figure 10.6). Similarly, following splenectomy as well as partial hepatectomy, the remnant grows across to occupy the space previously filled by the spleen as well as growing into the space resulting from removal of the right lobe of the liver (Figure 10.4).

HEPATIC PERFUSION

Controversy has existed for many years about the relevance of alterations in blood flow to the remnant following partial hepatectomy. As a result of the work of Mann and his colleagues,[29] it was postulated that an increase in flow to the remnant was the prime cause of the regenerative response. Increased perfusion results from diversion of all the blood in the portal vein and hepatic artery into the remnant. Associated with this diversion, an increase in portal pressure is found.[39] Following portacaval shunt-

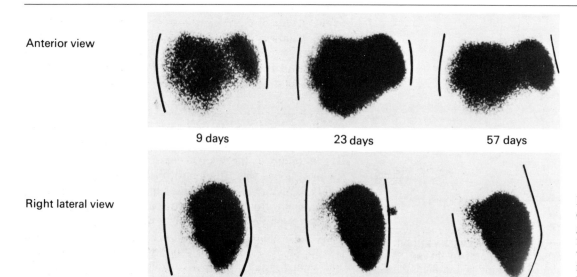

Figure 10.3 Further example of the early growth seen on radioisotope imaging, with little further increase in size after 23 days.

Figure 10.4 Gamma camera image in a girl of 9 years age 3 weeks after right hemihepatectomy and splenectomy. The heavy lines indicate the costal margins. Note that the liver remnant fills the regions previously occupied by both the spleen and the right lobe of the liver. (From ref. 7, with kind permission of the authors and the editor of *Gut*.)

ing, a decrease in liver size (atrophy) occurs, and when partial hepatectomy is performed following portacaval shunting the ability of the remnant to increase in *size* is severely inhibited. However, Weinbren[48] has shown that DNA synthesis and mitotic activity are still increased under these circumstances, indicating the presence of true hyperplasia. Diversion of portal venous blood with possible 'trophic' substances does not, therefore, deprive the remnant of its ability to regenerate. If such 'trophic' substances are responsible for the initiation and control of regeneration, these may still reach the remnant through the systemic circulation and ultimately the hepatic artery, even though they may suffer degradation and dilution in the process. The biochemical and molecular mechanisms initiating and promoting regeneration are detailed in Chapter 11.

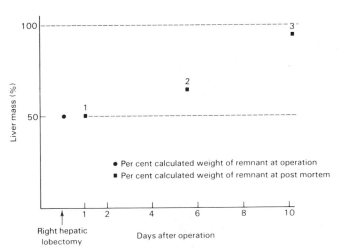

Figure 10.5 Estimations of the growth of the liver remnant in three patients who died at 1, 6 and 10 days after right hepatectomy.

Perfusion by both portal vein and hepatic artery, however, enables the full regenerative response to occur. Following portacaval shunting, partial hepatectomy produces an increased flow in the residual branches of the hepatic artery. Changes in perfusion of the remnant therefore still occur, though the increase is far less than that which occurs in the presence of an intact portal circulation. Following partial hepatectomy in the rat, a marked increase in 'specific' liver blood flow, i.e. ml/g, to the remnant was shown by both sacrificial uptake studies,[6,39] and in vivo techniques[16,21,26] (Figure 10.7). A similar pattern is seen in all these studies, although there are differences in the extent and timing of the increased perfusion. In Benacerraf's study[6] and Guest's[21] a delay of 16 and 4 h respectively occurred before maximal increases were seen. Both Rabinovici's study[39] and our own in vivo dynamic gamma camera study,[26] however, showed that maximal values were obtained *immediately* following hepatectomy. An *immediate* increase in perfusion of the remnant would appear the more probable event following occlusion of inflow to the resected lobes. Colloid uptake studies also show that the maximal increase occurs immediately following resection[24] (Figure 10.8). Delay in the demonstration of maximal perfusion in the other studies probably results from differences in technique.

The in vivo method of assessment of hepatic perfusion using the gamma camera and pinhole collimator is relatively simple and allows repeated examinations in the same animal (Figure 10.9). The isotope used, ^{99m}Tc, as a sulphur colloid, has a half-life of 6 h. Residual activity is insignificant 12 h after previous imaging, and repeated studies are therefore possible (Figure 10.10).

A compartmental mathematical model for the estimation of hepatic perfusion can be utilized for studying the changes produced by partial hepatectomy, hepatic

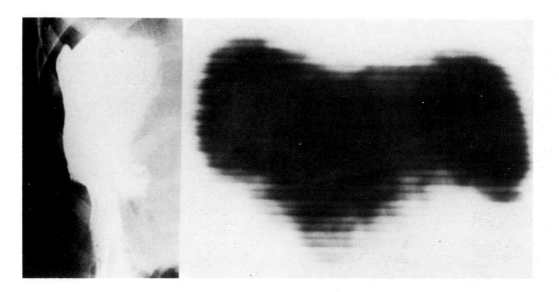

Figure 10.6 Sinogram in a patient who developed a subphrenic abscess following right hemihepatectomy, showing the globular enlargement of the remnant, which has grown to within 2 cm of the abdominal wall. This was confirmed at laparotomy. (From ref. 7, with kind permission of the authors and the editor of *Gut*.)

arterial ligation, portacaval diversion and transplantation (Figure 10.11).

In this model K_1 and K_2 represent the effective perfusion rates (in ml/min) of the liver and extrahepatic reticuloendothelial sites respectively. The effective perfusion rate is given by the product of the true perfusion rate and the extraction efficiency of the colloid, i.e. hepatic colloid trapping in a single passage.

This model is slightly simplified from the actual situation, since the fraction of the hepatic portal supply derived from the spleen has a reduced concentration of colloid due to splenic trapping. This simplification is valid as splenic perfusion is only 3% of total reticuloendothelial perfusion.[26]

Assuming that the colloid has been completely cleared from the blood at the end of imaging, measurement of the ratio of activity from the liver to that from the rest of the body enables the ratio K_1/K_2 to be calculated.

Since $(K_1 + K_2)/V$ and K_1/K_2 are both known, and assuming a value for the blood volume V of 5.93 ml/100 g body weight,[47] K_1 can be derived.

In this study, 1 mCi of ^{99m}Tc sulphur colloid (SC) was administered intravenously and extraction efficiency was measured separately in normal animals and also following partial hepatectomy. Anaesthetized animals were positioned under the gamma camera so that heart, spleen and liver could be imaged, and ^{99m}Tc SC was then injected into the tail vein. Figure 10.12 shows a typical hepatic colloid uptake curve in a normal and a partially hepatectomized animal.

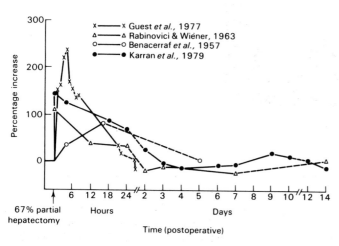

Figure 10.7 Change in 'specific' liver perfusion following 67% hepatectomy in the rat by both sacrificial[6,39] and in vivo techniques.[21,26] (From ref. 26, with kind permission of the authors and the editor of the *Journal of Nuclear Medicine*.)

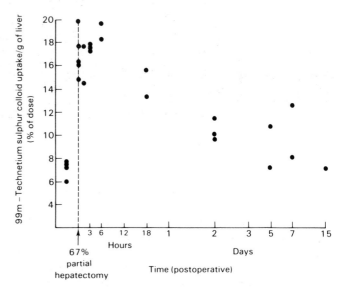

Figure 10.8 Change in hepatic uptake of colloid following 67% hepatectomy in the rat.

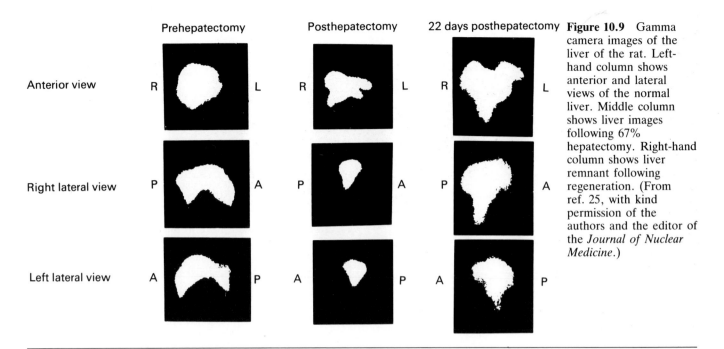

	Prehepatectomy	Posthepatectomy	22 days posthepatectomy
Anterior view	R	R	R
Right lateral view	P	P	P
Left lateral view	A	A	A

Figure 10.9 Gamma camera images of the liver of the rat. Left-hand column shows anterior and lateral views of the normal liver. Middle column shows liver images following 67% hepatectomy. Right-hand column shows liver remnant following regeneration. (From ref. 25, with kind permission of the authors and the editor of the *Journal of Nuclear Medicine*.)

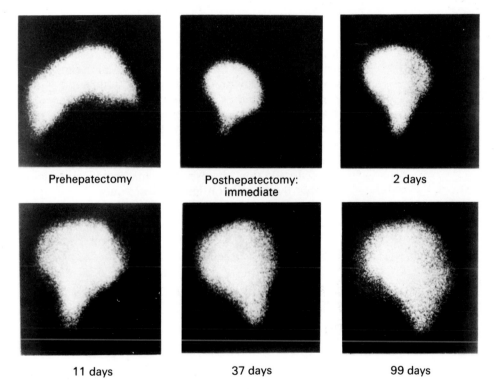

Prehepatectomy / Posthepatectomy: immediate / 2 days / 11 days / 37 days / 99 days

Figure 10.10 Sequential scans obtained following 67% hepatectomy (left lateral views).

The extraction efficiency of the liver can be estimated (Figure 10.13). Extraction efficiency in normal animals was 81%. This fell to 61% immediately after partial hepatectomy, but within 4 days extraction efficiency had returned to normal as regeneration proceeded (Table 10.1).

A liver uptake constant $[(K_1 + K_2)/V]$ can be calcu-

lated. The blood volume, V, following partial hepatectomy is assumed to be 10% less than normal as a result of blood loss.[7] True perfusion rates are then obtained by dividing the effective perfusion rate by the appropriate extraction efficiency.

Following 67% partial hepatectomy this method demonstrated an immediate increase in perfusion of each gram

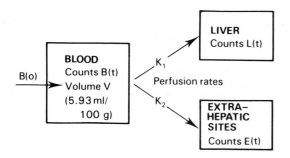

Figure 10.11 Compartmental model for measuring hepatic perfusion. (From ref. 26, with kind permission of the editor of the *Journal of Nuclear Medicine*.)

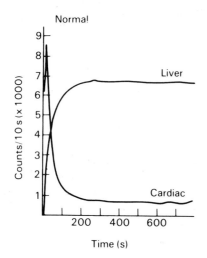

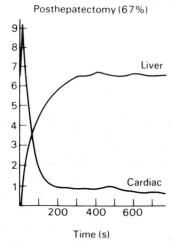

Figure 10.12 Dynamic liver scans using ^{99m}Tc sulphur colloid. Liver uptake curves in normal rat (above) and immediately post-hepatectomy (below). (From ref. 26, with kind permission of the authors and the editor of the *Journal of Nuclear Medicine*.)

of liver tissue of approximately 2.5-fold (from 2.15 to 5.25 ml min^{-1} g^{-1}), with only a slight reduction in *total* liver flow (from 25.12 to 22.46 ml min^{-1} g^{-1}). As partial hepatectomy is associated with a rise in portal pressure, it is clear that complete diversion of hepatic inflow into

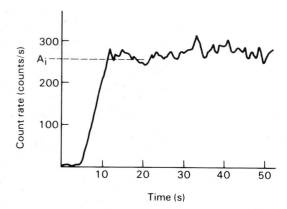

Figure 10.13 Colloid uptake in the liver following portal vein injection. By measuring extraction efficiency in this way, effective liver perfusion can be corrected to give actual blood flow. Such measurements are crucial to this technique of assessing blood flow in situations where reticuloendothelial function is altered such as in cirrhosis or, as in these experiments, immediately after extensive liver resection. (A_i = initial activity taken up by liver measured 5 seconds after end of injection.)

the remnant cannot be achieved. If this were to occur following two-thirds resection, the remnant would receive three times as much blood. The submaximal 2.5-fold increase in specific flow found by dynamic scintigraphy accords well with predicted changes, unlike the 4-fold increase suggested by one inert gas method.[21]

A particular advantage of dynamic scintigraphy over previously reported methods[6,39] is that serial blood sampling is unnecessary. It is also simpler to perform and allows more accurate measurement of time–activity variations. In addition, the use of the mathematical model to separate liver perfusion improves accuracy.

Using this technique in a portacavally shunted animal submitted to subsequent partial hepatectomy, increases in perfusion through the hepatic artery can be detected as previously mentioned.

DIFFERENTIAL ARTERIAL AND PORTAL VENOUS STUDIES IN THE RAT

The technique has been developed to differentiate hepatic arterial and portal venous components of liver blood flow.[17]

The dynamics of a colloid on first passage through the circulation following intravenous bolus injection are as follows (Figure 10.13). In its passage first through the heart and lungs and then through the arterial circulation to the rest of the body, the bolus of colloid gradually becomes diffused. The amount of colloid arriving at each organ on first passage is proportional to the perfusion of that organ. Colloid passing along the hepatic and splenic arteries is removed efficiently by these organs. Colloid passing through the mesenteric vessels to the gut, by contrast, reaches the liver through the portal vein a few seconds later. Colloid perfusing other organs, except bone

Table 10.1 Liver perfusion following partial hepatectomy in the rat

Group	Number of rats	Total counts Liver (%)	Spleen (%)	Carcass (%)	Efficiency (%)	Total liver perfusion K_1 (ml/mim)	Specific liver perfusion K_2 (ml/g/min)
Normal	11	89.71	2.44	7.82	81	25.12	2.15
Posthepatectomy							
Immediate	8	87.25	2.52	10.27	61	22.46	5.25
4 h	6	84.88	4.03	11.03	62.5	23.57	4.83
18 h	6	83.90	4.02	12.08	64	23.73	4.02
24 h	8	87.77	3.20	9.04	65.5	20.87	3.63
2 days	10	83.91	3.93	11.57	75.5	17.71	2.69
3 days	14	87.84	4.09	8.07	79	22.01	2.10
4 days	6	89.35	4.50	6.15	81	16.88	1.88
6 days	3	81.00	3.33	15.67		22.00	2.01
7 days	4	90.75	4.00	5.75		22.36	2.05
9 days	7	88.48	4.27	7.27		32.52	2.58
10 days	8	87.57	2.61	9.80		28.11	2.42
12 days	8	90.82	3.25	5.94		27.64	2.25
14 days	8	86.95	3.77	9.26		26.91	1.93

marrow, returns to the heart and some recirculates to the liver.

Separation of the two components of hepatic perfusion and their relative quantification depends on the following conditions:

1. Nearly all the colloid passing through the hepatic artery should reach the liver before the initial appearance of portal vein colloid (time t_a).
2. Nearly all portal vein colloid should reach the liver before significant hepatic arterial recirculation occurs (time t_p).
3. Hepatic extraction efficiency of colloid should be approximately 100%.
4. The splenic contribution to portal activity should be low. Colloid reaching the spleen is removed, so this part of portal supply will not be included in the measurement of colloid removed by the liver.

Normal hepatic extraction efficiency for ^{99m}Tc SC is 81%, and the ratio of perfusion of the liver to that of the spleen is 35 : 1. The ratio of hepatic arterial perfusion (K_a) to portal venous perfusion (K_p) is obtained from the relationship:

$$\frac{K_a}{K_p} = \frac{L(t_a)}{L(t_p) - L(t_a)}$$

A biphasic hepatic uptake curve is found in normal animals. The early phase, coincident with splenic uptake, achieves a brief plateau before an additional delayed increase is seen (Figure 10.14a). This early phase (assumed to be due to hepatic arterial inflow) constitutes $30 \pm 2\%$ of the total liver perfusion. Hepatic arterial ligation abolishes the early phase of hepatic uptake

(Figure 10.14b), whilst portacaval diversion eliminates the delayed phase of hepatic uptake (Figure 10.14c), confirming the temporal separation of the arterial and venous phases of hepatic perfusion shown by dynamic scintigraphy.

HUMAN STUDIES

Physiological

This technique has been applied to the assessment of physiological alterations in liver blood flow. Dynamic scintigraphy was performed in fasting healthy young adults and then repeated 1 h after a large meal of steak, chips (french fries), vegetables, a pudding, a glass of wine and a cup of sweet coffee (> 2000 kcal!). In Figure 10.15a it can be seen that the arterial phase (which is synchronous with splenic uptake) contributes approximately 45% of total liver uptake. Following the meal, the portal contribution to hepatic perfusion increases dramatically (Figure 10.15b). This represents an increase in total liver blood flow of approximately 60%. Arterial flow changes little, whilst the mesenteric fraction is greatly augmented. The ratio of arterial to portal venous inflow to the liver thus changes from approximately 45 : 55 in the fasting state to around 20 : 80 immediately after a meal.[46]

It is clear that this non-invasive technique has considerable potential in a wide variety of investigations. For example, the effect of many drugs on the splanchnic circulation is currently being investigated. Evaluation of the role of hormones in liver regeneration with particular reference to alterations in blood flow is also now possible.

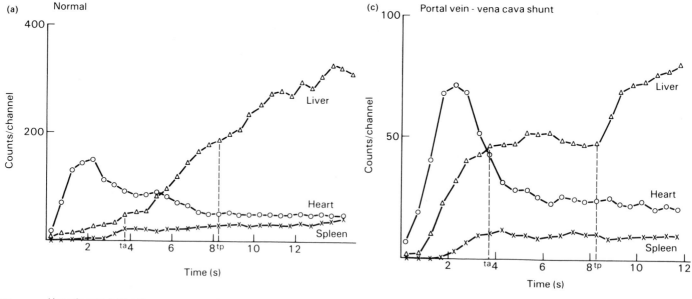

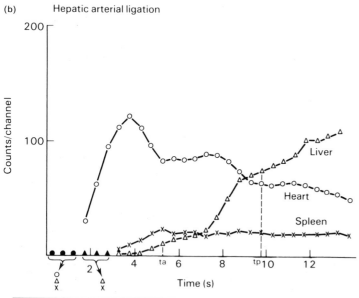

Figure 10.14 (a) Normal liver uptake curve demonstrating the end of arterial perfusion at time t_a and a delayed venous phase ending at time t_p when recirculation of colloid is seen. (b) Following ligation of the hepatic artery, the initial phase, assumed to be arterial, is abolished. (c) The delayed venous phase (from t_a to t_p) is abolished by portosystemic diversion, confirming the nature of this phase.

Pathological

The availability of a dynamic functional investigation is also of value in pathological states. For example, both experimental and clinical studies in mesenteric ischaemia and in cirrhosis have been undertaken. The effect of bowel infarction is illustrated in Figure 10.16. In addition, patients with diabetic mesenteric angiopathy have been found to have a diminished response to the feeding 'stress test'.

In cirrhosis the relationship between impaired reticuloendothelial function, as measured by colloid uptake, and alterations in *actual* liver blood flow have now been established in the animal model. Cirrhosis was induced by inhalation of carbon tetrachloride following pre-treatment with phenobarbitone. The severity of cirrhosis was graded histologically and the variations in colloid extraction following intraportal administration and actual liver

blood flow (ALBF) (where ELBF = ALBF × e) were assessed in different grades of cirrhosis. The effective liver blood flow (ELBF) measured by the uptake of activity is equal to the ALBF multiplied by the extraction efficiency (e) measured by intraportal injection of isotope.

It is of interest to observe that in the early stages of cirrhosis the depression of the ELBF (and thus the quality and quantity of uptake shown in scintigrams) is due almost exclusively to failure of colloid extraction (Figure 10.17). As the severity of cirrhosis increases, the ALBF also declines. There is a partial recovery in extraction efficiency coincident with histological evidence of regeneration. In more advanced disease, both the extraction efficiency and the ALBF fall markedly, producing the characteristic patchy uptake on static images mentioned in Chapter 21.

In a similar animal model of cirrhosis the changes in ELBF have been compared with the degree of portosystemic shunting, measured following the injection of

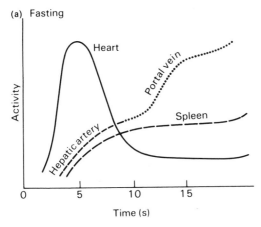

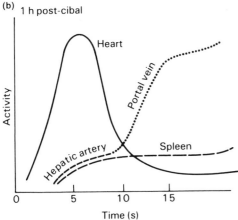

Figure 10.15 (a) Fasting dynamic liver curve. Arterial flow contributes approximately 50% of total flow in this situation. (b) Dynamic liver curve 1 h after a heavy meal. It can be seen that the total liver flow is greatly increased due to increased mesenteric flow (by about 60%). As a result, the arterial-to-portal ratio changes to approximately 20 : 80.

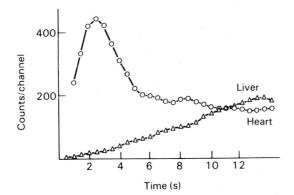

Figure 10.16 Depressed portal flow in a patient with laparotomy–confirmed evidence of small-bowel infarction.

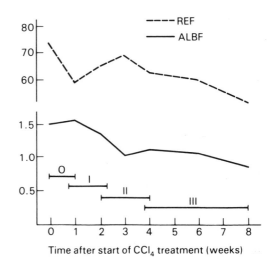

Figure 10.17 Reticuloendothelial function and liver blood flow in cirrhosis. I to III indicate the histological grades of severity of cirrhosis. It can be seen that with mild degrees of cirrhosis there is no fall in actual liver blood flow, and possibly even a slight increase. Diminished reticuloendothelial function, however, occurs rapidly with the onset of cirrhosis. Within a short time, some return of function occurs coincident with histological evidence of regeneration. Progression of this disease is associated with a fall in both function and blood flow. REF = reticuloendothelial function, measured by intraportal administration of a tracer dose of colloid (see Figure 10.13). ALBF = actual liver blood flow.

[57]Co-radiolabelled microspheres, and portal pressure.[32] A good correlation was found between the level of portal pressure and the degree of measured 'shunting' and there is an inverse relationship between the ELBF and 'shunting', although the latter does not account solely for the observed abnormalities in extraction efficiency.

The effect of certain drugs has also been studied. Cimetidine produces no significant effect on the measured ELBF, whereas when portal–systemic shunting is of the order of 20%, propranolol may increase the ELBF by an increase in colloid extraction.

In human studies the ability of the liver to undergo regenerative changes following the onset of cirrhosis makes dynamic scintigraphy a valuable technique for the investigation of basic pathophysiological events. In addition, this technique provides a direct means of assessing progression of, or recovery from, liver disease, whether induced by drugs, infection, trauma or other causes, and is worthy of further development and more widespread use. Other techniques such as single-photon emission computed tomography (SPECT) offer alternative non-invasive methods of studying liver regeneration.[23,45]

HISTOLOGICAL CHANGES

Following partial hepatectomy, histological changes can be detected in the remnant within a few hours. These changes are first seen in the region surrounding the

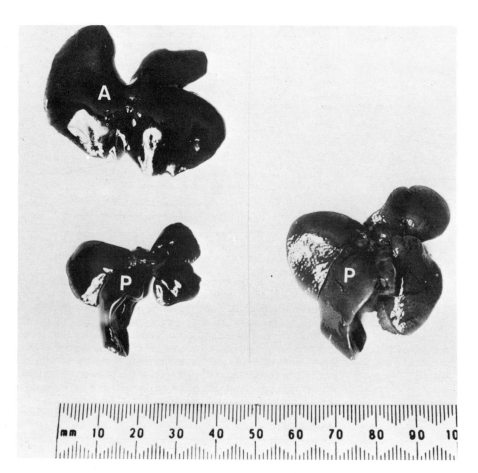

Figure 10.18 Increase in the size of the liver remnant of the rat 48 h after 67% hepatectomy (A = anterior, P = posterior lobes).

vascular inflow at the portal triad. Subsequently, they are seen to spread out from the triad until finally they surround the hepatic venous outflow.[19] This sequence of events emphasizes the importance of hepatic perfusion in the initiation and control of this remarkable phenomenon.

Following partial hepatectomy in the rat, the remnant becomes pale during the course of the first day owing to fatty infiltration. New constituents of protoplasm are formed and DNA replication commences. By 48 h the remnant has approximately doubled in size (Figure 10.18). Initially, mitotic activity lags behind the increase in weight, but after this initial delay the increase in cell population proceeds parallel with the increase in mass.[8] Regenerating liver 36 h after partial hepatectomy in the rat is shown in Figures 10.19 and 10.20.

Synthesis of DNA may be studied by the incorporation of tritiated thymidine. This radioactive precursor is taken up by parenchymal cells at greatly increased rates after 12 h following hepatectomy, and uptake reaches a peak at approximately 18 h. Doubling of DNA content is a prerequisite for mitosis. There is thus a lag before an increase in mitotic rate is seen and the peak of mitotic activity occurs some 30 h after resection (Figure 10.21).

A similar sequence of events occurs in ductal and sinusoidal cells except that these changes are delayed, with the peak in DNA synthesis occurring in both groups between 36 and 48 h after hepatectomy.

Although hepatocytes account for only 60–65% of the cell population,[9,43] they account for up to 95% of liver volume. Thus, growth of these cells produces immediate changes in the size of the remnant.

Within hours of hepatectomy, changes are visible in the hepatocytes surrounding the portal triad. These changes then involve adjacent cells until eventually hepatocytes around the terminal hepatic veins are affected. Ductular littoral and connective-tissue cells are relatively unaffected at this time.

The use of improved fixation techniques using glutaraldehyde suggests that many previously reported histological changes are probably artefactual.[15] The stress of hepatectomy possibly alters the susceptibility of tissue to fixation. Hypoxia, various toxins and other stressful conditions may also produce these changes. The endoplasmic reticulum, mitochondria and cell surfaces of hepatocytes are well preserved following hepatectomy, provided the tissues are fixed by the in situ perfusion technique using buffered glutaraldehyde. In these more refined preparations it is difficult to detect features that distinguish regenerating liver at 10 and 20 h after hepatectomy from the liver of normal sham-operated animals, apart from

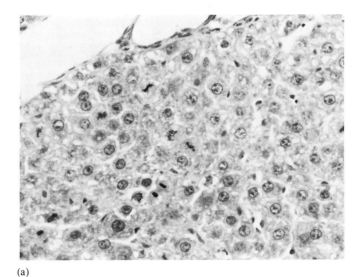

(a)

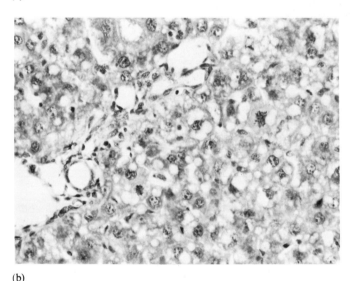

(b)

Figure 10.19 (a) Histological appearances of rat liver 24 h after partial hepatectomy. Note the large number of mitoses already visible. A portal tract is seen top left. (b) 66 h after partial hepatectomy. Mitoses are still visible and there is now prominent cytoplasmic vacuolation due to fatty change.

the accumulation of large droplets of lipid and a more prominent appearance of the smooth endoplasmic reticulum.

Over the first 10 h glycogen stores rapidly become depleted but then gradually reappear. Fat globules increase so that at 24 h the cellular pattern becomes distorted through compression of the sinusoidal spaces by these fat-laden hepatocytes. As already mentioned, other cellular structures remain comparatively unchanged at this time.

Non-specific changes, which are common to stressful situations such as hypoxia and biliary obstruction, include vacuolation, appearance of inclusion bodies, activation of lysosomes, loss of microvilli and disorganization of the endoplasmic reticulum.[1,3,4]

At 18–20 h after hepatectomy, DNA synthesis, as detected by autoradiography, reaches its peak in the periportal hepatocytes. Some 8 h later mitosis occurs. Gradually this sequence of events sweeps towards the terminal hepatic venous radicle.

Mitotic activity proceeds in a relatively asynchronous manner. Although mitosis is completed in individual cells within 1 h,[12] the peak of activity in the liver as a whole is spread over 12 h.[10] In the shortening of the cell life cycle from 21.5 to 16.15 h, the GI interval is the major variant determining the cell generation time. Control of cell proliferation is probably mediated during this phase.[13] During the early phases of regeneration at least some hepatocytes divide more than once, as demonstrated by double-labelling experiments. This fact is responsible for the production of the maximal initial growth rate, which subsequently declines. The regenerative response, as measured by 60-h [³H]thymidine infusion,[14,41,42,44] occurs diffusely throughout the liver remnant, and there is no evidence, therefore, of a microscopic 'focus' for the initiation of this phenomenon.

EFFECTS OF AGE ON REGENERATION

The age of the patient or animal is of importance in the regenerative response, not only with regard to recovery following major hepatic resection, but also because an inadequate regenerative response in patients more than 40 years old may be responsible for the high incidence of acute hepatic failure following viral hepatitis.[37] Several features of regeneration have been shown to differ with age. The maximal increase in DNA synthesis in rats, for example, is delayed by 7 days in old animals.[11] A similar delay in restoration of mass is found, with preoperative values being achieved at 3 weeks.[34] Differences are also seen in albumin synthesis, which occurs at an increased rate in old rats, although globulin synthesis is unchanged.[5,40] The increased albumin synthesis that occurs after hepatectomy also occurs later in old rats.[34] Following hepatectomy in old rats, the liver ribosomes have a lower specific activity than microsomes from livers of old control rats. In contrast, young rat liver microsomes continue albumin synthesis after hepatectomy at the same rate as young control liver microsomes, with increased synthesis seen 24 h after operation. This increased synthesis is delayed to 48 h in old rat liver microsomes.

The ferritin content of liver also differs between young and old rats.[35] The liver of old rats contains four times the amount of ferritin iron per gram and twice the amount of ferritin protein per gram of liver tissue. In addition, old rat liver ferritin contains twice as much iron as young rat liver ferritin.

It has also been shown that the proportion of polyploid hepatocytes increases with age,[38] so that at 2 years rat liver contains 10% diploids, 73% tetraploids and 17%

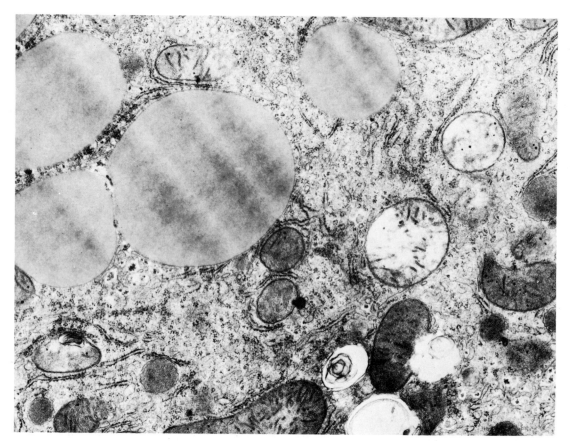

Figure 10.20
Electron micrograph of rat liver 36 h after partial hepatectomy, showing numerous fat droplets. × 8000.

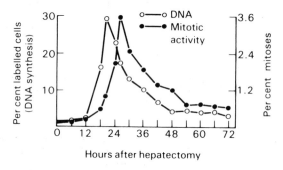

Figure 10.21 The increase in DNA synthesis in parenchymal cells precedes the increase in mitotic activity. (Based on ref. 20.)

octoploids, all of which are active in mitosis. This compares with 20–30% of binucleate hepatocytes, 70–80% tetraploid and 1–2% octaploid nuclei in normal adult rats.[9,33]

It seems probable that functional changes in the liver of old rats do not involve somatic mutations.[34]

The overall decrease in the regenerative response in old age is in harmony with the decrease in metabolic rate in man, which falls from 7 MJ/24 h (1700 kcal/24 h) in young males to less than 5 MJ/24 h (1300 kcal/24 h) with increasing age.[28]

REFERENCES

1. Abraham, R., Goldbert, L. & Grasso, P. (1967) Hepatic response to lysosomal effects of hypoxia, neutral red and chloroquine. *Nature*, **215**, 194–196.
2. Aronsen, K.F., Ericsson, B., Nosslin, B. *et al.* (1970) Evaluation of hepatic regeneration by scintillation scanning, cholangiography and angiography in man. *Annals of Surgery*, **171**, 567–574.
3. Bade, E.G. (1967) In *Control of Cellular Growth in Adult Organisms*. pp. 260–269. New York: Academic Press.
4. Bassi, M. & Bernelli-Zazzera, A. (1964) Ultrastructural cytoplasmic changes of liver cells after reversible and irreversible ischaemia. *Experimental and Molecular Pathology*, **3**, 332–350.
5. Beauchene, R.E., Roeder, L.M. and Barrows, C.H. (1970) The inter-relationships of age, tissue protein synthesis and proteinuria. *Journal of Gerontology*, **25**, 359.
6. Benacerraf, B., Bilbey, D., Biozzi, G. *et al.* (1957) The measurement of liver blood flow in partially hepatectomised rats. *Journal of Physiology*, **136**, 287–293.
7. Blumgart, L.H., Leach, K.G. & Karran, S.J. (1971) Observations on liver regeneration after right hepatic lobectomy. *Gut*, **12**, 922–928.
8. Brues, A.M., Drury, D.R. & Brues, M.C. (1936) A quantitative study of cell growth in regenerating liver. *Archives of Pathology*, **22**, 658–673.
9. Bucher, N.L.R. (1963) Regeneration of mammalian liver. *International Review of Cytology*, **15**, 245–300.
10. Bucher, N.L.R. & Malt, R.A. (1971) *Regeneration of the Liver and Kidney*. Boston: Little, Brown.
11. Bucher, N.L.R., Swaffield, M.N. & Di Troia, J.F. (1964) Influence of age upon incorporation of thymidine-2-C¹⁴ into DNA of regener-

ating rat liver. *Cancer Research*, **24**, 509–512.

12. Edwards, J.L. & Koch, A. (1964) Parenchymal and littoral cell proliferation during liver regeneration. *Laboratory Investigation*, **13**, 32–43.

13. Fabrikant, J.I. (1968) Kinetics of cellular proliferation in regenerating liver. *Journal of Cell Biology*, **36**, 551–565.

14. Fabrikant, J.I. (1969) Size of proliferating pools in regenerating liver. *Experimental Cell Research*, **55**, 277–279.

15. Fahimi, H.D. (1967) Perfusion and immersion fixation of rat liver with glutaraldehyde. *Laboratory Investigation*, **16**, 736–750.

16. Fleming, J.S., Karran, S.J., Eagles, C.J. & Ackery, D. (1977) A new in-vivo sequential technique for the measurement of effective liver blood flow in small animals. Proceedings of the European Society of Surgical Research. Warsaw. *European Surgical Research*, **9** (supplement 1), 175.

17. Fleming, J.S., Humphries, N.L.M., Karran, S.J. *et al.* (1981) In vivo assessment of hepatic-arterial and portal-venous components of liver perfusion: concise communication. *Journal of Nuclear Medicine*, **22**, 18–21.

18. Foster, J.H., Lawler, M.R., Welborn, M.B. *et al.* (1968) Recent experience with major hepatic resection. *Annals of Surgery*, **167**, 651–668.

19. Gebhardt, R. (1988) Different proliferative activity in vitro of periportal and perivenous hepatocytes. *Scandinavian Journal of Gastroenterology*, **23** (supplement 151), 8–18.

20. Grisham, J.W. (1962) Morphologic study of deoxyribonucleic acid synthesis and cell proliferation in regenerating rat liver; autoradiography with thymidine-H³. *Cancer Research*, **22**, 842–849.

21. Guest, J., Ryan, C.J., Benjamin, I.S. & Blumgart, L.H. (1977) Portacaval transposition and subsequent partial hepatectomy in the rat: effects on liver atrophy, hypertrophy, and regenerative hyperplasia. *British Journal of Experimental Pathology*, **58**, 140–146.

22. Higgins, G.M. & Anderson, R.M. (1931) Experimental pathology of the liver. I. Restoration of the liver of the white rat following partial surgical removal. *Archives of Pathology*, **12**, 186.

23. Jansen, P.L.M., Chamuleau, R.A.F.M., Van Leeuwen, D.J. *et al.* (1990) Liver regeneration and restoration of liver function after partial hepatectomy in patients with liver tumours. *Scandinavian J. Gastroenterology* **25**, 112–118.

24. Karran, S.J., Leach, K.G. & Blumgart, L.H. (1972) Radio-isotope investigation of protein synthesis and reticulo-endothelial activity following partial hepatectomy in the rat. *British Journal of Surgery*, **59**, 907.

25. Karran, S.J., Leach, K.G. & Blumgart, L.H. (1974) Assessment of liver regeneration in the rat using gamma camera. *Journal of Nuclear Medicine*, **15**(1), 10–16.

26. Karran, S.J., Eagles, C., Fleming, J. & Ackery, D. (1979) In-vivo measurement of liver perfusion in the normal and partially hepatectomised rat using Tc-99m sulfur colloid. *Journal of Nuclear Medicine*, **20**, 26–31.

27. Karran, S.J., Fleming, J.S. & Humphries, N.L.M. (1982) Non-invasive assessment of hepatic perfusion and of the relative arterial and portal components. In Mathie, R.T. (ed.) *Blood Flow Measurement in Man*, Ch. 15, pp. 155–167. Tunbridge Wells: Castle House Publications.

28. Kinney, J. (1979) Calorie and nitrogen requirements in catabolic states. In Karran, S.J. & Alberti, K.G.M.M. (eds) *Practical Nutritional Support*, Ch. 8, pp. 81–93. London: Pitman Medical.

29. Mann, F.C. (1944) Restoration and pathologic reactions of the liver. *Journal of Mount Sinai Hospital,* **11**, 65–74.

30. McDermott, W.V., Jr (1970) Circulatory changes associated with major hepatic resection. *Annals of the New York Academy of Sciences, **170**, 246–250.

31. McDermott, W.V., Jr, Greenberger, N.J., Isselbacher, K.J. & Webber, A. L. (1963) Major hepatic resection; diagnostic techniques and metabolic problems. *Surgery*, **54**, 56–66.

32. McLaren, M. (1985) Unpublished data.

33. Nadal, C. & Zajdela, F. (1966) Polyploidie somatique dans le foie de rat. I. Le rôle des cellules *binucléées* dans la genèse des cellules polyploides. *Experimental Cellular Research*, **42**, 99–116.

34. Obenrader, M., Chen, J., Ove, P. & Lansing, A.I. (1974) Functional regeneration in liver of old rats after partial hepatectomy. *Experimental Gerontology*, **9**, 181–190.

35. Ove, P., Obenrader, M.L. & Lansing, A.I. (1972) Synthesis and degradation of liver proteins in growing and old rats. *Biochimica et Biophysica Acta*, **277**, 211.

36. Pack, G.T., Islami, A.H., Hubbard, J.C. & Brasfield, R.D. (1962) Regeneration of human liver after major hepatectomy. *Surgery*, **52**, 617–623.

37. Peters, R.L. (1975) Viral hepatitis: a pathologic spectrum. *American Journal of the Medical Sciences*, **270**, 17–32.

38. Post, J. & Hoffman, J. (1972) In Popper, H. & Schaffner, F. (eds) *Progress in Liver Diseases*, Vol. 2, p. 155. New York: Grune & Stratton.

39. Rabinovici, N. & Wiener, E. (1963) Hemodynamic changes in the hepatectomized liver of the rat and their relationship to regeneration. *Journal of Surgical Research*, **3**, 3–8.

40. Salatka, K., Kresge, D., Harris, J.L. *et al.* (1971) Rat serum protein changes with age. *Experimental Gerontology*, **6**, 25.

41. Sigel, B., Baldia, L.B., Brightman, S.A. *et al.* (1968) Effect of blood flow reversal in liver autotransplants upon the site of hepatocyte regeneration. *Journal of Clinical Investigation*, **47**, 1231–1237.

42. Simpson, G.E.C. & Finckh, E.S. (1963) Pattern of regeneration of rat liver after repeated partial hepatectomies. *Journal of Pathology and Bacteriology*, **86**, 361–370.

43. Steiner, J.W., Perz, Z.M. & Taichman, L.B. (1966) Cell population dynamics in liver: review of quantitative morphological techniques applied to study of physiological and pathological growth. *Experimental and Molecular Pathology*, **5**, 146–181.

44. Stöcker, E. (1966) Der Proliferationsmodus in Niere und Leber. *Verhandlungen Deutschen Gesellschaft für Pathologie*, **50**, 53–74.

45. Van der Borght, T.M., Lambotte, L.E., Pauwels, S.A. & Dire, D.C. (1990) Uptake of thymidine labelled on carbon 2: a potential index of liver regeneration by positron emission tomography. *Hepatology*, **12**, 113–118.

46. Walmsley, B.H., Fleming, J.S. & Karran, S.J. (1982) A non-invasive stress for monitoring mesenteric haemodynamics. *European Surgical Research*, **14**, 91.

47. Wang, L. (1959) Plasma volume, cell volume, total blood volume and F. cells factor in the normal and splenectomized Sherman rat. *American Journal of Physiology*, **196**(1), 188–192.

48. Weinbren, K., Stirling, G.A. & Washington, S.L.A. (1972) Development of a proliferative response in liver parenchyma deprived of portal blood flow. *British Journal of Experimental Pathology*, **53** , 54–58.

49. Wood, C.B., Karran, S.J. & Blumgart, L.H. (1973) Metabolic changes following varying degrees of partial hepatectomy in the rat. *British Journal of Surgery*, **60**(8), 613–617.

CHAPTER 11

Regulatory Mechanisms in Hepatic Regeneration

Nancy L.R. Bucher and
Alastair J. Strain

INTRODUCTION

In the adult animal the liver is normally in a state of growth arrest, its energies channelled into an array of differentiated functions. In this state, usually termed G_0 all but about 0.01% of the cells are disengaged from the growth cycle manifested by continually proliferating cells.[9] The liver is readily stimulated to grow by an excess work load imposed by the body. This may arise from loss of functional liver tissue through physical, infectious or toxic injury or surgical ablation, or alternatively from metabolic overloading caused by pregnancy or extreme hormonal or nutritional imbalances.[37] (For reviews see Refs 18, 20, 21). The liver also grows when exposed to certain drugs whose action is unclear but appears to be associated with severe oxidative stress.[133,191]

The signals from the body indicating the need for more liver tissue are blood borne. The growth response is finely tuned: if the liver deficiency is small, the loss is restored

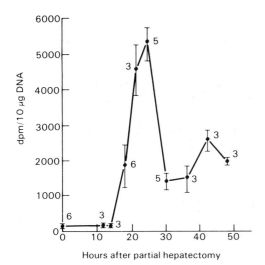

Figure 11.1 One-hour incorporation of [^{3}H]thymidine into hepatic DNA in 200-g male Sprague Dawley rats at intervals after partial hepatectomy. The vertical lines indicate the standard error of the mean and the numbers indicate the number of rats per point. Reprinted with permission from Bucher *et al.*[24] Copyright (1978) Pergamon Press.

slowly despite the high growth potential.[21] Moreover, the size of the liver is continually adjusted to the workload, increasing or diminishing as the need grows or slackens. It enlarges in severely diabetic animals, and returns to normal size following adequate insulin therapy.[210,211] Similarly, small liver transplants enlarge to assume a size appropriate to the recipient[104,209,237] and human liver segments transplanted into paediatric recipients are thought to enlarge with growth of the child.[53,63]

Interest in human liver growth has intensified recently as liver transplantation has become a commonplace treatment for end-stage liver disease. The very recent cloning of a human hepatocyte growth factor (hHGF), as well as isolation of similar factors from experimental animals (see later), have raised hopes for possible clinical therapeutic uses of such agents to promote liver regeneration and repair, although *in vivo* studies have not yet been done.

Although the liver regenerates in all of the species examined, including man, the rat is the one most intensively studied, probably in part because of the phenomenal rate of hepatic regeneration in this species. Following resection of the two main lobes—comprising 68% of the whole organ—changes in hepatocyte biochemistry begin almost immediately as the cells make the transition to the prereplicative or G_1 phase of the cell cycle. This phase terminates after 14–16 h at the onset of DNA synthesis, marking entry into the S-phase (Figure 11.1).

The rate of DNA synthesis rises sharply to a peak at 22–24 h, the time varying with age, nutritional status, and other factors. Mitosis follows a parallel course, peaking 6–8 h later than DNA synthesis.[83] The growth rate diminishes and ceases in a week or more as the size and cell

population of the liver remnant approximates that of the original organ.[65] The process is actually a compensatory hyperplasia; the excised lobes do not regrow, and proliferative activity occurs throughout the residual lobes, involving virtually all of the cells and preserving the histological architecture. The term regeneration, though widely accepted, is therefore misleading.

Most of the research has focused upon the early stages of regeneration (G_1 phase), where growth regulation is generally thought to occur. Once cells have entered upon DNA replication they usually progress through the remainder of the growth cycle, whereas if interrupted at early pre-replicative stages they may regress to a nonproliferating or G_0 state.[27] Transition from G_0 to G_1 and progression to S phase is therefore more than a one-step process, suggesting operation of more than a single regulator.

Additional evidence shows that the blood-borne signals from the body that control hepatic regeneration are indeed multiple and interact synergistically, and that they may act negatively or positively. Their precise identity remains elusive despite years of investigation. Present evidence supports various hormones and growth factors to be discussed in this review: some may serve as primary initiators and others as promoters, modulators or inhibitors of the growth process. Nutrients also have a role, if only indirect, because responsiveness to growth stimuli is influenced by the metabolic state of the cells. The converse problem—what causes the liver to shrink when the amplified cell complement is no longer needed—has been almost totally neglected. Cell attrition occurs through the poorly understood process of apoptosis.[45,244]

Studies in cultured cells of various types reveal that at least *in vitro* most of the known growth factors exhibit several seemingly unrelated functions and are influenced by the presence of other growth factors as well as by the metabolic state of the cells often reflecting conditions under which they are cultured.[82,180,206,240] Although much has been recently learned about the mechanism through which the actions of hormones and growth factors are implemented, they are still incompletely understood, even in the case of a well-known hormone such as insulin, which has been intensively studied for many years.

Hepatocytes, freshly isolated and maintained in culture, allow putative growth-regulatory factors to be assessed individually in a defined environment and their actions to be dissected without countervailing influences from the other cells of the body. Such work will be included when relevant. Although non-hepatocytes also participate in the regenerative process, their engagement is delayed and contribution to early regulatory events has not been observed (for possible involvement at a later stage see Ref. 65).

The background has been detailed in numerous reviews.[2,19,20,21,65,66,126,164,187] The experimental animal implied in the present review is the rat unless otherwise stated.

HEPATIC GROWTH REGULATORS

The numerous factors proposed as potential hepatic growth regulators can be grouped into several broad categories: (i) relatively low-molecular-weight substances including hormones and nutrients; (ii) polypeptide growth factors; (iii) larger molecules, including serum-derived or liver-derived (mainly protein) growth factors; (iv) inhibitory factors.

Work during the late 1960s and 1970s (see earlier editions of this book) stressed portal blood hepatotrophic factors, stemming from the observations that the liver atrophies when deprived of a portal blood supply and that mitotic activity in regenerating livers appears first in the areas receiving the incoming portal blood. The term 'hepatotrophic' has been loosely used to designate either or both hyperplasia and hypertrophy. Hyperplasia indicates an increase in cell number, or ploidy (as occurs in developing liver) and hypertrophy signifies increased size or protein content without an increase in DNA.[7] Atrophied livers, whether due to portal blood deprivation or to starvation, show slowing but little other impairment of regenerative capacity following partial hepatectomy.[212,239,242] In this review, liver growth will imply hyperplasia, as regeneration of this organ is basically a hyperplastic process.

HORMONES AND NUTRIENTS

Insulin and glucagon

Numerous intricate surgical manipulations in dogs and rats, including hepatic vascular transpositions (reviewed in Ref. 208) and liver isografts,[13,59–61] have implicated insulin in liver growth. In addition, continuous infusion of partially hepatectomized rats with anti-insulin serum depressed DNA synthesis,[23] and insulin treatment of alloxan-diabetic rats caused their intact livers to grow substantially. Even without insulin treatment, partial hepatectomy induced modest regenerative activity in diabetic animals.[8,245] It seems that although liver growth positively requires insulin, the small amount present in the portal veins of severely diabetic rats suffices.[16]

Glucagon seems also to have a role in liver growth. Under various conditions it can exert a growth-promoting influence, as for example when added (in pharmacological doses) to several empirically devised hormone mixtures, which when injected into normal rats induce a wave of proliferative activity in the liver.[86,112,199]

In partially hepatectomized rats and dogs previously deprived of all splanchnic viscera including the pancreas, hepatic DNA synthesis was greatly reduced and delayed but was dramatically restored to the control rate by simultaneous infusion of glucagon and insulin.[28,30,168,242] Neither hormone was effective alone.[28,30] Similarly, in mice with fulminant hepatic necrosis following a 100% lethal dose of A–59 murine hepatitis virus, survival was strikingly enhanced when both hormones were given in combination, but not separately.[64] Thus, synergistic interactions among growth promoters emerged as an important principle in hepatic growth regulation, now supported by numerous cell-culture studies in both hepatocytes and other cell types.

Generally, in portal venous blood, insulin decreases during the early period of hepatic regeneration, whereas glucagon undergoes a substantial increase,[22,31,125,150,223] except that in fasted rats insulin rises slightly.[46] These changes at least partly reflect the animal's nutritional status (see subsection on Nutrients). Hepatic extraction of both insulin and glucagon from the portal blood was enhanced during regeneration.[43] Although insulin binding to cell surface receptors changed little, glucagon binding was down-regulated by 40–60% by 24 hours.[125,165] These observations are consonant with roles for insulin and glucagon in regulating liver growth.

Insulin and glucagon are by no means the only regulators. In portal splanchnic eviscerated rats, even when partial hepatectomy was delayed for up to 22 hours to permit blood levels of these hormones to decay, small but significant regenerative activity was still evident.[30] Moreover, infusion of insulin and glucagon into rats with intact livers—either normal or eviscerated—even when given directly into the portal vein, caused no significant elevation of DNA synthesis.[29,77,222] On the other hand, combined insulin and glucagon treatment of rats additionally stimulated by partial hepatectomy approximately doubled the rate of DNA synthesis.[52,225]

In the studies involving glucagon the optimal doses were generally in the pharmacological range, whereas for insulin they were more nearly physiological. Although these doses at least follow the trends found in portal venous blood following partial hepatectomy—high glucagon relative to insulin—the requirement for seemingly excessive amounts of glucagon remains puzzling.

Insulin is widely regarded as an anabolic, growth-promoting hormone, in contrast to glucagon which at least in liver often has opposing, catabolic actions, particularly on carbohydrate and lipid metabolism. In certain instances, however, the actions of the two hormones are complementary.[36,109] The main function of the glucagon in such instances could be to maintain glucose supplies in the presence of high insulin levels, but other known effects, such as stimulation of amino-acid transport, activation or induction of specific enzymes, or phosphorylation of specific proteins, could be equally or more important.

The liver is recognized as a main target of insulin and glucagon action, although evidence cited so far does not prove that their effects upon hepatic growth observed *in vivo* result from direct action on the liver. Support for direct action comes from studies of freshly isolated adult rat hepatocytes in serum-free monolayer cultures.[15,78,110,138,173] The evidence for insulin is consistently positive, pointing to an essential, though largely permissive function. Although glucagon too usually serves as a promoter of liver growth, under some circumstances it may play a negligible or even an inhibitory role, probably depending on the prior metabolic state of the cells as well as its interactions with other hormones.[23,26]

At present it appears likely that both insulin and glucagon have physiological roles in regulating growth of adult liver. The results suggest that an essential growth stimulus is attributable to substances other than these two hormones, and can originate outside the pancreas and gastrointestinal tract.

Nutrients

The regulation of liver growth by particular hormones—especially insulin and glucagon but others also—depends in large part on the availability of specific nutrients whose transport into the hepatocytes and subsequent metabolic fate is largely hormone governed. Adequacy of nutrient availability is clearly essential for maximal regenerative activity, but within the animal mobilization of essential substances from other cells may preclude definitive conclusions about specific dietary requirements. The variable palatability of experimental diets and consequent consumption patterns also introduces divergencies.

Fasting caused a rapid loss of labile cell constituents, glycogen, protein and RNA.[3,58,85] A 48-h fast prior to partial hepatectomy delayed and diminished, but did not abolish, the regenerative responses.[213] Overfeeding of fat, protein or carbohydrate also had an inhibitory influence.[17,226] Infusion of glucose following partial hepatectomy[44,88] with or without a high-protein parenteral nutrient mixture (Nutramin), or a high-lipid mixture (Intralipid) inhibited the onset of regeneration. Nutramin alone did likewise, though to a lesser extent. On the contrary, rats infused with saline or Intralipid alone exhibited significantly higher activity.[88] When rats underwent a 90% instead of the usual 68% hepatectomy, and were then offered 20% glucose to drink, the glucose corrected the expected severe hypoglycaemia and nearly doubled the survival rate. Hypoglycemia was mild following 68% hepatectomy, and there was no mortality.[44]

An early pre-replicative event found in the liver remnant following partial hepatectomy was an increase in the free amino-acid pools.[67,163] Not only was more amino acid made available intracellularly, but translocation of amino acids across the plasma membrane was also enhanced.[121,197] There were eight or more distinct systems in normal hepatocytes for amino-acid transport, at least one of which responded to a wide variety of hormones, including insulin, glucagon, catecholamines, glucocorticoids, and growth and thyroid hormones.[107] Force-feeding of amino acids or branched-chain amino acids (but not their keto-analogues) somewhat depressed regeneration,[108] though regeneration began earlier in rats infused with a branch-chain-enriched mixture.[89,174]

Results of protein-free but otherwise complete diets upon cell replication after partial hepatectomy are at variance; depression of DNA synthesis was observed by several groups of investigators,[87,137,204,212] but not by others.[148,202] Caloric restriction in these animals caused further depression. The general conclusion appears to be that adequate intake of both calories and a complete protein or amino-acid mixture is required for a maximal rate of hepatic regeneration.

The importance of dietary protein also emerges from studies on the feeding schedule in relation to normal circadian oscillations in DNA synthesis and hepatic regeneration. In normal rats fed only during a brief, specified interval each day ('meal-fed rats'), a small daily peak of DNA synthesis occurred at about 12 h after the start of the feeding period; this periodicity in DNA labelling was abolished by a protein-free diet.[51] During regeneration, the circadian rhythm was superimposed on the growth response; the first wave of DNA synthesis always appeared at the same fixed interval after the partial hepatectomy, but the height of its peak depended upon the time of day. As regeneration progressed, the diminishing mitotic oscillations became in phase with the physiological circadian maxima.[6,21] In meal-fed rats, the peak rate of DNA synthesis was 2–3-fold higher than in ad libitum-fed controls, presumably owing to enhanced mitotic synchrony. Omission of the final 4-h feeding, which occurred some hours after the partial hepatectomy, reduced the peak rate by half.[22,103]

In rats adapted to controlled feeding and lighting schedules, intragastric α-hexachlorocyclohexane was used to stimulate liver cell proliferation, which was suppressed by fasting or protein deprivation and restored only by a protein-containing meal.[190] Results of a recent study of the kinetics of DNA synthesis in regenerating rat liver have postulated that there is a rapidly increasing subpopulation of cells which need a protein meal to allow passage to S phase. Unidentified hormones are suggested to mediate the effect.[103]

An early demonstration of the importance of dietary protein in regulating liver growth was when normal (non-hepatectomized) mice were changed from a low- to a high-protein diet, resulting in a burst of mitotic activity proportional to the protein content of the enriched diet.[122] When rats were changed from a protein-free to a 50% protein diet, a substantial rise in DNA synthesis began as early as 8 h after the dietary changes—a considerably shorter prereplicative interval than the 16–17 h seen in the case of partial hepatectomy.[197,198] It was necessary to precondition the animals by protein or amino-acid deprivation for several days for the change of diet to be effective. This increased cell proliferation was inhibited if the subsequent diet lacked particular amino acids; deletion of lysine, methionine or tryptophan reduced the DNA synthetic response by half, and deletion of isoleucine, threonine or valine by even more.

When rats maintained on a protein-free diet for several days were force-fed a casein hydrolysate (equivalent to a protein meal) and compared with fasted animals similarly force-fed, the insulin and glucagon concentrations in portal venous blood were found to follow a closely similar course in both groups, very much resembling the low-insulin and high-glucagon pattern seen after partial hepatectomy. The two groups differed strikingly, however, in that the protein-deprived/refed group underwent the expected large, early increase in DNA synthesis, whereas the fasted/refed animals showed no response. Both hormonal environment and the metabolic status of the cells are clearly important determinants in cellular responses to growth stimulation.[22]

To some extent, nutrients are able to regulate the growth of eukaryotic cells in culture in a manner reminiscent of 'stringent' amino acid controls in bacteria, but within the animal integrative hormonal signalling systems are more likely to play a dominant role.[90,91]

Thyroid hormones

Thyroid hormones have been reported to elicit a hypertrophic and hyperplastic response in the liver.[123,132,198–200] The rate of regeneration was reduced by half in thyroidectomized animals, and nuclear T_3 binding sites were similarly reduced.[57] Food deprivation also reduced receptor number, though to a lesser extent.

The T_3 and thyroxine concentrations in peripheral blood dropped following partial hepatectomy, whereas thyroid-stimulating hormone (TSH), after an initial fall, increased by 60–70%.[124]

T_3 was able to restore an 80% lowering of DNA synthesis in regenerating livers of thyroparathyroidectomized rats, but only in pharmacological doses[159,200] (for review see Ref. 201). In a similar study, others showed that the deficiency was overcome by a single dose of calcitonin.[177] The conclusion in a recent study of thyroparathyroidectomized rats is that the relative contribution of T_3 to liver regeneration is probably small.[159]

In hepatocyte cultures, growth enhancement by T_3 was observed by some investigators—although only under special conditions[127]—and not by others.[173] There is little support for a substantial effect.

Much of the stimulatory action of T_3 and thyroxine *in vivo* may be indirect and reflect extensive metabolic changes throughout the body.

Adrenal cortical hormones

Both adrenocorticotrophic hormone (ACTH) and glucocorticoids have been reported to induce liver enlargement, mainly due to cellular hypertrophy. Glucocorticoids, especially in pharmacological doses, tended to delay proliferative growth following partial hepatectomy or carbon tetrachloride intoxication; they had little or no effect on liver DNA increase in normally growing animals.[106,190,192]

Partial hepatectomy resulted in elevation of free and total plasma corticosterone levels, but no change in ACTH levels. The elevation might be at least partly due to reduced capacity of the liver remnant to inactivate the hormone.[243]

Surgical stress at any time from several hours to several days before partial hepatectomy significantly accelerated the rise in DNA synthesis caused by the hepatic resection. Pretreatment with growth hormone acted similarly and the combined procedures were additive. Treatment with cortisone, hydrocortisone or ACTH, however, was without accelerating effect.[149,187,205]

In adrenalectomized-orchidectomized rats, DNA synthesis differed little from similarly treated controls in one study,[228] but was retarded and diminished when adrenalectomized-orchidectomized animals received less rigorous glucose/saline supportive treatment. Pretreatment of these latter animals with growth hormone restored DNA synthesis to near normal.[187] Somewhat divergent results have been reported by others.[54]

Supplementation of hepatocyte cultures with glucocorticoids is widely employed to improve cell survival and function. Hydrocortisone has been reported to more than double the growth rate in hepatocyte cultures even without supplementation with other hormones or growth factors,[128] whereas more recently glucocorticoids were reported to inhibit EGF-stimulated hepatocytes in culture, even at moderate concentrations.[238] Glucocorticoid effects on growth generally vary with dosage and culture conditions, and no clear concept has emerged.

Parathyroid hormone, calcium and vitamin D

In parathyroidectomized or thyroparathyroidectomized rats, hepatic regeneration is greatly reduced. If blood calcium is briefly raised by calcium injection or treatment with parathyroid hormone even as late as 12 h after partial hepatectomy, DNA synthesis is restored to control values. Partial hepatectomy by itself causes a thyroid-dependent hypocalcaemia and hypophosphataemia which persists for at least 8 h. The secretion of both calcitonin and parathyroid hormone is increased during the early stages of liver regeneration.[129] The concentration of the intracellular calcium-binding protein calmodulin increased 3-fold at 6–8 h after partial hepatectomy, returning to normal by 18 h—that is, just before the onset of DNA synthesis.[131]

Additional work by the same group of investigators, involving functional parathyroid transplants, treatment with parathyroid hormone, or calcitonin, or the vitamin D metabolite 1-α,25-dihydroxycholecalciferol (1,25-(OH)$_2$-D3) pointed to extracellular Ca^{2+} ions as the probable regulators, whose concentrations are influenced by the other substances.[130,177] Hence, hepatocytes appeared to be activated by partial hepatectomy even in the hypocalcaemic, post-parathyroidectomy rat, and could reach an advanced pre-DNA synthetic stage of proliferative development. Further progression through the cell cycle, however, seemed to be calcium dependent.

These observations and many others involving Ca^{2+}, calmodulin, 1,25-(OH)$_2$-D3 and second-messenger systems including cyclic-AMP, arachidonic acid, prostaglandins and active substances resulting from breakdown of phosphatidylinositol 4,5-bisphosphate have been woven into an intricate hypothesis to explain step-by-step control of the progression of regenerating hepatocytes from G_0 growth arrest through DNA synthesis. An important central position in the scheme is assigned to calcium ions. Support for the concept is drawn from a variety of systems in addition to liver.[241]

There has been a recent surge of interest in 1,25-$(OH)_2$-D3, the major biologically active metabolite of vitamin D_3, which is actually a steroid hormone. Among other functions it is thought to have an essential role in regulating a set of replication-linked genes (c-*myc*, c-*myb* and histone H4) that are critical for rapid cell proliferation. An integrated analysis of combinations of genetic circuits that it regulates suggests that they may be collectively tied to a DNA replication–differentiation switch (for reviews see Refs. 145, 171). Additional new reports emphasize control of DNA polymerase-alpha by calcium and 1,25-$(OH)_2$-D3 in liver regeneration.[175,203]

The work summarized in this section largely deals with cells that are already re-engaged in the cell cycle, focusing primarily on growth regulatory influences during the pre-replicative period. Although this review centres on the signals that initiate liver growth, these studies seem relevant because of the importance of many still unknown synergistic interactions among hormones and growth factors and the widespread emphasis on calcium in signalling very early events associated with activation of growth in many cell types.

Prostaglandins

A few early studies present circumstantial evidence which is difficult to evaluate, implicating prostaglandins in liver regeneration. A few hours after partial hepatectomy a transient increase in prostaglandin E in the liver remnant, but not in peripheral blood, was attributed to an enhanced rate of synthesis on the basis of its inhibition by indomethacin, which inhibited DNA synthesis as well.[130, 146] Studies involving a wide spectrum of inhibitors of prostaglandin and thromboxane production during liver regeneration suggested that there is an early prostaglandin- or thromboxane-mediated process in stimulated hepatocytes that determines their later entry into mitosis and that this process is separate from the early events leading to DNA synthesis.[176]

Prolactin

Prolactin (PRL) administration to normal rats caused elevation of hepatic thymidine kinase (TK) and ornithine decarboxylase (ODC) activities. Both are known to rise dramatically during liver regeneration; repeated PRL injections led to a small, seemingly liver specific, increase in DNA synthesis.[33] Moreover, circulating PRL levels increased transiently immediately following partial hepatectomy.[32] Pituitary isografts in advance of the hepatectomy resulted in elevated endogenous PRL levels and

enhanced both TK and ODC activities. Liver weight, however, failed to increase, and the result was interpreted as negative,[101] although liver weight does not always correlate with DNA synthesis. PRL also induces increased ODC activity in several other tissues and it is not a specific hepatic mitogen.[231] It has failed to stimulate growth of hepatocyte cultures[181,220] and its status as a hepatic growth regulator seems equivocal.

Catecholamines

Evidence has accumulated that catecholamines may be effective early modulators of liver regeneration. (1) The specific α_1 adrenergic antagonist prazosin, injected at the time of partial hepatectomy, inhibited DNA synthesis in the regenerating liver, but by 72 h, DNA synthesis did not differ from controls, indicating that only early stages of regeneration were affected.[50] (2) A substantial adrenergic nerve supply can be demonstrated in the portal tracts with some extension into the hepatic acinus[10,35] and a great increase in the portal tract innervation is found in regenerated livers.[166] (3) DNA synthesis in regenerating livers is substantially reduced by surgical or chemical sympathetic denervation.[4,50,152] (4) Plasma catecholamine concentrations increased modestly 2 h after partial hepatectomy.[50]

The α_1 type adrenergic receptors that predominate in normal liver were found to shift largely to the β-type during liver regeneration.[1,14,188] This change also occurs in hypothyroidism or other conditions (reviewed in Ref. 114). Unlike prazosin, β-adrenoreceptor blockers were not inhibitory, nor were β-agonists stimulatory.[160] Early reports that β-adrenergic blocking agents interfered with the regenerative response may be attributable to the use of available but less selective compounds than prazosin, which is highly specific for α-receptors.[50]

In hepatocyte cultures conversion from α_1 to β-receptor-mediated functions also occurred. Alpha-1 receptors decreased in number by 30–40% during the first day, while β-receptors increased dramatically.[158,161,188] Consonant with the observations *in vivo*, norepinephrine enhanced EGF-stimulated hepatocyte DNA synthesis in culture.[78] This was specifically blocked by α_1 antagonists and not by β-blockers, nor were β-adrenergic agonists stimulatory.[49,224] Involvement of α_2 adrenoreceptors also appeared to be limited or negligible.[49] A down-regulation of EGF receptors occurred concomitantly with the norepinephrine enhancement of the EGF response.[48] In addition, norepinephrine selectively counteracted the growth inhibitory action of TGF-β[92,93] (see the section on Growth Inhibitory Factors).

Various actions of the α_1 adrenergic agonists on hepatocytes resemble those of glucagon, vasopressin and angiotensin II. All are known to be hormones which influence aspects of hepatic carbohydrate metabolism, suggesting their possible function as regulators of nutrient availability and utilization by the regenerating cells.

These parallels in interaction with hepatocytes point to

the likely importance of these hormones as modulators and enhancers of the regenerative response. The catecholamines have been the most thoroughly investigated and along with glucagon appear to be the more diverse and potent hepatocyte growth promoters in this hormone group.

Overall, there is now a substantial body of evidence favouring the view that catecholamines have an important role in hepatic growth regulation.

Vasopressin

Rat liver regeneration is substantially depressed in the hereditary vasopressin-deficient Brattleboro strain of rat and returns to near normal following infusion of exogenous hormone.[182] In primary adult rat hepatocyte cultures vasopressin directly augmented DNA synthesis induced with minimally stimulatory concentrations of growth factors, thus exerting a positive modulatory influence.[181, 216] Other studies suggest that vasopressin may not be important in liver growth, at least in species other than the rat. Although abundant high-affinity plasma membrane vasopressin receptors were found in rat hepatocytes,[69] they were barely detectable in rabbit and human liver[94,235] and no mitogenic response has been demonstrable in isolated adult human hepatocytes cultures.[94] It remains to be determined whether hormones such as norepinephrine or angiotensin that act in many respects like vasopressin carry out in other species whatever growth-promoting functions vasopressin exerts in the rat.

Oestrogens and androgens

The involvement of sex steroid hormones in control of liver growth is unclear. In early studies, gonadal hormones were thought to have small or negligible effects on liver regeneration.[21] Later, serum oestradiol levels were found to rise after 1 day to a maximum at 3 days after partial hepatectomy, with a corresponding fall in circulating androgens.[72] There were associated increases in total hepatic and nuclear accumulations of oestrogen receptors with reduced androgen receptor levels. Similar increases in serum oestradiol have recently been described following partial liver resection in patients with hepatic tumours.[73] Exogenous oestrogen administration has been reported to induce liver growth in experimental animals.[68] Furthermore, DNA synthesis in regenerating rat liver was reduced by administration of the oestrogen antagonist tamoxifen and the reduction was negated by co-injection with oestradiol.[76] Despite the early tamoxifen inhibition, liver regenerated fully within 10 days. In other studies, no changes were found in either liver weight, ODC or thymidine kinase activity in partially hepatectomized male rats following tamoxifen administration.[100]

In hepatocyte cultures, oestradiol enhanced DNA synthesis when given with rat serum,[76] but variously inhibited[76] or promoted[196] DNA synthesis when given with EGF.

Changes in oestrogen and androgen receptor content have recently been demonstrated in rat liver transplants.[102] The increasing therapeutic use of liver transplants has focused attention on the clinical relevance of oestrogen and androgen involvement in liver growth and function but interpretation of their role is complicated by the necessary inclusion of immunosuppressants.

On the whole, the evidence so far tends not to support oestrogens and androgens as important hepatic growth regulators.

POLYPEPTIDE GROWTH FACTORS

Epidermal growth factor (EGF) and transforming growth factor alpha (TGF-α)

Epidermal growth factor is a polypeptide first isolated from the submaxillary gland of the male mouse, where it is highly concentrated, but it can be synthesized and released by a number of other cells and tissues as well. Human EGF, originally known as urogastrone, differs from mouse EGF by only 20 of its 53 amino acids; their biological activities appear to be identical. EGF is a potent mitogen for numerous types of both epithelial and mesenchymal cells including those from the liver (for reviews, see Refs. 39, 40, 134).

Continuous intraperitoneal infusion of EGF into normal rats weakly stimulated DNA synthesis and mitosis in the liver, but was enhanced 10-fold by physiological doses of insulin or much less with glucagon.[23,24] Its seeming specificity for liver[24] may be due to the extraordinary ability of hepatocytes to sequester it,[207] essentially clearing it from the blood before it reaches the other organs. That EGF and insulin can directly stimulate hepatocytes to synthesize DNA, without intervention of signals from the rest of the body, was demonstrated in cell culture studies with serum-free medium.[138,173] These observations pointed to EGF as a possible physiological initiating signal for liver regeneration, subject to modulation by interactions with other hormones.

A recent report showed preferential accumulation of radioactive label in hepatocyte nuclei in regenerating liver following administration of ^{125}I-labelled EGF.[170] This suggested that EGF, its receptor, or both, may directly signal nuclear effectors to initiate DNA synthesis without the generally accepted requirement for intermediate processing and second messengers. Supportive evidence comes from new work with other cell types, but the significance for mitogenic signalling of EGF/EGF receptor presence in the nucleus remains to be fully established.[98]

Additional studies have utilised ^{125}I-labelled EGF binding to hepatic cell membranes to demonstrate a decrease in the number of EGF receptors detectable by 8 h post-hepatectomy, whereas insulin binding was unchanged.[62] The level of messenger RNA for the EGF receptor also fell at around 6–12 h, but then rose dramatically at 24 and 72 h post-hepatectomy.[99] A modest increase in responsiveness to EGF was observed in cultures of hepatocytes isolated from 12-h regenerating rat liver,[74] although other reports are at variance.[93]

There are divergent findings regarding circulating levels of EGF following partial hepatectomy. According to one report[47] the concentration rose between 6 and 18 h and fell again by 24 h, whereas in another report no differences from control rats were seen for up to 32 h.[162] In the latter study, however, intraperitoneal infusion of antiserum to EGF significantly reduced the regenerative response.[162] Moreover, EGF enhanced the stimulatory effect of insulin/glucagon on liver regeneration *in vivo*.[162]

In general, the accumulated evidence from *in vivo* experiments and hepatocyte cultures favours EGF as a possible primary hepatic growth regulator, but despite widespread studies in many different cell types, its physiological role within the animal remains enigmatic.

A recent significant development has been the identification of transforming growth factor alpha (TGF-α) as a possible stimulatory factor in the liver. TGF-α shares 30–40% amino-acid sequence homology to EGF and acts through the EGF receptor; it consequently mimics many of the biological actions of EGF. Although messenger RNA transcripts for TGF-α were undetectable in livers of normal and sham-hepatectomized rats, they appeared 8 h after partial hepatectomy, increasing 9-fold by 24 h,[142] the time when DNA synthesis is at its peak. Both the messenger RNA and the peptide were localized in hepatocytes, occurring in higher amounts in cells from regenerating liver. Moreover, TGF-α caused a 13-fold elevation of DNA synthesis in hepatocytes in primary culture, and was slightly more potent than epidermal growth factor in both rat and human hepatocytes.[97,142] The increase in TGF-α mRNA during the first day after partial hepatectomy coincided with an increase in EGF/TGF-α receptor mRNA and a decrease in receptor number.[62,95,99]

The previously mentioned increase in circulating EGF may be consonant with a rise in TGF-α instead, because the radio-receptor assay employed probably does not distinguish between EGF and TGF-α.[47] This rise in blood levels preceded the TGF-α messenger RNA elevation by 2 h, suggesting extrahepatic sources for the growth signal. Since EGF-stimulated hepatocyte cultures release TGF-α into the medium,[65,66] the discovery of TGF-α does not exclude a possible early requirement for EGF in signalling regeneration. Alternatively, TGF-α, if available from extrahepatic sources could fulfil this early requirement. The TGF-α originating in the liver may function as an autocrine regulator, promoting progression of regeneration after initiation by signals from the rest of the body.[65]

Overall, the evidence supporting a role for EGF or its homologue TGF-α in regulating liver regeneration is considerable, though much uncertainty remains.

Heparin-binding growth factors

Originally isolated from bovine pituitary and brain, heparin-binding growth factors (HBGF), also termed fibroblast growth factors (FGF), are mitogenic for a wide variety of cell types. Several variants are now known, the two major ones being HBGF-1 (acidic FGF) and HBGF-2 (basic FGF). They are polypeptides of similar molecular weight (15–16 kD) with 55% amino-acid sequence homology, but differ in their biological activities (reviewed in Refs 34, 230). Recently, specific messenger RNA transcripts for HBGF-1 were shown to rise from low but detectable levels in normal rat liver within 4 h after partial hepatectomy, reach a peak at 24 h, and remain elevated for 5 days.[105] This rise was accompanied by a substantial increase in the amount of immunoreactive peptide, at least at 48 h. HBGF-1 also exhibited growth stimulatory activity in rat hepatocyte cultures.[105] Expression of a 25-kD form of HBGF-2 has been shown to increase in regenerating rat liver.[167] These observations provide evidence of a role for HBGFs as possible extrahepatic initiators and/or additional autocrine growth mediators in the liver. As with TGF-α, their relevance to the initiating signals themselves is uncertain, since the increases in expression seem to be insufficiently early in the growth-induction process.

Growth hormone (GH) and insulin-like growth factors (IGFs)

Hypophysectomy was observed to retard hepatic regeneration (DNA synthesis) by about 15 h[169,234] and serum levels of GH were low.[150] GH administration accelerated and enhanced regeneration in non-hypophysectomized animals,[189] especially when given several hours or more in advance of liver resection.[149,187]

Insulin-like growth factors 1 and 2 (originally known as somatomedins, molecular weights 7 kD and 6.8 kD respectively) are synthesized in liver following administration or secretion of growth hormone and are thought to be its active principle.

In normal rats, plasma concentrations of total IGFs decreased by 75% within 4–6 h after partial hepatectomy and returned slowly to the original values during the next 5–6 days.[234] Others have reported that partially hepatectomized animals had higher total IGF activity than sham-operated controls over a 7-day period.[233] The discrepancy may in part be accounted for by differences in the assays used to measure IGF activity. Using a specific assay, further pair feeding studies showed a fall in plasma IGF-1 levels after partial hepatectomy which was attributable to diminished food intake, because circulating IGF-1 levels also fell in sham-hepatectomized rats fed an isocaloric diet.[184]

Although adult rat and human hepatocytes do not express IGF-1 receptors,[38,136] the recent demonstration of IGF-1 receptor expression in regenerating rat liver suggests that IGFs may mediate some effects on liver growth.[38] The changes occur more than 24 h after hepatectomy indicating little involvement in the growth-initiation phase.

The stimulatory influence of IGFs on adult rat hepatocytes in co-culture[111] is consistent with the previously recognized growth-enhancing effects of GH on the liver *in vivo*. We have consistently failed to demonstrate any growth-promoting effects of GH or IGFs on adult hepatocytes cultured alone.[181,220]

SERUM/PLASMA AND LIVER-DERIVED FACTORS __

During the 1980s several proteins that stimulate proliferation of hepatocytes in culture have been isolated from serum that are mostly larger molecules than the known hormones and growth factors. Additional factors have been extracted from liver, and are suggested to function in an autocrine mode. In all instances their activity has only been assessed in cultured cells, and their actions within the animal have been explored minimally, or not at all. Consequently their physiological function although likely to be important, remains to be definitively established.

Hepatocyte growth factor (HGF) from blood platelets

An observation that serum from normal rats stimulated proliferation of cultured hepatocytes more potently than sera from a number of other species,[214] coupled with the early report that serum is far more effective than plasma in stimulating growth in cultured cells,[5] led to the finding that rat blood platelets contained a potent mitogen for hepatocytes.[214] Partial characterization showed it to be a cationic protein, differing in physical properties and biological activity from the recognized human platelet-derived growth factor,[185,186,214] Subsequent investigators starting with platelets from over 1000 rats have succeeded in purifying this factor to homogeneity, designating it hepatocyte growth factor (HGF).[154,155] For full activation of HGF, mild proteolysis (thrombin treatment) was employed, which may partially explain differences among factors being studied elsewhere.

Hepatopoietins (HPTA and HPTB)

Two factors termed hepatopoietins A and B (HPTA and HPTB) have been identified in rat serum, and are more abundant in serum from rats 24–48 h after partial hepatectomy than from normal or sham-hepatectomized rats. Like HGF, they exhibit specificity for primary hepatocyte but not fibroblast or JM1 hepatoma cell cultures.[143,144]

HPTB was found to be a low-molecular-weight substance (< 3 kD) which interacted synergistically with HPTA in stimulating DNA synthesis in primary hepatocyte cultures.[144] Its precise characterization remains elusive.

HPTA, like HGF, also required proteolytic enzyme cleavage of a high-molecular-weight form for full activation.[229] A form recently isolated and purified from rabbit serum was found to be a protein comprising two subunits of 70 kD and 35 kD[246] sizes almost identical to those described for HGF. Very recently the amino-

terminal sequence of the light chain of this molecule was determined, and a monoclonal antibody was obtained. HPTA was localized in various tissues, including pancreatic acinar cells, brain neurones, salivary glands and Brunner's glands of the duodenum, but liver, spleen and kidney appeared negative.[247,248]

Human hepatocyte growth factor (hHGF)

A human hepatocyte growth-promoting activity originally identified in the serum of some patients with fulminant hepatic failure and probably not platelet derived[79] was purified and found to be an 85-kD protein comprising two subunits of approximately 60 kD and 33 kD. It was 10-fold more potent in stimulating DNA synthesis in isolated rat hepatocytes than EGF,[80] and was even more potent in adult human hepatocytes.[221] Of particular clinical interest, the hHGF level in plasma correlated closely with the degree of encephalopathy in patients with fulminant hepatic failure.[232]

Human HGF has been cloned, revealing the complete nucleotide and deduced amino-acid sequence for the two subunits.[147] In addition, this clone has recently been successfully expressed as a bioactive recombinant polypeptide with high potency on both rat and human hepatocytes.[221] The sequence proves to be identical not only to another human HGF sequence reported[153] but also with the N-terminal sequence of the light chain of HPTA.[247]

Independent studies from several groups have thus identified a common hepatic growth factor, and rapid progress in understanding its origin, the mechanisms through which its expression and release are controlled, and especially its likely role in liver regeneration are eagerly awaited.

Hepatic stimulatory substance (HSS)

Intraperitoneal injections of extracts of weanling and regenerating liver, but not normal rat liver augment growth of pre-stimulated liver.[116,118] Although also identified in mouse, dog, and pig,[71,75,227,236] purification of the active substance to homogeneity has not yet been achieved. It appears to be heat stable, non-dialysable, protease sensitive, unrelated to other known growth factors and hepatotrophic agents,[70,120] and to comprise between two and three subunits variably ranging from 12 to 50 kD.[70,75,119] *In vitro* HSS is inactive on non-hepatic epithelial cells and mesenchymal cells but stimulates growth of a variety of hepatoma cell lines.[70,115,117] Addition of EGF or serum factors is required to demonstrate its growth-promoting action in normal adult hepatocyte cultures.[115,116]

Although HSS may serve as a potentiating autocrine factor for liver growth, at present its possible role as a physiological growth modulator is difficult to evaluate.

Miscellaneous hepatotrophic factors

Numerous reports have identified additional substances with varying degrees of hepatotrophic potency either *in vivo* or *in vitro*. Active substances have been obtained from plasma/serum of patients following partial hepatic resections or with various liver diseases or from serum or proliferating animal livers.[55,56,81,113,151,193–195] Some have been well characterized, e.g. an albumin/bilirubin complex[55], others only partially so, and the way in which they may relate to the factors already discussed is unclear.

GROWTH INHIBITORY FACTORS _____

It was suggested long ago that negative growth controls may serve not only to maintain the normal state of growth arrest but also to modulate and/or terminate the process of liver regeneration or even to stimulate it (by their absence). This has led to a plethora of reports of factors present in serum or extracted from normally proliferating or neoplastic livers, exhibiting various liver growth-inhibitory properties either *in vivo* or *in vitro* (for review see Ref. 2). Much of the work has dealt with crude or non-hepatocyte-specific material.

Transforming growth factor beta (TGF-β)

TGF-β is a ubiquitous 25-kD polypeptide whose actions *in vivo* are unknown and *in vitro* are remarkably diverse depending upon the cell type, culture conditions and cytokines present. Its actions include inhibition or stimulation of cell proliferation, modulation of cell differentiation and regulation of numerous cellular functions (for reviews see Refs 135, 178 (general) and 215 (in liver)).

An intravenous injection of TGF-β 11 h post-hepatectomy delayed DNA synthesis substantially but injection at zero hours did not.[183] This inhibition was transient and reversible; hepatic DNA content was restored to normal by 5 days. Moreover, repeated administration for 5 days failed to suppress the recovery.[183]

TGF-β mRNA was low in livers of normal or sham-hepatectomized control rats, but rose several-fold in 4-h regenerating liver, increasing further around 18–20 h and peaking at 72 h, then falling. This mRNA was limited to the non-parenchymal (possibly endothelial) cells of the liver.[12,42] It was postulated that TGF-β might act as a paracrine growth inhibitor within the liver, maintaining a carefully regulated and limited growth response. The timing remains paradoxical; TGF-β mRNA rises and remains high during the period of maximal hepatocyte proliferative activity.

It was originally shown[157] and repeatedly confirmed[41,141,217] that TGF-β inhibited DNA synthesis with high potency in adult rat as well as adult human and fetal hepatocytes in culture,[97,219] and that the effect was reversible. Reports from several laboratories are varied and conflicting regarding changes in sensitivity to TGF-β of hepatocytes isolated from livers regenerating for different periods of time after partial hepatectomy.[12,42,93,217,]

[218] Responsiveness to TGF-β in other cultured cell types was found to be modifiable by various hormones and growth factors.[178] In normal and regenerating hepatocyte cultures norepinephrine increased the resistance to inhibition by TGF-β 5-fold[92,93] or more. It appears that interactions of a number of factors including growth-stimulatory hormones and growth factors influence reactions of hepatocyte cultures to TGF-β and at least some of the discrepancies may hinge on these interactions.

Other growth inhibitors

An inhibitor of hepatic proliferation, extracted from normal rat liver, has been identified, purified and designated hepatic proliferation inhibitor (HPI). It was found to have a molecular weight of 17–19 kD and an isoelectric point of 5.5.[96,140] Although similar to TGF-β in some properties, HPI reversibly inhibited a rat liver epithelial cell line which was irreversibly inhibited by TGF-β[139,141] and its inhibitory action was not blocked by anti-TGF-β antibodies.[96]

Rat platelets contain an additional hepatocyte growth inhibitor distinguished from platelet-derived TGF-β by its high molecular weight (> 200 kD) and acid and heat lability.[156]

CONCLUSIONS _____

Regulation of liver growth presents a problem of tantalizing complexity. Although the emphasis in this review has been upon hepatocytes and the factors that initiate and modulate their growth, non-parenchymal cells, which comprise about 40% of the hepatic cell population, participate in a highly coordinated fashion in the growth process. Following partial hepatectomy, they start proliferating many hours after the hepatocytes, suggesting that their engagement in regeneration may be secondary, depending upon direct signals from the already activated hepatocytes.

According to present concepts, a functional hepatic overload generates signals from the body which interact with receptor molecules on the hepatocyte surface. On the basis of studies in various cell types as well as hepatocytes, the binding of growth-initiating signals to their receptors triggers a cascade of events within the cell. This cascade involves second messengers, protein kinases and sequential activation and suppression of oncogenes and other growth-related genes, possibly leading to release of certain autocrine (and perhaps also paracrine) regulators. Ultimately, the cells progress through S phase, mitosis and cytokinesis. This is the broad overview: much remains to be elucidated. The large and rapidly expanding literature concerning these intracellular events is beyond the scope of this chapter.

A large body of evidence indicates that extracellular growth signals act at the G_0/G_1 phase of the cell cycle. The plethora of proposed extracellular signalling molecules reviewed in this chapter testifies to the uncertainty of their identity as true physiological regulators of liver growth. To pinpoint growth factors *in vivo* is not enough, even if it could be done conclusively; the signals are multiple and interact in ways that are incompletely understood. Cells must be exposed to growth signals for relatively long periods, even though certain responses that occur within seconds or minutes lead to DNA synthesis which does not begin until hours later.[27,39,179] Although these reactions can be obtained *in vivo*, clarification has largely come from studies involving cultures of many cell types, whose mechanisms for growth initiation and fine tuning differ in at least some respects from hepatocytes. Final unravelling of the complexities of growth signalling is unlikely to be accomplished within the animal.

The alternative to whole-animal studies is the *in vitro* approach, which has its own difficulties. Cells undergo drastic changes once removed from the body and placed in the artificial environment of a culture dish. Even relatively short-term survival and functioning of normal adult hepatocytes in primary cultures depend not only on adequacy of nutrient and hormone availability but also on interactions with other cells and the extracellular matrix.[11,25,84,172] In the absence of these, although the cells can initially respond to mitogens, many of their liver specific functions, such as synthesis of proteins produced mainly by hepatocytes, are rapidly lost, particularly in conventional cultures, but probably to a lesser extent in other cultures as well. This loss does not invalidate the valuable insights into mechanisms through which growth signal actions are implemented, now emerging from hepatocyte cultures. If, however, hepatocytes grow in response to demands for specific liver functions and hepatocytes in culture have lost most of these functions, identification of the true physiological growth signals from *in vitro* studies proves difficult (see Ref. 25 for fuller discussion). It is conceivable that cell responsiveness is so altered *in vitro* that growth could be induced by substances whose *in vivo* effects are unimportant, although the many parallels between mitogenic responses *in vitro* and *in vivo* make this seem unlikely.

Obviously, growth factor effectiveness must be evaluated in the animal as well as in culture. Even so, many of the suggested hepatocyte growth-signalling substances included in this review have been examined in both ways, but questions still remain.

Despite these caveats, several substances seem of particular interest as possible primary initiators, i.e. substances responsible for mobilizing hepatocytes from their G_o arrested state. These are: EGF, TGF-α, HBGFs and especially the relatively untested newly purified hepatocyte growth factor (HGF/HPTA). The role of EGF remains unclear despite intensive study. The more recently discovered TGF-α and HBGFs are effective hepatocyte growth stimulators and their production by hepatocytes during early regeneration may suggest their function in an autocrine mode as self-stimulating growth amplifiers;

alternatively or additionally, they may serve as signals from hepatocytes to potentiate growth in the non-parenchymal liver cell population. None of these factors acts only on liver cells. HGF/HPTA is a highly potent growth factor for hepatocytes, and its availability as a recombinant polypeptide[221] will enable rigorous testing of its cellular specificity, and indeed its *in vivo* physiological significance, to be evaluated.

Of the negative growth-signalling factors, TGF-β is the leading exponent. Its production is limited to non-hepatocytes and it appears to be maximally expressed during the period of highest regenerative activity. Although suggested to act as a paracrine regulator to deactivate regeneration as the liver cell complement nears completion, an alternative possibility is that its primary function is to promote the laying down of new extracellular matrix needed as the liver enlarges—indeed, enhancement of collagen production is a well-established TGF-β function.[178] It seems possible that for an organ as multifunctional as the liver, more than one set of growth signals may be required to meet the variety of possible functional needs. Perhaps more than one set of signals is required to set in motion two or more intracellular chains of events which must interact to activate DNA synthesis. The many possible modulators such as insulin, norepinephrine or TGF-β may have important ancillary roles in amplifying or damping the growth process. Specificity and potency of the growth stimulus may depend on receptor occupancy by key combinations of signals which may differ in response to differing functional demands of the body.

The final analysis depends upon a fuller understanding of the mechanisms through which the controlling signals operate. In this context, the growing research emphasis on the events resulting from growth signals binding to their receptors on the cell surface takes on an added significance. The preponderance of available data on induction and regulation of cell proliferation comes from fibroblasts which differ from hepatocytes in many respects, including the spectrum of growth factors to which they respond. With the rapidly mounting rate of hepatocyte research, however, new, more definitive answers to what factors control liver regeneration should not be far off.

. . . the trouble . . . is they ain't nothing but theories, after all, and theories don't prove nothing, they'll only give you a place to rest on a spell, when you are tuckered out, butting around and around trying to find out something . . ..

Mark Twain in *Tom Sawyer Abroad*

Acknowledgements

We gratefully acknowledge the support from USPHS Grant CA39099 awarded by the National Cancer Institute and Grant 2237 from the Council for Tobacco Research, USA (NLRB) the Nuffield Foundation, UK (AJS) and the Wellcome Trust (AJS).

REFERENCES

1. Aggerbeck, M., Ferry, N., Zafrani, E.S. *et al.* (1983) Adrenergic regulation of glycogenolysis in rat liver after cholestasis. *Journal of Clinical Investigation*, **71**, 476–486.
2. Alison, M.R. (1986) Regulation of hepatic growth. *Physiological Reviews*, **66**, 499–541.
3. Anthony, L.E. & Edozien, J.C. (1975) Experimental protein and energy deficiencies in the rat. *Journal of Nutrition*, **105**, 631–648.
4. Ashrif, S., Gillespie, J.S. & Pollock, D. (1974) The effects of drugs or denervation on thymidine uptake into rat regenerating liver. *European Journal of Pharmacology*, **29**, 324–327.
5. Balk, S.D. (1971) Calcium as a regulator of the proliferation of normal but not of transformed chick fibroblasts in a plasma-containing media. *Proceedings of the National Academy of Sciences of the USA*, **68**, 271–275.
6. Barbiroli, B. & Potter, V. (1971) DNA synthesis and interaction between controlled feeding schedules and partial hepatectomy in rats. *Science*, **172**, 738–740.
7. Barka, T. & Popper, H. (1967) Liver enlargement and drug toxicity. *Medicine*, **46**, 103–117.
8. Barra, R. & Hall, J.C. (1977) Liver regeneration in normal and alloxan-induced diabetic rats. *Journal of Experimental Zoology*, **201**, 93–100.
9. Baserga, R. (1985) *The Biology of Cell Reproduction*, Cambridge, Mass.: Harvard University Press.
10. Bioulac-Sage, P., Lafon, M.E., Saric, J. & Balabaud, C. (1990) Nerves and perisinusoidal cells in human liver. *Journal of Hepatology*, **10**, 105–112.
11. Bissell, D.M., Arenson, D.M., Maher, J.J. & Roll, F.J. (1987) Support of cultured hepatocytes by a laminin-rich gel. *Journal of Clinical Investigation*, **79**, 801–812.
12. Braun, L., Mead, J.E., Panzica, M. *et al.* (1988) Transforming growth factor β mRNA increases during liver regeneration: A possible paracrine mechanism of growth regulation. *Proceedings of the National Academy of Sciences of the USA*, **85**, 1539–1543.
13. Broelsch, C.E., Lee, S., Charters, A.C. *et al.* (1974) Regeneration of liver isografts transplanted in continuity with splanchnic organs. *Surgical Forum*, **25**, 394–396.
14. Bronstad, G. & Christoffersen, T. (1980) Increased effect of adrenaline on cyclic-AMP formation and positive β-adrenergic modulation of DNA synthesis in regenerating hepatocytes. *FEBS Letters*, **120**, 89–93.
15. Bronstad, G.O., Sand, T.E. & Christoffersen, T. (1983) Bidirectional concentration-dependent effects of glucagon and dibutyryl cyclic AMP and DNA synthesis in cultured adult rat hepatocytes. *Biochimica et Biophysica Acta*, **763**, 58–63.
16. Brown, J., Mullen, Y., Molner, I.G. & Clarke, W.R. (1976) Importance of hepatic portal route for control of diabetes. *Diabetes*, **25**, 338.
17. Brues, A.M., Drury, D.R. & Brues, M.C. (1936) A quantitative study of cell growth in regenerating liver. *Archives of Pathology*, **22**, 658–673.
18. Bucher, N.L.R. (1963) Regeneration of mammalian liver. *International Review of Cytology*, **15**, 245–300.
19. Bucher, N.L.R. (1987) Regulation of liver growth: Historical perspectives and future direction. In Rauckman, E.J. & Padilla, G.M. (eds) *The Isolated Hepatocyte: Use in Toxicology and Xenobiotic Transformations*, pp. 1–19. New York: Academic Press.
20. Bucher, N.L.R. (1982) Thirty years of liver regeneration: a distillate. In Sato, G.H., Pardee, A.B. & Sirbaska, D.A. (eds) *Cold Spring Harbor Conferences on Cell Proliferation*, vol. 9, pp. 15–24. New York: Cold Spring Harbor Laboratory.
21. Bucher, N.L.R. & Malt, R.A. (1971) *Regeneration of the Liver and Kidney*. Boston: Little, Brown.
22. Bucher, N.L.R., McGowan, J.A. & Patel, U. (1978) Hormonal regulation of liver growth. In Dirksen, E.R., Prescott, D.M. & Fox, C.F. (eds) *ICN/UCLA Symposia on Molecular and Cellular Biology*, vol. XII, pp. 661–670. New York: Academic Press.
23. Bucher, N.L.R., Patel, U. & Cohen, S. (1978) Hormonal factors concerned with liver regeneration. In *Ciba Foundation Symposium*, No. 55 (New series). *Hepatotrophic Factors*, pp. 95–107. New York: Elsevier/Excerpta Medica/North Holland.
24. Bucher, N.L.R., Patel, U. & Cohen, S. (1977) Hormonal factors and liver growth. In Weber, G. (ed.) *Advances in Enzyme Regulation*, vol. 16, pp. 205–213. New York: Pergamon Press.
25. Bucher, N.L.R., Robinson, G.S. & Farmer, S.R. (1990) Effects of extracellular matrix on hepatocyte growth and gene expression: implications for hepatic regeneration and the repair of liver injury. *Seminars in Liver Disease*, **10**, 11–19.
26. Bucher, N.L.R., Russell, W.E. & McGowan, J.A. (1982) Aspects of hormonal influence on liver growth. In Picazo, J. (ed.) *Glucagon in Gastroenterology and Hepatology*, pp. 141–151. Boston: MTP Press.
27. Bucher, N.L.R., Schrock, T.R. & Moolten, F.L. (1969) An experimental view of hepatic regeneration. *Johns Hopkins Medical Journal*, **125**, 250–257.
28. Bucher, N.L.R. & Swaffield, M.N. (1973) Regeneration of liver in rats in absence of portal splanchnic organs and a portal blood supply. *Cancer Research*, **35**, 3189–3194.
29. Bucher, N.L.R. & Swaffield, M.N. (1975) Synergistic action of glucagon and insulin in regulation of hepatic regeneration. In Weber, G. (ed.) *Advances in Enzyme Regulation*, vol. 13, pp. 281–293. New York and Oxford: Pergamon Press.
30. Bucher, N.L.R. & Swaffield, M.N. (1975) Regulation of hepatic regeneration in rats by synergistic action of insulin and glucagon. *Proceedings of the National Academy of Sciences of the USA*, **72**, 1157–1160.
31. Bucher, N.L.R. & Weir, G.C. (1976) Insulin, glucagon, liver regeneration, and DNA synthesis. *Metabolism*, **25**, 1423–1425.
32. Buckley, A.R., Putnam, C.W, Evans, R. *et al.* (1987) Hepatic protein kinase C: translocation stimulated by prolactin and partial hepatectomy. *Life Sciences*, **41**, 2827–2834.
33. Buckley, A.R., Putnam, C.W., Montgomery, D.W. & Russell, D.H. (1986) Prolactin administration stimulates rat hepatic DNA synthesis. *Biochemical and Biophysical Research Communications*, **138**, 1138–1145.
34. Burgess, W.H. & Maciag, T. (1989) The heparin-binding (fibroblast) growth factor family of proteins. *Annual Review of Biochemistry*, **58**, 575–606.
35. Burt, A.D., Tiniakos, D., MacSween, R.N.M. *et al.* (1989) Localization of adrenergic and neuropeptide tyrosine-containing nerves in the mammalian liver. *Hepatology*, **9**, 839–845.
36. Cahill, G. (1973) Glucagon. *New England Journal of Medicine*, **288**, 157–158.
37. Campbell, R.M., Fell, B.F. & Mackie, W.S. (1972) Ornithine decarboxylase activity, nucleic acid and cell turnover in the livers of pregnant rats. *Journal of Physiology*, **241**, 699–713.
38. Caro, J.F., Poulos, J., Ittoop, O. *et al.* (1988) Insulin-like growth factor I binding in hepatocytes from human liver, human hepatoma, and normal, regenerating, and fetal rat liver. *Journal of Clinical Investigation*, **81**, 976–981.
39. Carpenter, G., Stoscheck, C.M. & Soderquist, A.M. (1982) Epidermal growth factor. *Annals of the New York Academy of Sciences*, **397**, 11–17.
40. Carpenter, G. & Wahl, M.I. (1990) The epidermal growth factor family. In Sporn, M.B. & Roberts, A.B. (eds) *Handbook of Experimental Pharmacology*, chap. 4, pp. 69–171. New York: Springer-Verlag.
41. Carr, B.I., Hayashi, I., Branum, E.L. & Moses, H.L. (1986) Inhibition of DNA synthesis in rat hepatocytes by platelet-derived type β transforming growth factor. *Cancer Research*, **46**, 2330–2334.
42. Carr, B.I., Huang, T.H., Itakura, K. *et al.* (1989) TGFβ gene transcription in normal and neoplastic liver growth. *Journal of Cellular Biochemistry*, **39**, 477–487.
43. Caruana, J.A., Goldman, J.K., Camara, D.S. & Gage, A.A. (1981) Insulin, glucagon and glucose in the regeneration response of the liver. *Surgery, Gynaecology and Obstetrics*, **153**, 726–730.
44. Caruana, J.A., Whalen, D.A. Jr, Anthony, W.P. *et al.* (1986) Paradoxical effects of glucose feeding on liver regeneration and survival after partial hepatectomy. *Endocrinology Research*, **12**, 147–156.
45. Columbano, A., Ledda-Columbana, G.M., Coni, P.P. *et al.* (1985) Occurrence of cell death (apoptosis) during the involution of liver hyperplasia. *Laboratory Investigation*, **52**, 670–675.
46. Cornell, R.P. (1981) Hyperinsulinemia and hyperglucagonemia in

fasted rats during liver regeneration. *American Journal of Physiology*, **240**, E112–E118.

47. Cornell, R.P. (1985) Gut-derived endotoxin elicits hepatotrophic factor secretion for liver regeneration. *American Journal of Physiology*, **249**, R551–R562.

48. Cruise, J.L., Cotecchia, S. & Michalopoulos, G. (1986) Norepinephrine decreases EGF binding in primary rat hepatocyte cultures. *Journal of Cellular Physiology*, **127**, 39–44.

49. Cruise, J.L., Houck, K.A. & Michalopoulos, G.K. (1985) Induction of DNA synthesis in cultured rat hepatocytes through stimulation of α1 adrenoreceptor by norepinephrine. *Science*, **227**, 749–751.

50. Cruise, J.L., Knechtle, S.J., Bollinger, R. et al. (1987) α1-Adrenergic effects and liver regeneration. *Hepatology*, **7**, 1189–1194.

51. Dallman, P.R., Spirito, R.A. & Siimes, M.A. (1974) Diurnal patterns of DNA synthesis in the rat: modification by diet and feeding schedule. *Journal of Nutrition*, **104**, 1234–1241.

52. de Diego, J.A., Molina, L.M., Bujan, J. et al. (1986) Influence of the conjoint administration of insulin and glucagon upon hepatic regeneration. *Surgery, Gynaecology and Obstetrics*, **163**, 443–447.

53. de Hemptinne, B., Salizzoni, M., Yandza, T.C. et al. (1987) Indication, technique and results of liver graft volume reduction before orthotopic transplantation in children. *Transplantation Proceedings*, **19**, 3549–3551.

54. Desser-Wiest, L. (1975) Autosynchronization of rat liver cells with endogenous corticosterone after partial hepatectomy. *Cell and Tissue Kinetics*, **8**, 1–9.

55. Diaz-Gil, J.J., Gavilanes, J.G., Sanchez, G. et al. (1987) Identification of a liver growth factor as an albumin-bilirubin complex. *Biochemical Journal*, **243**, 443–448.

56. Diaz-Gil, J.J., Sanchez, G., Santamaria, L. et al. (1986) Liver DNA synthesis promoter activity detected in human plasma from subjects with hepatitis. *Hepatology*, **6**, 658–661.

57. Dillman, W.H., Schwartz, H.L. & Oppenheimer, J.H. (1978) Selective alterations in hepatic enzyme response after reduction of nuclear triiodothyronine receptor sites by partial hepatectomy and starvation. *Biochemical and Biophysical Research Communications*, **80**, 259–266.

58. Doljanski, P., Rosenthal, J. & Eisenberg, S. (1966) Liver regeneration in starved rats. *Experimental and Molecular Pathology*, **5**, 263–272.

59. Duguay, L.R., Charters, A.C., Lee, S. et al. (1975) Time course of liver regeneration after splanchnic organ ablation. *Surgical Forum*, **26**, 408–410.

60. Duguay, L.R. & Orloff, M.J. (1976) Regulation of liver regeneration by the pancreas in dogs. *Surgical Forum*, **27**, 355–356.

61. Duguay, R., Skivolocki, W.P. & Orloff, M.J. (1977) Regulation of liver regeneration by pancreatic hormones. *Gastroenterology*, **72**, 1053.

62. Earp, H.S. & O'Keefe, E.J. (1981) Epidermal growth factor receptor numbers decrease during rat liver regeneration. *Journal of Clinical Investigation*, **67**, 1580–1583.

63. Emond, J.C., Whitington, P.F., Thistlethwaite, J.R. et al. (1989) Reduced-size orthotopic liver transplantation: Use in the management of children with chronic liver disease. *Hepatology*, **10**, 867–872.

64. Farivar, M., Wands, J.R., Isselbacher, K.J. & Bucher, N.L.R. (1976) Effect of insulin and glucagon in fulminant murine hepatitis. *New England Journal of Medicine*, **295**, 1517–1519.

65. Fausto, N. (1990) Hepatic regeneration. In Zakim, D. & Boyer, T.D. (eds), *Hepatology*, 2nd edn, pp. 49–65. London: W.B. Saunders.

66. Fausto, N. & Mead, J.E. (1989) Regulation of liver growth: Protooncogenes and transforming growth factors. *Laboratory Investigation*, **60**, 4–13.

67. Ferris, G.M. & Clark, J.B. (1972) Early changes in plasma and hepatic free amino acids in partially hepatectomized rats. *Biochimica et Biophysica Acta*, **273**, 73–79.

68. Fisher, B., Gunduz, N., Saffer, E.A. & Zheng, S. (1984) Relation of oestrogen and its receptor to rat liver growth and regeneration. *Cancer Research*, **44**, 2410–2415.

69. Fishman, J.B., Dickey, B.F., Bucher, N.L.R. & Fine, R.E. (1985) Internalization, recycling and redistribution of vasopressin receptors in rat hepatocytes. *Journal of Biological Chemistry*, **260**, 12641–12646.

70. Fleig, W.E. & Hoss, G. (1989) Partial purification of rat hepatic

stimulator substance and characterization of its action on hepatoma cells and normal hepatocytes. *Hepatology*, **9**, 240–248.

71. Fleig, W.E., Lehmann, H., Wagner, H. et al. (1986) Hepatic regenerative stimulator substance in the rabbit: relation to liver regeneration after partial hepatectomy. *Journal of Hepatology*, **3**, 19–26.

72. Francavilla, A., Eagon, P.K., Dileo, A. et al. (1986) Sex hormone related functions in the regenerating male rat liver. *Gastroenterology*, **91**, 1263–1270.

73. Francavilla, A., Gavalien, J.S., Makawaka, L. et al. (1989) Estradiol and testosterone levels in patients undergoing partial hepatectomy. *Digestive Diseases and Sciences*, **34**, 818–822.

74. Francavilla, A., Ove, P., Polimeno, L. et al. (1986) Epidermal growth factor and proliferation in rat hepatocytes in primary culture isolated at different times after partial hepatectomy. *Cancer Research*, **46**, 1318–1323.

75. Francavilla, A., Ove, P., Polimeno, L. et al. (1987) Extraction and partial purification of a hepatic stimulatory substance in rats, mice, and dogs. *Cancer Research*, **47**, 5600–5605.

76. Francavilla, A., Polimeno, L., Dile, A. et al. (1989) The effect of estrogen and tamoxifen on hepatocyte proliferation in vivo and in vitro. *Hepatology*, **9**, 614–620.

77. Freise, J., Mueller, W.H. & Broelsch, C.E. (1982) Accumulation of insulin and glucagon in the liver (via portal vein catheter or with liposomes) does not stimulate liver cell regeneration after partial hepatectomy in normal or portacaval shunted rats. *Research in Experimental Medicine*, **180**, 31–39.

78. Friedman, D.L., Claus, T.H., Pilkis, S.J. & Pine, G. (1981) Hormonal regulation of DNA synthesis in primary cultures of adult rat hepatocyte—action of glucagon. *Experimental Cell Research*, **135**, 283–290.

79. Gohda, E., Tsubouchi, H., Nakayama, H. et al. (1986) Human hepatocyte growth factor in plasma from patients with fulminant hepatic failure. *Experimental Cell Research*, **166**, 139–150.

80. Gohda, E., Tsubouchi, H., Nakayama, H. et al. (1988) Purification and partial characterization of hepatocyte growth factor from plasma of a patient with fulminant hepatic failure. *Journal of Clinical Investigation*, **81**, 414–419.

81. Goldberg, M. (1985) Purification and partial characterization of a liver cell proliferation factor called hepatopoietin. *Journal of Cellular Biochemistry*, **27**, 291–302.

82. Gospodarowicz, D. & Moran, J.S. (1976) Growth factors in mammalian cell culture. *Annual Review of Biochemistry*, **45**, 531–558.

83. Grisham, J.W. (1962) A morphologic study of deoxyribonucleic acid synthesis of cell proliferation in regenerating rat liver; autoradiography with thymidine-^{3}H. *Cancer Research*, **22**, 842–849.

84. Guguen-Guillouzo, C. (1986) Role of homotypic and heterotypic cell interactions in expression of specific functions by cultured hepatocytes. In Guillouzo, A. & Guguen-Guillouzo, C. (eds) *Research in Isolated and Cultured Hepatocytes*, pp. 259–284. London: John Libbey Eurotext/INSERM.

85. Harrison, M.F. (1953) Effect of starvation on the composition of the liver cell. *Biochemical Journal*, **55**, 204–211.

86. Hasegawa, K. & Koga, M. (1977) Induction of liver cell proliferation in intact rats by amines and glucagon. *Life Sciences*, **21**, 1723–1728.

87. Hilton, J. & Sartorelli, A. (1970) Induction of microsomal drug metabolizing enzymes in regenerating liver. In Weber, G. (ed.) *Advances in Enzyme Regulation*, pp. 153–167. New York: Pergamon Press.

88. Holecek, M. & Simek, J. (1988) Effect of the infusion of glucose, intralipid and nutramin on the initiation of rat liver regeneration after partial hepatectomy. *Physiologia Bohemoslovenica*, **37**, 467–473.

89. Holecek, M., Simek, J., Kruf, M. et al. (1985) Effect of branched chain amino acids on liver regeneration after partial hepatectomy. *Physiologia Bohemoslovenica*, **34**, 359–366.

90. Holley, R.W. (1975) Control of growth of mammalian cells in cell culture. *Nature*, **258**, 487–490.

91. Holley, R.W. & Kiernan, J.A. (1974) Control of the initiation of DNA synthesis in 3T3 cells: low molecular weight nutrients. *Proceedings of the National Academy of Sciences of the USA*, **71**, 2942–2945.

92. Houck, K.A., Cruise, J.L. & Michalopoulos, G.K. (1988) Norepinephrine modulates the growth-inhibiting effect of transforming

growth factor β in primary rat hepatocyte cultures. *Journal of Cellular Physiology*, **135**, 551–555.

93. Houck, K.A. & Michalopoulos, G.K. (1989) Altered responses of regenerating hepatocytes to norepinephrine and transforming growth factor type β. *Journal of Cellular Physiology*, **141**, 503–509.

94. Howl, J., Ismail, T., Strain, A.J. *et al.* (1991) Characterization of the human liver vasopressin receptor. *Biochemical Journal*, in press.

95. Hseih, L.L., Peraino, C. & Weinstein, I.B. (1988) Expression of endogenous retrovirus-like sequences and cellular oncogenes during phenobarbital treatment and regeneration in rat liver. *Cancer Research*, **48**, 265–269.

96. Huggett, A.C., Krutzsch, H.C. & Thorgeirsson, S.S. (1987) Characterization of an hepatic proliferation inhibitor (HPI): Effect of HPI on the growth of normal liver cells—comparison with transforming growth factor beta. *Journal of Cellular Biochemistry*, **35**, 305–314.

97. Ismail, T., Strain, A.J. & McMaster, P. (1989) The role of transforming growth factors alpha and beta on DNA synthesis in normal adult human hepatocytes. *Hepatology*, **10**, 606.

98. Jiang, L.-W. & Schindler, M. (1990) Nucleocytoplasmic transport is enhanced concomitant with nuclear accumulation of epidermal growth factor (EGF) binding activity in both 3T3–1 and EGF receptor reconstituted NR–6 fibroblasts. *Journal of Cell Biology*, **110**, 559–568.

99. Johnson, A.C., Garfield, S.H., Merlino, G.T. & Pastan, I. (1988) Expression of epidermal growth factor receptor proto-oncogene mRNA in regenerating rat liver. *Biochemical and Biophysical Research Communications*, **150**, 412–418.

100. Kahn, D., Eagon, P.K., Porter, L.E. *et al.* (1989) Effect of tamoxifen on hepatic regeneration in male rats. *Digestive Diseases and Sciences*, **34**, 27–32.

101. Kahn, D., Gavaler, J.S., Makowka, L. *et al.* (1988) Does hyperprolactinemia effect hepatic regeneration independent of sex steroids. *Journal of Laboratory and Clinical Medicine*, **112**, 644–651.

102. Kahn, D., Zeng, Q., Makowka, L. *et al.* (1989) Orthotopic liver transplantation and the cytosolic estrogen–androgen receptor status of the liver. The influence of the sex of the donor. *Hepatology*, **10**, 861–866.

103. Kallenbach, M., Roome, N.O. & Schulte-Hermann, R. (1983) Kinetics of DNA synthesis in feeding-dependent and independent hepatocyte populations of rats after partial hepatectomy. *Cell Tissue Kinetics*, **16**, 321–332.

104. Kam, I., Lynch, S., Svanas, G. *et al.* (1987) Evidence that host size determines liver size: studies in dogs receiving orthotopic liver transplants. *Hepatology*, **7**, 362–366.

105. Kan, M., Huang, J., Mansson, P.E. *et al.* (1989) Heparin-binding growth factor type 1 (acidic fibroblast growth factor): A potential biphasic autocrine and paracrine regulator of hepatocyte regeneration. *Proceedings of the National Academy of Sciences of the USA*, **86**, 7432–7436.

106. Kaufmann, W.K., Kaufman, D.G., Rice, J.M. & Wenk, M.L. (1981) Reversible inhibition of rat hepatocyte proliferation by hydrocortisone and its effect on cell cycle-dependent hepatocarcinogenesis by *N*-methyl-*N*-nitrosourea. *Cancer Research*, **41**, 4653–4660.

107. Kilberg, M.S. (1982) Amino acid transport in isolated rat hepatocytes. *Journal of Membrane Biology*, **69**, 1–12.

108. Kirsch, R.E., Saunders, S.J. Frith, L.O. *et al.* (1979) The effects of intragastric feeding with amino acids on liver regeneration after partial hepatectomy in the rat. *American Journal of Clinical Nutrition*, **32**, 738–740.

109. Kleitzien, R.F., Pariza, M.W., Becker, J.E. & Potter, V.R. (1976) Hormonal regulation of amino acid transport and gluconeogenesis in primary cultures of adult rat liver parenchymal cells. *Journal of Cellular Physiology*, **89**, 641–646.

110. Koch, K.S. & Leffert, H.L. (1979) Increased sodium ion influx is necessary to initiate rat hepatocyte proliferation. *Cell*, **18**, 153–163.

111. Koch, K.S., Shapiro, P., Skelly, H. & Leffert, H.L. (1982) Rat hepatocyte proliferation is stimulated by insulin-like peptides in defined medium. *Biochemical and Biophysical Research Communications*, **109**, 1054–1060.

112. Koga, M. & Hasegawa, K. (1978) Induction of DNA synthesis in rat liver by combinations of saline and glucagon. *Dokkyo Journal of Medical Science*, **5**, 291–296.

113. Kubo, S., Matsui-Yuasa, I., Otani, S. *et al.* (1988) Characterization of liver regeneration stimulatory factor in human portal serum. *American Journal of Gastroenterology*, **83**, 1103–1107.

114. Kunos, G. & Ishac, E.J.N. (1987) Mechanism of inverse regulation of alpha1- and beta-adrenergic receptors. *Biochemical Pharmacology*, **36**, 1185–1191.

115. LaBrecque, D.R. (1979) The role of hepatotrophic factors in liver regeneration—a brief review including a preliminary report of the in vitro effects of hepatic regenerative stimulator substance. *Yale Journal of Biology and Medicine*, **52**, 49–60.

116. LaBrecque, D.R. & Bachur, N.R. (1982) Hepatic stimulator substance: physicochemical characteristics and specificity. *American Journal of Physiology*, **242**, G281–G288.

117. LaBrecque, D.R. & Bachur, N.R. (1982) In vitro stimulation of cell growth by hepatic stimulator substances. *American Journal of Physiology*, **242**, G289–G295.

118. LaBrecque, D.R. & Pesch, L.A. (1975) Preparation and partial characterization of hepatic regenerative stimulator substances (SS) from rat liver. *Journal of Physiology*, **248**, 273–284.

119. LaBrecque, D.R., Steele, G., Fogerty, S. *et al.* (1987) Purification and physical-chemical characterization of hepatic stimulator substance. *Hepatology*, **7**, 100–106.

120. LaBrecque, D.R., Wilson, M. & Fogerty, S. (1984) Stimulation of HTC hepatoma cell growth in vitro by hepatic stimulation substance. *Experimental Cell Research*, **150**, 419–429.

121. LeCam, A., Rey, J.F., Fehlman, M. *et al.* (1979) Amino acid transport in isolated hepatocytes after partial hepatectomy in the rat. *American Journal of Physiology*, **236**, E594–E602.

122. Leduc, E. (1949) Mitotic activity in the liver of the mouse during inanition followed by refeeding with different levels of protein. *American Journal of Anatomy*, **84**, 397–421.

123. Lee, K.L., Sun, S.C. & Miller, O.N. (1968) Stimulation of incorporation by triiodothyronine of thymidine-methyl-3H into hepatic DNA of the rat. *Archives of Biochemistry and Biophysics*, **125**, 751–757.

124. Leffert, H.L. & Alexander, N.M. (1976) Thyroid hormone metabolism during liver regeneration in rats. *Endocrinology*, **98**, 1205–1211.

125. Leffert, H.L., Alexander, N.M., Faloona, G. *et al.* (1975) Specific endocrine and hormonal receptor changes associated with liver regeneration in adult rats. *Proceedings of the National Academy of Sciences of the USA*, **72**, 4033–4036.

126. Leffert, H.L., Koch, K.S., Lad, P.J. *et al.* (1988) Hepatocyte regeneration, replication and differentiation. In Arias, I.M., Jacoby, W.B., Popper, H. *et al.* (eds) *The Liver: Biology and Pathobiology*, pp. 833–850. New York: Reven Press.

127. Leffert, H.L., Koch, K.S., Moran, T. & Rubalcava, B. (1979) Hormonal control of rat liver regeneration. *Gastroenterology*, **76**, 1470–1482.

128. Leffert, H.L., Moran, T., Boorstein, R. & Koch, K.S. (1977) Procarcinogen activation and hormonal control of cell proliferation in differentiated primary adult liver cell cultures. *Nature*, **267**, 58–61.

129. MacManus, J.P., Youdale, T. & Braceland, B.M. (1975) Evidence for the release of calcitonin and parathyroid hormone during liver regeneration in the rat. *Hormone and Metabolic Research*, **7**, 83–87.

130. MacManus, J.P. & Braceland, B.M. (1976) A connection between the production of prostaglandins during liver regeneration and the DNA synthetic responses. *Prostaglandins*, **11**, 609–620.

131. MacManus, J.P., Braceland, B.M., Rixon, R.H. *et al.* (1981) An increase in calmodulin during growth of normal and cancerous liver in vivo. *FEBS Letters*, **133**, 99–102.

132. Malamud, D. & Perrin, L. (1974) Stimulation of DNA synthesis in mouse pancreas by triiodothyronine and glucagon. *Endocrinology*, **94**, 1157–1160.

133. Marsman, D.S., Cattley, R.C., Conway, J.G. & Popp, J.A. (1988) Relationship of hepatic peroxisome proliferation and replicative DNA synthesis to the hepatocarcinogenicity of the peroxisome proliferators di(2-ethylhexyl)phthalate and [4-chloro-6-(2,3-xylidino)-2-pyrimidinyl [thio]acetic acid (Wy-14, 643) in rats. *Cancer Research*, **48**, 6739–6744.

134. Marti, U., Burwen, S.J. & Jones, A.L. (1989) Biological effects of epidermal growth factor, with emphasis on the gastrointestinal tract and liver: an update. *Hepatology*, **9**, 126–138.

135. Massague, J. (1987) The TGF-beta family of growth and differentiation factors. *Cell*, **49**, 437–438.

136. Massague, J. & Czech, M.P. (1982) The subunit structures of two distinct receptors for insulin-like growth factor I and II and their relationship to the insulin receptors. *Journal of Biological Chemistry*, **257**, 5038–5045.

137. McGowan, J.A., Atryzek, V. & Fausto, N. (1979) Effects of protein deprivation on the regeneration of rat liver after partial hepatectomy. *Biochemical Journal*, **180**, 25–35.

138. McGowan, J.A., Strain, A.J. & Bucher, N.L.R. (1981) DNA synthesis in primary cultures of adult rat hepatocytes in a defined medium: effects of epidermal growth factor, insulin, glucagon, and cyclic AMP. *Journal of Cellular Physiology*, **108**, 353–363.

139. McMahon, J.B., Farrelly, J.G. & Iype, P.T. (1982) Purification and properties of a rat liver protein that specifically inhibits the proliferation of non-malignant epithelial cells from rat liver. *Proceedings of the National Academy of Sciences of the USA*, **79**, 456–460.

140. McMahon, J.B. & Iype, P.T. (1980) Specific inhibition of proliferation of non-malignant rat hepatic cells by a factor from rat liver. *Cancer Research*, **40**, 1249–1254.

141. McMahon, J.B., Richards, W.L., del Campo, A.A. *et al.* (1986) Differential effects of transforming growth factor B on the proliferation of normal and malignant rat liver epithelial cells in culture. *Cancer Research*, **46**, 4665–4671.

142. Mead, J.E. & Fausto, N. (1989) Transforming growth factor alpha may be a physiological regulator of liver regeneration by means of an autocrine mechanism. *Proceedings of the National Academy of Sciences of the USA*, **86**, 1558–1562.

143. Michalopoulos, G., Cianciulli, H.D., Novotny, A.R. *et al.* (1982) Liver regeneration studies with rat hepatocytes in primary culture. *Cancer Research*, **42**, 4673–4682.

144. Michalopoulos, G., Houck, K.A., Dolan, M.L. & Luetteke, N.C. (1984) Control of hepatocyte replication by two serum factors. *Cancer Research*, **44**, 4414–4419.

145. Minghetti, P.P. & Normal, A. (1988) 1,25(OH)2-Vitamin D–3 receptors: gene regulation and genetic circuitry. *FASEB Journal*, **2**, 3043–3053.

146. Miura, Y. & Fukui, T. (1976) Pleiotypic responses of regenerating liver. *Advances in Enzyme Regulation*, **14**, 393–405.

147. Miyazawa, K., Tsubouchi, H., Naka, D. *et al.* (1989) Molecular cloning and sequence analysis of cDNA for human hepatocyte growth factor. *Biochemical and Biophysical Research Communications*, **163**, 967–973.

148. Montecuccoli, G., Novello, F. & Stirpe, F. (1972) Effect of protein deprivation on DNA synthesis in resting and regenerating rat liver. *Journal of Nutrition*, **102**, 507–514.

149. Moolten, F.L., Oakman, N.J. & Bucher, N.L.R. (1970) Accelerated response of hepatic DNA synthesis to partial hepatectomy in rats pretreated with growth hormone or surgical stress. *Cancer Research*, **30**, 2353–2357.

150. Morley, C.G.D., Kuku, S., Rubenstein, A.H. & Boyer, J.L. (1975) Serum hormone levels following partial hepatectomy in the rat. *Biochemical and Biophysical Research Communications*, **67**, 653–661.

151. Morley, C.G.D. & Kingdon, H.S. (1973) The regulation of cell growth. I. Identification and partial characterization of a DNA synthesis stimulating factor from the serum of partially hepatectomized rats. *Biochimica et Biophysica Acta*, **308**, 260–275.

152. Morley, C.G.D. & Royse, V.L. (1981) Adrenergic agents as possible regulators of liver regeneration. *International Journal of Biochemistry*, **13**, 969–973.

153. Nakamura, T., Nishizawa, T., Hagiya, M. *et al.* (1989) Molecular cloning and expression of human hepatocyte growth factor. *Nature*, **342**, 440–443.

154. Nakamura, T., Nawa, K., Ichihara, A. *et al.* (1987) Purification and subunit structure of hepatocyte growth factor from rat platelets. *FEBS Letters*, **224**, 311–316.

155. Nakamura, T., Teramoto, H. & Ichihara, A. (1986) Purification and characterization of a growth factor from rat platelets for mature parenchymal hepatocytes in primary cultures. *Proceedings of the National Academy of Sciences of the USA*, **83**, 6489–6493.

156. Nakamura, T., Teramoto, H., Tomita, Y. & Ichihara, A. (1986) Two types of growth inhibitor in rat platelets for primary cultured hepatocytes. *Biochemical and Biophysical Research Communications*, **134**, 755–763.

157. Nakamura, T., Tomita, Y., Hirai, R. *et al.* (1985) Inhibitory effect of transforming growth factor β on DNA synthesis of adult rat hepatocytes in primary culture. *Biochemical and Biophysical Research Communications*, **133**, 1042–1050.

158. Nakamura, T., Tomomura, A., Kato, S. *et al.* (1984) Reciprocal expression of alpha, and β-adrenergic receptors, but constant expression of glucagon receptor by rat hepatocytes during development and primary culture. *Journal of Biochemistry*, **96**, 127–136.

159. Nakata, R., Tsukamoto, I., Miyoshi, M. *et al.* (1987) Effect of thyroparathyroidectomy on the activities of thymidylate synthetase and thymidine kinase during liver regeneration after partial hepatectomy. *Clinical Science*, **72**, 455–461.

160. Nakata, R., Tsukamoto, I., Nanme, M. *et al.* (1985) Alpha-adrenergic regulation of thymidylate synthetase and thymidine kinase during liver regeneration after partial hepatectomy. *European Journal of Pharmacology*, **114**, 355–360.

161. Okajima, F. & Ui, M. (1982) Conversion of the adrenergic regulation of glycogen phosphorylase and synthase from an alpha to a beta type during primary culture of rat hepatocytes. *Archives of Biochemistry and Biophysics*, **213**, 658–668.

162. Olsen, P.S., Boesby, S., Kirkegaard, P. *et al.* (1988) Influence of epidermal growth factor on liver regeneration after partial hepatectomy in rats. *Hepatology*, **8**, 992–996.

163. Ord, M.G. & Stocken, L.A. (1972) Uptake of amino acids and nucleic acid precursors by regenerating rat liver. *Biochemical Journal*, **129**, 175–181.

164. Ord, M.J. & Stocken, L. (1984) *Cell and Tissue Regeneration*. New York: Wiley.

165. Pezzino, V., Vigneri, R., Cohen, D. & Goldfine, I.D. (1981) Regenerating rat liver: insulin and glucagon serum levels and receptor binding. *Endocrinology*, **108**, 2163–2169.

166. Pietralelli, R., Chamuleau, R.A.F.M., Speranza, V. & Lygidakis, N.J. (1987) Immunocytochemical study of the hepatic innervation in the rat after partial hepatectomy. *Histochemical Journal*, **19**, 327–332.

167. Presta, M., Statuto, M., Rusnati, M. *et al.* (1989) Characterization of Mr 25,000 basic fibroblast growth factor form in adult, regenerating and fetal rat liver. *Biochemical and Biophysical Research Communications*, **164**, 1182–1189.

168. Price, J.B. Jr, Takeshige, K., Max, M.H. & Voorhees, A.B. Jr (1972) Glucagon as the portal factor modifying hepatic regeneration. *Surgery*, **72**, 74–82.

169. Rabes, H.M. & Brandle, H. (1969) Synthesis of RNA, protein, and DNA in the liver of normal and hypophysectomized rats after partial hepatectomy. *Cancer Research*, **29**, 817–822.

170. Raper, S.E., Burwen, S.J., Barker, M.E. & Jones, A.L. (1987) Translocation of epidermal growth factor to the hepatocyte nucleus during rat liver regeneration. *Gastroenterology*, **92**, 1243–1250.

171. Reichel, H., Koeffler, H.P., Norman, A.W. (1989) The role of the vitamin D endocrine system in health and disease. *New England Journal of Medicine*, **320**, 980–991.

172. Reid, L.M., Narita, M., Fujita, M. *et al.* (1986) Matrix and hormonal regulation of differentiation in liver cultures. In Guillouzo, A. & Guguen-Guillouze, C. (eds) *Isolated and Cultured Hepatocytes*, pp. 225–258. Paris: Libbey Eurotext.

173. Richman, R.A., Claus, T.H., Pilkis, S.J. & Friedman, D.L. (1976) Hormonal stimulation of DNA synthesis in primary cultures of adult rat hepatocytes. *Proceedings of the National Academy of Sciences of the USA*, **73**, 3589–3593.

174. Rigotti, P., Peters, J.C., Tranberg, K.G. *et al.* (1986) Effects of amino acid infusions on liver regeneration after partial hepatectomy in the rat. *Journal of Parenteral and Enteral Nutrition*, **10**, 17–20.

175. Rixon, R.H., Isaacs, R.J. & Whitfield, J.F. (1989) Control of DNA polymerase-a activity in regenerating rat liver by calcium and 1α,25 (OH)2D3. *Journal of Cellular Physiology*, **139**, 354–360.

176. Rixon, R.H. & Whitfield, J.F. (1982) An early mitosis-determining event in regenerating rat liver and its possible mediation by

prostaglandins or thromboxane. *Journal of Cellular Physiology*, **113**, 281–288.

177. Rixon, R.H., MacManus, J.P., Whitfield, J.F. (1979) The control of liver regeneration by calcitonin, parathyroid hormone and 1 alpha, 25-dihydroxycholecalciferol. *Molecular and Cellular Endocrinology*, **15**, 79–89.

178. Roberts, A.B. & Sporn, M.B. (1990) The transforming growth factor betas: In Sporn, M.B. & Roberts, A.B. (eds) *Handbook of Experimental Pharmacology*, pp. 419–472. New York: Springer-Verlag.

179. Rozengurt, E. (1986) Early signals in the mitogenic response. *Science*, **234**, 161–166.

180. Ruoslahti, E. (1989) Proteoglycans in cell regulation. *Journal of Biological Chemistry*, **264**, 13369–13372.

181. Russell, W.E. & Bucher, N.L.R. (1983) Vasopressin as a regulator of liver growth. In Harris, R.A. & Cornell, N.W. (eds) *Isolation, Characterization and Use of Hepatocytes*, pp. 171–176. New York: Elsevier.

182. Russell, W.E. & Bucher, N.L.R. (1983) Vasopressin modulates liver regeneration in the Brattleboro rat. *American Journal of Physiology*, **245**, G321–G324.

183. Russell, W.E., Coffey, J.R., Ouellette, A.J. & Moses, H.L. (1988) Type β transforming growth factor reversibly inhibits the early proliferative response to partial hepatectomy in the rat. *Proceedings of the National Academy of Sciences of the USA*, **85**, 5126–5130.

184. Russell, W.E., D'Ercole, J. & Underwood, L.E. (1985) Somatomedin C/insulin-like growth factor I during liver regeneration in the rat. *American Journal of Physiology*, **248**, E618–E623.

185. Russell, W.E., McGowan, J.A. & Bucher, N.L.R. (1984) Partial characterization of an hepatocyte growth factor from rat platelets. *Journal of Cellular Physiology*, **119**, 183–192.

186. Russell, W.E., McGowan, J.A. & Bucher, N.L.R. (1984) Biological properties of an hepatocyte growth factor from rat platelets. *Journal of Cellular Physiology*, **119**, 193–197.

187. Sakamoto, Y., Jehn, D., Nicolson, M. *et al.* (1979) Acceleration of hepatic regeneration with prior stress and growth hormone. *Journal of Surgical Research*, **27**, 50–56.

188. Sandnes, D., Sand, T.E., Sager, G. *et al.* (1986) Elevated level of beta-adrenergic receptors in hepatocytes from regenerating rat liver. *Experimental Cell Research*, **165**, 117–126.

189. Schulte-Hermann, R. (1974) Induction of liver growth by xenobiotic compounds, and other stimuli. *Critical Review of Toxicology*, **3**, 79–158.

190. Schulte-Hermann, R. (1977) Two-stage control of cell proliferation induced in rat liver by α-hexachlorocyclohexane. *Cancer Research*, **37**, 166–171.

191. Schulte-Hermann, R., Leberl, C., Landgraf, H. & Parzifull, W. (1974) Liver growth and mixed-function oxidase activity: dose-dependent stimulatory and inhibitory effects of alpha hexachlorocyclohexane. *Naunyn-Schmiedeberg's Archives of Pharmacology*, **285**, 355–366.

192. Schulte-Hermann, R., Ochs, H., Bursch, W. *et al.* (1988) Quantitative structure-activity studies on effects of sixteen different steroids on growth and monooxygenases of rat liver. *Cancer Research*, **48**, 2462–2468.

193. Schwarz, L.C., Makowka, L., Falk, J.A. & Falk, R. (1985) The characterization and partial purification of hepatocyte proliferation factor. *Annals of Surgery*, **202**, 296–301.

194. Selden, C. & Hodgson, H.J.F. (1989) Further characterization of 'hepatotropin', a high molecular weight hepatotrophic factor in rat serum. *Journal of Hepatology*, **9**, 167–176.

195. Selden, C., Johnstone, R., Darby, H. *et al.* (1986) Human serum does contain a high molecular weight hepatocyte growth factor: studies pre- and post-hepatic resection. *Biochemical and Biophysical Research Communications*, **139**, 361–366.

196. Shi, Y.E. & Yager, J.D. (1989) Effects of the liver tumour promoter ethinyl estradiol on EGF-induced DNA synthesis and EGF receptor levels in cultured rat hepatocytes. *Cancer Research*, **49**, 3574–3580.

197. Short, J., Armstrong, N.B., Kolitsky, M.A. *et al.* (1974) Amino acids and the control of nuclear DNA replication in liver. In Clarkson, B., Baserga, R. (eds) *Control of Proliferation in Animal Cells* pp. 37–48. New York: Cold Spring Harbor Laboratory.

198. Short, J., Armstrong, N., Zemel, R. & Lieberman, I. (1973) A role for amino acids in the induction of deoxyribonucleic acid synthesis in liver. *Biochimica et Biophysica Acta*, **50**, 430–437.

199. Short, J., Brown, R.F., Husakova, A. *et al.* (1972) Induction of DNA synthesis in the liver of the intact animal. *Journal of Biological Chemistry*, **247**, 1757–1766.

200. Short, J., Klein, K., Kibert, L. & Ove, P. (1980) Involvement of the iodothyronines in liver and hepatoma cell proliferation in the rat. *Cancer Research*, **40**, 2417–2422.

201. Short, J. & Ove, P. (1983) Synthesis of an hypothesis advocating a prominent role for the thyroid hormones in mammalian liver cell proliferation in vivo. *Cytobios*, **38**, 39–49.

202. Short, J., Tsukada, K., Rudert, W.A. & Lieberman, I. (1975) Cyclic adenosine 3'5'-monophosphate and the induction of deoxyribonucleic acid synthesis in liver. *Journal of Biological Chemistry*, **250**, 3602–3606.

203. Sikorska, M., De Belle, I., Whitfield, J.F. *et al.* (1989) Regulation of the synthesis of DNA polymerase-a in regenerating liver by calcium and 1,25-dihydroxyvitamin D3. *Biochemistry and Cell Biology*, **67**, 345–351.

204. Siimes, M. & Dallman, P. (1974) Nucleic acid and polyamine synthesis in the rat during short term protein deficiency: response of the liver to partial hepatectomy. *Journal of Nutrition*, **104**, 47–58.

205. Simek, J., Erbenova, Z., Deml, F. & Dvorackova, I. (1968) Liver regeneration after partial hepatectomy in rats exposed before the operation to the stress stimulus. *Experientia*, **24**, 1166–1167.

206. Sporn, M.B. & Roberts, A.B. (1988) Peptide growth factors are multifunctional. *Nature*, **332**, 217–219.

207. St Hilaire, R.J., Hradek, G.T. & Jones, A.L. (1983) Hepatic sequestration and biliary secretion of epidermal growth factors: evidence for a high-capacity up-take system. *Proceedings of the National Academy of Sciences of the USA*, **80**, 3797–3801.

208. Starzl, T.E. & Terblanche, J. (1979) Hepatotrophic substances. *Progress in Liver Disease*, **6**, 135–151.

209. Starzl, T.E., Demetris, A.J. & Van Thiel, D. (1989) Liver transplantation. *New England Journal of Medicine*, **321**, 1092–1099.

210. Steiner, D.F. (1978) Insulin-induced liver hyperplasia: evidence for a negative liver-size-correcting process. In *Hepatotrophic Factors*. Ciba Foundation Symposium 55 (New Series), pp. 229–236.

211. Steiner, D.F., Chan, S.J., Terris, S. *et al.* (1978) Insulin as a cellular growth regulator. In *Hepatotrophic Factors*. Ciba Foundation Symposium 55 (New Series), pp. 217–228.

212. Stirling, G.A., Bourne, L.D. & Marsh, T. (1975) Effect of protein deprivation and a reduced diet on the regenerating rat liver. *British Journal of Experimental Pathology*, **56**, 502–508.

213. Stirling, G.A., Laughlin, J. & Washington, S.L.A. (1973) Effects of starvation on the proliferative response after partial hepatectomy. *Experimental and Molecular Pathology*, **19**, 44–52.

214. Strain, A.J., McGowan, J.A. & Bucher, N.L.R. (1982) Stimulation of DNA synthesis in primary cultures of adult rat hepatocytes by rat platelet-associated substances. *In Vitro*, **18**, 108–116.

215. Strain, A.J. (1988) Transforming growth factor-β and inhibition of hepatocellular proliferation. *Scandinavian Journal of Gastroenterology*, **23** (supplement 151), 37–45.

216. Strain, A.J. & Anderson, D. (1990) Lithium potentiates, vasopressin-, angiotensin II- and norepinephrine-induced DNA synthesis in rat hepatocytes. *Biochemical Society Transactions*, **18**, 455.

217. Strain, A.J., Frazer, A., Hill, D.J. & Milner, R.D.G. (1987) Transforming growth factor β inhibits DNA synthesis in hepatocytes isolated from normal and regenerating rat liver. *Biochemical and Biophysical Research Communications*, **145**, 436–442.

218. Strain, A.J. & Hill, D.J. (1990) Changes in sensitivity of hepatocytes isolated from regenerating rat liver to the growth inhibitory action of transforming growth factor beta. *Liver*, **10**, 282–290.

219. Strain, A.J., Hill, D.J. & Milner, R.D.G. (1986) Divergent action of transforming growth factor β on DNA synthesis in human foetal liver cells. *Cell Biology International Reports*, **10**, 855–860.

220. Strain, A.J. & Ingleton, P.M. (1990) Growth hormone and prolactin induced release of insulin-like growth factor I by isolated rat hepatocytes. *Biochemical Society Transactions*, **18**, 1206.

221. Strain, A.J., Ismail, T., Tsubouchi, H. *et al.* (1991) Native and recombinant human hepatocyte growth factors are highly potent

promoters of DNA synthesis in both human and rat hepatocytes. *Journal of Clinical Investigation*, in press.

222. Strecker, W., Goldberg, M., Feeny, D.A. & Ruhenstroth-Bauer, G. (1979) The influence of extended glucagon infusion on liver cell regeneration after partial hepatectomy in the rat. *Acta Hepato-Gastroenterologica*, **26**, 439–441.

223. Strecker, W., Silz, S., Ruhenstroth-Bauer, G. & Bottger, I. (1980) Insulin and glucagon in blood plasma of partially hepatectomised rats. *Zeitschrift für Naturforschung*, **35**, 65–71.

224. Takai, S., Nakamura, T., Komi, N. & Ichihara, A. (1988) Mechanism of stimulation of DNA synthesis induced by epinephrine in primary culture of adult rat hepatocytes. *Journal of Biochemistry*, **103**, 848–852.

225. Takatsuki, K., Fujiwara, K., Hayashi, S. *et al.* (1981) Acceleration of DNA synthesis in post-hepatectomised regenerating liver of normal rat by insulin and glucagon. *Life Sciences*, **29**, 2609–2615.

226. Talarico, K.S., Feller, D.D. & Neville, E.D. (1971) Mitotic response to various dietary conditions in the normal and regenerating rat liver. *Proceedings of the Society for Experimental Biology and Medicine*, **136**, 381–384.

227. Terblanche, J., Porter, K.A., Starzl, T.E. *et al.* (1980) Stimulation of hepatic regeneration after partial hepatectomy by infusion of cytosol extract from regenerating dog liver. *Surgery, Gynaecology and Obstetrics*, **151**, 538–544.

228. Terpstra, O., Malt, R.A. & Bucher, N.L.R. (1979) Negligible role of adrenal hormones in regulation of DNA synthesis in livers of partially hepatectomized rats. *Proceedings of the Society for Experimental Biology and Medicine*, **161**, 326–331.

229. Thaler, F.J. & Michalopoulos, G.K. (1985) Hepatopoietin A: Partial characterization and trypsin activation of a hepatocyte growth factor. *Cancer Research*, **45**, 2545–2549.

230. Thomas, K.A. (1988) Transforming potential of fibroblast growth factor genes. *Trends in Biochemical Sciences*, **13**, 327–328.

231. Thomson, M.J. & Richards, J.F. (1978) Ornithine decarboxylase and thymidine kinase activity in tissues of prolactin treated rats: effect of hypophysectomy. *Life Sciences*, **22**, 337–344.

232. Tsubouchi, H., Hirono, S., Gohda, E. *et al.* (1989) Clinical significance of human hepatocyte growth factor in blood from patients with fulminant hepatic failure. *Hepatology*, **9**, 875–881.

233. Unterman, T.G. & Phillips, L.S. (1986) Circulating somatomedin activity during hepatic regeneration. *Endocrinology*, **119**, 185–192.

234. Uthne, K. & Uthne, T. (1972) Influence of liver resection and regeneration on somatomedin (sulfation factor) activity in sera from normal and hypophysectomized rats. *Acta Endocrinologica*, **71**, 255–264.

235. Vandekerckhove, A., Miot, F., Keppens, S. & DeWulf, H. (1989) Lack of V_1 vasopressin receptors in rabbit hepatocytes. *Biochemical Journal*, **259**, 609–611.

236. Van Hoorn-Hickman, R.V., Kahn, D., Green, J. *et al.* (1981) Is there a regeneration stimulator substance in the effluent from perfused partially hepatectomized livers. *Hepatology*, **1**, 287–293.

237. Van Thiel, D.H., Gavaler, J.S., Kam, I. *et al.* (1987) Rapid growth of an intact human liver transplanted into a recipient larger than the donor. *Gastroenterology*, **93**, 1414–1419.

238. Vintermyr, O.K. & Doskeland, S.O. (1989) Characterization of the inhibitory effect of glucocorticoids on the DNA replication of adult rat hepatocytes growing at various cell densities. *Journal of Cellular Physiology*, **138**, 29–37.

239. Weinbren, K., Stirling, G.A. & Washington, S.L.A. (1972) Development of a proliferative response in liver parenchyma deprived of portal blood flow. *British Journal of Experimental Pathology*, **53**, 54–58.

240. Westermark, B. & Heldin, C.H. (1989) Growth factors and their receptors. *Current Opinion in Cell Biology*, **1**, 279–285.

241. Whitfield, J.F., Durkin, J.P., Franks, D.J. *et al.* (1987) Calcium, cyclic AMP and protein kinase C—partners in mitogenesis. *Cancer and Metastasis Reviews*, **5**, 205–250.

242. Whittemore, A.D., Kasuya, M., Voorhees, A.B. Jr & Price, J.B. Jr (1975) Hepatic regeneration in the absence of portal viscera. *Surgery*, **77**, 419–426.

243. Witek-Janusek, L. & Marcotta, S.F. (1981) Status of the pituitary–adrenocortical–liver axis following partial hepatectomy. *Proceedings of the Society for Experimental Biology and Medicine*, **166**, 210–215.

244. Wyllie, A.H., Kerr, J.F.R. & Currie, A.R. (1980) Cell death: the significance of apoptosis. *International Review of Cytology*, **68**, 251–306.

245. Younger, L.R., King, J. & Steiner, D.F. (1966) Hepatic proliferative response to insulin in severe alloxan diabetes. *Cancer Research*, **26**, 1408–1414.

246. Zarnegar, R. & Michalopoulos, G. (1989) Purification and biological characterization of human hepatopoietin A, a polypeptide growth factor for hepatocytes. *Cancer Research*, **49**, 3314–3320.

247. Zarnegar, R., Muga, S., Enghild, J. & Michalopoulos, G. (1989) NH_2-terminal amino acid sequence of rabbit hepatopoietin A. A heparin-binding polypeptide growth factor for hepatocytes. *Biochemical and Biophysical Research Communications*, **163**, 1370–1376.

248. Zarnegar, R., Muga, S., Rahija, R. & Michalopoulos, G. (1990) Tissue distribution of HPTA: a heparin-binding polypeptide growth factor for hepatocytes. *Proceedings of the National Academy of Sciences of the USA*, **87**, 1252–1256.

CHAPTER 12

The Physiology of the Gallbladder and Extrahepatic Biliary Tree

Pierce A. Grace, Ara Darzi & David Bouchier-Hayes

INTRODUCTION

Biliary physiology is characterized by a series of complex relationships between hepatic secretion and gallbladder modification of bile and the motility of the extrahepatic biliary tree, resulting in the delivery of bile to the duodenum. Various neural and hormonal agents modulate this process. The application of modern techniques to the study of biliary dynamics has allowed a composite picture of biliary physiology to emerge. This chapter examines recent developments in the understanding of biliary physiology and discusses the detailed events involved in the secretion and delivery of bile to the duodenum.

THE COMPOSITION OF BILE

Hepatic bile

Methods of obtaining human hepatic bile are unsatisfactory. Patients with T-tubes *in situ* will have had cholecystectomy for gallstones and studies on hepatic bile thus obtained are hampered by an impaired enterohepatic circulation. Diversion of more than 20% of bile flow from the common bile duct produces significant changes in the composition of biliary lipids in rhesus monkeys.[51] Thus, alternative methods for obtaining hepatic bile are needed.

The intestinal hormone cholecystokinin-pancreozymin (CCK-PZ) causes the gallbladder to discharge dark bile into the duodenum. Duodenal content subsequently becomes light yellow in colour and may represent hepatic bile. Moreover, bile lipid composition of fasting duodenal content is similar to that obtained after CCK-PZ-induced gallbladder evacuation. Thus, fasting duodenal content may be representative of hepatic biliary lipid secretion.[118]

Hepatic bile is made of water, electrolytes, lipids, proteins and bilirubin. The concentrations of electrolytes in hepatic bile resemble those in plasma, except that the bicarbonate concentration may be twice as high. The organic anion concentration distinguishes hepatic bile from plasma.

Normal human bile contains primary and secondary bile acids. The two principal primary bile acids formed in the liver are cholic and chenodeoxycholic acids. In the colon, bacteria convert cholic acid to deoxycholic acid and chenodeoxycholic acid to lithocholic acid (secondary bile acids). Bile acids are also conjugated with either glycine or taurine in the liver so that there are two subtypes of each bile acid.

Bile acids at a critical concentration will form aggregates known as micelles. In micelles the bile acid molecules are oriented so that the water-soluble portion of the molecule faces outwards while the lipid-soluble portion faces inwards. If the molecules are oriented in a radial manner, the interior becomes a lipid-soluble environment where very water-insoluble lipids such as cholesterol can be maintained in solution. Thus, in normal bile, bile acids, phospholipids and cholesterol probably exist as 'mixed micelles'. Ninety-eight per cent of phospholipid in hepatic bile is lecithin.[135] The rest consists of cephalin, sphingomyelin, and lysolecithin. The mean concentration of total phospholipid in hepatic bile is approximately 164 µg/ml.[68]

Proteins are present in hepatic bile as plasma proteins, biliary glycoproteins, immunoglobulins, and enzymes such as alkaline phosphatase, aspartate aminotransferase (AST), gamma glutamyl transferase (GGT), leucine aminopeptidase (LAP), and 5′ nucleotidase. The mean concenotration of protein in bile is approximately 0.04 mg/l.[20] It is possible that the glycoproteins in hepatic bile differ from those added by the gallbladder. Both AST and alkaline phosphatase are present in hepatic bile. Alkaline phosphatase exists in high-molecular-mass and low-molecular-mass forms with the high-molecular-mass form accounting for the majority of the enzyme in human bile and serum.[43] High-molecular-weight alkaline phosphatase, GGT, LAP, and 5′ nucleotidase are present in normal hepatic bile, presumably derived from hepatocyte (canalicular) plasma membrane. However, these enzymes do not constitute a homogeneous single complex but are separate entities, as determined by ion-exchange chromatography.[44] Their concentrations are dependent on bile acid secretion and the action of gastrointestinal hormones.[18]

Immunoglobulins G, M and A have been measured by radial immunodiffusion in hepatic bile. Normal levels have not yet been determined owing to the paucity of subjects studied. Secretory events of immunoglobulins will be discussed in the section on hepatocyte bile formation.

Bilirubin in human bile from both the liver and the gallbladder in normal subjects is present largely as bilirubin diglucuronoside, but about 22% of the total bile pigment is in the form of monoconjugated bilirubin.[68]

Gallbladder bile

Data on the composition of gallbladder bile have come from samples obtained from the fasted gallbladder by aspiration at laparotomy for non-biliary pathology, and considerable variation exists between individuals. The electrolyte concentration of gallbladder bile is significantly higher than that of hepatic bile, with the exceptions of chloride and bicarbonate. Animal data suggest that the pH of gallbladder bile is less than 7.0, owing to the secretion of hydrogen ion by the gallbladder mucosa.[25] The concentrations of bile acids and bilirubin in the gallbladder indicate that hepatic bile is concentrated by a factor of 10 by the absorption of water. While the concentrations of bile acids and sodium are increased and those of chloride and bicarbonate are decreased, the osmotically active concentrations remain unchanged owing to the formation of micelles. There is some evidence to indicate that some of the sodium and potassium is incorporated into the micelles.[120] The ratio of ionized calcium to total calcium in bile is much lower than in urine or plasma.[158] Most biliary calcium is bound to a substance with a molecular weight of 10 000, identical with the molecular weight of mixed micelles.[158]

Different methods of measuring concentrations of cholesterol give significantly different values. The Boehringer–Mannheim enzymatic method, utilizing cholesterol oxidase, underestimates cholesterol concentration by 23% compared to gas–liquid chromatography.[19] Glycine-conjugated bile acids predominate over taurine conjugates in gallbladder bile in a ratio of 2 : 1 or 3 : 1. Cholic and chenodeoxycholic acids constitute about 80% of bile acids, while deoxycholic acid accounts for most of the rest. Gallbladder bile from subjects without biliary tract disease contains seven different lecithins, each with its own fatty acid composition.[123] Lysolecithins, produced from lecithins by phospholipases in the wall of the gallbladder may have an aetiologic role in acalculous cholecystitis.[160]

Gallbladder epithelial phospholipases and lysophospholipases normally metabolize biliary lysolecithins to non-toxic substances.[160]

The factors favouring solubility of cholesterol in bile have been studied intensively. Using mixtures of bile acids, phospholipids, and cholesterol *in vitro*, the relationships between the mole percentages of the three lipids and the formation of cholesterol crystals were defined and the limits of a zone of micelle formation and a zone in which micelles and cholesterol crystals coexisted were established. Approximately 50% of normal subjects have supersaturated gallbladder bile.[29,30] *In vitro* studies have shown that bile acids account for about one-third of the solubilized cholesterol found in human gallbladder bile.[125] The lithogenic index or cholesterol saturation index is a ratio of the actual amount of cholesterol in moles percent in a given sample of bile to the maximum amount of cholesterol that can be dissolved in that sample. Thus, a lithogenic index of 1 falls on the line of maximum solubility of Admirand and Small's triangular coordinates. Lithogenic indices greater than 1 indicate supersaturated bile.[117] Significant imprecision exists in the measurement of the cholesterol saturation index.[178] A coefficient of variation of 4.1% has been observed in all subjects, with a 14.3% coefficient of variation in women.

A solubilizing effect of lecithin was noted independently of that of bile acids. Approximately 3 mM of lecithin solubilized an additional 1 mM concentration of cholesterol. Patients with cholesterol stones have a reduced molar lipid ratio. The molar lipid ratio is expressed as the sum of the bile acids and phospholipids divided by cholesterol in moles percent (i.e. bile acids + phospholipids/cholesterol). The ratio includes phospholipids as an important factor in the solubilization of cholesterol.[163] Other investigators found that cholesterol solubility *in vitro* increased proportionally with increasing bile acid concentrations. Deoxycholate showed greater cholesterol-dissolving power than did cholate.[85] Lecithin increased the cholesterol-dissolving power of bile acids.[162]

Proteins in gallbladder bile are derived in part from the blood and in part from the biliary tract and may contribute to the viscosity of bile. In bile from 11 normal subjects, the hexosamine concentration was 8.3 ± 5.3 mg/dl and a linear relationship was demonstrated between the hexosamine concentration and that of bilirubin.[21] Others have reported a crude glycoprotein concentration of 22.8 mg/dl in gallbladder bile.[116] Carbohydrates from bile glycoproteins may constitute over 15% of the total solids of gallbladder bile.[66] Biliary glycoproteins contribute 70–90% of the carbohydrate of bile; the remainder is due to the presence of plasma glycoproteins in bile.[146] Carbohydrates in biliary glycoproteins include galactose, fucose, *N*-acetylglucosamine, mannose, glucose, *N*-acetylgalactosamin, and *N*-acetylneuraminic acid.[99] The first three carbohydrate moieties make up 70–85% of biliary carbohydrate. Gallbladder bile glycoprotein concentration is greater in patients with radiolucent (cholesterol) stones than in normal subjects. Hepatic bile glycoprotein concen-

tration, however, is the same. This implies a secretion of glycoprotein from gallbladder epithelium in patients with gallstones.[100] Mucin secretion from gallbladder epithelium in rabbits may be by way of exocytosis, as noted by electron microscopy.[100] Serum proteins, including albumin, are present in gallbladder bile specimens from normal human subjects.[55,174] No clear differences have been shown in the bile protein composition between biles from patients with gallstones and from those without stones.

Total amylase activity in gallbladder bile approximates serum concentrations.[48] The amylase in gallbladder bile probably originates from the serum by way of a paracellular pathway in gallbladder epithelium.

FACTORS INFLUENCING THE COMPOSITION OF BILE

Sex and pregnancy

Gallbladder bile composition differs between men and women. The concentrations of total bile acids, chenodeoxycholic acid, and both glycine- and taurine-conjugated bile acids are significantly higher in women. On the other hand, the cholic acid/total bile acid ratio is higher in men. The ratio of glycine to taurine conjugates in women is about 2 : 1, while in men it is nearly 4 : 1. Administration of ethinyl oestradiol to young healthy men increases the cholesterol saturation index of bile within 7 days, with increases in cholesterol and phospholipid and a decrease in bile acid concentration.[3] Similarly, long-term oral contraceptive administration to young healthy women increases the cholesterol saturation index with increases in cholesterol but unchanged bile acid concentrations.[11]

Pregnancy may affect bile composition. A careful attempt to compare gallbladder bile from pregnant and non-pregnant women failed to establish a difference, but the methods for measuring bile acids were not acceptable by modern criteria. Bile aspirated from the gallbladders of pregnant guinea pigs at term had higher concentrations of bile acids and cholesterol than that from virgin females or postpartum animals.[81] In pregnant rabbits, there is an increase in the glycine/taurine conjugated bile acid ratio compared with non-pregnant rabbits.[90] In cats, oral administration of pure progesterone decreases the lithogenic index[150] while fasting decreases the concentration of bile acids and increases the concentration of phospholipids and cholesterol in hepatic bile from rhesus monkeys.[134]

Dietary factors

Long-term studies of the composition of normal human bile show a diurnal variation in biliary lipid composition.[117] Fasting increases the concentration of cholesterol in both hepatic and gallbladder bile. Modifications in the amount of fat in the diet do not alter the composition of hepatic bile in rhesus monkeys.[27,134] However, in human patients with T-tube drainage after cholecystectomy, increasing the lipid caloric intake increases the concentration of cholesterol in bile. Changes in the carbohydrate content of the diet have no effect on biliary lipids. However, reducing the cholesterol intake to zero significantly reduces the concentration of cholesterol, phospholipids and bile acids in duodenal aspirate.[47] A high-cholesterol diet fed to prairie dogs results in an increase in mucin secretion from the gallbladder.[99] Vitamin C may also play a role in biliary lipid composition. In guinea pigs, deficient and excessive vitamin C states induce decreased bile acid synthesis.[80,89]

Vegetarian diets or bran-supplemented diets (15 g of bran per day) change bile acid composition in man.[78,179] Both diets reduce deoxycholate concentrations in duodenal bile after CCK stimulation. A decrease in the dehydroxylating capacity of colonic bacteria in the presence of bran or the absence of animal fat is the presumed explanation. Deoxycholate is an inhibitor of chenodeoxycholate synthesis from cholesterol. Thus, since deoxycholate concentrations are reduced, the ability of bran to desaturate bile in patients with cholesterol gallstones may be related to increased chenodeoxycholate serum levels.[179]

Enterohepatic circulation

Interruption of the enterohepatic circulation by more than 20% of the normal flow through the common bile duct alters the composition of hepatic bile. Within 2–3 hours of interrupting the enterohepatic circulation in rhesus monkeys, the composition of bile begins to change. Between 3 and 4 hours, the relative proportions of the individual bile lipids are altered so that the bile becomes supersaturated with respect to cholesterol. However, after a few additional hours, an increase in the rate of synthesis of bile acids occurs and a new steady state is achieved, preserving cholesterol solubility. Interruption of the enterohepatic circulation lowers bile acid concentration more than that of lecithin or cholesterol.[51]

Vagotomy and cholecystectomy

Vagotomy and gastric drainage is associated with a significant rise in post-gallbladder evacuation duodenal bile cholesterol 1 year after surgery.[148] Truncal vagotomy, but not parietal cell vagotomy, results in a decrease in bile acid, cholesterol, and phospholipid outputs in cholecystectomized patients, but percentage saturation of cholesterol in bile remains unchanged from prevagotomy states in both groups.[149] In rhesus monkeys with cholecystectomy, hepatic bile composition was unchanged by truncal vagotomy after 4 months.[113] In dogs, vagotomy reduces the ratio of bile acid to cholesterol concentration in bile.[60] However, results in cats and rabbits have been at variance with these observations, and if vagotomy changes bile composition, it is likely that it does so on an extrahepatic basis.[60] The question of whether or not vagotomy is associated with an increased incidence of gallstones is unresolved.[151]

MECHANISM OF HEPATIC BILE FORMATION

Canalicular bile formation

Bile is formed invariably in the biliary canaliculi and modified by secretion and absorption in the gallbladder.[26] It has not yet been possible to determine the composition of bile in the canaliculi. Therefore, concepts of the mechanisms of hepatic bile secretion must be based upon indirect evidence. The large differences in concentration of bile acids and pigments between blood in the sinusoids and bile obtained from the hepatic ducts suggest that these substances are crossing the canalicular membrane against a concentration gradient. The electrical potential difference between bile and the peritoneal cavity in the rat was found to be -4.5 mV in the basal state. It became more negative when the bile acid concentration was increased by giving bile salts intravenously. The changes were even more marked when animals were depleted of bile acids by interruption of the enterohepatic circulation. These results may reflect changes in the potential difference (PD) at the canalicular level, because in the rat the bile ducts appear to contribute little to the modification of bile secretion or composition.[15] It is therefore likely that bile acids enter the canaliculi by an active transport mechanism.

Inhibitors of sodium transport such as ouabain have been shown to reduce bile flow without altering bile acid secretion.[56] This suggests that a bile acid-independent secretory mechanism for electrolyte transport across the canaliculi also involves active transport.

Once osmotically active substances enter the canaliculi, it can be predicted that water will follow and the volume of bile secreted will increase. Conversely, the administration of hypertonic solutions intravenously decreases the flow of bile and water and electrolyte secretion in parallel but does not alter the secretion of bile acids or bilirubin.[56]

Most investigators interested in the mechanisms of bile formation believe that it can be divided into two basic components, a bile salt-dependent fraction and a bile salt-independent fraction. Both, however, may be intimately linked through active sodium transport.

Bile salt-dependent canalicular bile formation

Secretion of bile salts across the canalicular hepatocyte plasma membrane is the major driving force for canalicular bile formation. Osmotic activity of bile salts in the canalicular fluid accounts for further secretion of water and electrolytes. Previous work had shown that bile flow increases linearly with the bile salt excretion rate, but data in the rat[5] and monkey[4] indicate a curvilinear relationship. Boyer postulates that the greater increments of change in bile flow at lower bile and excretory rates result from greater osmotic activity of bile acids below critical micellar concentrations.[16,57] The events that take place between presentation of bile salts in sinusoidal blood and their appearance in canalicular fluid are the major determinants of bile formation. These events may be divided into three parts: sinusoidal, intracellular, and canalicular.

At the sinusoidal level, the major driving force for bile acid uptake is Na^+-K^+ ATPase located on the basolateral membrane of hepatocytes. Hepatocyte uptake of bile acids is a saturable, specific process.[4,5,16] This implies receptor-mediated transport. The following sequence is the theoretical mechanism of bile acid hepatocyte uptake. A low sodium concentration is maintained within the hepatocyte by way of the Na^+-K^+ pump, which is dependent upon Na^+-K^+ ATPase activity. Carrier-mediated facilitated transport of sodium and an anion (e.g. bile acids) can thereby occur against an electrical gradient (i.e. the interior of the hepatocyte is approximately -40 mV).[17] Thus, negatively charged bile acids are transported against an electrical gradient as a result of the maintenance of a downward sodium gradient by Na^+-K^+ ATPase. Furosemide, an inhibitor of sodium-coupled ion transport, and ouabain, an inhibitor of the Na^+-K^+ pump, both retard sodium-dependent taurocholate uptake in isolated hepatocytes.[137]

Intracellular transfer of bile acids to canalicular fluid most likely occurs through vesicular transport and exocytosis but this has not been clearly established.[23] The mechanism of transfer of bile acids across the canalicular membrane is currently conjectural. It probably involves a combination of exocytosis,[23] electrochemical potential (with PD across the canalicular membrane of -32 mV inferred by indirect measurement)[24] and an intact canalicular microvillous architecture allowing for constant movement of bile downstream.[52,54] Phalloidin, a specific actin poison, produces flattening of the canalicular microvilli, which are normally maintained by the hepatocyte cytoskeleton (i.e. microfilaments). Phalloidin-treated animals develop classic histopathological signs of cholestasis (dilated canaliculi and loss of microvillous canalicular architecture).[52,54] Contraction of bile canaliculi has also been observed by time-lapse cinephotomicrography in cultured rat hepatocytes. Sequential canalicular contraction may be an important initiator of bile flow.[127]

Bile acid-independent canalicular bile secretion

The secretion of certain polysaccharides such as erythritol, mannitol and sucrose into bile occurs only at the level of the canaliculus and hence can be used as a measure of canalicular bile flow.[62] In dogs, the biliary clearance of mannitol was linearly related to the secretion of bile acids. Other experiments in the rat[5] and the rhesus monkey[4] indicate that bile flow varies in a curvilinear fashion with the bile acid excretion rate. However, when bile acid secretion was extrapolated to zero, a significant level of bile flow remained, implying a bile acid-independent canalicular bile secretion. Furthermore, the fact that mannitol clearance exceeded bile flow indicated significant absorption of water in the biliary tract distal to the canaliculi.

EXTRAHEPATIC BILIARY PHYSIOLOGY

THE BILE DUCTS

Bile flow into the duodenum is governed by a combination of hepatic secretion, gallbladder contraction and sphincter of Oddi motility. The biliary tract is a low-pressure system undergoing minimal pressure changes during fasting or after feeding, despite substantial changes in bile flow.[79,91] Bile secretion decreases when the common duct pressure rises above 10 cm of water, and with occlusion of the duct the pressure stabilizes at about 30 cm of water.[74] Thus, pressure is maintained at a relatively low level even in the presence of outflow obstruction.

THE GALLBLADDER

The pattern of emptying

The human gallbladder does not empty completely in response to food entering the duodenum, and there are frequent changes in its absolute storage volume and rate of emptying.[96] During the intestinal interdigestive period, partial emptying and refilling of the gallbladder occur synchronously with the migrating myoelectric complex (MMC). Thus, filling and emptying of the healthy gallbladder is analogous to the ebb and flow of the tide.

Gallbladder tone reflects the compliance of the smooth muscle and fibroelastic tissue within its wall. The static compliance of the gallbladder, measured by pressure–volume relationships, takes 12–16 hours to adjust to the volume of the organ.[94] Over shorter periods of 2–4 hours compliance remains relatively constant despite large changes in volume.[94] This property of slow tone adjustment permits re-filling during the period of increased bile secretion after gallbladder contraction. Gallbladder emptying is synchronous with stomach emptying and gallbladder refilling starts when gastric emptying is nearly complete.[97]

Lanzini and his associates have defined the events occuring in bile flow between meals.[96] Most hepatic bile is diverted into the gallbladder not only during fasting but also after meals. This storage process alternates at short intervals with ejection of bile from the gallbladder into the duodenum, similar to the action of a bellows. This property may be important for thorough mixing of its contents.

The role of cholecystokinin

Cholecystokinin (CCK) is released from the duodenum by luminal acid and nutrients, in particular fat and amino acids.[167] The half-life of CCK in plasma is about 2.5 minutes[167] and the kidney is its major site of uptake from the systemic circulation.[167] The predominant forms of CCK (CCK-8, CCK-33, CCK-39 and CCK-58) are all released by the upper gastrointestinal mucosa and it is probable that these forms of CCK are primarily responsible for stimulating gallbladder contraction and pancreatic secretion.

The presence of pancreatic enzymes (particularly trypsin) inhibits CCK release from the duodenum.[61,128] By contracting and thus stimulating bile flow, the gallbladder plays a role in the negative feedback suppression of CCK release by the upper intestine. Following diversion, bile salts inhibit the endogenous release of fat-stimulated CCK and neurotensin from the ileum.[67] Thus, a self-regulating feedback loop has been established for gallbladder emptying in response to duodenal food.

Infusions of CCK-8 cause the human gallbladder to contract,[104] and the degree of change in gallbladder volume is directly proportional to the level of CCK detected in the plasma.[104] The volume and intraluminal pressure of the gallbladder are inversely proportional to the circulating level of lipid-stimulated endogenous CCK.[63,180] Endogenous CCK is probably the main driving force behind gallbladder emptying.[63] Thus, CCK regulates the length of time that bile stays in the gallbladder exposed to the concentrating capability of its mucosa. CCK therefore regulates the bile acid/cholesterol saturation index by gallbladder volume change[88] rather than by altering the absorption of secretion of water and electrolytes across the gallbladder mucosa.[87]

Cholecystokinin acts directly on receptors in the muscle coat of the gallbladder.[154] Optimal binding of ^{125}I-CCK-33 occurs at pH 5.5 and requires the presence of magnesium.[154] The gallbladder muscle CCK receptor has been shown to have a molecular weight of 85 000–95 000, and there appears to be a wide range of binding capacity of CCK to its receptors between one gallbladder and another.[145] The response of the gallbladder to CCK is calcium-dependent and is inhibited by the addition of calcium channel blocking agents.[42] Removal of calcium from the extracellular fluid in gallbladder strip preparations decreases the contractile response to CCK by 80%.[42] Hypercalcaemia induced in normal volunteers by intravenous infusions of calcium chloride enhances CCK-stimulated gallbladder contraction *in vivo*.[114]

Gallbladder contraction in response to CCK is also mediated by cholinergic vagal nerve fibres. In dogs, truncal vagotomy reduces the sensitivity of the gallbladder to CCK (as measured by changes in intraluminal pressure).[103] However, truncal vagotomy may not alter the rate of gallbladder emptying.[84] In man, the post-contraction volume of the gallbladder is greater after complete vagotomy, suggesting a parasympathetic role in normal emptying.[84]

Vagal stimulation may also regulate the response of the gallbladder to CCK.[183] Sham feeding stimulates gallbladder emptying in up to 50% of people, suggesting a major role for vagal activity in gallbladder motility. This response is eliminated by cholinergic blockade with atropine, again suggesting that the vagus can stimulate the gallbladder to contract.[58] CCK receptors on cholinergic post-ganglionic parasympathetic neurones are much more important in mediating the response of the gallbladder to CCK than they are in mediating the response of pancreatic acini to this hormone.[155] Either hypersensitivity of the gallbladder to CCK or hyposensitivity of the sphincter of Oddi to CCK (resulting in the gallbladder contracting against a closed biliary system) may be the cause of acalculous biliary colic in the small group of patients whose symptoms can be reproduced by CCK infusion and who benefit from cholecystectomy.[101]

Other neurohumoral agents

Other gastrointestinal peptides and neurotransmitters have either cholecystokinetic actions (direct and/or CCK potentiating) or cholecystostatic actions (direct and/or CCK inhibiting). Gastrin-17 belongs to the same family of peptides as CCK. It causes gallbladder muscle contraction in some species, though much less potently than CCK[172] and not at all in man.[28] Secretin, released from the upper gut by the presence of acid, abolishes the net water absorption from bile in the gallbladder.[86] On its own, secretin has no effect on gallbladder muscle,[34,86] but it has been shown to potentiate the action of CCK on the gallbladder.[140] Substance P directly stimulates gallbladder contraction in both dogs and rabbits,[115] but its cholecystokinetic potency is only about 1/600 that of CCK.[109] Similarly, motilin is weakly cholecystokinetic, but this effect is limited to the quiescent period between meals.[161] The response of the gallbladder to neurotensin is species-specific. In dogs it causes gallbladder contraction with about 1/50 the potency of CCK.[64] In humans, neurotensin causes gallbladder relaxation *in vivo*, but this appears to be an indirect effect as neurotensin produces no response *in vitro*.[168] Histamine (H_1) receptor stimulation causes gallbladder muscle contraction, whereas stimulation of type 2 receptors (H_2) causes gallbladder muscle relaxation.[173]

Pancreatic polypeptide (PP) causes relaxation of the gallbladder and decreased intraluminal pressure,[1] which encourages refilling after contraction.[37] Infusions of CCK in humans bring about release of PP, as measured by radioimmunoassay.[110] PP levels remain elevated for up to 6 hours after a meal, suggesting that PP could play a role in the regulation of postprandial gallbladder filling.[37] Vasoactive intestinal peptide (VIP) decreases resting gallbladder pressure in a dose-dependent manner, eliminating spontaneous contractile activity.[140] VIP inhibits the contractile response of the gallbladder to CCK both *in vivo*[140, 156] and *in vitro*[109]. The gallbladder is supplied by three types of vagal nerve fibre: cholinergic, CCK-ergic and VIP-ergic. Thus, vagally regulated gallbladder tone and contraction is the net result of the interplay of stimulatory fibres (mediated by acetylcholine and CCK) and inhibitory fibres (mediated by VIP).[156] Besides diminishing the hepatic secretion of bile,[136] somatostatin is a potent inhibitor of gallbladder emptying in man, whether meal-stimulated, vagally-mediated or CCK-induced.[59] Peptide YY (PYY) has recently been shown to potentiate gallbladder relaxation and refilling after CCK-induced contraction,[38] and calcitonin gene-related peptide (CGRP)[76] and pancreastatin[75] inhibit CCK-induced gallbladder contraction in the guinea pig.

THE SPHINCTER OF ODDI

The sphincter of Oddi regulates bile flow into the duodenum, diverts hepatic bile into the gallbladder and prevents reflux of duodenal contents into the biliary tree.[24] The sphincter of Oddi is situated at the choledochoduodenal junction and is characterized physiologically by a high-pressure zone.[22,124] Physiological studies of the sphincter of Oddi have addressed three main areas: (1) the relationship between sphincter of Oddi activity and the activity of the surrounding duodenum; (2) the mechanism by which the sphincter controls the flow of bile into the duodenum; and (3) the factors that control sphincter of Oddi function.

Functional independence of the sphincter of Oddi

The relationship between the sphincter of Oddi and the upper gastrointestinal tract is complex. Early investigators[133] considered biliary flow to be solely dependent on changes in duodenal tone and muscular activity, while others held that the sphincter of Oddi was functionally independent of the duodenal musculature.[31,45,112] More recently, Mochinaga and colleagues have shown that in the fasted state gastroduodenal motor activity plays a role in the regulation of bile flow.[119] Using a canine model they observed that bile entered the duodenum only when the duodenal wall at the level of the choledochoduodenal junction was not contracting or when the amplitude of contraction was small compared with the maximum amplitude of contraction during phase III, the active phase of the MMC. They therefore suggested that when the duodenal wall contracts, it constricts the common bile duct and the choledochoduodenal junction to impede bile flow. Others have demonstrated a pylorocholecystic reflex[46] and a gastro-sphincter of Oddi reflex,[177] indicating a relationship between gastrointestinal and sphincter of Oddi motility. Both morphine and noradrenaline contract the sphincter but relax the duodenum.[129] These findings were confirmed by studying the effect of adrenaline and noradrenaline on the isolated terminal bile duct.[41] Ono and colleagues[126] simultaneously recorded bile flow and electrical activity from the sphincter and duodenum in humans. They found a negative correlation between bile flow and sphincter of Oddi electrical activity, i.e. bile

flowed into the duodenum only in the absence of sphincter electrical activity.

Bile flow into the duodenum

Several studies in animals and man show that the sphincter of Oddi exhibits spontaneous phasic contractions.[6,8,65,95,121,132,143] In man these phasic contractions occur at about 4 per minute and have a duration of 4–5 seconds.[65] Using a triple-lumen catheter with orifices spaced at 2-mm intervals from the distal end for manometric measurements, Toouli and his colleagues found that 60% of human phasic pressure waves propagate towards the duodenum, 14% propagate in a retrograde fashion towards the common bile duct, while 26% are simultaneous, i.e. propagate in both directions at once.[169] Species differences in phasic wave direction make the physiological purpose of this phenomenon unclear. In dogs the biliary sphincter may act as a pump to expel bile into the duodenum,[175] yet it has also been observed that flow through the common bile duct stops with each phasic contraction of the sphincter.[6,144,169] Moreover, in cats, increased sphincter activity is associated with increased resistance to flow through the choledochoduodenal junction.[129]

Using simultaneous cine-radiography, trans-sphincteric flow and electromyographic recordings of the opossum sphincter of Oddi, Toouli *et al.* have unravelled the mechanism of bile flow through the sphincter.[170] The main mechanism of common bile duct emptying in the opossum is antegrade contraction of the sphincter of Oddi. A wave of contraction begins at the junction of the bile duct and sphincter and strips the contents of the sphincter segment into the duodenum (the systolic phase). During sphincter contraction, no flow occurs from the bile duct into the sphincter segment. The sphincter then relaxes, and there is passive flow of bile from the duct into the sphincter segment (the diastolic phase). A wave of contraction then begins again at the ductal–sphincter junction, and the cycle repeats itself. The overall effect of antegrade phasic contractions is therefore to promote flow from the common bile duct into the duodenum. Initially, increased contractions are accompanied by increased flow across the sphincter; but when the contractions exceed a critical level, the diastolic interval is abolished and flow ceases. In the opossum, this phenomenon occurs when the frequency of contractions exceeds 8 per minute.[171]

Control mechanisms

The activity of the sphincter of Oddi is subject to many influences. Early investigators demonstrated neural influences on the sphincter of Oddi,[133] while more recently several hormones have been shown to affect sphincter function.[9,65,107,122] It is likely that humoral and neural stimuli are interlinked in affecting sphincter function.[7,8] Various pharmacological and physical agents also influence sphincter ativity while the response of the sphincter to food in the upper gastrointestinal tract probably represents the summation of many of these influences.

Hormonal factors

The response of the sphincter of Oddi to CCK was first described by Sandblom in 1935[142] and varies according to species. In man, CCK decreases phasic wave activity and reduces baseline pressure,[65] while a similar response is found in primates[95] and cats.[8] In these species the sphincter relaxes in response to CCK, thus facilitating the passive flow of bile from the common duct into the duodenum. However, in the rabbit,[143] opossum,[6] and prairie dog[49] the effect is to increase the phasic wave activity of the sphincter without affecting baseline pressure. In these species, increased sphincter of Oddi activity propels bile into the duodenum in response to CCK. Until recently, the inhibitory actions of CCK on the sphincter of Oddi were thought to be due to a direct action of the hormone on the sphincter muscle. New data indicate that the effects of CCK on the sphincter of Oddi are mediated by non-adrenergic, non-cholinergic neurones that inhibit the feline sphincter of Oddi. This effect masks a direct excitatory effect of CCK on the sphincter muscle.[8] In the opossum, on the other hand, excitation of the sphincter of Oddi by CCK appears to be mediated by a direct action of the hormone on the sphincter muscle.[79]

Other gastrointestinal hormones and peptides can also affect the sphincter of Oddi. Caerulein is a potent inhibitor of sphincter activity in a number of species.[2,13,107] Gastrin, which shares an identical carboxyterminal pentapeptide with CCK and caerulein, also influences the choledochal sphincter.[107] The potency of this hormone, however, is considerably less than that of CCK or caerulein. Agosti et al.[2] showed that human gastrin has only 10–40% of the activity of CCK in relaxing the sphincter of Oddi in the anaesthetized guinea pig. Secretin reduces sphincter resistance in the dog, probably indirectly by potentiating the action of CCK. Glucagon also decreases sphincter resistance in dogs[107] and man,[124] and it is often used to relax the sphincter to facilitate cannulation during ERCP.[79]

Recently motilin, serum levels of which fluctuate with phases of the interdigestive MMC, has also been found to influence the sphincter of Oddi.[79,122] In the dog[147] and opossum[35] phasic contractions exhibit cyclical variations in phase with the interdigestive MMC. Thus, the physiological role of motilin on the sphincter of Oddi may be to regulate this cyclical activity during the interdigestive period. The actions of motilin on the sphincter of Oddi may be mediated by an intramural excitatory pathway, which appears to consist of opiate, serotoninergic and cholinergic neurones.[7]

Pancreatic polypeptide (PP), peptide-YY (PYY) and neuropeptide-Y (NPY) all influence biliary motility. Both PP and PYY have been shown to enhance gallbladder filling in the prairie dog.[38,39] Tatemoto and Mutt reported that PYY stimulates gallbladder contraction *in vitro*[166]

but does not affect CCK-8-stimulated gallbladder contraction in the anaesthetized guinea pig.[165] Likewise, PYY does not influence resting gallbladder tension or CCK-stimulated gallbladder contraction in dogs[108] and prairie dogs.[69] None the less, PYY inhibits the increase in phasic contractions of the sphincter usually observed with CCK-8. Thus, PP and PYY may play a role in modulating biliary motility in the postprandial state by inhibiting bile flow into the duodenum and promoting gallbladder filling. Since NPY increases sphincter of Oddi activity and gallbladder pressure in the prairie dog,[106] it could be a neurotransmitter or neuromodulator regulating bile flow.

Neural factors

Perception of food causes a reduction in the resistance to bile flow through the choledochoduodenal junction,[133] indicating a neural influence on the biliary sphincter. Recent neurohistochemical studies have demonstrated both adrenergic and cholinergic neurones within the sphincter of Oddi of the cat and dog.[93] Persson[130] suggests that the cat gallbladder and sphincter contain contraction-mediating α-receptors and relaxation mediating β-adrenergic receptors. In the gallbladder β-receptors predominate, while in the sphincter α- and β-receptors are more evenly distributed. However, relaxation of the sphincter in response to adrenergic β-receptor stimulation occurs only when the α-receptors have previously been blocked with phenoxybenzamine.[130] Although both receptor types exist in sphincter smooth muscle, mainly α-adrenoreceptors are activated by sympathetic nerve stimulation. Thus, adrenergic stimulation causes the sphincter of Oddi to contract and the gallbladder to relax. This mechanism may be important during gallbladder filling by promoting the entry of bile into the gallbladder.

The biliary tract receives parasympathetic innervation from the vagus nerve.[138] Acetylcholine contracts both the gallbladder and the sphincter of Oddi in the cat and calf.[131,138] Cholinergic stimulation of the sphincter by bethanecol increases the frequency of phasic contractions in the opossum.[171] The function of the vagus nerve in sphincter of Oddi function remains obscure,[10,181] though recent work in the prairie dog has demonstrated increased resistance to flow through the sphincter after truncal vagotomy.[132] Vagal stimulation studies have also failed to define clearly the role of the vagus in biliary dynamics. Some investigators have reported sphincter contraction during vagal stimulation,[164] but others could not detect any response to either central or peripheral stimulation of the vagus.[164]

Behar and Biancani have suggested the presence of non-cholinergic, non-adrenergic neurones in the sphincter of Oddi.[8] Studying the feline sphincter of Oddi, they observed that CCK-induced sphincter relaxation was not antagonized by either adrenergic or cholinergic blockade. Either CCK has a direct action on sphincteric smooth muscle, therefore, or its effects are mediated by a different neurotransmitter. In support of such a neurological pathway, administration of tetrodotoxin (TTX), which blocks nerve transmission without affecting smooth muscle, completely antagonized the effects of CCK on the sphincter.[8]

Pharmacological factors

Morphine has long been known to increase resistance to bile flow. Studies in a number of species[129,175] have shown that the sphincter of Oddi is very sensitive to opiates, responding with marked contractions to low doses of morphine sulphate. In man, small doses of morphine increase the rate of phasic contraction of the sphincter of Oddi;[79] phasic wave amplitude and baseline pressure are also increased.[77] Pethidine also produces a marked rise in biliary pressure but its effect is only half that of morphine.[53] Amyl nitrate consistently relaxes the sphincter of Oddi in several species.[12,164] This inhibitory effect has been used clinically to distinguish sphincter spasm from stenosis.

Nifedipine, a calcium channel blocker, reduces baseline sphincter of Oddi pressure as well as the frequency, amplitude and duration of phasic contractions.[73] Intravenous butylscopolamine bromide will decrease sphincter of Oddi motility without affecting baseline pressure.[153] Alcohol administered either intravenously or into the duodenum causes a moderate decrease in baseline pressure without affecting sphincter motility.[153] Recent endoscopic manometry in humans given pentazocine has shown higher baseline pressures and increased amplitude of phasic contractions in the sphincter.[153] Fentanyl has also been associated with sphincter spasm during peroperative cholangiography,[33] whereas diazepam is without such effects.[124]

Various anaesthetic agents influence sphincter of Oddi function. Thus, small intravenous doses of barbiturate increase flow through the sphincter.[182] Xylazine and ketamine affect biliary tract motility in the prairie dog and should therefore be avoided during physiological studies of the sphincter.[70,141] Lastly, a study in dogs has shown inhibition of endogenous CCK release by several different anaesthetic agents (with the exception of α-chlorolose), which may therefore affect sphincter motility indirectly.[105]

Miscellaneous factors

Temperature affects sphincter of Oddi activity in rabbits, cold being inhibitory and elevation to 40°C being stimulatory.[144] Increasing the blood pressure in dogs by infusing saline elevates sphincter opening pressure, whereas hypotension produced by haemorrhage diminishes opening pressure.[164] Sphincter activity is also influenced by the degree of gallbladder filling.[49,121,182] In the prairie dog, distending the gallbladder increases sphincter activity and emptying it has the opposite effect, the so-called cholecystosphincter of Oddi reflex.[121] Recently a relationship has been demonstrated between sphincter of Oddi activity and the interdigestive or migrating myoelectric complex.[2,82] Two groups of investigators have shown in the conscious opossum that phasic contractions are synchronous with spike potentials in the sphincter and that both exhibit cyclical changes that correlate with the MMC.[2,82] Mochinaga has demonstrated a relationship between gastroduodenal motor activity and bile flow in dogs.[119]

Intraluminal stimuli

Early investigators observed that introduction of acid into the stomach increased resistance to bile flow entering the duodenum in the anaesthetized dog, whereas alkali achieved the reverse.[36] In patients with previous cholecystectomy, installation of dilute hydrochloric acid into the duodenum causes a transient increase in sphincter of Oddi resistance, which can be blocked with atropine.[50]

Fifty years ago, Best and Hicken[14] inferred from cholangiographic evidence that cream and olive oil relax the human sphincter of Oddi, but Doubilet could not confirm this finding in patients after cholecystectomy.[50] A more extensive investigation of cholecystectomy patients showed that an egg-yolk meal caused relaxation but olive oil did not; protein also caused slight relaxation of the sphincter, but carbohydrate had no effect.[12] Recent work in the prairie dog has shown that intraduodenal infusions of acidified saline[71] and sodium oleate[72] decrease sphincter of Oddi activity, whereas protein infusions stimulate sphincter activity.[177] Exogenous CCK consistently increases sphincter of Oddi activity in this species.[49] These conflicting data may be explained by evidence in rodents that CCK is not released after ingestion of fats but is released by protein.[102] Further investigations using modern techniques are needed to elucidate exactly which of the influences in the symphony that affects the sphincter of Oddi and promotes bile flow into the duodenum are activated by intraluminal stimulation of the upper gastrointestinal tract.

CONCLUSION

The production of bile and its delivery to the duodenum is essential for digestion and for survival of the individual. The physiology of this process is complex and relatively difficult to study. Recent advances in hormone and receptor assay techniques, ultrasonography and radiology as well as endoscopic manometry have given us new insights into biliary physiology. The events at cellular and subcellular levels are now being studied and further research in this area will be fruitful. More sophisticated analysis of bile production and composition will help us understand the pathology of gallstones and lead to more effective therapies, while already endoscopic manometry is uncovering a host of sphincter of Oddi abnormalities in patients with 'idiopathic' pancreatitis and the postcholecystectomy syndrome.

REFERENCES

1. Adrian, T.E., Mitchenere, P., Sagor, G. *et al.* (1982) Effect of pancreatic polypeptide on gallbladder pressure and hepatic bile secretion. *American Journal of Physiology*, **242**, G204–G207.
2. Agosti, A., Mantovani, P. & Mori, L. (1971) Actions of caerulein and related substances on the sphincter of Oddi. *Naunyn-Schmiedebergs Archiv für Pharmakologie*, **208**, 114–118.
3. Anderson, A., James, O.F.W., MacDonald, H.S. *et al.* (1980) The effect of ethinyl oestradiol on biliary lipid composition in young men. *European Journal of Clinical Investigation*, **10**, 77.
4. Baker, A.L., Wood, R.A.B., Moosa, A.R. *et al.* (1979) Sodium taurocholate modifies the bile acid independent fraction of canalicular bile flow in the rhesus monkey. *Journal of Clinical Investigation*, **64**, 312.
5. Balabaud, C., Kron, K.A. & Gumucio, J.J. (1977) The assessment of the bile salt nondependent fraction of canalicular bile water in the rat. *Journal of Laboratory and Clinical Medicine*, **89**, 393.
6. Becker, J.M., Moody, F.G. & Zinsmeister, A.R. (1982) Effect of gastrointestinal hormones on the biliary sphincter of the opossum. *Gastroenterology*, **82**, 1300–1307.
7. Behar, J. & Biancani, P. (1980) Effects of cholecystokinin and the octapeptide of cholecystokinin on the feline sphincter of Oddi and gallbladder. *Journal of Clinical Investigation*, **66**, 1231–1239.
8. Behar, J. & Biancani, P. (1988) Effects and mechanisms of action of motilin on the cat sphincter of Oddi. *Gastroenterology*, **95**, 1099–1105.
9. Behar, J. (1980) Effect of 5-hydroxytryptamine (5-HT) on the feline sphincter of Oddi (SO): Evidence for a PG inhibitory receptor. *Gastroenterology*, **78**, 1139 (Abstract).
10. Benevantano, T.C., Rosen, R.G. & Schein, C.J. (1969) The physiological effect of acute vagal section on canine biliary dynamics. *Journal of Surgical Research*, **9**, 331–334.
11. Bennion, L.J., Mott, D.M. & Howard, B.V. (1980) Oral contraceptives raise the cholesterol saturation of bile by increasing biliary cholesterol secretion. *Metabolism*, **29**, 18.
12. Bergh, G.S. (1942) The sphincter mechanism of the common bile duct in human subjects. Its reactions to certain types of stimulation. *Surgery*, **11**, 299–330.
13. Bertaccini, G., De Caro, G. & Endean, G. (1968) The actions of caerulin on the smooth muscle of the gastrointestinal tract and gallbladder. *British Journal of Pharmacology*, **4**, 291–310.
14. Best, R.R. & Hicken, N.F. (1938) Non operative management of remaining common duct stones. *Journal of the American Medical Association*, **110**, 1257–1261.
15. Binder, H.J. & Boyer, J.L. (1973) Bile salts: A determinant of the bile-peritoneal electrical potential differences in the rat. *Gastroenterology*, **65**, 943.
16. Blitzer, B.L. & Boyer, J.L. (1982) Cellular mechanisms of bile formation. *Gastroenterology*, **82**, 346.
17. Blitzer, B.L., Ratoosh, S.L. & Boyer, J.L. (1980) Inhibitors of Na⁺ coupled ion transport block taurocholate uptake by isolated rat hepatocytes. *Clinical Research*, **28**, 273A (Abstract).
18. Bode, J.C., Zelder, O. & Neuberger, H.O. (1973) Effect of taurocholate, dehydrocholate and secretion on biliary output of alkaline phosphatase and GOT. *Helvetica Medica Acta*, **37**, 143.
19. Bolton, C.H., Nicholls, J.S. & Heaton, K.W. (1980) Estimation of cholesterol in bile: Assessment of an enzymatic method. *Clinica Chimica Acta*, **105**, 225.
20. Bouchier, I.A.D. & Clamp, J.R. (1971) Glycoproteins in human bile. *Clinica Chimica Acta*, **35**, 219.
21. Bouchier, I.A.D., Copperband, S.R. & El-Kodsi, B.M. (1965) Mucus substances and viscosity of normal and pathological human bile. *Gastroenterology*, **49**, 343.
22. Bourke, J.B. & Ritchie, H.D. (1970) The pressure profile of the sphincter of Oddi in man and the pig. *British Journal of Surgery*, **57**, 848 (Abstract).
23. Boyer, J.L., Itabashi, M. & Huban, Z. (1973) Formation of pericanalicular vacuoles during sodium dehydrocholate choleresis— a mechanism for bile acid transport. In Paumgartner, G., Preisig, R. (eds) *The Liver: Quantitative Aspects of Structure and Function*. Basel: Karger.
24. Boyer, J.L. (1980) New concepts of mechanisms of hepatocyte bile formation. *Physiological Review*, **60**, 303.
25. Brooks, F.P. (1970) *Control of Gastrointestinal Function*, p. 184. New York: Macmillan.
26. Brooks, F.P. (1969) The secretion of bile. *American Journal of Digestive Diseases*, **14**, 4343.
27. Campbell, C.B., Cowley, D.J. & Dowling, R.H. (1972) Dietary factors affecting biliary lipid secretion in the rhesus monkey. A mechanism for the hypocholesterolaemic action of polyunsaturated fat? *European Journal of Clinical Investigation*, **2**, 332.
28. Cantor, P., Petrojijevic, L., Pedersen, J.F. *et al.* (1986) Cholecystokinetic and pancreozymic effect of O-sulfated gastrin compared with non-sulfated gastrin and cholecystokinin. *Gastroenterology*, **91**, 1154–1163.
29. Carey, M.C. & Small, D.M. (1973) Solubility of cholesterol (Ch) in aqueous bile-salt lecithin (L) solutions: Importance of metastability, lipid concentration and temperature. *Gastroenterology*, **64**, 706.
30. Carey, M.L. & Small, D.M. (1978) The physical chemistry of cholesterol solubility in bile. *Journal of Clinical Investigation*, **61**, 998.
31. Caroli, J., Porcher, P., Peguigot, G. *et al.* (1960) Contribution of cineradiography to study of the function of the human biliary tract. *American Journal of Digestive Diseases*, **5**, 677–696.
32. Chenderovitch, J., Phocas, E. & Rautureau, M. (1963) Effects of hypertonic solutions on bile formation. *American Journal of Physiology*, **205**, 863.
33. Chessick, K.C., Black, S. & Hoyer, S.J. (1975) Spasm and operative cholangiography. *Archives of Surgery*, **110**, 53–57.
34. Chowdhury, J.R., Berkowitz, J.M., Praissman, M. *et al.* (1975) Interaction between octapeptide-cholecystokinin, gastrin, and secretin on cat gallbladder in vitro. *American Journal of Physiology*, **229**, 1311–1315.
35. Coelho, J.C., Moody, F.G. & Senninger, N. (1985) A new method for correlating pancreatic and biliary duct pressures and sphincter of Oddi electromyography. *Surgery*, **97**, 342–349.
36. Cole, W.H. (1925) Relation of gastric content to the physiology of the common duct sphincter. *American Journal of Physiology*, **72**, 39–42.
37. Conter, R.L., Roslyn, J.J., DenBesten, L. *et al.* (1987) Pancreatic polypeptide enhances postcontractile gallbladder filling in the prairie dog. *Gastroenterology*, **92**, 771–776.
38. Conter, R.L., Roslyn, J.J. & Taylor, I.L. (1987) Effects of peptide YY on gallbladder motility. *American Journal of Physiology*, **252**, G736–G741.
39. Conter, R.L., Roslyn, J.J., Muller, E.L. *et al.* (1985) Effect of pancreatic polypeptide on gallbladder filling. *Journal of Surgical Research*, **38**, 461–467.
40. Conter, R.L., Roslyn, J.J. & Taylor, I.L. (1987) Effects of peptide YY on gallbladder filling. *American Journal of Physiology*, **252**, G736–741.
41. Crema, A. & Berte, F. (1963) Actions of sympathomimetic drugs on the isolated junction of the bile duct and duodenum. *British Journal of Pharmacology and Chemotherapy*, **20**, 221–229.
42. Crochelt, R.F. & Peikin, S.R. (1987) Effect of nifedipine and extracellular calcium on spontaneous and potassium-stimulated bovine gallbladder muscle contraction. *Gastroenterology*, **92**, 1799 (Abstract).
43. Crofton, P.M. & Smith, A.F. (1980) Alkaline phosphatase of high and low molecular mass in human serum and bile: A comparative study of kinetic properties. *Clinical Chemistry*, **26**, 451.
44. Crofton, P.M. & Smith, A.F. (1981) High molecular mass alkaline phosphatase in serum and bile: Physical properties and relationship with other high molecular mass enzymes. *Clinical Chemistry*, **27**, 860.
45. Cushieri, A., Hughes, J.H. & Cohen, M. (1972) Biliary pressure studies during cholecystectomy. *British Journal of Surgery*, **59**, 267–273.
46. Debas, H.T. & Yamagishi, T. (1979) Evidence for a pylorocholecystic reflex for gallbladder contraction. *Annals of Surgery*, **190**, 170–175.
47. Den Besten, L., Connor, W.E. & Bell, S. (1973) The effect of dietary cholesterol on the composition of human bile. *Surgery*, **73**, 266.

48. Donaldson, L.A., Joffe, S.N., McIntosh, W. *et al.* (1979) Amylase activity in human bile. *Gut*, **20**, 216.

49. Doty, J.E., Pitt, H.A., Kuchenbecker, S.L. *et al.* (1981) Effect of gallbladder filling and cholecystokinin on the prairie dog sphincter of Oddi. *Surgical Forum*, **32**, 148–150.

50. Doubilet, H. & Colp, R. (1937) Resistance of the sphincter of Oddi in the human. *Surgery, Gynecology and Obstetrics*, **64**, 622–633.

51. Dowling, R.H., Mack, E. & Small, D.M. (1971) Biliary lipid secretion and bile composition after acute and chronic interruption of the enterohepatic circulation in the rhesus monkey. *Journal of Clinical Investigation*, **50**, 1917.

52. Dublin, M., Maurice, M., Feldman, C. *et al.* (1978) Phalloidin induced cholestasis in the rat: Relation to changes in microfilaments. *Gastroenterology*, **75**, 450.

53. Economou, G. and Ward-McQuaid, J.N. (1971) A cross-over comparison of the effect of morphine, pethidine, pentazocine, and phenozocine on biliary pressure. *Gut*, **12**, 218–221.

54. Elias, E., Hruban, Z., Wade, J.B. *et al.* (1980) Phalloidin induced cholestasis: A microfilament mediated change in junctional complex permeability. *Proceedings of the National Academy of Sciences of the USA*, **77**, 2229.

55. Englert, E. (1970) The proteins of human gallbladder bile with and without gallstones. *Clinica Chimica Acta*, **29**, 319.

56. Erlinger, S., Dhumeaux, D., Berthelot, P. *et al.* (1970) Effect of inhibitors of sodium transport on bile formation in the rabbit. *American Journal of Physiology*, **219**, 416.

57. Erlinger, S. (1981) Hepatocyte bile secretion: Current views and controversies. *Hepatology*, **1**, 352.

58. Fisher, R.S., Rock, E. & Malmud, L.S. (1986) Gallbladder emptying response to sham feeding in humans. *Gastroenterology*, **90**, 1854–1857.

59. Fisher, R.S., Rock, E., Levin, G. *et al.* (1987) Effects of somatostatin on gallbladder emptying. *Gastroenterology*, **92**, 885–890.

60. Fletcher, D.M. & Clark, C.G. (1969) Changes in canine bile flow and composition after vagotomy. *British Journal of Surgery*, **56**, 103.

61. Folsch, U.R., Cantor, P., Wilms, H.M. *et al.* (1987) Role of cholecystokinin in the negative feedback control of pancreatic enzyme secretion in conscious rats. *Gastroenterology*, **92**, 449–458.

62. Forker, E.L. (1968) Bile formation in guinea pigs. Analysis with inert solutes of graded molecular radius. *American Journal of Physiology*, **215**, 56.

63. Fried, G.M., Ogden, W.D., Swierczek, J. *et al.* (1983) Release of cholecystokinin in conscious dogs: correlation with simultaneous measurements of gallbladder pressure and pancreatic protein secretion. *Gastroenterology*, **83**, 1113–1119.

64. Fujimura, M., Sakamoto, T., Khalil, T. *et al.* (1984) Physiologic role of neurotensin in gallbladder contraction in the dog. *Surgical Forum*, **35**, 192–194.

65. Geenan, J.E., Hogan, W.J.U., Doods, W.J. *et al.* (1980) Intraluminal pressure recording from the human sphincter of Oddi. *Gastroenterology*, **78**, 317–324.

66. Giles, R.B. Jr, Smith, J.E., Crowley, G. *et al.* (1960) A study of carbohydrates in human gallbladder bile. *Journal of Laboratory and Clinical Medicine*, **55**, 38.

67. Gomez, G., Lluis, F., Guo, Y.-S. *et al.* (1986) Bile inhibits release of cholecystokinin and neurotensin. *Surgery*, **100**, 363–368.

68. Gottfries, A.S., Nilsson, B., Samuelsson, B. *et al.* (1968) Phospholipids in human hepatic bile, gallbladder bile and plasma in cases with acute cholecystitis. *Scandinavian Journal of Clinical and Laboratory Investigation*, **21**, 168.

69. Grace, P.A., Couse, N. & Pitt, H.A. (1988) Peptide YY inhibits cholecystokinin-stimulated sphincter of Oddi activity in the prairie dog. *Surgery*, **1–4**, 546–552.

70. Grace, P.A., Webb, T.H., Romano, P.J. *et al.* (1987) Ketamine inhibits sphincter of Oddi phasic wave amplitude. *Current Surgery*, **44**, 403–405.

71. Grace, P.A., Romano, P.J. & Pitt, H.A. (1987) Duodenal acidification inhibits sphincter of Oddi motility in the prairie dog. *Journal of Surgical Research*, **43**, 68–74.

72. Grace, P.A. & Pitt, H.A. (1987) Cholecystectomy alters the hormonal response of the sphincter of Oddi. *Surgery*, **102**, 186–194.

73. Guelrud, M., Mendoza, S., Rossiter, G. *et al.* (1988) Effect of nifedipine on sphincter of Oddi motor activity: Studies in healthy volunteers and patients with biliary dyskinesia. *Gastroenterology*, **95**, 1050–1055.

74. Hallenbeck, G.A. (1967) Biliary and pancreatic intraductal pressures. In Code, C.F. (ed.) *The Handbook of Physiology*, section 6, The Alimentary Canal, Vol II, Secretion, pp 1007–1025. Washington, DC: American Physiological Society.

75. Hashimoto, T., Poston, G.J., Gomez, G. *et al.* (1988) The effect of pancreastatin on cholecystokinin stimulated gall-bladder contraction in vivo and in vitro. *Gastroenterology* (supplement) **94** A176 (Abstract).

76. Hasimoto, T., Poston, G.J., Greeley, G.H. Jr. *et al.* (1988) CGRP inhibits gallbladder contractility. *Surgery*, **104**, 419–423.

77. Helm, J.F., Venu, R.P., Geenen, J.E. *et al.* (1988) Effects of morphine on the human sphincter of Oddi. *Gut*, **29**, 1402–1407.

78. Hepner, G.W. (1975) Altered bile acid metabolism in vegetarians. *American Journal of Digestive Diseases*, **20**, 935.

79. Hogan, W.J., Dodds, W.J. & Geenen, J.E. (1983) The biliary tract. In Christensen, J. (ed.) *A Guide to Gastrointestinal Motility*, pp 157–197. Bristol: Wright. PSG.

80. Holloway, D.E. & Rivers, J.M. (1981) Influence of chronic ascorbic acid deficiency and excessive ascorbic acid intake in bile acid metabolism and bile composition in the guinea pig. *Journal of Nutrition*, **111**, 412.

81. Holtzbach, R.T., Marsh, M.E. & Halberg, M.C. (1971) The effect of pregnancy on lipid composition of guinea pig gallbladder bile. *Gastroenterology*, **60**, 288.

82. Honda, R., Toouli, J., Dodds, W.J. *et al.* (1982) Relationship of sphincter of Oddi spike bursts to gastrointestinal myoelectric activity in conscious opossums. *Journal of Clinical Investigation*, **69**, 770–778.

83. Hopton, D. & White, T.T. (1972) Effect of hepatic and celiac vagal stimulation on common bile duct pressure. *American Journal of Digestive Diseases*, **16**, 1095–1101.

84. Inberg, M.V. & Vuorio, M. (1969) Human gallbladder function after selective gastric and total abdominal vagotomy. *Acta Chirurgiae Scandinavica*, **135**, 625–633.

85. Inoue, T. & Juniper, K. Jr. (1973) The effect of sodium oleate on cholesterol solubility in bile salt-lecithin model systems. *American Journal of Digestive Diseases*, **18**, 1066.

86. Jansson, R. & Svanik, J. (1977) Effects of intravenous secretin and cholecystokinin on gallbladder net water absorption and motility in the cat. *Gastroenterology*, **72**, 639–643.

87. Jansson, R. (1978) Effects of gastrointestinal hormones on concentrating function and motility in the gallbladder. *Acta Physiologica Scandinavica Supplementum*, **456**, 1–38.

88. Jazrawi, R.R. & Northfield, T.C. (1986) Effects of a pharmacological dose of cholecystokinin on bile acid kinetics and biliary cholesterol saturation in man. *Gut*, **27**, 355–362.

89. Jenkins, S.A. (1980) Vitamin C status, serum cholesterol levels and bile composition in the pregnant guinea pig. *British Journal of Nutrition*, **43**, 95.

90. Johnson, J. & Kalant, N. (1972) Bile composition in the pregnant rabbit. *American Journal of Digestive Diseases*, **17**, 1.

91. Kern, M.K., Nakaya, M., Dodds, W.J. *et al.* (1986) Pressure kinetics of the biliary tract in conscious opossums. *Gastroenterology*, **91**, 1058 (Abstract).

92. Kutteh, W.H., Prince, S.J., Phillips, J.O. *et al.* (1982) Properties of immunoglobulin A in serum of individuals with liver diseases and in hepatic bile. *Gastroenterology*, **82**, 184.

93. Kyosola, K. (1979) Sympatho-adrenergic neural control of the sphincter of Oddi of the cat and dog. *Tohoku Journal of Experimental Medicine*, **127**, 113–117.

94. LaMorte, W.W., Schoetz, D.J. Jr, Birkett, D.H. *et al.* (1979) The role of the gallbladder in the pathogenesis of cholesterol gallstones. *Gastroenterology*, **77**, 580–592.

95. LaMorte, W.W., Gaca, J.M., Wise, W.E. *et al.* (1980) Choledochal sphincter relaxation in response to histamine in the primate. *Journal of Surgical Research*, **28**, 373–378.

96. Lanzini, A., Jazrawi, R.P. & Northfield, T.C. (1987) Simultaneous quantitative measurements of absolute gallbladder storage and emptying during fasting and eating in humans. *Gastroenterology*, **92**, 852–861.

97. Lawson, M., Everson, G.T., Klingensmith, W. *et al.* (1983) Co-

ordination of gastric and gallbladder emptying after ingestion of a regular meal. *Gastroenterology,* **85**, 866–870.

98. Lee, S.P., Lem, T.H. & Scott, A.J. (1979) Carbohydrate moieties of glycoproteins in human hepatic and gallbladder bile, gallbladder mucosa and gallstones. *Clinical Science,* **56**, 533.

99. Lee, S.P., LaMont, T. & Carey, M.C. (1981) Role of gallbladder mucus. Hypersecretion in the evolution of cholesterol gallstones. Studies in the prairie dog. *Journal of Clinical Investigation,* **67**, 1712.

100. Lee, S.P. (1980) The mechanism of mucus secretion by the gallbladder epithelium. *British Journal of Experimental Pathology,* **61**, 117.

101. Lennard, T.W.J., Farndon, J.R. & Taylor, R.M.R. (1984) Acalculous biliary pain: Diagnosis and selection for cholecystokinin test for pain reproduction. *British Journal of Surgery,* **71**, 368–370.

102. Liddle, R.A., Green, G.M., Conrad, C.K. *et al.* (1986) Proteins but not amino acids, carbohydrates, or fats stimulate CCK secretion in the rat. *American Journal of Physiology,* **251** (Gastrointest. Liver Physiol. 14) G243–G248.

103. Liedberg, G. (1969) The effect of vagotomy on gallbladder and duodenal pressures during rest and stimulation with cholecystokinin. *Acta Chirurgiae Scandinavica,* **135**, 695–700.

104. Lilja, P., Fagan, C.J., Wiener, I. *et al.* (1982) Infusion of pure cholecystokinin in humans. Correlation between plasma concentrations of cholecystokinin and gallbladder size. *Gastroenterology,* **83**, 256–261.

105. Lilja, P., Wiener, I., Inoune, K. *et al.* (1982) Effect of anesthetic agents on the release of cholecystokinin. *Surgical Forum,* **33**, 130–132.

106. Lillemoe, K.D., Webb, T.H. & Pitt, H.A. (1988) Neuropeptide Y: A candidate neurotransmitter for biliary motility. *Journal of Surgical Research,* **45**, 254–260.

107. Lin, T.M. & Spray, G.F. (1969) Effect of pentagastrin, cholecystokinin, caerulin and glucagon on the choledochal resistance and bile flow in dogs. *Gastroenterology,* **56**, 1178 (Abstract).

108. Lluis, F., Fujimura, M., Lonovics, J. *et al.* (1988) Peptide YY and gallbladder contraction. *Gastroenterology,* **94**, 1441–1446.

109. Lonovics, J., Varro, V. & Thompson, J.C. (1985) The effect of cholecystokinin and substance P antagonists on cholecystokinin- and substance P-stimulated gallbladder contraction. *Gastroenterology,* **88**, 1480 (Abstract).

110. Lonovics, J., Guzman, S., Devitt, P. *et al.* (1980) Release of pancreatic polypeptide in humans by infusion of cholecystokinin. *Gastroenterology,* **79**, 817–822.

111. Lonovics, J., Devitt, P., Rayford, P.L. *et al.* (1979) Actions of VIP, somatostatin and pancreatic polypeptide on gall-bladder tension and CCK-stimulated gallbladder contraction in vitro. *Surgical Forum,* **30**, 407–409.

112. Lueth, H.C. (1931) Studies on the flow of bile into the duodenum and the existence of a sphincter of Oddi. *American Journal of Physiology,* **99**, 237–252.

113. Mack, E., Chikako, S. and Patzer, E.M. (1981) Effect of truncal vagotomy and pyloroplasty on hepatic bile composition in the rhesus monkey. *Journal of Laboratory and Clinical Medicine,* **97**, 521.

114. Malagelada, J.-R., Holtermuller, K.H., Sizemore, G.W. *et al.* (1976) The influence of hypercalcemia on basal and cholecystokinin-stimulated pancreatic, gallbladder, and gastric functions in man. *Gastroenterology,* **71**, 405–408.

115. Mate, L., Sakamoto, T., Greeley, G.H. Jr *et al.* (1986) Effect of substance P on contractions of the gallbladder. *Surgery, Gynecology and Obstetrics,* **163**, 163–166.

116. Matsuhiro, T., Nemoto, T., Endo, M. *et al.* (1970) Glycoproteins and sulfated glycoproteins isolated from human bile. *Clinica Chimica Acta,* **30**, 645.

117. Metzger, A., Heymsfeld, S. & Grundy, S. (1972) The lithogenic index—a numerical expression for the relative lithogenicity of bile. *Gastroenterology,* **62**, 499.

118. Metzger, A.L., Adler, R., Heymsfield, S. *et al.* (1973) Diurnal variation in biliary lipid composition. *New England Journal of Medicine,* **288**, 333.

119. Mochinaga, N., Sarna, S.K., Condon, R.E. *et al.* (1988) Gastroduodenal regulation of common bile duct flow in the dog. *Gastroenterology,* **94**, 755–761.

120. Moore, E.W. & Dietschy, J.M. (1964) Na and K activity coefficients in bile and bile salts determined by glass electrodes. *American Journal of Physiology,* **206**, 1111.

121. Muller, E.L., Lewinski, M.A. & Pitt, H.A. (1984) The cholecystosphincter of Oddi reflex. *Journal of Surgical Research,* **36**, 377–383.

122. Muller, E.L., Grace, P.A., Conter, R.L. *et al.* (1987) Influence of motilin and cholecystokinin on sphincter of Oddi and duodenal motility. *American Journal of Physiology,* **253** (Gastrointest. Liver Physiol. 16), G679–G683.

123. Nakayama, F. & Kawamura, S. (1967) Composition of biliary lecithins. *Clinica Chimica Acta,* **17**, 53.

124. Nebel, O.T. (1975) Manometric evaluation of the papilla of Vater. *Gastrointestinal Endoscopy,* **21**, 126–128.

125. Neiderhiser, D.H. & Roth, H.P. (1968) Cholesterol solubilization by solutions of bile salts and bile salts plus lecithin. *Proceedings of the Society for Experimental Biology and Medicine,* **128**, 221.

126. Kno, K., Watanabe, N., Suzuki, K. *et al.* (1968) Bile flow mechanisms in man. *Archives of Surgery,* **96**, 869–874.

127. Oshio, C., Miyairi, M., Smith, C. *et al.* (1982) Temporal correlation of contractions in neighboring bile canaliculi. *Gastroenterology,* **82**, 1239.

128. Owyang, C., May, D. & Louie, D.S. (1986) Trypsin suppression of pancreatic enzyme secretion. Differential effect on cholecystokinin release and the enteropancreatic reflex. *Gastroenterology,* **91**, 637–643.

129. Persson, C.G.A. & Ekman, M. (1972) Effect of morphine, cholecystokinin and sympathomimetics on the sphincter of Oddi and intramural pressure in cat duodenum. *Scandinavian Journal of Gastroenterology,* **7**, 345–351.

130. Persson, C.G.A. (1972) Adrenergic, cholecystokinetic and morphine-induced effects on extra-hepatic biliary motility. *Acta Physiologica Scandinavica Supplementum,* **383**, 4–32.

131. Persson, C.G.A. (1971) Adrenoreceptor functions in the cat choledocho-duodenal junction in vitro. *British Journal of Pharmacology,* **42**, 447–461.

132. Pitt, H.A., Doty, J.E., DenBesten, L. *et al.* (1982) Altered sphincter of Oddi phasic activity following truncal vagotomy. *Journal of Surgical Research,* **32**, 598–607.

133. Potter, J.C. & Mann, F.C. (1926) Pressure changes on the biliary tract. *American Journal of Medical Science,* **171**, 202–217.

134. Redinger, R.N., Hermann, A.H. & Small, D.M. (1973) Primate biliary physiology. X. Effects of diet and fasting on biliary lipid secretion and relative composition and bile salt metabolism in the rhesus monkey. *Gastroenterology,* **64**, 610.

135. Reuben, A., Allen, R.M. & Boyer, J.L. (1982) Intrahepatic sources of "biliary-like" bile acid phospholipid, cholesterol micelles. *Gastroenterology,* **82**, 1241.

136. Ricci, G.L. & Fevery, J. (1981) Cholestatic action of somatostatin in the rat: Effect of the different fractions of bile secretion. *Gastroenterology,* **81**, 552–562.

137. Rollins, D.E., Freston, J.W. & Woodbury, D.M. (1980) Transport of organic anions into liver cells and bile. *Biochemical Pharmacology,* **29**, 1023.

138. Rothman, M.M. (1965) Anatomy and physiology of the gallbladder and bile ducts. *Gastroenterology,* **3**, 567–589.

139. Ryan, J. & Cohen, S. (1976) Interaction of gastrin I, secretin, and cholecystokinin on gallbladder smooth muscle. *American Journal of Physiology,* **230**, 553–556.

140. Ryan, J. & Cohen, S. (1977) Effect of vasoactive intestinal polypeptide on basal and cholecystokinin-induced gallbladder pressure. *Gastroenterology,* **73**, 870–872.

141. Ryan, T.D., Pellegrini, C.A., Broderick, W.C. *et al.* (1982) Effects of anaesthesia on biliary motility in the prairie dog. *Surgical Forum,* **33**, 209–213.

142. Sandblom, P., Voegtlen, W.L. & Ivy, I.C. (1935) The effect of CCK on the choledochoduodenal mechanism (sphincter of Oddi). *American Journal of Physiology,* **113**, 175–180.

143. Sarles, J.C., Devaus, M.A., Echinard, C. *et al.* (1976) Action of cholecystokinin and caerulein on the rabbit sphincter of Oddi. *Digestion,* **14**, 415–423.

144. Sarles, J.C., Midejean, A. & Deveaux, M.A. (1975) Electromyography of the sphincter of Oddi. *American Journal of Gastroenterology,* **63**, 221–231.

145. Schjoldager, B., Molero, X. & Miller, L.J. (1989) Functional and biochemical characterization of the human gallbladder muscularis cholecystokinin receptor. *Gastroenterology*, **96**, 1119–1125.

146. Schrager, J., Oates, M.D.G. & Rosbottom, A. (1972) The isolation and partial characterization of the principal biliary glycoprotein. *Digestion*, **6**, 338.

147. Scott, R.B., Strasberg, S.M., El-Sharkawi, Ty *et al.* (1984) Fasting canine biliary secretion and the sphincter of Oddi. *Gastroenterology*, **87**, 793–804.

148. Smith, D.C., MacKay, C. & McAllister, R.A. (1973) The effect of vagotomy and drainage on the composition of bile. *Scottish Medical Journal*, **18**, 65.

149. Smith, R.B., Edwards, J.P. & Johnston, D. (1981) Effect of vagotomy on exocrine pancreatic and biliary secretion in man. *American Journal of Surgery*, **141**, 40.

150. Snowball, S. & Taylor, W. (1981) Changes in biliary lipids of the conscious cat induced by a progestin-only oral contraceptive. *Proceedings of the Physiological Society*, July, 164.

151. Soloway, R.D. (1978) Gallstone disease. In Brooks, F.P. (ed.) *Gastrointestinal Pathophysiology*. New York: Oxford University Press.

152. Staritz, M., Poralla, T., Manns, M. *et al.* (1985) Investigation of the effect of modern morphine-like analgesics on the sphincter of Oddi. *Digestive Diseases and Science*, **30**, 796–801.

153. Staritz, M. (1988) Pharmacology of the sphincter of Oddi. *Endoscopy*, **20**, 171–174.

154. Steigerwalt, R.W., Goldfine, I.D. & Williams, J.A. (1984) Characterization of cholecystokinin receptors on bovine gallbladder membranes. *American Journal of Physiology*, **247**, G709–G714.

155. Strah, K.M., Pappas, T.N., Melendez, R.L. *et al.* (1986) Contrasting cholinergic dependence of pancreatic and gallbladder responses to cholecystokinin. *American Journal of Physiology*, **250**, G665–G669.

156. Strah, K.M., Melendez, R.L., Pappas, T.N. *et al.* (1986) Interactions of vasoactive intestinal polypeptide and cholecystokinin octapeptide on the control of gallbladder contraction. *Surgery*, **99**, 469–473.

157. Strasberg, S.M., Dorn, B.C., Redinger, R.N. *et al.* (1971) Effects of alteration of biliary pressure on bile composition—a method of study. *Gastroenterology*, **61**, 357.

158. Sutor, D.J. & Wilkie, L.I. (1977) Calcium in bile and calcium salts in gallstones. *Clinica Chimica Acta*, **79**, 119.

159. Sutor, D.J., Wilkie, L.I. & Jackson, M.J. (1980) Ionized calcium in pathological human bile. *Journal of Clinical Pathology*, **33**, 86.

160. Tagesson, C., Norrby, S. & Sjodahl, R. (1979) The pre-requisites for local lysolecithin formation in the human gallbladder. III. Demonstration of two different phospholipase A activities. *Scandinavian Journal of Gastroenterology*, **14**, 379.

161. Takahashi, I., Suzuki, T., Aizawa, I. *et al.* (1982) Comparison of gallbladder contractions induced by motilin and cholecystokinin in dogs. *Gastroenterology*, **82**, 419–424.

162. Tamasue, N., Inoue, T. & Juniper, K. Jr. (1973) Solubility of cholesterol in bile salt-lecithin model systems. *American Journal of Digestive Diseases*, **18**, 670.

163. Tandon, R.K., Srivastava, A.K., Bhaskar, A.K. *et al.* (1980) Lithogenicity of bile in Indian patients with cholesterol gallstones. *Indian Journal of Medical Research*, **71**, 907.

164. Tansey, M.J., Innes, D.L., Martin, J.S. *et al.* (1974) An evaluation of neural influences on the sphincter of Oddi in the dog. *Digestive Disease*, **19**, 423–437.

165. Tatemoto, I.K. (1982) Isolation and characterization of peptide YY (PYY), a candidate of gut hormone that inhibits pancreatic exocrine secretion. *Proceedings of the National Academy of Sciences of the USA*, **79**, 2514–2518.

166. Tatemoto, K. & Mutt, V. (1980) Isolation of two novel candidate hormones using a chemical method for finding naturally occurring polypeptides. *Nature*, **285**, 417–418.

167. Thompson, J.C., Fender, H.R., Ramus, N.I. *et al.* (1975) Cholecystokinin metabolism in man and dogs. *Annals of Surgery*, **182**, 496–504.

168. Thompson, J.C. (1985) The role of neurotensin in human gallbladder motility. *Annals of Surgery*, **201**, 678–689.

169. Toouli, J., Geenen, J.E., Hogan, W.J. *et al.* (1982) Sphincter of Oddi motor activity: A comparison between patients with common bile duct stones and controls. *Gastroenterology*, **82**, 111–117.

170. Toouli, J., Dodds, W.J., Honda, R. *et al.* (1983) Motor function of the opossum sphincter of Oddi. *Journal of Clinical Investigation*, **71**, 208–220.

171. Toouli, J. (1984) Sphincter of Oddi motility. *British Journal of Surgery*, **71**, 251–256.

172. Valenzuela, J.E., Walsh, J.H. & Isenberg, J.I. (1976) Effect of gastrin on pancreatic enzyme secretion and gallbladder emptying in man. *Gastroenterology*, **71**, 409–411.

173. Waldman, D.B., Zfass, A.M. & Makhlouf, G.M. (1977) Stimulatory (H1) and muscle inhibitory (H2) histamine receptors in gallbladder muscle. *Gastroenterology*, **72**, 932–936.

174. Wales, E.E. Jr, Englert, E. Jr, Winward, R.T. *et al.* (1969) Disc electrophoresis immunodiffusion of serum proteins in normal human gallbladder bile. *Proceedings of the Society for Experimental Biology and Medicine*, **132**, 146.

175. Watts, J.M. & Dunphy, J.E. (1966) The role of the common bile duct in biliary dynamics. *Surgery, Gynecology and Obstetrics*, **122**, 1207–1218.

176. Webb, T.A., Lillemoe, K.D. & Pitt, H.A. (1987) Intraduodenal protein stimulates resting but inhibits CCK-stimulated sphincter of Oddi motility. *Gastroenterology*, **92**, 1687 (Abstract).

177. Webb, T.H., Lillemoe, K.D. & Pitt, H.A. (1988) Gastro-sphincter of Oddi reflex. *American Journal of Surgery*, **155**, 193–198.

178. Whiting, M.J., Down, R.H.L. & Watts, J.McK. (1981) Precision and accuracy in the measurement of the cholesterol saturation index of duodenal bile. *Gastroenterology*, **80**, 533.

179. Wicks, A., Yeates, J. & Heaton, K. (1978) Bran and bile: Timecourse of changes in normal young men given a standard dose. *Scandinavian Journal of Gastroenterology*, **13**, 289.

180. Wiener, I., Inoue, K., Fagan, C.J. *et al.* (1981) Release of cholecystokinin in man. Correlation of blood levels with gallbladder contraction. *Annals of Surgery*, **194**, 321–327.

181. Williams, R.D. & Huang, T.T. (1969) The effect of vagotomy on biliary pressure. *Surgery*, **66**, 353–356.

182. Wyatt, A.P. (1967) The relationship of the sphincter of Oddi to the stomach, duodenum and gallbladder. *Journal of Physiology*, **193**, 225–241.

183. Yau, W.M. & Youther, M.L. (1984) Modulation of gallbladder motility by intrinsic cholinergic neurons. *American Journal of Physiology*, **247**, G662–G666.

CHAPTER 13

Bile Acids in Liver and Biliary Disease

Alan F. Hofmann

This chapter summarizes the metabolism and function of bile acids in the healthy human as well as in patients with liver disease. Inborn errors of bile acid biosynthesis are discussed, since therapy with exogenous bile acids is proving to be safe and effective. The role of bile acids in hepatocellular injury is discussed briefly, as is the use of bile acids as therapeutic agents for cholesterol gallstone disease and chronic cholestatic liver disease.

Two types of cells play a key role in bile acid metabolism. The first is the hepatocyte, which is the sole cell capable of performing the multiple enzymatic steps required for the biosynthesis of bile acids from cholesterol.

The hepatocyte also secretes bile acids into bile, a process which is the major factor responsible for the induction of bile flow. The hepatocyte removes bile acids from portal venous and hepatic arterial blood so efficiently that total bile acid levels in the systemic circulation remain at concentrations <10 μmol/l despite intestinal absorption rates during digestion averaging 100 μmol/min. The efficiency of hepatocyte uptake—70–90% first pass extraction by the liver—is balanced by equally efficient secretion of bile acids into the canaliculus, so that bile acid levels in the hepatocyte remain quite low.

The hepatocyte not only transports bile acids in an uphill manner, but also modulates bile acid biosynthesis according to the flux of bile acids through it. When the flux through the hepatocyte is decreased, biosynthesis from cholesterol increases in a classical 'negative feedback' manner. Thus, the hepatocyte functions as the site of bile acid biosynthesis, as a sensor of the flux of bile acid molecules, and as a polarized cell that pumps bile acids uphill against an enormous concentration gradient.

The transport of bile acid molecules through the hepatocyte and their secretion into canalicular bile has a number of direct and indirect effects. The most important of these effects is the generation of bile flow that results from the osmotic effects of the bile acid molecules secreted into the canaliculus. Another effect is the induction of vesicular secretion by the hepatocyte; the vesicles contain the two major classes of biliary lipids—phospholipids and cholesterol. Bile acids not only stimulate the secretion of lipid-rich vesicles into canalicular bile, but the secreted bile acids then solubilize the vesicles to form mixed micelles containing bile acids, phospholipid and cholesterol. Thus, canalicular secretion of bile acids is essential for cholesterol solubilization in bile. Bile acids also control, at least in part, cholesterol biosynthesis in the hepatocyte because any demand for increased bile acid biosynthesis must be accompanied by a parallel increase in the biosynthesis of cholesterol, the precursor of bile acids. Since increased cholesterol biosynthesis by the hepatocyte causes upregulation of the level of low-density lipoprotein (LDL) receptors on the sinusoidal surface of the hepatocyte, and since the level of LDL receptors is an important determinant of the plasma level of LDL (and LDL cholesterol), bile acid biosynthesis influences the level of plasma cholesterol.

The second cell type that plays a key role in bile acid metabolism is the ileal enterocyte, which actively transports bile acids from the intestinal lumen into the portal venous circulation, thus conserving bile acids that are secreted into the small intestine. After secretion into the canaliculus, bile acids pass down the biliary tree. They either enter the duodenum or, if the sphincter of Oddi is contracted, are stored in the gallbladder. When a meal is eaten, gallbladder contraction and relaxation of the sphincter of Oddi results in emptying of the stored bile acids into the small intestine. Here bile acids solubilize fatty acids and monoglycerides, which are formed by the action of pancreatic lipase on dietary triglyceride. The formation of mixed micelles of bile acids and these products of lipolysis increases the efficiency of fat absorption by accelerating diffusion of the lipolytic products up to the gut epithelium. Bile acids are not absorbed together with lipolytic products but pass distally to the terminal ileum, where they are efficiently extracted and transported by the ileal enterocytes. First pass ileal extraction is about 90% per meal.

Bile acids return to the liver in portal and arterial blood; they are efficiently extracted by the hepatocyte and are again secreted efficiently into the biliary tract. The repeated cycling of molecules from intestine to liver and back is termed the enterohepatic circulation. The relationship of the enterohepatic circulation to the hepatocyte is perhaps analogous to that of the flux of molecules to the substance being extracted in a solvent extraction apparatus. The enterohepatic circulation results in a continuous stream of surfactant or 'solvent' molecules, which not only induce bile to form but also form micelles in bile that solubilize or complex with amphipathic/lipophilic metabolic products. The end result of this flux of bile acid molecules is the delivery of undesired molecules from the hepatocyte to the intestinal lumen, from which they can be excreted.

Each of these functions and effects of bile acids is considered in more detail later in this chapter. The literature on bile acids in liver and biliary disease is vast, as this area has been the subject of research for more than a century. Many of the topics discussed here were subjects at recent symposia,[148,149,150] and several reviews[77,79] and monographs[37,67,137] are available.

BILE ACID EVOLUTION AND BILE ACID CHEMISTRY

EVOLUTION

From an evolutionary standpoint, bile acids first developed as a means of eliminating cholesterol. In the most ancient vertebrates (for example, cartilaginous fishes such as the shark), cholesterol, a sterol containing 27 carbon atoms (C_{27}), is hydroxylated in three or more positions to give bile alcohols. The resultant compounds, although hydrophilic, are still water-insoluble; solubility is achieved by sulphation of one or more of the hydroxyl groups. Such bile alcohol molecules are likely to form micelles in bile. However, they are unlikely to undergo enterohepatic cycling. In humans, bile alcohols are intermediates in the biosynthesis of bile acids. In patients with inborn errors of bile acid biosynthesis, bile alcohols are formed in large quantities and excreted in both bile and urine (see below).

In less ancient vertebrates (for example, reptiles, amphibians, some birds), cholesterol is converted to C_{27} bile acids; the side-chain, as that of cholesterol, contains eight carbon atoms and is analogous to iso-octanoic acid.[67,90] The side-chain is 6 carbon atoms long, and there is a methylene group present on the α (C-25) and the ε (C-21) carbon atoms. These C_{27} bile acids—sometimes termed 'primitive' or 'ancient' bile acids—are rendered water soluble by conjugation of the carboxylic acid group with the amino group of taurine in a peptide bond. (This kind of conjugation is termed an *N*-acyl linkage; bile acids conjugated with taurine are termed 'taurine amidates'.)

In modern vertebrates, cholesterol is converted to C_{24} bile acids; in these bile acids, the terminal three carbon atoms of the side-chain are oxidatively cleaved so that a carboxylic acid group is present at the 24 position. The side-chain is analogous to isopentanoic acid; the side chain is four atoms long and contains a methylene group present on the gamma carbon (C-21). Such bile acids are also conjugated with either taurine or glycine. It is thought that in most modern vertebrates, bile acids form micelles in the biliary tract and small intestine and undergo an enterohepatic circulation.

CHEMISTRY

From a chemical standpoint, the bile acid or bile alcohol molecule is best considered as consisting of two portions: (a) the nucleus with its hydroxyl substituents and (b) the aliphatic side-chain. The nucleus has 19 carbon atoms, 17 in the ring system and 2 in the angular methyl groups. The side-chain contains 5–8 carbon atoms, as discussed above, with a terminal hydroxyl group in bile alcohols and a terminal carboxylic acid group in bile acids; additional hydroxyl groups may be present in both bile acids and bile alcohols. The C_{24} bile acid skeleton, without substituents, is termed cholane; the C_{27} bile acid skeleton is termed cholestane.

STEROID NUCLEUS

Cholesterol has a double bond between the 5 and 6 carbon atoms, and during bile acid biosynthesis, this is isomerized to the 4,5 position and then stereospecifically reduced, so that the common natural bile acids are fully saturated molecules. The chemical structure of cholesterol and that of cholic acid are shown in Figure 13.1. Thus, the steroid nucleus of cholanes has the perhydrocyclopentanophenanthrene nucleus common to all perhydro steroids. The term perhydro means that no double bonds are present, that is, that the molecule is completely saturated. In modern vertebrates, the bile acid nucleus is curved because the A and B rings are in a *cis* configuration to each other. This occurs when the 5 hydrogen atom is in the β configuration; such compounds are termed 5β bile acids and are shown with a solid line at the 5 position. In ancient vertebrates, some of the biliary bile acids and bile alcohols are flat because the A/B ring juncture is *trans*. Such 5α bile acids are termed 'allo' bile acids.

During fetal development and in certain inborn errors of bile acid metabolism, bile acids are formed without the double bond of cholesterol being reduced. Such bile acids have a double bond either between the 4 and 5 carbon atoms or between the 5 and 6 positions; they are termed 'cholenic acids' and are flat molecules resembling allo bile acids.

Cholesterol has a 3β-hydroxy group that is epimerized to a 3α-hydroxy group during bile acid biosynthesis. The initial step in the biosynthesis of most natural bile acids is considered to be microsomal 7-hydroxylation by the enzyme cholesterol-7-hydroxylase. Accordingly, most natural bile acids have a 3α and a 7α hydroxyl group. The 3,7-dihydroxy bile acid, chenodeoxycholic acid, is a major primary bile acid in man. In man and many other mammals, there is additional hydroxylation at the 12 position to form cholic acid, which is in fact the bile acid most synthesized by the human hepatocyte. Other vertebrates may hydroxylate at the 1 or 6 or 16 position

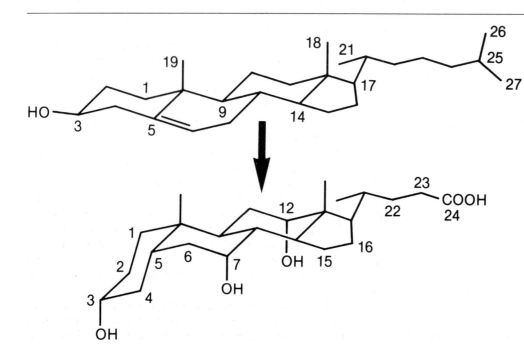

Figure 13.1 Molecular structure of cholesterol (above) and cholic acid (below). Cholesterol, a flat, insoluble, uncharged, unsaturated molecule, is converted by stereospecific saturation, epimerization of the 3-hydroxyl group, additional hydroxylation, and oxidative cleavage into a kinked, water-soluble, saturated, steroidal acid with surfactant properties.

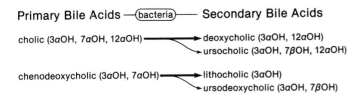

Figure 13.2 Left, location of hydroxyl substituents on the cholic acid and chenodeoxycholic acid, the two primary bile acids of man. Right, location of hydroxyl substituents on the major secondary bile acids in man formed by bacterial 7-dehydroxylation or 7-epimerization.

to form other trihydroxy bile acids. It seems likely that hydroxylation is limited to a single side of the molecule, so that one side of the molecule is hydrophobic and one side is hydrophilic (see below).

During their enterohepatic cycling, bile acids are exposed to bacterial enzymes which modify the nuclear substituents.[118] In the small intestine, any of the hydroxyl substituents may be oxidized to an oxo group. In the large intestine, the 7-hydroxyl group may be removed via a 3-oxo-$\Delta^4\Delta^6$ intermediate, or the oxo groups may be reduced to either the α or β hydroxy group. Thus, the major changes in the steroid nucleus involve oxidation–reduction–epimerization of any of the hydroxy groups and 7-dehydroxylation. The bacterial metabolites are absorbed in part and return to the liver where they may undergo biotransformation during transport. Biotransformation by hepatic enzymes in essence reverses biotransformation by bacterial enzymes. It includes rehydroxylation at the 7 position, stereospecific reduction of oxo bile acids, and epimerization of 3β-hydroxy bile acids.[46] Bile acids appearing in bile that were formed in part or completely by bacterial biotransformation are termed 'secondary bile acids' to distinguish them from those bile acids biosynthesized in the hepatocyte from cholesterol; these are termed 'primary bile acids'. The names and structures of the major secondary bile acids formed by 7-dehydroxylation or 7-epimerization are shown in Figure 13.2. The most common secondary bile acids occurring in man are deoxycholic acid—formed by bacterial 7-dehydroxylation of cholic acid—and lithocholic acid—formed by 7-dehydroxylation of chenodeoxycholic acid.[79] The distinction is not absolute, since epimerization of primary bile acids may occur in the liver.

Oxo (keto) bile acids are present in bile in trace amounts;[190] in general, these are absorbed as such from the intestine where they are formed by bacterial enzymes. Most are reduced during hepatic transport, but reduction is usually not complete and oxo bile acids spill over into bile. The cytosolic protein involved in bile acid transport within the hepatocyte has dehydrogenase activity, so in some instances it is possible for oxo bile acids to be formed within the hepatocyte, as well as by bacterial enzymes.[197]

In man, in contrast to many other mammals, the hepatocyte is incapable of 7-rehydroxylation. Accordingly, all deoxycholic acid (DCA) and lithocholic acid (LCA) absorbed from the colon appears unchanged in bile.

SIDE-CHAIN

The side-chain of cholesterol contains eight carbons, with branching at the C-20 and C-25 positions as illustrated in Figure 13.1. In bile acid biosynthesis, the initial side-chain hydroxylation occurs at C-26 followed by oxidation to the carboxylic acid group. Such oxidation is the final step in bile acid biosynthesis in those rather ancient vertebrates possessing C_{27} biliary bile acids, but in modern vertebrates, there is hydroxylation at C-27, elimination of a molecule of water to form an unsaturated compound, followed by oxidative cleavage to form a C_{24} acid; the process is a form of β-oxidation. In some marine mammals and birds, there is an additional hydroxylation at the C-23 (α) carbon or C-22 (β) carbon. In bile alcohols, one, two, three, or four hydroxy groups may be present at any of the positions between C-24 and C-27.

BILE ACID CONJUGATION

The pharmacologist R. T. Williams divided drug biotransformation into two types. Type I included biotransformation processes such as hydroxylation or oxidation; type II included conjugation processes such as glucuronidation, sulphation, amidation (with amino acids) or glycosylation.[215] The biosynthesis of bile acids or bile alcohols from cholesterol can be considered to be a series of sequential type I biotransformations; bile acid conjugation is a classical type II biotransformation.

Bile acid conjugation involves amidation with glycine or taurine, sulphation, glucuronidation, or glycosylation. Amidation denotes the formation of a peptide bond; this and ester glucuronidation or glycosylation with glucose or xylose can only occur on the side-chain, and they are mutually exclusive. Sulphation, either glucuronidation, or glycosylation are nuclear conjugation steps, occurring on the 3- or 7-hydroxyl groups; conjugates can be formed with two nuclear conjugating moieties and these may be the same or different. In addition, nuclear conjugations can occur as a single conjugation step or both nuclear and side-chain conjugation steps can occur on a bile acid molecule. A single dihydroxy bile acid can form at least 45 different conjugated derivatives!

The great preponderance of bile acids in human bile are glycine or taurine amidates. The only exception to this is lithocholic acid, the majority of which is present in bile with a sulphate on the 3 position and glycine or taurine on the side chain. Figure 13.3 shows the names and structures of the major conjugated bile acids found in human bile.

The virtual absence of other bile acid conjugates, such as glucuronates or sulfates, has two main explanations. First, unconjugated bile acids that are synthesized in or

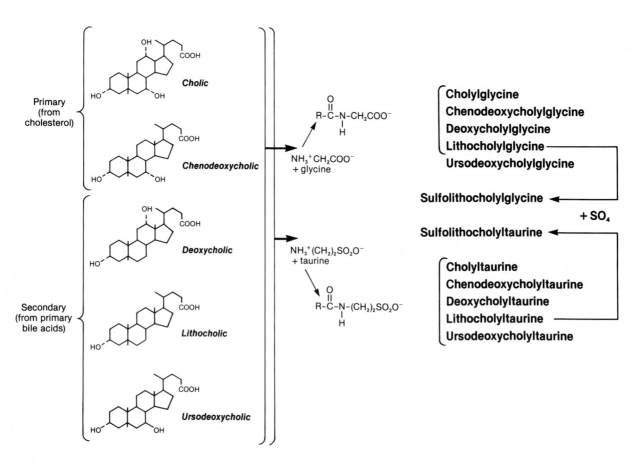

Figure 13.3 Names and chemical structures of major conjugated bile acids present in human bile. In the past, it was common practice to put the name of the amino acid first, for example, glycocholate or taurochenodeoxycholate.

transported into the hepatocyte are amidated in preference to nuclear glucuronidation or sulphation and such side-chain amidation precludes glucuronidation. Second, amidates are efficiently conserved by ileal absorption, whereas glucuronates or sulphates are not conserved, thus quickly leaving the circulating bile acid pool.[79]

Of all the amino acids present in the hepatocyte, only glycine or taurine are used for bile acid conjugation. Glycine and taurine amidates of bile acids differ from other amino acid amidates (such as leucine or lysine amidates) in being resistant to deconjugation by pancreatic carboxypeptidases.[91] Glucuronates and sulphates are also resistant to hydrolysis by pancreatic enzymes, since neither sulphatase nor glucuronidase is present among pancreatic enzymes. However, of these different classes of conjugates, only amidates are actively absorbed from the terminal ileum.

In the common trivial names of amidated bile acids, the amino acid moiety is used as a prefix before the name of the bile acid, which usually ends in '-ate' implying a salt. These names such as glycocholate, taurocholate, taurodeoxycholate, were proposed over a century ago when it was known that bile acids were conjugated to glycine or taurine but neither the structure of the bile acid nor the mode of linkage was known. Now that the

chemical structure of conjugated bile acids is fully known, it seems more appropriate to place the name of the bile acid first and the amino acid used for conjugation second, for example cholylglycine, cholyltaurine, or deoxycholyltaurine. Such a name indicates that the structure of bile acids is analogous to dipeptides, and also indicates that the ionizing moiety of the conjugate is not the bile acid moiety. At present, there is no agreement on trivial names for sulphates or glucuronide conjugates of bile acids.

There are two clinical situations and one pharmacological situation in which large amounts of bile acid conjugates, other than simple amidates, are formed. In cholestasis, bile acids are not only amidated with glycine or taurine on the side-chain, but also sulfated, and to a limited extent glucuronidated or glycosylated, on the nucleus.[192] In cerebrotendinous xanthomatosis, a rare inborn error of bile acid biosynthesis, bile alcohols, precursors of bile acids, are formed in large quantities.[14] These are glucuronidated or sulphated; amidation with glycine or taurine cannot occur because side-chain oxidation does not occur. When hyodeoxycholic acid is administered, it is not only amidated but glucuronidated at the 6 position; the resultant glucuronide does not undergo enterohepatic cycling.[169]

BILE ACID STRUCTURE–FUNCTION RELATIONSHIPS

Bile acids are functional molecules and their functions can be related to their physicochemical properties. The known functions of bile acids are: (1) induction of bile flow, (2) induction of biliary lipid secretion, (3) solubilization of biliary lipids, (4) solubilization of digestive lipids, (5) complexing of divalent cations such as Ca^{2+} and Fe^{2+}, and (6) negative feedback regulation of bile acid and cholesterol biosynthesis. The physicochemical properties are determined by the structure of the nucleus and the side-chain. For the nucleus, the determinants are the nature of the A/B ring juncture (whether *cis* or *trans*) and the number and type of substituents. For the side-chain, the determinants are the length (number of carbon atoms), the pattern of side-chain substituents, and the mode of conjugation.

UNCONJUGATED BILE ACIDS

It is useful to consider unconjugated bile acids first, even though under most circumstances the bile acids in bile are nearly all conjugated. The first consideration is aqueous solubility of the sodium salt. Bile acids are surfactants, and most surfactants show an abrupt and marked increase in solubility over some narrow temperature range. This is termed the critical micellar temperature (CMT) or Krafft point; it is that temperature at which the solubility of the monomer reaches the concentration at which micelle formation begins. What is important is whether the CMT is above or below body temperature. If the CMT is above body temperature, the molecule will be insoluble under physiological conditions.[86]

A bile acid with no nuclear substituents (sodium cholanoate) is completely insoluble (even at 100°C) because of its stable crystalline structure. The sodium salts of most bile acids with only a single hydroxy group have very limited solubility at body temperature, with CMT values ranging from 50 to 100°C. The common natural dihydroxy bile acids, chenodeoxycholic acid, deoxycholic acid, and ursodeoxycholic acid, are fully soluble at body temperature, whereas the sodium salts of two uncommon dihydroxy bile acids ($7\alpha,12\alpha$ and $3\alpha,6\beta$) have a CMT well above body temperature. Such compounds can be predicted to have calcium salts that are extremely insoluble at body temperature. The sodium salts of all trihydroxy bile acids that have been examined are highly soluble at body temperature.

Bile acids self-associate over a narrow range of concentration to form polymolecular aggregates called micelles. The natural bile acids have a hydrophilic face (α side) and a hydrophobic face (β side). In the natural bile acids, the hydrophobic side is large and the critical micellization concentration (CMC) value (in 0.15 M Na^+) is <10 mM. As the contiguous area of the hydrophobic side is decreased, the CMC increases.[86,162] The CMC of 5β bile acids also increases when α substituents are changed to

β substituents or to an oxo group, as this change in structure also diminishes the effective area of the hydrophobic face of the molecule. Extremely hydrophilic trihydroxy bile acids, such as $3\beta,7\beta,12\beta$-trihydroxy cholanoic acid, can be synthesized; in such bile acids, both sides of the molecule are hydrophilic and micellar aggregation does not occur. Dehydrocholate, the 3,7,12-trioxo bile acid, was originally also thought not to form micelles, but is now considered to form dimers at concentrations >40 mM. Table 13.1 summarizes physicochemical properties of some of the common unconjugated bile acids.

The molecular arrangement of the micelles formed by bile acids is not known, but is likely to be helical, based on the arrangements of bile acids in crystals[21] as well as X-ray studies of bile acid solutions.[22] The number of molecules in the aggregate varies according to bile acid structure (and also Na^+ concentration).[23] Hydrophilic trihydroxy bile acids form 'oligomers' containing 4 to 8 molecules; lipophilic dihydroxy bile acids form aggregates containing 20 to 40 molecules. Micellar solutions of bile acids are extremely efficient in solubilizing polar lipids such as phosphatidylcholine (or fatty acid–monoglyceride mixtures), and the resultant mixed micelles can solubilize other solutes such as cholesterol. The interactions of bile acid solutions with polar lipids is usually depicted by phase diagrams using triangular coordinates.

For many years, it has been common to assign hydrophobicity (or hydrophilicity) values to surfactants. Such values were based on a variety of physicochemical measurements such as CMC value, octanol/water partition coefficient, etc.[135] A similar approach has been used for bile acids based on retention time during reversed-phase partition chromatography.[7,73] By this criterion, monohydroxy bile acids are more hydrophobic than dihydroxy bile acids, which are more hydrophobic than trihydroxy bile acids. However, among dihydroxy bile acids, ursodeoxycholic acid (UDCA) is much more hydrophilic (and less hydrophobic) than CDCA or DCA. Figure 13.4 shows a chromatogram of the major bile acids present in human bile. Those eluting most rapidly are most hydrophilic.

Side-chain structure also influences the physicochemical properties of bile acids, which in turn influences function. Shortening the side-chain increases the CMC; the CMC rises exponentially as the side-chain is shortened. This relationship has been well documented experimentally for ionic surfactants.[183]

For any weak acid for which the protonated form has a low aqueous solubility, solubility increases logarithmically with increasing pH value of the solution. When the aqueous solubility reaches the CMC, insoluble material dissolves in the micelle and is in fact 'titrated' as the pH is increased. As a consequence, if solubility is plotted against pH for surfactants that are weak acids, aqueous solubility rises markedly over a narrow pH range. This pH range may be termed the 'critical micellar pH' and is thus analogous to the CMC and CMT. For unconjugated bile acids, this ranges from about pH 6 to pH 8, depending on the bile acid.[21,23,205]

Table 13.1 Physico-chemical properties of some common unconjugated bile acids.

	Nuclear substituents	Aqueous solubility[a] (μM)	CMC[b,f] (mM)	log P^c	$K'^{d,e}$
Dihydroxy					
Chenodeoxycholic	3αOH, 7αOH	27	4	2.20	2.05
Ursodeoxycholic	3αOH, 7βOH	19	7	0.95	1.05
Deoxycholic	3αOH, 12αOH	10	3	2.80	2.56
Hyodeoxycholic	3αOH, 6αOH	15	6	0.85	0.80
Trihydroxy					
Cholic	3αOH, 7αOH, 12αOH	273	11	1.08	0.72
Ursocholic	3αOH, 7βOH, 12αOH	1670	39	0.26	0.20
Hyocholic	3αOH, 6αOH, 7αOH	45	8	1.10	0.95

[a]The term 'aqueous solubility' denotes the solubility of the protonated form at pH <5. From Roda and Fini.[159]

[b]The CMC is a concentration at which self-association to form micelles occurs rapidly. From Roda *et al.*[162] (for 25°C). Data indicate values for total Na^+ concentration of 150 mM.

[c]Partition coefficient between n-octanol and water. The greater the value of *p*, the greater the lipophilicity of the bile acid. From Roda *et al.*[163]

[d]K' is the log of the relative retention volume by reversed phase chromatography with a C_{18} octadecylsilane stationary phase; with a C_8 column, the order of cholic acid and ursodeoxycholic acid is reversed. The higher the value of K', the greater the lipophilicity. Data from Roda *et al.*[163]

[e]The pK_a of all unconjugated bile acids is 5.0.

[f]Lithocholate has been omitted. This monohydroxy bile acid does not form micelles at 25°C, since its critical micellization temperature is above 60°.[85]

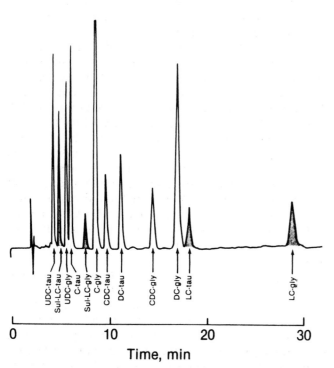

Figure 13.4 Chromatogram of major bile acids of human bile separated by reverse-phase partition chromatography. Those bile acids that are eluted first have least binding to the hydrophobic column and are termed 'hydrophilic'. The logarithm of the retention time is used as a measure of hydrophilicity, provided the state of ionization is held constant.

A final consideration in bile acid solubility is the solubility of the Ca^{2+} salt. Careful measurements have indicated that the K_{sp}, $[Ca^{2+}] \times [BA]^2$, for unconjugated dihydroxy bile acids are in the range of 10^{-8}.[65] Values for monohydroxy bile acids are lower; for trihydroxy bile acids, they are higher. Whether or not the K_{sp} is exceeded for surfactants such as bile acids depends on Ca^{2+} activity (which in turn depends on the Na^+ concentration of the system, as well as binding of Ca^{2+} by monomeric and micellar bile acid molecules) in relation to bile acid monomer concentration for micellar bile acid solutions. The monomer concentration is close to the CMC value of the system.

CONJUGATED BILE ACIDS

Unconjugated bile acids are substituted isopentanoic acid derivatives and, as any substituted aliphatic carboxylic acid, have pK_a values of about 5.0.[159] Conjugation of a bile acid with glycine or taurine lowers the pK_a value: glycine amidates have a pK_a value of about 3.8,[53] whereas taurine amidates have pK_a values <1.0.[86] The pK_a is not influenced by the pattern of nuclear substituents: all glycine amidated bile acids have an identical pK_a value, as do all taurine amidated bile acids.

It was noted above that the CMC value of a given bile acid decreases logarithmically as the side-chain is lengthened. Accordingly, it would be predicted that glycine or taurine amidates (being one nitrogen atom and one or two carbon atoms longer) would have lower CMC values than their corresponding unconjugated derivatives. In fact, measurements have indicated that amidation with glycine or taurine has little effect on the CMC because the additional lipophilicity of the methylene groups in the glycine or taurine appears to be balanced by the additional hydrophilicity of the amide bond.[162] The pK_a of bile acid glucuronides should be that of glucuronic acid—about 4.6. The pK_a of bile alcohol sulphates should be less than 1. The pK_a of bile acids with an α-hydroxy group on the side-chain is 3.8,[164] but such bile acids do not occur in nature in unconjugated form in bile, but rather as their taurine amidates.

There are several physicochemical consequences of amidation and these in turn lead to physiological consequences. Amidation decreases the pK_a of a given bile acid; this decreases the CMpH, so that a conjugated bile acid remains soluble at acidic pH. Conjugation with taurine greatly increases the resistance of a bile acid to precipitation by heavy-metal cations such as iron or calcium ions. Because of the lower pK_a value, conjugated bile acids are fully ionized at the pH conditions prevailing in hepatic bile and small intestinal content. Their complete ionization, especially for dihydroxy bile acids, greatly retards passive absorption across the enterocyte, promoting a high intraluminal concentration in the biliary tract and jejunum, which in turn facilitates lipid solubilization.[85] In the ileum the bile acid amidates are actively absorbed.

The effect of glucuronidation or sulphation on physico-chemical properties of bile acids has not been well studied because such conjugates are not available in quantity and purity. It seems likely that either glucuronidation or sulphation should not only increase aqueous solubility, but also should greatly increase the CMC value for a given bile acid. As noted, glucuronides and sulphates of bile acids (or bile alcohols) are neither hydrolysed by pancreatic enzymes nor actively absorbed from the ileum. Colonic absorption, if it occurs, will be passive and can occur only after bacterial hydrolysis of the ester or ether bonds.

Amidation does not greatly influence binding of bile acids to albumin.[161] The effect of sulphation and glucuronidation on albumin binding has not been studied.

BILE ACID METABOLISM IN HEALTHY MAN

The transport systems of the hepatocyte and ileoenterocyte, which cause bile acids to be efficiently extracted from portal blood and distal small intestinal content respectively, are responsible for the anatomical location of the circulating bile acids. A relatively constant mass of bile acids is secreted into bile and efficiently reabsorbed from the ileum. If a tracer dose of radioactive bile acid is injected, the mass of each of the common three circulating bile acids (cholic acid, chenodeoxycholic acid, deoxycholic acid) behaves as a single well-mixed 'pool' that can be described by first-order kinetics; that is, the decline of radioactivity from the pool is directly

proportional to the concentration of radioactivity in the pool. Accordingly, the technique of isotope dilution has been used to measure the mass of the exchangeable pool, in the same manner that labelled red cells are used to measure the plasma volume.[183] If the rate of radioactivity loss from the pool is determined by measuring the specific activity of biliary bile acids, the fractional turnover rate (FTR) of the injected bile acid can be determined. This technique, which was developed by Lindstedt,[117] requires isolation of bile acids from bile (or plasma) and determination of the specific activity (if radioactive bile acids are used) or atoms percent excess (if bile acids tagged with a stable isotope are used). Samples are obtained daily for several days. It has been widely used to measure the size of the constituent bile acid pools in man as well as the input of individual bile acids into the pool.

The basic equation is:

$$\text{Pool size (in g or } \mu\text{mol)} \times \text{FTR (in time}^{-1}) = \text{input rate (mass/time)}$$

The inputs of primary bile acids (cholic acid (CA) and CDCA) originate from *de novo* biosynthesis from cholesterol; in contrast, the inputs of the secondary bile acids, DCA and LCA, which are formed in the colon by bacterial 7-dehydroxylation of CA and CDCA, respectively, are the amount of newly formed DCA that is absorbed (for the first time) from the colon. In man, about twice as much CA as CDCA is synthesized.[83,84] In the colon, both bile acids are completely 7-dehydroxylated, CA to form DCA and CDCA to form LCA; and some fraction of the newly formed DCA or LCA is absorbed. Bacterial formation of DCA is essentially equivalent to CA biosynthesis, and bacterial formation of LCA is essentially equivalent to CDCA biosynthesis. The CA 'family' and the CDCA 'family' are not interconvertible; there is no 12-hydroxylation of CDCA to form CA or 12-dehydroxylation of CA to form CDCA.[79]

Using this technique, the total (exchangeable) bile acid pool in man has been shown to be 1.5–3.0 g in size (70–140 μmol/kg) and a majority of it to be composed of the two primary bile acids, CA and CDCA, each present in approximately equal proportions (30–40% each). Most of the remainder (20–35%) is DCA. A small fraction (<5%) is composed of LCA and UDCA, the latter being formed by bacterial epimerization of CDCA in the distal intestine.

The proportions of biliary bile acids are not identical to biosynthesis rates. Each individual bile acid pool (CA, CDCA, or DCA) is the quotient of input divided by the fractional turnover rate. The greater the fractional turnover rate, the smaller the pool for a given rate of biosynthesis. CA has a more rapid turnover rate than CDCA and, despite its being synthesized at nearly twice the rate of CDCA, the proportion of the two bile acids in biliary bile acids is nearly identical. DCA has a turnover rate similar to that of CDCA; its lower proportion in bile indicates that the input of newly formed DCA is less than that of CDCA in most individuals. In most individuals, about one-fifth to one-third of the DCA that is newly formed in the colon is absorbed.[121,191] In some older individuals, the proportion of DCA may exceed that of CDCA in biliary bile acids, indicating greater input from the colon.

The fractional turnover rate is largely determined by the efficiency of intestinal conservation, which is the sum of active and passive absorption. The intestinal conservation of CDCA and DCA is more efficient than that of CA for reasons that are discussed below.

The very small proportion of LCA and UDCA in bile has two explanations: first, input of these secondary bile acids is less than those of CA, CDCA, or DCA. Second, intestinal conservation is also less efficient. Figure 13.5 shows in schematic form the fate of DCA and LCA in man.

In the steady state, biosynthesis of bile acids from cholesterol is balanced by faecal loss. There is no appreciable urinary loss of bile acids for several reasons. First, efficient first pass hepatic extraction keeps the concentration of bile acids in $<10\ \mu$M in peripheral blood; second, bile acids entering the kidney are protein bound (75–99% depending on the bile acid), which diminishes their loss into the glomerular filtrate; and finally the natural bile acids that enter the glomerular filtrate are reabsorbed in the renal tubules by active and passive transport. Since bile acids are end metabolic products and since the steroid nucleus is not degraded by intestinal bacteria, the average rate of faecal bile acid excretion is identical to the average rate of hepatic biosynthesis. This assumption has been confirmed experimentally.[42,83]

BILE ACID CONJUGATION

After their biosynthesis, bile acids are amidated with glycine or taurine. Conjugation involves two enzymes, a Coenzyme A ligase, which is microsomal, and a cholyl CoA glycine : taurine transferase which is cytosolic. Peroxisomes also appear to be able to amidate bile acids with glycine or taurine.[46] The conjugating system prefers taurine, and the availability of hepatocyte taurine is rate-limiting.[66,208] Bile acid biosynthesis is believed to be localized to the perivenular cells,[200] and presumably amidation of newly biosynthesized bile acids also occurs in these cells. During enterohepatic cycling, there is considerable bacterial deconjugation of bile acids in the distal small intestine. The unconjugated bile acids thus formed are absorbed in part and are reconjugated during transport through the hepatocyte.[70] Such reconjugation should occur to a greater extent in the periportal cells, since these cells are involved in transporting the bile acids returning from the intestine. Calculations indicate that in the adult human, much more taurine and glycine are used for such 'reconjugation' of deconjugated bile acids than for conjugation of newly biosynthesized bile acids.[70,75]

In man, conjugation occurs to a greater extent with glycine than with taurine, unless taurine is administered in high doses. The taurine-conjugated bile acids undergo

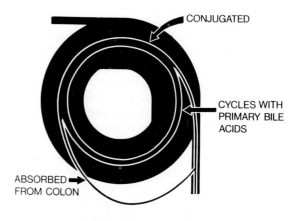

DEOXYCHOLIC ACID

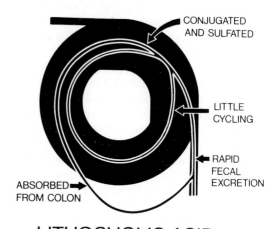

LITHOCHOLIC ACID

Figure 13.5 Schematic depiction of the absorption and enterohepatic cycling of deoxycholic acid (above) and lithocholic acid (below). About one-third to one-half of newly formed deoxycholic acid is absorbed from the colon and conjugated (with glycine or taurine) in the liver; the resultant conjugates circulate enterohepatically with primary bile acid conjugates. A smaller fraction of newly formed lithocholic acid is absorbed from the colon; in the liver it is not only conjugated with glycine or taurine, but also conjugated with sulphate to form sulpholithocholylglycine and sulpholithocholyltaurine. These sulphated derivatives are poorly absorbed from the small intestine, with the result that lithocholate undergoes little enterohepatic cycling.

less bacterial deconjugation than glycine-conjugated bile acids during enterohepatic cycling,[71] presumably because they are more resistant to bacterial deconjugation.[92] Accordingly, the proportion of bile acids conjugated with taurine in biliary bile acids may be slightly greater than the proportion of bile acids actually conjugated with taurine.[75] It has been customary to describe the proportion of bile acids conjugated with glycine or taurine as a ratio of glycine-conjugated bile acids to taurine-conjugated bile acids. This practice should be abandoned, as it can distort the molar proportion of conjugate type; for example, an increase in the proportion of glycine-conjugated bile acids from 75% to 90% causes the glycine-conjugate/taurine-conjugate ratio to increase from 3 to 9. The proportion of bile acids conjugated with glycine or taurine is determined by the taurine status of the hepatocyte, and not by bile acid factors.

Deconjugation of bile acid amidates during hepatocyte transport does not occur to any appreciable extent. Conjugation of newly formed bile acids and reconjugation is highly efficient, although traces of unconjugated bile acids can be isolated from bile.[124] In health, the natural di- and trihydroxy bile acids are almost exclusively conjugated with taurine or glycine and do not undergo sulphation or glucuronidation to any appreciable extent, with only one exception; namely LCA. The monohydroxy bile acid LCA, after amidation with glycine or taurine, undergoes sulphation to form sulpholithocholylglycine or sulpholitho-cholyltaurine.[30] Sulphation is not complete, and on the average only about half of the lithocholyl amidates in fasting-state bile are sulphated.[166] In some species, such as the dog, which are obligate taurine amidators, deficiency of taurine in the hepatocyte, which can be induced by a large intravenous load of bile acids, leads to secretion of the unconjugated bile acid[142] or a glucuronide[136] conjugate in bile.

Whether a bile acid is amidated with glycine or taurine or esterified with glucuronate on the side-chain is influenced strongly by the chemical structure of the side-chain, which in turn influences the K_m of the cholyl CoA ligase. Synthetically prepared C-23 nor bile acids (with one less carbon on the side-chain) have a high K_m for the CoA ligase;[103] as a consequence, such bile acids form glucuronides (either C-23-ester or C-3-ether) rather than glycine or taurine amidates.[219]

DYNAMICS OF ENTEROHEPATIC CYCLING _____

During overnight fasting, unconjugated bile acids are stored in the gallbladder because biliary secretory pressure exceeds the resistance of the cystic duct and gallbladder but is still less than the resistance of the contracted sphincter of Oddi. The gallbladder concentrates the bile by removing its inorganic electrolytes, so that with time the dominant anions are bile acid anions. The bile acid (and Na^+) concentration may reach 300 mM, although bile remains isotonic at all times. Since tonicity is determined by the number of particles in solution, micelle formation facilitates the formation of a highly concentrated, albeit isotonic bile.[94]

When a meal is ingested, cholecystokinin release causes simultaneous gallbladder contraction and relaxation of the sphinctor of Oddi. Bile is discharged into the duodenum. The secretion rate of bile acids into the duodenum has been estimated by marker perfusion techniques. It averages about 0.1 μmol min^{-1} kg^{-1} during the fasting state and increases three to eight times during digestion.[202]

Each of the lipid constituents of bile undergoes a different fate. Phospholipid (mostly phosphatidylcholine) is hydrolysed by pancreatic phospholipase to lysolecithin

and fatty acid which are efficiently absorbed. Cholesterol is absorbed in part (20–50%), and in part precipitated from solution. Bilirubin glucuronides remain in solution but are not absorbed.

Conjugated bile acids solubilize the products of fat digestion—fatty acids and monoglycerides—in mixed micelles and facilitate their diffusion to the enterocyte. The conjugated bile acids undergo little passive absorption in the small intestine. Absorption of the negatively charged bile acid anion cannot occur because the bile acid molecule is too large to pass paracellularly and, as it is charged, it cannot flip across the apical membrane of the enterocyte. Probably the most lipophilic conjugates (LCA, CDCA and DCA) that are conjugated with glycine undergo some absorption during moments when jejunal content becomes quite acid.[79] Duodenal absorption seems unlikely if the microclimate present on the epithelial surface is alkaline.

Conjugated bile acids are efficiently absorbed by an active transport system in the distal ileum. Based on animal studies, the transporter is a Na^+-coupled co-transport system driven by the Na^+K^+ATPase present on the basolateral membrane.[216] The efficiency of transport is about 90% per meal or 70% per day. A fraction (perhaps 20%) of the bile acids are deconjugated before absorption; deconjugated bile acids can be absorbed passively as well as actively. Exiting of the bile acid across the basolateral membrane of the ileal enterocyte involves an anion-exchange protein.[213] The sulphated amidates of LCA, in contrast to the other bile acids present in bile, do not undergo efficient ileal absorption; they pass together with the other unabsorbed bile acids across the ileocecal valve into the colon.[31]

In the colon, bile acids are deconjugated and 7-dehydroxylated to form DCA and LCA. Dehydroxylation involves strictly anaerobic bacteria and formation of a 3-oxo-4,6-diene intermediate that is formed intracellularly in the anaerobic bacteria mediating the 7-dehydroxylation step.[118] Epimers and oxo biotransformation products are also formed. Some DCA and LCA are absorbed passively and in the portal venous blood merge with the flux of other conjugated and unconjugated bile acids from the distal small intestine. A schematic description of the enterohepatic circulation of bile acids is shown in Figure 13.6.

HEPATOCYTE UPTAKE, INTRACELLULAR TRANSPORT, BIOTRANSFORMATION AND CANALICULAR SECRETION _____

Bile acid transport will be dealt with first, rather than bile acid biosynthesis, since most of the bile acid flux through the liver is composed of 'old' or 'used' bile acids, rather than newly synthesized ('new') bile acids.

Bile acids that enter portal venous blood from the intestine are albumin bound. Binding is less for CA and its amidates (c. 70%) than for CDCA or DCA and their corresponding amidates (>98%).[161] Among dihydroxy

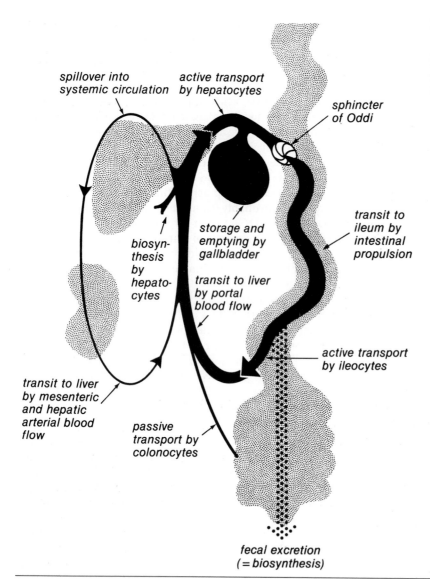

Figure 13.6 Schematic description of the enterohepatic circulation of primary and secondary bile acids in man. The small fraction of glycine-conjugated dihydroxy bile acids that is absorbed passively from the jejunum is not shown.

Figure labels: spillover into systemic circulation; active transport by hepatocytes; sphincter of Oddi; biosynthesis by hepatocytes; storage and emptying by gallbladder; transit to liver by portal blood flow; transit to ileum by intestinal propulsion; active transport by ileocytes; transit to liver by mesenteric and hepatic arterial blood flow; passive transport by colonocytes; fecal excretion (= biosynthesis).

bile acids, UDCA is less tightly bound than CDCA. The monohydroxy bile acid, LCA, is most tightly bound. Extensive studies of the relationship between bile acid structure and albumin binding involving bile acids ranging widely in HLB has not been performed, nor is it known whether binding involves a particular amino-acid sequence in the albumin molecule. The most hydrophobic bile acids are also bound to a small extent by plasma lipoproteins.[69] Whether the presence of bile acids in lipoproteins has any influence on lipoprotein metabolism is unknown.

Bile acids are efficiently extracted by the hepatocyte. Uptake of such bile acids involves three transport systems, one of which is considered to mediate a Na^+/bile acid co-transport system, which is near isolation and purification.[5,223] A second involves a Na^+-independent pathway.[223] Uptake of hydrophilic unconjugated bile acids appears to involve a bile acid/OH^- exchange system, which is a third transport system,[15] although this is disputed.[19] Figure 13.7 shows in schematic form some of the transport systems

involved in hepatic transport of bile acids.

Unconjugated lipophilic bile acids presumably enter the hepatocyte passively by simple partition into the lipid domains of the sinusoidal membranes.[3,206] Candidate bile acid molecules for such passive absorption are unconjugated monohydroxy and dihydroxy bile acids, such as LCA and CDCA.

Determinants of uptake

First, as noted before, bile acid uptake is strongly influenced by bile acid nuclear structure. For a given side-chain structure, the fractional extraction (FE) of hydrophilic bile acids is considerably greater than that of hydrophobic bile acids.[1,155] Second, it is influenced by side-chain charge, as mono-anionic and uncharged bile acids are rapidly taken up, whereas zwitterionic and cationic bile acids show little permeation into the hepatocyte.[6] Third, it is influenced by hepatic biotransformation, as bile acids

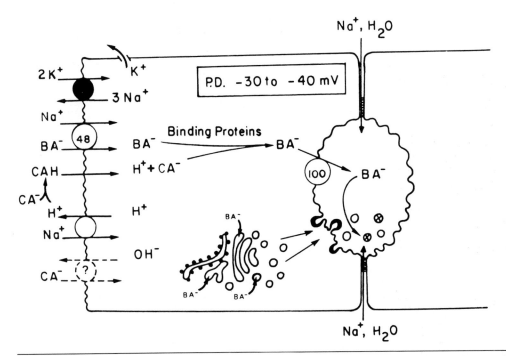

P.D. −30 to −40 mV

Binding Proteins

Figure 13.7 Membrane transport systems involved in the transport of bile acid molecules through the hepatocyte. Modified from Meier.[125] CA^-, cholate anion; BA^-, bile acid anion; PD, potential difference. The numbers denote the molecular weight (in kilodaltons) of the transport proteins involved.

(which do not form the Coenzyme A (CoA) derivative on entering the hepatocyte), appear to reflux back into plasma in the space of Disse, whereas the formation of a CoA derivative prevents or markedly slows such reflux.[26] Fourth, there are species effects, as bile acid uptake is often more rapid for a bile acid indigenous to a given mammalian species.[2]

Finally, albumin binding also influences the rate of uptake, as binding to albumin decreases the rate of bile acid uptake. Traditional pharmacological teaching has held that hepatic uptake of drugs and bile acids is linearly proportional to the concentration of the unbound species. Abundant work has now shown that, although albumin binding decreases the rate of uptake of a bile acid such as cholyltaurine, its uptake is considerably greater than that predicted from its unbound concentration.[57] Complex kinetic analyses have been reviewed,[56] with the hypothesis that there is a surface-mediated dissociation of the bile acid from its carrier molecule. This effect appears to be specific for albumin as it is not shown by some other proteins, and also for the hepatocyte as it is not exhibited by the enterocytes of the ileum. It probably involves membrane proteins, which may be transporters because the effect can be 'saturated', suggesting that a limited number of sites are mediating the dissociation.

Thus the rate of hepatic uptake of bile acids for a given flux of bile acids across the space of Disse appears to be influenced by the chemical structure of both the nucleus and the side-chain of the bile acid, by the species-dependent membrane transport rates, by albumin binding, and by surface-mediated dissociation from albumin. None the less, it should be noted that bile acid metabolism is relatively normal in the analbuminaemic rat.[195]

INTRACELLULAR TRANSPORT

Details of bile acid transport through the hepatocyte are poorly understood, but a recent excellent review summarizes current knowledge.[60] If overall concentrations are measured, values in the range of 50–100 µmol/l are obtained (cf. ref. 218). Such measurements, although valuable, do not distinguish contamination of cytosol by canaliculi in which the concentration of bile acids is likely to be 20–50 times higher; they also provide no information on the concentration of bile acids in individual organelles. Moreover, they do not consider the sinusoidal gradient, and it is not unreasonable to assume that the periportal hepatocytes that transport most bile acids have a higher intracellular concentration than the perivenular cells. Obviously, if a sample of liver tissue used for analyses contains non-parenchymal cells and these cells do not contain bile acids, the results will be falsely low. None the less, the current view is that the concentration of bile acid monomers in the hepatocyte is quite low (<30 µM) because of the efficiency of canalicular export in relation to the rate of sinusoidal import.

Bile acid-binding proteins

The hepatic cytosol contains proteins that bind bile acids avidly. These proteins are being purified and appear to possess enzymatic activity, e.g. sulphotransferase[196] and 3α- and 3β-hydroxysteroid dehydrogenase[197] activity. These activities result in the reduction of 3-oxo bile acids to 3α-hydroxy bile acids, the epimerization of 3β-hydroxy bile acids to 3α bile acids,[181] and the sulphation of lithocholyl amidates.[30]

In addition to a role in bile acid biotransformation,

these proteins are likely to have additional functions: for example, transport of bile acids from the sinusoidal membrane to the canalicular membrane (or for some bile acids back to the sinusoidal membrane) and retention of bile acids in the hepatic cytosol, i.e. inhibition of bile acid partitioning into organelles such as mitochondria. Whether the bile acid-binding proteins interact in a specific way with hepatocyte organelles is unknown. The movement of bile acids through the cytosol is considered to occur by diffusion of protein-bound and unbound bile acid monomers. Microtubules are involved to only a limited extent, since agents that disrupt microtubules do not abolish bile acid transport.[35]

CANALICULAR TRANSPORT

Canalicular transport of bile acids is also not well understood, but the development of improved techniques such as photoaffinity labelling of bile acids (cf. ref. 108) and isolation of canalicular membranes (cf. refs 95, 126) should accelerate progress in elucidating the mechanism of this powerful transport system that is responsible for bile acid-dependent flow. The high transcanalicular potential (30 mV) contributes to bile acid transport,[214] but the observed value for T_{max} in the rat (30 μmol min^{-1}kg^{-1})[104] has been thought to be too great to be explained by electrical forces alone.[141] It is likely that a pump or a co-transport system is involved. A putative carrier has been purified and used to develop antibodies;[59] cloning of this key molecule in bile formation is likely in the near future.

The canalicular transport system for bile acids transports bile acids with a negative charge on the side-chain whether they are conjugated with an amino acid or with glucuronate;[145] in contrast, 3-sulphated (and 3-glucuronidated) bile acids are transported by another canalicular carrier protein;[47,144] such bile acid conjugates are different topologically, since they have a charge on both the side-chain and the nucleus. Studies in rats with an inborn error of canalicular transport have characterized the broad specificity of this transport system, which appears to be an ATPase.[47,109,144] The T_{max} for transport of bile acids in rodents ranges from 15 to 30 μmol min^{-1} kg^{-1} for non-toxic bile acids.[104] In man, the highest value observed for bile acid secretion during meals is far lower (0.5–1.0 μmol min^{-1} kg^{-1}) but no data are available on the V_{max} for bile acid transport in man.

TRANSPORT IN THE BILIARY TRACT

Conjugated bile acids pass down the biliary tree and are either stored in the gallbladder or secreted into the intestine.[202] Under some circumstances, unconjugated bile acids may also be secreted into bile in appreciable proportions. For example C_{23} nor bile acids are not amidated, and if they are infused intravenously they are secreted in part in unconjugated form into the canaliculus.[146,219] The fate of unconjugated bile acids

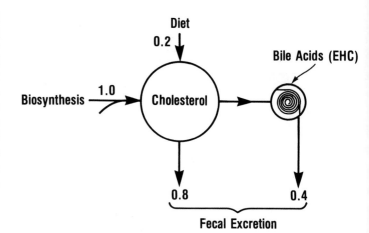

Figure 13.8 Cholesterol balance in man. Neutral sterol excretion is in faeces via biliary secretion. The efficiency of intestinal absorption of both dietary and biliary cholesterol is low—about 20–40%. Enterohepatic cycling of bile acids may be considered a 'delay term' in the intestinal elimination of cholesterol. On the other hand, the flux of bile acids through the liver promotes the elimination of cholesterol as such in bile.

entering the canaliculus depends on their lipophilicity. Mono- and dihydroxy bile acids are quite lipophilic, and it is likely they are absorbed by the biliary epithelial cells and return to the sinusoid in protonated form via the periductular capillary plexes. Such 'cholehepatic' cycling causes a bicarbonate choleresis, possibly because intraluminal carbonic acid donates the proton, permitting passive bile acid absorption.[146,219] Such cholehepatic cycling may explain the bicarbonate-rich choleresis induced by infusions of UDCA in the rat.[44] Unconjugated trihydroxy bile acids undergo much less passive absorption and induce only a weak choleresis.[143]

BILE ACID BIOSYNTHESIS

The mass of bile acids in the enterohepatic circulation is maintained by continuous bile acid biosynthesis from cholesterol. Were bile acid biosynthesis to stop, the bile acid pool would slowly disappear because of continuous intestinal loss. Cholesterol could not be eliminated; bile acid-dependent bile flow would cease; and fat-soluble vitamins could not be absorbed. Thus, bile acid biosynthesis is essential for health. Figure 13.8 illustrates the key role of bile acid biosynthesis as a means of cholesterol elimination.

Bile acid biosynthesis from cholesterol involves a number of complex steps in both the nucleus and the side-chain. Only selected aspects can be mentioned here and the major steps are illustrated in Figure 13.9 and have been recently reviewed.[14,177] The conversion of cholesterol to bile acids is a superb example of the capacity of the hepatocyte to convert an insoluble lipid into a water-soluble and amphipathic compound. This biotransform-

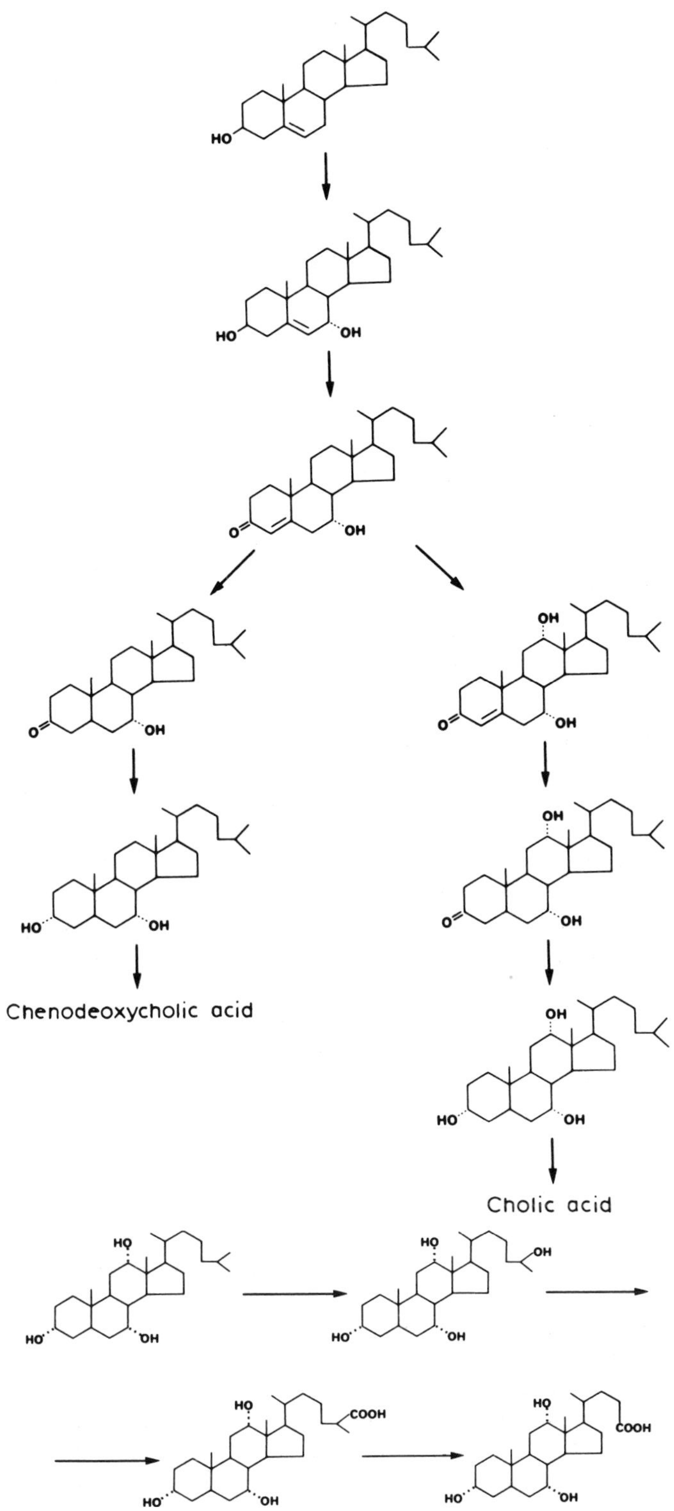

Figure 13.9 Major steps in bile acid biosynthesis.

ation involves at least five steps for the nucleus and at least five steps for the side-chain. Because these steps may occur in any order, there are 25 possible intermediates, which makes elucidation of the individual steps in bile acid biosynthesis extremely difficult for the biochem-

ist. The end result, a 'bile salt', has a saturated cholane nucleus, usually in the 5β (A–B *cis*) configuration, with at least one additional hydroxyl group. The side-chain is hydroxylated in the bile alcohols or converted to a carboxylic acid in the bile acids. The bile acids of mammals appear to represent the end of evolutionary development; their chemical structure has already been discussed.

The traditional method of investigating the pathways of bile acid biosynthesis was the injection of hypothetical (radioactive) intermediates and determination of the efficiency of their conversion to bile acids. The limitations of such a method are obvious because (a) the precursor may not exchange with the endogenous pool and thus not reach the appropriate enzymes, and (b) false precursors may be transformed by enzymes not involved in bile acid biosynthesis. None the less, these experiments have provided useful information, in clarifying the overall pathway of bile acid biosynthesis.

STEPS IN THE PATHWAY _____

Nuclear biotransformations

Cholesterol 7-hydroxylation to form 7α-hydroxy cholesterol is a microsomal process that is rate limiting and presumably essential for normal bile acid biosynthesis. This key enzyme has recently been cloned.[25] The 7α-hydroxy compound is converted via an isomerase and a reductase to a key intermediate cholest-7α-hydroxy-Δ^4-3-one. This unsaturated oxo derivative is a branch point, as it is the substrate for the 12-hydroxylase; 12-hydroxylation commits bile acid irreversibly to CA synthesis and distinguishes the CA 'family' from the CDCA 'family'.[118,177]

This Δ^4-3-oxo-7α-hydroxy derivative is then stereospecifically reduced to give the 5β bile acids in most ancient vertebrates. As a consequence of these hydroxylation, isomerization, oxidation, and reduction steps, the 'natural' bile acid nucleus is formed that has an α-hydroxy group at positions 3 and 7 in the CDCA family and at positions 3, 7 and 12 in the CA family. The nucleus is saturated with the A/B ring junction in a *cis* configuration. Such compounds were traditionally termed 'coprostanols', but today they are termed 5β-cholestane diols or triols.[90]

Side-chain biotransformations

The second key metabolic step, 26-hydroxylation, is believed to occur in the mitochondrion. This step, which is the first step of side-chain oxidation, is the key enzymatic defect in cerebrotendinous xanthomatosis. After 26-hydroxylation there is oxidation to form the C_{27} carboxylic acid and then a form of β-oxidation in the conventional manner. This step involves introduction of a double bond at C-24 followed by 24-hydroxylation and oxidative cleavage of a 3-carbon fragment, mediated by peroxisomal enzymes, to yield the 'modern' C_{24} bile acids.

The traditional paradigm was that nuclear biotransformations preceded side-chain biotransformations. If the side-chain were biotransformed without any nuclear changes, the result would be a 3β-hydroxy-Δ^5-cholenoic acid. Indeed this bile acid is synthesized by a hepatocellular carcinoma cell line[98] and is also a major constituent of amniotic fluid in man,[39] suggesting that during fetal life the enzymes for side-chain oxidation may mature more rapidly than the enzymes for nuclear biotransformations. This bile acid is also formed in cholestatic conditions,[194] proving that side-chain oxidation can proceed to completion despite any biotransformation of the cholesterol nucleus in some circumstances.

REGULATION OF BILE ACID BIOSYNTHESIS

The regulation of bile acid synthesis is not understood at a biochemical level. Grossly, it can be described as a negative feedback system in which the return of bile acids to the liver, or possibly the concentration of bile acids in the hepatocyte, inhibits bile acid synthesis. Bile acid synthesis can be diminished about 50% by bile acid feeding and probably decreases by 80–90% during cholestasis. With interruption of the enterohepatic circulation by biliary fistula or ileal dysfunction, bile acid synthesis increases 5- to 20-fold (cf. ref. 105). Attempts to demonstrate the negative feedback system using cell culture techniques have succeeded with pig hepatocytes but not with hepatocytes from other species.[110] The regulation may involve proteins with a relatively long half-life; this idea agrees with the biological observation that a compensatory increase in synthesis following interruption of the enterohepatic circulation does not occur for 6–20 hours. Recent studies in animals and man have indicated that the hydrophobic dihydroxy bile acids, CDCA and DCA, when fed chronically, are much more potent suppressors of bile acid biosynthesis than the hydrophilic dihydroxy bile acid, UDCA.[74,138] CA feeding also suppresses bile acid biosynthesis, although some of this effect may be mediated by DCA, to which it is converted by bacterial 7-dehydroxylation.[187]

Because bile acids are formed from cholesterol, any increase in bile acid synthesis must be accompanied by a corresponding increase in cholesterol biosynthesis (and/or increased input of dietary cholesterol) under steady-state conditions. Similarly, any decrease in bile acid synthesis must be accompanied by a corresponding decrease in cholesterol biosynthesis (and/or decreased input of dietary cholesterol). In animals such as the rat, cholesterol feeding causes increased bile acid synthesis, suggesting that cholesterol 7α-hydroxylase can be induced. It does not appear to be the case in man, and any increased absorption of dietary cholesterol is balanced by increased biliary secretion of cholesterol.

BILE ACID BIOTRANSFORMATION DURING BILE ACID TRANSPORT

In man, biotransformation of 'old' bile acids during hepatic transport is mostly limited to reamidation. A few

other biotransformation pathways should be mentioned. 3-Oxo bile acids are reduced stereospecifically to 3α-hydroxy bile acids and 3β-hydroxy ('iso') bile acids are oxidized and then stereospecifically reduced to 3α bile acids.[181] The biotransformation products have a lower CMC and are superior dispersants when compared to their precursors. The 7-oxo derivatives of CA and CDCA are stereospecifically reduced to the 7α-hydroxy derivative, at least in some species;[62] reduction is incomplete and some 7-oxo derivatives are secreted into bile. Finally, bile acids with shortened side-chains are likely to undergo little amidation, but undergo glucuronidation on either the nucleus or side-chain.[146,219]

EFFECTS OF BILE ACID TRANSPORT ON THE LIVER

INDUCTION OF BILE FLOW

Bile acids are secreted against a concentration gradient into the canalicular space, which may be considered a closed space surrounded by a semi-permeable membrane. Their osmotic effects induce the flow of water into the canaliculus across the paracellular junctions and possibly also across the canalicular membrane.[16,48] Since bile acids induce bile formation, they may be termed primary solutes. In addition to water, solutes that are sufficiently small to percolate through the paracellular junctions enter bile by convective flow (solvent drag). Diffusion also contributes at slow rates of bile flow. Solutes that enter bile passively may be termed secondary solutes.[80] Important secondary solutes are Ca^{2+}, N^+, K^+, Cl^-, HCO_3^-, glucose, amino acids and organic acids.

The pore size of the paracellular junctions of the mammalian liver is slightly larger than that of the intestinal mucosa. Erythritol is freely permeable, mannitol is less permeable, and sucrose has still less permeability. If bile flow is plotted against bile acid output, a straight line is observed with a slope of 10–14 μl/μmole bile acid or 5–7 μl/bile acid per osmotically active ion (bile acid anion plus the accompanying anion). This slope can be considered the choleretic 'potency' of bile acids to induce 'bile acid-dependent bile flow' and can be compared with a value of 3.3 μl water/μmol ion in isotonic NaCl. The remainder of water is 'obligated' by the secondary solutes in bile. Thus, since canalicular bile is always isotonic, the greater the entry of secondary solutes, the lower will be the concentration of bile acids in canalicular bile. Bile acids with a high CMC value (for example the trioxo derivative of CA, which only forms dimers at high concentrations) will induce more bile flow per bile acid molecule, since osmotic potency is a colligative property,

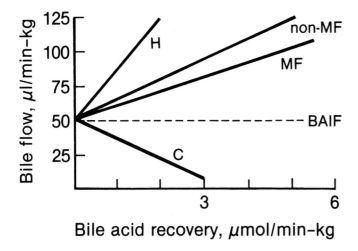

Figure 13.10 Major types of bile acid-dependent flow. Bile acid recovery in bile is shown as the horizontal axis; bile flow as the vertical axis. Natural bile acids which form micelles (micelle-forming, MF) induce about 10 μl/μmol bile acid recovered in bile. Bile acids that do not form micelles (non-MF) induce more bile flow, about 15 μl/μmol, since their osmotic effect is greater. Hypercholeretic (H) bile acids induce an anomalously high bile flow because they are reabsorbed from the ductules, and their osmotic activity is transferred to bicarbonate anions, which are not shown in the graph. Cholestatic (C) bile acids induce cholestasis, with both bile acid-dependent and bile acid-independent bile flow (BAIF) declining.

that is, it is related only to the number of molecules or aggregates in solution (cf. ref. 141). Figure 13.10 shows bile acid-dependent bile flow for different types of bile acids.

The slope of the bile flow/bile acid recovery curve has a positive intercept if extrapolated to zero bile acid recovery. This bile flow, which appears to be 'driven' by osmotically active substances, is defined as 'bile acid-independent flow' and is considered to result from canalicular secretion of substances, such as glutathione.[10] Secretion of water-containing lipid vesicles might also make a minor contribution to bile acid-independent bile flow. All of these substances that generate bile flow may be considered 'primary solutes'. At very low bile acid secretion rates, bile acids might be diluted below their CMC by the bile flow induced by these other primary solutes. If so, each bile acid molecule would induce slightly more osmotic water flow than bile acid molecules present as micelles.

There is a gradient of bile acid flux down the sinusoid. Probably the periportal hepatocytes secrete the most bile acids, and the perivenular cells the least. Accordingly, most bile acid-dependent bile flow originates at the periportal cells. The site of secretion of bile acid-independent bile flow is not known, but may well be the perivenular cells.

INDUCTION OF LIPID SECRETION

Besides inducing osmotic bile flow, bile acids also induce the secretion of lipid-rich vesicles from the hepatocyte. The vesicles contain cholesterol and phospholipid in a ratio averaging 0.3 in humans, a proportion that is much higher than that of most other mammals.[157] As a consequence of this high cholesterol/phospholipid ratio, human bile is extremely high in its cholesterol content. Secretion of cholesterol as such rather than by conversion to bile acids can be considered to be an ingenious, albeit hazardous, solution to cholesterol elimination, since less enzymes should be involved in vesicle assembly than in the conversion of cholesterol to bile acids, which requires at least ten enzymatic steps.

The biochemical and biophysical mechanisms of biliary lipid secretion are poorly understood.[24] The origin of the lipid is thought to be the Golgi apparatus. The phospholipid is predominantly phosphatidylcholine. It is derived from a pool specifically targeted for biliary secretion and has a characteristic fatty acid composition, even though this can be influenced by the composition of dietary fatty acids. The cholesterol is unlikely to be derived from any specific cholesterol pool, at least under conditions of normal biliary lipid secretion. Vesicular movement toward the canalicular pole of the hepatocyte is considered to involve microtubules, because agents that interfere with microtubule polymerization decrease induced biliary lipid secretion.[36] The vesicles may incorporate other organic anions, such as unconjugated bilirubin, but bilirubin diglucuronide is thought to be secreted into canalicular bile in a vesicle-independent manner.

In describing bile acid-induced biliary lipid secretion, it is convenient to use the expression linkage coefficients, which are defined as the ratio of secretion of phospholipid (in moles) to that of bile acid (in moles) (cf. ref. 38). The cholesterol/phospholipid ratio denotes vesicle lipid composition.

Factors influencing the phospholipid/bile acid ratio are not well understood. Extremely hydrophilic bile acids do not induce phospholipid secretion (cf. ref. 141). A variety of organic anions (ampicillin, bilirubin, ceftriaxone) cause a marked decrease in the phospholipid/bile acid ratio if given simultaneously with bile acids (reviewed in ref. 217). The locus of this effect is not known, but Verkade and his colleagues[207] have proposed that the effect is mediated inside the canaliculus, rather than inside the hepatocyte.

The cholesterol/phospholipid ratio can also be modified, but not greatly. It is increased by circumstances that cause increased input of cholesterol into the exchangeable cholesterol pool—obesity, rapid weight reduction in the obese patient, or cholesterol feeding.[64] It is decreased by circumstances that decrease the cholesterol input into the exchangeable cholesterol pool—administration of CDCA or UDCA and administration of inhibitors of HMG CoA reductase such as lovostatin and simvistatin (cf. ref. 43). Increases in the cholesterol/phospholipid ratio are associated with an increase in the risk for cholesterol gallstone formation; a decreased cholesterol/phospholipid ratio, if sufficient to desaturate bile, can induce the gradual dissolution of cholesterol gallstones if the stones are chronically exposed to unsaturated bile.

SOLUBILIZATION OF LIPID VESICLES INTO MIXED MICELLES

In addition to inducing bile flow and lipid-vesicle secretion, bile acids act on the lipid vesicles, converting them from their unilamellar bilayer arrangement to mixed micelles.[24] This process of conversion of vesicles to mixed micelles occurs rapidly as bile is flowing down the biliary tree. It continues as bile is stored in the gallbladder until equilibrium is reached. If the ratio of bile acids to lipid vesicles is sufficiently high, all of the vesicles will be transformed to mixed micelles. If the ratio of bile acids is inadequate to solubilize all of the vesicular lipid, vesicles will persist, even in gallbladder bile.

The two constituent lipids of the vesicles—phospholipid and cholesterol—are not solubilized at identical rates.[188] Phospholipid is solubilized preferentially, so that the vesicle becomes enriched in cholesterol. The cholesterol in the cholesterol-rich vesicle is at risk of formation of cholesterol monohydrate crystals, which is the first step in cholesterol gallstone formation or the formation of biliary sludge.

COMPLEXATION OF BILIARY Ca^{2+}

A final action of secreted bile acids is to complex Ca^{2+} ions, both as monomers and as micelles.[94,133,134] As a consequence of this binding by bile acids, the Ca^{2+} activity in bile is lowered considerably. Whether this Ca^{2+} complexation by bile acid monomers and micelles has an important physiological function is not known but it may prevent the formation of insoluble calcium salts of glycine dihydroxy bile salts, since the K_{sp} of the Ca^{2+} salt of the most common bile acid in bile (the glycine conjugate of CDCA) is only 2×10^{-9} M^3.[100] Hepatic bile is supersaturated with $CaCO_3$, but rapid Na^+/H^+ exchange by the gallbladder mucosa converts HCO_3^- to CO_2 and H_2O, so that gallbladder bile, during storage, has a progressively decreasing HCO_3^- concentration and as a result becomes unsaturated in $CaCO_3$ in model systems simulating hepatic bile that are supersaturated in $CaCO_3$.[158] The formation of $CaCO_3$ crystallization from supersaturated bile can be shown to be inhibited *in vitro* by an acidic protein isolated from gallstones.[182] This protein may inhibit $CaCO_3$ precipitation from supersaturated hepatic bile.

DEFECTS IN HEPATOCYTE TRANSPORT

To date, no primary defects in hepatic uptake of bile acids have been described. Such a defect might be quite subtle in its clinical presentation, as simulation of defective hepatic uptake in a pharmacokinetic model of the enterohepatic circulation results in increased plasma levels of bile acids with little change in net hepatic bile acid transport.[34] In addition, the redundancy of pathways for bile acid uptake implies that a defect in one transport pathway might be compensated for by adaptation of another. A primary defect in ileal transport of bile acids has been reported;[72] hepatic handling of bile acids in this condition has not been investigated but is not likely to be altered, since the ileal transport and hepatic transport proteins are clearly different.[122] Defects in the structure or activity of the cytosolic binding proteins have also not been identified.

In Byler's disease, a disease of neonatal cholestasis, there are elevated concentrations of bile acids in the hepatocyte yet low concentrations of bile acids in hepatic bile, suggesting defective canalicular transport. Indeed, in the healthy newborn, plasma bile acid levels are high and bile acid secretion rates are low, based on the concentrations present in the small intestinal lumen. Thus, 'physiological cholestasis' of the newborn is explained most simply as defective canalicular transport.[8]

A patient has been reported with cholestasis and absence of CDCA in bile, despite its presence in blood.[198] The authors suggested that the patient had a defect in the canalicular transporter for CDCA conjugates; however, to date, it has been generally assumed that there is only a single canalicular transporter for conjugated bile acids.

DEFECTS IN BILE ACID BIOSYNTHESIS

At least 10 enzymes are involved in bile acid biosynthesis from cholesterol; defects in bile acid biosynthesis are likely to be recognized with increasing frequency given the power of modern analytical techniques such as coupled gas chromatography–mass spectrometry (GCMS)[185] and high-performance liquid chromatography–mass spectrometry (HPLC/MS).[179] At least five defects are now recognized, and they can be classified according to whether the defect involves the nucleus or the side-chain. A recent review discusses these in considerable detail.[177]

Nuclear defects

A defect in the 3β-hydroxy-Δ^5 steroid dehydrogenase-isomerase pathway has been reported by Clayton *et al.*[27] in a child presenting with cholestasis and liver biopsy findings suggestive of giant cell hepatitis. There were large quantities of 3β,7α-dihydroxy- and 3β,7α,12α-trihydroxy-5-cholenoic acids in the urine, most as the sulphated non-amidated derivative.

A case of presumed 12-hydroxylase deficiency was reported by Dowling.[40] In this case there was a virtual absence of CA and it presented (in the adult) as severe chronic constipation. Presumably the CDCA in bile was efficiently 7-dehydroxylated to LCA, which is insoluble.

As yet a deficiency in cholesterol-7α-hydroxylase has not been reported. Such individuals could not form CA and CDCA by the usual route. They might form 3β-hydroxy-Δ⁵-cholenic acid and, if this were adequately secreted, cholesterol would be eliminated.

Side-chain defects

Cerebrotendinous xanthomatosis (CTX) a classic inborn error of metabolism, is being recognized with increasing frequency, with nearly 100 cases now known. The defect involves defective mitochondrial 26-hydroxylation of the 3,7-cholestane-di-ol.[118] As a consequence, biosynthesis of CDCA (and of CA to a lesser extent) is deficient; cholesterol synthesis is not suppressed and is markedly increased. The increased cholesterol synthesis leads to the accumulation of cholestane-diol, which is hydroxylated at multiple other sites, e.g. C-23, C-24 and C-25, to form bile alcohols, which are excreted in both urine and bile, mostly as glucuronides. The 3-oxo-7-hydroxy-4-cholest-en-one accumulates and undergoes hepatic 7-dehydroxyl-ation and subsequent reduction to form cholestanol, which accumulates in serum and tissues.[186] Treatment with CDCA completely reverses the biochemical defect, whereas treatment with UDCA does not.[151]

Zellweger's syndrome, a rare disease, presents with multiple developmental abnormalities in the newborn. Peroxisome formation is deficient, so that fatty acids and bile acids do not undergo β-oxidation. C₂₇ bile acids are present in bile and serum. The condition is usually fatal.[222] One case has been reported in which primary bile acid feeding corrected the biochemical defect and caused striking clinical improvement (C. Clerici, personal communication).

DEFECTS IN BILE ACID BIOTRANSFORMATION ____

Defective sulphation of bile acids has not been identified and must be extremely rare, as in the National Cooperative

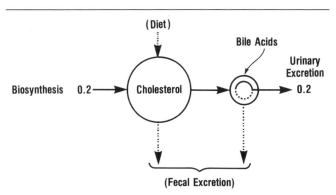

Figure 13.11 Bile acid metabolism in total hepatobiliary obstruction. Dietary cholesterol is not absorbed because of the absence of micelles in the intestinal lumen; biosynthesis falls. Cholesterol secretion in bile cannot occur; bile acids are sulphated and eliminated in urine, providing the sole means of eliminating cholesterol.

Gallstone Study no evidence of LCA accumulation occurred in more than 600 patients treated with CDCA.[54] Furthermore, some 30 000 patients have been treated with CDCA or UDCA for gallstone dissolution, and to date no well-documented case of LCA accumulation causing hepatotoxicity has been reported. Defective amidation of bile acids also has not been reported, but the clinical and biochemical features of the disease have been predicted.[87] The malady should present as an intestinal disease characterized by bile acid malabsorption, steatorrhoea, and fat-soluble vitamin malabsorption, since bile acids will be glucuronidated and rapidly excreted. Cholestasis should not be present. Plasma bile acids should consist solely of unconjugated CA.

BILE ACID METABOLISM IN LIVER AND BILIARY DISEASE

ALTERATIONS IN BILE ACID METABOLISM IN LIVER DISEASE _____

Cholestasis (see Chapter 15)

In severe cholestatic liver disease, primary bile acids accumulate in the hepatocyte. Secondary bile acids are not formed, since bile acids do not reach the intestine. If the biliary tree is obstructed extrahepatically, bile acids are likely to regurgitate into plasma through the paracellular junctions of the biliary ductules. Bile acid sulphation, especially of amidated CDCA, increases markedly. In addition, there is a slight increase in glucuronidation, presumably 3-ether glucuronidation, as bile acids continue to be amidated. 3-Glycosylation also occurs. Some 6-hydroxylation of CDCA occurs, forming hyocholic acid.[17] Plasma bile acids increase manyfold, and there is increased binding of bile acids by lipoproteins.[58] The concentration of non-protein-bound bile acid increases markedly, and glomerular filtration of bile acids increases manyfold. Sulphated bile acids are poorly reabsorbed from the renal tubule, and bile acid loss in urine increases greatly and in direct proportion to the degree of elevation of plasma bile acids. The major urinary bile acids are the sulphates of CDCA amidates.[156,192,204] Cholesterol and bile acid metabolism in complete cholestasis is shown in Figure 13.11.

In cholestasis, bile acid biosynthesis decreases by sev-eralfold, as does cholesterol biosynthesis. Since the demand for bile acid conjugation falls, bile acids become preferentially amidated with taurine. Because of the absence of bile acids in the small intestine, dietary cholesterol and fat-soluble vitamins are not absorbed. Cholesterol does not enter the intestine via bile, and presumably faecal bile acid loss is negligible. Thus, in the quasisteady state of complete biliary obstruction, the only input into the cholesterol pool is via hepatic cholesterol synthesis (which is markedly decreased), as well as tissue cholesterol synthesis; and the only output of cholesterol is by urinary excretion of bile acids in glucuronidated, sulphated, and unsulphated form.

A major function of bile acids is to induce the secretion of phospholipid/cholesterol vesicles into the canaliculus. With cholestasis these vesicles are likely to be exocytosed into plasma instead of bile, explaining the appearance of vesicles in plasma. These vesicles can adsorb lipoproteins and albumin to become what has been termed 'lipoprotein X' (see Chapter 4).

In mild cholestasis, bile acid secretion into the intestine is likely to be relatively unimpaired. Ileal absorption is efficient, and the fractional extraction by the small intestine probably increases, accompanied by decreased faecal excretion of bile acids. As cholestasis increases, ileal absorption can be so efficient that all secondary bile acids disappear from bile. Such ileal conservation of bile acids promotes liver injury.[81]

Parenchymal liver cell disease

In simple parenchymal liver disease, e.g. acute viral hepatitis, bile acid metabolism has not been well characterized. In cirrhosis the serum level of bile acids is moderately increased, bile acid secretion is reduced to a moderate amount, and urinary bile acids are increased severalfold[4,212] but bile remains the preponderant route of bile acid excretion. In cirrhosis there is a selective reduction in CA biosynthesis, suggesting decreased 12-hydroxylation;[211] neither the mechanism nor the significance of this effect is known.

In fulminant hepatic failure, bile acid uptake, amidation, and secretion into bile are markedly impaired.[89] Presumably, bile acid biosynthesis is also markedly decreased.

Detailed pharmacokinetic models of the metabolism and enterohepatic circulation of CA[88] and CDCA[131] metabolism in healthy man have been constructed. Such models include biotransformation (conjugation and deconjugation), hepatocyte and enterocyte transport, and inter-organ flow. It will be of interest to use such models to describe the changes in bile acid metabolism and distribution that occur in cholestatic liver disease and to a lesser extent in parenchymal liver disease. The effect of portal–systemic shunting is discussed below.

SERUM BILE ACID MEASUREMENTS _____

Physiological determinants

As a result of work from a number of laboratories, it is well established that in health the level of bile acids in systemic plasma (here termed 'serum bile acids') is determined by 'spillover' of bile acids reaching the liver from the intestine.[114,147,203] Because the fractional extraction (FE) of bile acids varies from 40% to 90%, the spillover (1 − FE) varies from 10% to 60%, and the pattern of serum bile acids is not identical to that of portal blood but is distorted predictably by the differing FE values for individual bile acids. The spillover of bile acids past the liver into the systemic circulation is independent of load; thus, the greater the load to the liver, the greater is the absolute amount of bile acids that reaches the systemic circulation. Because plasma volume is relatively constant, the serum bile acid level serves as a 'flowmeter' to indicate the flux of bile acids presented to the liver.

Serum bile acids are thus an enterohepatic entity, being determined not only by hepatic uptake but also by intestinal absorption. The rate of intestinal absorption of bile acids is determined by load (hepatic secretion and gallbladder emptying), intraluminal concentration (determined by water fluxes as well as by binding to food and/or food residues), and the kinetics of passive and active absorption from the intestine.[114] The pattern of bile acids absorbed depends on biliary bile acid composition and subsequent bacterial biotransformation. During overnight fasting, about half of the bile acids secreted by the liver are stored in the gallbladder;[202] if the gallbladder does not contract, there is progressive storage in the gallbladder during the overnight period, so that by morning most of the bile acid pool is stored in the gallbladder. When a meal is ingested, the gallbladder contracts, delivering its bile acids into the small intestine. The most lipophilic bile acid amidates (glycine amidates of CDCA and deoxycholic acid) undergo some passive absorption in the proximal small intestine, so that the early part of the postprandial elevation in serum bile acid levels is enriched in these amidates.[171] Most of the bile acid amidates pass to the terminal ileum, where they are actively absorbed; the postprandial peak of amidates of CA occurs about 120 minutes after a meal is ingested[171] and is illustrated in Figure 13.12.

If intestinal absorption is abrogated (e.g. by the fashioning of a biliary fistula), the serum bile acid levels become immeasurably low.[114] Thus, in the healthy person, reflux of bile acids from the hepatocyte makes a negligible contribution to serum bile acids. If a bile acid is injected intravenously, it is promptly extracted by the liver, so that the $T_{1/2}$ for plasma disappearance is only a few minutes.[32]

In complete cholestasis, bile acids reach the serum by reflux from the hepatocyte or the biliary ductules. In such conditions the plasma level reflects the relative rates of input from the liver and loss by excretion into urine. In incomplete cholestasis, serum bile acid levels are determined by intestinal, hepatic and renal factors.

Diagnostic utility (see Chapter 18)

There has been speculation for years that serum bile acid levels or patterns could provide useful diagnostic information. Early methods for measuring serum bile acid

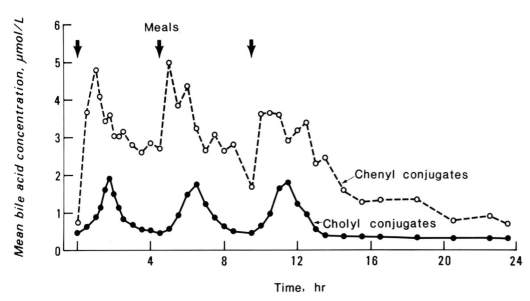

Figure 13.12 Diurnal pattern of plasma bile acids in response to three equicaloric liquid meals. The earlier rise of conjugates of chenodeoxycholic acid (chenodeoxycholyl conjugates) results from their passive absorption from the jejunum; cholyl conjugates are believed to be absorbed solely from the terminal ileum. Chenyl, chenodeoxycholyl.

concentrations were difficult and non-specific. With the development of chromatographic methods such as gas–liquid chromatography (GLC), it was possible to determine which serum bile acids increased in liver disease. This advance, in turn, was followed by the development of accurate and specific radioimmunoassays. The enzymatic method for measuring total serum bile acids based on a bacterial 3-hydroxysteroid dehydrogenase (HSD) has been modified in several ways to increase its sensitivity. For example, the reduced co-factor generation was coupled to oxidation of a fluorescent dye, a tetrazolium dye, or a bacterial luciferase (for review of available methods, see ref. 163). Finally, the powerful technique of mass spectroscopy has permitted exquisitely sensitive measurements of individual bile acids (after deconjugation) in serum.[178]

While this remarkable progress was being made in analytical methodology for measuring bile acids, other tests for detecting liver injury or for measuring hepatic function were also being developed and validated. These tests include those for liver injury (e.g. serum aminotransferases), tests for cholestasis (e.g. 5′-nucleotidase), as well as function tests (e.g. ICG and galactose elimination capacity clearance or the aminopyrine breath test).[13] Thus, any consideration of the utility (sensitivity and specificity) of serum bile acid measurements must be compared with that of other liver tests.

The consensus of a large number of careful studies using sensitive methods for measuring serum bile acids may be summarized as follows. (a) Serum bile acid measurements (SBAMs) as determined by a sensitive method such as radioimmunoassay are a good test; that is, the SBAMs have excellent sensitivity and moderate specificity for the presence of liver disease;[33,50] if a less sensitive method (e.g. enzymatic determination) is used, the test is still specific, although sensitivity is less. (b)

When patients are jaundiced because of liver disease, bile acids are invariably elevated; in contrast, patients with liver disease and normal serum levels of conjugated bilirubin may have elevated serum bile acid levels, suggesting that the serum bile acid level is a more sensitive test than the bilirubin level (cf. ref. 45). (c) The pattern of serum bile acids offers no useful diagnostic information as to the type of liver disease. (d) Fasting-state levels are in most instances as sensitive as postprandial elevations or elevations obtained after a meal or cholecystokinin (CCK)-induced gallbladder contraction. (e) Measurement of immunoreactive cholyl conjugates is as sensitive as measuring immunoreactive chenodeoxycholyl conjugates or immunoreactive total bile acids.[51,170] (f) Compared to aminotransferase levels, SBAMs are more specific (for liver disease) but less sensitive.[33,45,50,51,170]

Thus, the available information suggests that the addition of SBAMs to the conventional 'battery' of liver tests (aminotransferases, alkaline phosphatase, bilirubin) does *not* often provide important new diagnostic information. The question is whether SBAMs are ever useful. Three indications when SBAMs are likely to be cost-effective are (a) to exclude significant liver disease in (unconjugated) hyperbilirubinaemic conditions such as Gilbert's syndrome;[210] (b) to identify non-invasively and in a sensitive manner the presence of portal–systemic shunting as a sign of cirrhosis in patients in whom other common liver tests are within normal limits,[96,119] although this point remains controversial;[193] and (c) to 'stage' cirrhotic patients, in that SBAMs appear to offer predictive value for life expectancy.[120] Some studies (cf. refs. 106, 132), but not all have suggested that SBAMs can be used to distinguish chronic persistent hepatitis from chronic active hepatitis. Patients with chronic active hepatitis often have early cirrhosis and portal–systemic shunting, probably explaining these reports.

The pattern of serum bile acids provides no useful diagnostic information except in cases of inborn errors of bile acid biosynthesis, e.g. CTX and Zellweger's syndrome. The idea that the dihydroxy/trihydroxy ratio could be used to distinguish types of liver disease was based on insensitive analytical methods and has been shown to be erroneous. In patients with cirrhosis the CDCA (conjugates)/CA (conjugates) ratio exceeds that of patients with cholestasis, as was noted above, but there is considerable overlap in the values in the two groups of patients (cf. ref. 204). The mechanism responsible for this selective enrichment of plasma in CDCA conjugates is not known. One possibility is that 'capillarization' of the sinusoids (defined as a decrease in the size of the fenestrae of the endothelial cells) leads to a preferential reduction in the filtration rate of albumin-bound bile acids, since CDCA conjugates are more highly bound to albumin than CA conjugates and a smaller proportion should enter the space of Disse. Thus, the FE of CDCA conjugates should decrease to a greater extent than that of cholyl conjugates, and there would be preferential enrichment in the proportion of CDCA in systemic plasma.

Serum bile acid measurements are, in principle, a sensitive measure of portal–systemic shunting,[34] but one group has disputed this.[193] Simulation experiments[133] suggest that, if a total portal–systemic shunt were performed and hepatic arterial blood flow were increased so as to restore total hepatic blood flow to normal, the serum bile acid concentration would be increased about 4-fold (for a bile acid having an FE of 0.9). In the absence of a compensatory increase in hepatic arterial blood flow, portal–systemic shunting causes a progressive increase in the concentration of bile acids in the systemic circulation. Simulation experiments also suggest that an elevation of serum bile acid levels of more than 16-fold cannot be explained by shunting alone and requires the simultaneous presence of impaired hepatic uptake. From a practical standpoint these simulations suggest that a normal fasting-state serum bile acid level excludes extensive portal–systemic shunting in most patients. An intermediate elevation (2- to 16-fold) is ambiguous, indicating shunting and/or parenchymal damage; and a more than 16-fold elevation indicates unequivocal parenchymal damage. Time will tell whether these inferences from simulations have validity in the clinical situation.

When serum bile acid levels are elevated, increased concentrations of bile acids also occur in saliva and urine. Salivary concentration of bile acids correlates imperfectly with the concentration of unbound bile acids in serum, and there is little reason to recommend this measurement.[68] Urinary bile acids are the result of glomerular filtration and tubular reabsorption, but urinary bile acid outputs correlate highly with serum bile acid levels.[204] There seems no reason to recommend that any body fluid other than fasting-state serum be used for the measurement of bile acids.

Bile acid loading procedures

Because the serum bile acid concentration is an entero-hepatic entity, and the central input is largely determined by active absorption from the terminal ileum, workers have sought to eliminate this input as a variable. Two approaches have been used: (a) an intravenous load of a conjugated bile acid, e.g. the glycine amidate of CA;[107],[112] or (b) an oral load of an unconjugated bile acid such as CDCA or UDCA that is absorbed passively by the small intestine (cf. refs. 55, 102, 127). Neither of these techniques is likely to have clinical utility, for the following reasons. When bile acids are given intravenously, there may be local toxicity problems. Hepatic uptake occurs before complete mixing occurs, making kinetic analysis of the disappearance curves difficult, although a non-absorbable mixing marker may be used to increase precision.[20] A major problem is that the disappearance curve reflects (a) mixing, (b) blood flow to the liver, (c) the efficiency of hepatic extraction, which in turn is dependent on the flux of bile acids to the hepatocyte as well as intrinsic clearance. Thus, impaired disappearance may indicate a small volume of distribution, decreased hepatic blood flow, and/or decreased hepatic uptake. Clinical results have been disappointing.

Oral tolerance procedures suffer from the problem of the unpredictability of gastric emptying if material is ingested by mouth, as well as additional uncertainties in the rate of dissolution of the crystals of the bile acid. Because of this problem, accurate definition of the area under the curve (AUC) requires frequent measurements of serum bile acid concentrations. Hepatic uptake of unconjugated dihydroxy bile acids is passive, and thus the mechanism for hepatic uptake differs from that when a conjugated bile acid load is given intravenously. The bile acids that have been used (CDCA and UDCA) are extensively protein-bound, so that capillarization of the sinusoids might decrease hepatic uptake.

Despite this pessimistic assessment, such 'tolerance tests' may be of value for investigative purposes. If blood flow can be estimated independently, either an intravenous or an oral tolerance procedure might provide valuable information on hepatic uptake. The availability of a ^{75}Se-tagged bile acid (SeHCAT),[99] a substance whose metabolism is quite similar to that of cholyltaurine, makes measurement of plasma disappearance of bile acids extremely simple. This compound can also be used to measure transfer of conjugated bile acids from plasma into bile.

The future of SBAMs as routine laboratory determinations continues to be uncertain. SBAMs will continue to be of value for elucidating the fluxes of bile acid in the enterohepatic circulation, determining the bioavailability of orally administered bile acids (cf. refs. 165, 201), and determining the efficacy of bile acid sequestrants used to treat hypercholesterolaemia.[167] They may prove to be of value for detecting portal–systemic shunting or staging the cirrhotic patient but are likely to be performed by a specialized laboratory rather than a general clinical chemistry laboratory.

DEFECTIVE BILE ACID BIOTRANSFORMATIONS AS AN INDICATION OF HEPATIC DISEASE

The major types of bile acid biotransformation are conjugation, oxidation–reduction, and hydroxylation. No recent studies have examined the kinetics of hydroxylation or oxidation in liver disease. Horak *et al.*[89] injected cholate and cholyltaurine simultaneously and compared the rate of uptake, amidation, reflux into plasma, and biliary secretion in healthy volunteers with that of subjects with fulminant hepatic failure using a simple multicompartmental model. They showed that uptake, amidation, and biliary secretion were defective in fulminant hepatic failure. This approach requires multiple blood samples and definition of the chemical form of plasma radioactivity using chromatography, and is similar to the kinetic evaluation of BSP metabolism reported by Molino and Milanese.[130] Such techniques are elegant but difficult; they are helpful in elucidating the subtleties of the metabolism of cholephilic substances in patients with liver disease. They are unlikely, at least for the near future, to be useful in clinical hepatology.

BILE ACID CHOLESTASIS AND LIVER INJURY

The two lipophilic dihydroxy bile acids (CDCA and DCA) are cytotoxic to a variety of cells, such as erythrocytes, mast cells, or intestinal epithelial cells (reviewed in ref. 81). Amidation, in contrast to glucuronidation or sulphation, is not a detoxification step. Dihydroxy amidated bile acids are usually cytotoxic at concentrations above 1000 μm, and such concentrations are never obtained in the normal hepatocyte.

If dihydroxy bile acids are given intravenously or enterally at relatively low rates (2 μmol min^{-1} kg^{-1}), an immediate decrease in bile flow is observed, and occasional cell necrosis can be detected by microscopy (cf. ref. 128).

If monohydroxy bile acids are infused intravenously, immediate cholestasis is observed;[97,123,129,220] for reviews of cholestatic mechanisms, see refs 101, 140, 152, 184. If the monohydroxy bile acids, LCA or its precursors CDCA or UDCA, are administered chronically to animals that cannot detoxify LCA by hydroxylation or sulphation, liver cell necrosis and bile duct proliferation are induced (for review, see ref. 28). Thus, there is sound experimental evidence that under appropriate circumstances in the experimental animal, endogenous bile acids are cholestatic and hepatotoxic. The question is whether these observations relate to cholestasis or hepatocellular injury occurring in patients. A second question is by what mechanism(s) do bile acids induce cholestasis and liver cell injury.

The consensus of most workers is that endogenous bile acids will only rarely be involved as a primary causal

agent in acute (intrahepatic or chronic) cholestasis. Lithocholate is poorly absorbed from the colon and is readily sulphated, excreted into bile, and rapidly eliminated from the body. To date, an inborn error of sulphation of LCA has not been detected.

The one circumstance in which bile acids may be involved in the pathogenesis of acute (and chronic) cholestasis is the presence of an inborn error of bile acid biosynthesis in which bile acid precursors are formed. These may inhibit the canalicular secretory apparatus, perhaps by binding irreversibly to one or more of the canalicular transport proteins (cf. ref. 180).

Endogenous bile acids are also unlikely to be involved as a primary cause of chronic liver injury, except in the uncommon situation when high doses of CDCA are administered to gallstone patients in order to desaturate bile and induce cholesterol gallstone dissolution. CDCA has been shown to cause a dose-related increase in aminotransferase levels and to induce liver biopsy abnormalities in perhaps 5–10% of gallstone patients.[54] Thus, most gallstone patients can tolerate a marked enrichment in the proportion of CDCA (to >80%) of circulating bile acids without developing laboratory signs of hepatotoxicity. Oral administration of DCA has also induced abnormal liver tests in one healthy subject[113] and, presumably, if administered chronically to large numbers of patients, DCA would have a hepatotoxicity risk similar to that of CDCA.

Retention of endogenous bile acid within the hepatocyte because of cholestasis is presently considered to play a key role in the hepatocyte necrosis occurring in patients with obstruction to biliary secretion. In patients with severe cholestasis, secondary bile acids are not present in bile, so that the probable injurious agent is the primary bile acid, CDCA. CA is much less cytotoxic. The extent to which CDCA retention causes hepatocyte injury depends on its net uptake rate, intracellular binding and detoxification by sulphation or glucuronidation, and the susceptibility of key cell organelles to damage. The mechanism by which retained bile acids injure the hepatocyte has not been elucidated.

UDCA IN THE TREATMENT OF CHRONIC CHOLESTATIC LIVER DISEASE

UDCA has been used for about 15 years for cholesterol gallstone dissolution. Careful clinical studies by several groups in Japan performed some 30 years ago suggested that UDCA would improve liver tests in patients with chronic hepatitis or cholestatic liver disease (cited in ref. 80); such studies were not placebo-controlled. Leuschner and his colleagues administered UDCA to patients with chronic hepatitis and gallstones and observed that liver tests improved.[115] Shortly thereafter, Poupon and his colleagues reported that UDCA caused both symptomatic improvement and improvement in laboratory tests in 15 patients with primary biliary cirrhosis.[154] This exciting preliminary report has been confirmed in a double-blind controlled study by Leuschner and colleages,[116] as well as by a dose-ranging Italian study.[153] As yet, only very limited information is available as to the effect of UDCA on liver histology.

UDCA has also been shown to cause improvement in pruritus and laboratory signs of cholestasis in patients with primary sclerosing cholangitis.[176] UDCA has also been shown to reduce pruritus, improve growth, and improve liver tests in cholestatic disease in infants.[9] The disease conditions treated include bile duct atresia or paucity as well as neonatal hepatitis. Liver tests also improve in patients with chronic active hepatitis when patients receive UDCA, but the improvement in hepatitis patients is much less than that obtained using interferon. In most of these UDCA trials, the dose of UDCA employed has been similar to that used for cholesterol gallstone dissolution—8–10 mg kg^{-1} day^{-1}.

Whether UDCA treatment will alter the natural history of these chronic cholestatic liver diseases is not known at present. It is also not known whether therapy with UDCA will prove superior to or will be a useful adjunct to other therapies being tested such as methotrexate, cyclosporin (or its successors), or colchicine. Multicentre controlled trials are being planned and executed.

The present consensus is that UDCA administration leads to enrichment of the circulating bile acids in UDCA and a consequent reciprocal decrease in the proportion of CDCA, the cytotoxic endogenous bile acid. The depletion of CDCA is explained in part by competition for ileal transport by both the administered UDCA and its circulating conjugates.[54] In addition, it is hypothesized that UDCA (as well as its conjugates) may displace cytotoxic bile acids from sites inducing organelle injury in the hepatocyte. Addition of UDCA to the incubation medium decreases CDCA-induced injury to isolated human hepatocytes[63] or human erythrocytes.[93]

In my opinion, UDCA is likely to diminish that component of hepatocyte injury caused by retention of cytotoxic endogenous bile acids. If diseases such as primary biliary cirrhosis and sclerosing cholangitis have cell-mediated cytotoxicity as the primary event in pathogenesis, then the effect of UDCA will be to diminish liver injury but not to affect the fundamental steps in the disease process. It is also possible that bile acids such as UDCA have primary effects on the immune system or that retention of cytotoxic endogenous bile acids leads to stimulation of killer cell activity. If so, UDCA therapy will have multiple effects.

TREATMENT OF CHOLESTEROL GALLSTONES WITH UDCA (see Chapter 58) _____

Cholesterol gallstones are common in the older population and are more prevalent in fertile women as well as obese men or women. The presence of gallstones is usually established by ultrasound; oral cholecystography is used to document the radiolucency of the stones and define gallbladder concentrating and evacuating function. Additional information on gallstone composition can be obtained using computerized axial tomography.

The fundamental cause of the disease is the presence of bile that is supersaturated with cholesterol in the gallbladder; accelerated nucleation of cholesterol from bile and defective gallbladder evacuation also contribute.[78] The current recommendation of experts is that only patients with symptomatic gallstones should be treated, since the majority of patients with gallstones remain asymptomatic throughout life and do not appear to have morbidity because of the presence of gallstones in the gallbladder.[174] Recent epidemiological studies have confirmed that patients with asymptomatic gallstones develop symptomatic disease at an incidence rate of 1–3% per year.[11]

Administration of UDCA or CDCA, or a combination of the two, decreases cholesterol synthesis or absorption and enriches the circulating bile acid in the compound that has been administered. With time, bile becomes unsaturated in cholesterol in virtually all patients. If cholesterol gallstones are present and are lavaged by the unsaturated bile, gallstones will slowly dissolve.[49,160,173] The median rate is a decrease in stone diameter of about 0.7 mm/month.[175]

Medical dissolution of cholesterol gallstones is useful for patients with visible multiple small radiolucent gallstones present in the gallbladder.[82,111] Single stones are best treated by extracorporeal shockwave lithotripsy before medical therapy with UDCA/CDCA is initiated.[18,168] New techniques for percutaneous or endoscopic catheterization of the gallbladder are being developed and used with instillation of organic solvents to dissolve cholesterol gallstone rapidly.[199,221] All techniques that leave the gallbladder in place will be followed by gradual recurrence of mostly asymptomatic gallstones in the years after dissolution.[41,139,209] The recurrence rate of symptomatic gallstones has not yet been determined.

The traditional technique of cholecystectomy is being complemented by laparoscopic cholecystectomy, as well as by percutaneous endoscopic techniques commonly used in urological practice for the treatment of renal stones.

Extensive reviews on the physical chemistry and biology of gallstone formation,[76,189] and of medical therapy[12,29,61,172] are available.

ACKNOWLEDGEMENT _____

Portions of some of the text have been published in similar form elsewhere.[76] The author's work is supported by NIH grants DK21506 and DK32130, as well as grants-in-aid from Medstone International, Inc., Ciba-Geigy, Inc. and the Falk Foundation, e.V., Germany. The manuscript was prepared by Vicky Huebner, BS.

REFERENCES _____

1. Aldini, R., Roda, A., Morselli Labate, A.M. *et al.* (1982) Hepatic bile acid uptake: effect of conjugation, hydroxyl and keto groups, and albumin binding. *Journal of Lipid Research,* **23,** 1167–1173.

2. Aldini, R., Roda, A., Morselli Labate, A.M. *et al.* (1986) Species differences of the hepatic uptake of bile acids. *Italian Journal of Gastroenterology,* **19,** 1–4.

3. Aldini, R., Roda, A., Simoni, P. *et al.* (1989) Uptake of bile acids by perfused rat liver: evidence of a structure-activity relationship. *Hepatology,* **10,** 840–845.

4. Amuro, Y., Endo, T., Higashino, K. *et al.* (1981) Serum, fecal and urinary bile acids in patients with mild and advanced liver cirrhosis. *Gastroenterologica Japonica,* **16,** 506–513.

5. Ananthanarayanan, M., von Dippe, P. & Levy, D. (1988) Identification of the hepatocyte Na$^+$-dependent bile acid transport protein using monoclonal antibodies. *Journal of Biological Chemistry,* **263,** 8338–8343.

6. Anwer, M.S., O'Maille, E.R.L., Hofmann, A.F. *et al.* (1985) Influence of side-chain charge on hepatic transport of bile acids and bile acid analogues. *American Journal of Physiology,* **249,** G479–G488.

7. Armstrong, G.M.J. & Carey, M.C. (1982) The hydrophobic-hydrophilic balance of bile salts. Inverse correlation between reverse high performance liquid chromatographic mobilities and micellar cholesterol-solubilizing capacities. *Journal of Lipid Research,* **23,** 70–80.

8. Balistreri, W.F., Heubi, J.E. & Suchy, F.J. (1983) Immaturity of the enterohepatic circulation in early life: factors predisposing to "physiologic" maldigestion and cholestasis. *Journal of Pediatric Gastroenterology and Nutrition,* **2,** 346–354.

9. Balistreri, W.F., A-Kader, H.H., Heubi, J.E. *et al.* (1990) Ursodeoxycholic acid (UDCA) decreases serum cholesterol levels, ameliorates symptoms, and improves biochemical parameters in pediatric patients with chronic intrahepatic cholestasis. *Gastroenterology,* **98,** A566 (abstract).

10. Ballatori, N. & Truong, A.T. (1989) Relation between biliary glutathione excretion and bile acid-independent bile flow. *American Journal of Physiology,* **256,** G22–G30.

11. Barbara, L., Festi, D., Frabboni, R. *et al.* (1988) Incidence and risk factors for gallstone disease: the "Sirmione study". *Hepatology,* **8,** 1256 (abstract).

12. Bateson, M.C. (1986) *Gallstone Disease and Its Management.* Lancaster: MTP Press.

13. Beker, S. (1983) *Diagnostic Procedures in the Evaluation of Hepatic Diseases.* New York: Alan R. Liss.

14. Bjorkhem, I. (1985) Mechanism of bile acid biosynthesis in mammalian liver. In Danielsson, H. & Sjovall, J. (eds) *Sterols and Bile Acids,* pp. 231–278. Amsterdam: Elsevier.

15. Blitzer, B.L., Terzakis, C. & Scott, K.A. (1986) Hydroxyl-bile acid exchange: a new mechanism for the uphill transport of cholate by basolateral liver plasma membrane vesicles. *Journal of Biological Chemistry,* **261,** 12042–12046.

16. Boyer, J.L. (1980) New concepts of mechanisms of hepatocyte bile formation. *Physiological Reviews,* **60,** 303–320.

17. Bremmelgaard, A. & Sjövall, J. (1980) Hydroxylation of cholic, chenodeoxycholic, and deoxycholic acids in patients with intrahepatic cholestasis. *Journal of Lipid Research,* **21,** 1072–1081.

18. Burnett, D., Ertan, A., Jones, R. *et al.* (1989) Use of external shock-wave lithotripsy and adjuvant ursodiol for treatment of radiolucent gallstones: a national multicenter study. *Digestive Diseases and Sciences,* **34,** 1011–1015.

19. Caflisch, C., Zimmerli, B., Reichen, J. & Meier, P.J. (1990) Cholate uptake in basolateral rat liver plasma membrane vesicles and in liposomes. *Biochimica et Biophysica Acta,* **1021,** 70–76.

20. Calcraft, B., LaRusso, N.F., Hofmann, A.F. & Belobaba D.T.E. (1975) Development of a simple, safe, bile acid clearance test: the radiocholate clearance test. *Gastroenterology,* **69,** 812 (abstract).

21. Campanelli, A.R., Candeloro de Sanctis, S., Giglio, E. & Scaramuzza, L. (1987) A model for micellar aggregates of a bile salt: crystal structure of sodium taurodeoxycholate monohydrate. *Journal of Lipid Research,* **28,** 483–489.

22. Campanelli, A.R., Candeloro de Sanctis, S., Chiessi, E. *et al.* (1989) Sodium glyco- and taurodeoxycholate: possible helical models for conjugated bile salt micelles. *Journal of Physical Chemistry,* **93,** 1536–1542.

23. Carey, M.C. (1985) Physico-chemical properties of bile acids and their salts. In Danielsson, H. & Sjövall, J. (eds) *Sterols and Bile Acids,* pp. 345–403. Amsterdam: Elsevier.

24. Carey, M.C. & Cohen, D.E. (1987) Biliary transport of cholesterol in vesicles, micelles and liquid crystals. In Paumgartner, G., Stiehl, A. & Gerok, W. (eds) *Bile Acids and the Liver,* pp. 287–300. Lancaster: MTP Press.

25. Chiang, J.Y., Miller, W.F. & Lin, G.M. (1990) Regulation of cholesterol 7α-hydroxylase in the liver. Purification of cholesterol 7α-hydroxylase and the immunochemical evidence for the induction of cholesterol 7α-hydroxylase by cholestyramine and circadian rhythm. *Journal of Biological Chemistry,* **265,** 3889–3897.

26. Clayton, L.M., Gurantz, D., Hofmann, A.F. *et al.* (1989) The role of bile acid conjugation in hepatic transport of dihydroxy bile acids. *Journal of Pharmacology and Experimental Therapeutics,* **248,** 1130–1137.

27. Clayton, P.T., Leonard, J.V., Lawson, A.M. *et al.* (1987) Familial giant cell hepatitis associated with synthesis of 3β,7α-dihydroxy- and 3β,7α,12α-trihydroxy-5-cholenoic acids. *Journal of Clinical Investigation,* **79,** 1031–1038.

28. Cohen, B.I., Hofmann, A.F., Mosbach, E.H. *et al.* (1986) Differing effects of nor-ursodeoxycholic or ursodeoxycholic acid on hepatic histology and bile acid metabolism in the rabbit. *Gastroenterology,* **91,** 189–197.

29. Cohen, S. & Soloway, R.D. (1985) *Gallstones.* New York: Churchill Livingstone.

30. Cowen, A.E., Korman, M.G., Hofmann, A.F. & Cass, O.W. (1975) Metabolism of lithocholate in healthy man. I. Biotransformation and biliary excretion of intravenously administered lithocholate, lithocholylglycine, and their sulfates. *Gastroenterology,* **69,** 59–66.

31. Cowen, A.E., Korman, M.G., Hofmann, A.F. *et al.* (1975) Metabolism of lithocholate in healthy man. II. Enterohepatic circulation. *Gastroenterology,* **69,** 67–76.

32. Cowen, A.E., Korman, M.G., Hofmann, A.F. & Thomas, P.J. (1975) Plasma disappearance of radioactivity after intravenous injection of labeled bile acids in man. *Gastroenterology,* **68,** 1567–1573.

33. Cravetto, C., Molino, G., Biondi, A.M. *et al.* (1985) Evaluation of the diagnostic value of serum bile acids in the detection and functional assessment of liver diseases. *Annals of Clinical Biochemistry,* **22,** 596–605.

34. Cravetto, C., Molino, G., Hofmann, A.F. *et al.* (1988) Computer simulation of portal venous shunting and other isolated hepatobiliary defects of the enterohepatic circulation of bile acids using a physiological pharmacokinetic model. *Hepatology,* **8,** 866–878.

35. Crawford, J.M. and Gollan, J.L. (1988) Hepatocyte cotransport of taurocholate and bilirubin glucuronides: role of microtubules. *American Journal of Physiology,* **255,** G121–G131.

36. Crawford, J.M., Berken, C.A. & Gollan, J.L. (1988) Role of the hepatocyte microtubular system in the excretion of bile salts and biliary lipid: implications for intracellular vesicular transport. *Journal of Lipid Research,* **29,** 144–156.

37. Danielsson, H. & Sjovall, J. (1985) *Sterols and Bile Acids.* Amsterdam: Elsevier Science Publishers.

38. Danzinger, R.G., Nakagaki, M., Hofmann, A.F. & Ljungwe, E.B. (1984) Differing effects of hydroxy-7-oxotaurine-conjugated bile acids on bile flow and biliary lipid secretion in dogs. *American Journal of Physiology,* **246,** G166–G172.

39. Deleze, G., Paumgartner, G., Karlaganis, G. *et al.* (1978) Bile acid pattern in human amniotic fluid. *European Journal of Clinical Investigation,* **8,** 41–45.

40. Dowling, R.H. (1983) Bile acids in constipation and diarrhoea. In Barbara, L., Dowling, R.H., Hofmann, A.F. & Roda, E. (eds) *Bile Acids in Gastroenterology,* pp. 157–171. Lancaster: MTP Press.

41. Dowling, R.H., Gleeson, D.C., Hood, K.A. *et al.* (1987) Gallstone recurrence and postdissolution management. In Paumgartner, G., Stiehl, A. & Gerok, W. (eds) *Bile Acids and the Liver,* pp. 355–367. Lancaster: MTP Press.

42. Duane, W.C., Holloway, D.E., Hutton, S.W. *et al.* (1982) Compari-

son of bile acid synthesis determined by isotope dilution versus fecal acidic sterol output in human subjects. *Lipids*, **17**, 345–348.

43. Duane, W.C., Hunninghake, D.B., Freeman, M.L. *et al.* (1988) Simvastatin, a competitive inhibitor of HMG-CoA reductase, lowers cholesterol saturation index of gallbladder bile. *Hepatology*, **8**, 1147–1150.

44. Dumont, M., Erlinger, S. & Uchman, S. (1980) Hypercholeresis induced by ursodeoxycholic acid and 7-ketolithocholic acid in the rat: possible role of bicarbonate transport. *Gastroenterology*, **79**, 82–89.

45. Einarsson, K., Angelin, B., Bjorkhem, I. & Glaumann, H. (1985) The diagnostic value of fasting individual serum bile acids in anicteric alcoholic liver disease: relation to liver morphology. *Hepatology*, **5**, 108–111.

46. Elliott, W.H. (1985) Metabolism of bile acids in liver and extrahepatic tissues. In Danielsson, H. and Sjovall, J. (eds) *Sterols and Bile Acids*, pp. 303–329. Amsterdam: Elsevier Science Publishers.

47. Eng, C. & Javitt, N.B. (1983) Chenodeoxycholic acid-3-sulfate. Metabolism and excretion in the rat and hamster and effects on hepatic transport systems. *Biochemistry and Pharmacology*, **32**, 3555–3558.

48. Erlinger, S. (1988) Bile flow. In Arias, I.M., Jakoby, W.B., Popper, H. *et al.* (eds) *The Liver: Biology and Pathobiology*, pp. 643–661. New York: Raven Press.

49. Erlinger, S., Le Go, A., Husson, J.M. & Fevery, J. (1984) Franco-Belgian cooperative study of ursodeoxycholic acid in the medical dissolution of gallstones: a double-blind randomized dose-response study and comparison with chenodeoxycholic acid. *Hepatology*, **4**, 308–314.

50. Ferraris, R., Colombatti, G., Fiorentini, M.T. *et al.* (1983) Diagnostic value of serum bile acids and routine liver function tests in hepatobiliary diseases. *Digestive Diseases and Sciences*, **28**, 129–136.

51. Festi, D., Morselli Labate, A.M., Roda, A. *et al.* (1983) Diagnostic effectiveness of serum bile acids in liver diseases as evaluated by multivariate statistical methods. *Hepatology*, **3**, 707–713.

52. Fieser, L.F. & Fieser, M. (1959) *Steroids*. New York: Rienhold.

53. Fini, A. & Roda, A. (1987) Chemical properties of bile acids. IV. Acidity constants of glycine-conjugated bile acids. *Journal of Lipid Research*, **28**, 755–759.

54. Fisher, R.L., Hofmann, A.F., Converse, J.L. *et al.* (1990) Lack of relationship between hepatotoxicity and lithocholic acid sulfation during chenodiol therapy in the National Cooperative Gallstone Study. *Hepatology* (in review).

55. Foberg, U., Brostrom, C., Fryden, A. *et al.* (1987) Evaluation of an oral bile acid loading test for assessment of liver function in chronic hepatitis. A comparison with fasting serum bile acids and i.v. galactose elimination test. *Liver*, **7**, 116–122.

56. Forker, E.L. (1989) Hepatic transport of organic solutes. In Schultz, S.G. (ed.) *Handbook of Physiology. The Gastrointestinal System*, pp. 693–716. Bethesda: American Physiological Society.

57. Forker, E.L. & Luxon, B.A. (1985) Effects of unstirred Disse fluid, non-equilibrium binding, and surface mediated dissociation on hepatic removal of albumin bound organic anions. *American Journal of Physiology*, **248**, 709–717.

58. Fricker, G., Schneider, S., Gerok, W. & Kurz, G. (1987) Identification of different transport systems for bile salts in sinusoidal and canalicular membranes of hepatocytes. *Biological Chemistry Hoppe-Seyler*, **368**, 1143–1150.

59. Fricker, G., Landmann, L. & Meier, P.J. (1989) Extrahepatic obstructive cholestasis reverses the bile salt secretory polarity of rat hepatocytes. *Journal of Clinical Investigation*, **84**, 876–885.

60. Frimmer, M. & Ziegler, K. (1988) The transport of bile acids in liver cells. *Biochimica et Biophysica Acta*, **947**, 75–99.

61. Fromm, H. & Malavolti, M. (1988) Dissolving gallstones. *Advances in Internal Medicine*, **33**, 409–430.

62. Fromm, H., Carlson, G.L., Hofmann, A.F. *et al.* (1980) Metabolism in man of 7-ketolithocholic acid: precursor of cheno- and ursodeoxycholic acid. *American Journal of Physiology*, **239**, G161–G166.

63. Galle, P.R., Theilmann, L., Raedsch, R. *et al.* (1990) Ursodeoxycholate reduces hepatotoxicity of glycochenodeoxycholate in primary human liver cells. Part II. *Gastroenterology*, **98**, A588 (abstract).

64. Grundy, S.M. (1983) Mechanism of cholesterol gallstone formation. *Seminars in Liver Disease*, **3**, 97–111.

65. Gu, J.-J., Ton-Nu, H.-T. & Hofmann, A.F. (1988) Nuclear hydroxylation rather than glycine conjugation determines the solubility products of calcium bile salts. *Clinical Research*, **36**, 131A (abstract).

66. Hardison, W.G.M. (1978) Hepatic taurine concentration and dietary taurine as regulators of bile acid conjugation with taurine. *Gastroenterology*, **75**, 71–75.

67. Haslewood, G.A.D. (1967) *Bile Salts*. London: Methuen.

68. Hedenborg, G., Norlander, A. & Norman, A. (1987) Bile acids in serum, ultrafiltrate of serum and saliva from patients with cholestatic jaundice. *Scandinavian Journal of Clinical and Laboratory Investigation*, **47**, 82–89.

69. Hedenborg, G., Norman, A. & Ritzen, A. (1988) Lipoprotein-bound bile acids in serum from healthy men, postprandially and during fasting. *Scandinavian Journal of Clinical and Laboratory Investigation*, **48**, 241–245.

70. Hepner, G.P., Hofmann, A.F. & Thomas, P.J. (1972) Metabolism of steroid and amino acid moieties of conjugated bile acids in man. I. Cholylglycine. *Journal of Clinical Investigation*, **51**, 1889–1897.

71. Hepner, G.W., Sturman, J.A., Hofmann, A.F. & Thomas, P.J. (1973) Metabolism of steroid and amino acid moieties of conjugated bile acids in man. III. Cholyltaurine (taurocholic acid). *Journal of Clinical Investigation*, **52**, 433–440.

72. Heubi, J.E., Balistreri, W.F., Fondacaro, J.D. *et al.* (1982) Primary bile acid malabsorption: defective in vitro ileal active bile acid transport. *Gastroenterology*, **83**, 804–811.

73. Heuman, D.M. (1989) Quantitative estimation of the hydrophilic-hydrophobic balance of mixed bile salt solutions. *Journal of Lipid Research*, **30**, 719–730.

74. Heuman, D.M., Vlahcevic, Z.R., Bailey, M.L. & Hylemon, P.B. (1988) Regulation of bile acid synthesis. II. Effect of bile acid feeding on enzymes regulating hepatic cholesterol and bile acid synthesis in the rat. *Hepatology*, **8**, 892–897.

75. Hoffman, N.E. & Hofmann, A.F. (1974) Metabolism of steroid and amino acid moieties of conjugated bile acids in man. IV. Description and validation of a multicompartmental model. *Gastroenterology*, **67**, 887–897.

76. Hofmann, A.F. (1984) The physical chemistry of bile in health and disease. *Hepatology*, **4** (suppl.), 1S–252S.

77. Hofmann, A.F. (1988) Bile acids. In Arias, I.M., Jakoby, W.B., Popper, H. *et al.* (eds) *The Liver: Biology and Pathobiology*, pp. 553–572. New York: Raven Press.

78. Hofmann, A.F. (1988) Pathogenesis of cholesterol gallstones. *Journal of Clinical Gastroenterology*, **10** (suppl.), S1–S11.

79. Hofmann, A.F. (1989) Enterohepatic circulation of bile acids. In Schultz, S.G. (ed.) *Handbook of Physiology*. Section on the Gastrointestinal System, pp. 567–596. Bethesda: American Physiological Society.

80. Hofmann, A.F. (1989) Overview of bile secretion. In Schultz, S.G. (ed.) *Handbook of Physiology*. Section on the Gastrointestinal System, pp. 549–566. Bethesda: American Physiological Society.

81. Hofmann, A.F. (1989) Bile acid hepatotoxicity and the rationale of UDCA therapy in chronic cholestatic liver disease: some hypotheses. In Paumgartner, G., Stiehl, A., Barbara, L. & Roda, E. (eds) *Strategies for the Treatment of Hepatobiliary Diseases*, pp. 13–33. Boston: Kluwer Academic Publishers.

82. Hofmann, A.F. (1989) Medical dissolution of gallstones by oral bile acid therapy. *American Journal of Surgery*, **158**, 198–204.

83. Hofmann, A.F. & Cummings, S.A. (1983) Measurement of bile acid and cholesterol kinetics in man by isotope dilution: principles and applications. In Barbara, L., Dowling, R.H., Hofmann, A.F. & Roda, E. (eds) *Bile Acids in Gastroenterology*, pp. 75–117. Lancaster: MTP Press.

84. Hofmann, A.F. & Hoffman, N.E. (1974) Measurement of bile acid kinetics by isotope dilution in man. *Gastroenterology*, **67**, 314–323.

85. Hofmann, A.F. & Mysels, K.J. (1988) Bile salts as biological surfactants. *Colloids and Surfaces*, **30**, 145–173.

86. Hofmann, A.F. & Roda, A. (1984) Physicochemical properties of bile acids and their relationship to biological properties: an overview of the problem. *Journal of Lipid Research*, **25**, 1477–1489.

87. Hofmann, A.F. & Strandvik, B. (1988) Defective bile acid amidation: predicted biochemical and clinical features of a new inborn error of metabolism. *Lancet*, **2**, 311–313.

88. Hofmann, A.F., Molino, G., Milanese, M. & Belforte, G. (1983) Description and simulation of a physiological pharmacokinetic

model for the metabolism and enterohepatic circulation of bile acids in man. Cholic acid in healthy man. *Journal of Clinical Investigation,* **71**, 1003–1022.

89. Horak, W., Waldram, R., Murray-Lyon, I.M. *et al.* (1976) Kinetics of ^{14}C-cholic acid in fulminant hepatic failure, a prognostic test. *Gastroenterology,* **71**, 809–813.

90. Hoshita, T. (1985) Bile alcohols and primitive bile acids. In Danielsson, H. & Sjövall, J. (eds) *Sterols and Bile Acids,* pp. 279–302. Amsterdam: Elsevier Science Publishers.

91. Huijghebaert, S.M. & Hofmann, A.F. (1986) Pancreatic carboxy-peptidase hydrolysis of bile acid-amino acid conjugates: selective resistance of glycine and taurine amidates. *Gastroenterology,* **90**, 306–315.

92. Huijghebaert, S.M. & Hofmann, A.F. (1986) Influence of the amino acid moiety on deconjugation of bile acid amidates by cholylglycine hydrolase or human fecal cultures. *Journal of Lipid Research,* **27**, 742–752.

93. Heuman, D.M., Pandak, W.M., Hylemon, P.B. & Vlahcevic, Z.R. (1989) Conjugates of ursodeoxycholic acid (UDC) protect human red blood cells (RBC) *in vitro* against membrane-disrupting effects of more hydrophobic bile salts (BS). *Hepatology,* **10**, 728 (abstract).

94. Heuman, D.M., Moore, E.W. & Vlahcevic, Z.R. (1990) Formation and dissolution of gallstones. In Zakim, D. & Boyer, T.D. (eds) *Hepatology: A Textbook of Liver Disease,* pp. 1480–1516. Philadelphia: W.B. Saunders.

95. Inoue, M., Kinne, R., Tran, T. & Arias, I.M. (1984) Taurocholate transport by rat liver canalicular membrane vesicles: evidence for the presence of a Na$^+$ independent transport system. *Journal of Clinical Investigation,* **73**, 659–663.

96. Islam, S., Poupon, R.E., Barbare, J.C. *et al.* (1985) Fasting serum bile acid level in cirrhosis. A semi-quantitative index of hepatic function. *Journal of Hepatology,* **1**, 609–617.

97. Javitt, N.B. & Emerman, S. (1968) Effect of sodium taurolithocholate on bile flow and bile acid excretion. *Journal of Clinical Investigation,* **47**, 1002–1014.

98. Javitt, N.B., Pfeffer, R., Kok, E. *et al.* (1989) Bile acid synthesis in cell culture. *Journal of Biological Chemistry,* **264**, 10384–10387.

99. Jazrawi, R.P., Ferraris, R., Bridges, C. & Northfield, T.C. (1988) Kinetics for the synthetic bile acid ^{75}Selenohomocholic acid-taurine in humans: comparison with [^{14}C]taurocholate. *Gastroenterology,* **95**, 164–169.

100. Jones, C., Hofmann, A.F., Mysels, K.J. & Roda, A. (1986) The effect of calcium and sodium ion concentration on the properties of dilute aqueous solutions of glycine conjugated bile salts. *Journal of Colloid and Interface Science,* **114**, 452–470.

101. Kakis, G. & Yousef, I.M. (1978) Pathogenesis of lithocholate and taurolithocholate-induced intrahepatic cholestasis in rats. *Gastroenterology,* **75**, 595–607.

102. Kadohara, M., Kawasaki, H. & Hirayama, C. (1987) Serum bile acids and oral ursodeoxycholic acid tolerance test in the diagnosis of esophageal varices. *Gastroenterologia Japonica,* **22**, 614–620.

103. Kirkpatrick, R.B., Green, M.D., Hagey, L.R. *et al.* (1988) Effect of side chain length on bile acid conjugation: glucuronidation, sulfation, and CoA formation of nor-bile acids and their natural C$_{24}$ homologues by human rat liver fractions. *Hepatology,* **8**, 353–357.

104. Kitani, K., Kanai, S., Ohta, M. & Sato, Y. (1986) Differing transport maxima values for taurine-conjugated bile salts in rats and hamsters. *American Journal of Physiology,* **251**, G852–G858.

105. Koivisto, P., Lempinen, M. & Miettinen, T.A. (1987) Fecal bile acids related to small-bowel length before and after ileal exclusion. *Scandinavian Journal of Gastroenterology,* **22**, 691–695.

106. Korman, M.G., Hofmann, A.F. & Summerskill, W.H.J. (1974) Assessment of activity in chronic active liver disease: serum bile acids compared with conventional tests and histology. *New England Journal of Medicine,* **290**, 1399–1402.

107. Korman, M.G., LaRusso, N.F., Hoffman, N.E. & Hofmann, A.F. (1975) Development of an intravenous bile acid tolerance test: plasma disappearance of cholylglycine in health. *New England Journal of Medicine,* **292**, 1205–1209.

108. Kramer, W., Bickel, U., Buscher, H.P., Gerok, W. & Kurz, G. (1982) Bile-salt-binding polypeptides in plasma membranes of hepatocytes revealed by photoaffinity labelling. *European Journal of Biochemistry,* **129**, 13–24.

109. Kuipers, F., Enserink, M., Havinga, R. *et al.* (1988) Separate transport systems for biliary secretion of sulfated and unsulfated bile acids in the rat. *Journal of Clinical Investigation,* **81**, 1593–1599.

110. Kwekkeboom, J. (1990) *Regulation of Bile Acid Synthesis in Cultured Hepatocytes.* Kanters, Alblasserdam, Netherlands.

111. Lanzini, A. & Northfield, T.C. (1990) Review article: bile acid therapy. *Alimentary Pharmacology & Therapeutics,* **4**, 1–24.

112. LaRusso, N.F., Hoffman, N.E., Hofmann, A.F. & Korman, M.G. (1975) Validity and sensitivity of an intravenous bile acid tolerance test in patients with liver disease. *New England Journal of Medicine,* **292**, 1209–1214.

113. LaRusso, N.F., Szczepanik, P.A., Hofmann, A.F. & Coffin, S.B. (1977) Effect of deoxycholic acid ingestion on bile acid metabolism and biliary lipid secretion in normal subjects. *Gastroenterology,* **72**, 132–140.

114. LaRusso, N.F., Hoffman, N.E., Korman, M.G. *et al.* (1978) Determinants of fasting and postprandial serum bile acid levels in healthy man. *American Journal of Digestive Disease,* **23**, 385–391.

115. Leuschner, U., Leuschner, M., Sieratzki, J. *et al.* (1985) Gallstone dissolution with ursodeoxycholic acid in patients with chronic active hepatitis and two years follow-up. A pilot study. *Digestive Diseases and Sciences,* **30**, 642–649.

116. Leuschner, U., Fischer, H., Kurtz, W. *et al.* (1989) Ursodeoxycholic acid in primary biliary cirrhosis: results of a controlled double-blind trial. *Gastroenterology,* **97**, 1268–1274.

117. Lindstedt, S. & Norman, A. (1956) The turnover of bile acids in the rat: Bile acids and steroids 39. *Acta Physiologica Scandinavica,* **38**, 120–128.

118. Macdonald, I.A., Bokkenheuser, V.D., Winter, J. *et al.* (1983) Degradation of steroids in the human gut. *Journal of Lipid Research,* **24**, 675–700.

119. Mannes, G.A., Stellaard, F. & Paumgartner, G. (1982) Increased serum bile acids in cirrhosis with normal transaminases. *Digestion,* **25**, 217–221.

120. Mannes, G.A., Thieme, C., Stellaard, F. *et al.* (1986) Prognostic significance of serum bile acids in cirrhosis. *Hepatology,* **6**, 50–53.

121. Marcus, S.N. & Heaton, K.W. (1986) Intestinal transit, deoxycholic acid and the cholesterol saturation of bile—three inter-related factors. *Gut,* **27**, 550–558.

122. Marcus, S.N., Schteingart, C.D., Marquez, M.L. *et al.* (1991) Active absorption of conjugated bile acid in vivo: kinetic parameters and molecular specificity of the ileal transport system in the rat. *Gastroenterology* (in press).

123. Mathis, U., Karlaganis, G. & Preisig, R. (1983) Monohydroxy bile salt sulfates: tauro-3β-hydroxy-5-cholenoate-3-sulfate induced intrahepatic cholestasis in rats. *Gastroenterology,* **85**, 674–681.

124. Matoba, N., Une, M. & Hoshita, T. (1986) Identification of unconjugated bile acids in human bile. *Journal of Lipid Research,* **27**, 1154–1162.

125. Meier, P.J. (1988) Transport polarity of hepatocytes. *Seminars in Liver Disease,* **8**, 293–307.

126. Meier, P.J., Sztul, E.S., Reuben, A. & Boyer, J.L. (1984) Structural and functional polarity of canalicular and basolateral plasma membrane vesicles isolated in high yield from rat liver. *Journal of Cell Biology,* **98**, 991–1000.

127. Miescher, G., Paumgartner, G. & Preisig, R. (1983) Portal-systemic spillover of bile acids: a study of mechanisms using ursodeoxycholic acid. *European Journal of Clinical Investigation,* **13**, 439–445.

128. Miyai, K., Price, V.M. & Fisher, M.M. (1971) Bile acid metabolism in mammals. Ultrastructural studies on the intrahepatic cholestasis induced by lithocholic and chenodeoxycholic acids in the rat. *Laboratory Investigation,* **24**, 292–302.

129. Miyai, K., Richardson, A.L., Mayr, W. & Javitt, N.B. (1977) Subcellular pathology of rat liver in cholestasis and choleresis induced by bile salts. 1. Effects of lithocholic, 3β-hydroxy-5-cholenoic, cholic, and dehydrocholic acids. *Laboratory Investigation,* **36**, 249–258.

130. Molino, G. & Milanese, M. (1975) Structural analysis of compartmental models for the hepatic kinetics of drugs. *Journal of Laboratory and Clinical Medicine,* **85**, 865–878.

131. Molino, G., Hofmann, A.F., Cravetto, C. *et al.* (1986) Simulation

of the metabolism and enterohepatic circulation of endogenous chenodeoxycholic acid in man using a physiological pharmacokinetic model. _European Journal of Clinical Investigation,_ **16,** 397–414.

132. Monroe, P.S., Baker, A.L., Schneider, J.F. _et al._ (1982) The aminopyrine breath test and serum bile acids reflect histologic severity in chronic hepatitis. _Hepatology,_ **2,** 317–322.

133. Moore, E.W. (1984) The role of calcium in the pathogenesis of gallstones: Ca^{++} electrode studies of model bile salt solutions and other biologic systems (with a hypothesis on structural requirements for Ca^{++} binding to proteins and bile acids). _Hepatology,_ **4,** 228S–243S.

134. Moore, E.W., Celic, L. & Ostrow, J.D. (1982) Interactions between ionized calcium and sodium taurocholate: bile salts are important buffers for prevention of calcium-containing gallstones. _Gastroenterology,_ **83,** 1079–1089.

135. Mueller, B.W.M. (1978) Die Charakterisierung amphiphiler Substanzen. Versuch einer Literaturubersicht. _Deutsche Apotheker Zeitung,_ **118,** 404–409.

136. Munoz, J., Rege, R., Hagey, L.R. _et al._ (1990) Novel biotransformation and choleretic activity of ursodeoxycholic acid in the dog. _Gastroenterology,_ **98,** A613 (abstract).

137. Nair, P.P. & Kritchevsky, D. (1971; 1973; 1976) _The Bile Acids, Chemistry Physiology and Metabolism,_ Vol. 1: Chemistry; Vol. 2: Physiology and Metabolism; Vol. 3: Pathophysiology. New York: Plenum Press.

138. Nilsell, K., Angelin, B., Leijd, B. & Einarsson, K. (1983) Comparative effects of ursodeoxycholic acid and chenodeoxycholic acid on bile acid kinetics and biliary lipid secretion in humans. Evidence for different modes of action on bile acid synthesis. _Gastroenterology,_ **85,** 1248–1256.

139. O'Donnell, L.D.J. & Heaton, K.W. (1988) Recurrence and re-recurrence of gall stones after medical dissolution: a longterm follow up. _Gut,_ **29,** 655–658.

140. Oelberg, D.G. & Lester, R. (1986) Cellular mechanisms of cholestasis. _Annual Review of Medicine,_ **37,** 297–317.

141. O'Maille, E.R.L. & Hofmann, A.F. (1986) Relatively high biliary secretory maximum for non-micelle-forming bile acid: possible significance for mechanism of secretion. _Quarterly Journal of Experimental Physiology,_ **71,** 475–482.

142. O'Maille, E.R.L., Richards, T.G. & Short, A.H. (1965) Acute taurine depletion and maximal rates of hepatic conjugation and secretion of cholic acid in the dog. _Journal of Physiology (London),_ **180,** 67–79.

143. O'Maille, E.R.L., Kozmary, S.V., Hofmann, A.F. & Gurantz, D. (1984) Differing effects of norcholate and cholate on bile flow and biliary lipid secretion in the rat. _American Journal of Physiology,_ **246,** G67–G71.

144. Oude Elferink, R.P.J., Ottenhoff, R., Liefting, W. _et al._ (1989) Hepatobiliary transport of glutathione and glutathione conjugate in rats with hereditary hyperbilirubinemia. _Journal of Clinical Investigation,_ **84,** 476–483.

145. Oude Elferink, R.P.J., de Haan, J., Lambert, K.J. _et al._ (1989) Selective hepatobiliary transport of nordeoxycholate side chain conjugates in mutant rats with a canalicular transport defect. _Hepatology,_ **9,** 861–865.

146. Palmer, K.R., Gurantz, D., Hofmann, A.F. _et al._ (1987) Hypercholeresis induced by nor-chenodeoxycholate in the biliary fistula rodent. _American Journal of Physiology,_ **252,** G219–G228.

147. Paumgartner, G. (1986) Serum bile acids. Physiological determinants and results in liver disease. _Journal of Hepatology,_ **2,** 291–298.

148. Paumgartner, G., Gerok, W. & Stiehl, A. (1987) _Bile Acids and the Liver._ Lancaster: MTP Press.

149. Paumgartner, G., Stiehl, A. & Gerok, W. (1989) _Trends in Bile Acid Research._ Dordrecht: Kluwer Academic Publishers.

150. Paumgartner, G., Stiehl, A., Barbara, L. & Roda, E. (1990) _Strategies for the Treatment of Hepatobiliary Diseases._ Dordrecht: Kluwer Academic Publishers.

151. Pedley, T.A., Emerson, R.G., Warner, C.L. _et al._ (1985) Treatment of cerebrotendinous xanthomatosis with chenodeoxycholic acid. _Annals of Neurology,_ **18,** 517–518.

152. Phillips, M.J., Poucell, S. & Oda, M. (1986) Mechanisms of cholestasis. _Laboratory Investigation,_ **54,** 593–608.

153. Podda, M., Ghezzi, C., Battezzati, P.M. _et al._ (1988) Ursodeoxycholic acid for chronic liver diseases. _Journal of Clinical Gastroenterology,_ **10**(suppl. 2), S25–S31.

154. Poupon, R., Poupon, R.E., Calmus, Y. _et al._ (1987) Is ursodeoxycholic acid an effective treatment for primary biliary cirrhosis? _Lancet,_ **1,** 834–836.

155. Poupon, R., Chretien, Y., Parquet, M. _et al._ (1988) Hepatic transport of bile acids in the isolated perfused rat liver. Structure–kinetic relationship. _Biochemistry and Pharmacology,_ **37,** 209–212.

156. Raedsch, R., Lauterburg, B.H. & Hofmann, A.F. (1981) Altered bile acid metabolism in primary biliary cirrhosis. _Digestive Diseases and Sciences,_ **26,** 394–401.

157. Redinger, R.N. & Small, D.M. (1972) Bile composition, bile salt metabolism and gallstones. _Archives of Internal Medicine,_ **130,** 619–630.

158. Rege, R.V. & Moore, E.W. (1986) Pathogenesis of calcium-containing gallstones. Canine ductular bile, but not gallbladder bile, is supersaturated with calcium carbonate. _Journal of Clinical Investigation,_ **77,** 21–26.

159. Roda, A. & Fini, A. (1984) Effect of nuclear hydroxy substituents on aqueous solubility and acidic strength of bile acids. _Hepatology_ (suppl.) **4,** 72S–76S.

160. Roda, E., Bazzoli, F., Morselli Labate, A.M., _et al._ (1982) Ursodeoxycholic acid vs chenodeoxycholic acid as cholesterol gallstone-dissolving agents: a comparative randomized study. _Hepatology,_ **2,** 804–810.

161. Roda, A., Cappelleri, G., Aldini, R. _et al._ (1982) Quantitative aspects of the interaction of bile acids with human serum albumin. _Journal of Lipid Research,_ **23,** 490–495.

162. Roda, A., Hofmann, A.F. & Mysels, K.J. (1983) The influence of bile salt structure on self-association in aqueous solutions. _Journal of Biological Chemistry,_ **258,** 6362–6370.

163. Roda, A., Festi, D., Armanino, C. _et al._ (1989) Methodological and clinical aspects of bile acid analysis in biological fluids. _Progress in Clinical Biochemistry and Medicine,_ **8,** 131–173.

164. Roda, A., Grigolo, B., Minutello, A. _et al._ (1990) Physicochemical and biological properties of natural and synthetic C-22 and C-23 hydroxylated bile acids. _Journal of Lipid Research,_ **31,** 289–298.

165. Rossi, S.S., Clayton, L.M. & Hofmann, A.F. (1986) Determination of chenodiol bioequivalence using an immobilized multi-enzyme bioluminescence technique. _Journal of Pharmaceutical Science,_ **75,** 288–290.

166. Rossi, S.S., Converse, J.L. & Hofmann, A.F. (1987) High pressure liquid chromatographic analysis of conjugated bile acids in human bile: simultaneous resolution of sulfated and unsulfated lithocholyl amidates and the common conjugated bile acids. _Journal of Lipid Research,_ **28,** 589–595.

167. Rossi, S.S., Wayne, M.L., Smith, R.B. _et al._ (1989) Effect of the bile acid sequestrant colestipol on postprandial serum bile acid levels: evaluation by bioluminescent enzymatic analysis. _Alimentary Pharmacology & Therapeutics,_ **3,** 41–46.

168. Sackmann, M., Delius, M., Sauerbruch, T. _et al._ (1988) Shock-wave lithotripsy of gallbladder stones. The first 175 patients. _New England Journal of Medicine,_ **318,** 292–297.

169. Sacquet, F., Parquet, M., Riotto, M. _et al._ (1983) Intestinal absorption, excretion, and biotransformation of hyodeoxycholic acid in man. _Journal of Lipid Research,_ **24,** 604–613.

170. Samuelsson, K., Aly, A., Johansson C. _et al._ (1981) Evaluation of fasting serum bile acid concentration in patients with liver and gastrointestinal disorder. _Scandinavian Journal of Gastroenterology,_ **16,** 225–234.

171. Schalm, S.W., LaRusso, N.F., Hofmann, A.F. _et al._ (1978) Diurnal serum levels of primary conjugated bile acids. Assessment by specific radioimmunoassays for conjugates of cholic and chenodeoxycholic acid. _Gut,_ **19,** 1006–1014.

172. Schoenfield, L.J. (1988) Gallstones. _Clinical Symposia (Ciba-Geigy)_ **40,** 2–32.

173. Schoenfield, L.J., Lachin, J.M., the Steering Committee & the National Cooperative Gallstone Study Group (1981) Chenodiol (chenodeoxycholic acid) for dissolution of gallstones: The National Cooperative Gallstone Study. _Annals of Internal Medicine,_ **95,** 257–282.

174. Schoenfield, L.J., Carulli, N., Dowling, R.H. _et al._ (1989)

Asymptomatic gallstones: definition and treatment. *Gastroenterology International*, **2**, 25–29.

175. Senior, J.R., Johnson, M.F., DeTurck, D.M. *et al.* (1990) In vivo kinetics of radiolucent gallstone dissolution by oral ursodiol or chenodiol. *Gastroenterology* (in press).

176. Senior, J., O'Brien, C., Saul, S. *et al.* (1990) Ursodeoxycholic acid in the treatment of primary sclerosing cholangitis: the Philadelphia experience, 1988–9. In Paumgartner, G., Stiehl, A., Barbara, L. & Roda, E. (eds) *Strategies for the Treatment of Hepatobiliary Diseases*, pp. 97–103. Boston: Kluwer Academic Publishers.

177. Setchell, K.D.R. (1990) Disorders of bile acid synthesis. In Walker, W.A., Durie, P.R., Hamilton, J.R. *et al.* (eds) *Pediatric Gastrointestinal Disease, Pathophysiology, Diagnosis, Management*. Philadelphia: B. C. Dekker, Inc. (in press).

178. Setchell, K.D.R. & Matsui, A. (1983) Serum bile acid analysis. *Clinica Chimica Acta*, **127**, 1–17.

179. Setchell, K.D.R. & Vestal, C.H. (1989) Termospray ionization liquid chromatography-mass spectrometry: a new and highly specific technique for the analysis of bile acids. *Journal of Lipid Research*, **30**, 1459–1469.

180. Setchell, K.D.R., Suchy, F.J., Welsh, M.B. *et al.* (1989) A new inborn error in bile acid synthesis—Δ^4-3-oxosteroid-5β-reductase deficiency described in identical twins with neonatal hepatitis. In Paumgartner, G., Stiehl, A. & Gerok, W. (eds) *Trends in Bile Acid Research*, pp. 197–206. Boston: Kluwer Academic Publishers.

181. Shefer, S., Salen, G., Hauser, S. *et al.* (1982) Metabolism of iso-bile acids in the rat. *Journal of Biological Chemistry*, **257**, 1401–1406.

182. Shimizu, S., Sabsay, B., Veis, A. *et al.* (1989) Isolation of an acidic protein from cholesterol gallstones, which inhibits the precipitation of calcium carbonate in vitro. *Journal of Clinical Investigation*, **84**, 1990–1996.

183. Shinoda, K., Nakagawa, T., Tamamushi, B. & Isemure, T. (1963) *Colloidal Surfactants, Some Physical Chemistry Properties*. New York: Academic Press.

184. Simon, F.R. & Reichen, J. (1982) Bile secretory failure: recent concepts of the pathogenesis of intrahepatic cholestasis. *Progress in Liver Disease*, **7**, 179–194.

185. Sjövall, J. (1983) Gas chromatography-mass spectrometry in studies of steroids, bile acids and bile alcohols. *Proceedings of the Japanese Society of Medicine and Mass Spectrometry*, **8**, 29–46.

186. Skrede, S., Bjorkhem, I., Buchmann, M.S. *et al.* (1985) A novel pathway for biosynthesis of cholestanol with 7α-hydroxylated C27-steroids as intermediates, and its importance for the accumulation of cholestanol in cerebrotendinous xanthomatosis. *Journal of Clinical Investigation*, **75**, 448–455.

187. Stange, E.F., Scheibner, J. & Ditschuneit, H. (1989) Role of primary and secondary bile acids as feedback inhibitors of bile acid synthesis in the rat in vivo. *Journal of Clinical Investigation*, **84**, 173–180.

188. Strasberg, S.M. & Harvey, P.R.C. (1990) The pathogenesis of cholesterol gallstones: vesicles and substances affecting their stability in bile. In Paumgartner, G., Stiehl, A., Barbara, L. & Roda, E. (eds) *Strategies for the Treatment of Hepatobiliary Diseases*, pp. 109–118. Dordrecht: Kluwer Academic Publishers.

189. Strasberg, S.M. & Hofmann, A.F. (1990) Frontiers in gallstone formation: biliary cholesterol transport and precipitation. *Hepatology*, **12** (suppl.) 1S–244S.

190. Stellaard, F., Klein, P.D., Hofmann, A.F. & Lachin, J.M. (1985) Mass spectrometry identification of biliary bile acids in bile from gallstone patients before and during treatment with chenodeoxycholic acid. An ancillary study of the National Cooperative Gallstone Study (NCGS). *Journal of Laboratory and Clinical Medicine*, **105**, 504–513.

191. Stellaard, F., Pratschke, E. & Paumgartner, G. (1989) Effects of cholecystectomy on kinetics of primary and secondary bile acids. *Journal of Clinical Investigation*, **83**, 1541–1550.

192. Stiehl, A. (1977) Disturbances of bile acid metabolism in cholestasis. *Clinics in Gastroenterology*, **6**, 45–67.

193. Tabibian, N. & Reynolds, T.B. (1987) Serum bile acid determination for assessing patency of portosystemic shunts. Lack of value. *Archives of Internal Medicine*, **147**, 911–912.

194. Takikawa, H., Otsuka, H., Beppu, T. & Seyama Y. (1985) Determination of 3β-hydroxy-5-cholenoic acid in serum of hepato-biliary diseases—its glucuronidated and sulfated conjugates. *Biochemical Medicine*, **33**, 393–400.

195. Takikawa, H., Seyama, Y., Sugiyama, Y. & Nagase, S. (1985) Bile acid profiles in analbuminemia rats. *Journal of Biochemistry*, **97**, 199–203.

196. Takikawa, H., Stolz, A. & Kaplowitz, N. (1986) Purification of a 32.5 kDa monomeric sulfotransferase from rat liver with activity for bile acids and phenolic steroids. *FEBS Letters*, **207**, 193–197.

197. Takikawa, H., Stolz, A. & Kaplowitz, N. (1987) Cyclical oxidation–reduction of the C_3 position on bile acids catalyzed by rat hepatic 3α-hydroxysteroid dehydrogenase. I. Studies with the purified enzyme, isolated rat hepatocytes, and inhibition by indomethacin. *Journal of Clinical Investigation*, **80**, 852–860.

198. Tazawa, Y., Yamada, M., Nakagawa, M. *et al.* (1985) Bile acid profiles in siblings with progressive intrahepatic cholestasis: absence of biliary chenodeoxycholate. *Journal of Pediatric Gastroenterology and Nutrition*, **4**, 32–37.

199. Thistle, J.L., May, G.R., Bender, C.E. *et al.* (1989) Dissolution of cholesterol gallbladder stones by methyl tert-butyl ether administered by percutaneous transhepatic catheter. *New England Journal of Medicine*, **320**, 633–638.

200. Ugele, B., Kempen, H.J.M., Gebhardt, R. *et al.* (1989) Heterogeneous distribution of cholesterol 7α-hydroxylase among periportal and perivenous hepatocytes. In Paumgartner, G., Stiehl, A. & Gerok, W. (eds) *Trends in Bile Acid Research*, pp. 53–61. Dordrecht: Kluwer Academic Publishers.

201. van Berge Henegouwen, G.P. & Hofmann, A.F. (1977) Pharmacology of chenodeoxycholic acid. II. Absorption and metabolism. *Gastroenterology*, **73**, 300–309.

202. van Berge Henegouwen, G.P. & Hofmann, A.F. (1978) Nocturnal gallbladder storage and emptying in gallstone patients and healthy subjects. *Gastroenterology*, **75**, 879–885.

203. van Berge Henegouwen, G.P. & Hofmann, A.F. (1983) Systemic spill-over of bile acids. *European Journal of Clinical Investigation*, **13**, 433–437.

204. van Berge Henegouwen, G.P., Brandt, K.-H., Eyssen, H. & Parmentier, G. (1976) Sulfated and unsulfated bile acids in serum, bile and urine of patients with cholestasis. *Gut*, **17**, 861–869.

205. van Berge Henegouwen, G.P., Hofmann, A.F. & Gaginella, T.S. (1977) Pharmacology of chenodeoxycholic acid. I. Pharmaceutical properties. *Gastroenterology*, **73**, 291–299.

206. Van Dyke, R.W., Stephen, J.E. & Scharschmidt, B.F. (1982) Bile acid transport in cultured rat hepatocytes. *American Journal of Physiology*, **243**, G484–G492.

207. Verkade, H.J., Wolbers, M.J., Havinga, R., Uges, D.R.A., Vonk, R.J. & Kuipers, F. (1990) The uncoupling of biliary lipid from bile acid secretion by organic anions in the rat. *Gastroenterology*, **99**, 1485–1492.

208. Vessey, D.A. (1978) The biochemical basis for the conjugation of bile acids with either glycine or taurine. *Biochemical Journal*, **174**, 621–626.

209. Villanova, N., Bazzoli, F., Taroni, F. *et al.* (1989) Gallstone recurrence after successful oral bile acid treatment. A 12-year follow-up study and evaluation of long-term postdissolution treatment. *Gastroenterology*, **97**, 726–731.

210. Vierling, J.M., Berk, P.D., Hofmann, A.F. *et al.* (1982) Normal fasting-state levels of serum cholyl-conjugated bile acids in Gilbert's syndrome: an aid to the diagnosis. *Hepatology*, **2**, 340–343.

211. Vlahcevic, Z.R., Juttijudata, P., Bell, C.C., Jr & Swell, L. (1972) Bile acid metabolism in patients with cirrhosis. II. Cholic and chenodeoxycholic acid metabolism. *Gastroenterology*, **62**, 1174–1181.

212. von Bergmann, K., Mok, H.Y., Hardison, W.G.M. & Grundy, S.M. (1979) Cholesterol and bile acid metabolism in moderately advanced stable cirrhosis of the liver. *Gastroenterology*, **77**, 1183–1192.

213. Weinberg, S.L., Burckhardt, G. & Wilson, F.A. (1986) Taurocholate transport by rat intestinal basolateral membrane vesicles. Evidence for the presence of an anion exchange transport system. *Journal of Clinical Investigation*, **78**, 44–50.

214. Weinman, S.A., Graf, J. & Boyer, J.L. (1989) Voltage-driven, taurocholate-dependent secretion in isolated hepatocyte couplets. *American Journal of Physiology*, **256**, G826–G832.

215. Williams, R.T. (1959) *Detoxication Mechanisms*. London: Chapman & Hall.
216. Wilson, F.A. (1981) Intestinal transport of bile acids. *American Journal of Physiology*, **4**, G83–G92.
217. Xia, Y., Lambert, K.J., Schteingart, C.D. *et al.* (1990) Concentrative biliary secretion of ceftriaxone: inhibition of lipid secretion and precipitation of calcium ceftriaxone in bile. *Gastroenterology*, **99**, 454–465.
218. Yanagisawa, J., Ho, M., Ishibashi, M. *et al.* (1980) Microanalysis of bile acid in human liver by selected ion monitoring. *Analytical Biochemistry*, **104**, 75–86.
219. Yoon, Y.B., Hagey, L.R., Hofmann, A.F. *et al.* (1986) Effects of side-chain shortening on the physiological properties of bile acids: hepatic transport and effect on biliary secretion of 23-nor-ursodeoxycholate in rodents. *Gastroenterology*, **90**, 837–852.
220. Yousef, I.M., Tuchweber, B., Vonk, R.J. *et al.* (1981) Lithocholate cholestasis—sulfated glycolithocholate-induced intrahepatic cholestasis in rats. *Gastroenterology*, **80**, 233–241.
221. Zakko, S.F., Ramsby, G.R., Srb, S.M. & Guttermuth, C.F. (1990) Automatic computerized solvent litholysis (ACSL) for gallbladder stones: Experience with methyl tert-butyl ether (MTBE) and a microprocessor-assisted solvent transfer (MST) system. *Gastroenterology*, **98**, A647 (abstract).
222. Zellweger, H., Maertens, P., Superneau, D. & Wertelecki, W. (1988) History of the cerebrohepatorenal syndrome of Zellweger and other peroxisomal disorders. *Southern Medical Journal*, **81**, 357–364.
223. Zimmerli, B., Valantinas, J. & Meier, P.J. (1989) Multispecificity of Na^+-dependent taurocholate uptake in basolateral (sinusoidal) rat liver plasma membrane vesicles. *Journal of Pharmacology and Experimental Therapeutics*, **250**, 301–308.

CHAPTER 14

Bilirubin Metabolism and Hyperbilirubinaemic Disorders

Stephen Crane Hauser and John Gollan

Bilirubin is the principal waste product resulting from the degradation of haem in mammals. Its formation reflects the continuing turnover of haem and essential haemoproteins, such as haemoglobin, myoglobin and hepatic cytochromes. Under physiological conditions, the overall rate of bilirubin formation and the rate of haem synthesis are comparable. In humans, the relatively low plasma bilirubin concentration observed under physiological conditions (5.1 to 17.1 μmol/l; 0.3 to 1.0 mg/100 ml)[109] represents a balance between the rate of production and the hepatic clearance of bilirubin. Consequently, enhanced production of bilirubin or its impaired handling in the liver, caused by abnormalities of uptake, conjugation or secretion of the pigment into bile, are manifest by hyperbilirubinaemia. Jaundice (icterus) becomes clinically apparent as yellow coloration of the sclerae, mucous membranes and skin when the plasma bilirubin concentration has reached values in excess of 50 μmol/l (3 mg/100 ml). When hyperbilirubinaemia develops abruptly, the appearance of jaundice may lag one to two days behind the rise in plasma bilirubin concentration. Although hyperbilirubinaemia *per se* only rarely results in secondary tissue damage (in the form of encephalopathy, haemolysis or renal tubular dysfunction), it is of considerable clinical and pathophysiological interest as a manifestation of a variety of inherited and acquired disease processes. In addition, a basic understanding of bilirubin metabolism has direct application to the hepatic transport of other organic anions or xenobiotics which share similar pathways of metabolism and excretion.

In this chapter, consideration will be given primarily to the recent developments and evolving concepts in bilirubin metabolism, to the pathophysiology of jaundice, and to the various clinical disorders of bilirubin metabolism, with emphasis on the hereditary syndromes. Other comprehensive discussions of various aspects of bilirubin metabolism and hyperbilirubinaemia have recently been published.[25, 53,54,67,81,82,84,98,162,189,251,295,301,319,349,436,568,569,619,634,644, 648,650,784]

BILIRUBIN METABOLISM

PHYSICOCHEMICAL PROPERTIES OF BILIRUBIN

Bilirubin consists of four pyrrole rings linked by three carbon bridges (a central —CH_2— and two outer —CH groups). In the vast majority of naturally occurring mammalian bile pigments, the sequence of the four methyl, two vinyl and two propionic acid side-chains is the same, since they are formed by cleavage of the cyclic tetrapyrrole ferroprotoporphyrin IX (haem) at the α-methene bridge position (i.e. between the pyrrole rings bearing the vinyl groups). Spectroscopic and x-ray crystallographic studies have demonstrated that crystalline bilirubin-IXα is not a linear tetrapyrrole as typically illustrated in Figure 14.1a, but rather an involuted structure, with a ridge-tile conformation (Figure 14.1b).[115,461] The double bonds adjacent to the two outer rings are constrained to a Z,Z configuration, and the hydrophilic —COOH and —NH groups are linked by strong intramolecular hydrogen bonds, both in the solid state and in solution (at least in nonpolar solvents).[483] This hydrogen bonding shields the hydrophilic sites that could otherwise interact with polar solvents, and hence the naturally occurring bilirubin-IXα (Z,Z) is virtually insoluble in water (approximately 0.1 μmol/l at pH 7.4),[134] but is surprisingly lipid soluble and soluble in non-polar organic solvents such as chloroform and dimethylsulphoxide.[486] In alkaline solution, the six intramolecular bonds are opened and several hydrophilic sites are exposed, forming the divalent anion and giving rise to greatly enhanced solubility in polar solvents.

In strong acids or in moderately alkaline solutions, particularly in the presence of oxygen or light, the bilirubin-IXα anion may be cleaved at the central —CH_2— bridge and the nonidentical left and right halves may then spontaneously reunite at random (dipyrrole exchange). This leads to formation in vitro of the symmetric IIIα and XIIIα isomers,[487] both of which are found as minor constituents in commercial bilirubin preparations. In vitro, bilirubin glucuronides are also susceptible to dipyrrole exchange, so that two moles of bilirubin monoglucuronide

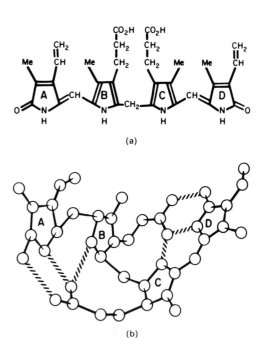

Figure 14.1 Structure of bilirubin-IXα. (a) Conventionally written structure. (b) Involuted hydrogen-bonded structure. In (b), the propionic acid groups of pyrrole rings B and C are linked to the nitrogens of the opposite pyrrole rings (interrupted lines). (Reprinted by permission of Elsevier Science Publishing Co., Inc. from Schmid.[644] Copyright 1978 by The American Gastroenterological Association.)

(BMG) can recombine to form one mole of unconjugated bilirubin and one of bilirubin diglucuronide (BDG). In mammals, very small amounts of haem may be cleaved at the non-α carbon bridge positions, giving rise to β-, γ- and δ-isomers of bilirubin-IX, which appear in trace amounts in the bile.[102,114] Characterization of these isomeric pigments has shown that, in contrast to bilirubin-IXα, they are unable to form intramolecular hydrogen bonds and, as a result of their increased polarity, are largely excreted in bile as unconjugated pigments.[101] It has been shown recently that rotation of either of the outer pyrrole rings of bilirubin-IXα at the double bonds gives rise to geometric isomers which differ physically from the normal Z,Z configuration.[137,493] Indeed, when bilirubin-IXα (Z,Z) is exposed to light of the appropriate wavelength (400–500 nm), it undergoes photoisomerization to the more polar and thermodynamically less stable Z,E, E,Z and E,E isomers.[437,489,697] Since intramolecular hydrogen bonding is absent in these geometric isomers, this appears to be the mechanism whereby unconjugated bilirubin-IXα is excreted in the bile of hyperbilirubinaemic infants[474] and Gunn rats during phototherapy[488,491,566,697] (see later).

Although bilirubin-IXα (Z,Z) accounts for most of the excreted bile pigments in mammals, it cannot be secreted into bile in its unconjugated form. This problem has been circumvented by the development of an efficient conjugating mechanism in the liver, which enzymatically converts the lipid-soluble, internally hydrogen-bonded pigment to more polar and readily excreted carbohydrate esters, particularly glucuronides. The esterification of bilirubin-IXα occurs on the propionic side-chains and disrupts the intramolecular hydrogen bonds of the COOH groups so that the central —CH$_2$— bridge is exposed, rendering the pigment less stable and more susceptible to autoxidation.[260] Physiological properties of the bilirubin-IXα conjugates and presumably of the water-soluble bilirubin isomers, such as IXβ, IXγ, IXδ and IXα (E,E), which do not form intramolecular hydrogen bonds, are strikingly different from those of bilirubin-IXα (Z,Z). In contrast to the water-soluble conjugates which are excreted as such in bile or urine, unconjugated bilirubin-IXα diffuses freely across most biological membranes such as the blood–brain barrier,[208] placenta,[492,640] and intestinal and gallbladder epithelium.[448,565] Thus, conjugation confers on the pigment the properties that inhibit its intestinal re-absorption and permit its elimination from the body. Moreover, bilirubin encephalopathy is never seen in conjugated hyperbilirubinaemia, regardless of the plasma level. Although bile pigments previously have been considered either potentially toxic or useless compounds, recent investigations raise the possible beneficial role of bilirubin as a potent endogenous antioxidant in mammalian tissues.[125,693,694]

SOURCES OF BILIRUBIN

Daily bilirubin production in adults measured by endogenous carbon monoxide (CO) production[172,438,439] or in turnover studies with radiolabelled bilirubin[61] averages 250–350 mg or 4.4 ± 0.7 (mean ± SE) mg/kg. Since haem is degraded in vivo to yield equimolar amounts of bilirubin and CO, the measurement of CO production in healthy persons reflects the total body haem turnover, whereas plasma bilirubin turnover measures only that pigment fraction which enters the plasma compartment prior to excretion and hence fails to account for the bilirubin fraction formed in the liver from turnover of intrinsic haem compounds, which is excreted directly into the bile.[189,393,417] Plasma bilirubin turnover studies yield values, therefore, which are slightly lower than those calculated from the rate of CO production.[63]

The prosthetic haem moiety of haemoglobin is the major source of bilirubin and in humans accounts for about 70% of the excreted pigment. All mammalian cells contain varying amounts of haem in the form of haemoproteins (e.g. mitochondrial and microsomal cytochromes) which are essential for aerobic metabolism. With the notable exception of the liver, the tissue concentrations of these haemoproteins are so low or their rates of turnover so slow (e.g. myoglobin) that their contribution to total bilirubin production is insignificant. Evidence for non-erythroid sources of bilirubin was first provided by injection of the haem precursor glycine, isotopically labelled, into humans.[320,469] The label was recovered in faecal stercobilin and, as expected, the major

Table 14.1 Sources of bilirubin

Origin	Bilirubin excretion after injection of radiolabelled haem precursor (glycine or δ-aminolaevulinic acid)
Catabolism of haemoglobin	
Senescent red blood cells (reticuloendothelial system: accounts for about 70% of total production)	Late peak (100–140 days)
Destruction of newly formed red cells (bone marrow or spleen)	Early-labelled bilirubin (ELB) fraction; second component
Blood extravasations, e.g. subcutaneous haematomas (macrophages)	Variable
Intravascular haemolysis (hepatocytes and renal tubules)	Variable
Turnover of non-erythroid haem and haemoproteins	
Cytochrome P450, tryptophan pyrrolase, catalase and other haemoproteins (hepatocytes)	ELB; first component
'Free' haem pool (hepatocytes and bone marrow)	ELB; initial phase of first component

peak of labelled stercobilin excretion corresponded to the destruction of senescent erythrocytes (100–140 days), but between 10 and 20% of the labelled pigment appeared within the first few days after administration of the glycine. Further studies established that production of this 'early-labelled bilirubin' (ELB) begins within minutes of administration of the labelled precursor, achieves maximum levels in 1–3 h, and subsequently declines asymptotically over a period of several days.[649] Using isotopically labelled δ-aminolaevulinic acid (ALA), which is preferentially incorporated into the haem of liver cells rather than into haemoglobin of maturing erythroid cells in bone marrow, the existence of at least two ELB components (Table 14.1) has been demonstrated.[608,611,694,798] The initial component appears to be derived largely from haemoproteins and haem in the liver, and the second component predominantly from the premature destruction of newly formed erythrocytes, either in the marrow or soon after their release into the circulation. The latter fraction appears to be responsible for only a minor fraction of the ELB in normal rats or humans.[607]

Initial estimates of the hepatic contribution to total bilirubin production in normal subjects ranged from 10 to 20%,[607] but recent observations suggest that this fraction may be greater than had previously been assumed, ranging between 23 and 37%.[65,393,417] Although it appears that the initial ELB component itself may comprise several phases, it has not yet been possible to equate these with specific haem or haemoprotein compounds in the liver. It is assumed that hepatic bilirubin is formed primarily from turnover of the microsomal cytochromes P450 and b_5, catalase, tryptophan pyrrolase and mitochondrial cytochrome b. *A priori*, cytochrome P450, which mediates the oxidative biotransformation of many lipophilic compounds,[291] would be expected to provide a major contribution, as it has been estimated in the rat that this haemoprotein accounts for at least 70% of the total haem synthesized in the liver.[485] Moreover, when hepatic cytochrome P450 synthesis is accelerated by treatment with xenobiotics, the shape and size of the ELB peak is significantly altered.[457,652] Catalase is the only other hepatic haemoprotein which is likely to provide a major contribution to ELB formation, since it has a relatively short biological half-life and is a tetramer containing four haem groups.[443] Analysis of the early phase of the ELB peak indicates that the hepatocytes[239,457] and the developing erythroid cells[799,800] contain small cytosolic pools of 'free' haem (Table 14.1), which have rapid turnover rates (60–90 min) exceeding those of any known haemoproteins.[89,518,694] This pool, which probably represents haem, newly formed in the mitochondria, in transit to the subcellular sites of haemoprotein synthesis,[642] acts both as a regulatory pool for new haem synthesis and a precursor pool for formation of hepatic haemoproteins.[90,318] When haem is administered intravenously, it is rapidly taken up by the liver and incorporated into the 'free' haem pool,[238] from where it is either converted to bilirubin[239] or incorporated into microsomal[183] or cytosolic[184,242] haemoproteins.

Although the latter component(s) of ELB is also derived largely from turnover of hepatic haem, the normally small erythropoietic fraction may increase in magnitude and distort the shape of the ELB peak when erythropoiesis is accelerated or abnormal. In clinical disorders associated with premature destruction of developing young erythroid cells ('ineffective erythropoiesis'),[339,609] such as the megaloblastic anaemias, iron deficiency anaemia, sideroblastic anaemia, thalassaemia minor, congenital erythropoietic porphyria and lead poisoning, between 30 and 80% of the faecal bile pigments may originate from this source. As might be expected, a decreased erythropoietic contribution to the ELB peak is observed in patients with aplastic anaemia.[37]

FORMATION OF BILIRUBIN

In humans, most normal erythrocytes are sequestered from the circulation after approximately 120 days by the reticuloendothelial cells (mononuclear phagocytic cells) of the spleen, liver, or bone marrow. Intracellular (extravascular) lysis follows within minutes and the degradation of haemoglobin then proceeds within the phagocytic cells. In haemolytic states or after splenectomy, the role of the hepatic sinusoidal cells in erythrocyte removal is enhanced.[91,378]

In contrast to intact senescent or modified red cells, which are sequestered and catabolized by the reticuloendothelial system, free haemoglobin, whether released into the plasma by intravascular haemolysis or administered intravenously, is taken up predominantly by hepatic parenchymal cells and converted to bile pigment.[91,354,796] The hepatic parenchymal cells are also largely responsible for uptake of the haem moiety of haptoglobin-bound haemoglobin, methaemoglobin, methaemalbumin, haemin, and haem-haemopexin.[87,517] It is likely that a fraction of the bilirubin formed in parenchymal cells, following the removal of haem from the circulation, is not secreted directly into bile, but first refluxes back into the plasma bilirubin pool, as occurs for the initial component of ELB[392,417] or following the infusion of haem[239] or biliverdin.[305] In the presence of severe intravascular haemolysis, when the plasma haptoglobin-binding capacity is exceeded, free haemoglobin is filtered by the glomeruli and then partially re-absorbed and degraded by the proximal tubular cells of the kidney.[143] Thus, the parenchymal cells of both the liver and kidney assume importance as sites of bilirubin formation in the presence of intravascular haemolysis.[586] The observation that significant haemoglobinaemia or methaemalbuminaemia is unusual in haemolytic states, whereas unconjugated hyperbilirubinaemia is relatively common, indicates that the rate of haem degradation generally exceeds the rate of haemoglobin release and probably also exceeds the maximum rate of bilirubin clearance by the liver.[649]

When haemoglobin is catabolized, the globin moiety is degraded and the products are returned to the amino acid pool. The remaining ferroprotoporphyrin ring is cleaved by oxidative cleavage of the α-meso-bridge carbon atom, which is eliminated as CO (Figure 14.2). The haem iron is transferred to iron-carrying proteins (i.e. transferrin and ferritin) and partially re-utilized for haem synthesis. A specific haem-cleaving enzyme, microsomal haem oxygenase,[416,716] has been identified and found to be most active in those tissues which are normally concerned with the degradation of haem. Haem oxygenase activity in the liver, spleen, bone marrow, macrophages, renal tubules and brain (choroid plexus) can be stimulated 3-fold to 20-fold by the administration of haem or haemoglobin.[366,586,667,718] This substrate-mediated enzyme induction provides an efficient adaptive mechanism to catabolize the increased amounts of haemoglobin released in haemolytic disorders or internal haemorrhage (e.g. subcutaneous, pleural or subarachnoid).

Haem oxygenase purified to apparent homogeneity from microsomes of pig[805,806] and bovine[810] spleen, and rat liver[807] has a minimum M_r of 32 000. The enzyme is synthesized on free polysomes and subsequently incorporated into rough and smooth microsomal membranes, the specific activity being higher in the latter.[668] Recent investigation suggests the existence of a second haem oxygenase which is functionally identical to but biochemi-

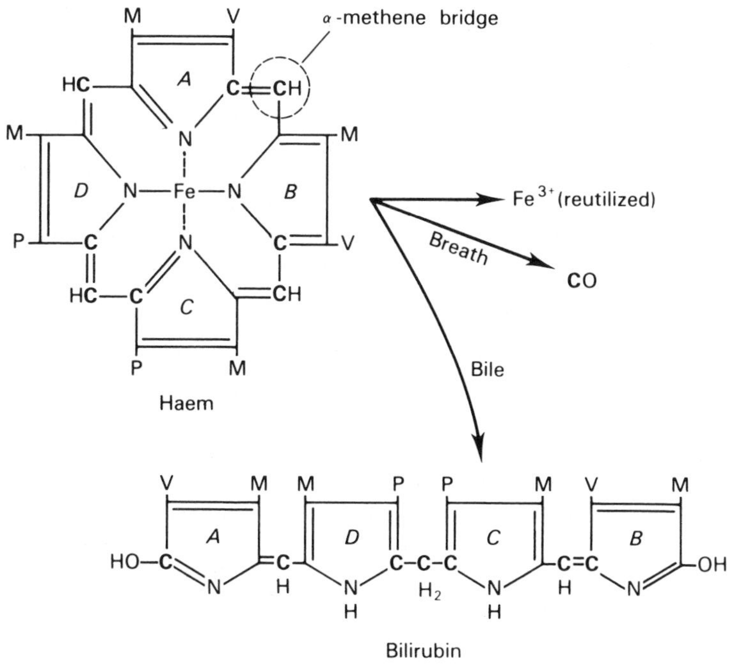

Figure 14.2 Conversion of protohaem IX to bilirubin-IXα. Cleavage of the α-methene bridge results in formation of equimolar amounts of iron carbon monoxide and bilirubin-IXα. (From Schmid,[643] with kind permission of the editor of *Transactions of the Association of American Physicians*.)

cally different from the first haem oxygenase.[193] Haem oxygenase appears to be distinct from cytochrome P450,[806,807] even though both are terminal oxidases of the microsomal electron transport system. The finding of an inverse relationship between the level of cytochrome P450 and haem oxygenase activity in a variety of experimental systems suggests that the former may be indirectly involved in haem catabolism. Microsomal haem oxygenase exhibits a relatively high degree of substrate specificity and tends to be most active with free haem or haem loosely associated with protein (e.g. methaemalbumin). In addition, the catalytic site of haem oxygenase recognizes some metalloporphyrins with central metal atoms other than iron;[404] thus, synthetic haem analogues, such as tin- and chromium-protoporphyrin[217,218,403,595] appear to act as competitive inhibitors of the haem oxygenase reaction (which is rate-limiting in the overall conversion of haem to bilirubin). Since these synthetic metalloporphyrins are not degraded to bilirubin, one possible consequence of this competitive inhibition, which has been observed in vitro in rat liver, spleen and kidney,[217] is diminished bilirubin formation. Another result of haem oxygenase blockade is a marked and rapid excretion of haem into bile.[675]

The administration of tin-protoporphyrin results in suppression of neonatal hyperbilirubinaemia in rat and monkey,[217,219] and this compound appears to persist in tissues, including the brain,[220] for prolonged periods[8] while remaining relatively innocuous.[404] In normal human volunteers, administration of tin-protoporphyrin decreased serum and biliary bilirubin concentrations and enhanced the excretion of endogenous haem in bile.[51,405] Not all metalloporphyrins behave alike: cobaltic-protoporphyrin inhibits haem oxygenase, but it also

induces haem oxygenase synthesis, and the latter action predominates.[630]

Further investigation of the mechanism responsible for the decrease in plasma bilirubin levels and more extensive evaluation of potential toxicity (e.g. photosensitization) are necessary before tin-protoporphyrin is indicated for treatment of severe neonatal jaundice.[490,691]

Activity of haem oxygenase is dependent on molecular oxygen (3 moles of O_2 are consumed per mole of haem degraded) and NADPH, with the latter being regenerated by microsomal NADPH-cytochrome c reductase.[717,808,811] Although some details of the haem oxygenase reaction remain uncertain, evidence obtained from in vitro model systems[650] animal studies using ^{18}O combined with mass spectrometric analysis,[140,141] systematic identification and characterization of the reaction intermediates[416,508,809] are consistent with the following concepts. In the enzymatic degradation of haemoproteins, haem is dissociated from its parent apoprotein, such as globin, and bound to haem oxygenase in the membrane of the endoplasmic reticulum to form a ferric haem–haem oxygenase complex (Figure 14.3). Histidine residues at the catalytic site may determine the orientation of the substrate and hence the stereospecific cleavage of the α-methene bridge.[812] The ferric haem bound to haem oxygenase is reduced to the ferrous state by NADPH-cytochrome c reductase. This is followed by binding of molecular oxygen to the ferrous haem iron,[142] yielding an oxygenated form of the complex. To initiate haem degradation, a second electron donated by the NADPH-cytochrome c reductase system is required to activate the bound oxygen, which is then utilized to oxidize the protoporphyrin ring.[808] The activated oxygen appears selectively to attack the α-methene bridge of the porphyrin to form α-hydroxyhaem. The next phase of

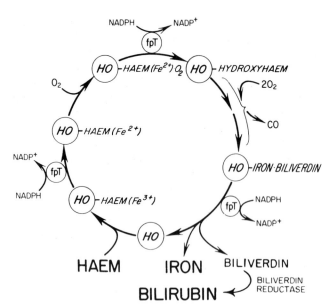

Figure 14.3 Postulated mechanism of haem degradation by the microsomal haem oxygenase system and cytosolic biliverdin reductase. HO = haem oxygenase; fpT = NADPH-cytochrome c reductase. (Modified from Kikuchi and Yoshida[416] with kind permission of the authors and the editor of *Trends in Biochemical Sciences*.)

the reaction sequence, which involves cleavage of the protoporphyrin ring and liberation of CO, is incompletely understood. Two molecules of oxygen are consumed in a sequential manner for the opening of the hydroxyhaem ring,[140,141] and an intermediate has been identified (not shown in Figure 14.3) which is formed from hydroxyhaem prior to the formation of the biliverdin–iron complex.[808] The structure of this intermediate has not been defined, and whether CO is liberated before or after its formation is unclear. It is apparent that all the steps in haem degradation up to formation of the biliverdin–iron complex may require molecular oxygen, which is activated by sequential binding to the ferrous haem iron.[416]

In the final step of the reaction, the biliverdin–iron complex is hydrolysed to biliverdin-IXα and iron. In most non-mammalian vertebrates (e.g. birds, reptiles and amphibia), haem degradation terminates at this step and the green-blue tetrapyrrole biliverdin is excreted in the unconjugated form into bile. In mammals, biliverdin is reduced at its central methene bridge to bilirubin by the cytosolic NADPH-dependent enzyme biliverdin reductase.[719] This enzyme has a stereochemical preference for the IXα isomer of biliverdin,[176] and has been purified to apparent homogeneity.[430] Since biliverdin reductase is most abundant in tissues with high haem oxygenase activities and always appears to be in excess, biliverdin is rarely detected in human plasma or bile. Recent observations suggest that the three enzymes catalysing the conversion of haem to bilirubin (i.e. microsomal haem oxygenase and NADPH-cytochrome c reductase and cytosolic biliverdin reductase) may exist as a ternary

complex located at the cytosol–endoplasmic reticulum interface.[811] Thus, without leaving the membranes of the endoplasmic reticulum, nascent biliverdin may be reduced to bilirubin where, in the liver, UDP-glucuronyltransferase catalyses its subsequent glucuronidation. In vivo studies have indicated that the total time required for the chemical transformations involved in the formation of biliverdin, its reduction to bilirubin, and the conjugation and excretion of bilirubin is of the order of 1–2 minutes.[141,302]

Discrepancies in the equimolar recovery of bilirubin and CO, or in the quantitative recovery of bilirubin from radiolabelled haem compounds, reflect the existence of alternate pathways of haem degradation which may become significant under certain circumstances. For example, a substantial discrepancy has been observed between cytochrome P450-haem turnover and CO recovery, both in intact animals and in primary rat hepatocyte culture.[88,328] Thus, the haem of microsomal cytochromes, particularly cytochrome P450, may be degraded in part by a pathway(s) which does not produce CO and, by implication, bilirubin. The mechanism(s) involved and the products formed have not been identified; a variety of systems may result in the destruction of cytochrome P450-haem without concomitant formation of either bile pigment or CO[204,324,707] or haem may be catabolized to dipyrrolic compounds and CO by NADPH-cytochrome c reductase.[323] Such non-bilirubin degradation mechanisms, involving selected haemoproteins, may give rise to the ill-defined dipyrrolmethenes (bilifuscins)[293,439,570,651] which have been identified in faeces and urine.[290]

PLASMA BILIRUBIN TRANSPORT

Unconjugated bilirubin is only sparingly soluble in aqueous solutions at physiological pH. In plasma, it is bound reversibly to albumin by a primary high-affinity site (most likely the lysine residue 240 of human albumin),[372] which has a reported binding constant at 37°C of 3×10^7 $(mol/l)^{-1}$.[129,373] Since the primary binding site is relatively hydrophobic, low concentrations of water-soluble organic anions that also bind to albumin do not readily displace bilirubin;[541] in addition, pH changes within the physiological range do not significantly alter the dissociation of bilirubin from this site.[540] Beyond a molar ratio of 1:1 (equivalent to a plasma bilirubin concentration of approximately 600 μmol/l; 35 mg/100 ml), bilirubin binds to albumin on at least two lower-affinity sites. Bilirubin can be displaced from these secondary sites by other organic anions, and small reductions in pH also result in an increased dissociation of the pigment from albumin.[531] The unbound or free bilirubin fraction in plasma, although exceedingly small, is conceptually of great physiological significance because only unbound bilirubin is thought to be available for transit across cell membranes such as the blood–brain barrier. Accurate, direct analytical methods for the determination of free bilirubin in plasma are not yet available;[470] indeed, the abundance of proposed methods and modifications for measuring bilirubin –albumin interactions and free bilirubin reflect the fact that none is precise, sensitive and routinely applicable. Recent reviews have considered the relative merits of the procedures using peroxidase, Sephadex chromatography, dye-binding or haematofluorometers.[127,130,138,163,407] Moreover, binding studies performed with crystalline human albumin preparations do not necessarily reflect the in vivo binding of bilirubin in hyperbilirubinaemic plasma.[376] Using the peroxidase technique,[375] it has been calculated that the plasma concentration of free bilirubin in normal adults is of the order of 0.12 nmol/l (7 pg/100 ml), and that the safe upper limit of free bilirubin in neonates, beyond which kernicterus may occur, is about 50 nmol/l (2.9 ng/100 ml).[127] This level of free bilirubin is achieved when approximately 80% of the albumin high-affinity binding sites are saturated with bilirubin.

Numerous compounds which compete with bilirubin for albumin binding promote the transfer of bilirubin into the brain and thereby increase the risk of kernicterus in jaundiced neonates. The long-chain fatty acids are amongst those compounds that compete with bilirubin for common binding sites on the albumin molecule. Although fatty acids are normally transported bound to albumin without interfering with bilirubin binding, increasing the molar ratio of fatty acids to albumin up to 4 : 1 progressively blocks the binding of bilirubin at the secondary sites, making it susceptible to displacement by water-soluble organic anions. At higher molar ratios of fatty acid to albumin (>5 : 1), there is also direct competition for binding between fatty acid and bilirubin at the secondary sites.[545] Since human breast milk contains high concentrations of fatty acids, the elevated levels of free fatty acids present in the plasma of breast-fed infants may result in the displacement of bilirubin from albumin.[803] Infusion of heparin into rats also causes a significant decrease in the plasma binding capacity for bilirubin (and salicylate).[780] This effect of heparin is probably due to the displacement of bound bilirubin by free fatty acids, whose plasma concentration is acutely increased by the heparin-induced activation or release of lipoprotein lipase. This potentially deleterious effect of heparin may be clinically pertinent when exchange transfusion of jaundiced neonates involves the use of heparinized blood.[781]

A large number of drugs apparently compete for the primary bilirubin binding site on albumin and hence potentially increase the risk of kernicterus in jaundiced newborn infants.[128,131,135,757] These compounds include certain sulphonamides (e.g. sulphafurazole [sulphisoxazole], but not sulphasalazine [Azulfidine]), antibiotics (e.g. penicillin derivatives, including ampicillin),[132] analgesics and non-steroidal anti-inflammatory agents (e.g. salicylate, indomethacin and phenylbutazone), food additives (e.g. parabens), x-ray contrast media for cholangiography, and diuretics (e.g. lasix [furosemide]).[164,665,770] Because albumin contains several binding regions, the interaction of a ligand with the molecule often results in

a conformational change that increases or decreases its affinity for ligands at other binding sites.[360,375,428] Some compounds, including the benzodiazepines, are bound strongly to albumin at different sites from bilirubin, but do not appear to displace bilirubin.[136] It is nevertheless important that all drugs used in newborns, during pregnancy or in lactating women should be considered with regard to their potential ability to displace bilirubin from albumin. The molecular mechanism of bilirubin encephalopathy is unclear and, although bilirubin binds to a variety of lipid membrane structures[233,527,631,778] and the activities of many membrane-bound enzymes are inhibited or accelerated in vitro in the presence of bilirubin,[407] no specific enzyme system or process has been identified whose dysfunction would account for bilirubin toxicity in vivo. Recent investigations into the age-dependent interaction of bilirubin with synaptosomal membranes suggest that inhibition of the phosphorylation of synapsin I may be important.[334,746]

Conjugated bilirubin is also transported in the plasma bound to albumin,[374] but its affinity for the protein appears to be somewhat less than that of the unconjugated pigment. This may explain the observation that the non-protein-bound fraction of conjugated bilirubin (which accounts for < 1% of the total plasma conjugated bilirubin in jaundiced patients), but not unconjugated bilirubin,[273] is freely filtered by the glomeruli; this filtered fraction is largely reabsorbed by the renal tubules[298] with the residual, non-reabsorbed component giving rise to the bilirubinuria which is characteristic in hepatocellular and cholestatic jaundice.

A previously unrecognized plasma bilirubin fraction has been identified by reverse-phase high-performance liquid chromatography and is very tightly and probably covalently bound to albumin.[280,442] This fraction reacts directly with the diazo reagent (indicative of conjugated pigment), but is removed by the deproteinizing step employed in most routine procedures for measurement of plasma bilirubin.[795] This non-dissociable albumin-bound bilirubin, which has variously been termed δ-fraction[442] BIL-ALB[769] or biliprotein,[494] is not detectable in the plasma of normal individuals or patients with unconjugated hyperbilirubinaemia (e.g. physiological neonatal jaundice, haemolysis or Gilbert's disease), but accounts for a varying proportion (8–90%) of the total plasma bilirubin in hepatobiliary conditions (e.g. acute and chronic hepatitis, cirrhosis) and cholestatic disorders (e.g. biliary obstruction, Dubin–Johnson syndrome).[97,769] The relative proportion of this fraction in plasma increases progressively with the duration of disease (Figure 14.4) owing to the fact that non-covalently bound bilirubin glucuronide, unlike the non-dissociable bile pigment–albumin complex, is freely available for hepatic uptake (and subsequent biliary excretion) or urinary excretion following glomerular filtration. The slow plasma clearance of biliprotein thus provides an explanation for the clinical observation that during recovery from jaundice, bilirubin often disappears from the urine, whereas the plasma remains

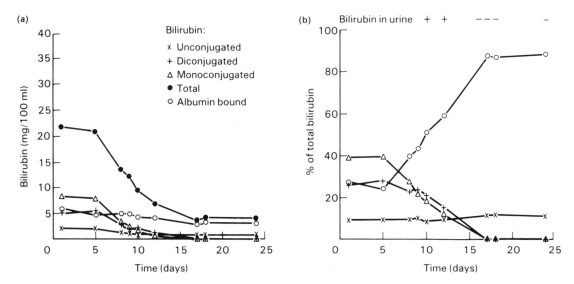

Figure 14.4 Total plasma bilirubin and subfractions in a patient recovering from postoperative jaundice associated with sepsis. (a) Absolute amounts of the bilirubin subfractions. (b) Bilirubin subfractions expressed as percentages of total bilirubin concentration. (Reprinted from Weiss *et al.*[769] by permission of the *New England Journal of Medicine.*)

icteric.[769] A recent study in animals with experimental cholestasis has demonstrated that the formation of bili-protein in vivo is non-enzymatic, and apparently is the result of acyl migration of bilirubin from a bilirubin–glucuronic acid ester to a nucleophilic site (e.g. NH₂ group) on albumin.[494] It now is apparent that at least four forms of δ-bilirubin exist in serum from cholestatic humans; both bilirubin monoglucuronide isomers (e.g. C-8 and C-12 bilirubin monoglucuronides) can bind covalently to albumin via the glucuronidated half of the molecule, and bilirubin diglucuronide can bind to albumin by either end of the molecule.[804] The irreversible covalent interaction of acyl glucuronides other than those of bilirubin (e.g. drugs) with albumin and their altered disposition in plasma may have considerable toxicological significance.[681]

Attention also has been focused on the possible role of alpha-fetoprotein in the transport of unconjugated bilirubin in the fetus and neonate. This fetal protein, which is produced in large quantities by fetal liver and yolk sac, is present in the plasma of adults in very low concentrations, except in association with hepatocellular carcinoma, regenerating liver or teratocarcinoma. The biological role of alpha-fetoprotein has yet to be determined, although structural and antigenic similarities to albumin suggest that it serves an albumin-like function in the transport of low-molecular-weight ligands. It has been shown that alpha-fetoprotein binds bilirubin with an affinity only slightly less than that of albumin[9,627,748] and that the two bilirubin binding sites on the molecule are in close proximity to, but distinct from, the fatty acid binding sites.[20,359] Despite these observations in vitro, it remains to be shown whether alpha-fetoprotein is involved in plasma transport and placental transfer of bilirubin in

the fetal period. Similarly, the relative importance of the recently identified role of high-density lipoprotein in plasma transport of bilirubin in rats remains to be determined.[706]

HEPATIC UPTAKE AND INTRACELLULAR TRANSPORT OF BILIRUBIN

Under normal circumstances, unconjugated bilirubin entering the plasma is rapidly cleared by the liver.[59,685] Fenestrations in the sinusoidal cells permit plasma proteins free access to the space of Disse and, hence, direct contact with the hepatocyte plasma membrane.[514] It has generally been assumed that bilirubin is separated from the carrier albumin prior to its uptake by the liver cell.[313] Alternatively, the sinusoidal surface of the cell membrane may initiate the uptake process by interacting with the albumin molecule on receptor sites which bind bilirubin and detach it from its carrier protein.[111,264,265,786] It has been postulated that if uptake is not driven predominantly by the plasma concentration of free bilirubin, it may be dependent on direct interaction between albumin and the sinusoidal surface.[32,266,538,727,766,767,768] This albumin receptor hypothesis may be summarized as follows: The albumin–ligand complex (bilirubin or other organic anion bound tightly to albumin) interacts specifically and saturably with an as yet uncharacterized binding site on the hepatocyte surface. This interaction favours more rapid dissociation of the ligand from albumin and its transfer to the cell surface, possibly by effecting a conformational change in the albumin molecule. The albumin molecule then dissociates rapidly from its putative receptor and returns to the circulation.[357,538] Although this hypothesis remains controversial[364,700] and validation of the model

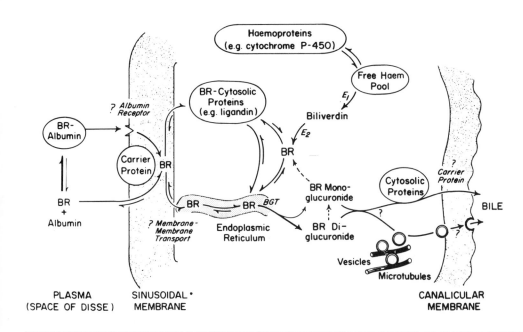

Figure 14.5 Scheme of bilirubin uptake, metabolism and intracellular transport in the hepatocyte incorporating recent conceptual advances. BR = bilirubin; E_1 = microsomal haem oxygenase system; E_2 = biliverdin reductase.

requires additional evidence, it would explain the efficient hepatic extraction of a variety of substances avidly bound to albumin.

Regardless of the initial mode of transfer of bilirubin from plasma to the hepatocyte, the uptake mechanism appears to be a carrier-mediated, saturable process that obeys Michaelis–Menten kinetics (Figure 14.5), and is shared, at least in part,[279] by a variety of other organic anions (e.g. sulphobromophthalein and indocyanine green) which exhibit mutually competitive inhibition.[313, 496,591,636,686] Bile acids, on the other hand, do not compete with bilirubin for hepatic uptake.[574] Sex steroids appear to modulate the hepatic uptake of organic anions (i.e. estrogens enhance uptake).[578] The finding in a mutant strain of Southdown sheep of impaired hepatic uptake of a variety of organic anions, including bilirubin,[181,507] supports the existence of a common carrier-mediated system which involves integral proteins of the sinusoidal plasma membrane. Several bilirubin and sulphobromophthalein (BSP) binding proteins have been identified in rat liver plasma membrane, although some divergence of opinion exists regarding their characteristics.[472,599,701,714, 725,787,819] Two groups of investigators have independently purified and partially characterized a protein with an M_r of approximately 54 000 which exhibits high affinity, saturable binding, and mutual competition for bilirubin, BSP and indocyanine green, but not taurocholate.[699,701, 787] There may be two distinct, but closely related binding proteins for BSP/bilirubin and other organic amines.[58] Although the binding affinities exceeded those reported for albumin and ligandin (see below), the role of specific carrier proteins in bilirubin and organic anion uptake in vivo has yet to be established.

The hepatic uptake system operates far below saturation at normal plasma bilirubin concentrations, and in experimental animals the maximal initial uptake rate has been shown to exceed greatly the steady-state excretory transport maximum; thus, the uptake of bilirubin does not appear to be the rate-limiting step in its excretion.[574] Direct experimental evidence obtained in animals has established that the flux of bilirubin and other organic anions across the plasma membrane is bidirectional.[239,313, 333,636] Compartmental analysis of radiolabelled bilirubin plasma disappearance curves suggests that, in normal individuals, about 40% of the bilirubin taken up by the hepatocytes in a single pass through the liver refluxes unchanged to the plasma.[61] In Gilbert's syndrome,[62,417] congenital non-haemolytic jaundice[110] and Gunn rats,[635] despite the presence of unconjugated hyperbilirubinaemia, the rate of hepatic bilirubin uptake is reported to be normal, although there is a corresponding increase in reflux to the plasma. Hence the initial hepatic uptake of bilirubin appears to be independent of its cytoplasmic binding and subsequent metabolism but, owing to the bidirectional flux, net uptake reflects the irreversible removal of pigment by intracellular metabolic pathways. Conjugated bilirubin is taken up by the liver even more rapidly than unconjugated bilirubin; the two compounds compete with one another and other organic anions for hepatic uptake, suggesting that the uptake mechanism for conjugated bilirubin may be the same as that for unconjugated bilirubin.[672]

Significant amounts of bilirubin have been shown to accumulate in the normal liver,[598,790] but the low polarity of the pigment argues against its existence in the free form. Once transferred across the plasma membrane into the hepatocyte, bilirubin is probably bound, in part, to the cytosolic protein ligandin,[76,402,453] which is also known as aminoazo dye-binding protein B,[415] Y-protein[453] or glutathione S-transferase B.[120,330,377,585] In addition to bilirubin, it binds a variety of ligands including carcinogens, haem, synthetic dyes, cholecystographic agents and hormones.[13] Cytoplasmic Z protein,[453] which is probably identical to aminoazo dye-binding protein A and fatty acid-binding protein,[537,539] has a lower binding affinity but greater binding capacity for bilirubin than does ligandin. The protein purified from human liver has an M_r of 11 000.[396] It appears likely that Z protein is involved principally with fatty acid transport, since it has a high affinity for long-chain fatty acids and is found in intestinal mucosa, liver, myocardium, and other tissues which take up and metabolize fatty acids; in fact, its role in the hepatic transport and storage of bilirubin remains unproven.[721] Preliminary evidence suggests that in patients with Gilbert's syndrome, hepatic content of ligandin is within the normal range,[259] but both hepatic and serum concentrations of Z protein are reduced.[396]

Ligandin is a basic protein with an M_r of 47 000, which constitutes 5% of the soluble protein in rat and human liver, and is also found to a lesser extent in kidney, small intestine and placenta.[733] Rat liver ligandin is composed of two polypeptide subunits[41,42,270] with a M_r of 22 000 (subunit A) and 25 000 (subunit B).[77] Whereas glutathione S-transferase B activity requires both subunits, the binding of bilirubin and BSP has been located on subunit A. The amino acid composition and sequence appear to be identical in the two subunits, except for a C-terminal extension of 30 amino acids on subunit B, which presumably prevents binding of bilirubin and BSP.[78,79] Opinions differ as to whether the two bilirubin binding sites on ligandin are structurally and functionally distinct and are at locations different from the sites for glutathione S-transferase activity.[76,78,123,199,677,734] Although glutathione S-transferases, similar to albumin and alpha-fetoprotein, exhibit binding sites for haem and bilirubin, there are distinct immunochemical differences between the glutathione S-transferases and both albumin and alpha-fetoprotein.[732]

The binding of bilirubin and other organic anions to ligandin is believed to decrease efflux of these substances from hepatocytes to plasma and hence influence net hepatic uptake, but ligandin does not appear to participate directly in the uptake process.[13,792] Phylogenetic studies suggest that ligandin evolved with terrestrial reptiles, birds and mammals and that its presence correlated with the appearance of selective hepatic organic anion uptake.[455] In newborn monkeys and humans, the 'maturation' of hepatic ligandin to adult levels during the first 5–10 days of life coincides with maturation of the hepatic uptake mechanism(s) for organic anions.[454] Drugs, such as phenobarbitone, that induce ligandin have been shown to accelerate the hepatic uptake of organic anions,[603] but phenobarbitone treatment has many additional effects on the liver, including stimulation of hepatic blood flow and bile secretion, which may be responsible for this effect. Nevertheless, findings in the isolated perfused liver pretreated with phenobarbitone[497] and in vivo in thyroidectomized rats, in which hepatic ligandin concentration is increased but hepatic blood flow is reduced,[792] support the concept that ligandin is involved in the regulation of

bilirubin efflux from the liver. Initially, the idea that ligandin may be involved in hepatic bilirubin uptake was difficult to reconcile with the observations that purified ligandin has a lower binding affinity than plasma albumin for bilirubin,[395] and that bilirubin migrates with albumin rather than ligandin on gel chromatography.[112] It is now established that the binding affinity of ligandin for bilirubin diminishes rapidly on fractionation of the isolated cytosol; thus ligandin prepared by moving-boundary sedimentation (in which lower-molecular-weight molecules remain associated with the protein) exhibits a much higher binding activity than that obtained by zonal centrifugation.[505] Moreover, in native cytosol, most ligandin is bound to reduced glutathione. In this complexed form, the cytosolic protein binds bilirubin more strongly than does albumin[467,506] and hence appears likely to limit organic anion efflux from the liver.

It is unclear whether ligandin facilitates the intracellular movement of bilirubin to the endoplasmic reticulum for glucuronidation and of bilirubin glucuronides to the canalicular membrane for excretion into bile, or whether it serves a storage function in situations of unconjugated and conjugated bilirubin excess. Immunocytochemical studies have localized ligandin to the cytosol, with highest concentrations occurring adjacent to endoplasmic reticulum.[155] This observation supports the recent finding that a portion of cellular glutathione S-transferase is associated with the microsomal membrane.[122,271,512,513] Presumably, both cytosolic and membrane-bound ligandin may influence the transport of bilirubin to the microsomal membrane and hence the rate of UDP-glucuronyltransferase-catalysed glucuronidation. Evidence for an alternative hypothesis, i.e. the intracellular transport of bilirubin by direct membrane transfer, has been found.[121,777,778] Equilibrium dialysis with lipid dispersions has suggested that a substantial portion of bilirubin and other hydrophobic compounds may be membrane bound in hepatocytes.[724] It also has been demonstrated that bilirubin incorporated into the membranes of unilamellar vesicles is glucuronidated more rapidly than bilirubin bound to the high-affinity sites of albumin or ligandin.[778] Hence, bilirubin may diffuse rapidly within the lateral plane of phospholipid membranes, and intracellular movement may occur by membrane–membrane transfer (Figure 14.5). Diffusional flux or transfer of bilirubin within hepatocytes may involve several processes, including free pigment in the aqueous phase (minimal), bilirubin bound to ligandin and possibly other cytosolic binding proteins, and pigment partitioned within intracellular membranes.[347,723,778] If this is a correct reflection of the situation in vivo, a portion of the bilirubin in hepatocytes may never enter the cytosolic phase, but rather may undergo transfer from one lipid membrane phase to another, at least up to the stage of microsomal glucuronidation.

Considerable insight into the processes of hepatic bilirubin transport and metabolism has been achieved by kinetic analysis and mathematical modelling of radiolabelled bilirubin disposition.[159,304,392,393,417] A large proportion of the newly formed bilirubin arising in the liver from turnover of hepatic haems refluxes in unconjugated form into the plasma before its conjugation and excretion into bile. Another fraction of bilirubin generated in the liver is excreted directly into bile, without prior passage through the plasma compartment.[394,417] Kinetic studies in rats suggest that for endogenously formed hepatic bilirubin, the rates of efflux from the liver to plasma and of excretion into bile are approximately 2- and 4-times higher than those for bilirubin taken up directly from plasma.[305] These findings most likely reflect differences in hepatic compartmentation of bilirubin arising from intra- and extrahepatic sources, and are consistent with the concept that bilirubin transported through the hepatocyte from plasma to bile does not appear to mix with pigment generated in intrahepatic compartments. Finally, kinetic studies in intact rats and isolated perfused liver led to the prediction and subsequent experimental verification that a small fraction of the bilirubin glucuronides formed in the liver normally undergoes hepatic deconjugation.[195,304] This observation may provide an explanation for the frequent finding of increased plasma unconjugated bilirubin levels in patients with cholestatic liver disease.

BILIRUBIN CONJUGATION

Under physiological conditions, bilirubin must be conjugated in order to be excreted into bile. In mammalian bile, most of the excreted bilirubin is conjugated and, with the exception of Gunn rats or patients with unconjugated hyperbilirubinaemia undergoing phototherapy,[459,489,566] only trace amounts of the hydrophobic unconjugated pigment are present. In Gunn rats, it has been suggested that the hepatic microsomal cytochrome P448-dependent monooxygenases may participate in the catabolism of bilirubin.[156,397] In addition, a mitochondrial bilirubin oxidase may play a role in the catabolism of bilirubin under circumstances in which the normal metabolic pathways to conjugate bilirubin are absent (e.g. the Gunn rat and Crigler–Najjar syndrome type I).[647,801]

Esterification on the carboxyl groups of one or both of the propionic acid side-chains of bilirubin-IXα (which are situated on the two central pyrrole rings) with glucuronyl or other carbohydrate moieties results in water-soluble compounds capable of rapid transport across the canalicular membrane into bile. Bilirubin differs from most other compounds that undergo glucuronidation in that it has two carboxyl groups which allow the formation of two different bilirubin monoglucuronide (BMG) isomers (i.e. the C-8 and C-12 BMG isomers) or a diglucuronide (BDG, Figure 14.6). In humans, BDG constitutes the major conjugate in bile (about 80%). Smaller quantities of the two bilirubin monoglucuronide isomers as well as trace amounts of other conjugates, such as bilirubin monoglucoside, bilirubin monoglucoside–monoglucuronide, and bilirubin xylosides, also have been detected in human bile.[96,250,254,306,307] Considerable species differ-

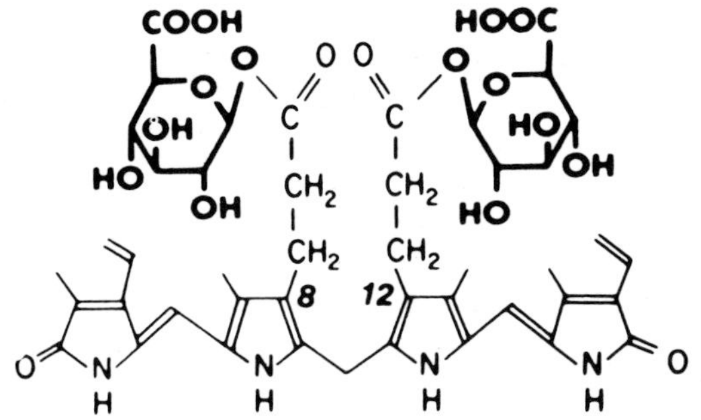

Figure 14.6 Structure of bilirubin-IXα diglucuronide. The two molecules of glucuronic acid attached to the propionic acid groups prevent intramolecular hydrogen bonding and thus account for the enhanced aqueous solubility.

ences exist in the nature and relative distribution of bilirubin conjugates,[256,260,311,353] for example, BDG predominates in the bile of monkeys, rats, dogs and cats, whereas bilirubin monoglucuronides are the major conjugate species in mice, sheep, pigs, rabbits and guinea pigs. With the exception of humans, monkeys, and rats, substantial proportions of bilirubin glucosides and xylosides are found in bile. Recent evidence suggests that the microsomal enzyme bilirubin UDP-glucuronyltransferase, rather than the availability of particular UDP-glycoside co-substrates, determines the pattern of bilirubin conjugates formed in each species.[684]

The chemical lability of both unconjugated and glucuronidated bilirubin, and difficulty in quantitation and isolation of the latter,[348,456] have greatly complicated studies of bilirubin conjugation. This instability can be attributed largely to the central methylene bridge of bilirubin-IXα (see Figure 14.1), which is susceptible to attack by electrophilic agents or oxidants to form two dipyrroles. Cleavage occurs in strong acid or moderately alkaline solution, with acceleration in the presence of oxygen or light, and is followed by random recombination of the two dipyrroles (i.e. dipyrrole exchange or scrambling) to form the symmetric IIIα and XIIIα isomers, as well as the asymmetric, native bilirubin-IXα.[487] Similarly, bilirubin glucuronides are prone to dipyrrole exchange, so that two moles of BMG can recombine to form one mole of BDG and one of unconjugated bilirubin. Bilirubin glucuronides also are susceptible to oxidation, with formation of green biliverdin derivatives, and, in bile, to an intramolecular rearrangement termed acyl 'shift'. The latter is due to the sequential migration of the acyl group of bilirubin from the native 1 position of the glucuronic acid molecule to the 2, 3 and 4 positions (forming 2-, 3- and 4-o-acylglucuronides). This acyl shift, which is accelerated at alkaline pH and occurs with storage of bile in vitro and during cholestasis,[103] may complicate the interpretation of analytical procedures such as the chromatographic separation of azo pigments.[254] In addition, the native 1-o-acylglucuronides are liable to cleavage of the glucuronide moiety by β-glucuronidase,

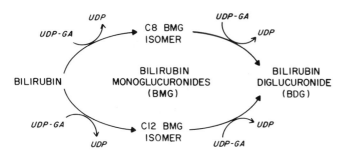

Figure 14.7 Pathways of bilirubin UDP-glucuronyltransferase-mediated formation of bilirubin monoglucuronide isomers and bilirubin diglucuronide from bilirubin. UDP-glucuronic acid (UDP-GA), which is synthesized from UDP-glucose in cytosol, is an essential co-substrate for each step.

whereas the 2-, 3- and 4-*o*-acylglucuronides are resistant.[678]

Despite these complexities and the potential pitfalls associated with studies of bilirubin glucuronides, a much clearer picture of the enzymatic mechanism of hepatic bilirubin glucuronidation has emerged. The liver is the major biological source of bilirubin glucuronides.[465] Hepatic UDP-glucuronyltransferases exist in multiple isoforms and catalyse the transfer of glucuronic acid to numerous acceptor substrates.[189,340] It is apparent that a single isoform of UDP-glucuronyltransferase, hepatic bilirubin UDP-glucuronyltransferase (bilirubin-GT), catalyses the transfer of glucuronic acid from UDP-glucuronic acid to bilirubin, resulting in the formation of both bilirubin monoglucuronide isomers, as well as bilirubin diglucuronide.[99,100,309,310,312,440,621,622] (Figure 14.7). This enzyme is capable of esterifying bilirubin with either glucuronic acid, glucose or xylose.[621,622,684] Recent enzyme kinetic studies suggest that both BMG isomers are synthesized at a single binding site on bilirubin-GT;[740] the ratio of C-8 and C-12 BMG isomer formation is species-dependent and approaches unity in man and monkey.[343] Although a plasma membrane enzyme mediating the dismutation or transglucuronidation of two BMG molecules to form BDG and bilirubin has been postulated, this mechanism is highly unlikely to be operative in vivo.[249]

Bilirubin-GT, like other UDP-glucuronyltransferase isoforms, is found primarily in the rough and smooth endoplasmic reticulum, and to a lesser extent in Golgi membranes and the nuclear envelope;[342] it has not been found in cytosol, or in lysosomal, peroxisomal, mitochondrial or plasma membranes.[340,342,620] Using the technique of chromatofocusing, Roy Chowdhury *et al.* have isolated as many as eight isoforms of UDP-glucuronyltransferase from rat liver.[622] Although many of these isoforms exhibited overlapping substrate specificities, peak V exhibited activity exclusively towards bilirubin. The molecular weight of this isoform was 53 kD, and its activity could be induced by phenobarbital or clofibrate administration. Previously, Burchell *et al.* isolated and purified a bilirubin-GT from rat liver with a molecular weight of 57 kD.[144] Recent evidence using radiation-inactivation analysis suggests that human bilirubin-GT may exist as a tetrameric enzyme, with BMG synthesis catalysed by a single subunit weighing 55 kD and BDG formation requiring catalysis by all four subunits of the 209 kD tetrameric enzyme.[580,583] Additional studies are needed to verify this hypothesis.

Investigation into the molecular biology of UDP-glucuronyltransferase has provided important data concerning the intimate relationship of this family of enzymes with its membrane environment.[147,341,379,581] At least some rat UDP-glucuronyltransferases possess amino-terminal and carboxyl-terminal amino acid sequences which are likely to function, respectively, as signal peptides and transmembrane-anchors.[476] Similar findings in studies of human liver UDP-glucuronyltransferase suggest a transmembrane orientation of the enzyme, which is stabilized by a highly charged carboxyl-terminal tail which protrudes from the membrane into the cytosol.[371] In addition, there is evidence for asparagine-linked glycosylation sites on some UDP-glucuronyltransferases. Monoclonal antibodies, which have recently been developed towards various epitopes of UDP-glucuronyltransferases,[581,583] should be helpful in future studies to define better the orientation and tertiary structure of UDP-glucuronyltransferases within the endoplasmic reticulum membrane.

Like all UDP-glucuronyltransferase isoforms, bilirubin-GT is a membrane-bound enzyme which is dependent on the presence of membrane phospholipids for activity. Any process which alters the composition or physical state of the microsomal membrane, such as delipidation, exposure to detergents or phospholipase treatment, has a profound effect on bilirubin-GT activity.[189,814] Dietary cholesterol supplementation, which increases the cholesterol content and decreases the fluidity of microsomal membranes, modifies UDP-glucuronyltransferase kinetics.[165] Moreover, the physical state of the membrane differentially modulates bilirubin-GT-catalysed formation of BMG isomers relative to that of BDG.[680]

Two hypotheses have been proposed to explain the mechanism(s) by which the activity of bilirubin-GT and other GT isoforms are regulated by its membrane environment. The compartmental model, introduced by Berry and Hallinan,[72] includes four assumptions. First, at least a portion of UDP-GT is located on the interior, cisternal side of the endoplasmic reticulum; thus, membrane perturbants increase UDP-GT activity by enhancing the access of substrate(s) to the enzyme. In support of this assumption, recent studies of the relationship of bilirubin-GT activity to microsomal membrane permeability have concluded that the active site of bilirubin-GT is on the luminal face of the endoplasmic reticulum.[739,741] Previous studies have demonstrated that non-penetrating protein-modifying agents, such as diazobenzenesulphonate, have no effect on glucuronidation, suggesting that the enzyme has no catalytic sites exposed on the cytosolic surface of the endoplasmic reticulum.[332] As discussed above, the exact location of bilirubin-GT in the endoplasmic reticulum is unknown, but from the amino acid analysis of purified UDP-GT preparations it is probably largely embedded in the phospholipid bilayer.[147] Based on this first assumption of the compartmentation model, glucuronidation of different substrates should be related to their physicochemical properties. Indeed, it has been observed that the sequential development of UDP-GT activity toward various substrates in newborn rats can be accounted for in part by the bulkiness or estimated planar thickness of the substrates.[340,555]

The second assumption of the compartmentation model states that the enzyme nucleotide diphosphatase resides in the same intracisternal location as UDP-GT and catalyses the hydrolysis of UDP, which is the potent inhibitory end-product of glucuronidation reactions. In fact, nucleotide diphosphatase has been shown to be loosely bound to the inner cisternal surface of the endoplasmic reticulum,[124] and studies using ^{31}P-nuclear magnetic resonance have documented rapid hydrolysis of UDP-GT-generated UDP to UMP and inorganic phosphate in this location.[258] Since UDP itself is unlikely to be capable of freely traversing the endoplasmic reticulum, its transformation to UMP is of great importance.

An integral component of the compartmentation model is the third assumption, the existence of a UDP-glucuronic acid membrane permease or transporter. The formation of UDP-glucuronic acid, which is the essential co-substrate for all glucuronidation reactions,[340] is catalysed from UDP-glucose by the cytosolic enzyme UDP-glucose dehydrogenase.[702] Like other bulky, charged, hydrophilic nucleotide-sugars, diffusion of UDP-glucuronic acid from the cytosol into the endoplasmic reticulum membrane is highly unlikely.[344] Numerous carrier-mediated transport systems have been described that shuttle charged nucleotide-sugars similar to UDP-glucuronic acid (i.e. UDP-galactose, GDP-fucose, UDP-xylose, UDP-*N*-acetylglucosamine and CMP-acetylneuraminic acid) from the cytosol into Golgi and/or endoplasmic reticulum membranes, where they function as substrates for glycosyltransferases.[39,72,536,577] The translocation of some of these nucleotide-sugars across Golgi membranes may involve an exchange with the corresponding nucleoside monophosphate (i.e. GDP-fucose and GMP[153,166]). Studies in our laboratory have provided direct evidence for a membrane transporter which mediates the access of UDP-glucuronic acid from the cytosol into the endoplasmic reticulum.[344] Using rat liver, uptake of UDP-glucuronic acid by membrane vesicles isolated from rough and smooth endoplasmic reticulum was extremely rapid, temperature dependent, and exhibited both saturability and a high degree of specificity. In addition, it was determined that UDP-glucuronic acid was transported into the membrane phase, rather than into the intravesicular space, unlike the transport processes described for other nucleotide-

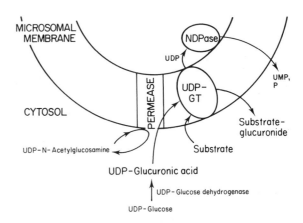

Figure 14.8 Putative structural organization of the UDP-glucuronosyltransferase (GT) enzyme system. Schematic illustration of the proposed membrane-bound carrier, or permease, which mediates the access of UDP-glucuronic acid from cytosol to its binding site or sites on UDP-GT in the microsomal membrane. Formation of UDP-glucuronic acid from UDP-glucose is catalysed by the cytosolic enzyme UDP-glucose dehydrogenase. UDP, a product of the UDP-GT-mediated glucuronidation reaction, is converted by nucleoside diphosphatase (NDPase) into uridine monophosphate (UMP) and phosphate (P).

sugars.[72,344,536] These data also suggest that the binding site(s) on UDP-GT for UDP-glucuronic acid resides within the membrane bilayer. Of interest, the K_m for this transporter was nearly an order of magnitude less than the apparent K_m for UDP-glucuronidation in vitro using microsomes isolated from primate or rat liver, whereas the V_{max} was comparable.[343,753] This suggests that the membrane transporter is characterized by both high capacity and high affinity (i.e. its K_m for UDP-glucuronic acid is considerably less than its intrahepatic concentrations, about 400 μM, in rat liver[344,355,818]) and thus is likely to be important in the regulation of glucuronidation reactions. Further work is necessary to isolate and characterize this membrane carrier.

The fourth and final assumption of the compartmentation model is that UDP-*N*-acetylglucosamine, which increases UDP-GT activity in vitro, enhances the transport activity of the UDP-glucuronic acid permease. This has not been proved directly but data from kinetic studies using microsomes isolated from primate (*Macaca fascicularis*) liver,[343,345] support this postulate. A proposed structural organization of the UDP-glucuronyltransferase system based on the available data in support of the compartmental model is illustrated schematically in Figure 14.8.

A second hypothesis, the conformational restraint model, has been proposed to explain the mechanism by which UDP-GT is regulated by its membrane microenvironment.[189,340,813] It is postulated that UDP-GT in its native, unperturbed membrane setting exhibits latency due to the constraining influence of associated phospholipids. Thus, perturbation of the membrane alters this constraint and, hence, the latency of catalytic activity is modified as the enzyme assumes different conformations. Depending on the nature of the perturbant and the duration of exposure, the modified UDP-GT conformation may exhibit either increased or decreased catalytic activity. A large body of kinetic data has been obtained which supports this model.[189,340,751,752,813] Using a purified, phospholipid-free UDP-GT preparation that lacks activity, a host of different kinetic forms can be generated by reconstituting the enzyme with lecithins that differ in the length and degree of unsaturation of their acyl chains, or with different species of phospholipid.[232] Further work is needed to understand better the complex relationships between UDP-GT and its membrane environment.[617] It is probable that components of both the compartmentation and conformational restraint models are necessary in order to account for all the experimental data.

The regulation of UDP-GT by its membrane environment is also dependent on the means by which hydrophobic substrates, such as bilirubin, reach their binding site(s) on the enzyme. Bilirubin is distributed within the hepatocyte in several locations, including a small unbound fraction in cytosol, bilirubin bound to ligandin (glutathione-S-transferase B) and other soluble binding proteins, and bilirubin partitioned into intracellular membranes.[189] The membrane pool of bilirubin appears to be delivered by membrane–membrane and lateral membrane transfer for glucuronidation more efficiently than bilirubin bound to cytosol or purified glutathione-S-transferases.[777,778] Moreover, the phospholipid composition and physical state of membranes containing the substrate (i.e. bilirubin) have been shown to influence UDP-GT activity.[777,779] Bilirubin substrate concentration has profound effects on bilirubin-GT activity; the ratio of BDG to BMG formation decreases progressively as bilirubin substrate concentration increases relative to that of the enzyme.[340,343] Thus, the capacity of bilirubin-GT for BDG synthesis is considerably lower than that for BDG formation. This provides a logical explanation for the finding in vivo that conditions associated with genetically reduced hepatic bilirubin-GT activity, such as Gilbert's syndrome and type 2 Crigler–Najjar syndrome, exhibit a proportionally increased amount of BMG relative to BDG in bile.[255,260,303,315] Similarly, the standard procedures for the in vitro assay of bilirubin-GT in liver microsomes or homogenates, which utilize bilirubin substrate concentrations in excess of those in normal liver, preferentially form BMG.[350,737] Subsequent studies have demonstrated abundant BDG synthesis in hepatic microsomes using lower bilirubin substrate concentrations than are recommended for the standard bilirubin-GT assay.[99,308,343] Interestingly, bilirubin substrate concentration does not affect formation of the C-8 BMG isomer relative to C-12 BMG in vivo.[343] This is consistent with data suggesting that both of the BMG isomers are synthesized at a single binding site.[740]

The availability and accessibility of the co-substrate, UDP-glucuronic acid, are crucial in the regulation of bilirubin-GT activity. Hypoxia, anaesthetic agents such as ether, and ethanol all diminish hepatic UDP-glucuronic acid levels and thereby reduce UDP-GT activity.[21,170,209,210,601] The hepatic concentration of UDP-glucuronic acid also may be depleted by the administration of large doses of drugs that are glucuronidated, such as acetaminophen.[358,594] It remains to be proved whether patients with diminished hepatic UDP-glucuronyltransferase activities (i.e. Gilbert's syndrome and the Crigler–Najjar syndromes) are more susceptible to acetaminophen or other drug toxicity.[205,206] Using a microsomal assay, we have demonstrated that UDP-glucuronic acid concentration has a profound effect on the synthetic rates of BDG relative to that of BMG, as well as the formation of the C-8 BMG isomer relative to that of C-12 BMG.[343] Finally, the physical properties of the microsomal membrane also may regulate UDP-glucuronic acid binding to UDP-GT, and thereby influence the activity of the enzyme.[310,356,680]

The cytosolic nucleotide-sugar, UDP-N-acetylglucosamine, greatly enhances UDP-GT activity in vitro toward virtually all substrates, including bilirubin, in concentrations that approach those in rat liver.[148,340,818] UDP-N-acetylglucosamine may function as an allosteric effector, increasing the affinity of UDP-GT for UDP-glucuronic acid, and lowering the K_m for UDP-glucuronic acid nearly 100-fold to approximately 0.5 mM, which is the presumed hepatic concentration of UDP-glucuronic acid in vivo.[754,818] The available evidence indicates that UDP-N-acetylglucosamine is not directly accessible to UDP-GT (or a binding site on the enzyme), suggesting that UDP-N-acetylglucosamine may enhance catalytic activity by facilitating the transport of UDP-glucuronic acid from the cytosol to the enzyme via the putative membrane transporter.[148,332,345] Contrary to these observations, one group of investigators, using a purified, delipidated UDP-GT reconstituted into model membranes, has suggested that the physical state of the membrane itself determines the sensitivity of UDP-GT to UDP-N-acetylglucosamine.[750] Finally, UDP-GT activation by UDP-N-acetylglucosamine has been postulated to be due to the dissociation of an oligomeric form of UDP-GT to more active monomers.[750] The mechanism(s) by which UDP-N-acetylglucosamine and other factors, such as divalent cations,[815] enhance UDP-GT activity obviously requires further work.[340] Other factors which undoubtedly are crucial in the regulation of UDP-GT activity include xenobiotics, drugs and hormones;[340] phenobarbital and clofibric acid in particular are capable of inducing bilirubin-GT activity.[105,340] Hormones such as testosterone, thyroxine, cortisol, glucagon and secretin also may influence UDP-GT activity.[178,277,340,445,604] Hormonal modulation of membrane lipid composition may be one of many factors accounting for age-related effects on UDP-GT activity.[45,118,340,400,444] Some, but not all studies, suggest that high bilirubin substrate concentrations are capable of inducing bilirubin-GT.[340,519] Finally, investigations into the complex regulatory effects of nutrition, bile salts, diurnal variations, and acinar heterogeneity on UDP-GT activity are in their infancy.[44,179,269,340,747,776]

Bilirubin-GT activity is extremely low in human fetal

liver; between 17 and 30 weeks of gestation, values are about 0.1% of the activity found in adults, increasing to about 1% of adult values between 30 and 40 weeks of gestation.[409] After birth, enzyme activity towards bilirubin in human liver increases at an exponential rate and attains adult levels by 14 weeks of age. This striking postnatal increase occurs following normal or premature birth[152] and hence appears to be due either to birth-related, rather than age-related, factors[409] or to the intrauterine milieu suppressing maturation of enzyme activity.[194] The observed changes in enzyme kinetics during the perinatal period[294] suggest that the postnatal rise in glucuronyl-transferase activity is unrelated to an increase in the number of active sites, but rather is due to maturation of the enzyme into a more highly regulated form. Kinetic differences between the enzyme from adult and from newborn liver (the newborn enzyme, for example, has a higher affinity for UDP-glucuronic acid) indicate that structural rearrangements of the enzyme may account for the apparent increase in activity occurring after birth.[294] Recently, data obtained with the use of immunoblot analysis has suggested that human bilirubin-GT may be absent in the fetus and, thus, it may develop postnatally.[185]

It has been shown that female rats have higher hepatic bilirubin-GT activity than male rats.[522,523] Castration of the female rats lowered bilirubin-GT activity, while castration of the males enhanced enzyme activity. If these findings can be applied to humans, they would provide an explanation for the observation that plasma bilirubin levels are higher in adult men than in women, as well as the increased prevalence of Gilbert's syndrome in men compared with women.

Bilirubin glucuronyltransferase activity has been demonstrated also in the renal cortex and gastrointestinal mucosa[223,338,628] and studies in hepatectomized animals confirmed that these tissues are the main sites of extrahepatic bilirubin formation.[268,624] Under physiological conditions, it is unlikely that extrahepatic conjugation of bilirubin is of importance, but it has been shown that grafting of normal rat kidneys into Gunn rats results in the conjugation and subsequent biliary excretion of a considerable portion of the plasma bilirubin pool.[261]

BILIARY SECRETION OF BILIRUBIN _____

Unlike the natural bilirubin-IXα (Z,Z), other isomers, including the artificial isomers IX-β, -γ and -δ[160] and the geometric isomers of bilirubin-IXα produced by photoisomerization,[459,491] all of which lack intramolecular hydrogen bonding, are excreted directly into bile without conjugation with carbohydrate moieties. Normal human bile contains only very small amounts of unconjugated bilirubin-IXα (less than 1% of total bilirubin in gallbladder bile), which appears to be excreted as such rather than representing conjugated bilirubin that has been hydrolysed by β-glucuronidase.[117,687] Small amounts of unconjugated bilirubin are also found in the bile of patients with Gilbert's and Crigler–Najjar syndromes.[256,647] Studies in

a patient with sickle cell disease and pigment gallstones demonstrate that unconjugated bilirubin output is hyperbolically related to bile salt output, although maximum excretion of unconjugated pigment represented only 3% of the total bilirubin output.[617] Since a similar hyperbolic relationship exists for biliary lipids, cholesterol and phospholipids, this has been taken as indirect evidence that unconjugated bilirubin is transported into bile in the form of mixed micelles or vesicles. This concept is supported by studies in Gunn rats, which have shown that the excretion of unconjugated bilirubin may be greatly enhanced by infusing either bile acids or conjugated bilirubin.[86,151]

Recent investigations have just begun to explore the mechanism(s) by which conjugated bilirubin is transported within the hepatocyte from the endoplasmic reticulum to the canalicular membrane. Circulating bilirubin glucuronides are very rapidly excreted into bile.[190] After intravenous administration of radiolabelled unconjugated bilirubin, it is difficult to recover conjugated bilirubin from hepatic subcellular fractions.[70] Using intravenous administration of tracer doses of purified radiolabelled biliverdin, bilirubin, BMG and BDG to intact normal or jaundiced homozygous Gunn rats, it has been demonstrated that bilirubin glucuronides formed in the liver both from endogenous (i.e. hepatic haem) and exogenous (extrahepatic) sources of bilirubin follow a similar excretory pathway.[190] BMG and BDG appear to traverse the hepatocyte by a transcellular pathway that is distinct from that for unconjugated bilirubin.[190] Whereas BMG formed endogenously is converted preferentially to BDG by microsomal bilirubin-GT, most circulating (exogenous) BMG is excreted unchanged. Thus, circulating bilirubin glucuronides are excreted independently of and more rapidly than those generated in the liver.[190]

It is likely that intracellular binding proteins, such as ligandin, play a role in facilitating the intracellular transport of bilirubin glucuronides to the canalicular membrane.[790] In addition, there is increasing evidence for the participation of bile salts and the microtubular system in this process.[633] It has been demonstrated that when steady-state transhepatic bile salt flux rates are increased, the microtubular system is crucial for efficient biliary excretion of bile salts, biliary lipid and bilirubin conjugates.[187,188] Both endogenously formed bilirubin conjugates and exogenous BMG and BDG taken up from plasma may be co-transported with bile salts to the canalicular membrane via a microtubular-dependent mechanism. It is unlikely that bilirubin conjugates and bile salts associate within the hepatocyte as mixed micelles; the concentrations of bile salts within the hepatocyte are well below their critical micellar concentrations.[674] It is possible that vesicles derived from intracellular organelles, such as endoplasmic reticulum and Golgi membranes, might facilitate the transport of both bilirubin conjugates and bile salts to the bile canaliculus via interactions with microtubules.[654]

By whatever mechanism bilirubin conjugates are transported to the canalicular membrane, it is apparent that their biliary secretion proceeds against a considerable concentration gradient and that the process overall displays saturation kinetics, and operates with a lower capacity than pigment uptake.[263] It has been assumed that secretion is rate limiting in the transport of bilirubin from plasma to bile,[313] although indirect evidence suggests that glucuronidation may, in fact, be the rate-limiting step.[520,606,742]

The secretion process probably involves a membrane carrier system which appears to be shared by a variety of endogenous and exogenous organic anions (e.g. sulpho-bromophthalein (BSP), rose bengal, indocyanine green (ICG) and cholecystographic dyes) but is functionally distinct from that for bile acids.[4,175,234,262,418] It is not clear whether there is a single membrane carrier which serves to concentrate a variety of structurally unrelated anions or whether there are multiple systems which are subject to allosteric interaction.[262,496] These hypothetical carriers may be genetically absent or defective in patients with the Dubin–Johnson syndrome and in mutant Corriedale sheep, in which the secretion of conjugated bilirubin and BSP is markedly defective, whereas bile acid transport is unimpaired.[4,204] In contrast to conjugated BSP, the excretion of unconjugated BSP is almost normal in mutant Corriedale sheep[30] and in Dubin–Johnson patients,[1] suggesting that at least two different canalicular carriers are involved in organic anion secretion.[30,478]

Despite the presence of separate secretory mechanisms for bile acids and for organic anions[676] these are not functionally independent of each other, since infusion of taurocholate substantially increases the maximum secretory rate (T_m) of bilirubin, BSP, ICG and iopanoic acid.[263,314] This effect on T_m, which is specific for bile acids and appears to correlate with their micelle-forming capacity,[229] is not produced by stimulants of bile salt-independent flow such as theophylline.[29,286] From these observations, Goresky[313] has proposed that, in addition to the canalicular membrane transport processes, the formation of mixed micelles at the canalicular surface or within the canalicular lumen may be an important determinant of net hepatic bilirubin transport. It has been postulated that the passive binding to micelles creates a 'sink' which reduces the luminal concentration of conjugated bilirubin in the non-micellar phase of bile, thus decreasing its availability for back-diffusion across the canalicular membrane. This association may create a net concentration gradient that favours flux of pigment into bile, thereby effectively reducing the energy barrier required for transport. Although the functional importance of micellar sequestration of bilirubin and other organic anions within the canalicular lumen has yet to be established, the concept is supported by the finding that conjugated bilirubin and BSP are present in bile almost entirely in the form of mixed micelles or macromolecular aggregates.[152,365,715,758] This hypothesis has been challenged by the failure to demonstrate an association between bile pigment and mixed lipid micelles in bile

containing bile acid concentrations in the physiological range;[275,602] alternatively, the observations may be attributable to bile acid-mediated alterations in the canalicular membrane.[301] Another hypothesis resulting from the observation that the T_m of bilirubin is increased by taurocholate infusion is that of a zonal gradient in the liver.[313,314] This is based on the concept that a concentration gradient for bile acids exists in the sinusoidal blood from the portal to the peripheral zone of the hepatic acinus, so that ordinarily only the more proximal, periportal hepatocytes are involved in the extraction and secretion of bile acids. During bile acid infusion, perivenular hepatocytes are progressively recruited for bile acid transport (which results in a flattened zonal profile for bile acid secretion). This postulated mechanism, which is supported by functional and morphological findings[325,391] would readily explain the observed increase in the T_m of bilirubin associated with taurocholate infusion.

w10 PHOTOBIOLOGY OF BILIRUBIN

Studies on the structure and photochemistry of bile pigments have demonstrated that excretion of unconjugated bilirubin in the bile of illuminated Gunn rats[566] or jaundiced newborns[475] is due largely to single-photon isomerization of bilirubin. Exposure of bilirubin to blue light in the 400–500 nm band causes either or both of the outer pyrrole rings of bilirubin-IXα (Z,Z geometric isomer) to 'flip over', resulting in formation of a mixture of geometric or configurational isomers (Z,E; E,Z; E,E), collectively termed photobilirubin (Figure 14.8).[173,463,464,698] These photoisomers of bilirubin-IXα are thermodynamically unstable, but are partially stabilized by binding to albumin; they have been separated by chromatography,[560,698,802] but have not been obtained in crystalline form. Physicochemical properties of photoisomers differ from those of 'ground-state' bilirubin (Z,Z) because the photoisomers cannot form the intramolecular hydrogen bonds characteristic of the Z,Z isomer. Consequently, photobilirubin is more polar than bilirubin (Z,Z) and therefore can be excreted in bile without the need of conjugation.

The E,Z photoisomer on exposure to light undergoes irreversible intramolecular cyclization of the C-3 vinyl group to an E,Z cycloform ('photobilirubin II').[116,362,696] Exposure to green light (500 nm) may facilitate the formation of this photoisomer.[321,557] An additional intramolecular cyclization may occur, resulting in an E,E cyclo form[367] (Figure 14.9). These structural isomers or lumirubins are considerably more stable than the configurational (geometric) isomers.[460]

These photoproducts are cleared from the circulation more rapidly than the E,Z and Z,E isomers[560,561,563] and have been detected in bile of illuminated Gunn rats[563,697] and newborn infants.[558] Accumulation of the E,Z-cyclobilirubin occurs in the presence of impaired liver function,[562] and it has been demonstrated that the azacyclopentadiene ring can be polymerized to form a bilifuscin-like brown substance that may be the pigment responsible

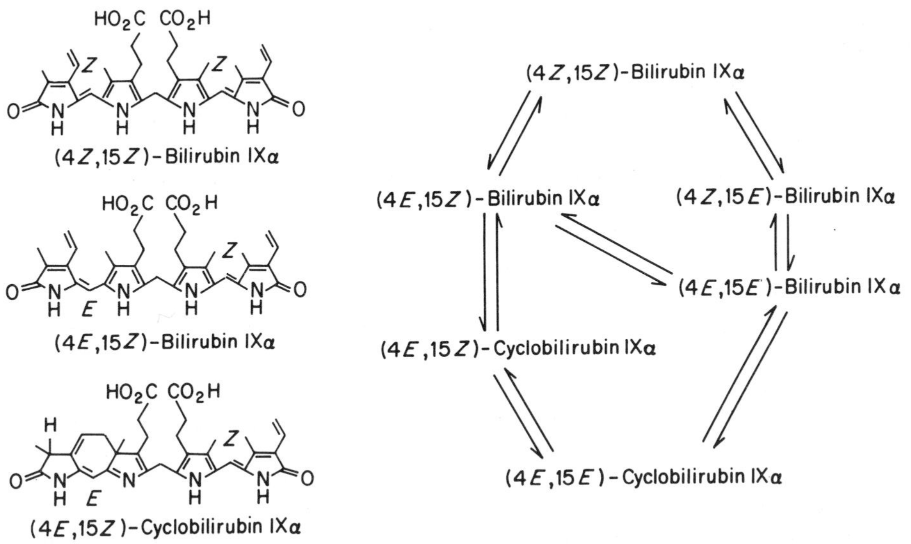

(4Z,15Z)-Bilirubin IXα

(4E,15Z)-Bilirubin IXα

(4E,15Z)-Cyclobilirubin IXα

(4Z,15Z)-Bilirubin IXα

(4E,15Z)-Bilirubin IXα (4Z,15E)-Bilirubin IXα

(4E,15E)-Bilirubin IXα

(4E,15Z)-Cyclobilirubin IXα

(4E,15E)-Cyclobilirubin IXα

Figure 14.9 Formation of geometric or photoisomers ('photobilirubin') from natural bilirubin-IXα (Z,Z). The bilirubin photoisomers are more polar than bilirubin-IXα (Z,Z) and hence are readily excreted into bile without prior conjugation. Once in bile, they rapidly revert to the stable Z,Z form.

for the discoloration observed in the bronze-baby syndrome (a major, albeit rare complication of phototherapy).[362,498] A number of photooxidation products have been identified in the urine of jaundiced neonates undergoing phototherapy, with and without the bronze-baby syndrome.[462] These photooxidation products, as well as abnormally high concentrations of serum porphyrins, may be important in the pathogenesis of this syndrome.[625]

Photoisomerization rather than photooxidation is believed to be the major mechanism resulting in removal of bilirubin from the organism exposed to phototherapy. Blue light has been postulated to cause photochemical excitation of bilirubin in the skin of jaundiced infants, resulting in the formation of photobilirubins I and II, which are rapidly released into the plasma. The observations that skin bleaches during phototherapy and that photobilirubin appears in bile only after a lag period following initiation of phototherapy,[491] suggest that photoisomerization involves relatively immobile bilirubin deposited in skin and perhaps in subcutaneous tissues, rather than in circulating plasma. As photoisomers are removed from the skin during illumination, they are replaced by fresh bilirubin, transferred from the plasma, which eventually results in a reduction of total plasma pigment concentration. Phototherapy is therapeutically efficacious until the plasma bilirubin concentration has decreased to about 85 μmol/l (5 mg/100 ml), after which little effect is observed with continued light exposure.[713] The various photoisomers formed during phototherapy have been identified in plasma of Gunn rats by absorbance-difference spectroscopy[489] and in icteric newborns by high-performance liquid chromatography[558] and fluorometric methods.[437] Geometric isomers of bilirubin in the blood of icteric newborns under phototherapy may reach 15% of the total plasma bilirubin concentration.[437]

Photobilirubin is taken up by the liver from plasma and appears to be excreted by the canalicular transport system(s) without prior conjugation, as are certain other hydrophilic organic anions such as indocyanine green.[383] Once in the bile, the unstable geometric isomers spontaneously revert to stable bilirubin-IXα (Z,Z),[489,697] which, in the intestine, presumably can undergo enterohepatic circulation. The structural isomers (lumirubins) are rapidly excreted into bile and appear more stable than the geometric isomers in the intestine.[230] Total removal of bilirubin from the body during phototherapy via stool and urine is dependent to a large extent on the formation of lumirubins.[231,564] Photoisomers produced in Gunn rats are excreted in bile independently of bilirubin and do not displace native bilirubin from its binding to plasma albumin,[489] although photobilirubin binds to albumin at the primary bilirubin binding site with an affinity only 2–3 times lower than that of bilirubin.[436,499] Since photobilirubin is produced even at the low light intensities of normal daylight, small amounts of photoisomers probably are formed and excreted in all icteric infants and patients with Crigler–Najjar disease if they are exposed to ambient visible light.[491]

FATE OF BILIRUBIN IN THE GASTROINTESTINAL TRACT

The absorption of conjugated bilirubin in both the gallbladder and intestine[83,448,449] is negligible because of its polar nature and molecular size. In healthy adults, the conjugates probably remain largely intact during transit through the small intestine, preventing appreciable enterohepatic circulation of bilirubin. In the presence of intestinal stasis or obstruction and in newborns, there is increased formation and absorption of unconjugated bilirubin; in the latter, this may contribute to neonatal hyperbilirubinaemia.[133,588]

Bilirubin glucuronides are hydrolysed to the unconjugated pigment, predominantly in the terminal ileum and colon, by bacterial β-glucuronidase. Bilirubin is reduced by the action of colonic bacteria to a complex series of colourless tetrapyrroles, collectively termed 'urobilinogen'.[227,760] It is not known whether deconjugation precedes reduction in the formation of urobilinogen. Urobilinogen can be formed from bilirubin in vitro by anaerobic cultures of *Clostridium, Bacteroides* or mixed faecal flora,[237,762] and the reaction appears to be mediated by enzymes bound to bacterial membranes.[729] Oral administration of broad-spectrum antibiotics greatly diminishes the formation of urobilinogen[760] and, in infants, lack of appropriate colonic flora during the first 2–6 months of life results in greatly reduced faecal urobilinogen excretion.[567] Normal adult faeces contain a mixture of urobilinogens and their corresponding orange-coloured oxidation products, urobilins.[761] The ultimate composition of faecal pigments is probably dependent primarily on the nature of the bacterial flora of the colon. In normal subjects, only about 50% of the daily bilirubin turnover can be recovered as faecal urobilinogen (measured by Ehrlich's aldehyde reaction). There is, therefore, a poor correlation between bilirubin production and faecal urobilinogen excretion, so that measurement of faecal urobilinogen is of limited diagnostic value.[107]

Urobilinogen undergoes an enterohepatic circulation, although less than 20% of the amount produced daily is re-absorbed because it is formed mostly in the colon where the absorption rate is low; about 90% of absorbed urobilinogen is promptly re-excreted by the liver into bile by the anionic transport system.[450,452] The remaining 10% in the systemic circulation is excreted in the urine (approximately 2% of daily urobilinogen production).[695] Urinary urobilinogen is increased in haemolytic disorders and in patients with hepatocellular disease and/or portosystemic shunts.[71] The mechanism of renal excretion involves glomerular filtration of the non-protein-bound plasma fraction (approximately 20% of the total plasma urobilinogen) followed by tubular re-absorption and secretion.[119,458] Urinary urobilinogen excretion is related to urine pH, higher values being recorded in alkaline than in acid urine, and a diurnal variation has also been demonstrated.[761]

DISORDERS OF BILIRUBIN METABOLISM

Laboratory methods

Despite methodological advances,[316,425,525] the routine determination of plasma bilirubin concentration is still most commonly achieved by one of several modifications of the diazo reaction or by direct spectrophotometry.[85] Although bilirubin has a characteristic absorption spectrum, with a maximum at 460 nm when bound to albumin (or 453 nm in chloroform, dimethyl sulphoxide or common organic solvents), the presence of turbidity, haemoglobin and dietary lipochromes in plasma may interfere with direct spectrophotometric readings. Despite these limitations, this method may be useful for the rapid and approximate estimation of total bilirubin concentration. In the more widely used diazo reaction, stable red-violet dipyrrolic azoderivatives are formed by the reaction of bilirubin with diazonium salts of aromatic amines, such as sulphanilic acid (van den Bergh reaction)[731] and the products formed are measured spectrophotometrically. The overall reaction is a multistep process[486] which leads to cleavage of the bilirubin molecule into formaldehyde and two diazotized dipyrroles (azopigments). Since bilirubin-IXα is asymmetrically substituted, it forms non-identical pairs of azopigments, which are sometimes referred to as 'vinyl' and 'isovinyl' azoderivatives.

In plasma, bilirubin-IXα reacts very slowly with diazotized sulphanilic acid, but the reaction is greatly accelerated by the addition of solvents such as methanol, ethanol, diphylline or caffeine benzoate ('indirect-reacting bilirubin'). These accelerators disrupt the intramolecular hydrogen-bonded structure of the unconjugated pigment, thereby facilitating reaction with the diazo reagent. In contrast, conjugated bilirubin in plasma reacts almost immediately without the addition of accelerators ('direct-reacting bilirubin'). In the method of Malloy and Evelyn[480] and its many modifications, methanol is employed as the accelerator. Although the sensitivity of this method is reduced by the required dilution of plasma (which is necessary to prevent protein precipitation), and the presence of lipaemia and haemolysis may cause errors,[86,671] it is widely used in clinical practice. The most satisfactory procedure currently available for the determination of unconjugated bilirubin in plasma appears to be that of Michaelsson, Nosslin and Sjölin,[509] based on the method of Jendrassik and Grof,[386] which uses diphylline or caffeine benzoate as the accelerator. The sensitivity of this method is enhanced by converting the azopigments from red to blue by the addition of alkali. Estimation of conjugated bilirubin is generally less accurate than that of unconjugated pigment (see below). Thus, in predominantly conjugated hyperbilirubinaemia, only an approximate value is obtained for both the conjugated and total bilirubin levels. The estimates obtained are adequate for most clinical purposes, since it is generally sufficient to ascertain the relative degree to which conjugated or unconjugated bilirubin predominates in the plasma.

A variety of modified diazo procedures have been advocated for the measurement of plasma bilirubin level,[335,466] and different accelerating agents have been proposed[468,535] but these do not represent a significant advance over existing techniques. Methods have also been developed using diazotized ethyl anthranilate or *p*-iodoaniline,[351,352,738] which yield azopigments that can readily be extracted into organic solvents for chromatographic separation and quantification. These methods are more sensitive than the classical diazo procedure and have been applied successfully in the analysis of individual bilirubin conjugates, but have not been widely adopted for routine clinical assays.

Since 1980, new specific methods for quantitating

unconjugated bilirubin and its mono- and diconjugates have been developed. A sensitive and precise assay involves conversion of bilirubin conjugates to their corresponding methyl esters by alkali-catalysed transesterification in methanol,[96] and separation of the ester derivatives by high-performance liquid chromatography (HPLC).[104] Using this approach, only unconjugated bilirubin was detectable in sera from healthy adults and individuals with Gilbert's syndrome.[524] In contrast, by diazo assay, a major portion of the pigment in the samples was direct-reacting (about 65%), illustrating the limited value of the direct-reacting fraction as an estimate of conjugated bilirubin in plasma at low total bilirubin levels. Further refinement of this procedure has shown that normal serum contains an average of 3.5% mono- and diconjugates.[521] In sera from patients with both cholestasis and parenchymal liver disease, unconjugated and conjugated bilirubin are increased, with monoconjugates either predominating[104] or present in similar concentration to diconjugates.[381] Why the pigment pattern found in the plasma of jaundiced patients should differ from that in normal bile (in which diconjugated bilirubin is the major pigment fraction) is unknown, but this may be related to differential hepatic deconjugation of bilirubin diglucuronide and monoglucuronides.[304] Finally, as determined by the alkaline methanolysis procedure, the concentration of bilirubin and its conjugates is lower than the total bilirubin level obtained using a conventional diazo procedure, reflecting the presence of non-bilirubin diazo-positive compounds in pathological plasma samples.[104]

A variety of other HPLC methods have been proposed which, unlike the alkaline methanolysis procedure, permit identification of the sugar conjugate moieties (e.g. glucuronide, glucoside) and hence direct measurement of the proportions of bilirubin conjugates in bile or serum.[380, 441,559,687,688] Because these specialized techniques are time-consuming, they have yet to be used to analyse plasma bilirubins, and as pure reference conjugates are unavailable, they have yet to gain widespread acceptance in clinical laboratories.

Pathophysiology of hyperbilirubinaemia

The plasma bilirubin in normal subjects is virtually all in the unconjugated form[52,521] and values obtained for conjugated bilirubin are largely spurious, representing artefacts inherent in the method employed (see above). The normal plasma bilirubin concentration (5.1–17.1 μmol/l [0.3–1.0 mg/100 ml]) varies directly with bilirubin turnover and inversely with hepatic bilirubin clearance.[53,109] Whether estimated by means of this relationship or determined directly,[593] the normal distribution is skewed, and slightly higher values have been observed in males than in females.[521] Black Americans have been found to have significantly lower mean serum bilirubin levels than whites of European origin, Latin Americans and Asians.[158] Individuals with a plasma unconjugated bilirubin level between 17 and 68 μmol/l (1

and 4 mg/100 ml) may have haemolysis, abnormal hepatic function, or both. The finding of concentrations persistently in excess of 68 μmol/l (4 mg/100 ml) implies reduced hepatic function, irrespective of the presence of haemolysis, since the maximum achievable rate of bilirubin production (eight times normal under steady-state conditions) seems to elevate plasma unconjugated bilirubin no higher than 60–68 μmol/l (3.5–4 mg/100 ml).[52] During acute haemolytic crises, such as occur in sickle cell disease or paroxysmal nocturnal haemoglobinuria, bilirubin production and plasma bilirubin may transiently exceed these levels.

Unconjugated hyperbilirubinaemia may be caused by accelerated pigment formation associated with haemolysis or 'ineffective erythropoiesis', or by defective hepatic uptake or conjugation of the pigment. Cholestasis due to impaired bile flow either at the canalicular or bile duct level results in accumulation of conjugated bilirubin in plasma (Table 14.2). Despite progress in understanding the nature of bile secretion, the mechanisms underlying defective canalicular bile flow have not yet been established. Nor is it known whether, in cholestasis, conjugated bilirubin refluxes to the plasma directly across the sinusoidal membrane or from damaged canaliculi via the paracellular pathway, or by a combination of these postulated defects. With the exception of familial hyperbilirubinaemias, the clinically important causes of jaundice attributable to liver disease probably involve both impairment of biliary secretion and hepatic deconjugation, although other defects in hepatic transport may exist, as well as an over-production of bilirubin. Similarly, the pathogenesis of hyperbilirubinaemia in extrahepatic bacterial infections is multifactorial.[43,337] Hence, in diffuse hepatocellular injury (e.g. hepatitis or cirrhosis), the plasma concentrations of both conjugated and unconjugated bilirubin are increased, with the former usually predominating, although the relative proportion of the two pigments is variable and of little diagnostic significance. Since the specific abnormalities in bilirubin metabolism that lead to jaundice in diffuse liver disease are unclear, the subsequent discussion will consider only those causes of hyperbilirubinaemia which are attributable to identifiable and recognizable defects.[296,379,554]

UNCONJUGATED HYPERBILIRUBINAEMIA

Increased bilirubin formation

Haemolysis

Haemolysis generally gives rise to a mild degree of hyperbilirubinaemia as discussed above. Although the plasma bilirubin level increases linearly in relation to bilirubin production, the plasma bilirubin concentration may still be near normal in patients with a 50% reduction in red cell survival, provided that hepatic bilirubin clearance is normal. Although the unconjugated fraction predominates in haemolytic jaundice,[381] increased plasma

Table 14.2 Causes of hyperbilirubinaemia and associated plasma bilirubin patterns

Disorder	Defect in bilirubin metabolism	Plasma bilirubin pattern		
		Unconjugated	Conjugated	Covalently bound
Haemolysis	↑ Production	+	− (rarely exceeds 68 μmol/l)	−
Haematomas	↑ Production (1 litre blood = 5 g bilirubin or 20 × daily production)	+	−	−
Ineffective erythropoiesis	↑ Production	+	−	−
Neonatal ('physiological') jaundice	↑ Production ↓ Glucuronyltransferase activity ↓ Cytosolic ligandin ↑ Intestinal bilirubin absorption	+ (100 μmol/l in full term, 170–205 μmol/l in premature)	−	−
Breast milk jaundice	Inhibition of glucuronyl-transferase activity? (pregnane-3α,20β-diol and long-chain fatty acids) ↑ Intestinal bilirubin absorption	+	− (up to 340–510 μmol/l)	−
Crigler–Najjar syndrome, type I	Absent glucuronyltransferase activity	+	− (usually > 340 μmol/l)	−
Crigler–Najjar syndrome, type II	Markedly decreased glucuronyltransferase activity	+	−	−
Gilbert's syndrome	↓ Glucuronyltransferase activity ↓ Hepatic uptake? Associated haemolysis (~50% of patients)	+	− (< 100 μmol/l, usually < 50 μmol/l)	−
Fasting hyperbilirubinaemia	↑ Production ↓ Hepatic clearance ↓ Hepatic uptake? ↓ Conjugation?	+	−	−
Dubin–Johnson syndrome	Impaired biliary secretion (membrane-carrier?)	+	+ (total usually < 85 μmol/l)	+
Rotor's syndrome and hepatic storage syndrome	↓ Hepatic uptake and storage? ↓ Biliary secretion?	+	+ (total usually < 85 μmol/l)	?
Intrahepatic cholestasis (canalicular or ductule damage)	↓ Biliary secretion Deconjugation → increased unconjugated bilirubin levels	+	+	+
Extrahepatic cholestasis (mechanical obstruction)	↓ Biliary secretion	+	+	+
Hepatocellular injury	↓ Biliary secretion (conjugation and other steps usually remain intact)			

levels of conjugated bilirubin (> 15% of the total plasma bilirubin) may be present in association with hepatic dysfunction[726] and in occasional patients with acute haemolytic crises, in whom the amount of bilirubin generated and conjugated may exceed the biliary secretory transport maximum for conjugated bilirubin.[632,683] Increased bilirubin production results in elevated excretion of faecal and urinary urobilinogen, but these parameters are of little value in the diagnostic evaluation of jaundice. Haemolysis due to hereditary abnormalities of erythrocytes (e.g. hereditary spherocytosis, pyruvate kinase deficiency, sickle cell disease) generally produces only a mild degree of jaundice which may present within a few days of birth or as recurrent episodes during later life, frequently in association with febrile illnesses. Cholelithiasis, reflecting precipitation of bilirubin, is the major complication of long-standing excessive bilirubin production.

Ineffective erythropoiesis

Ineffective erythropoiesis is associated with the premature destruction of defective red cells in the bone marrow or spleen and consequent augmentation of the erythropoietic component of 'early-labelled bilirubin'. Diagnosis of the various disorders of haem, haemoglobin or erythroid cell formation which give rise to ineffective erythropoiesis (see earlier) usually presents no difficulties. Jaundice is of a mild degree and the reticulocyte count is normal or only moderately increased, but elevated levels of faecal and urinary urobilinogen in the absence of a marked reduction in the survival of circulating red cells are characteristic of this condition.

Markedly increased ineffective erythropoiesis is the basis of a rare disorder known as 'primary shunt hyperbilirubinaemia[369] or 'idiopathic dyserythropoietic jaundice.[50] Since the former name incorrectly implies that bilirubin is formed directly from the pyrrolic precursors of haem and not via the breakdown of haem, the latter title is more appropriate. This heterogeneous group of disorders is frequently familial and characterized by the onset of asymptomatic jaundice in the second or third decades of life in the presence of a marked increase in faecal urobilinogen excretion and a normal or near normal red cell life span.[11,370,749] Israels[368] reviewed 11 such cases in which about half had splenomegaly, but hepatomegaly was absent and liver function tests were uniformly normal, apart from an elevated plasma unconjugated bilirubin concentration (20 to 136 μmol/l [1.2 to 8 mg/100 ml]). The presence of values exceeding 68 μmol/l (4 mg/100 ml) in some patients suggested the coexistence of defective hepatic bilirubin clearance. In the majority of patients, the disorder was further characterized by a reticulocytosis, normoblastic erythroid hyperplasia of bone marrow and increased iron turnover with diminished red cell incorporation, reflecting the state of ineffective erythropoiesis. The underlying defect responsible for the high rate of haem turnover within the marrow remains unknown. In addition, some cases exhibit an increased serum iron concentration and haemosiderosis of hepatic parenchymal

and Kupffer cells. A mild haemolytic anaemia with spherocytosis and increased osmotic fragility has also been described but, unlike congenital spherocytic anaemia, autohaemolysis and mechanical fragility tests were normal. Splenectomy resulted in a prolongation of red cell survival and a partial reduction in plasma bilirubin level, but marrow erythroid hyperplasia persisted and faecal urobilinogen excretion remained high. Although the prognosis of this rare, idiopathic form of ineffective erythropoiesis appears to be excellent, like other causes of enhanced bilirubin production, it predisposes to cholelithiasis.

Reduced hepatic clearance of bilirubin

The major aspects of the pathogenesis, diagnosis and treatment of non-haemolytic unconjugated hyperbilirubinaemia in the neonatal period have been reviewed by Cashore,[161,162] Johnson,[389] Lee,[446] Levine,[456] Newman and Maisels,[479,532] Seligman,[658] Thaler,[720] and Isherwood.[365]

'Physiological jaundice', a transient elevation of plasma unconjugated bilirubin to a mean of 103 to 137 μmol (6 to 8 mg/100 ml) during the first week of life, is the most common form. The cause of this condition is multifactorial (Table 14.2), reflecting accelerated erythrocyte breakdown, diminished hepatic ligandin, impaired bilirubin conjugation and possibly excretion by the newborn liver, and enhanced enterohepatic circulation of bilirubin. The quantitative contributions of these various factors have not been established.

Impaired hepatic bilirubin clearance, due specifically to reduced hepatic uptake or possible competition for binding to Z protein or ligandin, is associated with the administration of drugs such as rifampicin (and other rifamycin antibiotics),[2,154,414] bunamiodyl,[74] flavaspidic acid[333] and probenecid.[413] Plasma bilirubin concentration reverts rapidly to normal following discontinuation of the offending drug. Hepatic uptake of bilirubin and a variety of other organic anions is impaired in mutant Southdown sheep.[181] This condition is inherited as an autosomal recessive trait, and the animals exhibit chronic facial eczema due to phylloerythrin-mediated photosensitivity, a mild unconjugated hyperbilirubinaemia and abnormal renal function.[649]

A mutant strain of Wistar rat described by Gunn[326] and subsequently by Malloy and Lowenstein[481] has provided a unique experimental model for investigation of the underlying metabolic defect in type I Crigler–Najjar syndrome (which it closely resembles), of bilirubin metabolism in the newborn, and of the mechanism and efficacy of phototherapy. The major characteristics of the Gunn rat have been considered in detail by Schmid and McDonagh.[649] The disorder is inherited as an autosomal recessive trait,[326] and the absence of hepatic bilirubin UDP-glucuronyltransferase activity (see later for discussion of metabolic defect) gives rise to a severe unconjugated hyperbilirubinaemia (usually > 120 μmol/l [7 mg/100 ml]), which leads to tissue deposition of bilirubin and functional impairment of the central nervous system,[390] thyroid[306] and kidneys[150,543] (which are susceptible to analgesic-induced renal papillary necrosis).[336] Recent attempts to replace glucuronyltransferase in these mutant Gunn rats have been of interest because this would represent a significant therapeutic advance for patients with Crigler–Najjar type I syndrome. Such experiments have met with only limited success. When rat hepatoma cells[626] or normal rat kidney[261] were grafted into homozygous Gunn rats, the recipients acquired limited ability to conjugate endogenous bilirubin and excrete it in bile. Similarly, it has been claimed that the level of hyperbilirubinaemia was reduced in immunosuppressed Gunn rats following infusion of enzyme-replete hepatocytes into the portal vein,[322,705] but the results of this series of experiments were less convincing because they lacked essential controls. Reduction in serum bilirubin levels in Gunn rats after infusion into the portal vein of hepatocytes isolated from Wistar rats has been attributed to reduced red cell turnover and thus reduced bilirubin production.[794] Grafting normal liver tissue on to the liver of enzyme-deficient rats has produced conflicting results.[515,516] The attachment of Wistar rat hepatocytes to collagen-coated microcarriers followed by intraperitoneal transplantation into Gunn rats can result in the production of bilirubin glucuronides in bile, as well as decreased serum bilirubin levels.[773] Auxiliary liver transplantation also has produced promising results.[384]

Chronic non-haemolytic unconjugated hyperbilirubinaemia is a feature of several genetically transmitted syndromes in humans. This spectrum of disorders is distinguished primarily on the basis of the plasma bilirubin level, the response to phenobarbitone administration, and the presence or absence of bilirubin glucuronides in bile. While most patients can readily be categorized as having one of the three syndromes listed in Table 14.3, occasional patients manifest features which make precise classification difficult. The three syndromes may be defined as follows: (a) Crigler–Najjar type I syndrome,[192] an extremely rare and almost invariably fatal form of severe unconjugated hyperbilirubinaemia which is caused by a genetic defect in bilirubin conjugation similar to that found in homozygous Gunn rats; (b) Gilbert's syndrome,[288] a relatively common, benign and possibly heterogeneous condition presenting with a mild, fluctuating and often subclinical hyperbilirubinaemia, similar to that observed recently in Bolivian squirrel monkeys;[589] and (c) a condition characterized by an intermediate degree of hyperbilirubinaemia, arbitrarily defined as greater than 103 μmol/l (6 mg/100 ml), and clinical and biochemical features which merge with those of the other two syndromes. This last disorder is considered to be due to a partial defect in bilirubin conjugation and is commonly referred to as Crigler–Najjar type II syndrome.[16] Investigation of bilirubin metabolism in a number of non-human primates has contributed to our understanding of similar abnormalities in humans.[180]

Crigler–Najjar type I syndrome (congenital nonhaemolytic jaundice with glucuronyltransferase deficiency)

Clinicopathological features

In 1952, Crigler and Najjar[192] reported a familial form of severe non-haemolytic jaundice associated with neurological dysfunction. Six infants from three interrelated families were observed with markedly elevated plasma bilirubin concentration (445 to 770 μmol/l [26 to 45 mg/100 ml]), which appeared between the first and third postnatal days and persisted throughout life. The plasma bilirubin was all unconjugated, bilirubinuria was absent and there was no evidence of haemolysis. Hepatosplenomegaly was absent and hepatic histology and conventional liver function tests, including BSP clearance, were normal. Five of these icteric infants developed a neurological syndrome resembling kernicterus, which resulted in rapid deterioration and death by the age of 15 months. Autopsy examination of the brain in a 17-day-old infant revealed intense staining of the cerebral cortex and basal ganglia with bilirubin. The sixth affected child in this family group initially escaped overt neurological damage[168] and developed normally into the teens despite persistent hyperbilirubinaemia. Approaching the age of 15 and in the absence of an apparent precipitating event, this boy developed symptoms and signs closely resembling those of kernicterus which led to his death within 6 months.[113] In contrast to the autopsy findings in infants, pigment staining was not evident in the brain and the cerebral cortex was normal, but neuronal loss and gliosis of the thalamus and basal ganglia were evident.[276] In addition, bilirubin deposits were found in the renal papillae, intestinal mucosa, endocardium, connective tissue and perivascular adventitia. In a further patient born in the same kindred[168] and jaundiced since the second day of life, neuropsychiatric manifestations appeared at the age of 18 years in association with a rise in plasma bilirubin concentration to 680 μmol/l (40 mg/100 ml).[106] Despite the development of severe extrapyramidal abnormalities and grand mal seizures, her condition appeared to stabilize for about 12 months following a temporary reduction in plasma bilirubin level produced by exchange plasmapheresis.[64] Subsequently, her neurological status fluctuated somewhat and tended to correlate with plasma bilirubin levels (340 to 600 μmol/l); overall, her condition deteriorated inexorably and she died aged 23 years. Sporadic cases have also been recorded from other kindreds in whom neurological damage was absent during early childhood.[292,615] Since the original description of this syndrome, more than 60 additional patients have been reported from many different countries in association with a further 30 or so probable cases among family members of the propositi. In the vast majority of affected individuals, kernicteric brain damage and death ensued within 18 months of birth, although rarely patients survived beyond puberty before the development of bilirubin encephalopathy.[791]

Table 14.3 Characteristics of the chronic non-haemolytic unconjugated hyperbilirubinaemic syndromes

	Type I Crigler–Najjar syndrome	Type II Crigler–Najjar syndrome	Gilbert's syndrome
Incidence	Rare	Uncommon	< 7% of population Male to female ratio of 4 : 1
Mode of inheritance	Autosomal recessive	?Autosomal dominant with variable penetrance	?Autosomal dominant
Bilirubin UDP-glucuronyltransferase activity	Undetectable	Markedly decreased or absent	Decreased
Plasma bilirubin concentration (μmol/l [mg/100 ml])	308–855 (18–50), usually > 340 (> 20)	103–376 (6–22), usually < 340 (< 20)	< 103 (< 6), usually < 50 (< 3)
Age hyperbilirubinaemia recognized	< 3 days after birth	Usually 1st year of life: occasionally early adulthood	Usually early adulthood: may be associated with fasting
Clinical features	Jaundice and kernicterus in infants or early adulthood	Usually asymptomatic jaundice, kernicterus rare	Asymptomatic or nonspecific symptoms; occasional mild jaundice
Associated defects	None	?Decreased hepatic bilirubin uptake	Decreased hepatic uptake of bilirubin, BSP (< 40%) and ICG (< 20%) Mild haemolysis (< 50%) Impaired drug metabolism (see text)
Routine liver function tests, cholecystography, and liver histology	Normal	Normal	Normal
Bile	Usually pale yellow; a trace of unconjugated bilirubin and monoconjugates	Yellow: mostly bilirubin monoglucuronide	Normal colour; relative increase in monoglucuronide and decrease in diglucuronide
Effect of phenobarbitone on plasma bilirubin	None	Marked decrease	Decrease
Prognosis	Usually fatal in infancy or with later onset of neurological damage	Usually good; neurological damage rare	Good

Mode of inheritance

The familial nature of this syndrome has been widely established in kindreds other than that reported by Crigler and Najjar,[192] and a history of consanguinity is frequently obtained.[16,40] The available evidence indicates that the disorder is inherited as an autosomal recessive trait. This mode of inheritance is supported by excretion studies of compounds which undergo glucuronidation, such as salicylates[169] or menthol,[16,710] in non-icteric parents and siblings of patients. Despite the observation that formation of the glucuronides of these aglycones was generally reduced in the heterozygous carriers of the gene, none of these individuals exhibited an elevated plasma bilirubin concentration. Although it appears that the enzyme defect in carriers is usually not severe enough to interfere with pigment excretion, family studies using bilirubin as the test substrate have not been performed. Moreover, menthol excretion was normal in both parents of a black patient, but the mother was shown to have impaired hepatic clearance of radiobilirubin.[110] Although mild unconjugated hyperbilirubinaemia has been reported occasionally in relatives of patients,[447,647] this is observed far more frequently in association with the Crigler–Najjar type II syndrome (see below).

Laboratory findings

The evidence accumulated from many case studies indicates that bilirubin production is consistently normal. Hence, haemoglobin concentration, reticulocyte count, red cell survival,[110,774] magnitude and kinetics of the early-labelled bilirubin fraction,[611] plasma bilirubin turnover rate[66,110,647] and bone marrow structure are normal.

Light microscopic examination of the liver has generally revealed a normal appearance, although the presence of occasional and unexplained bile thrombi was observed by Crigler and Najjar.[192] On electron microscopy, subcellular structure also appears normal apart from prominence of the smooth endoplasmic reticulum[202,510] and minor, non-specific changes at the sinusoidal pole of the hepatocytes.[361]

Except for the elevated plasma bilirubin concentration, conventional liver function tests (including clearance of BSP) and cholangiography are uniformly normal. In the majority of cases, plasma bilirubin levels exceed 340 μmol/l (20 mg/100 ml), with all of the pigment in the unconjugated form.[647] The small amounts of direct-reacting bilirubin reported are probably artefactual and reflect the inadequate methodology (see earlier). Plasma bilirubin concentration may fluctuate, with a tendency to higher values in winter or during intercurrent illnesses.[647] Predictably, the urine contains no bilirubin, but a chloroform-soluble pigment has been found which may be similar to a presumed photoderivative of bilirubin obtained on ultrafiltration of plasma.[399] The faeces are normal in colour and the concentration of faecal urobilinogen is usually markedly reduced in both children[16,647] and adults.[703] Bile obtained from the gallbladder or following duodenal intubation is pale lemon-yellow. In a detailed examination of bile from patients, Fevery et al.[255] have confirmed that biliary excretion of bilirubin is markedly reduced (< 68 μmol/l [< 4 mg/100 ml]). It was shown also that the proportion of unconjugated bilirubin-IXα was increased to 30–57% of the total excreted bile pigment (< 1% in control subjects), although the actual amount of unconjugated bilirubin in bile was only one to seven times that observed in normal adults or patients with Gilbert's syndrome and constituted only a minor fraction of total bilirubin production. In addition, trace amounts of conjugated bilirubin were present in bile, predominantly in the form of bilirubin monoglucuronide. Glucose and xylose conjugates were also detectable.

Radiobilirubin kinetic studies in this syndrome showed a normal bilirubin production rate, greatly diminished hepatic bilirubin clearance (1–2% of normal) and a biological half-life of the pigment in excess of 156 hours.[66,110,191,647] The fractional transfer rate of bilirubin from plasma to liver was reduced to approximately half that of normal individuals. This finding may reflect saturation of either the intracellular binding sites or, less likely, the hepatic uptake process, as a result of the high plasma bilirubin levels. Isotopic studies also suggest that little more than half of the calculated extrahepatic bilirubin pool is present in extravascular tissues.[110,647] Removal by plasmapheresis of an amount of pigment equal to the total exchangeable bilirubin pool produced only a moderate and transient reduction in plasma bilirubin concentration,[64] suggesting that some tissues contain additional pigment deposits which do not readily exchange with bilirubin in the plasma. The tissue storage site of this excess pigment has not been determined. Only a small portion of the computed daily bile pigment turnover is eliminated in the form of bilirubin in the bile or as urobilinogen in the faeces. Studies on the effects of representative levels of indoor light on the biliary excretion of unconjugated bilirubin (e.g. photoisomers) in the Gunn rat indicate only a small contribution of this mechanism towards daily bilirubin turnover.[817] The major fraction of the bilirubin appears to be converted to polar diazo-negative derivatives that are excreted mainly in bile and to a lesser extent in urine.[647,682] These pigment catabolites probably resemble those excreted by the Gunn rat[566,647] and, at least in part, may represent dihydroxyl derivatives of bilirubin.[73] There is increasing evidence that specific microsomal cytochrome P450-dependent isoenzymes are involved, and that they may be induced, therefore, increasing bilirubin catabolism.[401]

The primary metabolic defect in Crigler–Najjar type I syndrome which leads to the markedly diminished hepatic bilirubin clearance involves the conjugation of bilirubin. In vitro assay of bilirubin UDP-glucuronyltransferase activity in liver biopsy specimens revealed complete absence of bilirubin glucuronide formation.[16,106,240,546,711] Glucuronide formation in vivo was also found to be reduced, but not absent, after administration of the following compounds that are normally excreted as glucuronides: N-acetyl-p-aminophenol[22] tetrahydrocortisol,[584] menthol,[710] chloral hydrate, trichloroethanol and salicylates,[169] o-aminophenol and 4-methylumbelliferone.[16] Thus, the genetic defect in hepatic glucuronide synthesis appears to be virtually complete for bilirubin, although trace amounts of bilirubin conjugates have been identified in the bile of some patients.[255] For several other aglycones, the defect seems to be less severe in that glucuronide formation and excretion are only partially reduced.

Studies in Gunn rat liver, which also has a greatly diminished ability to glucuronidate 2-aminophenol,[653] have shown that the addition of non-specific membrane perturbants, such as diethylnitrosamine[764] or alkyl ketones[435] enhances enzyme activity towards this substrate to a level comparable with that of normal rat liver. Similarly, enzyme activity with 2-aminophenol was restored in Gunn rat liver perfused with a medium containing pentan-3-one,[146] suggesting that the native enzyme is present in a functionally defective form. The diminished activity of UDP-glucuronyltransferase towards 4-nitrophenol in Gunn rats does not appear to be related to the elevated hepatic content of bilirubin.[168] Kinetic studies of the p-nitrophenol conjugating form of UDP-glucuronyltransferase suggested that the defect in Gunn rats is limited to an abnormal interaction between the enzyme and the UDP moiety of UDP-glucuronic acid and that this is due to an abnormality in the enzyme protein near the UDP-glucuronic acid binding site.[528] The existence of such a defect has been questioned since glucuronyltransferase from microsomes of normal and Gunn rats was found to be indistinguishable by immunological or electrophoretic methods.[765] Evidence obtained by separation of the UDP-glucuronyltransferase isoforms in Gunn rat liver has suggested that a defective subunit in the bilirubin glucuronidating isoform, and at least one other isoform, is responsible for the impaired glucuronide formation.[623,657]

Other more recent work suggests either absent or defective forms of bilirubin UDP-glucuronyltransferase as well as certain phenol-conjugating UDP-glucuronyltransferases in Gunn rats are involved.[623,657] Reduced mRNA levels have been observed in Gunn rats with phenol UDP-glucuronyltransferase deficiency, which may be due to posttranscriptional instability of the mRNA.[226] Preliminary studies suggest that some patients with Crigler–Najjar disease lack bilirubin UDP-glucuronyltransferase, whereas others possess defective bilirubin UDP-glucuronyltransferases.[735,736] Alternatively, the biochemical lesion in Gunn rats and Crigler–Najjar disease may reflect an inherited defect in the matrix structure of hepatic microsomes.[542] This hypothesis is based on the observations that infusion of dimethyl bilirubin (an esterified derivative of bilirubin) into homozygous Gunn rats led to biliary excretion of small amounts of bilirubin glucuronides, and that in vitro incubation of dimethyl bilirubin with microsomes from Gunn rats or liver from a patient with Crigler–Najjar type I disease resulted in apparent demethylation and glucuronidation of some of the pigment substrate.[542] Although some reservations regarding methodology and low pigment recovery can be raised, these findings suggest that the deficiency of bilirubin UDP-glucuronyltransferase activity is not due to a defective or absent enzyme, but to an alteration in the microenvironment of the endoplasmic reticulum. Detailed comparative analyses of the structure and physicochemical properties of the lipid bilayer of Gunn and Wistar rat microsomal membranes have not convincingly demonstrated any differences.[317,502,775] Furthermore, the demonstration that either Gunn or Wistar rat liver microsomes are equally effective environments for restoration of activity to highly purified bilirubin UDP-glucuronyltransferase[145] suggests that the enzyme is either absent or defective in Gunn rats and, presumably, in patients with Crigler–Najjar type I disease.

Treatment

A variety of innovative therapeutic modalities have been tried in an attempt to produce a sustained reduction of plasma bilirubin concentration, in the hope of preventing bilirubin encephalopathy, particularly in patients who survived the neonatal period. No form of treatment has been found to be consistently effective. As in the homozygous Gunn rat, phenobarbitone and other microsomal enzyme-inducing agents fail to stimulate bilirubin glucuronide formation or to reduce plasma bilirubin concentration in patients with Crigler–Najjar type I syndrome.[16,17,64,113] Failure to respond to phenobarbitone therapy has been advocated to distinguish patients with an absolute defect in bilirubin glucuronide formation from those considered to have a partial enzyme defect,[16] but this distinction does not appear to hold true in all

instances.[191,255] Several experimental manoeuvres, such as exchange transfusion or plasmapheresis[64,113,276,511] have been attempted in order to remove bilirubin from the body. These procedures remove substantial amounts of bilirubin and result in an acute, albeit transient reduction in plasma level which has been associated with dramatic clinical results in some cases;[64,791] the rapid rebound in plasma bilirubin and inherent practical problems limit the usefulness of this approach. Similarly, continuous extracorporeal perfusion through an affinity chromatography column containing albumin-covered agarose beads has proved successful in Gunn rats[637] and neonatal rhesus monkeys,[638] but major problems relating to the sterility, rheology and biocompatibility of such a system need to be overcome before it can be applied to humans.[639] From the observation that in normal individuals and patients with Gilbert's syndrome, hepatic bilirubin clearance is independent of pigment turnover, Berk et al.[66] subjected a patient with Crigler–Najjar type I syndrome (and Gunn rats) to repeated phlebotomy to reduce bilirubin turnover. Plasma bilirubin concentration remained essentially unchanged and this was found to be caused by an unexpected and unexplained reduction in plasma bilirubin clearance accompanying the fall in plasma bilirubin turnover. To prevent re-absorption and enterohepatic circulation of the small amount of unconjugated bilirubin which may be excreted in the bile, the potential value of orally administered binding agents such as agar or cholestyramine has been investigated. Although this approach has proved successful in neonatal jaundice[588] and in Gunn rats,[451,544] it has not been consistently beneficial in the treatment of Crigler–Najjar patients.[17,106,240,546]

The efficacy of phototherapy in the management of neonatal jaundice is well established[471] and this therapeutic modality has also been successful in reducing plasma bilirubin levels to below 170 μmol/l (10 mg/100 ml) in some infants with Crigler–Najjar type I syndrome.[5,316,406] Exposure for at least 12 h/day to an artificial light source (425–475 nm region of the visible spectrum) is necessary to maintain an adequate response. Apart from the practical problems involved some patients are resistant to phototherapy[106] and treatment may become ineffective after several years of intense exposure to light.[791] Moreover, little is known about possible long-term effects of such extensive illumination. It has been suggested that in hyperbilirubinaemic infants, the duration of daily phototherapy may be reduced by oral administration of cholestyramine,[17] making treatment at home a possibility.[546] This approach has proved ineffective in at least one reported adult case and its long-term efficacy has not been evaluated, so that it hardly appears to be a practical measure for life-long management of this condition. A case report in which chlorpromazine administration effectively reduced the plasma bilirubin level in a patient with Crigler–Najjar syndrome type I supports a role for inducers of specific microsomal cytochrome P450-dependent isoenzymes in treatment of these jaundiced patients.[398] Finally, liver transplantation has become the treatment of choice for patients with Crigler–Najjar type I syndrome, and for selected patients with Crigler–Najjar type II syndrome.[408,666,783]

Crigler–Najjar type II syndrome (congenital non-haemolytic jaundice with a partial defect in bilirubin conjugation)

Clinicopathological features

This condition was described in detail by Arias,[11] who reported a group of eight patients, aged 14 to 52 years. In half of these patients, jaundice was noted within the first year of life, and in the remaining four cases between the ages of 2 and 34 years. Jaundice was the only abnormal physical sign and, apart from the social problems imposed by chronic jaundice, most individuals led a relatively normal life. Although plasma bilirubin concentration ranged from 110 to 340 μmol/l (6.4 to 20 mg/100 ml), and virtually all of the pigment was in the unconjugated form, neurological manifestations, presumably due to bilirubin encephalopathy, were evident in only one patient.[387] This patient died at the age of 44, having been confined to a psychiatric institution for the last 20 years of her life; during this time, her neurological signs and plasma bilirubin level (250–375 μmol/l [15.8–22 mg/100 ml]) had remained relatively stable. At autopsy, the brain was reduced in weight and on histological examination showed degenerative changes consistent with kernicterus.[387] Subsequently, many more patients with this syndrome have been described.[56,649] Evidence of bilirubin encephalopathy was encountered much less frequently than in the more severe Crigler–Najjar type I syndrome, and the great majority of patients developed normally without signs of intellectual or extrapyramidal impairment.[16] Indeed, two of three icteric brothers, all over 50 years of age, with plasma bilirubin concentrations consistently in excess of 340 μmol/l (20 mg/100 ml) exhibited no neurological dysfunction, and the third had only minor and non-specific electroencephalographic changes.[303] Transient and reversible bilirubin encephalopathy has been observed in association with an increase in plasma bilirubin level related to prolonged fasting or an intercurrent illness.[309] Light microscopic examination of the liver has not revealed consistent morphological abnormalities, apart from occasional bile thrombi.[420] On electron microscopy, hypertrophy and hyperplasia of the smooth endoplasmic reticulum (SER) and prominence of the Golgi apparatus have been reported, particularly in the region of bile canaliculi,[303,772] although morphometric studies indicate that the surface density of the SER is comparable with that of normal subjects.[420]

Mode of inheritance

The frequent occurrence of Crigler–Najjar type II syndrome in families suggested that it is genetically determined but, unlike the type I syndrome, consanguinity appeared to be an infrequent association. Although jaundice may occur in successive generations, the exact pattern of inheritance has not been established. Some hold that the syndrome is transmitted as an autosomal dominant trait with incomplete penetrance.[11,80,679] This view is supported by the occurrence of significant hyperbilirubinaemia in three or four successive generations, and by the results of the menthol glucuronide test used as a screening procedure to identify carriers of the trait without hyperbilirubinaemia. For example, in a study of five families, reduced menthol glucuronide excretion was noted consistently on only one side of the family, and in no instance were abnormal test results found in both parents of a jaundiced patient.[16] Mild unconjugated hyperbilirubinaemia was present on the other side of the pedigree in two families in whom menthol glucuronide excretion was normal. This finding, together with the abnormal menthol glucuronide excretion noted in anicteric individuals presumed to be heterozygous for the type I syndrome,[710] indicates that the menthol excretion test fails to identify all carriers of the abnormal gene and hence its predictive value is limited. Since individuals with mild unconjugated hyperbilirubinaemia (Gilbert's syndrome) appear quite frequently in the families of patients with Crigler–Najjar type II syndrome,[303,363] others have postulated that the disorder is transmitted as a recessive trait. Crigler–Najjar type II syndrome is a very rare condition, whereas Gilbert's syndrome occurs in up to 7% of the population, so that this genetic interpretation may be an oversimplification. It has been suggested that two allelic genes may be involved, each being transmitted by a different parent, and that Gilbert's syndrome results when one or the other gene is present in a single dose.[363] It is evident that identification of the defect at a molecular level is required in order to establish the precise mode of inheritance of this syndrome.

Laboratory findings

Plasma unconjugated bilirubin levels usually range between 103 and 428 μmol/l (6–25 mg/100 ml), but values approaching 700 μmol/l (41 mg/100 ml) have been recorded in association with fasting or an intercurrent illness.[303,309] The plasma conjugated bilirubin fraction is normal and bilirubinuria is absent. Red cell survival and bilirubin production are normal, but hepatic bilirubin clearance is markedly diminished[95] and faecal urobilinogen excretion is moderately reduced. Bile obtained by duodenal aspiration or at laparotomy contains a considerable amount of bilirubin, but the bilirubin secretion rate is reduced in relation to the calculated pigment production rate.[309] Bilirubin monoglucuronide is the major bile pigment, with bilirubin diglucuronide and unconjugated bilirubin representing only minor fractions.[255,303,309,728] This pattern of bilirubin glucuronides excreted in bile is probably related to decreased UDP-glucuronyltransferase activity relative to the normal substrate load, since the enzyme has a greater capacity to synthesize bilirubin monoglucuronides than diglucuronide.[99,343] Bilirubin glucosides and xylosides are usually present in slightly higher proportion than in the bile of normal individuals, but formation of these conjugates far from compensates for the deficient glucuronide conjugation.[255] Bilirubin glucuronyltransferase activity in liver biopsy specimens is either not detectable[11,16,363,429] or greatly reduced.[303,728] With other aglycones, including *o*-aminophenol and *p*-nitrophenol, hepatic glucuronide formation was also found to be reduced.[11,16] In addition, glucuronide formation in vivo, measured by the menthol or salicylamide test, was diminished in most,[11,363,429] but not in all, cases.[16,772]

Treatment

It is now widely recognized that phenobarbitone and related drugs produce a dramatic fall in the plasma bilirubin concentration (frequently to less than 68 μmol/l [4 mg/100 ml]) in this syndrome, in contrast to patients with Crigler–Najjar type I syndrome.[16,303,682,797] Although in most instances phenobarbitone treatment is merely desirable, but not essential, for the management of this condition, many patients benefit cosmetically in terms of their social adjustment. Depending on the age of the patient, daily administration of 60–180 mg of phenobarbitone in divided doses usually brings about a progressive reduction in plasma bilirubin concentration over a period of 2–3 weeks, frequently to levels at which clinical jaundice is no longer recognizable. Therapy is effective regardless of when it is initiated in relation to the course of the disorder[303] and the pigment level gradually returns to pre-treatment values on withdrawal of the drug.[191] Results comparable to those with phenobarbitone have been obtained with oral administration of other microsomal enzyme-inducing agents, such as phenytoin, dicophane, glutethimide, phenazone (antipyrine), bucolome or the non-hypnotic barbiturate phetharbital.

It has been widely assumed that the response to phenobarbitone and related compounds is due to drug-mediated induction of hepatic microsomal glucuronyltransferase, particularly in view of the observation that hepatic enzyme activity and bilirubin transport capacity in heterozygous Gunn rats are substantially enhanced by phenobarbitone.[610] Similarly, in patients with acute hepatitis[246] or undergoing surgery,[94] activity of the enzyme was increased during phenobarbitone therapy. In patients with Crigler–Najjar type II syndrome, phenobarbitone has been shown to enhance significantly the hepatic clearance of bilirubin,[95] but with one possible exception no corresponding increase in bilirubin glucuronyltransferase activity[303] or in the surface density of the SER[420] could be demonstrated in the liver. Furthermore, it has been shown that, in patients with Gilbert's syndrome, phenobarbitone does not cause an increase in hepatic enzyme activity, despite the demonstrated reduction in plasma bilirubin level.[246] Thus, the weight of evidence indicates that Crigler–Najjar type II syndrome is due to a partial deficiency of hepatic bilirubin glucuronyltransferase activity, but based on available evidence, the dramatic reduction of hyperbilirubinaemia in response to phenobar-

bitone cannot be ascribed solely to induction of the enzyme.[303,429,772] The finding that bilirubin monoglucuronide remains the predominant pigment in bile while patients are receiving phenobarbitone therapy[303] remains unexplained.

Gilbert's syndrome (low-grade chronic hyperbilirubinaemia)

Clinicopathological features

In 1901, Gilbert and Lereboullet[288] described a syndrome of chronic, benign, intermittent jaundice, characterized by mild hyperbilirubinaemia in the absence of bilirubinuria or symptoms and signs of liver disease. The disorder was later shown to be distinct from haemolytic disease.[289] Although some of the original cases described by Gilbert probably had a state of compensated haemolysis, the term 'Gilbert's syndrome' has gained popular acceptance in the face of a variety of alternative proposals,[763] which include constitutional hepatic dysfunction,[177] familial non-haemolytic jaundice,[196] hereditary non-haemolytic bilirubinaemia,[6] and constitutional hyperbilirubinaemia.[24]

Since the introduction of routine biochemical screening, it has been apparent that mild elevation of plasma unconjugated bilirubin is not uncommon. The actual incidence is difficult to estimate and obviously depends on the value selected as the upper limit for normal plasma bilirubin concentration. Population studies have shown that, in general, men have a higher plasma bilirubin level than women[24,521,571] and that a clear bimodal distribution is frequently,[571,593] but not invariably, present.[24,744] On the basis of these and other investigations,[60,424] the incidence of Gilbert's syndrome appears to be approximately 3–7% of the population, with males predominating over females by a ratio of 2–7 : 1.[7,267,504,593]

The presence of hyperbilirubinaemia is recognized most often during the second and third decades of life. This observation and the predominance of Gilbert's syndrome in males may be related to hormone-induced changes in hepatic UDP-glucuronyltransferase activity that follow puberty.[522] Many older persons may be unaware of the abnormality until it is detected by incidental laboratory examination[267] or in the course of family studies.[593] Jaundice or scleral icterus is the only presenting symptom or abnormal physical finding in approximately 30% of patients. In some series, hyperbilirubinaemia was commonly an incidental finding in asymptomatic individuals,[60] whereas in others the disorder was associated with a variety of non-specific and protean symptoms, most frequently abdominal discomfort, fatigue or malaise.[593] In general, these symptoms do not correlate with the plasma bilirubin level and are, in fact, related to anxiety rather than to the underlying disorder in pigment metabolism. Since an increase in the level of plasma bilirubin in Gilbert's syndrome usually results from fasting[247,297,776] (see below), hyperbilirubinaemia in previously subclinical individuals may first be detected in association with caloric withdrawal due to an intercurrent febrile illness, 'morning sickness' of pregnancy, achalasia,[253] or postoperatively, especially following oral surgery.[596] Hyperbilirubinaemia may also be first noted in association with an acute haemolytic episode.[434] Many patients with Gilbert's syndrome are initially misdiagnosed as having acute or persistent hepatitis or cholelithiasis.[593] Consequently, the major importance of diagnosing this benign disorder is to distinguish it from more serious causes of hepatic dysfunction.

An essential component of the syndrome is that, on light microscopy, no significant abnormalities of liver structure are detectable. Although in a few individual cases a variety of minor and generally unimpressive histological abnormalities have been reported, the only finding noted by several investigators was accumulation of a lipofuscin-like pigment, predominantly around the terminal hepatic venules.[38,534,629] The histochemistry and ultrastructure of this pigment appear to differ from that found in the Dubin–Johnson syndrome. Electron microscopic studies have shown a variety of minor abnormalities,[139] the most consistent and notable finding has been gross hypertrophy of the smooth endoplasmic reticulum,[495] an observation reminiscent of Crigler–Najjar type II syndrome.[303] Morphological heterogeneity was evident in one series, with hypertrophy of the SER absent in about half of the patients,[200] while morphometric analysis of organelle structure has demonstrated an increase in the rough endoplasmic reticulum, mitochondrial membranes and cristae.[388] The functional relevance of these findings has to be determined.

Mode of inheritance

The occurrence of more than one case of mild unconjugated hyperbilirubinaemia within a given family has been recognized since the report of Gilbert and Lereboullet.[288] The heterogeneity of the disorder, as demonstrated by reduced red cell survival and mild abnormalities in hepatic clearance of BSP and/or ICG in some individuals (see below), has complicated many family studies so that the mode of inheritance has not been clearly defined. Many seemingly sporadic cases have been reported. Hence, the reported familial incidence of Gilbert's syndrome varies considerably in different series. A positive family history of hyperbilirubinaemia was obtained from only eight out of 58 patients studied by Foulk et al.,[267] whereas icterus was noted in three successive generations of a family reported by Baroody and Shugart.[34] In another series of 15 patients with Gilbert's syndrome, 55% of the siblings and 26% of the parents of the index cases had mild unconjugated hyperbilirubinaemia, and in a further study of 122 first-degree relatives of 42 patients, 27% of the siblings and 16% of the parents were found to have elevated bilirubin levels.[593] No affected relatives were observed in the kindred of 25 of the 42 patients. A higher incidence of hyperbilirubinaemia among relatives could be anticipated if plasma bilirubin levels were determined on repeated occasions or after fasting for 48 h. The accumulated evidence suggests that, in many cases, Gil-

bert's syndrome is probably inherited as an autosomal dominant and the patients are heterozygous for a single abnormal gene. Furthermore, the observation that cases of Gilbert's syndrome are occasionally found in families of Crigler–Najjar type II patients suggests that the two disorders may be genetically related.

Laboratory findings

Although by definition in Gilbert's syndrome the hyperbilirubinaemia is less than 103 μmol/l (6 mg/100 ml), the majority of patients exhibit a level below 50 μmol/l (3 mg/100 ml) and there is considerable daily and seasonal fluctuation. In a series of 58 patients reported by Foulk et al.,[267] and in another 55 observed by Powell et al.,[593] normal plasma bilirubin concentration was observed in 22% and 33%, respectively, of the patients at least once during the period of observation. In another series, the mean values obtained during the initial evaluation of patients ranged from 27 to 34 μmol/l (1.6 to 2 mg/100 ml).[60,297]

A variety of factors have been shown to produce fluctuations in plasma bilirubin concentration. Gilbert and Herscher[287] noted that in normal individuals, fasting resulted in a slight rise of plasma bilirubin. In subjects with Gilbert's syndrome, a 2- to 3-fold increase in plasma unconjugated bilirubin concentration is observed within 48 h of reducing the daily intake to 1.6 MJ (400 kcal) (Figure 14.10).[35,36,247,297] Twelve to 24 h after resuming a regular diet, plasma bilirubin returns to baseline level. Although fasting has also been shown to increase plasma unconjugated bilirubin levels in patients with liver disease or haemolysis, the magnitude of this rise is considerably less than that observed in Gilbert's syndrome.[243,572, 722] Findings in Gunn rats[299,300] and in patients with Crigler–Najjar type II syndrome and Gilbert's syndrome[36, 297,303] indicate that the degree of unconjugated hyperbili-

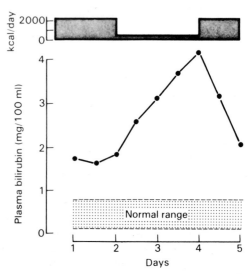

Figure 14.10 Effect of reduced caloric intake (400 kcal/day) for a period of 2 days on plasma bilirubin concentration in a patient with Gilbert's syndrome.

rubinaemia may be influenced by dietary composition as well as total caloric intake.[776] A normocaloric but lipid-free diet or intravenous infusion of glucose or amino acids increases hyperbilirubinaemia to an extent similar to that produced by fasting. Since addition of a small amount of lipid rapidly reverses the effect of these dietary manipulations and of fasting, it appears likely that in both situations the enhanced hyperbilirubinaemia may be attributable, at least in part, to lipid withdrawal. It is not known whether the mechanism responsible for the hyperbilirubinaemia is the same in fasting *per se* and in dietary lipid withdrawal.[300,776] Since similar dietary effects are observed in Gunn rats, it must be concluded that they are unrelated to hepatic bilirubin glucuronyltransferase activity because the enzyme is deficient in these animals. Kinetic studies have demonstrated a reduction in hepatic clearance of bilirubin both in fasting Gunn rats and in patients with Gilbert's syndrome,[108,417] and in Gunn rats fed a lipid-free diet.[300] Fasting does not appear to affect hepatic uptake of bilirubin significantly,[636] although the hepatic content of ligandin and Z protein is reduced.[690] With regard to changes in bilirubin production in fasting, the evidence is contradictory; enhanced catabolism of haem has been suggested by the finding of increased hepatic haem oxygenase activity[26,600] and carbon monoxide production,[433,473,500,600] and by the kinetic analysis of non-tracer doses of intravenous bilirubin.[553] Other investigators using kinetic methods have failed to find an increase in bilirubin production.[49,108,417] From the observation that plasma free fatty acid levels correlate with the rise in plasma bilirubin concentration both in fasting normal subjects[186] and in Gunn rats,[301] it has been proposed that fasting hyperbilirubinaemia may be due to lipolytic increase of bilirubin sequestered in adipose tissues. It has also been postulated that bilirubin conjugation may be decreased during fasting due to hepatic depletion of the co-substrate, UDP-glucuronic acid,[245] that intestinal absorption of unconjugated bilirubin may be enhanced during starvation,[278] and that the presence of bulk in the intestine may modify the fasting response, possibly by some neural or gut-endocrine mechanism.[605] It is evident that further investigation is necessary to clarify the complex mechanism(s) of fasting and dietary-induced hyperbilirubinaemia.[776]

Intravenous administration of nicotinic acid (50 mg) to patients with Gilbert's syndrome causes a 2- to 3-fold increase in plasma unconjugated bilirubin concentration within 3 hours of administration, whereas in normal individuals or in patients with haemolysis or liver disease, the rise is less impressive.[198,272,547,613] The underlying mechanism is unknown, but the observations that this response is largely prevented by prior splenectomy[272,329] and that nicotinic acid appears to increase erythrocyte fragility and splenic haem oxygenase activity[548] support the concept that splenic formation of bilirubin is enhanced. The haemolytic effect of nicotinic acid in Gilbert's syndrome is similar to that in controls and patients with haemolysis.[285] Nicotinic acid also has been shown to

compete with bilirubin for hepatic uptake[281,284,285] and to produce a transient inhibition of hepatic bilirubin glucuronyltransferase activity in heterozygous (anicteric) Gunn rats.[614] Although these effects may help explain the enhanced hyperbilirubinaemic response observed in Gilbert's syndrome, they do not account for the lack of a response in splenectomized patients. An exaggerated hyperbilirubinaemic response to nicotinic acid administration and caloric restriction has been reported in one series of patients to correlate with hypertrophy of the SER;[201] the responses in 12 of the 25 patients, those with normal hepatic morphology, did not differ significantly from controls. This association of morphological and functional heterogeneity requires confirmation, since the high proportion of normal (or negative) responses to fasting or nicotinic acid stimulation conflicts with other reported series.[198,243,297,572] The incidence and severity of prostaglandin-mediated side-effects secondary to nicotinic acid administration appear to be decreased by pre-treatment with indomethacin, without affecting the results of the test.[283]

Administration of phenobarbitone, glutethimide or clofibrate for 1–2 weeks reduces plasma unconjugated bilirubin concentration in patients with Gilbert's syndrome, frequently to normal levels.[93,431] Kinetic studies have shown that the reduction in plasma bilirubin is due both to accelerated hepatic bilirubin clearance and to reduced plasma bilirubin turnover.[95,105] Corticosteroid administration significantly reduces serum bilirubin concentration in patients with Gilbert's syndrome due to increased hepatic uptake and/or storage of bilirubin.[550]

Since virtually all plasma bilirubin is in the unconjugated form, bilirubinuria is absent. The faecal excretion of urobilinogen is usually normal, but it may be slightly decreased.[11,196] Hepatosplenomegaly is absent and conventional liver function tests are normal. It is now well documented that patients with Gilbert's syndrome have normal fasting, postprandial and postinfusion (i.e. intravenous glycocholate, cholate and chenodeoxycholate) plasma bile salt concentrations,[126,214,612,755] although an abnormal plasma clearance of orally administered ursodeoxycholic acid has been noted in one series.[551]

In about one-third of patients with Gilbert's syndrome, minor abnormalities of plasma BSP[57,75] and/or ICG disappearance[484,549] have been observed. reflecting a defect in hepatic anion transport. These abnormalities are probably due to defects in different stages of the hepatic uptake process. Similarly, it has been shown that in patients with Gilbert's syndrome the plasma half-life of tolbutamide is prolonged and its metabolic clearance is reduced.[160] Since tolbutamide is bound to ligandin but does not undergo glucuronidation, and clearance of the drug is generally enhanced by phenobarbitone administration, it would appear that hepatic uptake of this compound is defective in Gilbert's syndrome. Impaired elimination of selected drugs, including paracetamol (acetominophen),[213] has been attributed to the decrease in hepatic UDP-glucuronyltransferase activity. The plasma clearance of most drugs which undergo glucuronidation (e.g. the benzodiazepine derivatives oxazepam and lorazepam)[661] appears to be unaffected. The significance of reported changes in oxidation and acetylation are less clear,[477] although the prevalence of slow acetylators may be increased in patients with Gilbert's syndrome.[587] While these findings should be borne in mind when prescribing for patients with Gilbert's syndrome, significant clinical consequences of these abnormalities in drug metabolism have not been reported.

The pathogenesis of Gilbert's syndrome remains a source of controversy, largely because no single defect readily explains all of the observed abnormalities.[248,645] Kinetic studies with radiobilirubin have established that the mild unconjugated hyperbilirubinaemia is due to a reduction in hepatic bilirubin clearance to approximately 30% of normal,[62] resulting in increased retention of the pigment in plasma. In addition to this hepatic defect in pigment clearance, it has been found that up to 60% of patients have a mild and fully compensated state of haemolysis (detectable only by measuring ^{51}Cr-labelled red cell survival)[55,112,592] or dyserythropoiesis.[503] Reduced hepatic bilirubin clearance indicative of Gilbert's syndrome has been observed in association with hereditary spherocytosis, glucose-6-phosphate-dehydrogenase deficiency and a variety of non-spherocytic haemolytic anaemias.[55] Using radiolabelled haem precursors, increased hepatic haem production also has been demonstrated in four out of six patients with Gilbert's syndrome with a documented increase in bilirubin production; in the remaining two patients, haemolysis accounted for the enhanced bilirubin production.[816] Thus, patients with Gilbert's syndrome may have normal or increased bilirubin production, and the latter may be secondary either to accelerated erythroid or to hepatic haem turnover. In these instances, the coexistence of the two conditions is believed to be incidental rather than causal and the diagnosis of Gilbert's syndrome under these circumstances requires measurement of hepatic bilirubin clearance using sophisticated techniques.[55,816] The apparent prevalence of the combined appearance of the two abnormalities may simply reflect enhanced detection of Gilbert's syndrome due to the higher plasma bilirubin levels that result from the haemolysis- or dyserythropoiesis-related pigment overload. With the application of sophisticated methodology for analysis of serum bilirubin conjugates (alkaline methanolysis, TLC or HPLC), it is evident that either no or very little bilirubin conjugates are found in serum of patients with Gilbert's syndrome, whereas the serum of patients with haemolysis includes considerable quantities of bilirubin conjugates.[381,524,673] Whether patients with Gilbert's syndrome and haemolysis can be identified by their pattern of bilirubin conjugates in serum remains uncertain.

The mechanism underlying the reduction of bilirubin clearance in Gilbert's syndrome is not clear and remains a subject of considerable controversy. Measurement of ligandin concentration indicated that this intracellular binding protein is not reduced in the liver[259] or plasma.[730] From the analysis of kinetic studies with radiobilirubin, it has been suggested that a defect exists in the hepatic uptake as well as the microsomal conjugation of the pigment.[62,95] Whereas direct evidence for an uptake defect has not yet been obtained using tracer radiobilirubin, some, but not all, investigators have observed an uptake defect with non-tracer doses of bilirubin.[315,552] Hepatic bilirubin UDP-glucuronyltransferase activity measured in biopsy material is virtually always reduced.[14,19,46,92,246,297] With aglycones other than bilirubin, glucuronide formation in vitro or in vivo has been found to be unimpaired or reduced, depending on the substrate examined. Thus, in vitro glucuronidation of methyl umbelliferone has been reported as normal,[11,756] whereas that of paranitrophenol may be reduced significantly.[19] Similarly, in vivo conjugation of menthol,[285] salicylamide[33] and N-acetyl-p-aminophenol[646] is unimpaired, but urinary excretion of clofibrate glucuronide has been found to be diminished.[432]

The pathogenic significance of this partial and seemingly selective reduction in glucuronide formation and particularly of the reduced hepatic bilirubin UDP-glucuronyltransferase activity is unclear. The observation that enzyme inducers, such as phenobarbitone, decrease plasma bilirubin concentration and normalize the abnormal biliary pigment pattern (decrease in monoglucuronides with a relative increase in diglucuronide)[257,315] is consistent with the hypothesis that decreased glucuronidation alone is responsible for the decreased hepatic bilirubin clearance and the resultant hyperbilirubinaemia. Several findings are difficult to reconcile with the concept that reduced bilirubin glucuronyltransferase activity alone is responsible for the impaired hepatic clearance of the pigment in Gilbert's syndrome.[645] **(1)** Even the reduced hepatic enzyme activity is greatly in excess of the calculated enzyme activity in the whole liver required to conjugate all of the bilirubin produced in vivo. **(2)** Since enzyme activity in vitro is generally measured after digitonin activation (see earlier), it is difficult to determine to what extent this artificially perturbed enzyme level reflects the physiological situation. **(3)** The limitations of the conventional in vitro enzyme assay may also be responsible for the repeated observation that treatment with phenobarbitone or related drugs fails to produce a measurable increase in hepatic bilirubin glucuronyltransferase activity,[93,95,246] despite the associated reduction of plasma bilirubin concentration and improved hepatic pigment clearance. **(4)** The finding that hepatic bilirubin glucuronyltransferase activity may be reduced in chronic persistent hepatitis,[244] end-stage cirrhosis,[252] a variety of haemolytic disorders,[18] in several anicteric disorders such as non-cirrhotic portal fibrosis, extrahepatic portal vein obstruction or granulomatous involvement of the liver[197] and in a small proportion of patients with cholesterol gallstones[224] suggests that the reduced enzyme activity in Gilbert's syndrome may not represent the primary defect. **(5)** In a selected group of patients with hereditary spherocytosis and apparent Gilbert's syndrome, the initially low hepatic bilirubin clearance was found to increase or normalize following splenectomy.[68] This unexpected finding suggests that reduced hepatic bilirubin clearance is not an invariable finding and that occasionally it occurs only in the presence of an increased bilirubin load (i.e. latent Gilbert's syndrome that may be unmasked by haemolysis). (**6**) As mentioned above, patients with Gilbert's syndrome appear to have a moderately reduced rate of hepatic bilirubin uptake,[62] in contrast to patients with Crigler–Najjar syndrome type I[66] and homozygous Gunn rats,[636] where initial hepatic uptake of bilirubin is normal despite a lack of bilirubin glucuronyltransferase activity. This does not necessarily imply that the moderate reduction in uptake rate is the cause of the syndrome, since the intrinsic capacity of the hepatic uptake system enormously exceeds the normal net transport rate of bilirubin from blood to bile.[574,636] (**7**) A significant proportion of patients with Gilbert's syndrome exhibit abnormalities in hepatic transport of BSP, ICG, tolbutamide, rifamycin-SV[281,282] and/or oestrogens.[3] Since BSP is conjugated by a soluble hepatic enzyme and ICG is not conjugated prior to excretion, it is apparent that the reduction in glucuronyltransferase activity cannot account for these findings. It is thus evident that hepatic uptake of organic anions is defective, at least in a subgroup of patients with Gilbert's syndrome,[503] and that this abnormality is of variable selectivity. Considering the multiplicity of associated hepatic transport anomalies, the frequency of occult haemolysis, dyserythropoiesis or, possibly, increased hepatic haem turnover, and the apparent problems in ascribing the primary defect solely to reduced bilirubin glucuronyltransferase activity, it appears probable that Gilbert's syndrome represents a heterogeneous group of pathogenetic defects. Moreover, based on the demonstration that plasma bilirubin concentrations in a large population study did not exhibit a bimodal distribution,[24] it has been suggested that the high bilirubin levels observed in Gilbert's syndrome merely reflect the extreme upper values of normal expected from the skewed distribution curve. Although an apparent semantic argument, this observation implies that Gilbert's syndrome is not a clinical entity that can be clearly distinguished from normal.[645]

The diagnosis of Gilbert's syndrome is established primarily by exclusion of overt haemolysis and acquired liver disease. Further ascertainment of the diagnosis may be achieved by determining the effect of dietary restriction[297,572] or intravenous nicotinic acid administration[198,272,547] on the plasma bilirubin concentration. Either manipulation generally results in a 2- to 3-fold rise in plasma bilirubin concentration, although negative results are occasionally observed.[200,556] Other diagnostic manoeuvres which have been advocated are measurement of the effect of phenobarbitone on plasma bilirubin concentration[93] and administration of a tracer dose of radiobilirubin for estimation of the percentage of the dose remaining in the plasma after 4 h.[62] Percutaneous liver biopsy for both histological examination and determination of bilirubin glucuronyltransferase activity[92] is warranted in selected cases if the diagnosis remains in any doubt.

Treatment

Once the diagnosis is established, it is important to reassure the patient with regard to the benign and inconsequential nature of the disorder and the excellent prognosis. Although phenobarbitone, glutethimide and related drugs have been employed experimentally to reduce the hyperbilirubinaemia, there is little justification for the long-term use of these agents.

CONJUGATED HYPERBILIRUBINAEMIA _____

Dubin–Johnson syndrome (chronic idiopathic jaundice)

In 1954, Dubin and Johnson[222] and Sprinz and Nelson[689] independently described a benign disorder characterized by chronic or intermittent jaundice and a grossly pigmented liver (Table 14.4). Many additional cases have subsequently been reported in both sexes and in a wide variety of ethnic groups, including caucasians, blacks, Indians and Japanese.[69,149,221,423,704] The highest incidence of the disorder, about 1 per 1300, occurs in Persian Jews.[664]

Dubin[221] noted that jaundice was evident at birth or by the time of puberty in about half, and by the age of 20 in about two-thirds, of all afflicted individuals. Apart from chronic or recurrent jaundice of fluctuating intensity, most patients are asymptomatic, although some complain of vague right upper quadrant abdominal pain, weakness, nausea or vomiting. Many patients are anicteric at the time of diagnosis and their inherited abnormality is detected during the course of family studies for evaluation of a jaundiced relative. In women, subclinical hyperbilirubinaemia is often unmasked by pregnancy or the use of oral contraceptives.[174] For unclear reasons, a high frequency of fetal loss in pregnant Dubin–Johnson patients has been observed.[211] Physical examination is frequently normal except for slight icterus. In about 50% of cases, the urine is darker than normal and the liver is moderately enlarged and/or tender.[221] On visual examination, the liver is darkly pigmented; it has been variously described as green, slate blue, dark grey or even black in appearance and gross black discoloration of a liver biopsy is characteristic of this disorder. Although pigment may be observed occasionally in the phagocytic cells of lymph nodes and bone marrow, there is usually no generalized pigmentation of other tissues. The liver is histologically normal except for a conspicuous coarse-granular intracellular brown pigment which is most often limited to the perivenular areas (Figure 14.11). The pigment tends to be confined to parenchymal cells,[689] but small amounts may be present also in Kupffer cells.[221,782] On electron microscopy, abnormalities of pericanalicular microfilaments have been

Table 14.4 Characteristics of the hereditary conjugated hyperbilirubinaemias

	Dubin–Johnson syndrome	Rotor's syndrome	Hepatic storage syndrome
Incidence	Uncommon	Rare	Rare
Mode of inheritance	Autosomal recessive	Autosomal recessive	Not known
Plasma bilirubin concentration (μmol/l [mg/100 ml])	Occasionally up to 340 (20), but usually 35–85 (2–5); increased by oestrogens and pregnancy	Occasionally up to 340 (20), but usually 35–85 (2–5)	50–120 (3–7)
Age hyperbilirubinaemia recognized	Usually early adulthood (variable)	Usually childhood (variable)	Childhood
Clinical features	Asymptomatic or nonspecific symptoms; jaundice; occasional hepatosplenomegaly	Asymptomatic or nonspecific symptoms; jaundice	Asymptomatic jaundice
Routine liver function tests	Usually normal	Normal	Normal
Oral cholecystography	Gallbladder usually not visualized	Usually normal	Normal; delayed visualization of gallbladder
Gross appearance and histology of liver	Black-brown colour; pigment granules in perivenular hepatocytes	Normal	Normal
Plasma BSP disappearance	Slow initial disappearance (45 min retention < 20%); secondary rise at 90 min	Markedly slow initial disappearance (45 min retention 30–50%); no secondary rise	45 min retention; 36% in one case; no secondary rise
BSP transport maximum (T_m)	Markedly decreased	Moderately decreased (T_m also decreased for ICG)	Decreased
BSP hepatic storage capacity (S)	Normal	10% of normal (S also decreased for ICG)	Markedly decreased
Urinary coproporphyrin excretion	Normal total; > 80% coproporphyrin I (normal is 75% coproporphyrin III)	Increased total, proportion of coproporphyrin I elevated but < 80%	
Prognosis	Good	Good	Good

reported both in patients with Dubin–Johnson syndrome and with Rotor's syndrome.[712] Whether these cytoskeletal abnormalities are related causally to defective organic anion excretion or transport remains unclear. Apart from inconstant evidence of mitochondrial damage on electron microscopy,[228] the predominant finding is the aforementioned granular pigment which is present as dense membrane-enclosed bodies located primarily in the pericanalicular region.[534] It has been suggested that these are pigment-laden lysosomes.[526,660] Subcellular fractionation of liver tissue has shown increased activity of some lysosomal acid hydrolases and a selective deficiency of mitochondrial superoxide dismutase,[579] but the structural integrity of subcellular organelles seems generally preserved and the accumulation of pigment appears to represent a benign type of secondary lysosomal storage.[660] The observation that pigment disappears from the liver during the course of acute viral hepatitis, whereas the hepatic excretory defect for organic anions (see below)

persists, further supports the concept that the accumulation of pigment is the result, rather than the cause of the primary hepatic defect.[362,708,759] Furthermore, the degree of hepatic pigmentation is highly variable and is poorly correlated with plasma bilirubin concentration.[10,782] The chemical nature of the pigment remains unclear. Earlier investigators had assumed that the pigment belonged to the ill-defined group of lipofuscins,[221,222] but histochemical, spectroscopic and physicochemical analyses suggest that it is closely related to melanin.[2,236] Recent studies using electron spin resonance spectroscopy indicate that the pigment is not melanin and probably not a porphyrin, but is possibly made up of polymers of adrenaline (epinephrine) metabolites.[708,709,743]

The hyperbilirubinaemia is usually slight to moderate and exhibits considerable fluctuation.[221,664,689] Although values as high as 400 μmol/l (23 mg/100 ml) have been reported, most of the patients have plasma bilirubin levels of less than 86 μmol/l (5 mg/100 ml). Characteristically,

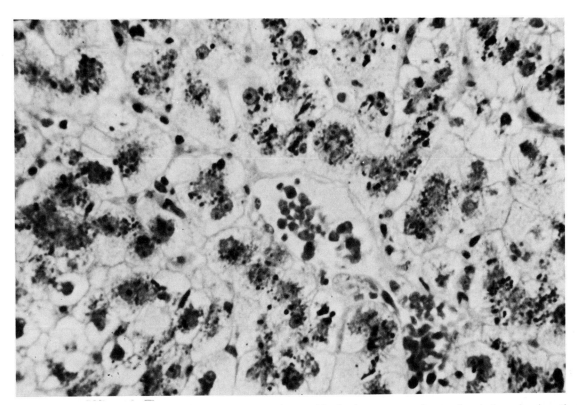

Figure 14.11 Hepatic histology in Dubin–Johnson syndrome. Dark pigment granules are located predominantly in hepatocytes around the terminal hepatic venule.

the plasma contains a significant fraction of 'direct-reacting' bilirubin (mean of 60%). The pattern of bilirubin conjugates in plasma (diconjugates > monoconjugates) is characteristic, and is dissimilar to that observed in acquired hepatobiliary disease.[616] The plasma also contains bilirubin glucuronides, which are presumed to have undergone acyl-shift[494] and to be bound covalently to albumin (see earlier).[769] The significant proportion of unconjugated bilirubin in plasma[616] may reflect diminished plasma bilirubin clearance[411] and/or enhanced hepatic deconjugation of bilirubin glucuronides.[304] Both conjugated bilirubin and urobilinogen are detectable in the urine of most patients.[221] Red cell survival and conventional liver function tests are generally normal.

Hepatic uptake of BSP and other organic dyes is normal or only mildly impaired, and the relative hepatic storage capacity of BSP is preserved.[530,664,771] The biliary excretion of both conjugated bilirubin[10] and BSP is markedly impaired, and the maximal hepatic secretory rate (T_m) for BSP approaches zero.[662,663] This results in prolonged hepatic storage of the dye.[423] Consequently, plasma BSP levels 45 min after a 5 mg/kg intravenous dose may be normal or only slightly increased but, because of the hepatic excretory defect, conjugated BSP refluxes from the liver into the plasma, producing a secondary rise in plasma concentration 60 to 90 min after injection. This peculiarity is demonstrable in more than 90% of all cases and is virtually pathognomonic for the Dubin–Johnson syndrome.[482,656,663] Studies in humans[1] and in the mutant

Corriedale sheep[30] which represents the ovine counterpart of the Dubin–Johnson syndrome indicate that whereas the biliary excretion of conjugated BSP is profoundly depressed, unconjugated BSP excretion remains relatively intact. With dibromosulphthalein, ICG and rose bengal, which do not require conjugation for excretion in bile, a secondary rise in plasma concentration is not observed.[235] Treatment with phenobarbitone frequently reduces the plasma level of conjugated bilirubin and increases the hepatic transport maximum of BSP, but this effect is inconstant.[501,662] Hepatic transport of conjugated oestrogens is defective,[3] but the biliary excretion of bile acids is unaffected and both fasting and postprandial plasma bile acid levels are normal.[171,174,327,385] In one series of patients, significantly elevated fasting plasma bile acid levels and impaired ursodeoxycholic acid tolerance were noted.[412,551] In addition, a woman with Dubin–Johnson syndrome has been reported with an elevated fasting conjugated cholate concentration and prolonged intravenous clearance of sodium glycocholate.[215] These reports suggest that some heterogeneity in this syndrome exists. In the majority of patients, oral cholecystography fails to outline the gallbladder or results in only faint opacification,[221] but intravenous administration of contrast medium may improve visualization. Similarly, ^{99m}Tc-labelled dimethyl iminodiacetic acid (HIDA) cholescintigraphy characteristically shows delayed or no visualization of the gallbladder and bile ducts with prompt, intense, homogeneous and prolonged visualization of the liver.[27]

An isolated deficiency of factor VII has been described in a significant proportion of patients with Dubin–Johnson syndrome in Israel,[659] but in family studies the two defects were found to segregate independently, suggesting that they are unrelated. The aminopyrine breath test was found to be normal in six patients with the Dubin–Johnson syndrome.[28]

Metabolic defects in the mutant Corriedale sheep are remarkably similar to those of the Dubin–Johnson syndrome.[30,182] The disorder is transmitted as an autosomal recessive trait and affected sheep have a mild conjugated hyperbilirubinaemia with greatly reduced biliary secretion of conjugated bilirubin, BSP, ICG, rose bengal and iodopanoic acid, but unimpaired hepatic transport of bile acids.[4,12,15,30,508] Heterozygote sheep do not appear to express biliary transport defects.[31] About 6 months after birth, brown-black pigment becomes apparent in the lysosomes of the hepatocytes around the terminal hepatic venule. The physicochemical properties of the pigment resemble those of melanin and it has been suggested that its formation may be related to defective biliary excretion of catecholamines.[12] Facial photosensitivity, which is an additional feature of this ovine disorder, results from the accumulation in plasma of phylloerythrin, a cyclic tetrapyrrole formed by bacterial degradation of chlorophyll in the gut. Recently, a mutant rat strain has been described with chronic conjugated hyperbilirubinaemia, defective transport of organic anions from liver to bile, and elevated urinary coproporphyrin isomer I excretion.[382] Other features of the Dubin–Johnson syndrome, such as abnormal liver morphology, are not present.

Patients with Dubin–Johnson syndrome have a unique and diagnostic abnormality of urinary coproporphyrin excretion. The urine of healthy individuals contains coproporphyrin isomers I and III, with about 75% in the isomer III form, reflecting the fact that porphyrins of the isomer III series are precursors in haem biosynthesis. In Dubin–Johnson syndrome, although total urinary coproporphyrin excretion is normal or only slightly increased, 84–90% of the total urinary coproporphyrin is the type I isomer.[47,421,426,427,788] In heterozygous carriers of the trait who are phenotypically normal, an intermediate urinary coproporphyrin isomer ratio is present (approximately 35% of coproporphyrin I).[48,421,788] In presumed heterozygotes, the range and overlap of values are too great for the isomer ratio to serve as an accurate diagnostic tool for detection of individual cases. The recent finding that uroporphyrinogen III cosynthetase activity is normal in both erythrocytes and liver of patients with Dubin–Johnson syndrome[669] and a study on the fate of injected δ-aminolaevulinic acid (precursor of hepatic haem),[422] both favour the concept that the altered urinary coproporphyrin excretion is not related to an abnormality in the relative production rates of porphyrinogen isomers I and III (i.e. there is no major enzymatic derangement in the haem synthetic pathway), but rather to defective biliary excretion of coproporphyrinogen III.

Family studies based on detection of presumptive carriers by determination of the urinary coproporphyrin isomer ratio indicated that Dubin–Johnson syndrome is inherited as an autosomal recessive trait.[48,225,788] This mode of inheritance is further supported by the high frequency of consanguinity noted in parents of affected individuals.[423] The primary defect appears to involve impaired biliary canalicular transport of organic anions, possibly due to an abnormality in the membrane carrier system.[30] Impaired biliary secretion has been demonstrated for conjugated bilirubin[221] and BSP,[1,482] ICG,[656] rose bengal,[782] and cholecystographic contrast media.[221] Since this benign disorder has a good prognosis with a normal life expectancy, no specific therapy is necessary other than reassurance. Female patients should be warned about the aggravating effect of oestrogen-containing preparations or pregnancy on the intensity of the jaundice.

Rotor's syndrome

In 1948, Rotor, Manahan and Florentin[618] described a benign disorder of familial non-haemolytic jaundice with direct-reacting bilirubin in a Filipino family. Some of these patients have been studied further by other investigators[573,789,793] and additional cases of the syndrome have been reported in both sexes and in other ethnic groups.[346,530,575,576,590,641,670,692,745,789] This disorder is seen much less commonly than the Dubin–Johnson syndrome from which it appears to differ pathophysiologically (Table 14.4).

Rotor's syndrome is characterized by chronic, relatively mild jaundice which fluctuates in intensity and is usually apparent before the age of 20 years. Although patients are usually asymptomatic, mild epigastric discomfort and weakness have been described, with occasional frank abdominal pain and fever. Hepatosplenomegaly is unusual, jaundice being the only abnormal physical finding. Both the gross and microscopic appearances of the liver are normal; pigmentation of the liver is conspicuously absent, but this is not a reliable feature by which to distinguish it from Dubin–Johnson syndrome, since the amount of hepatic pigmentation is highly variable in the latter condition.[10] With the exception of one reported family, evidence of haemolysis was lacking.[212] Conventional liver function tests are normal, apart from a predominantly conjugated hyperbilirubinaemia; plasma bilirubin concentration is usually elevated in the range of 34–86 μmol/l (2–5 mg/100 ml), with occasional values up to 400 μmol/l (23 mg/100 ml) being recorded. Bilirubinuria is evident, provided that the plasma level of conjugated bilirubin is sufficiently high. In contrast to Dubin–Johnson syndrome, the gallbladder is usually, although not invariably, visualized on oral cholecystography.

After intravenous injection of a single loading dose of bilirubin, plasma clearance of both bilirubin and conjugated bilirubin is reduced.[241,410,641] In addition, plasma clearance of BSP is markedly delayed in Rotor's syndrome, so that between 30 and 50% of the dye is usually retained in plasma 45 min after administration of a 5 mg/kg dose. In contrast to Dubin–Johnson syndrome, there is no reflux of conjugated BSP from the liver into the circulation and, hence, no secondary rise in plasma BSP 90 min after injection. Moreover, the computed hepatic storage capacity for BSP is only 10% of normal whereas the T_m is only modestly reduced.[410,793] Reduced plasma disappearance, T_m, and relative hepatic storage capacity of ICG,[34,529] ^{131}I-rose-bengal and ^{99m}Tc-IDA derivatives[241,274] have also been observed in Rotor's syndrome. The abnormalities in BSP and ICG transport in Rotor's syndrome differ from those in the Dubin–Johnson syndrome and suggest that Rotor's syndrome represents a defect in hepatic uptake and/or storage of organic anions.[241,274,410] Furthermore, the derangement in BSP transport resembles that of other hepatobiliary disorders,[655,771] so that it is not diagnostic for Rotor's syndrome. Analysis of urinary coproporphyrin excretion is a further means of differentiating this disorder from Dubin–Johnson syndrome.[670,785,789] Patients with Rotor's syndrome exhibit markedly increased (i.e. 6-fold) total urinary coproporphyrin excretion. Although more than 60% is excreted as the type I isomer, there is an absolute increase in coproporphyrin III excretion, in sharp contrast to the findings in Dubin–Johnson syndrome. A similar pattern of coproporphyrin isomer excretion is found in many cholestatic disorders[23] and this may simply reflect reduced biliary excretion of coproporphyrin with a concomitant shift to renal excretion.[597,785]

Pedigree analyses of families with Rotor's syndrome suggest an autosomal recessive mode of inheritance.[573,670] This is consistent with the more recent observations that phenotypically normal heterozygous carriers of the trait have a mildly elevated plasma retention of BSP at 45 min,[793] and usually, but not invariably,[692] a total urinary coproporphyrin excretion intermediate between that of normal subjects and of patients with the syndrome.[670,789]

Hepatic storage disease

A third type of congenital conjugated hyperbilirubinaemia associated with hepatic uptake and storage impairment

has been described by Dhumeaux and Berthelot.[207] Other presumed cases of this so-called 'hepatic storage disease' have been reported.[203,331,419] In this disorder, jaundice appeared early in childhood and the plasma bilirubin concentration fluctuated between 50 and 70 μmol/l (3 and 4.1 mg/100 ml), comprising around 50% conjugated bilirubin. Conventional liver function tests, plasma bile acid concentration and hepatic bilirubin UDP-glucuronyl-transferase activity were all normal. Hepatic histology was normal and intrahepatocytic pigment was lacking. The gallbladder was visualized on oral cholecystography, but only after a delay of 20 h.

The plasma disappearances of BSP, dibromo-sulphthalein, ICG and rose bengal were all significantly reduced. The most striking finding was a marked impairment of the relative hepatic storage capacity of BSP, and this defect was associated with a decrease in the biliary T_m. Although conjugated BSP was demonstrable in the plasma and urine, no distinct secondary rise of conjugated dye was evident in the plasma. These findings suggest that the primary defect is an impairment of hepatic uptake and/or storage of bilirubin and other organic anions. These hepatic transport abnormalities appear to be similar to those which have been described in the mutant Southdown sheep[181] and in all species of indigo snakes.[533] Because the ligandin and Z protein content of hepatocytes in the mutant Southdown sheep is normal,[453] and pheno-barbitone (which increases the hepatic ligandin concentration) modifies neither plasma bilirubin level nor BSP clearance in hepatic storage disease, it is unlikely that a deficiency of intracellular binding proteins is responsible. Although the defect in hepatic organic anion transport awaits clarification, on the basis of the available evidence the many similarities between hepatic storage disease and Rotor's syndrome makes it difficult to distinguish clearly the two syndromes.[241,419] Thus, the distinction between hepatic storage disease and Rotor's syndrome remains tentative.

ACKNOWLEDGEMENTS _____

We are indebted to Nancy Hegarty for editorial assistance in the preparation of this manuscript. Supported by National Institutes of Health Grant, DK36887.

REFERENCES _____

1. Abe, H. & Okuda, K. (1975) Biliary excretion of conjugated sulfobromophthalein (BSP) in constitutional conjugated hyperbilirubinemias. *Digestion*, 13, 272–283.
2. Acocella, G. & Billing, B.H. (1965) The effect of rifamycin-SV on bile pigment excretion in rats. *Gastroenterology*, 49, 526–530.
3. Adlercreutz, H. & Tikkanen, M.J. (1973) Defects in hepatic uptake and transport and biliary excretion of estrogens. *Médicine et Chirurgie Digestives*, 2, 59–65.
4. Alpert, S., Mosher, M., Shanske, A. & Arias, I.M. (1969) Multiplicity of hepatic excretory mechanisms for organic anions. *Journal of General Physiology*, 53, 238–247.
5. Altay, C. & Say, B. (1973) Phototherapy in nonobstructive nonhemolytic jaundice. *Pediatrics*, 51, 124–126.
6. Alwall, N. (1946) On hereditary nonhemolytic bilirubinemia. *Acta Medica Scandinavica*, 123, 560–595.

7. Alwall, N., Laurell, C.B. & Nilsby, J. (1946) Studies on heredity in cases of 'non-haemolytic hyperbilirubinaemia without direct van den Bergh reaction' (hereditary non-haemolytic bilirubinaemia). *Acta Medica Scandinavica*, 124, 114–125.
8. Anderson, K.E., Simionatto, C.S., Drummond, G.S. & Kappas, A. (1984) Tissue distribution and disposition of tin-protoporphyrin, a potent competitive inhibitor of heme oxygenase. *Journal of Pharmacology and Experimental Therapeutics*, 228, 327–333.
9. Aoyagi, Y., Ikenaka, T. & Ichida, F. (1979) α-Fetoprotein as a carrier protein in plasma and its bilirubin-binding ability. *Cancer Research*, 39, 3571–3574.
10. Arias, I.M. (1961) Studies of chronic familial non-hemolytic jaundice with conjugated bilirubin in the serum with and without an unidentified pigment in the liver cells. *American Journal of Medicine*, 31, 510–518.

11. Arias, I.M. (1962) Chronic unconjugated hyperbilirubinemia without overt signs of hemolysis in adolescents and adults. *Journal of Clinical Investigation,* **41,** 2233–2245.
12. Arias, I.M. (1968) Chronic idiopathic jaundice. In Beck, K. (ed.) *Ikterus,* pp. 65–71. Stuttgart: F.K. Schattauer Verlag.
13. Arias, I.M. & Jansen, P. (1975) Protein binding and conjugation of bilirubin in the liver cell. In Goresky, C.A. & Fisher, M.M. (eds) *Jaundice,* pp. 175–188. New York: Plenum Press.
14. Arias, I.M. & London, I.M. (1957) Bilirubin glucuronide formation in vitro; demonstration of a defect in Gilbert's disease. *Science,* **126,** 563–564.
15. Arias, I., Bernstein, L., Toffler, R. *et al.* (1964) Black liver disease in Corriedale sheep: a new mutation affecting hepatic excretory function. *Journal of Clinical Investigation,* **43,** 1249–1250.
16. Arias, I.M., Gartner, L.M., Cohen, M. *et al.* (1969) Chronic nonhemolytic unconjugated hyperbilirubinemia with glucuronyl transferase deficiency. Clinical, biochemical, pharmacologic and genetic evidence for heterogeneity. *American Journal of Medicine,* **47,** 395–409.
17. Arrowsmith, W.A., Payne, R.B. & Littlewood, J.M. (1975) Comparison of treatments for congenital non-obstructive nonhaemolytic hyperbilirubinaemia. *Archives of Disease in Childhood,* **50,** 197–201.
18. Auclair, C., Feldmann, G., Hakim, J. *et al.* (1976) Bilirubin and paranitrophenol glucuronyl transferase activities and ultrastructural aspect of the liver in patients with chronic hemolytic anemias. *Biomedicine,* **25,** 61–65.
19. Auclair, C., Hakim, J., Bowin, P. *et al.* (1976) Bilirubin and paranitrophenol glucuronyl transferase activities of the liver in patients with Gilbert's syndrome. *Enzyme,* **21,** 97–107.
20. Aussel, C. & Masseyeff, R. (1984) Interaction of retinoids and bilirubin with the binding of arachidonic acid to human alpha-fetoprotein. *Biochemical and Biophysical Research Communications,* **119,** 1122–1127.
21. Aw, T.Y. & Jones, D.P. (1984) Control of glucuronidation during hypoxia. Limitation by UDP-glucose pyrophosphorylase. *Biochemical Journal,* **291,** 707–712.
22. Axelrod, J., Schmid, R. & Hammaker, L. (1957) A biochemical lesion in congenital non-obstructive, non-haemolytic jaundice. *Nature,* **180,** 1426–1427.
23. Aziz, M.A., Schwartz, S. & Watson, C.J. (1964) Studies of coproporphyrin. VIII. Reinvestigation of the isomer distribution in jaundice and liver diseases. *Journal of Laboratory and Clinical Medicine,* **63,** 596–604.
24. Bailey, A., Robinson, D. & Dawson, A.M. (1977) Does Gilbert's disease exist? *Lancet,* **1,** 931–933.
25. Bakken, A.F. & Fog, J. (1975) *Metabolism and Chemistry of Bilirubin and Related Tetrapyrroles.* Oslo: Rikshospitalet.
26. Bakken, A.F., Thaler, M.M. & Schmid, R. (1972) Metabolic regulation of heme catabolism and bilirubin production. I. Hormonal control of hepatic heme oxygenase activity. *Journal of Clinical Investigation,* **51,** 530–536.
27. Bar-Meir, S., Baron, J., Seligsohn, U. *et al.* (1982) ⁹⁹ᵐTc-HIDA cholescintigraphy in Dubin–Johnson and Rotor syndromes. *Radiology,* **142,** 743–746.
28. Bar-Meir, S., Halpern, Z., Levy, R. *et al.* (1982) Aminopyrine breath test in Dubin–Johnson and Gilbert's syndrome. *Israel Journal of Medical Sciences,* **18,** 719–720.
29. Barnhart, J.L. & Combes, B. (1974) The effect of theophylline on hepatic excretory function. *American Journal of Physiology,* **227,** 194–199.
30. Barnhart, J.L., Gronwall, R.R. & Combes, B. (1981) Biliary excretion of sulfobromophthalein compounds in normal and mutant Corriedale sheep. Evidence for a disproportionate transport defect for conjugated sulfobromophthaleins. *Hepatology,* **1,** 441–447.
31. Barnhart, J.L., Gronwall, R.R. & Combes, B. (1983) Biliary excretion of infused conjugated sulfobromophthalein in sheep heterozygote for the transport defect present in mutant Corriedale sheep. *American Journal of Veterinary Research,* **44,** 2403–2404.
32. Barnhart, J.L., Witt, B.L., Hardison, W.G. & Berk, R.N. (1983) Uptake of iopanoic acid by isolated rat hepatocytes. *American Journal of Physiology,* **244,** G630–G636.
33. Barnville, H.T.F. & Misk, R. (1959) Urinary glucuronic acid excretion in liver disease and the effect of a salicylamide load. *British Medical Journal,* **1,** 337–340.
34. Baroody, W.G. & Shugart, R.T. (1956) Familial nonhemolytic icterus. *American Journal of Medicine,* **20,** 314–316.
35. Barrett, P.V.D. (1971) Hyperbilirubinemia of fasting. *Journal of the American Medical Association,* **217,** 1349–1353.
36. Barrett, P.V.D. (1975) Effects of caloric and noncaloric materials in fasting hyperbilirubinaemia. *Gastroenterology,* **68,** 361–369.
37. Barrett, P.V.D., Cline, M.J. & Berlin, N.I. (1966) The association of the urobilin 'early peak' and erythropoiesis in man. *Journal of Clinical Investigation,* **45,** 1657–1665.
38. Barth, R.F., Grimley, P.M., Berk, P.D. *et al.* (1971) Excess lipofuscin accumulation in constitutional hepatic dysfunction (Gilbert's syndrome). *Archives of Pathology,* **91,** 41–47.
39. Barthelson, R. & Roth, S. (1985) Topology of UDP-galactose cleavage in relation to *N*-acetyl-lactosamine formation in Golgi vesicles. Translocation of activated galactose. *Biochemical Journal,* **225,** 67–75.
40. Bartolozzi, G., Ciampoline, M., Salti, R. & Verrotti, M. (1969) La malattia di Crigler–Najjar: presentazione di un caso. *Minerva Pediatrica,* **21,** 2393–2406.
41. Beale, D., Ketterer, D., Carne, T. *et al.* (1982) Evidence that the Yₐ and Y_c subunits of glutathione-transferase B (ligandin) are the products of separate genes. *European Journal of Biochemistry,* **126,** 459–463.
42. Beale, D., Meyer, D.J., Taylor, J.B. & Ketterer, B. (1983) Evidence that the Y_b subunits of hepatic glutathione transferases represent two different but related families of polypeptides. *European Journal of Biochemistry,* **137,** 125–129.
43. Becker, S.D. & LaMont, J.T. (1988) Postoperative jaundice. *Seminars in Liver Disease,* **8,** 183–190.
44. Belanger, P.M., Lalande, M., LaBrecqut, G. *et al.* (1985) Diurnal variations in the transferases and hydrolases involved in glucuronide and sulfate conjugation of rat liver. *Drug Metabolism and Disposition,* **13,** 386–389.
45. Belina, H., Cooper, S.D., Farkas, R. *et al.* (1975) Sex differences in the phospholipid composition of rat liver microsomes. *Biochemical Pharmacology,* **24,** 301–303.
46. Bellet, H. & Raynaud, A. (1974) An assay of bilirubin UDP-glucuronyl transferase on needle-biopsies applied to Gilbert's syndrome. *Clinica Chimica Acta,* **53,** 51–55.
47. Ben-Ezzer, J., Rimington, C. & Shani, M. (1971) Abnormal excretion of the isomers of urinary coproporphyrin by patients with Dubin–Johnson syndrome in Israel. *Clinical Science,* **40,** 17–30.
48. Ben-Ezzer, J., Blonder, J., Shani, M. *et al.* (1973) Dubin–Johnson syndrome. Abnormal excretion of the isomers of urinary coproporphyrin by clinically unaffected family members. *Israel Journal of Medical Sciences,* **9,** 1431–1436.
49. Bensinger, I.A., Maisels, M.J., Carlson, D.E. & Conrad, M.E. (1973) Effect of low calorie diet on endogenous carbon monoxide production: normal adults and Gilbert's syndrome. *Proceedings of the Society for Experimental Biology and Medicine,* **144,** 417–419.
50. Berendsohn, S., Lowman, J., Sundberg, D. & Watson, C.J. (1964) Idiopathic dyserythropoietic jaundice. *Blood,* **24,** 1–18.
51. Berglund, L., Angelin, B., Blomstrand, R., Drummond, G. & Kappas, A. (1988) Sn-Protoporphyrin lowers serum bilirubin levels, decreases biliary bilirubin output, enhances biliary heme excretion and potently inhibits hepatic heme oxygenase activity in normal human subjects. *Hepatology,* **8(3),** 625–631.
52. Berk, P.D. (1975) Total body handling of bilirubin. In Goresky, C.A. & Fisher, M.M. (eds) *Jaundice,* pp. 135–157. New York: Plenum Press.
53. Berk, P.D. (1984) Pathophysiology, diagnosis and treatment of hereditary hyperbilirubinemias. In Williams, S.R. & Maddrey, W.C. (eds) *Butterworths International Medical Reviews: Gastroenterology,* Vol. 4, *Liver,* pp. 1–51. London: Butterworths.
54. Berk, P.D. & Berlin, N.I. (1977) *Chemistry and Physiology of Bile Pigments.* Fogarty International Center Proceedings No. 35. Washington, D.C. U.S. Government Printing Office.
55. Berk, P.D. & Blaschke, T.F. (1972) Detection of Gilbert's syndrome in patients with hemolysis. A method using radioactive chromium. *Annals of Internal Medicine,* **77,** 527–531.
56. Berk, P.D., Berlin, N.I. & Howe, R.B. (1974) Disorders of bilirubin metabolism. In Bondy, P.K. & Rosenberg, L. (eds) *Duncan's Diseases of Metabolism,* pp. 825–880A. Philadelphia: W.B. Saunders.

57. Berk, P.D., Blaschke, T.F. & Waggoner, J.G. (1972) Defective bromosulfophthalein clearance in patients with constitutional hepatic dysfunction (Gilbert's syndrome). *Gastroenterology*, **63**, 472–481.

58. Berk, P.D., Patel, S. & Isola, L.M. (1989) BSP/bilirubin- and organic anion-binding proteins, similar 54 kDA plasma membrane glycoproteins with high affinities for organic anions, are transcribed from different mRNA's. *Hepatology*, **10**, 631.

59. Berk, P.D., Potter, B.J. & Stremmel, W. (1987) Role of plasma membrane ligand-binding proteins in the hepatocellular uptake of albumin-bound organic anions. *Hepatology*, **7**, 165–176.

60. Berk, P.D., Wolkoff, A.W. & Berlin, N.J. (1975) Inborn errors of bilirubin metabolism. *Medical Clinics of North America*, **59**, 803–816.

61. Berk, P.D., Howe, R.B., Bloomer, J.R. & Berlin, N.I. (1969) Studies of bilirubin kinetics in normal adults. *Journal of Clinical Investigation*, **48**, 2176–2190.

62. Berk, P.D., Bloomer, J.R., Howe, R.B. & Berlin, N.I. (1970) Constitutional hepatic dysfunction (Gilbert's syndrome). A new definition based on kinetic studies with unconjugated radiobilirubin. *American Journal of Medicine*, **49**, 296–305.

63. Berk, P.D., Rodkey, F.L., Blaschke, T.F. *et al.* (1974) Comparison of plasma bilirubin turnover and carbon monoxide production in man. *Journal of Laboratory and Clinical Medicine*, **83**, 29–37.

64. Berk, P.D., Martin, J.F., Blaschke, T.F. *et al.* (1975) Unconjugated hyperbilirubinaemia. Physiologic evaluation and experimental approaches to therapy. *Annals of Internal Medicine*, **82**, 552–570.

65. Berk, P.D., Blaschke, T.F., Scharschmidt, B.F. *et al.* (1976) A new approach to quantitation of the various sources of bilirubin in man. *Journal of Laboratory and Clinical Medicine*, **87**, 767–780.

66. Berk, P.D., Scharschmidt, B.F., Waggoner, J.G. & White, S.C. (1976) The effect of repeated phlebotomy on bilirubin turnover, bilirubin clearance and unconjugated hyperbilirubinaemia in the Crigler–Najjar syndrome and the jaundiced Gunn rat: application of computers to experimental design. *Clinical Science and Molecular Medicine*, **50**, 333–348.

67. Berk, P.D., Jones, E.A., Howe, R.B. & Berlin, N.I. (1980) Disorders of bilirubin metabolism. In Bondy, P.K. & Rosenberg, L.E. (eds) *Metabolic Control and Disease*, 8th edn., pp. 1047–1088. Philadelphia: W.B. Saunders.

68. Berk, P.D., Berman, M.D., Blitzer, B.L. *et al.* (1981) Effect of splenectomy on hepatic bilirubin clearance in patients with hereditary spherocytosis. *Journal of Laboratory and Clinical Medicine*, **98**, 37–45.

69. Berkowitz, D., Entine, J. & Chunn, L. (1960) Dubin–Johnson syndrome: report of a case occurring in a Negro male. *New England Journal of Medicine*, **262**, 1028–1029.

70. Bernstein, L.H., Ezzer, J.B., Gartner, L. *et al.* (1966) Hepatic intracellular distribution of tritium-labelled unconjugated and conjugated bilirubin in normal and Gunn rats. *Journal of Clinical Investigation*, **45**, 1194–1201.

71. Bernstein, R.B., Troxler, R.F. & Lester, R. (1968) The effect of hepatobiliary disease on urobilinogen excretion. *Gastroenterology*, **54**, 150 (abstract).

72. Berry, C. & Hallinan, T. (1976) Summary of a novel, three-component regulatory model for uridine diphosphate glucuronyl-transferase. *Biochemical Society Transactions*, **4**, 650–652.

73. Berry, C.S., Zarembo, J.E. & Ostrow, J.D. (1972) Evidence for conversion of bilirubin to dihydroxyl derivatives in the Gunn rat. *Biochemical and Biophysical Research Communications*, **49**, 1366–1375.

74. Berthelot, P. & Billing, B.H. (1966) Effect of bunamiodyl on hepatic uptake of sulfobromophthalein in the rat. *American Journal of Physiology*, **211**, 395–399.

75. Berthelot, P. & Dhumeaux, D. (1978) New insights into the classification and mechanisms of hereditary, chronic, non-haemolytic hyperbilirubinaemias. *Gut*, **19**, 474–480.

76. Bhargava, M.M. & Arias, I.M. (1981) Ligandin. *Trends in Biochemical Sciences*, **6**, 131–133.

77. Bhargava, M.M., Listowsky, J. & Arias, J.M. (1978) Studies on subunit structure and evidence that ligandin is a heterodimer. *Journal of Biological Chemistry*, **253**, 4116–4119.

78. Bhargava, M.M., Listowsky, J. & Arias, I.M. (1978) Ligandin. Bilirubin binding and glutathione-S-transferase activity are independent processes. *Journal of Biological Chemistry*, **253**, 4112–4115.

79. Bhargava, M.M., Ohmi, N., Listowsky, I. & Arias, I.M. (1980) Structural, catalytic, binding and immunological properties associated with each of the two subunits of rat liver ligandin. *Journal of Biological Chemistry*, **233**, 718–723.

80. Billing, B.H. (1975) Genetics of unconjugated hyperbilirubinaemia. In Bakken, A.F. & Fog, J. (eds) *Metabolism and Chemistry of Bilirubin and Related Tetrapyrroles*, pp. 96–100. Oslo, Norway: Rikshospitalet.

81. Billing, B.H. (1978) Twenty-five years of progress in bilirubin metabolism (1952–1977). *Gut*, **19**, 481–491.

82. Billing, B.H. (1982) Bilirubin metabolism. In Schiff, L. & Schiff, E. (eds) *Diseases of the Liver*, 5th edn, pp. 349–378. Philadelphia: J.B. Lippincott.

83. Billing, B.H. (1986) Intestinal and renal metabolism of bilirubin including enterohepatic circulation. In Ostrow, J.D. (ed.) *Bile Pigments and Jaundice*, pp. 255–269. New York: Marcel Dekker.

84. Billing, B.H. (1987) Familial hyperbilirubinaemia. *Journal of Gastroenterology and Hepatology*, **2**, 67–75.

85. Billing, B., Haslam, R. & Wald, N. (1971) Bilirubin standards and the determination of bilirubin by manual and Technicon Autoanalyzer methods. *Annals of Clinical Biochemistry*, **8**, 21–30.

86. Billing, B.H., Jansen, F.H. & Bilton, E. (1973) The effect of bile depletion on the biliary excretion of unconjugated bilirubin and bilirubin conjugates. In Paumgartner, G. & Preisig, R. (eds) *The Liver. Quantitative Aspects of Structure and Function*, pp. 386–391. Karger: Basel.

87. Bissell, D.M. (1975) Formation and elimination of bilirubin. *Gastroenterology*, **69**, 519–538.

88. Bissell, D.M. & Guzelian, P.S. (1980) Degradation of endogenous hepatic heme by pathways not yielding carbon monoxide. Studies in normal rat liver and in primary hepatocyte culture. *Journal of Clinical Investigation*, **65**, 1135–1140.

89. Bissell, D.M. & Hammaker, L.E. (1976) Cytochrome P-450 heme and the regulation of δ-aminolevulinic acid synthetase in the liver. *Archives of Biochemistry and Biophysics*, **176**, 103–112.

90. Bissell, D.M. & Hammaker, L.E. (1977) Effect of endotoxin on tryptophan pyrrolase and δ-aminolaevulinate synthetase: evidence for an endogenous regulatory haem fraction in rat liver. *Biochemical Journal*, **166**, 301–304.

91. Bissell, D.M., Hammaker, L. & Schmid, R. (1972) Hemoglobin and erythrocyte catabolism in rat liver: the separate roles of parenchymal and sinusoidal cells. *Blood*, **40**, 812–822.

92. Black, M. & Billing, B.H. (1969) Hepatic bilirubin UDP-glucuron-yltransferase activity in liver disease and Gilbert's syndrome. *New England Journal of Medicine*, **280**, 1266–1271.

93. Black, M. & Sherlock, S. (1970) Treatment of Gilbert's syndrome with phenobarbitone. *Lancet*, **1**, 1359–1362.

94. Black, M., Perrett, R.D. & Carter, A.E. (1973) Hepatic bilirubin UDP-glucuronyltransferase activity and cytochrome P450 content in a surgical population, and the effects of preoperative drug therapy. *Journal of Laboratory and Clinical Medicine*, **81**, 704–712.

95. Black, M., Fevery, J., Parker, D. *et al.* (1974) Effect of phenobarbitone on plasma [^{14}C]bilirubin clearance in patients with unconjugated hyperbilirubinaemia. *Clinical Science and Molecular Medicine*, **46**, 1–17.

96. Blanckaert, N. (1980) Analysis of bilirubin and bilirubin mono- and diconjugates. Determination of their relative amounts in biological samples. *Biochemical Journal*, **185**, 115–128.

97. Blanckaert, N. & D'Argenio, G. (1982) Presence of bilirubins linked covalently to albumin in serum of patients with cholestasis. *Gastroenterology*, **82**, 1222 (abstract).

98. Blanckaert, N. & Schmid, R. (1982) Physiology and pathophysiology of bilirubin metabolism. In Zakim, D. & Boyer, T. (eds) *Hepatology*, pp. 246–296. Philadelphia: W.B. Saunders.

99. Blanckaert, N., Gollan, J.L. & Schmid, R. (1979) Bilirubin diglucuronide synthesis by a UDP-glucuronic acid-dependent enzyme system in rat liver microsomes. *Proceedings of the National Academy of Sciences, USA*, **76**, 2037–2041.

100. Blanckaert, N., Gollan, J. & Schmid, R. (1980) Mechanism of bilirubin diglucuronide formation in intact rats. Bilirubin diglucuronide formation in vivo. *Journal of Clinical Investigation*, **65**, 1332–1342.

101. Blanckaert, N., Heirwegh, K.P.M. & Zaman, Z. (1977) Comparison of the biliary excretion of the four isomers of bilirubin-IX in

Wistar and homozygous Gunn rats. *Biochemical Journal*, **164**, 229–236.

102. Blanckaert, N., Fevery, J., Heirwegh, K.P.M. & Compernolle, F. (1977) Characterization of the major diazo-positive pigments in bile of homozygous Gunn rats. *Biochemical Journal*, **164**, 237–249.

103. Blanckaert, N., Compernolle, F., Leroy, P. *et al.* (1978) The fate of bilirubin-IXα glucuronide in cholestasis and during storage in vitro: intramolecular rearrangement to positional isomers of glucuronic acid. *Biochemical Journal*, **171**, 203–214.

104. Blanckaert, N., Kabra, P.M., Farina, F.A. *et al.* (1980) Measurement of bilirubin and its mono- and diconjugates in human serum by alkaline methanolysis and high-performance liquid chromatography. *Journal of Laboratory and Clinical Medicine*, **96**, 198–212.

105. Blaschke, T.F., Berk, P.D., Rodkey, F.L. *et al.* (1974) Effects of glutethimide and phenobarbital on hepatic bilirubin clearance, plasma bilirubin turnover and carbon monoxide production in man. *Biochemical Pharmacology*, **23**, 2795–2806.

106. Blaschke, T.F., Berk, P.D., Scharschmidt, B.F. *et al.* (1974) Crigler–Najjar syndrome: an unusual course with development of neurologic damage at age eighteen. *Pediatric Research*, **8**, 573–590.

107. Bloomer, J.R., Berk, P.D., Howe, W.B. *et al.* (1970) Comparison of faecal urobilinogen excretion with bilirubin production in normal volunteers and patients with increased bilirubin production. *Clinica Chimica Acta*, **29**, 463–471.

108. Bloomer, J.R., Barrett, P.V., Rodkey, F.L. & Berlin, N.I. (1971) Studies on the mechanism of fasting hyperbilirubinaemia. *Gastroenterology*, **61**, 479–487.

109. Bloomer, J.R., Berk, P.D., Howe, R.B. & Berlin, N.I. (1971) Interpretation of plasma bilirubin levels based on studies with radioactive bilirubin. *Journal of the American Medical Association*, **218**, 216–220.

110. Bloomer, J.R., Berk, P.D., Howe, R.B. & Berlin, N.I. (1971) Bilirubin metabolism in congenital non-hemolytic jaundice. *Pediatric Research*, **5**, 256–264.

111. Bloomer, J.R., Berk, P.D., Vergalla, J. & Berlin, N.I. (1973) Influence of albumin on the hepatic uptake of unconjugated bilirubin. *Clinical Science and Molecular Medicine*, **45**, 505–516.

112. Blueger, A.F., Krupnikova, E.Z., Sondore, V. Yu. & Semushina, E.P. (1977) Study of the etiology and pathogenesis of low grade nonhemolytic unconjugated hyperbilirubinemia (Gilbert's disease). *Acta Hepato-Gastroenterologica*, **24**, 140–147.

113. Blumenschein, S.D., Kallen, R.J., Storey, B. *et al.* (1968) Familial non-hemolytic jaundice with late onset of neurological damage. *Pediatrics*, **42**, 786–792.

114. Blumenthal, S.G., Taggart, D.B., Ikeda, R.M. *et al.* (1977) Conjugated and unconjugated bilirubins in bile of humans and rhesus monkeys. Structure of adult human and rhesus monkey bilirubins compared with dog bilirubins. *Biochemical Journal*, **167**, 535–548.

115. Bonnett, R., Davies, J.E., Hursthouse, M.B. & Sheldrich, G.M. (1978) The structure of bilirubin. *Proceedings of the Royal Society of London. Series B: Biological Sciences*, **202**, 249–268.

116. Bonnett, R., Buckley, D.G., Hamzetash, D. *et al.* (1984) Photobilirubin II. *Biochemical Journal*, **219**, 1053–1056.

117. Boonyapisit, S.T., Trotman, B.W. & Ostrow, J.D. (1978) Unconjugated bilirubin, and the hydrolysis of conjugated bilirubin, in gallbladder bile of patients with cholelithiasis. *Gastroenterology*, **74**, 70–74.

118. Borghoff, S.J. & Birnbaum, L.S. (1985) Age-related changes in glucuronidation and deglucuronidation in liver, small intestine, lung and kidney of male Fischer rats. *Drug Metabolism and Disposition*, **13**, 62–67.

119. Bourke, E., Milne, M.D. & Stokes, G.S. (1965) Mechanisms of renal excretion of urobilinogen. *British Medical Journal*, **2**, 1510–1514.

120. Boyer, T.D. (1989) The glutathione S-transferases: An update. *Hepatology*, **9**, 486–496.

121. Boyer, T.D., Zakim, D. & Vessey, D.A. (1980) Direct, rapid transfer of estrone from liposomes to microsomes. *Journal of Biological Chemistry*, **255**, 627–631.

122. Boyer, T.D., Zakim, D. & Vessey, D.A. (1982) Studies of endogenous inhibitors of microsomal glutathione S-transferase. *Biochemical Journal*, **207**, 57–64.

123. Boyer, T.D., Vessey, D.A., Holcomb, C. & Saley, N. (1984) Studies of the relationship between the catalytic activity and binding of non-substrate ligands by glutathione S-transferases. *Biochemical Journal*, **217**, 179–185.

124. Brandan, E. & Fleisher, B. (1982) Orientation and role of nucleoside diphosphatase and 5′-nucleotidase in Golgi vesicles from rat liver. *Biochemistry*, **21**, 4640–4645.

125. Brass, C.A., Wrchota, E.M. & Gollan, J.L. (1989) Bilirubin is a potent inhibitor of lipid peroxidation in hepatic microsomal membranes. *Hepatology*, **10**(4), 609.

126. Briheim, G., Fryden, A. & Tobiasson, P. (1982) Serum bile acids in Gilbert's syndrome before and after reduced caloric intake. *Scandinavian Journal of Gastroenterology*, **17**, 877–880.

127. Brodersen, R. (1977) Prevention of kernicterus, based on recent progress in bilirubin chemistry. *Acta Paediatrica Scandinavica*, **66**, 625–634.

128. Brodersen, R. (1978) Free bilirubin in blood plasma of the newborn: effects of albumin, fatty acids, pH, displacing drugs and phototherapy. In Stern, L., Oh, W. & Früs-Hanson, B. (eds) *Intensive Care in the Newborn*, pp. 331–345. New York: Masson Publishing.

129. Brodersen, R. (1980) Binding of bilirubin to albumin. *CRC Critical Reviews in Clinical Laboratory Sciences*, **11**, 305–309.

130. Brodersen, R. (1980) Bilirubin transport in the newborn infant, reviewed with relation to kernicterus. *Journal of Pediatrics*, **96**, 349–356.

131. Brodersen, R. (1986) Aqueous solubility, albumin binding, and tissue distribution of bilirubin. In Ostrow, J.D. (ed) *Bile Pigments and Jaundice*, pp. 157–181. New York: Marcel Dekker.

132. Brodersen, R. & Ebbesen, F. (1983) Bilirubin-displacing effect of ampicillin, indomethacin, chlorpromazine, gentamicin and parabens in vitro and in newborn infants. *Journal of Pharmaceutical Sciences*, **72**, 248–253.

133. Brodersen, R. & Hermann, L.S. (1963) Intestinal reabsorption of unconjugated bilirubin. A possible contributing factor in neonatal jaundice. *Lancet*, **1**, 1242.

134. Brodersen, R. & Theilgaard, J. (1969) Bilirubin colloid formation in neutral aqueous solution. *Scandinavian Journal of Clinical and Laboratory Investigation*, **24**, 395–398.

135. Brodersen, R., Früs-Hansen, B. & Stern, L. (1983) Drug-induced displacement of bilirubin from albumin in the newborn. *Developmental Pharmacology and Therapeutics*, **6**, 217–229.

136. Brodersen, R., Sjödin, T. & Sjöholm, I. (1977) Independent binding of ligands to human serum albumin. *Journal of Biological Chemistry*, **252**, 5067–5072.

137. Brown, A.K. & McDonagh, A.F. (1980) Phototherapy for neonatal hyperbilirubinemia: efficacy, mechanism and toxicity. In Barness, L.A. (ed.) *Advances in Pediatrics*, Vol. 27, pp. 341–389. Chicago: Year Book Medical Publishers.

138. Brown, A.K., Eisinger, J., Blumberg, W.E. *et al.* (1980) A rapid fluorometric method for determining bilirubin levels and binding in the blood of neonates: comparisons with a diazo method and with 2-(4′-hydroxy-benzene)azobenzoic acid dye binding. *Pediatrics*, **65**, 767–776.

139. Brown, N.K. & Smuckler, E.A. (1970) Alkaptonuria and Gilbert's syndrome. Report of two affected siblings and hepatic ultrastructure in one sibling. *American Journal of Medicine*, **48**, 759–765.

140. Brown, S.B. & King, R.F. (1975) An 18O-double-labelling study of haemoglobin catabolism in the rat. *Biochemical Journal*, **150**, 565–567.

141. Brown, S.B. & King, R.F. (1978) The mechanism of haem catabolism. Bilirubin formation in living rats by [18O]oxygen labelling. *Biochemical Journal*, **170**, 297–311.

142. Brown, S.B. & Thomas, S.E. (1978) The mechanism of haem degradation in vitro—kinetic evidence for the formation of a haem-oxygen complex. *Biochemical Journal*, **176**, 327–330.

143. Bunn, H.F. & Jandl, J.H. (1969) The renal handling of hemoglobin. II. Catabolism. *Journal of Experimental Medicine*, **129**, 925–934.

144. Burchell, B. (1980) Isolation and purification of bilirubin UDP-glucuronyl-transferase from rat liver. *FEBS Letters*, **111**, 131–135.

145. Burchell, B. (1982) Reconstitution of purified Wistar rat liver bilirubin UDP-glucuronyltransferase into Gunn-rat liver microsomes. *Biochemical Journal*, **201**, 653–656.

146. Burchell, B. & Bock, K.W. (1980) Abolition of the apparent

deficiency of 2-aminophenol glucuronidation in perfused Gunn rat liver by pentan-3-one. *Biochemical Pharmacology,* **29,** 3204–3207.

147. Burchell, B., Jackson, M.R., Coarser, R.B. *et al.* (1987) The molecular biology of UDP-glucuronyltransferases. *Biochemical Society Transactions,* **15,** 581–584.

148. Burchell, B., Weatherill, P.J. & Berry, C. (1983) Evidence implicating that UDP-*N*-acetylglucosamine does not appear to stimulate hepatic microsomal UDP-glucuronosyltransferase by interaction with the catalytic unit of the enzyme. *Biochimica et Biophysica Acta,* **735,** 309–313.

149. Butt, H.R., Anderson, V.E., Foulk, W.T. *et al.* Studies of chronic idiopathic jaundice (Dubin–Johnson syndrome). II. Evaluation of a large family with the trait. *Gastroenterology,* **51,** 619–630.

150. Call, N.B. & Tisher, C.C. (1975) The urinary concentrating defect in the Gunn strain of rat. Role of bilirubin. *Journal of Clinical Investigation,* **55,** 319–329.

151. Callahan, E.W. & Schmid, R. (1969) Excretion of unconjugated bilirubin in the bile of Gunn rats. *Gastroenterology,* **57,** 134–137.

152. Campbell, M.T. & Wishart, G. (1980) The effect of premature and delayed birth on the development of UDP-glucuronosyltransferase activities towards bilirubin, morphine and testosterone in the rat. *Biochemical Journal,* **186,** 617–619.

153. Capasso, J.M. & Hirschberg, C.B. (1984) Mechanisms of glycosylation and sulfation in the Golgi apparatus: Evidence for nucleotide sugar/nucleoside monophosphate and nucleotide sulfate/nucleoside monophosphate antiports in the Golgi apparatus membrane. *Proceedings of the National Academy of Sciences of the USA,* **81,** 7051–7055.

154. Capelle, P., Dhumeaux, D., Mora, M. *et al.* (1972) Effect of rifampicin on liver function in man. *Gut,* **13,** 366–371.

155. Capron, F., Coltoff-Schiller, B., Johnson, A.B. *et al.* (1979) Immunocytochemical localization of hepatic ligandin and Z protein utilizing frozen sections for light and electron microscopy. *Journal of Histochemistry and Cytochemistry,* **27,** 961–966.

156. Cardenas-Vazquez, R., Yokosuka, O. & Billing, B.H. (1986) Enzymic oxidation of unconjugated bilirubin by rat liver. *Biochemistry Journal,* **236,** 625–633.

157. Carey, M.C. & Koretsky, A.P. (1979) Self-association of unconjugated bilirubin-IXα in aqueous solution at pH 10.0 and physical-chemical interactions with bile salt monomers and micelles. *Biochemical Journal,* **179,** 675–689.

158. Carmel, R., Wong, E.T., Weiner, J.M., Cage, S. & Johnson, M.D. (1985) Racial differences in serum total bilirubin levels in health and in disease (pernicious anemia). *Journal of the American Medical Association,* **253,** 3416–3418.

159. Carson, E.R. & Jones, E.A. (1979) Use of kinetic analysis and mathematical modeling in the study of metabolic pathways in vivo. Applications to hepatic organic anion metabolism. *New England Journal of Medicine,* **300,** 1016–1027 and 1078–1086.

160. Carulli, N., Ponz de Leon, M., Mauro, E. *et al.* (1976) Alteration of drug metabolism in Gilbert's syndrome. *Gut,* **17,** 581–587.

161. Cashore, W.J. (1988) Kernicterus and bilirubin encephalopathy. *Seminars in Liver Disease,* **8,** 163–167.

162. Cashore, W.J. & Stern, L. (1982) Neonatal hyperbilirubinaemia. *Pediatric Clinics of North America,* **29,** 1191–1203.

163. Cashore, W.J., Monin, P.J.P. & Oh, W. (1978) Serum bilirubin binding capacity and free bilirubin concentration: a comparison between sephadex G-25 filtration and peroxidase oxidation techniques. *Pediatric Research,* **12,** 195–198.

164. Cashore, W.J., Oh, W. & Brodersen, R. (1983) Bilirubin-displacing effect of furosemide and sulfisoxazole. *Development Pharmacology and Therapeutics,* **6,** 230–238.

165. Castuma, C.E. & Brenner, R.R. (1986) Effect of dietary cholesterol on microsomal membrane composition, dynamics and kinetic properties of UDP-glucuronyltransferase. *Biochimica et Biophysica Acta,* **855,** 231–242.

166. Cecchelli, R., Cacan, R. & Verbert, A. (1986) Mechanism of UDP-sugar transport into intracellular vesicles. Occurrence of UDP-GlcNAc/UDP and UDP-Gal/UDP antiports. *FEBS Letters,* **208,** 407–412.

167. Celier, C. & Foliot, A. (1984) Bilirubin content and 4-nitrophenol glucuronosyltransferase activity in Gunn rat liver. *Clinical Science,* **66,** 481–486.

168. Childs, B. & Najjar, V.A. (1956) Familial nonhemolytic jaundice with kernicterus: report of two cases without neurologic disease. *Pediatrics,* **18,** 369–377.

169. Childs, B., Sidbury, J.B. & Migeon, C.J. (1959) Glucuronic acid conjugation by patients with familial nonhemolytic jaundice and their relatives. *Pediatrics,* **23,** 903–913.

170. Christensson, P.I. & Eriksson, G. (1985) Effects of six anaesthetic agents on UDP-glucuronic acid and other nucleotides in rat liver. *Acta Anaesthesiologica Scandinavica,* **29,** 629–631.

171. Clarenburg, R. & Kao, G.C. (1973) Shared and separate pathways for biliary excretion of bilirubin and BSP in rats. *American Journal of Physiology,* **225,** 192–200.

172. Coburn, R.F., Williams, W.J. & Forster, R.E. (1964) Effect of erythrocyte destruction on carbon monoxide production in man. *Journal of Clinical Investigation,* **43,** 1098–1103.

173. Cohen, A.N. & Ostrow, J.D. (1980) New concepts in phototherapy: photoisomerization of bilirubin IXα and potential toxic effects of light. *Pediatrics,* **65,** 740–750.

174. Cohen, L., Lewis, C. & Arias, I.M. (1972) Pregnancy, oral contraceptives, and chronic familial jaundice with predominantly conjugated hyperbilirubinemia (Dubin–Johnson syndrome). *Gastroenterology,* **62,** 1182–1190.

175. Coleman, R. (1987) Biochemistry of bile secretion. *Biochemistry Journal,* **244,** 249–261.

176. Colleran, E. & O'Carra, P. (1977) Enzymology and comparative physiology of biliverdin reduction. In Berk, P.D. and Berlin, N.I. (eds) *Chemistry and Physiology of Bile Pigments,* pp. 69–80. Fogarty International Center Proceedings No. 35. Public Health Service National Institutes of Health.

177. Comfort, M.W. (1935) Constitutional hepatic dysfunction. *Proceedings of the Staff Meetings of the Mayo Clinic,* **10,** 57–61.

178. Constantopoulos, A. & Matsaniotis, N. (1978) Augmentation of uridine diphosphate glucuronyltransferase activity in rat liver by adenosine 3′,5′-monophosphate. *Gastroenterology,* **75,** 486–491.

179. Conway, J.G., Kauffman, F.C., Tsukuda, T. & Thruman, R.G. (1988) Glucuronidation of 7-hydroxycoumarin in periportal and pericentral regions of the lobule in livers from untreated and 3-methylcholanthrene-treated rats. *Molecular Pharmacology,* **33,** 111–119.

180. Cornelius, C.E. (1982) The use of nonhuman primates in the study of bilirubin metabolism and bile secretion. *American Journal of Primatology,* **2,** 343–354.

181. Cornelius, C.E. & Gronwall, R.R. (1968) Congenital photosensitivity and hyperbilirubinaemia in Southdown sheep in the United States. *American Journal of Veterinary Research,* **29,** 291–295.

182. Cornelius, C.E., Arias, I.M. & Osburn, B.I. (1965) Hepatic pigmentation with photosensitivity: a syndrome in Corriedale sheep resembling Dubin–Johnson syndrome in man. *Journal of the American Veterinary Medical Association,* **146,** 709–713.

183. Correia, M.A., Farrell, G.C., Schmid, R. *et al.* (1979) Incorporation of exogenous heme into hepatic cytochrome P-450 in vivo. *Journal of Biological Chemistry,* **254,** 15–17.

184. Correia, M.A., Farrell, G.C., Olson, S. *et al.* (1981) Cytochrome P-450 heme moiety. The specific target in drug-induced heme alkylation. *Journal of Biological Chemistry,* **256,** 5466–5470.

185. Coughtrie, M.W.H., Burchell, B., Leakey, J.E.A. & Hume, R. (1989) The inadequacy of perinatal glucuronidation: Immunoblot analysis of the developmental expression of individual UDP-glucuronosyltransferase isoenzymes in rat and human liver microsomes. *Molecular Pharmacology,* **34,** 729–735.

186. Cowan, R.E., Thompson, R.P.H., Kaye, J.P. & Clark, G.M. (1977) The association between fasting hyperbilirubinaemia and serum non-esterified fatty acids in man. *Clinical Science and Molecular Medicine,* **53,** 155–163.

187. Crawford, J.M. & Gollan, J.L. (1988) Hepatocyte cotransport of taurocholate and bilirubin glucuronides: role of microtubules. *American Journal of Physiology,* **255,** 121–131.

188. Crawford, J.M., Berken, C.A. & Gollan, J.L. (1988) Role of the hepatocyte microtubular system in the excretion of bile salts and biliary lipid: implications for intracellular vesicular transport. *Journal of Lipid Research,* **29,** 144–156.

189. Crawford, J.M., Hauser, S.C. & Gollan, J.L. (1988) Formation, hepatic metabolism, and transport of bile pigments: A status report. *Seminars in Liver Disease,* **8,** 105–118.

190. Crawford, J.M., Ransil, B.J., Potter, C.S., Westmoreland, S.V.

& Gollan, J.L. (1987) Hepatic disposition and biliary excretion of bilirubin and bilirubin glucuronides in intact rats. *Journal of Clinical Investigation*, **79**, 1172–1180.

191. Crigler, J.F. & Gold, N.I. (1969) Effect of sodium phenobarbital on bilirubin metabolism in an infant with congenital, nonhemolytic, unconjugated hyperbilirubinemia, and kernicterus. *Journal of Clinical Investigation*, **48**, 42–55.

192. Crigler, J.F. & Najjar, V.A. (1952) Congenital familial nonhemolytic jaundice with kernicterus. *Pediatrics*, **10**, 169–180.

193. Cruse, I. & Maines, M.D. (1988) Evidence suggesting that the two forms of heme oxygenase are products of different genes. *Journal of Biological Chemistry*, **263**, 3348–3353.

194. Cukier, J.O., Whitington, P.F. & Odell, G.B. (1981) Bilirubin, UDP-glucuronyltransferase of liver in postmature rats. A functional and morphologic comparison. *Laboratory Investigation*, **44**, 368–374.

195. Cuypers, H.T.M., Ter Haar, E.M. & Jansen, P.L.M. (1984) UDP-glucuronyltransferase-catalyzed deconjugation of bilirubin monoglucuronide. *Hepatology*, **4**, 918–922.

196. Dameshek, W. & Singer, K. (1941) Familial non-hemolytic jaundice: constitutional hepatic dysfunction with indirect van den Bergh reaction. *Archives of Internal Medicine*, **67**, 259–285.

197. Datta, D.V., Nair, R. & Nair, C.R. (1975) Estimation of hepatic bilirubin UDP-glucuronyl transferase in patients with noncirrhotic portal fibrosis and liver disease: significance and limitations. *Digestive Diseases*, **20**, 961–967.

198. Davidson, A.R., Rojas-Bueno, A., Thompson, R.P.H. & Williams, R. (1975) Reduced caloric intake and nicotinic acid provocation tests in the diagnosis of Gilbert's syndrome. *British Medical Journal*, **2**, 480.

199. Davis, D.R. & Yeary, R.A. (1980) Interaction of bilirubin and indocyanine green with the binding and conjugation of sulfobromophthalein by rat liver cytosol proteins. *Research Communications in Chemical Pathology and Pharmacology*, **27**, 373–388.

200. Dawson, J., Seymour, C.A. & Peters, T.J. (1979) Gilbert's syndrome: analytical subcellular fractionation of liver biopsy specimens. Enzyme activities, organelle pathology and evidence for subpopulations of the syndrome. *Clinical Science*, **57**, 491–497.

201. Dawson, J., Carr-Locke, D.L., Talbot, J.C. & Rosenthal, F.D. (1979) Gilbert's syndrome: evidence of morphological heterogeneity. *Gut*, **20**, 848–853.

202. De Brito, T., Borges, M.A. & Da Silva, L.C. (1966) Electron microscopy of the liver in non-hemolytic acholuric jaundice with kernicterus (Crigler–Najjar) and in idiopathic conjugated hyperbilirubinemia. (Rotor). *Gastroenterologia*, **106**, 325–335.

203. De Groote, J., Ramboer, C., Versieck, J. & Barbier, F. (1968) Pathologie isolée de la B.S.P. Etude chez quatre malades. *Revue Internationale d'Hépatologie*, **18**, 833–844.

204. De Matteis, F., Gibbs, A.H. & Unseld, A. (1977) Loss of haem from cytochrome P-450 caused by lipid peroxidation and 2-allyl-2-isopropylacetamatide. An abnormal pathway not involving production of carbon monoxide. *Biochemical Journal*, **168**, 417–422.

205. De Morais, S.M.F. & Wells, P.G. (1988) Deficiency in bilirubin UDP-glucuronyl transferase as a genetic determinant of acetaminophen toxicity. *Journal of Pharmacology and Experimental Therapeutics*, **247**, 323–331.

206. De Morais, S.M.F. & Wells, P.G. (1989) Enhanced acetaminophen toxicity in rats with bilirubin glucuronyl transferase deficiency. *Hepatology*, **10**, 163–167.

207. Dhumeaux, D. & Berthelot, P. (1975) Chronic hyperbilirubinemia associated with hepatic uptake and storage impairment. *Gastroenterology*, **69**, 988–993.

208. Diamond, I. & Schmid, R. (1966) Experimental bilirubin encephalopathy: the mode of entry of bilirubin ^{14}C into the central nervous system. *Journal of Clinical Investigation*, **45**, 678–689.

209. Dills, R.L. & Klaassen, C.D. (1984) Decreased glucuronidation of bilirubin by diethyl ether anesthesia. *Biochemical Pharmacology*, **33**, 2813–2814.

210. Dills, R.L., Howell, S.R. & Klaassen, C.D. (1987) Hepatic UDP-glucose and UDP-glucuronic acid synthesis rates in rats during a reduced energy state. *Drug Metabolism and Disposition*, **15**, 281–288.

211. Di Zoglio, J.D. & Cardillo, E. (1973) The Dubin–Johnson syndrome and pregnancy. *Obstetrics and Gynecology*, **42**, 560–563.

212. Dollinger, M.R., Brandborg, L.L., Sartor, V.E. & Bernstein, J.M. (1967) Chronic familial hyperbilirubinemia. Hepatic defect(s) associated with occult hemolysis. *Gastroenterology*, **52**, 875–881.

213. Douglas, A.P., Savage, R.L. & Rawlins, M.D. (1978) Paracetamol (acetaminophen) kinetics in patients with Gilbert's syndrome. *European Journal of Clinical Pharmacology*, **13**, 209–212.

214. Douglas, J.G., Beckett, G.J., Nimmo, A. *et al.* (1981) Bile salt measurements in Gilbert's syndrome. *European Journal of Clinical Investigation*, **11**, 421–423.

215. Douglas, J.G., Beckett, G.J., Percy-Robb, I.W. & Finlayson, N.D.C. (1980) Bile salt transport in the Dubin–Johnson syndrome. *Gut*, **21**, 890–893.

216. Doumas, B.T., Perry, B., Jendrzejczak, B. & Davis, L. (1987) Measurement of direct bilirubin by use of bilirubin oxidase. *Clinical Chemistry*, **33**, 1349–1353.

217. Drummond, G.S. & Kappa, A. (1981) Prevention of neonatal hyperbilirubinemia by tin protoporphyrin IX, a potent competitive inhibitor of heme oxidation. *Proceedings of the National Academy of Sciences of the USA*, **78**, 6466–6470.

218. Drummond, G.S. & Kappas, A. (1982) Suppression of hyperbilirubinemia in the rat neonate by chromium-protoporphyrin. *Journal of Experimental Medicine*, **156**, 1878–1883.

219. Drummond, G.S. & Kappas, A. (1982) Chemoprevention of neonatal jaundice: potency of tin-protoporphyrin in an animal model. *Science*, **217**, 1250–1252.

220. Drummond, G.S. & Kappas, A. (1986) Sn-Protoporphyrin inhibition of fetal and neonatal brain heme oxygenase. *Journal of Clinical Investigation*, **77**, 971–976.

221. Dubin, I.N. (1958) Chronic idiopathic jaundice. A review of fifty cases. *American Journal of Medicine*, **24**, 268–292.

222. Dubin, I.N. & Johnson, F.B. (1954) Chronic idiopathic jaundice with unidentified pigment in liver cells. A new clinicopathologic entity with a report of 12 cases. *Medicine*, **33**, 155–197.

223. Dutton, G.J. (1966) The biosynthesis of glucuronides. In Dutton, G.J. (ed.) *Glucuronic Acid, Free and Combined*, pp. 185–299. New York: Academic Press.

224. Duvaldestin, P., Mahu, J.-L., Metreau, J.-M. *et al.* (1980) Possible role of a defect in hepatic bilirubin glucuronidation in the initiation of cholesterol gallstones. *Gut*, **21**, 650–655.

225. Edwards, R.H. (1975) Inheritance of the Dubin–Johnson–Sprinz syndrome. *Gastroenterology*, **68**, 734–749.

226. ElAwady, M., Roy Chowdhury, J., Kesari, K.V. *et al.* (1989) Genetic deficiency of 3-methylcholanthrene-inducible UDP-glucuronosyltransferase in Gunn rats is associated with high gene transcription rate but low mRNA concentration. *Hepatology*, **10**, 650.

227. Elder, G., Gray, C.H. & Nicholson, D.G. (1972) Bile pigment fate in gastrointestinal tract. *Seminars in Hematology*, **9**, 71–90.

228. Enat, R. & Barzilai, D. (1975) Mitochondrial pathology in the liver in a patient with the Dubin–Johnson syndrome. *Israel Journal of Medical Sciences*, **13**, 1197–1205.

229. Engelking, L.R., Gronwall, R. & Anwer, M.S. (1980) Effect of dehydrocholic, chenodeoxycholic, and taurocholic acids on the excretion of bilirubin. *American Journal of Veterinary Research*, **41**, 355–361.

230. Ennever, J.F., Knox, I., Denne, S.C. & Speck, W.T. (1985) Phototherapy for neonatal jaundice: in vivo clearance of bilirubin photoproducts. *Pediatric Research*, **19**, 205–208.

231. Ennever, J.F., Costarino, A.T., Polin, R.A. & Speck, W.T. (1987) Rapid clearance of a structural isomer of bilirubin during phototherapy. *Journal of Clinical Investigation*, **79**, 1674–1678.

232. Erickson, R.H., Zakim, D. & Vessey, D.A. (1978) Preparation and properties of a phospholipid-free form of microsomal UDP-glucuronyltransferase. *Biochemistry*, **17**, 3706–3711.

233. Eriksen, E.F., Danielsen, H. & Brodersen, R. (1981) Bilirubin-liposome interaction. Binding of bilirubin dianion, protonization, and aggregation of bilirubin acid. *Journal of Biological Chemistry*, **256**, 4269–4274.

234. Erlinger, S. & Dhumeaux, D. (1974) Mechanisms and control of secretion of bile water and electrolytes. *Gastroenterology*, **66**, 281–304.

235. Erlinger, S., Dhumeaux, D., Desjeux, J.F. & Benhamou, J.P. (1973) Hepatic handling of unconjugated dyes in the Dubin–Johnson syndrome. *Gastroenterology*, **64**, 106–110.

236. Essner, E. & Novikoff, A.B. (1960) Human hepatocellular pigments and lysosomes. *Journal of Ultrastructural Research*, **3**, 374–391.

237. Fahmy, K., Gray, C.H. & Nicholson, D.C. (1972) The reduction of bile pigments by faecal and intestinal bacteria. *Biochimica et Biophysica Acta*, **264**, 85–97.

238. Farrell, G.C. & Correia, M.A. (1980) Structural and functional reconstitution of hepatic cytochrome P-450 in vivo. Reversal of allylisopropylacetamide-mediated destruction of hemoprotein by exogenous heme. *Journal of Biological Chemistry*, **255**, 10128–10133.

239. Farrell, G.C., Gollan, J.L. & Schmid, R. (1980) Efflux of bilirubin into plasma following hepatic degradation of exogenous heme. *Proceedings of the Society for Experimental Biology and Medicine*, **163**, 504–509.

240. Farrell, G.C., Gollan, J.L., Stevens, S.M. & Grierson, J.M. (1982) Crigler–Najjar type I syndrome: absence of hepatic bilirubin UDP-glucuronyl transferase activity and therapeutic response to light. *Australian and New Zealand Journal of Medicine*, **12**, 280–285.

241. Fedeli, G., Rapaccini, G.L., Anti, M. *et al.* (1983) Impaired clearance of cholephilic anions in Rotor syndrome. *Zeitschrift für Gastroenterologie*, **21**, 228–233.

242. Feigelson, P. & Greengard, O. (1961) A microsomal iron-porphyrin activator of rat liver tryptophan pyrrolase. *Journal of Biological Chemistry*, **236**, 153–157.

243. Felsher, B.F. & Carpio, N.M. (1975) Caloric intake and unconjugated hyperbilirubinemia. *Gastroenterology*, **69**, 42–47.

244. Felsher, B.F. & Carpio, N.M. (1979) Chronic persistent hepatitis and unconjugated hyperbilirubinemia. *Gastroenterology*, **76**, 248–252.

245. Felsher, B.F., Carpio, N.M. & Van Couvering, K. (1979) Effect of fasting and phenobarbital on hepatic UDP-glucuronic acid formation in the rat. *Journal of Laboratory and Clinical Medicine*, **93**, 414–427.

246. Felsher, B.F., Craig, J.R. & Carpio, N. (1973) Hepatic bilirubin glucuronidation in Gilbert's syndrome. *Journal of Laboratory and Clinical Medicine*, **81**, 829–837.

247. Felsher, B.F., Rickard, D. & Redeker, A.G. (1970) The reciprocal relation between caloric intake and the degree of hyperbilirubinaemia in Gilbert's syndrome. *New England Journal of Medicine*, **283**, 170–172.

248. Fevery, J. (1981) Pathogenesis of Gilbert's syndrome. *European Journal of Clinical Investigation*, **11**, 417–418.

249. Fevery, J. (1985) The bilirubin diglucuronide controversy. *Journal of Hepatology*, **1**, 437–442.

250. Fevery, J. & Blanckaert, N. (1986) What can we learn from analysis of serum bilirubin? *Journal of Hepatology*, **2**, 113–121.

251. Fevery, J. & Heirwegh, K.P.M. (1980) Liver and biliary tract physiology. I. In Javitt, N.B. (ed.) *International Review of Physiology*, Vol. 21, pp. 171–220. Baltimore: University Park Press.

252. Fevery, J., De Groote, J. & Heirwegh, K.P.M. (1973) Quantitation of hepatic bilirubin conjugation. In Paumgarten, G. & Preisig, R. (eds) *The Liver. Quantitative Aspects of Structure and Function*, pp. 203–209. Basel: Karger.

253. Fevery, J., Heirwegh, K.P.M. & De Groote, J. (1974) Unconjugated hyperbilirubinaemia in achalasia. *Gut*, **15**, 121–124.

254. Fevery, J., Van Damme, B., Michiels, R. *et al.* (1972) Bilirubin conjugates in bile of man and rat in the normal state and in liver disease. *Journal of Clinical Investigation*, **51**, 2482–2492.

255. Fevery, J., Blanckaert, N., Heirwegh, K.P.M. *et al.* (1977) Unconjugated bilirubin and an increased proportion of bilirubin monoconjugates in the bile of patients with Gilbert's syndrome and Crigler–Najjar disease. *Journal of Clinical Investigation*, **60**, 970–979.

256. Fevery, J., Van De Vijver, M., Michiels, R. & Heirwegh, K.P.M. (1977) Comparison in different species of biliary bilirubin-IXα conjugates with the activities of hepatic and renal bilirubin-IXα-uridine diphosphate glycosyltransferases. *Biochemical Journal*, **164**, 737–746.

257. Fevery, J., Blanckaert, N., Leroy, P. *et al.* (1983) Analysis of bilirubins in biological fluids by extraction and thin-layer chromatography of the intact tetrapyrroles: Application to bile of patients with Gilbert's syndrome, hemolysis, or cholelithiasis. *Hepatology*, **3**, 177–183.

258. Finch, S.A.E., Slater, T.F. & Stier, A. (1979) Nucleotide metabolism by microsomal UDP-glucuronyltransferase and nucleoside diphosphatase as determined by ^{31}P nuclear magnetic resonance spectroscopy. *Biochemical Journal*, **177**, 925–930.

259. Fleischner, G., Kamisaka, K., Habig, W. *et al.* (1975) Human ligandin: characterization and quantitation. *Gastroenterology*, **69**, 821 (abstract).

260. Fog, J. & Jellum, E. (1963) Structure of bilirubin. *Nature*, **198**, 88–89.

261. Foliot, A., Christoforov, B., Petite, J.P. *et al.* (1975) Bilirubin UDP-glucuronyltransferase activity of Wistar rat kidney. *American Journal of Physiology*, **229**, 340–343.

262. Forker, E.L. (1975) Canalicular anion-transport, pathogenetic mechanisms, and a steady-state distributed model for measuring kinetics. In Goresky, C.A. & Fisher, M.M. (eds) *Jaundice*, pp. 229–240. New York: Plenum.

263. Forker, E.L. (1977) Mechanisms of hepatic bile formation. *Annual Review of Physiology*, **39**, 323–347.

264. Forker, E.L. (1985) Lumpers vs distributers. *Hepatology*, **5**, 1236–1237.

265. Forker, E.L. & Ghiron, C. (1988) ESR, albumin, and the riddle of organic anion uptake by the liver. *American Journal of Physiology*, **254**, G463–G464.

266. Forker, E.L. & Luxton, B.A. (1981) Albumin helps mediate removal of taurocholate by rat liver. *Journal of Clinical Investigation*, **67**, 1517–1522.

267. Foulk, W.T., Butt, H.R., Owen, C.A. *et al.* (1959) Constitutional hepatic dysfunction (Gilbert's syndrome): its natural history and related syndromes. *Medicine*, **38**, 25–46.

268. Franco, D., Préaux, A.M., Bismuth, H. & Berthelot, P. (1972) Extrahepatic formation of bilirubin glucuronides in the rat. *Biochimica et Biophysica Acta*, **286**, 55–61.

269. Freilich, H.S., Ziurys, J.C. & Gollan, J.L. (1985) Modulation of hepatic UDP-glucuronyltransferase activity by bile salts: Potential physiologic and clinical applications (abstract). *Gastroenterology*, **88**, 1659.

270. Frey, A.B., Friedberg, T., Oesch, F. & Kreibich, G. (1983) Studies on the subunit composition of rat liver glutathione *S*-transferases. *Journal of Biological Chemistry*, **258**, 11321–11325.

271. Friedberg, T., Bentley, P., Stasiecki, P. *et al.* (1979) The identification, solubilization, and characterization of microsome-associated glutathione *S*-transferases. *Journal of Biological Chemistry*, **254**, 12028–12033.

272. Fromke, V.L. & Miller, D. (1972) Constitutional hepatic dysfunction (CHD: Gilbert's disease); a review with special reference to a characteristic increase and prolongation of the hyperbilirubinemic response to nicotinic acid. *Medicine*, **51**, 451–464.

273. Fulop, M., Sandson, J. & Brazeau, P. (1965) Dialyzability, protein binding and renal excretion of plasma conjugated bilirubin. *Journal of Clinical Investigation*, **44**, 666–680.

274. Galli, G., Focacci, C., Maini, C.O. *et al.* (1982) The hepatic excretion of ^{131}I-rose bengal and ^{99m}Tc-IDA derivatives in Rotor's syndrome. *European Journal of Nuclear Medicine*, **7**, 311–317.

275. Garcia-Marin, J.J. & Esteller, A. (1984) Biliary inter-relationship between phospholipid, bilirubin and taurocholate in the anaesthetized rat. *Clinical Science*, **67**, 499–504.

276. Gardner, W.A. & Konigsmark, B. (1969) Familial nonhemolytic jaundice: bilirubinosis and encephalopathy. *Pediatrics*, **43**, 365–376.

277. Gartner, L.M. & Arias, I.M. (1972) Hormonal control of hepatic bilirubin transport and conjugation. *American Journal of Physiology*, **222**, 1091–1099.

278. Gartner, L.M. & Lee, K.S. (1977) Effect of starvation and milk feeding on intestinal bilirubin absorption. *Gastroenterology*, **77**, A13 (abstract).

279. Gartner, U., Stockert, R.J., Levine, W.G. & Wolkoff, A.W. (1982) Effect of nafenopin on the uptake of bilirubin and sulfobromophthalein by isolated perfused rat liver. *Gastroenterology*, **83**, 1163–1169.

280. Gautam, A., Seligson, H., Gordon, E. *et al.* (1984) Irreversible binding of conjugated bilirubin to albumin in cholestatic rats. *Journal of Clinical Investigation*, **73**, 873–877.

281. Gentile, S., Marmo, R., Persico, M. *et al.* (1984) Plasma clearance of nicotinic acid and rifamycin-SV, and their interaction in Gilbert's

syndrome: application of a compartmental model. _Hepato-gastroenterology_, **31**, 72–75.

282. Gentile, S., Persico, M., Baldini, G. et al. (1985) The implication of bilitranslocase function in the impaired rifamycin SV metabolism in Gilbert's syndrome. _Clinical Science_, **68**, 675–680.

283. Gentile, S., Rubba, P., Persico, M. et al. (1985) Improvement of the nicotinic acid test in the diagnosis of Gilbert's syndrome by pretreatment with indomethacin. _Hepato-gastroenterology_, **32**, 267–269.

284. Gentile, S., Tiribelli, C., Baldini, G. et al. (1985) Sex differences of nicotinate-induced hyperbilirubinemia in Gilbert's syndrome. _Journal of Hepatology_, **1**, 417–429.

285. Gentile, S., Tiribelli, C., Persico, M. et al. (1986) Dose dependence of nicotinic acid-induced hyperbilirubinemia and its dissociation from hemolysis in Gilbert's syndrome. _Journal of Laboratory and Clinical Medicine_, **107**, 166–171.

286. Gibson, G.E. & Forker, E.L. (1974) Canalicular bile flow and bromosulfophthalein transport maximum: the effect of a bile salt-independent cholerectic. SC-2644. _Gastroenterology_, **66**, 1046–1053.

287. Gilbert, A. & Herscher, M. (1906) Sur les variations de la cholémie physiologique. _Presse Médicale_, **14**, 209–211.

288. Gilbert, A. & Lereboullet, P. (1901) La cholémie simple familale. _Semaine Medicale (Paris)_, **21**, 241–245.

289. Gilbert, A., Lereboullet, P. & Herscher, M. (1907) Les trois cholémies congénitales. _Bulletins et Mémoires de la Société Médicale des Hôpitaux de Paris_, **24**, 1203–1210.

290. Gilbertson, A.S., Lowry, P.T., Hawkinson, V. & Watson, C.J. (1959) Studies on the dipyrrylmethene ('fuscin') pigments. 1. The anabolic significance of the fecal mesobilifuscin. _Journal of Clinical Investigation_, **38**, 1166–1174.

291. Gillette, J.R., Davis, D.D. & Sasame, H.A. (1972) Cytochrome P-450 and its role in drug metabolism. _Annual Review of Pharmacology_, **12**, 57–84.

292. Girotti, F., Finocchi, G., Sartori, L. & Boscherini, B. (1969) Congenital non-haemolytic jaundice in a four-year-old girl without disease of the central nervous system. _Helvetica Paediatrica Acta_, **24**, 399–403.

293. Goldstein, G.W., Hammaker, L. & Schmid, R. (1968) The catabolism of Heinz bodies: an experimental model demonstrating conversion to non-bilirubin catabolites. _Blood_, **31**, 388–395.

294. Goldstein, R.B., Vessey, D.A., Zakim, D. et al. (1980) Perinatal developmental changes in hepatic UDP-glucuronyltransferase. _Biochemical Journal_, **186**, 841–845.

295. Gollan, J.L. & Schmid, R. (1982) Bilirubin update: formation, transport, and metabolism. In Popper, H. & Schaffner, F. (eds) _Progress in Liver Diseases_, Vol. VII, pp. 261–283. New York: Grune and Stratton.

296. Gollan, J.L. & Knapp, A.B. (1985) Bilirubin metabolism and congenital jaundice. _Hospital Practice_, **20**, 83–106.

297. Gollan, J.L., Bateman, C. & Billing, B.H. (1976) Effect of dietary composition on the unconjugated hyperbilirubinaemia of Gilbert's syndrome. _Gut_, **17**, 335–340.

298. Gollan, J.L., Dallinger, K.J. & Billing, B.H. (1978) Factors influencing excretion of conjugated bilirubin in the isolated kidney. _Clinical Science and Molecular Medicine_, **54**, 381–389.

299. Gollan, J.L., Hatt, K.J. & Billing, B.H. (1975) The influence of diet on unconjugated hyperbilirubinaemia in the Gunn rat. _Clinical Science and Molecular Medicine_, **49**, 229–235.

300. Gollan, J.L., Hole, D.R. & Billing, B.H. (1979) The role of dietary lipid in the regulation of unconjugated hyperbilirubinemia in Gunn rats. _Clinical Science_, **57**, 327–337.

301. Gollan, J.L., Keeffe, E.B. & Scharschmidt, B.F. (1980) Cholestasis and hyperbilirubinemia. In Gitnick, G.L. (ed.) _Current Hepatology_, Vol. 1, pp. 277–312. Boston: Houghton Mifflin.

302. Gollan, J.L., McDonagh, A.F. & Schmid, R. (1977) Biliverd IXα: a new probe of hepatic bilirubin metabolism. _Gastroenterology_, **72**, 1186 (abstract).

303. Gollan, J.L., Huang, S.N., Billing, B.H. & Sherlock, S. (1975) Prolonged survival in three brothers with severe type 2 Crigler–Najjar syndrome. Ultrastructural and metabolic studies. _Gastroenterology_, **68**, 1543–1555.

304. Gollan, J., Hammaker, L., Licko, V. & Schmid, R. (1981) Bilirubin kinetics in intact rats and isolated perfused liver. Evidence for hepatic deconjugation of bilirubin glucuronides. _Journal of Clinical Investigation_, **67**, 1003–1015.

305. Gollan, J.L., Hammaker, L., Schmid, R. & Licko, V. (1982) Transport differences between exogenously administered and endogenously formed hepatic bilirubin. _Gastroenterology_, **82**, 1229 (abstract).

306. Gomba, Sz., Gautier, A., Lemarchand-Béraud, Th. & Gardiol, D. (1976) Pigmentation and dysfunction of Gunn rat thyroid. Correlation between morphological and biochemical data. _Virchows Archiv. B. Cell Pathology_, **20**, 41–54.

307. Gordon, E.R., Chan, T.-H., Samodai, K. & Goresky, C.A. (1977) The isolation and further characterization of the bilirubin tetrapyrroles in bile-containing human duodenal juice and dog gallbladder bile. _Biochemical Journal_, **167**, 1–8.

308. Gordon, E.R. & Goresky, C.A. (1980) The formation of bilirubin diglucuronide by rat liver microsomal preparations. _Canadian Journal of Biochemistry_, **58**, 1302–1310.

309. Gordon, E.R., Shaffer, E.A. & Sass-Kortsak, A. (1976) Bilirubin secretion and conjugation in the Crigler–Najjar syndrome type II. _Gastroenterology_, **70**, 761–765.

310. Gordon, E.R., Sommerer, U. & Goresky, C.A. (1983) The hepatic microsomal formation of bilirubin glucuronide. _Journal of Biological Chemistry_, **258**, 15028–15036.

311. Gordon, E.R., Goresky, C.A., Chang, T.-H. & Perlin, A.S. (1976) The isolation and characterization of bilirubin diglucuronide, the major bilirubin conjugate in dog and human bile. _Biochemical Journal_, **155**, 477–486.

312. Gordon, E.R., Meier, P.J., Goresky, C.A. & Boyer, J.L. (1984) Mechanism and subcellular site of bilirubin diglucuronide formation in rat liver. _Journal of Biological Chemistry_, **259**, 5500–5506.

313. Goresky, C.A. (1975) The hepatic uptake process: its implications for bilirubin transport. In Goresky, C.A. & Fisher, M.M. (eds) _Jaundice_, pp. 159–174. New York: Plenum Press.

314. Goresky, C.A., Haddad, H.H., Kluger, W.S. et al. (1974) The enhancement of maximal bilirubin excretion with taurocholate-induced increments in bile flow. _Canadian Journal of Physiology and Pharmacology_, **52**, 389–403.

315. Goresky, C.A., Gordon, E.R., Shaffer, E.A. et al. (1978) Definition of a conjugation dysfunction in Gilbert's syndrome: studies of the handling of bilirubin loads and of the pattern of bilirubin conjugates excreted in bile. _Clinical Science and Molecular Medicine_, **55**, 63–71.

316. Gorodischer, R., Levy, G., Krasner, J. & Yaffe, S.J. (1970) Congenital nonobstructive nonhemolytic jaundice: effect of phototherapy. _New England Journal of Medicine_, **282**, 375–377.

317. Gourley, G.R., Mogilevsky, W. & Odell, G.B. (1983) Hepatic microsomal composition studies in the Gunn rat. _Biochimica et Biophysica Acta_, **750**, 419–423.

318. Grandchamp, B., Bissell, D.M., Licko, V. & Schmid, R. (1981) Formation and disposition of newly synthesized heme in adult rat hepatocytes in primary culture. _Journal of Biological Chemistry_, **256**, 11677–11683.

319. Gray, C.H. (1983) The bile pigments 1933–1983. _Trends in Biochemical Sciences_, **8**, 381–383.

320. Gray, C.H., Neuberger, A. & Sneath, P.H. (1950) Studies in congenital porphyria. 2. Incorporation of ¹³N in the stercobilin in the normal and in the porphyric. _Biochemical Journal_, **47**, 87–92.

321. Greenberg, J.W., Malhotra, V. & Ennever, J.F. (1987) Wavelength dependence of the quantum yield for the structural isomerization of bilirubin. _Photochemistry and Photobiology_, **46**, 453–456.

322. Groth, C.G., Arborgh, B., Björken, C. et al. (1977) Correction of hyperbilirubinemia in the glucuronyltransferase-deficient rat by intraportal hepatocyte transplantation. _Transplantation Proceedings_, **9**, 313–316.

323. Guengerich, F.P. (1978) Destruction of heme and hemoproteins mediated by liver microsomal reduced nicotinamide adenine dinucleotide phosphate-cytochrome P-450 reductase. _Biochemistry_, **17**, 3633–3639.

324. Guengerich, F.P. & Strickland, T.W. (1977) Metabolism of vinylchloride: destruction of the heme of highly purified liver microsomal cytochrome P-450 by a metabolite. _Molecular Pharmacology_, **13**, 993–1004.

325. Gumucio, J.J., Balabaud, C., Miller, D.L. *et al.* (1978) Bile secretion and liver cell heterogeneity in the rat. *Journal of Laboratory and Clinical Medicine*, **91**, 350–362.

326. Gunn, C.H. (1938) Hereditary acholuric jaundice in a new mutant strain of rats. *Journal of Heredity*, **29**, 137–139.

327. Gutstein, S., Alpert, S. & Arias, I.M. (1968) Studies of hepatic excretory function. IV. Biliary excretion of sulfobromophthalein sodium in a patient with the Dubin–Johnson syndrome and a biliary fistula. *Israel Journal of Medical Sciences*, **4**, 36–40.

328. Guzelian, R.S. & Swisher, R.W. (1979) Degradation of cytochrome P-450 haem by carbon tetrachloride and 2-allyl-2-isopropylaceta-mide in rat liver in vivo and in vitro. *Biochemical Journal*, **184**, 481–489.

329. Gydell, K. (1959) Nicotinic acid induced hyperbilirubinemia and hypersideremia. *Acta Medica Scandinavica*, **164**, 305–320.

330. Habig, W.H., Pabst, M.J., Flieschner, G. *et al.* (1974) The identity of glutathione *S*-transferase B with ligandin, a major binding protein of liver. *Proceedings of the National Academy of Sciences, USA*, **71**, 3879–3882.

331. Hadchouel, P., Charbonnier, A., Lageron, A. *et al.* (1971) A propos d'une nouvelle forme d'ictère chronique idiopathique. Hypothese physiopathologique. *Revue Médico-Chirurgicale des Maladies du Foie*, **46**, 61–68.

332. Haeger, B., DeBrito, R. & Hallinan, T. (1980) Diazoben-zenesulfphonate selectively abolishes stimulation of glucuronid-ation by UDP-*N*-acetylglucosamine. *Biochemistry Journal*, **192**, 971–974.

333. Hammaker, L. & Schmid, R. (1967) Interference with bile pigment uptake in the liver by flavaspidic acid. *Gastroenterology*, **53**, 31–37.

334. Hansen, T.W.R., Bratlid, D. & Walaas, S.I. (1988) Bilirubin decreases phosphorylation of synapsin I, a synaptic vesicle-associ-ated neuronal phosphoprotein, in intact synaptosomes from rat cerebral cortex. *Pediatric Research*, **23**, 219–223.

335. Hargreaves, T. (1969) Neonatal serum bilirubin estimation. *Clinica Chimica Acta*, **26**, 331–337.

336. Harper, G.S. & Axelsen, R.A. (1982) Salicylate-induced renal papillary necrosis in the Gunn rat. *Laboratory Investigation*, **47**, 258–264.

337. Harris, R.L., Musher, D.M., Blook, K. *et al.* (1987) Manifestations of sepsis. *Archives of Internal Medicine*, **147**, 1895–1906.

338. Hartmann, F. & Bissell, D.M. (1982) Metabolism of heme and bilirubin in rat and human small intestinal mucosa. *Journal of Clinical Investigation*, **70**, 23–29.

339. Haurani, F.I. & Tocantins, L.M. (1961) Ineffective erythropoiesis. *American Journal of Medicine*, **31**, 519–531.

340. Hauser, S.C. & Gollan, J.L. (1986) UDP-glucuronyltransferase and the conjugation of bilirubin. In Ostrow, J.D. (ed.) *Bile Pigments and Jaundice*, pp. 211–241. New York: Marcel Dekker.

341. Hauser, S.C. & Gollan, J.L. (1990) Mechanistic and molecular aspects of hepatic bilirubin, glucuronidation. In *Progress in Liver Diseases*, Popper, H. & Schaffner, F. (eds) **9**, 225–235. Philadel-phia: W.B. Saunders.

342. Hauser, S.C., Ziurys, J.C. & Gollan, J.L. (1984) Subcellular distribution and regulation of hepatic bilirubin UDP-glucuronyl-transferase. *Journal of Biological Chemistry*, **259**, 4527–4533.

343. Hauser, S.C., Ziurys, J.C. & Gollan, J.L. (1986) Regulation of bilirubin glucuronide synthesis in primate (*Macaca fascicularis*) liver: Kinetic analysis of microsomal bilirubin UDP-glucuronyl-transferase. *Gastroenterology*, **91**, 287–296.

344. Hauser, S.C., Ziurys, J.C. & Gollan, J.L. (1988) A membrane transporter mediates access of uridine 5′-diphosphoglucuronic acid from the cytosol into the endoplasmic reticulum of rat hepatocytes: Implications for glucuronidation reactions. *Biochimica et Biophys-ica Acta*, **967**, 149–157.

345. Hauser, S.C., Ransil, B.J., Ziurys, J.C. *et al.* (1988) Interaction of uridine 5′-diphosphoglucuronic acid with microsomal UDP-glucuronosyltransferase in primate liver: The facilitating role of uridine 5′-diphospho-*N*-acetylglucosamine. *Biochimica et Biophys-ica Acta*, **967**, 141–148.

346. Haverback, B.J. & Wirtschafter, S.K. (1960) Familial non-hemo-lytic jaundice with normal liver histology and conjugated bilirubin. *New England Journal of Medicine*, **262**, 113–117.

347. Hayward, D., Schiff, D., Fedunec, S. *et al.* (1986) Bilirubin diffusion through lipid membranes. *Biochimica et Biophysica Acta*, **8600**, 149–153.

348. Heirwegh, K.P.M. & Blanckaert, N. (1982) Analytical chemistry of rubins. In Heirwegh, K.P.M. & Brown, S.B. (eds) *Bilirubin. Vol. I: Chemistry*, pp. 125–151. Boca Raton, Florida: CRC Press.

349. Heirwegh, K.P.M. & Brown, S.B. (1982) (Eds) *Bilirubin. Vol. I: Chemistry*, pp. 1–158; *Vol. 2: Metabolism*, pp. 1–226. Boca Raton, Florida: CRC Press.

350. Heirwegh, K.P.M., Van de Vijver, M. & Fevery, J. (1972) Assay and properties of digitonin-activated bilirubin uridine diphosphate glucuronyltransferase from rat liver. *Biochemical Journal*, **129**, 605–618.

351. Heirwegh, K.P.M., Van Hees, G.P., Leroy, P. *et al.* (1970) Heterogeneity of bile pigment conjugates as revealed by chroma-tography of their ethyl anthranilate azopigments. *Biochemical Journal*, **120**, 877–890.

352. Heirwegh, K.P.M., Fevery, J., Meuwissen, J.A.T.P. *et al.* (1974) Recent advances in the separation and analysis of diazo-positive bile pigments. *Methods of Biochemical Analysis*, **22**, 205–250.

353. Heirwegh, K.P.M., Fevery, J., Michiels, R. *et al.* (1975) Separation by thin-layer chromatography and structure elucidation of bilirubin conjugates isolated from dog bile. *Biochemical Journal*, **145**, 185–199.

354. Hershko, C., Cook, J.D. & Finch, C.A. (1972) Storage iron kinetics. II. The uptake of hemoglobin iron by hepatic parenchymal cells. *Journal of Laboratory and Clinical Medicine*, **80**, 624–634.

355. Hjelle, J.J., Hazelton, G.A. & Klaassen, C.D. (1985) Acetamin-ophen decreases adenosine 3′-phosphate 5′-phosphosulfate and uridine diphosphoglucuronic acid in liver. *Drug Metabolism and Disposition*, **13**, 35–41.

356. Hochman, Y., Kelly, M. & Zakim, D. (1983) Modulation of the number of ligand binding sites of UDP-glucuronyltransferase by the gel to liquid-crystal phase transition of phosphatidylcholines. *Journal of Biological Chemistry*, **258**, 6509–6516.

357. Horie, T., Mizuma, T., Kasai, S. & Awazu, S. (1988) Confor-mational change in plasma albumin due to interaction with isolated rat hepatocyte. *American Journal of Physiology*, **254**, G465–G470.

358. Howell, S.R., Hazelton, G.A. & Klaassen, C.D. (1986) Depletion of hepatic UDP-glucuronic acid by drugs that are glucuronidated. *Journal of Pharmacology and Experimental Therapeutics*, **236**, 610–614.

359. Hsia, J.C., Er, S.S., Tan, C.T. *et al.* (1980) α-Fetoprotein binding specificity for arachidonate, bilirubin, docosahexaenoate, and pal-mitate. A spin label study. *Journal of Biological Chemistry*, **255**, 4224–4227.

360. Hsia, J.C., Er, S.S., Tab, C.T. & Tinker, D.O. (1982) Human serum albumin: an allosteric domain model for bilirubin binding specificity. An enantiomeric spin label study. *Journal of Biological Chemistry*, **257**, 1724–1729.

361. Huang, P.W.H., Rozdilsky, B., Gerrard, J.W. *et al.* (1970) Crigler–Najjar syndrome in four of five siblings with postmortem findings in one. *Archives of Pathology*, **90**, 536–542.

362. Hunter, F.M., Sparks, R.D. & Flinner, R.L. (1964) Hepatitis with resulting mobilization of hepatic pigment in a patient with Dubin–Johnson syndrome. *Gastroenterology*, **47**, 631–635.

363. Hunter, J.O., Thompson, R.P.H., Dunn, P.M. & Williams, R. (1973) Inheritance of type 2 Crigler–Najjar hyperbilirubinaemia. *Gut*, **14**, 46–49.

364. Inoue, M., Okajima, K., Nagase, S. & Morino, Y. (1983) Plasma clearance of sulfobromophthalein and its interaction with hepatic binding proteins in normal and analbuminemic rats: is plasma albumin essential for vectorial transport of organic anions in the liver? *Proceedings of the National Academy of Sciences of the USA*, **80**, 7654–7658.

365. Isherwood, D.M. & Fletcher, K.A. (1985) Neonatal jaundice: investigation and monitoring. *Annals of Clinical Biochemistry*, **22**, 109–128.

366. Ishizawa, S., Yoshida, T. & Kikuchi, G. (1983) Induction of heme oxygenase in rat liver. *Journal of Biological Chemistry*, **258**, 4220–4225.

367. Isobe, K., Itoh, S., Onishi, S. *et al.* (1983) Kinetic study of photochemical and thermal conversion of bilirubin IX alpha and its photoproducts. *Biochemical Journal*, **209**, 695–700.

368. Israels, L.G. (1970) The bilirubin shunt and shunt hyperbilirubinemia. In Popper, H. & Schaffner, F. (eds) *Progress in Liver Diseases*, Vol. III, pp. 1–12. New York: Grune & Stratton.
369. Israels, L.G. & Zipursky, A. (1962) Primary shunt hyperbilirubinaemia. *Nature*, **193**, 73–74.
370. Israels, L.G., Suderman, H.J. & Ritzmann, S.E. (1959) Hyperbilirubinemia due to an alternate path of bilirubin production. *American Journal of Medicine*, **27**, 693–702.
371. Jackson, M.R., McCarthy, L.R., Harding, D. *et al.* (1987) Cloning of a human liver microsomal UDP-glucuronosyltransferase cDNA. *Biochemistry Journal*, **242**, 581–588.
372. Jacobsen, C. (1978) Lysine residue 240 of human serum albumin is involved in high-affinity binding of bilirubin. *Biochemical Journal*, **171**, 453–459.
373. Jacobsen, J. (1969) Binding of bilirubin to human serum albumin. Determination of the dissociation constants. *FEBS Letters, 5*, 112–114.
374. Jacobsen, J. (1970) Dimerisation of bilirubin diglucuronide and formation of a complex of bilirubin and the diglucuronide. *Scandinavian Journal of Clinical and Laboratory Investigation*, **26**, 395–398.
375. Jacobsen, J. & Brodersen, R. (1983) Albumin-bilirubin binding mechanism. *Journal of Biological Chemistry*, **258**, 6319–6326.
376. Jacobsen, J. & Wennberg, R.P. (1974) Determination of unbound bilirubin in the serum of newborns. *Clinical Chemistry*, **20**, 783–789.
377. Jakoby, W.B. (1978) The glutathione *S*-transferases: a group of multifunctional detoxification proteins. *Advances in Enzymology and Related Areas of Molecular Biology*, **46**, 383–414.
378. Jandl, J.H., Jones, A.R. & Castle, W.B. (1957) The destruction of red cells by antibodies in man. 1. Observations on the sequestration and lysis of red cells altered by immune mechanism. *Journal of Clinical Investigation*, **36**, 1428–1459.
379. Jansen, P.L.M. & Onde Elferink, R.P.J. (1988) Hereditary hyperbilirubinemias: A molecular and mechanistic approach. *Seminars in Liver Disease*, **8**, 168–178.
380. Jansen, P.L.M. & Tangerman, A. (1980) Separation and characterization of bilirubin conjugates by high-performance liquid chromatography. *Journal of Chromatography*, **182**, 100–104.
381. Jansen, P.L.M., Cuypers, H.T. & Peters, W.H.M. (1984) Quantitation of bilirubin conjugates with high-performance liquid chromatography in patients with low total serum bilirubin levels. *European Journal of Clinical Investigation*, **14**, 295–300.
382. Jansen, P.L.M., Peters, W.H. & Lamers, W.H. (1985) Hereditary chronic conjugated hyperbilirubinemia in mutant rats caused by defective hepatic anion transport. *Hepatology*, **5**, 573–579.
383. Jansen, P.L.M., Peters, W.H.M. & Meijer, D.K.F. (1987) Hepatobiliary excretion of organic anions in double-mutant rats with a combination of defective canalicular transport and uridine 5'-diphosphate-glucuronyltransferase deficiency. *Gastroenterology*, **93**, 1094–1103.
384. Jansen, P.L.M., Hess, F., Peters, W.H.M. *et al.* (1989) Auxiliary liver transplantation in jaundiced rats with UDP-glucuronyltransferase deficiency and defective hepatobiliary transport. *Journal of Hepatology*, **8**, 192–200.
385. Javitt, N.B., Kondo, T. & Kuchiba, K. (1978) Bile acid excretion in Dubin–Johnson syndrome. *Gastroenterology*, **75**, 931–932.
386. Jendrassik, L. & Gref, P. (1938) Vereinfachte photometrische Methoden zur Bestimmung des Blutbilirubins. *Biochemische Zeitschrift*, **297**, 81–89.
387. Jervis, G.A. (1959) Constitutional nonhemolytic hyperbilirubinemia with findings resembling kernicterus. *AMA Archives of Neurology and Psychiatry*, **81**, 55–64.
388. Jezequel, A.M., Moscu, P.G., Koch, M.M. & Orlandi, F. (1981) The fine morphology of unconjugated hyperbilirubinemia revised with stereometry. In Okolicsanyi, L. (ed.) *Familial Hyperbilirubinemia*, pp. 121–131. Chichester: John Wiley.
389. Johnson, J.D. (1975) Neonatal nonhemolytic jaundice. *New England Journal of Medicine*, **292**, 194–197.
390. Johnson, L., Sarmento, F., Blanc, W.A. & Day, R. (1959) Kernicterus in rats with an inherited deficiency of glucuronyl transferase. *AMA Journal of Diseases of Children*, **97**, 591–608.
391. Jones, A.L., Schmucher, D.L., Mooney, J.S. *et al.* (1976) Morpho-
metric analysis of rat hepatocytes after total biliary obstruction. *Gastroenterology*, **71**, 1050–1060.
392. Jones, E.A., Carson, E.R. & Berk, P.D. (1986) Quantitation of bilirubin metabolism in vivo: Kinetic studies and mathematical modelling. In Ostrow, J.D. (ed.) *Bile Pigments and Jaundice*, pp. 439–474. New York: Marcel Dekker.
393. Jones, E.A., Shrager, R., Bloomer, J.R. *et al.* (1972) Quantitative studies of the delivery of hepatic synthesized bilirubin to plasma utilizing δ-aminolevulinic acid-4-^{14}C and bilirubin-^{3}H in man. *Journal of Clinical Investigation*, **51**, 2450–2458.
394. Jones, E.A., Bloomer, J.R., Berk, P.D. *et al.* (1977) Quantitation of hepatic bilirubin synthesis in man. In Berk, P.D. & Berlin, N.J. (eds) *The Chemistry and Physiology of Bile Pigments*, pp. 189–205. DHEW Publication No. (NIH) 77-1100, Government Printing Office, Washington, D.C.
395. Kamisaka, K., Listowsky, J. & Arias, I.M. (1973) Circular dichroism studies of Y protein (ligandin), a major organic anion binding protein in liver, kidney, and small intestine. *Annals of the New York Academy of Sciences*, **226**, 148–153.
396. Kamisaka, K., Maezawa, H., Inagaki, T. & Okano, K. (1981) A low molecular weight binding protein (Z protein) from human hepatic cytosol: purification and quantitation. *Hepatology*, **1**, 221–227.
397. Kapitulnik, J. & Ostrow, J.D. (1977) Stimulation of bilirubin catabolism in jaundiced Gunn rats by an inducer of microsomal mixed function monooxygenases. *Proceedings of the National Academy of Sciences of the USA*, **75**, 682–685.
398. Kapitulnik, J., Bircher, J. & Hadorn, H.B. (1989) Chlorpromazine (CPZ) reduces plasma bilirubin (BR) levels in Crigler–Najjar syndrome type I (CNS-I). *Hepatology*, **10**, 704.
399. Kapitulnik, J., Kaufmann, N.A., Goitein, K. *et al.* (1974) A pigment found in Crigler–Najjar syndrome and its similarity to an ultrafiltrable photo-derivative of bilirubin. *Clinica Chimica Acta*, **57**, 231–237.
400. Kapitulnik, J., Weil, E., Rabinowitz, R. *et al.* (1987) Fetal and adult human liver differ markedly in the fluidity and lipid composition of their microsomal membranes. *Hepatology, 7*, 55–60.
401. Kapitulnik, J., Hardwick, J.P., Ostrow, J.D. *et al.* (1987) Increase in a specific cytochrome P-450 isoenzyme in the liver of congenitally jaundiced Gunn rats. *Biochemistry Journal*, **242**, 297–300.
402. Kaplowitz, N. (1980) Physiological significance of glutathione *S*-transferases. *American Journal of Physiology*, **239**, G439–G444.
403. Kappas, A. & Drummond, G.S. (1986) Control of heme metabolism with synthetic metalloporphyrins. *Journal of Clinical Investigation*, **77**, 335–339.
404. Kappas, A., Drummond, G.S., Simionatto, C.S. & Anderson, K.E. (1984) Control of heme oxygenase and plasma levels of bilirubin by a synthetic heme analogue, tin-protoporphyrin. *Hepatology*, **4**, 336–341.
405. Kappas, A., Simionatto, C.S., Drummond, G.S. *et al.* (1985) The liver excretes large amounts of heme into bile when heme oxygenase is inhibited competitively by Sn-protoporphyrin. *Proceedings of the National Academy of Sciences of the USA*, **82**, 896–900.
406. Karon, M., Imach, D. & Schwartz, A. (1970) Effective phototherapy in congenital nonobstructive, nonhemolytic jaundice. *New England Journal of Medicine*, **282**, 377–380.
407. Karp, W.B. (1979) Biochemical alterations in neonatal hyperbilirubinemia and bilirubin encephalopathy: a review. *Pediatrics*, **64**, 361–368.
408. Kaufman, S.S., Wood, R.P., Shaw, B.W., Jr. *et al.* (1986) Orthotopic liver transplantation for type I Crigler–Najjar Syndrome. *Hepatology*, **6**, 1259–1262.
409. Kawade, N. & Onishi, S. (1981) The prenatal and postnatal development of UDP-glucuronyltransferase activity towards bilirubin and the effect of premature birth on this activity in the human liver. *Biochemical Journal*, **196**, 257–260.
410. Kawasaki, H., Kimura, N., Irisa, T. & Hirayama, C. (1979) Dye clearance studies in Rotor's syndrome. *American Journal of Gastroenterology*, **71**, 380–388.
411. Kawasaki, H., Kuchiba, K., Kondo, T. *et al.* (1979) Unconjugated bilirubin kinetics in Dubin–Johnson syndrome. *Clinica Chimica Acta*, **92**, 87–92.
412. Kawasaki, H., Yamanishi, Y., Kishimoto, Y. *et al.* (1981) Abnor-

mality of oral ursodeoxycholic acid tolerance test in the Dubin–Johnson syndrome. *Clinica Chimica Acta,* **112**, 13–19.

413. Kenwright, S. & Levi, A.G. (1973) Impairment of hepatic uptake of rifamycin antibiotics by probenecid, and its therapeutic implications. *Lancet,* **2**, 1401–1405.

414. Kenwright, S. & Levi, A.G. (1974) Sites of competition in the selective hepatic uptake of rifamycin-SV, flavaspidic acid, bilirubin, and bromosulphthalein. *Gut,* **15**, 220–226.

415. Ketterer, B., Ross-Mansell, P. & Whitehead, J.K. (1967) The isolation of carcinogen-binding protein from livers of rats given 4-di-methylaminoazobenzene. *Biochemical Journal,* **103**, 316–324.

416. Kikuchi, G. & Yoshida, T. (1980) Heme degradation by the microsomal heme oxygenase system. *Trends in Biochemical Sciences,* **5**, 323–325.

417. Kirshenbaum, G., Shames, D.M. & Schmid, R. (1976) An expanded model of bilirubin kinetics: effect of feeding, fasting, and phenobarbital in Gilbert's syndrome. *Journal of Pharmacokinetics and Biopharmaceutics,* **4**, 115–155.

418. Klaasen, C.D. & Watkins, J.B. (1984) Mechanisms of bile formation, hepatic uptake, and biliary excretion. *Pharmacology Review,* **36**, 1–67.

419. Knoflach, P., Horak, W., Kerstan, E. & Thaler, H. (1979) Benign chronic conjugated hyperbilirubinaemia: Rotor syndrome or hepatic storage impairment? *Zeitschrift für Gastroenterologie,* **17**, 32–37.

420. Koch, M.M., Lorenzini, I., Freddara, U. *et al.* (1978) Type 2 Crigler–Najjar syndrome. Quantitation of ultrastructural data and evolution under therapy with phenytoin. *Gastroenterologie Clinique et Biologique,* **2**, 831–842.

421. Kondo, T., Kuchiba, K. & Shimizu, Y. (1976) Coproporphyrin isomers in Dubin–Johnson syndrome. *Gastroenterology,* **70**, 1117–1120.

422. Kondo, T., Kuchiba, K. & Shimizu, Y. (1979) Metabolic fate of exogenous delta-aminolevulinic acid in Dubin–Johnson syndrome. *Journal of Laboratory and Clinical Medicine,* **94**, 421–428.

423. Kondo, T., Kuchiba, K., Ohtsuka, Y. *et al.* (1974) Clinical and genetic studies on Dubin–Johnson syndrome in a cluster area in Japan. *Japanese Journal of Human Genetics,* **18**, 378–392.

424. Kornberg, A. (1942) Latent liver disease in persons recovered from catarrhal jaundice and in otherwise normal medical students as revealed by the bilirubin excretion test. *Journal of Clinical Investigation,* **21**, 299–308.

425. Kosaka, A., Yamamoto, C., Morishita, Y. & Nakane, K. (1987) Enzymatic determination of bilirubin fractions in serum. *Clinical Biochemistry,* **20**, 451–458.

426. Koskelo, P. & Mustajoki, P. (1980) Altered coproporphyrin-isomer excretion in patients with the Dubin–Johnson syndrome. *International Journal of Biochemistry,* **12**, 975–978.

427. Koskelo, P., Toivonen, I. & Adlercreutz, H. (1967) Urinary coproporphyrin isomer distribution in the Dubin–Johnson syndrome. *Clinical Chemistry,* **13**, 1006–1009.

428. Kragh-Hansen, U. (1981) Molecular aspects of ligand binding to serum albumin. *Pharmacological Reviews,* **33**, 17–46.

429. Kreek, M.J. & Sleisenger, M.H. (1968) Reduction of serum unconjugated bilirubin with phenobarbitone in adult congenital nonhemolytic unconjugated hyperbilirubinaemia. *Lancet,* **2**, 73–78.

430. Kutty, R.K. & Maines, M.D. (1981) Purification and characterization of biliverdin reductase from rat liver. *Journal of Biological Chemistry,* **256**, 3959–3962.

431. Kutz, K., Kandler, H., Gugler, R. & Fevery, J. (1984) Effect of clofibrate on the metabolism of bilirubin, bromosulphophthalein and indocyanine green and on the biliary lipid composition in Gilbert's syndrome. *Clinical Science,* **66**, 389–397.

432. Kutz, K., Schulte, A., Jensen, C. & Gugler, R. (1977) Impaired drug conjugation in subjects with Gilbert's syndrome. *Gastroenterology,* **73**, 1229 (abstract).

433. Kutz, K., Egger, R., Bachofen, H. & Preisig, R. (1977) Effect of fasting on endogenous carbon monoxide production in normal subjects and those with Constitutional Hepatic Dysfunction (Gilbert's syndrome). In Berk, P.D. & Berlin, N.I. (eds) *Chemistry and Physiology of Bile Pigments,* pp. 156–167. Washington, D.C.: Public Health Service, National Institutes of Health.

434. Lake, A.M., Truman, J.T., Bode, H.H. *et al.* (1978) Marked

hyperbilirubinemia with Gilbert's syndrome and immunohemolytic anemia. *Journal of Pediatrics,* **73**, 812–814.

435. Lalani, El-N.M.A. & Burchell, B. (1979) Stimulation of defective Gunn-rat liver uridine diphosphate glucuronyltransferase activity in vitro by alkyl ketones. *Biochemical Journal,* **177**, 993–995.

436. Lamola, A.A., Flores, J. & Blumberg, W.E. (1983) Binding of photobilirubin to human serum albumin. Estimate of the affinity constant. *European Journal of Biochemistry,* **132**, 165–169.

437. Lamola, A.A., Blumberg, W.E., McClead, R. & Fanaroff, A. (1981) Photoisomerized bilirubin in blood from infants receiving phototherapy. *Proceedings of the National Academy of Sciences, USA,* **78**, 1882–1886.

438. Landaw, S.A. (1975) Carbon monoxide production as a measurement of heme catabolism. In Goresky, C.A. & Fisher, M.M. (eds) *Jaundice,* pp. 103–127. New York: Plenum Press.

439. Landaw, S.A., Callahan, E.W. & Schmid, R. (1970) Catabolism of heme in vivo: comparison of the simultaneous production of bilirubin and carbon monoxide. *Journal of Clinical Investigation,* **49**, 914–925.

440. Lathe, G.H. & Walker, W. (1957) An enzyme defect in human neonatal jaundice and in Gunn's strain of jaundiced rats. *Biochemical Journal,* **67**, 9P.

441. Lauff, J.L., Kasper, M.E. & Ambrose, R.T. (1981) Separation of bilirubin species in serum and bile by high performance reversed-phase liquid chromatography. *Journal of Chromatography,* **226**, 391–402.

442. Lauff, J.J., Kasper, M.E., Wu, T.W. & Ambrose, R.T. (1982) Isolation and preliminary characterization of a fraction of bilirubin in serum that is firmly bound to protein. *Clinical Chemistry,* **28**, 629–637.

443. Lazarow, P.B. & de Duve, C. (1973) The synthesis and turnover of rat liver peroxisomes. Biochemical pathway of catalase synthesis. *Journal of Cell Biology,* **59**, 491–506.

444. Leakey, J.E.A., Hume, R. & Burchell, B. (1987) Development of multiple activities of UDP-glucuronyltransferase in human liver. *Biochemical Journal,* **243**, 859–861.

445. Leakey, J.E.A., Althans, Z.R., Bailey, J.R. *et al.* (1985) Dexamethasone increases UDP-glucuronyltransferase activity towards bilirubin, oestradiol and testosterone in foetal liver from rhesus monkey during late gestation. *Biochemical Journal,* **225**, 183–188.

446. Lee, K. & Gartner, L.M. (1983) Management of unconjugated hyperbilirubinemia in the newborn. *Seminars in Liver Disease,* **3**, 52–64.

447. Lelong, M., Colin, J., Alagille, D. *et al.* (1961) Ictère familial non-hémolytique avec ictère nucléaire (maladie de Crigler–Najjar). *Archives Francaises de Pediatrie,* **18**, 272–275.

448. Lester, R. & Schmid, R. (1963) Intestinal absorption of bile pigments. II. Bilirubin absorption in man. *New England Journal of Medicine,* **269**, 178–182.

449. Lester, R. & Schmid, R. (1963) Intestinal absorption of bile pigments. I. The enterohepatic circulation of bilirubin in the rat. *Journal of Clinical Investigation,* **42**, 736–746.

450. Lester, R. & Schmid, R. (1965) Intestinal absorption of bile pigments. III. The enterohepatic circulation of urobilinogen in the rat. *Journal of Clinical Investigation,* **44**, 722–730.

451. Lester, R., Hammaker, L. & Schmid, R. (1962) A new therapeutic approach to unconjugated hyperbilirubinaemia. *Lancet,* **2**, 1257.

452. Lester, R., Schumer, W. & Schmid, R. (1965) Intestinal absorption of bile pigments. IV. Urobilinogen absorption in man. *New England Journal of Medicine,* **272**, 939–943.

453. Levi, A.G., Gatmaitan, Z. & Arias, I.M. (1969) Two hepatic cytoplasmic protein fractions, Y and Z, and their possible role in the hepatic uptake of bilirubin sulfobromophthalein, and other anions. *Journal of Clinical Investigation,* **48**, 2156–2167.

454. Levi, A.G., Gatmaitan, Z. & Arias, I.M. (1970) Deficiency of hepatic organic anion binding protein, impaired organic anion uptake by liver and 'physiologic' jaundice in newborn monkeys. *New England Journal of Medicine,* **284**, 1136–1139.

455. Levine, R.I., Reyes, H., Levi, A.J. *et al.* (1971) Phylogenetic study of organic anion transfer from plasma into the liver. *Nature: New Biology,* **231**, 277–279.

456. Levine, R.L. (1988) Neonatal jaundice. *Acta Paediatrica Scandinavica,* **77**, 177–182.

457. Levitt, M., Schacter, B.A., Zipursky, A. & Israels, L.G. (1968) The nonerythropoietic component of early bilirubin. *Journal of Clinical Investigation*, **47**, 1281–1294.

458. Levy, M., Lester, R. & Levinsky, N.G. (1968) Renal excretion of urobilinogen in the dog. *Journal of Clinical Investigation*, **47**, 2117–2124.

459. Lightner, D.A. (1977) The photoreactivity of bilirubin and related pyrroles. *Photochemistry and Photobiology*, **26**, 427–436.

460. Lightner, D.A. & McDonagh, A.F. (1984) Molecular mechanisms of phototherapy for neonatal jaundice. *Accounts of Chemical Research*, **17**, 417–424.

461. Lightner, D.A., Gawronski, J.K. and Gawronska, K. (1985) Conformational enantiomerism in bilirubin. Selection by cyclodextrins. *Journal of American Chemistry Society*, **107**, 2456–2461.

462. Lightner, D.A., Linnane, W.P. III & Ahlfors, C.E. (1984) Bilirubin photooxidation products in the urine of jaundiced neonates receiving phototherapy. *Pediatric Research*, **18**, 696–700.

463. Lightner, D.A., Woolridge, T.A. & McDonagh, A.F. (1979) Photobilirubin: an early bilirubin photoproduct detected by absorbance difference spectroscopy. *Proceedings of the National Academy of Sciences of the USA*, **76**, 29–32.

464. Lightner, D.A., Woolridge, T.A. & McDonagh, A.F. (1979) Configurational isomerization of bilirubin and the mechanism of jaundice phototherapy. *Biochemical and Biophysical Research Communications*, **86**, 235–243.

465. Lipschitz, W.L. (1939) Mechanism of the biological formation of conjugated glucuronic acids. *Journal of Biological Chemistry*, **129**, 333–358.

466. Lipsitz, P.J. & London, M. (1973) A rapid total bilirubin test using sodium hypochlorite. *Journal of Laboratory and Clinical Medicine*, **81**, 625–631.

467. Listowsky, I., Gatmaitan, Z. & Arias, I.M. (1978) Ligandin retains and albumin loses bilirubin binding capacity in liver cytosol. *Proceedings of the National Academy of Sciences of the USA*, **75**, 1213–1216.

468. Lolekha, P.H. & Limpavithayakul, K. (1977) Promoting ability of 5 accelerating agents for diazotization of several types of bilirubin samples. *Clinical Chemistry*, **23**, 778–779.

469. London, I.M., West, R., Shemin, D. & Rittenberg, D. (1950) On the origin of bile pigment in normal man. *Journal of Biological Chemistry*, **184**, 351–358.

470. Lucey, J.F. (1982) Bilirubin and brain damage—a real mess (editorial). *Pediatrics*, **69**, 381–382.

471. Lucey, J.F., Ferreiro, M. & Hewitt, J. (1968) Prevention of hyperbilirubinemia of prematurity by phototherapy. *Pediatrics*, **41**, 1047–1054.

472. Lunazzi, G., Tiribelli, C., Gazzin, B. & Sottocasa, G. (1982) Further studies on bilitranslocase, a plasma membrane protein involved in hepatic organic anion uptake. *Biochimica et Biophysica Acta*, **685**, 117–122.

473. Lundh, B., Johansson, M.-B., Mercke, C. & Cavallin-Ståhl, E. (1972) Enhancement of heme catabolism by caloric restriction in man. *Scandinavian Journal of Clinical and Laboratory Investigation*, **30**, 421–427.

474. Lundh, H.T. & Jacobsen, J. (1972) Influence of phototherapy on unconjugated bilirubin in duodenal bile of newborn infants with hyperbilirubinaemia. *Acta Paediatrica Scandinavica*, **61**, 693–696.

475. Lundh, H.T. & Jacobsen, J. (1974) Influence of phototherapy on the biliary bilirubin excretion pattern in newborn infants with hyperbilirubinemia. *Journal of Pediatrics*, **85**, 262–267.

476. Mackenzie, P.I. (1986) Rat liver UDP-glucuronosyltransferase. Sequence and expression on a cDNA encoding a phenobarbital-inducible form. *Journal of Biological Chemistry*, **261**, 6119–6125.

477. Macklon, A.F., Savage, R.L. & Rawlins, M.D. (1979) Gilbert's syndrome and drug metabolism. *Clinical Pharmacokinetics*, **4**, 223–232.

478. Mahu, J.-L., Duvaldestin, P., Dhumeaux, D. & Berthelot, P. (1977) Biliary transport of cholephilic dyes: evidence for two different pathways. *American Journal of Physiology*, **232**, E445–E450.

479. Maisels, K.J. (1988) Neonatal jaundice. *Seminars in Liver Disease*, **8**, 148–162.

480. Malloy, H. & Evelyn, K. (1937) The determination of bilirubin with the photoelectric colorimeter. *Journal of Biological Chemistry*, **119**, 481–490.

481. Malloy, H. & Lowenstein, L. (1940) Hereditary jaundice in the rat. *Canadian Medical Association Journal*, **42**, 122–125.

482. Mandema, E., de Fraiture, W.H., Nieweg, H.O. & Arends, A. (1960) Familial chronic idiopathic jaundice (Dubin–Sprinz disease), with a note on bromsulphalein metabolism in this disease. *American Journal of Medicine*, **28**, 42–50.

483. Manitto, P. & Monti, D. (1976) Free-energy barrier of conformational inversion of bilirubin. *JCS Chemical Communications*, 122–123.

484. Martin, J.F., Vierling, J.M., Wolkoff, A.W. *et al.* (1976) Abnormal hepatic transport of indocyanine green in Gilbert's syndrome. *Gastroenterology*, **70**, 385–391.

485. Marver, H.S. & Schmid, R. (1972) The porphyrias. In Stanbury, J.B., Wyngaarden, J.B. & Fredrickson, D.S. (eds) *The Metabolic Basis of Inherited Disease*, pp. 1087–1140. New York: McGraw-Hill.

486. McDonagh, A.F. (1979) Bile pigments. Bilatrienes and 5,15-biladienes. In Dolphin, D. (ed.) *The Porphyrins*, Vol. VI, pp. 293–491. New York: Academic Press.

487. McDonagh, A.F. & Asissi, F. (1972) The ready isomerization of bilirubin-IXα in aqueous solution. *Biochemical Journal*, **129**, 797–800.

488. McDonagh, A.F. & Lightner, D.A. (1988) Phototherapy and photobiology of bilirubin. *Seminars in Liver Disease*, **8**, 272–283.

489. McDonagh, A.F. & Palma, L.A. (1980) Hepatic excretion of circulating bilirubin photoproducts in the Gunn rat. *Journal of Clinical Investigation*, **66**, 1182–1185.

490. McDonagh, A.F. & Palma, L.A. (1985) Tin-protoporphyrin: a potent photosensitizer of bilirubin destruction. *Photochemistry and Photobiology*, **42**(3), 261–264.

491. McDonagh, A.F., Palma, L.A. & Lightner, D.A. (1980) Blue light and bilirubin excretion. *Science*, **208**, 145–151.

492. McDonagh, A.F., Palma, L.A. & Schmid, R. (1981) Reduction of biliverdin and placental transfer of bilirubin and biliverdin in the pregnant guinea pig. *Biochemical Journal*, **194**, 273–282.

493. McDonagh, A.F., Palma, A.L., Trull, F.R. & Lightner, D.A. (1982) Phototherapy for neonatal jaundice. Configurational isomers of bilirubin. *American Chemical Society*, **104**, 6865–6869.

494. McDonagh, A.F., Palma, L.A., Lauff, J.J. & Wu, T.-W. (1984) Origin of mammalian biliprotein and rearrangement of bilirubin glucuronides in vivo in the rat. *Journal of Clinical Investigation*, **74**, 763–770.

495. McGee, J.O'D., Allan, J.G., Russell, R.I. & Patrick, R.S. (1975) Liver ultrastructure in Gilbert's syndrome. *Gut*, **16**, 220–224.

496. Meijer, D.K.F. (1987) Current concepts on hepatic transport of drugs. *Journal of Hepatology*, **4**, 259–268.

497. Meijer, D.K.F., Vonk, R.J., Keulemans, K. & Weitering, J.G. (1977) Hepatic uptake and biliary excretion of dibromosulphthalein. Albumin dependence, influence of phenobarbital and nafenopin pretreatment and the role of Y and Z protein. *Journal of Pharmacology and Experimental Therapeutics*, **202**, 8–21.

498. Meisel, P., Jahrig, D., Theel, L. *et al.* (1982) The bronze baby syndrome: consequence of impaired excretion of photobilirubin? *Photobiochemistry and Photobiophysics*, **3**, 345–352.

499. Meisel, P., Biebler, K.E., Gens, A. & Jaehrig, K. (1983) Albumin binding of photobilirubin II. *Biochemical Journal*, **213**, 25–29.

500. Mercke, C., Cavallin-Stähl, E. & Lundh, B. (1975) Diurnal variation in endogenous production of CO. Effect of caloric restriction. *Acta Medica Scandinavica*, **198**, 161–164.

501. Merdler, C., Burke, M., Shani, M. *et al.* (1976) The effect of phenobarbital on patients with Dubin–Johnson syndrome. *Digestion*, **14**, 394–399.

502. Meredith, C.G., Muhoberac, B.B., Gray, J.P. *et al.* (1986) Hepatic oxidative drug metabolism and the microsomal milieu in a rat model of congenital hyperbilirubinemia. *Biochemical Pharmacology*, **35**, 3831–3837.

503. Metreau, J.M., Yvart, J., Dhumeaux, D. & Berthelot, P. (1978) Role of bilirubin overproduction in revealing Gilbert's syndrome: is dyserythropoiesis an important factor? *Gut*, **19**, 838–843.

504. Meulengracht, E. (1947) A review of chronic intermittent juvenile jaundice. *Quarterly Journal of Medicine*, **16**, 83–98.

505. Meuwissen, J.A.T.P., Ketterer, B. & Heirwegh, K.P.M. (1977) Role of soluble binding proteins in overall hepatic transport of bilirubin. In Berk, P.D. & Berlin, N.I. (eds) *Chemistry and Physiology of Bile Pigments*, pp. 323–337. Bethesda, MD: National Institutes of Health.

506. Meuwissen, J.A.T.P., Zeegers, M., Srai, K.S. & Ketterer, B. (1977) Effect of glutathione on the activity of bilirubin-binding proteins from rat liver cytosol. *Biochemical Society Transactions*, **5**, 1404–1407.

507. Mia, A.S., Gronwall, R.R. & Cornelius, C.E. (1970) Bilirubin-^{14}C turnover studies in normal and mutant Southdown sheep with congenital hyperbilirubinemia. *Proceedings of the Society for Experimental Biology and Medicine*, **133**, 955–959.

508. Mia, A.S., Gronwall, R.R. & Cornelius, C.E. (1970) Unconjugated and conjugated bilirubin transport in normal and mutant Corriedale sheep with Dubin–Johnson syndrome. *Proceedings of the Society for Experimental Biology and Medicine*, **135**, 33–37.

509. Michaelsson, M., Nosslin, B. & Sjölin, S. (1965) Plasma bilirubin determination in the newborn infant. *Pediatrics*, **35**, 925–931.

510. Minio-Paluello, F., Gautier, A. & Magnenat, P. (1968) L'ultrastructure du foie humain dans un cas de Crigler–Najjar. *Acta Hepato-splenologica*, **15**, 65–71.

511. Mooney, R.A., Smith, C.H. & Zakowsky, H.S. (1983) Free bilirubin measurements in a patient with Crigler–Najjar syndrome after crush injury. *Journal of Pediatrics*, **103**, 262–265.

512. Morgenstern, R. & De Pierre, W. (1983) Microsomal glutathione transferase. Purification in unactivated form and further characterization of the activation process, substrate specificity and amino acid composition. *European Journal of Biochemistry*, **134**, 591–597.

513. Morgenstern, R., Guthenberg, C. & DePierre, J.W. (1982) Microsomal glutathione S-transferase. *European Journal of Biochemistry*, **126**, 243–248.

514. Motta, P. (1975) A scanning electron microscopic study of the rat liver sinusoid: endothelial and Kupffer cells. *Cell and Tissue Research*, **164**, 371–385.

515. Mukherjee, B. & Krasner, J. (1973) Induction of an enzyme in genetically deficient rats after grafting of normal liver. *Science*, **182**, 68–70.

516. Mukherjee, B. & Krasner, J. (1979) Survival of transplanted normal hepatic cells in bilirubin UDP-glucuronyl transferase-deficient Gunn rat liver. *Research Communications in Chemical Pathology and Pharmacology*, **24**, 159–168.

517. Muller-Eberhard, U. & Liem, H.H. (1974) Hemopexin, the heme-binding serum β-glycoprotein. In Allison, A.C. (ed.) *Structure and Function of Plasma Proteins*, Vol. I, pp. 35–53. London: Plenum Press.

518. Muller-Eberhard, U. & Vincent, S.H. (1985) Concepts of heme distribution within hepatocytes. *Biochemical Pharmacology*, **34**, 719–725.

519. Munoz, M.E., Esteller, A. & Gonzalez, J. (1987) Substrate induction of bilirubin conjugation and biliary excretion in the rat. *Clinical Science*, **73**, 371–375.

520. Munoz, M.E., Gonzalez, J. & Esteller, A. (1987) Effect of glucose administration on bilirubin excretion in the rabbit. *Experientia*, **43**, 166–168.

521. Muraca, M. & Blanckaert, N. (1983) Liquid-chromatographic assay and identification of mono- and diester conjugates of bilirubin in normal serum. *Clinical Chemistry*, **29**, 1767–1771.

522. Muraca, M. & Fevery, J. (1984) Influence of sex and sex steroids on bilirubin uridine diphosphate-glucuronosyl-transferase activity of rat liver. *Gastroenterology*, **87**, 308–313.

523. Muraca, M., De Groote, J. & Fevery, J. (1983) Sex differences of hepatic conjugation of bilirubin determine its maximal biliary excretion in non-anaesthetized male and female rats. *Clinical Science*, **64**, 85–90.

524. Muraca, M., Fevery, J. & Blanckaert, N. (1987) Relationships between serum bilirubins and production and conjugation of bilirubin. *Gastroenterology*, **92**, 309–317.

525. Muraca, M., Fevery, J. & Blanckaert, N. (1988) Analytic aspects and clinical interpretation of serum bilirubins. *Seminars in Liver Disease*, **8**, 137–147.

526. Muscatello, U., Mussini, J. & Agnolucci, M.T. (1967) The Dubin–Johnson syndrome: an electron microscopic study of the liver cell. *Acta Hepato-Splenologica*, **14**, 162–170.

527. Nagaoka, S. & Cowger, M.L. (1978) Interaction of bilirubin with lipids studied by fluorescence quenching method. *Journal of Biological Chemistry*, **253**, 2005–2011.

528. Nakata, D., Zakim, D. & Vessey, D.A. (1976) Defective function of a microsomal UDP-glucuronyltransferase in Gunn rats. *Proceedings of the National Academy of Sciences of the USA*, **73**, 289–292.

529. Namihisa, T. & Nambu, M. (1977) Rotor's and Dubin–Johnson syndromes. *New England Journal of Medicine*, **297**, 560.

530. Namihisa, T. & Yamaguchi, K. (1973) The constitutional hyperbilirubinemia in Japan: studies on 139 cases reported during the period from 1963 to 1969. *Gastroenterologia Japonica*, **8**, 311–321.

531. Nelson, T., Jacobsen, J. & Wennberg, R.P. (1974) Effect of pH on the interaction of bilirubin with albumin and tissue culture cells. *Pediatric Research*, **8**, 963–967.

532. Newman, T.B. & Maisels, M.J. (1989) Bilirubin and brain damage: What do we do now? *Pediatrics*, **83**, 1062–1065.

533. Noonan, N.E., Olsen, G.A. & Cornelius, C.E. (1979) A new animal model with hyperbilirubinemia. The indigo snake. *Digestive Diseases and Sciences*, **24**, 521–524.

534. Novikoff, A.B. & Essner, E. (1960) The liver cell. *American Journal of Medicine*, **29**, 102–131.

535. Novros, J.S., Koch, T.R. & Knoblock, E.C. (1979) Improved method for accurate quantitation of total and conjugated bilirubin in serum. *Clinical Chemistry*, **25**, 1891–1899.

536. Nuwayhid, N., Glaser, J.H., Johnson, J.C. et al. (1986) Xylosylation and glucuronosylation reactions in rat liver Golgi apparatus and endoplasmic reticulum. *Journal of Biological Chemistry*, **261**, 12936–12941.

537. Ockner, R., Manning, J.A. & Kane, J.P. (1982) Fatty acid binding protein. *Journal of Biological Chemistry*, **257**, 7872–7878.

538. Ockner, R.K., Weisiger, R.A. & Gollan, J.L. (1983) Hepatic uptake of albumin-bound substances: albumin receptor concept. *American Journal of Physiology*, **245**, G13–G18.

539. Ockner, R.K., Manning, J.A., Poppenhausen, R.B. & Ho, W.R.L. (1972) A binding protein for fatty acids in cytosol of intestinal mucosa, liver, myocardium and other tissues. *Science*, **177**, 56–58.

540. Odell, G.B. (1965) Influence of pH on the distribution of bilirubin between albumin and mitochondria. *Proceedings of the Society for Experimental Biology and Medicine*, **120**, 352–354.

541. Odell, G.B. (1966) The distribution of bilirubin between albumin and mitochondria. *Journal of Pediatrics*, **68**, 164–180.

542. Odell, G.B., Cukier, J.O. & Gourley, G.R. (1981) The presence of a microsomal UDP-glucuronyl transferase for bilirubin in homozygous jaundiced Gunn rats and in the Crigler–Najjar syndrome. *Hepatology*, **1**, 307–315.

543. Odell, G.B., Natzschka, J.C. & Storey, G.N. (1967) Bilirubin nephropathy in the Gunn strain of rat. *American Journal of Physiology*, **212**, 931–938.

544. Odell, G.B., Bolen, J.L., Poland, R.L. et al. (1974) Protection from bilirubin nephropathy in jaundiced Gunn rats. *Gastroenterology*, **66**, 1218–1224.

545. Odell, G.B., Cukier, J.O., Ostrea, E.M. et al. (1977) The influence of fatty acids on the binding of bilirubin to albumin. *Journal of Laboratory and Clinical Medicine*, **89**, 295–307.

546. Odièvre, M., Trivin, F., Eliot, N. & Alagille, D. (1978) Case of congenital nonobstructive, nonhaemolytic jaundice. Successful long-term phototherapy at home. *Archives of Disease in Childhood*, **53**, 81–82.

547. Ohkubo, H. & Okuda, K. (1984) The nicotinic acid test in constitutional conjugated hyperbilirubinemias and effects of corticosteroid. *Hepatology*, **4**, 1206–1208.

548. Ohkubo, H., Musha, H. & Okuda, K. (1979) Studies on nicotinic acid interaction with bilirubin metabolism. *Digestive Diseases and Sciences*, **24**, 700–704.

549. Ohkubo, H., Okuda, K. & Iida, S. (1981) A constitutional unconjugated hyperbilirubinemia combined with indocyanine green intolerance: a new functional disorder? *Hepatology*, **1**, 319–324.

550. Ohkubo, H., Okuda, K. & Iido, S. (1981) Effects of corticosteroids on bilirubin metabolism in patients with Gilbert's syndrome. *Hepatology*, **1**, 168.

551. Ohkubo, H., Okuda, K., Iida, S. & Makino, I. (1981) Ursodeoxy-

cholic acid oral tolerance test in patients with constitutional hyperbilirubinemias and effect of phenobarbital. *Gastroenterology*, **81**, 126–135.

552. Okolicsanyi, L., Ghidini, O., Orlando, R. *et al.* (1978) An evaluation of bilirubin kinetics with respect to the diagnosis of Gilbert's syndrome. *Clinical Science and Molecular Medicine*, **54**, 539–547.

553. Okolicsanyi, L., Orlando, R., Venuti, M. *et al.* (1981) A modeling study of the effect of fasting on bilirubin kinetics in Gilbert's syndrome. *American Journal of Physiology*, **240**, R266–R271.

554. Okolicsanyi, L., Nassuato, F., Muraca, M. *et al.* (1988) Epidemiology of unconjugated hyperbilirubinemia: revisited. *Seminars in Liver Disease*, **8**, 179–182.

555. Okulicz-Kozaryn, I., Schaefer, M. & Batt, A.-M. (1981) Sterochemical heterogeneity of hepatic UDP-glucuronosyltransferase activity in rat liver microsomes. *Biochemical Pharmacology*, **30**, 1457–1461.

556. Olsson, R. & Lindstedt, G. (1980) Evaluation of tests for Gilbert's syndrome. *Acta Medica Scandinavica*, **207**, 425–428.

557. Onishi, S., Itoh, S. & Isobe, K. (1986) Wavelength-dependence of the relative rate constants for the main geometric and structural photoisomerization of bilirubin IX alpha bound to human serum albumin. *Biochemical Journal*, **236**, 23–29.

558. Onishi, S., Isobe, K., Itoh, S. *et al.* (1980) Demonstration of a geometric isomer of bilirubin-IXα in the serum of a hyperbilirubinaemic newborn infant and the mechanism of jaundice phototherapy. *Biochemical Journal*, **190**, 533–536.

559. Onishi, S., Itoh, S., Kawade, N. *et al.* (1980) An accurate and sensitive analysis by high-pressure liquid chromatography of conjugated and unconjugated bilirubin-IXα in various biological fluids. *Biochemical Journal*, **185**, 281–284.

560. Onishi, S., Kawade, N., Itoh, S. *et al.* (1980) High-pressure liquid chromatographic analysis of anaerobic photoproducts of bilirubin-IXα in vitro and its comparison with photoproducts in vivo. *Biochemical Journal*, **190**, 527–532.

561. Onishi, S., Kawade, N., Itoh, S. *et al.* (1981) Kinetics of biliary excretion of the main two bilirubin photoproducts after injection into Gunn rats. *Biochemical Journal*, **198**, 107–112.

562. Onishi, S., Miura, I., Isobe, K. *et al.* (1984) Structure and thermal interconversion of cyclobilirubin IXα. *Biochemical Journal*, **218**, 667–676.

563. Onishi, S., Ogino, T., Yokoyama, T. *et al.* (1984) Biliary and urinary excretion rates and serum concentration changes of four bilirubin photoproducts in Gunn rats during total darkness and low or high illumination. *Biochemical Journal*, **221**, 717–721.

564. Onishi, S., Isobe, K., Itoh, S. *et al.* (1986) Metabolism of bilirubin and its photoisomers in newborn infants during phototherapy. *Journal of Biochemistry*, **100**, 789–795.

565. Ostrow, J.D. (1967) Absorption of bile pigments by the gallbladder. *Journal of Clinical Investigation*, **46**, 2035–2052.

566. Ostrow, J.D. (1971) Photocatabolism of labeled bilirubin in the congenitally jaundiced Gunn rat. *Journal of Clinical Investigation*, **50**, 707–718.

567. Ostrow, J.D. (1974) Bilirubin and jaundice. In Becker, F.F. (ed.) *The Liver, Normal and Abnormal Functions*, pp. 303–369. New York: Marcel Dekker.

568. Ostrow, J.D. (ed.) (1986) *Bile Pigments and Jaundice*. New York: Marcel Dekker.

569. Ostrow, J.D. (1988) Therapeutic amelioration of jaundice: Old and new strategies. *Hepatology*, **8**(3), 683–689.

570. Ostrow, J.D., Jandl, J.H. & Schmid, R. (1962) The formation of bilirubin from hemoglobin in vivo. *Journal of Clinical Investigation*, **41**, 1628–1637.

571. Owens, D. & Evans, J. (1975) Population studies in Gilbert's syndrome. *Journal of Medical Genetics*, **12**, 152–156.

572. Owens, D. & Sherlock, S. (1973) Diagnosis of Gilbert's syndrome: role of reduced caloric intake test. *British Medical Journal*, **3**, 559–563.

573. Pascasio, F.M. & de la Fuente, D. (1969) Rotor–Manahan–Florentin syndrome: clinical and genetic studies. *Philippine Journal of Internal Medicine*, **7**, 151–157.

574. Paumgartner, G. & Reichen, J. (1976) Kinetics of hepatic uptake of unconjugated bilirubin. *Clinical Science and Molecular Medicine*, **51**, 169–176.

575. Peck, O.C., Rey, D.F. & Snell, A.M. (1960) Familial jaundice with free and conjugated bilirubin in the serum and without liver pigmentation. *Gastroenterology*, **39**, 625–627.

576. Pereira Lima, J.E., Utz, E. & Roisenberg, I. (1966) Hereditary nonhemolytic conjugated hyperbilirubinemia without abnormal liver cell pigmentation. A family study. *American Journal of Medicine*, **40**, 628–633.

577. Perez, M. & Hirschberg, C.B. (1986) Transport of sugar nucleotides and adenosine 3′-phosphate 5′-phosphosulfate into vesicles derived from the Golgi apparatus. *Biochimica et Biophysica Acta*, **864**, 213–222.

578. Persico, M., Bellentani, S., Marchegiano, P. *et al.* (1988) Sex steroid modulation of the hepatic uptake of organic anions in rat. *Journal of Hepatology*, **6**, 343–349.

579. Peters, T.J. & Seymour, C.A. (1978) The organelle pathology and demonstration of mitochondrial superoxide dismutase deficiency in two patients with Dubin–Johnson–Sprinz syndrome. *Clinical Science and Molecular Medicine*, **54**, 549–553.

580. Peters, W.H.M. & Jansen, P.L.M. (1986) Microsomal UDP-glucuronyltransferase-catalyzed bilirubin diglucuronide formation in human liver. *Journal of Hepatology*, **2**, 182–194.

581. Peters, W.H.M. & Jansen, P.L.M. (1988) Immunocharacterization of UDP-glucuronyltransferase isoenzymes in human liver, intestine and kidney. *Biochemical Pharmacology*, **37**, 564–567.

582. Peters, W.H.M., Jansen, P.L.M. & Nauta, N. (1984) The molecular weights of UDP-glucuronyltransferase determined with radiation-inactivation analysis. A molecular model of bilirubin UDP-glucuronyltransferase. *Journal of Biological Chemistry*, **259**, 11701–11705.

583. Peters, W.H.M., Allebes, W.A., Jansen, P.L.M. *et al.* (1987) Characterization and tissue specificity of a monoclonal antibody against human uridine 5′-diphosphate-glucuronosyltransferase. *Gastroenterology*, **93**, 162–169.

584. Peterson, R.E. & Schmid, R. (1957) A clinical syndrome associated with a defect in steroid glucuronide conjugation. *Journal of Clinical Endocrinology and Metabolism*, **17**, 1485–1488.

585. Pickett, C.B., Telakowski-Hopkins, C.A., Ding, G. *et al.* (1984) Rat liver glutathione *S*-transferases. *Journal of Biological Chemistry*, **259**, 5182–5188.

586. Pimstone, N.R., Engel, P., Tenhunen, R. *et al.* (1971) Inducible heme oxygenase in the kidney: a model for the homeostatic control of hemoglobin catabolism. *Journal of Clinical Investigation*, **50**, 2042–2050.

587. Platzer, R., Kupfer, A., Bircher, J. & Preisig, R. (1978) Polymorphic acetylation and aminopyrine demethylation in Gilbert's syndrome. *European Journal of Clinical Investigation*, **8**, 219–223.

588. Poland, R.L. & Odell, G.B. (1971) Physiologic jaundice: the enterohepatic circulation of bilirubin. *New England Journal of Medicine*, **284**, 1–6.

589. Portman, O.W., Chowdhury, J.R., Chowdhury, N.R. *et al.* (1984) A nonhuman primate model of Gilbert's syndrome. *Hepatology*, **4**, 175–179.

590. Porush, J.G., Delman, A.J. & Feuer, M.M. (1962) Chronic idiopathic jaundice with normal liver histology. *Archives of Internal Medicine*, **109**, 102–109.

591. Potter, B.J., Blades, B.F., Shepard, M.D. *et al.* (1987) The kinetics of sulfobromophthalein uptake by rat liver sinusoidal vesicles. *Biochimica et Biophysica Acta*, **898**, 159–171.

592. Powell, L.W., Billing, B.H. & Williams, H.S. (1967) The assessment of red cell survival in idiopathic unconjugated hyperbilirubinaemia (Gilbert's syndrome) by the use of radioactive diisopropylfluorophosphate and chromium. *Australasian Annals of Medicine*, **16**, 221–225.

593. Powell, L.W., Hemingway, E., Billing, B.H. & Sherlock, S. (1967) Idiopathic unconjugated hyperbilirubinemia (Gilbert's syndrome). A study of 42 families. *New England Journal of Medicine*, **277**, 1108–1112.

594. Price, V.F. & Jollow, D.J. (1988) Mechanism of decreased acetaminophen glucuronidation in the fasted rat. *Biochemical Pharmacology*, **37**, 1067–1075.

595. Qato, M.K. & Maines, M.D. (1985) Prevention of neonatal

hyperbilirubinemia in non-human primates by Zn-protoporphyrin. *Biochemical Journal,* **226,** 51–57.

596. Quinn, N.W. & Gollan, J.L. (1975) Jaundice following oral surgery: Gilbert's syndrome. *British Journal of Oral Surgery,* **12,** 285–288.

597. Rapaccini, G.L., Topi, G.C., Anti, M. *et al.* (1986) Porphyrins in Rotor's syndrome: A study on an Italian family. *Hepatogastroenterology,* **33,** 11–13.

598. Raymond, G.D. & Galambos, J.T. (1971) Hepatic storage and excretion of bilirubin in man. *American Journal of Gastroenterology,* **55,** 135–144.

599. Reichen, J. & Berk, P.D. (1979) Isolation of an organic anion binding protein from rat liver plasma membrane fractions by affinity chromatography. *Biochemical and Biophysical Research Communications,* **91,** 484–489.

600. Reichen, J., Hoilien, C., Sheldon, G.F. & Kirshenbaum, G. (1983) A novel method for continuous monitoring of bilirubin production in unstressed rats. *American Journal of Physiology,* **244,** G336–G340.

601. Reinke, L.A., Moyer, M.J. & Notley, K.A. (1986) Diminished rates of glucuronidation and sulfation in perfused rat liver after chronic ethanol administration. *Biochemical Pharmacology,* **35,** 439–447.

602. Reuben, A., Howell, K.E. & Boyer, J.L. (1982) Effects of taurocholate on the size of mixed lipid micelles and their associations with pigment and proteins in rat bile. *Journal of Lipid Research,* **23,** 1039–1052.

603. Reyes, H., Levi, A.J. & Arias, J.M. (1971) Studies of Y and Z, two hepatic cytoplasmic organic anion-binding proteins: effect of drugs, chemicals, hormones and cholestasis. *Journal of Clinical Investigation,* **50,** 2242–2252.

604. Ricci, G.L. & Fevery, J. (1979) Stimulation by secretin of bilirubin UDP-glycosyltransferase activities and of cytochrome P-450 concentration in rat liver. *Biochemical Journal,* **182,** 881–884.

605. Ricci, G.L. & Ricci, R.R. (1984) Effect of an intraluminal food-bulk on low calorie induced hyperbilirubinaemia. *Clinical Science,* **66,** 493–496.

606. Ricci, G.L., Michiels, R., Fevery, J. & De Groote, J. (1984) Enhancement by secretin of the apparently maximal hepatic transport of bilirubin in the rat. *Hepatology,* **4,** 651–657.

607. Robinson, S.H. (1968) The origins of bilirubin. *New England Journal of Medicine,* **279,** 143–149.

608. Robinson, S.H. (1972) Formation of bilirubin from erythroid and nonerythroid sources. *Seminars in Hematology,* **9,** 43–53.

609. Robinson, S.H. & Tsong, M. (1970) Hemolysis of 'stress' reticulocytes: a source of erythropoietic bilirubin formation. *Journal of Clinical Investigation,* **49,** 1025–1034.

610. Robinson, S.H., Yannoni, C. & Nagasawa, S. (1971) Bilirubin excretion in rats with normal and impaired bilirubin conjugation: effect of phenobarbital. *Journal of Clinical Investigation,* **50,** 2606–2613.

611. Robinson, S.H., Lester, R., Crigler, J.F. & Tsong, M. (1967) Early-labeled peak of bile pigment in man. Studies with glycine-^{14}C and δ-aminolevulinic acid-^{3}H. *New England Journal of Medicine,* **277,** 1323–1329.

612. Roda, A., Roda, E., Sama, C. *et al.* (1982) Serum primary bile acids in Gilbert's syndrome. *Gastroenterology,* **82,** 77–83.

613. Rollinghoff, W., Paumgartner, G. & Preisig, R. (1981) Nicotinic acid test in the diagnosis of Gilbert's syndrome: correlation with bilirubin clearance. *Gut,* **22,** 663–668.

614. Rosental, E. & Thaler, M.M. (1977) Inhibition of bilirubin conjugation and induction of hyperbilirubinemia by nicotinic acid. *Gastroenterology,* **73,** 1244.

615. Rosenthal, I.M., Zimmerman, H.J. & Hardy, N. (1965) Congenital nonhemolytic jaundice with disease of the central nervous system. *Pediatrics,* **18,** 378–386.

616. Rosenthal, P., Kabra, P., Blanckaert, N. *et al.* (1981) Homozygous Dubin–Johnson syndrome exhibits a characteristic serum bilirubin pattern. *Gastroenterology,* **81,** 50 (abstract).

617. Rotenberg, M. & Zakim, D. (1989) Effect of phospholipids on the thermal stability of microsomal UDP-glucuronosyltransferase. *Biochemistry,* **28,** 8577–8582.

618. Rotor, A.B., Manahan, L. & Florentin, A. (1948) Familial non-hemolytic jaundice with direct van den Bergh reaction. *Acta Medica Philippina,* **5,** 37–48.

619. Roy Chowdhury, J., Wolkoff, A.W. & Arias, A.M. (1988) Heme and bile pigment metabolism. In Arias, A.M., Jakoby, W.B., Popper, H. *et al.* (eds) *The Liver, Biology and Pathology,* pp. 419–450. New York: Raven Press.

620. Roy Chowdhury, J., Novikoff, P.M., Roy Chowdhury, N. *et al.* (1985) Distribution of UDP-glucuronosyltransferase in rat tissue. *Proceedings of the National Academy of Sciences of the USA,* **82,** 2990–2994.

621. Roy Chowdhury, N., Arias, I.M., Lederstein, M. *et al.* (1986) Substrates and products of purified rat liver bilirubin UDP-glucuronosyltransferase. *Hepatology,* **6,** 123–128.

622. Roy Chowdhury, J., Roy Chowdhury, N., Falany, C.N. *et al.* (1986) Isolation and characterization of multiple forms of rat liver UDP-glucuronate glucuronosyltransferase. *Biochemistry Journal,* **233,** 827–837.

623. Roy Chowdhury, N., Gross, F., Moscioni, A.D. *et al.* (1987) Isolation of multiple normal and functionally defective forms of uridine diphosphate-glucuronosyltransferase from inbred Gunn rats. *Journal of Clinical Investigation,* **79,** 327–334.

624. Royer, M., Noir, B.A., Sfarcich, D. & Nanet, H. (1974) Extrahepatic bilirubin formation and conjugation in the dog. *Digestion,* **10,** 423–434.

625. Rubaltelli, F.F., Jori, G. & Reddi, E. (1983) Bronze baby syndrome: A new porphyrin-related disorder. *Pediatric Research,* **17,** 327–330.

626. Rugstad, H.E., Robinson, S.H., Yannoni, C. & Tashjian, A.H. (1970) Transfer of bilirubin uridine diphosphate-glucuronyltransferase to enzyme-deficient rats. *Science,* **170,** 553–555.

627. Ruoslahti, E., Estes, T. & Seppälä, M. (1979) Binding of bilirubin by bovine and human α-fetoprotein. *Biochimica et Biophysica Acta,* **578,** 511–519.

628. Rush, G.F. & Hook, J.B. (1984) Characteristics of renal UDP-glucuronyl-transferase. *Life Sciences,* **35,** 145–153.

629. Sagild, U., Dalgaard, O.Z. & Tygstrup, N. (1962) Constitutional hyperbilirubinemia with unconjugated bilirubin in the serum and lipochrome-like pigment granules in the liver. *Annals of Internal Medicine,* **56,** 308–314.

630. Sardana, M.K. & Kappas, A. (1987) Dual control mechanism for heme oxygenase: Tin (IV)-protoporphyrin potently inhibits enzyme activity while markedly increasing content of enzyme protein in liver. *Proceedings of the National Academy of Sciences of the USA,* **84,** 2464–2468.

631. Sato, H. & Kashiwamata, S. (1983) Interaction of bilirubin with human erythrocyte membranes. *Biochemical Journal,* **210,** 489–496.

632. Schalm, L. & Weber, A.P. (1964) Jaundice with conjugated bilirubin in hyperhaemolysis. *Acta Medica Scandinavica,* **176,** 549–555.

633. Scharschmidt, B.F. (1986) Biliary secretion of bile pigments. In Ostrow, J.D. (ed.) *Bile Pigments and Jaundice,* pp. 243–253. New York: Marcel Dekker.

634. Scharschmidt, B.F. & Gollan, J.L. (1979) Current concepts of bilirubin metabolism and hereditary hyperbilirubinemia. In Popper, H. & Schaffner, F. (eds) *Progress in Liver Diseases,* Vol. VI, pp. 187–212. New York: Grune & Stratton.

635. Scharschmidt, B.F. & Schmid, R. (1978) The micellar sink: a quantitative assessment of the association of organic anions with mixed micelles and other macromolecular aggregates in rat bile. *Journal of Clinical Investigation,* **62,** 1122–1132.

636. Scharschmidt, B.F., Waggoner, J.G. & Berk, P.D. (1975) Hepatic organic anion uptake in the rat. *Journal of Clinical Investigation,* **56,** 1280–1292.

637. Scharschmidt, B.F., Plotz, P.H., Berk, P.D. *et al.* (1974) Removing substances from blood by affinity chromatography. II. Removing bilirubin from the blood of jaundiced rats by hemoperfusion over albumin-conjugated agarose beads. *Journal of Clinical Investigation,* **53,** 786–795.

638. Scharschmidt, B.F., Martin, J.F., Shapiro, L.J. *et al.* (1977) Hemoperfusion through albumin-conjugated agarose gel for the treatment of neonatal jaundice in premature rhesus monkeys. *Journal of Laboratory and Clinical Medicine,* **89,** 101–109.

639. Scharschmidt, B.F., Martin, J.F., Shapiro, L.J. *et al.* (1977) The use of calcium chelating agents and prostaglandin E₁ to estimate platelet and white blood cell losses resulting from hemoperfusion through uncoated charcoal, albumin-agarose gel, and neutral and cation exchange resins. *Journal of Laboratory and Clinical Medicine,* **89,** 110–119.

640. Schenker, S., Dawber, N.H. & Schmid, R. (1964) Bilirubin metabolism in the fetus. *Journal of Clinical Investigation,* **43,** 32–39.

641. Schiff, L., Billing, B.H. & Oikawa, Y. (1959) Familial nonhemolytic jaundice with conjugated bilirubin in the serum. A case study. *New England Journal of Medicine,* **260,** 1315–1318.

642. Schmid, R. (1973) Synthesis and degradation of microsomal hemoproteins. *Drug Metabolism and Disposition,* **1,** 256–258.

643. Schmid, R. (1976) Pyrrolic victories. *Transactions of the Association of American Physicians,* **84,** 64–76.

644. Schmid, R. (1978) Bilirubin metabolism: state of the art. *Gastroenterology,* **74,** 1307–1312.

645. Schmid, R. (1983) Disorders of bilirubin metabolism. In Bianchi, L., Gerok, W., Landmann, L. *et al.* (eds) *Liver in Metabolic Diseases,* pp. 369–378. Lancaster: MTP Press.

646. Schmid, R. & Hammaker, L. (1959) Glucuronide formation in patients with constitutional hepatic dysfunction (Gilbert's syndrome). *New England Journal of Medicine,* **260,** 1310–1314.

647. Schmid, R. & Hammaker, L. (1963) Metabolism and disposition of C¹⁴-bilirubin in congenital non-hemolytic jaundice. *Journal of Clinical Investigation,* **42,** 1720–1734.

648. Schmid, R. & McDonagh, A.F. (1975) The enzymatic formation of bilirubin. *Annals of the New York Academy of Sciences,* **244,** 533–552.

649. Schmid, R. & McDonagh, A.F. (1978) Hyperbilirubinemia. In Stanbury, J.B., Wyngaarden, J.B. & Frederickson, D.S. (eds) *The Metabolic Basis of Inherited Disease,* pp. 1221–1257. New York: McGraw-Hill.

650. Schmid, R. & McDonagh, A.F. (1979) Formation and metabolism of bile pigments in vivo. In Dolphin, D. (ed.) *The Porphyrins,* Vol. VI, pp. 257–292. New York: Academic Press.

651. Schmid, R., Brecher, G. & Clemens, T. (1959) Familial hemolytic anemia with erythrocyte inclusion bodies and a defect in pigment metabolism. *Blood,* **14,** 991–1007.

652. Schmid, R., Marver, H.S. & Hammaker, L. (1966) Enhanced formation of rapidly labeled bilirubin by phenobarbital: hepatic microsomal cytochromes as a possible source. *Biochemical and Biophysical Research Communications,* **24,** 319–328.

653. Schmid, R., Axelrod, J., Hammaker, L. & Swarm, R.L. (1958) Congenital jaundice in rats, due to a defect in glucuronide formation. *Journal of Clinical Investigation,* **37,** 1123–1130.

654. Schnapp, B.J., Vale, R.D., Sheetz, M.P. *et al.* (1985) Single microtubules from squid axoplasm support bidirectional movement of organelles. *Cell,* **40,** 455–462.

655. Schoenfield, L.J., Foulk, W.T. & Butt, H.R. (1964) Studies of sulfobromophthalein sodium (BSP) metabolism in man. 1. In normal subjects and patients with hepatic disease. *Journal of Clinical Investigation,* **43,** 1409–1418.

656. Schoenfield, L.J., McGill, D.B., Hunton, D.B. *et al.* (1963) Studies of chronic idiopathic jaundice (Dubin–Johnson syndrome). 1. Demonstration of hepatic excretory defect. *Gastroenterology,* **44,** 101–111.

657. Scragg, I., Celier, C. & Burchell, B. (1985) Congenital jaundice in rats due to the absence of hepatic bilirubin UDP-glucuronyltransferase enzyme protein. *FEBS Letters,* **183,** 37–42.

658. Seligman, J.W. (1977) Recent and changing concepts of hyperbilirubinemia and its management in newborn. *Pediatric Clinics of North America,* **24,** 509–528.

659. Seligsohn, U., Shani, M., Ramot, B. *et al.* (1970) Dubin–Johnson syndrome in Israel. II. Association with factor-VII deficiency. *Quarterly Journal of Medicine,* **39,** 569–584.

660. Seymour, C.A., Neale, G. & Peters, T.J. (1977) Lysosomal changes in liver tissue from patients with the Dubin–Johnson–Sprinz syndrome. *Clinical Science and Molecular Medicine,* **52,** 241–248.

661. Shader, R.I., Divoll, M. & Greenblatt, D.J. (1981) Kinetics of oxazepam and lorazepam in two subjects with Gilbert's syndrome. *Journal of Clinical PsychoPharmacology,* **1,** 400–402.

662. Shani, M., Seligsohn, U. & Ben-Ezzer, J. (1974) Effect of phenobarbital on liver functions in patients with Dubin–Johnson syndrome. *Gastroenterology,* **67,** 303–308.

663. Shani, M., Gilon, E., Ben-Ezzer, J. & Sheba, C. (1970) Sulfobromophthalein tolerance test in patients with Dubin–Johnson syndrome and their relatives. *Gastroenterology,* **59,** 842–847.

664. Shani, M., Seligsohn, U., Gilon, E. *et al.* (1970) Dubin–Johnson syndrome in Israel. I. Clinical, laboratory, and genetic aspects of 101 cases. *Quarterly Journal of Medicine,* **39,** 549–567.

665. Shankaran, S. & Poland, R.L. (1977) Displacement of bilirubin from albumin by furosemide. *Journal of Pediatrics,* **90,** 642–646.

666. Shevell, M.I., Adelson, J.W., Laberge, J.-M. & Guttman, F.M. (1987) Crigler–Najjar syndrome type I: Treatment by home phototherapy followed by orthotopic hepatic transplantation. *Journal of Pediatrics,* **110,** 429–431.

667. Shibahara, S., Yoshida, T. & Kikuchi, G. (1978) Induction of heme oxygenase by hemin in cultured pig alveolar macrophages. *Archives of Biochemistry and Biophysics,* **188,** 243–250.

668. Shibahara, S., Yoshida, T. & Kikuchi, G. (1980) Intracellular site of synthesis of microsomal heme oxygenase in pig spleen. *Journal of Biochemistry,* **88,** 45–50.

669. Shimizu, Y., Kondo, T., Kuchiba, K. & Urata, G. (1977) Uroporphyrinogen III cosynthetase in liver and blood in the Dubin–Johnson syndrome. *Journal of Laboratory and Clinical Medicine,* **89,** 517–523.

670. Shimizu, Y., Naruto, H., Ida, S. & Kohakura, M. (1981) Urinary coproporphyrin isomers in Rotor's syndrome: a study in eight families. *Hepatology,* **1,** 173–178.

671. Shull, B.C., Lees, H. & Li, P.K. (1980) Mechanism of interference by hemoglobin in the determination of total bilirubin. 1. Method of Malloy–Evelyn. *Clinical Chemistry,* **26,** 22–25.

672. Shupeck, M., Wolkoff, A.W., Scharschmidt, B.F. & Waggoner, J.G. (1978) Studies of the kinetics of purified conjugated bilirubin-³H in the rat. *American Journal of Gastroenterology,* **70,** 259–264.

673. Sieg, A., Stiehl, A., Raedsch, R. *et al.* (1986) Gilbert's syndrome: diagnosis by typical serum bilirubin pattern. *Clinica Chimica Acta,* **154,** 41–48.

674. Simion, F.A., Fleischer, B. & Fleischer, S. (1984) Subcellular distribution of bile acids, bile salts and taurocholate binding sites in rat liver. *Biochemistry,* **23,** 6459–6466.

675. Simionatto, C.S., Anderson, K.E., Drummond, G.S. & Kappas, A. (1985) Studies on the mechanism of Sn-protoporphyrin suppression of hyperbilirubinemia. *Journal of Clinical Investigation,* **75**(2), 513–521.

676. Simon, F.R., Sutherland, E.M. & Gonzalez, M. (1982) Regulation of bile salt transport in rat liver. *Journal of Clinical Investigation,* **70,** 401–411.

677. Simons, P.C. & Vander Jagt, D.L. (1980) Bilirubin binding to human liver ligandin (glutathione *S*-transferase). *Journal of Biological Chemistry,* **255,** 4740–4744.

678. Sinclair, K.A. & Caldwell, J. (1982) The formation of β-glucuronidase resistant glucuronides by the intramolecular rearrangement of glucuronic acid conjugates at mild alkaline pH. *Biochemical Pharmacology,* **31,** 953–957.

679. Sleisenger, M.H., Kahn, I., Barniville, H. *et al.* (1967) Nonhemolytic unconjugated hyperbilirubinemia with hepatic glucuronyl transferase deficiency: a genetic study in four generations. *Transactions of the Association of American Physicians,* **80,** 259–266.

680. Smith, D.J. & Gordon, E.R. (1987) Role of the physical state of the hepatic microsomal membrane in the formation of bilirubin diglucuronide. *Journal of Hepatology,* **4,** 1–7.

681. Smith, P.C., McDonagh, A.F. & Benet, L.Z. (1984) Covalent binding of zomepiric acyl glucuronide to albumin in healthy human volunteers. *Hepatology,* **4,** 1059 (abstract).

682. Smith, P.M., Middleton, J.E. & Williams, R. (1967) Studies on the familial incidence and clinical history of patients with chronic unconjugated hyperbilirubinaemia. *Gut,* **8,** 449–453.

683. Snyder, A.L., Satterlee, W., Robinson, S.H. & Schmid, R. (1967) Conjugated plasma bilirubin in jaundice caused by pigment overload. *Nature,* **213,** 93.

684. Sommerer, U., Gordon, E.R. & Goresky, C.A. (1988) Microsomal specificity underlying the differing hepatic formation of bilirubin

glucuronide and glucose conjugates by rat and dog. *Hepatology,* **8**, 116–124.

685. Sorrentino, D. & Berk, P.D. (1988) Mechanistic aspects of hepatic bilirubin uptake. *Seminars in Liver Disease,* **8**, 119–136.

686. Sorrentino, D., Stremmel, W. & Berk, P.D. (1987) The hepatocellular uptake of bilirubin: Current concepts and controversies. *Molecular Aspects of Medicine,* **9**, 405–428.

687. Spivak, W. & Carey, M. (1985) Reverse-phase h.p.l.c. separation, quantitation and preparation of bilirubin and its conjugates from native bile: quantitative analysis of the intact tetrapyrroles based on h.p.l.c. of their ethyl anthranilate azoderivatives. *Biochemical Journal,* **225**, 787–805.

688. Spivak, W. & Yuey, W. (1986) Application of a rapid and efficient h.p.l.c. method to measure bilirubin and its conjugates from native bile and in model bile systems. *Biochemical Journal,* **234**, 101–109.

689. Sprinz, H. & Nelson, R.S. (1954) Persistent nonhemolytic hyperbilirubinemia associated with lipochrome-like pigment in liver cells: report of 4 cases. *Annals of Internal Medicine,* **41**, 952–962.

690. Stein, L.B., Mishkin, S., Fleischner, G. *et al.* (1976) Effect of fasting on hepatic ligandin, Z protein, and organic anion transfer from plasma in rats. *American Journal of Physiology,* **231**, 1371–1376.

691. Stevenson, D.K., Rodgers, P.A. & Vreman, H.J. (1988) The use of metalloporphyrins for the chemoprevention of neonatal jaundice. *American Journal of Diseases in Children,* **143**, 353–356.

692. Stiel, D., Lunzer, M. & Poulos, V. (1982) Urinary coproporphyrin excretion in Rotor's syndrome: a family study. *Australian and New Zealand Journal of Medicine,* **12**, 594–597.

693. Stocker, R., Glazer, A.N. & Ames, B.N. (1987) Antioxidant activity of albumin-bound bilirubin. *Proceedings of the National Academy of Sciences of the USA,* **84**, 5918–5922.

694. Stocker, R., Yamamoto, Y., McDonagh, A.F. *et al.* (1987) Bilirubin is an antioxidant of possible physiological importance. *Science,* **235**, 1043–1046.

695. Stoll, M.S. (1982) Formation, metabolism, and properties of pyrrolic compounds appearing in the gut. In Heirwegh, K.P.M. & Brown, S.B. (eds) *Bilirubin, Vol. 2: Metabolism,* pp. 103–131. Boca Raton, Florida: CRC Press.

696. Stoll, M.S., Vicker, N. & Gray, C.H. (1982) Concerning the structure of photobilirubin II. *Biochemical Journal,* **201**, 179–188.

697. Stoll, M.S., Zenone, E.A. & Ostrow, J.D. (1981) Excretion of administered and endogenous photobilirubins in the bile of the jaundiced Gunn rat. *Journal of Clinical Investigation,* **68**, 131–141.

698. Stoll, M.S., Zenone, E.A., Ostrow, J.D. & Zarembo, J.E. (1979) Preparation and properties of bilirubin photoisomers. *Biochemical Journal,* **183**, 139–146.

699. Stremmel, W. & Berk, P.D. (1986) Hepatocellular uptake of sulfobromophthalein and bilirubin is selectively inhibited by an antibody to the liver plasma membrane sulfobromophthalein/bilirubin binding protein. *Journal of Clinical Investigation,* **78**, 822–826.

700. Stremmel, W., Potter, B.J. & Berk, P.D. (1983) Studies of albumin binding to rat liver plasma membranes. Implications for the albumin receptor hypothesis. *Biochemica et Biophysica Acta,* **756**, 20–27.

701. Stremmel, W., Gerber, M.A., Glezerov, V. *et al.* (1983) Physicochemical and immunohistological studies of a sulfobromophthalein- and bilirubin-binding protein from rat liver plasma membrane. *Journal of Clinical Investigation,* **71**, 1796–1805.

702. Strominger, J.L., Kalcker, H.M., Axelrod, J. *et al.* (1954) Enzymatic oxidation of uridine diphosphate glucose to uridine diphosphate glucuronic acid. *Journal of the American Chemistry Society,* **76**, 6411–6412.

703. Sugar, P. (1961) Familial nonhemolytic jaundice. Congenital, with kernicterus. *Archives of Internal Medicine,* **108**, 189–195.

704. Suri, V.P., Chatterjee, T. & Sagaraya, K. (1966) Dubin–Johnson syndrome. *Journal of the Indian Medical Association,* **47**, 32–34.

705. Sutherland, D.E.R., Mattas, A.J., Steffes, M.W. *et al.* (1977) Transplantation of liver cells in an animal model of congenital enzyme deficiency disease: the Gunn rat. *Transplant Proceedings,* **9**, 317–320.

706. Suzuki, N., Yamaguchi, T. & Nakajima, H. (1988) Role of high-density lipoprotein in transport of circulating bilirubin in rats. *Journal of Biological Chemistry,* **263**, 5037–5043.

707. Svingen, B.A., Buege, J.A. & O'Neal, F.O. (1979) The mechanism of NADPH-dependent lipid peroxidation. The propagation of lipid peroxidation. *Journal of Biological Chemistry,* **254**, 5892–5899.

708. Swartz, H.M., Sarna, T. & Varma, R.R. (1979) On the nature and excretion of the hepatic pigment in the Dubin–Johnson syndrome. *Gastroenterology,* **76**, 958–964.

709. Swartz, H.M., Sarna, T. & Varma, R.R. (1979) The pigment in Dubin–Johnson syndrome. *Gastroenterology,* **77**, 821 (abstract).

710. Szabó, L. & Ebrey, P. (1963) Studies on the inheritance of Crigler–Najjar syndrome by the menthol test. *Acta Paediatrica Hungarica,* **4**, 153–158.

711. Szabó, L., Kovacs, Z. & Ebrey, P.B. (1962) Crigler–Najjar's syndrome. *Acta Paediatrica Hungarica,* **3**, 49–70.

712. Tajima, J. & Kuroda, H. (1988) Pericanalicular microfilaments of hepatocytes in patients with familial non-hemolytic hyperbilirubinemia. *Gastroenterologia Japonica,* **23**, 273–278.

713. Tan, K.L. (1982) The pattern of bilirubin response to phototherapy for neonatal hyperbilirubinaemia. *Pediatric Research,* **16**, 670–674.

714. Tanno, M., Yamada, H., Muraki, T. *et al.* (1982) Partial isolation and characterization of bromosulphophthalein-binding protein from rat liver plasma membranes. *Gastroenterologia Japonica,* **17**, 135–143.

715. Tazuma, S. & Holzbach, R.T. (1987) Transport in bile of conjugated bilirubin and other organic anions: Relation to biliary lipid structures. *Proceedings of the National Academy of Sciences of the USA,* **84**, 2052–2056.

716. Tenhunen, R., Marver, H.S. & Schmid, R. (1968) The enzymatic conversion of heme to bilirubin by microsomal heme oxygenase. *Proceedings of the National Academy of Science of the USA,* **61**, 748–755.

717. Tenhunen, R., Marver, H.S. & Schmid, R. (1969) Microsomal heme oxygenase. Characterization of the enzyme. *Journal of Biological Chemistry,* **244**, 6388–6394.

718. Tenhunen, R., Marver, H.S. & Schmid, R. (1970) The enzymatic catabolism of hemoglobin: stimulation of microsomal heme oxygenase by hemin. *Journal of Laboratory and Clinical Medicine,* **75**, 410–421.

719. Tenhunen, R., Ross, M.E., Marver, H.S., Schmid, R. (1970) Reduced nicotinamide-adenine dinucleotide phosphate dependent biliverdin reductase: partial purification and characterization. *Biochemistry,* **9**, 298–303.

720. Thaler, M.M. (1977) Jaundice in the newborn. Algorithmic diagnosis of conjugated and unconjugated hyperbilirubinemia. *Journal of the American Medical Association,* **237**, 58–62.

721. Theilmann, L., Stollman, Y.R., Arias, I.M. & Wolkoff, A.W. (1984) Does Z-protein have a role in transport of bilirubin and bromosulfophthalein by isolated perfused rat liver? *Hepatology,* **4**, 923–926.

722. Thomsen, R.F., Hardt, F. & Juhl, E. (1981) Diagnosis of Gilbert's syndrome. Reliability of the calories restriction and phenobarbital stimulation tests. *Scandinavian Journal of Gastroenterology,* **16**, 699–703.

723. Tipping, E. & Ketterer, B. (1981) The influence of soluble binding proteins on lipophile transport and metabolism in hepatocytes. *Biochemical Journal,* **195**, 441–452.

724. Tipping, E., Ketterer, B. & Christodoulides, L. (1979) Interactions of small molecules with phospholipid bilayers. Binding to egg phosphatidylcholine of some organic anions (bromosulphophthalein, oestrone sulphate, haem, and bilirubin) that bind to ligandin and aminoazo-dye-binding protein A. *Biochemical Journal,* **180**, 327–337.

725. Tiribelli, C., Lunazzi, G., Luciani, M. *et al.* (1978) Isolation of a sulfobromophthalein-binding protein from hepatocyte plasma membrane. *Biochimica et Biophysica Acta,* **523**, 105–112.

726. Tisdale, W.A., Klatskin, G. & Kinsella, E.D. (1959) The significance of the direct-reacting fraction of serum bilirubin in hemolytic jaundice. *American Journal of Medicine,* **26**, 214–227.

727. Trevisan, A., Gudat, F., Guggenheim, R. *et al.* (1982) Demonstration of albumin receptors on isolated human hepatocytes by light and scanning electron microscopy. *Hepatology,* **2**, 832–835.

728. Trotman, B.W., Shaw, L., Roy Chowdhury, R. *et al.* (1983) Effect of phenobarbital on serum and biliary parameters in a patient with Crigler–Najjar syndrome, type II and acquired cholestasis. *Digestive Diseases and Sciences,* **28**, 753–762.

729. Troxler, R.F., Dawber, N.H. & Lester, R. (1968) Synthesis of urobilinogen by broken cell preparations of intestinal bacteria. _Gastroenterology,_ **54**, 568–574.

730. Tsuru, M., Kamisaka, K., Hirano, M. & Kameda, H. (1978) Quantification of human serum ligandin by radioimmunoassay. _Clinica Chimica Acta,_ **84**, 251–254.

731. Van den Bergh, H.A.A. & Müller, P. (1916) Über eine direkte und indirekte Diazoreaktion auf Bilirubin. _Biochemische Zeitschrift,_ **77**, 93–103.

732. Vander Jagt, D.L. & Garcia, K.B. (1987) Immunochemical comparisons of proteins that bind heme and bilirubin: human serum albumin, alpha-fetoprotein and glutathione _S_-transferases from liver, placenta and erythrocyte. _Comparisons of Biochemical Physiology,_ **87B**, 527–531.

733. Vander Jagt, D.L., Wilson, S.P. & Heidrich, J.E. (1981) Purification and bilirubin binding properties of glutathione _S_-transferase from human placenta. _FEBS Letters,_ **136**, 319.

734. Vander Jagt, D.L., Wilson, S.P., Dean, V.L. & Simons, P.C. (1982) Bilirubin binding to rat liver ligandins (glutathione _S_-transferases A and B). _Journal of Biological Chemistry,_ **257**, 1997–2001.

735. Van Es, H.H.G., Goldhoorn, B.G., Oude Elferink, R.P.J. _et al._ (1988) Immunological characterization of UDP-glucuronyltransferase (UDPGT) deficiencies in man and in rat. _Hepatology,_ **8**, 1278.

736. Van Es, H.H.G., Roy Chowdhury, J., Oude Elferink, R.P.J. _et al._ (1989) Two distinct molecular defects in Crigler–Najjar syndrome, type I: Parallel abnormalities in two Gunn rat strains. _Gastroenterology,_ **96**, A695.

737. Van Roy, F.P. & Heirwegh, K.P.M. (1968) Determination of bilirubin glucuronide and assay of glucuronyltransferase with bilirubin as acceptor. _Biochemical Journal,_ **107**, 507–518.

738. Van Roy, F.P., Meuwissen, J.A.T.P., de Meuter, F. & Heirwegh, K.P.M. (1971) Determination of bilirubin in liver homogenates and serum with diazotized _p_-iodoaniline. _Clinica Chimica Acta,_ **31**, 109–118.

739. Vanstapel, F. & Blanckaert, N. (1987) Endogenous esterification of bilirubin by liver microsomes. Evidence for an intramicrosomal pool of UDP-glucose and lumenal orientation of bilirubin UDP-glycosyltransferase. _Journal of Biological Chemistry,_ **262**, 4616–4623.

740. Vanstapel, F. & Blanckaert, N. (1987) On the binding of bilirubin and its structural analogues to hepatic microsomal bilirubin UDP-glucuronyltransferase. _Biochemistry,_ **26**, 6074–6082.

741. Vanstapel, F. & Blanckaert, N. (1988) Topology and regulation of bilirubin UDP-glucuronyltransferase in sealed native microsomes from rat liver. _Archives of Biochemical Biophysiology,_ **263**, 216–225.

742. Van Steenbergen, W. & Fevery, J. (1982) Maximal biliary secretion of bilirubin in the anaesthetized rat: dependence on UDP-glucuronosyltransferase activity. _Clinical Science,_ **62**, 521–528.

743. Varma, R.R. & Sarna, T. (1983) Hepatic pigments in Dubin–Johnson syndrome and mutant Corriedale sheep are not melanin. _Gastroenterology,_ **84**, 1401 (abstract).

744. Vaughan, J.M. & Haselwood, G.A.D. (1938) The normal level of plasma bilirubin. _Lancet,_ **1**, 133–135.

745. Vaughan, J.P., Marubbio, A.T., Maddocks, I. & Cooke, R.A. (1970) Chronic idiopathic jaundice in Papua and New Guinea: a report of nine patients with Dubin–Johnson's or Rotor's syndrome. _Transactions of the Royal Society of Tropical Medicine and Hygiene,_ **64**, 287–292.

746. Vazquez, J., Garcia-Calvo, M., Valdivieso, F. _et al._ (1988) Interaction of bilirubin with the synaptosomal plasma membrane. _Journal of Biological Chemistry,_ **263**, 1255–1265.

747. Vermeulen, J.P., Ziurys, J.C. & Gollan, J.L. (1986) Hepatic cytochrome P-450 and UDP-glucuronyltransferase activities are rapidly modulated by bile salts (abstract). _Hepatology,_ **6**, 1178.

748. Versee, V. & Barel, A.O. (1979) Interactions of rat α-foetoprotein with bilirubin. _Biochemical Journal,_ **179**, 705–707.

749. Verwilghen, R., Verhaegen, H., Waumans, P. & Beert, J. (1969) Ineffective erythropoiesis with morphologically abnormal erythroblasts and unconjugated hyperbilirubinaemia. _British Journal of Haematology,_ **17**, 27–33.

750. Vessey, D.A. & Kempner, E.S. (1989) In situ structural analysis of microsomal UDP-glucuronyltransferases by radiation inactivation. _Journal of Biological Chemistry,_ **264**, 1–5.

751. Vessey, D.A. & Zakim, D. (1971) Regulation of microsomal enzymes by phospholipids. II. Activation of hepatic uridine diphosphate-glucuronyltransferase. _Journal of Biological Chemistry,_ **246**, 4649–4656.

752. Vessey, D.A. & Zakim, D. (1972) Regulation of microsomal enzymes by phospholipids. V. Kinetic studies of hepatic uridine diphosphate-glucuronyltransferase. _Journal of Biological Chemistry,_ **247**, 3023–3028.

753. Vessey, D.A., Goldenberg, J. & Zakim, D. (1973) Differentiation of homologous forms of hepatic microsomal UDP-glucuronyltransferase. II. Characterization of the bilirubin conjugating form. _Biochimica et Biophysica Acta,_ **309**, 75–82.

754. Vessey, D.A., Goldenberg, J. & Zakim, D. (1973) Kinetic properties of microsomal UDP-glucuronyltransferase. Evidence for cooperative kinetics and activation by UDP-_N_-acetylglucosamine. _Biochimica et Biophysica Acta,_ **309**, 58–66.

755. Vierling, J.M., Berk, P.D., Hofmann, A.F. _et al._ (1982) Normal fasting-site levels of serum cholylconjugated bile acids in Gilbert's syndrome: an aid to the diagnosis. _Hepatology,_ **2**, 340–343.

756. Wakisaka, G., Ichida, F., Kuge, T. _et al._ (1961) Clinical and enzymological observation on cases with Gilbert's disease. _Japanese Archives of Internal Medicine,_ **8**, 634–648.

757. Walker, P.C. (1987) Neonatal bilirubin toxicity. A review of kernicterus and the implications of drug-induced bilirubin displacement. _Clinical Pharmacokinetics,_ **13**, 26–50.

758. Ware, A.J., Carey, M.C. & Combes, B. (1976) Solution properties of sulfobromophthalein sodium (BSP) compounds alone and in association with sodium taurocholate (TC). _Journal of Laboratory and Clinical Medicine,_ **87**, 443–456.

759. Ware, A.J., Eigenbrodt, E.H., Shorey, J. & Combes, B. (1972) Viral hepatitis complicating the Dubin–Johnson syndrome. _Gastroenterology,_ **63**, 337–339.

760. Watson, C.J. (1969) Gold from dross: the first century of the urobilinoids. _Annals of Internal Medicine,_ **70**, 839–851.

761. Watson, C.J. & Weimer, M. (1959) Composition of the urobilin group in urine, bile, and feces and the significance of variations in health and disease. _Journal of Laboratory and Clinical Medicine,_ **54**, 1–25.

762. Watson, C.J., Campbell, M. & Lowry, P.T. (1958) Preferential reduction of conjugated bilirubin to urobilinogen by normal fecal flora. _Proceedings of the Society for Experimental Biology and Medicine,_ **98**, 707–711.

763. Watson, K.J.R. & Gollan, J.L. (1989) Gilbert's syndrome. _Baillière's Clinical Gastroenterology,_ **3**, 337–355.

764. Weatherill, P.J. & Burchell, B. (1978) Reactivation of a pure defective UDP-glucuronyltransferase from homozygous Gunn rat liver. _FEBS Letters,_ **87**, 207–211.

765. Weatherill, P.J., Kennedy, S.M.E. & Burchell, B. (1980) Immunochemical comparison of UDP-glucuronyltransferase from Gunn- and Wistar-rat livers. _Biochemical Journal,_ **191**, 155–163.

766. Weisiger, R., Gollan, J. & Ockner, R. (1980) An albumin receptor on the liver cell may mediate hepatic uptake of sulfobromophthalein and bilirubin: bound ligand, not free, is the major uptake determinant. _Gastroenterology,_ **79**, 1065 (abstract).

767. Weisiger, R., Gollan, J. & Ockner, R. (1981) Receptor for albumin on the liver cell surface may mediate uptake of fatty acids and other albumin-bound substances. _Science,_ **211**, 1048–1051.

768. Weisiger, R.A. (1985) Dissociation from albumin: A potentially rate-limiting step in the clearance of substances by the liver. _Proceedings of the National Academy of Sciences of the USA,_ **82**, 1563–1567.

769. Weiss, J.S., Gautam, A., Lauff, J.J. _et al._ (1983) The clinical importance of a protein-bound fraction of serum bilirubin in patients with hyperbilirubinemia. _New England Journal of Medicine,_ **309**, 147–150.

770. Wennberg, R.P., Rasmussen, L.F. & Ahlfors, C.E. (1977) Displacement of bilirubin from human albumin by 3 diuretics. _Journal of Pediatrics,_ **90**, 647–650.

771. Wheeler, H.O., Meltzer, J.I. & Bradley, S.E. (1960) Biliary transport and hepatic storage of sulfobromophthalein sodium in

the unanaesthetized dog, in normal man, and in patients with hepatic disease. *Journal of Clinical Investigation,* **39**, 1131–1141.

772. Whelton, M.J., Krustev, L.P. & Billing, B.H. (1968) Reduction in serum bilirubin by phenobarbital in adult unconjugated hyperbilirubinemia. Is enzyme induction responsible? *American Journal of Medicine,* **45**, 160–164.

773. Whiting, J., Roy Chowdhury, J., Feldman, D., Levenson, S.M., Roy Chowdhury, N. & Demetriou, A.A. (1986) Prolonged survival and function of transplanted hepatocytes in Gunn and analbuminemic rats. *Gastroenterology,* **90**, 1800.

774. Whitington, G.L. (1960) Congenital nonhemolytic icterus with damage to the central nervous system. Report of a case in a Negro child. *Pediatrics,* **25**, 437–440.

775. Whitington, P.F., Black, D.D., Struve, W. & Dockter, M.E. (1985) Evidence against an abnormal hepatic microsomal lipid matrix as the primary genetic defect in the jaundiced Gunn rat. *Biochimica et Biophysica Acta,* **812**, 774–778.

776. Whitmer, D.I. & Gollan, J.L. (1983) Mechanisms and significance of fasting and dietary hyperbilirubinemia. *Seminars in Liver Disease,* **3**, 42–51.

777. Whitmer, D.I., Russell, P.E. & Gollan, J.L. (1987) Membrane-membrane interactions associated with rapid transfer of liposomal bilirubin to microsomal UDP-glucuronyltransferase. Relevance for hepatocellular transport and biotransformation of hydrophobic substrates. *Biochemistry,* **244**, 41–47.

778. Whitmer, D., Zuirys, J. & Gollan, J. (1984) Hepatic microsomal glucuronidation of bilirubin in unilamellar liposomal membranes. Implications for intracellular transport of lipophilic substrates. *Journal of Biological Chemistry,* **259**, 11969–11975.

779. Whitmer, D.I., Russell, P.E., Ziurys, J.C. *et al.* (1986) Hepatic microsomal glucuronidation of bilirubin is modulated by the lipid microenvironment of membrane-bound substrate. *Journal of Biological Chemistry,* **261**, 7170–7177.

780. Wiegand, U.W. & Levy, G. (1979) Effect of heparin injection on plasma protein binding of bilirubin and salicylate in rats. *Journal of Pharmaceutical Sciences,* **68**, 1483–1486.

781. Wiegand, U.W., Soda, D.M. & Levy, G. (1980) Effect of heparin on bilirubin clearance in rats: pharmacokinetic consequences of extensive hepatic extraction of plasma protein binding inhibitors. *Journal of Pharmaceutical Sciences,* **69**, 1228–1230.

782. Wolf, R.L., Pizette, M., Richman, A. *et al.* (1960) Chronic idiopathic jaundice: a study of two afflicted families. *American Journal of Medicine,* **28**, 32–41.

783. Wolff, H., Otto, G. & Giest, H. (1986) Liver transplantation in Crigler–Najjar syndrome. A case report. *Transplantation,* **42**, 84.

784. Wolkoff, A. (1983) Bilirubin metabolism and hyperbilirubinemia. *Seminars in Liver Disease,* **3**, 1–86.

785. Wolkoff, A.W. (1983) Inheritable disorders manifested by conjugated hyperbilirubinemia. *Seminars in Liver Disease,* **3**, 65–72.

786. Wolkoff, A.W. (1987) The role of an albumin receptor in hepatic organic anion uptake: The controversy continues. *Hepatology,* **7**, 777–779.

787. Wolkoff, A.W. & Chung, C.T. (1980) Identification, purification and partial characterization of an organic anion binding protein from rat liver cell plasma membrane. *Journal of Clinical Investigation,* **65**, 1152–1161.

788. Wolkoff, A.W., Cohen, L.E. & Arias, I.M. (1973) The inheritance of the Dubin–Johnson syndrome. *New England Journal of Medicine,* **288**, 113–117.

789. Wolkoff, A.W., Wolpert, E., Pascasio, F.N. & Arias, I.M. (1976) Rotor's syndrome: A distinct inheritable pathophysiologic entity. *American Journal of Medicine,* **60**, 173–179.

790. Wolkoff, A.W., Ketley, J.N., Waggoner, J.G. *et al.* (1978) Hepatic accumulation and intracellular binding of conjugated bilirubin. *Journal of Clinical Investigation,* **61**, 142–149.

791. Wolkoff, A.W., Chowdhury, J.R., Gartner, L.A. *et al.* (1979) Crigler–Najjar syndrome (Type I) in an adult male. *Gastroenterology,* **76**, 840–848.

792. Wolkoff, A.W., Goresky, C.A., Sellin, J. *et al.* (1979) Role of ligandin in transfer of bilirubin from plasma into liver. *American Journal of Physiology,* **236**, E638–E648.

793. Wolpert, E., Pascasio, F.M., Wolkoff, A.W. & Arias, I.M. (1977) Abnormal sulfobromophthalein metabolism in Rotor's syndrome

and obligate heterozygotes. *New England Journal of Medicine,* **296**, 1099–1101.

794. Woods, R.J. & Parbhoo, S.P. (1981) An explanation for the reduction in bilirubin levels in congenitally jaundiced Gunn rats after transplantation of isolated hepatocytes. *European Journal of Surgical Research,* **13**, 278–284.

795. Wu, T.-W. (1983) Delta bilirubin: the fourth fraction of bile pigments in human serum. *Israel Journal of Chemistry,* **23**, 241–247.

796. Wyman, J.F., Gollan, J.L., Settle, W. *et al.* (1986) Incorporation of hemoglobin-heme into rat hepatic hemoproteins: tryptophan pyrrolase and cytochrome P-450. *Biochemical Journal,* **238**, 837–846.

797. Yaffe, S.J., Levy, G., Matsuzawa, T. & Baliah, T. (1966) Enhancement of glucuronide-conjugating capacity in a hyperbilirubinemic infant due to apparent enzyme induction by phenobarbital. *New England Journal of Medicine,* **275**, 1461–1466.

798. Yamamoto, T., Skanderberg, J., Zipursky, A. & Israels, L.G. (1965) The early appearing bilirubin: evidence for two components. *Journal of Clinical Investigation,* **44**, 31–41.

799. Yannoni, C.Z. & Robinson, S.H. (1975) Early-labelled haem in erythroid and hepatic cells. *Nature,* **258**, 330–331.

800. Yannoni, C.Z. & Robinson, S.H. (1976) Early labeled heme synthesis in normal rats and rats with iron deficiency anemia. *Biochimica et Biophysica Acta,* **428**, 533–549.

801. Yokosuka, O. & Billing, B. (1987) Enzymatic oxidation of bilirubin by intestinal mucosa. *Biochimica et Biophysica Acta,* **923**, 268–274.

802. Yokoyama, T., Ogino, T., Onishi, S. *et al.* (1984) Significance of the endo-vinyl group of bilirubin in photochemical reactions. *Biochemical Journal,* **220**, 377–383.

803. Yong, F.-C. & Cheah, S.-S. (1977) Breast milk jaundice: an in vitro study of the effect of free fatty acids on the bilirubin-serum albumin complex. *Research Communications in Chemical Pathology and Pharmacology,* **17**, 679–688.

804. Yoshida, H., Inagaki, T., Hirano, M. & Sugimoto, T. (1987) Analyses of azopigments obtained from the delta fraction of bilirubin from mammalian plasma (mammalian biliprotein). *Biochemical Journal,* **248**, 79–84.

805. Yoshida, T. & Kikuchi, G. (1977) Heme oxygenase purified to apparent homogeneity from pig spleen microsomes. *Journal of Biochemistry,* **81**, 265–268.

806. Yoshida, T. & Kikuchi, G. (1978) Purification and properties of heme oxygenase from pig spleen microsomes. *Journal of Biological Chemistry,* **253**, 4224–4229.

807. Yoshida, T. & Kikuchi, G. (1979) Purification and properties of heme oxygenase from rat liver microsomes. *Journal of Biological Chemistry,* **254**, 4487–4491.

808. Yoshida, T., Noguchi, M. & Kikuchi, G. (1980) Oxygenated form of heme-heme oxygenase complex and requirement for second electron to initiate heme degradation from the oxygenated complex. *Journal of Biological Chemistry,* **255**, 4418–4420.

809. Yoshida, T., Noguchi, M. & Kikuchi, G. (1982) The step of carbon monoxide liberation in the sequence of heme degradation catalyzed by the reconstituted microsomal heme oxygenase system. *Journal of Biochemical Chemistry,* **257**, 9345–9348.

810. Yoshinaga, T., Sassa, S. & Kappas, A. (1982) Purification and properties of bovine spleen heme oxygenase. *Journal of Biological Chemistry,* **257**, 7778–7785.

811. Yoshinaga, T., Sassa, S. & Kappas, A. (1982) The occurrence of molecular interactions among NADPH-cytochrome c reductase, heme oxygenase, and biliverdin reductase in heme degradation. *Journal of Biological Chemistry,* **257**, 7786–7793.

812. Yoshinaga, T., Sassa, S. & Kappas, A. (1982) A comparative study of heme degradation by NADPH-cyctochrome c reductase alone and by the complete heme oxygenase system. *Journal of Biological Chemistry,* **257**, 7794–7802.

813. Zakim, D. & Vessey, D.A. (1982) The role of the microsomal membrane in modulating the activity of UDP-glucuronyltransferase. In Martonosi, A.N. (ed.) *Membranes and Transport,* Vol. 1. New York: Plenum Press.

814. Zakim, D., Cantor, M. & Eibl, H. (1988) Phospholipids and UDP-glucuronosyltransferase. Structure/function relationships. *Journal of Biological Chemistry,* **263**, 5164–5169.

815. Zakim, D., Goldenberg, J. & Vessey, D.A. (1973) Effects of

metals on the properties of hepatic microsomal uridine diphosphate glucuronyltransferase. *Biochemistry,* **12**, 4068–4074.

816. Zeneroli, M.L., Piaggi, V., Cremonini, C. *et al.* (1982) Sources of bile pigment overproduction in Gilbert's syndrome: studies with non-radioactive bilirubin kinetics and with δ-(3.5-^{3}H) aminolaevulinic acid and (2-^{14}C) glycine. *Clinical Science,* **62**, 643–649.

817. Zenone, E.A., Stoll, M.S. & Ostrow, J.D. (1982) The effect of elimination of environmental light on the metabolism of unconjugated bilirubin in the Gunn rat. *Digestive Diseases and Sciences,* **27**, 1117–1120.

818. Zhivkov, V.I. & Tosheva, R.T. (1986) Uridine diphosphate sugars: Concentration and rate of synthesis in tissues of vertebrates. *International Journal of Biochemistry,* **18**, 1–6.

819. Ziegler, K., Frimmer, M. & Fasold, H. (1984) Further characterization of membrane proteins involved in the transport of organic anions in hepatocytes. *Biochimica et Biophysica Acta,* **769**, 117–129.

Cholestasis

Fenton Schaffner

Cholestasis, an important component of many diseases of the liver and biliary tract, is discussed in various parts of this book under each of the respective diseases. The emphasis in this chapter is on the definition, mechanisms and features of cholestasis. Information about these aspects of cholestasis is accumulating so rapidly that only some of the latest references at the time of writing can be included. The diseases with cholestasis are listed in this chapter primarily for purposes of aiding in the differential diagnosis. The mechanisms of cholestasis are described in the light of available knowledge of the molecular basis of bile secretion to aid in the understanding of pathogenesis, diagnosis and management of clinical disorders. A brief review of diagnosis and therapy, supplementing material to be found in other chapters, concludes this one.

DEFINITION OF CHOLESTASIS

The term cholestasis was first used in the mid-1920s to describe stagnation of bile in the gallbladder and larger bile ducts. The use of the term was extended in 1950 to include visualization of bile in liver tissue on histological examination, in dilated bile canaliculi, in the cytoplasm of hepatocyes and in Kupffer cells and other macrophages. The ability to see bile in liver tissue depends on the technique used. Some bile is always in transit in normal hepatocytes and biliary passages but cholestasis implies an excess of morphologically demonstrable bile. Electron microscopically, cholestasis is associated with characteristic alterations of the bile canaliculi, the Golgi apparatus, the cytoskeleton and mitochondria. These ultrastructural findings are particularly important in experimental rodents, in which bile thrombi do not form even in severe cholestasis (except in neonatal rats or after overload with bilirubin, combined with manganese).[45] The morphological observations provided a basis for making clinical–pathological correlations and thereby the term cholestasis could be applied without morphological confirmation. Functionally, cholestasis is impairment of secretion of all the compounds of bile into the canaliculi by hepatocytes. Selective secretory defects of organic anions like conjugated bilirubin and exogenous dyes, features of the Dubin–Johnson and Rotor syndromes, therefore are not included. The early stages of primary biliary cirrhosis (see Chapter 33) are less readily excluded. Bile presumably regurgitates through the altered bile ducts in the early stage of chronic non-suppurative destructive cholangitis to raise the level of all biliary substances in the blood without electron microscopic or functional evidence of disturbed secretion of bile by the hepatocytes.[199]

Clinically, cholestasis is recognized by the appearance in blood of increased amounts of all the components of bile. The concentrations of the various components and the activities of the various enzymes do not rise in a parallel fashion. For instance, the increase in the serum bilirubin may be less than that of other substances and jaundice may be absent although bilirubinuria occurs at some time in almost all instances. Obstruction to the flow of bile in the larger bile ducts, leading to mechanical cholestasis, can now be demonstrated by various imaging procedures including the use of endoscopy. The development of these techniques has greatly simplified the differential diagnosis of cholestasis.

CLASSIFICATION OF CHOLESTASIS

The two main categories of cholestasis are the one produced by demonstrable mechanical obstruction in the extrahepatic and large intrahepatic bile ducts and the other in which such an obstruction cannot be demonstrated. The mechanism(s) by which cholestasis is produced without obstruction has not been established and the term 'intrahepatic cholestasis' is usually applied to describe this common feature of many liver diseases. Some ambiguity arises in that intrahepatic cholestasis may be the result of widespread obstruction of small bile ducts throughout the liver as is seen in sclerosing cholangitis or biliary atresia (see later). Nevertheless, the term intrahepatic cholestasis has no substitute.

EXTRAHEPATIC BILIARY OBSTRUCTION

Any obstacle to the flow of bile in the common hepatic duct or common bile duct produces cholestasis, usually with dilatation of the ducts above the obstacle (hydrohepatosis). Factors other than simple retention of all biliary constituents, which can be experimentally produced by a choledochocaval fistula, contribute to the abnormalities observed in extrahepatic biliary obstruction.[94] Jaundice is usually present in this form of cholestasis but it may be inconspicuous or even absent, while the activities of enzymes like alkaline phosphatase, considered to be markers of cholestasis, are greatly increased (dissociated jaundice). The main reason for the enhanced enzyme activity seems to be increased enzyme protein synthesis.[112,206] When obstruction is sudden, aminotransferase activities rise steeply, before alkaline phosphatase does, but fall within a few days to normal or nearly so despite deepening jaundice.[171] The concentration of serum IgA also rises due to impaired biliary secretion of the polymeric form of the protein. IgA levels have been said to be more sensitive indicators of the degree of cholestasis due to obstruction than serum alkaline phosphatase activity.[185] Pruritus may occur with any form of cholestasis, as may elevated serum cholesterol levels, although the latter occurs much less regularly. Chills and fever, abdominal pain and jaundice (Charcot's triad) with septicaemia result from bacterial infection in the stagnated bile or 'ascending' cholangitis, which can lead to formation of cholangitic abscesses.[146] Severe dysfunction of the sinus node of the heart can occur in obstructive jaundice[11] perhaps owing to the presence of digoxin-like factors in serum, which may also explain the bradycardia which often accompanies cholestatic jaundice.[43] The common causes of bile duct obstruction are gallstones, tumours, inflammatory lesions of the bile ducts and pancreatic diseases, plus several unusual causes.

Gallstones

Stones in the common bile duct lead the list of causes of biliary obstruction. They may initially become impacted anywhere in the course of the duct system, but most often this occurs at the papilla of Vater. Relaxation of spasm of the duct and subsidence of oedema of the duct wall eventually loosen the impaction and the stone may pass into the duodenum or move back up the duct. A loose stone in the common bile duct causes incomplete obstruction, often without jaundice but recognizable by increased alkaline phosphatase activity. A ball-valve effect of the stone produces fluctuations in the degree of cholestasis, especially the serum bilirubin level. Because obstruction by a stone is of short duration or is incomplete and because inflammation and, later, fibrosis develops in the wall of the duct due to cholangitis, dilatation of the intrahepatic ducts is often missing. A stone in the cystic duct or gallbladder does not produce cholestasis except when it is located near the common duct. Oedema and inflammation in these circumstances may compromise the lumen of the common duct. Stones in the common hepatic duct and its branches are uncommon and, as a rule, develop only if an area of narrowing, such as a stricture or tumour, is present or if they were retained after cholecystectomy was performed.

Tumours

Cholestasis due to carcinoma of the papilla of Vater occasionally fluctuates as obstruction is temporarily relieved by sloughing of the carcinomatous tissue, usually accompanied by bleeding. Tumours in and around the extrahepatic bile ducts produce cholestasis. Pedunculated intrinsic benign tumours, such as papillomas or leiomyomas, can cause cholestasis which varies in intensity when the tumour changes position; papillomatous tumours of the papilla of Vater can do the same thing. Benign papillomatosis of the bile duct is a rare entity causing cholestasis; it has a high recurrence rate after removal and can involve intrahepatic ducts.[23] Malignant tumours, primarily carcinomas of the duct, produce unremitting and progressive cholestasis until some manipulative intervention occurs. Extrinsic malignant tumours extending from organs near the liver like the stomach or pancreas also cause obstruction as they invade the wall of the bile duct, preventing the duct from being pushed aside in the loose connective tissue of the lesser omentum. Enlarged lymph nodes need not produce obstruction if they do not invade and fix the duct, even if the nodes are in large clusters. Most instances of cholestasis in leukaemias and lymphomas have an intrahepatic basis. The exceptions are chloroma, histiocytic non-Hodgkin's lymphoma and occasionally Hodgkin's disease when the tumour has invaded the duct. Metastatic carcinoma in hilar lymph nodes infrequently produces cholestasis because the bile duct is not fixed until spread occurs into the hilar connective tissue and the tumour invades the duct wall. Diagnosis of malignant biliary obstruction by endoscopic or percutaneous cholangiography[247] provides the opportunity for non-surgical palliation by insertion of various endoprostheses.[51]

Inflammatory lesions of the bile ducts

These lesions may result in strictures, a frequent cause of extrahepatic biliary obstruction. Surgical misadventure was thought to be the common cause of these strictures, frequently complicated by infection. The degree of obstruction varies but it usually is incomplete. Some of these strictures may indeed have followed ligation of the duct, insertion of a T-tube or compromise of the blood supply of the duct. However, some are the result of sclerosing cholangitis which either existed prior to the surgery or was caused by the surgery. Primary sclerosing cholangitis, in the absence of surgery, is being recognized more frequently, owing to routine blood screening[114,250] (see Chapter 37). Sclerosing cholangitis has been associated with HLA-DR-w52a, indicating a genetic predisposition for the development of the disease.[270] A study of the natural history of a group of patients with sclerosing cholangitis led to the conclusion that this disease is generally progressive regardless of how early it is detected.[269] It is associated with inflammatory bowel disease in about two-thirds of the cases, but also with use of some drugs like fluorodeoxyuridine[134,173] or methysergide.[33,125,127] Formalin flushing of bile ducts after resection of echinococcus cysts can also cause sclerosing cholangitis. Similar changes leading to biliary cirrhosis have been seen in experimental animals after formalin injection of the bile ducts.[15] Patients with the acquired immunodeficiency syndrome (AIDS) may develop sclerosing cholangitis if they have been infected with the cytomegalovirus and/or with *Cryptosporidium*. Sclerosing cholangitis involves the extrahepatic ducts alone in about 15% of the cases, while both intrahepatic and extrahepatic ducts are involved in the rest. Rare instances of purely intrahepatic sclerosing cholangitis have been reported. Sclerosing cholangitis may be a transient, relapsing or progressive disease. Unremitting cholestasis with unremitting jaundice usually indicates a bad prognosis and time for consideration of liver transplantation.[7] Acalculous cholecystitis may be the result of sclerosing cholangitis involving the gallbladder. Obstruction of the hepatic duct by a benign fibrosing process called the Mirizzi syndrome[223] and fibrosis of or near the sphincter of Oddi[31] may be variants of sclerosing cholangitis as may be proliferative cholangitis.[122] Extrahepatic biliary atresia with or without involvement of the intrahepatic ducts, and paucity of intrahepatic ducts, often with other anomalies (Alagille syndrome) are diseases of infancy and childhood[159,222] (see Chapter 44).

Pancreatic diseases

Diseases of the pancreas, particularly carcinoma of the head and pancreatitis, may cause extrahepatic biliary obstruction. Pancreatitis as a cause is more frequently recognized by endoscopic or percutaneous cholangiography, when smooth tapering of the end of the common bile duct is seen. Jaundice has been reported in up to a quarter of cases of acute pancreatitis and in over 40% some obstruction of the pancreatic portion of the common bile duct has been noted.[136] Similarly, in chronic pancreatitis both inflammation and fibrosis distort and kink the common bile duct.[252] Pseudocysts and retention cysts may also produce obstructive jaundice.[213] Cholestasis may be protracted in chronic pancreatitis but secondary biliary cirrhosis has not been seen.[49] Cholestasis due to alcoholic pancreatitis can be separated from intrahepatic cholestasis due to alcohol by aminotransferase activities, in that a high AST/ALT ratio indicates intrahepatic cholestasis.[27]

Unusual causes

Several conditions can produce mechanical biliary obstruction but the conditions themselves or the instances of obstruction are uncommon. These include choledochal cysts,[254] strategically located amoebic and bacterial abscesses (Chapter 37), diverticula of the duodenum, parasitic infestations such as ascariasis or fascioliasis (Chapter 61) and haemobilia.[129,150,236] The belief that the inspissated bile syndrome in infants can produce extrahepatic biliary obstruction has been challenged. Inspissated bile in the biliary passages in this syndrome is the result of an underlying disease usually associated with increased red-cell breakdown. The hepatic alterations, including morphological evidence of cholestasis, are also expressions of the underlying disease and are not produced mechanically. Whether dyskinesia or spasm of the sphincter of Oddi causes cholestasis is not established.

INTRAHEPATIC MECHANICAL OBSTRUCTION _____

Narrowing and kinking of intrahepatic bile ducts can be produced by several processes and can result in focal cholestasis in that part of the parenchyma drained by a distorted duct. Jaundice rarely results because the remaining part of the liver is able to compensate for the local biliary obstruction. Biochemical evidence of obstruction with elevation of alkaline phosphatase activity depends on the size and number of ducts obstructed. Obstruction of one main hepatic duct at the bifurcation of the common hepatic duct at the hilum of the liver by either ligation or tumour is not associated with hyperbilirubinaemia as long as the liver is otherwise normal and the other main hepatic duct is not involved. Under these circumstances, however, pruritus does occur, alkaline phosphatase activity rises and hypercholesterolaemia may develop. Minor stresses to the liver or beginning involvement of the other duct results in jaundice. Conditions producing focal cholestasis with or without biochemical evidence of cholestasis include any fibrosing lesion such as cirrhosis, abscesses, granulomas and metastatic tumours. Jaundice can result in any of these from a small contribution of hepatocellular dysfunction. Nodular regenerative hyperplasia has also been associated with cholestasis.[48] Cystic fibrosis is associated with steatosis and plugging of bile ducts and ductules by inspissated mucus, proliferation of ductules and periductular fibrosis. PAS staining of the mucous material is diagnostic. Focal biliary cirrhosis develops in 25% of the survivors of this disease but less than 3% develop end-stage liver disease with portal hypertension. Cholestasis is not part of the disease except in infancy and occasionally in the end stage and it is not an aetiologic factor in the disease (see Chapter 44).[102] Less common conditions in which mechanical intrahepatic biliary obstruction is extensive enough to produce jaundice are listed below. More extensive discussion of each can be found in appropriate chapters in this book.

Carcinoma of the bifurcation of the common hepatic duct (see Chapter 60)

This lesion, discussed before, has the features of a tumour in the extrahepatic bile duct although it is technically intrahepatic. Different degrees of involvement in both branches account for variations in the clinical picture as well as for the different morphological changes in the right and left lobes of the liver.

Infantile obstructive cholangiopathy (see Chapters 44 and 45)

Bile duct abnormalities causing obstructive cholestasis in infancy fall into three categories.[46]

(1) *Extrahepatic bile duct atresia* is fetal in about one-third of cases and perinatal in two-thirds. The fetal type is characterized by conjugated hyperbilirubinaemia becoming apparent while physiological jaundice is still present. The perinatal form has a jaundice-free interval of a few weeks before conjugated hyperbilirubinaemia develops. The former type may be associated with multiple anomalies while the latter is not. Extrahepatic atresia is the result of fibrous obliterating cholangitis. Biliary atresia may or may not have an intrahepatic atretic component and may also be accompanied by multinucleate giant hepatocytes. It occurs most frequently after viral infections in the mother during pregnancy, particularly reovirus type 3,[82] rubella and cytomegalovirus disease.[68] The probability of intrauterine infection suggests that atresia is an acquired lesion. It has been seen in only one of a set of monozygotic twins.[156] However, it may also be associated with trisomy 18. About 1 in 14 000 children are born with or develop extrahepatic biliary atresia.[100] The therapeutic approach has long been the construction of a portoenterostomy—

the Kasai procedure; however, in most centres this operation has a long-term success rate of only about 50%. Earlier surgery, within the first weeks of life, has been urged as the only way to improve these statistics.[99,152] Intrahepatic problems following portoenterostomy may be the result of involvement of the intrahepatic ducts with the same process as the extrahepatic duct or may be the result of incomplete drainage of the intrahepatic duct system.[205,248] Serum type III procollagen peptide may be a useful marker indicating progressive hepatic fibrosis.[233] The fibrosis appears to be related at least in part to ductular cell proliferation and may be mediated by activation of clones of connective-tissue cells.[44] Ultimately, those patients in whom portoenterostomy has failed are candidates for liver transplantation.[5,61] Because of the difficulties sometimes encountered in transplantation as a result of prior surgery, transplantation is occasionally recommended as the initial procedure.[61]

(2) *Intrahepatic bile duct atresia*, ductopenia or paucity of bile ducts[243] possibly is also the result of loss of existing ducts. Two varieties with prolonged survival exist, arteriohepatic dysplasia or Alagille's syndrome associated with mental retardation, ataxia, cardiac and digital or facial abnormalities[4] and a non-syndromatic form.[109] Renal abnormalities have also been seen[230] and several hepatocellular carcinomas have been reported in patients who survived into adult life.[183] An interstitial deletion of the short arm of chromosome 20 has been found in patients with Alagille syndrome.[277] Idiopathic ductopenia leading to biliary cirrhosis has also been described in adults.[135] Zellweger's syndrome, the congenital absence of peroxisomes, results in abnormal cholesterol metabolism and in some instances, a paucity of bile ducts.

(3) *Ductal plate malformation* is a developmental anomaly in which ducts are not formed (agenesis) or the ductal plate from which ducts are formed does not mature properly. Only agenesis causes infantile cholestasis, while the other malformations, including infantile polycystic disease, Meyenberg's complexes or bile duct hamartomas, Caroli's disease, congenital hepatic fibrosis and choledochal cysts, usually do not.

Intrahepatic cholangitis

Both intrahepatic suppurative and primary sclerosing cholangitis are causes of intrahepatic biliary obstruction and have been discussed before.

Periductal and periductular fibrosis

This lesion, which can obstruct the flow of bile out of the liver acinus, occurs in late primary biliary cirrhosis and in secondary biliary cirrhosis, particularly in extrahepatic biliary obstruction lasting longer than 1 year. The lesion is seldom uniform throughout the liver but it may become severe enough to cause jaundice and functional sequelae (see below). Its development may herald the need for liver transplantation. When the periductal fibrosis is extensive and has resulted from a stricture or sclerosing cholangitis, attempts at balloon dilatation, stenting or surgical correction fail. Graft versus host disease, especially after bone marrow transplantation[214] and the disappearing bile duct syndrome (a form of rejection after liver tranplantation[67]) are associated with biliary obstruction due to destruction of small bile ducts and resemble accelerated primary biliary cirrhosis.[198] Rare patients with hepatic sarcoidosis can develop a picture of primary biliary cirrhosis but the condition is not associated with mitochondrial antibodies and is histologically easily recognized.[175]

Metastatic carcinoma

Jaundice, largely cholestatic, is common in the terminal stages of metastatic disease of the liver. Occasionally, however, it is the first symptom of a cancer. Primary hepatocellular carcinoma is less frequently a cause of cholestasis. Whether the jaundice is produced by a primary or secondary tumour and whether it develops early or late depend on the extent and location of the tumour deposits. Some of the jaundice is explained by mechanical obstruction of a sufficient number of intrahepatic bile ducts. When biliary drainage fails to relieve the jaundice, this explanation is inadequate and a metabolic hepatocellular reason has to be presumed.

INTRAHEPATIC CHOLESTASIS WITHOUT OBSTRUCTION

Jaundice with conjugated hyperbilirubinaemia and the histological manifestations of cholestasis has presented one of the most difficult diagnostic problems in liver disease. While the aetiology is known in most instances, the mechanism of the cholestasis, which is discussed later, remains problematical. Cholestasis may be a component of hepatitis or cirrhosis of different aetiologies in which other manifestations of hepatocellular damage are present to a variable degree. Less frequently, the structural, functional and clinical manifestations of cholestasis predominate or are present alone. Hepatocellular organelles, including the bile canalicular membrane, may be altered by cholestasis or by the aetiological agent or indirectly by injury to the hepatocyte caused by either. Separation of the primary manifestations of cholestasis from those due to other factors is difficult although desirable in diagnosis and management.

Pure intrahepatic cholestasis

The aetiology of this form should be included in the diagnosis when it is known. It is most often seen in infants, especially premature ones,[209] from many causes.[52] Liver biopsy can be helpful in sorting out the various aetiologies. Breast feeding can be a common cause.[203] It can also occur in adolescent children, during pregnancy and in the elderly. It can also occur in hyperthyroidism at any age.[255] Multiple factors usually complicate or trigger the cholestatic phenomenon.

Cholestasis in infection

Pure cholestasis complicating lobar pneumonia was once common but is now a rare phenomenon; the prognosis was grave at a time when antimicrobial therapy did not exist. Increased activity of enzymes like gamma glutamyl transferase may be the result of medications given rather than of cholestasis. Urinary tract infections in children can cause cholestasis, while in adults such Gram-negative infections rarely do. Endotoxins cause cholestasis in tissue culture and may be responsible for it during sepsis as well as for disseminated intravascular coagulation. Prostaglandin E_2 and leukotriene D_4 cause cholestasis in rats.[101] They act synergistically and are both produced under conditions associated with cholestasis like sepsis or severe injury. The toxic shock syndrome is accompanied by cholestasis and alterations in the small bile ducts.[87]

Alpha-1-antitrypsin deficiency (see Chapter 43)

This is a frequent cause of neonatal cholestasis, but the mechanism is not understood and it is not necessarily associated with hepatitis. The cholestasis spontaneously disappears in most babies, and only a few develop cirrhosis later in childhood or adult life.

Parenteral alimentation

Total parenteral alimentation in children[16,66] and in adults[242] may lead to cholestasis. Among the several factors held to be responsible are bacterial overgrowth,[30,253] altered bile acid metabolism,[71,132] immaturity or low birth weight in children,[148,193] and abnormalities in the handling of lipids and amino acids. Phenobarbital administration has been said to be helpful in treating this condition by some[220] and to be ineffective by others.[83]

Haemolysis

Slender bile thrombi can be found in the perivenular zone in many forms of moderate to severe haemolysis from any cause and canalicular changes typical of cholestasis can be found by electron microscopy. The conjugated hyperbilirubinaemia which can develop during severe haemolysis is largely the result of this cholestasis. Since secretion of bilirubin into the canaliculus is the rate-limiting step in its removal from the hepatocyte, any interference with this process causes retention of bilirubin. Indeed, the highest levels of serum bilirubin recorded with a large proportion of the direct-reacting form occur during haemolysis, especially if renal plasma flow is also compromised. Whether the excessive load of bilirubin itself causes the cholestasis is unknown, but bilirubin injected into experimental animals is cholestatic, especially if manganese is also given.[45] Severe cholestasis can occur in patients with sickle cell crisis and may mimic biliary obstruction from gallstones. Histologically, bile stasis may be impressive.

Postoperative cholestasis (see Chapter 52)

Jaundice following surgery results from many factors, including breakdown of transfused red blood cells, spontaneous haemolysis, shifts in the distribution of bilirubin, hypoxia and shock. Jaundice may be severe if many units of blood have been transfused. The elevation of the serum bilirubin level is the most striking abnormality and in many instances may be the only one, suggesting that the defect is a temporary inability of the liver to secrete organic anions other than bile acids. Bilirubin levels generally fall to normal by the time the patient is discharged home.

Cholestasis in congestion

Acute as well as chronic passive congestion of the liver may be associated with cholestasis, not clearly related to the degree of congestion. The extent of the cholestasis does not correlate with the amount of hepatocellular necrosis that is often present. That increased venous pressure mechanically interferes with bile flow cannot be supported. Hypoxia and pressure on hepatocytes may be factors. The congestion need not be cardiac in origin and cholestasis is seen in the Budd–Chiari syndrome and in constrictive pericarditis. Pulmonary infarcts may be associated with jaundice in part due to haemolysis of the accumulated blood, although injection of blood into tissues in amounts equivalent to that in an infarct does not produce jaundice. Tissue breakdown products and endotoxaemia may play a role. Similar factors may operate in shock when cholestasis is present; however, jaundice out of proportion to the degree of cholestasis is usually the result of decreased plasma flow.

Amyloidosis (see Chapter 37)

Alkaline phosphatase activity is frequently elevated in diffuse or parenchymal amyloidosis in contrast to the portal or perivascular form. Jaundice, however, is uncommon and when it is present it can be attributed to interference with the microcirculation as well as by compression of hepatocytes by amyloid.[69,179]

Malignancies

Although carcinomas and lymphomas may obstruct bile flow sufficiently to produce cholestasis, this explanation does not account for all instances of jaundice or its occasional severity. Therefore, a metabolic component, hypothetical in nature, has been suggested. Cholestasis may be a paraneoplastic syndrome in carcinoma of the kidney without liver involvement.[105] While jaundice may

also occur in Hodgkin's disease and in some other lymphomas in the terminal stages of disease, it is seen in about 10% of cases of Hodgkin's disease without lymphoma in the liver. This latter cholestasis resolves after the Hodgkin's disease has been appropriately treated. Some of the pruritus in Hodgkin's disease may be explained by cholestasis. By contrast, rapidly progressive cholestasis in Hodgkin's disease can result from extensive destruction of small bile ducts in the liver by the tumour. Cholestatic jaundice is an early phenomenon in histiocytic medullary reticulosis to which severe haemolysis contributes as it may in lymphomas (see Chapters 8 and 41).

Cholestatic viral hepatitis

Cholestasis may be the only alteration in rare instances of liver disease caused by any one of the hepatitis viruses.[229] The differential diagnosis in these instances is usually not difficult and the aetiology is established by the detection of appropriate viral markers and by the demonstration of a patent bile duct system with the help of cholangiography.

Drug-induced cholestasis

Administration of several drugs may be followed by pure cholestasis without any other clinical, laboratory or histological manifestations[180] (see Chapter 46). The list of drugs continues to grow longer and has included some physiological substances such as oestradiol,[1] somatostatin[119] and chenodeoxycholic acid.[177]

Cholestasis in pregnancy (see Chapter 42)

Uncomplicated pregnancy, particularly in the last trimester, may be accompanied by pruritus and biochemical manifestations of cholestasis, including mild jaundice, despite a histologically normal liver by light microscopy.[78] This phenomenon tends to recur with each pregnancy as well as following the use of oral contraceptives. Recurrent cholestasis of pregnancy is sometimes familial, being inherited as a Mendelian dominant trait with inhibition of expression of the phenotype in males.[98] It has been seen in twins.[86] Pruritus of pregnancy is a milder form of the condition. Abnormal oestrogen metabolism or increased sensitivity to these steroids appears to be the cause of cholestasis.[76] Cholestasis of pregnancy can be reversed by administration of high doses of *S*-adenosyl-L-methiononine,[77] as can experimental oestrogen-induced cholestasis.[21] Steatorrhea often accompanies cholestasis of pregnancy but its degree was not correlated with the high risk of premature deliveries and fetal distress seen in this condition.[188] Cholestatic jaundice in pregnancy can result from other causes, viral hepatitis being the commonest. The incidence of cholestasis in pregnancy has been estimated from the literature to be about 1 in 1500 pregnancies, of which about 40% are thought to be due to viral hepatitis. As markers for hepatitis C and hepatitis E (the transfusion-related and enteric forms of non-A, non-B hepatitis) have become available, more precise data will be forthcoming. Choledocholithiasis is the second commonest, but far less frequent, cause of cholestasis in pregnancy, while chronic active hepatitis and alcoholic hepatitis are rare, presumably because conception is infrequent. Cholestasis from drugs, urosepsis and haemolysis are uncommon causes. Early primary biliary cirrhosis may be unmasked by the development of cholestasis during pregnancy when bilirubin and alkaline phosphatase do not return to normal after delivery.[199] Acute fatty liver of pregnancy is usually associated with mild cholestasis clinically while it may be striking histologically.

Cholestasis may also occur in the toxaemia of pregnancy although it is not a major manifestation. Activities of alkaline phosphatase may be elevated but jaundice is infrequent. Even in fatal eclampsia, jaundice is primarily haemolytic and is accompanied by intravascular coagulation and the deposition of fibrin thrombi in hepatic sinusoids.

Idiopathic recurrent cholestasis

This rare disorder is usually familial and autosomal recessive in character with poor penetrance. As many as half the cases may be sporadic without a family history. The condition is marked by repeated attacks of intrahepatic cholestasis occurring at fairly regular intervals, from several months to several years apart. A few women with this syndrome began with recurrent cholestasis of pregnancy. Each attack starts with anorexia, pruritus and weight loss without colic or high fever. Serum bilirubin levels may rise to 342 μmol/l (20 mg/dl) and alkaline phosphatase and aminotransferase activities may be several times the upper limit of normal. The latter recedes rapidly while the former remains elevated after bilirubin has returned to normal. Serum bile acid levels are very high but serum proteins are not changed except for elevation of β-globulin. Histologically, perivenular cholestasis without hepatocellular changes and with mild portal inflammation is seen. Electron microscopically, only the changes of cholestasis are found. After several attacks mild portal fibrosis may remain. Jaundice with itching may last up to 3 months. Between attacks everything is normal clinically, biochemically and histologically. The attacks begin in early adult life but a few patients experience them in childhood.

Abnormal bile acid metabolism has been said to be the cause of the condition[17,153] but nothing consistently abnormal has been found in the few cases examined. No therapy seems capable of preventing attacks. Cholestyramine is useful for control of pruritus if it is given early and as maintenance therapy between attacks.[18] Phenobarbital and corticosteroids have been used but with questionable effect. Preliminary reports have suggested that ursodeoxycholic acid may be useful in preventing attacks of cholestasis in this condition.[261,262]

Progressive familial cholestasis

Several families have been described in which cholestasis begins in childhood or early adult life and progresses in a few years to hepatic failure and death, often with cirrhosis.[191] S-adenosylmethionine therapy has proved to be ineffective and even hepatotoxic.[62] One such family, named Byler, was among the first reported and the name Byler's disease has been applied to the group although the condition is not identical in all families. At the onset jaundice may be intermittent but it gradually becomes unremitting. Serum bile acid levels are high and a defect in bile acid metabolism has been held responsible[74] but has not been demonstrated. No characteristic light- or electron-microscopic changes have been seen except for those related to cholestasis. Cirrhosis may not be evident for years. No therapy has proved useful although some patients may become candidates for liver transplantation. A benign chronic form of familial cholestasis has also been described.

Cholestasis in hepatitis

Diffuse hepatocellular damage with inflammation and disturbed liver function is 'hepatitis' in a generic sense, although the hepatocytic damage is more important in most instances than the inflammatory reaction. The necro-inflammatory component is combined with a cholestatic one in most acute and chronic liver diseases. Agents causing hepatitis induce both components, each to a variable degree, in a spectrum from anicteric to cholestatic hepatitis.

Acute viral hepatitis (see Chapter 30)
During the course of acute viral hepatitis, cholestatic manifestations are usually far overshadowed by hepatocellular damage. Healing, however, begins with improvement of hepatocytic function before bile formation recovers. Thus, the patient may feel better with a return of appetite and a drop in serum amino-transferase activity while serum bilirubin and alkaline phosphatase activity remain elevated, sometimes for several weeks. Eventually bile secretion is restored. Alkaline phosphatase activity is the last test result to return to normal and this may take several months after the patient has fully recovered. If liver biopsies are performed serially (which rarely, if ever, is indicated) hepatocellular damage with necrosis and inflammation is seen initially. As this subsides, bile thrombi, bile staining of hepatocytes and bile pigment in macrophages remain in the perivenular zone. When cholestatic features are prominent clinically, they are readily recognized histologically, and by the same token, if little evidence of cholestasis is noted clinically, little is seen histologically. Viral hepatitis is more likely to be cholestatic in infancy and puberty, during pregnancy and in older persons. Also, the more prominent cholestasis is, the longer the patient remains jaundiced. Hepatitis A and E (enteric non-A, non-B) are often more cholestatic than hepatitis B and C. Cholestasis, even when protracted,

is not a harbinger of chronicity. Epidemics of cholestatic hepatitis of unknown aetiology have been described; the long-term prognosis in these cases has been good.

Chronic hepatitis (see Chapter 31)

Cholestasis in chronic hepatitis can be transient, intermittent, unremitting or a terminal occurrence. Transient or intermittent cholestasis can result from a flare-up of the activity of the chronic hepatitis or can be caused by haemolysis, medications or intercurrent infections, even another acute hepatitis. These episodes do not seem to have special prognostic significance. On the contrary, unremitting or progressive jaundice is a bad prognostic sign with survival limited to a year or so. No therapy short of transplantation is effective. Cholestasis as a terminal event can result from hepatic failure, poor hepatic perfusion, hypoxia, associated renal failure, primary hepatocellular carcinoma, medications and unrelated biliary obstruction. The cholestasis is usually a manifestation of impending demise but not its cause.

Alcoholic hepatitis (see Chapter 34)

Infrequently, alcoholic liver disease presents clinically and with laboratory findings of cholestasis. Fever, abdominal pain and leukocytosis usually accompany this syndrome and occasionally prompts surgical exploration. Cholangiography and liver biopsy, in that order, readily establish the correct diagnosis. Tissue cholestasis in liver biopsy specimens from patients with acute alcoholic hepatitis was a significant indicator of a poor prognosis.[268] The most common cause of obstructive jaundice in the alcoholic is pancreatitis, while intrahepatic cholestasis results from alcoholic hepatitis. Zieve's syndrome with hypertriglyceridaemia and haemolysis in alcoholics may be associated with a high level of direct-reacting bilirubin and perivenular cholestasis. When haemolysis complicates cholestasis, the alkaline phosphatase activity is elevated less than the bilirubin level would suggest. Such haemolysis may be severe when many burr or spur forms of erythrocytes are present.

Drug hepatitis (see Chapter 46)

The most frequent type of hepatic drug reaction with jaundice is cholestatic hepatitis in which the cholestasis predominates. Cholestatic drug hepatitis is usually accompanied by fever, anorexia, malaise and hepatic tenderness. Histologically, parenchymal and portal inflammation distinguish this lesion from pure cholestasis but the hepatitic component is of shorter duration than the cholestatic one so that only pure cholestasis remains late in the course. The same drug may produce severe hepatitis with little cholestasis in one patient and severe cholestasis in another.

Cholestasis in cirrhosis

Cholestasis may be an important component of cirrhosis of any variety at any stage. The degree of cholestasis may vary histologically throughout the liver and may involve some nodules or even parts of nodules preferentially. Focal cholestasis may lead to the destruction of nodules. Cholestasis is also a component of some cases of metabolic liver diseases such as Wilson's disease, alpha-1-antitrypsin deficiency in children, Niemann–Pick disease, galactosaemia, late type IV glycogen storage disease, Wolman's disease, tyrosinosis and familial hepatosteatosis, all primarily in children.[73]

Primary biliary cirrhosis (see Chapter 33)

Early in its course cholestasis is not a component of this disease, although many of the components of bile are elevated in the blood. Regurgitation of bile occurs through damaged bile ducts as part of non-suppurative destructive cholangitis. Therefore the disease appears to be one of cholestasis in the laboratory but not histologically. Primary biliary cirrhosis can present with true cholestasis accompanied by jaundice, dark urine, acholic stools and pruritus in patients who are developing the disease but in addition are given drugs capable of producing cholestasis or are pregnant. Histologically under these circumstances typical perivenular cholestasis is found. All resolves when the offending drug is withdrawn or pregnancy terminates. However, high levels of alkaline phosphatase activity persist and ultimately prompt the search for the correct diagnosis. Late in the course of primary biliary cirrhosis when many small intrahepatic bile ducts are destroyed and the picture of intrahepatic mechanical obstruction develops, as described earlier, periportal cholestasis is seen histologically with accumulation of much copper and copper-binding protein in the periportal hepatocytes. The patient becomes progressively more jaundiced as this mechanical cholestasis continues, yet in many instances true cirrhosis has not developed.

Multifactorial cholestasis

Cholestasis can be the result of a variety of contributing factors such as infection, medications, parenteral alimentation, shortened red blood cell survival, intravascular coagulation and multiple blood transfusions. Since renal function often is also reduced, serum bilirubin levels may be elevated far more than the activity of alkaline phosphatase is increased. Endotoxin and products of the metabolism of prostaglandins and related compounds may contribute or even initiate both cholestasis and renal impairment.[22,70] The cholestasis often seen after liver transplantation is partly the result of ischaemic injury during cold perfusion, partly rejection, partly medications and partly clearance of excess pretransplant bilirubin.[251]

MECHANISMS OF CHOLESTASIS

Descriptions of the mechanism and consequences of cholestasis were first based on light- and electron-microscopic studies of the morphological alterations.

MORPHOLOGICAL FEATURES OF ACUTE CHOLESTASIS

These histological changes can be divided into primary or essential manifestations and secondary or accompanying ones. The secondary features are of greater importance in recognizing the cause of the cholestasis than the essential features, which are the same for all forms of cholestasis. The most important essential feature is a change of the bile canaliculus. This structure is a modified portion of the plasma membrane constituting about 13% of the total plasma membrane. Early in cholestasis, the perivenular canaliculi dilate and contain bile thrombi in their lumens. Since the perivenular zone is composed of several zones 3 of different acini, the degree of cholestasis may not be concentric but is paravenular rather than perivenular. Bile pigment staining in the cytoplasm of hepatocytes and bile-stained granules in macrophages appear as cholestasis persists. Macrophages may also contain engulfed bile thrombi. Hepatocytes in the cholestatic perivenular zone may have an eosinophilic ground-glass appearance to their cytoplasm because of increased smooth endoplasmic reticulum. Binucleated hepatocytes may be numerous, indicating regeneration or hypertrophy. Tubular hepatocytes or pseudoductules result from dilatation of a canaliculus as part of cholestasis or from regeneration.[161] The former type often has a bile thrombus in the lumen.

On transmission electron microscopy, the earliest lesion is shortening and disappearance of canalicular microvilli followed by canalicular dilatation (Figure 15.1). Even in normal individuals, portions of bile canaliculi may have similar abnormalities suggesting variations in function of different segments of the canaliculus. Blebs may form on the canalicular plasma membrane and project into the lumen, in some instances appearing to fill the lumen. The microvilli at the junction of two cells (one extending from each cell) persist after all the others have disappeared. These microvilli and the tight junction binding neighbouring cells to one another remain intact until and unless disruption of the liver cell plate occurs. Bile thrombi in the dilated canalicular lumens vary in appearance; they may be fibrillar, granular, homogeneous, crystalline or lamellar with whorl formation (Figure 15.2a). Most often they are mixed in composition. The differences are due to variations in the age of the thrombi and in contributions of bile pigment, phospholipids and components of the plasma membrane. Bile thrombi and blebs have been said to constitute an obstruction to the flow of bile, but this is doubtful in view of the extensive intercommunications of the bile canalicular network. Dilated bile canaliculi have diverticular outpouchings into the hepatocytic cytoplasm.

This appearance is common in the neonatal liver and may be an indication of new formation of canaliculi. The turnover of canalicular membranes is increased in cholestasis and can also be induced by long-term administration of oestrogens.[89] While bile thrombi are predominantly in zone 3, canalicular dilatation extends throughout the acinus but the degree of dilatation varies greatly, even in the same canaliculus. This probably depends on the hepatocyte forming the canalicular wall and suggests variation in the degree of cholestasis in adjacent canaliculi, even in the perivenular zone. Canaliculi with normal lumens can be found, even in severe cholestasis. The number of canaliculi is increased but hepatocellular size and the volume of the intracellular space are reduced, perhaps permitting easier exchange between blood and bile.[241]

Variations are also seen within the hepatocytes in cholestasis. The pericanalicular cytoplasm bordering the canaliculus is more dense and broader than normal (Figure 15.1). This portion of the cytoplasm contains few cytoplasmic vacuoles but has bundles of microfilaments which appear to be aggregates of the normal network of microfilaments surrounding the canaliculus and extending into the microvilli similar to the terminal web of the intestinal epithelium (Figure 15.1, inset). The function of these smooth muscle fibrils is to provide peristaltic contractions to the canaliculi, an action dependent on calcium ions and calmodulin.[215,245,246] These contractions are needed to develop the high secretory pressure required for bile flow.[75] Cytokeratin intermediate filaments have been demonstrated to play a role in the formation of bile canaliculi as well as in the hepatic uptake, transhepatic transport and secretion into bile of substances like fluorescein diacetate and horseradish peroxidase.[267] Some of these processes require conjugation with ubiquitin. Cell-to-cell communication is necessary for coordinated peristalsis and is either chemical or electrical. The vesicles and cisternae of the Golgi zone, located between the nucleus and the canaliculus, are large, and the vesicles often contain electron-dense granules (Figure 15.1). The smooth endoplasmic reticulum appears to be increased but morphometric studies in rats with ligated bile ducts have produced conflicting results. The volume of both smooth and rough endoplasmic reticulum is unchanged but the surface area of both doubles. This is reflected chemically in an increase of the microsomal fraction of the total liver without alterations in the protein/phospholipid ratio, but with a significant reduction in cytochrome P-450.[200] Activities of some but not all the drug-metabolizing enzymes remain normal.[118] The number of lysosomes is increased, as can be seen under the light microscope by an increase in diastase-resistant PAS-positive granules. Normally, lysosomal constituents, regardless of origin, are excreted into the bile, perhaps with the help of microtubules.[210] The lamellated or whorl-like electron dense material, presumably phospholipids, is surrounded by a membrane (Figure 15.2b). Less dense and granular or fibrillar material not membrane-bound may represent

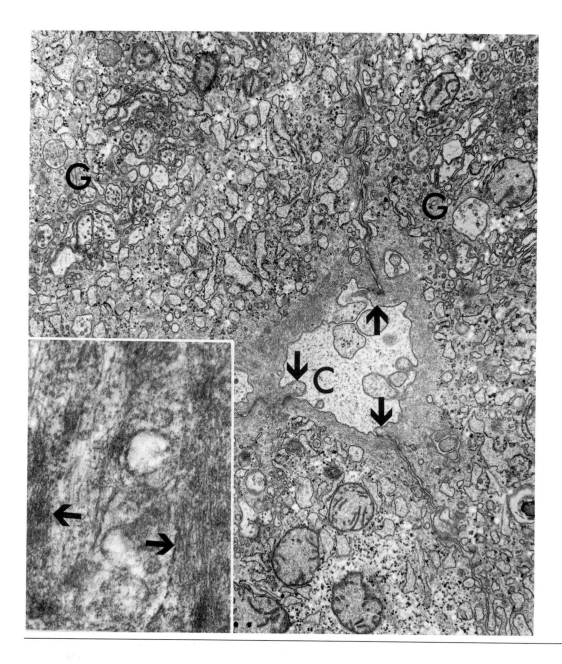

Figure 15.1 Intrahepatic cholestasis with dilated bile canaliculus (C) which has lost its microvilli except at the junction of neighbouring cells (arrows). The cytoplasm around the dilated canaliculus is more dense than normal, in part due to aggregated microfilaments (arrows, inset). The Golgi zones (G) are irregular and dilated and the numerous vesicles contain dense particles. (Glutaraldehyde/osmium tetroxide fixed, lead citrate stained, ×12 500; inset ×100 000; reproduced at 95%).

bilirubin. The tight junction between neighbouring hepatocytes remains intact even in severe cholestasis (Figure 15.1) but the number of strands that make up the tight junction may be reduced, as seen on freeze-fracture scanning electron microscopy. These changes indicate an increase in permeability or leakiness of the tight junction (see Chapter 20). The tight junction is disrupted when the hepatocyte undergoes necrosis. The pericellular space, an extension of the space of Disse is lengthened and the size of gap junctions, the pathway of intercellular communication, is reduced. The amount of the 26 kD gap junction protein decreases after bile duct ligation and hepatic lysosomal membranes contain less of this protein.[232] These findings support the idea that proteins are degraded during cholestasis rather than being dispersed.

Cine studies, particularly in hepatocyte couplets in culture,[25,176] indicate that canalicular peristalsis is impaired in cholestasis[178] as is suggested by the aggregation of contractile microfilaments around the canaliculus in both human and experimental cholestasis.[2]

The localization of bile thrombi in the perivenular zone, as far as possible from the site of obstruction in extrahepatic biliary obstruction, can be explained in several ways. Some bile continues to be secreted by hepatocytes even in complete biliary obstruction. The rate of bile flow in the acinus is slowest in the perivenular zone and faster near the entry of the canalicular system into the bile duct. The slower perivenular flow allows for greater reabsorption of water, probably through the leaky tight junction and is more likely to lead to inspissation. Moreover, bile salts essential for the solubility of hydrophobic biliary constituents are excreted mainly in the periportal zone.[90] Bile thrombi form in the periportal area in or near the limiting plate of hepatocytes when small bile ducts are destroyed or obstructed by portal fibrosis. Under these circumstances, flow is slowest immediately behind the obstruction. Hepatocellular alterations may also play a role in perivenular cholestasis. This zone is more vulnerable to injury because it has the lowest oxygen tension. The perivenular hepatocytes also have more smooth endoplasmic reticulum responsible for microsomal biotransformation. The morphological changes of cholestasis are readily reversible if experimental bile duct obstruction is relieved within 2 weeks but not after this.[257] The appearance of the mitochondrial cristae is said to be useful in assessing reversibility. Enlarged, pigment-laden macrophages persist after biliary decompression.

Cholestasis is a hepatocytic alteration initiated by increased biliary pressure in biliary obstruction and by metabolic processes in the intrahepatic form. Whether a cholestatic factor produced by lymphocytes in the form of a lymphokine is an ultimate pathogenetic factor in many or all instances of cholestasis[116,154,155] remains to be confirmed. The identity of the morphological features seen by various techniques in all types of cholestasis suggests that the same basic process operates and explains why morphological analysis may not assist in differential diagnosis. The same holds true for biochemical parameters of cholestasis, although they do reflect its intensity and duration.

PATHOGENESIS OF PERIVENULAR CHOLESTASIS

This, the most common distribution of cholestasis, results from an alteration in the formation of bile by hepatocytes. Metabolic and osmotic factors are more important than hydrodynamic ones such as blood and bile pressures, in contrast to renal glomerular filtration. Indeed, cholestasis is independent of the effects its causes may have on the microcirculation. Increasing sinusoidal outflow resistance or the rate of perfusion in the isolated liver did not produce cholestasis,[37] although cholestasis is common but not always present in passive congestion from any cause. Bile reaching the intestine receives contributions from several different sources. The largest contribution is from a fraction dependent on bile salt secretion from the hepatocytes, which is greatest postprandially. As bile salt secretion diminishes so does bile flow but it never ceases. That fraction of bile flow which does not appear to be dependent on bile salt secretion is called the bile salt-independent fraction but the amount is small, about half of basal or fasting bile flow, and the driving forces are not all known. Indeed, whether zero bile salt secretion ever exists with bile still flowing is conjectural. Osmotic forces may drag some water and inorganic cations and anions between hepatocytes across tight junctions into bile canaliculi. The extent of leakiness of tight junctions varies under many physiological and pathological circum-

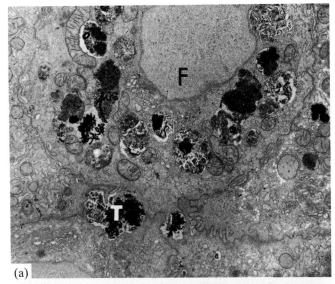

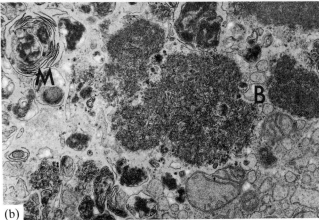

Figure 15.2 (a) Hepatocyte (F) showing extensive feathery degeneration of the cytoplasm and a bile thrombus (T) in a dilated bile canaliculus in intrahepatic cholestasis. (Glutaraldehyde/osmium tetroxide fixed, lead citrate stained, ×7000; reproduced at 67%). (b) Detail of feathery degeneration of hepatocellular cytoplasm; showing myelin-like figures (M) which are surrounded by a thin membrane and amorphous aggregation of granular material free in the cytoplasm and presumed to be bilirubin (B) (×22 000; reproduced at 67%).

stances and the volume of fluid contributed via this pathway is not certain. The biliary tree itself can add and remove components from the bile, including water. The larger bile ducts and the gallbladder secrete a glycoprotein-rich mucus from goblet cells and adnexal glands. All the fluid contributions are diminished or cease in severe cholestasis except formation of mucus which amounts to about 1 ml/day.

Transmembrane transport mechanisms

To maintain intrahepatocellular homeostasis as well as to provide the hepatocytes with the materials with which to form bile, several mechanisms exist in the sinusoidal plasma membrane and in the canalicular membrane. These include ion pumps, ion channels, transporters, receptors, carriers, and signal transducers, with the energy for most of these derived from ATP. The inorganic ions moved are Na^+, K^+, H^+, Cl^-, HCO_3^-, Ca^{2+} and Mg^{2+}, with Na^+ being the most important as far as bile formation is concerned. A given ion may move in or out of the cell via some pathways but may move in only one direction in others. The energy is released from ATP by various ATPases, most of which are on the sinusoidal membrane but some are also on the canalicular membrane. The most important is the Na^+/K^+-ATPase located on the sinusoidal and the lateral membranes, its function being to remove sodium from the cell and bring potassium into it.[19,172] That Na^+/K^+-ATPase is on the canalicular membrane also has been claimed[202,260] and denied.[207,225] The Na^+, K^+-ATPase activity in canalicular membranes probably is of basolateral origin.[273] Bile salts, after attachment to receptors on the plasma membrane,[212] mainly in the periportal zone,[90] move into the cell along with Na^+[239] in a symport[58] or cotransport[104] system. The symport needs a sodium gradient,[24] which is created by the removal of sodium from the cell by the Na^+/K^+-ATPase.[55,238] Some of the sodium, however, is used for the bile salt-independent bile flow and thus the bile salt-dependent and independent flows are coupled.[59,88,141,202] Chloride pumps and bicarbonate secretion also contribute to bile salt-independent bile flow, although bicarbonate enters the hepatocyte via a Na^+/HCO_3^- cotransport system found on the sinusoidal membranes but not on the canaliculus.[186] Calcium movement in and out of the hepatocyte and into the canaliculus is carrier mediated and is driven by an ATPase which is independent of Mg^{2+} at least on the canalicular membrane.[20] When a hypocalcemic medium is perfused through the isolated liver, cholestasis results along with a decrease in hepatocellular volume.[276] This suggests that in this model, cholestasis is produced by disturbed osmotic equilibrium which impairs ion transport. Changes in pH due to the fluxes of the inorganic anions and cations and the organic anions are kept to a minimum by proton transport systems or antiports which are primarily pumps to move hydrogen ions, an energy-requiring process depending on a specific proton translocating ATPase. The sodium–proton exchange also occurs at the basolateral and not the canalicular membrane.[158] One Na^+/H^+ antiport is an 82-kD protein found in rat liver mitochondria.[140] Most of the ions move through channels in proteins in the plasma membrane. These proteins contain guanosine and are called G-proteins; their channels can be opened and closed by various endogenous or exogenous substances attaching to or leaving surface receptors.[26] The chloride channel is an interesting example.[54] On the cytoplasmic side of the membrane, signal transducers like the inositol phosphates and GTP along with some cytoskeletal elements direct material to the endoplasmic reticulum or the Golgi apparatus or the bile canaliculus. Organic anions other than bile salts get into the hepatocyte with the help

of specific receptors and carrier proteins within the plasma membrane. Some carriers transport whole classes of substances such as fatty acids, while others may be for single substances like bilirubin, although exogenous dyes seem to utilize the same pathway. How most of the components of bile are moved across the canalicular membrane is not known. Some are carried to the canalicular membrane in small vesicles directly from the sinusoidal surface. These include immunoglobulin A and horseradish peroxidase[95] while others go through the Golgi complex or lysosomes. Cholesterol for biliary excretion is also carried in vesicles.[237] Some biliary components may be moved by simple diffusion down a concentration gradient or sink created by the formation of micelles of bile salts. Micelle formation is not necessary for the transmembrane translocation of bile salts but an active transport system at the canaliculus is responsible.[168] Some ions are secreted by pumps since ATPases are located on the canalicular membrane. Epinephrine, by virtue of its alpha-adrenergic action, stimulates bile formation at the level of the canaliculus,[120] while somatostatin reduces bile flow.[137]

Bile salt-independent bile flow

This flow, ascribed to pressure rather than bile acid flux,[231] mainly develops in the perivenular region and does not contain bilirubin, other organic ions or exogenous dyes.[84,224] It is greater in rodents and rabbits than in man, in whom it is about 0.16 ml/min and represents 30–60% of basal bile flow. Basal secretion by hepatocytic couplets has been estimated to be 3.8 ± 1.3 fl/min; it rises fourfold after addition of bile salts and the secretion rate after bile salts is correlated with canalicular surface area before stimulation.[80] It is inhibited by ouabain and ethacrynic acid and, in contrast to bile salt-dependent flow, is increased by phenobarbital and theophylline. Glutathione may serve as a driving force of bile salt-independent bile flow.[10] The attempt to quantify the contribution to bile salt-independent bile flow made by paracellular fluid movement revealed that small inert molecules as well as macromolecules could gain either transcellular or paracellular access to bile depending on their charge.[93]

Bile salt-dependent bile flow

This portion of canalicular bile secretion rises on stimulation of bile flow by food. Bile salts enter the hepatocyte by crossing the canalicular membrane with the help of two membrane protein transporters, one of which requires cotransport with sodium. Some bile salts traverse the hepatocyte to the canaliculus in tiny vesicles[123,196] but this is not an important pathway. Taurocholate stimulates the transcytotic vesicular pathway through the hepatocyte.[265] This transit is not inhibited by colchicine and is probably not dependent on microtubules. Transcellular cytosolic transport, the major pathway, involves a carrier protein.[147] Vesicular transport is important for moving some proteins like immunoglobulin A into and through the hepatocytes and into the bile.[187] The Golgi zone may be the major terminus for most of these vesicles.[65] Cholestasis induced by ethinyl oestradiol does not affect vesicular transport.[85] Microfilaments and microtubules of the cytoskeleton, and the movement of calcium in and out of cells and organelles, regulated in part by calmodulin, probably play a role. Taurocholate and bilirubin glucuronide move through the hepatocyte by a cotransport mechanism which requires the aid of microtubules.[40] Thus, how bile salts move through the hepatocytes is not fully understood. Bile salts cross the canalicular membrane with the help of a 100-kD transport protein.[207] A 100 kD protein has been isolated from canalicular membranes which probably is responsible for transmembrane transport of bile acids into the bile.[274] The driving force seems to be the potential difference across the membrane. Glutathione may play a role in this secretion. Once in the canaliculus the bile salts aggregate to form micelles. This creates a micellar 'sink' providing a gradient along which the bile salts can move into the bile from the hepatocytes. Micelle formation may also create an osmotic gradient which moves water in or out of bile, mainly along the paracellular pathway across the tight junction.

Bile salt-dependent flow depends on the availability of bile salts for transport. Availability is determined by the blood level of bile salts, which is dependent on the enterohepatic circulation and by an active saturable transport system coupled with the Na^+/K^+-ATPase-dependent pump. Uptake is more efficient for trihydroxy bile salts than for dihydroxy ones and for conjugated bile salts than for unconjugated ones. Under normal circumstances hepatic uptake is more efficient than biliary excretion. The hepatocellular synthesis of bile salts is normally not quantitively significant in bile flow but it can be increased severalfold by removing bile salts from the enterohepatic circulation by external biliary drainage or by bile salt sequestrants like cholestyramine. The free cholesterol pool for bile salt synthesis is functionally unrelated to the pool from which VLDL and biliary cholesterol originate.[162]

Bile ductular flow

The bile ductules under normal circumstances both reabsorb an electrolyte-containing fluid and secrete one which is rich in bicarbonate. Ductular function does not develop until after birth[227] and the number of ducts does not reach normal until near the end of gestation.[110] Thus, premature babies may have a paucity of bile ducts with poor function of those present. Some of the electrolyte and water exchange takes place by a countercurrent mechanism since bile is slowly flowing in one direction and blood in adjacent arterioles and venules is flowing rapidly in the other direction. This exchange helps conserve needed cations and anions and modifies the composition of bile as it moves toward the intestine. The secretion is stimulated by secretin[117] and other hormones like vasoactive intestinal peptide[164] and provides an increment

of 150 ml/day in man to yield a total average bile flow of 600 ml/day. During cholestasis, only reabsorption may be occurring with uptake of components of bile like bilirubin and bile salts. The amount of bile flow in complete obstruction is equal to the rate of water reabsorption or about $0.2 \ ml^{-1} \ min^{-1} \ g^{-1}$ liver.[226] This reabsorption supports the observations of continued hepatocellular secretion even though no bile reaches the intestine; a hepatocellular–ductular circulation is thus operative. Hepatocytes in all zones of the acinus participate in secretion after experimental bile duct ligation and the proliferated bile ductules all participate in reabsorption.[29] The possibility of ductular cell metaplasia to hepatocytes has been proposed and also questioned.[275] Support for the concept of metaplasia comes from the demonstration of neuroendocrine features of some ductular cells in cholestasis; granules in these cells may play a regulatory role in ductular metaplasia.[271]

Bile salt metabolism in initiation of cholestasis

Both bile salt-dependent and independent flows may be inhibited in cholestasis; agents such as lithocholate and oestrogens diminish both. Impairing bile salt-independent flow by ethinyl oestradiol reduces the number of strands in the tight junction, thereby increasing its leakiness. Thus, reduction of bile salt-independent flow may reduce bile salt-dependent flow by lowering the sodium gradient. Diminishing bile salt-dependent flow by any means produces the structural changes characteristic of cholestasis. That cholestasis reflects impaired bile salt secretion was first illustrated by experiments with lithocholate which produced the structural and functional features of cholestasis. Whether this cholestasis is the result of deposition of lithocholate in the canalicular plasma membrane, thereby increasing its stiffness and also its cholesterol content or is the result of lithocholate being a poor micelle former either inside the cell or in the canalicular lumen is not known. Newborns are less susceptible to lithocholate-induced cholestasis probably because the immature liver has a reduced capacity to secrete this bile acid.[235] The cholestatic potency of taurolithocholate is less when it is perfused backward in the isolated liver possibly because of increased biotransformation in the perivenular zone and because the reduction in bile flow is greater with periportal canalicular changes than with perivenular ones.[14]

While the study of lithocholate cholestasis had major heuristic value in emphasizing the role of bile salts in cholestasis, the theory that primary alterations of bile salt metabolism cause cholestasis now has little support. Bile salts are formed from cholesterol by the microsomal biotransformation system in the smooth endoplasmic reticulum. Preferential formation of dihydroxy bile salts and synthesis of monohydroxy bile salts were postulated to occur in cholestasis and monohydroxy bile salts were found in the meconium and urine of neonates with cholestasis.[8] However, alterations of microsomal biotransformation with reduced haemoprotein synthesis but with normal degradation occur later in cholestasis. Thus, the alterations of the endoplasmic reticulum are the result rather than the cause of cholestasis. Nevertheless, permeability of the endoplasmic reticulum to calcium changes before any structural damage is noted.[6,36] Whether the increased calcium is from intracellular and extracellular sources is argued but changes in organelle calcium concentrations may be important factors in cholestasis.

An important factor in the initiation of cholestasis is the reduction of the amount of bile salts available to the hepatocytes in hepatocellular injury. Damage to the sinusoidal and lateral plasma membranes of the hepatocytes impairs uptake of bile salts from the portal blood. Furthermore, the transport proteins for bile salts on the membranes and within the cytoplasm may be decreased. Thus, the enterohepatic circulation is not only interrupted by reduced canalicular bile secretion but also by reduced hepatic bile salt uptake. Cholate and chenodeoxycholate blood levels are increased in cholestasis, in part because of reduced uptake but also because of leakage from hepatocytes. Secretion into the blood can occur as a result of loss of polarity of hepatocytes and leakage can occur across loosened tight junctions. The bioelectric sinusoidal-canalicular barrier is rapidly dissipated after bile duct ligation although sinusoidal bile salt uptake continues; this provides evidence for loss of polarity of the hepatocyte with resulting secretion back into the blood.[38] Most of the excess bile salts are sulphated in the liver and excreted in the urine. Sulphation increases bile flow and may protect against the toxic effect of high concentrations of bile salts.[259] The net reduction in the amount of bile salts available to the hepatocytes from reduced uptake is exaggerated by reduction in bile salt synthesis from cholesterol due to hepatocellular damage possibly caused by the detergent action of bile salts bound to specific intracellular sites.

Sites of initiation of cholestasis

Cholestasis may begin because of changes in the sinusoidal or canalicular plasma membrane, the cytoskeleton of the hepatocyte, the tight junction, the endoplasmic reticulum just discussed, or in bile ducts and ductules (Table 15.1). The probability is that cholestasis may begin at one site under one circumstance from a single change with all the other changes following the first one.[207] Under different circumstances another site may be where cholestasis is initiated. Thus, deciding cause and effect may be difficult.

Alterations in the plasma membrane

The plasma membranes have different receptors for some of the substances to be excreted into the bile, transport proteins, several ion pumps and ion channels. The canalicular membrane has some but not all of these components and has been less well studied because of difficulties in purification. Nevertheless, changes have been found in the

Table 15.1 Possible sites of initiation of cholestasis

1. No bile acid transport into the bile canaliculus
   (a) Deficient 100-kD carrier protein
   (b) Deficient energy (potential/glutathione) for transport
   (c) Inadequate gradient across canaliculus

2. Altered canalicular membrane
   (a) Membrane fluidity decreased
   (b) Membrane permeability changed
   (c) Inhibition of ion exchange (Cl^-/HCO_3^-)

3. Cytoskeletal changes
   (a) Actin microfilament disruption/aggregation
       (i) Diminished peristaltic activity
       (ii) Canalicular dilatation
   (b) Microtubular malfunction/depolymerization

4. Cytoplasmic changes
   (a) Loss of cell polarity
   (b) Inhibition of transcytotic vesicle pathway
   (c) Hypoactive endoplasmic reticulum
   (d) Malfunction of Golgi apparatus
   (e) Increased lysosomal activity

5. Sinusoidal membrane alterations
   (a) Diminished activity of Na^+/K^+-ATPase
   (b) Diminished proton antiport (Na^+/H^+) activity
   (c) Reduced Na^+-dependent bile acid transport
   (d) Reduced Na^+-independent bile acid transport

6. Leaky tight junctions

7. Proliferated ductules with increased permeability

canalicular membrane histochemically and biochemically. Ectoenzymes in the membrane like magnesium-dependent ATPase and 5′-nucleotidase are reduced, while alkaline phosphatase is increased. These enzymes are located in the deeper layers of the glycocalyx, the carbohydrate-rich covering of the canalicular microvilli. The enzyme gamma glutamyl transferase rises earlier in intrahepatic cholestasis than in obstructive jaundice and is visualized on canaliculi after it appears in ductules.[28] The increase of gamma glutamyl transferase in serum occurring in cholestasis may be of biliary cell origin rather than from hepatocytes, the presumed source of alkaline phosphatase.[263] Reduction in the amount of the 100-kD bile salt carrier protein, dissipation of the potential difference across the membrane and diminution of membrane fluidity are all possible first events in cholestasis.

Na^+/K^+-ATPase activity and the fluidity of the sinusoidal plasma membrane are reduced in cholestasis.[216] The sialic acid content is increased and the amount and proportions of cholesterol and phospholipid are altered.[111] Increased cholesterol seems to be one of the main changes of the canalicular membrane although different substances producing cholestasis do not all have the same effect. Thus, the function of the canalicular membrane is reduced in cholestasis, partly by a change in transport systems, partly by a change in fluidity[115] or permeability,[217] partly by reduction of membrane-associated enzyme activity and partly by diminution of the driving forces within the hepatocyte as well as by raised intraluminal pressure and alterations of paracellular flow. Since all these mechanisms may be interrelated, they are all probably operative in cholestasis and any one may be the site of initiation depending on the responsible agent.

Changes in microfilaments
The cytoskeleton below the plasma membrane consists of rigid intermediate filaments, microtubules and contractile microfilaments of actin and myosin.[201,256] The cytoskeleton not only facilitates biliary secretion by peristaltic action but also maintains the shape and tone of the plasma membrane. When membranes are reorganized in tissue culture, magnesium ATPase is lost and re-established at the new canaliculus; microfilament but not microtubule function is needed for this reorganization.[79] Microfilament function may be more important in the canalicular portion of the plasma membrane than in the rest of it. Cytochalasin B, which specifically alters microfilaments, produces cholestasis[108,149] and cholestatic analogues of sex steroids inhibit microfilament action. Microfilaments are aggregated in bundles in the pericanalicular cytoplasm and in ductular cells in human and experimental cholestasis from many causes.[2,63,103] Microtubules have been related to lipid secretion at the canalicular membrane. Intermediate filaments increase in hepatocytes after biliary obstruction, especially around the dilated canaliculi but not in ductules.[166]

Leaky tight junctions
The tight junction between hepatocytes permits passage of some small molecules. It is normally composed of several strands which are closely interconnected but which surround the canalicular membrane in a parallel fashion.[128] The strands effectively seal the canaliculus, although some water and small ions or molecules may traverse the tortuous path the strands create in the junction.[47,192] Normally the strands average five in number, but in cholestasis they are reduced to an average of two and are not as tightly aggregated. Therefore, water and small solutes can more easily travel from the canaliculus back to the bloodstream.[57]

Cytoskeleton fibres condense at the tight junction, which also has an adjacent mitochondrion suggesting a local energy-dependent process. Phalloidin increases the visibility of actin filaments around the tight junction.[56] It weakens the plasma membrane, producing invaginations into hepatocytes and local protrusions from isolated cells depending on the hydrostatic pressure. Phalloidin influences the tight junction, permitting more fluid to enter or leave the bile canaliculus from or to the perisinusoidal space. This fluid seems to move mainly out of the bile in cholestasis. The leaky tight junction may be the site of increased permeability of the bile canaliculus and biliary pressure appears to be the most specific determinant of this permeability.[231] The movement of fluid at this site might explain the preservation of microvilli

at the tight junction as well as shortening of the intercellular space. The changes described in tight junctions in experimental cholestasis have also been found in human intrahepatic cholestasis.[143]

Portal and bile duct changes
Bile ducts, ductules and portal tracts are usually altered in cholestasis. The microcirculation in the portal tracts may be changed, with arterial flow increasing over venous flow. Oedema often develops and may create a mechanical obstructive component by compressing ducts or ductules. Ductules appear distorted in protracted cholestasis and they have cytoplasmic vacuoles which frequently contain bile, as evidence of their reabsorbing capability even in complete obstruction. The hepatoductular circulation provides sufficient bile flow in the periportal region to prevent stagnation of bile and bile thrombi here. Bile ducts and ductules increase in prolonged cholestasis. Proliferating ductules either sprout from ducts as a reaction to inflammation (when they are flattened cylinders on three-dimensional reconstruction), or by lengthening in response to increased intraluminal pressure. When the proliferative stimulus is removed, the extra ductular cells are rapidly removed by apoptosis with shedding of the cellular pieces into the bile.[12] Lengthening involves small ducts also and produces tortuosity. The bile ducts are mainly on the periphery of the portal tract in biliary obstruction, while proliferated bile ductules fill and enlarge the portal tract in stage 2 of primary biliary cirrhosis. Proliferated ductules are first surrounded by inflammatory exudate and later by thickened collagen bundles. The stimulus for the proliferation and alteration of the ductules is not known. Ultrastructural changes are found in lithocholate-induced cholestasis at a time when the canalicular changes are recovering. Ductular proliferation and alterations, as well as periductular inflammation and fibrosis, develop with prolonged administration of lithocholate.

Causes of bile canalicular dilatation
The most important factor in bile canalicular dilatation, the hallmark of cholestasis, is reduced membrane tone, either from cytoskeletal—mainly microfilament—failure or changes in membrane fluidity owing to alteration of the lipid composition. The slowing of bile flow is another factor in which bile thrombi and membrane blebs may contribute. Impairment of flow in ductules and ducts in the portal tracts because of oedema, inflammation or fibrosis may cause dilatation late. Increasing bile flow by administration of bile salts may also cause dilatation.

Mechanical factors within the liver which may contribute to cholestasis include compression of bile ducts in swollen, inflamed or fibrotic portal tracts, increased tortuosity of the proliferated biliary system and bile duct destruction as part of viral hepatitis, biliary cirrhosis or transplantation rejection. The combination of all these may convert metabolic intrahepatic cholestasis into obstructive jaundice.[181]

Cholestasis from medication (see Chapter 46)

So many drugs of different types have produced cholestasis that it is not possible even to list them here. Several mechanisms operate in cholestatic drug reactions.[121,211] Anabolic and oestrogenic steroids compete for organic anion secretion, inhibit the Na$^+$/K$^+$-ATPase pump and possibly other pumps, stimulate biotransformation, deposit in the canalicular membrane and stiffen it, change actin polymerization and distribution and increase tight junction permeability. Changes in membrane fluidity caused by oestrogens can also be caused by spironolactone; however, bile flow is not affected, suggesting that this is not the major determinant of oestrogen cholestasis. Chlorpromazine and related drugs, particularly their metabolites, also reduce ATPase activity,[115,228] complex with bile salts to disturb micelle formation and interfere with calcium movement.[201] Chlorpromazine, in addition, reduces cholesterol in the sinusoidal membrane and dilates the endoplasmic reticulum and canaliculi in cultured hepatocytes.[107] Experimental cholestasis induced by somatostatin reduces secretion of bile salts and bile flow but not bilirubin output,[119] suggesting that the pathway for bilirubin transfer into bile is different from that for bile salts and therefore that cholestasis involves change in more than one pathway.[189]

Chronic or at least very protracted cholestasis can be initiated by several drugs such as chlorpromazine, prochlorperazine,[133] thiobendazole,[139] and troleandomycin.[124] Combinations of drugs that can affect the liver like chlorpromazine and valproic acid can lead to progressive cholestatic liver disease, ultimately requiring transplantation[7] as did thiobendazole alone.[139]

EFFECT OF CHOLESTASIS ON HEPATOCYTES

Although the mechanism of cholestasis remains obscure, the consequences are better understood. Of major importance is retention of bile salts and bilirubin in the hepatocytes. Phospholipid retention leads to deposition of myelin-figures in the cytoplasm but probably is more a morphological marker than injurious; the same is true for cholesterol crystals in the cytosol. Bilirubin in the intracellular concentrations found in cholestasis decreases oxygen uptake by hepatic mitochondria and uncouples oxidative phosphorylation. Bilirubin in brain cells depresses phosphorylation of synaptic proteins and nuclear histones.[157] Haemoprotein synthesis is decreased and haem catabolism is increased.[200] The function of cytochrome P-450[180] is decreased as is aminopyrine demethylase,[258] but the results of the aminopyrine breath test do not correlate with the severity of cholestasis.[9] Hepatic mitochondrial cytochromes are decreased, which may relate to altered carbohydrate metabolism. The alteration in carbohydrate metabolism is in part related to a

reduction in the number of β-adrenoceptors and inhibition of adrenaline (epinephrine)-stimulated glycogenolysis by propranolol in the bile duct-ligated rat[3] and is in part due to pancreatic endocrine dysfunction.[165] Glycogenolysis in the normal rat liver, by constrast, is inhibited by α-adrenergic blockers such as phentolamine. Bile salt excess causes curling of mitochondrial cristae before jaundice develops. Mitochondrial aspartate aminotransferase is increased in extrahepatic cholestasis and in alcohol-induced liver injury, probably reflecting the mitochondrial damage seen in both conditions.[92]

Bile salt retention is probably the most important consequence of cholestasis. Competitive binding of dihydroxy and trihydroxy bile salts to microsomes, as shown in experimental animals, inhibits biotransformation of drugs in cholestasis. Greater concentrations of bile salts lead to a dose-dependent detergent action on microsomes. Dihydroxy bile salts are more effective detergents than trihydroxy bile salts and unconjugated ones more than conjugated ones. Exposure of microsomes to bile salts *in vitro* results in their gradual disintegration with reduction of cytochrome P-450, inhibition of its reductase, destruction of its lipoprotein-binding site, and transformation into an inactive form. Since determination of bile salts in liver tissue does not reflect the relative amounts in cytoplasm, blood and bile, the observation that the hepatic bile salt concentration in rats with ligated bile ducts reaches only levels causing competitive binding may not reflect what is occurring at specific intracellular sites. After prolonged biliary obstruction in man, levels of dihydroxy bile salts are high enough to have a detergent action.

Cholestasis affects the rough endoplasmic reticulum in addition to the smooth form. Synthesis of some proteins, particularly of lipoproteins, is increased in rats. This may account also for the high amounts of cholesterol-rich lipoprotein-X (LP-X), the microsomal synthesis of which is raised in cholestasis.[197,249] This lipoprotein artefactually raises the blood level of high-density lipoproteins, often to strikingly high values. Excess bile salts also solubilize canalicular membrane components, particularly phospholipids, leading to the appearance in the blood of abnormal membranous components. Solubilization also explains in part the increased release to the blood of ectoenzymes such as alkaline phosphatase. Study of the isoenzymes of alkaline phosphatase showed that one is derived from membranes but another arises in the cytoplasm,[204] the synthesis of the latter being enhanced after bile duct ligation.[206] The membrane alkaline phosphatase is the major protein phosphatase of the plasma membrane[32] and some of the hepatocytic dysfunction may be the result of loss of this enzyme activity.

The histological change in the cytoplasm in cholestasis is rarefaction of the cytoplasm with formation of a network of brown strands called feathery degeneration. The rarefactions correspond electron microscopically to myelin-like figures. This lesion, which involves isolated cells in perivenular cholestasis, is explained by the detergent action of bile salts since its intensity parallels the tissue content of dihydroxy bile salts. An identical lesion is seen in renal tubules with bile salt retention. Another effect, representing hydration more than feathery degeneration, is caused by alterations in the tubulin of microtubules. The swollen appearance of such hepatocytes is similar to those in alcoholic liver injury, in which an antitubulin effect has been demonstrated, resulting in retention of proteins secreted by the hepatocyte. Moreover, cytoplasmic deposits of Mallory's hyalin are noted in prolonged cholestasis. Hyalin has been produced in mice by griseofulvin, which can also cause cholestasis and alters the activities of some microsomal enzymes. Mallory's hyalin consists mainly of aggregated intermediate filaments either produced in excess or inadequately utilized; chemically it is mainly cytokeratin.

Feathery degeneration proceeds to single cell necrosis associated with focal reactive inflammation. This inflammatory reaction caused by cholestasis can be differentiated from that in viral hepatitis by its restriction to the cholestatic zone. Intralobular inflammation, usually perivenular, is accompanied by reactive portal inflammation. Ductular alterations with proliferation as well as fibrosis are caused by the effects of cholestasis itself and of portal inflammation. The portal reaction persists after subsidence of cholestasis of any aetiology and is the lesion seen between episodes of recurrent benign cholestasis. This 'cholangiolitis' is the result of cholestasis, and not its cause, in almost all situations.

Eventually, portal and periportal fibrosis can develop in any form of cholestasis. The first type of collagen to appear in both man and experimental animals is the more pliable type III, which largely corresponds to reticulin, soon followed by the formation of hard, doubly refractile type I collagen which causes scarring fibrosis around bile ducts and ductules. If severe enough, the scarring interferes mechanically with ductular and ductal bile flow and produces a mechanical intrahepatic obstructive component in any prolonged cholestasis. Periportal or zone 1 cholestasis results. This varies in intensity throughout the liver but is more uniform around the portal tract than perivenular cholestasis is around the efferent veins. Destruction of the layer of hepatocytes around the portal tracts, with relatively little but often neutrophilic leukocytic inflammation (biliary piecemeal necrosis), leads to apparent enlargement of the portal tracts. The lesion need not be associated with conspicuous bile pigment accumulation, although it shows 'feathery degeneration' and is presumably 'cholate-stasis'. Copper and copper-binding proteins, demonstrable by staining with rhodanine or orcein respectively, accumulate in the periportal cells. Periportal cholestasis associated with portal and periportal scarring is the lesion seen in later stages of primary biliary cirrhosis, in other conditions associated with bile duct lesions and in rare instances of sarcoidosis.[175] It may account for residual impairment of biliary secretion following successful surgical correction of extrahepatic mechanical obstruction. It probably represents the end stage of

prolonged cholestasis, which is initially free of liver cell injury or obstruction, for instance in hereditary infantile cholestasis. All these conditions, including uncorrected or infected biliary obstruction, strictures, sclerosing cholangitis and atresia, eventually terminate in biliary cirrhosis from which the original aetiology cannot be ascertained.

Periportal cholestasis must be distinguished from ductal cholestasis, which is often associated with dense bile deposits or microliths in ductules. This results from dehydration or reduced blood flow in the agonal period, usually in liver disease, but does not necessarily reflect jaundice. It is also characteristic of septicaemia. Cellular immunity is defective in cholestasis[195] and procoagulant activity is increased[208] both resulting from dysfunction of macrophages and monocytes directly due to the cholestasis. This may contribute to the high incidence of infection in obstructive jaundice.

DIAGNOSIS

Cholestasis often presented diagnostic problems which took many days to resolve, at considerable expense and the use of invasive procedures. Different strategies have been recommended, including a single target strategy exploring one diagnostic hypothesis only,[131] decision theory,[130] clinical decision analysis,[190] and computer models.[81,138] This attempt at devising various protocols has brought the warning 'keep your eye on the welfare of the patient rather than on the diagnostic process'.[240] Here the individual components of the diagnostic approach to the patient are reviewed and a simplified scheme is offered to serve as a guide for the clinician.

CLINICAL OBSERVATIONS

Cholestasis by itself does not produce the usual clinical manifestations of acute and chronic liver disease such as malaise and fatiguability. The only specific systemic manifestation in cholestasis is pruritus, which was originally thought to be due to intradermal deposition of bile salts. Trihydroxy bile salts were held responsible, but later dihydroxy ones were incriminated. Biochemical and clinical studies have cast doubt on this mechanism of pruritus.[34,72] The pruritus of cholestasis may be the result of increased availability of endogenous opiate ligands at central opiate receptors.[266]

The history in the jaundiced patient is of great help in ascertaining factors pointing to viral hepatitis, alcohol intake, and exposure to drugs or chemicals. Chills and fever, anorexia and loss of taste for cigarettes are not diagnostic. A family history of gallstones or anaemia favours gallstone disease. Cutaneous stigmata of liver disease suggest intrahepatic disease. Right upper quadrant pain and also back pain point to an obstructive disorder. A grossly enlarged and very tender liver is seldom seen in extrahepatic obstruction, while a mass or an enlarged gallbladder is the most significant feature indicating either obstruction or tumour.

LABORATORY FINDINGS (see Chapter 18) _____

Since the basic lesion in cholestasis is the same in the mechanical form and in the metabolic one, the likelihood of developing a biochemical laboratory test to separate the two is small. Most test results reflect the intensity and degree of cholestasis rather than its aetiology. Testing for conjugated rather than direct bilirubin in neonates may be more helpful in following developing or resolving cholestasis.[169] The most reliable laboratory indicator of cholestasis is increased activity of alkaline phosphatase. Attempts have been made to determine specific isoenzymes.[219] Elevation of the isoenzyme associated with hyperbilirubinaemia suggests an intrahepatic cause.[244] Alkaline phosphatase activity is not always significantly elevated in malignant obstruction. Elevation out of proportion to bilirubin suggests primary biliary cirrhosis, granulomatosis, a space-occupying lesion, obstruction of one main bile duct, or a stone in the common duct. It also may be a manifestation of a systemic infection.[64] Elevation of bilirubin without an appropriate increase in alkaline phosphatase activity suggests an increased supply of bilirubin from haemolysis, Dubin–Johnson or Rotor's syndrome, or the early stages of viral hepatitis. Gamma glutamyl transferase activity parallels that of alkaline phosphatase except in alcoholics, where gamma-GT may be more elevated, while in jaundice due to sex steroids or pregnancy it tends to be normal. The activities of leucine aminopeptidase and 5′-nucleotidase also usually parallel that of alkaline phosphatase, except that the former is elevated in pancreatic diseases even without cholestasis. When measured in rat serum and liver after bile duct ligation, the activities of alkaline phosphatase, gamma-GT, and 5′-nucleotidase do not parallel each other. Simultaneous elevation of liver and bone alkaline phosphatase raises the suspicion of a malignant lesion with bone metastases. The activities of aminotransferases, aspartate aminotransferase (AST) more than alanine aminotransferase (ALT), are elevated in pure cholestasis, although far less than that of alkaline phosphatase. Relatively high aminotransferase activities are found in early cholestasis and stone obstruction and then decline rapidly. Serum protein partition is not significantly altered in pure cholestasis. Gamma globulin need not be elevated but, in prolonged cholestasis, beta globulins rise. Total cholesterol is often high, while cholesterol esters are not reduced. Many other biochemical tests have been recommended, but most of them, like determination of LP-X, have little value in the separation of aetiological factors. Some hints may be obtained from older tests. For instance, the sedimentation rate is low in viral hepatitis but normal or high in other liver and biliary tract diseases. Very high levels suggest malignancy or bacterial infections. Leukocytosis characterizes infected biliary obstruction, alcoholic hepatitis, and massive hepatic necrosis. Hyper-glycaemia suggests pancreatic carcinoma in the absence of long-standing diabetes. Serum bile salt levels are greatly increased in cholestasis. Glycocholate and taurocholate levels increase earliest, while conjugated chenodeoxycholate become higher as hepatocellular function becomes impaired by protracted cholestasis. Deoxycholate levels decrease while lithocholate levels remain unchanged. Binding to serum proteins of glycocholate and, less so, of glycochenodeoxycholate is reduced in cholestasis, binding of the former being inversely related to the serum bilirubin level.[35]

HISTOLOGICAL FEATURES (see Chapter 19) _____

Large bile duct obstruction is suggested by oedema of the portal tracts, tortuosity of bile ducts and ductules, location of ductules with cuboidal epithelium close to the margin of the portal tracts, and numerous fibroblasts and segmented leukocytes in the portal tracts. None of these findings is pathognomonic.

The following features are of little diagnostic significance in cholestasis: perivenular or peripheral feathery degeneration, ductular proliferation and alteration, vacuolization of peripheral hepatocytes, intraparenchymal foam cells and any type of inflammation. More reliable are features developing after prolonged obstruction. These include extravasation of bile from bile ducts, often with granuloma formation, and biliary necrotic foci or bile infarcts near the portal tracts. Small extravasations of bile in the parenchyma, as well as small or 'micro' bile infarcts remote from portal tracts, also occur in various forms of intrahepatic cholestasis, particularly in late primary biliary cirrhosis. Segmented leukocytes intermixed with mononuclear inflammatory cells around proliferated bile ductules do not point to any specific aetiology. They indicate infection only if they are the prominent infiltrating cells within the epithelium or lumen of the bile ducts. If neutrophil leukocytes are absent, the intensity of the portal inflammation serves as a preliminary indicator. A conspicuous reaction in the first 3 weeks of jaundice favours intrahepatic cholestasis; it is absent only in the form induced by sex steroids. By contrast, intense portal inflammation after 3 weeks of cholestasis suggests large bile duct obstruction, since in both viral and drug-induced cholestasis the portal inflammation has usually subsided. However, errors in the histological evaluation are common. Enthusiasm for histological differential diagnosis of cholestasis has waned with the development of more decisive physical imaging techniques, especially percutaneous or endoscopic cholangiography and sonography.[145]

Two specific problems deserve mention. First, with direct-reacting hyperbilirubinaemia without histological cholestasis and with normal hepatocytic structure, an early stage of primary biliary cirrhosis or Rotor's syndrome should be considered. Secondly, cholestasis in a biopsy specimen in the absence of jaundice suggests a nearby tumour.

PHYSICAL IMAGING METHODS (see Chapters 22, 23, 24 and 25) _____

Cholestasis established by clinical and laboratory examinations without recognized aetiology calls for a series of procedures, depending on the availability of equipment and the skill of the examiner. These include cholangiography, either endoscopic retrograde cholangiopancreatography (ERCP)[144] or percutaneous transhepatic cholangiography using a thin flexible needle.[160] The latter localizes the upper end of the obstruction, which is important for surgical relief but the former is being more widely used.[218] Transjugular cholangiography is also possible. Ultrasonography, an inexpensive non-invasive and risk-free procedure, is increasingly being used as an initial study.[42,167] A randomized controlled trial showed ultrasound to be superior to computed tomography. Ultrasound may often be all that is needed for diagnosis, especially if real-time techniques are used.[151,167] The roles of magnetic resonance imaging and positron emission tomography have not been established in the differential diagnosis of jaundice. Radioisotope scanning after injection of dyes secreted in the bile in sufficient quantity to be visualized in the presence of incomplete obstruction may localize the cause of the cholestasis or disclose the patency of the biliary tree.[113] Non-excretion of radionuclide on cholescintigraphy usually means complete obstruction.[171] Technetium scanning with biopsy into a cold area, computed tomography and selected coeliac angiography are useful. Simultaneous use of hepatobiliary scintigraphy and the string test is helpful in the evaluation of neonatal cholestasis.[194] Laparoscopy is recommended by those with experience in the procedure. Radiological studies with barium should not be performed since the barium may interfere with the more definitive procedures. Exploratory laparotomy can no longer be justified.

LIVER BIOPSY (see Chapter 19) _____

A high percentage of biopsy differential diagnoses of cholestasis are correct when made by experienced pathologists. While the risk of biliary peritonitis with liver biopsy in extrahepatic biliary obstruction is small, the greater accuracy and greater safety of the imaging procedures make liver biopsy in cholestasis a procedure that should be conducted only after mechanical obstruction has been excluded.

A SIMPLE PROTOCOL FOR APPROACHING THE CLINICAL PROBLEM OF CHOLESTASIS _____

(1)   Check urine for bilirubin and serum for direct and indirect reacting bilirubin.

(2)   If bilirubin is mainly indirect-reacting (unconjugated) and the urine is free of bilirubin, screen for haemolysis (reticulocytes, haptoglobin). If no haemolysis is found, further investigation is unnecessary and a diagnosis of a variant of Gilbert's disease can be made.

(3)   If the urine contains bilirubin and the serum bilirubin is mainly direct-reacting, check AST, ALT, alkaline phosphatase, gamma-GT, serum protein electrophoresis, and acute hepatitis markers and mitochondrial, smooth muscle and antinuclear antibodies.

(a) If everything but the bilirubin is normal, undertake a liver biopsy to look for the pigment of the Dubin–Johnson syndrome.

(b) If the activities of the aminotransferases are greater than 5 times normal after a week but that of alkaline phosphatase is less than 3 times normal and gamma globulin is normal with negative immunological studies, the cholestasis is probably due to viral, chemical (drug), or alcoholic hepatitis. A liver biopsy facilitates recognition of alcoholic hepatitis. If the gamma globulin level is high, especially IgG, a liver biopsy should be carried out to diagnose chronic hepatitis with or without cirrhosis.

(c) If the activities of the aminotransferases are less than 5 times normal after a week but that of alkaline phosphatase (and gamma-GT) are more than 3 times normal, a variant of intrahepatic cholestasis should be distinguished from large bile duct obstruction. Pruritus is a usual complaint, and serum cholesterol is elevated. Sonography, and endoscopic or percutaneous cholangiography should be used until an obstruction is found or the biliary tree is seen to be normal. Computed tomography should be used only if an abnormality found by sonography cannot be clearly defined. An upper gastrointestinal radiological study with barium is not likely to be helpful, and in most cases should not be ordered. Under any circumstances, barium studies should be delayed until the imaging studies are complete. If no obstruction is found, the diagnosis is intrahepatic cholestasis. A liver biopsy should be performed to see whether alcoholic or viral hepatitis is present, and the drug history should be re-investigated.

(d) If the diagnostic features in (c) are present with a normal biliary tree, and mitochondrial antibody is found, IgM should be determined, and a liver biopsy should be obtained to diagnose primary biliary cirrhosis.

(e) Scanning or sonographic areas suggestive of a space-occupying lesion, in addition to the features described in (c), should lead to directed liver biopsy to detect metastases.

THERAPY

Therapeutic or palliative drainage to relieve biliary obstruction can be carried out surgically[174] as well as percutaneously[106] or endoscopically,[39,91] or combined[234] but its ultimate value has been challenged.[163] Various endoscopic approaches may be preferable for geriatric patients, in whom the mortality rate of surgical intervention is high.[41] The endoscopically placed biliary stents may become clogged, usually with bacteria.[122] This leads to diagnostic problems in explaining increasing cholestasis and may require replacement of the stent. No effective therapy exists for intrahepatic cholestasis. Phenobarbital reduces the bilirubin level in some forms of jaundice, especially in infants. High doses of S-adenosyl methionine has been said to reverse the cholestasis of pregnancy.[77] This substance restores bile flow, Na⁺,K⁺-ATPase activity and membrane fluidity in ethinyl oestradiol-induced cholestasis[21] and protected rats against alpha-naphthyl-isothiocyanate-induced cholestasis.[50] Short-term administration of S-adenosyl methionine by mouth improved the clinical and laboratory features of cholestasis in patients with various liver diseases as shown in a double-blind, placebo-controlled study.[264] Corticosteroids do not influence the course of the disease but often reduce the bilirubin level in any variety of jaundice.[77] They may alter bilirubin metabolism by increasing production of non-pigmented metabolites and by increasing shortened red-cell survival. Ursodeoxycholic acid, a naturally occurring bile acid now being extensively tested in primary biliary cirrhosis[13,182] is also being tested in other forms of cholestatic jaundice.[184,261,262] The widespread use of urso-deoxycholic acid in cholestatic liver diseases has raised concern about its relation to lithocholic acid which can cause cholestasis as well as hepatocellular toxicity. Co-infusion of ursodeoxycholic acid and lithocholic acid prevented lithocholate cholestasis and hepatotoxicity which should minimize fear of long-term adverse effects of ursodeoxycholic acid administration.[272] Tin protoporphyrin lowers serum bilirubin by interfering with its synthesis via reduction of haem oxygenase activity.[53] Hyperbilirubinaemia in the neonate has been treated with

phototherapy or exchange transfusions. Attempts are being made to lower serum bilirubin levels with the use of an immobilized bilirubin detoxifying enzyme placed in an extracorporeal circuit.[126] Whether this treatment will be useful in cholestasis needs to be established. Cholestyramine relieves pruritus, presumably by binding bile salts in the gut, but it is not recommended when the serum bilirubin level is above 171 μmol/l (10 mg/dl). Hypolipidaemic drugs such as clofibrate are contraindicated in liver disease; in primary biliary cirrhosis they have a paradoxical hypercholesterolaemic effect. Anabolic steroids, although they relieve itching, accentuate jaundice. Fat-soluble vitamins can be given parenterally or orally in a water-soluble form. The preferred preparation of vitamin D is 25-hydroxycholecalciferol or 1,25-dihydroxycholecalciferol. The liver is responsible for 25-hydroxylation of vitamin D, a function depressed in some liver diseases in addition to malabsorption of the vitamin. Calcium supplements may also be needed in chronic cholestasis. However, the bone disease of primary biliary cirrhosis, which is mainly osteoporosis, responds poorly to 25-hydroxyvitamin D and calcium.[96,142] By contrast, this therapy may be useful in preventing the bone disease of chronic childhood cholestasis.[97] Whether fluoride is helpful in preventing the bone changes secondary to cholestasis remains to be established. Absorption of vitamins A and K may also be impaired, and parenteral administration may be needed. Vitamin E supplements are useful in prolonged cholestasis, particularly in the presence of neuromuscular abnormalities. The postoperative renal failure that occasionally develops in patients with obstructive jaundice, possibly due to systemic endotoxaemia, may be prevented by use of lactulose, which binds to endotoxin in the gut.[170]

REFERENCES

1. Adinolfi, L.E., Utili, R., Gaeta, G.B. et al. (1984) Cholestasis induced by estradiol-17 β-D-glucuronide: mechanisms and prevention by sodium taurocholate. Hepatology, 4, 30–37.
2. Adler, M., Chung, K.W. & Schaffner, F. (1980) Pericanalicular hepatocytic and ductular microfilaments in cholestasis in man. American Journal of Pathology, 98, 603–616.
3. Aggerbeck, M., Ferry, N., Zafram, E.-S. et al. (1983) Adrenergic regulation of glycogenolysis in rat liver after cholestasis. Journal of Clinical Investigation, 71, 476–486.
4. Alagille, D., Estrada, A., Hadchouel, M. et al. (1987) Syndromatic paucity of intralobular bile ducts (Alagille syndrome or arterio-hepatic dysplasia): A review of 80 cases. Journal of Pediatrics, 110, 195–200.
5. Andrews, W.S., Wanek, W., Fyock, B. et al. (1989) Pediatric liver transplantation. A 3-year experience. Journal of Pediatric Surgery, 24, 77–82.
6. Anwer, M.S., Engelking, L.R., Nolan, K., Sullivan, D., Zimniak, P. & Lester, R. (1988) Hepatotoxic bile acids increase cytosolic Ca²⁺ activity of isolated rat hepatocytes. Hepatology, 8, 887–891.
7. Bach, N., Thung, S.N., Schaffner, F. & Tobias, H. (1989) Exaggerated cholestasis and hepatic fibrosis following simultaneous administration of chlorpromazine and sodium valproate. Digestive Diseases and Sciences, 34, 1303–1307.
8. Back, P. & Walter, K. (1980) Developmental pattern of bile and metabolism as revealed by bile acid analysis of meconium. Gastroenterology, 78, 671–676.
9. Baker, A.L., Krager, P.S., Kotake, A.N. & Schoeller, D.A. (1987) The aminopyrine breath test does not correlate with histologic disease severity in patients with cholestasis. Hepatology, 7, 464–467.
10. Ballatori, N. & Truong, A.T. (1989) Relation between biliary glutathione excretion and bile acid-independent bile flow. American Journal of Physiology, 256, G22–G30.
11. Bashour, T.T., Antonini, C., Sr & Fisher, J. (1985) Severe sinus node dysfunction in obstructive jaundice. Annals of Internal Medicine, 103, 384–385.
12. Bathal, P.S. & Gall, J.A.M. (1985) Deletion of hyperplastic biliary epithelial cells by apoptosis following removal of the proliferative stimulus. Liver, 5, 311–325.
13. Battan, A.K., Salen, G., Arora, R. et al. (1989) Effect of ursodeoxycholic acid on bile acid metabolism in primary biliary cirrhosis. Hepatology, 10, 414–419.
14. Baumgartner, U., Hardison, W.G.M. & Miyai, K. (1987) Reduced cholestatic potency of taurolithocholate during backward perfusion of rat liver. Laboratory Investigation, 56, 576–582.
15. Bedossa, P., Houry, S., Bacei, J. et al. (1989) A longitudinal study of histologic and immunohistologic changes in an experimental model of sclerosing cholangitis. Virchows Archiv A Pathologic Anatomy, 414, 165–171.
16. Benjamin, D.F. (1981) Hepatobiliary dysfunction in infants and children associated with long-term total parenteral nutrition. A clinico-pathologic study. American Journal of Clinical Pathology, 76, 276–283.
17. Bijleveld, C.M.A., Vonk, R.J., Kuipers, F. et al. (1989) Benign recurrent intrahepatic cholestasis: Altered bile acid metabolism. Gastroenterology, 97, 427–432.
18. Bijleveld, C.M.A., Vonk, R.J., Kuipers, F. et al. (1989) Benign recurrent intrahepatic cholestasis: A long-term follow-up study of two patients. Hepatology, 9, 532–537.

19. Blitzer, B.L. & Boyer, J.L. (1982) Cellular mechanisms of bile formation. *Gastroenterology*, **82**, 346–357.

20. Blitzer, B.L., Hostetler, B.R. & Scott, K.A. (1989) Hepatic adenosine triphosphate-dependent Ca^{2+} transport is mediated by distinct carriers on rat basolateral and canalicular membranes. *Journal of Clinical Investigation*, **83**, 1319–1325.

21. Boelsterli, U.A., Rakhit, G. & Balazs, T. (1983) Modulation by S-adenosyl-1-methionine of hepatic Na^+, K^+-ATPase, membrane fluidity, and bile flow in rats with ethinyl estradiol-induced cholestasis. *Hepatology*, **3**, 12–17.

22. Boelsterli, U.A., Abernathy, C.O., Balazs, T. & Zimmerman, J.H. (1982) Effects of endotoxin tolerance on hepatic excretory function: in vivo study. *Toxicology Letters* **11**, 207–212.

23. Böttger, T., Sorgeer, K. & Junginger, T.H. (1989) Die progressive Papillomatose der intra- und extrahepatischen Gallenwege. *Der Chirurg*, **60**, 110–114.

24. Boyer, J.L., Allen, R.M. & Ng, O.C. (1983) Biochemical separation of Na^+, K^+-ATPase from a 'purified' light density 'canalicular'-enriched plasma membrane fraction from rat liver. *Hepatology*, **3**, 18–28.

25. Boyer, J.L., Gautam, A. & Graf, J. (1988) Mechanisms of bile secretion: Insights from the isolated rat hepatocyte couplet. *Seminars in Liver Disease*, **8**, 308–316.

26. Brown, A.M. & Birnbaumer, L. (1989) Ion channels and G proteins. *Hospital Practice*, **24**, 189–204.

27. Buehler, H., Muench, R., Schmid, M. & Amman, R. (1985) Cholestasis in alcoholic pancreatitis. Diagnostic value of the transaminase ratio for differentiation between extra- and intra-hepatic cholestasis. *Scandinavian Journal of Gastroenterology*, **20**, 851–856.

28. Busachi, X., Mebis, J., Broeckaert, L. & Desmet, V. (1981) Histochemistry of γ-glutamyl transpeptidase in human liver biopsies. *Pathological Research Practice*, **172**, 99–108.

29. Buscher, H.-P., Miltonberger, C., MacNelly, S. & Gerok, W. (1989) The histoautoradiographic localization of taurocholate in rat liver after bile duct ligation. Evidence for ongoing secretion and reabsorption processes. *Journal of Hepatology*, **8**, 181–191.

30. Capron, J.-P., Gineston, J.-L., Herve, M.-A. & Braillon, A. (1983) Metronidazole in prevention of cholestasis associated with total parenteral nutrition. *Lancet*, **i**, 446–447.

31. Cardewell, R.J., Phillips, E. & Thomford, N.R. (1989) Idiopathic benign stricture of the common bile duct. *American Journal of Gastroenterology*, **84**, 56–58.

32. Chan, J.R.A. & Stinson, R.A. (1986) Dephosphorylation of phosphoproteins of human liver plasma membranes by endogenous and purified liver alkaline phosphatases. *Journal of Biological Chemistry*, **261**, 7635–7639.

33. Chapman, R.W.G., Arborgh, B.A.M., Rhodes, J.M. *et al.* (1980) Primary sclerosing cholangitis: a review of its clinical features, cholangiography, and hepatic histology. *Gut*, **21**, 870–877.

34. Chianale, J., Glasinovic, J.C., Lopez, J. *et al.* (1982) Evolucion del prurito en la cholestasia del embarazo y su relacion con la concentracion serica de acidos biliares. *Revista de Medicina de Chile*, **110**, 538–541.

35. Chitranukroh, A. & Billing, B.H. (1983) Changes in the binding of radioactive conjugated bile salts to serum proteins in cholestatic jaundice. *Clinical Science*, **65**, 77–84.

36. Combettes, L., Berthon, B., Claret, M. & Erlinger, S. (1989) Selective permeabilization of the endoplasmic reticulum by monohydroxylated bile acids in liver. *Hepatology*, **9**, 663–664 (letter).

37. Corasanti, J.G., Smith, N.D., Gordon, E.R. & Boyer, J.L. (1989) Protein kinase C agonists inhibit bile secretion independently of effects on the microcirculation in the isolated perfused rat liver. *Hepatology*, **10**, 8–13.

38. Cotting, J., Zysset, T. & Reichen, J. (1989) Biliary obstruction dissipates bioelectric sinusoidal-canalicular barrier without altering taurocholate uptake. *American Journal of Physiology*, **256**, G312–G318.

39. Cotton, P.B. (1982) Duodenoscopic placement of biliary prostheses to relieve malignant obstructive jaundice. *British Journal of Surgery*, **69**, 501–503.

40. Crawford, J.M. & Gollan, J.L. (1988) Hepatocyte cotransport of taurocholate and bilirubin glucuronides: role of microtubules. *American Journal of Physiology*, **255**, G121–G131.

41. Croker, J.R. & Vallon, A.G. (1985) Endoscopic management of

obstructive jaundice in the geriatric patient. *Geriatric Medicine Today*, **4**, 41–49.

42. Cronan, J.B. (1986) US diagnosis of choledocho-lithiasis: a reappraisal. *Radiology*, **161**, 133–134.

43. Day, C.P. & James, O.F.W. (1989) Digoxin-like factors in liver disease. *Journal of Hepatology*, **9**, 281–284.

44. DeFreitas, L.A.R., Chevallier, M., Louis, D. & Grimaud, J.-A. (1986) Human extrahepatic biliary atresia: portal connective tissue activation related to ductular proliferation. *Liver*, **6**, 253–261.

45. DeLamirande, E., Tuchweber, B. & Plaa, G.L. (1982) Morphological aspects of manganese-bilirubin induced cholestasis. *Liver*, **2**, 22–27.

46. Desmet, V.J. (1987) Cholangiopathies: Past, present and future. *Seminars in Liver Disease*, **7**, 67–76.

47. Desmet, V.J. & DeVos, R. (1982) Tight junctions in the liver. In Popper, H. & Schaffner, F. (eds) *Progress in Liver Diseases*, vol. 7, pp. 31–50. New York: Grune & Stratton.

48. Diaz de Otazu, R., Garcia-Campos, F., Basterra, G. & Lopez-Barbarin, J.M. (1986) Nodular regenerative hyperplasia and focal nodular hyperplasia of the liver associated with severe cholestasis. *Liver*, **6**, 30–34.

49. DiBisceglie, A.M., Paterson, A.C. & Segal, I. (1985) The liver in biliary obstruction due to chronic pancreatitis. *Liver*, **5**, 189–195.

50. DiPadova, C., DiPadova, F., Tritapepe, R. & Stramentinoli, G. (1985) S-adenosyl-L-methionine protection against naphthyl-isothiocyanate-induced cholestasis in the rat. *Toxicology Letters*, **29**, 1312–1316.

51. Dooley, J.S., Dick, R., George, P. *et al.* (1984) Percutaneous transhepatic endoprosthesis for bile duct obstruction. Complications and results. *Gastroenterology*, **86**, 905–909.

52. Dosi, P.C., Raut, A.J., Chelliah, B.P. *et al.* (1985) Perinatal factors underlying neonatal cholestasis. *Journal of Pediatrics*, **106**, 471–474.

53. Drummond, G.S. & Kappas, A. (1982) Chemoprevention of neonatal jaundice: potency of tin protoporphyrin in an animal model. *Science*, **217**, 1250–1252.

54. Dubinsky, W.B. (1989) The physiology of epithelial chloride channels. *Hospital Practice*, **24**, 69–82.

55. Duffy, M.C., Blitzer, B.L. & Boyer, J.L. (1983) Direct determination of the driving forces for taurocholate uptake into rat liver plasma membrane vesicles. *Journal of Clinical Investigation*, **73**, 1470–1481.

56. Elias, E., Hruban, Z., Wade, J.B. & Boyer, J.L. (1980) Phalloidin induced cholestasis: a microfilament-mediated change in junctional complex permeability. *Proceedings of the National Academy of Sciences of the USA*, **77**, 2229–2233.

57. Elias, E., Iqbal, S., Knutton, S. *et al.* (1983) Increased tight junction permeability: a possible mechanism of oestrogen cholestasis. *European Journal of Clinical Investigation*, **13**, 383–390.

58. Erlinger, S. (1981) Hepatocyte bile secretion: current views and controversies. *Hepatology*, **1**, 352–359.

59. Erlinger, S. (1982) Does Na^+-K^+-ATPase have any role in bile secretion? *American Journal of Physiology*, **243**, G243–G247.

60. Eriksson, S. & Larsson, C. (1983) Familial benign chronic intrahepatic cholestasis. *Hepatology*, **3**, 391–398.

61. Esquivel, C.O., Koneru, B., Karrer, F. *et al.* (1987) Liver transplantation before one year of age. *Journal of Pediatrics*, **110**, 545–548.

62. Everson, G.T., Ahnen, D., Harper, P.C. & Krawitt, E.L. (1989) Benign recurrent intrahepatic cholestasis: Treatment with S-adenosyl methionine. *Gastroenterology*, **96**, 1354–1357.

63. Fallani, M., Ballardini, G., Bianchi, F.B. & Pisi, E. (1988). Modulation of biliary tree microfilament system in longstanding cholestasis. In Gentilini, P. & Dianzani, M.U. (eds) *Pathophysiology of the Liver*, pp. 121–129. New York: Elsevier.

64. Fang, M.H., Ginsberg, A.L. & Dobbins, W.O., III (1980) Marked elevation in serum alkaline phosphatase activity as a manifestation of systemic infection. *Gastroenterology*, **78**, 592–597.

65. Farquhar, M.G. (1983) Multiple pathways of exocytosis, endocytosis and membrane recycling: validation of a Golgi route. *Federation Proceedings*, **42**, 2407–2413.

66. Farrel, M.K. & Balistreri, W.F. (1986) Parenteral nutrition and hepatobiliary dysfunction. *Clinics in Perinatology* **13**, 197–212.

67. Fennell, R.H., Shikes, R.H. & Vierling, J.M. (1983) Relationship of pretransplant hepatobiliary disease to bile duct damage occuring in the liver allograft. *Hepatology*, **3**, 84–89.

68. Finegold, M.J. & Carpenter, R.J. (1982) Obliterative cholangitis due to cytomegalovirus: a possible precursor of paucity of intrahepatic bile ducts. *Human Pathology*, **13**, 662–665.

69. Finkelstein, S.D., Fornaiser, V.L. & Pruzanski, W. (1981) Intrahepatic cholestasis with predominant pericentral deposition in systemic amyloidosis. *Human Pathology*, **12**, 470–472.

70. Fletcher, M.S., Westwick, J. & Kakkar, V.V. (1982) Endotoxin, prostaglandin and renal fibrin deposition in obstructive jaundice. *British Journal of Surgery*, **69**, 625–629.

71. Fouin-Fortunet, H., LeQuernec, L., Erlinger, S. *et al.* (1982) Hepatic alterations during total parenteral nutrition in patients with inflammatory bowel disease: a possible consequence of lithocholate toxicity. *Gastroenterology*, **82**, 932–937.

72. Freedman, M.R., Holzbach, R.T. & Ferguson, D.R. (1981) Pruritus in cholestasis: no direct causative role for bile acid retention. *American Journal of Medicine*, **70**, 1011–1016.

73. Freese, D. (1982) Intracellular cholestatic syndrome of infancy. *Seminars in Liver Disease*, **2**, 255–270.

74. Freese, D.K. & Hanson, R.F. (1983) Neonatal cholestatic syndromes associated with alterations in bile acid synthesis. *Journal of Pediatric Gastroenterology and Nutrition*, **2**, 374–380.

75. French, S.W. (1985) Role of canalicular contraction in bile flow. *Laboratory Investigation*, **53**, 245–249.

76. Frezza, M., Chiesa, L., Ricci, C. *et al.* (1985) Gallbladder volume and contraction in non-pregnant women previously affected with intrahepatic cholestasis of pregnancy. *Italian Journal of Gastroenterology*, **17**, 311–313.

77. Frezza, M., Pozzato, G., Chiesa, L. *et al.* (1984) Reversal of intrahepatic cholestasis of pregnancy in women after high dose S-adenosyl-L-methionine administration. *Hepatology*, **4**, 274–278.

78. Fulton, I.C., Douglas, J.G., Hutchon, D.J.R. & Beckett, G. J. (1983) Is normal pregnancy cholestatic? *Clinica Chimica Acta*, **130**, 171–176.

79. Gautam, A., Ng, O.-C. & Boyer, J.L. (1987) Isolated rat hepatocyte couplets in short-term culture: Structural characteristics and plasma membrane reorganization. *Hepatology*, **7**, 216–223.

80. Gautam, A., Ng, O.-C., Strazzabosco, M. & Boyer, J.L. (1989) Quantitative assessment of canalicular bile formation in isolated hepatocyte couplets using microscopic optical planimetry. *Journal of Clinical Investigation*, **83**, 565–573.

81. Girardin, S.-M. M.-F., LeMinor, M. & Alperovitch, A. (1985) Computer-aided selection of diagnostic tests in jaundiced patients. *Gut*, **26**, 961–967.

82. Glaser, J.H. & Morecki, R. (1987) Reovirus type 3 and neonatal cholestasis. *Seminars in Liver Disease*, **7**, 100–107.

83. Gleghorn, E.E., Merritt, R.J., Subramanian, N. & Ramos, A. (1986) Phenobarbital does not prevent total parenteral nutrition-associated cholestasis in noninfected neonates. *Journal of Parenteral and Enteral Nutrition*, **10**, 282–283.

84. Golan, J.L. & Schmid, R. (1982) Bilirubin update: formation, transport and metabolism. In Popper, H. & Schaffner, F. (eds) *Progress in Liver Diseases*, vol. 7, pp. 261–283. New York: Grune and Stratton.

85. Goldsmith, M.A., Huling, S. & Jones, A.L. (1983) Hepatic handling of bile salts and protein in the rat during intrahepatic cholestasis. *Gastroenterology*, **84**, 978–986.

86. Gonzalez, M.C., Reyes, H., Arrese, M. *et al.* (1989) Intrahepatic cholestases of pregnancy in twin pregnancies. *Journal of Hepatology*, **9**, 84–90.

87. Gourley, G.R., Chesney, P.J., Davis, J.P. & Odell, G.B. (1981) Acute cholestasis in patients with toxic-shock syndrome. *Gastroenterology*, **81**, 928–931.

88. Graf, J. (1983) Canalicular bile salt-independent bile formation: concept and clues from electrolyte transport in rat liver. *American Journal of Physiology*, **244**, G233–G246.

89. Grosser, V., Robenek, H., Rassat, J. & Themann, H. (1982) Ultrastructural study of cholestasis induced by longterm treatment with estradiol valerate. *Virchows Archiv B Cell Pathology*, **40**, 365–378.

90. Gumucio, J.J. & Miller, D. L., (1982) Zonal hepatic function: solute-hepatocyte interactions within the liver acinus. In Popper, H. & Schaffner, F. (eds) *Progress in Liver Diseases*, vol. 7, pp. 17–30. New York: Grune and Stratton.

91. Hagenmuller, F. & Classen, M. (1982) Therapeutic endoscopic and percutaneous procedures for biliary disorders. In Popper, H. & Schaffner, F. (eds) *Progress in Liver Diseases*, vol. 7, pp. 299–317. New York: Grune and Stratton.

92. Hanny, P., Ink, O., Goenner, S. *et al.* (1989) Activite serique de l'aspartate aminotransferase mitochondriale et cholestase extra-hepatique. *Gastroenterologie et Clinical Biologie*, **13**, 66–70.

93. Hardison, W.G.M., Lowe, P.J. & Shanahan, M. (1989) Effect of molecular charge on para- and transcellular access of horseradish peroxidase into rat bile. *Hepatology*, **9**, 866–871.

94. Hardison, W.G.M., Weiner, R.G., Hatoff D.E. & Miyai, K. (1983) Similarities and differences between models of extrahepatic biliary obstruction and complete biliary retention without obstruction in the rat. *Hepatology*, **3**, 383–390.

95. Hashieh, I.A., Remy, L., Mathieu, S. & Gerolami, A. (1989) The effects of monensin on the transport of horseradish peroxidase into intracellular lumina in cultured rat hepatocytes. *Hepatology*, **10**, 61–65.

96. Herlong, H.F., Recker, R.R. & Maddrey, W.C. (1982) Bone disease in primary biliary cirrhosis: histologic features and response to 25-hydroxyvitamin D. *Gastroenterology*, **83**, 103–108.

97. Heubi, J.B., Hollis, B.W., Specker, B. & Tsang, R.C. (1989) Bone disease in chronic childhood cholestasis. 1. Vitamin D absorption and metabolism. *Hepatology*, **9**, 258–264.

98. Holzbach, R.T., Sivak, D.A. & Braun, W.E. (1983) Familial recurrent intrahepatic cholestasis of pregnancy: a genetic study providing evidence for transmission of a sex-limited, dominant trait. *Gastroenterology*, **85**, 175–179.

99. Houwen, R.H.J., Zwierstra, R.B., Severijnen, R.S.V.M. *et al.* (1989) Prognosis of extrahepatic biliary atresia. *Archives of Disease in Childhood*, **64**, 214–218.

100. Howard, E.R. & Tan, K.C. (1989) Biliary atresia. *British Journal of Hospital Medicine*, **41**, 123–130.

101. Huber, M. & Keppler, D. (1990) Eicosanoids and the liver. In Popper, H. & Schaffner, F. (eds) *Progress in Liver Diseases*, vol. 9, pp. 117–141. Philadelphia: Saunders.

102. Hultcrantz, R., Mengarelli, S. & Strandvik, B. (1986) Morphological findings in the livers of children with cystic fibrosis: A light and electron microscopical study. *Hepatology*, **6**, 881–889.

103. Imanari, H., Kuroda, H. & Tamura, K. (1981) Microfilaments around the bile canaliculi in patients with intrahepatic cholestasis. *Gastroenterologia Japonica*, **16**, 168–173.

104. Inoue, M., Kinne, R., Tran, T. & Arias, J.M. (1982) Taurocholate transport by rat liver sinusoidal membrane vesicles: evidence for sodium cotransport. *Hepatology*, **2**, 572–579.

105. Jakobovits, A.E., Crimmins, F.B., Sherlock, S. *et al.* (1981) Cholestasis as a paraneoplastic manifestation of carcinoma of the kidney. *Australian and New Zealand Journal of Medicine*, **11**, 64–67.

106. Joseph, P.K., Bizer, L.S., Sprayregen, S.S. & Gliedman, M.L. (1986) Percutaneous transhepatic biliary drainage. Results and complications in 81 patients. *Journal of the American Medical Association*, **255**, 2763–2767.

107. Jung, W., Gebhardt, R. & Robanck, H. (1985) Primary culture of rat hepatocytes as a model of canalicular development, biliary secretion, and intrahepatic cholestasis. *Virchows Archiv B Cell Pathology*, **49**, 349–363.

108. Kacich, R.L., Renston, R.H. & Jones, A.L. (1983) Effects of cytochalasin D and colchicine on the uptake, translocation and biliary secretion of horseradish peroxidase and [^{14}C]sodium taurocholate in the rat. *Gastroenterology*, **85**, 385–394.

109. Kahn, E., Daum, F., Markowitz, J. *et al.* (1986) Nonsyndromatic paucity of bile ducts: Light and electron microscopic evaluation of sequential liver biopsies in early childhood. *Hepatology*, **6**, 890–901.

110. Kahn, E., Markowitz, J., Aiges, H. & Daum, F. (1989) Human ontogeny of the bile duct to portal space ratio. *Hepatology*, **110**, 21–23.

111. Kakis, G., Phillips, M.J. & Yousef, I.M. (1980) The respective roles of membrane cholesterol and of sodium-potassium adenosine tri-phosphatase in the pathogenesis of lithocholate-induced cholestasis. *Laboratory Investigation*, **43**, 73–81.

112. Kaplan, M.M., Ohkubo, A., Quaroni, E.G. & Szetu, D. (1983) Increased synthesis of rat liver alkaline phosphatase by bile duct ligation. *Hepatology*, **3**, 368–376.

113. Kaplun, L., Weissmann, H.S., Rosenblatt, R.R. & Freeman, L.M. (1985) The early diagnosis of common bile duct obstruction using

cholescintigraphy. *Journal of the American Medical Association,* **254**, 2431–2434.

114. Keeffe, E.B. (1989) Diagnosis of primary sclerosing cholangitis in a blood donor with elevated serum alanine aminotransferase. *Gastroenterology,* **96**, 1358–1359.
115. Keeffe, E.G., Blankenship, N.M. & Scharschmidt, B.F. (1980) Alteration of rat liver plasma membrane fluidity and ATPase activity by chlorpromazine hydrochloride and its metabolites. *Gastroenterology,* **79**, 222–231.
116. Kioka, K., Mizoguchi, Y., Kodama, C. *et al.* (1988) Determination of serum cholestatic factor level by ELISA in drug-induced allergic hepatitis. *Gastroenterologia Japonica,* **23**, 624–628.
117. Knuchel, J., Krähenbühl, S., Zimmermann, A. & Reichen, J. (1989) Effects of secretin on bile formation in rats with cirrhosis of the liver: structure–function relationship. *Gastroenterology,* **97**, 950–957.
118. Kolde, G., Herwig, J. & Themann, H. (1981) Normoactive hypertrophic endoplasmic reticulum in taurolithocholate-induced cholestasis in rats. *Virchows Archiv B Cell Pathology,* **37**, 103–108.
119. Kortz, W.J., Meyers, W.C., Schirmer, B.D. & Jones, R.S. (1983) Somatostatin-induced cholestasis can be independent of portal blood flow. *Surgery,* **93**, 649–652.
120. Krell, H., Jaeschke, H. & Pfaff, E. (1985) Regulation of canalicular bile formation by α-adrenergic action and external ATP in the isolated perfused liver. *Biochemical and Biophysical Research Communications,* **131**, 139–145.
121. Krell, H., Metz, J., Jaeschke, H. *et al.* (1987) Drug-induced intrahepatic cholestasis: characterization of different pathomechanisms. *Archives of Toxicology,* **60**, 124–130.
122. Krukowski, Z.H., McPhie, J.L., Farquharson, G.H. & Matheson, N.A. (1983) Proliferative cholangitis (cholangitis glandularis proliferans). *British Journal of Surgery,* **70**, 166–171.
123. Lamri, Y., Roda, A., Dumont, M. *et al.* (1988) Immunoperoxidase localization of bile salts in rat liver cells. *Journal of Clinical Investigation,* **82**, 1173–1182.
124. Larrey, D., Amouyal, G., Dana, G. *et al.* (1987) Prolonged cholestasis after troleandomycin-induced hepatitis. *Journal of Hepatology,* **4**, 327–329.
125. LaRusso, N.F., Wiesner, R.H., Ludwig, J. & MacCarty, R.L. (1984) Primary sclerosing cholangitis. *New England Journal of Medicine,* **310**, 899–903.
126. Lavin, A., Sung, C., Klibanov, A.M. & Langer, R. (1985) Enzymatic removal of bilirubin from blood: A potential treatment for neonatal jaundice. *Science,* **230**, 543–545.
127. Lefkowitch, J.H. (1982) Primary sclerosing cholangitis. *Archives of Internal Medicine,* **142**, 1157–1160.
128. Legarde, S., Elias, E., Wade, J.N. & Boyer, J.L. (1981) Structural heterogeneity of hepatocyte 'tight' junctions: a quantitative analysis. *Hepatology,* **1**, 193–303.
129. Lewis, D.R., Jr, Jung, H. & Cannon, J.J. (1982) Biliary obstruction secondary to hepatic artery aneurysm. Cholangiographic appearance and diagnostic considerations. *Gastroenterology,* **82**, 1446–1451.
130. Lindberg, G., Nilsson, L.H. & Thulen, L. (1983) Decision theory as an aid in the diagnosis of cholestatic jaundice. *Acta Chirurgica Scandinavica,* **149**, 521–529.
131. Lindberg, G., Björkman, A. & Helmers, C. (1983) A description of diagnostic strategies in jaundice. *Scandinavian Journal of Gastroenterology,* **18**, 257–265.
132. Lirussi, F., Vaja, S., Murphy, G.M. & Dowling, R.H. (1989) Cholestasis of total parenteral nutrition: Bile acid and bile lipid metabolism in parenterally nourished rats. *Gastroenterology,* **96**, 493–501.
133. Lok, A.S.-F. & Ng, I.O.L. (1988) Prochlorperazine-induced chronic cholestasis. *Journal of Hepatology,* **6**, 369–373.
134. Ludwig, J., Kim, C.H., Wiesner, R.H. & Krom, R.A.F. (1989) Floxuridine-induced sclerosing cholangitis: An ischemic cholangiopathy? *Hepatology,* **9**, 215–218.
135. Ludwig, J., Wiesner, R.H. & LaRusso, N.F. (1988) Idiopathic adulthood ductopenia. A cause of chronic cholestatic liver disease and biliary cirrhosis. *Journal of Hepatology,* **7**, 193–199.
136. Macquart-Moulin, C., Cornee, J., Sahel, F. *et al.* (1980) Jaundice and chronic pancreatitis. *Digestion,* **20**, 410–415.
137. Magnusson, I., Einarsson, K., Angerin, B. *et al.* (1989) Effects of

somatostatin on hepatic bile formation. *Gastroenterology,* **96**, 206–212.

138. Malchow-Møller, A., Thomsen, C., Matzen, P. *et al.* (1986) Computer diagnosis in jaundice: Baye's rule founded on 1002 consecutive cases. *Journal of Hepatology,* **3**, 154–163.
139. Manivel, J.C., Bloomer, J.R. & Snover, D.C. (1987) Progressive bile duct injury after thiobendazole administration. *Gastroenterology,* **93**, 245–249.
140. Martin, V.H., Beavis, A.D. & Garlid, K.D. (1984) Identification of an 82 000-dalton protein responsible for K^+/H^+ antiport in rat liver mitochondria. *Journal of Biological Chemistry,* **259**, 2062–2065.
141. Mathisen, Ø. & Raeder, M. (1983) Mechanism of hepatic bicarbonate secretion and bile acid independent bile secretion. *European Journal of Clinical Investigation,* **13**, 193–200.
142. Matloff, D.S., Kaplan, M.M., Neer, R.M. *et al.* (1982) Osteoporosis in primary biliary cirrhosis: effects of 25-hydroxyvitamin D_3 treatment. *Gastroenterology,* **83**, 97–102.
143. Matsumoto, H. (1982) Morphologic changes of the tight junction in human liver with intrahepatic cholestasis. *Acta Hepatologica Japonica,* **23**, 271–278.
144. Matzen, P., Malchow-Møller, A., Lejerstofte, J. *et al.* (1982) Endoscopic retrograde cholangiopancreatography and transhepatic cholangiography in patients with suspected obstructive jaundice. A randomized study. *Scandinavian Journal of Gastroenterology,* **17**, 731–735.
145. Matzen, P., Malchow-Møller, A., Brun, B. *et al.* (1983) Ultrasonography, computed tomography and cholescintigraphy in suspected obstructive jaundice—a prospective comparative study. *Gastroenterology,* **84**, 1492–1497.
146. McGarrity, T.J. & Jeffries, G.H. (1987) New options for managing ascending cholangitis. *Journal of Critical Illness,* **2**, 39–50.
147. Meier, P.J. (1989) The bile salt secretory polarity of hepatocytes. *Journal of Hepatology,* **9**, 124–129.
148. Merritt, R.J. (1989) Cholestasis associated with total parenteral nutrition. *Journal of Pediatric Gastroenterology and Nutrition,* **5**, 9–22.
149. Mesland, D.A.M., Los, G. & Spiele, H. (1981) Cytocholasin B disrupts the association of filamentous web and plasma membrane in hepatocytes. *Experimental Cell Research,* **135**, 431–435.
150. Messer, J., Solano, C., Romeu, J. & Dave, P.B. (1984) An unusual case of obstructive jaundice. *American Journal of Gastroenterology,* **79**, 152–153.
151. Metges, P.J., Flageat, J., Hernandez, C. *et al.* (1982) Place de l'échotomographie dans le diagnostic des ictères obstructifs. *Médicine et Chirurgie Digestives,* **11**, 337–343.
152. Mieli-Vergani, G., Howard, E.R., Portman, B. & Mowat, A.P. (1989) Late referral for biliary atresia-missed opportunities for effective surgery. *Lancet,* **1**, 421–423.
153. Minuk, G.Y. & Schaffer, E.A. (1987) Benign recurrent intrahepatic cholestasis. Evidence for an intrinsic abnormality in hepatocyte secretion. *Gastroenterology,* **93**, 1187–1193.
154. Miyajima, K., Mizoguchi, Y., Tsutsui, H., *et al.* (1986) Studies on the effects of cholestatic factor on immunoglobulin-A excretion in bile. *Japanese Journal of Gastroenterology,* **89**, 1993–1997.
155. Mizoguchi, Y., Kato, H., Tsutsui, H. *et al.* (1985) Possible participation of cholestatic factor in the pathogenesis of intrahepatic cholestasis in alcoholic liver disease. *Japanese Journal of Gastroenterology,* **82**, 441–449.
156. Moore, T.C. & Hyman, P.E. (1985) Extrahepatic biliary atresia in one human leukocyte antigen identical twin. *Pediatrics,* **76**, 604–605.
157. Morphis, L., Constantopoulos, A. & Matsaniotis, N. (1982) Bilirubin-induced modulation of cerebral protein phosphorylation in neonate rabbits in vivo. *Science,* **218**, 156–158.
158. Mosely, R.H., Meier, P.J., Aronson, P.S. & Boyer, J.L. (1986) Na-H exchange in rat liver basolateral but not canalicular plasma membrane vesicles. *American Journal of Physiology,* **250**, G35–G43.
159. Mowat, A.P. (1983) Jaundice in the newborn. *Practical Gastroenterology,* **7**, 8–17.
160. Mueller, P.R., van Sonnenberg, E. & Simeone, J.F. (1982) Fine-needle transhepatic cholangiography: indications and usefulness. *Annals of Internal Medicine,* **97**, 567–572.

161. Nagore, N., Howe, S., Boxer, L. & Scheuer, P.J. (1989) Liver cell rosettes: structural differences in cholestasis and hepatitis. *Liver*, **9**, 43–51.

162. Nervi, F., Marinovic, I., Rigotti, A. & Ulloa, N. (1988) Regulation of biliary cholesterol secretion. Functional relationship between the canalicular and sinusoidal secretory pathways in the rat. *Journal of Clinical Investigation*, **82**, 1818–1825.

163. Norlander, A., Kalin, B. & Sundblad, R. (1982) Effect of percutaneous transhepatic drainage upon liver function and postoperative mortality. *Surgery Gynecology and Obstetrics*, **155**, 161–166.

164. Nyberg, B., Einersson, K. & Sonnenfeld, T. (1989) Evidence that vasoactive intestinal peptide induces ductular secretion of bile in humans. *Gastroenterology*, **96**, 920–924.

165. Obata, H. & Koga, A. (1988) Glucose intolerance and pancreatic endocrine dysfunction in dogs with obstructive jaundice. *Gastroenterologica Japonica*, **23**, 666–672.

166. Okanoue, T., Ohta, M., Kachi, K. *et al.* (1988) Intermediate filaments of hepatocytes and biliary epithelial cells in bile duct obstruction: Transmission and scanning electron microscopy study. *Gastroenterologica Japonica*, **23**, 428–434.

167. Okuda, K. & Tsuchiya, Y. (1982) Ultrasonography of the biliary tract. In Popper, H. & Schaffner, F. (eds) *Progress in Liver Diseases*, vol. 7, pp. 285–297. New York: Grune & Stratton.

168. O'Maille, E.R.L. & Hofmann, A.F. (1986) Relatively high biliary secretory maximum for non-micelle-forming bile acid. Possible evidence for mechanism of secretion. *Quarterly Journal of Experimental Physiology*, **71**, 475–482.

169. Ou, C.-N., Buffone, G.J. & Calomeni, P.J.H. (1986) Conjugated bilirubin versus direct bilirubin in neonates. *American Journal of Clinical Pathology*, **85**, 613–616.

170. Pain, J.A. & Bailey, M.E. (1986) Experimental and clinical study of lactulose in obstructive jaundice. *British Journal of Surgery*, **73**, 775–778.

171. Patwardhan, R.V., Smith, O.J. & Farmelant, M.H. (1987) Serum transaminase levels and cholescintigraphic abnormalities in acute biliary tract obstruction. *Archives of Internal Medicine*, **147**, 1249–1253.

172. Paumgartner, G. and Paumgartner, D. (1982) Current concepts of bile formation. In Popper, H. & Schaffner, F. (eds) *Progress in Liver Diseases*, vol. 7, pp. 207–220. New York: Grune & Stratton.

173. Pettavel, J., Gardiol, D., Bergier, N. & Schnyder, P. (1988) Necrosis of main bile ducts caused by hepatic artery infusion of 5-fluoro-2-deoxyuridine. *Regional Cancer Treatment*, **1**, 83–92.

174. Pelligrini, C.A., Allegra P., Bongard, F.S. *et al.* (1987) Risk of biliary surgery in patients with hyperbilirubinemia. *American Surgeon*, **154**, 111–117.

175. Pereira-Lima, J. & Schaffner, F. (1987) Chronic cholestasis in hepatic sarcoidosis with clinical features resembling primary biliary cirrhosis. *American Journal of Medicine*, **83**, 144–148.

176. Phillips, M.J., Oshio, C., Miyairi, M. *et al.* (1982) A study of bile canalicular contractions in isolated hepatocytes. *Hepatology*, **2**, 763–768.

177. Phillips, M.J., Fisher, R.L., Anderson, D.W. *et al.* (1983) Ultrastructural evidence of intrahepatic cholestasis before and after chenodeoxycholic acid therapy in patients with cholelithiasis: the National Cooperative Gallstone Study. *Hepatology*, **3**, 209–220.

178. Phillips, M.J., Oshio, C., Miyairi M. & Smith, C.R. (1983) Intrahepatic cholestasis as a canalicular motility disorder. Evidence using cytochalasin. *Laboratory Investigation*, **48**, 205–211.

179. Pirovino, M., Altorfer, J., Maranta, E. *et al.* (1982) Icterus vom Typ der intrahepatischen Cholestase bei Amyloidose der Leber. *Zeitschrift für Gastroenterologie*, **82**, 310–317.

180. Plaa, G.L. & Hewitt, W.R. (1982) Biotransformation products in cholestasis. In Popper H. & Schaffner F. (eds) *Progress in Liver Diseases*, vol. 7, pp. 179–194. New York: Grune & Stratton.

181. Popper, H. (1981) Cholestasis: the future of a past and present riddle. *Hepatology*, **1**, 187–191.

182. Poupon, R., Chretien, Y., Poupon, R.E. *et al.* (1987) Is ursodeoxycholic acid an effective treatment for primary biliary cirrhosis? *Lancet*, **1**, 834–836.

183. Rabinovitz, M., Imperial, J.C., Schade, R.R. & Van Thiel, D.H. (1989) Hepatocellular carcinoma in Alagille's Syndrome: A family study. *Journal of Pediatric Gastroenterology and Nutrition*, **8**, 26–30.

184. Raedsch, R. & Stiehl, A. (1989) Ursodesoxycholsaure—Ein neues therapiekonzept bei cholestatischen Leberkrankheiten. *Klinische Wochenschrift*, **67**, 265–268.

185. Rank, J. & Wilson, I.D. (1983) Changes in IgA following varying degrees of biliary obstruction in the rat. *Hepatology*, **3**, 241–247.

186. Renner, C.L., Lake, J.R., Scharschmidt, B.F. *et al.* (1989) Rat hepatocytes exhibit basolateral Na^+/HCO_3^- cotransport. *Journal of Clinical Investigation*, **83**, 1225–1235.

187. Renston, R.H., Maloney, D.V., Jones, A.L. *et al.* (1980) Bile secretory apparatus: evidence for a vesicular transport mechanism for proteins in the rat, using horseradish peroxidase and (^{125}I)-insulin. *Gastroenterology*, **78**, 1373–1388.

188. Reyes, H., Radrigan, M.E., Gonzalez, M.C. *et al.* (1987) Steatorhea in patients with intrahepatic cholestasis of pregnancy. *Gastroenterology*, **93**, 584–590.

189. Ricci, G.L., Cornelis, M., Fevery, J. & DeGroote, J. (1983) Maximum hepatic bilirubin transport in the rat during somatostatin-induced cholestasis and taurocholate choleresis. *Journal of Laboratory and Clinical Medicine*, **101**, 835–846.

190. Richter, J.M., Silverstein, M.D. & Schapiro, R. (1983) Suspected obstructive jaundice: a decision analysis of diagnostic strategies. *Annals of Internal Medicine*, **99**, 46–51.

191. Riely, C.A. (1987) Familial intrahepatic cholestatic syndromes. *Seminars in Liver Disease*, **7**, 119–133.

192. Robenek, H., Heiweg, J. & Themann, H. (1981) A quantitative freeze fracture analysis of gap and tight junctions in normal and cholestatic human liver. *Virchows Archiv B Cell Pathology*, **38**, 39–56.

193. Robertson, J.F.R., Garden, O.J. & Shenkin, A. (1986) Intravenous nutrition and hepatic dysfunction. *Journal of Parenteral and Enteral Nutrition*, **10**, 172–176.

194. Rosenthal, P., Miller, J.H. & Sinatra, F.R. (1989) Hepatobiliary scintigraphy and the string test in the evaluation of neonatal cholestasis. *Journal of Pediatric Gastroenterology and Nutrition*, **8**, 292–296.

195. Rougheen, P.T., Drath, D.B., Kulkarni, A.D. & Rowlands, B.J. (1987) Impaired nonspecific cellular immunity in experimental cholestasis. *Annals of Surgery*, **5**, 578–582.

196. Ruifrok, P.G., Meijer, D.K.F. (1982) Sodium ion-coupled uptake of taurocholate by rat liver plasma membrane vesicles. *Liver*, **2**, 28–34.

197. Sabesin, S.J. (1982) Cholestatic lipoproteins—their pathogenesis and significance. *Gastroenterology*, **83**, 704–709.

198. Saito T., Fujiwara, M., Nomoto, M. *et al.* (1988) Histologic studies on the hepatic lesions induced by graft-versus-host reaction in MHC class II disparate hosts compared with primary biliary cirrhosis. *American Journal of Pathology*, **135**, 301–307.

199. Schaffner, F. & Popper, H. (1982) Clinical–pathologic relations in primary biliary cirrhosis. In Popper, H. & Schaffner, F. (eds) *Progress in Liver Diseases*, vol. 7, pp. 529–554. New York: Grune & Stratton.

200. Schachter, B.A., Joseph, E. & Firneisz, G. (1983) Effect of cholestasis produced by bile duct ligation on hepatic heme and hemoprotein metabolism in rats. *Gastroenterology*, **84**, 227–235.

201. Scharschmidt, B.F. (1983) Cholestasis-Medical Staff Conference, University of California, San Francisco. *Western Journal of Medicine*, **138**, 233–242.

202. Schenck, D.B. & Leffert, H.L. (1983) Monoclonal antibodies to rat Na^+,K^+-ATPase block enzymatic activity. *Proceedings of the National Academy of Sciences of the USA*, **80**, 5281–5285.

203. Schneider, A.P., II (1986) Breast milk jaundice in the newborn. A real entity. *Journal of the American Medical Association*, **255**, 3270–3274.

204. Schönau, E., Herzog, K.H. & Böhles, H.-J. (1986) Clinical relevance of alkaline phosphatase isoenzyme determinations by high performance liquid chromatography. *Journal of Clinical Chemistry and Clinical Biochemistry*, **24**, 641–646.

205. Schweizer, P. (1985) Langzeitergebnisse in der Behandlung der extrahepatischen Gallengangsatresie. *Zeitschrift fur Kinderchirurgie*, **40**, 263–267.

206. Seetharam, S., Sussman, N.L., Komoda, T. & Alpers, D.H. (1986) The mechanism of elevated alkaline phosphatase activity after bile duct ligation in the rat. *Hepatology*, **6**, 374–380.

207. Sellinger, M. & Boyer, J.L. (1982) Physiology of bile secretion

and cholestasis. In Popper, H. & Schaffner, F. (eds) *Progress in Liver Diseases*, vol. 9, pp. 237–259. Philadelphia: Saunders.

208. Semeraro, N., Montemurro, P., Chetta, G. *et al.* (1989) Increased procoagulant activity of peripheral blood monocytes in human and experimental obstructive jaundice. *Gastroenterology*, **96**, 892–898.

209. Senger, H., Boehm, G., Beyreiss, K. & Braun, W. (1987) Cholestasis in late metabolic acidosis of prematurely born infants. *Journal of Clinical Chemistry and Clinical Biochemistry*, **25**, 413–418.

210. Sewell, R.B., Barham, S.S., Zinsmeister, A.M. & LaRusso, N.F. (1984) Microtubule modulation of biliary excretion of endogenous and exogenous lysosomal constituents. *American Journal of Physiology*, **246**, G8–G15.

211. Simon, F.R. & Reichen, J. (1982) Bile secretory failure: recent concepts of the pathogenesis of intrahepatic cholestasis. In Popper, H. & Schaffner, F. (eds) *Progress in Liver Diseases*, vol. 7, pp. 195–206. New York: Grune & Stratton.

212. Simon, F.R., Sutherland, E.M. & Gonzalez, M. (1982) Regulation of bile acid transport in rat liver. Evidence that increased maximum bile salt secretion capacity is due to increased cholic acid receptors. *Journal of Clinical Investigation*, **70**, 401–411.

213. Skellenger, M.E., Patterson, D., Foley, N.T. & Jordan, P.H. (1983) Cholestasis due to compression of the common bile duct by pancreatic pseudocysts. *American Journal of Surgery*, **145**, 343–348.

214. Sloane, J.P., Farthing, M.J.G. & Powles, R.L. (1980) Histopathologic changes in the liver after allogeneic bone marrow transplantation. *Journal of Clinical Pathology*, **33**, 344–450.

215. Smith, C.R., Oshio, C., Miyairi, M. *et al.* (1985) Coordination of the contractile activity of bile canaliculi. Evidence from spontaneous contractions in vitro. *Laboratory Investigation*, **53**, 270–274.

216. Smith, D.J. & Gordon, E.R. (1988) Role of liver plasma membrane fluidity in the pathogenesis of estrogen-induced cholestasis. *Journal of Laboratory and Clinical Medicine*, **112**, 679–685.

217. Smith, N.D. & Boyer, J.L. (1982) Permeability characteristics of bile ducts in the rat. *American Journal of Physiology*, **243**, G52–G57.

218. Sochendra, N., Grimm, H., Berger, B. & Nam, V.C. (1989) Malignant jaundice: results of diagnostic and therapeutic endoscopy. *World Journal of Surgery*, **13**, 171–177.

219. Sørenson, S., Matzen, P. & Bögh, I. (1981) Electrophoretic separation of alkaline phosphatase isoenzymes compared with alkaline phosphatase and γ-glutamyltransferase in hepatobiliary disease. *Scandinavian Journal of Gastroenterology*, **16**, 885–889.

220. South, M. & King, A. (1987) Parenteral nutrition-associated cholestasis: Recovery following phenobarbitone. *Journal of Parenteral and Enteral Nutrition*, **11**, 208–209.

221. Speer, A.G., Cotton, P.B., Rode, J. *et al.* (1988) Biliary stent blockage with bacterial biofilm. A light and electron microscopic study. *Annals of Internal Medicine*, **108**, 543–546.

222. Spivak, W. & Grand, R.J. (1983) General configuration of jaundice in the newborn. *Journal of Pediatric Gastroenterology and Nutrition*, **2**, 381–392.

223. Starling, J.R. & Matallona, R.H. (1980) Benign mechanical obstruction of the common hepatic duct (Mirizzi syndrome). *Surgery*, **88**, 737–740.

224. Stremmel, W., Tavoloni, N. & Berk, P.D. (1983) Uptake of bilirubin by the liver. *Seminars in Liver Disease*, **3**, 1–10.

225. Sztul, E.S., Biemesderfer, D., Caplan, M.J. *et al.* (1987) Localization of Na^+,K^+-ATPase α-subunit to the sinusoidal and lateral but not canalicular membranes of rat hepatocytes. *Journal of Cell Biology*, **104**, 1239–1248.

226. Tavaloni, N. (1985) Role of ductular bile water reabsorption in canine bile secretion. *Journal of Laboratory and Clinical Medicine*, **106**, 154–161.

227. Tavaloni, N. (1986) Bile secretion and its control in the newborn puppy. *Pediatrics Research*, **20**, 203–208.

228. Tavaloni, N. & Boyer, J.L. (1980) Relationship between hepatic metabolism of chlorpromazine and cholestatic effects in the isolated perfused rat liver. *Journal of Pharmacology and Experimental Therapeutics*, **214**, 269–274.

229. Teixeira, M.R., Weller, I.V.D., Murray, A. *et al.* (1982) The pathology of hepatitis A in man. *Liver*, **2**, 53–60.

230. Tolia, V., Dubois, R.S., Watts, F.B., Jr & Perrin, E. (1987) Renal abnormalities in paucity of interlobular bile ducts. *Journal of Pediatric Gastroenterology and Nutrition*, **6**, 971–976.

231. Toyota, N., Miyai, K. & Hardison, W.G.M. (1984) Effect of biliary pressure versus high bile acid flux on the permeability of hepatocellular tight junctions. *Laboratory Investigation*, **50**, 536–542.

232. Traub, O., Drüge, P.M. & Willecke, K. (1983) Degradation and resynthesis of gap junction protein in plasma membranes of regenerating liver after partial hepatectomy or cholestasis. *Proceedings of the National Academy of Sciences of the USA*, **80**, 755–759.

233. Triveda, P., Cheeseman, P., Portmann, B. & Mowat, A.P. (1986) Serum type III procollagen peptide as a noninvasive marker of liver damage during infancy and childhood in extrahepatic atresia, idiopathic hepatitis of infancy and α-1-antitrypsin deficiency. *Clinica Chimica Acta*, **161**, 137–146.

234. Tsang, T.-K., Crampton, A.R., Bernstein, J.R. *et al.* (1987) Percutaneous-endoscopic biliary stent placement. A preliminary report. *Annals of Internal Medicine*, **106**, 389–392.

235. Tuchweber, B., Perea, A. & Yousef, I.M. (1983) Lithocholic acid-induced cholestasis in newborn rats. *Toxicology Letters*, **19**, 107–112.

236. Uflacker, R., Wholey, M.H., Amaral, N.M. & Lima, S. (1982) Parasitic and mycotic causes of biliary obstruction. *Gastrointestinal Radiology*, **7**, 173–179.

237. Ulloa, N., Garrido, J. & Nervi, F. (1987) Ultracentrifugal isolation of vesicular carriers of biliary cholesterol in native human and rat bile. *Hepatology*, **7**, 235–244.

238. Van Dyke, R.W. & Scharschmidt, B.F. (1983) (Na,K)-ATPase-mediated cation pumping in cultured rat hepatocytes. *Journal of Biological Chemistry*, **258**, 12912–12919.

239. Van Dyke, R.W., Stephens, J.E. & Scharschmidt, B.F. (1982) Effects of ion substitution on bile acid-dependent and -independent bile formation by rat liver. *Journal of Clinical Investigation*, **70**, 505–517.

240. Vennes, J.A. & Bond, J.H. (1983) Approach to the jaundiced patient. Editorial. *Gastroenterology*, **84**, 1615.

241. Vital, A., Bioulac-Sage, P., Iron, A. & Balabaud, C. (1982) Morphologic structure of bile canaliculi after bile duct ligation in the rat. *Archives of Pathology and Laboratory Medicine*, **106**, 464–467.

242. Wagman, L.D., Burt, M.E. & Brennan, M.F. (1982) The impact of total parenteral nutrition on liver function tests in patients with cancer. *Cancer*, **49**, 1249–1257.

243. Waldschmidt, J., Charissis, G. & Schier, F. (eds) (1988) *Cholestasis in Neonates*: Springer Verlag.

244. Warnes, T.W., Hine, P., Kay, G. & Smith, A. (1981) Intestinal alkaline phosphatase in bile: evidence for enterohepatic circulation. *Gut*, **22**, 493–498.

245. Watanabe, S., Miyazaki, A., Namihisa, T. & Phillips, M.J. (1985) Ca^{2+} and calmodulin are involved in the mechanism of bile canalicular contraction of cultured hepatocytes. *Acta Hepatologica Japonica*, **16**, 1346–1350.

246. Watanabe, S., Smith, C.R. & Phillips, M.J. (1985) Coordination of the contractile activity of bile canaliculi. Evidence from calcium microinjection of triplet hepatocytes. *Laboratory Investigation*, **53**, 275–279.

247. Weismüller, J., Gail, K. & Seifert, E. (1983) Maligner extrahepatischer Gallenwegsverschluss. *Deutsche Medizinische Wochenschrift*, **108**, 203–209.

248. Werlin, S.L., Sty, J.R., Starshak, R.J. *et al.* (1985) Intrahepatic biliary tract abnormalities in children with corrected extrahepatic biliary atresia. *Journal of Pediatric Gastroenterology and Nutrition*, **4**, 537–541.

249. Wieland, H., Meissner-Heins, H., Heins, C. & Seidel, D. (1982) Die Bedeutung des Lipoprotein-X-cholesterin in der Differentialdiagnostik der Cholestase. *Klinische Wochenschrift*, **60**, 343–348.

250. Wiesner, R.H., Grambsch, P.M., Dickson, E.R. *et al.* (1989) Primary sclerosing cholangitis: Natural history, prognostic factors and survival analysis. *Hepatology*, **10**, 430–436.

251. Williams, J.W., Vera, S., Peters, T.G. *et al.* (1986) Cholestatic jaundice after hepatic transplantation. A nonimmunologically mediated event. *American Journal of Surgery*, **151**, 65–70.

252. Wisloff, F., Jakobsen, J. & Osnes, M. (1982) Stenosis of the

common bile duct in chronic pancreatitis. *British Journal of Surgery*, **69**, 52–54.

253. Wolf, A. & Pohlandt, F. (1989) Bacterial infection: The main cause of acute cholestasis in newborn infants receiving short-term parenteral nutrition. *Journal of Pediatric Gastroenterology and Nutrition*, **8**, 297–303.

254. Yamaguchi, M. (1980) Congenital choleductal cyst. Analysis of 1433 patients in the Japanese literature. *American Journal of Surgery*, **140**, 653–656.

255. Yao, J.D.C., Gross, J.B., Ludwig, J. & Purnell, D.C. (1989) Cholestatic jaundice in hyperthyroidism. *American Journal of Medicine*, **86**, 619–620.

256. Yasuura, S., Veno, T., Watanabe, S. *et al.* (1989) Immunocyto-chemical localization of myosin and phalloidin-treated rat hepato-cytes. *Gastroenterology*, **97**, 982–989.

257. Yokoi, H. (1983) Morphologic changes of the liver in obstructive jaundice and its reversibility—with special reference to morpho-metric analysis of ultrastructure of the liver in dogs. *Acta Hepato-logica*, **24**, 1381–1391.

258. Younes, M., Pauli, V., Korb, G. & Siegers, C.-P. (1985) Effect of subchronic cholestasis on microsomal mixed-function oxidases and the glutathione-conjugating enzyme system in rat liver. *Phar-macological Research Communications*, **17**, 841–846.

259. Yousef, I.M., Tuchweber, B., Mignault, D. & Weber, A. (1989) Effect of coinfusion of cholic acid and sulfated cholic acid on bile formation in rats. *American Journal of Physiology*, **256**, G62–G66.

260. Yousef, I.M., Tuchweber, B., Weber, A. & Ray, C.R. (1984) Where is Na⁺,K⁺-ATPase located in the liver cell plasma mem-brane? *New England Journal of Medicine*, **86**, 1632–1633.

261. Bijleveld, C.M.A., Vonk, R.J. & Kuipers, F. (1989) Treatment of patients with benign recurrent intrahepatic cholestasis. *Hepatology*, **10**, 1031.

262. Bircher, J. (1989) Treatment of patients with benign recurrent intrahepatic cholestasis. *Hepatology*, **10**, 1030.

263. Bulle, F., Mavier, P., Zafrani, E.S. *et al.* (1990) Mechanism of γ glutamyl transpeptidase release in serum during intrahepatic and extrahepatic cholestasis in the rat: A histochemical, biochemical and molecular approach. *Hepatology*, **11**, 545–550.

264. Frezza, M., Surrenti, C., Manzillo, G. *et al.* (1990) Oral S-adenosylmethionine in the symptomatic treatment of intrahepatic cholestasis. A double-blind, placebo-controlled study. *Gastroenter-ology*, **99**, 211–215.

265. Hayakawa, T., Cheng, O., Ma, A. & Boyer, J.L. (1990) Taurochol-ate stimulates vesicular pathways labeled by horseradish peroxidase in the isolated perfused rat liver. *Gastroenterology*, **99**, 216–228.

266. Jones, E.A. & Bergasa, N.V. (1990) The pruritus of cholestasis: From bile acids to opiate agonists. *Hepatology*, **11**, 884–887.

267. Kawahara, H., Cadrin, M., Perry, G. *et al.* (1990) Role of cytokeratin intermediate filament in transhepatic transport and canalicular secretion. *Hepatology*, **11**, 435–448.

268. Nissenbaum, M., Chedid, A., Mendenhall, C. *et al.* (1990) Prognos-tic significance of cholestatic alcoholic hepatitis. *Digestive Diseases and Sciences*, **35**, 891–896.

269. Porayko, M.K., Wiesner, R.H., LaRusso, N.F. *et al.* (1990) Patients with asymptomatic primary sclerosing cholangitis fre-quently have progressive disease. *Gastroenterology*, **99**, 1594–1602.

270. Prochazka, E.J., Terasaki, P.I., Park, M.S. *et al.* (1990) Association of primary sclerosing cholangitis with HLA-DRw52a. *The New England Journal of Medicine*, **322**, 1842–1844.

271. Roskams, T., van den Oord, J.J., De Vos, R. & Desmet, V.J. (1990) Neuroendocrine features of reactive bile ductules in cholestatic liver disease. *American Journal of Pathology*, **137**, 1019–1025.

272. Scholmerich, J., Baumgartner, U., Miyai, K. & Gerok, W. (1990) Tauroursodeoxycholate prevents taurolithocholate-induced cholestasis and toxicity in rat liver. *Journal of Hepatology*, **10**, 280–283.

273. Sellinger, M., Barrett, C., Malle, P. *et al.* (1990) cryptic Na⁺, K⁺-ATPase activity in rat liver canalicular plasma membranes: Evidence for its basolateral origin. *Hepatology*, **11**, 223–229.

274. Sippel, C.J., Ananthanarayanan, M. & Suchy, F.J. (1990) Isolation and characterization of the canalicular membrane bile acid transport protein of rat liver. *American Journal of Physiology*, **258**, G728–G737.

275. Slott, P.A., Liu, M.H. & Tavaloni, N. (1990) Origin, pattern and mechanism of bile duct proliferation following biliary obstruction in the rat. *Gastroenterology*, **99**, 466–477.

276. Stammler, L., Reichen, J., Oehler, R. *et al.* (1990) Decreased hepatocellular volume and intact morphology of tight junctions in calcium deprivation-induced cholestasis. *Journal of Hepatology*, **10**, 318–326.

277. Zhang, F., Deleuze, J.-F., Aurias, A. *et al.* (1990) Interstitial deletion of the short arm of chromosome 20 in arteriohepatic dysplasia (Alagille syndrome). *The Journal of Pediatrics*, **116**, 73–77.

Haem Metabolism and the Porphyrias

D.M. Bissell

Porphyrins are planar molecules with four pyrrole rings joined by carbon bridges to form a macrocycle, the centre of which readily binds transition metals (Figure 16.1). As complexes with iron, magnesium or cobalt, they act as the prosthetic group for molecules essential to life (Figure 16.1). The presence of these structurally closely related compounds in both the plant and animal kingdoms suggests that they must have arisen early in evolution. Indeed, they are linked by the fact that all three metalloporphyrins have a common precursor in uroporphyrinogen III.[148]

In mammals, porphyrins function exclusively as metal complexes, primarily with iron as haem and with cobalt as vitamin B_{12}. Free porphyrins serve no biologically useful function in humans. They are produced in minute amounts and then only as accidental side-products of haem synthesis. The pathway of haem synthesis normally operates at high efficiency; intermediates are utilized nearly completely so that less than 1% escape from the biosynthetic route to appear in blood and undergo excretion. The appearance of increased amounts of porphyrins or porphyrin precursors in urine or faeces implies a disturbance in haem synthesis. These biochemical disturbances, when expressed clinically, give rise to specific disease patterns which collectively are termed *porphyria*. The underlying abnormality of haem synthesis may be hereditary or acquired and may reflect alteration of any one of the several individual steps in haem formation (see below). Excess excretion of porphyrins also occurs in asymptomatic individuals, representing either latent porphyria or benign porphyrinuria. The latter is seen in a variety of acute and chronic illnesses and is generally without clinical significance. Fortunately, with the methods currently available for quantitating the individual porphyrins and porphyrin precursors in body fluids, the interpretation of porphyrin studies is usually straightforward. The first published cases of porphyria were recognized as having more than a single aetiology. Mathias Petry (1892–1925), whose urine provided Hans Fischer with the material needed for the characterization of uroporphyrin,[78] suffered from a severe congenital, pre-sumably hereditary, form. In other instances, the occurrence of porphyria was clearly toxin-related, as in the numerous cases following the introduction (in 1888) of the hypnotic, sulphomethane (Sulphonal). In the latter cases, there was no evidence for a hereditary sensitivity to the drug. The spectrum of the porphyrias was enlarged still further in the 1930s with the description of a type that involved excretion of a compound that was colourless in urine but gave a red reaction with Ehrlich's reagent. Waldenström suggested correctly that the compound was a pyrrole precursor of haem, and it was later identified as porphobilinogen.[222] Patients with pyrroluria experienced severe abdominal pains, often associated with a peripheral neuropathy and psychological disturbances, and these symptoms were frequently elicited or markedly exacerbated by administration of barbiturates. The unique sensitivity to barbiturates in these patients was recognized as hereditary. This condition is known today as acute intermittent porphyria, a misnomer in view of the fact that the characteristic abnormality is increased excretion of a pyrrole, not a porphyrin. Nevertheless, the designation is widely accepted and serves to group this disease correctly with the closely related 'true' porphyrias.

In addition to the above forms of porphyria, types were described which were discrete in some respects but overlapped with those previously described. This situation led to some confusion in the classification and nomenclature of the porphyrias. However, important developments over the past 50 years have provided a secure basis for delineating most, if not all, of these diseases. These include elucidation of the pathway of haem biosynthesis, studies of its regulation and measurement of the enzymes catalysing specific steps in the pathway. Animal models with congenital or chemically-induced porphyria have provided much of the insight in these areas. Such work has been reviewed and will not be described in detail here.[154,220] However, a summary of current concepts will be given below, inasmuch as an understanding of haem biosynthesis and its regulation is essential to a coherent view of the porphyrias.

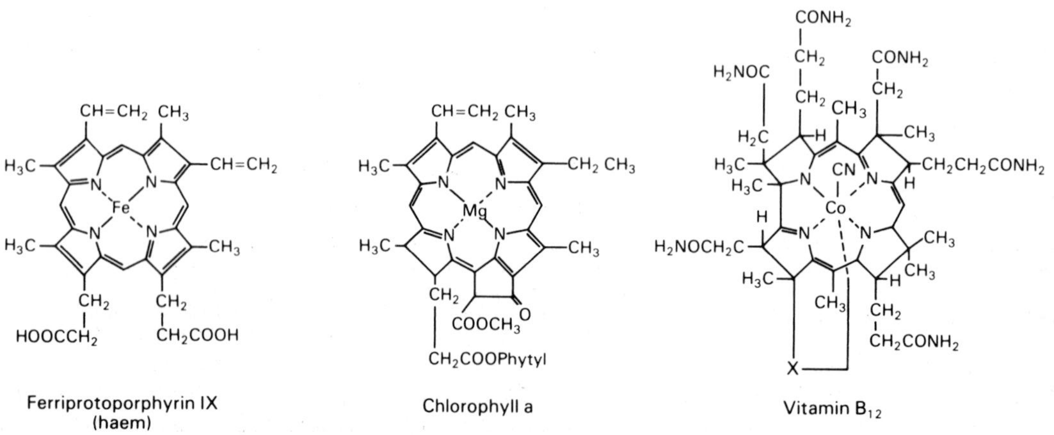

Ferriprotoporphyrin IX (haem)

Chlorophyll a

Vitamin B_{12}

Figure 16.1
Biologically important metalloporphyrins.

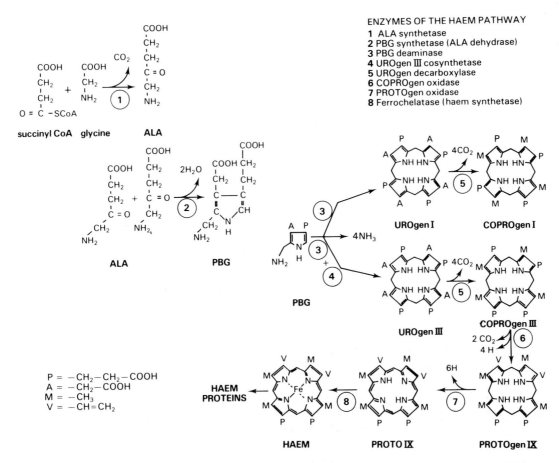

ENZYMES OF THE HAEM PATHWAY
1 ALA synthetase
2 PBG synthetase (ALA dehydrase)
3 PBG deaminase
4 UROgen III cosynthetase
5 UROgen decarboxylase
6 COPROgen oxidase
7 PROTOgen oxidase
8 Ferrochelatase (haem synthetase)

P = —CH₂—CH₂—COOH
A = —CH₂—COOH
M = —CH₃
V = —CH=CH₂

Figure 16.2 The pathway of haem synthesis. ALA = δ-aminolaevulinic acid; PBG = porphobilinogen; UROgen = uroporphyrinogen; COPROgen = coproporphyrinogen; PROTOgen = protoporphyrinogen; PROTO = protoporphyrin.

HAEM BIOSYNTHESIS

Formation of δ-aminolaevulinic acid (ALA)

As shown in Figure 16.2, glycine and succinic acid provide the constituent carbons for haem. One mol of glycine and 1 mol of succinyl CoA, derived from the tricarboxylic acid cycle, combine in the presence of pyridoxal phosphate to form ALA. The reaction is catalysed by the mitochondrial enzyme, ALA synthetase, and the product, ALA, is considered to be the first compound of the pathway committed to haem synthesis, although its metabolism by minor alternate routes occurs.[154] This reaction is rate-limiting for the formation of haem in the liver and possibly in other tissues; therefore, ALA synthetase plays a key role in regulating the pathway, as will be discussed below.

Formation of porphobilinogen

Porphobilinogen, the pyrrole subunit of the porphyrin ring, is formed by condensation of 2 mol of ALA, with elimination of water, in a reaction catalysed by the

cytosolic enzyme porphobilinogen synthetase (ALA dehydrase). The enzyme contains sulphydryl groups, is activated in vitro by sulphydryl-reducing agents, is particularly sensitive to inhibition by lead and requires zinc.[76]

Examination of rates of product formation in vitro by ALA synthetase and porphobilinogen synthetase suggests that the latter enzyme is present in relative abundance and therefore is unlikely to be involved significantly in regulation of the rate of haem synthesis. Both ALA and porphobilinogen are soluble in aqueous solution at physiological pH, are colourless and non-fluorescent and, therefore, impart no unusual hue to urine.

Formation of uroporphyrinogen

Condensation of 4 mol of porphobilinogen and ring closure yields the first porphyrin-like compound of the haem pathway, uroporphyrinogen. As depicted in Figure 16.3, the true intermediates in haem synthesis (up to protoporphyrin) are *porphyrinogens*, reduced porphyrins containing six additional hydrogen atoms. They are colourless, non-fluorescent compounds which are readily converted in the presence of light and air to the corresponding

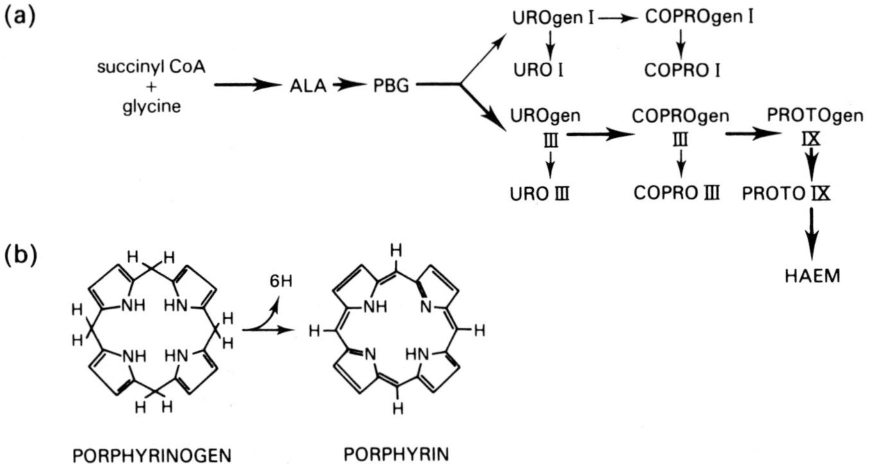

(a)

(b)

PORPHYRINOGEN   PORPHYRIN

Figure 16.3 The relationship of porphyrinogens and porphyrins to the haem synthesis pathway. (a) Formation of different porphyrinogens and porphyrins. (b) Oxidation of a porphyrinogen to a porphyrin. ALA=δ-aminolaevulinic acid; PBG=porphobilinogen; UROgen=uroporphyrinogen; URO=uroporphyrin. COPROgen=coproporphyrinogen; COPRO=coproporphyrin; PROTOgen=protoporphyrinogen; PROTO=protoporphyrin.

porphyrin by an irreversible oxidation (Figure 16.3). The resulting porphyrins, with the exception of protoporphyrin, cannot be re-incorporated into the pathway and undergo elimination from the organism. A feature of porphobilinogen with important biological consequences is its asymmetry, conferred by two different side-chains, one an acetic and the other a propionic group (Figure 16.2). Because of the asymmetry, condensation of 4 mol of porphobilinogen may theoretically yield four possible isomeric forms: a regular (head-to-tail) arrangement, with strictly alternating acetic and propionic acid groups (type I), or an arrangement in which two opposite pyrrole substituents are reversed (type II), a single pyrrole is reversed (type III) or two adjacent pyrroles are reversed (type IV). Of these, only types I and III are found in nature (Figure 16.2), and only the isomer III series serve as intermediates in haem synthesis.

This striking isomeric specificity for uroporphyrinogen is achieved in a reaction of intriguing complexity. The principal enzyme of the reaction catalyses the head-to-tail condensation of four pyrrole units, releasing 1 mol of ammonia from each pyrrole added (Figure 16.2). The enzyme is variously termed uroporphyrinogen I synthetase, porphobilinogen deaminase, or, as currently recommended, hydroxymethylbilane synthase (EC 4.3.1.8). The actual product of the reaction is the linear tetrapyrrole, hydroxymethylbilane, which undergoes spontaneous cyclization as it leaves the enzyme, forming uroporphyrinogen I. As shown in Figure 16.2, the I-isomer porphyrins constitute an abortive pathway. Formation of the physiologically 'correct' III isomer requires a second enzyme, uroporphyrinogen III cosynthetase (uroporphyrinogen III synthase, EC 4.2.1.75), acting in concert with the principal enzyme. The cosynthetase effects a reversal of the final pyrrolic unit of the linear tetrapyrrole on the enzyme complex, so that with ring closure and formation of the porphyrin, the final pyrrole substituent (ring D) and ring A condense in a head-to-head relationship.[5]

Separation and assay of PBG deaminase and uroporphyrinogen III cosynthetase in vitro suggest that in normal liver the latter activity is present in relative excess. This may ensure that porphobilinogen is carried through to uroporphyrinogen III, with minimal formation of the biologically useless I-isomer series.

Formation of coproporphyrinogen

Uroporphyrinogen is converted to coproporphyrinogen by sequential decarboxylation of the four acetyl side chains of the molecule. Intermediate porphyrins containing seven, six or five carboxyl groups are found in small amounts in normal urine. A single enzyme, uroporphyrinogen decarboxylase, mediates all four decarboxylations of both the isomer III and I compounds.[53,110]

Formation of protoporphyrinogen

Conversion of coproporphyrinogen III to protoporphyrinogen IX (coproporphyrinogen I is not further metabolized) involves decarboxylation and dehydrogenation of two of the propionic side chains on adjacent pyrrole units, yielding vinyl groups. The latter modification, mediated by coproporphyrinogen oxidase, confers additional asymmetry on the molecule. By rearrangement of the four constituent pyrroles the number of possible isomers increases to 15; these were arbitrarily designated as I to XV by Fischer and Orth[77] without regard to the biosynthetic precursors of specific isomers. Isomer IX of protoporphyrinogen belongs to the III series of uro- and coproporphyrin and is the only naturally occurring isomer of protoporphyrinogen.

Formation of haem

Finally, protoporphyrinogen is oxidized to protoporphyrin, and iron is inserted to form ferriprotoporphyrin IX, or haem. The oxidation of protoporphyrinogen was formerly believed to be non-enzymatic, because it occurs readily in vitro in the presence of air. However, in the reducing atmosphere of cells, spontaneous oxidation may be prevented, and studies suggest that the process is enzymatically mediated.[179] The insertion of iron is catalysed by a mitochondrial enzyme activity termed ferrochelatase. Although this process can also occur non-enzymatically in vitro, the evidence for an enzymatically mediated catalysis under physiological conditions is convincing.[27]

SUBCELLULAR AND EXTRACELLULAR TRANSPORT OF HAEM AND HAEM PRECURSORS

The pathway of haem synthesis takes in both the mitochondrial and cytosolic portions of the cell, and the final product, haem, undergoes distribution to multiple subcellular compartments and, at least in the case of hepatic parenchymal cells, transport out of the cell. The initial enzyme of the pathway, ALA synthetase, is formed on the rough endoplasmic reticulum and subsequently passes to mitochondria where it catalyses the formation of ALA. Thus, potential points of regulation of this key enzyme exist at the level of transcription of specific messenger RNA, translation on the rough endoplasmic reticulum, post-translational modification, its transport into mitochondria, and direct negative feedback of its activity in mitochondria. With the formation of ALA, the haem pathway leaves the mitochondrion since the next three enzymes—porphobilinogen synthetase, uroporphyrinogen synthetase–cosynthetase and uroporphyrinogen decarboxylase—are located in the extramitochondrial cytosol. The product of the latter reaction, coproporphyrinogen, reenters the mitochondrion where coproporphyrinogen oxidase, protoporphyrinogen oxidase and ferrochelatase catalyse the formation of haem.

A substantial portion of newly synthesized haem passes from the mitochondrion to combine with protein acceptors on the endoplasmic reticulum. Presumably, haem proteins in other sites (microbodies or cytosol) similarly draw on mitochondrial haem. In addition, haem may be transferred out of the cell, either into plasma or directly into bile.[18]

An unsolved and largely unexplored problem in haem metabolism concerns the manner in which constituents and intermediates of the pathway are translocated within the cell. The presence of haem-carrying proteins in liver cytosol has been postulated;[112,233] specific transport mechanisms for haem precursors similarly may reasonably be inferred, although these lack direct confirmation. Their significance lies in the fact that they represent potential points of regulation of haem synthesis in addition to the specific enzymes of the pathway.

In plasma, ALA and porphobilinogen appear to be only loosely associated with protein, so that they undergo efficient elimination by the kidneys. Haem is transported on albumin or on the β-glycoprotein, haemopexin.[161] In most species, the affinity of haem for haemopexin is measurably greater than for albumin, although plasma albumin is present in 30- to 40-fold greater concentration than is haemopexin and therefore may be quantitatively the more important carrier. Porphyrins are associated with the same serum proteins but with less affinity than haem.

PHYSIOLOGICAL EFFECTS OF HAEM PRECURSORS

Although haem synthesis is highly efficient, small amounts of intermediates escape the pathway and enter the circulation. In porphyria, these amounts are substantially increased. Their distribution in body tissues or excreta (hence their detection) reflects to a large extent their physical properties. In general, the intermediates of haem synthesis, viewed in their biosynthetic sequence, comprise increasingly lipophilic compounds. Up to and including uroporphyrin, the intermediates of the pathway contain sufficient ionizable groups to be relatively water soluble at physiological pH, and to be filtered by renal glomeruli and appear in urine. The decarboxylation of uroporphyrinogen, however, and formation of subsequent intermediates involve progressive removal of ionizable groups, with a parallel increase in lipophilicity. As a result, coproporphyrin is excreted preferentially into bile, and hence appears in faeces, although substantial amounts also appear in urine. Protoporphyrin is excreted solely by the faecal route.

Porphyrins are red-purple in colour and are fluorescent, in contrast to ALA and porphobilinogen which are colourless and non-fluorescent. The fluorescence reflects the fact that porphyrins undergo excitation by light, the effect being maximal with light of wavelength of about 400 nm, which corresponds to the absorption maximum for porphyrins. Relaxation of 'excited-state' porphyrins back to ground state occurs spontaneously. The released energy appears in vitro as a fluorescent emission with a peak intensity at about 600 nm (the precise wavelength varies for the different porphyrins and can be used for their quantification).[177] Porphyrins exposed to light in vivo (in skin or epidermal capillaries) undergo a similar excitation but in relaxing to ground state produce active molecules—possibly complement-derived peptides[128,129] or singlet oxygen[206]—which initiate inflammation and/or cause direct tissue damage. The nature of the light-induced damage varies with the type of porphyrin, probably because of differences in the subcutaneous distribution of uro-, copro- or protoporphyrin. Accordingly, the clinical manifestations of photosensitivity differ among the various porphyrias but include urticaria, oedema, bullae or ulceration and possibly haemolysis.[206] By contrast, those porphyrias associated with overproduction of only ALA or porphobilinogen exhibit no photosensitivity.

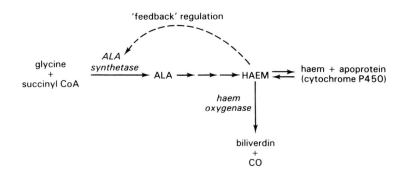

Figure 16.4 A postulated model for end-product regulation of haem synthesis in the liver. From Bissell and Hammaker (1976),[16] with kind permission of the authors and the editor of *Archives of Biochemistry and Biophysics*.

REGULATION OF HEPATIC HAEM SYNTHESIS

ROLE OF ALA SYNTHETASE

Studies in animals and in cell culture have established that in normal liver the rate-determining step in haem synthesis is the formation of ALA, which directly reflects the activity of the enzyme catalysing this reaction, ALA synthetase. The activity fluctuates rapidly (within several minutes) in response to changes in the cellular requirements for haem. Consistent with this rapid response is the relatively short half-life of the enzyme and its messenger RNA in both avian and mammalian liver.[228] Thus, a homeostatic mechanism exists for adjusting the level of haem synthesis to the needs of the organism. Based on cogent, albeit circumstantial, evidence, a haem 'pool' serving this regulatory function has been postulated, as indicated in Figure 16.4. This pool appears to consist of haem-in-transit and is fed by endogenous synthesis as well as being in equilibrium with cytochrome-associated haem.[196] In addition, exogenously administered haem, in part, may enter the pool, effecting a reduction in the activity of ALA synthetase, as shown in experimental animals given haem intraperitoneally or intravenously.[144] Conversely, a manipulation that results in withdrawal of haem from the regulatory pool, e.g. new synthesis of apocytochrome, results in stimulation of ALA synthetase activity. Administration of barbiturate to experimental animals constitutes a model for the latter sequence of events. The initial event after administration of phenobarbital to rats is formation of apocytochrome P450 followed by stimulation of the haem synthetic pathway.[40,182]

The precise way in which haem alters the activity of ALA synthetase is uncertain. Evidence has been obtained for a decrease in enzyme synthesis (haem acting as a corepressor), direct (feedback) inhibition of the enzyme itself or post-translational interaction of haem and ALA synthetase, which prevents transfer of the enzyme from cytosol to mitochondria. Any one or a combination of these mechanisms could be operative in vivo.[85]

In addition to serving the biosynthesis of tissue haem proteins, haem in the regulatory pool presumably also undergoes degradation to bile pigment. Haem degradation involves irreversible oxidative cleavage of the porphyrin ring, and the α-methane bridge carbon is released as carbon monoxide (Figure 16.4). In liver, the process appears to be mediated by a microsomal enzyme, haem oxygenase, which is present in the parenchymal cell fraction of the liver as well as in sinusoidal lining cells.[17] After administration of a haem load to experimental animals, hepatic haem oxygenase activity increases, apparently serving to eliminate excess intracellular haem.[213] It is not known whether haem oxygenase may be stimulated in the absence of an increased haem load and thereby deplete intracellular hepatic haem. Although the activity increases after administration of a variety of non-haem substances, this response may reflect shifts in intracellular haem and presentation of an 'endogenous' haem load to the enzyme.[15] Experimental porphyria in rats is associated with subnormal activity of hepatic haem oxygenase.[189]

ROLE OF CYTOCHROME P450

All tissues, other than erythrocytes, exhibit aerobic metabolism and therefore require mitochondrial cytochromes. Presumably all such cells synthesize haem to meet the need for cytochrome formation. Requirements for haem synthesis vary widely among individual tissues, reflecting the type of haem protein present in a tissue, its concentration and its half-life. Haem formation in bone marrow is active because of the relatively large amounts required for haemoglobin synthesis, although the turnover of haemoglobin is slow (the red-cell life span in humans is 120 days and in the rat is 57 days). In the liver, 50% of newly synthesized haem is utilized in the formation of cytochrome P450. Although the amount of cytochrome P450 in liver is only a very small fraction of the amount of haemoglobin in the organism, the half-life of cytochrome P450 is short (in the rat its decay is biphasic, with an average half-life of about 16 h). The haem requirement for hepatic cytochrome P450 in the rat can be estimated at approximately 10% of that for haemoglobin. Therefore, synthesis of cytochrome P450 appears to account for the high rate of haem synthesis in the liver, and changes in the production of cytochrome P450 would be expected to exert major changes in the rate of hepatic haem synthesis. The liver contains a number of haem proteins in addition to cytochrome P450, which collectively undoubtedly affect the rate of haem synthesis. Individually, however, none of these is comparable either in concentration or rate of turnover to cytochrome P450.

An important characteristic of cytochrome P450 is its inducibility by its substrates (administered drugs or lipophilic endogenous substances such as gonadal steroids). Ultimately, induction brings about accelerated removal (and/or inactivation) of the substrate from the organism. This response requires new synthesis of cytochrome P450, a process which in turn requires increased haem synthesis. Normal liver meets this demand with increased activity of ALA synthetase and new production of haem precursors. In porphyric individuals, the flow of precursors may be partially blocked by a defective or deficient enzyme, thus limiting the capacity for increasing haem synthesis. In such an individual, depletion of the haem pool may occur, so that ALA synthetase is de-repressed and the defective enzymatic step becomes rate-determining for haem synthesis. Under these conditions, the intermediates prior to the block accumulate, spilling over into the circulation and appearing in urine or faeces. This type of porphyria may be regarded as a *haem-deficient* condition; characteristically, it is exacerbated by the administration of inducers of cytochrome P450 (of which barbiturates are the archetype). The haem-deficient porphyrias may be contrasted with porphyrias with a normal capacity for haem synthesis which are unaffected by inducers of cytochrome P450: these may be termed *haem-compensated*. This distinction is important in the diagnosis and management of the various porphyrias.

CLASSIFICATION OF THE PORPHYRIAS

The porphyrias may be classified according to pathogenesis (hereditary or acquired) or according to tissue localization (bone marrow or liver) (Table 16.1). With regard to the latter, presumably all cells in the body synthesize haem, as noted above, and thus all potentially may be affected by a genetic defect in the haem pathway. The liver and marrow are major sites of haem synthesis and therefore also of porphyrin production. The kidneys synthesize substantial haem;[14] their contribution to porphyrin formation has not been quantified.[48] Thus, at present, porphyrin overproduction is attributed to either the bone marrow or liver, although the porphyric state may have important consequences in tissues not contributing quantitatively to the overproduction of porphyrins or porphyrin precursors. Indeed, neural dysfunction is prominent in acute intermittent porphyria and may be an expression of the genetic defect in this tissue (see below).

The specific enzyme defect associated with each porphyria is listed in Table 16.1. In the case of the hepatic porphyrias, the position of the defect in the haem pathway is shown in Figure 16.5, as well as the individual pattern of excretion of precursors associated with each type. Of the three porphyrias that comprise the haem-deficient group (Table 16.1), the pattern of precursor excretion provides the principal means for their differentiation, their main clinical features being essentially identical, as will be discussed.

PATHOLOGY OF THE PORPHYRIAS

The liver commonly contains an excess of porphyrins or their precursors. Porphyrins can be demonstrated in liver tissue by their red fluorescence in ultraviolet light, but this technique does not specify the nature of the porphyria. Specific and diagnostic inclusions are seen in hepatocytes by light and electron microscopy in both protoporphyria[21, 139,147] and porphyria cutanea tarda[41,106] (see below). By electron microscopy, liver tissue from patients with acute intermittent porphyria exhibits a variety of changes in mitochondrial and cytosolic structures.[168] Significant chronic liver disease is rare except in association with porphyria cutanea tarda and protoporphyria, although micronodular cirrhosis has been described in a young adult female with congenital erythropoietic porphyria.[111]

ERYTHROPOIETIC PORPHYRIA

Extensive discussion of erythropoietic porphyria is beyond the scope of this chapter; the reader is referred to a detailed review.[154] In brief, *congenital erythropoietic porphyria* is a rare, recessively inherited disease, with less than 100 cases in the world literature. The classical form involves severe photosensitivity and anaemia from infancy. Disfiguring cutaneous damage occurs, with loss of nasal tissue, ears, lips and digits. The underlying defect is a deficiency of uroporphyrinogen III cosynthetase, which results in a marked excess of isomer I uroporphyrin in plasma and urine. The bone marrow is the site of porphyrin overproduction. Haemolytic anaemia is present, with circulating normoblasts and reticulocytes that contain uroporphyrin and are fluorescent under blue-light excitation. Suggested therapies, based on single case reports, are hypertransfusion to suppress the patient's own bone marrow,[175] haematin,[224] chloroquine,[105] and oral administration of activated charcoal, the last to bind porphyrin within the bowel lumen and enhance its excretion.[172] Avoidance of light is important in theory but difficult in practice; the activating wavelength passes through window glass and is present in incandescent light. Topical sunscreens provide little or no protection.[146]

A second form with an identical clinical presentation but a different enzymatic defect has been described and termed hepatoerythropoietic porphyria. It involves a severe deficiency of uroporphyrinogen decarboxylase and has been viewed as homozygous porphyria cutanea tarda (see below).[73,217] Dyserythropoiesis has been reported,[116] and all affected individuals appear to have increased erythrocyte porphyrins. The pattern of porphyrin overproduction differs from that of the classic form in that urine uroporphyrin, while markedly elevated, is predominantly isomer III rather than I, and erythrocytes contain protoporphyrin (as zinc protoporphyrin) rather than uroporphyrin. The basis

Table 16.1 Classification of the porphyrias.

	Synonym	Inheritance	Enzyme defect	Haem status
Hereditary erythropoietic				
Congenital	Günther's disease	Recessive	Uroporphyrinogen III cosynthetase (?)	Compensated
Protoporphyria	Erythropoietic or protoporphyria	Dominant (?)	Ferrochelatase	Compensated (?)
Hereditary hepatic				
Acute intermittent	Swedish porphyria, pyrroloporphyria	Dominant	PBG deaminase	Deficient
Coproporphyria		Dominant	Coproporphyrinogen oxidase	Deficient
Variegate	South African porphyria	Dominant	Undetermined (protoporphyrinogen oxidase?)	Deficient
ALAuria		Recessive	Porphobilinogen synthetase	Deficient (?)
Acquired				
Intoxications (heavy metals, hexachlorobenzene, etc.)			Variable	Variable

for the latter abnormality is unknown. Increased zinc protoporphyrin is associated otherwise with iron deficiency or heavy-metal intoxication. Therapy for this form is uncertain. If (as seems likely), porphyrin overproduction originates primarily in the liver, hypertransfusion would have no benefit. Orally administered charcoal was beneficial in one patient.[172]

Finally, it should be noted that, while congenital photosensitivity is the rule, relatively mild forms exist, with the diagnosis first being made only in adulthood. Such individuals present with the signs of porphyria cutanea tarda.[57]

PROTOPORPHYRIA

Protoporphyria is characterized by a variable (usually mild) cutaneous photosensitivity, which is manifest minutes after exposure of the skin to sunlight and consists of a stinging, burning sensation and oedema (solar urticaria). With repeated exposure, thickening and fibrosis of the skin may occur.[138] The cutaneous reaction is quite distinct from the bullous lesion of congenital erythropoietic porphyria or porphyria cutanea tarda. This may reflect the fact that plasma protoporphyrin is elevated in protoporphyria, whereas uroporphyrin is increased in

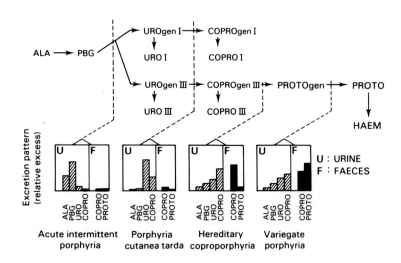

Figure 16.5 Patterns of precursor excretion in the major hereditary hepatic porphyrias. The vertical dashed line for each type of porphyria indicates the point in the haem pathway at which defective enzymatic activity has been identified or is presumed to exist (see also Table 16.1). Abbreviations are as in Figure 16.3.

the other conditions. In vitro studies have shown that protoporphyrin combined with irradiation is markedly more active than uroporphyrin in stimulating release of mediators, such as serotonin, from mast cells.[127]

The underlying defect is a deficiency of ferrochelatase (haem synthase).[27,31] The frequency of protoporphyria in one population group (in the Netherlands) has been estimated at 2 in 100 000.[226] The inheritance of the condition previously was believed to be autosomal dominant with incomplete penetrance accounting for the lack of expression in successive generations. This is supported by studies of the distribution of the protoporphyrinogen oxidase deficiency within affected families.[27] However, recessive inheritance within a three-allele system also has been proposed.[226] In this system, "*f*" is the normal gene; "*F−*" is an abnormal gene in an individual without fluorescent erythrocytes; and "*F+*" is an abnormal gene with fluorescent erythrocytes. The genotype *F−F+* is classic protoporphyria. Neither parent (*fF−* and *fF+*) is affected, but one has fluorescent red cells. Among other possible genotypes, *F−F−* has not been characterized; *F+F+* has typical protoporphyria.[46]

Investigations

The characteristic porphyrin abnormality is a moderate-to-marked increase in plasma and faecal protoporphyrin, with a lesser increase in coproporphyrin. Urinary porphyrins are normal. Immature erythrocytes in the marrow exhibit an evanescent red fluorescence under excitation with light of approximately 400 nm wavelength, and a portion of circulating erythrocytes (primarily reticulocytes) are similarly fluorescent in most affected individuals, a finding which is useful in screening for the disease.[43] Patients either have a normal haemoglobin or are only mildly anaemic,[50] suggesting that protoporphyrin is produced in excess of requirements for haem formation.

The relative contribution of erythroid tissue and liver to the overproduction of protoporphyrin apparently varies among individual patients. In some studies, leakage of protoporphyrin from erythrocytes accounts entirely for the excess porphyrin in plasma and stool.[174] In other patients, however, a significant portion of the excreted protoporphyrin originates in the liver,[198] where its production appears to be sensitive to administered haem.[23,122] Whether these divergent findings reflect an underlying heterogeneity of this type of porphyria or only variation in its biochemical expression is unclear at the present time.

Because of its relative lipophilicity (see above), protoporphyrin does not appear in urine but, rather, is excreted solely in faeces. Thus all circulating protoporphyrin either must pass through the liver into bile or undergo excretion by direct transmucosal transfer from plasma to the intestinal lumen. The high throughput of porphyrin in liver is associated with a variety of disturbances. Protoporphyrin-containing gallstones occur in approximately 10% of persons with protoporphyria.[24,50]

Pathology

Deposition of porphyrin in bile canaliculi, hepatocytes and sinusoidal cells occurs, accompanied by inflammatory cells and fibrosis.[22] The porphyrins can be readily visualized on light microscopy as numerous dark-brown pigment deposits that exhibit a distinctive bright-red birefringence with a dark central Maltese cross when examined under polarized light.[20,44] An equally distinctive appearance is seen using electron microscopy.[34,147] Numerous long, slender, curved rod-like crystals arranged singly in sheaves or as a tangled mass can be found free within the hepatocyte cytoplasm or within lysosomes of Kupffer cells. Biochemical analysis of the crystals in a liver from a patient with protoporphyria has confirmed that they are protoporphyrin.[21] As the inflammatory lesion progresses, the excretory capacity of the liver declines, leading to increased levels of plasma protoporphyrin. Routine liver function tests may be only mildly abnormal. However, with the appearance of jaundice, rapid progression to liver failure and death is observed. For this reason, in patients with liver function abnormalities—particularly those with protoporphyrin in plasma >50 μg/dl or in erythrocytes >1000 μg/dl—liver biopsy is recommended to assess the stage and activity of the hepatopathy.[22]

Liver transplantation was successful in one patient although probably not curative, since the bone marrow in this individual was the source of the excess porphyrin.[190]

Treatment

Betacarotene is effective in increasing tolerance to sunlight,[146] apparently by blocking active intermediates (see above) in porphyrin-induced tissue damage, and, apart from the rare patients in whom hepatic complications develop, the prognosis of the disease is good.

Cholestyramine has been administered to patients with porphyric liver disease, with the rationale that the drug binds protoporphyrin in the intestine,[20] interrupting its enterohepatic circulation and facilitating its excretion from the body; activated charcoal also has been given on the same basis.[84] Their efficacy is uncertain, with only anecdotal reports available. Administered haematin appears to suppress formation of protoporphyrin in some, but not all, patients with protoporphyria. The effect on hepatic function is still unclear, although serum bilirubin levels may decline.[23] Long-term benefit presumably would require chronic haematin therapy, an approach which at present is impractical due to the need for its intravenous administration. Red-cell transfusions may lead to reduced levels of circulating protoporphyrin and improvement of the hepatic disease. In patients with iron deficiency, administration of iron produces mixed results, with lowering of blood porphyrins in some cases[90] but aggravation in others.[232] The basis for the differing response to iron is unclear.

Table 16.2 Clinical presentation of acute attacks of haem-deficient porphyria.

Symptoms	%	Physical findings	%
Abdominal pain	90	Tachycardia	83
Vomiting	80	Hypertension	55
Constipation	80	Motor neuropathy	53
Pain in limbs	51	Pyrexia	38
Pain in back	50	Leucocytosis	20
Confused state	32	Bulbar involvement	18
Urinary frequency	30	Sensory loss	15
Dysuria	28	Cranial nerve	
Abnormal behaviour	23	involvement	9
Seizures	12	Proteinuria	8
Diarrhoea	8	Hepatomegaly	5
Stupor	7		
Coma	6		

Data from Eales' study of 80 patients with variegate porphyria.[64] The presentation of acute intermittent porphyria[207,222] and of hereditary coproporphyria[33] is similar.

HEPATIC PORPHYRIAS WITH HAEM DEFICIENCY: ACUTE INTERMITTENT PORPHYRIA, HEREDITARY COPROPORPHYRIA AND VARIEGATE PORPHYRIA

Although these porphyrias are distinct genetic entities, they will be described as a group because they are indistinguishable in terms of their main clinical features. Each involves an enzyme defect that results in a potential—or actual—deficiency of hepatic haem synthesis, which may account for the many clinical characteristics they have in common. These porphyrias differ primarily with regard to their respective patterns of haem precursor excretion, which are of importance for screening of carriers and account also for the presence of cutaneous symptoms in hereditary coproporphyria and variegate porphyria.

Clinical presentation

Acute attacks are accompanied by the manifestations listed in Table 16.2. Abdominal pain, often colicky and severe, is a frequent symptom, characteristically lasting for several days; it may mimic acute inflammation of a hollow viscus. Many patients complain of severe constipation for a considerable period of time, beginning in some cases in puberty. Nausea and vomiting are frequent. Neurological symptoms are protean, ranging from headache and psychiatric disturbances to paraesthesias and paralysis. A family history may elicit information concerning relatives who succumbed to an obscure 'neurological' disease that, in retrospect, was probably porphyria.

Physical examination may reveal abdominal tenderness and diminished bowel sounds, although the findings are characteristically less impressive than the symptoms; rebound tenderness is distinctly unusual. Attacks are accompanied almost invariably by sinus tachycardia, which parallels disease activity in many patients. Approximately one-third of patients present with altered mental status.

The Klüver–Bucy syndrome has been reported in a patient with an acute attack.[97] The complete syndrome consists of aggressive oral tendencies and hypersexuality; it has been attributed to a temporal lobe lesion on the basis of studies in monkeys. While the syndrome is rare as an overt psychosis, subtle abnormalities of the same type may be observed not uncommonly during acute attacks. Patients often exhibit an hysterical affect, which in the context of a requirement for narcotic analgesics may be interpreted as manipulative, drug-seeking behaviour. While patients receiving potent narcotics for frequent recurrent attacks are at risk for addiction, as a rule the abnormal behaviour clears rapidly as the attack resolves.

Grand mal seizures may be a component of the acute presentation and, when persistent or recurring, represent a particularly difficult management problem (see below). Motor and sensory neurological abnormalities may develop rapidly during the early phase of an attack.[9] These begin with proximal weakness and may progress in severe cases to quadriplegia and respiratory failure. Death is usually due to respiratory failure and the complications associated with its management.

Investigations

Laboratory studies are useful in differentiating acute porphyric attacks from other intraabdominal crises (Table 16.3). The total leukocyte count is usually within normal limits and, even when elevated, the differential cell count is normal. An abdominal radiograph may reveal distended bowel loops. Dark urine, when it is present, should suggest the diagnosis. Hyponatraemia may also occur, possibly due to inappropriate secretion of antidiuretic hormone; it may develop rapidly in patients receiving large volumes of dextrose in water as part of their therapy and may be responsible for acute mental changes unrelated to porphyria *per se*. The spinal fluid either is normal or exhibits a minimal pleocytosis consistent with seizure activity. In the absence of other causes of liver disease, routine liver function studies reveal only a modest increase in serum transaminase activity.[207] An increase in total serum cholesterol (related to increased low density lipoprotein) is also observed[207] and may occur more often in symptomatic than in asymptomatic patients;[164] its cause is obscure. Total serum thyroxine is elevated in many patients, and this, with other manifestations, suggests a hyperthyroid state. However, the increase reflects elevation only of thyroid-binding globulin and other parameters of thyroid function are normal; this appears to occur more often in females than in males with porphyria.[207]

Table 16.3 Normal values for the laboratory determination of porphyrins and porphyrin precursors.

	Urine (24 h)	Faeces (dry wt)	Erythrocytes
ALA	<57 μmol (<7.5 mg)	—	—
Porphobilinogen	<9 μmol (<2.0 mg)	—	—
Uroporphyrin	12–60 nmol (0.01–0.05 mg)	trace	<23 nmol/l (<1.5 μg/dl)
Coproporphyrin	76–382 nmol (0.05–0.25 mg)	<76 nmol/g (<50 μg/g)	
Protoporphyrin	—	<215 nmol/g (<120 μg/g)	<1.3 μmol/l (<75 μg/dl)

The ranges for δ-aminolaevulinic acid and porphobilinogen are those for the procedure of Davis and Andelman,[47] which is available in kit form (Bio-Rad Laboratories, Richmond, California). The measurement includes both ALA and aminoacetone, the latter normally being present in only small amounts.[145] Porphyrin analyses were carried out according to Schwartz *et al.*,[199] the normal ranges are those utilized by the author and are similar to those of Meyer and Schmid[154] and Elder, Gray and Nicholson.[69]

Pathogenesis

Enzyme defects (Table 16.1)

The defect in acute intermittent porphyria has been studied in several laboratories and consists of a 50% reduction in PBG deaminase activity.[208] The enzyme has been purified[3,157] and its gene localized to human chromosome 11.[151] The purified enzyme consists of five charge isomers (designated A to E) which represent native enzyme (A) or enzyme-substrate complexes comprising native enzyme plus one to four linked pyrrole units (B to E).[3]

PBG deaminase, as a cytosolic protein, is present in erythrocytes as well as in nucleated cells, and in most carriers, a deficiency is detectable in erythrocytes. In some families, however, the erythrocyte activity is normal,[94,163] suggesting at least two forms of acute intermittent porphyria. An additional level of heterogeneity is suggested by analysis of genetic carriers for cross-reactive immunological material (CRIM) representing PBG deaminase that is catalytically inactive. In 85% of carriers, enzyme activity and protein were similarly decreased (CRIM-negative cases), but a minority were CRIM-positive.[51]

This clinical and immunological evidence for genetic heterogeneity has been confirmed in recent molecular studies. Cloning and sequencing of the PBG deaminase gene demonstrate that two forms of mRNA are produced, one in all cells and one restricted to erythroid cells.[37,92,94] They are products of a single gene containing two different transcriptional initiation sites (Figure 16.6). The 'general' (G) transcript undergoes processing that eliminates the second exon. The 'erythropoietic' (E) transcript is controlled by the region of DNA immediately upstream (5') of the second exon[156] and apparently is active only in erythroid cells.[94] Analysis of one family in which erythrocyte PBG deaminase is normal revealed a mutation of the splice sequence between the first exon and first intron (Figure 16.6, arrow*). Failure of proper splicing at this point very likely would prevent formation of a usable G-transcript but would have no effect on the E-transcript, which is initiated distally. Thus, the mutation

appears to account for those cases in which the enzyme defect is present in liver but not in erythrocytes.[94] A search for the genetic basis of CRIM-positive and CRIM-negative carriers revealed one CRIM-positive individual with an mRNA of reduced size. On sequence analysis, a mutation was found at a distal splice junction (Figure 16.6, arrow**), such that processing of the primary transcript resulted in loss of exon 12.[93] It is postulated that this mRNA translates a protein that is catalytically inactive but immunoreactive and stable. Because of its position in a distal region of the gene, the mutation affects both G and E mRNA and thus is expressed in erythrocytes as well as liver. A different splicing defect has been reported in one CRIM-negative individual.[234] Such data indicate the substantial genetic diversity that must exist within the currently recognized types of porphyria. DNA analysis will facilitate the identification of latent carriers[126,133] using methodology such as polymerase chain reaction to amplify a diagnostic mutation.[93] This approach is less ambiguous than measurement of enzyme activity and soon may be cost-effective.

In hereditary coproporphyria (Figure 16.5), relatively few individuals have been studied, in part because coproporphyrinogen oxidase is mitochondrial and therefore requires blood leucocytes or skin fibroblasts for its assay. In these cells, decreases of 50% or more in enzyme activity have been recorded in affected individuals.[71]

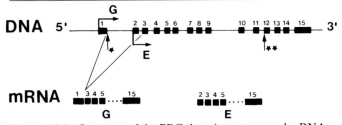

Figure 16.6 Structure of the PBG deaminase gene and mRNAs for the general (G) and erythroid (E) forms. The two start sites of transcription are marked by right-angle arrows labelled G and E respectively. Filled boxes, numbered 1 to 15, indicate transcribed regions (exons) that appear in the mature mRNA. The representation of the gene is roughly to scale.[37]

Studies of patients with variegate porphyria have implicated deficiencies of both protoporphyrinogen oxidase
and ferrochelatase in the pathogenesis of this type of
porphyria.[10,32] In studies of South Africans, both enzymes
appeared to be deficient.[203] In other studies, only protoporphyrinogen oxidase was abnormal[165] or, in one, both
protoporphyrinogen oxidase and PBG deaminase.[152]
These varying data may be traceable to the use of different
assay methods or to genetic heterogeneity. Linkage analysis places the responsible trait on human chromosome
14.[12]

The pattern of transmission for all three of these
porphyrias is autosomal dominant, affected persons being
heterozygous for the altered gene. Once it was speculated
that a double dose of the abnormal gene was incompatible
with life. However, several apparent homozygotes for
hereditary coproporphyria and variegate porphyria have
been described. They differ from heterozygotes clinically
in displaying photosensitivity from an early age, even
within days of birth,[91,162,165] and often growth retardation
with skeletal abnormalities. An unexpected feature of all
cases reported to date (also in homozygous porphyria
cutanea tarda or hepatoerythropoietic porphyria and in
homozygous δ-aminolaevulinic aciduria) is the presence
of elevated erythrocyte protoporphyrin, which is not
found in the heterozygous parents or in typical cases of
variegate porphyria. While its basis is unknown, it may
serve as a useful pointer to the diagnosis of persons
with lifelong bullous photosensitivity. Affected individuals
demonstrate a severe deficiency of the appropriate enzyme
(coproporphyrinogen oxidase or protoporphyrinogen
oxidase).

Drug sensitivity

In known carriers of these defects the biochemical manifestations of disease vary from minimal to marked,
reflecting the importance of secondary factors in the
clinical disease. A fixed capacity for haem synthesis will
be of little consequence if the demand for haem remains
within that capacity. Many patients with porphyria, in
fact, appear to enjoy a haem-compensated state, are
asymptomatic and exhibit minimally increased excretion of
haem precursors. However, an endogenous or exogenous
challenge to the haem synthetic system may rapidly induce
a haem-deficient state. Many acute attacks follow the
unwitting administration of drug inducers of cytochrome
P450. 'Spontaneous' attacks also occur (more frequently,
it appears, in acute intermittent porphyria than in the
other two forms), reflecting the importance of endogenous
factors. Acute attacks are more frequent in women
than in men, and first attacks are rare before puberty.
Pregnancy may exacerbate the condition in some women,
and cyclical attacks associated with menstruation have
been described.[229] These findings emphasize the importance of hormonal changes in the pathogenesis of acute
attacks, possibly related to the fact that gonadal steroids
are metabolized in part by cytochrome P450 and may
stimulate endogenously the rate of hepatic haem synthesis.

Exogenous progesterone induces cytochrome P450 in
experimental animals, and exogenous hormones (oral
contraceptives) have provoked acute attacks in some
patients with porphyria.

Neurological dysfunction

Most, if not all, of the symptoms and findings of acute
attacks suggest neurological dysfunction, including
abdominal pain which may result from a neurogenic
motility disorder of the bowel.[9] Hyperactivity of the
sympathetic nervous system may account for tachycardia
and constipation which are frequently seen. Increased
excretion of catecholamines has been documented in
persons during attacks of acute intermittent porphyria,
as have abnormalities in the uptake of noradrenaline
(norepinephrine) by platelets from individuals with this
disorder.[6] The aetiology of neurological dysfunction in
these types of porphyria remains a major unresolved
problem. To date, attention has centred on ways in which
elevated circulating levels of porphyrins or porphyrin
precursors might affect the nervous system. While the
haem-deficient porphyrias differ with respect to the pattern of precursor overproduction, they all exhibit excess
excretion of ALA and porphobilinogen, and these compounds characteristically undergo striking increases during
acute attacks in all three types of porphyria. In addition,
in two diseases unrelated to porphyria—heavy metal
intoxication and hereditary tyrosinaemia—acute abdominal manifestations occur in association with increased
urinary excretion of ALA and are similar to those with
porphyria.[130] Furthermore, 'neurological' symptoms are
absent in those porphyrias involving overproduction of
porphyrins but not ALA or porphobilinogen, i.e. the
haem-compensated porphyrias (Table 16.1). While these
findings suggest that increased plasma ALA may alter
neural function, correlation between the plasma level of
ALA or porphobilinogen and the severity of symptoms
is poor. In a study of a patient with acute porphyria,
charcoal haemoperfusion and haemodialysis removed substantial amounts of ALA and porphobilinogen from the
circulation but failed to improve symptoms.[118] Moreover,
attempts to demonstrate direct toxicity of ALA to neural
tissues, either in vivo or in vitro, have produced results
that are either negative or inconclusive, despite the use
of pharmacological concentrations of ALA. An alternative
possibility is that neurological dysfunction reflects intrinsic
haem deficiency at the cellular level, either because cells
of the nervous system, like the liver, are sensitive to
inducers of cytochrome P450 or because they require
exogenous haem. The latter might normally be supplied
by the liver (see p. 401) but decrease during an acute
attack associated with intrahepatic haem depletion (see
below). Finally, acute deficiency of hepatic haem may
lead indirectly to altered neurological function. An early
manifestation of experimentally induced hepatic haem
deficiency (in the rat) is reduced activity of the haem-
dependent enzyme tryptophan pyrrolase. This results in
elevation of plasma tryptophan, increased tryptophan

uptake by the brain, and increased brain levels of 5-hydroxytryptamine (serotonin).[131,132] These experimental findings raise the possibility that neurological symptoms in acute hepatic porphyria may be due in part to local overproduction of tryptophan-derived neurotransmitters. Extrapolation of the results to humans, however, awaits studies of tryptophan metabolism in acute porphyria. Increased excretion of 5-hydroxyindoleacetic acid has been described in one family with acute intermittent porphyria.[135]

The efficacy of intravenous haematin in the treatment of acute porphyric symptoms is consistent with any of these postulated pathophysiological mechanisms. Administered haem would be expected to suppress ALA synthetase, reducing overproduction of ALA and porphobilinogen;[144] it could supply the nervous system directly with haem and, in repleting hepatic haem, it would restore tryptophan pyrrolase to full activity, with reduction of circulating tryptophan and decreased metabolism of this amino acid by extrahepatic tissues such as brain.[132]

Diagnosis

Acute porphyric attacks

An initial attack of porphyria in which 'classic' manifestations readily suggest the diagnosis is a rare event. Commonly, only a part of the symptom complex is present, unaccompanied by abnormal physical findings. Such patients are often told that their complaints are psychosomatic; the less fortunate are those thought to have a surgically correctable abdominal condition. While the diagnosis may be suggested by history and physical examination, definitive evaluation virtually always requires appropriate laboratory investigation. Decisions as to the laboratory tests to be ordered depend on the type of porphyria under consideration, since the principal precursor excess (as well as its route of excretion) differs among the three haem-deficient porphyrias (Figure 16.5). Elevation of urinary porphobilinogen is characteristic of acute intermittent porphyria, faecal coproporphyrin of hereditary coproporphyria and faecal protoporphyrin of variegate porphyria. During an acute attack of any of the three, urinary porphobilinogen will be elevated, and this can be assessed qualitatively by means of the Watson–Schwartz test in which porphobilinogen forms a pink complex with Ehrlich's reagent.[223] The test is positive in virtually all patients suffering acute attacks, although its sensitivity is insufficient for detecting asymptomatic carriers. It is also specific when performed properly. In this regard, it should be emphasized that extraction of the pink complex with chloroform or butanol is essential to a correct interpretation of the colour reaction. The porphobilinogen complex will remain in the aqueous phase after extraction with organic solvents, whereas a number of other substances in urine (notably, urobilinogen, indoles and phenazopyridine) which also yield a red reaction with Ehrlich's reagent are extractable with organic solvents. Other causes of false-positive tests have been noted but are relatively infrequent.[69] A modification of the Ehrlich's procedure (the Hoesch test) has been re-evaluated.[123] It eliminates the necessity for extraction of the pink reaction product.

Tests for the carrier state

In screening for carriers of acute intermittent porphyria, urinary porphobilinogen is measured by a column chromatographic procedure originally introduced by Mauzerall and Granick.[149] The column method is both quantitative and, with few exceptions, specific. Urine from persons taking large amounts of phenothiazines may contain chromogens which are eluted from the column together with porphobilinogen and interfere with the analysis.[183] The sensitivity of the column procedure permits measurement of urinary porphobilinogen in normal individuals. Porphobilinogen excretion exceeds the normal range in 70% of persons with acute intermittent porphyria, regardless of the presence or absence of symptoms of the disease. In a proportion of affected individuals, and in most prepubertal carriers, the urinary findings are normal. For this reason, negative results based on urine analysis alone carry a definite measure of uncertainty. In acute intermittent porphyria, this difficulty can be circumvented in part by assay of the hereditary enzyme defect, i.e. decreased activity of PBG deaminase. The enzyme, being cytosolic, is present in mature erythrocytes and therefore may be measured in red-cell haemolysates. The genetically determined decrease in activity is expressed regardless of the age of the individual. The original assay method has undergone modifications,[141,155] and the determination is suitable for routine clinical use.[107,121,170,194] Cultured skin fibroblasts and amniotic cells from affected individuals also display diminished activity of PBG deaminase.[30,153,193] While porphyric individuals exhibit, on average, 50% of normal activity, occasional determinations with erythrocytes from affected individuals fall into the low-normal range. In persons with a reticulocytosis, enzyme activity may be elevated. The activity is highest in young red cells and progressively declines as erythrocytes age in the circulation. In other instances, relatively high enzyme activity in porphyrics may be genetically determined, and unaffected family members display approximately twice the activity of porphyric members.[194] It has been reported that enzyme activity rises during acute attacks,[114] although not all studies are in agreement.[191] A possible basis for the finding is that during acute attacks the concentration of substrate (porphobilinogen) generally rises and the enzyme–substrate complex appears to be more stable than free enzyme.[8] Finally, as noted above, one variant involves normal erythrocyte uroporphyrinogen I synthetase activity.[94,163] In such families, analysis of DNA is a useful adjunct to urine studies. The combined use of urinary analysis, enzyme assay and pedigrees yields an unequivocal identification of carriers in at least 90% of persons studied.[121]

Deficient activity of coproporphyrinogen oxidase in hereditary coproporphyria has been documented.[33,71]

Table 16.4 Drug usage in persons with haem-deficient porphyria (acute intermittent porphyria, hereditary coproporphyria and variegate porphyria).

May precipitate acute attacks[a]	Believed to be safe
Barbiturates	Aspirin
Griseofulvin	Bromides
Sulphonamides	Chlorpromazine
Glutethimide	Corticocosteroids
Hydantoins	Diazepam
Sodium valproate	Dicoumarol
Carbamazepine	Digoxin
Meprobamate	Diphenhydramine
Oestrogens	Ether
Ergot preparations	Guanethidine
Methyldopa	Pethidine (meperidine)
Chloroquine	Morphine
Chlorpropamide	Neostigmine
Chlordiazepoxide	Nitrous oxide
Tolbutamide	Penicillins
Ethanol	Propranolol
Halothane	Tetracyclines
Chloramphenicol	
Pyrazinamide	

Data in part from Moore.[158]
[a] Listed in decreasing order of importance as precipitants of acute attacks.

Consistent with this, elevated faecal coproporphyrin excretion appears to be present in all affected individuals, so that estimation of coproporphyrinogen oxidase activity may be unnecessary as a screening procedure. In variegate porphyria, measurement of faecal protoporphyrin is the appropriate test for carriers.[49]

Management

Prevention of attacks

In the management of the haem-deficient porphyrias, prevention of attacks is of paramount importance. This requires screening of families with a known case and education of affected family members about circumstances that may precipitate acute attacks. Information concerning hazardous drugs should be provided; Table 16.4 lists compounds that have been implicated in acute attacks of porphyria. Barbiturates are the most frequent offenders, reflecting in part their widespread use. Also in Table 16.4 is a short list of agents that have been administered without ill effects to persons with haem-deficient porphyria. Although these should not provoke acute attacks, porphyrics may be unusually sensitive to 'usual' doses. For example, propranolol appears to be efficacious in some patients, alleviating tachycardia and hypertension,[7] but even in small doses may cause profound hypotension in others.[26] Also, hepatic metabolism of drugs may be significantly protracted in persons with acute intermittent porphyria.[2]

Fasting has been implicated in producing acute attacks in a number of individuals. The basis for the effect is unclear. Fasting in experimental animals increases the activity of ALA synthetase and produces an exaggerated response to inducers of haem synthesis.[144] Carriers of porphyria should be advised that stringent dieting is dangerous and that caloric intake should be maintained, if possible, during periods of anorexia due to viral illness or other cause. Surgical operations pose a hazard because of the routinely imposed preoperative fast; if the fast cannot be modified, caloric intake should be maintained with intravenous solutions. On the other hand, caloric intake in excess of normal needs is discouraged; there is no evidence that a high-carbohydrate diet prevents acute attacks, and weight-control problems are frequent.

Acute attacks

The management of acute porphyric attacks includes supportive care, judicious use of analgesics, administration of carbohydrate and intravenous haematin. (In the context of this discussion, 'haem', 'haematin' and 'haemin' should be regarded as equivalent terms. Haematin and haemin are the hydroxide and chloride salts, respectively, of haem. Since only the hydroxide is soluble in aqueous solution, haem is prepared as haematin (at pH 8.0) for intravenous injection. In plasma, the compound undoubtedly exists as haem, bound to plasma protein with the hydroxyl replaced by a protein ligand.) Pain symptoms in some patients are controlled with chlorpromazine; other patients will require pethidine (meperidine). The latter, because of its addicting potential, should be used for short periods only; indeed, given the remitting nature of acute attacks, chronic administration of pethidine should not only be unnecessary but should suggest that the pain symptoms are due to causes other than porphyria.

Glucose is given by whatever route is most convenient, although it is usually necessary to use the intravenous route, with the aim of giving at least 2.2 mol/24 h (400 g/24 h). The rationale for glucose therapy is the fact that the effect of fasting on ALA synthetase in animals (described above) is reversed promptly after administration of glucose,[28,221] and the efficacy of glucose infusions has been documented in individual clinical reports.[207]

The treatment of seizures during an acute porphyric attack is controversial.[202] Although diazepam has been used successfully—and without apparent aggravation of the porphyria—parenteral magnesium has been proposed as a non-porphyrogenic alternative.[212] Close monitoring of tendon reflexes and serum magnesium are essential; the therapeutic range for serum magnesium is 1 to 3 mmol/1 (2 to 6 mEq/l).[79] Experience with this form of therapy in porphyria is extremely limited. Chronic seizure disorders in porphyrics are a difficult problem in that the most commonly employed pharmacological agents (barbiturates, hydantoins and related compounds) are contraindicated because of their known ability to induce porphyric attacks. Similarly, carbamazepine, clonazepam and sodium valproate either are inducers of haem synthesis in experimental systems or have been observed to induce acute attacks in humans and therefore should be considered dangerous.[29,125] Bromides have been used without incident in porphyrics and are effective, although careful monitoring of therapeutic levels is required.[140] Haematin (see below) probably controls seizures related to porphyria, although its effect is exerted only slowly (3 to 5 days after its initiation); as noted below, it is not useful in chronic therapy.[13]

Intravenous haematin Administration of haematin should be undertaken in those patients with acute attacks showing progressive deterioration despite the above regimen. The mortality of acute porphyric attacks was formerly placed as high as 25%. Modern techniques of intensive care undoubtedly have brought about a reduction in that figure and haematin therapy promises to reduce it still further. Haematin may be administered safely to patients in amounts large enough to suppress endogenous hepatic haem synthesis (most of the administered haem is degraded rapidly and irreversibly to bile pigment, leaving only a small fraction of the dose to mix with the intracellular haem 'pool', where it exerts a regulatory effect). The initial studies of haematin therapy were carried out in patients with respiratory failure and little chance of survival. Nevertheless, striking successes with this group occurred, encouraging more extensive trials.

Several reports now convincingly document the efficacy of haematin administration in acute porphyria.[13,124,225] The reported negative or equivocal results[101,150] may be due to failure to utilize freshly prepared haematin (see below) or to a wrong diagnosis. In known carriers of acute hepatic porphyria presenting with pain, it may not be possible in every instance to establish whether symptoms are due to porphyria or to other causes. Measurement of urinary porphobilinogen is helpful only if the values are substantially increased above the individual patient's baseline level and/or increasing over a period of days. Although a clinical response to haematin is not yet accepted as a differential test, it may ultimately prove very useful in distinguishing porphyric from non-porphyric symptoms in this situation.

Haematin is prepared by dissolving crystalline haemin in sodium carbonate solution (10 g/l) at a concentration of about 10 mg/ml. The solution is adjusted with HCl to pH 8.0 and sterilized by membrane filtration (0.20 μm filter). It should be infused as soon as is practicable, since it decays in aqueous solution. If storage is required, prepared solutions may be refrigerated but should be discarded after 12 h. The infusion is given via a large vein to minimize the irritant effects of the slightly alkaline solution; a chemical phlebitis occurs as a minor side-effect in about 4% of cases.[124] The maximal recommended dose of haematin is 3 mg/kg at 12-h intervals;[59] smaller doses may suffice in many patients.[13] It should be noted that, while haematin will promptly (within 96 h) abort acute attacks, its effect on the biochemical manifestations of the disease is transient. Suppression of porphobilinogen

is achieved only as long as plasma haem is elevated. For this reason, and also because it requires intravenous administration, haematin is unsuited for chronic therapy. Fortunately, the clinical remission induced by haematin usually persists despite the return of porphobilinogen excretion to elevated values. A lyophilized haematin preparation,[88,124] which can be reconstituted immediately prior to administration, is available from Abbott Laboratories (Chicago, Illinois). Oral administration is ineffective,[124] probably because the intestinal mucosa contains haem-degrading activity.[181]

Haematin appears to be safe, provided that the published guidelines with regard to maximal dose are adhered to.[59] In one case of transient renal failure, the patient received an usually large dose.[58] Haematin administration has been associated with thrombocytopenia, reduced activity or concentration of several clotting factors, and clinically significant bleeding.[87,159] In one patient, heparin aggravated the thrombocytopenia.[87] The anticoagulant effects generally correlate with plasma haematin concentration, being maximal 10 min after haematin administration, substantially diminished at 5 h and undetectable at 48 h.[87] The anticoagulant appears to be a degradation product of haematin.[88] The prepared material is unstable, undergoing oxidative decay in bicarbonate solution or in plasma. Thus, it should be administered as soon as it is prepared and should be used with caution in patients with known bleeding tendencies and in those receiving other anticoagulants or undergoing surgical procedures.

An alternative preparation is haem arginate (Normosang®, Medica, Helsinki), which is marketed in Europe and available in the United States on an investigational basis. In a number of trials, its efficacy has been equal to that of haematin,[52,100,166,167,218] and it is stable in solution.[204,214] The preparation contains 40% 1,2-propanediol and 10% ethanol;[214] side-effects other than local phlebitis at the site of the infusion (reported also with haematin) have not been observed.[214,219]

Other haem analogues have been explored as well. Haem-albumin is one such preparation and is commercially available (Behringwerke).[80] Its advantages over haematin are unclear, particularly in that it contains an additional human blood product. Tin-protoporphyrin and tin-mesoporphyrin competitively inhibit haem oxygenase, the enzyme that converts haem to bile pigment. They also suppress chemically induced porphyria in animals.[82] As agents for treating acute porphyria, they offer the theoretical advantage of blocking haem oxygenase (or, at least, not inducing the enzyme), which could extend their antiporphyric effect. However, if induction of haem oxygenase occurs with haematin administration to humans, it appears to have no detectable effect on the half-life of circulating haematin or on its clinical efficacy.[124] Moreover, in initial human studies, tin-protoporphyrin brought about only a modest (non-significant) decrease in porphobilinogen excretion,[83] which raises questions about its efficacy at the doses used. Finally, it has the singular disadvantage of rendering recipients photosensitive.[83]

In short, haem arginate appears to be the best of the current agents. Until it is released in the United States, physicians there should continue to use haematin (Panhematin®, Abbott).

Subacute symptoms

Patients who have had acute attacks (and often known carriers who have not) may have recurrent subacute complaints, typically without physical findings but suggestive of porphyric symptomatology.[13] Urinary porphyrin studies generally are not helpful, unless porphobilinogen excretion is found to be normal or only slightly elevated (less than 10 mg/24 h), in which case a porphyric aetiology for the symptoms is unlikely. Treatment is empirical, with due regard for medication that may precipitate acute attacks (Table 16.4). In the few studies conducted to date, haematin has been of no demonstrable benefit.[13] In some carriers of acute intermittent porphyria, symptoms occur in a monthly cycle, usually peaking just prior to menstruation. It may be difficult clinically to differentiate porphyria from severe premenstrual syndrome. In a few patients, a 'pre-emptive' dose of haematin given at the expected onset of symptoms, has proved helpful.[13] In others, ovulatory suppression has alleviated symptoms.[1] Contraceptive steroids carry the risk of inducing acute porphyria. Because of this, analogues of luteinizing hormone-releasing hormone (LHRH) are under study. As peptides, these agents should have no porphyria-inducing action, and they have been effective in early studies.[1,200]

Prognosis

Neurological deficits comprise the most important residue of acute attacks of porphyria of the haem-deficient type. While these are highly variable in extent and severity, a large measure of recovery can be expected in nearly all patients.[185] Repeated acute attacks are uncommon, particularly if a precipitating agent has been identified, and occur in less than 20% of patients.[207] It has been stated that the prevalence of carriers of acute hepatic porphyria is unusually high among psychiatric inpatients,[216] implying an association with chronic mental illness. The statistical validity of these observations remains to be established. The general experience is that, while psychosis is seen as a component of an acute attack, it resolves with recovery. Progressive mental deterioration has not occurred in long-term follow-up.

In a retrospective Finnish study of deceased individuals with acute intermittent porphyria or variegate porphyria, the prevalence of hepatocellular carcinoma was higher than that of the general population.[109] Whether this is related to porphyria *per se* or to other factors remains a question. To complicate the issue, a case of hepatocellular carcinoma presenting with the biochemical findings of acute hepatic porphyria (apparently as a paraneoplastic syndrome) has also been reported.[171] On the whole, hepatocellular carcinoma appears to be rare as a complication of acute hepatic porphyria (although not of porphyria cutanea tarda—see below).

Differentiation of the haem-deficient porphyrias

Cutaneous and urinary manifestations

The overproduction of precursors in acute intermittent porphyria, hereditary coproporphyria or variegate porphyria reflects the site in the haem pathway at which the flow of intermediates has been partially blocked (Figure 16.5); haem precursors prior to the block in each case spill over into plasma. The presence of excess *porphyrins* in hereditary coproporphyria and variegate porphyria— but not in acute intermittent porphyria—is responsible for differences in the clinical presentation of the three conditions. In about 80% of patients with variegate porphyria and 25% of those with hereditary coproporphyria, circulating porphyrins cause cutaneous photosensitivity and/or increased fragility of exposed skin areas. The skin lesions consist of a bullous eruption, indistinguishable from that of porphyria cutanea tarda, leading eventually to ulceration and chronic scarring, typically involving the extensor surface of the hands and also the face. By contrast, persons with acute intermittent porphyria experience no photosensitivity whatsoever. Overproduction of porphyrins also gives the urine an abnormal colour, which varies from wine-red to brownish. Because porphyrins are not usually elevated in acute intermittent porphyria, the colour of the urine is often unaltered. Urine that has been standing (particularly if exposed to sunlight) may darken noticeably, however, reflecting non-enzymatic conversion of porphobilinogen to uroporphyrin-like compounds of undetermined structure.

Geographical and racial distribution

These three porphyrias have distinctive geographical and racial associations, which may be useful in their differential diagnosis. The prevalence of acute intermittent porphyria appears to be less than one case per 10 000 persons, except in isolated, inbred groups[222] both in Europe and in the white population of the United States; the disease appears to be unusual in non-white populations. Variegate porphyria is extremely common in the Cape area of South Africa, but it is less common than acute intermittent porphyria in Europe and the United States. The prevalence of variegate porphyria has been estimated at 0.3% of the Afrikaner population of South Africa, where the disease was introduced in 1688 by a Dutch immigrant to the Cape.[49] Hereditary coproporphyria appears to be distributed in a pattern similar to that of acute intermittent porphyria. However, large numbers of cases have not been reported, possibly because it appears to be more often latent and clinically less severe when symptomatic than is acute intermittent porphyria.[89] The differentiation of these types by laboratory diagnosis (virtually always required) has been described earlier.

HEREDITARY δ-AMINOLAEVULINIC ACIDURIA

This form of porphyria is characterized by a deficiency of PBG synthetase. From analysis of reaction kinetics, the enzyme appears to be present in substantial excess relative to the needs of the haem synthetic pathway.[69] Heterozygote carriers exhibit a 50% reduction in enzyme activity and are asymptomatic.[11] Homozygotes, however, with less than 3% of normal activity have intermittent acute symptoms similar to those occurring in the other acute haem-deficient porphyrias.[62,63] Onset in infancy has been reported.[81,215] Laboratory analysis reveals marked hyperexcretion of ALA in the urine as well as increased urine coproporphyrin and erythrocyte protoporphyrin. The basis for the latter two abnormalities is unclear. The overall pattern is similar to that of lead poisoning or other heavy-metal intoxication, which must be ruled out. It is unknown whether a haem-deficiency is present. Haematin was ineffective as therapy in the reported juvenile cases.[81,215]

HAEM-COMPENSATED PORPHYRIA: PORPHYRIA CUTANEA TARDA

Incidence

In Europe and the United States porphyria cutanea tarda is probably seen more frequently than any other form of porphyria. For this reason, its differentiation from the haem-deficient porphyrias is important, given the very different management of these conditions. It is classified as a haem-compensated type because it is associated with normal excretion of ALA and porpholibinogen and is unaffected by barbiturates or other inducers of cytochrome P450.

Clinical presentation

The sole clinical manifestations of this form of porphyria are dark urine and cutaneous photosensitivity. The condition arises most often in persons with underlying liver disease, usually related to excessive ethanol intake. The onset typically is insidious, with bulla formation and unusual fragility of sun-exposed skin (in particular the back of the hands). Patients may be unaware of the association with sun exposure. With repeated light-induced injury, chronic lesions evolve, consisting of facial hyperpigmentation, hypertrichosis and discoid or sclerodermoid changes.[96] The skin lesions resemble those of variegate porphyria (see above) and their severity is roughly proportional to the degree of porphyrin overproduction (as reflected in urinary porphyrin content). Unlike the haem-deficient porphyrias, porphyria cutanea tarda carries no associations with a neurological syndrome, with

attacks of abdominal pain or psychosis. Similar cutaneous symptoms are absent in acute intermittent porphyria; in variegate porphyria or hereditary coproporphyria they are secondary in importance to the 'neurological' symptom complex. About 15% of affected individuals have diabetes mellitus.[96] Also, several cases have occurred in persons infected with the human immunodeficiency virus.[103,134] The basis for the latter association, if statistically significant, is unknown.

Investigations

Examination of haem precursors in urine and faeces conclusively differentiates between these porphyrias (see Figure 16.5). The urine contains markedly elevated concentrations of uroporphyrin I and also coproporphyrin I, the excretion of uroporphyrin typically exceeding 960 nmol/24 h (800 μg/24 h) (see Table 16.3 for normal values) when cutaneous symptoms are present.[74] The cutaneous symptoms of the disease are due to increased circulating concentrations of uroporphyrin acting by the mechanisms discussed on p. 401. The liver contains high concentrations of uroporphyrin, biopsy samples exhibiting red fluorescence under Woods-light (near-ultraviolet) excitation.

Pathology

The cutaneous histopathology is notable for deposition of PAS-positive material at the dermal–epidermal junction and reduplication of the basement membrane around dermal vessels.[96] The latter change is characteristic but does not distinguish true porphyria from 'pseudoporphyria' (see below).

The pathological changes of chronic liver disease of varying aetiology (frequently alcohol-related) may be seen.[169] In addition, demonstrable iron deposition is present in most patients, distributed to hepatocytes as well as sinusoidal cells.[136] In one study,[41] no consistent distinction could be made between biopsies from alcoholics compared with non-alcoholics, suggesting that there was liver damage specific to porphyria cutanea tarda, possibly accelerated by excessive alcohol consumption. With care, numerous fine doubly refractile but water-soluble acicular crystals can be found in hepatocytes: these appear to be pathognomonic for porphyria cutanea tarda.[41,106]

Pathogenesis

Porphyria cutanea tarda in the past was viewed as an acquired disease only. Familial clustering of cases was observed but was infrequent and could be explained on an environmental basis. The close association with acquired liver disease, as well as the fact that exposure to toxins was clearly implicated in some cases (see below), provided further support for this viewpoint. However, studies of the haem synthetic pathway undertaken in the mid-1970s provided evidence for a genetic component. The pattern of urinary haem precursors characterizing the disease (uroporphyrin present in marked excess) suggests impaired conversion of uroporphyrinogen to coproporphyrinogen. Indeed, assay of liver biopsy samples from several patients with porphyria cutanea tarda revealed a significant deficiency of uroporphyrinogen decarboxylase, the enzyme required for this conversion.[70,75,115] In some instances, the deficiency was expressed in erythrocytes as well as in liver, and family studies of erythrocyte activity showed the deficiency to be present in first-degree relatives, consistent with autosomal dominant inheritance.[115] Other cases were studied, however, in which a deficiency of the hepatic enzyme was present but levels in erythrocytes from patients were normal as well as erythrocytes from family members.[70] These findings have been confirmed,[56] with the result that two types of porphyria cutanea tarda, termed 'hereditary' and 'sporadic', have been postulated. The sporadic type is believed to be acquired, although the present data are insufficient for excluding a hereditary basis. In untreated patients, the amount of immunoreactive uroporphyrinogen decarboxylase (CRIM) exceeds the catalytically active. With iron-depletion therapy, the abnormality clears,[72] unlike the deficiency in the familial form of the disease, which is unaffected by iron-depletion.[75] This response was interpreted as evidence for an acquired lesion. However, it does not explain why only a few patients among those at risk (with siderosis, ethanolism or other environmental exposure) actually manifest the disease. In vitro, uroporphyrinogen decarboxylase from patients with familial porphyria cutanea tarda is more sensitive to inhibition by iron than is the enzyme from normals,[160] suggesting the presence of a structural alteration. The gene has been cloned.[188] A search for restriction-site polymorphisms associated with an enzyme deficiency has been unrewarding, to date[99] but a mutation causing a splicing defect (analogous to that presented in Figure 16.6, above) has been identified in some families.[231] In hepatoerythropoietic porphyria with a severe deficiency of uroporphyrinogen decarboxylase (homozygous for the lesion), a single amino-acid mutation has been documented associated with rapid degradation of the enzyme.[54,55] As in acute intermittent porphyria, substantial genetic heterogeneity can be anticipated.

These studies suggest that deficiency of *hepatic* uroporphyrinogen decarboxylase is present in all individuals with porphyria cutanea tarda. However, it is apparent that, in the clearly genetic type, only a small proportion of carriers express the disease.[115] Thus, the enzymatic defect is a necessary, but not the sole, determinant of clinical symptoms.[67] Supporting this inference are data indicating the importance of environmental factors in the pathogenesis of this disease. A commonly observed finding in persons with porphyria cutanea tarda is hepatic siderosis with iron deposited in parenchymal as well as sinusoidal cells.[136] Most importantly, virtually all patients with the disease respond to iron depletion therapy (see below). These findings provide cogent evidence for the role of iron in the pathogenesis of porphyria cutanea tarda. On the other hand, hepatic iron deposition is usually quantitatively minor and does not correlate with the severity of porphyria. Cutaneous porphyria is rarely observed in individuals with massive hepatic iron overload, as in idiopathic haemochromatosis or transfusional siderosis. Although liver disease is a common accompaniment of porphyria cutanea tarda, the two are unrelated in terms of stage or severity.

New insight into the role of iron in porphyria cutanea tarda and the mechanism of its effects on hepatic haem synthesis may emerge from data linking this porphyria with hereditary haemochromatosis. Plasma iron values and estimates of body iron stores in porphyria cutanea tarda[136] closely resemble those in heterozygous carriers of haemochromatosis.[65] Transferrin saturation is moderately increased, with a mean value of 60%, and total hepatic non-haem iron averages 76 μg/100 mg wet weight of tissue in males (normal—12 μg/100 mg; heterozygous haemochromatosis—96 μg/100 mg; and homozygous haemochromatosis—877 μg/100 mg). Iron stores in patients with porphyria cutanea tarda average 2–4 g, based on the amount of iron removed by a phlebotomy prior to clinical responses, a value that is moderately increased but well below that associated with symptomatic (homozygous) haemochromatosis.[65] Serum ferritin—while not elevated in the absence of active liver disease—decreases during therapy as in haemochromatosis.[187,210] Finally, HLA markers denoting haemochromatosis are also present in excess in patients with porphyria cutanea tarda, consistent with their being heterozygous for haemochromatosis.[66] These findings suggest that a single dose of the gene for haemochromatosis and deficiency of uroporphyrinogen decarboxylase occur together in persons with porphyria cutanea tarda and may be required for the expression of clinical disease. This postulate may explain the peculiar epidemiological features of porphyria cutanea tarda, from which it is apparent that neither abnormal iron metabolism nor uroporphyrinogen decarboxylase deficiency alone is sufficient for producing disease. It would also represent a striking example of clinical manifestations associated with the heterozygous state of haemochromatosis—otherwise entirely subclinical[65]—and may provide fresh insight into the disturbances of cellular iron metabolism in haemochromatosis.

Based in part on experimental studies in animals,[68] a variety of chemicals have been implicated in the pathogenesis of porphyria cutanea tarda. While ethanol figures prominently in this disease, oestrogens,[67,98] cyclophosphamide[143] and polyhalogenated aromatic hydrocarbons[195] also cause symptoms in some patients. Whether these act in concert with iron is unclear. In experimental porphyria, the effect of aromatic hydrocarbons is significantly greater in animals pretreated with iron than in controls.[205]

Differential diagnosis

The differentiation of porphyria cutanea tarda from the acute porphyrias with cutaneous symptoms (hereditary coproporphyria and variegate porphyria) is important and, with the appropriate laboratory tests, is straightforward (see above).

Congenital erythropoietic porphyria in mild form may present in adults with cutaneous manifestations identical to those of porphyria cutanea tarda.[57] Its differential feature is a marked increase in erythrocyte uroporphyrin.

Hepatoerythropoietic porphyria—apparently a homozygous form of porphyria cutanea tarda—presents in infancy and resembles congenital erythropoietic porphyria (see above). Its differential feature is the presence of uroporphyrin III in marked excess in urine and zinc-protoporphyrin in erythrocytes.

Porphyrin-producing hepatic tumours in a setting of chronic liver disease may underlie cutaneous manifestations in some patients. In a review,[95] all patients with this disorder were greater than 60 years of age, and their urinary and faecal porphyrin patterns were often atypical for porphyria cutanea tarda. Thus, screening tests for tumours are probably unnecessary in porphyria cutanea tarda in relatively young patients. There are five reported cases of porphyria cutanea tarda in association with lymphomas.[117]

Persons undergoing chronic haemodialysis for renal failure may display the cutaneous findings of porphyria cutanea tarda.[86,178] Evaluation involves measurement of plasma porphyrins,[108] which are elevated in virtually all patients on dialysis, presumably because porphyrins are not readily filtered.[201] In most patients with cutaneous symptoms, the level of porphyrins is well below that associated with porphyria cutanea tarda and is assumed to be unrelated to the porphyria. The syndrome in these patients has been termed 'bullous dermatosis of dialysis' or 'pseudoporphyria'. Some patients, however, have strikingly elevated plasma porphyrins, predominantly uroporphyrin, and probably represent true porphyria cutanea tarda. Successful therapy with plasma exchange[60] or desferrioxamine has been reported.[180] Even though such patients invariably are anaemic, cautious phlebotomy has been tried with evident positive results.[184] Erythropoietin also has been used successfully, with the rationale that the haematopoietic stimulus causes mobilization of hepatic storage iron similar to that produced by phlebotomy in the usual case of porphyria cutanea tarda.[230]

An array of pharmaceuticals will cause the cutaneous picture of porphyria cutanea tarda in the absence of elevated porphyrins; some are weak photosensitizers.[176] Chronic sun exposure is another cause of 'pseudoporphyria'.[176]

Lupus erythematosus may present with photosensitivity and cutaneous pathology similar to that of porphyria cutanea tarda; the two conditions also may coexist in the same patient.[38,42] Their differentiation is important, in that the antimalarials used in lupus may precipitate a severe hepatic reaction in porphyrics (see below); conversely, phlebotomy therapy is contraindicated in patients with lupus who are anaemic or leucopenic. For patients with combined disease, plasmapheresis may be effective in reducing porphyrin levels.

Management

Patients should discontinue iron, drugs which may be aggravating the condition, and also alcohol.[98] While improvement may result from these manipulations alone, serial phlebotomy is usually undertaken and is virtually always effective.[104] Provided that the patient maintains a satisfactory haemoglobin level, one unit of blood (500 ml) may be removed biweekly until a response occurs, as judged by decreasing urinary porphyrin excretion. The cutaneous manifestations of the disease resolve as urinary uroporphyrin excretion drops below 1200 nmol/24 h (1000 µg/24 h). The time between initiation of phlebotomy therapy and response varies widely among individual patients but averages several months.[74] The duration of the response is similarly unpredictable; uroporphyrin excretion may remain low for years without further phlebotomy, particularly if factors aggravating the condition have been identified and eliminated. For patients unable to tolerate phlebotomy and significantly disabled by cutaneous symptoms, therapy with chloroquine may be undertaken. Although serious hepatotoxic reactions to chloroquine have been described in patients with porphyria cutanea tarda, 'low-dose' treatment (125–250 mg chloroquine phosphate twice weekly) appears relatively safe,[142,211] at least in the short term, and as effective as phlebotomy.[35] The long-term effects are unknown. Chloroquine administration results in depletion of hepatic stores of uroporphyrin, apparently by complexing in situ with the porphyrin.[197] An alternative to chloroquine is plasmapheresis.[96] The use of desferrioxamine by continuous infusion provides another form of iron depletion therapy.[186]

The role of screening procedures in the families of affected persons is unclear at present. Assay of erythrocyte uroporphyrinogen decarboxylase activity would differentiate the sporadic and hereditary types according to present concepts. However, in view of the fact that only a small proportion of hereditary carriers become symptomatic and that the clinical disease is readily treated, extensive screening may not be justified. The assay itself is complex and available as a research procedure only. Should further studies verify the occurrence of the haemochromatosis gene in families with porphyria cutanea tarda, screening for this disease (by HLA testing and/or studies of iron status) may be indicated, with the aim of an early diagnosis of homozygous individuals.

Prognosis

The cutaneous signs of blistering and fragility clear as porphyrin excretion falls; facial hyperpigmentation and hypertrichosis resolve slowly but improve after 18 to 24 months; discoid changes in some patients persist indefinitely.[96] Long-term remission requires that aggravating factors be avoided, with strict limitations on alcohol intake. In persons resistant to treatment, the possibility of a tumour should be considered.[96] The associated liver disease may improve with elimination of alcohol and reduction of hepatic iron stores.

ACQUIRED PORPHYRIA

Toxins

Polychlorinated aromatic hydrocarbons

Chemically induced disturbances of haem metabolism fall into two groups. One pattern involves a predominant increase in urinary uroporphyrin, resembling porphyria cutanea tarda. There is no elevation of ALA or porphobilinogen. Chlorinated aromatic hydrocarbons are the principal cause, the most notorious being hexachlorobenzene, which was responsible for a poisoning involving roughly 4000 people in Turkey in the late 1950s.[45,195] The toxin was ingested and caused the signs of severe porphyria cutanea tarda, which were present for years in many cases.[45] Although other toxic exposures producing porphyria are documented,[137] few have approached the Turkish one in terms of severity. Despite widespread concern, there is little evidence that exposure to persistent chemicals such as 2,3,7,8-tetrachloro-dibenzo-p-dioxin (TCDD) (a by-product and contaminant of herbicides) causes porphyria. In several studies of apparent industrial exposure of workers to halogenated aromatic hydrocarbons, minor elevation of urine uroporphyrin, or an increase in the ratio of uroporphyrin to coproporphyrin, was found.[19,102,209] Such changes were rarely of magnitude sufficient to cause cutaneous signs of porphyria. Chloracne, which is attributed to toxin exposure, was manifested by a number of workers but was unrelated to urine uroporphyrin levels.[19] The clinical and diagnostic significance of these minimal alterations is difficult to assess. Changes in urine uroporphyrin occur with ethanol use, moderately excessive hepatic iron, latent liver disease of any cause, and a hereditary predisposition to porphyria cutanea tarda, among other factors. In most reports of toxin exposure, studies of control groups are lacking. Where healthy controls have been examined, the prevalence of 'abnormal' porphyrin excretion has been surprisingly high.[102,209]

The other pattern of porphyrin excretion reported as a sign of toxin exposure is increased urine coproporphyrin, generally as an isolated abnormality. However, as 'secondary coproporphyrinuria' (see below), it is non-specific and of little diagnostic significance.

Lead

Intoxication with lead results in increased urinary excretion of ALA, together with lesser increases in coproporphyrin. This pattern reflects inhibition of porphobilinogen synthetase by lead, which may react with sulphydryl groups on the enzyme or displace zinc, which appears to be essential for normal enzyme activity. Presumably, partial inhibition of coproporphyrinogen oxidase also occurs, accounting for the increased excretion of urinary coproporphyrin. In erythrocytes of lead-poisoned individuals, decreased activity of porphobilinogen synthetase correlates well with blood lead concentrations.[192] Although abdominal pain and neurological deficits occur with lead intoxication, the disorder can be distinguished readily from acute intermittent porphyria by the absence of increased urinary porphobilinogen.

In addition to porphobilinogen synthetase, ferrochelatase activity in erythroid cells appears to be inhibited in lead intoxication. As a result, protoporphyrin in circulating erythrocytes is substantially increased.[173] A similar increase occurs in iron deficiency.[119] In both conditions, the porphyrin appears to be trapped within the cell as a metal chelate (zinc protoporphyrin), so that it fails to diffuse into plasma and therefore does not cause symptoms of cutaneous photosensitivity.[120] Faecal excretion of protoporphyrin in these disorders is normal. In these respects, the signs of iron deficiency or lead intoxication differ strikingly from those of protoporphyria (see above). The increased protoporphyrin can be quantitated by a simple one-step extraction procedure which lends itself to rapid and sensitive clinical screening.[25,36,173]

SECONDARY PORPHYRINURIA

Mildly increased urinary excretion of coproporphyrin—*without* an increase in ALA or porphobilinogen—is commonly observed during the course of viral hepatitis[4] and may accompany a variety of toxic insults to the liver. Presumably it reflects either minimally impaired haem synthesis or diversion of coproporphyrin from excretion in bile to the urinary route. Similar abnormalities of porphyrin excretion have been described in occasional patients representing a wide range of clinical problems including diabetes mellitus, Hodgkin's disease, leukaemia, haemolytic anaemia, myocardial infarction and hereditary hyperbilirubinaemia.[61] In all of these circumstances, the porphyrinuria is not accompanied by clinical manifestations of porphyria. The main clinical significance of this benign porphyrinuria is that it may be misconstrued as evidence for a hereditary condition.

In persons with hereditary conjugated hyperbilirubinaemia (Rotor syndrome), urinary coproporphyrin is moderately elevated, and the ratio of coproporphyrin isomers I and III (which is normally 1:4) is altered to about

$3:2.^{227}$ In the clinically similar, but genetically distinct, Dubin–Johnson syndrome, total urinary coproporphyrin is normal but the isomer ratio is markedly shifted to approximately $9:1.^{113}$ Measurement of coproporphyrin isomers has proved useful as a non-invasive approach to the diagnosis of these conditions.

CONCLUSION

The porphyrias are abnormalities of haem synthesis in which haem precursors—ALA, porphobilinogen or porphyrins—are overproduced and appear in increased amounts in blood, urine or faeces. Several types of porphyria occur, differing in pathogenesis (hereditary or acquired), organ involvement (bone marrow or liver) and the presence or absence of a relative haem deficiency in affected tissues. These distinctions form the basis for classifying the various porphyrias, as well as providing a rationale for the clinical and laboratory characteristics of the individual types.

Congenital erythropoietic porphyria is a rare disease which appears to involve only the bone marrow and is characterized by severe photosensitivity from early childhood.

Protoporphyria involves overproduction of protoporphyrin, predominantly by erythroid cells but also by liver. In the vast majority of cases, the clinical manifestations are dermatological only. However, in persons in whom overproduction is striking, massive deposition of protoporphyrin in the liver has occurred, followed by rapidly progressive hepatic failure.

Acute intermittent porphyria, hereditary coproporphyria and *variegate porphyria* comprise the *hepatic haem-deficient porphyrias*. While each type is associated with a distinct, inherited enzymatic defect, the abnormality in all cases potentially compromises the synthetic capacity of the liver for haem. This fact may account for the similar clinical manifestations of these diseases. The major symptom complex consists of neuropsychiatric abnormalities and is commonly precipitated by drug inducers of hepatic haem synthesis, notably barbiturates. Cutaneous photosensitivity is present in variegate porphyria and to a lesser extent in hereditary coproporphyria; it is absent in acute intermittent porphyria. Treatment with haematin infusions represents a major therapeutic advance which promises to reduce substantially the mortality of acute attacks.

Porphyria cutanea tarda is a *haem-compensated porphyria* characterized by cutaneous photosensitivity and excessive excretion of urinary uroporphyrin, without increased ALA or porphobilinogen and without neurological symptoms. An enzyme abnormality appears to act in concert with environmental factors (including iron and acquired liver disease) to produce clinical manifestations. Effective treatment is provided by serial phlebotomy, which reduces the burden of iron in the liver.

Acquired porphyrias result from specific intoxications (e.g. hexachlorobenzene, lead).

All of the above must be differentiated from *secondary* (asymptomatic) *porphyrinuria*, which may accompany acquired liver disease as well as a variety of acute and chronic illnesses. The urinary porphyrin findings in these instances typically consist of an isolated minor increase in coproporphyrin, a pattern which is readily distinguished from those associated with porphyrias.

REFERENCES

1. Anderson, K.E. (1989) LHRH analogues for hormonal manipulation in acute intermittent porphyria. *Seminars in Hematology,* **26**, 10–15.
2. Anderson, K.E., Alvares, A.P., Sassa, S. & Kappas, A. (1976) Studies in porphyria. V. Drug oxidation rates in hereditary hepatic porphyria. *Clinical Pharmacology and Therapeutics,* **19**, 47–54.
3. Anderson, P.M. & Desnick, R.J. (1980) Purification and properties of uroporphyrinogen I synthase from human erythrocytes. Identification of stable enzyme-substrate intermediates. *Journal of Biological Chemistry,* **255**, 1993–1999.
4. Aziz, M.A., Schwartz, S. & Watson, C.J. (1964) Studies of coproporphyrin. VIII. Reinvestigation of the isomer distribution in jaundice and liver diseases. *Journal of Laboratory and Clinical Medicine,* **63**, 596–604.
5. Battersby, A.R., Fookes, C.J.R., Matcham, G.W.J. & McDonald, E. (1980) Biosynthesis of the pigments of life: formation of the macrocycle. *Nature,* **285**, 17–21.
6. Beal, M.F., Atuk, N.O., Westfall, T.C. & Turner, S.M. (1977) Catecholamine uptake, accumulation, and release in acute porphyria. *Journal of Clinical Investigation,* **60**, 1141–1148.
7. Beattie, A.D., Moore, M.R., Goldberg, A. & Ward, R.L. (1973) Acute intermittent porphyria: response of tachycardia and hypertension to propranolol. *British Medical Journal,* **3**, 257–260.
8. Beaumont, C., Grandchamp, B., Bogard, M., de Verneuil, H. & Nordmann, Y. (1986) Porphobilinogen deaminase is unstable in the absence of its substrate. *Biochimica et Biophysica Acta,* **882**, 384–388.
9. Becker, D.M. & Kramer, S. (1977) The neurological manifestations of porphyria: a review. *Medicine,* **56**, 411–423.
10. Becker, D.M., Viljoen, J.D., Katz, J. & Kramer, S. (1977) Reduced ferrochelatase activity: a defect common to porphyria variegata and protoporphyria. *British Journal of Haematology,* **36**, 171–179.
11. Bird, T.D., Hamernyik, P., Nutter, J.Y. & Labbe, R.F. (1979) Inherited deficiency of delta-aminolevulinic acid dehydratase. *American Journal of Human Genetics,* **31**, 662–668.
12. Bissbort, S., Hitzeroth, H.W., du Wentzel, D.P., Van den Berg, C.W., Senff, H., Wienker, T.F. & Bender, K. (1988) Linkage between the variegate porphyria (VP) and the alpha-1-antitrypsin (PI) genes on human chromosome 14. *Human Genetics,* **79**, 289–290.
13. Bissell, D.M. (1988) Treatment of acute hepatic porphyria with hematin. *Journal of Hepatology,* **6**, 1–7.
14. Bissell, D.M. & Guzelian, P.S. (1980) Degradation of endogenous hepatic heme by pathways not yielding carbon monoxide. Studies in normal rat liver and in primary hepatocyte culture. *Journal of Clinical Investigation,* **65**, 1135–1140.
15. Bissell, D.M. & Hammaker, L.E. (1976) Cytochrome P-450 heme and the regulation of hepatic heme oxygenase activity. *Archives of Biochemistry and Biophysics,* **176**, 91–102.
16. Bissell, D.M. & Hammaker, L.E. (1976) Cytochrome P-450 heme and the regulation of δ-aminolevulinic acid synthetase in the liver. *Archives of Biochemistry and Biophysics,* **176**, 103–112.
17. Bissell, D.M., Hammaker, L. & Schmid, R. (1972) Hemoglobin and erythrocyte catabolism in rat liver: the separate roles of parenchymal and sinusoidal cells. *Blood,* **40**, 812–822.
18. Bissell, D.M., Liem, H.H. & Muller-Eberhard, U. (1979) Secretion of haem by hepatic parenchymal cells. *Biochemical Journal,* **184**, 689–694.

19. Bleiberg, J., Wallen, M., Brodkin, R. & Applebaum, I.L. (1964) Industrially acquired porphyria. *Archives of Dermatology*, **89**, 793–797.

20. Bloomer, J.R. (1979) Pathogenesis and therapy of liver disease in protoporphyria. *Yale Journal of Biology and Medicine*, **52**, 39–48.

21. Bloomer, J.R. (1982) Evidence that hepatic crystalline deposits in a patient with protoporphyria are composed of protoporphyrin. *Gastroenterology*, **82**, 569–573.

22. Bloomer, J.R. (1988) The liver in protoporphyria. *Hepatology*, **8**, 402–407.

23. Bloomer, J.R. & Pierach, C.A. (1982) Effect of hematin administration to patients with protoporphyria and liver disease. *Hepatology*, **2**, 817–821.

24. Bloomer, J.R., Phillips, M.J., Davidson, D.L. & Klatskin, G. (1975) Hepatic disease in erythropoietic protoporphyria. *American Journal of Medicine*, **58**, 869–882.

25. Blumberg, W.E., Eisinger, J. Lamola, A.A. & Zuckerman, D.M. (1977) The hematofluorometer. *Clinical Chemistry*, **23**, 270–274.

26. Bonkowsky, H.L. & Tschudy, D.P. (1974) Hazard of propranolol in treatment of acute porphyria. *British Medical Journal*, **4**, 47–48.

27. Bonkowsky, H.L., Bloomer, J.R., Ebert, P.S. & Mahoney, M.J. (1975) Heme synthetase deficiency in human protoporphyria. Demonstration of the defect in liver and cultured skin fibroblasts. *Journal of Clinical Investigation*, **56**, 1139–1148.

28. Bonkowsky, H.L., Collins, A., Doherty, J.M. & Tschudy, D.P. (1973) The glucose effect in rat liver: studies of δ-aminolevulinate synthase and tyrosine amino-transferase. *Biochimica et Biophysica Acta*, **320**, 561–576.

29. Bonkowsky, H.L., Sinclair, P.R., Emery, S. & Sinclair, J.F. (1980) Seizure management in acute hepatic porphyria: risks of valporate and clonazepam. *Neurology*, **30**, 588–592.

30. Bonkowsky, H.L., Tschudy, D.P., Weinbach, E.C. *et al.* (1975) Porphyrin synthesis and mitochondrial respiration in acute intermittent porphyria: studies using cultured human fibroblasts. *Journal of Laboratory and Clinical Medicine*, **85**, 93–102.

31. Bottomley, S.S., Tanaka, M. & Everett, M.A. (1975) Diminished erythroid ferrochelatase activity in protoporphyria. *Journal of Laboratory and Clinical Medicine*, **86**, 126–131.

32. Brenner, D.A. & Bloomer, J.R. (1980) The enzymatic defect in variegate porphyria. Studies with human cultured skin fibroblasts. *New England Journal of Medicine*, **302**, 765–769.

33. Brodie, M.J., Thompson, G.G., Moore, M.R. *et al.* (1977) Hereditary coproporphyria. Demonstration of the abnormalities in haem biosynthesis in peripheral blood. *Quarterly Journal of Medicine*, **46**, 229–241.

34. Bruguera, M., Esquerda, J.E., Mascaro, J.M. & Pinol, J. (1976) Erythropoietic protoporphyria. A light, electron and polarisation microscopical study of the liver in three patients. *Archives of Pathology and Laboratory Medicine*, **100**, 587–589.

35. Cainelli, T., Padova, C. Di., Marchesi, L. *et al.* (1983) Hydroxychloroquine versus phlebotomy in the treatment of porphyria cutanea tarda. *British Journal of Dermatology*, **108**, 593–600.

36. Chisolm, J.J., Mellits, E.D., Keil, J.E. & Barrett, M.B. (1974) A simple protoporphyrin assay-microhematocrit procedure as a screening technique for increased lead absorption in young children. *Journal of Pediatrics*, **84**, 490–496.

37. Chretien, S., Cubart, A., Beaupain, D., Raich, N., Grandchamp, B., Rosa, J., Goossens, M. & Romeo, P.H. (1988) Alternative transcription and splicing of the human porpholilinogen deaminase gene result either in tissue-specific or in housekeeping expression. *Proceedings of the National Academy of Sciences of the USA*, **85**, 6–10.

38. Clemmensen, O. & Thomsen, K. (1982) Porphyria cutanea tarda and systemic lupus erythematosus. *Archives of Dermatology*, **118**, 160–162.

39. Conley, C.L. & Chisolm, J.J., Jr. (1979) Recovery from hepatic decompensation in protoporphyria. *The Johns Hopkins Medical Journal*, **145**, 237–240.

40. Correia, M.A. & Meyer, U.A. (1975) Apocytochrome P-450: reconstitution of functional cytochrome with hemin in vitro. *Proceedings of the National Academy of Sciences of the USA*, **72**, 400–404.

41. Cortes, J.M., Oliva, H., Paradinas, F.J. & Hernandez-Guio, C. (1980) The pathology of the liver in porphyria cutanea tarda. *Histopathology*, **4**, 471–485.

42. Cram, D.L., Epstein, J.H. & Tuffanelli, D.L. (1973) Lupus erythematosus and porphyria. Coexistence in seven patients. *Archives of Dermatology*, **108**, 779–784.

43. Cripps, D.J. & MacEachern, W.N. (1971) Hepatic and erythropoietic porphyria. *Archives of Pathology*, **91**, 497–505.

44. Cripps, D.J. & Scheuer, P.J. (1965) Hepatobiliary changes in erythropoietic protoporphyria. *Archives of Pathology*, **80**, 500–508.

45. Cripps, D.J., Goemen, A. & Peters, H.A. (1980) Porphyria turcica. Twenty years after hexachlorobenzene intoxication. *Archives of Dermatology*, **116**, 46–50.

46. Crosby, D.L., Wheeler, C.E. & Cheesborough, J.D. (1989) An unusual case of erythropoietic protoporphyria. *Archives of Dermatology*, **125**, 846–847.

47. Davis, J.R. & Andelman, S.L. (1967) Urinary delta-aminolevulinic acid (ALA) levels in lead poisoning. I. A modified method for the rapid determination of urinary delta-aminolevulinic acid using disposable ion exchange chromatography columns. *Archives of Environmental Health*, **15**, 53–59.

48. Day, R.S., Eales, L. & Disler, P.B. (1981) Porphyrias and the kidney, *Nephron*, **28**, 261–267.

49. Dean, G. (1971) *The Porphyrias, A Story of Heredity and Environment*, 2nd edn. London: Pitman Medical.

50. DeLeo, V.A., Poh-Fitzpatrick, M., Mathews-Roth, M. & Harber, L.C. (1976) Erythropoietic protoporphyria: ten years' experience. *American Journal of Medicine*, **60**, 8.

51. Desnick, R.J., Ostasiewicz, L.T., Tishler, P.A. & Mustajoki, P. (1985) Acute intermittent porphyria: characterization of a novel mutation in the structural gene for porphobilinogen deaminase. *Journal of Clinical Investigation*, **76**, 865–874.

52. Devars du Mayne, J.F., Deybach, J.C., Phung, L., Likforman, J., Tenhunen, R., Cerf, M. & Nordmann, Y. (1986) Crises aigues de porphyries hepatiques. *La Presse Médicale*, **15**, 1673–1676.

53. de Verneuil, H., Sassa, S. & Kappas, A. (1983) Purification and properties of uroporphyrinogen decarboxylase from human erythrocytes. A single enzyme catalyzing the four sequential decarboxylations of uroporphyrinogens I and III. *Journal of Biological Chemistry*, **258**, 2454–2460.

54. De Verneuil, H., Grandchamp, B., Beaumont, C., Picat, C. & Nordmann, Y. (1986) Uroporphyrinogen decarboxylase structural mutant (Gly 281 → Glu) in a case of porphyria. *Science*, **234**, 732–734.

55. De Verneuil, H., Grandchamp, B., Romeo, P.H., Raich, N., Bequmont, C., Goossens, M., Nicolas, H. & Nordmann, Y. (1986) Molecular analysis of uroporphyrinogen decarboxylase deficiency in a family with two cases of hepatoerythropoietic porphyria. *Journal of Clinical Investigation*, **77**, 431–435.

56. de Verneuil, H., Nordmann, Y., Phung, N. *et al.* (1978) Familial and sporadic porphyria cutanea: two different diseases. *International Journal of Biochemistry*, **9**, 927–931.

57. Deybach, J.-C., de Verneuil, H., Phung, N. *et al.* (1981) Congenital erythropoietic porphyria (Günther's disease): enzymatic studies on two cases of late onset. *Journal of Laboratory and Clinical Medicine*, **97**, 551–558.

58. Dhar, G.J., Bossenmaier, I., Cardinal, R. *et al.* (1978) Transitory renal failure following rapid administration of a relatively large amount of hematin in a patient with acute intermittent porphyria in clinical remission. *Acta Medica Scandinavica*, **203**, 437–443.

59. Dhar, G.J., Bossenmaier, I., Petryka, Z.J. *et al.* (1975) Effects of hematin in hepatic porphyria. Further studies. *Annals of Internal Medicine*. **83**, 20–30.

60. Disler, P., Day, R., Burman, N. *et al.* (1982) Treatment of hemodialysis-related porphyria cutanea tarda with plasma exchange. *American Journal of Medicine*, **72**, 989–993.

61. Doss, M. (1987) Porphyrinurias and occupational disease. *Annals of the New York Academy of Sciences*, **514**, 204–221.

62. Doss, M., Benkmann, H.-G. & Goedde, H.-W. (1986) Delta-aminolevulinic acid dehydrase (porphobilinogen synthase) in two families with inherited enzyme deficiency. *Clinical Genetics*, **30**, 191–198.

63. Doss, M., Schneider, J., von Tiepermann, R. & Brandt, A. (1982) New type of acute porphyria with porphobilinogen synthase (δ-aminolevulinic acid dehydratase) defect in the homozygous state. *Clinical Biochemistry*, **15**, 52–55.

64. Eales, M. (1963) Porphyria as seen in Cape Town: a survey of

250 patients and some recent studies. *South African Journal of Laboratory and Clinical Medicine,* **9**, 151–162.

65. Edwards, C.Q., Skolnick, M.H. & Kushner, J.P. (1981) Hereditary hemochromatosis: contributions of genetic analyses. *Progress in Hematology,* **12**, 43–71.

66. Edwards, C.Q., Griffen, L.M., Goldgar, D.E., Skolnick, M.H. & Kushner, J.P. (1989) HLA-linked hemochromatosis alleles in sporadic porphyria cutanea tarda. *Gastroenterology,* **97**, 972–981.

67. Elder, G.H. (1977) Porphyrin metabolism in porphyria cutanea tarda. *Seminars in Hematology,* **14**, 227–242.

68. Elder, G.H. & Sheppard, D.M. (1982) Immunoreactive uroporphyrinogen decarboxylase is unchanged in porphyria caused by TCDD and hexachlorobenzene. *Biochemical and Biophysical Research Communications,* **109**, 113–120.

69. Elder, G.H., Gray, C.H. & Nicholson, D.C. (1972) The porphyrias: a review. *Journal of Clinical Pathology,* **25**, 1013–1033.

70. Elder, G.H., Lee, G.B. & Tovey, J.A. (1978) Decreased activity of hepatic uroporphyrinogen decarboxylase in sporadic porphyria cutanea tarda. *New England Journal of Medicine,* **229**, 274–278.

71. Elder, G.H., Evans, J.O., Thomas, N. et al. (1976) The primary enzyme defect in hereditary coproporphyria. *Lancet* **2**, 1217–1219.

72. Elder, G.H., Salamanca, R.E., Urquhart, A.J., Munoz, J.J. & Bonkovsky, H.L. (1985) Immunoreactive uroporphyrinogen decarboxylase in the liver in porphyria cutanea tarda. *Lancet* **2**, 229–232.

73. Elder, G.H., Smith, S.G., Herrero, C. et al. (1981) Hepatoerythropoietic porphyria: a new uroporphyrinogen decarboxylase defect or homozygous porphyria cutanea tarda? *Lancet,* **1**, 916–919.

74. Epstein, J.H. & Redeker, A.G. (1968) Porphyria cutanea tarda. A study of the effect of phlebotomy. *New England Journal of Medicine,* **279**, 1301–1304.

75. Felsher, B.F., Carpio, N.M., Engleking, D.W. & Nunn, A.T. (1982) Decreased hepatic uroporphyrinogen decarboxylase activity in porphyria cutanea tarda. *New England Journal of Medicine,* **306**, 766–769.

76. Finelli, V.N., Murthy, L., Peirano, W.B. & Petering, H.G. (1974) δ-Aminolevulinate dehydratase, a zinc dependent enzyme. *Biochemical and Biophysical Research Communications,* **60**, 1418–1424.

77. Fischer, H. & Orth, H. (1934 and 1937) *Die Chemie des Pyrrols,* Vols I and II. Leipzig: Akademische Verlag.

78. Fischer, H., Hilmer, H., Lindner, F. & Putzer, B. (1925) Zur Kenntnis der naturerlichen Porphyrine: Chemische Befunde bei einem Fall von Porphyrinurie (Petry). *Zeitschrift für Physiologische Chemie,* **150**, 44–101.

79. Flowers, C.E., Jr, Easterling, W.E., Jr, White, F.D. et al. (1962) Magnesium sulphate in toxemia of pregnancy. *Obstetrics and Gynecology,* **19**, 315–327.

80. Fuchs, T. & Ippen, H. (1987) Behandlung der akut intermittierenden porphyrie mit einem neuen, an albumin gebundenen lyophilisierten hamatin. *Deutsche Medizinische Wochenschrift,* **112**, 1302–1305.

81. Fujita, H., Sassa, S., Lundgren, J., Holmberg, L., Thunell, S. & Kappas, A. (1987) Enzymatic defect in a child with hereditary hepatic porphyria due to homozygous delta-aminolevulinic acid dehydratase deficiency: immunochemical studies. *Pediatrics,* **80**, 880–885.

82. Galbraith, R.A., Drummond, G.S. & Kappas, A. (1985) Sn-protoporphyrin suppresses chemically induced experimental hepatic porphyria. *Journal of Clinical Investigation,* **76**, 2436–2439.

83. Galbraith, R.A. & Kappas, A. (1989) Pharmacokinetics of tin-mesoporphyrin in man and the effects of tin-chelated porphyrins on hyperexcretion of heme pathway precursors in patients with acute inducible porphyria. *Hepatology,* **9**, 882–888.

84. Gandhi, S.N. & Pimstone, N.R. (1983) Charcoal is superior to cholestyramine in blocking enterohepatic circulation of porphyrins: a major therapeutic tool in porphyria. *Gastroenterology,* **84**, 1372.

85. Gidari, A.S. & Levere, R.D. (1977) Enzymatic formation and cellular regulation of heme synthesis. *Seminars in Hematology,* **14**, 145–168.

86. Gilchrest, B., Rowe, J.W. & Mihm, M.C., Jr (1975) Bullous dermatosis of hemodialysis. *Annals of Internal Medicine,* **83**, 480–483.

87. Glueck, R., Green, D., Cohen, I. & Ts'ao, C. (1983) Hematin: unique effects on hemostasis. *Blood,* **61**, 243–249.

88. Goetsch, C.A. & Bissell, D.M. (1986) Instability of hematin used in the treatment of acute hepatic porphyria. *New England Journal of Medicine,* **315**, 235–238.

89. Goldberg, A., Rimington, C. & Lochhead, A. (1967) Hereditary coproporphyria. *Lancet,* **1**, 632–636.

90. Gordeuk, V.R., Brittenham, G.M., Hawkins, C.W., Mukhtar, H. & Bickers, D.R. (1986) Iron therapy for hepatic dysfunction in erythropoietic protoporphyria. *Annals of Internal Medicine,* **105**, 27–31.

91. Grandchamp, B., Phung, N. & Nordmann, Y. (1977) Homozygous case of hereditary coproporphyria. *Lancet,* **2**, 1348–1349.

92. Grandchamp, B., de Verneuil, H., Beaumont, C., Chretien, S., Walter, O. & Nordmann, Y. (1987) Tissue-specific expression of porphobilinogen deaminase. Two enzymes from a single gene. *European Journal of Biochemistry,* **162**, 105–110.

93. Grandchamp, B., Picat, C., de Rooij, F., Beaumont, C., Wilson, P., Deybach, J.C. & Nordmann, Y. (1989) A point mutation G-to-A in exon 12 of the porphobilinogen deaminase gene results in exon skipping and is responsible for acute intermittent porphyria. *Nucleic Acids Research,* **17**, 6637–6649.

94. Grandchamp, B., Picat, C., Mignotte, V., Wilson, J.H.P., TeVelde, K., Sandkuyl, L., Romeo, P.H., Goossens, M. & Nordmann, Y. (1989) Tissue-specific splicing mutation in acute intermittent porphyria. *Proceedings of the National Academy of Sciences of the USA,* **86**, 661–664.

95. Grossmann, M.E. & Bickers, D.R. (1978) Porphyria cutanea tarda, a rare cutaneous manifestation of hepatic tumors. *Cutis,* **21**, 782–784.

96. Grossman, M.E., Bickers, D.R., Poh-Fitzpatrick, M.B. et al. (1979) Porphyria cutanea tarda. Clinical features and laboratory findings in 40 patients. *American Journal of Medicine,* **67**, 277–286.

97. Guidotti, T.L., Charness, M.E. & Lamon, J.M. (1979) Acute intermittent porphyria and the Klüver–Bucy syndrome. *Johns Hopkins Medical Journal,* **145**, 233–235.

98. Haberman, H.F., Rosenberg, F. & Menon, I.A. (1975) Porphyria cutanea tarda: comparison of cases precipitated by alcohol and estrogens. *Journal of the Canadian Medical Association,* **113**, 653–655.

99. Hansen, J.L., O'Connell, P., Romana, M., Romeo, P.-H. & Kushner, J.P. (1988) Familial porphyria cutanea tarda: hybridization analysis of the uroporphyrinogen decarboxylase locus. *Human Heredity,* **38**, 283–286.

100. Herrick, A., McLellan A., Brodie, M. J., McColl, K.E.L., Moore, M.R. & Goldberg, A. (1987) Effect of haem arginate therapy on porphyrin metabolism and mixed function oxygenase activity in acute hepatic porphyria. *Lancet,* **2**, 1178–1179.

101. Herrick, A.L., Moore, M.R., McColl, K.E.L., Cook, A. & Goldberg, A. (1989) Controlled trial of haem arginate in acute hepatic porphyria. *Lancet,* **1**, 1295–1297.

102. Hill, R.H. (1985) Effects of polyhalogenated aromatic compounds on porphyrin metabolism. *Environmental Health Perspectives,* **60**, 139–143.

103. Hogan, D., Card, R.T., Ghadially, R., McSheffrey, J.B. & Lane, P. (1989) Human immunodeficiency virus infection and porphyria cutanea tarda. *Journal of the American Academy of Dermatology,* **20**, 17–20.

104. Ippen, H. (1961) Allgemeinsymptome der späten Hautporphyrie (Porphyria cutanea tarda) als Hinweise für deren Behandlung. *Deutsche Medizinische Wochenschrift,* **86**, 127–133.

105. Ippen, H., Tillmann, W., Seubert, S. & Seubert, A. (1978) Porphyria erythropoetica congenita Gunther und Chloroquin. *Klinische Wochenschrift,* **56**, 623–624.

106. James, K.R. (1980) Demonstration of intracytoplasmic needle-like inclusions in hepatocytes of patients with porphyria cutanea tarda. *Journal of Clinical Pathology,* **33**, 899–900.

107. Johansson, L., Thunell, S. & Wetterberg, L. (1984) A filter paper dry blood spot procedure for acute intermittent porphyria population screening by use of whole blood uroporphyrinogen-I-synthase assay. *Clinica Chimica Acta,* **137**, 317–331.

108. Kalb, R.E., Grossman, M.E. & Poh-Fitzpatrick, M.B. (1985) Correlation of serum and urinary porphyrin levels in porphyria cutanea tarda. *Archives of Dermatology,* **121**, 1289–1291.

109. Kauppinen, R. & Mustajoki, P. (1988) Acute hepatic porphyria and hepatocellular carcinoma. *British Journal of Cancer,* **57**, 117–120.

110. Kawanishi, S., Seki, Y. & Sano, S. (1983) Uroporphyrinogen decarboxylase. Purification, properties, and inhibition by polychlorinated biphenyl isomers. *Journal of Biological Chemistry,* **258**, 4285–4292.
111. Kench, J.D., Langley, F.A. & Wilkinson, J.F. (1955) Biochemical and pathological studies of congenital porphyria. *Quarterly Journal of Medicine,* **22**, 285–294.
112. Ketterer, B., Srai, K.S. & Christodoulides, L. (1976) Haem-binding proteins of the rat liver cytosol. *Biochimica et Biophysica Acta,* **428**, 683–689.
113. Koskelo, P., Toivonen, I. & Aldercreutz, H. (1967) Urinary coproporphyrin isomer distribution in the Dubin–Johnson syndrome. *Clinical Chemistry,* **13**, 1006–1009.
114. Kostrzewska, E. & Gregor, A. (1986) Increased activity of porphobilinogen deaminase in erythrocytes during attacks of acute intermittent porphyria. *Annals of Clinical Research,* **18**, 195–198.
115. Kushner, J.P., Barbuto, A.J. & Lee, G.R. (1976) An inherited enzymatic defect in porphyria cutanea tarda. Decreased uroporphyrinogen decarboxylase activity. *Journal of Clinical Investigation,* **58**, 1089–1097.
116. Kushner, J.P., Pimstone, N.R., Kjedlsberg, C.R., Pryor, M.A. & Huntley, A. (1982) Congenital erythropoietic porphyria, diminished activity of uroporphyrinogen decarboxylase and dyserythropoiesis. *Blood,* **59**, 725–737.
117. Lai, C.-L., Wu, P.-C., Lin, H.-J. & Wong, K.-L. (1984) Case report of symptomatic porphyria cutanea tarda associated with histocytic lymphoma. *Cancer,* **53**, 573–576.
118. Laiwah, A.C.Y., Junor, B., MacPhee, G.J.A. *et al.* (1983) Charcoal haemoperfusion and haemodialysis in acute intermittent porphyria. *British Medical Journal,* **287**, 1746–1747.
119. Lamola, A.A. & Yamane, T. (1974) Zinc protoporphyrin in the erythrocytes of patients with lead intoxication and iron deficiency anemia. *Science,* **186**, 936–938.
120. Lamola, A.A., Piomelli, S., Poh-Fitzpatrick, M.B. *et al.* (1975) Erythropoietic protoporphyria and lead intoxication: the molecular basis for difference in cutaneous photosensitivity. II. Different binding of erythrocyte protoporphyrin in hemoglobin. *Journal of Clinical Investigation,* **56**, 1528–1535.
121. Lamon, J.M., Frykholm, B.C. & Tschudy, D.P. (1979) Family evaluations in acute intermittent porphyria using red cell uroporphyrinogen I synthetase. *Journal of Medical Genetics,* **16**, 134–139.
122. Lamon, J.M., Poh-Fitzpatrick, M.B. & Lamola, A.A. (1980) Hepatic protoporphyrin production in human protoporphyria. Effects of intravenous hematin and analysis of erythrocyte protoporphyrin distribution. *Gastroenterology,* **79**, 115–125.
123. Lamon, J., With, T.K. & Redeker, A.G. (1974) The Hoesch test: bedside screening for urinary porphobilinogen in patients with suspected porphyria. *Clinical Chemistry,* **20**, 1438–1440.
124. Lamon, J.M., Frykholm, B.C., Hess, R.A. & Tschudy, D.P. (1979) Hematin therapy for acute porphyria. *Medicine,* **58**, 252–269.
125. Larson, A.W., Wasserstrom, W.R., Felsher, B.F. & Shih, J.C. (1978) Posttraumatic epilepsy and acute intermittent porphyria: effects of phenytoin, carbamazepine, and clonazepam. *Neurology,* **28**, 824–828.
126. Lee, J.S., Anvret, M., Lindsten, J., Lannfelt, L., Gellerfors, P., Wetterberg, L., Floderus, Y. & Thunell, S. (1988) DNA polymorphisms within the porphobilinogen deaminase gene in two Swedish families with acute intermittent porphyria. *Human Genetics,* **79**, 379–381.
127. Lim, H.W., Gigli, I. & Wasserman, S.I. (1987) Differential effects of protoporphyrin and uroporphyrin on murine mast cells. *Journal of Investigative Dermatology,* **88**, 281–286.
128. Lim, H.W., Poh-Fitzpatrick, M.B. & Gigli, I. (1984) Activation of the complement system in patients with porphyrias after irradiation in vivo. *Journal of Clinical Investigation,* **74**, 1961–1965.
129. Lim, H.W., Perez, H.D., Poh-Fitzpatrick, M. *et al.* (1981) Generation of chemotactic activity in serum from patients with erythropoietic protoporphyria and porphyria cutanea tarda. *New England Journal of Medicine,* **304**, 212–216.
130. Lindblad, B., Lindstedt, S. & Steen, G. (1977) On the enzymic defects in hereditary tyrosinemia. *Proceedings of the National Academy of Sciences of the USA,* **74**, 4641–4645.
131. Litman, D.A. & Correia, M.A. (1983) L-Tryptophan: a common denominator of biochemical and neurological events of acute porphyria? *Science,* **22**, 1031–1033.
132. Litman, D.A. & Correia, M.A. (1985) Elevated brain tryptophan and enhanced 5-hydroxytryptamine turnover in acute hepatic heme deficiency: clinical implications. *Journal of Pharmacology and Experimental Therapeutics,* **232**, 337–345.
133. Llewellyn, D.H., Kalsheker, N.A., Harrison, P.R., Picat, C., Romeo, P.H., Elder, G.H., Grandchamp, B., Nordmann, Y. & Goossens, M. (1987) DNA polymorphism of human porphobilinogen deaminase gene in acute intermittent porphyria. *Lancet,* **2**, 706–708.
134. Lobato, M.N. & Berger, T.G. (1988) Porphyria cutanea tarda associated with the acquired immunodeficiency syndrome. *Archives of Dermatology,* **124**, 1009–1010.
135. Ludwig, G.D. & Epstein, I.S. (1961) A genetic study of two families having the acute intermittent type of porphyria. *Annals of Internal Medicine,* **55**, 81–93.
136. Lundvall, O., Weinfeld, A. & Lundin, P. (1970) Iron storage in porphyria cutanea tarda. *Acta Medica Scandinavica,* **188**, 37–53.
137. Lynch, R.E., Lee, G.R. & Kushner, J.P. (1975) Porphyria cutanea tarda associated with disinfectant misuse. *Archives of Internal Medicine,* **135**, 549–552.
138. Magnus, I.A., Jarret, A., Prankerd, T.A.J. & Rimington, C. (1961) Erythropoietic protoporphyria—a new porphyria syndrome with solar urticaria due to protoporphyrinaemia. *Lancet,* **2**, 448–451.
139. MacDonald, D.M. (1981) The histopathology and ultrastructure of liver disease in erythropoietic protoporphyria. *British Journal of Dermatology,* **104**, 7–17.
140. Magnussen, C.R., Doherty, J.M., Hess, R.A. & Tschudy, D.P. (1975) Grand mal seizures and acute intermittent porphyria. The problem of differential diagnosis and treatment. *Neurology,* **25**, 1121–1125.
141. Magnussen, C.R., Levine, J.B., Doherty, J.M. *et al.* (1974) A red cell enzyme method for the diagnosis of acute intermittent porphyria. *Blood,* **44**, 857–868.
142. Malkinson, F.D. & Levitt, L. (1980) Hydroxychloroquine treatment of porphyria cutanea tarda. *Archives of Dermatology,* **116**, 1147–1150.
143. Manzione, N.C., Wolkoff, A.W. & Sassa, S. (1988) Development of porphyria cutanea tarda after treatment with cyclophosphamide. *Gastroenterology,* **95**, 1119–1122.
144. Marver, H.S. (1969) The role of heme in the synthesis and repression of microsomal protein. In Gillette, J.R., Conney, A.H., Cosmides, G.J. *et al.* (eds) *Microsomes and Drug Oxidations,* pp. 495–515. New York: Academic Press.
145. Marver, H.S., Tschudy, D.P., Perlroth, M.G. *et al.* (1966) The determination of aminoketones in biological fluids. *Analytical Biochemistry,* **14**, 53–60.
146. Mathews-Roth, M.M. (1987) Photoprotection by carotenoids. *Federation Proceedings,* **46**, 1890–1893.
147. Matilla, A. & Molland, E.A. (1974) A light and electron microscopic study of the liver in a case of erythrohepatic protoporphyria and in griseofulvin-induced porphyria in mice. *Journal of Clinical Pathology,* **27**, 698–709.
148. Mauzerall, D. (1976) Chlorophyll and photosynthesis. *Philosophical Transactions of the Royal Society of London. Series B: Biological Sciences,* **273**, 287–294.
149. Mauzerall, D. & Granick, S. (1956) The occurrence and determination of delta-aminolevulinic acid and porphobilinogen in urine. *Journal of Biological Chemistry,* **219**, 435–446.
150. McColl, K.E.L., Moore, M.R., Thompson, G.G. & Goldberg, A. (1981) Treatment with haematin in acute hepatic porphyria. *Quarterly Journal of Medicine,* **198**, 161–174.
151. Meisler, M., Wanner, L., Eddy, R.E. & Shows, T.B. (1980) The UPS locus encoding uroporphyrinogen I synthase is located on human chromosome 11. *Biochemical and Biophysical Research Communications,* **95**, 170–176.
152. Meissner, P.N., Day, R.S., Moore, M.R., Disler, P.B. & Harley, E. (1986) Protoporphyrinogen oxidase and porphobilinogen deaminase in variegate porphyria. *European Journal of Clinical Investigation,* **16**, 257–261.
153. Meyer, U.A. (1973) Intermittent acute porphyria. Clinical and

biochemical studies of disordered heme biosynthesis. *Enzyme*, **16**, 334–342.

154. Meyer, U.A. & Schmid, R. (1978) The porphyrias. In Stanbury, J.B., Wyngaarden, J.B. & Frederickson, D.S. (eds) *The Metabolic Basis of Inherited Disease*, pp. 1166–1220. New York: McGraw-Hill.

155. Meyer, U.A., Strand, L.J., Doss, M. *et al.* (1972) Intermittent acute porphyria—demonstration of a genetic defect in porphobilinogen metabolism. *New England Journal of Medicine*, **286**, 1277–1282.

156. Mignotte, V., Elequet, J.F., Raich, N. & Romeo, P.H. (1989) Cis- and trans-acting elements involved in the regulation of the erythroid promoter of the human porphobilinogen deaminase gene. *Proceedings of the National Academy of Sciences of the USA*, **86**, 6548–6552.

157. Miyagi, K., Kaneshima, M., Kawakami, J. *et al.* (1979) Uroporphyrinogen I synthase from human erythrocytes: separation, purification, and properties of isoenzymes. *Proceedings of the National Academy of Sciences of the USA*, **76**, 6172–6176.

158. Moore, M.R. (1980) International review of drugs in acute porphyria. *International Journal of Biochemistry*, **12**, 1089–1097.

159. Morris, D.L., Dudley, M.D. & Pearson, R.D. (1981) Coagulopathy associated with hematin treatment for acute intermittent porphyria. *Annals of Internal Medicine*, **95**, 700–701.

160. Mukerji, S.K., Pimstone, N.R. & Tan, K.T. (1985) A potential biochemical explanation for the genesis of porphyria cutanea tarda. *Federation of European Biochemical Societies Letters*, **189**, 217–220.

161. Muller-Eberhard, U. & Liem, H.H. (1974) Hemopexin, the heme-binding serum β-glycoprotein. In Allison, A.C. (ed.) *Structure and Function of Plasma Proteins*, pp. 35–53. London: Plenum Press.

162. Murphy, G.M., Hawk, J.L.M., Magnus, I.A., Barrett, D.F., Elder, G.H. & Smith, S.G. (1986) Homozygous variegate porphyria: two similar cases in unrelated families. *Journal of the Royal Society of Medicine*, **79**, 361–364.

163. Mustajoki, P. (1981) Normal erythrocyte uroporphyrinogen I synthase in a kindred with acute intermittent porphyria. *Annals of Internal Medicine*, **95**, 162–166.

164. Mustajoki, P. & Nikkilä, E.A. (1984) Serum lipoprotein in asymptomatic acute porphyria: no evidence for hyperbetalipoproteinemia. *Metabolism*, **33**, 266–269.

165. Mustajoki, P., Tenhunen, R., Niemi, K.M., Nordmann, Y., Kaariainen, H. & Norio, R. (1987) Homozygous variegate porphyria: a severe skin disease of infancy. *Clinical Genetics*, **32**, 300–305.

166. Mustajoki, P., Tenhunen, R., Pierach, C. & Volin, L. (1989) Heme in the treatment of porphyrias and hematological disorders. *Seminars in Hematology*, **26**, 1–9.

167. Mustajoki, P., Tenhunen, R., Tokola, O. & Gothoni, G. (1986) Haem arginate in the treatment of acute hepatic porphyrias. *British Medical Journal*, **293**, 538–539.

168. Ostrowski, J., Kostrzewska, E., Michalak, T. *et al.* (1983) Abnormalities in liver function and morphology and impaired aminopyrine metabolism in hereditary hepatic porphyrias. *Gastroenterology*, **85**, 1131–1137.

169. Ostrowski, J., Michalak, T., Zawirska, B., Kostrzewska, E., Blaszczyk, M. & Gregor, A. (1984) The function and morphology of the liver in porphyria cutanea tarda. *Annals of Clinical Research*, **16**, 195–200.

170. Peterson, L.R., Hamernyik, P., Bird, T.D. & Labbe, R.F. (1976) Erythrocyte uroporphyrinogen I synthase activity in diagnosis of acute intermittent porphyria. *Clinical Chemistry*, **22**, 1835–1840.

171. Pierach, C.A., Bossenmaier, G.C., Cardinal, R.A. & Weimer, M.K. (1984) Pseudo-porphyria in a patient with hepatocellular carcinoma. *American Journal of Medicine*, **76**, 545–548.

172. Pimstone, N.R., Gandhi, S.N. & Mukerji, S.K. (1987) Therapeutic efficacy of oral charcoal in congenital erythropoietic porphyria. *New England Journal of Medicine*, **316**, 390–393.

173. Piomelli, S. (1973) A micromethod for free erythrocyte porphyrins: the FEP test. *Journal of Laboratory and Clinical Medicine*, **81**, 932–940.

174. Piomelli, S., Lamola, A.A., Poh-Fitzpatrick, M.B. *et al.* (1975) Erythropoietic protoporphyria and lead intoxication: the molecular basis for difference in cutaneous photosensitivity. I. Different rates of disappearance of protoporphyrin from the erythrocytes, both in vivo and in vitro. *Journal of Clinical Investigation*, **56**, 1519–1527.

175. Piomelli, S., Poh-Fitzpatrick, M.B., Seaman, C., Skolnick, L.M.

& Berdon, W.E. (1986) Complete suppression of the symptoms of congenital erythropoietic porphyria by long-term treatment with high-level transfusions. *New England Journal of Medicine*, **314**, 1029–1031.

176. Poh-Fitzpatrick, M.B. & Ellis, D.L. (1989) Porphyria-like bullous dermatosis after chronic intense tanning and/or sunlight exposure. *Archives of Dermatology*, **125**, 1236–1238.

177. Poh-Fitzpatrick, M.B. & Lamola, A.A. (1976) Direct spectrofluorometry of diluted erythrocytes and plasma: a rapid diagnostic method in primary and secondary porphyrinemias. *Journal of Laboratory and Clinical Medicine*, **87**, 362–370.

178. Poh-Fitzpatrick, M.B., Masullo, A.S. & Grossman, M.E. (1980) Porphyria cutanea tarda associated with chronic renal disease and hemodialysis. *Archives of Dermatology*, **116**, 191–195.

179. Poulson, R. (1976) The enzymic conversion of protoporphyrinogen IX to protoporphyrin IX in mammalian mitochondria. *Journal of Biological Chemistry*, **251**, 3730–3733.

180. Praga, M., deSalamanca, R.E., Andres, A., Nieto, J., Oliet, A., Perpina, J. & Morales, J.M. (1987) Treatment of hemodialysis-related porphyria cutanea tarda with deferoxamine. *New England Journal of Medicine*, **316**, 547–548.

181. Raffin, S.B., Woo, C.H., Roost, K.T. *et al.* (1974) Intestinal absorption of hemoglobin iron-heme cleavage by mucosal heme oxygenase. *Journal of Clinical Investigation*, **54**, 1344–1352.

182. Rajamanickam, C., Satyanarayana Rao, M.R. & Padmanaban, G. (1975) On the sequence of reactions leading to cytochrome P-450 synthesis—effect of drugs. *Journal of Biological Chemistry*, **250**, 2305–2310.

183. Reio, L. & Wetterberg, L. (1969) False porphobilinogen reactions in the urine of mental patients. *Journal of the American Medical Association*, **207**, 148–150.

184. Riccioni, N., Donati, G., Soldani, S., Scatena, P. & Aracabasso, G.D. (1987) Treatment of hemodialysis-related porphyria cutanea tarda with small repeated phlebotomies. *Nephron*, **46**, 125–127.

185. Ridley, A. (1969) The neuropathy of acute intermittent porphyria. *Quarterly Journal of Medicine*, **38**, 307–333.

186. Rocchi, E., Bigertini, P., Cassanelli, M., Pietrangelo, A., Borghi, A., Pantaleoni, M., Jensen, J. & Ventura, E. (1986) Iron removal therapy in porphyria cutanea tarda: phlebotomy versus slow subcutaneous desferrioxamine infusion. *British Journal of Dermatology*, **114**, 621–629.

187. Rocchi, E., Gibertini, P., Cassanelli, M., Pietrangelo, A., Borghi, A. & Ventura, E. (1986) Serum ferritin in the assessment of liver iron overload and iron removal therapy in porphyria cutanea tarda. *Journal of Laboratory and Clinical Medicine*, **107**, 36–42.

188. Romeo, P.-H., Dubart, A., Grandchamp, B., De Verneuil, H., Rosa, J., Nordmann, Y. & Goossens, M. (1984) Isolation and identification of a cDNA clone coding for rat uroporphyrinogen decarboxylase. *Biochemistry*, **81**, 3346–3350.

189. Rothwell, J.D., LaCroix, S. & Sweeney, G.D. (1973) Evidence against a regulatory role for heme oxygenase in hepatic heme synthesis. *Biochimica et Biophysica Acta*, **304**, 871–874.

190. Samuel, D., Boboc, B., Bernuau, J., Bismuth, H. & Benhamou, J.-P. (1988) Liver transplantation for protoporphyria: evidence for the predominant role of the erythropoietic tissue in protoporphyrin. *Gastroenterology*, **95**, 816–819.

191. Sassa, S. & Kappas, A. (1989) Lack of effect of pregnancy or hematin therapy on erythrocyte porphobilinogen deaminase activity in acute intermittent porphyria. *New England Journal of Medicine*, **321**, 192–193.

192. Sassa, S., Granick, S. & Kappas, A. (1975) Effect of lead and genetic factors on heme biosynthesis in the human red cell. *Annals of the New York Academy of Sciences*, **244**, 419–440.

193. Sassa, S., Solish, G., Levere, R.D. & Kappas, A. (1975) Studies in porphyria. IV. Expression of the gene defect of acute intermittent porphyria in cultured human skin fibroblasts and amniotic cells: prenatal diagnosis of the porphyric trait. *Journal of Experimental Medicine*, **142**, 722–731.

194. Sassa, S., Granick, S., Bickers, D.R. *et al.* (1974) A microassay for uroporphyrinogen I synthase, one of three abnormal enzyme activities in acute intermittent porphyria, and its application to the study of the genetics of this disease. *Proceedings of the National Academy of Sciences of the USA*, **71**, 732–736.

195. Schmid, R. (1960) Cutaneous porphyria in Turkey. *New England Journal of Medicine*, **263**, 397–398.

196. Schmid, R. (1973) Synthesis and degradation of microsomal hemoproteins. *Drug Metabolism and Disposition*, **1**, 256–258.

197. Scholnick, P.L., Marver, H.S. & Epstein, J. (1973) The molecular basis of the action of chloroquine in porphyria cutanea tarda. *Journal of Investigative Dermatology*, **61**, 226–232.

198. Scholnick, P., Marver, H.S. & Schmid, R. (1971) Erythropoietic protoporphyria: evidence for multiple sites of excess protoporphyrin formation. *Journal of Clinical Investigation*, **50**, 203–207.

199. Schwartz, S., Berg, M.H., Bossenmaier, I. & Dinsmore, H. (1960) Determination of porphyrins in biological materials. *Methods of Biochemical Analysis*, **8**, 221–293.

200. Semon, C., Dupond, J.L., Mallet, H., Grandmottet-Cambefort, C. & Humbert, P. (1986) Traitement d'une porphyrie aigue intermittente avec attaques cycliques par un agoniste LH-RH administre par voie nasale. *Annales d'Endocrinologie (Paris)*, **47**, 399–402.

201. Seubert, S., Seubert, A., Rumpf, K.W. & Kiffe, H. (1985) A porphyria cutanea tarda-like distribution pattern of porphyrins in plasma, hemodialysate, hemofiltrate, and urine of patients on chronic hemodialysis. *Journal of Investigative Dermatology*, **85**, 107–109.

202. Shedlofsky, S.I. & Bonkowsky, H.L. (1984) Seizure management in the hepatic porphyrias: results from a cell-culture model of porphyria. *Neurology*, **34**, 399.

203. Siepker, L.J. & Kramer, S. (1985) Protoporphyrin accumulation by mitogen stimulated lymphocytes and protoporphyrinogen oxidase activity in patients with porphyria variegata and erythropoietic protoporphyria: evidence for deficiency of protoporphyrinogen oxidase and ferrochelatase in both. *British Journal of Haematology*, **60**, 65–74.

204. Sievers, G., Hakli, H. Luhtala, J. & Tenhunen, R. (1987) Optical and EPR spectroscopy studies on haem arginate, a new compound used for treatment of porphyria. *Chemical-Biological Interactions*, **63**, 105–114.

205. Smith, A.G. & Francis, J.E. (1983) Synergism of iron and hexachlorobenzene inhibits hepatic uroporphyrinogen decarboxylase in inbred mice. *Biochemical Journal*, **214**, 909–913.

206. Spikes, J.D. (1975) Porphyrins and related compounds as photodynamic sensitizers. *Annals of the New York Academy of Sciences*, **244**, 496–508.

207. Stein, J.A. & Tschudy, D.P. (1970) Acute intermittent porphyria: a clinical and biochemical study of 46 patients. *Medicine*, **49**, 1–16.

208. Strand, L.J., Felsher, B.F., Redeker, A.G. & Marver, H.S. (1970) Enzymatic abnormalities in heme biosynthesis in intermittent acute porphyria: decreased hepatic conversion of porphobilinogen to porphyrins and increased δ-aminolevulinic acid synthetase activity. *Proceedings of the National Academy of Sciences of the USA*, **67**, 1315–1320.

209. Strik, J.J.T.W.A., Doss, M., Schraa, G., Robertson, L.W., von Tiepermann, R. & Harmsen, E.G.M. (1979) Coproporphyrinuria and chronic hepatic porphyria type A found in farm families from Michigan (U.S.A.) exposed to polybrominated biphenyls (PBB). In Strik, J.J.T.W.A. & Koeman, J.H. (eds) *Chemical Porphyria in Man*, pp. 29–53. Amsterdam: Elsevier/North Holland.

210. Sweeney, G.D. & Jones, K.G. (1979) Porphyria cutanea tarda: clinical and laboratory features. *Canadian Medical Association Journal*, **120**, 803–807.

211. Taljaard, J.F.F., Shanley, B.C., Stewart-Wynne, E.G. *et al.* (1972) Studies on low dose chloroquine therapy and the action of chloroquine in symptomatic porphyria. *British Journal of Dermatology*, **87**, 261–269.

212. Taylor, R.L. (1981) Magnesium sulfate for AIP seizures. *Neurology*, **31**, 1371–1372.

213. Tenhunen, R., Marver, H.S. & Schmid, R. (1970) The enzymatic catabolism of hemoglobin: stimulation of microsomal heme oxygenase by hemin. *Journal of Laboratory and Clinical Medicine*, **75**, 410–421.

214. Tenhunen, R., Tokola, O. & Linden, I.-B. (1987) Haem arginate: a new stable haem compound. *Journal of Pharmacy and Pharmacology*, **39**, 780–786.

215. Thunell, S., Holmberg, L. & Lundgren, J. (1987) Aminolaevulinate dehydratase porphyria in infancy: a clinical and biochemical study. *Journal of Clinical Chemistry and Clinical Biochemistry*, **25**, 5–14.

216. Tishler, P.V., Woodward, B., O'Connor, J., Holbrook, D.A., Seidman, L.J., Hallett, M. & Knighton, D.J. (1985) High prevalence of intermittent acute porphyria in a psychiatric patient population. *American Journal of Psychiatry*, **142**, 1430–1436.

217. Toback, A.C., Sassa, S., Poh-Fitzpatrick, M.B., Schechter, J., Zaider, E., Harber, L.C. & Kappas, A. (1987) Hepatoerythropoietic porphyria: clinical, biochemical and enzymatic studies in a three-generation family lineage. *New England Journal of Medicine*, **316**, 645–650.

218. Tokola, O., Linden, I.-B. & Tenhunen, R. (1987) The effects of haem arginate and haematin upon the allylisopropylacetamide induced experimental porphyria in rats. *Pharmacology & Toxicology*, **61**, 75–78.

219. Tokola, O., Tenhunen, R., Volin, L. & Mustajoki, P. (1986) Pharmacokinetics of intravenously administered haem arginate. *British Journal of Clinical Pharmacology*, **22**, 001–005.

220. Tschudy, D.P. & Bonkowsky, H.L. (1972) Experimental porphyria. *Federation Proceedings*, **31**, 147–159.

221. Tschudy, D.P., Welland, F.H., Collins, A. & Hunter, G. (1964) The effect of carbohydrate feedings on the induction of δ-aminolevulinic acid synthetase. *Metabolism*, **13**, 396–405.

222. Waldenström, J. (1957) The porphyrias as inborn errors of metabolism. *American Journal of Medicine*, **22**, 758–773.

223. Watson, C.J. & Schwartz, S. (1941) A simple test for urinary porphobilinogen. *Proceedings of the Society for Experimental Biology and Medicine*, **47**, 393–394.

224. Watson, C.J., Bossenmaier, I.B., Cardinal, R. & Patryka, Z.J. (1974) Repression by hematin of porphyrin biosynthesis in erythrocyte precursors in congenital erythropoietic porphyria. *Proceedings of the National Academy of Sciences of the USA*, **71**, 278–282.

225. Watson, C.J., Pierach, C.A., Bossenmaier, I. & Cardinal, R. (1977) Postulated deficiency of hepatic heme and repair by hematin infusions in the 'inducible' hepatic porphyrias. *Proceedings of the National Academy of Sciences of the USA*, **74**, 2118–2120.

226. Went, L.N. & Klasen, E.C. (1984) Genetic aspects of erythropoietic protoporphyria. *Annals of Human Genetics*, **48**, 105–117.

227. Wolkoff, A.W., Wolpert, E., Pascasio, F.N. & Arias, I.M. (1976) Rotor's syndrome: a distinct inheritable pathophysiologic entity. *American Journal of Medicine*, **60**, 172–179.

228. Yamamoto, M., Hayashi, N. & Kikuchi, G. (1982) Evidence for the transcriptional inhibition by heme of the synthesis of δ-aminolevulinate synthase in rat liver. *Biochemical and Biophysical Research Communications*, **105**, 985–990.

229. Zimmerman, T.S., McMillin, J.M. & Watson, C.J. (1966) Onset of manifestations of hepatic porphyria in relation to the influence of female sex hormones. *Archives of Internal Medicine*, **118**, 229–240.

230. Andersen, K.E., Goeger, D.E., Carson, R.W., Lee, S.M.K., & Stead, R.B. (1990) Erythropoietin for the treatment of porphyria cutanea tarda in a patient on long-term hemodialysis. *New England Journal of Medicine*, **322**, 315–317.

231. Garey, J.R., Harrison, L.M., Franklin, K.F. *et al.* (1990) Uroporphyrinogen decarboxylase: a splice site mutation causes the deletion of exon 6 in multiple families with porphyria cutanea tarda. *Journal of Clinical Investigation*, **86**, 1416–1422.

232. Milligan, A., Graham-Brown, R.A.C., Sarkany, I. & Baker, H. (1988) Erythropoietic protoporphyria exacerbated by oral iron therapy. *British Journal of Dermatology*, **119**, 63–66.

233. Muller-Eberhard, U. & Nikkilä, H. (1989) Transport of tetrapyrroles by proteins. *Seminars in Hematology*, **26**, 86–104.

234. Scobie, G.A., Llewellyn, D.H., Urquhart, A.J. *et al.* (1990) Acute intermittent porphyria caused by a C→T mutation that produces a stop codon in the porphobilinogen deaminase gene. *Human Genetics*, **85**, 631–634.

CHAPTER 17

The Liver and Response to Drugs

Charles F. George, Richard H. George & Colin W. Howden

FACTORS INFLUENCING THE RESPONSE TO DRUGS

Drugs may exert their pharmacological and therapeutic effects in one of several ways.[128] Firstly, they may mimic or block the effects of endogenous hormones and neurotransmitter substances including acetylcholine, noradrenaline and enkephalins through an interaction with specific drug receptors. Secondly, they can affect the activity of certain enzymes, monoamine oxidase for example, in a more or less specific manner. Alternatively, they may have a non-specific action on cellular function in cell membranes and affect ionic fluxes, a property which is shared by anaesthetic agents.

Whatever the precise mechanism and locus of action, the magnitude of a drug's operation is usually related to its free concentration in extracellular fluid[13,19,39,40,226] and the latter is in equilibrium with the concentration of free drug in plasma water. The most important factors affecting drug action are the dose, the proportion of this which reaches the systemic circulation, its distribution volume in the body, protein binding and the rate of elimination,[111] all of which may be influenced by hepatic function.

PHARMACOKINETIC FACTORS

Absorption

Whatever the route of administration, the major factors which govern drug absorption are the formulation, its physicochemical characteristics and the surface area available. For injected drugs, the local blood supply is also important in determining the rate and amount absorbed. With orally administered treatment, gastric and intestinal motility have similar consequences.[144]

Bioavailability of orally administered drugs
With the exception of a few whose molecular size is sufficiently small to allow them to pass between intercellular gaps, and others, like levodopa, which are absorbed by active transport, drugs are absorbed by passive diffusion across mucosal barriers. Most lipid-soluble drugs that are non-ionized at intestinal pH are well absorbed.[160] Despite this, the proportion of the dose which reaches the systemic circulation unchanged (bioavailability) may be low. Figure 17.1 shows the sites which limit the bioavailability of drugs and hence their effectiveness. For many the liver (site 6) is the most important of these.

For example, the anti-anginal, antihypertensive, β-adrenoceptor antagonist propranolol is almost completely absorbed after oral administration[255,306] but its bioavailability is low. This phenomenon has been extensively studied[102,116,303,307] and the explanation resides in the liver, which extracts and biotransforms this and other drugs as they pass through it on their way to the systemic circulation. This phenomenon, which is frequently referred to as a 'first-pass effect', is lacking after the creation of a portacaval anastomosis.[92,139,303]

An example of this occurrence for propranolol after intravenous dosing is shown in Figure 17.2. The hepatic extraction of propranolol (E) was derived from the equation

$$E = \frac{(A - H)}{A} \times 100$$

where A was the concentration in arterial blood and H the concentration in hepatic venous blood, and it amounted to over 80%. Thus, when given orally (Figure 17.3), a substantial proportion of the dose is removed by the liver before it reaches the systemic circulation (Figure 17.4).

Other drugs which exhibit a large hepatic first-pass effect include the β-adrenoceptor antagonists, alprenolol,[1] labetalol,[161,230] metoprolol[170] and oxprenolol,[218] and many of the calcium channel blocking drugs including verapamil,[93] nicardipine[84] and nifedipine,[60,356] as well as the antiarrhythmic compounds, lignocaine,[118,139,324] encainide and lorcanide.[181] In addition, a number of CNS active compounds undergo first-pass metabolism: they include the analgesics, morphine,[113] pentazocine,[27] pethidine[182,219] and propoxyphene[373] as well as the tricyclic antidepressants such as imipramine[132] and nortriptyline.[133,145] Further details can be found in the succeeding tables and in reviews by George,[113] Howden et al.[163] and Williams and Mamelok.[367]

Distribution volume

After reaching the systemic circulation, drugs become distributed to the tissues according to their physicochemical characteristics, binding to plasma proteins (see below) and blood flow. The volume of distribution of a drug is a theoretical measurement based upon the assumption that instantaneous mixing occurs throughout the body. Thus, the volume of distribution (V_d) is calculated from the dose divided by the concentration in blood and can be obtained in two ways.

Firstly, a concentration–time curve for the drug in blood can be constructed and the concentration at zero time estimated by extrapolating the second exponential in Figure 17.5 to obtain the apparent volume of distribution ($V_d(a)$). This parameter is useful in calculating loading doses of drugs as well as infusion rates. It is also of fundamental importance in determining the rate of drug elimination (see below).

Alternatively, the volume of distribution can be calculated at steady state ($V_d(ss)$). This can be regarded as the volume of distribution that would be attained if the drug were infused intravenously until a steady concentration in blood was attained.[260] $V_d(ss)$ is a better measurement than $V_d(a)$ because the former is dependent only on the distribution volume and the distribution rate constant, whereas the latter is affected also by the elimination process itself.[171,285]

Drug distribution volumes vary widely. Some, such as heparin, are confined in plasma water because of their

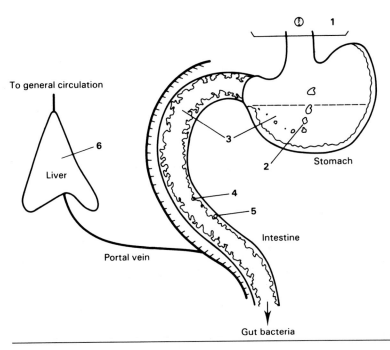

Figure 17.1 Sites at which the bioavailability of orally administered drugs may be reduced. Site 1—compliance. Site 2—disintegration and dissolution. Site 3—gastric and intestinal motility. Site 4—physicochemical characteristics of the drug. Site 5—metabolism by intestinal enzymes. Site 6—hepatic metabolism at the first pass.

high molecular weight and ionization; others, like antipyrine, are distributed throughout body water,[51] whereas lipid-soluble drugs like propranolol have a V_d of several litres/kg[306] because they are widely distributed and concentrated in the tissues, especially those of brain, liver and lung.[148]

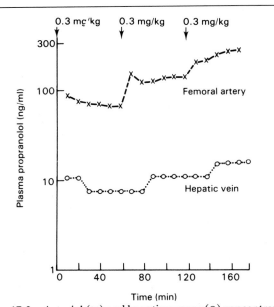

Figure 17.2 Arterial ($\times$) and hepatic venous ($\circ$) concentrations of propranolol after three doses of ($-$)-propranolol, 0.3 mg/kg i.v. in the dog, each followed by continuous infusion to maintain a constant arterial level. The extraction of propranolol is similar at each of the three levels. From George *et al.* (1976)[116] with kind permission of the editor of *Journal of Pharmacokinetics and Biopharmaceutics*.

Protein binding

Many drugs are carried in the blood bound to non-specific sites on plasma proteins. Albumin is the most important protein for the majority of acidic drugs and some basic compounds, although the latter tend to bind preferentially to alpha$_1$ acid glycoprotein.[262] For other drugs, curare for example, binding to globulin is very important.[19] Drug bound to protein is in equilibrium with that free in plasma water, but only the latter exerts a pharmacological and therapeutic effect (see above). The amount of drug bound to protein is determined by the number of binding sites available, which varies for different drugs, their affinity

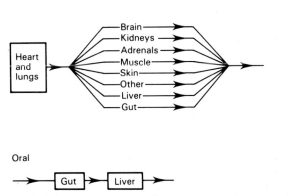

Figure 17.3 The effects of dosing by two different routes with a drug which undergoes extensive metabolism at the first pass in the liver. For intravenously administered drugs, the liver is in parallel with other organs and the rate of removal of drugs from the circulation is dependent upon liver blood flow. In contrast, when given orally, virtually all of the drug is presented to the liver, and intrinsic metabolism will determine the bioavailability.

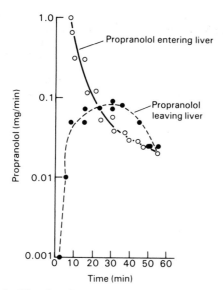

Figure 17.4 Kinetics of propranolol administered via the portal vein of a dog. ○ represents the amount of propranolol entering the liver and ● that leaving the liver. During the first five minutes of the experiment, extraction was almost 100% and the total systemic availability was approximately 30%. From George *et al.* (1976),[116] with kind permission of the editor of *Journal of Pharmacokinetics and Biopharmaceutics.*

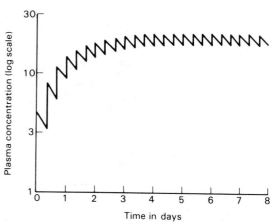

Figure 17.6 Concentration–time profile for a drug during repetitive dosing. A steady state is achieved after approximately five half-lives have elapsed. At this time fluctuation from one day to the next in concentrations does not differ.

for the drug and its concentration.[184] Plasma protein binding is an important factor in determining drug distribution and the rate of elimination. Only the unbound fraction is available for distribution: thus, for example, the greater the degree of binding of sulphonamides to albumin, the greater is the proportion that remains in the blood and the lower the concentration that enters cerebrospinal fluid.[109] Similarly, the distribution of most

antibiotics into the tissues is closely related to their binding on plasma proteins.[22] Drugs and drug metabolites can displace one another from binding to plasma proteins and the resultant increase in free concentration will lead to a temporary increase in their effects.[14,50,184]

For most drugs, except those which show a high hepatic extraction,[101] only free drug can be eliminated. Because of this, protein binding will lessen the removal of drugs and delay their elimination.[15,206,244] Details of the extent to which large numbers of drugs are bound to plasma proteins can be found in the review by Koch-Weser and Sellers.[184]

Rates of elimination

The rate of elimination of a drug from the body will determine its duration of action.[201] In addition, together with the frequency of administration, the rate of elimination determines the concentration in blood during regular dosing, which is frequently known as the steady-state concentration (Figure 17.6). For many water-soluble drugs, including digoxin,[79] chlorpropamide,[290] aminoglycosides[142,191] and atenolol,[223] the kidney is the most important route of elimination. However, others which are largely non-ionized at physiological pH are extensively reabsorbed from the kidney. Thus, for the majority of drugs the duration and intensity of action are largely determined by the speed at which they are metabolized in the body by the enzymes in the liver microsomes.[67]

Drug metabolism in the liver

Although metabolism can occur at several sites in the liver, including mitochondria and the cytosol, for the majority of drugs the smooth endoplasmic reticulum (Figure 17.7) is the most important. In the endoplasmic reticulum, enzymes attached to lipid layers of the membranes catalyse the metabolism of drugs to more water-

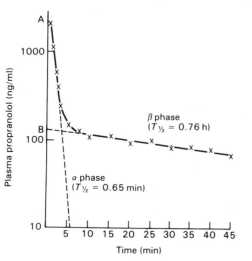

Figure 17.5 Concentration–time curve for intravenously administered propranolol. The log-linear plot can be resolved into two exponentials, and extrapolation of the second exponential or β-phase to zero time allows calculation of the volume of distribution. From George (1978),[112] with kind permission of the publisher, Kimpton.

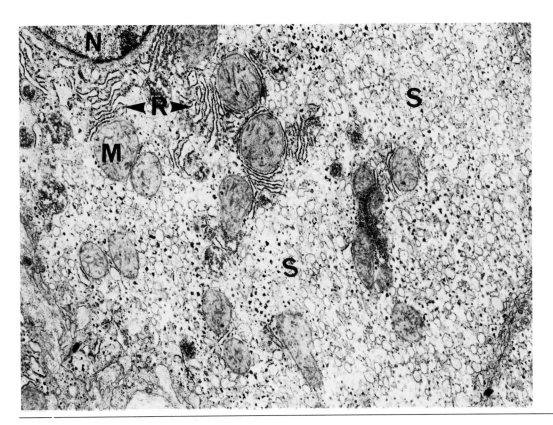

Figure 17.7 Electron micrograph of an hepatocyte showing smooth endoplasmic reticulum. (S) M=mitochondrion; N=nucleus; R=ribosomes.

soluble compounds, which are subsequently eliminated either in bile or in urine (see below). Experimentally, separation of the smooth endoplasmic reticulum can be achieved by ultracentrifugation at $1 \times 10^5 \, g$. This produces a pellet of membranes known as the microsomal fraction. Metabolism of drugs by this fraction is usually referred to as 'microsomal enzyme metabolism'.

Among the enzymes located in the endoplasmic reticulum are cytochrome P450, so called because of its striking absorption peak at 450 nm in the presence of carbon monoxide;[100] flavin enzymes, responsible for reduction of azo and nitro groups; esterases; and transferases. Pathways of drug metabolism in the microsomal system can broadly be categorized into two main types: firstly, preconjugation or phase I reactions, which serve to append or reveal suitable chemical groups such as OH, NH_2 and COOH within the drug; and secondly, conjugation, synthetic, or phase II reactions, in which groupings revealed by phase I reactions are coupled to endogenous compounds such as glucuronic acid and sulphate (Table 17.1). Phase II reactions may occur without prior oxidation, reduction or hydrolysis if suitable groupings already exist.

Most phase I metabolites are generated by a common hydroxylating enzyme system, cytochrome P450. This system was first described by Estabrook, Cooper and Rosenthal[100] and further elucidated by the same group, initially in the adrenal cortex.[250] Later, however, the same enzyme system was found to be present and more active in the liver.[97,279] This enzyme system has the capacity to

transport electrons to a cytochromal acceptor and in the process an oxygen atom is donated to the drug:

$$X + 2e^- + 2H^+ = O_2 \rightarrow X{:}O + H_2O$$

One of the two electrons is used for the reduction of one atom of oxygen to water and the second oxygen atom is incorporated into the substrate. The electron donor is reduced by NADPH and the electrons are picked up by a flavin protein known as cytochrome P450 reductase.[172] Thereafter, the electrons flow from the reduced flavin enzymes to cytochrome P450 (Figure 17.8). The activity of the cytochrome P450 system is, in part, genetically determined[7,349,359] but is also under the influence of environmental factors including substances present in the diet and various medicines (see below).[67]

Generally, phase I reactions led to a diminution of the pharmacological activity, but there are important exceptions to this rule. They include the red dye, prontosil, and the antidepressant, imipramine, which are converted to the active metabolites, sulphanilamide and desipramine, respectively.[75] Toxic metabolites of phenacetin and paracetamol may also be generated by this system.[233]

Cytochrome P450

At one time, cytochrome P450 was thought to be a single enzyme with a very broad chemical specificity. Further research has shown that there is in reality a family of isoenzymes with overlapping specificities.[136,175,208] Nearly

Table 17.1 Pathways of drug elimination in man.

Phase	Reaction	Enzyme	Examples
I	Oxidation of aliphatic and aromatic groups etc.	Cytochrome P450 Flavin monooxygenases	Barbiturates Meprobamate Phenytoin Phenothiazines Chlordiazepoxide Antihistamines Phenacetin Antipyrine Mefanamic acid Steroids Diazoxide
	Reduction of azo, nitro and sulphoxide groups, etc.	Cytochrome P450 Flavin enzymes Xanthine oxidase Aldehyde oxidase	Prontosil Chloramphenicol Chloramphenicol Chloralhydrate Sulindac
	Hydrolysis	Esterases Amidases	Esters Procaine Lignocaine Indomethacin Atropine substitutes
II	Glucuronide synthesis	Glucuronyl-transferase	Paracetamol Chloramphenicol
	Glycine conjugation	Transacylase	Salicylate
	Ethereal sulphate synthesis	Sulphokinase	Isoprenaline
	Methylation	Catechol-*O*-methyltransferase	Isoprenaline
	Acetylation	*N*-Acetyl-transferase	Isoniazid Sulphamethazine
	Mercapturic acid synthesis	Glutathione-transferases	Paracetamol

Other phase II reactions include conjugation with other amino acids, e.g. glutamate and thiocyanate formation

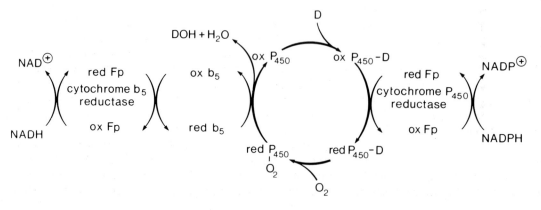

Figure 17.8 The cytochrome P450 hydroxylating system.

20 human isoenzymes have been cloned and characterized/ sequenced in full, but many more forms may exist. A nomenclature has been developed which allows the categorization of the growing number of primary amino-acid sequences.[241] Thus, the P450 gene superfamily has been subdivided into families, subfamilies and individual P450s. Families are identified by the use of a Roman numeral; subfamilies by capital letters, and the individual (trivial) P450s are denoted by the use of Arabic numerals. They include debrisoquine 4-hydroxylase (IID6), S-mephenytoin 4-hydroxylase (IIC9), nifedipine oxidase (III4A) and arachidonic acid epoxygenase. For a fuller description of these and other cytochromes, readers are referred to reviews[129,292] on the purification and characterization of hepatic microsomal cytochrome P450s.

Two well-defined sources of variability in human drug response have been identified, namely debrisoquine 4-hydroxylase and S-mephenytoin 4-hydroxylase.[91,166–168, 194] Between 5% and 10% of the population show impaired metabolism of debrisoquine (and 20 or so other compounds) and this deficiency is inherited in an autosomal recessive manner.[270] Poor metabolizers of debrisoquine are more susceptible to its effects and will develop postural hypotension when treated with it. Other substrates for this enzyme include sparteine and the anti-arrhythmics, encainide and propafenone, several β-adrenoceptor blockers including alprenolol, bopindolol, bufuralol, metoprolol, penbutolol, propranolol and timolol. In addition, some antidepressants, including clomipramine, desmethylimipramine and nortriptyline, are metabolized by this enzyme.[56] Deficient metabolism of these compounds explains many adverse effects which were previously regarded as being 'idiosyncratic', e.g. vomiting with bufuralol and adverse effects from perhexiline and phenformin.

The isoenzymes of cytochrome P450 show differences in their responses to environmental factors, including substances present in the diet and various medicines[67,137] (see below). Drugs may affect the activity of the P450 cytochrome system in one of two ways. Firstly, the amount and activity of the enzyme may be increased by drugs which are referred to as inducers of microsomal oxidation.[97,279,315] They include barbiturates, glutethimide, dichloralphenazone, haloperidol, alcohol and griseofulvin.[80,331] When an inducer of microsomal oxidation is introduced into the treatment of the patient stabilized on another drug which is metabolized by hepatic microsomal enzymes, the effect is gradually to increase the rate of inactivation of the latter.[48] Thus, to maintain the previous pharmacological and therapeutic effects it may be necessary to increase the dose severalfold. Secondly, drugs may inhibit the action of hepatic microsomal enzymes: these include methylphenidate, chloramphenicol, disulfiram, allopurinol, alcohol/dextropropoxyphene[80,251] and cimetidine.[319,320]

The discovery of the various isoenzymes of cytochrome P450 has clarified our understanding of why some substances selectively induce[24] or inhibit the metabolism of certain drugs. Thus, rifampicin has a relatively specific action to increase the activity of steroid-metabolizing enzymes[90,331,347] and cigarette smoking increases the pre-systemic metabolism of propranolol but not of nifedipine.[280,350] By contrast, cimetidine inhibits the metabolism of both propranolol and nifedipine. Despite the comparative lack of substrate specificity, the inhibitory action of cimetidine is stereoselective in the case of R-warfarin[61] and R-nicoumalone.[119] Other drugs, such as verapamil, exhibit stereoselective presystemic (first-pass) metabolism.[89,351] It is, therefore, likely to exhibit stereoselective inhibition of its metabolism. The metabolism of debrisoquine and other compounds can also be selectively inhibited by quinidine, which has the effect (even in single doses) of converting 'extensive metabolizers' to 'poor metabolizers'.[168,198]

The generation of toxic metabolites can also be dependent upon the presence of a normally functioning cytochrome P450 and exacerbated by inducing agents.[233,342] Thus, the toxicity of paracetamol (acetaminophen) relates to the generation of an electrophile which binds covalently to protein thiol groups and causes hepatotoxicity. These processes are enhanced by previous exposure to enzyme-inducing compounds such as the barbiturates.[233] Similarly, a metabolite of halothane binds selectively to amino groups.[294]

Another cytochrome P450-dependent form of toxicity is that created by the generation of free radicals which preferentially attack unsaturated fatty acids in membranes and lead to lipid peroxidation.[342] For halothane the relative contribution of this effect in vivo is uncertain. Clinically, halothane toxicity appears to be immune-mediated and antibodies with the potential for causing liver damage can be demonstrated in the serum of patients recovering from halothane hepatitis (see Chapter 52).[177]

In addition to these clear influences of cytochrome P450 in determining the magnitude and duration of drug response, as well as adverse effects, this group of enzymes is also important in chemical carcinogenesis and cancer chemotherapy.[137]

Synthetic, conjugation or phase II reactions

These are listed in Table 17.1. Glucuronic acid conjugation is probably the most widespread and versatile synthetic reaction in the liver: glucuronic acid can be transferred to many chemical groupings including hydroxyls (alcoholic, phenolic and hydroxyl amino), carboxyl, amino and sulphydryl.[313] In contrast, sulphate conjugation occurs only on hydroxyl groupings, usually phenolic. Methylation can occur on hydroxyl, sulphydryl and amino groupings. Conjugation with amino acids may also be important; aspirin, for example, is normally conjugated with glycine.

A few phase II reactions take place in the cytosol. Among the enzymes located therein, N-acetyl-transferase is responsible for the acetylation of isoniazid, hydralazine, sulphonamides and procainamide. The activity of this enzyme is genetically determined in an autosomal recessive manner and patients are either fast or slow acetylators.[254] The proportion of the genotypes varies among ethnic groups; about 95% of Eskimos are fast acetylators, whereas among caucasians the proportion is less than half.

Metabolism outside the liver

Finally, hydrolysis of some drugs takes place in the blood, where non-specific esterases exist in plasma. These are responsible for the hydrolysis of drugs including succinylcholine, procaine and procainamide. The activity of this plasma esterase (pseudocholinesterase) is genetically determined and the trimodal distribution of activity suggests an autosomal, autonomous inheritance.[254] Pseudocholinesterase is synthesized within the liver, which is, therefore, important in terminating the action of some neuromuscular blocking drugs.

Fate of metabolites formed within the liver

After the formation of polar metabolites within the liver they are excreted in either bile or urine.

Biliary excretion of drugs has been the subject of an extensive review by Smith.[312] Most of our understanding of the basic mechanisms involved stems from animal experiments. In man, ethical considerations have precluded the widespread use of radiolabelled drugs for metabolic studies so that reliance has been placed on bile collections made from patients with T-tube drainage after surgery on the biliary tree. Such data do not provide an accurate quantitative guide to normal biliary excretion of drugs because of the underlying disease, which may induce variable degrees of hepatic damage and obstruction to bile flow. Furthermore, the collection of bile may be incomplete and most studies have been based on single doses of drugs.

Normal bile contains bile salts, lecithin and cholesterol as stable ionic mixed micelles. For drugs to be excreted in this manner they must have a molecular structure which possesses affinities for both the aqueous and lipid domains of the micelle. This conclusion is based on the very slow elimination of non-polar compounds such as dieldrin which cannot be metabolized by the liver[312] and the fact that highly polar compounds, for example the aminoglycoside antibiotics such as gentamicin (which have large numbers of amino and hydroxyl groups), are not excreted in the bile. However, trapping of some drugs can occur in mixed micelles and may, in part, explain the secretion of compounds into the bile against an apparent concentration gradient.

Another important determinant of whether a drug is eliminated in bile is its molecular weight. There are significant species differences in the patterns and pathways of drug elimination. Biliary excretion tends to be relatively unimportant in man because the threshold for elimination by this route lies at a molecular weight of around 500, in contrast to rats, in which the threshold occurs at 325.[154] Thus, glucuronidation has two important effects: firstly,

since glucuronides are strong acids, such metabolites are highly water soluble (at physiological pH the carboxyl group of the conjugate is almost completely ionized and readily inserts into water by attracting dipoles in the vicinity); and secondly, addition of the glucuronide grouping increases the molecular weight of the drug by 176, which may facilitate excretion into the bile.

Among the drugs which undergo biliary excretion in man is fusidic acid, a tetracyclic turpene which is extensively metabolized by the liver so that less than 1% appears in the bile as unchanged drug.[125] Although the fusidic acid molecule already possesses polar groups in the form of hydroxyl groups in the 3 and 11 positions and a carboxyl at C-21, the oxidated metabolites (Figure 17.9) show enhanced polarity. These have comparable micellar properties to sodium taurocholate and are capable of solubilizing lecithins.[59] Rifampicin is also excreted in the bile after undergoing partial O-dealkylation in the liver; the metabolite, 25-desacetylrifampicin, is more polar and is largely excreted in the faeces via the bile.[331]

Other compounds which are eliminated in bile include digitoxin[57] and Sulindac.[329] However, a proportion of these drugs is reabsorbed from the small intestine, a process referred to as enterohepatic recirculation.

Methods of estimating the rate of drug elimination in man

With the exception of alcohol, phenytoin in high doses[282] and phenylbutazone,[76] the majority of drugs are removed in an exponential fashion, which implies that a fixed proportion of the dose is removed in unit time: this type of removal is said to obey first-order kinetics. It contrast with that of alcohol, of which a fixed amount is removed in unit time, about 10 mg/h,[130] and which thus exhibits zero-order kinetics. For the majority of drugs, if the logarithm of the blood concentration is plotted against time (by the method of least squares), a straight-line relationship will be obtained. From this, the time taken to fall from a concentration of 2X to X units can be calculated (Figure 17.5). In practice, the usual way of estimating the half-life ($t_{1/2}$) is from the slope of the regression, which is equal to:

$$\frac{-k_{el}}{2.3}$$

where k_{el} is the overall first-order elimination rate constant and has the dimensions of either min^{-1} or h^{-1}, and 2.3 represents log$_e$ 10. The half-life $t_{1/2}$ is then equal to

$$\frac{0.693}{k_{el}}$$

$t_{1/2}$ has been by far the most widely used estimate of drug elimination but is subject to numerous errors since it assumes that the β-phase of the concentration–time curve (see Figure 17.5) represents only drug elimination. This is frequently not the case since $t_{1/2}$ calculated in this way

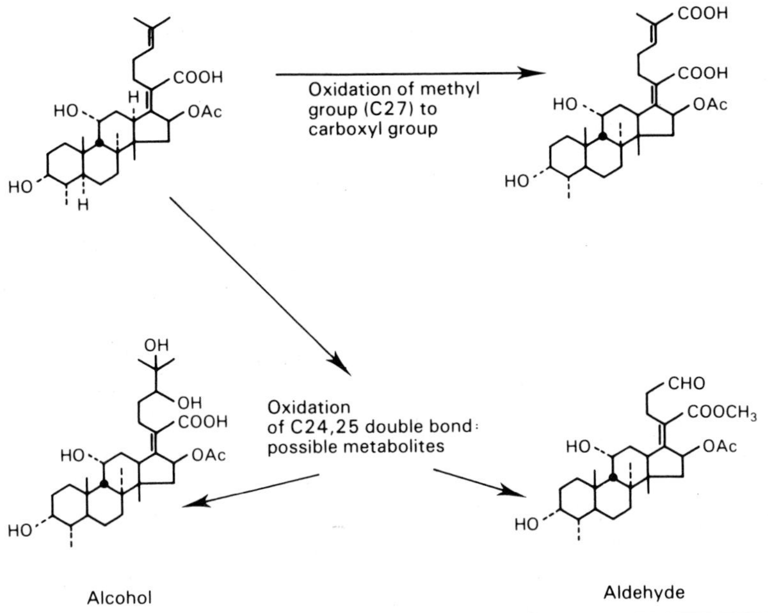

Figure 17.9 Metabolism of fusidic acid.

may lengthen on successive doses,[81] which suggests that distribution to the tissues (where access is slow) may contribute to the β-phase and the overall k_{el}. *Clearance (Cl)* represents a more precise estimate of the body's efficiency to remove a drug since it refers to the total volume of blood or plasma from which a drug is irreversibly removed in unit time. This is particularly important when trying to estimate changes produced by liver disease, where changes in protein binding, blood flow and capacity for metabolism may not necessarily be reflected in the $t_{1/2}$.

$$Cl = V_d \frac{0.693}{t_{1/2}}$$

Alternatively, clearance can be estimated from the ratio of the injected dose to the area under the concentration–time curve from the zero to time infinity.

Estimating P450 activity

There are comparatively few situations where it is possible to study or estimate drug metabolism directly in man: the indirect measurements described above will usually have to suffice. However, in recent years, the activity of hepatic cytochrome P450 has been estimated in samples of liver obtained either by needle biopsy[53,308] or by wedge biopsy at surgical operation.[76] In addition, 'banks' of human liver material have been established,[352] which has allowed a detailed study of metabolic reactions to be performed *in vitro*, e.g. on lignocaine.[152]

PHARMACODYNAMICS _____

Strictly speaking, pharmacodynamics refers to studies of the response to a given concentration of drug at the target organ or effector tissue, but since it is not usually possible to measure the concentration in the tissue itself, pharmacodynamics will be defined in this chapter as 'a study of the response to a given concentration of a drug in the blood'.

Surprisingly few well-conducted pharmacodynamic studies have been undertaken in either health or disease. Furthermore, relatively little is known about individual differences in response to the same concentration of drug in the blood.[112,314] There is, however, evidence for individual differences in receptor sensitivity and increasing information on alterations in response to drugs with ageing. Despite this paucity of information, pharmacodynamic factors should be remembered when considering the potential response of an individual to drugs. Changes relating to hepatic disease are discussed in the following section, by Howden *et al.*[163] and by Roberts *et al.*[287]

LIVER DISEASE AND THE RESPONSE TO DRUGS

Despite the obvious importance of the liver in the handling of drugs, there have been few well-controlled studies on the effects of hepatic disease. However, from the foregoing discussion it should be apparent that liver disease could affect the response to drugs in a number of ways: firstly, the bioavailability, half-life or clearance of a drug may change; secondly, the unbound fraction may increase, thereby altering the pharmacological effects; and finally, the response of the end organ may vary.

Much of the work done previously has assumed that patients with liver disease represent a homogeneous group. This is clearly erroneous and in the present review liver disease will be subdivided into (a) acute liver disease due to toxins, e.g. paracetamol overdosage and acute viral hepatitis (AVH), and (b) chronic liver disease, that is, chronic hepatitis and cirrhosis. The severity of chronic liver disease varies from one patient to another, and whether the illness is compensated or not is among the more important factors which will determine the response to drugs. Thus, patients who are jaundiced, hypoproteina-emic or show evidence of encephalopathy will tend to respond differently from others who are well compen-sated. Finally, most hospital patients and a high proportion of those in general practice will be receiving drug treat-ment. Inevitably, some of these therapies will have an effect on drug protein binding and on the activity of the microsomal enzyme oxidizing system. Concurrent or recent drug therapy may, therefore, mask the effects of liver disease[199] or possibly aggravate it.[270]

BIOAVAILABILITY AND LIVER DISEASE

Absorption

There are no reliable data on drug absorption in hepatic disease. It might, however, be anticipated that absorption of some drugs would be reduced in patients with obstruc-tive jaundice. Furthermore, interruption of the entero-hepatic circulation could alter the half-life of digitoxin and some antibiotics. The ion-exchange resin cholestyramine, which has been used to treat pruritus associated with biliary obstruction,[73] can also reduce the reabsorption of drugs which undergo an enterohepatic recirculation, thereby reducing their half-lives.[57]

Metabolism at the first pass

The best evidence for an alteration in the bioavailability produced by hepatic disease exists for propranolol,[303] lignocaine[139] and verapamil[92] and relates to subjects or dogs in whom a portacaval anastomosis has been created. Similar changes should be expected in patients with cirrhosis and oesophageal varices or other portosystemic anastomoses.

Numerous pharmacokinetic studies have been under-taken in patients with both acute and chronic liver disease in the past 10 years. Many of these are detailed in succeeding tables, but they have, in addition, been reviewed by George,[113] George and Shand,[115] Howden et al.[163] and Williams and Mamelok.[366]

Altered volumes of distribution

Extensive data are now available on the volumes of distribution of analgesics,[12,42,182,227] anticonvulsants,[35] anticoagulants,[369] minor tranquillizers,[45,180,309] cardio-active drugs including lignocaine,[108,324,337,338,367] proprano-lol[43] and barbiturates.[49,221] (See tables for individual drug data.) From these it would appear that there is no alteration in the volume of distribution of drugs in acute viral hepatitis. In contrast, the volume of distribution is usually increased in patients with cirrhosis, particularly in those whose serum albumin concentrations are depressed.

The most prominent changes are seen with lignocaine[337] and propranolol.[43]

Protein binding

Protein binding may be significantly reduced in the following circumstances, particularly where a drug is heavily bound to plasma proteins, for example phenylbuta-zone,[355] phenytoin,[5] diazepam[180] and tolbutamide.[335] There is usually a good correlation between the serum albumin concentration and the degree of protein binding, which will, therefore, be reduced in the presence of hypoalbuminaemia. In addition, an elevated serum biliru-bin in jaundiced patients may displace drugs from their binding to sites on plasma proteins. Finally, binding may be particularly lowered in patients who, in addition to being jaundiced and having a lowered serum albumin concentration, are uraemic—the hepatorenal syndrome[248] (see Chapter 51).

Elimination half-life

This is by far the most widely studied parameter in liver disease. Little change has been demonstrated in the half-lives of most drugs during acute viral hepatitis, except in patients who are severely ill. However, diazepam is an exception and shows a prolonged half-life in this situation,[180] as does pethidine.[227] In contrast, the half-lives of many drugs are prolonged in patients with cirrhosis or chronic active hepatitis, particularly those who are hypoalbumina-emic, jaundiced and show a diminished clearance of indocyanine green.[42,44] Data relating to individual drugs can be found in the tables.

Clearance

This parameter has been measured only comparatively recently in patients with liver disease but is probably the most sensitive index of overall dysfunction. Thus, the clearance of phenazone,[11] pethidine[227] and lignocaine[367] is depressed during attacks of acute viral hepatitis but increases during recovery. However, clearance tends to be disturbed to a greater degree in patients with chronic liver disease, the extent varying according to the serum albumin, bilirubin and indocyanine green clearance.[42,44] Data relating to individual drugs can be found in the tables.

INDIVIDUAL DRUGS

Anti-inflammatory analgesics

Paracetamol (acetaminophen). The half-life of paracet-amol is unchanged in the great majority of patients with liver disease, including Gilbert's syndrome[83,344] and those with cirrhosis,[108] in whom the half-life averages 2.8±0.3 h compared with the normal 2.0±0.4 h. Only in patients with severe liver damage due to paracetamol overdosage is there any clinically significant prolongation of the half-life[269] (see Table 17.2 and Forest et al.[107]).

Phenazone (antipyrine). Although not much used as an anti-inflammatory analgesic, phenazone has been widely studied as a 'model drug' because of its distribution throughout the body water, total dependence on liver metabolism for elimination and uniformly low degree of protein binding. Data relating to studies published prior to 1985 are detailed in Table 17.2. Since then Birnie et al.[32] have published data for 104 patients with cirrhosis in whom the half-life was 21.7±1.6 h compared to 11.8±11.6 h in 37 controls (P<0.01).

Phenylbutazone. This powerful non-steroidal anti-inflammatory drug is now seldom used because of its high incidence of bone marrow toxicity. The protein binding of phenylbutazone is diminished in patients with hepatic disease.[355] This may, in part, account for the failure of Brodie et al.[52] and Hvidberg et al.[165] to demonstrate prolongation of its half-life in patients with cirrhosis. A prolonged half-life was demonstrated by Levi et al.[199] but only in those patients who were not receiving drugs known to induce microsomal enzyme oxidation (see Table 17.2).

Naproxen. The mean elimination half-life of this non-steroidal anti-inflammatory drug was 14.1 h in a group of controls but 20.4 h in a group of patients with a variety of liver disorders.[58]

Salicylamide. Salicylamide shows a major increase in its concentration–time curve following oral administration to patients with cirrhosis.[240] Presumably this reflects diminished glucuronidation in liver disease. However, sulphation of this drug occurs in the wall of the intestine and is dose dependent. Thus, the extent of the increased bioavailability in patients with liver disease should also exhibit dose dependency.

Opioid analgesics and antagonists

Morphine. Although there is some evidence for an increased sensitivity to morphine in patients with cirrhosis,[196] there are few data on its pharmacokinetics in liver disease. Plasma protein binding, volume of distribution, elimination half-life and clearance were unaltered in a small group of patients with stable cirrhosis,[256] but protein binding was significantly depressed in hepatic failure[248] (see Table 17.3).

Naloxone. Naloxone is a specific competitive antagonist of morphine of two of its receptors. It undergoes significant presystemic metabolism in the gut wall and liver[114] and has a high systemic clearance.[105] It is to be anticipated that the clearance will be diminished and the half-life substantially prolonged in patients with cirrhosis.

Pentazocine. Pentazocine also exhibits extensive first-pass metabolism.[113] There is a reduction in systemic clearance by approximately 46% in cirrhotic patients[240, 266] and the half-life is about doubled. However, the bioavailability after oral administration is increased some 2½-fold.[240, 266]

Pethidine (meperidine). Extensive pharmacokinetic studies have been undertaken on pethidine in patients with liver disease.[182,227,266,267] Some of these data are summarized in Table 17.3. Pethidine is best avoided in patients with hepatic disease because, after parenteral injection, there is a highly significant reduction in its systemic clearance and a prolongation of the half-life.[266, 267] Furthermore, there is an increase in its bioavailability after oral administration from around 50% to in excess of 80%.[227, 267]

Propoxyphene. Propoxyphene, like pentazocine and pethidine, undergoes extensive first-pass metabolism.[373] Thus, it would be expected to show major changes in its pharmacokinetics in patients with cirrhosis.

Anticonvulsants

Chlormethiazole. Chlormethiazole has been used not only as a hypnotic but also as an anticonvulsant/sedative in patients with delirium tremens. Its pharmacokinetics have been studied by Moore et al.[237] and Pentikainen et al.[258] It exhibits extensive first-pass metabolism with a high systemic clearance rate. Thus, in patients with liver disease, there is a significant diminution in its rate of clearance after parenteral injection from 18.1±1.2 ml kg^{-1} min^{-1} to 12.8±1.7. But, after oral administration, there is a massive (10-fold) increase in bioavailability in cirrhotics. Thus, despite its value in the management of delirium tremens, the drug must be used with caution in patients with severe liver disease.[258]

Phenobarbitone (see Table 17.4). Phenobarbitone is only partially metabolized in the liver, and renal excretion can therefore compensate to some degree for alterations in hepatic metabolism. Nevertheless, the half-life is prolonged in patients with cirrhosis and to a lesser degree in patients with acute viral hepatitis.[9]

Phenytoin (see Table 17.4). The unbound fraction is increased in patients with hepatic disease.[5,35,162,248] Since the pharmacological and therapeutic effects relate to the free concentration, patients with hepatic disease tend to have their epilepsy controlled at lower total plasma phenytoin concentrations than usual. Furthermore, intoxication is particularly likely to occur in patients with liver disease.[174,195] There are, however, few data on the half-life of phenytoin in liver disease.

Table 17.2 Drug class: anti-inflammatory analgesics.

Type of patient	No.	Dose	Route	Protein binding (%)	V_d (l/kg)	$t_{1/2}$ (h)	Cl (ml min^{-1}kg^{-1})	Reference
Paracetamol (acetaminophen)								
Paracetamol overdosage	17	N.K.	o	—	—	7.6 ± 0.8	—	Prescott et al.[269]
Healthy normals	17	—	—	—	—	2.0 ± 0.4	—	
Cirrhotics (15) + 2 others	17	1.5 g	o	—	—	2.9 ± 0.3	—	Forrest et al.[108]
Phenazone (antipyrine)								
Controls	20	1 g	i.v.	—	—	11.9 (5.3–13.9)	—	Brodie et al.[52]
Cirrhotics	9	1 g	i.v	—	—	9.0 (3.3–11.9)	—	
Controls	6	1.2 g	o	—	33.3 ± 2.8	—	38.4 ± 4.4	Branch et al.[42]
Chronic liver disease								
Albumin > 3 g/100 ml	5	1.2 g	o	—	33.6 ± 2.4	—	27.1 ± 2.1	
Albumin < 3 g/100 ml	9	1.2 g	o	—	41.3 ± 3.2	—	10.3 ± 1.6	
Chronic active hepatitis	1	18 mg/kg	o	—	—	137	—	Adjepon-Yamoah et al.[4]
Controls	9	15 mg/kg	i.v.	—	36.9 ± 9.3	7.9 ± 1.7	58.6 ± 16.6	Andreasen et al.[12]
Cirrhotics	11	15 mg/kg	i.v.	—	38.5 ± 7.3	31.8 ± 19.5	18.5 ± 11.8	
Halothane hepatitis	1							
Biliary obstruction	1							
Cirrhotics	5	15 mg/kg	i.v.	—	—	—	9.6 ± 1.9	Andreasen and Ranek[11]
Cirrhotics with encephalopathy	13	15 mg/kg	i.v.	—	—	—	4.6 ± 1.4	
AVH	1	15 mg/kg	i.v.	—	—	—	5.9	
5/12 later							54.5	
Cirrhotics (17) + 2 others	19	18 mg/kg	o	—	—	30.3 ± 6.8	—	Forrest et al.[108]
Phenylbutazone								
Controls	10	800 mg	o	—	—	72.2 (44–114)	—	Brodie et al.[52]
Cirrhotics	11	800 mg	o	—	—	50.6 (31.7–122)	—	
Normals	36	400–600 mg	o	—	—	78.1 ± 14.6	—	Levi et al.[191]
Liver disease (no inducing drugs)	34	400–600 mg	o	—	—	100 ± 29.2	—	
Liver disease (on inducing drugs)	61	400–600 mg	o	—	—	54.3 ± 18.4	—	
Normals (on inducing drugs)	19	400–600 mg	o	—	—	57.2 ± 17.4	—	
Controls	8	—	—	94 ± 1.1	—	—	—	Wallace and Brodie[355]
Chronic hepatic disease	6	—	—	90 ± 2.0	—	—	—	
Salicylic acid								
Controls	6	1.3 g	i.v.	—	—	6.1 (4.7–9.0)	—	Brodie et al.[52]
Cirrhotics	8	1.3 g	i.v.	—	—	6.6 (3.3–10.3)	—	

V_d = volume of distribution; $t_{1/2}$ = half-life in blood or plasma; Cl = clearance; i.v. = intravenous; o = oral; AVH = acute viral hepatitis; N.K. = not known.

Table 17.3 Drug class: opioid analgesics.

Type of patient	No.	Dose	Route	Protein binding (%)	V_d (l/kg)	$t_{1/2}$ (h)	Cl (ml min^{-1}kg^{-1})	Reference
Morphine								
Normals	—	—	—	35.1	—	—	—	Olsen *et al.*[248]
Hepatic failure	2	—	—	25.0 (21.2–28.8)	—	—	—	
Pethidine								
Normals	8	0.8 mg/kg	i.v.	64.3 ± 13.5	4.17 ± 1.33	3.21 ± 0.80	1316 ± 383	Klotz *et al.*[182]
Cirrhotics	10	0.8 mg/kg	i.v.	64.9 ± 5.8	5.76 ± 2.55	7.04 ± 0.92	664 ± 293	
Normals	15	—	—	58.3 ± 8.2	5.94 ± 2.65	3.37 ± 0.82	1261 ± 527	McHorse *et al.*[227]
AVH	14	—	—	56.0 ± 11.8	5.56 ± 1.8	6.99 ± 2.74	649 ± 278	
In recovery	(5)	—	—	—	—	3.25 ± 0.8	—	

V_d = volume of distribution; $t_{1/2}$ = half-life in blood or plasma; Cl = clearance; i.v. = intravenous; AVH = acute viral hepatitis.

Table 17.4 Drug class: anticonvulsants.

Type of patient	No.	Dose	Route	Protein binding (%)	V_d (l/kg)	$t_{1/2}$ (h)	Cl (ml min^{-1}kg^{-1})	Reference
Phenobarbitone								
Normals	8		—	—	—	86 ± 3	—	
Cirrhotics	9	0.85–2.55 mg/kg	—	—	—	130 ± 15		Alvin *et al.*[9]
AVH	8		—	—	—	104 (60–177)		
Phenytoin								
Normals	—	—	—	10.6 ± 1.3 (free)	—	—	—	Hooper *et al.*[164]
Hepatic disease	—	—	—	15.9 ± 6.0 (free)	—	—	—	
Normals	—	—	—	8.3 ± 0.8 (free)	—	—	—	Affrime and Reidenberg[5]
Cirrhotics	8	—	—	11.7 ± 6.2 (free)	—	—	—	
AVH								
Acute	5	250 mg	i.v.	12.6 (free)	0.68	13.2	2.55	Blaschke *et al.*[35]
Recovery	—	—	—	9.9 (free)	0.63	13.5	2.22	
Hepatic failure	2	—	—	76.3 (63–89.6)	—	—	—	Olsen *et al.*[248]
Hepatorenal syndrome	3	—	—	77.5 ± 2.2	—	—	—	

V_d = volume of distribution; $t_{1/2}$ = half-life in blood or plasma; Cl = clearance; i.v. = intravenous; AVH = acute viral hepatitis.

Anticoagulants (see Chapter 8)

The half-life of dicoumarol is prolonged in patients with cirrhosis[52] and an accentuation of its hypoprothrombinaemic effects has been seen following exposure to carbon tetrachloride,[18,209] a hepatotoxin which is known to impair oxidative enzymes in liver microsomes by decreasing the amount of cytochrome P450.[293] However, the half-life of phenprocoumon is unchanged in cirrhotics[150] and the pharmacokinetics of warfarin are unchanged in patients with acute viral hepatitis[369] (see Table 17.5).

Anti-asthma drugs

Theophylline. The half-life of theophylline is substantially prolonged in patients with cirrhosis[213,263,272,322] (see Table 17.6).

Corticosteroids (Table 17.6). The fate of corticosteroids in liver disease has been reviewed by Uribe and Go[345] and Uribe *et al.*[346] In general, it would appear that the changes (if any) are small. Thus the half-life of prednisolone is slightly prolonged in patients with chronic liver disease[268] but total serum concentrations are depressed following oral administration of prednisone owing, presumably, to decreased 11β-hydroxy-dehydrogenase activity. In addition, Davis *et al.*[77] noted a marked interindividual variation in plasma prednisolone levels when prednisone was given to patients with chronic active hepatitis. The frequency of side-effects due to prednisone is doubled when the serum albumin concentrations are less than 25 g/l.

We conclude that prednisolone is the corticosteroid of choice in patients with liver disease. Its activity is increased in patients with hepatic disease when serum protein concentrations are lowered.

Table 17.5 Drug class: anticoagulants.

Type of patient	No.	Dose	Route	Protein binding (%)	V_d (l/kg)	$t_{1/2}$ (h)	Cl (ml min^{-1}kg^{-1})	Reference
Dicoumarol								
Controls	19	0.3 g	i.v.	—	—	30.7 (7.2–100)	—	Brodie et al.[52]
Cirrhotics	6	0.3 g	i.v.	—	—	50.6 (15.5–100)	—	
Phenprocoumon								
Cirrhotics	3	20 mg	i.v.	—	—	138.7 (103–160)	—	Heni et al.[147]
	2	10 mg	i.v.	—	—	132 (128–136)	—	
Normals						150		
Warfarin								
AVH	5	15 mg	o	—	0.19 ± 0.04	23 ± 5	6.1 ± 0.9	Williams et al.[369]
Acute recovery	—	15 mg	o	—	0.21 ± 0.02	25 ± 3	6.1 ± 0.7	

V_d = volume of distribution; $t_{1/2}$ = half-life in blood or plasma; Cl = clearance; i.v. = intravenous; o = oral; AVH = acute viral hepatitis.

Table 17.6 Drug class: anti-asthma compounds.

Type of patient	No.	Dose	Route	Protein binding (%)	V_d (l/kg)	$t_{1/2}$ (h)	Cl (ml min^{-1}kg^{-1})	Reference
Theophylline								
Normals	5	2.8 mg/kg	i.v.			9.19 ± 1.5		Piafsky et al.[264]
Cirrhotics	4	2.8 mg/kg	i.v.	No change		30.0 ± 17.8		
Normals	—	5.6 mg/kg	i.v.		—	6.68 (2.77–12.4)		Rangno et al.[272]
Cirrhotics	—	5.6 mg/kg	—			30.8 (11.5–55.8)		
Controls	—	193 mg			0.41	7.70	0.63	Staib et al.[322]
Cirrhotics (compensated)	—	193 mg	—		0.45	11.90	0.65	
Cirrhotics (uncompensated)	—	193 mg	—		0.59	65.40	0.12	
AVH	—	193 mg	—		0.58	19.20	0.35	
Cholestasis	—	193 mg	—		0.58	14.40	0.65	
Prednisolone								
Controls	3	—	—	—		2.92 (2.5–3.25)		Powell and Axelsen[269]
Chronic liver disease	3	—	—	—		3.69 (3.25–4.16)		
Normals	8	—	—	53.5 ± 5.2	—	—		
Active chronic hepatitis	9	—	—	46.6 ± 5.8	—	—		
Inactive chronic hepatitis	7	—	—	54.3 ± 4.1	—	—		
AVH	6	—	—	50.4 ± 7.0	—	—		

V_d = volume of distribution; $t_{1/2}$ = half-life in blood of plasma; Cl = clearance; i.v. = intravenous; AVH = acute viral hepatitis.

Minor tranquillizers

Chlordiazepoxide. Two studies of chlordiazepoxide pharmacokinetics have been undertaken in patients with cirrhosis. Although there are substantial differences in the two studies, both showed reduced clearance values and substantial prolongation of the elimination half-life.[288,300] The same is true for patients with alcoholic hepatitis in whom a 45% reduction in clearance and a 143% increase in elimination half-lives were found after an oral dose of 25 mg.[238]

Diazepam. Unwanted CNS effects of diazepam are considerably more frequent in patients with reduced serum albumin concentrations.[135] In patients with normal serum albumin concentrations, 2.9% have unwanted CNS depression, compared with 9.3% in those with severe hypoalbuminaemia (<30 g/l). This finding accords with reduced binding of diazepam reported by Klotz *et al.*[180] and Thiessen *et al.*[335] Furthermore, only 17.9±5.8 mg of intravenous diazepam was required as a premedication for endoscopy in patients with liver disease, compared with 27±12.1 mg in normals,[45] and individual doses showed a strong correlation with the serum albumin concentration. Details of some of the pharmacokinetic alterations seen for diazepam in liver disease are given in Table 17.7 and in reference 10. Like many other benzodiazepines, diazepam is converted to active metabolites and one of these, desmethyldiazepam, also shows a prolongation of its half-life in patients with cirrhosis or fibrosis of the liver.[179] By contrast, a further metabolite, oxazepam, shows little alteration in its metabolism in this situation.[309]

Diazepam can produce substantial reductions in arterial blood gas tensions during upper gastrointestinal endoscopy[361] and it can be used for that purpose in patients with hepatic disease provided dosage adjustments are made. Recent studies suggest that patients most at risk are those with pre-existing portosystemic encephalopathy, who can be identified by their abnormal Reitan trailmaking tests[379] (performed before drug treatment).[225]

Although patients with cirrhosis show a significant prolongation in diazepam half-life and reduction in clearance, there is no significant alteration to these measurements in patients with cholestasis.[151]

Lorazepam. The pharmacokinetics of lorazepam have been studied in cirrhotic patients by Kraus *et al.*[188] who showed a prolongation of the half-life from 21.7±7.6 h to 41.2±24.5 h, and an increased distribution volume (which reflected diminished binding from 93.2±1.8% to 88.6±2.5%). However, there was no change in the disposition of this drug in patients with acute viral hepatitis.

Midazolam. This short-acting benzodiazepine is being used increasingly for sedation during gastrointestinal endoscopy and other procedures. Its half-life in controls is 1.6 h but is extended to 4.8 h in patients with cirrhosis. Clearance is reduced from 10.4 to 5.4 ml min^{-1} kg^{-1} in patients with cirrhosis.[211]

Oxazepam. Oxazepam would appear to be the preferred benzodiazepine for use in patients with liver disease since there are only minor alterations in its pharmacokinetics[309] (see Table 17.7).

Major tranquillizers

Few data are available on phenothiazines and butyrophenones in hepatic disease. There is, however, no evidence for prolongation of the chlorpromazine half-life in patients with cirrhosis[222] (see Table 17.8).

Oral hypoglycaemic agents

Data are confined to tolbutamide (see Table 17.9) and they are conflicting. Ueda *et al.*[343] have claimed that the half-life of tolbutamide was prolonged in five of ten cirrhotic patients whom they studied. These findings were challenged by Nelson[242] because of a failure to take account of the normal range of variability. However, it seems likely that the pharmacological effect may be slightly increased owing to a reduction in protein binding.[343]

In patients with acute viral hepatitis there was a 48% prolongation of elimination half-life and a 31% reduction in clearance.[368] Among the various oral hypoglycaemic agents, tolbutamide seems particularly prone to give rise to problems in patients with liver disease.[301]

Cardioactive drugs

Digitoxin. There are few data on the handling of digitoxin in liver disease. Nevertheless, Storstein *et al.*[327] found no increased incidence of toxicity in patients with reduced liver function and the half-life was slightly reduced to 4.4 days in patients with chronic active hepatitis.[326]

Digoxin. There is no evidence of an alteration in half-life of this drug.[215,381] It is possible that its distribution volume may be altered, but there are no data on this point.

Encainide. This anti-arrhythmic agent has a high hepatic extraction and is extensively metabolized by oxidation. In patients with cirrhosis its clearance is much reduced.[26]

Lignocaine. Data showing that the handling of this drug is abnormal in patients with acute viral hepatitis and markedly altered in those with chronic hepatic disease are extensive (see Table 17.10). This drug must therefore be used with extreme caution in patients with liver disease.

Table 17.7 Drug class: tranquillizers (benzodiazepines).

Type of patient	No.	Dose	Route	Protein binding (%)	V_d (l/kg)	$t_{1/2}$ (h)	Cl (ml min^{-1}kg^{-1})	Reference
Diazepam								
Normals	5	0.1 mg/kg	i.v.	97.8 ± 1.0	1.13 ± 0.28	46.6 ± 14.2	44.8 ± 9.1	Klotz *et al.*[180]
Cirrhotics	9	0.1 mg/kg	i.v.	95.3 ± 1.8	1.74 ± 0.21	105.6 ± 15.2	24.8 ± 12.7	
AVH	8	10 mg	o	—	—	74.5 ± 27.5	—	
CAH	4	10 mg	o	—	—	59.7 ± 23.0	—	
Controls	5	27 ± 5.4 mg	i.v.	—	0.98 ± 0.41	43 ± 7.2	15.1 ± 6.9	Branch *et al.*[45]
Chronic liver disease								
No ascites	10	17.9 ± 1.5 mg	i.v.	—	0.69 ± 0.44	48.7 ± 38.3	10.6 ± 6.2	
With ascites	7	17.9 ± 1.5 mg	i.v.	—	0.59 ± 0.29	77.4 ± 11.4	6.0 ± 3.9	
Normals	21	—	—	98.5 ± 0.4	—	—	—	Thiessen *et al.*[335]
Alcoholics	14	—	—	97.8 ± 1.2	—	—	—	
Controls	—	0.1 mg/kg	—	—	—	53.1	15.1	Hepner[151]
Mixed chronic liver disease	—	0.1 mg/kg	—	—	—	116.0	9.8	—
Cholestasis	—	0.1 mg/kg	—	—	—	59.0	16.9	—
Oxazepam								
Young normals	8	45 mg[a]	o	86.7 ± 4.7	52.5 ± 15.6	5.1 ± 1.4	112.5 ± 32.8	Schull *et al.*[309]
AVH	7	45 mg	o	86.0 ± 3.8	62.0 ± 22.0	5.3 ± 0.8	137.4 ± 55.6	
Middle-aged normals	8	45 mg[a]	o	89.6 ± 4.5	70.6 ± 13.6	5.6 ± 0.8	136.0 ± 49.5	
Cirrhotics	6	45 mg	o	87.6 ± 3.5	76.5 ± 29.9	5.8 ± 1.2	155.5 ± 52.7	

[a]Except two who received 15 mg orally.
V_d = volume of distribution; $t_{1/2}$ = half-life in blood or plasma; Cl = clearance; i.v. = intravenous; o = oral; AVH = acute viral hepatitis; CAH = chronic active hepatitis.

Table 17.8 Drug class: tranquillizers (phenothiazines).

Type of patient	No.	Dose	Route	Protein binding (%)	V_d (l/kg)	$t_{1/2}$ (h)	k_{el}/h
Chlorpromazine							
Normals	13	25 mg	i.v.	—	—	31	0.053
Cirrhotics	24						
On inducing drugs	7	25 mg	i.v.	—	—	7	0.078
No drugs	14			—	—	14	0.078

V_d = volume of distribution; $t_{1/2}$ = half-life in blood or plasma; k_{el}/h = overall first-order elimination rate constant (see text); i.v. = intravenous.
Data from Maxwell *et al.*[222]

Lorcainide. Lorcainide is another class I anti-arrhythmic agent which shows blood flow-dependent kinetics and extensive first-pass metabolism.[113] These kinetics are highly abnormal in patients with cirrhosis of the liver.[181]

Procainamide. There is a marked increase in elimination half-life in patients with cirrhosis.[87]

Tocainide. Although this drug has a low hepatic extraction, its half-life is more than doubled in patients with cirrhosis owing partly to an increase in its distribution volume.[249]

β-Adrenoceptor antagonists. β-Adrenoceptor antagonists can be classified into three main groups according to their solubility in lipid. Some, e.g. alprenolol, labetalol,

metroprolol, oxprenolol and propranolol are soluble in lipid. They undergo extensive first-pass metabolism, have short half-lives and are cleared from the circulation at a rate which depends upon hepatic blood flow.[113,115] Thus, the pharmacokinetics of propranolol and other lipid-soluble β-adrenoceptor antagonists are highly abnormal in liver disease. Bioavailability is increased,[161,277,303,374] the clearance is reduced and the half-life is prolonged.[43] The latter abnormality is due, in part, to diminished protein binding[101] and reduced hepatic blood flow (there is a close correlation between the clearance of propranolol and that of indocyanine green[43]) plus shunting through portosystemic anastomoses. Finally, the intrinsic clearance rate by metabolism is important[304,305,364] and is reduced by cirrhosis. The pharmacological effects, which depend upon the free concentration in plasma,[226] may be increased

Table 17.9 Drug class: oral hypoglycaemics.

Type of patient	No.	Dose	Route	Protein binding (%)	V_d (l/kg)	$t_{1/2}$ (h)	Cl (ml min^{-1}kg^{-1})	Reference
Tolbutamide								
Normals	7	20 mg/kg	i.v.	—	—	4.4 ± 0.7	—	Ueda et al.[343]
Cirrhotics	10	20 mg/kg	i.v.	—	—	Normal in 5; 9.3 in 5 (7.8 ± 11.2)	—	
Unspecified liver disease	10	0.5 g	o	—	—	6.0 (3.2–10.0)	—	Nelson[242]
Normals	21	50 µg/ml	—	97.9 ± 0.3	—	—	—	Thiessen et al.[335]
		300 µg/ml	—	95.2 ± 0.6	—	—	—	
Alcoholics	14	50 µg/ml	—	96.3 ± 2.6	—	—	—	
		300 µg/ml	—	88.1 ± 8.5	—	—	—	

V_d = volume of distribution; $t_{1/2}$ = half-life in blood or plasma; Cl = clearance; i.v. = intravenous; o = oral.

Table 17.10 Drug class: cardioactive drugs.

Type of patient	No.	Dose	Route	Protein binding (%)	V_d (l/kg)	$t_{1/2}$ (h)	Cl (ml min^{-1}kg^{-1})	Reference
Digoxin								
Cirrhotics	3	1 mg	i.v.	—	—	33.6 ± 38.4 (normal 30–40)	—	Marcus and Kapadia[215]
AVH	15	0.375–0.75 mg	i.v.	—	—	—	—	Zilly et al.[381]
Lignocaine								
Normals	10	50 mg	i.v.	—	1.70 ± 0.21	1.80 ± 0.17	701 ± 41	Thomson et al.[338]
Liver disease (alcoholic)	8	50 mg	—	—	2.22 ± 0.94	5.72 ± 3.90	368 ± 180	
Normals	10	50 mg	—	—	1.32	1.8	10.0	Thomson et al.[337]
Liver disease (alcoholic)	8	50 mg	—	—	2.31	4.9	6.0	
Normals	4	400 mg	o	—	—	1.40 ± 0.26	—	Adjepon-Yamoah et al.[4]
CAH	1	400 mg	—	—	—	19.1	—	
AVH	6	1 mg/kg	i.v.	56 ± 8 (free)	3.1 ± 1.8	2.67 (1.1–7.2)	13.0 ± 3.9/kg	Williams et al.[367]
AVH in recovery	—	—	—	49 ± 12 (free)	2.0 ± 0.5	1.5 (1.2–3.5)	20.0 ± 3.9/kg	
Cirrhotics 16, CAH 3, Others 2	21	400 mg	o	—	—	6.6 ± 1.1	—	Forrest et al.[108]
Propranolol (+) isomer					V_d (l)			
Normals	6	40 mg	i.v.	—	221.5 (121–286)	2.9 (2.1–3.8)	919.7 (512–1326)	Branch et al.[43]
Cirrhotics 12, CAH 6, Others 2	20	40 mg	i.v.	—	460.1 (183–787)	15.6 (2.8–35.4)	463.2 (137–1086)	
Quinidine								
Normals	7	5 µ/ml		14.1 ± 4.6 (free)	—	—	—	Affrime and Reidenberg[5]
Alcoholics	10			51.5 ± 16.0 (free)	—	—	—	

V_d = volume of distribution; $t_{1/2}$ = half-life in blood or plasma; Cl = clearance; i.v. = intravenous; o = oral; AVH = acute viral hepatitis; CAH = chronic active hepatitis.

further because of hypoalbuminaemia and jaundice. Thus, despite recent claims[197] that propranolol may be of use in preventing bleeding from oesophageal varices in patients who have established cirrhosis, it will have increased pharmacological effects[16] and may precipitate encephalopathy.[276,334]

By contrast, the water-soluble β-adrenoceptor antagonists, which include atenolol, nadolol and sotalol, are unlikely to display any change in their half-lives in patients with liver disease. There are insufficient data available on the intermediate group of compounds, for example acebutolol, pindolol and timolol, to allow firm conclusions to be drawn concerning their likely fate in patients with liver disease. However, it is unlikely that major changes in metabolism and excretion will occur.

Quinidine. The protein binding of quinidine is considerably reduced in patients with alcoholic liver disease and this necessitates reduction in the dosage.[5]

Verapamil. Verapamil is another agent with antiarrhythmic and anti-anginal properties which exhibits first-pass metabolism of a stereo-selective nature. Normally, the bioavailability is low (10–22%)[297] but is greatly increased in patients with cirrhosis.[286,317,376] There is some controversy about the half-life but after single doses this is thought to be between 2 and 5 hours. In patients with cirrhosis there is a considerable prolongation to an average of 13.6 hours.[286,317]

The dihydropyridines. The pharmacokinetics of both nicardipine and nifedipine are altered markedly in liver disease.[84,178]

Frusemide. The pharmacokinetics of frusemide in liver disease have been studied by Allgulander *et al.*[8] and by Sawnhey *et al.*[295] This drug is normally extensively bound to proteins, but in hepatic cirrhosis with hypoalbuminaemia the free concentration in plasma rises (thus increasing its pharmacological effect).

Clofibrate. This agent is now rarely used except in the treatment of certain hyperlipidaemias because of its potential for causing carcinoma of the gastrointestinal tract.[360] There is no significant change in its pharmacokinetics in hepatic disease.[138]

Barbiturates

The effects of liver disease on the pharmacokinetics of individual barbiturate drugs are summarized in Tables 17.4 and 17.11 and in the review by Williams and Mamelok.[367] The half-life of amylobarbitone is prolonged and its clearance diminished, particularly in patients with reduced serum albumin concentrations;[221] similar findings have been reported for hexobarbitone in acute viral hepatitis.[49] Similar findings have been reported for hexobarbitone in acute viral hepatitis[49] and cirrhotics have a

considerable prolongation of elimination half-life,[380] but the kinetics of this drug are not significantly altered in patients with cholestasis.[283] However, the removal of pentobarbitone appears to be 'more rapid' in patients with cirrhosis.[302] The anaesthetic induction agent, thiopentone, has a prolonged duration of action in patients with hepatic disease (mean 488.5 seconds compared with 151.5 seconds) after a 4 mg/kg i.v.[308] Thus, the dose required to produce anaesthesia for 60 minutes was 0.54 g in patients with severe liver damage compared with 1.04 g in normal subjects.[86] This is probably due to diminished protein binding in patients with hepatic disease.[117]

Neuromuscular blocking drugs

The requirements for (+)-tubocurarine are also reduced in patients with hepatic disease,[86] owing to diminished hydrolysis.[106,224,353] Similarly, the rate of procaine hydrolysis is reduced from 0.66 ± 0.14 minutes to 2.3 ± 0.9 minutes.[278]

Data relating to these and a few other drugs, published mainly in abstract form, are summarized by Closson.[62]

Anti-ulcer drugs

Cimetidine. The drug is eliminated largely unchanged in the urine. In cirrhosis, the non-renal clearance is reduced and its elimination half-life is increased. Plasma clearance is dramatically reduced when renal function is also impaired.[318]

Ranitidine. The kinetics of ranitidine do not seem to be significantly altered in patients with cirrhosis.[311]

Omeprazole. This is an irreversible inhibitor of the gastric H^+/K^+-ATPase (or 'proton pump'). In cirrhosis, the clearance of omeprazole is greatly reduced and the half-life is increased.[228]

Antibiotics

Penicillins (see Table 17.12). Among the penicillins, azlocillin, furazocillin, mezlocillin and piperacillin (the acyluredopenicillins) exhibit dose dependent pharmacokinetics, the half-life increasing the large doses.[25] The proportion of these penicillins excreted in urine correlates directly with dosage. Significant metabolism of some penicillins occurs in the liver,[64,131,277] with 10–20% of a dose being excreted as penicilloic acid or other derivatives. Metabolites of piperacillin have not been detected.[78] Rapid urinary excretion of unmetabolized penicillins permits normal therapeutic dosage in patients with liver disease whose renal function is good.[357] Most penicillins are secreted in small amounts in bile as active drug. In normals, 29.9% of mezlocillin is excreted in the bile compared to only 4.4% in patients with severe liver

Table 17.11 Drug class: barbiturates.

Type of patient	No.	Dose	Route	Protein binding (%)	V_d (l)	$t_{1/2}$ (h)	Cl (ml min^{-1}kg^{-1})	Reference
Amylobarbitone								
Normals	10	3.23 mg/kg	i.v.	60.7 ± 5.3	91.3 ± 32.3	21.1 ± 3.9	92.0 ± 22.1	Mawer *et al.*[221]
Mixed liver disease								
Normal albumin	5	3.23 mg/kg	i.v.	60.5 ± 2.4	114 ± 43.4	17.7 ± 4.1	118.9 ± 28.0	
Low albumin	5	3.23 mg/kg	i.v.	31.0 ± 13.8	79.5 ± 40.0	39.4 ± 14.8	41.0 ± 11.4	
Hexobarbitone								
Normals	14	2.97–	i.v.	—	1.1 ± 0.12 kg	4.35 ± 1.15	3.57 ± 0.83 kg	Breimer *et al.*[49]
AVH	13	7.32 mg/kg	—	—	1.1 ± 0.40 kg	8.17 ± 3.09	1.94 ± 0.85 kg	
Pentobarbitone								
Controls	35	—	—	—	—	—	—	Sessions *et al.*[302]
Liver disease (17 cirrhotics)	21	—	—	—	—	'More rapid'	—	
Thiopentone								
Normals	10	—	—	72 (28 ± 0.9% free)	—	—	—	Ghoneim and Pandya[117]
Cirrhotics	10	—	—	47 (53 ± 2.1% free)	—	—	—	

V_d = volume of distribution; $t_{1/2}$ = half-life in blood or plasma; Cl = clearance; i.v. = intravenous; AVH = acute viral hepatitis.

impairment.[140] Approximately 20% of piperacillin is excreted by the biliary route,[78] which explains the findings that in end-stage renal failure the half-life did not exceed 6 hours.[78] When liver dysfunction is associated with renal failure, the half-life of piperacillin is extended to 11 hours. Because a lower percentage of most penicillins is excreted into bile, their half-lives are longer in anuric patients, but here again concurrent liver dysfunction affects the half-life. Thus, Hoffman, Cestero and Bullock[159] found that in five oliguric patients with severe hepatic dysfunction the mean half-life of carbenicillin was 23.2±2.9 h, some 7.5 h longer than in those with oliguric renal failure alone.

Clearly care must be taken to prevent toxicity from penicillins occurring in patients with hepatorenal failure. Two penicillins should be avoided in patients with liver disease: talampicillin, which is hydrolysed in part by the liver to ampicillin and an ester moiety.[183] and nafcillin, which is largely excreted via the bile.[246]

Cephalosporins and cephamycins (see Table 17.12). While hepatic metabolism of most cephalosporins is slight, 40% of cefotaxime undergoes desacetylation to a microbiologically active metabolite.[299] Thirty to forty per cent of cephalothin, 40% of cephapirin and 20% of cephacetrile also undergo desacetylation.[370] Great differences are noted in the biliary concentrations of different cephalosporins.[216] The major route of elimination of most cephalosporins is the kidney but less than 30% of ceftriaxone[220] and cefoperazone[63] are excreted unchanged by this route. Cochet *et al.*[63] found that the half-life of cefoperazone was increased 3-fold in patients with liver disease, although increased renal excretion was noted in

these individuals. These two cephalosporins should be used with caution in patients with hepatic disease.

Table 17.12 shows those cephalosporins which are metabolized extensively, those in which significant amounts are excreted in bile and representative examples of oral and parenteral drugs.

Other β-lactams. Two-thirds of aztreonam (a monobactam) is excreted unchanged in urine and a further 7% as an inactive metabolite. Approximately 12% is excreted in bile.[332] The serum half-life is significantly longer in patients with alcoholic cirrhosis and dosage should be reduced by 20–25%.[212]

When administered alone, imipenem (a carbapenem) is mainly excreted in urine as a metabolite, owing to hydrolysis in the brush border of the proximal renal tubular epithelium. Following concurrent administration of cilastatin, which prevents hydrolysis, between 60% and 75% of imipenem is excreted unchanged in the urine and less than 2% in faeces.[243]

Aminoglycosides. The aminoglycosides are excreted unchanged as a function of the glomerular filtration rate; no adjustment of the dosage is required in liver disease without concomitant renal failure.

Chloramphenicol and thiamphenicol (see Table 17.13). Although they are chemically related, the pharmacokinetics of these drugs differ markedly. Less than 10% of chloramphenicol is excreted unchanged in the urine, compared with 50–70% of thiamphenicol. Thiamphenicol

Table 17.12 Drug class: antibiotics (penicillins and cephalosporins).

Type of patient	No.	Dose	Route	Protein binding (%)	$t_{1/2}$ (h)	Renal excretion (% dose given)	Common duct bile concentration (mg/l)	Reference
Penicillins								
Ampicillin[a]								
Normals	5	500 mg	o	20	0.8–1.0		22.3 (10–36)	Acocella et al.[2]
Normals		600 mg	i.v.	—	1.3	92	—	Lewis and Jusko[203]
Cirrhotics	9	600 mg	i.v.	—	1.3	66	—	Lewis and Jusko[203]
Amoxycillin[a]								
Normals	—	500 mg	o	25	1.0–1.3	50–64	9.5(1–53)	Barza and Weinstein[21]
Normals	6	500 mg	o	—	—	49.1 ± 13.4 plus 24.7 ± 10.7 penicilloic acid	—	Cole et al.[64]
Azlocillin	10	1 g	i.v.	30–50	0.89	59.4	—	
Normals	10	2 g	i.v.	30–50	0.98	75.5	1137	Bergan[25]
	10	5 g	i.v.	30–50	1.53	74.7	—	
Cholestatic jaundice	6	4 g	i.v.	—	3.15 ± 0.82	71.4	—	Kuhlman et al.[190]
Carbenicillin								
Normals	5	2 g	i.v.	50	1.0 ± 0.25	85	14–33	Hoffman et al.[159]
Hepatic dysfunction	9	2 g	i.v.	—	1.9 ± 0.6	—	—	
Cloxacillin[a]								
Normals	—	500 mg	o	93	0.5	41	—	Giusti[121]
Flucloxacillin	—	500 mg	o	88–93.2			29–65	Takenaka and Sakai[333]
Normals	6	500 mg	o	—	40.6 ± 30.1 plus 3.7 ± 5.1 penicilloic acid			Cole et al.[64]
Mecillinam								
Normals	15	200 mg	i.v.	10–15	0.81	58	—	Mitchard et al.[232], Rohalt et al.[289]
Normals	42	800 mg	i.v.	—	—	—	Mean 49	Hares et al.[147]
Obstructed	11	800 mg	i.v.	—	—	—	Mean 8	Hares et al.[147]
Mezlocillin	10	1 g	i.v.	27–42	0.96	33.5	—	
Normals	10	2 g	i.v.	27–42	0.79	47.2	—	Bergan[25]
Normals	10	5 g	i.v.	27–42	1.21	54.8	—	
Normals	14	2 g	i.v.	—	1–1.6	75	42–8800	Gundert-Remy et al.[141]
Penicillin G[a]								
Normals	—	3 MU	i.v.	60	0.7	58–85	10–20	Kosmidis et al.[186]
Piperacillin	5	1 g	i.v.	—	0.60	74.1	—	
Normals	5	2 g	i.v.	—	0.90	81.4	—	Tjandramaga et al.[339]
Normals	5	4 g	i.v.	—	1.02	79.8	—	
Normals	5	1 g	i.v.	—	—	—	467(31–920)	Giron et al.[120]
Normals	5	4 g	i.v.	16	1.02	80		de Schepper et al.[78]
Ticarcillin	—	3 g	i.v.	—	—	—	Mean 100	Aikewa et al.[6]
	1	—	i.v.	—	—	—	164	Ervin and Bullock[98]
	6	5 g	i.v.	—	1.3	94.3	—	Davies et al.[74]
Cephalosporins								
Cefoperazone								
Normals	4	1 g	i.v.	—	—	—	1290(273–3100)	Nakamura et al.[239]
Normals	8	2 g	i.v.	—	1.6	25(12 h)	—	Cochet et al.[63]
Hepatic dysfunction	6	2 g	i.v.	—	4.3	70(12 h)	—	

Table 17.12 Continued.

Type of patient	No.	Dose	Route	Protein binding (%)	$t_{1/2}$ (h)	Renal excretion (% dose given)	Common duct bile concentration (mg/l)	Reference
Cefotaxime								
Normals	43	1 g	i.m.	30–45	0.9–1.3	58	—	Esmieu et al.[99]
Normals	4	1 g	i.v.	47	0.8	54.5 plus 28.7 desacetyl metabolite	—	Harding et al.[146]
Normals	2	1 g	i.m.	—	0.9–1.1	55–60	12–14	Kosmidis et al.[187]
Normals	2	—	—	—	—	—	39.7–77.4 plus (78.6–101.2 desacetyl metabolite)	White et al.[358]
Biliary disease	14	15 mg/kg	i.v.	—	1.7 plus desacetyl 3.1 metabolite	—	25.1	Shyu et al.[310]
Acute liver disease	6	1 g	i.v.	—	0.7–3.3	—	—	Wise et al.[372]
Acute hepatocellular necrosis	5	1 g	i.v.	—	1.58 (0.7–3.3)	—	—	Wright and Wise[377]
Cefoxitin								
Normals	2	2 g	i.v.	—	—	—	227	Geddes et al.[110]
Normals	—	—	—	73	0.7	98	—	Schrogie et al.[299]
Ceftazidime								
Normals	4	500 mg	i.v.	17	1.7	89	—	Harding et al.[146]
Normals	5	2 g	i.v.	—	—	—	36.3 ± 4.0	Brogard et al.[55]
Cirrhosis	1	2 g	i.v.	—	—	—	11.9	Brogard et al.[55]
Cephalothin								
Normals	—	—	—	65	0.6	52	12	Schrogie et al.[299]
Normals	7	1 g	i.v.	—	—	—	4(1–17)	Ratzan et al.[274]
Cephazolin								
Normals	15	0.5 g	i.v.	70	0.49	91.5	—	Paradelis[253]
Normals	10	1 g	i.v.	—	—	—	95.3	Cunha et al.[68]
Normals	8	1 g	i.v.	—	—	—	31(5–168)	Ratzan et al.[274]
Other β-lactams								
Aztreonam								
Normals	6	1 g	i.v.	—	1.9	62.4	—	MacLeod et al.[212]
Normals	4	500 mg	i.v.	69.5	1.6	67.3	—	Swabb et al.[332]
Biliary disease	14	1 g	i.v.	—	—	—	42.9 (9.7–88.2)	Martinez et al.[217]
Alcoholic cirrhosis	6	1 g	i.v.	—	3.2	75.5	—	MacLeod et al.[212]
Primary biliary cirrhosis	6	1 g	i.v.	—	2.2	54.4	—	MacLeod et al.[212]
Imipenem (combined with cilastatin)	4	500 mg	i.v.	10–20	1.0	70 (active) + 29 (metabolites)	—	Norrby et al.[245]
Normals	6	500 mg	i.v.	—	—	—	1.32 (0.3–3.3)	Graziani et al.[134]

[a]Data calculated from more than one source.
$t_{1/2}$ = half-life in blood or plasma; o = oral; i.v. = intravenous.

is handled normally in patients with cirrhosis[18] but chloramphenicol is not. In patients with severely impaired liver function the rate of conjugation with glucuronic acid is reduced, resulting in prolongation of its serum half-life.[18,193] The half-life is similarly prolonged in neonates, especially premature infants, owing to defective conjugation by the immature liver. Accumulation of free drug produces the 'grey baby syndrome'; this syndrome has also been reported in adults.[336] Increased hepatic metabolism occurs when phenobarbitone is administered concur-

Table 17.13 Drug class: antibiotics (chloramphenicol, thiamphenicol and tetracyclines).

Type of patient	No.	Dose	Route	Protein binding (%)	$t_{1/2}$ (h)	Renal excretion (% dose given)	Common duct bile concentration (mg/l)	Reference
Chloramphenicol								
Normals	4	10 mg/kg	i.v.	60	2.29 (1.72–2.82)	Total 75–90	—	Azzollini et al.[18]
	18	500 mg	i.v.	—	2.9	Active 5–15	—	Azzollini et al.[18]
Normal adult	1	1 g	o	—	—	—	46	Glazko et al.[123]
Premature								
neonate <7 day	15	50 mg/kg	i.m.	—	24	—	—	
>7 day	5	50 mg/kg	i.m.	—	14	—	—	Hodgman and
<7 day	3	25 mg/kg	i.v.	—	15–22	—	—	Burns[156]
>7 day	2	50 mg/kg	i.v.	—	8–15	—	—	
Cirrhosis	8	10 mg/kg	i.v.	—	4.05 (2.19–6.42)	—	—	Azzollini et al.[18]
Cirrhosis	11	500 mg	i.v.	—	5	Total 73	—	Kunin et al.[193]
Thiamphenicol								
Normals	4	10 mg/kg	i.v.	0–10	2.0 (1.57–2.43)	50–70	—	Azzollini et al.[18]
Cirrhosis	9	10 mg/kg	i.v.	—	1.92 (1.4–2.7)	—	—	Azzollini et al.[18]
Acute hepatitis	9	20 mg/kg	i.v.	—	—	61	—	Olderhausen et al.[247]
Tetracycline	10	1 g	o	65	10.8	60	0.5–4	Acocella et al.[3]
Doxycycline	10	200 mg	o	90	16.7	33	—	Doluisio and Dittert[81]
Minocycline	10	600 mg	o	75	14.3	6	—	Macdonald et al.[210]

$t_{1/2}$ = half-life in blood or plasma; i.v. = intravenous; o = oral.

rently.[252] Suhrland and Weisberger[330] showed definite erythropoietic depression in 8 of 16 patients with hepatic insufficiency who received chloramphenicol 2 g daily for 10–28 days. The suggestion was that only unmetabolized chloramphenicol is toxic to the marrow; certainly the mean free drug levels of 19 mg/l in cirrhotics with impaired red cell production was significantly higher than the mean level of 3–9 mg/l in patients with normal erythropoiesis. The relationship of direct toxicity to chloramphenicol-induced marrow aplasia is not clear. Nevertheless, with the availability of alternative drugs there can be few indications for chloramphenicol in patients with liver disease. In the neonate, serum levels should be monitored routinely.

Tetracyclines (see Table 17.13). The fact that only 31% of minocycline and 70% of doxycycline can be recovered from faeces and urine in an active form[210] is suggestive of significant hepatic metabolism of these drugs. Hepatic metabolism is enhanced by induction of microsomal enzymes with anticonvulsants, as shown by the reduced half-life of doxycycline from 15.1 h in normals to 7.4 h in patients receiving drugs.[257] Despite reports by

Bernard, Yin and Simon[28] that serum levels of minocycline are unaffected by hepatic disease, special care must be taken to avoid their accumulation in severe hepatocellular failure because tetracyclines are potent antimetabolites and are potentially hepatotoxic.[207] Erythromycin seems a safer choice for the treatment of chlamydial and rickettsial infections in patients with liver disease.

Lincosamides: clindamycin, lincomycin (see Table 17.14). Excretion of clindamycin is significantly impaired in patients with liver disease; in hepatitis the half-life may be prolonged to 14 h compared to the normal 3 h.[46]

Accumulation of clindamycin may be hepatotoxic, resulting in raised serum alkaline phosphatase, aspartate aminotransferase and alanine aminotransferase.[104,365] Single case studies suggest that clindamycin may be a cause of drug hepatitis.[95] Although other workers have not experienced problems using clindamycin in patients with liver disease,[153] elevated levels could contribute to liver damage[96] and caution is clearly indicated.

The simplest approach is to use alternative antibiotics for the treatment of staphylococcal and anaerobic infections. If used in severe liver disease, a reduction in the

Table 17.14 Drug class: antibiotics (clindamycin and lincomycin).

Type of patient	No.	Dose	Route	Protein binding (%)	$t_{1/2}$ (h)	Renal excretion (% dose given)	Common duct bile concentration (mg/l)	Reference
Clindamycin								
Normals	6	300 mg	i.m.	—	3 (2.4–4.2)	15	—	Brandl et al.[46]
	7	300 mg	i.v.	79	3.42 ± 0.45	—	—	Avant et al.[17]
Normals	9	8 mg/kg	i.v.	—	—	—	44(25–88)	Moesgaard et al.[234]
Obstructed	18	8 mg/kg	i.v.	—	—	—	9(0–40)	Moesgaard et al.[234]
Acute hepatitis	6	300 mg	i.m.	—	7.3 (2.98–14.16)	—	—	Brandl et al.[46]
Hepatic dysfunction	2	Varied	i.v.	—	—	33	48–50	Williams et al.[365]
Cirrhosis	2	300 mg	i.v.	79	4.46 ± 0.93	—	—	Avant et al.[17]
Lincomycin								
Normals	6	600 mg	i.m.	72	4.85 (4.45–5.67)	6–15	—	Bellamy et al.[23]
Hepatic insufficiency	9	600 mg	i.m.	—	8.96 (6.11–11.80)	—	—	Medina et al.[231]

$t_{1/2}$ = half-life in blood or plasma; i.m. = intramuscular; i.v. = intravenous.

dosage of clindamycin is required and levels should be monitored by serial blood assays.

The use of lincomycin in patients with liver disease is less well documented; nevertheless, the evidence indicates impaired excretion.[23]

Macrolides (see Table 17.15). Little unchanged erythromycin is excreted by the kidney. This suggests extensive secretion by the liver, some as the des-*N*-methyl derivative.[214] Up to 20% of roxithromycin is excreted in the bile as metabolites.[229] As yet, there are no data on the metabolism of spiramycin in man, although it is known to achieve biliary concentrations in excess of those in serum.[200] There are conflicting data on the effect of alcoholic liver disease on the pharmacokinetics of erythro-

mycin[143,189] but the half-life of roxithromycin is significantly extended.[229,259]

Following administration of erythromycin base or salts, a benign increase in transaminases occurs in up to 10% of patients.[176,261] Additionally, erythromycin estolate causes potentially severe but uncommon cholestatic liver injury, the ester linkage of the 2'-position of the erythromycin molecule with lauryl sulphate being responsible.[85,340] Secondary or tertiary amines present on the molecule of many macrolides (but not spiramycin or josamycin) are dealkylated and oxidized by hepatic cytochrome P450 into nitrosalkane derivatives which then form stable complexes with cytochrome P450. This leads to decreased metabolism and to drug interactions with ergotamine, warfarin and theophylline.[261]

Table 17.15 Drug class: antibiotics (erythromycin and fusidic acid).

Type of patient	No.	Dose	Route	Protein binding (%)	$t_{1/2}$ (h)	Renal excretion (% dose given)	Common duct bile concentration (mg/l)	Reference
Erythromycin								
Normals	14	125–500 mg	o	90	1.18	6–7	200–500	Wiegand and Chun[362]
Normals	13	200–500 mg	o	—	—	(parenteral)	6–800	Twiss et al.[341]
Normals	6	500 mg	o	—	6.6	—	—	Kroboth et al.[189]
Chronic liver disease	8	500 mg	o	—	4.5	—	—	Kroboth et al.[189]
Fusidic acid								
Normals	10	500 mg	o	95	8	<1	—	Godtfredsen et al.[126] Godtfredsen[124]

$t_{1/2}$ = half-life in blood or plasma; o = oral.

Table 17.16 Drug class: antibiotics (co-trimoxazole).

Type of patient	No.	Dose	Route	Protein binding (%)	$t_{1/2}$ (h)	Renal excretion (% dose given)	Common duct bile concentration (mg/l)	Reference
Co-trimoxazole								
Normals	6	2 tabs	o	—	—	—	161 (128–200)	Neuman et al.[243]
Hepatic dysfunction	6	2 tabs	o	—	—	—	50 (15.5–150)	
Sulphamethoxazole								
Normals	13	1800 mg	o	62	12.1 (7.9–17.4)	57 (24 h)	—	Rieder and Schwartz[284]
Hepatic dysfunction	7	1800 mg	o	—	12.3 (9.3–15.1)	47.7 (24 h)	—	
Trimethoprim								
Normals	13	320 mg	o	42–46	11.5 (8.4–13.5)	40.7 (24 h)	—	Rieder and Schwartz[284]
Hepatic dysfunction	7	320 mg	o	—	14.3 (6.6–23.7)	25.3 (24 h)	—	

$t_{1/2}$ = half-life in blood or plasma; o = oral.

Fusidic acid. Less than 1% of fusidic acid is excreted unchanged in the urine, indicating extensive metabolism by the liver.[124] Although fusidic acid is remarkably non-toxic, some impairment of sulphobromophthalein excretion occurs[378] and there are anecdotal reports of jaundice. The drug should therefore be used with extreme caution in patients with hepatic failure.

Sulphonamides. The capacity to acetylate sulphonamides is distributed bimodally. In rapid acetylators, conjugated drug accounts for over 70% of the drug in the urine.[273] Less than 1% of older sulphonamides is excreted in bile, but up to 6.3% of long-acting compounds is excreted by this route.

Co-trimoxazole (see Table 17.16). Chemical assays have shown that although the sulphamethoxazole component of co-trimoxazole is excreted normally in patients with liver disease, the half-life of trimethoprim may be prolonged to twice normal in patients with severe hepatic damage.[284] The same workers found that following a single oral dose of co-trimoxazole the maximum plasma levels of both sulphamethoxazole and trimethoprim were lower by an average factor of 1.6–2.0 in patients with liver disease compared to normal controls. The suggested explanation was impaired absorption secondary to changes in the bile. The alternative possibility, that the lower plasma levels reflect an increased distribution volume, is untenable if the findings by Hitzenberger et al.[155] of a reduced volume of distribution of trimethoprim in patients with cirrhosis (1.0 versus 1.71/kg) are correct.

Lower than normal maintenance doses should be given to prevent accumulation of trimethoprim when co-trimoxazole is being used parenterally in patients with severe

parenchymal damage. There is no reliable information on patients receiving oral therapy but similar precautions would seem sensible.

Metronidazole and tinidazole. Metronidazole is partially metabolized in the liver by oxidation of the hydroxy group on the side-chain or by conjugation with glucuronic acid.[169] Significant amounts are excreted into the bile,[173] mean levels of 28 mg/l being reported.[264] Only 15–20% of the drug is excreted unchanged in the urine.[271] There is little information at present on the biliary excretion of tinidazole but a small proportion is excreted in the form of metabolites in urine.[375]

There are few data on the use of these drugs in liver disease except in schistosomiasis,[72] where no clinically significant alteration in pharmacokinetics was seen. These data, together with the fact that both drugs penetrate tissues and are bactericidal, suggest that they are the drugs of choice for the treatment of anaerobic infections in patients with hepatic dysfunction. However, the ability of these drugs to produce the 'Antabuse syndrome' must be remembered and toxic psychoses have been reported when metronidazole was given to alcoholic patients receiving disulfiram.[291]

Urinary antibacterials

Quinolones (see Table 17.17). Nalidixic acid and its hydroxy-metabolite account for 15% of the drug in the urine and the remaining 85% is excreted as inactive conjugates.[323]

Urinary metabolites account for 10% of the dose of ciprofloxacin and ofloxacin, 20% of norfloxacin and 55% of pefloxacin. Pefloxacin is also partly metabolized to

Table 17.17 Drug class: antibiotics (quinolones).

Type of patient	No.	Dose	Route	Protein binding (%)	$t_{1/2}$ (h)	Renal excretion (% dose given)	Common duct bile concentration (mg/l)	Reference
Ciprofloxacin								
Normals	6	500 mg	o	35	3.9	30.6	—	Wise *et al.*[371]
Normals	12	500 mg	o	—	—	—	16.0 (total active compounds 21.2)	Brogard *et al.*[54]
Enoxacin								
Normals	7	600 mg	o	43	6.2	61.2	—	Wise *et al.*[371]
Nalidixic acid	—	—	—	90	1.5	—	—	—
Norflaxacin								
Normals	6	400 mg	o	15	4.28 (3.35–5.94)	32	—	Eandi *et al.*[88]
Acute hepatitis	3	400 mg	o	—	5.47 (4.51–6.05)	33	—	Eandi *et al.*[88]
Oflaxacin								
Normals	4	600 mg	o	8–30	7.0	73	—	Wise *et al.*[371]
Pefloxacin								
Normals	3	800 mg	o	—	—	—	Mean 19 (total active 23)	Montay *et al.*[236]
Normals	12	8 mg/kg	i.v.	25	11.0 ± 2.64	—	—	Danan *et al.*[71]
Cirrhosis	16	8 mg/kg	i.v.	—	35.1 (11.2–90.7)	—	—	Danan *et al.*[71]

$t_{1/2}$ = half-life in blood or plasma; o = oral; i.v. = intravenous.

norfloxacin. Small amounts of quinolones are excreted by the biliary route.

The half-life of pefloxacin was found to be significantly prolonged in patients with cirrhosis[71] and combined hepatorenal disease exaggerates the problem.[236] Impaired liver function leads only to slight increases in the half-lives of ciprofloxacin and norfloxacin.[88] Prolongation of ofloxacin's half-life was reported by Vulterini *et al.*[354] in patients with advanced cirrhosis, despite the limited metabolism of this drug. Pefloxacin and nalidixic acid should be used with caution in patients with liver dysfunction.

Nitrofurantoin. Only about a third of nitrofurantoin is excreted in the urine in an active form. Inactivation apparently occurs in all body tissues, but the liver plays a major role.[157] Rare cases of hepatotoxicity have been reported[29] and allergic-type hepatitis associated with antinuclear factor has also been reported. In the absence of data, alternative agents should be administered whenever possible to patients with liver disease.

Anti-fungals

5-Fluorocytosine (see Table 17.18). Ninety per cent of the drug is recovered unchanged in urine within 48 hours. A small amount is metabolized to 5-fluorouracil.[69] A report of the administration of the drug to a single patient with cirrhosis showed serum levels of 5-fluorocytosine to be unchanged.[36] Hepatic dysfunction is not, therefore, a contraindication to the use of 5-fluorocytosine.

Amphotericin B. The metabolic fate of this drug is uncertain. The long half-life with continued detection in the urine up to 7 days after administration suggests that metabolism is not an important means of disposal but that it is bound within the body and slowly released from this site.[31] There is no reason, on present evidence, to avoid this drug on grounds of liver disease.

Imidazoles (see Table 17.18). Following intravenous injection, 25% of miconazole is excreted in the urine as inactive metabolites. Hoeprich and Goldstein[158] were unable to detect active drug in the urine.

Ketoconazole is metabolized by the liver and largely excreted by the biliary route. Therapy is associated with an indiosyncratic form of liver damage in approximately 1 in 15 000 individuals. Primary hepatocellular damage is the most common form, but cholestatic jaundice and mixed reactions also occur.[205] Although mild liver disease did not affect the pharmacokinetics of ketoconazole in patients studied by Heel *et al.*[149] or lead to its accumulation in a patient with hepatic insufficiency treated by Brass *et*

Table 17.18 Drug class: antibiotics (antifungal agents).

Type of patient	No.	Dose	Route	Protein binding (%)	$t_{1/2}$ (h)	Renal excretion (% dose given)	Common duct bile concentration (mg/l)	Reference
5-Fluorocytosine								
Normal	10	2 g	o	—	2.89	87	—	Schonebeck et al.[298]
Miconazole								
Normal	4	600 mg/day	i.v.	81–93	24 ± 2.8	—	—	Lewi et al.[202]
Normal	14	600–3600 mg/day	i.v.	90	20	—	—	Stevens et al.[325]
Amphotericin B								
Normal	15	45 mg/day	i.v.	91–95	24	2–5	—	Bindschadler and Bennett[31]
Normal	13	Various	i.v.	—	—	—	7.3	Collette et al.[65]
Fluconazole								
Normal	—	50 mg	o i.v.	12	24.4 ± 3.1 / 30.2 ± 3.8	80	—	Brammer and Tarbitt[41]
Ketoconazole	24	200 mg	o	—	7.5–7.9	—	—	Huang et al.[164]
	—	200 mg	o	99	—	2–4	—	Heel et al.[149]

$t_{1/2}$ = half-life in blood or plasma; o = oral; i.v. = intravenous.

al.,[47] it is contraindicated in patients with pre-existing liver disease because of the potential for toxicity.

Approximately 80% of fluconazole is excreted unchanged in urine and a further 11% as metabolites.[41] It is estimated that between 0.8% and 14.6% of the daily excretion is via the biliary route.[65]

Miconazole and fluconazole appear to be generally safe but, in the absence of data, patients with liver dysfunction should be treated with caution.

Antitubercular drugs (see Chapter 46; Table 17.19)

Ethambutol. Of the ethambutol which is absorbed from the gut, approximately 75% is excreted unchanged in the urine; the remainder is excreted in urine as the aldehyde and dicarboxylic acid metabolites. No data are available on the handling of the drug in the presence of hepatic dysfunction, but in view of the small proportion of the drug which is metabolized it seems unlikely that liver disease would significantly increase the risk of toxicity from ethambutol.

Isoniazid. Isoniazid is acetylated in the liver by a similar process to sulphonamides, so a person is either a rapid or a slow acetylator of both these drugs.[273] Elevated transaminases have been reported frequently and clinical hepatotoxicity occurs occasionally. Chronic liver disease in itself does not appear to predispose to further damage by this drug[33] and is not a contraindication to its use.

Pyrazinamide. The drug accumulates in jaundiced patients who are given conventional doses.[328] Its use can only be justified in patients with pre-existing liver disease in desperate situations, when no alternative is available.

Rifampicin. Rifampicin is extensively metabolized by the liver and can cause mild hepatotoxicity, which may subside with continuation of treatment. It may accumulate in the presence of liver disease or biliary obstruction and patients with pre-existing liver disease are at greater risk of developing other toxic manifestations.[30] Alternative drugs should be used in such subjects.

Antivirals (see Table 17.20)

Adenine arabinoside. This drug is deaminated in the liver and 40–50% is excreted as hypoxanthine derivatives in the urine. It has been used to treat patients with chronic active hepatitis without hepatotoxicity.[70] It is likely therefore to be safe in patients with liver dysfunction.

Acycloguanosine. Seventy per cent is excreted unchanged in the urine, together with its 9-carboxymethoxymethyl metabolite. Hepatitis has not been reported in early clinical studies. Its activity is dependent on the presence of viral thymidine synthetase to activate the drug and its activity against the human cell is a thousandfold lower than that for the virus. Although data are lacking for its use in hepatic dysfunction, in the light of its selective action there seems to be no reason to withhold treatment in serious herpetic infections.

Table 17.19 Drug class: antibiotics (antitubercular agents).

Type of patient	No.	Dose	Route	Protein binding (%)	$t_{1/2}$ (h)	Renal excretion (% dose given)	Common duct bile concentration (mg/l)	Reference
Ethambutol								
Normal	10	25 mg/kg	o	—	6	70	—	Place and Thomas[265]
Isoniazid								
Normal	6	600 mg	o	None	3.24 ± 0.14	5–25	—	Acocella et al.[3]
Chronic liver disease	7	600 mg	o	—	6.74 ± 0.33	—	—	Acocella et al.[3]
Pyrazinamide								
Normal	27	1.5 g/day	o	—	6.1	34	—	Ellard[94]
Rifampicin								
Normal	2	250 mg	i.v.	—	—	—	1200–2400	Acocella et al.[2]
Normal	6	600 mg	o	75–85	2.8 ± 0.22	5–24	—	Acocella et al.[3]
Chronic liver disease	7	600 mg	o	—	5.42 ± 0.55	—	—	Acocella et al.[3]

$t_{1/2}$ = half-life in blood or plasma; o = oral; i.v. = intravenous.

Table 17.20 Drug class: antiviral agents.

Type of patient	No.	Dose	Route	Protein binding (%)	$t_{1/2}$ (h)	Renal excretion (% dose given)	Common duct bile concentration (mg/l)	Reference
Acyclovir								
Normals	20	5 mg/kg	i.v.	9–22	2.5 ± 0.6	67 ± 15.3	—	Barry and Blum[20]
Adenine arabinoside								
Normals	—	1 mg/kg	i.m.	3	3–5	50	—	Glazko et al.[122]
Amantadine								
Normals	—	2–4 mg/kg	o	67	11.8 ± 2.1	62–93	—	Koppell and Tenczer[185]
Ganciclovir								
Normals	13	5 mg/kg	i.v.	1–2	3.6 ± 1.4	73.2 ± 31	—	Somadossi et al.[316]
Zidovudine								
Normals	22	1–7.5 mg/kg	i.v.	—	1.1	18.5 ± 5	—	Blum et al.[37]

$t_{1/2}$ = half-life in blood or plasma; o = oral; i.v. = intravenous.

Amantidine.   Amantidine is excreted largely unchanged in urine, but 5–15% of the dose undergoes acetylation before excretion.[185] No data exist about its handling in hepatic disease.

Ganciclovir.   In studies by Somadassi et al.[316] 70% of ganciclovir was excreted unchanged in the urine. Early clinical experience suggests that modification to dosage is not necessary in patients with liver disease.

Zidovudine.   Approximately 90% of zidovudine is excreted in urine, but only 18% of this is unchanged, the remainder being in the form of an inactive glucuronide.[37]

Because of the high degree of metabolism and short half-life in normal individuals, caution should be exercised when treating patients with hepatic impairment.

Drugs not studied to date

Several attempts have been made to devise pharmacokinetic models for the effects of liver disease on drug handling: these have been summarized by Wilkinson and Shand,[364] Wilkinson and Schenker[363] and Blaschke.[34]

Although the models produced by these authors have some value, they are no substitute for studies of individual drug pharmacokinetics in various disease states.[75] Nevertheless, the following conclusions may be drawn. Hepatic disease may lead to increased bioavailability of orally administered drugs if they undergo a high clearance at the first pass. The distribution volume tends to be increased in patients with chronic hepatic disease, particularly those with reduced serum albumin concentrations. Protein binding is also reduced in patients who are hypoalbuminaemic, jaundiced and/or uraemic, leading to increased pharmacological and therapeutic effects. The elimination half-lives of drugs which are metabolized by the microsomal enzymes and the metabolic clearances are usually unchanged in acute viral hepatitis, but considerable alterations can occur in patients with decompensated chronic liver disease. These changes are accompanied by a reduction in serum albumin and reduced clearance of indocyanine green or portosystemic encephalopathy. Smaller than normal doses of most drugs should be used in such patients.

Cytochrome P450 activity in liver disease

Studies of this and other enzyme activity in liver disease are comparatively few. The first, by Doshi, Luisada-Opper and Leevy,[82] concerned microsomal pentobarbital hydroxylase activity in acute viral hepatitis. The second studied the cytochrome P450 content in patients with severe hepatitis and cirrhosis.[296] Subsequently, N-oxidation of dimethyl aniline and oxidative demethylation of aminopyrine were studied by Gold and Ziegler.[127] All three studies confirmed that enzymic activity is preserved in hepatitis except in the most severe cases when P450 content may fall to 50% of normal values. P450 activity may be increased in areas of regenerating tissue.

The situation is more complicated in the presence of hepatic cirrhosis. Cytochrome P450 content is diminished[38,53,103] to an extent depending on the severity of the disease.[53,321] Arylhydroxylase activity is diminished but the extent depends not only on the degree of liver damage but also on smoking habits and caffeine ingestion.[53] By contrast, ethylmorphine demethylase activity is preserved even in patients with evidence of hepatocellular destruction, and NADPH–cytochrome c reductase activity remains unimpaired even in severe liver damage.

PHARMACODYNAMICS

Altered pharmacodynamic responses have been clearly demonstrated for three groups of drugs in hepatic diseases: anticoagulants, sedatives and diuretics.

Anticoagulants

The ability to synthesize the vitamin K_1-dependent clotting factors II, VII, IX and X in patients with severe liver disease is reduced. Thus, their sensitivity to oral anticoagulants of either the coumarin or indanedione series is increased.[348]

Sedatives

Morphine tolerance is diminished in patients with hepatic cirrhosis, particularly those who have previously had episodes of portosystemic encephalopathy.[196] These authors attributed the changes to an increased sensitivity of the CNS to morphine, but it is equally possible that they reflect the diminished protein binding demonstrated by Olsen, Bennett and Porter.[248] However, patients with cirrhosis are more susceptible to the effects of chlorpromazine[275] and this is almost certainly due to an altered end-organ response.[222] The increased sensitivity to diazepam[45] may be explained by pharmacokinetic changes.

Diuretics

Whilst there is no doubt of the usefulness of these agents in the treatment of patients with oedema due to hepatic disease, they are extremely hazardous.[66] Encephalopathy is likely to develop in up to 20% of patients treated with frusemide and great care must be taken to give adequate potassium replacement therapy.

Acknowledgement

We wish to thank Mrs F.D. Lowman, who typed the original manuscript.

REFERENCES

1. Ablad, B., Ervik, M., Hallgren, J. *et al.* (1972) Pharmacological effects and serum levels of orally administered alprenolol in man. *European Journal of Clinical Pharmacology,* **5,** 44–52.
2. Acocella, G., Mattiussi, R., Nicolis, F.B. *et al.* (1968) Biliary excretion of antibiotics in man. *Gut,* **9,** 536–545.
3. Acocella, G., Bonollo, L., Garimoldi, M. *et al.* (1972) Kinetics of rifampicin and isoniazid administered alone and in combination to normal subjects and patients with liver disease. *Gut,* **13,** 47–53.
4. Adjepon-Yamoah, K.K. Nimmo, J & Prescott, L.F. (1974) Gross impairment of hepatic drug metabolism in a patient with chronic liver disease. *British Medical Journal,* **iv,** 387–388.
5. Affrime, M. & Reidenberg, M.M. (1975) The protein binding of some drugs in plasma from patients with alcoholic liver disease. *European Journal of Clinical Pharmacology,* **8,** 267–269.
6. Aikawa, N., Ishibiki, H., Takami, H. *et al.* (1977) A basic and clinical evaluation of ticarcillin in surgical field. *Chemotherapy,* **25,** 2699–2713.

7. Alexanderson, B., Price Evans, D.A. & Sjoqvist, F. (1969) Steady-state levels of nortriptyline in twins: influence of genetic factors and drug therapy. *British Medical Journal,* **iv,** 764–768.
8. Allgulander, C., Beermann, B. & Sjogren, A. (1980) Frusemide pharmacokinetics in patients with liver disease. *Clinical Pharmacokinetics,* **5,** 570–575.
9. Alvin, J., McHorse, T., Hoyumpa, A. *et al.* (1975) The effect of liver disease in man on the disposition of phenobarbital. *Journal of Pharmacology and Experimental Therapeutics,* **192,** 224–235.
10. Andreasen, P.B., Hendel, J., Griesen, G. & Hvidberg, E.F. (1976) Pharmacokinetics of diazepam in disordered liver function. *European Journal of Clinical Pharmacology,* **10,** 115–20.
11. Andreasen, P.B. & Ranek, L. (1975) Liver failure and drug metabolism. *Scandinavian Journal of Gastroenterology,* **10,** 293–297.
12. Andreasen, P.B., Ranek, L., Statland, B.E. & Tygstrup, N. (1974) Clearance of antipyrine-dependence on quantitative liver function. *European Journal of Clinical Investigation,* **4,** 129–134.

13. Anton, A.H. (1960) The relation between the binding of sulfonamides to albumin and their antibacterial efficacy. *Journal of Pharmacology and Experimental Therapeutics*, **129**, 282–290.

14. Anton, A.H. (1973) Increasing activity of sulfonamides with displacing agents: a review. *Annals of the New York Academy of Sciences*, **226**, 273–292.

15. Anton, A.H. & Boyle, J.J. (1964) Alteration of the acetylation of sulphonamides by protein binding, sulphinpyrazone and suramin. *Canadian Journal of Physiology and Pharmacology*, **42**, 809–817.

16. Arthur, M.J.P., Tanner, A.R., Patel, C. *et al.* (1985) Pharmacology of propranolol in patients with cirrhosis and portal hypertension. *Gut*, **26**, 14–19.

17. Avant, G.R., Schenker, S. & Alford, R.H. (1975) The effect of cirrhosis on the disposition and elimination of clindamycin. *American Journal of Digestive Diseases*, **20**, 223–230.

18. Azzolini, F., Gazzaniga, A., Lodola, E. & Natangelo, R. (1972) Elimination of chloramphenicol and thiamphenicol in subjects with cirrhosis of the liver. *International Journal of Clinical Pharmacology, Therapy and Toxicology*, **6**, 130–134.

19. Baraka, A. & Gabali, F. (1968) Correlation between tubocurarine requirements and plasma protein pattern. *British Journal of Anaesthetics*, **40**, 89–93.

20. Barry, D.W. & Blum, M.R. (1983) Antiviral drugs: acyclovir. In Turner, P. & Shand, D. (eds) *Recent Advances in Clinical Pharmacology*, pp. 57–80. Edinburgh: Churchill Livingstone.

21. Barza, M. & Weinstein, L. (1976) Pharmacokinetics of the penicillins in man. *Clinical Pharmacokinetics*, **1**, 297–308.

22. Barza, M., Samuelson, T. & Weinstein, L. (1974) Penetration of antibiotics into fibrin loci in vivo. II. Comparison of nine antibiotics: effect of dose and degree of protein binding. *Journal of Infectious Diseases*, **129**, 66–72.

23. Bellamy, H. Jr, Bates, B.B. & Reinarz, J.A. (1966) Lincomycin metabolism in patients with hepatic insufficiency: effect of liver disease on lincomycin serum concentration. In Hobby, G.L. (ed.) *Antimicrobial Agents and Chemotherapy*, pp. 36–41. Michigan: The American Society for Microbiology.

24. Benford, D.J., Bridges, J.W., Boobis, A.R. *et al.* (1981) The selective activation of cytochrome P450 dependent microsomal hydroxylases in human and rat liver microsomes. *Biochemical Pharmacology*, **30**, 1702–1703.

25. Bergan, T. (1981) Overview of acylureidopenicillin pharmacokinetics. *Scandinavian Journal of Infectious Diseases*, **29** (supplement), 33–48.

26. Bergstrand, R.H., Wang, T., Roden, D.M. *et al.* (1986) Encainide disposition in patients with chronic cirrhosis. *Clinical Pharmacology and Therapeutics*, **40**, 148–154.

27. Berkowitz, B.A., Asling, J.H., Shnider, S.M. & Way, E.L. (1969) Relationship of pentazocine plasma levels to pharmacologic activity in man. *Clinical Pharmacology and Therapeutics*, **10**, 320–328.

28. Bernard, B., Yin, E.J. & Simon, H.J. (1971) Clinical pharmacological studies with minocycline. *Journal of Clinical Pharmacology*, **11**, 332–348.

29. Bhagwat, A.G. & Warren, R.E. (1969) Hepatic reaction to nitrofurantoin. *Lancet*, **ii**, 1369.

30. Binda, G., Domenichini, E., Gottardi, A. *et al.* (1971) Rifampicin, a general review. *Arzneimittel Forschung*, **21**, 1907–1978.

31. Bindschadler, D.D. & Bennett, J.E. (1969) A pharmacologic guide to the clinical use of amphotericin B. *Journal of Infectious Diseases*, **120**, 427–436.

32. Birnie, G.G., Thompson, G.G., Cooke, A. & Brodie, M.J. (1987) Antipyrine and indocyanine green kinetics in the prediction of the natural history of liver disease. *British Journal of Clinical Pharmacology*, **27**, 615P–616P.

33. Black, M. (1974) Isoniazid and the liver. *American Review of Respiratory Diseases*, **110**, 1–3.

34. Blaschke, T.F. (1977) Protein binding and kinetics of drugs in liver diseases. *Clinical Pharmacokinetics*, **2**, 32–44.

35. Blaschke, T.F., Meffin, P.J. Melmon, K.L. & Rowland, M. (1975) Influence of acute viral hepatitis on phenytoin kinetics and protein binding. *Clinical Pharmacology and Therapeutics*, **17**, 685–691.

36. Block, E.R. (1973) Effect of hepatic insufficiency on 5-fluorocytosine concentrations in serum. *Antimicrobial Agents and Chemotherapy*, **3**, 141–142.

37. Blum, M.R., Liao, S.H.T., Good, S.S. *et al.* (1988) Pharmacokinetics and bioavailability of Zidovudine in humans. *American Journal of Medicine*, **85** (supplement 2A), 189–194.

38. Boobis, A.R., Brodie, M.J., Kahn, G.C. *et al.* (1980) Monooxygenase activity of human liver in microsomal fractions of needle biopsy specimens. *British Journal of Clinical Pharmacology*, **9**, 11–19.

39. Booker, H.E. & Darcey, B. (1973) Serum concentrations of free diphenylhydantoin and their relationship to clinical intoxication. *Epilepsia*, **14**, 177–184.

40. Borgå, O., Hamberger, B., Malmfors, T. & Sjoqvist, F. (1970) The role of plasma protein binding in the inhibitory effect of nortriptyline on the neuronal uptake of norepinephrine. *Clinical Pharmacology and Therapeutics*, **11**, 581–588.

41. Brammer, K.W. & Tarbit, M.H. (1987) A review of fluconazole (UK–49,858) in laboratory animals and man. In Fromtling, R.A. (ed) *Recent Trends in the Discovery, Development and Evaluation of Antifungal Agents*. Barcelona: Prous Science Publishers, S.A.

42. Branch, R.A., Herbert, C.M. & Read, A.E. (1973) Determinants of serum antipyrine half-lives in patients with liver disease. *Gut*, **14**, 569–573.

43. Branch, R.A., James, J. & Read, A.E. (1976) A study of factors influencing drug disposition in chronic liver disease, using the model drug (+)-propranolol. *British Journal of Clinical Pharmacology*, **3**, 243–249.

44. Branch, R.A., James, J.A. & Read, A.E. (1976) The clearance of antipyrine and indocyanine green in normal subjects and in patients with chronic liver disease. *Clinical Pharmacology and Therapeutics*, **20**, 81–89.

45. Branch, R.A., Morgan, M.H., James, J. & Read, A.E. (1976). Intravenous administration of diazepam in patients with chronic liver disease. *Gut*, **17**, 975–983.

46. Brandl, R., Arkenau, C., Simon, C., Malerczyk, V. & Eidelloth, G. (1972) The pharmacokinetics of clindamycin in the presence of impaired liver and kidney function. *Deutsche Medizinische Wochenschrift*, **91**, 1051–1059.

47. Brass, C., Galgiani, J.N., Blaschke, T.F. *et al.* (1982) Disposition of ketoconazole, an oral antifungal in humans. *Antimicrobial Agents and Chemotherapy*, **21**, 151–158.

48. Breckenridge, A., Orme, M. L'E., Davies, L., Thorgeirsson, S.S. & Davies, D.S. (1973) Dose-dependent enzyme induction. *Clinical Pharmacology and Therapeutics*, **14**, 514–520.

49. Breimer, D.D., Zilly, W. & Richter, E. (1975) Pharmacokinetics of hexobarbital in acute hepatitis and after apparent recovery. *Clinical Pharmacology and Therapeutics*, **18**, 433–440.

50. Brodie, B.B. (1967) Idiosyncrasy and intolerance. In Wolstenholme, G.E.W. & Porter, R. (eds) *Drug Responses in Man*, pp. 188–213. London: J. & A. Churchill.

51. Brodie, B.B. & Axelrod, J. (1950) The fate of antipyrine in man. *Journal of Pharmacology and Experimental Therapeutics*, **98**, 97–104.

52. Brodie, B.B., Burns, J.J. & Weiner, M. (1959) Metabolism of drugs in subjects with Laennec's cirrhosis. *Medicina Experimentalis*, **1**, 290–292.

53. Brodie, M.J., Boobis, A.R., Bulpitt, C.J. & Davies, D.S. (1981) Influence of liver disease and environmental factors on hepatic monooxygenase activity in vitro. *European Journal of Clinical Pharmacology*, **20**, 39–46.

54. Brogard, J.M., Jehl, F., Monteil, H. *et al.* (1985) Comparison of high-pressure liquid chromatography and microbiological assay for the determination of biliary elimination of ciprofloxacin in humans. *Antimicrobial Agents and Chemotherapy*, **28**, 311–314.

55. Brogard, J.M., Jehl, F., Paris-Bockel, D. *et al.* (1987) Biliary elimination of ceftazidime. *Journal of Antimicrobial Chemotherapy*, **19**, 671–678.

56. Brosen, K. (1990) Recent developments in hepatic drug oxidation: implications for clinical pharmacokinetics. *Clinical Pharmacokinetics*, **18**, 220–239.

57. Caldwell, J.H. & Greenberger, N.J. (1970) Cholestyramine enhances digitalis excretion and protects against lethal intoxication. *Journal of Clinical Investigation*, **49**, 16a.

58. Calvo, M.V., Dominguez-Gil, A., Macias, J.G. & Diez, J.L. (1980) Naproxen disposition in hepatic and biliary disorders. *International Journal of Clinical Pharmacology, Therapeutics and Toxicology*, **18**, 242–246.

59. Carey, M.C. & Small, D.M. (1971) Micellar properties of sodium

fusidate, a steroid antibiotic structurally resembling the bile salts. *Journal of Lipid Research,* **12,** 604–613.

60. Challenor, V.F., Waller, D.G., Renwick, A.F. *et al.* (1987) The trans-hepatic extraction of nifedipine. *British Journal of Clinical Pharmacology,* **24,** 473–477.

61. Choonara, I.A., Cholerton, S., Haynes, B.P. *et al.* (1986) Stereoselective interaction between the R enantiomer of warfarin and cimetidine. *British Journal of Clinical Pharmacology,* **21,** 271–277.

62. Closson, R.G. (1977) Terminal half-lives of drugs studied in patients with hepatic diseases. *American Journal of Hospital Pharmacy,* **34,** 520–524.

63. Cochet, B., Belaieff, J., Allaz, A.F. *et al.* (1981) Decreased extrarenal clearance of cefoperazone in hepatocellular disease. *British Journal of Clinical Pharmacology,* **11,** 389–390.

64. Cole, M., Kenig, M.D. & Hewitt, V.A. (1973) Metabolism of penicillins to penicilloic acids and 6-aminopenicillanic acid in man and its significance in assessing penicillin absorption. *Antimicrobial Agents and Chemotherapy,* **3,** 463–468.

65. Collette, N., Van De Auwera, P., Lopez, A.P. *et al.* (1989) Tissue concentrations and bioactivity of amphoterecin B in cancer patients treated with amphoterecin B-deoxycholate. *Antimicrobial Agents and Chemotherapy,* **33,** 362–365.

66. Conn, H.O. (1972) The rational management of ascites. *Progress in Liver Disease,* **4,** 269–288.

67. Conney, A.H. (1967) Pharmacological implications of microsomal enzyme induction. *Pharmacology Reviews,* **19,** 317–366.

68. Cunha, B.A., Ristuccia, A.M., Jonas, M. *et al.* (1981) Tissue penetration characteristics of ceftizoxime and cefazolin in human bile and gallbladder wall. *Journal of Antimicrobial Chemotherapy,* **10,** (Supplement C), 117–120.

69. Daisio, R.B., Lakings, D.E. & Bennett, J.E. (1978) Evidence for conversion of 5-fluorocytosine to 5-fluorouracil in humans: possible factors in 5-fluorocytosine clinical toxicity. *Antimicrobial Agents and Chemotherapy,* **14,** 903–908.

70. Damjanivic, V. & Brumfitt, W. (1980) Prophylaxis and treatment of viral hepatitis. *Journal of Antimicrobial Chemotherapy,* **6,** 11–32.

71. Danan, G., Montay, G., Cunci, R. & Erlinger, S. (1985) Pefloxacin kinetics in cirrhosis. *Clinical Pharmacology and Therapeutics,* **38,** 439–442.

72. Daneshmend, T.K., Homeida, M., Kaye, C.M. *et al.* (1982) Disposition of oral metronidazole in hepatic cirrhosis and in hepatosplenic schistosomiasis. *Gut,* **23,** 807–813.

73. Datta, D.V. & Sherlock, S. (1963) Treatment of pruritus of obstructive jaundice with cholestyramine. *British Medical Journal,* **i,** 216–219.

74. Davies, B.E., Humphrey, M.J., Langley, P.F. *et al.* (1982) Pharmacokinetics of ticarcillin in man. *European Journal of Clinical Pharmacology,* **23,** 167–172.

75. Davies, D.S. (1972) Drug metabolism and poisoning. *Medicine,* **4,** 287–293.

76. Davies, D.S. & Thorgeirsson, S.S. (1971) Mechanism of hepatic drug oxidation and its relationship to individual differences in rates of oxidation in man. *Annals of the New York Academy of Sciences,* **179,** 411–420.

77. Davis, M., Williams, R., Chakraborty, J. *et al.* (1978) Prednisone or prednisolone for the treatment of chronic active hepatitis? A comparison of plasma availability. *British Journal of Clinical Pharmacology,* **5,** 501–505.

78. de Schepper, P.J., Tjandramega, T.B., Mullie, A. *et al.* (1982) Comparative pharmacokinetics of piperacillin in normals and in patients with renal failure. *Journal of Antimicrobial Chemotherapy,* **9** (supplement B), 49–57.

79. Doherty, J.E., Flanigan, W.J., Patterson, R.M. & Dalrymple, G.V. (1969) The excretion of tritiated digoxin in normal human volunteers before and after unilateral nephrectomy. *Circulation,* **40,** 555–561.

80. Dollery, C.T., George, C.F. & Orme, M. L'E. (1974) Drug interactions affecting cardiovascular therapy. In Cluff, L.E. & Petrie, J.C. (eds) *Clinical Effects of Interaction Between Drugs,* pp. 117–151. Amsterdam: Excerpta Medica.

81. Doluisio, J.T. & Dittert, L.W. (1969) Influence of repetitive dosing of tetracycline on biologic half-life in serum. *Clinical Pharmacology and Therapeutics,* **10,** 690–701.

82. Doshi, J., Luisada-Opper, A. & Leevy, C.M. (1972) Microsomal pentobarbital hydroxylase activity in acute viral hepatitis. *Proceed-*

ings of the Society for Experimental Biology and Medicine, **140,** 492–495.

83. Douglas, A.P., Savage, R.L. & Rawlins, M.D. (1978) Paracetamol (acetominophen) kinetics in patients with Gilbert's syndrome. *European Journal of Clinical Pharmacology,* **13,** 209–212.

84. Dow, R.J. & Graham, D.J.M. (1986) A review of the human metabolism and pharmacokinetics of nicardipine hydrochloride. *British Journal of Clinical Pharmacology,* **22,** 195S–202S.

85. Dujovne, C.A., Shoeman, D., Bianchine, J. & Lasagna, L. (1972) Experimental bases for the different hepatoxicity of erythromycin preparations in man. *Journal of Laboratory and Clinical Medicine,* **79,** 832–844.

86. Dundee, J.W. (1952) Thiopentone narcosis in the presence of hepatic dysfunction. *British Journal of Anaesthetics,* **24,** 81–100.

87. Du Souich, P. & Erill, S. (1977) Metabolism of procainamide and p-aminobenzoic acid in patients with chronic liver disease. *Clinical Pharmacology and Therapeutics,* **22,** 588–595.

88. Eandi, M., Viano, I., Dinola, F. *et al.* (1983) Pharmacokinetics of norflaxacin in healthy volunteers and patients with renal and hepatic damage. *European Journal of Clinical Microbiology,* **2,** 253–259.

89. Echizen, H., Brecht, T., Niedergesass, S. *et al.* (1985) The effect of dextro-, levo-, and racemic verapamil on atrioventricular conduction in humans. *American Heart Journal,* **109,** 210–217.

90. Edwards, O.M., Courtenay-Evans, R.J., Galley, J.M. *et al.* (1974) Changes in cortisol metabolism following rifampicin therapy. *Lancet,* **ii,** 549–551.

91. Eichelbaum, M. (1986) Polymorphic oxidation of debrisoquine and sparteine. *Progress in Clinical and Biological Research,* **214,** 157–167.

92. Eichelbaum, M., Albrecht, M., Kliems, G. *et al.* (1980) Influence of meso-caval shunt surgery on verapamil kinetics, bioavailability and response. *British Journal of Clinical Pharmacology,* **10,** 527–529.

93. Eichelbaum, M., Mikus, G. and Vogelgesang, B. (1984) Pharmacokinetics of (+)-, (−)- and (±)-verapamil after intravenous administration. *British Journal of Clinical Pharmacology,* **17,** 453–458.

94. Ellard, G.A. (1969) Absorption, metabolism and excretion of pyrazinamide in man. *Tubercle,* **50,** 144–158.

95. Elmore, M., Rissing, J.P., Rink, L. & Brooks, G.F. (1974) Clindamycin-associated hepatotoxicity. *American Journal of Medicine,* **57,** 627–630.

96. Eng, R.H.K., Gorski, S., Person, A. *et al.* (1981) Clindamycin elimination in patients with liver disease. *Journal of Antimicrobial Chemotherapy,* **8,** 277–281.

97. Ernster, L. & Orrenius, S. (1965) Substrate induced synthesis of the hydroxylating enzyme system of liver microsomes. *Federation Proceedings,* **24,** 1190–1199.

98. Ervin, F.R. & Bullock, W.E. (1976) Clinical and pharmacological studies of ticarcillin in gram-negative infections. *Antimicrobial Agents and Chemotherapy,* **9,** 94–101.

99. Esmieu, F., Guibert, J., Rosenkilde, H.C. *et al.* (1980) Pharmacokinetics of cefotaxime in normal human volunteers. *Journal of Antimicrobial Chemotherapy,* **6** (supplement A), 83–92.

100. Estabrook, R.W., Cooper, D.Y. & Rosenthal, O. (1963) The light reversible carbon monoxide inhibition of the steroid C21-hydroxylase system of the adrenal cortex. *Biochemische Zeitschrift,* **338,** 741–755.

101. Evans, G.H., Nies, A.S. & Shand, D.G. (1973) The disposition of propranolol. III: Decreased half-life and volume of distribution as a result of plasma binding in man, monkey, dog and rat. *Journal of Pharmacology and Experimental Therapeutics,* **186,** 114–122.

102. Evans, G.H., Wilkinson, G.R. & Shand, D.G. (1973) The disposition of propranolol. IV. A dominant role for tissue uptake in the dose-dependent extraction of propranolol by the perfused rat liver. *Journal of Pharmacology and Experimental Therapeutics,* **186,** 447–454.

103. Farrell, G.C., Cooksley, W.G.E. & Powell, L.W. (1979) Drug metabolism in liver disease: activity of hepatic microsomal metabolizing enzymes. *Clinical Pharmacology and Therapeutics,* **26,** 483–492.

104. Fass, R.J., Scholand, J.F., Hodges, G.R. & Saslaw, S. (1973) Clindamycin in the treatment of serious anaerobic infections. *Annals of Internal Medicine,* **78,** 853–859.

105. Fishman, J., Roffwarg, H. & Hellman, L. (1973) Disposition of naloxone-7,8 ³H in normal and narcotic dependent men. *Journal of Pharmacology and Experimental Therapeutics,* **187,** 575–589.

106. Foldes, F.F., Swerdlow, M., Lipschitz, E. *et al.* (1956) Comparison of the respiratory effects of suxamethonium and suxethonium in man. *Anaesthesiology,* **17,** 559–568.

107. Forrest, J.A.H., Adrigenssens, P., Finlayson, N.D.C. & Prescott, L.F. (1979) Paracetamol metabolism in chronic liver disease. *European Journal of Clinical Pharmacology,* **15,** 427–431.

108. Forrest, J.A.H., Finlayson, N.D.C., Adjepon-Yamoah, K.K. & Prescott, L.F. (1977) Antipyrine, paracetamol and lignocaine elimination in chronic liver disease. *British Medical Journal,* i, 1384–1387.

109. Garrod, L.P. & O'Grady, F.W. (1971) *Antibiotic and Chemotherapy.* Edinburgh and London: Churchill Livingstone.

110. Geddes, A.M., Schnurr, L.P., Ball, A.P. *et al.* (1977) Cefoxitin: a hospital study. *British Medical Journal,* i, 1126–1128.

111. George, C.F. (1976) Diseases of the alimentary system: absorption, distribution and metabolism of drugs; effects of disease of the gut. *British Medical Journal,* ii, 742–744.

112. George, C.F. (1978) *Topics in Clinical Pharmacology.* London: Kimpton.

113. George, C.F. (1979) Drug kinetics and hepatic blood flow. *Clinical Pharmacokinetics,* **4,** 433–448.

114. George, C.F. (1981) Drug metabolism by the gastrointestinal mucosa. *Clinical Pharmacokinetics,* **6,** 259–274.

115. George, C.F. & Shand, D.G. (1982) Presystemic drug metabolism in the liver. In George, C.F., Shand, D.G. & Renwick, A.G. (eds) *Presystemic Drug Elimination,* pp. 69–77. London: Butterworths.

116. George, C.F., Orme, M.L'E., Buranapong, P. *et al.* (1976) Contribution of the liver to overall elimination of propranolol. *Journal of Pharmacokinetics and Biopharmaceutics,* **4,** 17–27.

117. Ghoneim, M.M. & Pandya, H. (1975) Plasma protein binding of thiopental in patients with impaired renal or hepatic function. *Anesthesiology,* **42,** 545–549.

118. Gibaldi, M., Boyes, R.W. & Feldman, S. (1971) Influence of first-pass effect on availability of drugs on oral administration. *Journal of Pharmaceutical Sciences,* **60,** 1338–1340.

119. Gill, T.S., Hopkins, K.J., Bottomley, J. *et al.* (1989) Cimetidine-nicoumalone interaction in man: stereochemical considerations. *British Journal of Clinical Pharmacology,* **27,** 469–474.

120. Giron, J.A., Meyers, B.R. & Hirschman, S.Z. (1981) Biliary concentrations of piperacillin in patients undergoing cholescystectomy. *Antimicrobial Agents and Chemotherapy,* **19,** 309–311.

121. Giusti, D.L. (1973) A review of the clinical use of antimicrobial agents in patients with renal and hepatic insufficiency. I. The penicillins. *Drug Intelligence and Clinical Pharmacy,* **7,** 62–74.

122. Glazko, A.J., Chang, T., Drach, J.C. *et al.* (1975) Species differences in the metabolic disposition of adenine arabinoside. In Pavan-Langston, D., Buchanan, R.A. & Alford, C.A. (eds) *Adenine Arabinoside: An Antiviral Agent,* pp. 111–133. New York: Raven Press.

123. Glazko, A.J., Wolf, L.M., Dill, W.A. & Bratton, A.C. (1949) Biochemical studies on chloramphenicol (chloromycetin). *Journal of Pharmacology and Experimental Therapeutics,* **96,** 445–459.

124. Godtfredsen, W.O. (1967) *Fusidic Acid and Some Related Antibiotics.* Copenhagen: Leo Pharmaceutical Products.

125. Godtfredsen, W.O. & Vangedal, S. (1966) On the metabolism of fusidic acid in man. *Acta Chemica Scandinavica,* **20,** 1599–1607.

126. Godtfredsen, W.O., Roholt, K. & Tybring, L. (1962) Fucidin, a new orally active antibiotic. *Lancet,* i, 928–931.

127. Gold, M.S. & Ziegler, D.M. (1973) Dimethylaniline N-oxidase and aminopyrine *N*-demethylase activities of human liver tissue. *Xenobiotica,* **3,** 179–189.

128. Goldstein. A., Aranow, L. & Kaplan, S.M. (1974) *Principles of Drug Action,* 2nd edn. New York, Evanston and London: Harper & Row.

129. Gonzalez, F.J. (1990) Molecular genetics of the P450 superfamily. *Pharmacology and Therapeutics,* **45,** 1–38.

130. Goodman, L.S. & Gilman, A. (1975) *The Pharmacological Basis of Therapeutics,* 5th edn. New York: Macmillan.

131. Graber, H., Arr, M. & Csiba, A. (1979) Biotransformation of azlocillin and mezlocillin. *Acyclureidopenicillins. International Symposium, Vienna, 1979,* pp. 75–77. Amsterdam: Excerpta Medica.

132. Gram, L.F. & Christiansen, T. (1975) First-pass metabolism of imipramine in man. *Clinical Pharmacology and Therapeutics,* **17,** 555–563.

133. Gram, L.F. & Overo, K.F. (1975) First pass metabolism of nortriptyline in man. *Clinical Pharmacology and Therapeutics,* **18,** 305–314.

134. Graziani, A.L., Gibson, G.A. & MacGregor, R.R. (1987) Biliary excretion of imipenem-cilastatin in hospitalized patients. *Antimicrobial Agents and Chemotherapy,* **31,** 1718–1721.

135. Greenblatt, D.J. & Koch-Weser, J. (1974) Clinical toxicity of chlordiazepoxide and diazepam in relation to serum albumin concentration: a report from the Boston Collaborative Drug Surveillance Program. *European Journal of Clinical Pharmacology,* **7,** 259–262.

136. Guengerich, F.P. (1979) Isolation and purification of cytochrome P_{450} and the existence of multiple forms. *Pharmacology and Therapeutics,* **6,** 99–121.

137. Guengerich, F.P. (1983) Roles of cytochrome P450 enzymes in chemical carcinogenesis and cancer chemotherapy. *Cancer Research,* **48,** 2946–2954.

138. Gugler, R., Kurten, J.W., Jensen, C.J. *et al.* (1979) Clofibrate disposition in renal failure and acute and chronic liver disease. *European Journal of Clinical Pharmacology,* **15,** 341–347.

139. Gugler, R., Lain, P. & Azarnoff, D.L. (1975) Effect of portacaval shunt on the disposition of drugs with and without first pass effect. *Journal of Pharmacology and Experimental Therapeutics,* **195,** 416–423.

140. Gundert-Remy, J., Förster, D. & Schact, P. (1978) Pharmakokinetische Untersuchungen von Mezlocillin unter besonderer Berücksichtigung der Galleausscheidung. In Spitzy, K.H. (ed.) *Berichte über das Internationale symposium Acyclureidopenicilline, Stuttgart,* pp. 137–143. Munchen: Verlag für angewandte Wissenschaften.

141. Gundert-Remy, U., Roster, D., Schacht, P. & Weber, E. (1982) Kinetics of mezlocillin in patients with biliary T tube drainage. *Journal of Antimicrobial Chemotherapy,* **9** (supplement A), 65–75.

142. Gyselnyck, A.M., Forrey, A. & Cutler, R. (1971) Pharmacokinetics of gentamicin: distribution and plasma and renal clearance. *Journal of Infectious Diseases,* **124** (supplement 124), 70–76.

143. Hall, K.W., Nightingale, C.M., Gibaldi, M. *et al.* (1982) Pharmacokinetics of erythromycin in normal and alcoholic liver disease subjects. *Journal of Clinical Pharmacology,* **22,** 321–325.

144. Hamlyn, A.N., McKenna, K. & Douglas, A. (1977) Gastric emptying in coeliac disease. *British Medical Journal,* **1,** 1257–1258.

145. Hammer, W. & Sjoqvist, F. (1967) Plasma levels of monomethylated tricyclic antidepressants during treatment with imipramine-like compounds. *Life Sciences,* **6,** 1895–1903.

146. Harding, S.M., Monro, A.J., Thornton, J.E. *et al.* (1981) The comparative pharmacokinetics of ceftazidime and cefotaxime in healthy volunteers. *Journal of Antimicrobial Chemotherapy,* **8** (supplement B), 263–272.

147. Hares, M.M., Hegarty, A., Tomkyns, J. *et al.* (1982) A study of biliary excretion of mecillinam in patients with biliary disease. *Journal of Antimicrobial Chemotherapy,* **9,** 217–222.

148. Hayes, A. & Cooper, R.G. (1971) Studies on the absorption, distribution and excretion of propranolol in rat, dog and monkey. *Journal of Pharmacology and Experimental Therapeutics,* **176,** 302–311.

149. Heel, R.C., Brogden, R.N., Carmine, A. *et al.* (1982) Ketoconazole: A review of its therapeutic efficacy in superficial and systemic fungal infections. *Drugs,* **23,** 1–36.

150. Heni, N., Lehnhardt, G. & Glogner, P. (1976) Elimination kinetics of phenprocoumon (Marcoumar) in liver cirrhosis and after premedication with phenobarbital. *International Journal of Clinical Pharmacology and Biopharmaceutics,* **13,** 253–261.

151. Hepner, G.W., Vesell, E.S., Lipton, A. *et al.* (1977) Disposition of aminopyrine, antipyrine, diazepam and indocyanine green in patients with liver disease or on anticonvulsant therapy. *Journal of Laboratory and Clinical Medicine,* **90,** 440–456.

152. Hermansson, J., Glaumann, H., Karlen, B. & Von Bahr, C. (1980) Metabolism of lidocaine in human liver in vitro. *Acta Pharmacologia et Toxicologia,* **47,** 49–52.

153. Hinthorn, D.R., Baker, L.H., Romig, D.A. *et al.* (1976) Use of

clindamycin in patients with liver disease. *Antimicrobial Agents and Chemotherapy,* **9,** 498–501.

154. Hirom, P.C., Milburn, P., Smith, R.L. & Williams, R.T. (1972) Species variations in the threshold molecular-weight factor for the biliary excretion of organic amines. *Biochemical Journal,* **129,** 1071–1077.

155. Hitzenberger, G., Bonelli, J., Korn, A. & Pesendorfer, F. (1974) Pharmacokinetics of cotrimoxazole in patients with impaired liver function. *Proceedings of the 8th International Congress of Chemotherapy,* **1,** 692–695.

156. Hodgman, J.E. & Burnes, L.E. (1961) Safe and effective chloramphenicol dosages for premature infants. *American Journal of Diseases in Children,* **101,** 140–148.

157. Hoener, B.A. & Patterson, S.E. (1981) Nitrofurantoin disposition. *Clinical Pharmacology and Therapeutics,* **29,** 808–816.

158. Hoeprich, P.D. & Goldstein, E. (1974) Miconazole therapy for coccidiomycosis. *Journal of the American Medical Association,* **230,** 1153–1157.

159. Hoffman, T.A., Cestero, R. & Bullock, W.E. (1970) Pharmacodynamics of carbenicillin in hepatic and renal failure. *Annals of Internal Medicine,* **73,** 173–178.

160. Hogben, C.A.M., Tocco, D.J., Brodie, B.B. & Schanker, L.S. (1959) On the mechanism of intestinal absorption of drugs. *Journal of Pharmacology and Experimental Therapeutics,* **125,** 275–282.

161. Homeida, M., Jackson, L. & Roberts, C.J.C. (1978) Decreased first-pass metabolism of labetalol in chronic liver disease. *British Medical Journal,* **ii,** 1048–1050.

162. Hooper, W.D., Bochner, F., Eadie, M.J. & Tyrer, J.H. (1974) Plasma protein binding of diphenylhydantoin. Effects of sex hormones, renal and hepatic disease. *Clinical Pharmacology and Therapeutics,* **15,** 276–282.

163. Howden, C.W., Birnie, G.G. & Brodie, M.J. (1989) Drug metabolism in liver disease. *Pharmacology and Therapeutics,* **40,** 439–474.

164. Huang, Y.C., Collaizzi, J.L., Bierman, R.H. *et al.* (1986) Pharmacokinetics and dose proportionality of ketoconazole in normal volunteers. *Antimicrobial Agents and Chemotherapy,* **30,** 206–210.

165. Hvidberg, E.F., Andreasen, P.B. & Ranek, L. (1974) Plasma half-life of phenylbutazone in patients with impaired liver function. *Clinical Pharmacology and Theapeutics,* **15,** 171–177.

166. Idle, J.R. & Smith, R.L. (1979) Polymorphisms of oxidation at carbon centers of drugs and their clinical significance. *Drug Metabolism Reviews,* **9,** 301–317.

167. Inaba, T., Jurima, M., Nakano, M. & Kalow, W. (1984) Mephenytoin and sparteine pharmacokinetics in Canadian caucasians. *Clinical Pharmacology and Therapeutics,* **36,** 670–676.

168. Inaba, T., Tyndale, R.E. & Mahon, W.A. (1986) Quinidine: potent inhibition of sparteine and debrisoquine oxidation in vivo. *British Journal of Clinical Pharmacology,* **22,** 109–110.

169. Ings, R.M.J., Law, G.L. & Parnell, E.W. (1966) The metabolism of metronidazole. *Biochemical Pharmacology,* **15,** 515–519.

170. Johnsson, G., Regardh, C.-G. & Solvell, L. (1975) Combined pharmacokinetic and pharmacodynamic studies in man of the adrenergic B₁-receptor antagonist metoprolol. *Acta Pharmacologia et Toxicologia,* **36** (Supplement V), 31–44.

171. Jusko, W.J. & Gibaldi, M. (1972) Effects of change in elimination on various parameters of the two-compartment open model. *Journal of Pharmaceutical Sciences,* **61,** 1270–1273.

172. Kamin, H., Siler Masters, B.S., Gibson, Q.H. & Williams, C.H. (1965) Microsomal TPNH-cytochrome-C-reductase. *Federation Proceedings,* **24,** 1164–1171.

173. Kane, P.O., McFadzean, J.A. & Squires, S. (1961) Absorption and excretion of metronidazole. Part II. Studies on primary failures. *British Journal of Venereal Diseases,* **37,** 276–277.

174. Karlin, J.M. & Kutt, H. (1970) Acute diphenylhydantoin intoxication following halothane anesthesia. *Journal of Pediatrics,* **76,** 941–944.

175. Kato, R. (1979) Characteristics and differences in the hepatic mixed function oxidases of different species. *Pharmacology and Therapeutics,* **6,** 41–98.

176. Keller, H. & Bircher, J. (1980) Miscellaneous antibiotics. In Dukes, M.N.G. (ed.) *Meyler's Side Effects Of Drugs,* 9th edn. pp. 452–473. Amsterdam: Exerpta Medica.

177. Kenna, J.G., Satoh, H., Christ, D.D. & Pohl, L.R. (1988) Metabolic basis for a drug hypersensitivity: antibodies in sera from patients with halothane hepatitis recognize liver neoantigens that contain the trifluoroacetyl group derived from halothane. *Journal of Pharmacology and Experimental Therapeutics,* **245,** 1103–1109.

178. Kleinbloesem, C.H., Van Harten, J., Wilson, J.P.H. *et al.* (1986) Nifedipine kinetics and hemodynamic effects in patients with liver cirrhosis after intravenous and oral administration. *Clinical Pharmacology and Therapeutics,* **40,** 21–28.

179. Klotz, U., Antonin, K.H., Brugel, H. & Bieck, P.R. (1977) Disposition of diazepam and its major metabolite desmethyl diazepam in patients with liver disease. *Clinical Pharmacology and Therapeutics,* **21,** 430–436.

180. Klotz, U., Avant, G.R., Hoyumpa, A. *et al.* (1975) The effects of age and liver disease on the disposition and elimination of diazepam in adult man. *Journal of Clinical Investigation,* **55,** 347–359.

181. Klotz, U., Fischer, C., Müller-Seydlitz, P. *et al.* (1979) Alterations in the disposition of differently cleared drugs in patients with cirrhosis. *Clinical Pharmacology and Therapeutics,* **26,** 221–227.

182. Klotz, U., McHorse, T.S., Wilkinson, G.R. & Schenker, S. (1974) The effect of cirrhosis on the disposition and elimination of meperidine in man. *Clinical Pharmacology and Therapeutics,* **16,** 667–675.

183. Knudsen, E.T. & Harding, J.W. (1975) A multicentre comparative trial of talampicillin and ampicillin in general practice. *British Journal of Clinical Practice,* **29,** 255–266.

184. Koch-Weser, J. & Sellers, E.M. (1976) Binding of drugs to serum albumin. *New England Journal of Medicine,* **294,** 311–316.

185. Koppel, C. & Tenczer, J. (1985) A revision of the metabolic disposition of amantidine. *Biomedical Mass Spectrometry,* **12,** 499–501.

186. Kosmidis, J., Williams, J.D., Andrews, J. *et al.* (1972) Amoxycillin pharmacology, bacteriology and clinical studies. *British Journal of Clinical Practice,* **26,** 341–346.

187. Kosmidis, J., Stathakis, Ch., Mantopoulos, K. *et al.* (1980) Clinical pharmacology of cefotaxime including penetration into bile, sputum, bone and cerebrospinal fluid. *Journal of Antimicrobial Chemotherapy,* **6** (supplement A), 147–151.

188. Kraus, J.W., Desmond, P.V., Marshall, J.P. *et al.* (1978) Effects of ageing and liver disease on disposition of lorazepam. *Clinical Pharmacology and Therapeutics,* **24,** 411–419.

189. Kroboth, P.D., Brown, A., Lyon, J.A. *et al.* (1982) Pharmacokinetics of single dose erythromycin in normal and alcoholic liver disease subjects. *Antimicrobial Agents and Chemotherapy,* **21,** 135–140.

190. Kuhlman, J., Sommer, H. & Forster, D. (1984) Elimination of Azlocillin in patients with cholestasis. In *Proceedings of the IVth Mediterranean Congress of Chemotherapy, Rhodes,* pp. 332–333.

191. Kunin, C.M. (1967) A guide to use of antibiotics in patients with renal disease. *Annals of Internal Medicine,* **67,** 151–158.

192. Kunin, C.M., Craig, W.A., Kornguth, M. & Monson, R. (1973) Influence of binding on the pharmacologic activity of antibiotics. *Annals of the New York Academy of Sciences,* **226,** 214–224.

193. Kunin, C.M., Glazko, A.J. & Finland, M. (1959) Persistence of antibiotics in blood of patients with acute renal failure. II. Chloramphenicol and its metabolic products in the blood of patients with severe renal disease or hepatic cirrhosis. *Journal of Clinical Investigation,* **38,** 1498–1508.

194. Kupfer, A. & Preisig, R. (1984) Pharmacogenetics of mephenytoin: a new drug hydroxylation polymorphism in man. *European Journal of Clinical Pharmacology,* **26,** 753–759.

195. Kutt, H., Winters, W. Scherman, R. & McDowell, F. (1964) Diphenylhydantoin and phenobarbital toxicity: the role of liver disease. *Archives of Neurology,* **11,** 649–656.

196. Laidlaw, J., Read, A.E. & Sherlock, S. (1961) Morphine tolerance in hepatic cirrhosis. *Gastroenterology,* **40,** 389–396.

197. Lebrec, D., Poynard, T., Hillon, P. & Benhamou, J.P. (1981) Propranolol for prevention of recurrent gastrointestinal bleeding in patients with cirrhosis. A controlled study. *New England Journal of Medicine,* **305,** 1371–1374.

198. Leemann, T., Dayer, P. & Meyer, U.A. (1986) Single-dose quinidine treatment inhibits metoprolol oxidation in extensive metabolizers. *European Journal of Clinical Pharmacology,* **29,** 739–741.

199. Levi, A.J., Sherlock, S. & Walker, D. (1968) Phenylbutazone and

isoniazid metabolism in patients with chronic liver disease in relation to previous drug therapy. *Lancet,* **1**, 1275–1279.

200. Levrat, M., Brette, R. & Truchot, R. (1984) L'elimination biliare des antibiotiques. *Revue Internationale d'Hepatologie,* **14**, 137–169.

201. Levy, G. (1966) Kinetics for pharmacologic effects. *Clinical Pharmacology and Therapeutics,* **7**, 362–372.

202. Lewi, P.J., Boelaert, J., Daneels, R. *et al.* (1976) Pharmacokinetic profile of intravenous miconazole in man. *European Journal of Clinical Pharmacology,* **10**, 49–54.

203. Lewis, G.P. & Jusko, W.J. (1975) Pharmacokinetics of ampicillin in cirrhosis. *Clinical Pharmacology and Therapeutics,* **18**, 475–484.

204. Lewis, G.P., Jick, H., Slone, D. & Shapiro, S. (1971) The role of genetic factors and serum protein binding in determining drug response as revealed by comprehensive drug surveillance. *Annals of the New York Academy of Sciences,* **179**, 729–738.

205. Lewis, J.H., Zimmerman, H.J., Benson, G.D. & Ishak, K.G. (1984) Hepatic injury associated with ketoconazole therapy: Analysis of 33 cases. *Gastroenterology,* **86**, 503–513.

206. Letteri, J.M., Mellk, H., Louis, S. *et al.* (1971) Diphenylhydantoin metabolism in uremia. *New England Journal of Medicine,* **285**, 648–652.

207. Lloyd-Still, J.D., Grand, R.J. & Vawter, G.F. (1974) Tetracycline hepatotoxicity in the differential diagnosis of postoperative jaundice. *Journal of Pediatrics,* **84**, 366–370.

208. Lu, A.Y.H. & West, S.B. (1979) Multiplicity of mammalian microsomal cytochromes P$_{450}$. *Pharmacological Reviews,* **31**, 277–295.

209. Luton, E. (1965) Carbon tetrachloride exposure during anticoagulant therapy. *Journal of the American Medical Association,* **964**, 1386–1387.

210. Macdonald, H., Kelly, R.G., Allen, S.E. *et al.* (1973) Pharmacokinetic studies on minocycline in man. *Clinical Pharmacology and Therapeutics,* **14**, 852–861.

211. MacGilchrist, A.J., Birnie, G.G., Cook, A. *et al.* (1986) Pharmacokinetics and pharmacodynamics of intravenous midazolam in patients with severe alcoholic cirrhosis. *Gut,* **27**, 190–195.

212. Macleod, C.M., Barkley, E.A. & Payne, J.A. (1984) Effects of cirrhosis on kinetics of Aztreonam. *Antimicrobial Agents and Chemotherapy,* **26**, 493–497.

213. Mangione, A., Imhoff, T.E., Lee, R.V. *et al.* (1978) Pharmacokinetics of theophylline in hepatic disease. *Chest,* **73**, 616–622.

214. Mao, J.C.H. & Tardrew, P.L. (1965) Demethylation of erythromycins by rabbit tissues in vitro. *Biochemical Pharmacology,* **14**, 1049–1058.

215. Marcus, F.I. & Kapadia, G.G. (1964) The metabolism of tritiated digoxin in cirrhotic patients. *Gastroenterology,* **47**, 517–524.

216. Maroske, D., Knothe, H. & Rox, A. (1976) Die Lebergewebekonzentration von Cephradin und Cephacetril sowie deren Gallenausscheidung. *Journal for the Clinical Study and Treatment of Infections,* **4**, 159–165.

217. Martinez, O.V., Levi, J.V. & Devlin, R.G. (1984) Biliary excretion of Aztreonam in patients with biliary tract disease. *Antimicrobial Agents and Chemotherapy,* **25**, 358–361.

218. Mason, W.D. & Winer, N. (1976) Pharmacokinetics of oxprenolol in normal subjects. *Clinical Pharmacology and Therapeutics,* **20**, 401–412.

219. Mather, L.E., Tucker, G.T., Pflug, A.E. *et al.* (1975) Meperidine kinetics in man, intravenous injection in surgical patients and volunteers. *Clinical Pharmacology and Therapeutics,* **17**, 21–30.

220. Maudgal, D.P., Maxwell, J.D., Lees, L.J. & Wild, R.N. (1982) Biliary excretion of amoxycillin and ceftriaxone after intravenous administration in man. *British Journal of Clinical Pharmacology,* **14**, 213–217.

221. Mawer, G.E., Miller, N.E. & Turnberg, L.A. (1972) Metabolism of amylobarbitone in patients with chronic liver disease. *British Journal of Pharmacology,* **44**, 549–560.

222. Maxwell, J.D., Carrella, M., Parkes, J.D. *et al.* (1972) Plasma disappearance and cerebral effects of chlorpromazine in cirrhosis. *Clinical Science,* **43**, 143–151.

223. McAinsh, J. (1977) Pharmacokinetics of atenolol. *Postgraduate Medical Journal,* **53** (supplement 3), 74–78.

224. McArdle, B. (1940) The serum choline esterase in jaundice and diseases of the liver. *Quarterly Journal of Medicine,* **9**, 107–119.

225. McConnell, J.B., Curry, S.H., Davis, M. & Williams, R. (1982) Clinical effects and metabolism of diazepam in patients with chronic liver disease. *Clinical Science,* **63**, 75–80.

226. McDevitt, D.G., Frisk-Holmberg, M., Hollifield, J.W. & Shand, D.G. (1976) Plasma binding and the affinity of propranolol for a beta-receptor in man. *Clinical Pharmacology and Therapeutics,* **20**, 152–157.

227. McHorse, T.S., Wilkinson, G.R., Johnson, R.F. & Schenker, S. (1975) Effect of acute viral hepatitis on the disposition and elimination of meperidine. *Gastroenterology,* **68**, 775–780.

228. McKee, R.F., MacGilchrist, A.J., Garden, O.J. *et al.* (1988) The antisecretory effect and pharmacokinetics of omeprazole in chronic liver disease. *Alimentary Pharmacology and Therapeutics,* **2**, 429–438.

229. McLean, A., Sutton, J.A., Salmon, J. & Chatelet, D. (1988) Roxithromycin—pharmacokinetic and metabolism study in humans. *British Journal of Clinical Practice,* **42** (supplement 55), 52–53.

230. McNeill, J.J., Anderson, A.E. & Louis, W.J. (1979) Pharmacokinetics of labetalol in hypertensive subjects. *British Journal of Clinical Pharmacology,* **8**, 163S–166S.

231. Medina, A., Fiske, N., Hjelt-Harvey, I. *et al.* (1963) Absorption, diffusion, excretion of a new antibiotic, lincomycin. *Antimicrobial Agents and Chemotherapy,* **4**, 189–196.

232. Mitchard, M., Andrews, J., Kendall, M.J. & Wise, R. (1977) Mecillinam serum levels following intravenous injection: a comparison with pivmecillinam. *Journal of Antimicrobial Chemotherapy,* **3** (supplement B), 83–88.

233. Mitchell, J.R., Jollow, D.J., Potter, W.Z. *et al.* (1973) Acetaminophen-induced hepatic necrosis. I. Role of drug metabolism. *Journal of Pharmacology and Experimental Therapeutics,* **187**, 211–217.

234. Moesgaard, F., Nielsen, M.L. & Scheibel, J.H. (1980) Excretion of clindamycin in bile in common duct obstruction. *World Journal of Surgery,* **4**, 755–760.

235. Montay, G., Bariety, J., Jacquot, C. *et al.* (1984) Pharmacokinetics of the antibacterial pefloxacin in hepatic and renal disease. *Chemotherapia,* **4** (supplement 2), 501–502.

236. Montay, G., Goueffon, Y. & Roquet, F. (1984). Absorption, distribution, metabolic fate and elimination of pefloxacin mesylate in mice, rats, dogs, monkeys and humans. *Antimicrobial Agents and Chemotherapy,* **25**, 463–472.

237. Moore, R.G., Triggs, E.J., Shanks, C.A. & Thomas, J. (1975) Pharmacokinetics of chlormethiazole in humans. *European Journal of Clinical Pharmacology,* **8**, 353–357.

238. Morgan, D.D., Robinson, J.D. & Mendenhall, C.L. (1981) Clinical pharmacokinetics of chlordiazepoxide in patients with alcoholic hepatitis. *European Journal of Clinical Pharmacology,* **19**, 279–285.

239. Nakamura, T., Hashimoto, I., Sawada, Y. *et al.* (1980) Cefoperazone concentration in bile and gallbladder wall after intravenous administration. *Antimicrobial Agents and Chemotherapy,* **18**, 980–982.

240. Neal, E.A., Meffin, P.J., Gregory, P.B. & Blaschke, T.F. (1979) Enhanced bioavailability and decreased clearance of analgesics in patients with cirrhosis. *Gastroenterology,* **77**, 96–102.

241. Nebert, D.W., Adesnik, M., Coon, M.J. *et al.* (1987) The P450 gene superfamily: recommended nomenclature. *DNA,* **6**, 1–11.

242. Nelson, E. (1964) Rate of metabolism of tolbutamide in test subjects with liver disease or with impaired renal function. *American Journal of Medical Sciences,* **248**, 657–659.

243. Neuman, M., Kazmierczak, A. & Cachin, M. (1971) The serum biliary and urinary antibacterial levels of trimethoprim-sulfamethoxazole in relation to the liver function. *Proceedings of the 7th International Congress of Chemotherapy,* **1**, 85–87.

244. Newbould, B.B. & Kilpatrick, R. (1960) Long-acting sulphonamides and protein-binding. *Lancet,* **i**, 887–891.

245. Norrby, S.R., Rogers, J.D., Ferber, F. *et al.* (1984) Disposition of radiolabelled imipenem and cilastation in normal human volunteers. *Antimicrobial Agents and Chemotherapy,* **26**, 707–714.

246. Nunes, H.L., Pecoro, C.C., Judy, K. *et al.* (1964) Turnover and distribution of nafcillin in tissues and body fluids of surgical patients. In Sylvester, J.C. (ed.) *Antimicrobial Agents and Chemotherapy,* pp. 237–249. Michigan: The American Society for Microbiology.

247. Olderhausen, H.F., Menz, H.P., Hartman, I. *et al.* (1974) Serum levels and elimination of thiamphenicol in patients with impaired

liver function and with renal failure on dialysis. *Postgraduate Medical Journal*, **50** (supplement 5), 44–46.

248. Olsen, G.D., Bennett, W.M. & Porter, G.A. (1975) Morphine and phenytoin binding to plasma proteins in renal hepatic failure. *Clinical Pharmacology and Therapeutics*, **7**, 677–684.

249. Oltmanns, D., Pottage, A. & Endell, W. (1983) Pharmacokinetics of tocainide in patients with combined hepatic and renal dysfunction. *European Journal of Clinical Pharmacology*, **25**, 787–790.

250. Omura, T., Sato, R., Cooper, D.Y. *et al.* (1965) Function of cytochrome P-450 of microsomes. *Federation Proceedings*, **24**, 1181–1189.

251. Orme, M.L'E., Breckenridge, A. & Cook, P. (1976) Warfarin and distalgesic interaction. *British Medical Journal*, **i**, 200.

252. Palmer, D.L., Despopoulos, A. & Rael, E.D. (1972) Induction of chloramphenicol metabolism by phenobarbital. *Antimicrobial Agents and Chemotherapy*, **1**, 112–115.

253. Paradelis, S.G. (1975) Absorption and excretion studies of cephalosporins in human subjects. In Williams, J.D. & Geddes, A.M. (eds) *Chemotherapy (Penicillins and Cephalosporins)*, pp. 283–292. London: Plenum Press.

254. Paterson, J.W. (1972) Pharmacogenetics in relation to poisoning. *Medicine* (1st series), **4**, 294–300.

255. Paterson, J.W., Conolly, M.E., Dollery, C.T. *et al.* (1970) The pharmacodynamics and metabolism of propranolol in man. *European Journal of Clinical Pharmacology*, **2**, 127–133.

256. Patwardhan, R.V., Johnson, R.F., Hoyumpa, A. *et al.* (1981) Normal metabolism of morphine in cirrhosis. *Gastroenterology*, **81**, 1006–1011.

257. Pentilla, O., Neuvonen, P.J., Aho, K. & Lehtovaara, R. (1974) Interaction between doxycycline and some antiepileptic drugs. *British Medical Journal*, **2**, 470–472.

258. Pentikainen, P.J., Neuvonen, P.J., Tarpila, S. & Syvalahti, E. (1978) Effect of cirrhosis of the liver on the pharmacokinetics of chlormethiazole. *British Medical Journal*, **2**, 861–863.

259. Peritri, P. & Mazzei, T. (1987) Pharmacokinetics of roxythromycin in renal and hepatic failure and drug interactions. *Journal of Antimicrobial Chemotherapy*, **20** (supplement B), 107–112.

260. Perrier, D. & Gibaldi, M. (1973) Relationship between plasma or serum drug concentration and amount of drug in the body at steady state upon multiple dosing. *Journal of Pharmacokinetics and Biopharmaceutics*, **1**, 17–22.

261. Pessayre, D., Larrey, D., Funck-Brentano, C. & Benhamou, J.P. (1985) Drug interactions and hepatitis produced by some macrolide antibiotics. *Journal of Antimicrobial Chemotherapy*, **16** (supplement A), 181–194.

262. Piafsky, K.M., Borga, O., Odar-Cederlof, L. *et al.* (1978) Increased plasma protein binding of propranolol and chlorpromazine mediated by disease-induced elevations of plasma α_1-acid glycoprotein. *New England Journal of Medicine*, **299**, 1435–1439.

263. Piafsky, K.M., Sitar, D., Rangno, R.E. & Ogilvie, R.I. (1975) Disposition of theophylline in chronic liver disease. *Clinical Pharmacology and Therapeutics*, **17**, 241.

264. Pieri, F., Andre, L.J. & Abed, L. (1969) Étude du métabolisme du métronidazole chez l'homme: demonstration de la présence de cet amoebicide dans la bile. *Médecine Tropicale*, **29**, 375–376.

265. Place, V.A. & Thomas, J.P. (1963) Clinical pharmacology of ethambutol. *American Review of Respiratory Disease*, **87**, 901–904.

266. Pond, S.M., Tong, T., Benowitz, N.L. & Jacob, P. (1980) Enhanced bio-availability of pethidine and pentazocine in patients with cirrhosis of the liver. *Australia & New Zealand Journal of Medicine*, **10**, 515–519.

267. Pond, S.M., Tong, T., Benowitz, N.L. *et al.* (1981) Pre-systemic metabolism of meperidine to normeperidine in normal and cirrhotic subjects. *Clinical Pharmacology and Therapeutics*, **30**, 183–188.

268. Powell, L.W. & Axelsen, E. (1972) Corticosteroids in liver disease: studies on the biological conversion of prednisone to prednisolone and plasma protein binding. *Gut*, **14**, 690–696.

269. Prescott, L.F., Wright, N., Roscoe, P. & Brown, S.S. (1971) Plasma-paracetamol half-life and hepatic necrosis in patients with paracetamol overdosage. *Lancet*, **i**, 519–522.

270. Price Evans, D.A., Mahgoub, A., Sloan, T.P. *et al.* (1980) A family and population study of the genetic polymorphism of debrisoquine oxidation in a white British population. *Journal of Medical Genetics*, **17**, 102–105.

271. Ralph, E.D., Clarke, J.T., Libke, R.D. *et al.* (1974) Pharmacokinetics of metronidazole as determined by bioassay. *Antimicrobial Agents and Chemotherapy*, **6**, 691–696.

272. Rangno, R.E., Piafsky, K.M., Sitar, D. & Ogilvie, R.I. (1976) The clinical pharmacology of theophylline and its pharmacokinetics in pulmonary edema and cirrhosis. *Arzneimittel Forschung*, **26**, 1268–1269.

273. Rao, K.V.N., Mitchison, D.A., Nair, N.G.K. *et al.* (1970) Sulphadimidine acetylation test for classification of patients as slow or rapid inactivators of isoniazid. *British Medical Journal*, **iii**, 495–497.

274. Ratzan, K.R., Ruiz, C. & Irvin, G.L. (1974) Biliary tract excretion of cefazolin, cephalothin and cephaloridine in the presence of biliary tract disease. *Antimicrobial Agents and Chemotherapy*, **6**, 426–431.

275. Read, A.E., Laidlaw, J. & McCarthy, C.F. (1969) Effects of chlorpromazine in patients with hepatic disease. *British Medical Journal*, **ii**, 497–499.

276. Reding, P. (1982) Risk of hepatic encephalopathy in patients taking propranolol for portal hypertension. *Lancet*, **ii**, 550.

277. Regardh, C.-G., Jordo, L., Ervik, M. *et al.* (1981) Pharmacokinetics of metoprolol in patients with hepatic cirrhosis. *Clinical Pharmacokinetics*, **6**, 375–388.

278. Reidenberg, M.M., James, M. & Dring, L.G. (1972) The rate of procaine hydrolysis in serum of normal subjects and diseased patients. *Clinical Pharmacology and Therapeutics*, **13**, 279–284.

279. Remmer, H. & Merker, H.J. (1965) Effect of drugs on the formation of smooth endoplasmic reticulum and drug-metabolizing enzymes. *Annals of the New York Academy of Sciences*, **123**, 79–97.

280. Renwick, A.G., LeVie, J., Challenor, V.F. *et al.* (1987) Factors affecting the pharmacokinetics of nifedipine. *European Journal of Clinical Pharmacology*, **32**, 351–355.

281. Renzini, G., Ravagnan, G., Oliva, B. & Salvetti, E. (1974) Cephradine microbiological activity in vitro and in vivo serum and tissue levels. *Medicamentos de Actualidad*, **10**, 75–83.

282. Richens, A. & Houghton, G.W. (1975) Effect of drug therapy on the metabolism of phenytoin. In Schneider, H., Janz, D., Gardner-Thorpe, G. *et al.* (eds) *Clinical Pharmacology of Anti-epileptic Drugs*, pp. 87–110. Berlin: Springer-Verlag.

283. Richter, E., Breimer, D.D., & Zilly, W. (1980) Disposition of hexobarbital in intra- and extrahepatic cholestasis in man and the influence of drug metabolism-inducing agents. *European Journal of Clinical Pharmacology*, **17**, 197–202.

284. Rieder, J. & Schwartz, D.E. (1975) Pharmakokinetik der Wirkstoffkombination Trimethoprim + Sulfamethoxazol bei Leberkranken im Vergleich zu Gesunden. *Arzneimittel Forschung: Drug Research*, **25**, 656–666.

285. Riegelman, S., Loo, J. & Rowland, M. (1968) Concept of a volume of distribution and possible errors in evaluation of this parameter. *Journal of Pharmaceutical Sciences*, **57**, 128–133.

286. Rietbrock, I., Woodcock, B.G., Kirsten, R. *et al.* (1979) Altered kinetics of verapamil in liver disease and in intensive-care patients. *Proceedings of the British Pharmacological Society, Dublin*, July 17–20th, 1979.

287. Roberts, R.K., Desmond, P.V. & Schenker, S. (1979) Drug prescribing in hepatobiliary disease. *Drugs*, **17**, 198–212.

288. Roberts, R.K., Wilkinson, G.R., Branch, R.A. & Schenker, S. (1978) Effect of age and parenchymal liver disease on the disposition and elimination of chlordiazepoxide (librium). *Gastroenterology*, **75**, 479–485.

289. Roholt, K. (1977) Pharmacokinetic studies with mecillinam and pivmecillinam. *Journal of Antimicrobial Chemotherapy*, **3** (supplement B), 71–81.

290. Rothfeld, E.L., Crews, A.H., Ribot, S. & Bernstein, A. (1965) Severe hypoglycemia. Result of renal retention of chlorpropamide. *Archives of Internal Medicine*, **115**, 468–469.

291. Rothstein. E. & Clancy, D.D. (1969) The toxicity of disulfiram combined with metronidazole. *New England Journal of Medicine*, **280**, 1006–1007.

292. Ryan, D.E. & Levin, W. (1990) Purification and characterization of hepatic microsomal P-450. *Pharmacology and Therapeutics*, **45**, 153–239.

293. Sasame, H.A., Castro, J.A. & Gillette, J.R. (1968) Studies on the destruction of liver microsomal cytochrome P-450 by carbon

tetrachloride administration. *Biochemical Pharmacology*, **17**, 1759–1768.

294. Satoh, H., Fukuda, Y., Anderson, D.K. *et al.* (1985) Immunological studies on the mechanism of halothane induced hepatotoxicity: immunohistochemical evidence of trifluoroacetylated hepatocytes. *Journal of Pharmacology and Experimental Therapeutics*, **233**, 857–862.

295. Sawnhey, V.K., Gregory, P.B., Swezey, S.E. & Blaschke, T.F. (1981) Furosemide disposition in cirrhotic patients. *Gastroenterology*, **81**, 1012–1016.

296. Schoene, B., Fleischmann, R.A., Remmer, H. & Oldershausen, H.F.V. (1972) Determination of drug metabolizing enzymes in needle biopsies of human liver. *European Journal of Clinical Pharmacology*, **4**, 65–73.

297. Schomerus, M., Spiegelhalder, B., Stieren, B. & Eichelbaum, M. (1976) Physiological disposition of verapamil in man. *Cardiovascular Research*, **10**, 605–612.

298. Schonebeck, J., Polak, A., Fernex, M. & Scholer, H.J. (1973) Pharmacokinetic studies on the oral antimycotic agent 5-fluorocytosine in individuals with normal and impaired kidney function. *Chemotherapy*, **18**, 321–336.

299. Schrogie, J.J., Rogers, J.D., Yeh, K.C. *et al.* (1979) Pharmacokinetics and comparative pharmacology of cefoxitin and cephalosporins. *Reviews of Infectious Diseases*, **1**, 90–97.

300. Sellers, E.M., Greenblatt, D.J., Giles, H.G. *et al.* (1979) Chlordiazepoxide and oxazepam disposition in cirrhosis. *Clinical Pharmacology and Therapeutics*, **26**, 240–246.

301. Seltzer, H.S. (1972) Drug-induced hypoglycaemia. A review based on 473 cases. *Diabetes*, **21**, 955–966.

302. Sessions, J.T., Minkel, H.P., Bullard, J.C. & Ingelfinger, F.J. (1954) The effect of barbiturates in patients with liver disease. *Journal of Clinical Investigation*, **33**, 1116–1127.

303. Shand, D.G. & Rangno, R.E. (1972) The disposition of propranolol. 1. Elimination during oral absorption in man. *Pharmacology*, **7**, 159–168.

304. Shand, D.G., Evans, G.H. & Nies, A.S. (1971) The almost complete hepatic extraction of propranolol during intravenous administration in the dog. *Life Sciences*, **10**, 1417–1421.

305. Shand, D.G., Kornhauser, D.M. & Wilkinson, G.R. (1975) Effects of route of administration and blood flow on hepatic drug elimination. *Journal of Pharmacology and Experimental Therapeutics*, **195**, 424–432.

306. Shand, D.G., Nuckolls, E.M. & Oates, J.A. (1970) Plasma propranolol levels in adults with observations in four children. *Clinical Pharmacology and Therapeutics*, **11**, 112–120.

307. Shand, D.G., Rangno, R.E. & Evans, G.H. (1972) The disposition of propranolol. II. Hepatic elimination in the rat. *Pharmacology*, **8**, 344–352.

308. Shideman, F.E., Kelly, A.R., Lee, L.E. *et al.* (1949) The role of the liver in the detoxication of thiopental (Pentothal) in man. *Anesthesiology*, **10**, 421.

309. Shull, H.J., Wilkinson, G.R., Johnson, R. & Schenker, S. (1976) Normal disposition of oxazepam in acute viral hepatitis and cirrhosis. *Annals of Internal Medicine*, **84**, 420–425.

310. Shyu, W.C., Nightingale, C.H., Quintiliani, R. *et al.* (1984) Biliary excretion of Cefotaxime. *Current Therapeutic Research*, **35**, 727–734.

311. Smith, I.L., Ziemniak, J.A., Bernhard, H. *et al.* (1984) Ranitidine disposition and systemic availability in hepatic cirrhosis. *Clinical Pharmacology and Therapeutics*, **35**, 487–494.

312. Smith, R.L. (1973) *The Excretory Function of Bile*. London: Chapman & Hall.

313. Smith, R.L. & Caldwell, J. (1977) Drug metabolism in non-human primates. In Parke, D.V. & Smith, R.L. (eds) *Drug Metabolism from Microbe to Man*, pp. 331–356. London: Taylor & Francis.

314. Smith, S.E. & Rawlins, M.D. (1973) *Variability in Human Drug Response*. London: Butterworth.

315. Snyder, R. & Remmer, H. (1979) Classes of hepatic microsomal mixed function oxidase inducers. *Pharmacology and Therapeutics*, **7**, 203–244.

316. Sommadossi, J.P., Bevan, R., Ling, T. *et al.* (1988) Clinical pharmacokinetics of ganciclovir in patients with normal and impaired renal function. *Review of Infectious Diseases*, **10** (supplement 3), 507–514.

317. Somogyi, A., Albrecht, M., Kliems, G. *et al.* (1981) Pharmacokinetics, bioavailability and ECG response of verapamil in patients with liver cirrhosis. *British Journal of Clinical Pharmacology*, **12**, 51–60.

318. Somogyi, A. & Gugler, R. (1983) Clinical pharmacokinetics of cimetidine. *Clinical Pharmacokinetics*, **8**, 463–495.

319. Somogyi, A. & Gugler, R. (1982) Drug interactions with cimetidine. *Clinical Pharmacokinetics*, **7**, 23–41.

320. Somogyi, A. & Muirhead, M. (1987) Pharmacokinetic interactions of cimetidine. *Clinical Pharmacokinetics*, **12**, 321–366.

321. Sontaniemi, E.A., Pelkonen, R.O. & Puukka, M. (1980) Measurement of hepatic drug-metabolising enzyme activity in man. Comparison of three different assays. *European Journal of Clinical Pharmacology*, **17**, 267–274.

322. Staib, A.H., Schuppan, D., Lissner, R. *et al.* (1980) Pharmacokinetics and metabolism of theophylline in patients with liver disease. *International Journal of Clinical Pharmacology, Therapeutics and Toxicology*, **18**, 500–502.

323. Stamey, T.A., Nemoy, N.J. & Higgins, M. (1969) The clinical use of nalidixic acid. A review and some observations. *Investigative Urology*, **6**, 585–592.

324. Stenson, R.E., Constantino, R.T. & Harrison, D.C. (1971) Interrelationships of hepatic blood flow, cardiac output and blood levels of lidocaine in man. *Circulation*, **43**, 205–211.

325. Stevens, D.A., Levine, H.B. & Deresinski, S.C. (1976) Miconazole in coccidioidomycosis. *American Journal of Medicine*, **60**, 191–202.

326. Storstein, L. & Amlie, J. (1975) Digitoxin pharmacokinetics in chronic active hepatitis. *Digestion*, **12**, 353.

327. Storstein, O., Hansteen, V., Hatle, L. *et al.* (1977) Studies on digitalis. XIII. A prospective study of 649 patients on maintenance treatment with digitoxin. *American Heart Journal*, **93**, 434–443.

328. Stottmeier, K.D., Bream, R.E. & Kubica, G.P. (1968) The absorption and excretion of pyrazinamide. *American Review of Respiratory Disease*, **98**, 70–74.

329. Strong, H.A., Warner, N.J., Renwick, A.G. & George, C.F. (1985) Sulindac metabolism: the importance of an intact colon. *Clinical Pharmacology and Therapeutics*, **38**, 387–393.

330. Suhrland, L.G. & Weisberger, A. (1963) Chloramphenicol toxicity in liver and renal disease. *Archives of Internal Medicine*, **112**, 747–753.

331. Sunahara, S. & Nakagawa, H. (1972) Metabolic study and controlled clinical trials of rifampin. *Chest*, **61**, 526–532.

332. Swabb, E.A., Singhvi, S.M., Leitz, M.A. *et al.* (1983) Metabolism and pharmacokinetics of Aztreonam in healthy subjects. *Antimicrobial Agents and Chemotherapy*, **24**, 394–400.

333. Takenaka, H. & Sakai, K. (1969) Laboratory and clinical studies of flucloxacillin. *Chemotherapy*, **17**, 1428–1433.

334. Tarver, D., Walt, R.P., Dunk, A.A. *et al.* (1983) Precipitation of hepatic encephalopathy by propranolol in cirrhosis. *British Medical Journal*, **287**, 585.

335. Thiessen, J.J., Sellers, E.M., Denbeigh, P. & Dolman, L. (1976) Plasma protein binding of diazepam and tolbutamide in chronic alcoholics. *Journal of Clinical Pharmacology*, **16**, 345–351.

336. Thompson, W.L., Anderson, S.E., Lipsky, J.J. & Lietman, P.S. (1975) Overdose of chloramphenicol. *Journal of the American Medical Association*, **234**, 149–150.

337. Thomson, P.D., Melmon, K.L., Richardson, J.A. *et al.* (1973) Lidocaine pharmacokinetics in advanced heart failure, liver disease, and renal failure in humans. *Annals of Internal Medicine*, **78**, 499–508.

338. Thomson, P.D., Rowland, M. & Melmon, K.L. (1971) The influence of heart failure, liver disease and renal failure on the disposition of lidocaine in man. *American Heart Journal*, **82**, 417–421.

339. Tjandramaga, T.B., Mullie, A., Verbesselt, R. *et al.* (1978) Piperacillin: human pharmacokinetics after intravenous and intramuscular administration. *Antimicrobial Agents and Chemotherapy*, **14**, 829–837.

340. Tolman, K.G., Sannella, J.J. & Feston, J.W. (1974) Chemical structure of erythromycin and hepatotoxicity. *Annals of Internal Medicine*, **81**, 58–60.

341. Twiss, J.R., Berger, W.V., Gillette, L. *et al.* (1956) The biliary excretion of erythromycin (Ilotycin). *Surgery, Gynecology and Obstetrics*, **102**, 355–357.

342. UCLA Conference. Drug-induced hepatotoxicity. *Annals of Internal Medicine,* **104,** 826–829.

343. Ueda, H., Sakurai, T., Ota, M. *et al.* (1963) Disappearance rate of tolbutamide in normal subjects and in diabetes mellitus, liver cirrhosis and renal disease. *Diabetes,* **12,** 414–419.

344. Ullrich, D., Sieg, A., Blune, R. *et al.* (1987) Normal pathways for glucuronidation, sulphation and oxidation of paracetamol in Gilbert's syndrome. *European Journal of Clinical Investigation,* **17,** 237–240.

345. Uribe, M. & Go, V.L.W. (1979) Corticosteroid pharmacokinetics in liver disease. *Clinical Pharmacokinetics,* **4,** 233–240.

346. Uribe, M., Summerskill, W.H.J. & Go, V.L.W. (1982) Comparative serum prednisone and prednisolone concentrations following the administration to patients with chronic active liver disease. *Clinical Pharmacokinetics,* **7,** 452–459.

347. van Marle, W., Woods, K.L. & Beeley, L. (1979) Concurrent steroid and rifampicin therapy. *British Medical Journal,* **i,** 1020.

348. Verstraete, M. & Verwilghen, R. (1976) Haematological disorders. In Avery, G.S. (ed.) *Principles and Practice of Clinical Pharmacology and Therapeutics,* Ch. XXII, pp. 661–716. Edinburgh and London: Churchill Livingstone.

349. Vesell, E.S., Passananti, G.T., Greene, F.E. & Page, J.G. (1971) Genetic control of drug levels and of the induction of drug-metabolizing enzymes in man: individual variability in the extent of allopurinol and nortriptyline inhibition of drug metabolism. *Annals of the New York Academy of Sciences,* **179,** 752–773.

350. Vestal, R.E., Wood, A.J.J., Branch, R.A. *et al.* (1979) Effects of age and cigarette smoking on propranolol disposition. *Clinical Pharmacology and Therapeutics,* **26,** 8–15.

351. Vogelgesang, H., Echizen, H., Schmidt, E. & Eichelbaum, M. (1984) Stereoselective first-pass metabolism of highly cleared drugs: studies of the bioavailability of L- and D-verapamil examined with a stable isotope technique. *British Journal of Clinical Pharmacology,* **18,** 733–740.

352. von Bahr, C., Groth, C.G., Jansson, H. *et al.* (1980) Drug metabolism in human liver in vitro: establishment of a human liver bank. *Clinical Pharmacology and Therapeutics,* **27,** 711–725.

353. Vorhaus, L.J. & Kark, R.M. (1953) Serum cholinesterase in health and disease. *American Journal of Medicine,* **14,** 707–719.

354. Vulterini, S., Bologna, E., Campo, S. & Fostini, R. (1985) Ofloxacin: clinical and pharmacokinetic study in health and disease. In Ishagami, J. (ed.) *Recent Advances in Chemotherapy,* Vol. 2, pp. 1791–1792. Tokyo: University of Tokyo Press.

355. Wallace, S. & Brodie, M.J. (1976) Decreased drug binding in serum from patients with chronic hepatic disease. *European Journal of Clinical Pharmacology,* **9,** 429–432.

356. Waller, D.G., Renwick, A.G., Gruchy, B.S. & George, C.F. (1984) The first-pass metabolism of nifedipine in man. *British Journal of Clinical Pharmacology,* **18,** 951–954.

357. Wenk, M. & Follath, F. (1986) Azlocillin serum levels on repetitive dosage in patients with normal and abnormal renal function. *Chemotherapy,* **32,** 205–208.

358. White, L.O., Holt, H.A., Rever, D.P. *et al.* (1980) Separation and assay of cefotoxime (HR 756) and its metabolites in serum, urine and bile. In Nelson, J.D. & Grassi, C. (eds) *Proceedings 19th ICAAC: Boston,* vol. 1, pp. 153–154. Washington: American Society of Microbiology.

359. Whittaker, J.A. & Price Evans, D.A. (1970) Genetic control of phenylbutazone metabolism in man. *British Medical Journal,* **iv,** 323–328.

360. W.H.O. Cooperative Trial on primary prevention of ischaemic heart disease using clofibrate to lower serum cholesterol: mortality follow-up. (1980) *Lancet,* **2,** 379–385.

361. Whorwell, P.J., Smith, C.L. & Foster, K.J. (1976) Arterial blood gas tensions during upper gastrointestinal endoscopy. *Gut,* **17,** 797–800.

362. Wiegand, R.G. & Chun, A.H.C. (1972) Serum protein binding of erythromycin and erythromycin 2'-propionate ester. *Journal of Pharmaceutical Sciences,* **61,** 425–428.

363. Wilkinson, G.R. & Schenker, S. (1976) Effects of liver disease on drug disposition in man. *Biochemical Pharmacology,* **25,** 2675–2681.

364. Wilkinson, G.R. & Shand, D.G. (1975) A physiological approach to hepatic drug clearance. *Clinical Pharmacology and Therapeutics,* **18,** 377–390.

365. Williams, D.N., Crossley, K., Hoffman, F. & Sabath, L.D. (1975) Parenteral clindamycin phosphate: pharmacology with normal and abnormal liver function and effect on nasal staphylococci. *Antimicrobial Agents and Chemotherapy,* **7,** 153–158.

366. Williams, R.L. & Mamelok, R.D. (1980) Hepatic disease and drug pharmacokinetics. *Clinical Pharmacokinetics,* **5,** 528–547.

367. Williams, R.L., Blaschke, T.F., Meffin, P.J. *et al.* (1976) Influence of viral hepatitis on the disposition of two compounds with high hepatic clearance: lignocaine and indocyanine green. *Clinical Pharmacology and Therapeutics,* **20,** 290–299.

368. Williams, R.L., Blaschke, T.F., Meffin, P.J. *et al.* (1976) Influence of acute viral hepatitis on disposition and plasma binding of tolbutamide. *Clinical Pharmacology and Therapeutics,* **21,** 301–309.

369. Williams, R.L., Schary, W.L., Blaschke, T.F. *et al.* (1976) Influence of acute viral hepatitis on disposition and pharmacologic effect of warfarin. *Clinical Pharmacology and Therapeutics,* **20,** 90–97.

370. Wise, R. (1982) Penicillins and cephalosporins: Antimicrobial and pharmacological properties. *Lancet,* **ii,** 140–143.

371. Wise, R., Lister, D., McNulty, C.A.M. *et al.* (1986) The comparative pharmacokinetics of five quinolones. *Journal of Antimicrobial Chemotherapy,* **18** (supplement D), 71–81.

372. Wise, R., Wright, N. & Wills, P.J. (1981) Pharmacology of cefotaxime and its desacetyl metabolite in renal and hepatic disease. *Antimicrobial Agents and Chemotherapy,* **19,** 526–531.

373. Wolen, R.L., Gruber, C.M., Kiplinger, G.F. & Scholz, N.E. (1971) Concentration of propoxyphene in human plasma following oral, intramuscular and intravenous administration. *Toxicology and Applied Pharmacology,* **19,** 480–492.

374. Wood, A.J.J., Kornhauser, D.M., Wilkinson, G.R. *et al.* (1978) The influence of cirrhosis on steady-state blood concentrations of unbound propranolol after oral administration. *Clinical Pharmacokinetics,* **3,** 478–487.

375. Wood, B.A., Faulker, J.K. & Monro, A.M. (1982) The pharmacokinetics, metabolism and tissue distribution of tinidazole. *Journal of Antimicrobial Chemotherapy,* **10** (Supplement A), 43–57.

376. Woodcock, B.G., Rietbrock, I., Vohringer, H.F. & Rietbrock, N. (1981) Verapamil disposition in liver disease and intensive care patients: kinetics. Clearance and apparent blood flow relationships. *Clinical Pharmacology and Therapeutics,* **29,** 27–34.

377. Wright, N. & Wise, R. (1981) Pharmacokinetics and metabolism of cefotaxime. In Mouton, R.P. (ed.) *Proceedings of Symposium, Utrecht,* pp. 59–74. Amsterdam: Exerpta Medica.

378. Wynn, V. (1965) Metabolic effects of steroid antibiotic fusidic acid. *British Medical Journal,* **i,** 1400–1404.

379. Zeegan, R., Drinkwater, J.E. & Dawson, A.M. (1970) A method for measuring cerebral dysfunction in patients with liver disease. *British Medical Journal,* **ii,** 633–636.

380. Zilly, W., Breimer, D.P. & Richter, E. (1978) Hexobarbital disposition in compensated and decompensated cirrhosis of the liver. *Clinical Pharmacology and Therapeutics,* **23,** 525–534.

381. Zilly, W., Richter, E. & Rietbrock, N. (1975) Pharmacokinetics and metabolism of digoxin- and β-methyl-digoxin-12a-^{3}H in acute hepatitis. *Clinical Pharmacology and Therapeutics,* **17,** 302–309.

PART 2

DIAGNOSIS AND MANAGEMENT

CHAPTER 18

Assessment of Liver Function

Rudi Preisig, Niels Tygstrup & Christopher Price

The liver has a central role in the metabolism of carbohydrates, lipids, proteins, hormones and vitamins, as well as a role as a storage and excretory organ. Consequently, it is not surprising that whole batteries of biochemical measurements have been proposed as 'liver function tests', although not all of these tests relate to the function of the organ. In addition, a variety of exogenous compounds, processed primarily by the liver, have been administered and the fate of the parent compound and/or its metabolites measured in blood, breath or urine in an attempt to assess the functional capacity of the liver. Some of these tests have stood the test of time but, rather than giving an historic overview, this chapter will concentrate on tests of proven value in a format reflecting the way in which the tests may be used:

1. *Search tests*: measurements generally applied for screening healthy people or for confirming (or ruling out) a clinical suspicion of specific liver disease.
2. *Diagnostic tests*: used in patients with clinically, biochemically, and/or histologically documented liver disease in order to arrive at an aetiological diagnosis.
3. *Quantitative function tests*: designed for estimation of severity of the disease, used as a basis for prognosis, and employed for assessing the effects of therapy.

Although these tests may be a reasonable sequence for use in clinical medicine, the history, presenting symptoms and physical signs may provide sufficient information to allow 'jumping' of unnecessary investigations. Furthermore, some selected tests from groups 1 to 3 may also provide important information for assessing results of specific treatments (e.g. ferritin levels measuring the effects of phlebotomy in haemochromatosis) or for determining a given point in time of the natural course of the disease (e.g. fall in aminotransferases and appearance of antibodies in viral hepatitis).

SEARCH TESTS

Except for the screening of healthy people (for insurance examinations, occupational medicine), search tests are usually employed in patients. The most important settings are (1) to confirm a clinical suspicion of the presence of liver disease; (2) to provide background information potentially important for assessing the clinical course (e.g. preoperative evaluation, evaluation prior to drug treatment; (3) to follow the evolution of the liver disease; (4) to arrive at a differential diagnosis (e.g. cholestatic vs non-cholestatic liver disease).

Long before the introduction of automated laboratory equipment it was realized[143] that the sensitivity (defined as the ratio of true positives over true negatives plus false negatives) of any single, commonly available search test was insufficient for reliably determining the presence or absence of liver disease. As a consequence, 'batteries' of tests are usually performed. This procedure, though more costly, has the added benefit of increasing the specificity (ratio of true negatives over true negatives plus false positives). Thus, if more than one test is positive, the probability of the presence of liver disease is very high (Figure 18.1), but abnormal results of a single test (e.g. total serum bilirubin) are found in a larger proportion of normal subjects.[14] The combination of an increased serum bilirubin, an elevated AST or ALT, and an elevated alkaline phosphatase has a predictive accuracy (ratio of true positives over true positives plus false positives) for the presence of liver disease of greater than 90%.[63]

Commonly used search tests are listed in Table 18.1. It must be emphasized that serum bilirubin and virtually all enzymes (with the exception of 5'-nucleotidase) are non-specific in the sense that extrahepatic factors may

have an important influence (in terms of release and/or metabolism) on their serum concentrations.[45] Since rates of disappearance from the bloodstream and volume of distribution are largely unknown, pharmacokinetic interpretation of these blood levels is not possible.

Serum bilirubin, transaminases and enzymes indicative of cholestasis are the most commonly used tests for monitoring patients with liver disease. During follow-up, transaminases play a key role, e.g. in assessing 'activity' of a chronic active hepatitis, implying inflammatory infiltration with associated hepatocellular necrosis. Conversely, the effect of corticosteroids on the hepatic inflammatory lesions in autoimmune hepatitis is best documented by a fall in aminotransferases.[61] Similar considerations apply to enzymes of cholestasis in the follow-up of patients with cholestatic liver diseases and the use of gamma-glutamyltransferase in monitoring abstinence from alcohol.

Serum bilirubin

In recent years, an enormous scientific effort has been devoted to clarifying the handling of bile pigments in the body. Unfortunately, this knowledge has brought little advance to the clinical application of bilirubin measurements. There are three potential causes of an increased total serum bilirubin concentration: increased production, decreased uptake, and/or conjugation and decreased biliary excretion. Within the context of suspected liver disease, the increased total serum bilirubin does little more than confirm the presence of subclinical or clinical jaundice.[91]

Fractionation of bilirubin into its conjugated and unconjugated moieties has no place within the 'search tests'. Its limited application is discussed in the section on diagnostic tests.

Serum aminotransferases

These enzymes are present in high concentration within hepatocytes: AST (a mitochondrial and cytosolic enzyme) is distributed throughout the liver acinus, ALT (a cytosolic enzyme) is predominantly within the periportal zone (zone 1). The presence of AST in extrahepatic tissues, especially muscle, heart and kidney, creates occasional problems in interpretation, but otherwise increased serum levels imply disturbed integrity of hepatocytic membranes (leakage) or cellular necrosis. Serum levels of these enzymes may be grossly elevated in all forms of acute (often more than 10 times upper limit of normal) or chronic hepatitis (often 3-6 times upper limit of normal), with the ALT elevation often being the greater. In acute hepatocellular necrosis due to chemical or vascular injury, when levels can be more than 20 times the upper limit of normal,[31] the elevation of AST is often the greater. In contrast to drug-induced or viral liver disease, alcoholic liver disease is often associated with an AST elevation greater than that

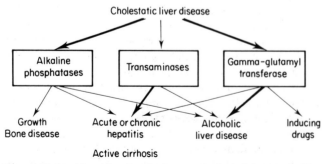

Figure 18.1 Algorithm for the interpretation of changes in liver enzyme tests commonly used in the differential diagnosis of suspected bile duct obstruction.

Table 18.1 Search tests

Test	Normal range (SI units)	Comments on abnormal results
Serum bilirubin		Confirming jaundice
Total	4–17 μmol/l	Assessing severity in PBC
Unconjugated	<0.3 μmol/l	Gilbert's syndrome (Dubin–Johnson)
Aspartate aminotransferase (AST)	11–41 U/l	Hepatocellular leakage or necrosis
Alanine aminotransferase (ALT)	10–37 U/l	AST/ALT > 1 in alcoholic liver damage
Alkaline phosphatase[a]	36–108 U/l	Cholestasis
	30–135 U/l	
	50–275 U/l	
Gamma-glutamyl transferase	11–64 U/l	Cholestasis or induction
5'-Nucleotidase	1–18 U/l	Cholestasis
Total serum bile acids	0–6 μmol/l	Cholestasis/portosystemic shunt
Serum albumin	550–830 μmol/l (30–44 g/l)	Decreased synthetic function, increased turnover or loss, pathological redistribution
Prothrombin time	70–130%	Decreased synthetic function
Hyaluronidase	10–100 ug/l	Fibrotic liver disease

[a] Reference range highly dependent on methodology.

of ALT.[9] This may be due to the release of mitochondrial aspartate aminotransferase[108] while also reflecting varying distribution of the aminotransferases within the liver. Relatively short-lived (days) increases may be observed following acute extrahepatic biliary obstruction, presumably related to the damaging effect of regurgitated bile acids, and during acute circulatory failure[46] as a result of tissue anoxia. Conversely, stable compensated cirrhosis is often associated with normal or near-normal amino transferases.

Generally, ALT is a more sensitive and specific indicator of hepatocellular damage than is AST[81] and has been employed in epidemiological studies,[1,123] but in certain conditions there may be a preferential increase in AST.

Enzymes indicative of cholestasis

The enzymes alkaline phosphatase, gamma-glutamyltransferase and 5'-nucleotidase are all regarded as indicators of cholestasis, presumably due to increased synthesis and release stimulated by the retention of bile acids.[91] For alkaline phosphatase it has been clearly shown that bile duct obstruction leads to *de novo* synthesis of the enzyme at the canalicular face of the hepatocyte[77] and that the serum contains two forms of the enzyme, with the appearance of a form similar to the enzyme present in bile[76,116] The following points should be borne in mind.

Alkaline phosphatase (ALP) constitutes a group of enzymes capable of hydrolysing organic phosphate esters at alkaline pH to yield inorganic phosphate. These enzymes originate not only from the liver, but also from bone (reflecting the osteoblastic activity), from the intestine and from the placenta. Although separation of the enzymatic activities is possible,[76] in the clinical setting confirmation of an increased serum ALP as indicator

of cholestasis may be achieved in most situations by simultaneous determination of gamma-glutamyl transferase and/or 5'-nucleotidase. However, a normal serum 5'-nucleotidase does not always rule out hepatic origin for a raised alkaline phosphatase.[65] The highest levels of ALP are observed with extrahepatic biliary obstruction, but there is considerable overlap with elevated serum concentrations seen as a consequence of inflammatory (hepatitis, granulomas) or infiltrative (metastatic) liver disease.

Gamma-glutamyltransferase (GGT) is found in high concentrations in the kidney, pancreas and liver. In the latter it is primarily localized in membranes of bile canaliculi and of the smooth endoplasmic reticulum. The enzyme catalyses the transfer of the gamma-glutamyl residue to other peptides and to amino acids. GGT is the most sensitive biochemical indicator for the presence of liver disease and is certainly the most sensitive indicator of cholestasis. In contrast to ALP, normal levels are observed during growth, during pregnancy and in subjects with bone disease except in some patients on long-term anticonvulsant therapy. Its interpretation is complicated by the fact that enzyme induction from drugs or chronic excessive alcohol consumption results in increased GGT levels[111] and these are claimed to be the most sensitive test for detecting liver involvement in a suspected alcoholic.[53] However, the parallel increase of ALP and GGT is highly indicative of cholestasis.

5'-Nucleotidase (5NT) hydrolyses nucleotide phosphates with a phosphate residue in the 5-prime position of the pentose. It is the most specific of the cholestatic enzymes, being located in liver membranes, almost exclusively on the bile canalicular side.[91] 5NT is of particular value in adding to the specificity of the other cholestatic enzymes, differentiating liver from bone disease (in the case of ALP) and induction from cholestasis (in the case of GGT), although this is not totally reliable.[65]

Serum bile acids (SBA)

Bile acids are synthesized in the liver from cholesterol. The first products are cholate and chenodeoxycholate (primary bile acids). Following biliary excretion into the gut, deoxycholate (and small amounts of lithocholate) are formed by bacterial 7α-dehydroxylation (secondary bile acids) and reabsorbed into the blood stream (so called enterohepatic circulation). In the liver, epimerization of secondary bile acids leads to tertiary bile acids.[12] Commercially available radioimmunoassays are usually directed against the glycine- or taurine-conjugated forms of the primary bile acids cholate and chenodeoxycholate and the results, called 'serum conjugated bile acids', do not reflect total serum bile acids. They are usually measured in the fasting subject, since estimation of postprandial level confers no major advantage.[55]

Elevated levels of serum bile acid are generally regarded as a very specific indicator of the presence of liver disease except in situations where there is excessive bacterial growth in the small intestine. Despite earlier contrary claims, serum bile acids are less sensitive than other tests, such as the aminotransferases, in the detection of liver disease,[74] but in certain situations they may be of additional help. Thus, compensated cirrhotics with normal aminotransferases may be detected on the basis of increased SBA, since SBA levels are augmented by portosystemic shunting.[97] Augmented SBA represent the earliest indicator of cholestasis of pregnancy; normal levels may help in differentiating Gilbert's syndrome from structural liver disease.[149]

Indicators of synthetic function

Albumin, and several other transport proteins, as well as essential components (Factors I, II, V, VII, X) of the blood coagulation system (measured as prothrombin time) and several acute-phase proteins are synthesized exclusively in the liver.[142] Despite the relatively high frequency of abnormal results, interpretation is hampered by the following facts.

Albumin has a long half-life of 20 days, which may even be increased in the presence of liver disease, thus precluding its use as an indicator of acute injury. Further, serum levels may be low owing to loss into urine, the gut or into a third compartment (ascites). Finally, the sensitivity of serum albumin measurements is relatively low owing to the large reserve capacity of the liver in producing this protein.

Pre-albumin, retinol binding protein and transferrin all have shorter half-lives of 2, 0.5 and 8 days respectively and serum levels may fall more rapidly than albumin with acute injury. As in the case of albumin they are all, so-called, negative acute phase proteins and decreases in serum levels will be seen in many conditions associated with an acute-phase response.

The clotting factors determining prothrombin time are short-lived (hours), making the test suited for evaluating acute liver injury. Because of the complexity of the coagulation system, the sensitivity of the test is not very high; its specificity is low in the presence of malabsorption, since Factors II, VII and X are vitamin K-dependent.

Acute-phase proteins: many proteins produced by the liver constitute the so-called acute-phase proteins, synthesis being modulated during the acute-phase response. The rate of synthesis of proteins such as C-reactive protein, alpha-1-antitrypsin, alpha-1-antichymotrypsin, alpha-1-acid glycoprotein, and haptoglobin is increased in the acute phase response, while that of the transport proteins, referred to above, decreases.[82] Thus, the changes in serum levels of these proteins in patients with liver disease may reflect more than one pathological aetiology.

Indicators of fibrosis (see Chapter 32)

Among the tests suggested for assessment of fibrosis, procollagen type III peptide (PIIIP), hyaluronate (Hy), and laminin have been most extensively studied.[45,47,57] Both PIIIP cleaved off the procollagen molecule during synthesis of collagen type III, hyaluronate (a polysaccharide synthesized by mesenchymal cells), and laminin (a non-collagenous high-molecular-mass glycoprotein of basement membranes) can be estimated in serum using radioimmunoassay. Present evidence suggests that serum hyaluronate and laminin levels[80] may be more useful in distinguishing fibrotic from non-fibrotic liver disease (Figure 18.2) and the diagnostic efficiencies are reported as being very similar.[45,80] The similarity of results with the two latter tests are interesting as they reflect quite different metabolic pathways.

Urine pigments

It is well known that an increase in urine bilirubin can precede changes in the serum level and consequently the urine test using a dipstick method is a useful screening test in the primary care environment.[74] The absence of urobilinogen in the urine as an indicator of bile duct obstruction is less helpful. One report of the use of urine bilirubin and urobilinogen testing to determine the need for additional biochemical tests produced a high proportion of false negative results.[15]

DIAGNOSTIC TESTS

Ideally, the prerequisite for employing diagnostic tests is a clinical suspicion and/or biochemical, radiological or histological confirmation of the presence of liver disease. In clinical practice, some of the diagnostic tests are often performed simultaneously with search tests, when history and clinical findings allow a presumptive diagnosis (viral hepatitis, cirrhosis, etc.) to be made. Routine diagnostic tests are listed in Table 18.2. Most specific diagnostic tests such as hepatitis A IgM antibody titres are not 'liver function tests' and are discussed in conjunction with the specific diagnosis.

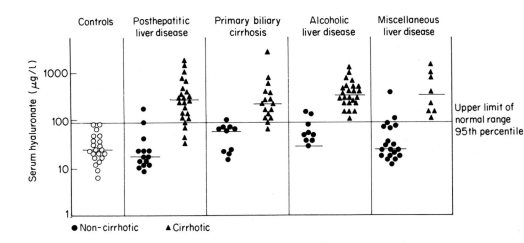

Figure 18.2 Serum hyaluronate levels in normal controls and in patients with biopsy documented chronic liver diseases. On the basis of histology, the latter have been subdivided into those with and without cirrhosis.

Table 18.2 Diagnostic tests

Test	Normal range (SI units)	Comments on abnormal results
Serum iron concentration	8–31 μmol/l	Combination of increased ferritin and increased transferrin saturation highly suggestive of haemochromatosis
Transferrin saturation	< 50%	
Serum ferritin	10–250 μg/l	
Serum caeruloplasmin	1.1–2.9 μmol/l (0.25–0.55 g/l)	Combination of low caeruloplasmin, low total serum copper and increased urinary copper highly suggestive of Wilson's disease
Serum copper	11–24 μmol/l	
Urinary copper excretion	0.15–0.8 μmol/24 h	
Serum alpha-1-antitrypsin	25–64 μmol/l (0.9–1.8 g/l)	Low serum level suggestive of alpha-1-antitrypsin deficiency
Serum alpha-fetoprotein	< 0.29 nmol/l (< 30 μg/l)	Increased levels highly suggestive of hepatocellular carcinoma

Unconjugated bilirubin

Estimation of unconjugated bilirubin (as the difference between the total and the conjugated form) is required for arriving at a definitive diagnosis where a familial non-haemolytic hyperbilirubinaemia is suspected. In the most frequent form, the Gilbert–Meulengracht syndrome, the unconjugated moiety is largely responsible for the increase in total serum bilirubin. During a provocative test (following 24 h fasting or following administration of nicotinic acid) the additional increase in serum bilirubin is almost exclusively due to the unconjugated fraction[132] (Figure 18.3).

Ferritin, transferrin saturation and serum iron concentration

Ferritin (storage protein) and transferrin (transport protein) saturation measurements are the key elements for diagnosing idiopathic haemochromatosis (see Chapter 36). Transferrin saturation is calculated as the ratio of serum iron and total iron binding capacity. Increases in serum ferritin levels are also found in a variety of liver diseases as a result of hepatocellular damage.[117] A serum

ferritin level increased above 200 μg/l together with a transferrin saturation of >50% is highly suggestive of idiopathic haemochromatosis,[10] but the 'gold standard' for a definitive diagnosis remains the hepatic iron content measured in a liver biopsy specimen.

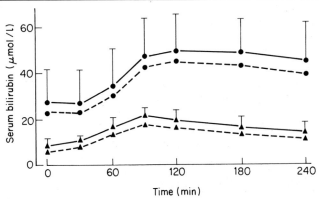

Figure 18.3 Total (——) and unconjugated (---) serum bilirubin in normal controls (solid triangles) and subjects with Gilbert–Meulengracht's syndrome (solid circles) following administration of 50 mg nicotinic acid.

Caeruloplasmin, serum copper and urinary copper excretion

A caeruloplasmin level of <0.2 g/l is suggestive of Wilson's disease (see Chapter 35). Reliance cannot be placed on this single test, since reduced synthesis of this protein may be a sequel of chronic liver disease. Therefore, measurement of total serum copper (which is reduced) and a 24-h urinary copper excretion (which is increased) are important components of the diagnostic approach.[155] Here, too, measurement of the copper content in a liver biopsy specimen is the definitive step for establishing the diagnosis of Wilson's disease.

Alpha-1-antitrypsin

Serum levels of alpha-1-antitrypsin will be low in homozygous alpha-1-antitrypsin deficiency and may be reduced to 10% of normal serum levels (see Chapter 43). They are unreliable for detection of the heterozygote. In all instances phenotyping by isoelectric focusing is required.

Alpha-fetoprotein

High serum levels (usually >500 IU/ml) of alpha-fetoprotein are strongly suggestive of primary liver cancer (see Chapter 39), particularly in subjects with pre-existing liver disease due to hepatitis B infection or due to idiopathic haemochromatosis.[139]

Lipid storage diseases

Biochemical tests in serum and urine are of little value in the diagnosis of the lipid storage diseases and the changes in routine tests can be very variable (see Chapter 44). It is worth noting that a persistently elevated tartrate-resistant acid phosphatase level is often present in Gaucher's disease. The diagnosis of Gaucher's disease may be confirmed using cultured skin fibroblasts or leucocytes and a method capable of detecting heterozygotes and homozygotes using a fluorogenic substrate for the estimation of leucocyte glucocerebrosidase has been described.[112] Cultured skin fibroblasts are also required for the diagnosis of Niemann–Pick disease, a disorder associated with deposition of sphingomyelin in the reticuloendothelial system; again a fluorogenic substrate has been developed for the detection of sphingomyelinase.

Glycogen storage diseases

The diagnosis of glycogen storage diseases is accomplished by direct enzyme assays using liver tissue or cultured skin fibroblasts. The various enzyme deficiencies are discussed in greater detail in Chapter 44.

QUANTITATIVE ASSESSMENT OF LIVER FUNCTION

Quantitative assessment of liver function aids estimation of prognosis, which may be important for making decisions in relation to patient management (e.g. liver transplantation). The understanding of liver function has not changed much during the last century. The liver is partly considered as a central organ in metabolic homeostasis, partly as a filter protecting the organism from harmful substances absorbed from the gut, and as the site of synthesis of many important proteins (Figure 18.4). Most present knowledge of liver functions is related to these aspects. Knowledge about the 'intrinsic' functions, responsible for maintenance of the structural and functional integrity of the liver, is only slowly developing.

Functions involved in maintaining metabolic homeostasis have been extensively studied in the biochemical literature, but this has had little impact on quantitative assessment of liver function, possibly with the exception of the synthesis of albumin and coagulation factors. Most current methods for quantitative assessment of liver function are related to various types of detoxification of endogenous (e.g. bilirubin) and exogenous (e.g. xenobiotic) substances.

Two main problems restrict rational assessment of liver function: the hepatic uptake and release of components is not easily directly quantitated, and the clinical consequences of failing liver function are vague and nonspecific. The so-called liver function tests such as the level of bilirubin, albumin and coagulation factors are liver function tests only to the extent to which they reflect the ability of the liver to eliminate or produce these components. Thus, the serum level of a compound is a result of the amount produced minus the amount eliminated and its volume of distribution at any given time. Furthermore, a functional reserve exists in many instances whereby there is considerable disease progression before the reserve capacity is exceeded.

In contrast to diagnostic tests, which can be assessed by comparison with the definitive diagnosis, usually made by histology, there is no 'gold standard' for validation of quantitative liver function tests. New tests are usually validated from their correlation with other tests, and statistically significant correlation is considered as a positive result. Significant correlation presumes that the results reflect a common factor, which sometimes has been designated the 'functional liver mass'. Correlation does not ascertain that the common causal factor is one of major clinical significance. It is likely, for instance, that the reduced ability of the liver to excrete bromsulphthalein, bilirubin and other organic anions is a phenomenon with limited clinical consequences, e.g. in certain cholestatic conditions, while in other conditions it may reflect a globally reduced 'functional liver mass'. Examples of quantitative liver function tests are given in Table 18.3.

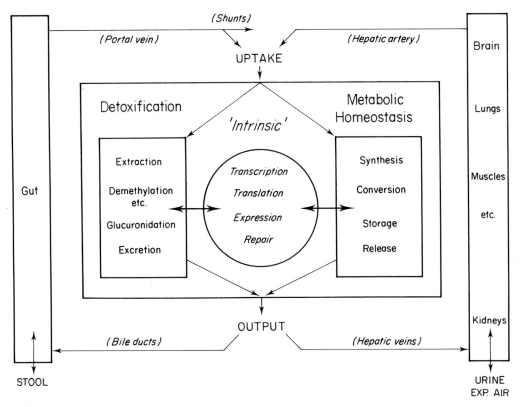

Figure 18.4 A schematic concept of liver functions, with distinction between detoxification, typically in the endoplasmic reticulum, metabolic homeostasis, typically in the cytoplasm, and functional regulation mediated by genes in the nucleus.

Blood tests

Among the commonly used liver tests, serum bilirubin, serum albumin, coagulation factors II, VII, X (prothrombin) and bile acids can be related to liver function. They are based on single blood samples, which makes them attractive for routine use because they cause little inconvenience to the patient and can be assayed quickly and relatively cheaply. On the other hand, the information they give is limited because actual blood levels usually depend on factors other than the quantity of liver function.

Bilirubin

Although jaundice is still the most obvious indicator of liver disease, the relation between quantitative liver function and hyperbilirubinaemia is an indirect one. Uptake of bilirubin from plasma is a hepatocyte plasma membrane function, and conjugation is a function of the smooth endoplasmic reticulum, but there is little evidence that these functions are reduced in parenchymal liver disease, where mainly conjugated bilirubin is increased.

Bilirubin has been found to have prognostic significance in fulminant hepatitis in some[26,38] but not in other studies.[32,121] It is an element in the prognostic scores suggested by Child and Turcotte[25] and by Pugh et al.[118] which in several studies was related to survival in cirrhosis.[70,95,129] The increase in bilirubin over time has prognostic significance in cirrhosis in general[30] and particularly in primary biliary cirrhosis.[138] Furthermore, it is a significant element in Cox regression models of the prognosis in cirrhosis in general,[113,129,135,150] for short-term survival[70] in primary biliary cirrhosis with[27,126] and without[127] inclusion of histological observations, for alcoholic cirrhosis[144] and for compensated cirrhosis.[52] Bilirubin values have great weight in a time-dependent

Table 18.3 Quantitative liver function tests

Estimated function	Type of test	Adverse effects[a]	Reference
Metabolic capacity	Galactose elimination	0	143
	ICG max. removal rate	2	110
	BSP storage	3	156
Microsomal function	Aminopyrine demethylation	1	16
	Antipyrine clearance	1	42
	Caffeine clearance	0	124
Functional hepatic perfusion	ICG clearance	2	110
	Galactose clearance	0	146
	Sorbital clearance	0	99
Excretory function	BSP clearance (k_2)	3	69
	BSP T_{max}	3	156

[a] 0 = No serious adverse effects. 1 = Theoretical risk of drug reaction. 2 = Exceedingly rare anaphylactic reaction. 3 = Very rare, but fatal reaction described.

prognostic index[29] based on longitudinal observations. A rise in bilirubin is a bad prognostic sign in cirrhosis.

Albumin

Albumin is one of the liver-specific proteins and quantitatively one of the most important ones. Serum albumin is generally accepted as part of the 'liver test battery'. Albumin turnover rate is relatively slow, so that changes in the rate of synthesis are reflected by the serum concentration only with some delay. Furthermore, the hepatic albumin synthesis rate is only one of the determinants of serum albumin, the others being rate of degradation, loss into the gut and urine, and volume of distribution.[60] All three factors may contribute to the well-established role of serum albumin as a prognostic indicator in advanced, chronic liver disease, in contrast to fulminant liver failure.[26] In the latter case, other proteins with shorter turnover times may be of value, such as coagulation factors (see below) prealbumin, transferrin or heat-stable alpha-glycoprotein.[79]

Like bilirubin, serum albumin is an element of the prognostic scores. It is a significant variable in the regression analysis studies mentioned above, except the study on compensated cirrhosis[52] and in two studies[135,144] where it was replaced by pseudocholinesterase, which is highly correlated with serum albumin.

Prothrombin

Prothrombin time (coagulation factors II, VII, and X) is quickly prolonged in liver damage because of the short half life of these factors. For factor VII this is only a few hours. Low values, not directly related to liver function, may be caused by malabsorption of vitamin K, by consumption coagulopathy, and treatment with anticoagulants. Direct determination of, e.g., Factor VII levels is possible, but has only been evaluated as a quantitative liver function test in a small series of patients with fulminant liver failure[41] with encouraging results, and Factor V was demonstrated to be a powerful predictor of survival by both univariate and multivariate analysis in fulminant hepatitis B.[11]

Prothrombin has for a long time been accepted as a prognostic indicator in fulminant hepatitis,[32,120,145] the latter study finding two-thirds surviving with prothrombin index >25% against one-fifth with lower values. Other studies have failed to confirm this,[67] possibly owing to the influence of disseminated intravascular coagulation.[66] In a multivariate analysis, based on routine tests and clinical observations, prothrombin contributed significantly,[26] whereas in univariate analysis it discriminated less well between survivors and non-survivors than did bilirubin.

Prothrombin was significantly different in cirrhotic patients surviving less than, compared with more than 3 months.[159] In the Pugh score, prothrombin time replaces nutrition of the Child–Turcotte score. In regression studies

on cirrhosis, prothrombin is less frequently among the significant variables than albumin. Stepwise discriminant analysis of 1-year survival in alcoholic liver disease included prothrombin, but regression analysis did not.[107] In a study of 1155 cirrhotic patients prothrombin contributed significantly in decompensated as well as in compensated cases, whereas bilirubin and albumin did not[36] and it also replaced albumin in the above-mentioned study of compensated cirrhosis.[52] In PBC it was included in the model without[127] but not in that with histology.[27] Prothrombin was included in a time-dependent (i.e. based on consecutive determinations) index of the therapeutic effect of prednisone in cirrhosis,[29] but not in a similar index based on observations at entry into the study,[28] confirming that prothrombin is a better indicator of short-term than of long-term prognosis. The direction and/or rate of change of the prothrombin level may yield important additional information.

Bile acid

Bile acid assay is less common. Several types of analysis have been proposed (fasting or postprandial values, conjugated/unconjugated bile acids, primary/secondary bile acids) and fairly simple radioimmunoassays have been developed. Bile acids are synthesized in the liver, yet the serum concentration is usually increased in liver disease owing to incomplete extraction of reabsorbed bile acids from the portal blood (intra- or extrahepatic shunts), or to defects in the canalicular excretion. In the latter respect bile acids share the conditions of bilirubin and probably give practically the same information. In chronic hepatitis a relation has been found between the bile acid level and bridging necrosis in the liver biopsy[100] and a better relation to reduced function than to shunting, assessed from mephenytoin metabolites.[6] Other studies indicate that shunts play a major role for bile acid elevation in patients with cirrhosis.[97,105] By univariate analysis, total conjugated primary bile acids in the serum discriminated better between 1-year survivors and non-survivors with cirrhosis than bilirubin, albumin and prothrombin.[88]

Conjugation of bile acids was found by Horak et al.[67] to have prognostic significance in fulminant hepatitis. This was confirmed for cholic acid conjugation,[26] which when entered into a discriminant score made the contribution of bilirubin and prothrombin insignificant.

Tolerance tests

Study of the activity of a given hepatic metabolic pathway usually requires administration of a test substance and subsequent collection and analysis of blood or other body fluids. For this reason, tolerance tests are rarely accepted for routine use, even if much has been done to make them simpler without losing much sensitivity. It probably must be accepted that the quantitative assessment of liver function is a complex matter which cannot be answered reliably by simple means.

Aminopyrine breath test

Ingestion or intravenous injection of ^{14}C-methyl-labelled antipyrine results in $^{14}CO_2$ in the breath, which can be taken as a measure of demethylation in the endoplasmic P450 system.[85] Several intermediate steps are involved which may influence the result.[71] In animal studies the test correlates with liver[83] and hepatocyte[122] volume, and it predicts survival in experimental cirrhosis,[58] but in this situation it is not correlated with hepatocyte mass.

Results of the breath test are given in arbitrary units, i.e. they cannot be compared directly with kinetic constants of other processes. The amount of radioactivity given by performing the test is considered to be insignificant.[64] As with other substances metabolized in this system, enzyme induction[40,83] or inhibition[131] may influence the result. Comparison of exhaled $^{14}CO_2$ in 2 hours with aminopyrine blood clearance showed a correlation coefficient of about 0.9,[64] indicating that about 80% of the variation in $^{14}CO_2$ output is determined by the blood clearance. Later studies indicate 30 min to be the optimum sampling time[98] for minimizing the influence of enzyme induction and inhibition, which may be more pronounced in patients with cirrhosis than in normal subjects.[101]

The test result is significantly correlated with albumin,[64] bromsulphthalein[16,64] and galactose elimination[16,98] and systemic clearance of Indocyanine Green,[98] but only weakly correlated with prothrombin time.[21] A relation has been demonstrated between aminopyrine breath test and histological severity in alcoholic cirrhosis,[21] necroinflammatory changes in cirrhosis,[137] and bridging necrosis in chronic hepatitis[100] but not with presence or absence of cirrhosis in patients with cholestasis due to PBC, sclerosing cholangitis and large duct obstruction,[8] or with development of liver damage following intestinal bypass surgery.[7]

By univariate analysis the aminopyrine breath test was found to be of prognostic significance in acute paracetamol intoxication[134] and also in cirrhosis[3,9,64,95,137] except in one study.[63] Two multivariate studies on survival in cirrhosis failed to include aminopyrine breath test in the final model.

Antipyrine clearance

Antipyrine elimination from the blood follows first-order kinetics[56] and it is converted to a number of metabolites in the microsomal system.[37] In experimental studies the elimination has been found to follow Michaelis–Menten kinetics,[19] and the measured clearance equals the V_{max}/K_m ratio, i.e. the intrinsic hepatic clearance, which is independent of the hepatic blood flow.[160] Disadvantages of the test—excluding the dependence on induction and inhibition, which it shares with other substances metabolized in the microsomal system[148]—are that acute changes cannot be measured (the test lasts for 24 h), that it cannot be repeated at intervals of less than a week (owing to induction by the test dose), and the (theoretical) risk of drug reactions. It is weakly protein bound, and antipyrine clearance can be determined by a simple, non-invasive, self-administered test based on oral administration and collection of saliva.[42]

Antipyrine clearance has been used to evaluate hepatotoxic effects of methotrexate given to patients with psoriasis,[109] and to follow restoration of liver function after transplantation.[93] It is highly correlated to galactose elimination capacity,[18,89,145] to bromsulphthalein,[34] and to caffeine clearance.[89] In fulminant hepatitis it was of value in univariate analysis for prediction of survival[120] but did not contribute significantly by multivariate analysis.[26] It seems that high antipyrine clearance invariably indicates a good prognosis, whereas low values may be seen in both lethal and non-lethal cases.[145]

Clearance studies with acceptable sample size of survival in cirrhosis have not been published, but the test reflects the degree of hepatic incapacity[18] and renal sodium retention[161] in patients with cirrhosis. Neither antipyrine clearance nor galactose elimination were significantly correlated with psychometric tests in patients with portocaval anastomosis.[125]

Caffeine clearance

This test, introduced originally as a breath test[158] reflects P450 metabolism. The number of metabolites is high, but the rate-limiting step is N-demethylation.[3] Specific activity in breath measured 120 min after intravenous injection correlates well with caffeine plasma clearance.[124] Measurement of caffeine in saliva[75] increases the acceptability of the test, particularly in children.[13] The clearance showed a hyperbolic relation to fasting caffeine concentration, which therefore was suggested as a simple measure of liver function. This has been found not to be the case unless the caffeine intake during the preceding days was strictly controlled.[89] The metabolism is not induced by phenobarbital, but is by smoking.[73] Caffeine clearance is significantly correlated with antipyrine clearance,[24,89] galactose elimination[89,124] and bromsulphthalein clearance.[124]

In 110 patients with cirrhosis, 24 with PBC, caffeine clearance was significantly lower in patients who died within 30 months than in survivors,[86] and it was claimed to be of special value in predicting the need for liver transplantation.[24] Multivariate studies including caffeine clearance have not been published.

Other xenobiotics

Formation of a lignocaine metabolite in liver donors was found to give information on the chance of survival of the graft, one-fourth being rejected against two-thirds by the selected value of discrimination.[104] Galactose elimination and Indocyanine Green clearance were not of value in predicting graft survival. A breath test using phenacetin[17] and a breath test of mitochondrial function using ketoisocaproic acid[84] have been described but not clinically evaluated. The latter test is stimulated by ethanol and inhibited by salicylate.

Galactose elimination

Galactose tolerance, introduced as a liver function test in 1906, has been studied in a number of modifications, especially intravenous tests which avoid the variations in intestinal absorption of galactose. When given in sufficiently high dose, and with adequate sampling of blood and urine, the elimination capacity[143] as an expression of 'functional liver mass' can be estimated with good reproducibility.[59] It is an invasive test requiring technical assistance for intravenous administration and repeated blood sampling, which limits its use in large-scale studies. However, it is innocuous and the result can be obtained quickly so that it is well suited for following acute changes. Acute alcohol ingestion inhibits galactose elimination, and the patient must have been abstinent for 24 h. A breath test has been developed[140] which correlated with hepatocyte mass,[58] but the relation between galactose elimination rate and CO_2 production from galactose may depend on extrahepatic factors which make the test unreliable, e.g. diabetic patients.[115] Apart from correlation with other tests mentioned above, it is correlated with bromsulphthalein,[16,124] with Indocyanine Green intrinsic clearance,[78,98] with prealbumin level[128] and tryptophan elimination,[133] and with the Child–Turcotte score in cirrhotics.[128] Furthermore, the galactose elimination capacity was used to demonstrate a significant reduction in the liver function of kidney graft recipients.[48]

In fulminant liver failure it was significantly different in surviving versus non-surviving patients, with increasing values after admission invariably a signal of survival.[120] It seems to be of particular value for the early identification of fatal cases[145] (i.e. with high priority for transplantation). Following partial hepatectomy in man[72] galactose elimination and caffeine clearance are reduced to 60 and 50% respectively but after 3 months liver volume and caffeine clearance are restored to 75% and galactose elimination to 100%.

Prognostic significance in cirrhosis has been shown in three studies by univariate analysis,[2,87,95] but was not found in one.[86] Repeated determinations in five patients with PBC predicted the time of death to within ±2 months by extrapolation.[33] In cirrhotic patients with hepatocellular carcinoma (HCC), galactose elimination was reduced further than in those without HCC,[20] and in patients with alcoholic cirrhosis it deteriorated more rapidly in drinking than in abstinent cases.[90]

Galactose elimination did not contribute significantly in multivariate analysis of survival in fulminant liver failure[26] and in two studies on cirrhosis, using the Child–Turcotte or Pugh scores,[54] whereas one showed a slight contribution.[95]

Bromosulphthalein elimination

This has been widely studied, either as the retention test or estimation of elimination constants after intravenous bolus injection, or determination of storage and transport maximum during continuous infusion.[69,156] Like bilirubin and other organic anions its elimination largely reflects biliary excretion, and it has primarily been used for diagnostic purposes. The substance has been withdrawn from the market in many countries owing to rare but fatal anaphylactic reactions, and the test is therefore not generally available. Its correlation with other quantitative tests, mentioned above, essentially emanates from chronic, non-cholestatic liver disease.

Rose Bengal, which has properties very similar to bromsulphthalein, is also used infrequently now.

Indocyanine Green

Indocyanine Green (ICG), another organic anion, has replaced bromsulphthalein for estimation of hepatic blood flow. It is extracted with high efficiency by the liver and excreted unchanged in the bile. It is used either as a bolus injection for measurement of elimination constants, or as continuous infusion for estimation of clearance. Owing to the high extraction, the clearance (amount infused/arterial concentration) is high and dependent on the hepatic blood flow.[160] For quantitative assessment of liver function, the 'intrinsic' clearance (amount infused/(arterial-hepatic venous concentration)) should be determined,[78] but the need for sampling of hepatic venous blood limits its use. The correlation with other quantitive tests is mentioned above. It has been positively correlated with the Child–Turcotte score in cirrhosis.[9]

Univariate analysis of survival in cirrhosis has shown significantly different Indocyanine Green clearance, whether measured by bolus injection or continuous infusion and as systemic or intrinsic clearance. In patients with surgical portocaval shunt it was not related to survival or to development of encephalopathy.[114] In several multivariate studies, Indocyanine Green did not contribute significantly after inclusion of the Child–Turcotte or the Pugh score.[2,54,94,95]

Clearance of sorbital

The clearance of the natural polyol sorbital also provides an estimate of the function of the normal liver.[99] In addition, measurement of the bioavailability—after enteral and parenteral administration—can provide an estimate of intra- and extrahepatic shunting in chronic liver disease.[22] The clinical utility of tests based on sorbital has not been demonstrated so far.

Urea synthesis

Urea synthesis is a specific liver function, and the rate may be estimated by measuring urinary urea output, even if this slightly underestimates production rate. Urea is broken down by urease activity of the intestinal flora to ammonia, which is resynthesized to urea in the liver.[154] The hepatic urea synthesis rate is regulated by substrate concentration (mainly alpha-amino acids) and by hormones (especially glucagon and insulin), which therefore should be taken into account to obtain a reliable relation between urea synthesis and liver function.[151]

Urinary urea excretion has been found to be of prognostic value in fulminant hepatic failure[103] and cirrhosis with hepatic coma[152] and correlates with the Child–Turcotte score in cirrhosis.[43] Urea production after a protein load, attempting to saturate the synthesis processes,[130] is correlated with the Child–Turcotte score and the risk of developing encephalopathy.[4,125] Measurement of urea production during amino acid infusion estimates production relative to substrate concentration.[151] This 'clearance' is closely correlated with galactose elimination.[153] Multivariate analysis of urea synthesis determinations and survival has not been published.

Other applications

Quantitative liver function tests have been, and should be, used for other purposes than estimation of spontaneous survival in groups of liver patients. The aminopyrine breath test has been used as a predictor of the favourable effect of prednisolone treatment in chronic active hepatitis,[50] and the galactose test and others have been used to show that reduction of hepatic blood flow by vasopressin[119] and beta blockade[96] does not reduce liver function. Furthermore, the gradual deterioration of liver function with age has been demonstrated by aminopyrine and caffeine breath tests, and most consistently with galactose elimination,[136] which was also correlated with the decrease in liver volume.

Lately great interest has been devoted to selection of patients for liver transplantation. The problem has two aspects which are related but not identical: the expected survival without transplantation, and the expected survival with transplantation. The first question is studied by assessing patients for transplantation with a prognostic index developed in a previous cohort of patients and comparing predicted and actual survival.[39,102] Both studies showed significantly better survival in the patients with a transplant than predicted from their prognostic index. In principle this approach is identical with using historical controls for evaluation of therapeutic effect, and it is open to the same criticism, but is probably the best alternative to a randomized trial. The second question is primarily one of the relation between reduced liver function and surgical risk, which the Child–Turcotte score was originally proposed to answer concerning portocaval anastomosis.

Assessment of surgical risk

Surgical intervention in patients with chronic liver disease is associated with an increased risk.[5] A reliable preoperative assessment of the surgical risk is particularly desirable

prior to hepatic resections[23] or shunt procedures which result in further reduction of hepatic function. Three studies suggest that quantitation of liver function preoperatively may yield important clues to outcome. A study analysing surgical intervention in general showed that an aminopyrine breath test below 2.3% was associated with high postoperative mortality, whereas the Child–Turcotte score had little predictive power.[51] Likewise, in patients with extrahepatic obstruction the clearance of antipyrine provided an estimate of the outcome,[92] and the maximum rate of ICG removal yielded a reliable estimate of surgical risk related to tumour resection of the liver.[106] Galactose elimination was found to be a useful estimate of the need for surgery (shunt procedure or transplantation) in Budd–Chiari syndrome.[62]

Liver transplantation is a major surgical procedure which requires special risk evaluation. Stepwise discriminant analysis has shown serum creatinine to be the most significant test, much more than bilirubin.[35] Other studies[44] have confirmed the high significance of kidney function, and the relatively low significance of routine liver tests.[141] The results of such studies naturally depend highly on the selection of patients for transplantation and therefore may vary between centres.

CONCLUSIONS

It will be clear from the foregoing discussion that the relationship between function, pathology and diagnostic tests is, in many instances, tenuous. Biochemical tests have been shown to be valuable in the detection and confirmation of liver disease. Biochemical tests, on the other hand, have a limited role to play in routine differential diagnosis, being a minor partner in the full diagnostic armamentarium of the hepatologist. In certain circumstances, where the pathophysiology of the disease is understood, biochemical tests can, and do, provide the confirmatory diagnostic test.

The developments of dynamic function in recent years have provided valuable data while not gaining widespread acceptance in routine practice. The results have confirmed the central role of the liver, its large reserve capacity, and the multifactorial nature of biochemical changes in pathological states. Despite this apparent dilemma, the simple maxim of knowing the question being asked and the limitations of the answer is paramount.

REFERENCES

1. Aach, R.D., Szmuness, W., Mosley, J.W. *et al.* (1981) Serum alanine aminotransferase of donors in relation to the risk of non-A non-B hepatitis. The transfusion transmitted virus study. *New England Journal of Medicine*, **304**, 989–994.

2. Albers, I., Hartmann, H., Bircher, J. & Creutzfeldt, W. (1989) Superiority of the Child–Pugh classification to quantitative liver function tests for assessing prognosis of liver cirrhosis. *Scandinavian Journal of Gastroenterology*, **24**, 269–276.

3. Aldridge, A., Parsons, W.D. & Neims, A.H. (1977) Stimulation

of caffeine metabolism in the rat by 3-methylcholanthrene. *Life Sciences*, **21**, 967–974.

4. Ansley, J.D., Isaacs, J.W., Rikkers, L. *et al.* (1978) Quantitative tests of nitrogen metabolism in cirrhosis; relation to other manifestations of liver disease. *Gastroenterology*, **75**, 570–579.

5. Aranha, G.V., Sontag, S.J. & Greenlee, H.B. (1982) Cholecystectomy in cirrhotic patients: A formidable operation. *American Journal of Surgery*, **143**, 55–60.

6. Arns, P.A., DiBesceglie, A., Waggoner, J.G. *et al.* (1988) Elev-

ation of bile acids in liver disease are more closely related to reductions in hepatic function than development of portasystemic shunts. *Hepatology*, **8**, 87.

7. Baker, A.L., Krager, P.S., Glagov, S. & Schoeller, D. (1983) Aminopyrine breath test. Prospective comparison with liver histology and liver chemistry tests following jejunoileal bypass performed for refractory obesity. *Digestive Diseases and Sciences*, **28**, 405–410.

8. Baker, A.L., Krager, P.S., Kotake, A.N. & Schoeller, D.A. (1987) The aminopyrine breath test does not correlate with histologic disease severity in patients with cholestasis. *Hepatology*, **7**, 464–467.

9. Barbare, J.C., Poupon, R.E., Jaillon, P. *et al.* (1985) Intrinsic hepatic clearance and Child–Turcotte classification for assessment of liver function in cirrhosis. *Journal of Hepatology*, **1**, 253–259.

10. Bassett, M., Halliday, J.W. & Powell, L.W. (1984) Genetic hemochromatosis. *Seminars in Liver Disease*, **4**, 217–227.

11. Bernuau, J., Goudeau, A., Poynard, T. *et al.* (1986) Multivariate analysis of prognostic factors in fulminant hepatitis B. *Hepatology*, **6**, 648–651.

12. Berry, W. & Reichen, J. (1983) Bile acid metabolism: Its relation to clinical disease. *Seminars in Liver Disease*, **3**, 330–340.

13. Bianchetti, M.G., Kraemer, R., Passweg, J. *et al.* (1988) Use of salivary levels to predict clearance of caffeine in patients with cystic fibrosis. *Journal of Pediatric Gastroenterology and Nutrition*, **7**, 688–693.

14. Billing, B.H. (1983) A 1983 assessment of the value of bile pigment determinations in the diagnosis of jaundice. *Postgraduate Medical Journal*, **59**, 19–25.

15. Binder, L., Smith, D., Kupka, T. *et al.* (1989) Failure of prediction of liver function test abnormalities with the urine urobilinogen and urine bilirubin assays. *Archives of Pathology and Laboratory Medicine*, **113**, 73–76.

16. Bircher, J., Küpfer, A., Gikalov, I. & Preisig, R. (1976) Aminopyrine demethylation measured by breath analysis in cirrhosis. *Clinical Pharmacology and Therapeutics*. **20**, 484–492.

17. Breen, K.J., Bury, R.W., Calder, J.V. *et al.* A (14C) phenacetin breath test to measure hepatic function in man. *Hepatology*, **4**, 47–52.

18. Buch Andreasen, P., Ranek, L., Statland, B.E. & Tygstrup, N. (1974) Clearance of antipyrine-dependence of quantitative liver function. *European Journal of Clinical Investigation*, **4**, 129–134.

19. Buch Andreasen, P., Tonnesen, K., Rabol, A. & Keiding, S. (1977) Michaelis–Menten kinetics of phenazone elimination in the perfused pig liver. *Acta Pharmacologica et Toxicologica*, **40**, 1–13.

20. Buzzelli, G., Meacci, E., Smorlesi, C., *et al.* (1987) Galactose loading tests in patients with hepatocellular carcinoma. *Italian Journal of Gastroenterology*, **19**, 95–97.

21. Carlisle, R., Galambos, J.T. & Warren, W.D. (1979) The relationship between conventional liver tests, quantitative function tests and histopathology in cirrhosis. *Digestive Diseases and Sciences*, **24**, 358–362.

22. Cavanna, A., Molino, G., Ballarè, M. *et al.* (1987) Non-invasive evaluation of portal-systemic shunting in man by D-sorbitol bioavailability. *Journal of Hepatology*, **5**, 154–161.

23. Chandler, J.G., van Meter, C.H., Kaiser, D.L. & Mills, S.E. (1985) Factors affecting immediate and long-term survival after emergent and elective splanchnic-systemic shunts. *Annals of Surgery*, **201**, 476–487.

24. Cheng, S.C.W., Murphy, T.L., Smith, M.T. *et al.* (1988) Serial caffeine and antipyrine clearances in the assessment of disease progression with particular reference to liver transplantation. *Hepatology*, **8**, 1403.

25. Child, C.G.III & Turcotte, J.G. (1964) Surgery and portal hypertension. In Child, C.G.III (ed.) *The Liver and Portal Hypertension*, p. 50. Philadelphia: W.B. Saunders.

26. Christensen, E., Bremmelgaard, A., Bahnsen, M. *et al.* (1984) Prediction of fatality in fulminant hepatic failure. *Scandinavian Journal of Gastroenterology*, **19**, 90–96.

27. Christensen, E., Neuberger, J., Crowe, J. *et al.* (1985) Beneficial effect of azathioprine and prediction of prognosis in primary biliary cirrhosis. Final results of an international trial. *Gastroenterology*, **89**, 1084–1091.

28. Christensen, E., Schlichting, P., Andersen, P. *et al.* (1985) A therapeutic index that predicts the individual effects of prednisone in patients with cirrhosis. *Gastroenterology*, **88**, 156–165.

29. Christensen, E., Schlichting, P., Andersen, P. *et al.* (1986) Updating prognosis and therapeutic effect evaluation in cirrhosis with Cox's multiple regression model for time-dependent variables. *Scandinavian Journal of Gastroenterology*, **21**, 163–174.

30. Christensen, E., Schlichting, P., Fauerholdt, L. *et al.* (1986) Changes of laboratory variables with time in cirrhosis: Prognostic and therapeutic significance. *Hepatology*, **5**, 843–853.

31. Clermont, R.J. & Chalmers, T.C. (1967) The transaminase tests in liver disease. *Medicine*, **46**, 197–207.

32. Colombi, T.A. (1970. Early diagnosis of fatal hepatitis. *Digestion*, **3**, 129–145.

33. Cotting, J., Widmer, T., Bircher, J. *et al.* (1987) Accurate prediction of death by serial determination of galactose elimination capacity (GEC) in primary biliary cirrhosis. *Hepatology*, **7**, 124 (Abstract).

34. Couet, C., Brissot, P., Messner, M. *et al.* (1984) Fractional clearance of bromosulfonephthalein and metabolic clearance of antipyrine. Correlative study in liver diseases. *Annals of Gastroenterology and Hepatology (Paris)*, **20**, 1–6.

35. Cuervas-Mons, V., Millan, I., Gavaler, J.S. *et al.* (1986) Prognostic value of preoperatively obtained clinical and laboratory data in predicting survival following orthoptic liver transplantation. *Hepatology*, **6**, 922–927 (Abstract).

36. D'Amico, G., Morabito, A., Pagliaro, L. & Marubini, E. (1986) Liver study group of V Cervello Hospital. Survival and prognostic indicators in compensated and decompensated cirrhosis. *Digestive Diseases and Sciences*, **31**, 468–475.

37. Danhof, M. & Breimer, P.P. (1979) Studies on the different metabolic pathways of antipyrine in man. *British Journal of Clinical Pharmacology*, **8**, 529–537.

38. Davis, M.A., Peters, R.L., Redeker, A.G. & Reynolds, T.B. (1968) Appraisal of the mortality in acute fulminant viral hepatitis. *New England Journal of Medicine*, **278**, 1248–1253.

39. Dickson, E.R., Grambsch, P.M., Marcus, B.M. *et al.* (1988) Transplantation markedly improves survival in PBC patients: Application of the Mayo model on Pittsburg transplant patients. *Gastroenterology*, **94**, A535.

40. Dollery, C.T., Frase, H.S., Mucklow, C.J. & Bulpitt, C.J. (1979) Contribution of environmental factors to variability in human drug metabolism. *Drug Metabolism Review*, **9**, 207–220.

41. Dymock, I.W., Tucker, J.S., Woolf, I.L. *et al.* (1975) Coagulation studies as a prognostic index in acute liver failure. *British Journal of Haematology*, **29**, 385–395.

42. Dessing, M., Poulsen, H.E., Buch Andreasen, P. & Tygstrup, N. (1982) A simple method for determination of antipyrine clearance. *Clinical Pharmacology and Therapeutics*, **32**, 392–396.

43. Einarsson, K., Angelin, B. & Glaumann, H. (1985) Plasma disappearance of 14C-glycocholic acid as a test of liver dysfunction. Relation to liver histology. *Scandinavian Journal of Gastroenterology*, **20**, 175–178.

44. Elias, E. & McMaster, P. (1987) Liver transplantation: Indicators and pre-operative risk factors. *Schweizerische Medicinische Wochenschrift*, **117**, 1053–1060.

45. Engström-Laurent, A., Lööt, L., Nyberg, A. *et al.* (1985) Increased serum levels of hyaluronate in liver disease. *Hepatology*, **5**, 638–642.

46. Fortson, W.C., Tedesco, F.J., Starnes, E.C. *et al.* (1985) Marked elevation of serum transaminase activity associated with extrahepatic biliary tract disease. *Journal of Clinical Gastroenterology*, **7**, 502–505.

47. Frei, A., Zimmermann, A. & Weigand, K. (1984) The N-terminal propeptide of collagen type III in serum reflects activity and degree of fibrosis in patients with chronic liver disease. *Hepatology*, **4**, 830–834.

48. Frey, F.J., Schaad, H.J., Renner, B.L. *et al.* (1989) Impaired liver function in stable renal allograft recipients. *Hepatology*, **9**, 606–613.

49. Galambos, J.T. & Wills, C.E. (1978) Relationship between 505 paired liver tests and biopsies in 242 obese patients. *Gastroenterology*, **74**, 1191–1195.

50. Galizzi, J., Long, R.G., Billing, B.H. & Sherlock, S. (1978) Assessment of the (14C) aminopyrine breath test in liver disease. *Gut*, **19**, 40–45.

51. Gill, R.A., Goodman, M.W., Golfus, G.R. *et al.* (1983) Amino

pyrine breath test predicts surgical risk for patients with liver disease. *Annals of Surgery*, **198**, 701–704.

52. Gins, P., Quintero, E. Arroyo, V. *et al.* (1987) Compensated cirrhosis: Natural history and prognostic factors. *Hepatology*, **7**, 122–128.

53. Gluud, C., Andersen, I., Dietrichson, O. *et al.* (1981) Gamma glutamyltransferase, aspartate aminotransferase and alkaline phosphatase as markers of alcohol consumption in out-patient alcoholics. *European Journal of Clinical Investigation*, **11**, 171–176.

54. Gluud, C., Henriksen, J.H. & Nielsen, G. (1988) Prognostic indicators in alcoholic cirrhotic men. *Hepatology*, **8**, 222–227.

55. Greenfield, S.M., Soloway, R.D., Carithers, R.J. Jr. *et al.* (1986) Evaluation of postprandial serum bile acid response as a test of hepatic function. *Digestive Diseases and Sciences*, **31**, 785–791.

56. Greisen, G. & Andreasen, P.B. (1976) Two compartment analysis of plasma elimination of phenazone in normals and in patients with cirrhosis of the liver. *Acta Pharmacologica et Toxicologica*, **38**, 49–58.

57. Gressner, A.M. & Tittor, W. (1986) Serum laminin - its concentrations increases with portal hypertension in cirrhotic liver disease. *Klinische Wochenschrift*, **64**, 1240–1248.

58. Gross, J.B., Reichen, J., Zeltner, T.B. & Zimmermann, A. (1987) The evolution of changes in quantitative liver function tests in a rat model of biliary cirrhosis: Correlation with morphometric measurement of hepatocyte mass. *Hepatology*, **7**, 457–463.

59. Gross, J.B. & Rundquist, R. (1988) Reproducibility of galactose clearance measurements in normal subjects. *Hepatology*, **8**, 194 (Abstract).

60. Hasch, E., Jarnum, S. & Tygstrup, N. (1967) Albumin synthesis rate as a measure of liver function in patients with cirrhosis. *Acta Medica Scandinavica*, **182**, 83–92.

61. Hegarty, J.E., Nouri Aria, K.T., Portmann, B. *et al.* (1983) Relapse following treatment withdrawal in patients with autoimmune chronic active hepatitis. *Hepatology*, **3**, 685–689.

62. Henderson, J.M., Warren, W.D., Millikan, W.J. *et al.* (1990) Surgical options, hematologic evaluation, and pathologic changes in Budd–Chiari syndrome. *American Journal of Surgery*, **159**, 41–50.

63. Henry, D.A., Kitchingman, G. & Langman, M.J.S. (1985) 14C aminopyrine breath analysis and conventional biochemical tests as predictors of survival in cirrhosis. *Digestive Diseases and Sciences*, **30**, 813–818.

64. Hepner, G.W. & Vesell, E.S. (1975) Quantitative assessment of hepatic function by breath analysis after oral administration of 14C aminopyrine. *Annals of Internal Medicine*, **83**, 632–638.

65. Hills, P.G. & Sammons, H.G. (1987) An assessment of 5'-nucleotidase as a liver function test. *Quarterly Journal of Medicine*, **36**, 457–468.

66. Hillenbrand, P., Parbhoo, S.P., Jedrychowski, A. & Sherlock, S. (1974) Significance of intravascular coagulation and fibrinolysis in acute hepatic failure. *Gut*, **15**, 83–88.

67. Horak, W., Waldram, R., Murray-Lyon, I.M. *et al.* (1976) Kinetics of 14C-cholic acid in fulminant hepatic failure: A prognostic test. *Gastroenterology*, **71**, 809–813.

68. Hultcrantz, R., Glaumann, H., Lindberg, G. & Nilsson, L.H. (1986) Liver investigation in 149 asymptomatic patients with moderately elevated activities of serum aminotransferases. *Scandinavian Journal of Gastroenterology*, **21**, 109–113.

69. Häcki, J., Bircher, J. & Preisig, R. (1976) A new look at the plasma disappearance of sulfobromophthalein (BSP): Correlation with the BSP transport maximum and the hepatic plasma flow in man. *Journal of Laboratory and Clinical Medicine*, **88**, 1019–1031.

70. Infante-Rivard, C., Esnaola, S. & Villeneuve, J.-P. (1987) Clinical and statistical validity of conventional prognostic factors in predicting short-term survival among cirrhotics. *Hepatology*, **7**, 660–664.

71. Irving, C.S., Schoeller, D.A., Nakamura, K.I. *et al.* (1983) The amino pyrine breath test as a measure of liver function. A quantitative description of its metabolic basis in normal subjects. *Journal of Laboratory and Clinical Medicine*, **100**, 356–373.

72. Jansen, P.M.L., Chamuleau, R.A.F.M., van Leuven, D.J. *et al.* (1990) Liver regeneration and restoration of liver function after partial hepatectomy in patients with liver tumors. *Scandinavian Journal of Gastroenterology*, **25**, 112–118.

73. Joeres, R., Klinker, H., Heusler, H. *et al.* (1988) Influence of smoking on caffeine elimination in healthy volunteers and in patients with alcoholic liver cirrhosis. *Hepatology*, **8**, 575–579.

74. Johnson, P.J. & McFarlane, I.G. (1989) *The Laboratory Investigation of Liver Disease*, pp.308. London, Baillière Tindall.

75. Jost, G., Wahlländer, A., Mandach, U. & Preisig, R. (1987) Overnight salivary caffeine clearance: A liver function test suitable for routine use. *Hepatology*, **7**, 338–344.

76. Kaplan, M.M. (1986) Serum alkaline phosphatase — another piece is added to the puzzle. *Hepatology*, **6**, 526–528.

77. Kaplan, M.M., Ohkubo, A., Quaroni, E.G. & Sze-Tu, D. (1983) Increased synthesis of rat liver alkaline phosphatase by bile duct ligation. *Hepatology*, **3**, 368–376.

78. Keiding, S. & Skak, C. Methodological limitations of the use of intrinsic hepatic clearance of ICG as a measure of liver cell function. *European Journal of Clinical Investigation*, **18**, 507–511.

79. Kobayashi, K., Kameda, S., Sugimoto, S. *et al*, (1978) The measurement of serum protein with rapid turnover for early diagnosis of fatal hepatitis. *Acta Hepatogastroenterologica*, **25**, 287–291.

80. Kropf, J., Gressner, A.M. & Negwer, A. (1988) Efficacy of serum laminin measurement for diagnosis of fibrotic liver diseases. *Clinical Chemistry*, **34**, 2026–2030.

81. Laker, M.F. (1990) Liver function tests. *British Medical Journal*, **301**, 250–251.

82. Laurell, C.-B. (1985) Acute phase proteins — a group of protective proteins. In Price, C.P. & Alberti, K.G.M.M. (eds) *Recent Advances In Clinical Biochemistry* Vol.3, pp.103–124. Edinburgh: Churchill Livingstone.

83. Lauterburg, B.H. & Bircher, J. (1973) Hepatic microsomal drug metabolizing capacity measured in vivo by breath analysis. *Gastroenterology*, **65**, 556 (Abstract).

84. Lauterburg, B.H., Cap, L. & Michaletz, P.A. (1988) Assessment of mitochondrial dysfunction produced by ethanol and uncoupling of oxidate phosphorylation in vivo: Validation of a breath test using 14C-keto-iso-caproic acid (Kica). *Hepatology*, **8**, 47.

85. Lauterburg, B.H., Sautter, V., Preisig, R. & Bircher, J. (1976) Hepatic functional deterioration after portacaval shunt in the rat. Effects on sulfobromophthalein transport-maximum, indocyanine green clearance and galactose elimination capacity. *Gastroenterology*, **71**, 221–227.

86. Lautz, H.U., Schmidt, F.W., Schmidt, E. *et al.* (1988) Quantitative liver function tests as predictors of survival in hepatic and primary biliary cirrhosis. *Hepatology*, **8**, 1414 (Abstract).

87. Lindskov, J. (1982) The quantitative liver function as measured by the galactose elimination capacity. II. Prognostic value and changes during disease in patients with cirrhosis. *Acta Medica Scandinavica*, **212**, 303–308.

88. Mannes, G.A., Thieme, Chr., Stellaard, F. *et al.* (1986) Prognostic significance of serum bile acids in cirrhosis. *Hepatology*, **6**, 50–53.

89. Marchesini, G., Checchia, G.A., Grossi, G. *et al.* (1988) Caffeine intake, fasting plasma caffeine and caffeine clearance in patients with liver diseases. *Liver*, **8**, 241–246.

90. Marchesini, G., Fabbri, A., Bugianesi, E. *et al.* (1990) Analysis of the deterioration rates of liver function in cirrhosis, based on galactose elimination capacity. *Liver*, **10**, 65–71.

91. McIntyre, N. (1983) The limitations of conventional liver function tests. *Seminars in Liver Disease*, **3**, 265–274.

92. McPherson, G.A.D., Benjamin, I.S., Boobis, A.R. & Blumgard, L.H. (1985) Antipyrine elimination in patients with obstructive jaundice: A predictor of outcome. *American Journal of Surgery*, **149**, 140–143.

93. Mehta, M.U., Venkataramanan, R., Burckart, G.J. *et al.* (1986) Antipyrine kinetics in liver disease and liver transplantation. *Clinical Pharmacology and Therapeutics*, **39**, 372–377.

94. Merkel, C., Bolognesi, M., Finucci, G.F. *et al.* (1989) Indocyanine green intrinsic clearance as a prognostic index of survival in patients with cirrhosis. *Journal of Hepatology*, **9**, 16–22.

95. Merkel, C., Gatta, A., Bolognesi, M. *et al.* (1988) Prognostic value of galactose elimination capacity, aminopyrine breath test, and ICG clearance in cirrhosis: Comparison with the Pugh score. *Hepatology*, **8**, 1402 (Abstract).

96. Merkel, C., Sacerdoti, D., Finucci, G.F. *et al.* (1986) Effect of

nadolol on liver haemodynamics and function in patients with cirrhosis. _British Journal of Clinical Pharmacology_, **21**, 713–719.

97. Miescher, G., Paumgartner, G. & Preisig, R. (1983) Portal-systemic spill-over of bile acids: a study of mechanisms using ursodeoxycholic acid. _European Journal of Clinical Investigation_, **13**, 439–445.

98. Miotti, T., Bircher, J. & Preisig, R. (1988) The 30-minute aminopyrine breath test; Optimization of sampling times after intravenous administration of 14C-aminopyrine. _Digestion_, **39**, 241–250.

99. Molino, G., Cavanna, A., Avagnina, P. _et al._ (1987) Hepatic clearance of D-sorbitol. Noninvasive test for evaluating functional liver plasma flow. _Digestive Diseases and Sciences_, **32**, 753–758.

100. Monroe, P.S., Baker, A.L., Schneider, J.F. _et al._ (1982) The aminopyrine breath test and serum bile acids reflect histologic severity in chronic hepatitis. _Hepatology_, **2**, 317–322.

101. Nelson, D.C., Avant, G.R., Speeg, K.V. Jr. _et al._ (1985) The effect of cimetidine on hepatic drug elimination in cirrhosis. _Hepatology_, **5**, 305–309.

102. Neuberger, J., Altman, D.G., Christensen, E. _et al._ (1986) Use of a prognostic index in evaluation of liver transplantation for primary biliary cirrhosis. _Transplantation_, **41**, 713–716.

103. Nusinovici, V., Crubille, C., Opolon, P. _et al._ (1977) Hepatitis fulminates avec coma. Rue de 137 cas. –II. Évolution et prognostique. _Gastroenterologie Clinique et Biologique_, **1**, 875–886.

104. Oellerich, M., Burdelski, M., Ringe, B. _et al._ (1989) Lignocaine metabolite formation as a measure of pre-transplant liver function. _Lancet_, **1**, 640–642.

105. Ohkubo, H., Okuda, K., Iida, S. _et al._ (1983) Role of portal and splenic vein shunts and impaired hepatic extraction in the elevated serum bile acids in liver cirrhosis. _Gastroenterology_, **86**, 514–520.

106. Okamoto, E., Kyo, A., Yamanaka, N. _et al._ (1984) Prediction of the safe limits of hepatectomy by combined volumetric and functional measurements in patients with impaired hepatic function. _Surgery_, **95**, 586–592.

107. Orrego, H., Israel, Y., Blake, J.E. & Medline, A. (1983) Assessment of prognostic factors in alcoholic liver disease: Toward a global quantitative expression of severity. _Hepatology_, **3**,, 896–905.

108. Panteghini, M., Falsetti, F., Chiari, E. & Malchiodi, A. (1983) Determination of aspartate aminotransferase isoenzymes in hepatic diseases — a preliminary report. _Clinica Chimica Acta_, **128**, 133–140.

109. Paramsothy, J., Strange, R., Sharif, H. _et al._ (1988) The use of antipyrine clearance to measure liver damage in psoriatic patients receiving methotrexate. _British Journal of Dermatology_, **119**, 761–765.

110. Paumgartner, G. (1975) The handling of indocyanine green by the liver. _Schweizerische Medicinische Wochenschrift_, **105** (supplement) 5–30.

111. Penn, R. & Worthington, D.J. (1983) Is serum glutamyl transferase a misleading test? _British Medical Journal_, **1**, 531–535.

112. Peters, S.P., Lee, R.E. & Glew, R.H. (1975) A microassay for Gaucher's disease. _Clinica Chimica Acta_, **60**, 391–396.

113. Pignon, J.P., Poynard, T., Naveau, S. _et al._ (1986) Analyse multidimensionnelle selon le modèle de Cox de la survie de patients atteints de cirrhose alcoolique. _Gastroenterologie Clinique et Biologique_, **10**, 461–467.

114. Pomier-Layrargues, G., Huet, P.-M., Infante-Rivard, C. _et al._ (1988) Prognostic value of indocyanine green and lidocaine kinetics for survival and chronic hepatic encephalopathy in cirrhotic patients following elective end-to-side portacaval shunt. _Hepatology_, **8**, 1506–1510.

115. Preisig, R., Grimm, L. & Bircher, J. (1979) Galactose breath test: Differences in rate limitation between liver normals, cirrhotics, and diabetics. _Gastroenterology_, **76**, 1296–1299.

116. Price, C.P. & Sammons, H.G. (1976) An interpretation of the serum alkaline phosphatase isoenzyme patterns in patients with obstructive liver disease. _Journal of Clinical Pathology_, **29**, 976–980.

117. Prieto, J., Barry, M. & Sherlock, S. (1975) Serum ferritin in patients with iron overload and with acute and chronic liver disease. _Gastroenterology_, **68**, 525–533.

118. Pugh, R.N.H., Murray-Lyon, I.M., Dawson, J.L. _et al._ (1973) Transection of the oesophagus for bleeding oesophageal varices. _British Journal of Surgery_, **60**, 646–649.

119. Ramsce Jacobsen, K., Ranek, L. & Tygstrup, N. (1969) Liver function and blood flow in normal man during infusion of vasopressin. _Scandinavian Journal of Clinical and Laboratory Investigation_, **24**, 279–284.

120. Ramsce, K., Buch Andreasen, P. & Ranek, L. (1980) Functioning liver mass in uncomplicated and fulminant acute hepatitis. _Scandinavian Journal of Gastroenterology_, **15**, 65–72.

121. Ranek, L., Andreasen, P.B. & Tygstrup, N. (1976) Galactose elimination capacity as a prognostic index in patients with fulminant liver failure. _Gut_, **17**, 959–964.

122. Reichen, J., Arts, B., Schafroth, U. _et al._ (1987) Aminopyrine N-demethylation by rats with liver cirrhosis evidence for the intact cell hypothesis. A morphometric-functional study. _Gastroenterology_, **93**, 719–726.

123. Reichling, J.J. & Kaplan, M.M. (1988) Clinical use of serum enzymes in liver disease. _Digestive Diseases and Sciences_, **33**, 1601–1614.

124. Renner, E., Weitholtz, H., Huguenin, P. _et al._ (1984) Caffeine: A model compound for measuring liver function. _Hepatology_, **4**, 38–46.

125. Rikkers, L., Jenko, P., Rudman, D. & Freides, D. (1978) Subclinical hepatic encephalopathy: Detection, prevalence and relationship to nitrogen metabolism. _Gastroenterology_, **75**, 462–469.

126. Roll, J., Boyer, J.L., Barry, D. & Klatskin, G. (1983) The prognostic importance of clinical and histologic features in asymptomatic and symptomatic primary biliary cirrhosis. _New England Journal of Medicine_, **308**, 1–7.

127. Rolland Dickson, E., Grambsch, P.M., Fleming, T.R. _et al._ (1989) Prognosis in primary biliary cirrhosis: Model for decision making. _Hepatology_, **10**, 1–7.

128. Rondana, M., Milani, L., Merkel, C. _et al._ (1987) Value of prealbumin plasma level as liver test. _Digestion_, **37**, 72–78.

129. Rossi, L., Milani, A., Marra, L. & Siciliano, M. (1986) Grading scores and survivorship functions in liver cirrhosis: A comparative statistical analysis of various predictive models. _Hepatogastroenterology_, **33**, 240–243.

130. Rudman, D., DiFulco, T.J., Galambos, J.T. _et al._ (1973) Maximal rates of excretion and synthesis of urea in normal and cirrhotic subjects. _Journal of Clinical Investigation_, **52**, 2241–2249.

131. Röllinghoff, W. & Paumgartner, G. (1982) Inhibition of drug metabolism by cimetidine in man: Dependence on pretreatment microsomal liver function. _European Journal of Clinical Investigation_, **12**, 429–432.

132. Röllinghoff, W., Paumgartner, G. & Preisig, R. (1981) Nicotinic acid test in the diagnosis of Gilbert's syndrome: correlation with bilirubin clearance. _Gut_, **22**, 663–668.

133. Rössle, M., Herz, R., Hiss, W. & Gerok, W. (1983) Der Tryptophan-Belas-tungstest als Funktionsparameter bei Lebererkrankungen (Tryptophan loading test as a function parameter in liver diseases) _Klinische Wochenschrift_, **61**, 277–283.

134. Saunders, J.B., Wright, N. & Lewis, K.O. (1980) Predicting outcome of paracetamol poisoning by using 14C-aminopyrine breath test. _British Medical Journal_, **280**, 279–280.

135. Schlichting, P., Christensen, E., Andersen,, P.K. _et al._ (1983) Prognostic factors in cirrhosis identified by Cox's regression model. _Hepatology_, **3**, 889–895.

136. Schnegg, M. & Lauterburg, B.H. (1986) Quantitative liver function in the elderly assessed by galactose elimination capacity, aminopyrine demethylation and caffeine clearance. _Journal of Hepatology_, **3**, 164–171.

137. Schneider, J.F., Baker, A.L., Haines, N.W. _et al._ (1980) Aminopyrine N-demethylation: A prognostic test of liver function in patients with alcoholic liver disease. _Gastroenterology_, **79**, 1145–1150.

138. Shapiro, J.M., Smith, H. & Schaffner, F. (1979) Serum bilirubin: A prognostic factor in primary biliary cirrhosis. _Gut_, **20**, 137–140.

139. Sheu, J.C., Sung, J.L., Chen, D.S. _et al._ (1985) Growth rate of asymptomatic hepatocellular carcinoma and its clinical implications. _Gastroenterology_, **89**, 259–266.

140. Shreeve, W.W., Shoop, J.D., Ott, D.G. & McInteer, B.B. (1976) Test for alcoholic cirrhosis by conversion of 14C- or 13C-galactose to expired CO_2. _Gastroenterology_, **71**, 98–101.

141. Stock, P.G., Estrin, J.A., Fryd, D.S. _et al._ (1987) Prognostic

perioperative factors predicting the outcome of liver transplantation. *Transplantation Proceedings*, **XIX**, 2427–2428.

142. Tavill, A.S. (1972) The synthesis and degradation of liver-produced proteins. *Gut*, **13**, 225–241.

143. Tygstrup, N. (1966) Determination of the hepatic elimination capacity (Lm) of galactose by single injection. *Scandinavian Journal of Clinical and Laboratory Investigation*, **18** (supplement 2), 118–125.

144. Tygstrup, N., Andersen, P. Kragh. & Riegels Thomsen, B.L. Prognostic evaluation in alcoholic cirrhosis. *Acta Medica Scandinavica (Supplement)*, **703**, 149–156.

145. Tygstrup, N. & Ranek, L. (1986) Assessment of prognosis in fulminant hepatic failure. *Seminars in Liver Disease*, **6**, 129–137.

146. Tygstrup, N. & Winkler, K. (1958) Galactose blood clearance as a measure of hepatic blood flow. *Clinical Science*, **17**, 1–9.

147. Van Ness, M.M. & Diehl, A.M. (1989) Is liver biopsy useful in the examination of patients with chronically elevated liver enzymes? *Annals of Internal Medicine*, **111**, 473–478.

148. Vesell, E.S. (1979) The antipyrine test in clinical pharmacology: Conceptions and misconceptions. *Clinical Pharmacology and Therapeutics*, **26**, 275–286.

149. Vierling, J.M., Berk, P.D., Hofman, A.F. *et al.* (1982) Normal fasting-state levels of serum cholyl-conjugated bile acids in Gilbert's syndrome: an aid to diagnosis. *Hepatology*, **2**, 340–343.

150. Villeneuve, J.-P., Infante-Rivard, C., Ampelas, M. *et al.* (1986) Prognostic value of the aminopyrine breath test in cirrhotic patients. *Hepatology*, **6**, 928–931.

151. Vilstrup, H. (1980) Synthesis of urea after stimulation with amino acids: Relation to liver function. *Gut*, **21**, 990–995.

152. Vilstrup, H., Gluud, C., Hardt, F. *et al.* (1990) Branched chain enriched amino acid versus glucose treatment of hepatic encephalopathy. A double-blind study of 65 patients with cirrhosis. *Hepatology*, **10**, 291–296.

153. Vilstrup, H., Iversen, J. & Tygstrup, N. (1986) Glucoregulation in acute liver failure. *European Journal of Clinical Investigation*, **16**, 193–197.

154. Walser, M. & Bodenlos, L.J. (1959) Urea metabolism in man. *Journal of Clinical Investigation*, **38**, 1617–1626.

155. Walshe, J.M. (1984) Copper: its role in the pathogenesis of liver disease. *Seminars in Liver Disease*, **4**, 252–263.

156. Wheeler, H.O., Meltzer, J.I. & Bradley, S.E. (1960) Biliary transport and hepatic storage of sulphobromophthalein sodium in the unanesthetized dog, in normal man and in patients with hepatic diseases. *Journal of Clinical Investigation*, **39**, 1131–1144.

157. Whitehead, T.P. & Wotton, D.P. (1974) Biochemical profiles for hospital patients. *Lancet*, **2**, 1439–1443.

158. Wietholtz, H., Voegelin, M., Arnaud, M.J. *et al.* (1981) Assessment of the cytochrome P-448 dependent liver enzyme system by a caffeine breath test. *European Journal of Clinical Pharmacology*, **21**, 53–59.

159. Winkel, P., Juhl, E. & Tygstrup, N. (1970) The prognostic value of clinical and laboratory data in patients with cirrhosis. *Scandinavian Journal of Gastroenterology* (supplement 7), 181–187.

160. Winkler, K., Keiding, S. & Tygstrup, N. (1973) Clearance as a quantitative measure of liver function. In *The Liver. Quantitative Aspects of Structure and Function*, p.144. Basel: Karger.

161. Wood, L.J., Massie, D., McLean, A.J. & Dudley, F.J. (1988) Renal sodium retention in cirrhosis; Tubular site and relation to hepatic dysfunction. *Hepatology*, **8**, 831–836.

CHAPTER 19

Liver Biopsy: Methods, Diagnostic Value and Interpretation

G.H. Millward-Sadler & P.J. Whorwell

Although first used before the turn of the century, the technique of liver biopsy did not become firmly established until the 1940s. Refinements in techniques have led to its being widely accepted as a routine part of the investigation of a patient with liver disease in any general hospital. This wide use must not, however, detract from the fact that it remains a potentially hazardous procedure that should not be lightly undertaken.

INDICATIONS

1. Diagnosis of primary liver disease.
2. Assessment of progression of disease and response to therapy.
3. Confirmation of malignant disease.
4. Staging and diagnosis of lymphomas.
5. Diagnosis of metabolic disease, such as glycogen storage disease.
6. Diagnosis of multisystem disease, such as sarcoidosis, amyloidosis or haemochromatosis.
7. Diagnosis of pyrexia of unknown origin and uncommon infections. In addition to histology, the biopsy may be cultured and stained for specific organisms such as tubercle bacilli.
8. Assessment of advisability of the use of potentially hepatotoxic drugs such as methotrexate in psoriasis.

PRECAUTIONS AND CONTRAINDICATIONS

A skilled operator is required, as not only is this more likely to result in an adequate biopsy specimen but the patient's cooperation is considerably enhanced by a confident, assured attendant.

A clotting profile, which should at least include the prothrombin ratio and platelet count, must be obtained shortly before biopsy. If any abnormality is detected, biopsy should be delayed until it has been corrected by the appropriate use of vitamin K or clotting factor concentrates. It should be borne in mind that dysproteinaemias and some drugs can lead to platelet dysfunction, despite a normal count. We are prepared to biopsy a patient with a platelet count greater than 80 000 000/1 and a prothrombin ratio of 1.3 or below. It is usual to group and cross-match two units of blood beforehand.

In any situation where a space-occupying lesion of the liver is suspected, previous ultrasound and a colloid liver scan may indicate the nature of the lesion and its location, thus enabling a specific area to be aimed for. The diagnostic yield when sampling for suspected malignancy can be increased from approximately 50% of cases[31] by taking two biopsies from different angles.[25]

Greater accuracy, up to between 83 and 100%, can be achieved with guided biopsy under ultrasonographic or computed tomographic (CT) control.[17,39,129] Hydatid cyst or haemangioma are usually regarded as absolute contraindications to biopsy. Most haemangiomas can be correctly diagnosed with a combination of ultrasonographic, CT or magnetic resonance imaging, but in doubtful cases percutaneous biopsy has been performed safely, using a fine needle.[17,27,132] Percutaneous biopsy of a hydatid cyst is contraindicated because of the risk of anaphylaxis but has been inadvertently performed without complications.[11]

Biopsy in the presence of biliary obstruction is rarely necessary and has an increased risk of biliary peritonitis but, when indicated, the risks are not unacceptable.[92,133] Our practice is to refrain from biopsying anyone shown by ultrasound or cholangiography to have dilated ducts. We are also relatively reluctant to biopsy patients who have had previous biliary surgery, particularly if it was in any way complicated.

It is more difficult to obtain a good specimen from biopsy of the liver in the presence of ascites and there is a corresponding increased risk of complications. It has been claimed that these can be reduced if the procedure in such patients is performed under ultrasonographic or CT control.[94] Passive congestion of the liver is associated with an increased risk of haemorrhage and the congestion should be minimized before biopsy. A series of biopsies without complication in this situation has been reported.[126]

PROCEDURE

Types of needles

The original needles consisted of a trocar and cannula with a bore of up to 3 mm.[55] It soon became apparent that the incidence of haemorrhage could be reduced by decreasing the size of the bore.[64] Safety was also adversely affected by the slow speed of the manoeuvre, which was revolutionized by the introduction of the 'one-second' technique by Menghini.[86] He designed a needle with an oblique tip, slightly convex towards the outside, which has an internal nail to prevent the biopsy being drawn up into the syringe. The needles come in sizes of 1.0, 1.5 and 2.0 mm in diameter, the 1.5 mm version being the most commonly used. There have been several modifications of the Menghini needle, and we use the one introduced by Klatskin, in which the whole circumference of the tip is sharpened. We also prefer to use the needle without the nail, as otherwise this may lead to crushing artefact when the biopsy impacts on it. In addition, there is immediate confirmation that a biopsy has been obtained, and undue fragmentation does not occur.

The other needle in common use is the Vim–Silverman or its disposable derivative, the Trucut.[110] In the former, a trocar and cannula are introduced into the liver, the trocar is removed and a split cannula with a tendency to spring open is advanced through the other cannula into the liver. The split cannula is then closed by advancing the outside one over it, and after rotation of the two they are withdrawn. No suction is required, but distortion can be considerable. The main advantage of this technique is that it is usually possible to obtain biopsies from fibrotic livers in which the Menghini needle has failed. Today the Trucut modification, in which the inside cannula has a 2-cm notch cut out of one side and the sliding cannula has a cutting edge, is more often used. In addition a number of mechanical devices have recently been developed that automatically perform the manoeuvre involved in taking a Trucut type biopsy.

It has been suggested that the addition of an outer plastic sheath to a Trucut needle allows biopsy in high-risk patients.[22,111] The sheath is left in situ following the biopsy and, using fluoroscopy, the biopsy tract can then be embolized.

Fine needle liver biopsy

Biopsy needles are designated as 'fine' when the external diameter is less than 1 mm.[73] The risks of a needle biopsy increase when the external diameter exceeds 1.2 mm.[57] The use of fine needle biopsy has increased over the past 10 years, particularly for providing a tissue diagnosis on focal liver lesions. Liver biopsy using a 0.7 mm external diameter needle has been advocated for cytodiagnosis[75] or where repeat biopsies are needed for such purposes as enzyme estimations. It has greater safety than standard biopsy techniques: a cutting fine needle has a slightly higher complication rate but this is compensated by the increased diagnostic yield from the biopsy.[17,84] Fine needle biopsy has advantages if all that is required is tissue confirmation of malignancy, although focal benign lesions can also be diagnosed.[17,35] Cytological examinations of the fluid/blood aspirated with a routine biopsy will increase the diagnostic yield by an additional 15%.[46]

Preparation

Although there have been recent reports of outpatient liver biopsy,[62,104,127] we prefer the patient to be admitted to hospital for biopsy. Premedication is not usually necessary, although an intramuscular injection of diazepam or midazolam will calm the unduly anxious patient. Sedation should never be so extensive that patient cooperation is lost. The patient should lie flat on the edge of the bed with one head-pillow and the right hand placed behind the head. Except when it is necessary to biopsy a specific area, the intercostal route should be used. The site for biopsy is selected by percussing out the borders of the liver and then choosing the area of maximum dullness on expiration in the mid-axillary line. This usually involves traversing either the eighth, ninth or tenth intercostal space.

Technique

After cleansing the skin with a suitable antiseptic, local anaesthetic is introduced at the biopsy site and infiltrated down to and including the liver capsule. A small incision is made in the skin to facilitate entry of the biopsy needle. At this point the bleeding time should be noted and, if unacceptable, the procedure should be abandoned despite a normal clotting screen. The forthcoming events should then be explained and rehearsed with the patient, with particular emphasis given to the importance of breath-holding. The patient should also be warned that there may be some local and perhaps shoulder-tip pain. The needle should be placed on a 10-ml syringe, which is filled

with 6 ml of sterile normal saline. With the patient breathing quietly, the needle is advanced until it is felt to give into the space overlying the liver. Two millilitres of saline is injected to clear any debris from the needle. The patient is told to breathe out and then stop breathing. Two millilitres of suction is applied to the syringe and the needle can then be rapidly advanced in and out of the liver in one movement. The appearance of blood in the syringe at the time of the biopsy should not cause alarm and is not indicative of subsequent haemorrhage. On withdrawal, the biopsy appears in the barrel of the syringe and is easily removed by withdrawing the plunger and pouring the contents into a suitable dish, which should have a small piece of gauze in the bottom. It can then be transferred into specimen container(s) appropriate for the investigation(s) required. In situations where malignant disease is suspected, a second pass of the needle in a different direction is justified, particularly if the first biopsy appears macroscopically normal (see Chapter 39). After the biopsy, the patient is asked to lie on the right side for 2 hours and remain in bed for 24 hours. Regular recordings of pulse and blood pressure should be made for the first few hours.

Transvenous liver biopsy

This technique was first developed in 1964[32] for obtaining tissue when percutaneous biopsy is contraindicated. The patients usually have a severe bleeding diathesis or ascites and it is considered that a biopsy would positively contribute to diagnosis or management. The technique involves a jugular puncture with subsequent fluoroscopic guidance of the catheter into a small hepatic vein. After wedging the catheter, a needle is advanced into the liver and either suction is applied or a Trucut technique used to obtain the biopsy.

An adequate biopsy can be obtained in about 65% of patients with fibrotic disease and many more with non-fibrotic disorders.[12,67] A transfemoral approach has also been employed.[87] The biopsies were smaller using this route but the frequency of haematoma at the venepuncture site was considerably less than with the transjugular approach.

Plugged liver biopsy

The percutaneous liver biopsy technique has been modified to permit the procedure in patients with a major bleeding diathesis. The principle is to plug the biopsy track once the core of tissue has been removed. This may be done using a needle with a plastic sheath which is left *in situ* after the needle is withdrawn. It can then be used as a guide to embolize the track before being removed.[22,111] Alternatively, a specifically designed biopsy needle may be used which delivers steel coils into the track once the biopsy has been taken.[2]

Liver biopsy in children

This is increasingly used and is safe, providing that the child is appropriately sedated and properly restrained.[51] A general anaesthetic may be required if a biopsy is particularly necessary in an uncooperative child. The subcostal route is used, depending on the liver size, and a Menghini needle is usually employed. Movement of the liver may be minimized by an assistant who pushes it upwards from below the costal margin.

Fetal liver biopsies can now be obtained in utero. This is done under direct vision using a fetoscope and can be performed after about 18 weeks of gestation.[112]

Liver biopsy with imaging

Computed tomography or ultrasound to aid liver biopsy are increasingly being used.[143] They have two main advantages. One is to allow targeting of the needle to specific lesions[129] or to improve success rate in difficult situations such as abnormal anatomy or ascites.[39,94] The other is that it probably improves safety by often allowing fewer passes of the needle to achieve an adequate biopsy and enabling avoidance of potentially dangerous structures (see Chapter 23).

COMPLICATIONS

Almost all complications of liver biopsy occur within 24 hours and the majority within the first 2 hours of the procedure. A higher rate of complications has been found in patients with cirrhosis or malignancy and was also associated with the use of a Trucut compared with a Menghini needle.[106]

Pain

Some pain may be experienced at the site of biopsy and there is sometimes shoulder-tip pain secondary to diaphragmatic irritation. If there is any bleeding into the pleural cavity there may be some pleuritic-type pain with an associated friction rub. Post-biopsy pain was a complaint in 11 of 108 patients but no abnormality was found on ultrasound examination.[50]

Intrahepatic haematoma

The incidence of intrahepatic haematoma following needle biopsy of the liver has been reported to be as high as 23%,[90] but the more common experience indicates that it is less, and usually much less, than 10%.[21,37,83,103,109,] [134] Raines et al.[109] in a prospective study of 40 patients undergoing needle biopsy of the liver, found 3 (7%) to have a solitary filling defect on a post-biopsy liver scan. Except for a fall in haematocrit, and in one case some transitory pain, none of the patients experienced any other effects. In a larger series of 108 patients examined by ultrasound 2–4 hours after using a 1.6 mm diameter biopsy needle, evidence of haematoma was seen in 1% of patients.[50] The overall experience suggests that the incidence is approximately 1% of all needle biopsy procedures if the liver is examined by ultrasound. The low incidence of intrahepatic haematoma—0.059% of 68 276 biopsies, in the large study by Piccinino et al.[106] probably reflects the low usage of ultrasound to screen for this complication. A much lower incidence of haematoma is claimed for fine needle biopsies in a large series of 2091 cases.[17] Intrahepatic haematomas may very rarely cause biliary obstruction.[19]

Haemorrhage

This is the most common complication and cause of death.[106] Terry[136] estimated that significant bleeding complicated 0.2% of biopsies. The largest series reported, consisting of 68 276 biopsy procedures gathered from a multicentre questionnaire, found an incidence of 0.32%. In this series the highest incidence of haemorrhage was associated with use of the Trucut needle in patients with malignancy or cirrhosis.[106] The risk is still present with fine needle biopsies, although reduced. Haemoperitoneum complicated 6 of 2091 fine needle biopsy procedures and in addition one patient had haematobilia. Only one patient required transfusion. In this study the complications were more commonly associated with the use of a cutting needle.[17]

Arterio-venous fistulae are claimed to be relatively common after liver biopsy.[100] One patient who died of haemorrhage following percutaneous liver biopsy was shown to have an arterio-portal-peritoneal fistula. Attempts to embolize the fistula with Gelfoam failed.[63] *The risk* of haemorrhage can be minimized provided the precautions previously described are taken. Haemorrhage is occasionally unavoidable, particularly if a deep breath is taken at the moment of biopsy or some major vessel is punctured. Strict observations should give an early indication of bleeding, and if blood transfusion fails to stabilize the situation, laparotomy has to be considered.

Perforation of other organs

Gallbladder, lung, colon and kidney have all been inadvertently punctured. The total incidence is low (0.204%) and the gallbladder is the most common organ involved.[80,106] Transit through the costophrenic angle can more frequently give rise to complications of pneumothorax, haemothorax and pleural effusion, although these only rarely require treatment.[34,106] A pneumoscrotum has been described as a further complication of pneumothorax secondary to the biopsy procedure.[34]

Biliary peritonitis

Biliary leakage may complicate perforation of the gallbladder or biopsies in patients with obstructed, dilated intrahepatic ducts. This complication is potentially lethal, and if suspected is an indication for early laparotomy and decompression. None the less, in a study of 68 276 biopsies, none of the 15 patients who developed biliary peritonitis required surgery.[106]

Needle fracture

Purow, Grosberg and Wapnik[108] reported fracture of the biopsy needle during the procedure with retention of the broken end. They were able to obtain more information on three similar incidents. The fracture site was approximately level with the tip of the nail when *in situ* and may be of significance if metal fatigue was responsible in any way. A further four cases have been reported from a large multicentre study of the complications of liver biopsy. A Menghini needle was involved in all four cases: although the Trucut needle was not involved with this complication, it was only used in a total of just over 10% of procedures.[106]

Mortality

Haemorrhage and peritonitis account for the majority of deaths complicating liver biopsy. One of the highest figures, of 1%, was given by Snapper in 1951,[131] although at about the same time Gallison and Skinner[38] suggested the figure was 0.35%. Two large reviews of 10 600 and 20 016 patients gave figures of 0.12 and 0.17%,[135,147] but more recent reviews of 79 381 and 68 276 biopsies have respectively given figures of 0.015%[72] and 0.009%.[106] It seems likely that the current rate of mortality is closer to 0.01% than the original figure of 0.1%.

THE LIVER BIOPSY

MACROSCOPIC FEATURES

A limited amount of information is available from macroscopic appearances.

Architecture

A normal architecture can be identified in a cylinder of liver when a regular dark brown/pale brown mottling is seen. This results from the perivenular distribution of lipofuscin.

Abnormal fibrosis is seen as a grey-white tissue that is usually narrower than the rest of the biopsy. In a micronodular cirrhosis this fibrous tissue may predominate and a few tiny nodules of pale brown parenchyma may be embedded within it. A macronodular cirrhosis may not be identified grossly but a fragmented biopsy is suggestive of a cirrhosis.

Pigments

Lipofuscin has been mentioned; as a 'wear and tear' pigment it shows zonal emphasis around the terminal hepatic venule and its presence indicates lack of regeneration. Other pigments may also be seen and these include bile, haemosiderin and the Dubin–Johnson pigments. Bile will produce a green to dark green colour in the biopsy which with any zonal accentuation will be reflected as a mottled green pattern. In haemochromatosis the iron is present in such excess that the biopsy may be a uniform dark brown, but lesser degrees of iron retention may show a dark brown/light brown mottling that is very similar to lipofuscin deposition. By light microscopy, the iron pigmentation is distinguished by its periportal distribution and staining reactions. Dubin–Johnson pigment may be suspected in a very dark brown or almost black liver.

Miscellaneous

The most frequently identified abnormality is fatty liver, which is seen as a very pale cream cylinder of liver. Tumour may closely resemble fibrosis in gross appearance and indeed many tumours are desmoplastic, but a glistening, slightly mucoid and pearly-grey appearance suggests carcinoma. The presence of flecks of yellowing necrosis may be seen grossly within areas of tumour and sometimes there is a cylinder of liver with which to contrast the abnormal appearances. Primary tumours of the liver may have these gross appearances on biopsy but hepatocellular carcinoma may be tan, yellow or yellow-green and fragmented. These appearances may mimic a cirrhosis with multiple fragmented tiny nodules.

TECHNIQUES

The specimen

Most of the specimen should be fixed in 10% formalin for routine histology, but small portions may be fixed in 2–4% glutaraldehyde for electron microscopy or snap-frozen for storage in liquid nitrogen. If there is a suspicion of infection, a piece may be sent for culture.

The specimen must be handled with great care, especially for light microscopy and ultrastructural examination. Squeezing by forceps should be avoided; instead, the biopsy should be gently lifted out on the paper or gauze from the container and transferred to fixative.

Fixation

The properties of the various fixatives have been reviewed by Hopwood[52] and Glauert.[41]

A perfect fixative does not exist, but a 10% solution of neutral buffered formol-saline has fewest disadvantages and several advantages. Carnoy's, Helly's and Zenker's fixatives are excellent for histological and especially nuclear detail, but unfortunately are unsatisfactory for the orcein or immunoperoxidase techniques and are preferably avoided[88] (Table 19.1). Fixation in formalin requires at least 4 hours for small biopsies at ambient temperatures but is quicker at higher temperatures (37°C). For formalin fixation, it should be appreciated that:

1. Fixation is progressive and not complete for several days.
2. Penetration of the fixative is limited.
3. The process involves interaction of aldehyde with the amino groups in tissue proteins and requires a great excess by volume ($\times$ 20) of fixative.

These are minor points for a small needle biopsy, but

Table 19.1 Effect of fixative on demonstration of HBsAg

Fixative	Orcein	Immunoperoxidase[a]
Formalin pH 7	+ + + +	+ + + +
Bouin	+ + +	+ +
Carnoy	−	+
Zenker	+ +	+
Helly	+	−

[a]Peroxidase antiperoxidase (PAP) technique standardized for our laboratory at rabbit anti-HBs 1/10, swine antirabbit IgG 1/20, and rabbit PAP at 1/200.

become of increasing importance for wedge biopsies of liver, hepatic (lobar) resections and the occasional removal of liver during transplantation.

For ultrastructural studies, glutaraldehyde (electron microscopy grades) remains the fixative of choice, but good detail is preserved after fixation in buffered paraformaldehyde of adequate osmolarity and this has been recommended as an appropriate general fixative for combined light microscopy with transmission and scanning electron microscopic studies.[45] We use a 4.5% solution of glutaraldehyde with a cacodylate buffer (at pH 7.4) and keep the solution at 4°C for up to 4 weeks. Phosphate buffer may be substituted for cacodylate.

Intrinsic enzyme activity is normally demonstrated on frozen sections which are then processed for electron microscopy, but some can also be demonstrated after fixation. There is great variation in the effect of a fixative on various enzymes and in the effect of various fixatives on a particular enzyme.[114]

Processing

After fixation, routine histopathology processing schedules are adequate. These will dehydrate the specimen in a series of graded alcohols, clear in chloroform or toluene, and impregnate with hot paraffin wax. Thin epoxy resin sections may also be prepared from thick sections of paraffin-embedded material[14] or, alternatively, if facilities are available a methacrylate embedding procedure may be employed by which sections 1–2 μm thick may be cut.[68] A method combining freeze-drying with methacrylate embedding enables histochemistry to be performed on biopsies while preserving excellent morphological detail.[95]

Other techniques

Diagnostic techniques, apart from those required for standard light and electron microscopy, can be used but usually require fresh or snap-frozen liver. Culture of the specimen for bacteria or viruses,[148] assays of enzymes,[71, 124,125,141] metals[7,33] or other hepatocellular constituents,[66] and frozen sections of liver for histochemistry,[30] for fluorescence of porphyrins,[76] immunofluorescence or, very rarely, for a rapid histopathological diagnosis may all be employed as indicated by clinical circumstances.

Immunofluorescence has been widely employed in liver for the demonstration of virus antigens such as hepatitis

A and B (see Chapters 30 and 31), serum immunoglobulins and products of the hepatocyte such as albumin and alpha-1-antitrypsin.[128] With the advent of the immunoperoxidase technique, many of these fluorescent preparations have been superseded. The disadvantages of fluorescence are the requirements of fresh and therefore potentially infected and infective material, the use of specialized fluorescence microscopy, the lack of a permanent record unless photographs are taken, and poor correlation with diagnostic histopathology. The immunoperoxidase technique overcomes these handicaps but is limited by the stability of antigen in the fixative and in the processing to paraffin blocks. In many instances, loss of antigenicity can be restored by pretreatment of the sections with proteolytic enzymes such as pronase and trypsin. Immunogenicity of hepatitis B surface antigen is lost on prolonged storage of tissue in formalin but can be restored by this method while extracellular antigens such as immunoglobulins and components of complement have been identified in renal glomeruli following careful protease digestion.[79]

The immunoperoxidase technique has revolutionized diagnostic histopathology because it combines specificity with sensitivity and morphological discrimination. Its very specificity means that it supplements rather than replaces standard diagnostic morphology.

In situ hybridization techniques can be applied to routinely processed sections of a liver biopsy. The principle of the technique is based on the specific complementary pairing of DNA or RNA bases to each other. By attaching a label that is morphologically identifiable to a short (~50 base sequence) segment of a single DNA or RNA strand, a matching complementary strand can be identified and located in the tissue section. The method was first developed in 1970[13] and is now applicable to all formalin-fixed and paraffin-embedded tissues.[65] A major value of the technique will be in the identification of viruses within the liver[15,91] and in the correlation of both their presence and their patterns of expression with specific diseases and pathological processes.

The polymerase chain reaction[10] allows the selective amplification of short sequences of DNA or RNA which can then be identified and cloned by more conventional procedures. Only 5 pg of DNA are required for the technique to be successful. It therefore provides enhanced sensitivity but very strict attention to detail is required to avoid contamination and careful controls are necessary to maintain specificity. Again viruses in the liver can be very successfully revealed by this technique,[74,142] but morphological localization with point discrimination is not possible with this method.

STAINING

We prefer not to section liver biopsies serially but instead to cut a small series of 10–15 consecutive sections, 3–4 μm thick. They are stained with haematoxylin and eosin (H&E), silver impregnation,[44] periodic acid–Schiff after diastase digestion (DPAS), orcein,[128] and Perl's Prussian blue. A further series of sections is cut if the clinical information or the biopsy features suggest a focal lesion which is not apparent on the first set of sections. Tissue can thus be preserved for additional investigations using techniques such as electron probe analysis or the polymerase chain reaction as required.

Routinely employed special stains should demonstrate detail not seen or only poorly seen in routine H&E sections. Trichrome preparations of varying hues (Masson, Goldner, Mallory, Picro-Mallory, Martius Scarlet Blue, etc.) can also be used. They are aesthetically attractive and photogenic but rarely provide information that is not available from an H&E, a reticulin preparation, or the orcein stain. They are of value for the easy differentiation of parenchyma and connective tissue, for the demonstration of fibrin thrombi, and for photography.

Reticulin preparations
Omission of gold toning from the reticulin preparation results in collagen in portal tracts and in the wall of the terminal hepatic venule staining a dark golden brown, while sinusoid reticulin is grey black. Collapsed reticulin remains black but collagen that forms within the parenchyma stains as the portal tracts. A counterstain such as neutral red may be employed but is not necessary. Alcian blue has also been used in combination with non-toned preparations to demonstrate connective-tissue mucins.[77]

Iron
The Perls' Prussian blue technique is a reliable histochemical stain for iron and often demonstrates it in scanty amounts in periportal hepatocytes. A grading system of 0 to 4 can be employed[121] which reliably identifies symptomatic and latent haemochromatosis.[33] This stain is also useful in that other pigments, such as lipofuscin and bile, are not obscured unless there is gross excess of iron. A light counterstain such as neutral red is usually employed.

Periodic acid–Schiff (PAS)
Glycogen can be demonstrated histochemically in formalin-fixed paraffin-processed liver by the PAS technique. This is unreliable because of its solubility in aqueous media. For a definitive demonstration, alcohol-based reagents must be used either on frozen sections or on tissue fixed and processed in non-aqueous media. Specificity of the reaction for glycogen is confirmed by prior diastase (or amylase) digestion of the section but quantitation of the glycogen present is suspect unless these precautions are taken. Even then any reduction in glycogen has to be gross before it is detectable. The generalized intense staining of glycogen also obscures other positively-stained non-glycogen structures in the biopsy. Consequently, a section stained by the PAS technique after diastase digestion is the more valuable preparation since then ceroid pigment, globules and basement membranes can be identified when present.

Ceroid pigment is a phagocytosed granular material within Kupffer cells that is frequently intensely PAS positive. It is closely allied to the lipofuscins, having similar light microscopic appearances and staining reactions. The main distinction is that lipofuscin is positive in Schmorl's reaction and ceroid is negative. This pigment is a consequence of death of hepatocytes and occurs in both viral hepatitis and a focus of non-specific necrosis. During the evolution of extrahepatic bile duct obstruction, bile is found in Kupffer cells and is accompanied by PAS-positive pigment. With relief of the obstruction the bile rapidly disappears, but this pigment may persist.

Globules of PAS-positive diastase-resistant material may be present in hepatocytes. When present in periportal hepatocytes they are regarded as diagnostic of alpha-1-antitrypsin deficiency until proved otherwise (see Chapter 43). These globules may be very small and appear more as a coarse granularity, particularly in association with the heterozygous deficiency state (Plate 19.8). On other occasions palely stained globules may be seen in hepatocytes adjacent to zones of necrosis. Immunocytochemical techniques demonstrate that these are also globules of alpha-1-antitrypsin. They also contain other proteins such as albumin and are probably autophagolysosomes. They do not have the same genetic implication as periportal globules and disappear with resolution of the hepatocellular damage.

Nuclei of hepatocytes may be vacuolated as a result of cytoplasmic invagination. This occurs in normal liver and in many conditions associated with non-specific changes in the liver, such as diabetes mellitus and psoriasis. Glycogen may occur in these but occasionally some of the vacuoles are intensely PAS positive after diastase digestion. The significance of this is not known.

Basement membranes within portal tracts, particularly around bile ducts and ductules, can be demonstrated by the PAS stain. No disorders of the bile duct basement membrane equivalent to those of the renal glomerulus are described.

Other infiltrations within the liver such as amyloid may be positive and the mucin in adenocarcinomas can be identified.

Orcein
The orcein technique also provides specific diagnostic information. It is one of several stains which can demonstrate hepatocytes containing hepatitis B surface antigen (HBsAg).[128] The most frequently used alternative to orcein for this demonstration is aldehyde fuchsin. A trichrome modification for HBsAg has been described.[47]

None of these staining techniques is particularly sensitive for detecting HBsAg, especially when compared with immunocytochemical methods. Orcein will demonstrate a copper-binding protein in periportal hepatocytes and elastic fibres in the portal tracts and terminal hepatic veins.

HBsAg positive hepatocytes (Figure 19.1) contain a discrete area of positively stained but finely honeycombed brown to brown-black cytoplasm. The smallest positive

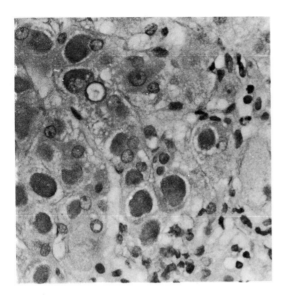

Figure 19.1 Positive cytoplasmic staining for HBsAg by orcein. Note the clear rim of cytoplasm under the plasma membrane. Patient with cirrhosis and HBsAg positive chronic active hepatitis. Orcein, × 800.

areas are simply a perinuclear rim of stained cytoplasm but even when large they rarely reach the plasma membrane. Care must be taken as acidophil degenerate cells take up the stain non-specifically and various other positively stained features must be distinguished (see below).

Ceroid pigments are stained brown but are readily identified by their granularity and position in Kupffer cells. Their identity can be confirmed if necessary by their other staining reactions.[102]

Copper-binding protein (Figure 19.2) is demonstrated as blue-black granules within periportal hepatocytes. These copper-binding proteins within hepatocytes are increased in conditions of chronic cholestasis, such as biliary atresia and the later stages of primary biliary cirrhosis.[115,130] There is good correlation between the orcein demon-

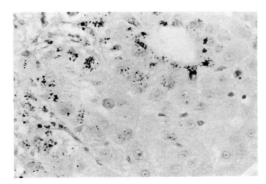

Figure 19.2 Numerous blue-black granules within periportal hepatocytes demonstrated by orcein staining and representing copper-binding protein. Orcein, × 500.

stration of copper-binding protein and the demonstration of copper by the rhodanine technique.[53]

Elastic fibres can be stained brown-black by the orcein technique. The connective tissue of the portal tracts contains coarse irregular serpiginous elastic fibres that extend up to the parenchymal interface of a normal portal tract. Scar tissue in cirrhosis and other chronic liver diseases also contains positively stained fibrils but these differ from the more coarse serpiginous elastic fibres of the portal tract, being finer, straighter and more aligned. It is therefore usually quite easy to identify the original architecture using this staining procedure. Consequently, small portal tracts with mild fibrosis can be distinguished and separated from a normal conducting portal tract of equivalent calibre and the pattern of architectural distortion in cirrhosis can be related to the original skeleton. The type 3 collagen (reticulin) in the sinusoids is not stained and this is of value in distinguishing passive collapse of the reticulin found in acute hepatocellular damage from the active fibrosis of chronic liver disease.[120]

HISTOLOGY

Despite the helpful and sometimes diagnostic features provided by these additional stains, most biopsy interpretation relies on sections stained with haematoxylin and eosin. The main objectives of a liver biopsy are to provide or confirm a diagnosis, to offer a prognosis and to study the effects of treatment. Furthermore, the biopsy should be critically evaluated initially without clinical details and a presumptive diagnosis with differential diagnosis made. Only then should comparison and correlation with clinical details and investigations be made. Meaningful discussion often results. In all instances it is essential to examine the biopsy in a systematic and logical manner.

Architecture

Firstly the architecture of the biopsy should be established. This is usually obvious either with a regular arrangement of portal tracts to the terminal hepatic venules or alternatively with abnormal fibrous bands and regenerative nodules of cirrhosis, but occasionally difficulty may be encountered. Sometimes this is because the portal tracts on the edge of the biopsy have been torn out of the specimen by a blunt biopsy needle. On other occasions part of a large macronodule may have been biopsied. Features which may then help when present are slender abnormal bands of fibrous tissue, an abnormal cell plate pattern (Figure 19.3), an excess of efferent veins in the biopsy frequently with an abnormal approximation to fibrous bands, and absence of lipofuscin in hepatocytes. In difficult cases, careful examination of the individual components of the acinus is required.

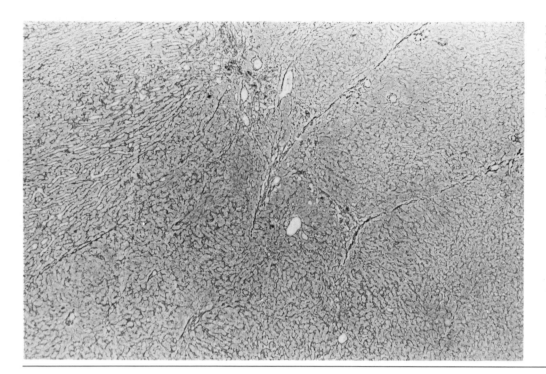

Figure 19.3 A macronodular multiacinar cirrhosis showing very slender bands of fibrous tissue, an excess of efferent veins and an abnormal cell plate pattern, × 20.

Portal tracts

Large portal tracts present no problem with identification but smaller ones may be difficult to separate from bands of fibrous tissue containing a few bile ductules. Even in obvious portal tracts the individual structures should be identified and any abnormalities noted. The relative size and calibre of the bile duct, artery and vein should be studied: portal vein thrombosis may be reflected in the biopsy only by branches of smaller calibre relative to their accompanying bile ducts and arteries. Bile ducts may be hypoplastic[1] as well as atretic or, in acquired large duct obstruction, dilated. Characteristic changes also occur in primary biliary cirrhosis (see Chapter 33) and chronic hepatitis (see Chapter 31). The nature of the stroma should be noted: the collagen becomes more dense and hyaline with increasing age and becomes oedematous in bile duct obstruction.

The quality and location of any inflammatory infiltrate should be identified. Neutrophils around peripheral proliferating bile ductules indicate obstruction to bile ducts but when present in the lumen of the bile duct indicate a cholangitis. Likewise, an inflammatory infiltrate within the artery or vein wall indicates a corresponding arteritis or endophlebitis. Both are relatively rare events: branches of the hepatic artery can be involved by polyarteritis nodosa and are claimed to be more frequently involved in acute rather than subacute bacterial endocarditis; portal endophlebitis usually indicates portal pyaemia due to sepsis within the portal venous drainage. A mixed lymphocytic and macrophage infiltrate is a common reactive component in portal tracts and distinction between this, chronic persistent hepatitis and pericholangitis can be extremely difficult if not impossible. Indeed, sometimes no clear histological distinction can be made between the

pericholangitis and non-specific reactive inflammatory infiltrate. The presence of plasma cells in more than scanty numbers is suggestive of significant liver disease or a complication. For instance, plasma cells are present in acute viral hepatitis in the early stages of the disease. If they persist when evidence of active parenchymal damage has subsided then they indicate possible transition to chronicity. If plasma cells are seen in portal tracts in large bile duct obstruction, an ascending cholangitis is frequently present. Ceroid-laden macrophages usually persist in portal tracts after resolution elsewhere and can be demonstrated up to 4–6 months after the clinical onset of an acute viral hepatitis.

Piecemeal necrosis

The features of piecemeal necrosis are more fully discussed in Chapter 31. Conceptually it is the morphological representation of a lymphocyte-mediated attack on hepatocytes (Plates 19.1 and 19.2). The infiltrate on the edges of the portal tracts and fibrous septa is composed of lymphocytes with varying proportions of macrophages, plasma cells and other cells. The cells are also to be found in the periportal sinusoids and, with careful scrutiny, in the space of Disse in close association with the hepatocytes. Hepatocytes show varying degrees of degenerative change. Fibrosis and bile ductular proliferation are frequent secondary changes at the interface and single or small groups of hepatocytes are isolated by the process. It is very difficult morphologically to distinguish piecemeal necrosis from the inflammatory spillover into periportal sinusoids that can occur in acute viral hepatitis.[6] The presence of maximal parenchymal damage occurring around the terminal hepatic vein and a large amount of granular ceroid pigment in clusters of Kupffer cells can

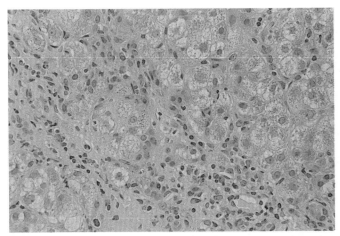

Plate 19.1 Piecemeal necrosis: an abnormal fibrous band passes obliquely from top left to lower right. Within it are many mononuclear cells including plasma cells as well as an isolated group and single hepatocytes. Proliferating bile ductules are forming at the parenchymal/stromal interfaces. Many hepatocytes show ballooning degeneration. (H & E ×300).

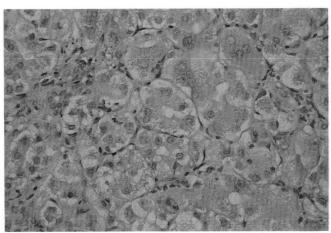

Plate 19.3 Regeneration: clusters of 6–8 hepatocytes are forming rosettes with a tiny central lumen and are demarcated from other hepatocytes by basement membrane. Some multinucleate hepatocytes are also present. (H & E ×500).

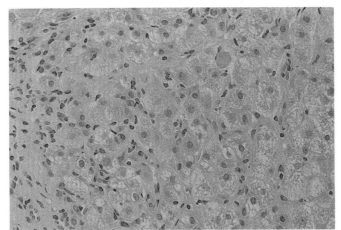

Plate 19.2 Piecemeal necrosis: lymphocytes, plasma cells and macrophages extend from the fibrous septum on the left into the parenchyma and are in close contact with the hepatocytes. The cell pattern is disrupted by a combination of ballooning degeneration and regenerative twinning of cell plates. Note the acidophil body, top right, as the round, more deeply eosinophilic body that in this instance lacks a nucleus. (H & E ×300).

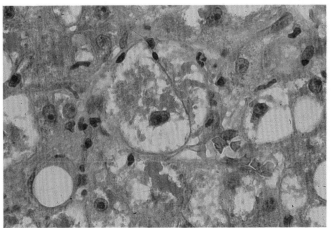

Plate 19.4 Mallory bodies: an enlarged swollen hepatocyte in the centre of the field has a very dense hyalin, irregular rope-like eosinophilic cytoplasmic inclusion just above the nucleus. Most of the cytoplasm is non-staining. Neutrophils are beginning to cluster around the cell membrane. Similar dense hyalin bodies are present in other hepatocytes. (H & E ×500).

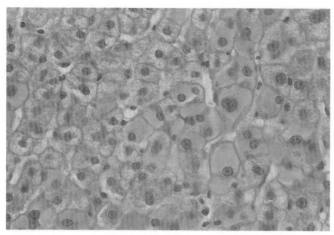

Plate 19.5 Ground-glass hepatocytes: these hepatocytes are enlarged by a large volume of glassy, palely eosinophilic cytoplasm. More deeply stained and granular cytoplasm is displaced to the periphery. Compare with the more normal hepatocytes in the left upper quadrant. (H & E ×300).

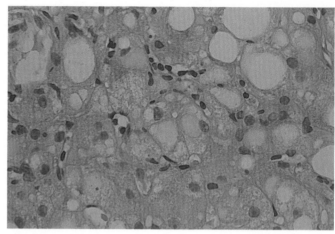

Plate 19.7 Fibrinogen storage disease: ground-glass hepatocytes.

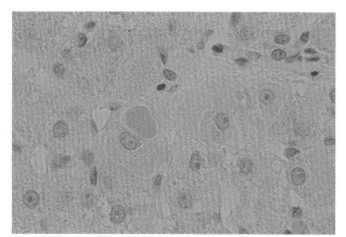

Plate 19.6 Lafora bodies: ground-glass hepatocytes in myoclonic epilepsy have cytoplasmic inclusions that stain positively with colloidal iron. (Colloidal iron ×500. Courtesy of Dr Ian Talbot, St. Mark's Hospital, London).

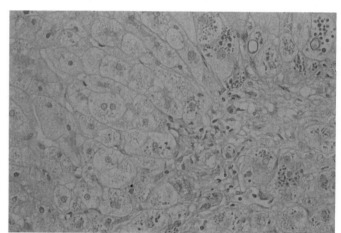

Plate 19.8 Globules of alpha-1-antitrypsin: intensely stained red globules of alpha-1-antitrypsin are present in periportal hepatocytes. The globules are of various sizes: in some biopsies only small numbers of the very smallest globules may be present. (PAS after diastase digestion ×300).

be helpful. They are characteristic features in acute viral hepatitis and should indicate caution in interpreting the periportal inflammatory infiltrate (see Chapter 30).

Parenchyma

The limiting plate

Examination of the architecture begins with the limiting plate which is simply the concentric layer of hepatocytes opposed to the connective tissue of the portal tracts. This plate is interrupted by the opening of vessels into the sinusoids but is comprehensively distorted in many liver diseases ranging from piecemeal necrosis (Plates 19.1 and 19.2) to bile duct obstruction.

Acinus

From the limiting plate, anastomosing radial plates of hepatocytes pass to the efferent vein. This pattern is altered readily in many conditions ranging from focal necroses to regeneration and is most reliably identified in reticulin preparations. The anatomical location of such lesions is important and particular attention should be paid to the hepatocytes around the terminal hepatic vein. Damage here is emphasized in acute viral hepatitis, alcoholic liver disease and some cases of drug-induced hepatitis, but is minor in bile duct obstruction and pure drug-induced cholestasis.

Regeneration is reflected in the liver by increased mitotic activity, twinning of the cell plates and increased nuclear pleomorphism and multinucleate hepatocytes. Mitotic activity is transient and therefore frequently not morphologically visualized. Twinning of cell plates can be found most often in periportal zones but will occur anywhere in the acinus in response to a focus of necrosis (Figure 19.4). Extensive regeneration in one area can result in compression of closely adjacent sinusoids (Figure 19.5). The nuclei in the twinned plates are often aligned along the sinusoidal margin of the cell and then give the plate a distinctive appearance. The regenerating areas of liver may also show rosette formation (Plate 19.3). These are suggested to be remodelled cylinders of hepatocytes surviving the episode of hepatocellular damage.[96] Rosettes may also be found in severe cholestasis but these are clusters of hepatocytes which form around a central bile-filled canaliculus. Less florid changes such as the number of binucleate hepatocytes, variation in nuclear size and staining, and the presence and distribution of intracellular pigments should be systematically sought. Increased numbers of binucleate and trinucleate hepatocytes and increased variation in nuclear pleomorphism are found with increasing age. These changes also result from renegeration following hepatocellular damage and persist after other signs of regeneration have disappeared. An increased variation in size and number of hepatocyte nuclei for the age of the patient may therefore give an indication of previous disease within the liver. Bizarre nuclear morphology within clusters of hepatocytes has been found within non-neoplastic areas of livers containing hepatocellular carcinoma and termed liver cell dysplasia. The relevance and prognostic significance of dysplasia in relation to hepatocellular carcinoma is disputed.[21,113]

Hepatocytes

These should be carefully examined and types of degeneration identified. These are rarely specific for one disease and it is usually a combination of the types of degeneration and its distribution that indicate the different diagnoses.

Fatty change This is a very common finding particularly in small amounts around the terminal hepatic vein. Severe degrees are most commonly found in alcoholic liver disease in Western society. Periportal fatty change suggests malnutrition or cachexia or rarely phosphorus poisoning (see Chapters 6 and 37).

Ballooning (hydropic) degeneration Hepatocytes are swollen to twice normal size or more (Plates 19.1 and 19.2). The nucleus may be normal in appearance but degenerative changes ranging from pyknosis to nuclear inclusions may be found.[118] It is central in position and surrounded by a cuff of granular cytoplasm. Fine strands of cytoplasm radiate from this cuff to the plasma membrane. There is no staining between the strands and this gives an appearance of peripheral pallor to the cell. The plasma membrane is often sharply defined but focal defects may be seen along its length. Electron microscopically there is striking dilatation of both rough and smooth endoplasmic reticulum, swelling of mitochondria and a loss of ribosomes and glycogen.[105] Many hepatocytes may be involved and cell death may occur by lysis.

Feathery degeneration Feathery degeneration is similar to ballooning degeneration by light microscopy but has different ultrastructural features. The cell is enlarged and the cytoplasm is rarefied. Perinuclear cytoplasm extends as wispy irregular strands out to the plasma membrane. Bile is usually present within the cell both as discrete granules and as brown staining of the strands of cytoplasm. Electron microscopically the cytoplasmic vacuolation is not due to hydropic distension of the endoplasmic reticulum as ballooning degeneration but to the presence of electron-dense myelin-like whorls of phospholipid. The lesion is due to the action of retained bile salts and feathery degeneration is therefore a common finding in all forms of prolonged cholestasis of both biliary and hepatocellular origin (see Chapter 15). Usually this form of degeneration is an inconspicuous or minor form of cell damage when the problem is primarily hepatocellular but it may be prominent in cirrhosis particularly if the patient is decompensating.

Acidophil degeneration (Plate 19.2) Acidophil degeneration is the morphological manifestation of apoptosis which is a process of cell death found in many tissues. Apoptosis is involved in normal regulatory mechanisms

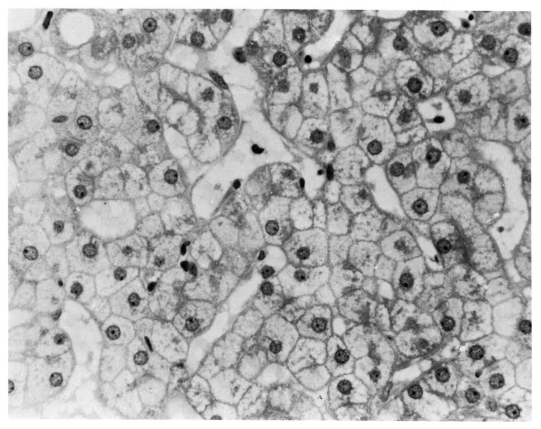

Figure 19.4 Abnormal cell plate pattern resulting from regeneration. The plates are two cells thick and where they meet they form 'knots' of hepatocytes. Haematoxylin and eosin, × 800.

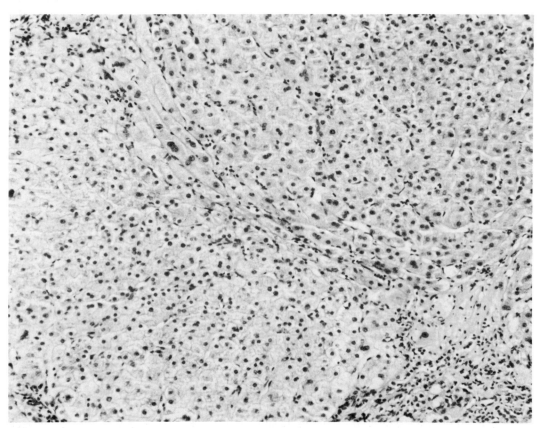

Figure 19.5 Abnormal cell plate pattern from regeneration. Asynchronous growth between two areas of parenchyma has resulted in a line of compression. This pattern most commonly occurs in cirrhosis. Haematoxylin and eosin, × 400.

but is considerably enhanced in pathological states.[123] In the liver, acidophil degeneration is seen as a small single shrunken hepatocyte with intensely stained deeply eosinophilic cytoplasm. The cell outline may be angulated at points of residual contact with other hepatocytes but often is rounded and then is completely separated by a clear space from its neighbours. The nucleus, if still present, shows pyknosis, karyorrhexis or both. Electron microscopically the cells are relatively electron-dense with residual organelles compacted together. Membranes of the endoplasmic reticulum are without a lumen, glycogen and ribosomes are absent, and surface microvilli and intercellular junctions are characteristically sparse. Mitochondria, by contrast, appear relatively well preserved.[105] Acidophil bodies are characteristically found in acute viral hepatitides including yellow fever—where they have been eponymously entitled Councilman bodies (Chapter 30). They also are seen in drug-induced hepatitis and are a common lesion in patients receiving both rifampicin and isoniazid.[122] They are also found in chronic liver disease and indicate activity of the inflammatory process; as such they are a hallmark for chronic lobular hepatitis (see Chapter 31).

Mallory bodies (Plate 19.4) are intracytoplasmic inclusions characterized by their dense homogenous hyalin appearance. Their shape varies from an irregular elongated serpentine to a rounded or oval non-membrane bound body. Electron microscopically they are dense aggregates of non-membrane-bound intermediate filaments that entrap other cell organelles (see Chapter 20).

They may be found in any established cirrhosis, in chronic cholestasis,[40] in primary biliary cirrhosis, in Wilson's disease,[117] in Indian childhood cirrhosis,[99] following intestinal bypass operations for obesity,[82] in diabetes mellitus[36] and sometimes in Weber–Christian disease[61] as well as in alcoholic liver disease. When combined with fatty change and ballooning degeneration of hepatocytes and localized to hepatocytes around the terminal hepatic vein, the pattern is almost pathognomonic for alcohol. Diabetic hepatitis is the major differential diagnosis.[97]

Cytoplasmic inclusions. Cytoplasmic inclusions other than Mallory bodies may also be found within hepatocytes. The most commonly seen are ground-glass hepatocytes which have a large volume of homogeneous finely stippled eosinophilic cytoplasm displacing mitochondria and rough endoplasmic reticulum to the periphery of the cell (Plate 19.5). The cell volume is usually increased. Electron microscopically the ground-glass change corresponds to hyperplastic smooth endoplasmic reticulum. Ground-glass hepatocytes occur in a wide variety of conditions.[3,137] They are a common finding in patients receiving enzyme-inducing drugs such as barbiturates, in alcoholics (where alcohol also acts as an enzyme inducer) and in patients who are chronic Hepatitis B carriers.[49] In this latter instance the ground-glass cytoplasm is rich in hepatitis B surface antigen and can be positively stained by immuno-

cytochemical and orcein staining techniques (see Figure 19.1). By contrast, drug-induced ground-glass hepatocytes are orcein negative and are usually located around the terminal hepatic vein.

Cytoplasmic inclusions closely resembling ground-glass hepatocytes are also seen in other conditions. Alcoholics treated with cyanamide (disulphiram),[140] myoclonic epilepsy (Lafora's disease) and Type IV glycogenosis,[54] all have such inclusions but these differ by being PAS positive and diastase resistant (Plate 19.6). The inclusions of myoclonic epilepsy and of Type IV glycogenosis can be confirmed by digestion with amylopectinase: by contrast with myoclonic epilepsy the inclusions in Type IV storage disease do not stain positively with colloidal iron. Cyanamide-induced inclusions can be identified from the clinical history.

Fibrinogen storage disease[18] has ground-glass inclusions that are weakly PAS positive (Plate 19.7); these may be clearly differentiated by their positive immunocytochemical staining for fibrinogen.

Occasionally the inclusions of alpha-1-antitrypsin deficiency can be seen on H&E stained preparations as bright round hyaline eosinophilic globules which are intensely PAS positive (Plate 19.8). Any doubt about their nature can be resolved by their positive immunocytochemical staining for alpha-1-antitrypsin.

Pigments

Pigments within hepatocytes are most commonly iron, lipofuscin and bile. Iron is easily identified by its periportal location and specific staining reactions and bile and lipofuscin are located around the terminal hepatic vein. Lipofuscin has fairly uniform refractile golden-brown granules and has characteristic staining reactions.[102] Electron microscopically, granules are membrane bound, irregularly lobulate, complex particles with varied electron-dense and electron-lucent areas (Chapter 2). It is a 'wear and tear' pigment noted for its absence in regenerating liver cells. It has significance, therefore, in suggesting that cirrhosis is not present in biopsies where identification of the architecture is otherwise equivocal. Dubin–Johnson pigment within hepatocytes superficially resembles lipofuscin but its chemical nature is not determined.[135]

Bile is more variable in appearance and may range from brown through yellow to green in colour. Definitive identification of bile is made by finding it within canaliculi.

Copper and copper-binding protein are found in the normal fetal and neonatal liver but rapidly disappear after birth. In adult liver their presence is pathological, representing Wilson's disease or chronic intrahepatic obstruction to the flow of bile at either canalicular or bile duct/ductular level. Copper can be specifically demonstrated by the very sensitive rubeanic acid technique or the sensitive and more reliable rhodanine technique.[53] Copper-binding protein is most simply demonstrated by the orcein technique[115] as blue-black granules in periportal or paraseptal hepatocytes (see Figure 19.2). Sometimes it can be seen on routine H&E stains as fine perinuclear

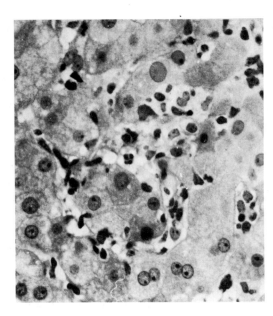

Figure 19.6 Sinusoids filled with inflammatory cells and proliferating Kupffer cells. Haematoxylin and eosin, × 1000.

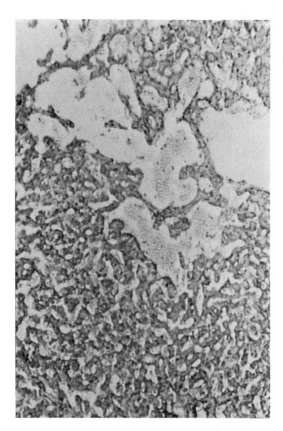

Figure 19.7 Focal sinusoidal ectasia: sudden widening of the sinusoids with associated atrophy of hepatocytes. Haematoxylin and eosin, × 250.

brown-grey granules which may be very weakly PAS positive after diastase digestion. Specific and diagnostic inclusions can be found in hepatocytes in protoporphyria[9, 78] and porphyria cutanea tarda.[26,56] The crystals found in porphyria cutanea tarda can be difficult to demonstrate without careful attention to technical detail. Although the pigment in protoporphyria closely resembles, and frequently is associated with cholestasis, it can be readily and specifically identified by its Maltese cross structure in polarized light.

Sinusoids

These narrow channels are usually less than half the width of a hepatocyte. Identification of relative width is helpful as apparent occlusion of the sinusoids indicates pathological change in the liver. This may be damage to hepatocytes such as fatty change or ballooning degeneration, or focal proliferation of sinusoidal cells as occurs in viral hepatitis (Figure 19.6), or twinning of cell plates as in regeneration (see Figure 19.4). The first two are usually obvious, so that bland obliteration of the sinusoidal space should result in a careful search for regenerative activity. Unfortunately, over-enthusiastic aspiration using a nail within the Menghini needle, or subsequent forceful expulsion with the stylet, can produce a similar artefact.

Conversely, dilatation of sinusoids (Figure 19.7) may be associated with loss of hepatocytes, passive venous congestion, infarcts of Zahn,[146] metastases within the liver (see Chapter 39), and drugs.[144] Passive venous congestion produces perivenular dilatation, while portal vein occlusion (infarct of Zahn) will be multiacinar and affect all zones of an acinus. The sinusoidal ectasia associated with the contraceptive pill and with metastases is usually

random in the acinus but a periportal pattern has been associated with the contraceptive pill.[144]

Congested sinusoids are rarely identified in a biopsy as the blood readily escapes from such small fragments of tissue. Persistence of many red cells in sinusoids, particularly dilated ones, is unusual. Two possible causes are erythrophagocytosis by Kupffer cells, as occurs in some haemolytic anaemias, and engorgement of the space of Disse. Originally described as pathognomonic for veno-occlusive disease of the liver[70] this has also been identified in left ventricular failure without right heart failure.[24]

Cells Cells within the sinusoids should be noted. Malignant cells ranging from carcinoma to hairy cell leukaemia, reactive (or infected) cells as in infectious mononucleosis, and aberrant normal or hyperplastic tissue as in extramedullary haemopoiesis may all occur. Endothelial cells and Kupffer cells are usually inconspicuous, but the latter especially may show hyperplasia and phagocytic activity in response to hepatocellular damage and death (see Figure 19.6) or may contain extraneous pigments such as Thorotrast,[29] malarial or schistosomal pigment or melanin. Thorotrast is a refractile granular pigment (Figure 19.8) that fluoresces when stained with alcoholic morin. Schistosomal and malarial pigments are granular, black, and doubly refractile in polarized light. Schistosomal and malarial pigments are both haematoidins and are probably

(a)

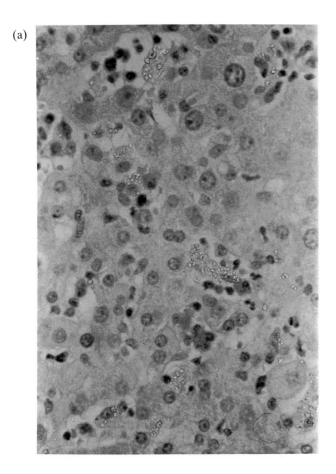

(b)

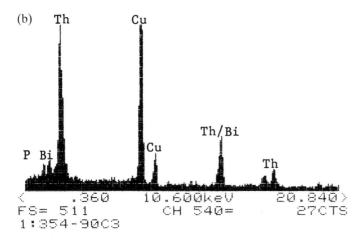

Figure 19.8 (a) Thorotrast: aggregates of refractile but non-staining granular pigment are present in sinusoidal macrophages. Haematoxylin and eosin, × 300. (b) X-ray probe analysis of a thin section of part of the biopsy shows the presence of thorium. The peaks of copper are from the specimen grid.

identical. Malignant melanoma metastatic to the liver can sometimes be suspected because Kupffer cells are rich in phagocytosed melanin.

Kupffer cells may have a foamy cytoplasm. Most commonly this is due to the phagocytosis of fat from

degenerate hepatocytes—particularly when there is severe fatty change in hepatocytes but it is also a feature in the many rare disorders of lipid metabolism and in the mucopolysaccharidoses.[54] These can be most commonly distinguished morphologically with electron microscopic techniques.[105] Other storage disease inclusions may be present. Cystinosis is particularly characteristic by its refractile and doubly refractile crystalline inclusions.[54] These are soluble in aqueous fixatives and processing and can only be demonstrated if non-aqueous fixation and processing or frozen sections are used. Otherwise the Kupffer cells will only have a foamy vacuolated appearance. Again electron microscopy is helpful.[145]

The space of Disse This normally lacks morphologically visible basement membrane but this is rapidly deposited in incipient and chronic liver disease (see Chapters 2 and 32). It is also a common site for deposition of amyloid (Chapter 37), which can be seen as an acellular eosinophilic zone between the hepatocyte and sinusoidal lumen. With increasing degrees of amyloidosis, hepatocytes become atrophic, but in the earliest stages special techniques such as Congo red staining may be required to demonstrate it.

Terminal hepatic vein

Last, but not least, the efferent vein should be identified. It has already been noted that an excess of efferent veins may be found in a macronodular cirrhosis, but important information is provided in differentiating acute liver disease. Hepatocytes around the efferent terminal hepatic vein are most frequently involved in cholestatic liver disease and show maximal damage in viral, drug and alcoholic liver disease (Figures 19.9 and 19.10). The efferent vein may be occluded by fibrosis in veno-occlusive disease and in alcoholic liver disease.[43] Veno-occlusive lesions are a common finding in cirrhosis at autopsy. More than 70% of cirrhotic livers have been recorded as showing veno-occlusive disease regardless of the primary aetiology,[98] although Burt and MacSween could only find such lesions in 22% of the 50 consecutive cirrhotic livers they studied at autopsy.[16] Recognition of a lesion in a biopsy is much more difficult and may explain why the lesion was found only in 10% of 256 liver biopsies from patients with alcoholic liver disease.[16]

Prolapse of hepatocytes through the wall of the terminal hepatic vein has been described in association with prolonged androgenic steroid therapy.[101]

DIAGNOSIS

Diagnosis in liver biopsies varies between primary and secondary liver lesions and the presence of focal or diffuse changes in the liver. Of these the most important distinction is between focal and diffuse liver disease as the latter is more reliably present and the sampling error

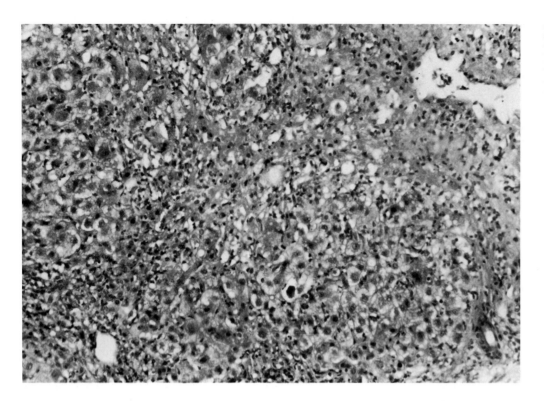

Figure 19.9 Parenchymal disarray in acute viral hepatitis. Terminal hepatic venule top right and portal tract bottom left. Haematoxylin and eosin, ×250

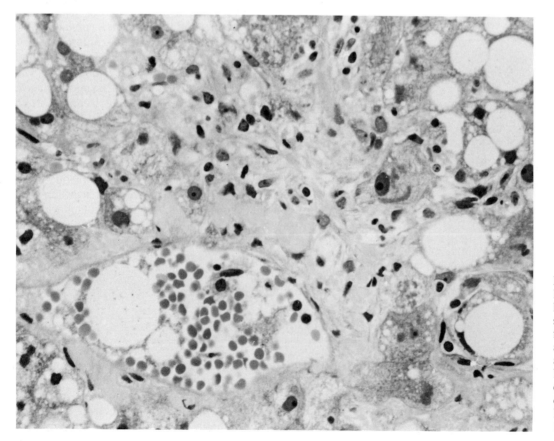

Figure 19.10 Alcoholic liver disease. The hepatic vein is surrounded by dense fibrous tissue which is also extending into adjacent sinusoids. Hepatocytes show fatty change and some also contain Mallory bodies. Haematoxylin and eosin, × 1200.

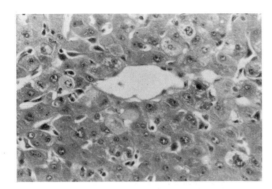

Figure 19.11 Acute bile duct obstruction. Cholestasis is present around the terminal hepatic venule. Note the lack of hepatocellular damage. Haematoxylin and eosin, × 500.

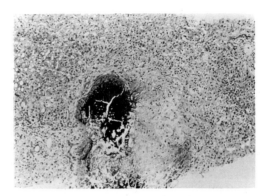

Figure 19.12 Bile infarct: a lake of extracellular bile within the parenchyma surrounded by a pale zone of histiocytes and degenerate hepatocytes. Haematoxylin and eosin, × 20.

may be considerable with focal lesions. With focal lesions, therefore, a normal or 'non-specific' biopsy does not necessarily exclude the clinical diagnosis.

Diffuse lesions

These are some of the major indications for liver biopsy and include the differential diagnosis of jaundice (Chapter 28) and the confirmation and differential diagnosis of cirrhosis (Chapter 32).

Jaundice

There are many causes of jaundice but the common differential in acute liver disease includes viral hepatitis, drug-induced jaundice and large bile duct obstruction. Congenital disorders of bilirubin metabolism affecting children or young adults can usually be readily separated by their clinical and biochemical features, sometimes in association with a biopsy (see Chapter 14). Cholestasis is considered in more detail in Chapter 15.

The emphasis in acute viral hepatitis (see also Chapter 30) is on panacinar hepatocellular damage including ballooning and acidophil degeneration with accentuation of the cell damage around efferent veins (see Figure 19.9). Cholestasis is present as bile within hepatocytes and canaliculi, but usually does not reflect the degree of hyperbilirubinaemia. Portal tracts may be expanded but the emphasis is on a mononuclear cell inflammatory infiltrate and there is rarely any significant bile ductule proliferation. There is generalized hyperplasia of Kupffer cells, particularly around efferent veins where they are also hypertrophied and laden with phagocytosed debris. These cells may fill a sinusoid and the features are associated with hepatocellular damage and death.

In obstruction to the biliary tree, cholestasis is the earliest feature and correlates with the degree of hyperbilirubinaemia.[20,92,93,107] Again, it is identified within hepatocytes and canaliculi around the terminal hepatic venule, but there is no significant hepatocellular damage (Figure 19.11). Any that is present is consequent upon the cholestasis and therefore occurs as a relatively late event. Bile damaged hepatocytes show feathery degeneration.

Within the first week cholestasis may be the only notable feature, so that for any accurate biopsy interpretation the duration of jaundice is critical clinical information.

After the first week changes also occur in portal tracts. These initially become rounded in cross-section and the cells and fibres of the stroma more widely separated as a result of oedema. The bile duct is distended and later the epithelium shows considerable distortion as a result of focal degeneration and regeneration. A multilayered epithelium may thus form while at the same time parts of the duct wall are degenerate and lined by epithelial cells with flattened contours and pyknotic nuclei.

An inflammatory reaction initially is scanty and confined to a few neutrophils which may be easily overlooked. As the numbers of neutrophils increase they concentrate along the margins of the portal tracts and characteristically around the bile ductules. Lymphocytes and macrophages appear but remain central within the tract. Plasma cells, if present, indicate a complication, particularly a cholangitis: otherwise an alternative diagnosis should be sought.

As the obstruction progresses so the portal tracts expand by the formation of new fibrous tissue. Proliferating bile ductules at the edge of the tract[107] are prominent in this fibrosis. They are frequently angulate and may be perpendicular to the parenchymal interface.

Occasionally bile infarcts within the parenchyma and bile granulomas within the portal tracts may be found. These are attributed to the escape of bile into the tissues and are virtually pathognomonic for obstruction (Figure 19.12). In long-standing cases the bile disappears and a network of reticulin fibres and macrophages remains. Within the portal tract, escape of bile from bile duct results in a foreign body giant cell granulomatous reaction usually positioned against the bile duct. This should not be confused with the granuloma associated with primary biliary cirrhosis.

Ancillary stains assist by the negative information they provide. The normality of the zone around the terminal hepatic vein in obstruction is clearly demonstrated in the reticulin preparations, while the absence of focal Kupffer cell proliferation can be seen on diastase PAS preparations. PAS-positive pigment is present within the Kupffer cells but their distribution is uniform around the efferent vein, and numbers diminish drastically in the mid-zone and even more in the periportal areas. Focal clusters of Kupffer cells reflect a response to hepatocyte death and are usually a late event in obstruction. These features are helpful in distinguishing between obstruction and the cholestatic variety of viral hepatitis (see Chapter 30).

These classical features are now rarely seen because, with the advent of ERCP, percutaneous transhepatic cholangiography and ultrasound, biopsy is relatively contraindicated in bile duct obstruction. Biopsies are much more likely to be taken in 'odd' cases or those showing complications.

When obstruction to the major ducts is intermittent, the degree of bile retention may be minimal and overshadowed by the portal tract changes of fibrosis with bile ductule proliferation and surrounding neutrophils. A similar lack of cholestasis may be seen with focal intrahepatic obstruction. Then not only may the portal tract changes be relatively emphasized but there may be considerable variation between portal tracts with some apparently unaffected or only mildly affected.

The evolution of the changes is difficult to time because the onset of obstruction is rarely known accurately in a patient. Experimentally, ligation of the common bile duct in rats results in mitotic activity in bile duct epithelium detectable by autoradiography within 48 hours. By the eighth day the proportion of bile ductules by volume has approximately doubled and gradually increases thereafter. New fibrous tissue is formed after the bile ductule proliferation and apparently in response to it.[58]

Although the morphology of drug-induced jaundice is varied and complex (see Chapter 46), very few drugs mimic the portal tract changes of biliary obstruction. When there is only cholestasis with minimal or no inflammation or hepatocellular damage, distinction between drug-induced jaundice and large bile duct obstruction can be impossible without knowledge of the duration of jaundice. Clinical or biochemical features of jaundice of more than 2 weeks' duration without portal tract changes are unlikely to be due to large bile duct

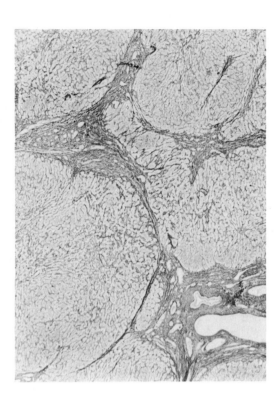

Figure 19.14 Macronodular cirrhosis with portal tract bottom right, slender bands of abnormal fibrous tissue and abnormal cell plate patterns. A needle biopsy demonstrating only the right half of the figure may show mild fibrosis only. Wedge biopsy. Reticulin, × 20.

obstruction. Drugs most likely to create diagnostic confusion are the anabolic and 17α-substituted steroids and those drugs producing a cholestatic hepatitis: chief among these are the phenothiazines.

Distinction between viral hepatitis and drug hepatitis can be extremely difficult and sometimes impossible.[8] Points in favour of a drug-induced hepatitis are the more sharply circumscribed focal or even zonal distribution of the hepatocellular degenerative changes, fatty change in hepatocytes, and minimal reactive mesenchymal and inflammatory changes away from the degenerate hepatocytes.

Cirrhosis

This is considered in Chapter 32. The value of needle biopsy varies with the type of needle and the technique employed. Cutting needles such as Vim–Silverman and Trucut are not deflected by the connective tissue and so are more accurate. Blunt needles such as the Menghini needle core out the softer parenchyma and slide along connective-tissue bands. Cirrhosis may then be underdiagnosed.[119]

Generally a micronodular cirrhosis (Figure 19.13) shows uniformity throughout the liver and is not affected by sampling. The most difficult problem is to establish when, for instance, severe central hyaline sclerosis in an alcoholic is or is not an early micronodular cirrhosis. In a macronod-

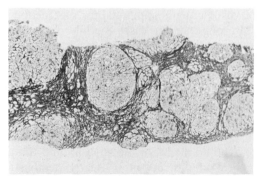

Figure 19.13 Micronodular cirrhosis. Numerous tiny nodules are identified within a needle biopsy, × 10.

ular multiacinar cirrhosis (Figures 19.3 and 19.14) with
areas of apparently normal architecture, sampling error
can be considerable and, in the absence of obvious
regenerative nodules, diagnosis is difficult. The presence
of slender bands of fibrous tissue (Figures 19.3 and 19.14)
the abnormal cell plate patterns (see Figure 19.5) and the
excess of efferent veins are important features in these
cases. In such cases there should also be an absence of
lipofuscin around these efferent veins. Conversely, its
presence suggests a lack of regeneration, implies an
'ageing' hepatocyte and indicates that the efferent vein is
anatomically a hepatic venule.

Focal lesions

A significant proportion of the liver biopsies performed
in routine clinical practice is for a tissue diagnosis in non-
hepatic diseases that involve the liver. There may be
diffuse involvement of the liver as in amyloidosis and
malaria but focal lesions are more common. Consequently,
considerable sampling error occurs and examination of
multiple levels of the biopsy may be necessary. There is
thus a conflict between the examination of biopsies for
focal lesions and the need for retention of tissue for
additional diagnostic techniques, such as the search for
organisms in tuberculosis or the immunoperoxidase
method for viruses, proteins or other antigens.

The accurate identification of focal lesions when present
is usually simple:[42,116,129] metastatic liver disease rarely
presents diagnostic problems except for identification of
its origin. Likewise, epithelioid granulomas are not difficult to identify but their aetiology can rarely be determined
from the morphology. Many causes have been described
(see Chapter 37) but the most common in the UK are
sarcoidosis, sarcoidal reaction to tumour, tuberculosis,
drug reactions and primary biliary cirrhosis. Despite this,
a significant proportion remains undiagnosed.

Sometimes secondary changes related to a focal lesion
may be identified. The presence of neutrophils around
proliferating bile ductules in some but not all portal tracts
suggests a focal intrahepatic lesion involving a branch of
the biliary tree. Focal sinusoidal ectasia may be identified
where sinusoids in one area are dilated and hepatocytes
are small and atrophic (see Figure 19.7). This feature has
various associations such as severe wasting illness, drugs,
cirrhosis and vascular disturbances, but is also seen
sometimes around metastases. Its architectural localization may indicate a particular association, such as the
periportal ectasia described with the contraceptive pill.[144]
The perivenular sinusoidal dilatation from heart failure is
similar but identified by its regular distribution and even
appearance. When focal sinusoidal ectasia is the only
abnormality in a biopsy, particularly when metastatic liver
disease is suspected clinically, multiple levels through the
specimen must be examined for microscopic deposits of
tumour in portal tract or sinusoids.

Focal lesions may also be primary within the liver.
Apart from hepatocellular carcinoma, adenoma and focal

nodular hyperplasia, small microhamartomas of the biliary
tree (von Meyenburg complexes) may also be found.
They are most commonly an incidental finding and bear
no relationship to other hepatic changes but they may be
associated with congenital hepatic fibrosis,[60] even in
adults,[28,81] and polycystic liver.[85]

PROGNOSTIC FEATURES

Making a specific diagnosis inevitably implies a prognosis
for the patient, but occasionally additional features in the
biopsy may indicate the further natural history of the
disease more clearly. This has been most intensively
investigated and debated in acute viral hepatitis, where
such features as bridging hepatic necrosis (Figure 19.15),
excessive numbers of plasma cells, bile duct lesions,
piecemeal necrosis, impaired hepatocyte regeneration and
the presence of complement in hepatocytes have all been
suggested to be of adverse prognostic significance (see
Chapter 30).

Similarly prognostic features may be found in other
conditions. In alcoholics the presence of perivenular
fibrosis is a bad prognostic sign indicating inevitable
progression to cirrhosis if drinking continues[139] (see Figure
19.10), while the presence of granulomas in primary
biliary cirrhosis[69] or the absence of bile ducts in childhood
alpha-1-antitrypsin deficiency[48] may be favourable features.

A slightly different use is to predict the outcome of
a portoenterostomy performed for extrahepatic biliary
atresia. Here a core of tissue is removed from the porta
hepatis and a loop of bowel is anastomosed to the raw
surface of the liver. The presence of tiny bile ductules
within this excised core indicates an increased chance of
successful bile drainage.[59]

RESPONSE TO THERAPY

The restricted use of liver biopsy for assessing the results
of therapy reflects as much the limited range of therapeutic
manoeuvres available in liver disease as the sampling
error and consequent variation that occur in biopsy
material. The most obvious use is to assess the reduction
in iron (or copper) overload in response to venesection
or chelation therapy. Iron in particular can be assessed
in a semiquantitative fashion by histochemical techniques
and shows a reasonable correlation with liver iron measured biochemically.[33] The effects of venesection can then
be accurately followed and treatment suspended when
demonstrable iron is grade 1 or less, although continual
reassessment may be necessary (see Chapter 36).

The biopsy is also used to assess the effects of steroid
therapy in chronic active hepatitis. Piecemeal necrosis,
particularly its lymphocytic component, sometimes subsides dramatically on steroid therapy. Unfortunately, any
reduction in activity may simply reflect the geographical

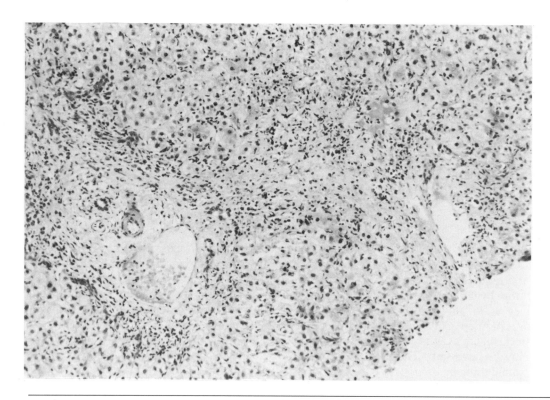

Figure 19.15 Bridging hepatic necrosis in acute viral hepatitis. The portal tract (left) and efferent vein (right) are bridged by a zone of collapsed reticulin. Haematoxylin and eosin, × 250.

variation of activity within the liver that is a feature of this disease and consequently a misleading impression of therapeutic response may be obtained. Nevertheless, by so employing liver biopsy, workers at the Mayo Clinic assessed the relative merits of steroids and azathioprine and found a combination of the two to be most effective.[5]

It can be used to follow the consequences of a portoenterostomy performed for extrahepatic biliary atresia. In such a patient recently there was initial clinical improvement. A follow-up liver biopsy 3 months later demonstrated continuing bile duct obstruction and at subsequent

re-exploration a mass of clot and mucin within the enterostomy was removed. A further biopsy has demonstrated a dramatic decrease in activity, although considerable scarring is now present.

Liver biopsy is used to anticipate the complications of methotrexate therapy for psoriasis.[4] Prolonged administration of methotrexate, particularly orally, can result in cirrhosis.[89] The development of the cirrhosis cannot be predicted by clinical features or liver function tests. Consequently, if this therapy is employed, regular liver biopsy is mandatory.

REFERENCES

1. Alagille, D., Odièvre, M., Gautier, M. & Domergues, J.P. (1975) Hepatic ductular hypoplasia associated with characteristic facies, vertebral malformations, retarded physical, mental and skeletal development and cardiac murmur. *Journal of Pediatrics*, **86**, 63–71.
2. Allison, D.J. & Adam, A. (1988) Percutaneous liver biopsy and track embolization with steel coils. *Radiology*, **169**, 261–263.
3. Alonso-Marti, C., Moreno, A., Barat, A. *et al.* (1990) Co-existence of hepatocyte ground-glass inclusions from several causes. *Histopathology*, **16**, 304–307.
4. Ashton, R.E., Millward-Sadler, G.H. & White, J.E. (1982) Complications in methotrexate treatment of psoriasis with particular reference to liver fibrosis. *Journal of Investigative Dermatology*, **79**, 229–232.
5. Baggenstoss, A.H., Soloway, R.D., Summerskill, W.H.J. *et al.* (1972) Chronic active liver disease. The range of histologic lesions, their response to treatment and evolution. *Human Pathology*, **3**, 183–198.
6. Baptista, A., Bianchi, L., De Groote, J. *et al.* (1988) The diagnostic significance of periportal hepatic necrosis and inflammation. *Histopathology*, **12**, 569–580.
7. Barry, M. & Sherlock, S. (1971) Measurement of liver-iron concentration in needle biopsy specimens. *Lancet*, **1**, 100–103.
8. Bianchi, L., De Groote, J., Desmet, V.J. *et al.* (1974) Guidelines for diagnosis of therapeutic drug induced liver injury in liver biopsies. Review by an international group. *Lancet*, **1**, 854–857.
9. Bloomer, J.R. (1982) Evidence that hepatic crystalline deposits in a patient with protoporphyria are composed of protoporphyrin. *Gastroenterology*, **82**, 569–573.
10. Brechot, C. (1990) Polymerase chain reaction. A new tool for the study of viral infections in hepatology. *Journal of Hepatology*, **11**, 124–129.
11. Bret, P.M., Fond, A., Bretagnolle, M. *et al.* (1988) Percutaneous aspiration and drainage of hydatid cysts in the liver. *Radiology*, **168**, 617–620.
12. Bull, H.J.M., Gilmore, I.T., Bradley, R.D. *et al.* (1983) Experience with transjugular liver biopsy. *Gut*, **24**, 1057–1060.
13. Buorgiorno-Nardelli, M. & Amaldi, F. (1970) Autoradiographic detection of molecular hybrids between rRNA and DNA in tissue sections. *Nature*, **225**, 946–948.
14. Burns, J. (1970) Preparations of thin epoxy resin sections from thick sections of paraffin-embedded material. *Journal of Clinical Pathology*, **23**, 643–645.
15. Burrell, C.J., Gowans, E.J., Jibert, A.R. *et al.* (1982) Hepatitis B virus DNA detection by *in situ* cytohybridization: implications for viral replication strategy and pathogenesis of chronic hepatitis. *Hepatology*, **2**, 858–918.

16. Burt, A.D. & MacSween, R.N.M. (1986) Hepatic vein lesions in alcoholic liver disease: retrospective biopsy and necropsy study. *Journal of Clinical Pathology,* **39,** 63–67.

17. Buscarini, L., Fornari, F., Bolandi, L. *et al.* (1990) Ultrasound-guided fine-needle biopsy of focal liver lesions: techniques, diagnostic accuracy and complications. A retrospective study on 2091 biopsies. *Journal of Hepatology,* **11,** 334–338.

18. Callea, F., de Vos, R., Togni, R. *et al.* (1986) Fibrinogen inclusions in liver cells: a new type of ground-glass hepatocyte. Immune, light and electron microscopic characterisation. *Histopathology,* **10,** 65–74.

19. Chiprut, R.O., Greenwald, R.A., Morris, S.J. *et al.* (1978) Intrahepatic hematoma resulting in obstructive jaundice. *Gastroenterology,* **74,** 124–127.

20. Christoffersen, P. & Poulsen, H. (1970) Histological changes in human liver biopsies following extrahepatic biliary obstruction. *Acta Pathologica et Microbiologica Scandinavica. Supplement,* **212,** 150–157.

21. Chossegros, P., Trepo, C., Marion, D. & Hanss, M. (1988) Hepatic hematomas after transparietal liver biopsy (Letter). *Gastroenterology,* **95,** 848–849.

22. Chuang, V.P. & Alspaugh, J.P. (1988) Sheath needle for liver biopsy in high risk patients. *Radiology,* **166,** 261–262.

23. Cohen, C. & Berson, S.D. (1986) Liver cell dysplasia in normal, cirrhotic and hepatocellular patients. *Cancer,* **57,** 1535–1538.

24. Cohen, J.A. & Kaplan, M.M. (1978) Left-sided heart failure presenting as hepatitis. *Gastroenterology,* **74,** 583–587.

25. Conn, H.O. (1972) Rational use of liver biopsy in the diagnosis of hepatic cancer. *Gastroenterology,* **62,** 142–146.

26. Cortes, J.M., Oliva, H., Paradinas, F.J. & Hernandez-Guio, C. (1980) The pathology of the liver in porphyria cutanea tarda. *Histopathology,* **4,** 471–485.

27. Cronan, J.J., Esparza, A.R. & Dorfman, G.S. (1988) Cavernous hemangioma of the liver: role of percutaneous biopsy. *Radiology,* **166,** 135–138.

28. Daroca, P.J., Tuthill, R. & Reed, R.J. (1975) Cholangiocarcinoma arising in congenital hepatic fibrosis. *Archives of Pathology,* **99,** 592–595.

29. da Silva Horta, J., Abbatt, J.D., da Motta, L.C. & Roriz, M.L. (1965) Malignancy and other late effects following administration of Thorotrast. *Lancet,* **2,** 201–205.

30. Desmet, V.J., Bullens, A.M., De Groote, J. & Heirwegh, K.P.M. (1968) A new diazo reagent for specific staining of conjugated bilirubin in tissue sections. *Journal of Histochemistry and Cytochemistry,* **16,** 419–427.

31. Dixon, A.G. & Barnes, W.A. (1973) Liver biopsy in patients with malignancy: a post mortem study. *Laboratory Investigation,* **28,** 405.

32. Dotter, C.T. (1964) Catheter biopsy. Experimental technic for transvenous liver biopsy. *Radiology,* **82,** 312–314.

33. Edwards, C.Q., Carroll, M., Bray, P. & Cartwright, G.E. (1977) Hereditary haemochromatosis. Diagnosis in siblings and children. *New England Journal of Medicine,* **297,** 7–13.

34. Engelhard, D., Ornoy, A. & Deckelbaum, R.J. (1981) Pneumoscrotum complicating percutaneous liver biopsy. *Gastroenterology,* **80,** 390–392.

35. Evander, A., Ihse, I., Lunderquist, A. *et al.* (1980) Percutaneous cytodiagnosis of carcinoma of the pancreas and bile duct. *Annals of Surgery,* **188,** 90–92.

36. Falchuk, K.R., Fiske, S.C., Haggitt, R.C. *et al.* (1980) Pericentral hepatic fibrosis and intracellular hyalin in diabetes mellitus. *Gastroenterology,* **78,** 535–541.

37. Ferrari, A., Cassanelli, M. & Barbolini, G. (1988) Hematomas after percutaneous liver biopsy (Letter). *Gastroenterology,* **94,** 250.

38. Gallison, D.T. Jr. & Skinner, D. (1950) Bile peritonitis complicating needle biopsy of liver. *New England Journal of Medicine,* **243,** 47–50.

39. Gazelle, G.S. & Haaga, J.R. (1989) Guided percutaneous biopsy of intraabdominal lesions. *American Journal of Roentgenology,* **153,** 929–935.

40. Gerber, A.M., Orr, W., Denk, H. *et al.* (1973) Hepatocellular hyalin in cholestasis and cirrhosis: its diagnostic significance. *Gastroenterology,* **64,** 89–98.

41. Glauert, A.M. (1975) *Fixation Dehydration and Embedding of Biological Specimens.* Amsterdam: North-Holland Publishing Co.

42. Glenthoj, A., Sehested, M. & Torp-Pedersen, S. (1989) Diagnostic reliability of histological and cytological fine needle biopsies from focal liver lesions. *Histopathology,* **15,** 375–383.

43. Goodman, Z.D. & Ishak, K.G. (1982) Occlusive venous lesions in alcoholic liver disease. A study of 200 cases. *Gastroenterology,* **83,** 786–796.

44. Gordon, H. & Sweets, H.H. Jr. (1936) Simple method for silver impregnation of reticulum. *American Journal of Pathology,* **12,** 545–552.

45. Grisham, J.W., Nopanitaya, W. & Compagno, J. (1976) Scanning electron microscopy of the liver: a review of methods and results. In Popper, H. & Schaffner, F. (eds) *Progress in Liver Diseases,* Vol. V, pp. 1–23. New York: Grune & Stratton.

46. Grossman, B., Goldstein, M.J., Koss, L.G. *et al.* (1972) Cytological examination as an adjunct to liver biopsy in the diagnosis of hepatic metastases. *Gastroenterology,* **62,** 56–60.

47. Gubetta, L., Rizzetto, M., Crivelli, O. *et al.* (1977) A trichrome stain for the intrahepatic localisation of the hepatitis B surface antigen (HBsAg). *Histopathology,* **1,** 277–288.

48. Hadchouel, M. & Gautier, M. (1976) Histopathologic study of the liver in the early cholestatic phase of αIAT deficiency. *Journal of Pediatrics,* **89,** 211–215.

49. Hadziyannis, S., Gerber, M.A., Vissoulis, C. & Popper, H. (1973) Cytoplasmic Hepatitis B antigen in 'ground-glass' hepatocytes of carriers. *Archives of Pathology,* **96,** 327–330.

50. Hederstrom, E., Forsberg, L., Floren, C-H. & Prytz, H. (1989) Liver biopsy complications monitored by ultrasound. *Journal of Hepatology,* **8,** 94–98.

51. Hong, R. & Schubert, W.K. (1960) Menghini needle biopsy of the liver. *American Journal of Diseases of Children,* **100,** 42–46.

52. Hopwood, D. (1969) Fixatives and fixation: a review. *Histochemical Journal,* **1,** 323–360.

53. Irons, R.D., Schenk, E.A. & Lee, J.C.K. (1977) Cytochemical methods for copper. Semiquantitative screening procedure for identification of abnormal copper levels in liver. *Archives of Pathology and Laboratory Medicine,* **101,** 298–301.

54. Ishak, K.G. & Sharp, H.L. (1987) Metabolic errors and liver disease. In MacSween, R.N.M., Anthony, P.P. & Scheuer, P.J. (eds) *Pathology of the Liver,* 2nd edn, pp. 99–180. Edinburgh: Churchill Livingstone.

55. Iversen, P. & Roholm, K. (1939) On aspiration biopsy of the liver, with remarks on its diagnostic significance. *Acta Medica Scandinavica,* **102,** 1–16.

56. James, K.R. (1980) Demonstration of intracytoplasmic needle-like inclusions in hepatocytes of patients with porphyria cutanea tarda. *Journal of Clinical Pathology,* **33,** 899–900.

57. Jennings, P.E., Coral, A., Donald, J.J. *et al.* (1989) Ultrasound guided core biopsy. *Lancet,* **1,** 1369–1371.

58. Johnstone, J.M. & Lee, E.G. (1976) A quantitative assessment of the structural changes in the rat's liver following obstruction of the common bile duct. *British Journal of Experimental Pathology,* **57,** 85–94.

59. Kasai, M., Watanabe, I. & Ohi, R. (1975) Follow-up studies of long-term survivors after portoenterostomy for 'non-correctable' biliary atresia. *Journal of Pediatric Surgery,* **10,** 173–182.

60. Kerr, D.N.S., Harrison, C.V., Sherlock, S. & Miles-Walker, R. (1961) Congenital hepatic fibrosis. *Quarterly Journal of Medicine,* **30,** 91–117.

61. Kimura, H., Kako, M., Yo, K. & Oda, T. (1980) Alcoholic hyalin (Mallory Bodies) in a case of Weber–Christian disease: electron microscopic observations of liver involvement. *Gastroenterology,* **78,** 807–812.

62. Knauer, C.M. (1978) Percutaneous biopsy of the liver as a procedure for outpatients. *Gastroenterology,* **74,** 101–102.

63. Korula, J., Fried, J., Weissman, M. *et al.* (1989) Fatal haemorrhage from an arterio-portal-peritoneal fistula after percutaneous liver biopsy. *Gastroenterology,* **96,** 244–246.

64. Krarup, N.B. (1949) Aspiration biopsy of the liver with special reference to the method of Iversen–Roholm. *Acta Medica Scandinavica. Supplement,* **234,** 199–209.

65. Kretschmer, C., Jones, D.B., Morrison, K. *et al.* (1990) Tumor

necrosis factor α and lymphotoxin production in Hodgkin's disease. *American Journal of Pathology*, **137**, 341–351.

66. Laurell, S. & Lundquist, A. (1971) Lipid composition of human liver biopsy specimens. *Acta Medica Scandinavica*, **189**, 65–68.

67. Lebrec, D., Goldfarb, G., Degott, C. *et al.* (1982) Transvenous liver biopsy. An experience based on 1000 hepatic tissue samplings with this procedure. *Gastroenterology*, **83**, 338–340.

68. Lee, R.L. (1977) 2-hydroxyethyl methacrylate embedded tissue—a method complementary to routine paraffin embedding. *Medical Laboratory Sciences*, **34**, 231–239.

69. Lee, R.G., Epstein, C., Jauregin, H. *et al.* (1981) Granulomas in primary biliary cirrhosis: a prognostic feature. *Gastroenterology*, **81**, 983–986.

70. Leopold, J.G., Parry, T.E. & Storring, F.K. (1970) A change in the sinusoid trabecular structure of the liver with hepatic venous outflow block. *Journal of Pathology*, **100**, 87–98.

71. Levin, B., Dobbs, R.H., Burgess, A. & Palmer, T. (1969) Hyperammonaemia. A variant type of deficiency of liver ornithine transcarbamylase. *Archives of Disease in Childhood*, **44**, 162–169.

72. Lindner, H. (1967) Grenzen und Gefahren der perkutanen Leberbiopsie mit der Menghi-Ninadel. *Deutsch Medizinische Wochenschrift*, **92**, 1751–1757.

73. Livraghi, T., Damascelli, B., Lombardi, C. & Spagnoli, I. (1983) Risk in fine-needle abdominal biopsy. *Journal of Clinical Ultrasound*, **11**, 77–81.

74. Lo, Y.-M.D., Mehal, W.Z. & Fleming, K.A. (1989) In vitro amplification of Hepatitis B virus sequences from liver tumour DNA and from paraffin wax embedded tissues using the polymerase chain reaction. *Journal of Clinical Pathology*, **42**, 840–846.

75. Lundquist, A. (1970) Liver biopsy with a needle of 0.7 mm outer diameter. *Acta Medica Scandinavica*, **188**, 471–474.

76. Lundvall, O. & Enerbäck, L. (1969) Hepatic fluorescence in porphyria cutanea tarda studied in fine needle aspiration biopsy smears. *Journal of Clinical Pathology*, **22**, 704–709.

77. Lyon, H. & Prento, P. (1973) Alcian blue-silver impregnation. A method differentiating between acid carbohydrates, reticulin fibres and collagen fibres. *Acta Pathologica et Microbiologica Scandinavica, Section A*, **81**, 6–8.

78. MacDonald, D.M. (1981) The histopathology and ultrastructure of liver disease in erythropoietic protoporphyria. *British Journal of Dermatology*, **104**, 7–17.

79. MacIver, A.G., Giddings, J. & Mepham, B.L. (1979) Demonstration of extracellular immunoproteins in formalin fixed renal biopsy specimens. *Kidney International*, **16**, 632–636.

80. Madden, R.E. (1961) Complications of needle biopsy of the liver. *Archives of Surgery*, **83**, 781–788.

81. Manes, J.L., Kissane, J.M. & Valdes, A.J. (1977) Congenital hepatic fibrosis, liver cell carcinoma and adult polycystic kidneys. *Cancer*, **39**, 2619–2623.

82. McGill, D.B., Humphreys, S.R., Baggenstoss, A.H. & Dickson, E.R. (1972) Cirrhosis and death after jejunoileal shunt. *Gastroenterology*, **63**, 872–877.

83. Malone, D.E., McCormick, P.A., O'Donoghue, D.P. & MacErlean, D.P. (1988) Hematomas after percutaneous liver biopsy (Letter). *Gastroenterology*, **94**, 249.

84. Martino, C.R., Haaga, J.R., Bryan, P.J. *et al.* (1984) CT-guided liver biopsies: Eight years experience. *Radiology*, **152**, 755–757.

85. Melnick, P.J. (1955) Polycystic liver. Analysis of seventy cases. *Archives of Pathology*, **59**, 162–172.

86. Menghini, G. (1958) One-second needle biopsy of the liver. *Gastroenterology*, **35**(2), 190–199.

87. Mewissen, M.W., Lipchik, E.O., Schreiber, G.R. & Varma, R.R. (1988) Liver biopsy through the femoral vein. *Radiology*, **169**, 842–843.

88. Millward-Sadler, G.H. & Giddings, J. (1978) Unpublished observations.

89. Millward-Sadler, G.H. & Ryan, T.J. (1974) Methotrexate induced liver disease in psoriasis. *British Journal of Dermatology*, **90**, 661–667.

90. Minuk, G.Y., Sutherland, L.R., Wiseman, D.A., *et al.* (1987) Prospective study of the incidence of ultrasound-detected intrahepatic and subcapsular hematomas in patients randomized to 6 or 24 hours of bed rest after percutaneous liver biopsy. *Gastroenterology*, **92**, 290–293.

91. Monath, T.P., Ballinger, M.E., Miller, B.R. & Salaun, J.J. (1989) Detection of yellow fever viral RNA by nucleic acid hybridisation and viral antigen by immunocytochemistry in fixed human liver. *American Journal of Tropical Medicine and Hygiene*, **40**, 663–668.

92. Morris, J.S., Gallo, G.A., Scheuer, P.J. & Sherlock, S. (1975) Percutaneous liver biopsy in patients with large bile duct obstruction. *Gastroenterology*, **68**, 750–754.

93. Movitt, E.R. & Davis, A.E. (1954) Extrahepatic biliary obstruction: experience with needle biopsy of the liver. *Annals of Internal Medicine*, **40**, 952–962.

94. Murphy, F.B., Barefield, K.P., Steiberg, H.V. & Bernadino, M.E. (1988) CT- or sonographic-guided biopsy of the liver in the presence of ascites: frequency of complications. *American Journal of Roentgenology*, **151**, 485–486.

95. Murray, G.I. & Ewen, S.W.B. (1989) A new approach to enzyme histochemical analysis of biopsy specimens. *Journal of Clinical Pathology*, **42**, 767–771.

96. Nagore, N., Howe, S., Boxer, L. & Scheuer, P.J. (1989) Liver cell rosettes: structural differences in cholestasis and hepatitis. *Liver*, **9**, 43–51.

97. Nagore, N. & Scheuer, P.J. (1988) The pathology of diabetic hepatitis. *Journal of Pathology*, **156**, 155–160.

98. Nakanuma, Y., Ohta, G. & Doishita, K. (1985) Quantitation and serial section observations of focal veno-occlusive lesions of hepatic veins in liver cirrhosis. *Virchows Archiv A*, **405**, 429–438.

99. Nayak, N.C., Sagreiya, K. & Ramalingaswami, V. (1969) The nature and significance of cytoplasmic hyalin of hepatocytes. *Archives of Pathology*, **88**, 631–637.

100. Okuda, K., Musha, H., Nakajima, Y. *et al.* (1978) Frequency of intrahepatic arteriovenous fistula as a sequela to percutaneous needle puncture of the liver. *Gastroenterology*, **74**, 1204–1207.

101. Paradinas, F.J., Bull, T.B., Westaby, D. & Murray-Lyon, I.M. (1977) Hyperplasia and prolapse of hepatocytes into hepatic veins during long-term methyltestosterone therapy: possible relationships of these changes to the development of peliosis hepatis and liver tumours. *Histopathology*, **1**, 225–246.

102. Pearse, A.G.E. (1972) *Histochemistry*, 3rd edn. Edinburgh: Churchill Livingstone.

103. Pelckmans, P.A., Pen, J.H., Michielsen, P.P. & van Maercke, Y.M. (1988) Hematomas after percutaneous liver biopsy (Letter). *Gastroenterology*, **94**, 249.

104. Perrault, J., McGill, D.B., Ott, B.J. & Taylor, W.F. (1978) Liver biopsy: complications in 1000 inpatients and outpatients. *Gastroenterology*, **74**, 103–106.

105. Phillips, M.J., Poucell, S., Patterson, J. & Valencia, P. (1987) *The Liver. An Atlas and Text of Ultrastructural Pathology*. New York: Raven Press.

106. Piccinino, F., Sagnelli, E., Pasquale, G. *et al.* (1986) Complications following percutaneous liver biopsy. A multicentre retrospective study on 68,276 biopsies. *Journal of Hepatology*, **2**, 165–173.

107. Poulsen, H. & Christoffersen, P. (1970) Histological changes in liver biopsies from patients with surgical bile duct disorders. *Acta Pathologica et Microbiologica Scandinavica, Section A*, **78**, 571–579.

108. Purow, E., Grosberg, S.J. & Wapnick, S. (1977) Menghini needle fracture after attempted liver biopsy. *Gastroenterology*, **73**, 1404–1405.

109. Raines, D.R., van Heertum, R.L. & Johnson, L.F. (1974) Intrahepatic hematoma: a complication of percutaneous liver biopsy. *Gastroenterology*, **67**, 284–289.

110. Rake, M.O., Murray-Lyon, I.M., Ansell, I.D. & Williams, R. (1969) Improved liver-biopsy needle. *Lancet*, **2**, 1283.

111. Riley, S.A., Ellis, W.R., Irving, H.C. *et al.* (1984) Percutaneous liver biopsy with plugging of needle track: a safe method for use in patients with impaired coagulation. *Lancet*, **2**, 436.

112. Rodeck, C.H., Pembrey, M.R., Patrick, A.D. *et al.* (1982) Fetal liver biopsy for prenatal diagnosis of ornithine carbamyl transferase deficiency. *Lancet*, **2**, 297–300.

113. Roncalli, M., Borzio, M., de Biagi, G. *et al.* (1986) Liver cell dysplasia in cirrhosis. *Cancer*, **57**, 1515–1521.

114. Sabatini, D.D., Bensch, K. & Barrnett, R.J. (1963) Cytochemistry and electron microscopy. The preservation of cellular ultrastructure and enzymatic activity by aldehyde fixation. *Journal of Cell Biology*, **17**, 19–58.

115. Salaspuro, M. & Sipponen, P. (1976) Demonstration of an intra-

cellular copper binding protein by orcein staining in long-standing cholestatic liver disease. *Gut,* **17,** 787–790.

116. Sangalli, G., Livraghi, T. & Giordano, F. (1989) Fine needle biopsy of hepatocellular carcinoma: improvement in diagnosis by microhistology. *Gastroenterology,* **96,** 524–526.
117. Schaffner, F., Sternlieb, I., Barka, T. & Popper, H. (1962) Hepatocellular changes in Wilson's disease. Histochemical and electron microscopic studies. *American Journal of Pathology,* **41,** 315–328.
118. Schaffner, F. (1970) The structural basis of altered hepatic function in viral hepatitis. *American Journal of Medicine,* **49,** 658–668.
119. Scheuer, P.J. (1970) Liver biopsy in the diagnosis of cirrhosis. *Gut,* **11,** 275–278.
120. Scheuer, P.J. & Maggi, G. (1980) Hepatic fibrosis and collapse: histological distinction by orcein staining. *Histopathology,* **4,** 487–490.
121. Scheuer, P.J., Williams, R. & Muir, A.R. (1962) Hepatic pathology in relatives of patients with haemochromatosis. *Journal of Pathology and Bacteriology,* **84,** 53–64.
122. Scheuer, P.J., Lal, S., Summerfield, J.A. & Sherlock, S. (1974) Rifampicin hepatitis. *Lancet,* **1,** 421–425.
123. Searle, J., Harmon, B.V., Bishop, C.J. & Kerr, J.F.R. (1987) The significance of cell death by apoptosis in hepatobiliary disease. *Journal of Gastroenterology and Hepatology,* **2,** 77–96.
124. Seymour, C.A. & Peters, T.J. (1977) Enzyme activities in human liver biopsies: assay methods and activities of some lysosomal and membrane-bound enzymes in control tissue and serum. *Clinical Science and Molecular Medicine,* **52,** 229–239.
125. Seymour, C., Neale, G. & Peters, T.J. (1977) Lysosomal changes in liver tissue from patients with the Dublin–Johnson–Sprinz syndrome. *Clinical Science and Molecular Medicine,* **52,** 241–248.
126. Sherlock, S. (1951) The liver in heart failure: relation of anatomical, functional and circulatory changes. *British Heart Journal,* **13,** 273–293.
127. Sherlock, S., Dick, R. & van Leeuwen, D.J. (1985) Liver biopsy today—the Royal Free Hospital experience. *Journal of Hepatology,* **1,** 75–85.
128. Shikata, T., Uzawa, T., Yoshiwara, N., Akatsuka, T. & Yamazaki, S. (1974) Staining methods of Australia antigen in paraffin section. *Japanese Journal of Experimental Medicine,* **44,** 25–36.
129. Sholli, G., Fornari, F., Civardi, G. *et al.* (1990) Role of ultrasound guided fine needle aspiration biopsy in the diagnosis of hepatocellular carcinoma. *Gut,* **31,** 1303–1305.
130. Sipponen, P. (1976) Orcein positive hepatocellular material in long-standing biliary diseases. I. Histochemical characteristics. *Scandinavian Journal of Gastroenterology,* **11,** 545–552.
131. Snapper, I. (1951) Liver biopsy. *Review of Gastroenterology,* **18,** 649–650.

132. Solbiati, L., Livraghi, T., Pra, L.D. *et al.* (1985) Fine needle biopsy of hepatic hemangioma with sonographic guidance. *American Journal of Roentgenology,* **144,** 471–474.
133. Spellburg, M.A. & Bermudez, F. (1977) Value and safety of percutaneous liver biopsy in obstructive jaundice. *American Journal of Gastroenterology,* **67,** 444–448.
134. Spinzi, G.C., Terruzzi, V. & Minoli, G. (1988) Hematomas after percutaneous liver biopsy (Letter). *Gastroenterology,* **94,** 249–250.
135. Swartz, H.M., Sarna, T. & Varma, R.R. (1979) On the nature and excretion of the hepatic pigment in the Dubin–Johnson syndrome. *Gastroenterology,* **76,** 958–964.
136. Terry, R. (1952) Risks of needle biopsy of the liver. *British Medical Journal,* **1,** 1102–1105.
137. Thomsen, P., Poulsen, H. & Petersen, P. (1976) Different types of ground glass hepatocytes in human liver biopsies: morphology, occurrence and diagnostic significance. *Scandinavian Journal Gastroenterology,* **11,** 113–119.
138. Triger, D.R., Millward-Sadler, G.H., Czaykowski, A.A. *et al.* (1976) Alpha-1-antitrypsin deficiency and liver disease in adults. *Quarterly Journal of Medicine,* **45,** 51–72.
139. Van Waes, L. & Lieber, C.S. (1977) Early perivenular sclerosis in alcoholic fatty liver: an index of progressive liver injury. *Gastroenterology,* **73,** 646–650.
140. Vasquez, J.J., Guillen, F.J., Zozaya, J. & Lahoz, M. (1983) Cyanamide induced liver injury. A predictable lesion. *Liver,* **3,** 225–230.
141. Wagner, R., Huijing, F. & Porter, E. (1971) Hepatic gluconeogenesis due to phosphorylase deficiency. Limitations of enzyme studies on liver biopsy specimens. *American Journal of Medicine,* **51,** 685–691.
142. Weiner, A.J., Kuo, G., Bradley, D.W. *et al.* (1990) Detection of Hepatitis C viral sequences in non-A, non-B hepatitis. *Lancet,* **335,** 1–3.
143. Whitmire, L.F., Galambos, J.T., Phillips, V.M. *et al.* (1985) Imaging guided percutaneous hepatic biopsy: diagnostic accuracy and safety. *Journal of Clinical Gastroenterology,* **6,** 511–515.
144. Winkler, K. & Poulson, H. (1975) Liver disease with periportal sinusoidal dilatation. A possible complication to contraceptive steroids. *Scandinavian Journal of Gastroenterology,* **10,** 699–704.
145. Witzleben, C.L., Monteleone, J.A. & Rejent, A.J. (1972) Electron microscopy in the diagnosis of cystinosis. *Archives of Pathology,* **94,** 362–365.
146. Woolling, K.R., Baggenstoss, A.H. & Weir, J.F. (1951) Infarcts of liver. *Gastroenterology,* **17,** 479–493.
147. Zamcheck, N. & Klausenstock, O. (1953) Liver biopsy (concluded). II. The risk of needle biopsy. *New England Journal of Medicine,* **249,** 1062–1069.
148. Zuckerman, A.J. (1970) *Virus Diseases of the Liver.* London: Butterworths.

CHAPTER 20

Some Aspects of Ultrastructural Pathology

A-M. Jezequel

In the past decade much has been learned about the liver's response to injury and the significance of some elementary alterations has begun to emerge. A great part of our information comes from experimental studies but a body of knowledge has also been obtained through studies on human material. This chapter will cover mainly the latter and will focus on some areas which have aroused a special interest in recent years. Specific pathological situations are considered in other chapters. For more extensive reviews, the reader is referred to the papers by Jezequel and Orlandi,[44] Trump et al.,[100] Schaffner,[85] Schaffner and Popper[86] and Phillips et al.[71]

The most conspicuous alteration of the single hepatocyte is shrinkage necrosis, in which the cell loses all relationship with the neighbouring hepatocytes and tends to become round in shape, with smooth contours and disappearance of microvilli, leading to an appearance similar to that described in apoptosis.[88] The cytoplasm is electron dense, deprived of glycogen, and the usual organization of cytoplasmic organelles is lost. However, stacks of rough endoplasmic reticulum, mitochondria and lysosomes retain their structural features. The nucleus becomes pyknotic with increased density of the chromatin. The denaturation of cytoplasmic proteins with an increased affinity for eosin leads to the formation of 'acidophilic' or 'eosinophilic' bodies seen under the light microscope. Such cell remnants can be seen free in the parenchyma, or engulfed in the cytoplasm of fixed or circulating macrophages, or sometimes inside neighbouring hepatocytes. They are a usual feature during acute hepatitis, both viral or drug-induced, and have been given the name of Councilman-like bodies[52] (Figure 20.1). Other forms of necrosis can be observed, such as the necrosis which follows ischaemia and is associated with prominent mitochondrial swelling and formation of intracytoplasmic vacuoles,[3] or the feathery degeneration observed during cholestasis.[26,74] These represent gross alterations of the liver cell and are usually accompanied by the presence of an inflammatory reaction or an infiltration of the portal tracts, with or without collagen proliferation. Electron-microscopic studies have shown that cellular alterations do not need to involve the whole hepatocyte. Although hepatic response to injury rarely produces specific structural changes, a pattern of response involving particular organelles or groups of organelles can be expected in a number of circumstances.

NUCLEUS

Except for gross alterations occurring in pyknosis and during the formation of acidophilic bodies, ultrastructural alterations in liver cell nuclei are rarely observed in human pathology. Modifications in size and shape with occasional cytoplasmic invaginations occur in tumour cells or in regenerating nodules[71] but do not have characteristic

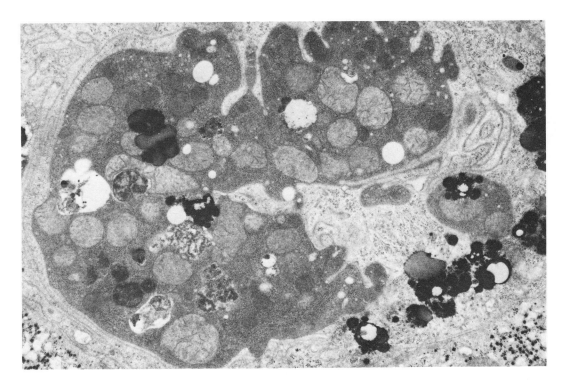

Figure 20.1
Councilman-like body in drug-induced hepatitis (chloramphenicol). Some components of hepatocytes—rough ER, mitochondria and lipofuscin granules—can be identified in the dense cytoplasm. No nucleus is visible in the plane of section. The cell remnants appear engulfed in a macrophage (x 9000).

features. Nuclear abnormalities, with enlarged nucleoli associated with proliferation of rough endoplasmic reticulum and formation of cytolysomes, are frequent in hereditary tyrosinaemia; the alterations are similar to those observed in experimental intoxication with ethionine.[87] Inclusions of viral origin may be found during infections with viruses of the herpes group.[71] Eosinophilic inclusions which give a 'sanded' appearance to the nuclei may be seen in chronic hepatitis B and are due to the presence of excess viral core material in the nucleoplasm.[6,36,37] Peculiar inclusions have also been described in non-A non-B hepatitis.[71]

ENDOPLASMIC RETICULUM

Changes in the configuration of the endoplasmic reticulum are among the most prominent cytoplasmic alterations; they are often the earliest changes observed in various experimental situations in animals[49,94] or after administration of a number of drugs in man.[43,44,71] As discussed in Chapter 2, the rough endoplasmic reticulum is the site of protein synthesis, while the 'biotransformation' of chemicals is a major function of the complex enzymatic system located in smooth endoplasmic reticulum. The main function is to render 'foreign' compounds (drugs, pesticides, environmental pollutants, carcinogens, synthetic or endogenous steroids)[13] more polar and thus more readily excretable. However, active (toxic) metabolites may be formed during the process and may be responsible for the hepatotoxicity of some drugs. Among the mechanisms leading to cell necrosis, great importance has been given to the covalent, irreversible binding of metabolites with cytoplasmic proteins,[64] but covalent binding may occur during the metabolism of various substances and is not necessarily a harmful process.[77] At the moment the 'point of no return' of cellular alterations remains unknown.

A conspicuous increase in the smooth endoplasmic reticulum in hepatocytes may follow the administration of some drugs and has been extensively studied, especially after administration of phenobarbitone in animals. This increase has been considered a major criterion of some drug-induced liver cell alterations[71] and is usually accompanied by an increase in drug-metabolizing enzymes.[78] Morphometric studies show that in the rat there is an early and short-lived increase in the membranes of the rough endoplasmic reticulum which returns to normal values by the fifth day of treatment, whereas the smooth membranes continue to increase. The increase in the smooth endoplasmic reticulum has been positively correlated with the increase in drug-metabolizing enzymes such as cytochrome P450.[91] Such an increase in smooth membranes is not specifically correlated with enzyme induction. Several substances produce the same response as phenobarbitone;[13] others stimulate a more limited number of pathways and, like 3-methylcholanthrene, may increase a variant of cytochrome P450 (P448) without causing quantitative changes of the smooth membranes.[21] Conversely as observed in D-galactosamine-induced hepatitis,[58] an increase in smooth membranes may not be accompanied by changes in microsomal enzyme activity.

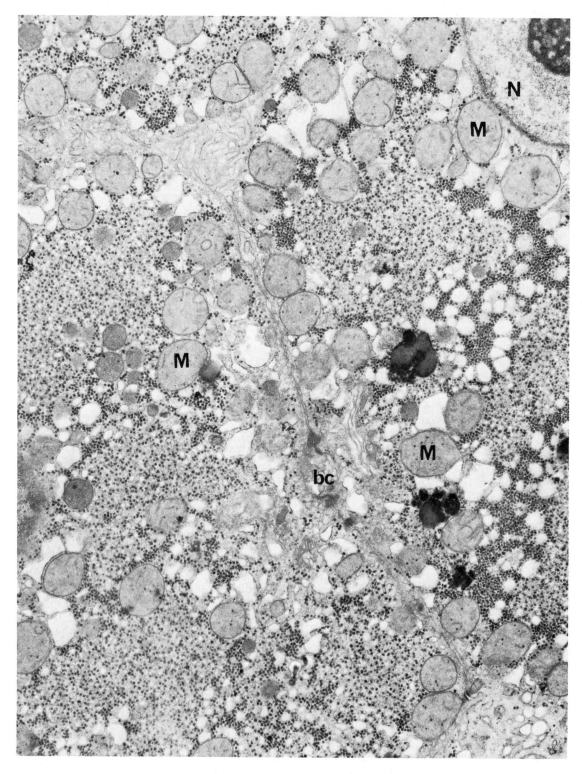

Figure 20.2 Low-power view of hepatic parenchyma in a patient under long-term anticonvulsant therapy. In the three hepatocytes present in the field, the smooth endoplasmic reticulum is prominent and other cell components appear normal. N = nucleus; bc = bile canaliculus; M = mitochondrion (x 11 250).

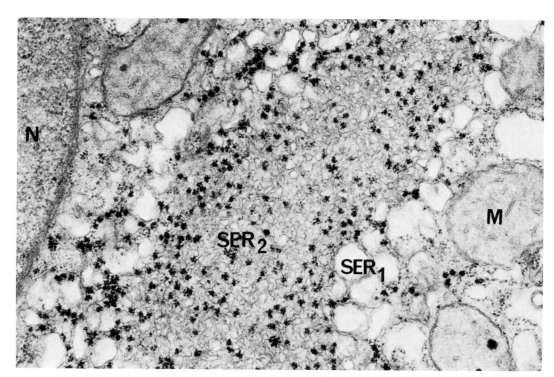

Figure 20.3 Same patient as in Figure 20.1 . Part of a hepatocyte shows large clumps of densely packed smooth membranes (SER$_2$) next to vesicles with a wide lumen (SER$_1$). The respective increase of each component was eightfold and threefold as measured by quantitative morphometry.[44] N = nucleus; M = mitochondrion (x 30 000).

In man, changes in the distribution or amount of endoplasmic reticulum have often been described, but the evaluation of such changes has often been hampered by the lack of baseline data. As previously mentioned, human hepatocytes contain a relatively large amount of smooth endoplasmic reticulum; the finding of 'increased' smooth membranes in humans should therefore be interpreted with caution. Quantitative studies have shown that an increase in smooth membranes does occur in the hepatocytes of patients under treatment with drugs inducing microsomal drug-metabolizing enzymes. This was especially evident in patients undergoing long-term anticonvulsant therapy (Figures 20.2 and 20.3) where an eightfold increase in smooth endoplasmic reticulum was measured.[48] The activity of the microsomal enzyme NADPH cytochrome *c* reductase was significantly increased in all subjects.[48] A discrete increase also occured in a patient with Crigler–Najjar type II syndrome treated with phenytoin.[56] The pattern of proliferation of the smooth endoplasmic reticulum in man is somewhat different from the pattern observed in the rat: at low magnification it assumes the 'pepper and salt' appearance first described in patients under therapy with rifampicin.[46] This is due to the formation of scattered foci of densely packed smooth membranes. A proliferation of the smooth endoplasmic reticulum has been described following the administration of ethanol in the rat and in man, together with an increase in various drug-metabolizing enzymes, [62,83] but quantitative studies have suggested that a degranulation of the rough endoplasmic reticulum may have occurred.[67] Others have found an inconstant increase[57] or even a true decrease[19] of the smooth endoplasmic reticulum. The discrepancies may lie in the experimental procedure itself, interspecies variations, lack of a standardized diet or difficulties in recognizing intra-acinar variations. An increase in the endoplasmic reticulum may also be related to altered turnover of membranous components, due to interactions with a drug or its metabolites. Many examples have been reported in experimental conditions. In man, a similar phenomenon may occur in drug-induced phospholipidosis,[14,41] or in the alcoholic hepatitis-like reaction following therapy with perhexiline maleate.[5] According to a hypothesis suggested by studies on perfused rat liver, chlorpromazine-induced cholestasis could be due to a binding of chlorpromazine to membrane phospholipids with consequent widespread alterations in membrane properties.[35]

A peculiar alteration in the endoplasmic reticulum may be observed in the hepatocytes of subjects with HBsAg-positive hepatitis (Figure 20.4), giving rise to the 'ground-glass' appearance of liver cells under the light microscope. This is due to the formation of a rich network of the cisternae of the smooth reticulum which contain rod-like structures, showing in cross-section as tubules about 35 nm in diameter and occasionally containing a small core. These elements are thought to represent excess formation of viral protein coat.[36–38,72,92] This structural change can be estimated at the level of the light microscope by immunohistochemistry or with special staining,[89] but the number of altered hepatocytes is highly variable and has not been correlated with any feature of the disease. Hepatocytes showing eosinophilic cytoplasm with a rim of basophilic material may be observed after steroid administration (Figure 20.5) due to the increased amount of smooth endoplasmic reticulum and the crowding of mitochondria and rough endoplasmic reticulum along the

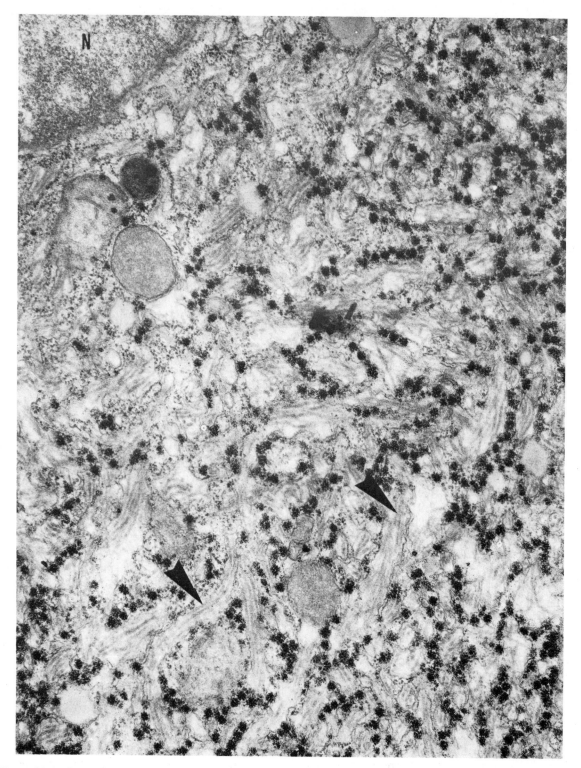

Figure 20.4 Part of the cytoplasm of a hepatocyte showing disruption of the normal architecture. Numerous filamentous structures 35 nm in diameter (arrowheads) fill the cisternae of the endoplasmic reticulum and are seen in longitudinal, oblique or cross-sections. These filaments represent excess production of hepatitis B virus protein coat (HBsAg). N = nucleus (x 35 000).

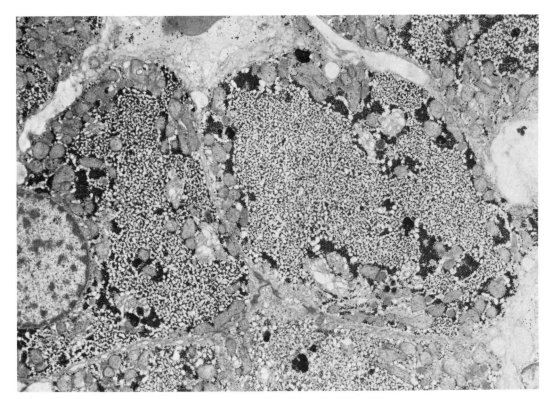

Figure 20.5
'Margination' of mitochondria in a group of hepatocytes from a patient receiving anabolic steroids. The smooth membranes occupy most of the cytoplasm while the mitochondria and rough endoplasmic reticulum are concentrated along the cell membrane and around the nucleus (x 6000).

nuclear and peripheral cell membrane.[66] 'Ground-glass' hepatocytes may be seen in other situations where an increase in the smooth endoplasmic reticulum occurs, such as following the administration of barbiturates or other microsomal enzyme inducers. In these cases, intracisternal rods are not present and special staining is negative.[72,99,107]

Changes in the endoplasmic reticulum are a prominent feature in subjects with alpha-1-antitrypsin deficiency, whether they are homozygotes or heterozygotes. In these patients, hepatocytes contain globules of PAS-positive, diastase-resistant material, which is moderately electron dense, shows a finely granular structure and is contained within enlarged cisternae. The inclusion bodies have been localized in both the rough and the smooth endoplasmic reticulum[20,109] and have been shown to contain asialo alpha-1-antitrypsin[42] (Figure 20.6). Despite prominent morphological alterations in the endoplasmic reticulum of these patients, the hepatic microsomal enzymes involved in aminopyrine demethylation are not impaired.[60] A new type of ground-glass-like hepatocyte has been recently described and related to accumulation of fibrinogen in endoplasmic reticulum, as demonstrated by immune light and electron microscopy.[10] The content of dilated cisternae shows as finely granular or fluffy material (Figure 20.7). These alterations are likely related to an hereditary disorder leading to impaired intracellular transport of fibrinogen.[10] In patients undergoing antitumour therapy, hepatic steatosis is a common observation, accounting for the hepatomegaly often present in these subjects. This may be accompanied by a variety of

alterations in the endoplasmic reticulum, with formation of large distended cisternae filled with light fluffy material (Figure 20.8). The administration of vincristine, an antimicrotubular agent, leading to impairment of secretory activity and retention of secretory products in the liver cell, might account for this alteration, offering an example of drug-induced endoplasmic reticulum storage disease.

MITOCHONDRIA

Apparent swelling of mitochondria or 'bizarre' shapes are not necessarily evidence of degenerative changes but may reflect an adaptive phenomenon, as suggested after administration of cortisone.[104] In these conditions the increase in the volume density of the mitochondria is accompanied by a numerical decrease so that the total volume per cell remains constant. In man, megamitochondria, often containing crystalloid material, occur in a number of circumstances[93] and appear especially prominent in alcoholics.[59,82,101] It is well established that megamitochondria and alcoholic hyalin (see below) are distinct entities.[40] Enlarged mitochondria with an expanded matrix are present in Reye's syndrome in nearly all hepatocytes at the onset of the illness and return to normal during recovery,[39,68] but the changes are not 'characteristic' as claimed by some workers. A comparison of liver ultrastructure in Reye's syndrome and congenital abnormalities of the urea cycle demonstrated that the mitochondrial alterations seen in Reye's syndrome cannot be explained by ornithine transcarbamylase deficiency.[61]

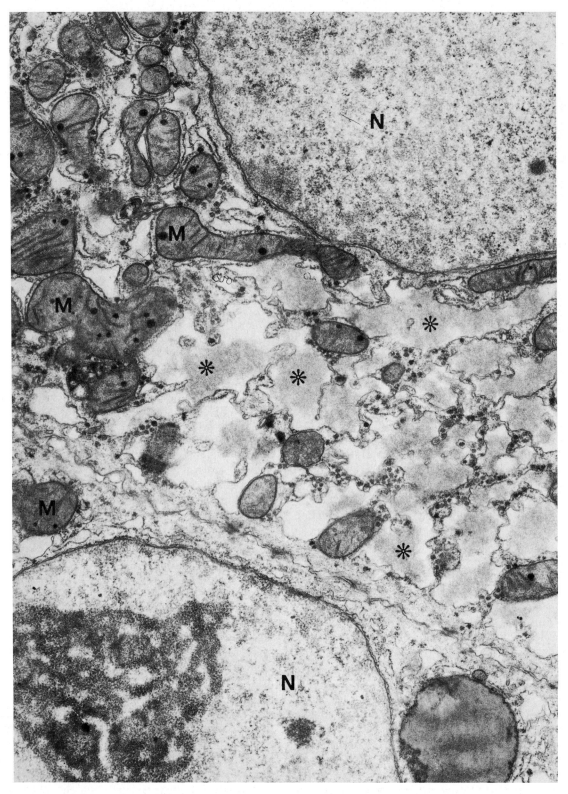

Figure 20.6 Alpha-1-antitrypsin deficiency. In the middle part of the picture the cytoplasm of the hepatocyte contains numerous cisternae of rough endoplasmic reticulum; these are slightly distended and contain characteristic amorphous deposits (asterisks). These correspond to the PAS-positive globules seen under the light microscope. N = nucleus; M = mitochondrion (x 25 000).

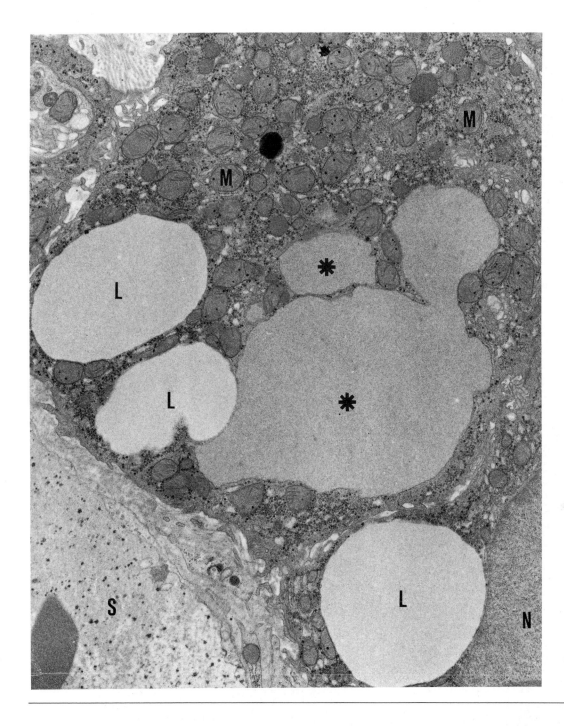

Figure 20.7 Fibrinogen storage disease in adult liver. The picture shows part of a hepatocyte containing lipid droplets (L) and two cytoplasmic inclusions filled with fine fluffy material (asterisks). These inclusions are delimited by membranes of the rough endoplasmic reticulum and contain fibrinogen as demonstrated by immunohistochemistry. All other organelles appear normal.
N = nucleus;
M = mitochondria;
S = sinusoid (x 11 500, reproduced at 85%).

Swelling and pleomorphism of mitochondria are a well known feature of alcoholic liver disease[71] and also occur when thyroid function is altered.[54] Although various hypotheses have been proposed, the nature of these alterations is not understood at the moment. In intra- or extrahepatic cholestasis, changes in the conformation of cristae with 'curling' are frequently observed[17,73] (Figure 20.9). Morphometric studies have shown that this configurational change is associated with an increase in the surface density of mitochondrial cristae.[11,47] The significance of this alteration is not known but it is of interest that similar qualitative and quantitative changes have been observed in patients with uncomplicated cholelithiasis, i.e. in the absence of jaundice.[55] This suggests that disturbances in bile salts and cholesterol metabolism may be responsible for changes in the molecular structure of mitochondrial membranes and consequently in their enzymatic properties. Much emphasis has been placed on mitochondrial changes during halothane hepatitis, such as variations in size and shape of mitochondria or breaks in the outer envelope,[53,102] which could help in differentiating between acute viral hepatitis and unexplained postoperative hepatitis. The presence of such specific features was not confirmed in a survey which included a

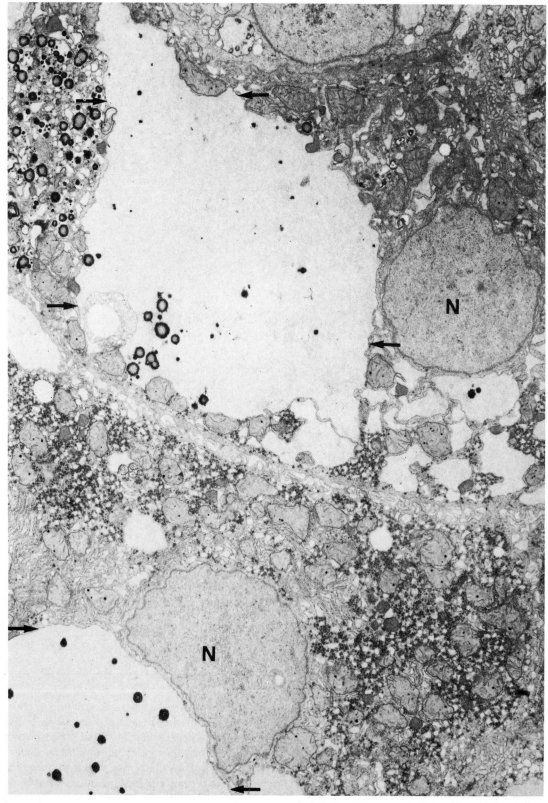

Figure 20.8 The two hepatocytes in the field exhibit profound alterations in the cisternae of the rough endoplasmic reticulum. These are distended to a variable extent; in the upper part of the picture they form large cysts occupying two-thirds of the cell. The distension of the endoplasmic reticulum may result from a blockade of secretory functions of the liver cell, due to interference of vincristine with the microtubular system. As shown by microanalysis, the dense granules dispersed throughout are sites of precipitation of calcium. N = nucleus. (x 8000).

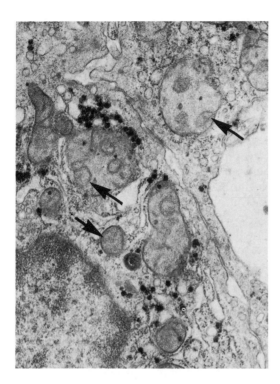

Figure 20.9 Liver biopsy from a patient with extrahepatic cholestasis showing curled or circular cristae in numerous mitochondria (arrows) (x 17 500).

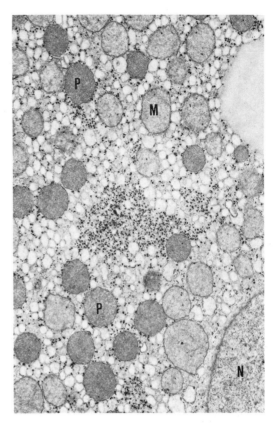

Figure 20.10 Increased number of peroxisomes (P) in a patient under therapy with 6-mercaptopurine. The ratio of peroxisomes to mitochondria is about 1:1. M = mitochondrion; N = nucleus (x 10 500). From Jezequel (1976),[43] with kind permission of the publisher, Plenum Press.

large number of patients.[106] By a mechanism which appears to apply to a large number of compounds, it has been suggested that the toxic effects of halothane could be mediated through the binding of its metabolites with microsomal phospholipids, which could in turn trigger the formation of antigenic complexes.[12,33] Mitochondrial abnormalities, together with a variety of cytoplasmic alterations, are frequently observed in patients with Wilson's disease[94] and are dealt with in Chapter 35.

PEROXISOMES

Changes in the number or structure of peroxisomes have been observed, especially in experimental conditions. Until now, the proliferation of peroxisomes which occurs following administration of hypolipidaemic agents or other substances to animals[32,34,76,96] has not been reported to the same extent in man. Only in patients receiving 6-mercaptopurine does there seem to be a numerical increase in peroxisomes[43] (Figure 20.10). The presence of electron-dense material in peroxisomes in cholestasis has been reported by various authors[17,47] and has also been observed in patients with cholelithiasis.[55] This core-like material is amorphous in appearance (Figure 20.11) and lacks the crystalloid configuration described in one case of benign recurrent cholestasis.[8] A variety of inclusions are occasionally observed in the peroxisomes

in normal individuals (see Chapter 2). The absence of peroxisomes is a characteristic feature associated with Zellweger's syndrome,[29,71] whereas malformed peroxisomes are present in Refsum's disease and other varieties of peroxisomal diseases.[28]

LYSOSOMES AND RESIDUAL BODIES

As previously mentioned, cellular lysis does not need to involve the whole hepatocyte and the occurrence of focal cytoplasmic degradation is not an uncommon phenomenon. In focal cytoplasmic degradation, only a segment of the cell is affected, so that a defined area of the cytoplasm, containing a variety of organelles, becomes progressively surrounded by a membranous system arising from the endoplasmic reticulum, and is later entrapped into autophagic vacuoles or 'cytolysosomes' (Figure 20.12). The products of complete or incomplete lysis will become part of the various 'residual bodies'. This may be part of a pathological or a physiological process.[1,30,44,97] Apart from the process of autophagocytosis and the formation of cytolysosomes, storage of various substances may occur by temporary or permanent impairment of lysosomal enzymatic activity. Evidence of genetic alter-

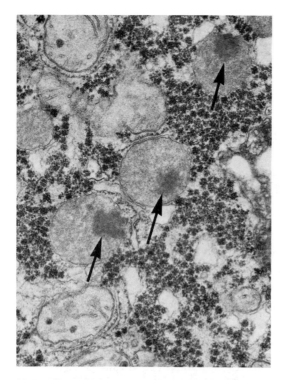

Figure 20.11 Part of a hepatocyte in a patient with extrahepatic cholestasis, showing numerous peroxisomes containing an amorphous, core-like material (arrows) (x 30 000).

ations in the synthesis or activation of lysosomal enzymes has led to the concept of 'inborn lysosomal disease'. This has been applied to some storage diseases (glycogenoses, polysaccharidoses, lipidoses, etc.). The EM findings in lysosomal storage diseases have been reviewed extensively.[71] In type II glycogenosis (Pompe's disease) excess glycogen is deposited in the liver, mainly as monoparticulate elements inside lysosomes, and is accumulated by an autophagic process.[4,31,63] In mucopolysaccharidoses such as Hurler's and pseudo-Hurler's diseases, enlarged lysosomes in the hepatocytes contain fluffy, electron-lucent material, which is different from the ultrastructural features observed in the brain.[31] In fucosidosis, features similar to those present in Hurler's disease have been observed together with numerous intralysosomal dense lamellar deposits.[31] Pericanalicular dense bodies containing dense laminated material have also been described in some hepatocytes of children with Tay–Sachs disease[103] or in Fabry's disease,[31] whereas in Niemann–Pick disease numerous inclusions filled with dense membranous material are distributed throughout hepatocytes[103] (Figure 20.13). All these alterations have in common an inherited defect of one or more lysosomal enzymes with consequent accumulation of undigested products (Figures 20.14 and 20.15). Similar changes may be produced by temporary overload or inefficiency of lysosomal enzymes in some pathological situations (Figures 20.16 and 20.17). This may explain the unusual, lysosome-associated formations observed in hepatocytes of subjects under long-term

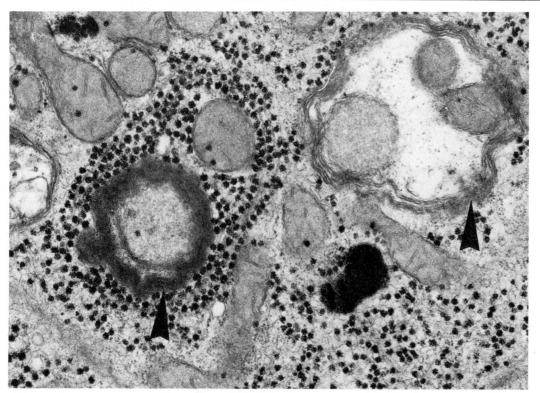

Figure 20.12 Part of a hepatocyte in a patient under treatment with 6-mercaptopurine. Cytolysosomes (arrowheads) are present and contain various cytoplasmic components surrounded by a multi-layered envelope. From Jezequel and Orlandi (1972),[4] with kind permission of the publisher, Academic Press (x 17 500).

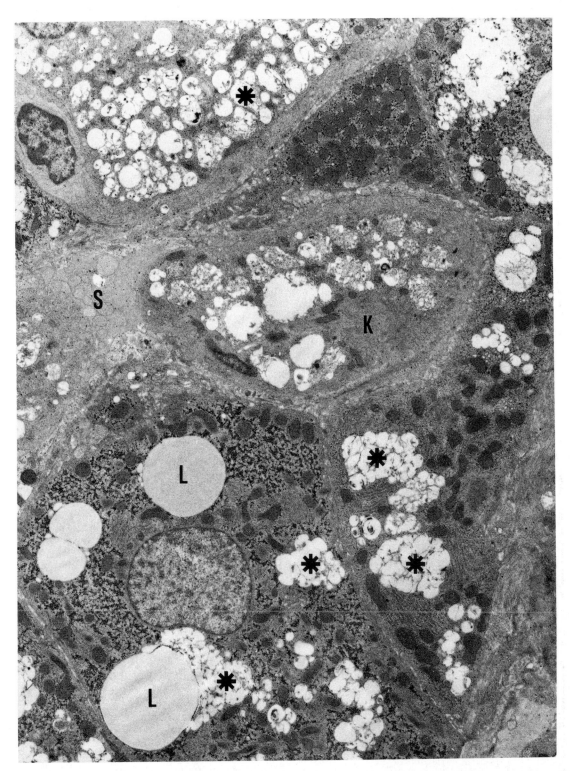

Figure 20.13 General view of hepatic parenchyma in a child with Niemann-Pick disease. All hepatocytes are filled with group of finely lamellar residual bodies (asterisks), at times closely apposed to lipid droplets (L). Complex residual bodies are also present in non-hepatocytes, presumably Kupffer cells (K). S = sinusoid (x 11 500, reproduced at 93%).

anticonvulsant therapy[45] and in patients with untreated cholelithiasis[55] (Figure 20.18). In these situations, an alteration in cholesterol metabolism and the formation of abnormal membranous components have been hypothesized. A similar mechanism could explain the changes observed in 'phospholipidosis'[41] or following therapy with perhexiline maleate[5] or amiodarone.[75,90] Lysosomal overload is also involved in the formation of 'siderosomes' or iron-laden lysosomes. Ferritin particles, sometimes in crystalline arrays, non-ferritin iron, carbohydrates, lipids and protein have been identified in haemochromatosis and systemic iron overload.[50,51,79,80] This localization is not specific since excess storage iron also occurs in the cytoplasmic matrix and in the lysosomes of phagocytic cells throughout the body.[80]

MALLORY BODIES

The term 'alcoholic hyalin' which is often used to describe Mallory bodies implies some specificity of this alteration. Hyalin has been observed in a variety of conditions: cirrhosis of various aetiologies—including primary biliary cirrhosis—as well as in unrelated pathological situations[23, 27,75,90,105,108] (Figure 20.19). The presence of hyalin in

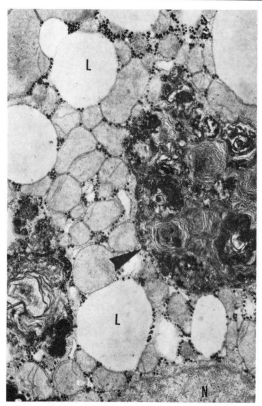

Figure 20.14 Part of a hepatocyte in a child with lipid storage disease. The cytoplasm contains numerous lipid droplets (L) of various sizes and large electron-dense bodies with a complex lamellar structure (arrowheads), presumably of lysosomal origin. N = nucleus (x 10 500).

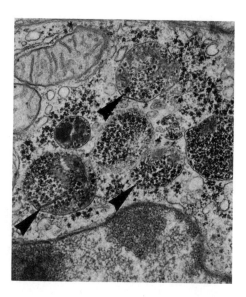

Figure 20.15 Part of a hepatocyte showing residual bodies (arrowheads) loaded with glycogen, as observed in type II glycogenosis. (x 16 000). Courtesy of Dr J.P. Benhamou.

perivenular hepatocytes together with intact acinar architecture has been claimed to be pathognomonic of alcoholic liver injury.[27] The conditions associated with the presence of Mallory bodies in man have been recently reviewed and cover a variety of situations, including a number of cases involving drug-induced liver injury.[2] The first extensive ultrastructural study of Mallory bodies was published in 1964[7] and has been expanded with the description of three types of 'alcoholic hyalin',[108] i.e. bundles of filaments in parallel arrays, clusters of randomly oriented fibrils and granular or amorphous substance. It has been suggested that Mallory bodies are made up of actin-like filaments capable of binding antiactin antibodies.[65] A comparative study of griseofulvin-induced Mallory bodies in mice and hyperplastic actin-rich microfilaments induced by phalloidin has not confirmed this hypothesis, but tends to suggest that Mallory bodies are related to the prekeratin subclass of intermediate (10 nm) filaments.[16] Their formation might result from an antitubulin action of griseofulvin (in mice) or of alcohol (in man)[25] or of other compounds. The immunological similarity of hyalin in a variety of hepatic conditions has been demonstrated by immunocytochemistry,[69] suggesting a common involvement of the cytoskeleton.

PLASMA MEMBRANE

Alterations in the plasma membrane have often been invoked in the pathogenesis of various diseases, especially in cholestasis. Evidence of structural changes rests on biochemical or immunological rather than morphological data. The formation of blebs or localized swelling of microvilli, with occasional shedding of parts of the cytoplasm at the sinusoidal or the canalicular pole of the

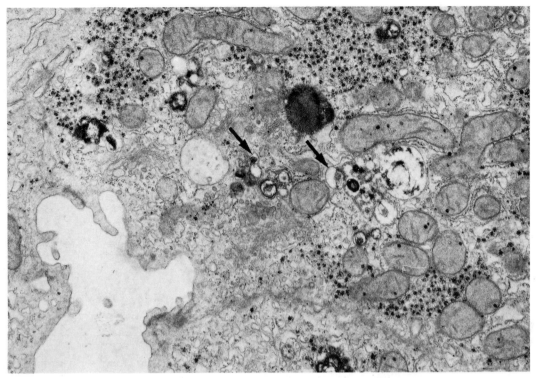

Figure 20.16 Part of a hepatocyte in a patient under treatment with 6-mercaptopurine. Numerous multilobulated dense bodies are evident. They contain heterogeneous ring-shaped osmiophilic material associated with bile retention (arrows). The lumen of the bile canaliculus is distended and lacks microvilli. From Jezequel and Orlandi (1972),[44] with kind permission of the publisher, Academic Press (x 17 500).

hepatocytes, is often observed in cholestasis[17,73,74] but is not a specific change (Figure 20.20). Large pinocytic vacuoles may form from deep invaginations of the cell surface, especially in hypoxic conditions.[84] Invaginations of the cell membrane at the level of the space of Disse seem also to occur in peliosis[81,98] and may be secondary to the profound changes occurring in the vascular bed. In human peliosis, the formation of large cytoplasmic blebs bulging into the space of Disse and even in the sinusoidal lumen is accompanied by cystic dilatation of vascular spaces, including the subendothelial compartment.[110]

More meaningful may be the modifications observed in membrane-associated cytoplasmic components from the 'cytoskeleton', such as actin-like microfilaments, which may play a role in membrane flow, transport and bile secretion into the canaliculus (Figure 20.21). Such modifications have been implicated in the pathogenesis of cholestasis,[22,24,70] but it has been suggested that these could be secondary rather than primary events, and may be due to a toxic action of bile salts on the canalicular membrane.[9]

Changes at the level of the tight junctions have been described in various situations, for instance after bile duct ligation or in various models of intrahepatic cholestasis. In freeze-fracture studies each tight junction of the normal canaliculus is formed as a parallel series of four to five lines which occasionally link or have aberrant strands moving at right angles away from the canalicular lumen[15] (Figure 20.22). During cholestasis, the strands of the tight junction lose their parallel, ordinate arrangement, are reduced in number and show an increased number of breaks along their length (Figure 20.23). This suggests that the permeability of the tight junctional area, and consequently of the 'paracellular pathway' is enhanced.[18] The cohesion between hepatocytes is retained as shown by transmission electron microscopy, even where there is an extreme dilatation of the bile canaliculi.[18]

In summary, abnormal features of hepatocytes involving single organelles or groups of organelles, and not appreciable with the light microscope, may be recognized by electron microscopy. This increases our understanding of the structure and function of the liver cell, and helps to elucidate the mechanism of some pathological processes.

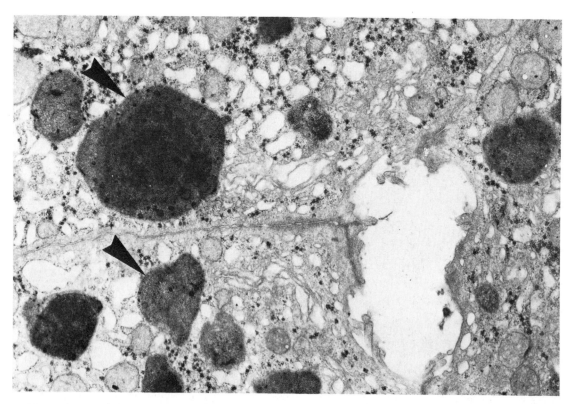

Figure 20.17 Large heterogeneous granules, limited by a single membrane (arrowheads), are present in the juxtacanalicular areas of hepatocytes in a patient with Dubin–Johnson syndrome. The lumen of the bile canaliculus is distended and microvilli are rare. The junctional complexes around the canalicular lumen are normal (x 18 200).

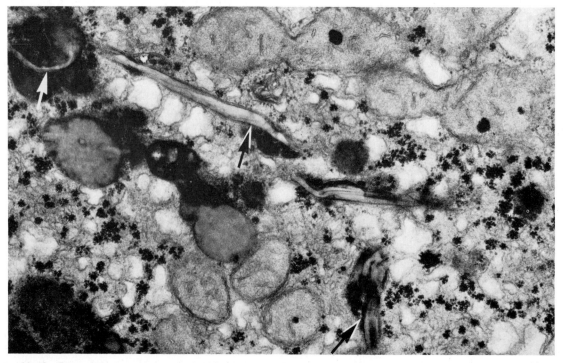

Figure 20.18 Part of the cytoplasm of a hepatocyte in a patient under long-term anticonvulsant therapy. Numerous ribbon-like formations (arrows) extending into the cytoplasm are associated with the lipofuscin granules. They are variable in width and in length, and show a dense limiting membrane surrounding an electron-lucent core (x 30 000).

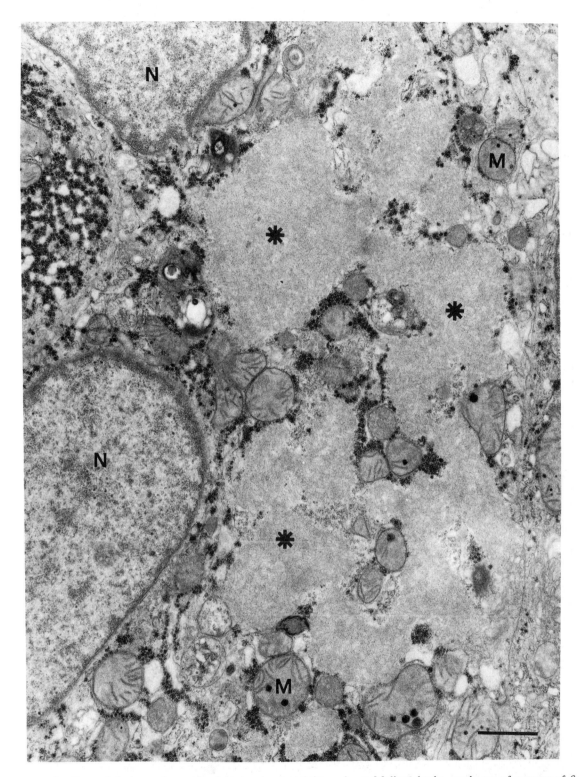

Figure 20.19 Part of the cytoplasm of a hepatocyte containing a large Mallory body, made up of a mass of fine filaments seen at various planes of section (asterisks). No limiting membrane is present at the interface between the mass of filaments and the cytoplasmic matrix. N = nucleus, M = mitochondria. (x 17 500, reproduced at 90%).

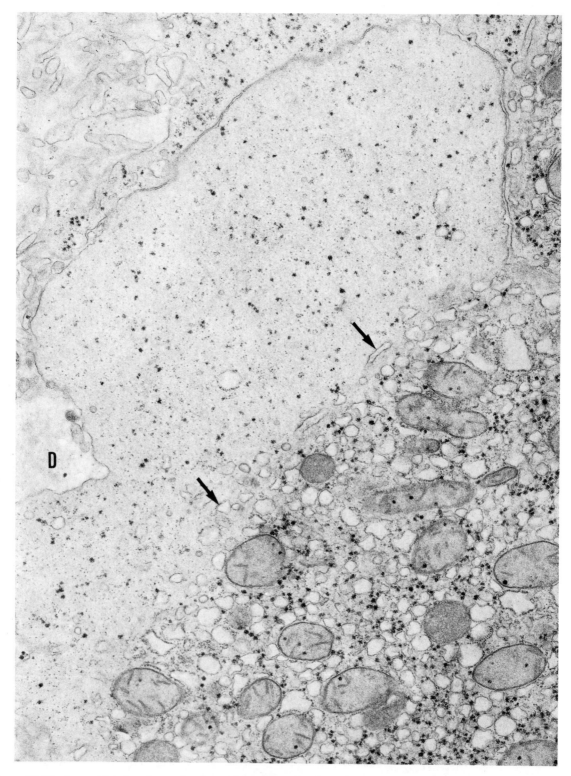

Figure 20.20 Large bleb forming at the sinusoidal surface of an hepatocyte in normal human liver. A row of vesicles (arrows) separate the cytoplasm from the bleb. It is possible that the ultimate fusion of vesicles causes the separation of blebs from the hepatocytes and their elimination into the sinusoidal lumen as free cellular debris, containing only a few ribosomes and glycogen particles. D = space of Disse. From Jezequel and Orlandi (1972),[44] with kind permission of the publisher, Academic Press (x 19 000).

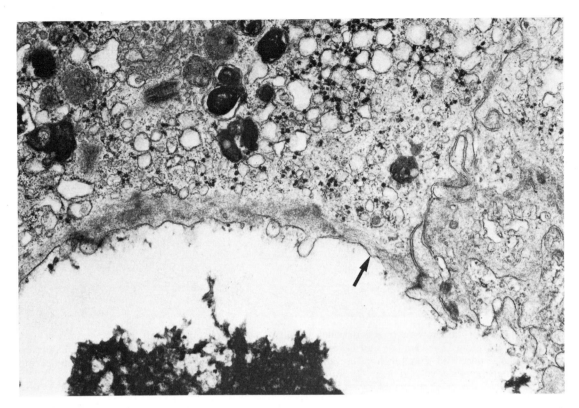

Figure 20.21 Alterations of the canalicular membrane in a patient with cholestasis. Microvilli are rare and microfilaments can be seen in the pericanalicular area (arrow). The bile canaliculus (lower margin) contains a large thrombus and there is evidence of intracytoplasmic bile retention (x 20 000).

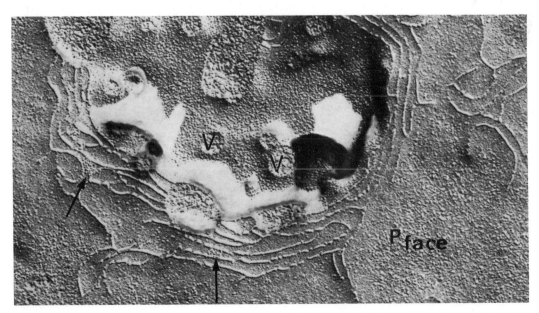

Figure 20.22 Liver from normal rat showing a bile canaliculus surrounded by the parallel strands of the tight junctional area. P_{face} = protoplasmic face; V = bile canalicular microvilli. Arrows indicate small gap junctional areas (x 60 000). From De Vos and Desmet (1981),[15] with kind permission of the authors and the editor of *Pathology, Research and Practice*.

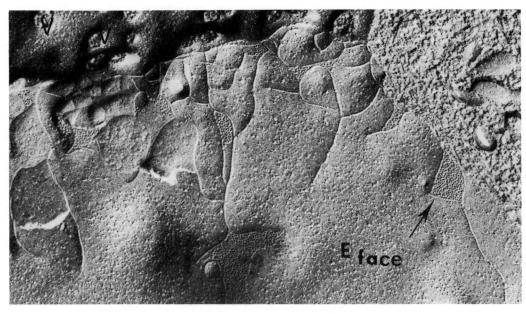

Figure 20.23 Detail of the irregular tight junctional network of an oestradiol-treated rat. The strands of the tight junctional areas are reduced in number and have lost their parallel, ordinate arrangement. E_{face} = external face; V = bile canalicular microvilli. Gap junctions are arrowed. From De Vos and Desmet (1981),[15] with kind permission of the authors and the editor of *Pathology, Research and Practice*.

REFERENCES

1. Arstila, A.U. & Trump, B.F. (1968) Studies on cellular autophagocytosis. The formation of autophagic vacuoles in the liver after glucagon administration. *American Journal of Pathology*, **53**, 687–733.
2. Babany, G., Uzzan, F., Larrey, D. *et al.* (1989) Alcoholic-like liver lesions induced by nifedipine. *Journal of Hepatology*, **9**, 252–255.
3. Bassi, M. & Bernelli-Zazzera, A. (1964) Ultrastructural cytoplasmic changes of liver cells after reversible and irreversible ischemia. *Experimental and Molecular Pathology*, **3**, 332–350.
4. Baudhuin, P., Hers, H.G. & Loeb, H. (1964) An electron microscopic and biochemical study of type II glycogenosis. *Laboratory Investigation*, **13**, 1139–1152.
5. Beaugrand, M., Chousterman, M., Callard, P. *et al.* (1977) Hépatites au maléate de perhexiline (Pexid) évoluant vers la cirrhose malgré l'arret du traitement (2 cas). *Gastroenterologie Clinique et Biologique*, **1**, 745–750.
6. Bianchi, L. & Goudat, F. (1976) Sanded nuclei in hepatitis B. Eosinophilic inclusions in liver cell nuclei due to excess in hepatitis B core antigen formation. *Laboratory Investigation*, **35**, 1–5.
7. Biava, C. (1964) Mallory alcoholic hyalin : a heretofore unique lesion of hepatocellular ergastoplasm. *Laboratory Investigation*, **13**, 301–320.
8. Biempica, L., Gutstein, S. & Arias, I.M. (1967) Morphological and biochemical studies of benign recurrent cholestasis. *Gastroenterology*, **52**, 521–535.
9. Boyer, J.L., Layden, T.J. & Hruban, Z. (1977) Mechanism of cholestasis.Taurolithocholate alters canalicular membrane composition, structure and permeability. In Popper, H., Bianchi, L. & Reutter, W. (eds) *Membrane Alterations as Basis of Liver Injury*, pp. 353–369. Lancaster: MTP Press.
10. Callea, F., De Vos, R., Togni, R. *et al.* (1986) Fibrinogen inclusions in liver cells: a new type of ground-glass hepatocyte. Immune light and electron microscopy. *Histopathology*, **10**, 65–73.
11. Capurso, L., Koch, M.M., Freddara, U. *et al.* (1975) Contribution of morphometry to the study of cholestasis in man. *Digestion*, **12**, 294.

12. Carney, F.M. & Van Dyke, R.A. (1972) Halothane hepatitis. A critical review. *Anesthesia and Analgesia*, **51**, 135–160.
13. Conney, A.H. (1967) Pharmacological implications of microsomal enzyme induction. *Pharmacological Reviews*, **19**, 317–366.
14. de la Iglesia, F., Feuer, G., Takada, A. & Matsuda, Y. (1974) Morphological studies on secondary phospholipidosis in human liver. *Laboratory Investigation*, **30**, 539–549.
15. De Vos, R. & Desmet, V.J. (1981) Morphology of liver cell tight junctions in ethinyl estradiol induced cholestasis. *Pathology, Research and Practice*, **171**, 381–383.
16. Denk, H., Franke, W.W., Eckerstorfer, R., *et al.* (1979) Formation and involution of Mallory bodies ("alcoholic hyalin") in murine and human liver revealed by immunofluorescence microscopy with antibodies to prekeratin. *Proceedings of the National Academy of Sciences of the USA*, **76**, 4112–4116.
17. Desmet, V.J. (1972) Morphological and histochemical aspects of cholestasis. In Popper, H. & Schaffner, F. (eds) *Progress in Liver Diseases*, vol.3, pp. 97–132. New York: Grune & Stratton.
18. Desmet, V.J. & De Vos, R. (1982) Tight junctions in the liver. In Popper, H. & Schaffner, F. (eds) *Progress in Liver Diseases*, vol.7, pp. 31–50. New York: Grune & Stratton.
19. Dobbins, W.O., III, Rollins, E.L., Brooks, S.G. & Fallon, M.J. (1972) A quantitative morphological analysis of ethanol effect upon rat liver. *Gastroenterology*, **62**, 1020–1033.
20. Feldman, G., Bignon, J., Chahinian, P. *et al.* (1974) Hepatocyte ultrastructural changes in alpha-1-antitrypsin deficiency. *Gastroenterology*, **67**, 1214–1224.
21. Fouts, J.R. & Rogers, L.A. (1965) Morphological changes in the liver accompanying stimulation of drug metabolizing enzyme activity by phenobarbital, chlordane, benzypyrene or metylcholanthrene in rats. *Journal of Pharmacology and Experimental Therapeutics*, **147**, 112–119.
22. French, S.W. (1976) Is cholestasis due to microfilament failure? *Human Pathology*, **7**, 243–244.
23. French, S.W. (1981) The Mallory bodies: structure, composition and pathogenesis. *Hepatology*, **1**, 76–81.

24. French, S.W. & Davies, P.L. (1975) Ultrastructural localization of actin-like filaments in rat hepatocytes. *Gastroenterology*, **68**, 765–774.

25. French, S.W., Sim, J.S. & Caldwell, M.G. (1977) Thick microfilaments (intermediate filaments) and chronic alcohol ingestion. In Popper, H., Bianchi, L. & Reutter, W. (eds) *Membrane Alterations as Basis of Liver Injury*, pp. 311–325. Lancaster: MTP Press.

26. Gall, E.A. & Dabrogorki, O. (1964) Hepatic alterations in obstructive jaundice. *American Journal of Clinical Pathology*, **41**, 126–139.

27. Gerber, M.A., Orr, W., Denk, H. *et al.* (1973) Hepatocellular hyalin in cholestasis and cirrhosis: its diagnostic significance. *Gastroenterology*, **64**, 89–98.

28. Goldfischer, S.L. (1988) Peroxisomal diseases. In Arias, I.M. *et al.* (eds), *The Liver: Biology and Pathology*, 2nd Edn., pp. 255–267. New York: Raven Press.

29. Goldfischer, S.L., Moore, C.L., Johnson, A.B. *et al.* (1973) Peroxisomal and mitochondrial defects in the cerebrohepatorenal syndrome. *Science*, **182**, 62–64.

30. Goldfischer, S.L., Novikoff, A.B., Albala, A. & Biempica, L. (1970) Hemoglobin uptake by rat hepatocytes and its breakdown within lysosomes. *Journal of Cell Biology*, **44**, 513–530.

31. Hers, H.G. & Van Hoof, F. (1970) The genetic pathology of lysosomes. In Popper, H. & Schaffner, F. (eds) *Progress in Liver Disease*, vol.3, pp. 185–205. New York: Grune & Stratton.

32. Hess, R., Staubli, W. & Reiss, W. (1965) Nature of the hepatomegalic effect produced by ethylchlorophenoxyisobutyrate in the rat. *Nature*, **208**, 856–858.

33. Howard, L.C., Brown, D.R. & Blake, D.A. (1973) Subcellular binding of halothane 1-^{14}C in mouse liver and brain. *Journal of Pharmaceutical Science*, **62**, 1021–1023.

34. Hruban, Z., Gotoh, N., Slesers, A. & Chou, S. (1974) Structure of hepatic microbodies in rats treated with acetylsalicylic acid, clofibrate and dimethrin. *Laboratory Investigation*, **30**, 64–75.

35. Hruban, Z., Tavoloni, N., Reed, J.S. & Boyer, J.L. (1978) Ultrastructural changes during cholestasis induced by chlorpromazine in the isolated perfused rat liver. *Virchows Archiv, Abteilung B*, **26**, 289–306.

36. Huang, S.N. & Groh, V. (1973) Immunoagglutination electron microscopic study on virus-like particles and Australian antigen in liver tissue. *Laboratory Investigation*, **4**, 353–366.

37. Huang, S.N., Millman, I., O'Connell, A. *et al.* (1972) Virus-like particles in Australian-antigen associated hepatitis: an immunoelectronmicroscopic study of human liver. *American Journal of Pathology*, **67**, 453–470.

38. Huang, S.N., Groh, V., Beaudoin, J.G. *et al.* (1974) A study of the relationship of virus-like particles and Australian antigen in the liver. *Human Pathology*, **5**, 209–222.

39. Iancu, T.C., Mason, W.H. & Neustein, H.B. (1977) Ultrastructural abnormalities of liver cells in Reye's syndrome. *Human Pathology*, **8**, 421–431.

40. Iseri, O.A. & Gottlieb, L.S. (1971) Alcoholic hyalin and megamitochondria as separate and distinct entities in liver disease associated with alcoholism. *Gastroenterology*, **60**, 1027–1035.

41. Ito, S. & Tsukada, Y. (1973) Clinical-pathological and electron microscopical studies on a coronary dilating agent: 4-4-diethylamino-ethoxiexestrol-induced liver injuries. *Acta Hepato-gastroenterologica*, **20**, 204–215.

42. Jeppsson, J.O., Larsson, C. & Eriksson, S. (1975) Characterization of alpha-1-antitrypsin in the inclusion bodies from the liver in alpha-1-antitrypsin deficiency. *New England Journal of Medicine*, **293**, 576–580.

43. Jezequel, A.M. (1976) Ultrastructural changes induced by drugs in the liver. In Taylor, W. (ed.) *The Hepatobiliary System*, pp. 179–203. London: Plenum Press.

44. Jezequel, A.M. & Orlandi, F. (1972) Fine morphology of the human liver as a tool in clinical pharmacology. In Orlandi, F. & Jezequel, A.M. (eds) *Liver and Drugs*, pp. 145–192. London: Academic Press.

45. Jezequel, A.M. & Orlandi, F. (1976) Unusual residual bodies in human liver cells. *Journal of Ultrastructure Research*, **57**, 87–93.

46. Jezequel, A.M., Orlandi, F. & Tenconi, L.I. (1971) Changes of the smooth endoplasmic reticulum induced by rifampicin in human and guinea-pig hepatocytes. *Gut*, **12**, 984–987.

47. Jezequel, A.M., Librari, M.L., Mosca, P.G. & Novelli, G. (1983) The human liver in extrahepatic cholestasis. Ultrastructural morphometric data. *Liver*, **3**, 303–314.

48. Jezequel, A.M., Librari, M.L., Mosca, P.G. *et al.* (1984) Changes induced in human liver by long-term anticonvulsant therapy. Functional and ultrastructural data. *Liver*, **4**, 307–317.

49. Jones, A.L. & Schmucker, D.L. (1977) Current concepts of liver structure as related to function. *Gastroenterology*, **73**, 833–851.

50. Kent, G. (1965) Iron storage diseases and the liver. In Popper, H. & Schaffner, F. (eds) *Progress in Liver Diseases*, vol.2, pp. 253–271. New York: Grune & Stratton.

51. Kerr, D.N.S. & Muir, A.R. (1960) A demonstration of the structure and deposition of ferritin in the human liver cell. *Journal of Ultrastructure Research*, **3**, 313–319.

52. Klion, F.M. & Schaffner, F. (1966) The ultrastructure of the acidophilic "Councilman-like" bodies in the liver. *American Journal of Pathology*, **48**, 755–767.

53. Klion, F.M., Schaffner, F. & Popper, H. (1969) Hepatitis after exposure to halothane. *Annals of Internal Medicine*, **71**, 467–477.

54. Klion, F.M., Segal, R. & Schaffner, F. (1971) The effect of altered thyroid function on the ultrastructure of the human liver. *American Journal of Medicine*, **50**, 317–324.

55. Koch, M.M., Freddara, U., Lorenzini, I. *et al.* (1978) A stereological and biochemical study of the human liver in uncomplicated cholelithiasis. *Digestion*, **18**, 162–177.

56. Koch, M.M., Lorenzini, I., Freddara, U. *et al.* (1978) Type 2 Crigler–Najjar syndrome. Quantification of ultrastructural data and evolution under therapy with phenytoin. *Gastroenterologie Clinique et Biologique*, **2**, 831–842.

57. Koff, S., Carter, E.A., Lui, S. & Isselbacher, K.L. (1970) Prevention of the ethanol-induced fatty liver in the rat by phenobarbital. *Gastroenterology*, **59**, 50–61.

58. Koff, R.S., Davidson, L.J., Gordon, G. & Sabesin, S. (1973) D-Galactosamine hepatotoxicity. III. Normoactive smooth endoplasmic reticulum and modification by phenobarbital. *Experimental and Molecular Pathology*, **19**, 168–177.

59. Lane, B.P. & Lieber, C.S. (1966) Ultrastructural alterations in human hepatocytes following ingestion of ethanol with adequate diets. *American Journal of Pathology*, **49**, 593–603.

60. Larsson, C. & Eriksson, S. (1977) Liver function in asymptomatic adult individuals with severe alpha-1-antitrypsin deficiency. *Scandinavian Journal of Gastroenterology*, **12**, 543–546.

61. Latham, P.S., LaBrecque, D.R., McReynolds, J.W. & Klatskin, G. (1984) Liver ultrastructure in mitochondrial urea cycle enzyme deficiencies and comparison with Reye's syndrome. *Hepatology*, **4**, 404–407.

62. Lieber, C.S. (1973) Hepatic and metabolic effects of alcohol. *Gastroenterology*, **65**, 821–846.

63. McAdams, A.J. & Wilson, H.E. (1966) The liver in generalized glycogen storage disease. *American Journal of Pathology*, **49**, 99–111.

64. Mitchell, J.R. & Jollows, D.J. (1975) Metabolic activation of drugs to toxic substances. *Gastroenterology*, **68**, 390–410.

65. Nenci, I. (1975) Identification of actin-like protein in alcoholic hyalin by immunofluorescence. *Laboratory Investigation*, **32**, 257–260.

66. Orlandi, F. & Jezequel, A.M. (1962) Electron microscopy of the human liver after methandrostenolone administration. In Martini, G.A. (ed.) *Aktuelle Probleme der Hepatologie*, pp. 41–47. Stuttgart: G. Thieme Verlag.

67. Oudea, M.C., Collette, M. & Oudea, P. (1973) Morphometric study of ultrastructural changes induced in rat liver by chronic alcohol intake. *American Journal of Digestive Diseases*, **18**, 398–402.

68. Partin, J.C., Schubert, W.K. & Partin, J.S. (1971) Mitochondrial structure in Reye's syndrome (encephalopathy and fatty degeneration of the viscera). *New England Journal of Medicine*, **285**, 1339–1343.

69. Peters, M., Tinberg, H.M. & Govindarajan, S. (1982) Immunocytochemical identity of hepatocellular hyalin in alcoholic and non-alcoholic liver diseases. *Liver*, **2**, 361–368.

70. Phillips, M.J., Oda, M., Mak, E. *et al.* (1975) Microfilament dysfunction as a possible cause of intrahepatic cholestasis. *Gastroenterology*, **69**, 48–58.

71. Phillips, M.J., Poucell, S., Patterson, J. & Valencia, P. (1987) *The Liver. An Atlas and Text of Ultrastructural Pathology*. New York: Raven Press.

72. Popper, H. (1975) The ground-glass hepatocyte as a diagnostic hint. *Human Pathology*, **6**, 517–520.

73. Popper, H. & Schaffner, F. (1970) Pathophysiology of cholestasis. *Human Pathology*, **1**, 1–24.

74. Popper, H., Schaffner, F. & Denk, H. (1976) Molecular pathology of cholestasis. In Taylor, W. (ed.) *The Hepatobiliary System*, pp. 605–629. London: Plenum Press.

75. Poucell, S., Ireton, J., Valencia-Mayoral, P. *et al.* (1984) Amiodarone-associated phospholipidosis and fibrosis of the liver. *Gastroenterology*, **86**, 926–936.

76. Reddy, J.K., Azarnoff, D.L., Svoboda, D.H. & Prasad J.D. (1974) Nafenopin-induced hepatic microbody (peroxisomes) proliferation and catalase synthesis in rats and mice. Absence of sex difference in response. *Journal of Cell Biology*, **61**, 344–358.

77. Remmer, H. & Bock, K.W. (1974) The role of the liver in drug metabolism. In Schaffner, F., Sherlock, S. & Leevy, C.M. (eds) *The Liver and its Diseases*, pp. 34–42. New York: Intercontinental Medical Book Co.

78. Remmer, H. & Merker, H.J. (1963) Drug-induced changes in the endoplasmic reticulum; association with metabolizing enzymes. *Science*, **142**, 1657–1658.

79. Richter, G.W. (1960) The nature of storage iron in idiopathic hemochromatosis and in hemosiderosis. *Journal of Experimental Medicine*, **112**, 551–570.

80. Richter, G.W. (1978) The iron loaded cell. The cytopathology of iron storage. A review. *American Journal of Pathology*, **91**, 361–404.

81. Ross, R.C., Kovacks, K. & Horvath, E. (1972) Ultrastructure of peliosis hepatis in a percutaneous biopsy. *Pathologia Europaea*, **7**, 273–282.

82. Rubin, E. & Lieber, C.S. (1967) Early fine structural changes in the human liver induced by alcohol. *Gastroenterology*, **52**, 1–13.

83. Rubin, E., Hutterer, F. & Lieber, C.S. (1968) Ethanol increases smooth endoplasmic reticulum and drug metabolizing enzymes. *Science*, **159**, 1469–1471.

84. Schaffner, F. (1970) Oxygen supply and the hepatocyte. *Annals of the New York Academy of Sciences*, **170**, 67–77.

85. Schaffner, F. (1974) Some unresolved ultrastructural problems encountered in the study of the liver and its diseases. In Schaffner, F., Sherlock, S. & Leevy, C.M. (eds) *The Liver and its Diseases*, pp. 7–18. New York: Intercontinental Medical Book Co.

86. Schaffner, F. & Popper, H. (1975) Electron microscopy of the liver. In Schiff, L. (ed.) *Diseases of the Liver*, 4th edn., pp. 51–85. Philadelphia: Lippincott.

87. Scotto, J.M., Stralin, H.G. & Landrieu, P. (1977) Etude ultrastructurale du foie dans deux cas de tyrosienémie héréditaire. *Gastroenterologie Clinique et Biologique*, **1**, 139–149.

88. Searle, J., Harmon, B.V., Bishop, C.J. *et al.* (1987) The significance of cell death by apoptosis in hepatobiliary disease. *Journal of Gastroenterology & Hepatology*, **2**, 77–96.

89. Shikata, T., Uzawa, T., Yoshiwara, N. *et al.* (1974) Staining methods of Australia antigen in paraffin section. Detection of cytoplasmic inclusion bodies. *Japanese Journal of Experimental Medicine*, **44**, 25–36.

90. Simon, J.B., Manley, P.N., Brien, J.F. & Armstrong, P.W. (1984) Amiodarone hepatotoxicity simulating alcoholic liver disease. *New England Journal of Medicine*, **311**, 167–172.

91. Staubli, W., Hess, R. & Weibel, E.R. (1969) Correlated morphometric and biochemical studies on the liver cell. II. Effect of phenobarbital on rat hepatocytes. *Journal of Cell Biology*, **42**, 92–112.

92. Stein, O., Fainaru, M. & Stein, Y. (1972) Visualization of virus-like particles in endoplasmic reticulum of hepatocytes of Australia antigen carriers. *Laboratory Investigation*, **26**, 262–269.

93. Steiner, J.W., Jezequel, A.M., Phillips, M.J. *et al.* (1965) Some aspects of the ultrastructural pathology of the liver. In Popper, H. & Schaffner, F. (eds) *Progress in Liver Diseases*, vol.2, pp. 303–372. New York: Grune & Stratton.

94. Stenger, R.J. (1970) Organelle pathology of the liver. The endoplasmic reticulum. *Gastroenterology*, **58**, 554–574.

95. Sternlieb, I. & Scheinberg, I.H. (1974) Wilson's disease. In Schaffner, F., Sherlock, S. & Leevy, C.M. (eds) *The Liver and its Diseases*, pp. 328–336. New York: Intercontinental Medical Book Co.

96. Svoboda, D.J. & Azarnoff, D.L. (1966) Response of hepatic microbodies to a hypolipidemic agent, ethylchlorophenoxyisobutyrate (CPIB). *Journal of Cell Biology*, **30**, 442–450.

97. Swift, H. & Hruban, Z. (1964) Focal degradation as a biological process. *Federation Proceedings*, **23**, 1026–1037.

98. Taxy, J.B. (1978) Peliosis: a morphological curiosity becomes an iatrogenic problem. *Human Pathology*, **9**, 331–340.

99. Thomsen, P., Poulsen, H. & Petersen, P. (1977) Different type of ground glass hepatocytes in human liver biopsies. Morphology, occurence and diagnostic significance. *Scandinavian Journal of Gastroenterology*, **11**, 113–119.

100. Trump, B.F., Dees, J.H. & Shelburne, J.D. (1973) The ultrastructure of human liver cell and its common patterns of reaction of injury. In Gall, E.A. & Mostofi, F.K. (eds) *The Liver*, pp. 80–120. Baltimore: Williams & Wilkins.

101. Uchida, T., Kronborg, I. & Peters, R.L. (1984) Giant mitochondria in the alcoholic liver diseases. Their identification, frequency and pathologic significance. *Liver*, **4**, 29–38.

102. Uznalimoglu, B., Yardley, J.H. & Boitnott, J.K. (1970) The liver in mild halothane hepatitis. *American Journal of Pathology*, **61**, 457–478.

103. Volk, B.W., Wellmann, K.F. & Wallace, B.J. (1970) Hepatic changes in various lipidosis: electron microscopic and histochemical studies. In Popper, H. & Schaffner, F. (eds) *Progress in Liver Diseases*, vol. 3, pp. 206–221. New York: Grune & Stratton.

104. Wiener, J., Loud, A.V., Kimberg, D.V. & Spiro, D. (1968) A quantitative description of cortisone-induced alterations in the ultrastructure of rat liver parenchymal cells. *Journal of Cell Biology*, **37**, 47–61.

105. Wiggers, K.D., French, S.W., French, B.A. & Carr, B.N. (1973) The ultrastructure of Mallory body filaments. *Laboratory Investigation*, **29**, 652–658.

106. Wills, E.J. & Walton, B. (1978) A morphological study of unexplained hepatitis following halothane anesthesia. *American Journal of Pathology*, **91**, 11–32.

107. Winkler, K., Junge, U. & Creutzfeldt, W. (1977) Ground-glass hepatocytes in unselected liver biopsies. Ultrastructure and relationship to Hepatitis B antigen. *Scandinavian Journal of Gastroenterology*, **11**, 167–170.

108. Yakoo, H., Minick, O.T., Batti, F. & Kent, G. (1972) Morphologic variants of alcoholic hyalin. *American Journal of Pathology*, **69**, 25–40.

109. Yunis, E.J., Agostini, R.M. & Glew, R.H. (1976) Fine structural observations on the liver in alpha-1 antitrypsin deficiency. *American Journal of Pathology*, **82**, 265–286.

110. Zafrani, E.S., Cazier, A., Baudelot, A.M. & Feldmann, G. (1984) Ultrastructural lesions of the liver in human peliosis. *American Journal of Pathology*, **114**, 349–359.

Radionuclide Imaging

Duncan M. Ackery

Radionuclides have been used for several decades to study the morphology and function of the liver and its related structures.[38] Diagnostic imaging investigations require the administration of a radioactive pharmaceutical followed by measurement of gamma radiation emitted from the body. This is simple for the patient and involves minimal risk. Nowadays radionuclide procedures are complemented by other imaging investigations[2,82] such as ultrasound, computed tomography, and nuclear magnetic resonance (see Chapters 22–24). These mainly demonstrate hepatic structure and anatomical relationships, whereas radionuclides give images of liver function. Function may be impaired by focal or diffuse disease.

INSTRUMENTATION AND TECHNIQUE

Distribution of radioactivity within the liver is measured by a scintillation detector placed close to the skin surface. A gamma camera is almost always used for this. It consists of a collimated sodium iodide crystal for detecting gamma photons and a series of photomultiplier tubes, with associated electronics, to analyse the detected events as a spatial distribution. The final image is displayed on photographic or polaroid film. Pulses can also be passed through an analogue-to-digital converter to a computer for image analysis and quantification. The gamma camera does not move during the procedure (the term 'gamma image' is therefore more appropriate than 'scan') and usually a measurement of several minutes is required to give a statistically acceptable result.

Two types of radiopharmaceutical are used for routine investigation: colloid preparations that are taken up by Kupffer cells of the hepatic sinusoids; or chemicals and dyes that are actively transported by hepatocytes. Liver concentration of these agents is related to hepatic blood flow and the capacity of the liver to extract the radiopharmaceutical from the circulation. The product of hepatic perfusion and extraction efficiency is termed 'effective liver blood flow'.

The optimal photon energy for gamma camera imaging is around 200 keV. To minimize the patient radiation dose, the physical half-life of the radionuclide label should be short (a few hours) and there should be no beta emission. Technetium-99*m* is ideal in these respects, with monochromatic photon emission at 140 keV, a 6-h half-life, and no beta radiation. It is available from a [99]Mo generator, and is used to label a variety of colloids and other chemicals of pharmaceutical grade. For labelled colloid preparations, 80 MBq of ^{99m}Tc is the recommended adult dose, and this is taken up by the liver and spleen over a period of 10–15 min following intravenous administration. [198]Au and ^{111}In colloids may also be used but give a greater radiation dose to the patient and are more expensive.

Hepatocyte function and biliary excretion can be assessed using derivatives of iminodiacetic acid (IDA) labelled with [99m]Tc.[54] These are rapidly cleared by the liver and secreted promptly into the biliary tract. They can be used to show gallbladder function and biliary drainage. Radiation doses for the various radionuclide procedures are generally no greater than those for common radiographic investigation.

For the radiocolloid procedure, imaging is carried out in the anterior, posterior, and right and left lateral positions. These give a comprehensive examination of both the liver and the spleen. The anterior view gives the best overall impression of liver morphology, and shows the relationship to the costal margin and to palpated masses. The posterior image shows the lumbar surface of the right hepatic lobe and its relationship to the right kidney. It is used for the measurement of splenic length. The left lobe of the liver is not shown in this projection as it lies anteriorly and much of the photon emission is attenuated by the spine. The right lateral view is used to mark the position of focal lesions within the right lobe prior to needle biopsy. The left lateral position views the lateral aspect of the spleen with the left lobe of the liver lying anterior to it. Appropriate anatomical landmarks should accompany all images. Typical normal appearances are given in Figure 21.1.

INTERPRETATION OF THE RADIOCOLLOID IMAGE

Having inspected the images for technical quality and artefacts, interpretation is based upon organ size and shape, uniformity of colloid distribution, and the relative uptake of activity in liver, spleen and bone marrow.[39]

Hepatic enlargement

Palpation of the abdomen may give a misleading impression of increased liver size, especially if the right hemidiaphragm is low.[35,100] With practice, hepatomegaly can be readily recognized from inspection of the gamma camera image. Calculation of liver volume using mathematical modelling gives no greater accuracy.[86] Normal splenic length, taken from the posterior aspect, should be no more than 13 cm in the adult.[69] Liver enlargement is usually the consequence of hepatic focal or diffuse disease, but the liver may be large without pathological change, e.g. when a Riedel's lobe is present (Figure 21.2). Rarely an infiltrated liver may show no enlargement.

Hepatic morphology

A wide variety of shapes has been reported for the normal liver,[66] and an awareness of these can reduce the incidence of false positive reporting of focal disease from radionuclide images.[27,47,74] The gallbladder fossa or porta hepatis can appear as a solitary defect in the normal pattern of colloid uptake, and thinning of the left lobe in the midline by the spine, indentation of the right lobe by the ribs, and notching of the superior surface of the right lobe at the site of the confluence of the hepatic veins may all give a misleading pattern. Owing to its greater volume, the right lobe has a higher count rate than the left, and the position of the falciform ligament is often clearly shown. The liver may migrate to the left hypochondrium after splenectomy,[16] or into the chest with congenital or post-traumatic diaphragmatic eventration.[97,119] It may also be displaced by intraperitoneal fluid or by the bowel. Cases of doubt should be referred for confirmation by other imaging investigations.

Uniformity of uptake

Normal liver should show even radiocolloid distribution, and any departure from this pattern indicates potential disease. Well-defined intrahepatic foci are almost always pathological. Diffuse hepatic disease impairs both blood flow and reticuloendothelial function, so that poor and patchy distribution of radiocolloid results. In this case preferential uptake is shown by the spleen, which may be large due to portal hypertension, and by bone marrow. Bone marrow concentration is relatively too low to be shown in normal subjects.

FOCAL HEPATIC DISEASE

Radiocolloid imaging has been shown to be a particularly effective procedure for identifying space-occupying lesions within the liver.[66,67,78] Its resolution is approximately equivalent to that of ultrasound, computed tomography and nuclear magnetic resonance, but it does not have the specificity of these techniques.[57,104] Also, it does not show the interrelationship of the liver to other abdominal structures. Difficulties in interpretation arising from normal variant morphology can lead to false positive reporting and overdiagnosis of focal disease. Table 21.1 provides a useful guide to the possible causes for a solitary focal lesion.

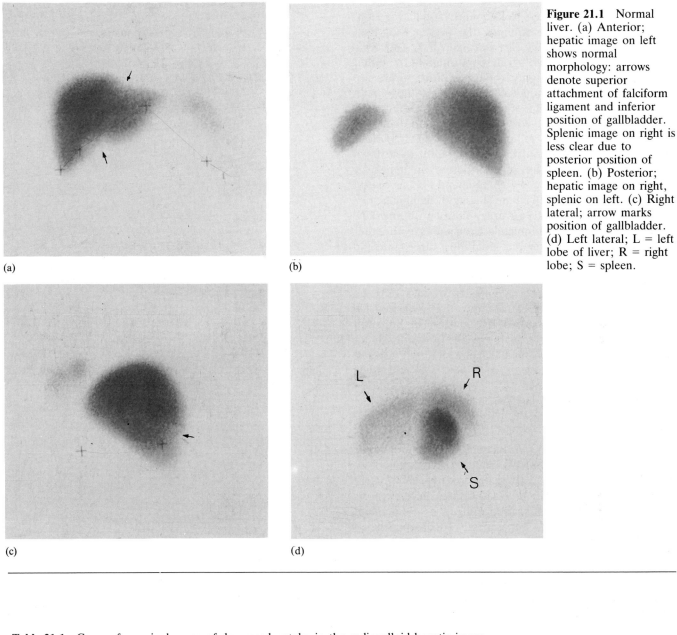

(a)

(b)

(c)

(d)

Figure 21.1 Normal liver. (a) Anterior; hepatic image on left shows normal morphology: arrows denote superior attachment of falciform ligament and inferior position of gallbladder. Splenic image on right is less clear due to posterior position of spleen. (b) Posterior; hepatic image on right, splenic on left. (c) Right lateral; arrow marks position of gallbladder. (d) Left lateral; L = left lobe of liver; R = right lobe; S = spleen.

Table 21.1 Causes for a single area of decreased uptake in the radiocolloid hepatic image

Common	Less common	Rare
Metastatic neoplasms	Cirrhosis	Haemangioma
Pyogenic abscess	Primary hepatic neoplasm	Focal nodular hyperplasia
False positive causes	Trauma	Hamartoma
	Lymphoma	Hepatic vein thrombosis
	Post-radiotherapy	Amyloidosis
	Cysts:	Viral hepatitis
	Simple	Gumma
	Hydatid	
	Abscess:	
	Amoebic	
	Tuberculous	
	Actinomycotic	
	Arteriovenous malformations	

Modified from Holder *et al.*[25]

The radiocolloid image is frequently used as a non-invasive method for determining the presence of liver metastases.[36] Its accuracy lies between 75% and 85% when compared to histological confirmation by either needle biopsy or laparotomy.[62] False positive results are common in severely jaundiced patients or those with hepatic dysfunction from other causes. The diagnostic accuracy has not changed with recent improvements in gamma camera and radiopharmaceutical technology although radionuclide emission tomography has shown some promise.[10] Detection of small lesions is limited by the spatial resolution of the technique and for this reason it is of less value for the routine staging of malignancy.[21,] [23,77,93] Greater diagnostic accuracy may be obtained by the combination of radionuclide procedures with other imaging investigation such as angiography, ultrasound and computed tomography.[33,53]

In spite of its limitations, the radiocolloid study often demonstrates the presence of metastases and avoids the necessity for exploratory laparotomy. It is indicated for patients with clinical hepatomegaly, or when liver function tests are abnormal. It can give guidance for subsequent needle biopsy, which can have a large sampling error if carried out without image assistance.[14] A multifocal pattern (Figures 21.3 and 21.4), taken within the clinical context, is usually diagnostic of secondary malignancy, although greater specificity is obtained by ultrasound and computed tomography.

Other hepatic tumours may be detected by radionuclide imaging but show no distinctive features. Primary hepatocellular carcinoma (HCC) is uncommon but may present at any age. In the adult it usually arises in a cirrhotic liver, which makes identification difficult as radiocolloid uptake is uneven due to generalized reticuloendothelial dysfunction.[52] Confirmation is required by biochemistry, ultrasound and computed tomography.[106] Angiography is necessary for selecting patients for hepatic lobectomy in this condition[29] (see Chapter 25). Haemangioma shows as a space-occupying lesion, often on the hepatic surface. Specific identification is required[103] to avoid the hazard of needle biopsy. Radionuclide vascular studies may help in this (see below). Focal nodular hyperplasia shows either normal or patchy colloid uptake.[108]

The radiocolloid image is used in the investigation of patients with signs of sepsis. Intrahepatic pyogenic abscess[84,92] (Figure 21.5), and subdiaphragmatic lesions are visible if large, and the image can guide surgical exploration. Amoebic abscess[15] usually shows as a clearly defined lesion (Figure 21.6), and radiocolloid investigation should be undertaken in patients with unexplained fever who have travelled in regions of the world with high risk for amoebiasis.

Cysts of the liver, which can be solitary or multiple, give an identical appearance whether simple or of parasitic origin. Furthermore, the image appearances may be very similar to those of multiple metastases (Figure 21.7). Differentiation is obtained by ultrasound. A specific image

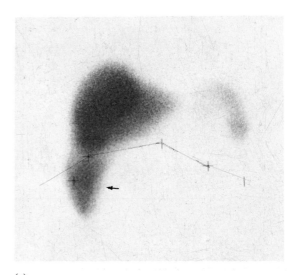

(a)

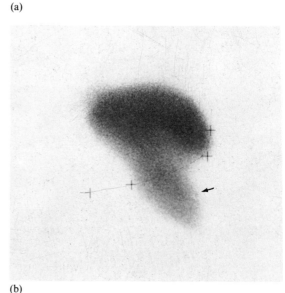

(b)

Figure 21.2 Normal liver with Riedel's extension to right lobe (arrowed). (a) Anterior. (b) Right lateral.

diagnosis is necessary to avoid the dangers of needle biopsy of an hydatid cyst.

Special techniques

As the radiocolloid technique does not discriminate between the different causes for focal disease, alternative radiopharmaceuticals have been tried in an attempt to improve diagnostic specificity.

Assessment of lesion vascularity is obtained by measuring the 'first pass' of radioactivity after rapid bolus intravenous administration. This technique is similar to contrast angiography and may show an early 'blush' of activity in vascular lesions[111] (see 'Dynamic Studies'). Alternatively, a radiopharmaceutical is administered which remains within the circulation and shows increased blood pooling in a vascular lesion.[61] Radionuclides of

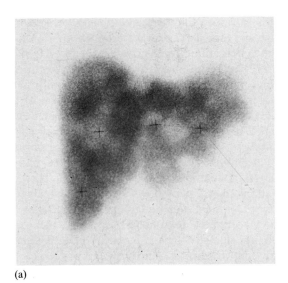

(a)

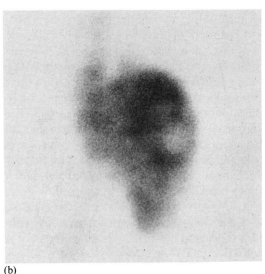

(b)

Figure 21.3 Carcinoma of the breast. (a) Anterior and (b) right lateral views showing multiple hepatic deposits.

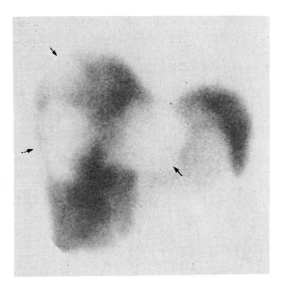

Figure 21.4 Carcinoma of the colon. Large deposits shown in the right and left hepatic lobes.

Autologous white cells labelled either with ^{111}In or ^{99m}Tc-hexamethyl propylene amine oxime (HMPAO) are also used for identifying inflammatory lesions in the liver.[22]

These procedures increase the specificity of the routine colloid image, but alone they seldom give a precise diagnosis. They have been replaced to a large extent by ultrasound and other imaging investigations which give better lesion characterization.

Radionuclide methods may also be used to monitor the distribution of degradable starch microspheres in the liver when these are used to enhance the efficacy of hepatic arterial administration of chemotherapy agents[8] (see Chapter 40).

TRAUMA

The liver and spleen may be affected by external injury or by penetrating wounds. Radionuclide screening has been shown to be useful in defining the extent of injury,[20,31] particularly in those with closed trauma, and can be done without too much difficulty as an emergency procedure, even in seriously injured patients. This enables assessment prior to angiography. Large intrahepatic lesions, concave defects on the liver margin, organ displacement, and minor patchy losses have been reported. Nuclide imaging also provides a simple way to assess subsequent hepatic regeneration.[18,49]

DIFFUSE PARENCHYMAL DISEASE

Irregular and patchy hepatic uptake of radiocolloid is observed in many disorders which alter normal hepatic function and architecture. The mechanisms for these appearances include impairment of normal hepatic macrophage function, alterations in blood flow, and replacement of liver parenchyma by fibrous tissue. When hepatic

indium which label transferrin, or ^{99m}Tc-labelled human serum albumin or red cells are used for this purpose.

A second approach is to administer a radiopharmaceutical which is actively concentrated in tumours or inflammatory lesions. ^{75}Se-selenomethionine behaves as a substrate for protein synthesis and may show increased concentration in primary and secondary hepatic malignancy compared with normal liver parenchyma.[12,48] Uptake by individual tumours is variable and may require digital subtraction of the colloid image to enhance lesion detection. Selective concentration of ^{67}Ga citrate by tumours[83] and abscess cavities is also used[17,46,55] but the results are unpredictable. Gallium concentration in normal liver, and in large intestine may be misleading. Colonic cleansing is required prior to imaging at, usually, 48 h following intravenous ^{67}Ga administration. Although ^{67}Ga is expensive, it is used more commonly than other pharmaceuticals for characterizing focal hepatic lesions.

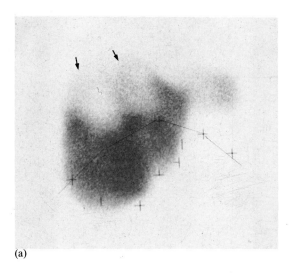

(a)

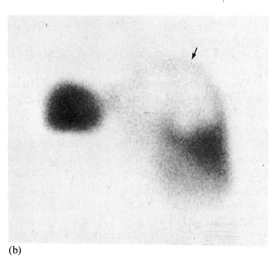

(b)

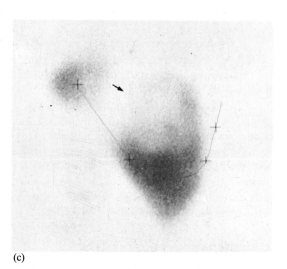

(c)

Figure 21.5 Pyogenic hepatic abscess. (a) Anterior; (b) posterior, and (c) right lateral views, showing multifocal abscess cavity (arrows).

function is impaired, the macrophages of spleen, bone marrow and lung clear a larger proportion of radiocolloid from the circulation. The characteristic image appearance (Figure 21.8) is an enlarged liver, usually with irregular distribution of radiocolloid, splenomegaly with increased radiocolloid uptake, and a higher proportion of activity in bone marrow. The lungs seldom show increased concentration. These appearances reflect the functional deficit which takes place with cirrhosis, acute and chronic hepatitis, portal fibrosis, and extensive metastatic replacement, and are not characteristic of any one of these. Fatty infiltration on its own shows hepatic enlargement with otherwise minimal functional impairment. The loss of function correlates reasonably well with the extent of histological change shown at biopsy.[30] The relative uptake of activity in the spleen and liver expressed as a quantitative ratio may be used to study progression of disease and response to therapy.

The non-specific appearance of images in many generalized disorders of the liver limit the diagnostic contribution of the radiocolloid procedure. The liver and spleen may show general enlargement in Hodgkin's disease and with other lymphomas (Figure 21.9) even in the absence of obvious focal infiltration. Radionuclide imaging has been disappointing in staging these diseases.[60] Obstructive jaundice may secondarily impair Kupffer cell function,[1] giving patchy radiocolloid distribution, but a more focal defect at the porta hepatis due to distension of the large bile ducts may also be shown in jaundiced patients. The liver may be reduced in size in patients with advanced cirrhosis, or with portal vein obstruction, but occlusion of the portal vein usually does not give the high splenic activity expected in cirrhosis. Although the liver may also be small, with right lobe atrophy in schistosomiasis, image appearances are variable in this condition, and splenic enlargement with increased uptake may not be present.[44] A more characteristic appearance occurs in some patients with the Budd–Chiari syndrome. A focal region of high uptake is sited centrally in the anterior image, and posteriorly in the right lateral. This is because the caudate lobe is spared the effect of occlusion by independent drainage direct into the inferior vena cava.[102] Superior vena caval occlusion shows a similar appearance when intravenous colloid is given at the arm, and collateral circulation diverts activity via the umbilical vein into small segments of the liver.[40] Thrombosis of smaller hepatic veins, unlike the Budd–Chiari syndrome, gives a more generalized patchiness of uptake which can be confused with metastatic infiltration. Other generalized liver disorders which cause local hepatic necrosis and fibrosis may also give an appearance of focal disease.[114] These so-called 'pseudotumours' are particularly common in cirrhosis and may be mistaken for malignancy.

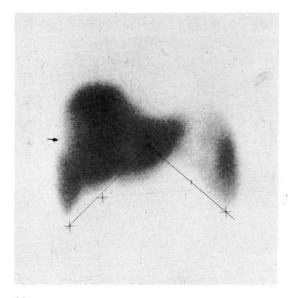

(a)

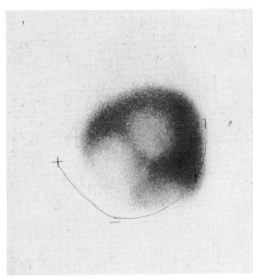

(b)

Figure 21.6 Amoebic hepatic abscess. (a) Anterior and (b) right lateral views showing confluent abscess cavities in the right lobe with little obvious hepatic enlargement. (c) and (d) Same views one week later after metronidazole therapy, showing reduction in size of abscess and liver.

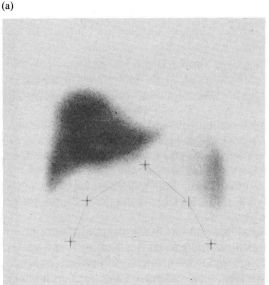

(c)

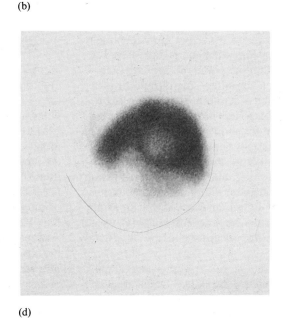

(d)

DYNAMIC STUDIES

This term refers to serial measurements of hepatic or splenic radioactivity with time. This is done either with a simple probe counter or a gamma camera with computer acquisition. Time activity histograms, constructed by integrating counts in the region of an organ from stored images, are used to study the kinetics of labelled compounds in health and disease. Liver blood flow and biliary function can be studied by this procedure.

HEPATIC BLOOD FLOW _____

The fundamental principle underlying radionuclide imaging procedures is that concentration of radioactivity takes place following the intravenous administration of a radiopharmaceutical. Uptake of a radiopharmaceutical depends

upon regional cardiac output to the tissue under examination and on the extraction efficiency by the tissue. The product of these two factors is often called the 'Effective Organ Blood Flow'.

Hepatic blood flow may be estimated by a variety of techniques. Extraction of a radiopharmaceutical can be measured using the Fick Principle, but this requires direct sampling from the hepatic veins and cannot be used for clinical purposes. Alternatively, the clearance of a radioactive tracer, such as radiocolloid, from peripheral blood can be determined by multiple blood sampling[6] and the effective blood flow can be calculated from the product of the rate constant of clearance from the vascular compartment and the blood volume. This method assumes single-compartment kinetics with no variation in extraction efficiency. In fact, following injection of radiocolloid, clearance takes place according to a three-compartment

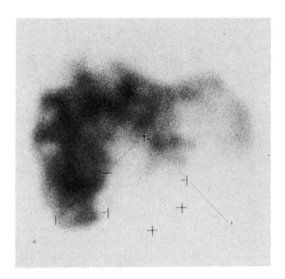

Figure 21.7 Multiple cysts in enlarged liver.

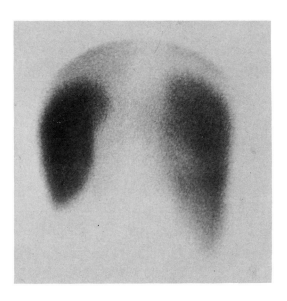

Figure 21.9 Non-Hodgkins lymphoma. Posterior view showing generalized increase in size of liver and spleen.

model.[19] When this is applied to in vivo gamma camera measurements[85] the first compartment is taken to represent the particle distribution pool, the second that of particle turnover at the macrophage membrane and the third the intracellular space of Kuppfer cells, reflecting the time course of phagocytosis and metabolic degradation.

It has been appreciated for some time that early images of the haemodynamic phase of hepatic radionuclide imaging can add discrimination to the diagnostic interpretation[41,101,110,117] and this has stimulated an increasing interest in the use of 'first pass' radionuclide techniques. From these the degree of vascularity of focal lesions compared to that of normal hepatic parenchymal tissue can be demonstrated. More recently the use of digital

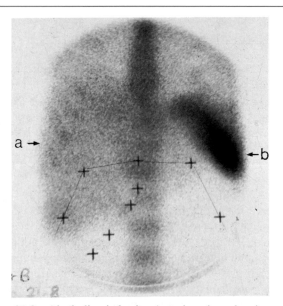

Figure 21.8 Alcoholic cirrhosis. Anterior view showing poor radiocolloid uptake in enlarged liver (a), high uptake in moderately enlarged spleen (b), and uptake in marrow of spine and ribs.

methods with fast on-line acquisition of data has permitted quantitative analysis of activity–time curves from which the arterial and portal components of hepatic flow can be determined.

Mathematical modelling[63] and gamma camera measurements of the rate of colloid clearance and total uptake by the liver, spleen and extrahepatic tissues have been used for estimating total hepatic blood flow without the necessity for blood sampling.[50,89] These may then be combined with the estimates of relative component flow.[109]

Hepatic blood flow, and its fractional contribution from the hepatic artery and portal vein, may vary under different physiological conditions.[6] A fourfold variation in liver blood flow under normal conditions in animals has been attributed to irregularity of flow through the sinusoids, and this is supported by changes in sinusoid flow observed directly in the trans-illuminated liver. Both upright posture and exercise cause a relative drop in the cardiac output to the liver. Flow in the mesenteric circulation increases following feeding both in absolute terms and in the proportion perfusing the liver. This proportion rises from 59% to 76% of total flow between fasting and taking a standard meal.[109] For these reasons it is recommended that clinical studies are undertaken in the supine position, after a period of rest, and after overnight fasting.

FIRST PASS TECHNIQUES

Most radionuclide techniques for observing hepatic haemodynamics use a gamma scintillation camera. This may be sited above the supine subject with the field of view including the heart, lung bases, major abdominal blood vessels, liver, spleen and kidneys. Alternatively, the camera is positioned under the bed, allowing better visualization of the posterior hepatic right lobe and kidneys. The radiopharmaceutical is drawn up in a small (under 0.5 ml) volume and administered rapidly as a bolus into an antecubital vein. This is followed by a saline flush which assists the rapid transit of the activity through the heart and into the systemic circulation. The most convenient method of delivery is through an indwelling venous line using a three-way tap.

Data on an on-line computer is obtained in two stages; in the first stage the data are acquired on the first pass of radiocolloid into the liver, from which the arterial and portal components of hepatic blood flow are determined. In the second stage the rate of colloid clearance is measured, which gives an index of hepatic reticuloendothelial flow.

RADIOPHARMACEUTICALS FOR DYNAMIC STUDIES

Either pertechnetate (^{99m}Tc) or colloids may be used. During the first pass of pertechnetate into the liver the counts rise to a peak and then drop as activity is removed in the venous outflow. Colloid is extracted by reticuloendothelial macrophages found primarily in the liver (Kupffer cells) and to a lesser extent in the spleen and bone marrow. In health more than 80% of activity is cleared from the circulation during the first pass. Extraction varies with colloid particles of different sizes, and is impaired in liver disease. The time–activity curve over the liver for radiocolloid does not show a decline due to venous washout and continues to rise. Radiocolloid arriving at the liver in the portal vein has almost entirely passed through the mesenteric circulation. Activity which has taken the splenic route will be removed by the spleen. The proportional portal flow when measured with radiocolloid may be referred to as the 'mesenteric fraction'.

Radiocolloid has certain advantages over pertechnetate for measuring the arterial and portal components of flow.[79] The clearance of most of the activity from the splenic circulation improves the temporal separation of arterial and portal phases as the mesenteric pathways are longer than those for the spleen. Also, the uptake of colloid by the liver simplifies the choice of appropriate regions of interest, and following the haemodynamic study a conventional hepatic image can be obtained. The use of pertechnetate and technetium-labelled colloid in the same subject permits assessment of the relative contributions of extrahepatic and intrahepatic circulations and that of reticulendothelial extraction.[45]

Other radiopharmaceuticals that may be used to investigate hepatic haemodynamics include labelled microspheres, which are extracted in the first passage through a capillary bed and thus require direct arterial or portal injection. The clearance of ^{133}Xe from hepatic parenchyma has also been used to measure liver blood flow in animals and patients. The gas is dissolved in saline solution and administered directly into the hepatic artery or portal circulation (via dilatation and cannulation of the obliterated umbilical vein). This is followed by continuous measurement by a collimated probe or gamma camera to give the time–activity clearance curve. This is a double exponential function the fast component of which represents blood flow.

MEASUREMENT OF THE RELATIVE HEPATIC ARTERY AND PORTAL VEIN PERFUSION

Of the two afferent hepatic vascular systems, the hepatic artery supplies approximately 25–30% of the total. Rapid data acquisition following a bolus administration can be used to separate hepatic and portal arrival of activity, and to determine the relative contribution of each to hepatic perfusion.[50]

These measurements may be made by direct administration of radiopharmaceutical into the hepatic artery by catheterization, or into the portal system via percutaneous splenic puncture, cannulization of the umbilical vein, or direct injection of microspheres into the portal vein.[32,51,73] Such techniques are invasive and do not measure the fractionated perfusion. Animal studies of relative cardiac output by each route can be carried out using intracardiac injection of labelled microspheres with arterial sampling.[68]

Alternatively, non-invasive studies can be carried out using pertechnetate or labelled colloid. Following rapid bolus injection of radiopharmaceutical into a peripheral vein, activity passes through the heart and into the systemic circulation. Activity appears in the liver first through the hepatic artery, followed by that arriving in the portal venous system. Different analytical methods have been described to measure the proportionate flow via the two routes. This principle was first investigated by Taplin[101] and later by Biersack, who calculated the relative arterial and portal contributions to flow from the areas under the biphasic time–activity curve.[4,5]

Hepatic perfusion index (HPI)

In this method the gradient of the time activity curve is measured for the two components of flow. A rapid bolus (0.2–0.5 ml) of activity is administered. Either pertechnetate or technetium-labelled colloid may be used. Rapid gamma camera images are taken to include the heart, liver, lung bases, spleen and kidneys. Data are stored for 100 sec following injection. Sequential frames of the study are added and regions of interest are drawn for the left ventricle, right hepatic lobe, right lung, spleen and kidneys. Particular care is taken to avoid major vessels and other regions of high background within the chosen region for the liver. Time–activity curves are plotted for the six regions.[90] An improved method of analysis[91] corrects for the error which results in the early part of the portal phase due to washout of activity from the arterial component. This is done by estimating hepatic washout from the downslope of the splenic time–activity curve following the peak. The HPI is then calculated as the true portal component divided by the sum of the arterial and true portal components.

A variation of the technique acquires data from the posterior aspect, which minimises the statistical inaccuracy in counts from the kidneys.[79] The left kidney is shown to be more reliable than the right for the estimation.[81] The Hepatic Perfusion Index can also be reliably measured in small animals,[75] and the results have been validated by comparison with absolute flows using a microsphere technique.[68]

Hepatic arterial ratio (HAR)

In this method patients are positioned supine over a large field of view gamma camera fitted with a high-sensitivity collimator.[118] 150 MBq of technetium sulphur colloid are administered as a rapid intravenous bolus. Sequential posterior images are recorded for 5 min, initially at 2-s and later at 6-s intervals. Quantitative anterior and posterior images of the liver and spleen are recorded after maximum colloid clearance. After construction of activity–time curves from appropriate regions of interest the arterial component of hepatic flow is calculated by fitting the initial rise of the splenic curve to the hepatic curve. The arterial percentage of hepatic flow is then calculated from the relative heights of the hepatic uptake curve and the arterial component at 5 min, applying a correction for the colloid removed from the portal circulation by the spleen. The rate of clearance of tracer is determined by a simple clearance index obtained from the cardiac blood pool activity at 30 and 120 s.

Mesenteric fraction (MF)

Using this method the temporal separation of the two phases of hepatic perfusion is given by comparison with activity in the cardiac blood pool, the spleen and left kidney.[26] The fractional perfusion is given by the relative heights of the liver activity–time curve as with the HAR method. The patient is positioned supine beneath a gamma camera and technetium-labelled colloid is administered in a bolus.

To calculate the mesenteric fraction the end of the arterial phase in the liver is taken from a mean of the half-peak decline value of cardiac activity, the plateau value of splenic activity, and the peak activity in the left kidney. Similarly, three estimates are taken from the heart, spleen and left kidney to establish the termination of the portal phase.

Colloid arriving at the liver via the portal vein will comprise only that which has passed through the mesenteric circulation; activity in the splenic artery having been extracted in the spleen. The method has been validated by measurements in experimental animals following ligation of the hepatic artery and portocaval anastomosis.[25]

Comparison of different techniques and errors

The various methods of analysis used to determine the contribution of flow to the liver via the hepatic artery and portal vein use different assumptions and variables. Both physiological and physical factors may affect the result.[105] Considerable variations for the values of HPI are obtained depending on the number of data points used in the determination of the flow gradient or the number of smoothing operations to which the data are subjected. The use of an extracted tracer is recommended, and it is possible that the currently considered abnormal ranges for HPI may be poor indicators of the fractional flow.

In a study of the variability between different observers using the HPI analysis for patients with colorectal malignancy, better agreement was obtained when the left renal peak activity was used to define the end of the arterial phase than the right.[114] Indices of relative arterial perfusion depend upon the regions chosen for analysis and the extent of this has been calculated.[9] Parametric imaging improves the choice of selection of regions of interest and the separation of hepatic activity from that in overlying tissues.

EXPERIMENTAL AND CLINICAL STUDIES OF LIVER BLOOD FLOW

HEPATIC MALIGNANCY _____

Conventional radionuclide colloid imaging does not detect metastases of less than about 2 cm, particularly if they lie deep in the liver. Because metastases in the liver are primarily nourished by hepatic arterial blood, it has been proposed that the arterial component of flow might be proportionately increased with early metastatic involvement. A significant increase in the fraction of hepatic arterial blood to the liver has been shown in patients with positive laparotomy even when no metastases were visible by conventional radionuclide imaging.[58] The Hepatic Perfusion Index was found to be increased in patients with occult metastatic disease with a diagnostic sensitivity of 96% and specificity of 72% as judged by the finding of metastases 1 year later.[59] In 150 patients with primary carcinoma of the gastrointestinal tract the Hepatic Perfusion Index was elevated in 94% of those with liver metastases at laparotomy and in 87% of those with occult metastases which became overt within 3 years.[13]

It remains unclear whether the apparent rise in hepatic arterial contribution is not in fact due to a reduction in portal flow to the liver. It has been shown that metastases from colorectal carcinoma which spread to the liver via the portal vein preferentially block the portal inflow to the liver.[73] In the rat liver, into which micrometastases have been inoculated via the portal vein, the Hepatic Perfusion Index rises over a 6-day period. Hepatic arterial flow, as determined by intraventricular injection of labelled microspheres, did not alter and portal flow was proportionately reduced.[75] On the other hand, using the mesenteric fraction technique it has been shown[42] that the absolute arterial flow increases proportionately with the amount of hepatic replacement by colorectal metastases.

CIRRHOSIS

A number of different methods have been described to measure the severity of diffuse liver disease from quantification of the radionuclide colloid image. Initially this was done by simply summing the counts in the liver and spleen and expressing a ratio of activity. Increasingly impaired hepatic function was indicated by a reduced liver : spleen ratio. A significant reduction in liver uptake rate of colloid has been shown in cirrhotic patients compared to normals, but not for those with alcoholic hepatitis.[72] This is supported by other studies.[24,56,99,118] In animals there is a close correlation between rise in portal pressure and shunting, measured by the diversion away from the liver of radiolabelled microspheres injected into the portal vein. Beta-1-blocking drugs reduce liver blood flow in normal rats and have a variable effect in cirrhotic animals, probably reflecting the balance between changes in cardiac output and hepatic perfusion.[70] In humans the mesenteric fraction shows some overlap of cirrhotics with a healthy group, but better discrimination is obtained when data for mesenteric fraction were combined with liver : spleen ratios measured as a geometric mean.[71] Patients who had recently bled from varices showed a greater reduction in values. Patients who have bled and have a low initial value of mesenteric fraction have a significant risk of rebleeding despite active prophylactic treatment.[37] In an attempt to estimate the degree of shunting of the portal circulation, studies have been undertaken in cirrhotic patients using simultaneous technetium-labelled colloid and pertechnetate.[64] The results permit calculation of a 'trapping index' which has been found to be a reliable indicator of the risk of bleeding.

LIVER GRAFT REJECTION

Measurement of the portal contribution to hepatic flow can be used to monitor the status of patients following hepatic transplantation.[65] In general the transplant has a lower portal contribution than normal liver. The level drops below 55% with acute rejection but remains above this value in post-transplant hepatitis.

PORTAL OCCLUSION AND MESENTERIC ISCHAEMIA

A good correlation is shown between measurement of mesenteric fraction and the degree of portal shunting using direct portal injection of labelled microspheres in experimental animals in which portal hypertension has been produced by progressive portal vein ligation.[11] The results suggest that non-invasive radionuclide methods

could be used clinically for assessing the extent of portal flow prior to hepatic arterial embolization,[28] and for estimating the degree of mesenteric ischaemia in patients with symptoms of intestinal ischaemia.

HEPATIC REGENERATION FOLLOWING SURGERY

After partial resection in children and young adults the remaining liver grows rapidly to its original mass by about 3–4 weeks. Measurements of hepatic blood flow with radiocolloid have been used to show the haemodynamic changes after resection in animals.[50]

In summary, dynamic studies provide simple non-invasive procedures for measuring hepatic haemodynamics. So far these procedures have shown clinical promise rather than any routine place in the management of hepatic disorders. The relative arterial component has been shown to increase in cirrhosis, hepatic metastases and mesenteric ischaemia. There is therefore a possible place for the monitoring of patients with cirrhosis or following hepatic transplantation, for assessing of the adequacy of perfusion prior to embolization, and in the early detection of hepatic malignancy.

HEPATOBILIARY STUDIES

The investigation of jaundice with radionuclides has for many years depended on the administration of ^{131}I-labelled rose bengal. This dye is concentrated by hepatocytes and excreted into bile, and the time course of activity has been used to measure hepatic function and biliary patency. This has been useful in distinguishing between the different causes of neonatal jaundice.[95] The radiation dose of ^{131}I has permitted only low activities to be given to patients. This results in low counts and inferior images which cannot show biliary anatomy or the level of extrahepatic biliary obstruction. These limitations of ^{131}I have been overcome by the introduction of hepatobiliary agents which can be labelled with [99m]Tc.[87,116] Of these the ^{99m}Tc-labelled *N*-substituted iminodiacetic acids (IDA agents) are most useful. These undergo good biliary concentration even when bilirubin levels are elevated.[80] The IDA radiopharmaceuticals are rapidly concentrated by hepatocytes following intravenous administration and are secreted promptly into the biliary tract. The high photon flux available with ^{99m}Tc ensures good images of the main biliary ducts and the gallbladder, and enables the flow of activity into the duodenum to be shown (Figure 21.10). These agents are also cleared to a small extent by the kidneys and, when hepatic function is impaired, activity in the urinary tract can give a misleading impression of intestinal transit. They are of value in investigating jaundiced patients and in measuring biliary flow. They can be useful in showing intermittent extrahepatic obstruction when ultrasound gives no evidence of duct dilatation, in assessing biliary patency

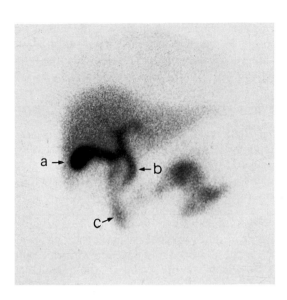

Figure 21.10 Normal hepatobiliary system. ^{99m}Tc-IDA concentrated in liver and gallbladder (a), common duct (b), and duodenum (c).

following surgery, and in demonstrating biliary leaks. They have also been shown to be both sensitive and specific for the diagnosis of acute cholecystitis.[34,76,112] In this condition the radiopharmaceutical is not concentrated in the gallbladder owing to cystic duct obstruction, and this appearance discriminates accurately between acute gallbladder inflammation and other causes for upper abdominal pain. The results for chronic cholecystitis are less successful.

PAEDIATRIC INVESTIGATIONS

The non-invasive nature of radionuclide investigation makes it particularly suited for the investigation of children. With reassurance and mild sedation the child can

be persuaded to lie quietly under the gamma camera, and images of good quality can be obtained with minimal administered activity. A converging collimator can be used to give image magnification and enhanced spatial resolution.

Indications for paediatric studies include investigation of hepatosplenomagaly, identification of intra- and extra-hepatic lesions, assessment of congenital abnormalities, and studies of neonatal jaundice. These are carried out using ^{99m}Tc-labelled pharmaceuticals.

RADIATION DOSIMETRY

The absorbed radiation dose received by a patient during a radionuclide procedure should be carefully considered when balancing the potential risks of the examination against the clinical benefit. Radiation dose is minimized by the selection of radionuclides with short physical half-life, and no beta emission. Generally, radiation doses for radionuclide procedures are no greater than those for common radiographic procedures[43,98] and are also acceptable for paediatric investigation.[107]

SUMMARY

Advances in diagnostic imaging over recent years make it necessary to define precisely the place of radionuclide liver and biliary studies so that unnecessary investigation is avoided.[88] The sensitivity for detection of focal hepatic disease is similar to that of ultrasound and computed tomography, but both these techniques have better diagnostic specificity and are able to demonstrate the relationship of the liver to other abdominal viscera.[3,113] Radionuclides can give a quantitative assessment of overall hepatic function in diffuse hepatic disorders which supplements but is unlikely to replace biochemistry and histology for diagnostic purposes.

REFERENCES

1. Agnew, J.E., James, O. & Bouchier, I.A.D. (1975) Liver and pancreas scanning in extrahepatic obstructive jaundice (with special reference to tumours of the bile and hepatic ducts). *British Journal of Radiology*, **48**, 190–199.
2. Ashare, A.B. (1980) Radiocolloid live scintigraphy. A choice and an echo. *Radiologic Clinics of North America*, **18**, 315–320.
3. Biello, D.R., Levitt, R.G., Siegel, B.A. *et al.* (1978) Computed tomography and radionuclude imaging of the liver: a comparative evaluation. *Radiology*, **127**, 159–163.
4. Biersack, H.J., Thelen, M., Schulz, D. *et al.* (1977) Die sequenttielle hepatospleno-szintigraphie zur quantitativen beurteilung der leberdurchblutung. *Fortschritte auf dem Gebiete der Rontgenstrahlen und der Nuklearmedizin*, **126**, 47–52.
5. Biersack, H.J., Torres, J., Thelen, M. (1981) Determination of liver and spleen perfusion by quantitative sequential scintigraphy: results in normal subjects and in patients with portal hypertension. *Clinical Nuclear Medicine*, **6**, 218–220.
6. Bradley, E.L. (1974) Measurement of hepatic blood flow in man. *Surgery*, **75**, 783–789.
7. Bradley, S.E. (1949) Variations in hepatic blood flow in man during health and disease. *New England Journal of Medicine*, **240**, 456–461.
8. Britten, A., Flowerdew, A., Hunt, T. *et al.* (1989) A gamma camera method to monitor the use of degradable starch microspheres in hepatic arterial chemotherapy. *European Journal of Nuclear Medicine*, **15**, 649–654.
9. Britten, A.J., Fleming, J.S., Flowerdew, A.D.S. *et al.* (1989) Regional indices of relative hepatic arterial perfusion from dynamic liver scintigraphy: the variability of indices and the use of parametric imaging. *Nuclear Medicine Communications*, **11**, 29–36.
10. Burdine, J.A., Murphy, P.H. & DePuey, E.G. (1979) Radionuclide computed tomography of the body using routine radiopharmaceuticals. II. Clinical applications. *Journal of Nuclear Medicine*, **20**, 108–114.
11. Burge, D.M., Holbrook, A.G., Karran, S.J. (1987) Non invasive assessment of portosystemic shunting in extrahepatic portal hypertension in rats. *Journal of Paediatric Surgery*, **22**, 211–214.
12. Coakley, A.J. & Wraight, E.P. (1980) Selenomethionine liver scanning in the diagnosis of hepatoma. *British Journal of Radiology*, **53**, 538–543.
13. Cooke, D.A., Parkin, A., Wiggins, P. *et al.* (1987) Hepatic perfusion index and the evolution of liver metastases. *Nuclear Medicine Communications*, **8**, 970–974.

14. Conn, H.O. (1972) Rational use of liver biopsy in the diagnosis of hepatic cancer. *Gastroenterology*, **62**, 142–146.

15. Cuaron, A., Sepulveda, B. & Landa, L. (1965) Topographic distribution of amoebic abscesses studies by liver scanning. *International Journal of Applied Radiation and Isotopes*, **16**, 603–609.

16. Custer, J.R. & Shafter, R.B. (1975) Changes in the liver scan following splenectomy. *Journal of Nuclear Medicine*, **16**, 194–195.

17. Damron, J.R., Beihn, R.M., Selby, J.B. & Rosenbaum, H.D. (1974) Gallium-technetium subtraction scanning for the localization of subphrenic abscess. *Radiology*, **113**, 117–122.

18. Deland, F.H. & Wagner, N.H. (1968) Regeneration of the liver after hepatectomy. *Journal of Nuclear Medicine*, **9**, 587–589.

19. Dobson, E.L. & Jones, H.B. (1952) The behaviour of intravenously injected particulate material; the rate of disappearance from the blood stream as a measure of liver blood flow. *Acta Medica Scandinavica*, **144**, Suppl. 273.

20. Evans, G.W., Curtin, F.G., McCarthy, H.F. & Kiernan, J.H. (1972) Scintigraphy in traumatic lesions of liver and spleen. *Journal of the American Medical Association*, **6**, 665–667.

21. Evans, R.A., Bland, K.I., McMurtrey, M.J. & Ballantyne, A.J. (1980) Radionuclide scans not indicated for clinical stage 1 melanoma. *Surgery, Gynecology and Obstretrics*, **150**, 532–534.

22. Fawcett, H.D., Lantieri, R.L., Frankel, A. & McDougall, I.R. (1980) Differentiating hepatic abscess from tumor: combined 111 In white blood cell and 99mTc liver scans. *American Journal of Roentgenology*, **135**, 53–56.

23. Fee, H.J., Prokop, E.K., Cameron, J.L. & Wagner, H.N. (1974) Liver scanning in patients with suspected abdominal tumours. *Journal of the American Medical Association*, **230**, 1675–1677.

24. Ferguson, W.R., Laird, J.D. & Cranley, K. (1981) Early dynamic studies as an adjunct to liver scintigraphy in the investigation of diffuse liver disease. *Journal of Nuclear Medicine*, **22**, P88.

25. Fleming, J.S., Humphries, N.L.M., Karran, S.J. et al. (1981) In vivo assessment of hepatic-arterial and portal-venous components of liver perfusion: concise communication. *Journal of Nuclear Medicine*, **22**, 18–21.

26. Fleming, J.S., Ackery, D.M., Walmsley, B.H. et al. (1983) Scintigraphic estimation of arterial and portal blood supplies to the liver. *Journal of Nuclear Medicine*, **24**, 1108–1113.

27. Freeman, L.M., Meng, C.H., Johnson, P.M. et al. (1969) False positive liver scans caused by disease processes in adjacent organs and structures. *British Journal of Radiology*, **42**, 651–656.

28. Flowerdew, A.D.S., McLaren, M.I., Fleming, J.S. et al. (1987) Liver tumour blood flow and responses to arterial embolization measured by dynamic hepatic scintigraphy. *British Journal of Cancer*, **55**, 269–273.

29. Gammill, S.L., Takahishi, M., Jingu, K. et al. (1975) A comparison of scans and angiograms in selecting patients with hepatomas for hepatic lobectomy. *American Journal of Roentgenology, Radium Therapy and Nuclear Medicine*, **123**, 522–530.

30. Geslien, G.E., Pinsky, S.M., Poth, R.K. & Johnson, M.C. (1976) The sensitivity and specificity of 99m Tc-sulphur colloid liver imaging in diffuse hepatocellular disease. *Radiology*, **118**, 115–119.

31. Gilday, D.L. & Alderson, P.O. (1974) Scintigraphic evaluation of liver and spleen injury. *Seminars in Nuclear Medicine*, **4**, 357–370.

32. Gross, G., Goldberg, H.I. & Shames, D.M. (1976) A new approach to evaluating hepatic blood flow in the present intrahepatic portal systemic shunting. *Investigative Radiology*, **11**, 146–149.

33. Grossman, Z.D., Winstow, B.W., Bryan P.J. et al. (1977) Radionuclide imaging, computed tomography and grey-scale ultrasonography of the liver: a comparative study. *Journal of Nuclear Medicine*, **18**, 327–332.

34. Hall, A.W., Wisby, M.L., Hutchinson, F. et al. (1981) The place of hepatobiliary isotope scanning in the diagnosis of gallbladder disease. *British Journal of Surgery*, **68**, 85–90.

35. Halpern, S., Coel, M., Ashburn, W. et al. (1974) Correlation of liver and spleen size. *Archives of Internal Medicine*, **134**, 123–124.

36. Hatfield, P.M. (1975) Role of liver scanning in the diagnosis of hepatic metastases. *Medical Clinics of North America*, **59**, 247–276.

37. Holbrook, A.G., Burge, D., Fleming, J.S. et al. (1987) Dynamic hepatic scintigraphy in the prediction of recurrent variceal bleeding. *British Journal of Surgery*, **74**, 527.

38. Holder, L.E. & Saenger, E.L. (1975) The use of nuclear medicine in evaluating liver disease. *Seminars in Roentgenology*, **10**, 215–222.

39. Holder, L.E., Ashare, A.B., Tomsicke, T. et al. (1975) The gamut approach to scintigram interpretation—diagnostic aid and teaching method. *Journal of Nuclear Medicine*, **16**, 1121–1124.

40. Holmquest, D.L. & Burdin, J.A. (1973) Caval-portal shunting as a cause of a focal increase in radiocolloid uptake in normal livers. *Journal of Nuclear Medicine*, **14**, 348–351.

41. Houston, A.S. & Macleod, M.A. (1980) Processing of liver dynamic studies with technetium-labelled sulphur colloid. *British Journal of Radiology*, **53**, 87–92.

42. Hunt, T.M., Flowerdew, A.D.S., Britten, A.J. et al. (1989) An association between haemodynamic parameters obtained by dynamic liver scintigraphy and percentage hepatic replacement with tumour. *Annals of the Royal College of Surgeons*, **71**, 11–14.

43. ICRP Publications 17 (1969) Protection of the patient in radionuclide investigations. Report prepared for the International Commission on Radiological Protection 1969. Oxford, New York: Pergamon Press.

44. Iio, M., Iuchi, M., Kitani, K. et al. (1971) Scintigraphic evaluation of the liver with schistosomiasis japonica. *Journal of Nuclear Medicine*, **12**, 655–659.

45. Izzo, G., Diluzio, S., Guerris, M. et al. (1983) On the interpretation of the early part of the liver time activity curve: double tracer experiment. *European Journal of Nuclear Medicine*, **8**, 101–104.

46. James, O., Wood, E.J. & Sherlock, S. (1974) ^{67}Ga scanning in the diagnosis of liver disease. *Gut*, **15**, 404–410.

47. Johnson, P.M. & Sweeney, W.A. (1967) The false positive hepatic scan. *Journal of Nuclear Medicine*, **8**, 451–460.

48. Kaplan, E. & Domingo, M. (1972) 75Se-selenomethionine in hepatic focal lesions. *Seminars in Nuclear Medicine*, **2**, 139–149.

49. Karran, S.J., Leach, K.G. & Blumgart, L.H. (1974) Assessment of liver regeneration in the rat using the gamma camera. *Journal of Nuclear Medicine*, **15**, 10–16.

50. Karran, S.J., Eagles, C.J., Fleming, J.S. & Ackery, D.M. (1979) In vivo measurement of liver perfusion in the normal and partially hepatectomized rat using Tc-99m sulfur colloid. *Journal of Nuclear Medicine*, **20**, 26–31.

51. Kashiwagi, T., Kamada, T. & Abe, H. (1974) Dynamic studies on the portal hemodynamics by scintiphotosplenoportography: the visualization of portal venous system using ^{99m}Tc. *Gastroenterology*, **67**, 668–673.

52. Kido, C. (1975) Primary liver cancer (angiography and scintigraphy). *Australasian Radiology*, **19**, 129–139.

53. Kim, D.K., McSweeney, S.D. & Yeh, J. (1975) Tumours of liver as demonstrated by scan and laparotomy. *Surgery, Gynecology and Obstetrics*, **141**, 409–410.

54. Klingensmith, W.C., Fitzberg, A.R., Spitzer, V.M. et al. (1980) Clinical comparison of ^{99m}Tc-diethyl-IDA and ^{99m}Tc-PIPIDA for evaluation of the hepatobiliary system. *Radiology*, **134**, 195–199.

55. Lavender, J.P., Lowe, J., Barker, J.R. et al. (1971) Gallium-67 citrate scanning in neoplastic and inflammatory lesions. *British Journal of Radiology*, **44**, 361–366.

56. Leng, B., O'Driscoll, M.P., Majeed, F.A. et al. (1987) Hepatic perfusion index in cirrhotic livers—investigation of imaging and analytical procedures. *Nuclear Medicine Communications*, **8**, 1001–1010.

57. Lerona, P.T., Go, R.T. & Cornell, S.H. (1974) Limitations of angiography and scanning in diagnosis of liver masses. *Radiology*, **112**, 139–145.

58. Leveson, S.H., Wiggins, P.A., Nausiru, T.A. et al. (1982) Improving the detection of hepatic metastases by the use of dynamic flow scintigraphy. *British Journal of Cancer*, **47**, 719–721.

59. Leveson, S.H., Wiggins, P.A., Giles, G.R. et al. (1985) Deranged liver blood flow patterns in the detection of liver metastases. *British Journal of Surgery*, **72**, 128–130.

60. Lipton, M.J., Denardo, G.L., Silverman, S. & Glatstein, E. (1972) Evaluation of the liver and spleen in Hodgkin's disease. 1. The value of hepatic scintigraphy. *American Journal of Medicine*, **52**, 356–361.

61. Lubin, E. & Lewitus, Z. (1972) Blood pool scanning in investigating hepatic mass lesion. *Seminars in Nuclear Medicine*, **2**, 128–132.

62. Lunia, S., Parthasarathy, S., Barkshi, S. & Bender, M.A. (1975) An evaluation of ^{99m}Tc-sulfur colloid liver scintiscans and their usefulness in metastatic work-up: a review of 1,424 studies. *Journal of Nuclear Medicine*, **16**, 62–65.

63. Magrini, A., Izzo, G., Guerrisi, M. *et al.* (1985) A new approach to non-invasive quantitative study of hepatic haemodynamics using radiocolloids in vivo. *Clinical Physics and Physiological Measurement,* **6,** 179–204.

64. Mairiang, E.O., Parkin, A., Robinson, P.J. *et al.* (1986) Noninvasive indices of liver blood flow in patients with complications of cirrhosis. *Nuclear Medicine Communications,* **7,** 268–269.

65. Martin-Comin, J., Mora, J., Figueras, J. *et al.* (1988) Calculation of portal contribution to hepatic blood flow with ^{99m}Tc-microcolloids: a non-invasive method to diagnose liver graft rejection. *Journal of Nuclear Medicine,* **29,** 1776–1780.

66. McAfee, J.G., Ause, R.G. & Wagner, H.N. (1965) Diagnostic value of scintillation scanning of the liver. *Archives of Internal Medicine,* **116,** 95–110.

67. McCready, V.R. (1972) Scintigraphic studies of space-occupying liver disease. *Seminars in Nuclear Medicine,* **2,** 108–127.

68. McDevitt, D.G. & Nies, A.S. (1976) Simultaneous measurement of cardiac output and its distribution with microspheres in the rat. *Cardiovascular Research,* **10,** 494–498.

69. McIntyre, P.A. (1972) Diagnostic significance of the spleen scan. *Seminars in Nuclear Medicine,* **2,** 278–287.

70. McLaren, M., Braye, S., Fleming, J. *et al.* (1987) Changes in blood flow, portal pressure and shunting during the development of cirrhosis in response to beta-blockade. *Gut,* **28,** 663–667.

71. McLaren, M.I., Fleming, J.S., Walmsley, B.H. *et al.* (1985) Dynamic liver scanning in cirrhosis. *British Journal of Surgery,* **72,** 394–396.

72. Miller, J., Diffey, B.L. & Fleming, J.S. (1979) Measurement of colloid clearance rate as an adjunct to static liver imaging. *European Journal of Nuclear Medicine,* **4,** 1–5.

73. Mooney, B., Grime, J.S., Taylor, I. & Critchley, M. (1983) Portal scanning for liver metastases in colorectal carcinoma. *Clinical Radiology,* **34,** 657–659.

74. Nishiyama, H., Lewis, J.T., Ashare, A.B. & Saenger, E.L. (1975) Interpretation of radionuclide liver images: do training and experience make a difference? *Journal of Nuclear Medicine,* **15,** 11–16.

75. Nott, D.M., Grime, J.S., Yates, J. *et al.* (1987) A model of the hepatic perfusion index in the rat. *Nuclear Medicine Communications,* **8,** 990–994.

76. O'Callaghan, J.D., Verow, P.W., Hopton, D. & Craven, J.L. (1980) The diagnosis of acute gallbladder disease by technetium-99m-labelled HIDA hepatobiliary scanning. *British Journal of Surgery,* **67,** 805–808.

77. Operchal, J.A., Bowen, R.D. & Grove, R.B. (1976) Efficacy of radionuclide procedures in staging bronchogenic carcinoma. *Journal of Nuclear Medicine,* **17,** 530.

78. Oster, Z.H., Larson, S.M., Strauss, H.W. & Wagner, H.N. (1975) Analysis of scanning in a general hospital. *Journal of Nuclear Medicine,* **16,** 450–453.

79. Parkin, A., Robinson, P.J., Baxter, P. *et al.* (1983) Liver perfusion scintigraphy—method, normal range and laparotomy correlation in 100 patients. *Nuclear Medicine Communications,* **4,** 395–402.

80. Pauwels, S., Piret, L., Schoutens, A. *et al.* (1980) Tc-99m-Diethyl-IDA imaging: clinical evaluation in jaundiced patients. *Journal of Nuclear Medicine,* **21,** 1022–1028.

81. Perkins, A.C., Whalley, D.R., Ballantyre, K.C. *et al.* (1987) Reliability of the hepatic perfusion index for the detection of liver metastases. *Nuclear Medicine Communications,* **8,** 982–989.

82. Petasnick, J.P., Ram, P., Turner, D.A. & Fordham, E.W. (1979) The relationship of computed tomography, gray-scale ultrasonography, and radionuclide imaging in the evaluation of hepatic masses. *Seminars in Nuclear Medicine,* **9,** 8–21.

83. Pinsky, S.M. & Henkin, R.E. (1979) Gallium-67 tumor scanning. *Seminars in Nuclear Medicine,* **6,** 397–409.

84. Ranson, J.H., Madayag, M.A., Localio, S.A. & Spencer, F.C. (1975) New diagnostic and therapeutic techniques in the management of pyogenic liver abscesses. *Annals of Surgery,* **181,** 508–518.

85. Reske, S.N., Vyska, K. & Feinendegen, L.E. (1981) In vivo assessment of phagocytic properties of Kupffer cells. *Journal of Nuclear Medicine,* **22,** 405–410.

86. Rollo, R.D. & Deland, F.H. (1968) The determination of liver mass from radionuclide images. *Radiology,* **91,** 1191–1194.

87. Ronai, P.M. (1977) Hepatobiliary radiopharmaceuticals: defining their clinical role will be galling experience. *Journal of Nuclear Medicine,* **18,** 488–490.

88. Rothschild, M.A. (1976) Hepatic radionuclide imaging: an effective diagnostic procedure! *American Journal of Digestive Diseases,* **21,** 655–659.

89. Rutland, M.D. (1984) An analysis of the uptake of 99Tcm-sulphur colloid by the liver and spleen. *Nuclear Medicine Communications,* **5,** 593–602.

90. Sarper, R., Fajmam, W.A., Rypins, E.B. *et al.* (1981) A non-invasive method for measuring portal venous/total hepatic blood flow by hepatosplenic radionuclide angiography. *Radiology,* **141,** 179–184.

91. Sarper, R. & Tarcan, Y.A. (1983) An improved method of estimating the portal venous fraction of total hepatic blood flow from computerized radionuclide angiography. *Radiology,* **147,** 559–562.

92. Schraibman, I.G. (1974) Non-parasitic liver abscess. *British Journal of Surgery,* **61,** 709–712.

93. Sears, H.F., Gerber, F.H., Sturtz, D.L. & Fouty, W.J. (1975) Liver scan and carcinoma of the breast. *Surgery, Gynecology and Obstetrics,* **140,** 409–411.

94. Sherriff, S.B., Smart, R.C. & Taylor, I. (1977) Clinical study of liver blood flow in man measured by 133Xe clearance after portal vein injection. *Gut,* **18,** 1027–1031.

95. Silverberg, M., Rosenthal, L. & Freeman, L.M. (1973) Rose bengal excretion studies as an aid in the differential diagnosis of neonatal jaundice. *Seminars in Nuclear Medicine,* **3,** 69–80.

96. Smith, A. & Clarke, M.B. (1976) The determination of hepatic blood flow in the rat using xenon-133. *International Journal of Applied Radiation and Isotopes,* **27,** 201–210.

97. Soucek, C.D. (1975) Foramen of Morgagni hernia diagnosed by liver scan. *Journal of Nuclear Medicine,* **16,** 261–263.

98. Spencer, R.P., Hosian, F. & Spitznagle, L.A. (1976) Kinetic and dosimetry of radiopharmaceuticals in evaluating liver, gall bladder and spleen. In Cloutier, R.J. (ed.) A Radiopharmaceutical Dosimetry Symposium: Proceedings of Conference held at Oak Ridge, Tennessee, pp. 256–266. U.S. Department of Health, Education and Welfare.

99. Stewart, C., Sakimura, I., Siegel, M.E. *et al.* (1984) The hepatic-arterial/portal-venous scintiangiogram in alcoholic hepatitis. *Journal of Nuclear Medicine,* **25,** P67.

100. Sullivan, S., Krasner, N. & Williams, R. (1976) The clinical estimation of liver size: a comparison of techniques and an analysis of the source of error. *British Medical Journal,* **2,** 1042–1043.

101. Taplin, G.V. (1971) Dynamic studies of liver function with radioisotopes. In *Dynamic Studies with Radioisotopes in Medicine: Proceedings,* pp. 373–392. Vienna: International Atomic Energy Agency.

102. Tavill, A.S., Wood, E.J., Kreel, L. *et al.* (1975) The Budd-Chiari syndrome: correlation between hepatic scintigraphy and the clinical, radiological and pathological findings in nineteen cases of hepatic venous outflow obstruction. *Gastroenterology,* **68,** 509–518.

103. Taylor, R.D., Anderson, P.M., Winston, M.A. & Blahd, W.H. (1976) Diagnosis of hepatic hemangioma using multiple radionuclide and ultrasound techniques. *Journal of Nuclear Medicine,* **17,** 362–364.

104. Taylor, K.J., Sullivan, D.C., Rosenfield, A.T. *et al.* (1977) Grayscale ultrasound and isotope scanning: complementary techniques for imaging the liver. *American Journal of Roentgenology,* **128,** 277–281.

105. Tindale, W.B. & Barber, D.C. (1987) The effect of methodology and tracer identity on a non-invasive index of liver blood flow. *Nuclear Medicine Communications,* **8,** 973–981.

106. Tonami, N., Aburano, T. & Hisada, K. (1975) Comparison of alpha-fetoprotein radioimmunoassay method and liver scanning for detecting primary hepatic cell carcinoma. *Cancer,* **36,** 466–470.

107. Treves, S. & Spencer, R.P. (1973) Liver and spleen scintigraphy in children. *Seminars in Nuclear Medicine,* **3,** 55–68.

108. Uszler, J.M. & Swanson L.A. (1975) Focal nodular hyperplasia of the liver: case report. *Journal of Nuclear Medicine,* **16,** 831–832.

109. Walmsley, B.H., Fleming, J.S., Ackery, D.M. & Karran, S.J. (1987) Noninvasive assessment of absolute values of hepatic haemodynamics using radiocolloid scintigraphy. *Nuclear Medicine Communications,* **8,** 613–621.

110. Waxman, A.D., Apau, R. & Siemsen, J.K. (1972) Rapid sequential liver imaging. *Journal of Nuclear Medicine,* **13,** 522–524.

111. Waxman, A.D., Finck, E.J. & Siemsen, J.K. (1974) Combined

contrast and radionuclide angiography of the liver. *Radiology,* **113**, 123–129.

112. Weissmann, H.S., Frank, M.S., Bernstein, L.H. *et al.* (1979) Rapid and accurate diagnosis of acute cholecystitis with 99mTc-HIDA cholescintigraphy. *American Journal of Roentgenology,* **132**, 523–528.

113. Weissmann, H.S., Frank, M., Rosenblatt, R. *et al.* (1979). Cholescintigraphy, ultrasonography and computerized tomography in the evaluation of biliary tract disorders. *Seminars in Nuclear Medicine,* **9**, 22–35.

114. Whalley, D.R., Perkins, A.C., Ballantyre, K.C. & Hardcastle, J.D. (1987) Validity of the hepatic perfusion index for the detection of liver metastases. *Nuclear Medicine Communications,* **8**, 271–272.

115. Winston, M.A. & Shapiro, M. (1974) Pseudotumors in acute hepatitis. *Journal of Nuclear Medicine,* **15**, 1039–1040.

116. Wistow, B.W., Subramanian, G., van Heertum, R.L. *et al.* (1977) An evaluation of ^{99m}Tc-labelled hepatobiliary agents. *Journal of Nuclear Medicine,* **18**, 455–461.

117. Witek, J.T. & Spencer, R.P. (1974) Clinical correlation of hepatic flow studies. *Journal of Nuclear Medicine,* **16**, 71–72.

118. Wraight, E.P., Barber, R.W. & Ritson, A. (1982) Relative hepatic arterial and portal flow in liver scintigraphy. *Nuclear Medicine Communications,* **3**, 273–279.

119. Yeung, W.C., Haines, J.E. & Larson, S.M. (1976) Diagnosis of posterolateral congenital diaphragmatic (Bochdalek) hernia by liver scintigram: case report. *Journal of Nuclear Medicine,* **17**, 110–112.

CHAPTER 22

Ultrasound Imaging

K.C. Dewbury, H.B. Meire & J. Herbetko

Diagnostic procedures using ultrasound are painless, harmless, relatively inexpensive and have no contraindications at the intensities used. Ultrasound can perhaps offer more diagnostic information about the liver than for any other organ. In this chapter its main diagnostic uses and some indication as to its current limitations are given.

BASIC PRINCIPLES

Diagnostic ultrasound scanners utilize very short pulses (about one-millionth of a second) of high-frequency sound, usually two to five million cycles per second. At this very high frequency, sound can be focused into a fine beam a few millimetres in diameter, and when this beam impinges on the interface between two structures of different density and elasticity a proportion of it is reflected, as in marine echo sounding. Diagnostic scanners employ a transducer which acts as a transmitter and receiver of the sound. The sound transmitted from the transducer takes the form of a fine beam, which is scanned to interrogate the structures within a thin slice of the patient.

The scanning action may be performed either manually or automatically. In the older, manually operated static scanners the transducer is held in contact with the patient and moved by hand in a linear fashion over the area of interest. The returning echoes are compiled into a static image of the structures beneath the transducer's path. These static scanners produced high-resolution images but required considerable operator expertise and could not be used to observe moving structures. Modern diagnostic ultrasound makes use of real-time scanners. These devices vary widely in design but consist of either mechanical or electronic mechanisms to steer the ultrasound beam through the plane of interest. The majority of real-time scanners perform the scanning so rapidly that a continuously changing or 'real-time' image is displayed. This permits observation of tissue movements and also rapid surveying of the anatomy. They have resulted in an increase in speed with which an examination can be performed and their image quality has progressively improved. The major limitation is the small field of view. This may lead to problems in interpreting and demonstrating frozen images.

Electronic real-time scanners consist of a linear array of transducers which are fired in sequence. The resulting image is rectangular in shape, the width of the image being determined by the length of the transducer array. Many mechanical systems have been devised to produce a sector image, commonly with a sector angle of 90°. The small area of contact between the transducer and the patient, combined with the shape of the field of view, makes these devices ideal for imaging the liver. When scanning a patient, the transducer is held in contact with the skin and moved over the region of interest. To ensure good acoustic contact between transducer and skin, the skin is coated with gel or another suitable coupling medium. Electronic devices record the position of the transducer and also calculate the precise position of any tissue discontinuities (interfaces) from which echoes are received. The received echoes are displayed as dots on the screen, the position of each dot corresponding to the locus of the interface which gave rise to that echo. In general, there are more echoes from heterogeneous tissues than from homogeneous tissues. Stronger echoes are received from interfaces between tissues with large differences in acoustic impedence. More homogeneous tissues cause lower-amplitude echoes which are displayed as grey dots; the lower the amplitude the darker the grey. Fluid-filled spaces generate no echoes and so appear black. As the transducer is moved over the patient, an image is built up of all the interfaces contained within the thin slice of the patient over which the transducer has been moved.

The limitations of the system result from total reflection of sound at gas–soft tissue or bone–soft tissue interfaces. In practice, therefore, ultrasound cannot 'see' through gas or bone and, when the liver is examined, the interposition of ribs or bowel gas between liver and transducer has to be avoided. This is possible in over 90% of patients, failures occurring in patients with high diaphragms, low ribs or excessive upper abdominal bowel gas.

SCANNING TECHNIQUE

It is preferable to examine the liver with the patient maintaining suspended deep inspiration. Since each scan takes only about one second to perform, this is generally possible. If the patient has pulmonary emphysema or hepatomegaly, inspiration may be unnecessary. No patient preparation is required except for attempts at reducing bowel gas in patients who have had a failed examination from this cause.

Since each scan examines only a thin slice of liver, it is essential to perform many adjacent scans to image the whole volume of the organ. Most operators employ a series of longitudinal scans initially, each of these corresponding to the lateral view of a parasagital section. It is generally advisable to perform transverse scans also, to facilitate imaging of the extreme lateral portion of the right lobe and to verify the nature of structures seen on the longitudinal scans. By convention, the transverse scans are displayed as if the section is viewed from the foot of the bed, perhaps because the apparatus was developed by a gynaecologist! Ultrasound imaging of the liver using real-time apparatus permits significant departure from the protocol described above. This is of particular value when trying to identify tubular structures such as the intrahepatic biliary radicals. Such structures can be followed throughout multiple image planes and their connections identified in order to confirm their precise nature. It is also possible to survey almost the entire liver volume with a real-time scanner; this is impossible with a B scanner since there are invariably non-visualized spaces between the scan planes.

NORMAL ULTRASOUND APPEARANCES

Knowledge of the normal ultrasound appearances in the upper abdomen is essential to the understanding of the pathological variations discussed in the following sections. The best assessment of the liver parenchyma is made in the longitudinal scan. The liver parenchyma produces a soft, even, low-level echo pattern, which is interspersed with higher-level echoes from the portal vein walls (Figure 22.1). These vascular echoes form rings or parallel lines depending on the plane in which the vessel is cut by the ultrasound beam. Hepatic veins within the liver are seen as echo-free rings or tubular structures with no surrounding bright echoes.[6] In addition to the left and right lobes of the liver, the caudate lobe is also seen lying cephalad and posterior to the portal vein and anterior to the inferior vena cava. In our experience this lobe may rarely show a lower reflectivity than from the remainder of the liver. The superior and posterior surface of the liver is clearly defined by the diaphragm, identified as a thin, bright bow. The posterior surface is usually also partly defined by the right kidney, well seen through the ultrasound 'window' of the liver. The inferior surface forms a smooth concave border under which the gallbladder is usually found. The inferior surface of the liver may be partially obscured by colonic gas. The normal gallbladder is a smooth, pear-shaped, echo-free sac.

On technically good scans it is always possible to identify a large number of vascular structures in the

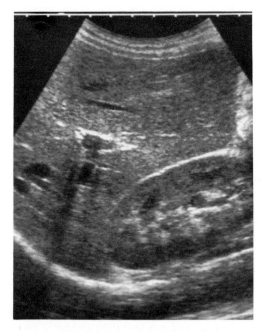

Figure 22.1 A longitudinal scan through the right lobe of liver and kidney. The normal texture of the liver is interspersed with the high-level echoes from the portal vein walls and the lower reflectivity from the hepatic veins.

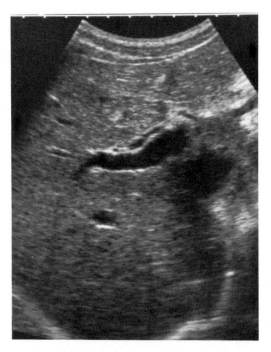

Figure 22.2 A transverse scan through the right lobe of the liver showing the right main portal vein. The fine tubular structure above it is the right hepatic duct.

abdomen, both intra- and extrahepatic. The extrahepatic portal venous system is best seen on the transverse scan. At the level of the first lumbar vertebra the inferior vena cava and aorta lie anteriorly to the right and left of the spine. Just anterior to the aorta a small echo-free ring surrounded by a bright cuff of echoes represents the superior mesenteric artery. Anterior to these vessels the splenic and then portal veins are seen passing across the midline to enter the liver anterior to the inferior vena cava. At this point the right portal vein usually extends onwards into the hepatic parenchyma (Figure 22.2). On a longitudinal scan just to the right of the aorta, the superior mesenteric vein is seen running up to join the splenic vein, so forming the portal vein.

The body of the pancreas lies parallel to the splenic vein and a little below and anterior to it. The superior mesenteric artery and superior mesenteric vein pass through the head of the pancreas, the majority of the head lying above and anterior to these vessels (Figure 22.3). Identification of these landmarks on longitudinal and transverse scans aids in the accurate localization of the pancreas, allowing its visualization in some 80% of normal patients.[31] For visualization of head, body and tail on a single section, an oblique scan may be more suitable than a transverse scan.

The normal extrahepatic biliary tree can be reliably identified with a modern ultrasound scanner. The junction between the right hepatic duct and common hepatic duct can be identified anterior to the right branch of the portal vein in the majority of patients. In addition, the more distal segments of the left and right hepatic ducts can be

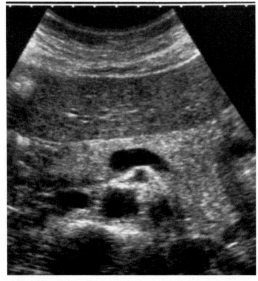

Figure 22.3 A transverse scan through the pancreas. Note this has a slightly higher reflectivity than the adjacent left lobe of the liver. The pancreatic head encloses the superior mesenteric artery and vein, and pancreas lies on vena cava and aorta.

identified as they run along the anterior margins of the respective branches of the portal venous system. The use of real-time scanners and the left lateral decubitus position for the patient permits identification and measurement of the common bile duct in more than 80% of patients[9]

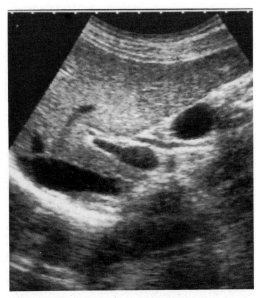

Figure 22.4 A longitudinal oblique scan over the mid line showing a portion of the normal common hepatic and common bile duct passing anterior to the portal vein.

(Figure 22.4). The normal intrahepatic biliary radicles should have diameters of 2 mm or less, whereas the common hepatic duct should not exceed 6 mm in diameter in the normal patient. After cholecystectomy there may be a slight increase in the duct diameter, particularly if the cholecystectomy was performed after an episode of obstructive jaundice. In these patients, diameters greater than 1 cm should be regarded as pathological.

DIAGNOSIS OF LIVER DISEASE

Patients are generally referred for liver ultrasound examinations for one or more of the following reasons:

1. Confirmation of hepatomegaly and determination of its cause
2. Further investigation of an abnormal isotope image
3. Confirmation or exclusion of hepatic metastases after diagnosis of primary malignancy
4. Investigation of jaundice

Hepatomegaly

In a patient with suspected hepatomegaly, non-hepatic causes must first be excluded. The common cause is a low, flat diaphragm secondary to pulmonary emphysema and this is very easily seen at ultrasound examination. Non-hepatic masses inferior to the liver may also be detected and can generally be shown to be extrahepatic. Lesions arising in the upper pole of the right kidney displace the liver anteriorly and inferiorly and may be clinically indistinguishable from genuine hepatomegaly. A Reidel's lobe is easily identified by ultrasound and can

be shown to be of the same echo consistency as the remainder of the liver.

Clinical assessment of liver size is subjective, whereas ultrasound images yield objective measurements. However, the shape of the liver varies considerably from one patient to another and its volume will depend on the patient's build. It is therefore difficult to confirm or exclude hepatomegaly with absolute confidence in any patient without making liver volume measurements. In practice an adequate assessment of liver size can be made by eye, based on a series of longitudinal scans. If necessary, an accurate measurement of liver volume can be made by taking serial longitudinal scans at known intervals, measuring the area of liver seen on each, and adding all the areas together after allowing for slice thickness (scan spacing).[7] This technique is useful for monitoring changes in liver volume during therapy but is seldom necessary for the actual diagnosis of hepatomegaly.

The disease process which may cause hepatomegaly may also be present in normal or small-sized livers; the different forms of liver disease which can be demonstrated or diagnosed by ultrasound are discussed below.

Focal disease

This may be unifocal or multifocal, benign or malignant, and may have been previously diagnosed by other techniques or initially diagnosed at the time of the ultrasound examination.

Isotope scanning detects focal disease as 'cold' areas, but can usually give no further differential diagnosis. Ultrasound imaging, however, will reliably differentiate many forms of focal disease.

Benign disease

The commonest benign abnormality seen in our patients is a simple cyst, which has been detected in approximately 2.5% of the population.[13] These are usually single, though occasionally three or four may be present. They are seen as clearly-defined, echo-free spaces with thin walls and accentuation of the echoes from distal structures. Their size can be accurately measured and followed by serial scans if required. When these cysts are seen, especially if they are multiple, the kidneys and pancreas should also be examined for cysts. The polycystic liver is unlikely to be diagnosed initially by ultrasound, but we have seen localized areas of this disease in patients with polycystic kidneys.

Hydatid cysts are not often seen in the United Kingdom but are common in some countries. They may be multiple, usually have thick walls (which may be laminated) and frequently daughter cysts may be seen within the main cyst. Not uncommonly, a hydatid cyst will present as a single, simple, thin-walled cyst and thus this diagnosis can never be ruled out by ultrasound when a cyst is detected.

Rarely metastases may become cystic; these will be discussed in the following section.

Ultrasound is the best radiological technique for detecting liver abscesses and monitoring their response to treatment.[11] In addition, diagnostic or therapeutic aspiration or catheter drainage can be undertaken under real-time guidance. Abscesses differ from simple cysts in having thicker, ill-defined walls with irregular inner margins (Figure 22.5). They are usually hyporeflective relative to the liver but can appear bright if they contain gas. The quantity of fluid present, its reflectivity and the wall thickness will depend on the stage in the natural history of the disorder at which the scan is performed. There is no reliable way of distinguishing bacterial from amoebic abscesses although the latter often lack significant wall echoes, are round or oval, well-defined and usually peripherally sited. This may relate to amoebic access via the portal veins lodging in the peripheral venules. Bacterial abscesses are commonly a result of spread from the biliary tree and are multiple in about 10% of cases.[25] The other primary site is the large bowel.

Cavernous haemangiomas are the commonest benign liver tumour. They are noted usually as incidental findings and may be multiple. They vary in size from a few millimetres to several centimetres and have a characteristic uniformly high reflectivity (Figure 22.6). They are well-defined and when greater than 2.5 centimetres may attenuate sound poorly, which results in enhancement of distal structures.[52] More often no distal effect is seen. Usually a confident diagnosis may be made on ultrasound appearances. Occasionally, it may be necessary to confirm that these are not metastases. In the majority of cases, echogenic metastases are multiple and the patient will have a known carcinoma elsewhere which will often be colonic. It may be necessary to biopsy small lesions or

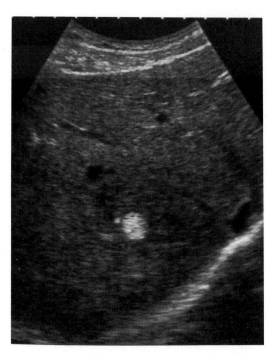

Figure 22.6 A transverse scan through the right lobe of the liver showing a small reflective haemangioma.

perform dynamic computed tomography in those larger than 1.5 cm. Follow-up with a further ultrasound scan at 4–6 months is an alternative option since, unlike metastases, haemangiomas rarely change their size, shape or reflectivity.[16]

A rare but interesting group of vascular tumours–infantile haemangioendotheliomas, are seen in the liver during infancy.[51] Massive vascular shunting can occur, resulting in their occasional presentation in cardiac failure. There is hepatomegaly and there may be associated cutaneous haemangiomas. Although well defined, these do not generally have the appearance of adult haemangiomas on ultrasound but rather have a non-homogeneous, irregular appearance with mixed reflectivity. In addition, large draining veins may be seen or even some enlargement of the proximal abdominal aorta due to increased flow through the hepatic artery. Ultrasound is particularly useful in subsequent scans since the natural history of these lesions is to decrease in size over 6 months until they are no longer visible.

Focal nodular hyperplasia and liver cell adenoma are two unusual non-malignant focal abnormalities. They are commoner in women and adenomas have an association with the oral contraceptive pill. There is some overlap in their ultrasonic appearances. Both are normally solitary, well defined, often hypoechoic and homogeneous in appearance. Ultrasound is said to be 100% sensitive in detecting focal nodular hyperplasia, but when uptake is seen with radioisotope colloid scanning, this is usually diagnostic.[41]

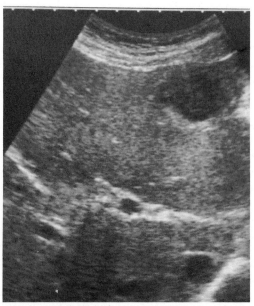

Figure 22.5 An oblique scan through the upper part of the liver showing a small abscess 3 cm in diameter. This has slightly irregular walls and contains low-level reflections. Pus was aspirated.

Malignant disease

Primary hepatocellular carcinoma

Primary hepatocellular carcinoma (HCC) is a rare disorder in the United Kingdom and the United States but its incidence is higher in parts of Africa and East Asia. Differentiation from metastases and other tumours is extremely difficult with any imaging modality. Their ultrasonic appearances are variable and there are no acoustic criteria specific for this disorder. Tumours less than 3 cm in diameter are usually hypoechoic, while larger ones vary from highly reflective lesions to a cystic appearance. Multiple tumour foci occur in almost one-third of cases.[59]

It has been suggested that lesions which display a complex 'mosaic' pattern and have posterior enhancement with lateral shadowing are statistically more likely to be HCC than metastases but in practice, biopsy is the only reliable means of diagnosis.[59]

In this context, ultrasound is most useful in confirming or excluding a focal hepatic lesion when for example, rapid clinical deterioration occurs in a patient with cirrhosis.

Metastases

The liver with its large blood supply is a common site for metastatic disease and ultrasound is the most sensitive way of detecting this, particularly when lesions are multiple. In technically suitable patients, ultrasound has proved to be more sensitive than computed tomography, angiography, and radionuclide imaging.[54] Unfortunately, metastases of

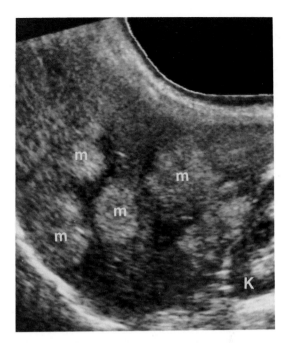

Figure 22.8 A longitudinal scan through the right lobe of the liver showing multiple echogenic metastases from a carcinoma of the colon (m). K = kidney.

several centimetres can be missed in obese patients. Lesions of similar reflectivity to the liver parenchyma or diffuse involvement may not be immediately recognizable on ultrasound as malignant disease. In these cases, hepatomegaly, distortion of vascular structures within the liver, or irregularity or nodularity of its free edge are alerting factors in an otherwise 'normal' scan.

Metastases vary considerably in their ultrasonic appearance but certain characteristics provide pointers to the organ of origin, allowing further investigations to be tailored accordingly. Unfortunately, none of these correlate precisely with the tumour type. Reflectivity is the most useful of these. Most metastases are hyporeflective appearing darker than areas of normal liver tissue. Often multiple, they most commonly arise from breast, bronchus or lymphoma but many other sites of origin have this same appearance (Figure 22.7).

Of hyperreflective lesions, 54% were colonic in origin and 25% arose from HCC in one series.[53] Many other intra-abdominal adenocarcinomas produce high-amplitude echogenic metastases. Even so, when this appearance is seen in a patient with an unknown primary tumour, investigation of the colon with either barium enema or colonoscopy is normally recommended (Figure 22.8).

Occasionally, both high- and low-amplitude lesions occur from the same primary tumour. This may be related to differences in their vascularity but the presence of haemorrhage or necrosis in some deposits will also alter their echo pattern.[22] This leads to the second characteristic that can aid in localization of the primary tumour, namely the presence of fluid. These metastases may be truly cystic

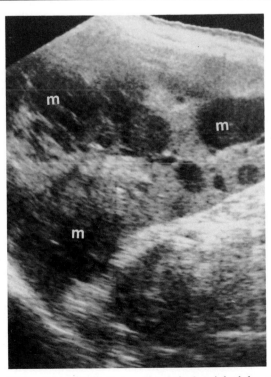

Figure 22.7 A longitudinal scan through the right lobe of the liver showing multiple echo-poor metastases (m).

in nature or, as mentioned above, this may result from ischaemic necrosis or haemorrhage.

Sarcomatous metastases and in particular leiomyosarcomas are said to undergo degenerative necrosis proportionally more often than metastatic carcinoma and it may be difficult without biopsy, to differentiate these lesions from abscesses.[58]

The walls of truly cystic metastases are usually thick and irregular and there may be nodules of tissue within them. When their walls are thin, differentiation from a benign cyst may be difficult particularly as this may be an incidental finding in a patient with a primary tumour elsewhere. In cases where doubt exists, follow up with serial interval scans may be useful. True cystic metastases are rare but occur with carcinoma of the ovary (Figure 22.9).

The third characteristic is the presence of shadowing from calcification. Ultrasound will be more sensitive than plain radiography in its detection.[5] In adults, calcified metastases are more commonly seen from carcinoma of the colon and less frequently from other tumours including ovary, breast and osteosarcoma; in children, secondaries from a neuroblastoma can calcify.

Diffuse liver disease

With diseases of hepatocellular origin the changes seen on ultrasound are either textural, as seen in fatty infiltration, or anatomical, with hepatomegaly, decrease in

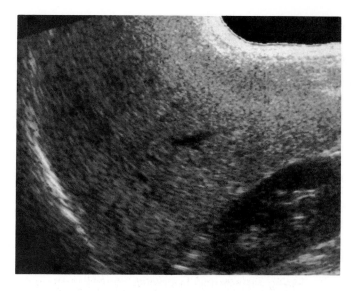

Figure 22.10 A longitudinal scan through the right lobe of the liver in a patient with cirrhosis and acute alcoholic hepatitis. Note loss of normal visualization of normal portal vein walls and the contrast between the bright liver and the apparently dark kidney.

size of the liver or irregularity of the liver edge. In many cases, the appearances will be completely normal. Ultrasound is particularly useful in separating true from apparent hepatomegaly.

Fatty change

There are multiple causes of fatty change within the liver, including obesity, ethanol abuse, diabetes mellitus and steroid therapy and parenteral nutrition amongst others.

Ultrasonically, the characteristic appearance is that of a 'bright' liver with a fine textural pattern showing poor beam penetration.[14] This results in some difficulty in visualizing the more posterior parts of the liver. Liver brightness in fatty infiltration accentuates the normal difference between the renal cortex and hepatic parenchyma. Additionally, the normal bright walls of the portal veins become poorly seen. These changes increase with the degree of fatty infiltration which, although usually diffuse, may produce focal or patchy change.

Cirrhosis

The high reflectivity and increased attenuation of fatty change often precedes or accompanies hepatic cirrhosis (Figure 22.10). When this is not present, early cases may show a coarse 'pin head' pattern of reflectivity.[10,21,49]

It is this irregular textural appearance together with nodularity of the liver surface that is the hallmark of cirrhosis[28] (Figure 22.11). The liver may be enlarged, normal or small but a significant finding may be the increase in size of the caudate lobe relative to the right lobe.[20,35] This enlargement can cause compression of the inferior vena cava. Ultrasound has been compared to arterial portography in its sensitivity in detecting the

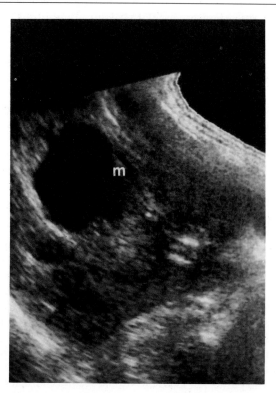

Figure 22.9 A longitudinal scan of right lobe of liver showing a large cystic metastasis (m) from a carcinoma of the ovary.

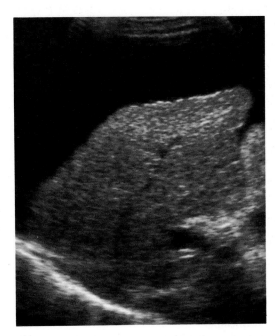

Figure 22.11 A scan in a patient with cirrhosis and ascites. The ascites outlines the liver edge showing the nodularity typical of cirrhosis.

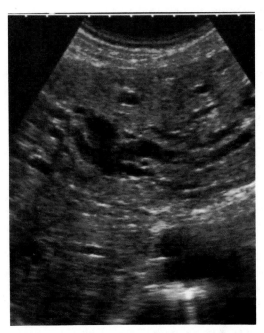

Figure 22.12 A transverse scan through the liver showing the typical radiating pattern of dilated ducts.

patency of the portal vein.[38] There may be enlargement of the portal vein itself. Doppler studies will show reduced flow or even reversal of flow when portal hypertension is of a sufficient degree. This is discussed in more detail later.

Ascites is a common accompaniment of cirrhosis and ultrasound is very sensitive in detecting even small amounts.[10] Fluid tends to collect in the fissure between the kidney and liver, the hepatorenal angle, and appears as an echo-free collection with smooth, well-defined interfaces with these adjacent organs. With larger amounts, bowel is seen to float freely within the fluid. Simple echo-free fluid is usually a transudate. Exudative fluid often appears complex, with internal echoes caused by debris or septae and is the result of inflammatory or neoplastic processes. These findings must be interpreted with some caution as the ultrasonic appearances are non-specific.

Ultrasound has little to offer in the search for the aetiology of cirrhosis, except perhaps in the case of severe congestive cardiac failure (cardiac cirrhosis), where clear distention of the hepatic veins and inferior vena cava is seen. In these cases, there is minimal attenuation from the liver parenchyma.

Hepatitis
While 50% of cases of acute viral hepatitis show no abnormality on ultrasound, the remainder will have combinations of smooth hepatomegaly, a decrease in hepatic reflectivity (again using the right kidney as a reference), and a resultant relative increase in reflectivity of portal vein walls. Thickening of the gallbladder wall and the

presence of biliary sludge are additional findings. Regeneration nodules may be seen in patients with submassive hepatic necrosis and must be distinguished from tumours. These changes of decreased reflectivity are not specific for hepatitis and also occur in patients with other inflammatory liver conditions and in congestive cardiac failure. They have recently been reported in healthy subjects.[17]

JAUNDICE AND THE BILIARY TREE

The major role of ultrasound in the patient presenting with jaundice is to distinguish those with extrahepatic biliary obstruction with dilated ducts from those with hepatocellular causes (see Chapter 28). The first group usually require surgical or interventional management while the second are treated medically. Ultrasound may also provide additional information on the aetiology in both groups.

Although the normal non-dilated biliary tree can be visualized in most patients, the intrahepatic radicals show a characteristic pattern when dilated. The accuracy of diagnosis of moderate to severe obstruction approaches 100%. False negative examinations may occur in early acute obstruction when the bilirubin level is below 100 μmol/l (6 mg/dl).[29] The criterion for the diagnosis of bile duct dilatation is the recognition of tubular, branching, fluid filled structures radiating out from the porta hepatis (Figure 22.12). The distended biliary tree is usually best seen in the longitudinal scan where the dilated ducts have rather short courses and are seen to run parallel to the portal veins, giving the appearance of a double channel. Multiple branch points may be seen and the directional changes are rather sharp and angular. Acoustic enhancement beyond the dilated ducts commonly occurs.

The normally prominent portal system is best seen in transverse scans. The vessels form smooth curves and acoustic enhancement does not occur beyond the individual veins. A particular tubular structure should, wherever possible, be traced back to either the common bile duct (CBD) or portal vein. Biliary radicals measuring 3 mm or more and a CBD measuring 6 mm or more indicate dilatation.[4] In the post-cholecystectomy patient, this diameter may normally be larger.[54]

A diagnosis of obstruction is made on the identification of dilated biliary radicals in a jaundiced patient. The next step is to define the level of obstruction. In practice, this entails identification of the CBD. Transverse or oblique scans usually show the dilated upper CBD lying nearly parallel and anterolateral to the portal vein. Scans closer to the longitudinal plane may show the lower CBD lying anterior to the inferior vena cava. The site of obstruction is most conveniently classified into two groups: (a) at the level of the porta hepatis; and (b) in the lower CBD or pancreas. In our experience, the accuracy of identifying the level of obstruction into these two groups is over 70%, the main limiting factor being the presence of gas in the duodenal bulb or pyloric antrum, which may obscure much of the CBD. If the level of obstruction is clearly shown, ultrasound will indicate the cause in approximately 50%. In the majority of cases this will be a stone or stricture.

Biliary calculi are visualized as echogenic foci since they strongly reflect the ultrasound beam. As a consequence, little energy is left to pass beyond the stone, which gives rise to the characteristic shadow seen distally. This acoustic shadow is sometimes more obvious than the calculus itself. Calculi may be found at any level in the biliary tree (Figure 22.13). In general, the higher they are lodged, the easier they are to see, but in practice the majority of stones causing obstruction lodge in the region of the ampulla. In this difficult area, a stone may best be seen in the transverse scan as a bright spot in the head of the pancreas—the so called 'target' sign. Differentiation from an ampullary carcinoma may not be possible since this tumour can present with obstruction when still small.

Tumours

Numerous tumours may cause biliary obstruction. Pancreatic carcinoma is the commonest, where small tumours may cause low obstruction and larger tumours extend up to the porta hepatis. As described earlier, the normal pancreas appears as a smooth homogeneous structure with reflectivity slightly above that of the normal liver. Pancreatic carcinomas are shown as an irregular heterogeneous mass with areas of high and low echo amplitudes (Figure 22.14a,b). Tumours in the head of the pancreas larger than 4 cm can usually be recognized, although smaller lesions may also be seen. Unfortunately, it may

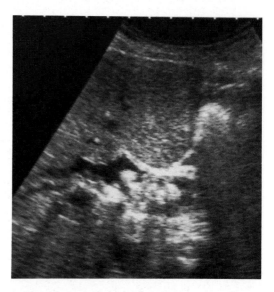

Figure 22.13 A longitudinal oblique scan through a slightly dilated common bile duct which is full of high reflections from contained calculi.

not always be possible to distinguish this appearance from that seen in chronic pancreatitis, particularly if localized to a single area. The management of these patients with small lesions visualized on ultrasound is difficult, since computed tomography often provides useful anatomical information but is again unhelpful in making a pathological diagnosis. Fine-needle aspiration of small lesions, if positive for carcinoma, will usually result in laparotomy and resection, but a negative biopsy or one showing inflammation does not exclude malignancy and laparotomy may be necessary.[15]

In addition to pancreatic tumours, a pseudocyst in the head of the pancreas may also cause biliary obstruction. Pseudocysts almost always occur in association with generalized acute pancreatitis. The pancreas is enlarged and, being oedematous, returns lower-level echoes than normal. The pseudocyst is identified as a localized cystic area (Figure 22.15). It is most commonly rounded but may have a more irregular shape and debris is commonly seen within it. The detection of pseudocysts with ultrasound approaches 100%.[46] Serial scans will show the progress of the cyst, which may abruptly change in size if it discharges spontaneously into a neighbouring viscus. Again the therapeutic insertion of a drainage catheter may be possible.

Almost 90% of cholangiocarcinomas occur at either the confluence of the right and left intrahepatic bile ducts in the porta hepatis (Klatskin tumours) or in the common hepatic or distal common bile duct.[24] They are uncommonly seen in the intrahepatic biliary tree itself.

Since the site of origin predisposes to early presentation with jaundice, when the tumour is relatively small, its identification is often difficult.[40] This is still the case when the level of change in calibre of the ducts from dilated to normal or reduced size is identified. In addition,

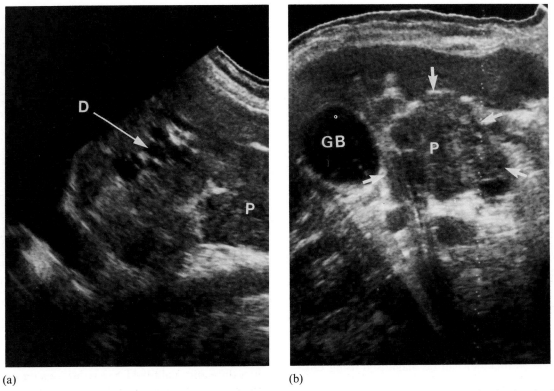

(a)   (b)

Figure 22.14 (a) A longitudinal and (b) a transverse scan showing an irregular lobular mass in the head of the pancreas (P). This has the typical appearance of a typical pancreatic carcinoma. D = dilated duct; GB = gallbladder.

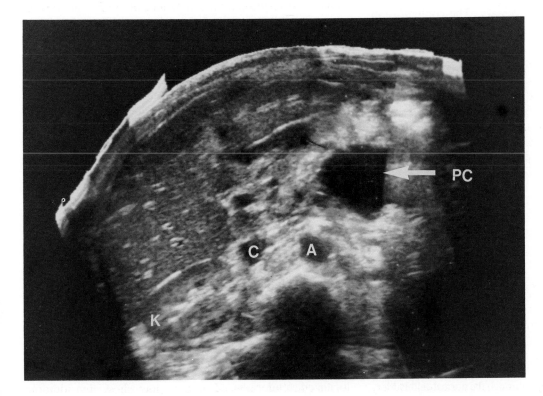

Figure 22.15 A transverse scan showing a pseudocyst of the pancreas (PC). C = inferior vena cava; A = aorta; K = kidney.

cholangiocarcinomas most commonly present as tapering, stenotic lesions infiltrating along the duct. This makes their identification difficult, but when they are recognized increased echogenicity in almost 80% of cases is present.[8,] [33,45,60] The distinction between primary sclerosing cholangitis (PSC) and tumour may be difficult, particularly as the tumour may complicate established PSC.

THE GALLBLADDER

It is generally accepted that in all cases of suspected disease of the gallbladder, ultrasonography should be the investigation of choice and additionally will often be the only one necessary.[19,30] Occasionally, this may need to be supplemented with oral cholecystography or cholescintigraphy. By far the commonest pathology of the gallbladder is cholelithiasis[43,44] which occurs in 11% of the population.[2] Gallstones were seen in 8.2% of male and 9.4% of female Italian civil servants screened by ultrasound. By far the commonest pathology of the gallbladder is cholelithiasis.[43,44] Many other important diseases of the gallbladder can be diagnosed using ultrasound.

The gallbladder can be satisfactorily outlined in 95% of normal fasting subjects (Figure 22.16). As the gallbladder is most frequently located lying obliquely under the free edge of the liver, its position in relation to external landmarks varies considerably. It may be deep to the free edge of the liver or superficially located just beneath the skin. In this subcutaneous position, for optimum visualization, a change in probe frequency from 3.5 MHz to 5 MHz may be necessary. The configuration

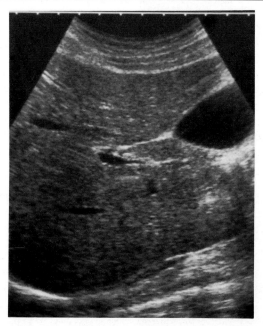

Figure 22.16 A longitudinal scan through the normal gallbladder.

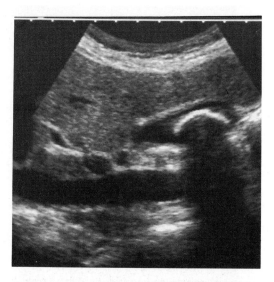

Figure 22.17 A longitudinal scan through the gallbladder containing a single large calculus. Note the strong distal acoustic shadowing.

of the gallbladder varies from a simple pear-shaped sac when the entire gallbladder may be seen on one scanning section, to a complex folded shape, when scanning from multiple directions and in multiple planes may be necessary to exclude disease. The typical appearance of gallstones has been described above, and when these are located within the gallbladder and surrounded by echo-free bile they are considerably easier to detect than when in the bile ducts themselves (Figure 22.17). This may not be the case when the gallbladder is diseased, or contracted in the non-fasted patient, or where optimal visualization is not possible because of obscuring gas, fat or abdominal scarring. In these instances the presence of gallstones may be confirmed by turning the patient onto their side and noting any gravitational change that will occur with non-impacted stones.

Cholecystitis

While the normal gallbladder wall in the fasting state measures 3 mm or less, in almost all cases of acute cholecystitis there is thickening to at least 5 mm. In 90% of cases, gallstones are present, usually obstructing the cystic duct and causing some degree of gallbladder distention.[39,55] In the acute presentation, a halo of oedema may be seen surrounding the wall of the gallbladder (Figure 22.18). In emphysematous cholecystitis, the high reflectivity of gas may be seen in the gallbladder wall or even in the gallbladder itself.

With tenderness in the right upper quadrant, it is often possible to locate this with pin-point accuracy to the exact position of the gallbladder. Although not always present, this ultrasonic 'Murphy's' sign is strong supporting evidence for acute cholecystitis. Empyema of the gallbladder presents with a markedly distended viscus in addition to localized tenderness. The bile may show considerable

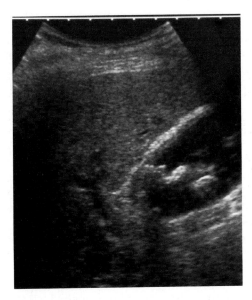

Figure 22.18 Scan through the gallbladder in acute cholecystitis. The gallbladder wall is oedematous showing a halo appearance. There are multiple stones in the gallbladder.

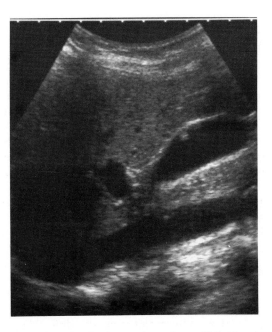

Figure 22.19 Longitudinal scan through a gallbladder showing a small polyp arising from the anterior wall. Clinically this was an incidental finding.

reflectivity from its purulent content, but we have also aspirated thick pus from anechoic bile in this situation.

With repeated episodes of acute or subacute cholecystitis, the gallbladder may become fibrotic and contracted. At this stage it can be difficult to identify confidently, only being recognized from the bright echoes and strong acoustic shadowing of associated calculi. Care must be taken to differentiate this appearance from shadowing due to gas in the hepatic flexure of the colon. Thickening of the gallbladder wall occurs in several other conditions and is certainly not confined to cholecystitis. Since incidental gallstones are common, the two findings do not necessarily imply the one diagnosis. Thickening may also be present in hepatitis, ascites, hypoproteinaemic states and infiltrations of the wall and has been reported in acalculus patients suffering from AIDS. These patients may also have dilated common bile ducts, possibly related to repeated opportunistic infection.[42]

Tumours of the gallbladder

Malignant tumours of the gallbladder are uncommon and their diagnosis by any technique is difficult, partly owing to the gallbladder contraction that occurs. Small benign polyps of the gallbladder measuring a few millimetres across can be seen sufficiently often to be reported as incidental findings (Figure 22.19). They can be mistaken for gallstones because they are reflective lesions adjacent to the wall. Unlike the majority of gallstones, they have no distal shadow and do not alter their position with gravity as the patient moves. Distinction is always possible with technically good scans.

Carcinoma

The gallbladder is the commonest site of carcinoma in the biliary system. It is more often seen as an ill-defined, infiltrating lesion, sometimes extending into the gallbladder lumen or into the liver itself than as a discrete mass involving the gallbladder wall. There may also be metastatic spread in the liver at the time of presentation. Carcinoma must be suspected in the older patient when poor views of an irregular, contracted gallbladder are obtained, and since it is uncommon for it to occur in the absence of gallstones the initial diagnosis is often that of acute cholecystitis. Calcification, present in the gallbladder wall in up to 25% of cases, will not generally be separable on ultrasound from shadowing caused by calculi.[56]

Although there is wide variation in the size of the normal gallbladder, marked distension is usually obvious. Unlike chronic cholecystitis where the gallbladder wall is contracted and non-distensible, the most distended gallbladders are seen in patients with long-standing obstruction secondary to pancreatic or ampullary carcinomas. The intrahepatic bile ducts as well as the common bile duct will also be distended but it is the additional recognition of a distended gallbladder that may suggest the correct diagnosis.

In the young child or infant, a choledochal cyst is readily diagnosed when an echo-free lesion in the right upper quadrant separate from the gallbladder is seen. This usually involves the CBD and may also involve the intrahepatic ducts. Radioisotope imaging confirms its continuity with the proximal bile ducts. Ultrasound is a convenient way of monitoring resolution following surgical decompression.

Biliary sludge

The characteristic appearance of biliary sludge is of an echogenic zone which layers out beneath the echo-free bile above producing a fluid/fluid level. It should not be confused with multiple small gallstones or milk of calcium bile since it produces no distal shadowing. With changes in patient position this sludge can be seen to slowly slide to the most dependent portion of the gallbladder. Sludge has been shown to consist of precipitates of mucus, calcium bilirubinate and cholesterol crystals. It is predominantly found when there is biliary stasis as seen with cholecystitis or extrahepatic biliary obstruction but is also seen in fasting or parenterally fed patients. It is occasionally a precursor of gallstones.[26]

Adenomyomatosis

Proliferative thickening of the gallbladder wall with mucosal outpouchings (Rokitansky–Aschoff sinuses) may be segmental or diffuse and it can be difficult in milder cases to identify with ultrasound. In areas where thickening is present, these intramural diverticula may be seen as hyporeflective interruptions when they contain bile, or as echogenic foci when there is biliary sludge or small calculi within them.[12] When oral cholecystography was the first-line investigation for suspected gallstones, adenomyomatosis was more frequently detected. Its pathological significance has been questioned although it is seen in association with gallstones.[38]

HEPATIC DOPPLER STUDIES

INTRODUCTION

Doppler examination of the major hepatic vessels is now possible using the recently developed 'duplex scanners' which combine a high-quality real-time imaging system with a steerable Doppler beam. These systems are capable of extracting Doppler ultrasound information from any specific location within a conventional two-dimensional image.

Using a duplex scanner, conventional two-dimensional scanning is initially performed in the normal manner and the target vessel is identified. The anatomical approach to the vessel must be optimized to obtain as small an angle as possible between the direction of the examining ultrasound beam and the orientation of the long axis of the vessel. In practice satisfactory Doppler signals can be obtained with beam/vessel angles of less than 70°.

When the vessel of interest has been identified an electronic cursor is placed on the vessel and the Doppler sequence is initiated. The Doppler-shifted echoes returning from the blood cells moving within the blood vessel are then collected and the degree to which their frequency has been altered is determined by a process known as 'spectrum analysis'. The resulting frequency shifts are displayed graphically with velocity information on the vertical axis and time on the baseline.

It is possible to compute a number of mathematical indices from this display. The most frequently used are the time-averaged mean velocity (TAV), the pulsatility index (PI) and the resistance index (RI).[57] The first of these is a useful guide of the mean blood velocity in a vessel and, in theory at least, when multiplied by the cross-sectional area of the vessel permits estimation of the volume blood flow. Regrettably there are several major sources of error in the computation of blood flow and, at the present time, the resulting computed volume flow measurements seem to be of no clinical value over and above the basic velocity values.

The pulsatility and resistance indices are normally used to assess the flow in arteries. As a general rule they are reduced if the peripheral vascular bed supplied by the artery shows decreased resistance to blood flow and vice versa. When the pulsatility index is applied to the hepatic vein waveform, increasing stiffness of the liver dampens the waveform and gives rise to a reduction in pulsatility, the converse of what happens on the arterial side. The degree to which these indices change in these two circulations may prove useful for the diagnosis and grading of liver disease.

CLINICAL USES OF LIVER DOPPLER

Portal vein

In the normal patient there is continuous forward flow in the portal vein, often with a little modulation due to arterial pulsation or respiration. In the fasting state the time-averaged mean velocity is usually in the range of 10–12 cm/s (Figure 22.20).[48] After a meal the portal flow increases to about four times the fasting level. About half of this rise is accommodated by an increase in the vessel cross-sectional area, the rest is seen by a rise in the TAV value to approximately 25 cm/s. Arterial pulsations transmitted from the splanchnic circulation are more commonly seen after a meal.

Portal vein blood flow may be reduced or reversed in patients with liver disease[3] but the incidence of this has probably been greatly overstated in many medical textbooks. The majority of patients with mild to moderate liver disease exhibit normal portal vein blood flow, though there may be some reduction in the postprandial increase.

In cases of more severe liver disease the time-averaged mean velocity may be reduced and, provided the patients are examined during the fasting state, the severity of the liver disease can be gauged from the degree of flow reduction (Figure 22.21). Volume flow studies in these patients are, however, usually normal as the portal hypertension increases the vessel diameter.

If the liver disease becomes more severe, the increased pressure within the portal circulation fails to compensate for the increasing resistance to flow in the liver and portal vein flow may cease. Further increase in the severity of

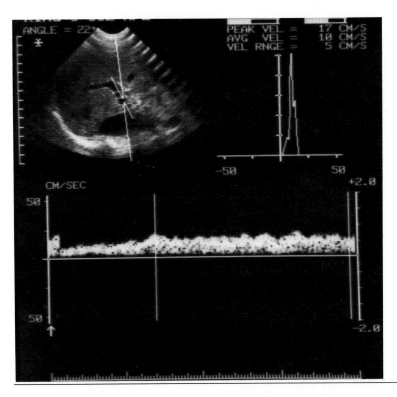

Figure 22.20 Normal fasting portal vein flow. The TAV is 12 cm/s.

the disease may lead to arterioportal shunting with reversed flow in the portal vein.[27]

Many patients with portal hypertension develop splenomegaly with consequent increase in splenic vein flow. This may be sufficiently great to overcome the increased flow resistance into the liver and forward flow in the portal vein may be re-established. Spleen size must therefore always be taken into account when assessing portal vein flow.

It can be seen from the preceding discussions that the dynamics and pathophysiology of portal flow are rather complex and that a single velocity or volume flow measure-

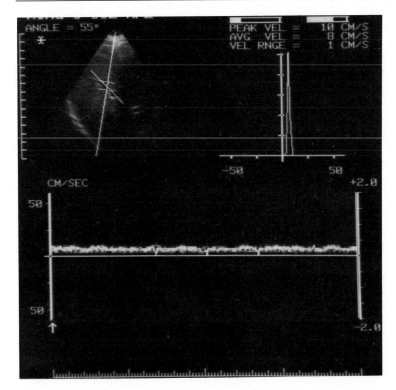

Figure 22.21 Reduced portal flow velocity in a patient with cirrhosis.

ment may be very misleading. Where possible, serial studies should be performed and the Doppler findings must always be interpreted with a full knowledge of the patient's clinical state.

In patients with surgically created portosystemic shunts, blood flow within the portal vein should be reversed if both the shunt and portal vein remain patent.[1,3,32] Doppler ultrasound of the portal vein is therefore a useful technique for the assessment of shunt patency even if the shunt itself cannot be directly visualized. If the shunt subsequently fails and the portal vein remains patent, forward flow may again be established within the portal vein. The subcutaneous section of mesoatrial shunts is very accessible to high-frequency ultrasound scanning and confirmation of flow in these shunts is readily achieved with suitable Doppler apparatus.

Occasionally the reduction of portal vein flow in patients with liver disease may precipitate thrombosis of the portal vein. This can also be readily diagnosed by Doppler investigation.

In the Budd–Chiari syndrome the main hepatic veins are occluded. In the acute phase and if all vessels are occluded, the blood can only leave the liver via the portal vein and established continuous reverse flow will be detected. If one or more of the hepatic veins remain patent, low-velocity forward flow may persist and in patients with long-standing Budd–Chiari syndrome the umbilical vein may recanalize, permitting forward flow in the main portal vein to be re-established while flow in the left and right branches remains reversed.

If the portal vein is occluded by a fresh and complete thrombus, there is no flow detectable within the vessel. If the thrombosis occurred at a very early age, numerous collateral channels develop, which has been termed 'cavernous transformation'. The appearance of this condition can be confusing on ultrasound imaging and Doppler studies in this situation reveal low-velocity flow within the numerous small vessels detectable at the porta hepatis.[37,47] In general the flow velocity will be between 2 and 7 cm/s (TAV).

In adult patients portal vein thrombosis may undergo complete resolution and the re-establishment of portal vein flow can be confirmed by Doppler studies.

Confusion may occur on ultrasound imaging if tumour has entered the portal vein, as frequently occurs in patients with HCC.[34] The ultrasound appearances on imaging are indistinguishable from portal vein thrombosis, but the tumour seldom completely occludes the vessel lumen, although it may appear so on the image. Doppler studies in this situation will usually reveal flow around the margins of the tumour, thus permitting its differentiation from actual vessel thrombosis.

Doppler ultrasound is seldom of value in the diagnosis of liver tumours. Some liver tumours develop arterioportal shunts and may cause a reduction or even reversal in portal vein blood flow. Haemangiomas may also drain into the portal circulation but may equally well be supplied by it and give rise to abnormal increase in portal vein velocity.

Careful study of the blood flow velocities within the different branches of the portal vein may permit the operator to identify exactly which vessel the tumour is draining into, as flow in the other vessels will be normal in direction and velocity. It is doubtful whether this information will often be of diagnostic value.

Hepatic artery

The Doppler signal from a normal hepatic artery is shown in Figure 22.22. Flow is in the forward direction throughout the whole of the cardiac cycle with relatively high velocity during cardiac diastole. This is the typical arterial trace from a vessel supplying a low resistance circulation and is similar to that seen in the normal brain and kidney.

The large majority of adults with liver disease show remarkably little change in the hepatic artery velocity waveform. In many patients with very severe cirrhosis the associated reduction in the portal vein blood flow is compensated for by an increase in the arterial flow with an increase in diastolic flow and reduction in the PI and RI values (Figure 22.23).

In paediatric patients with secondary biliary cirrhosis there may be a progressive increase in the pulsatility index as the severity of the cirrhosis increases (Figure 22.24). In very severe cases diastolic flow reversal may occur.

The majority of liver tumours have no effect on hepatic artery blood flow. Highly vascular tumours may give rise to increased arterial flow with a consequent reduction in the pulsatility index. This is particularly so in vascular tumours, especially in the paediatric age group. It is doubtful that Doppler ultrasound advances the diagnosis in these cases. If the tumour has been demonstrated to be highly vascular and arterial embolization is undertaken, the degree of success achieved by the embolization can be assessed and monitored by serial Doppler examinations. Revascularization occurs surprisingly quickly after major embolizations or arterial ligation. This may be within days after an embolization and 3–4 weeks after arterial ligation.

Hepatic vein

The Doppler waveform obtained from the hepatic vein in the normal patient is complex. It can be seen that flow is not in a continuous forward direction but is modulated with occasional flow reversal. The majority of flow is in a direction away from the probe and down towards the vena cava and therefore appears below the zero line in the normal tracing (Figure 22.25). The reason for this modulation is the passage of the normal atrial and ventricular systolic pressure waves from the right heart back into the vena cava and up into the hepatic veins.

Most types of liver disease give rise to an increase in liver stiffness which prevents the liver from expanding to accommodate the blood dammed back into the hepatic

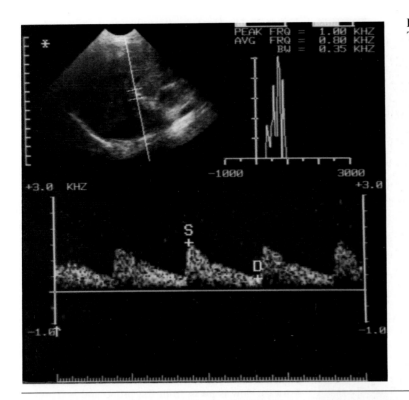

Figure 22.22 The normal hepatic artery waveform. There is continuous forward flow with an RI of 0.73.

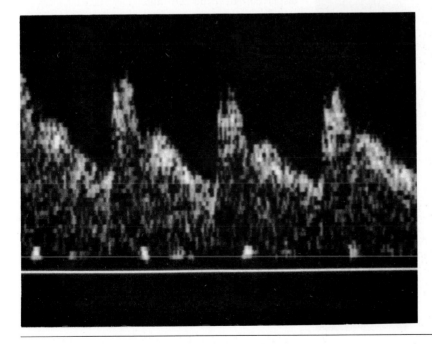

Figure 22.23 Hepatic artery flow in a patient with portal vein occlusion. The flow is increased, especially in diastole, with the RI reduced to 0.46.

veins during atrial and ventricular systole (Figure 22.26). The degree of flattening of the waveform is roughly proportional to the severity of the liver disease.

Many forms of heart disease give rise to increased pressure waves within the heart and the majority of these are conducted back into the IVC. They may therefore give rise to increased pulsatility in the hepatic veins if the liver is normal. If there is coexistent liver and heart disease it is possible that the excessive pressure waves

may result in an apparently normal hepatic vein tracing even in the presence of moderate liver stiffness.

In the Budd–Chiari syndrome the main hepatic veins may be detectable on imaging and thrombosis can be confirmed by failure to detect a Doppler signal from the vessels. There may be different degrees of venous occlusion in this disorder and the disease not uncommonly spares at least one liver segment. If partial recanalization of the veins occurs, low-velocity unmodulated forward

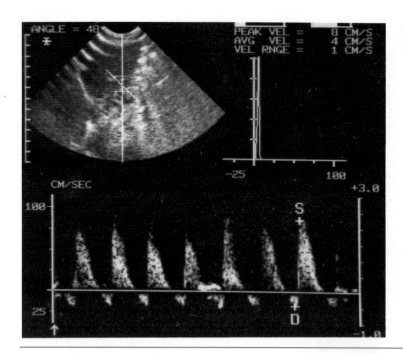

Figure 22.24 Hepatic artery flow in a child with secondary biliary cirrhosis. The RI and PI are greatly increased and there is reversed flow in diastole.

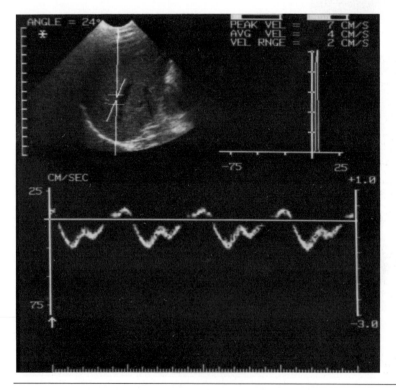

Figure 22.25 The normal right hepatic vein tracing. Forward flow is away from the probe and is therefore displayed below the zero line.

flow may be detected. If isolated peripheral segments remain patent, it is not unusual to find low-velocity reverse flow in some of these segments.

Umbilical vein

The umbilical vein is normally not patent and cannot be reliably detected by ultrasound imaging. In patients with established portal hypertension the umbilical vein may recanalize and be identified on imaging as an aberrant vascular channel. The vascular anatomy on imaging usually allows a correct diagnosis to be made, but Doppler permits confirmation of the correct diagnosis by the detection of hepatofugal flow within the recanalized vessel (Figure 22.27).[18]

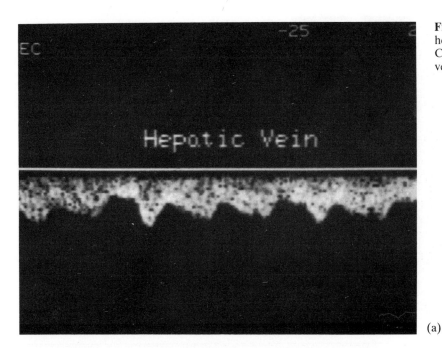

Figure 22.26 (a) Moderate flattening of the hepatic vein waveform in cirrhosis. (b) Complete hepatic vein waveform flattening by a very stiff liver.

(a)

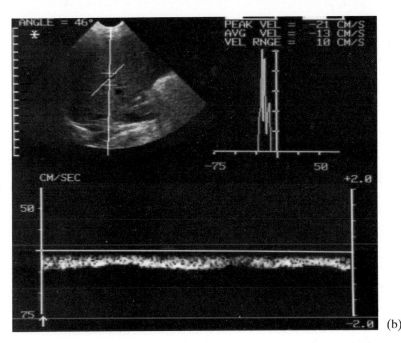

(b)

SUMMARY

Duplex Doppler ultrasound of the hepatic circulation permits the acquisition of considerable physiological information from the liver. The hepatic vein waveform is generally the most sensitive but non-specific indicator of the presence of liver disease, and the degree of departure from the normal pattern may allow estimation of the severity of the disease.

Examination of the portal vein signal permits the detection and grading of more severe cases of liver disease, enables the ultrasonologist to assess the adequacy

of shunting procedures and permits confirmation of vessel patency before and after liver transplantation.

Examination of the hepatic artery waveform is seldom of direct value but does allow the estimation of the degree of vascularity of hepatic tumours and can assess the success of therapeutic embolization. It may be useful in the assessment of the severity of paediatric secondary biliary cirrhosis and is an invaluable non-invasive test for arterial patency after transplantation.

Since many of the disease processes mentioned above are not associated with any alteration in the size or

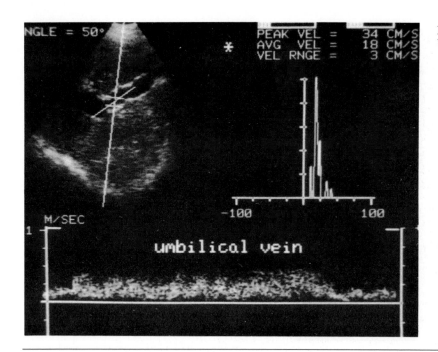

Figure 22.27 A patent umbilical vein confirmed by Doppler study.

appearance of the liver on conventional ultrasound imaging, Doppler ultrasound undoubtedly enables ultrasonologists to detect and to some extent characterize disease processes which they might otherwise miss.

CONCLUSIONS

The advent of ultrasound has provided an excellent first-line investigative tool in examining the liver and biliary system. It is highly accurate in distinguishing extrahepatic biliary obstruction from other causes of jaundice, is good

at detecting metastatic spread of tumour to the liver and in many other cases points to the next investigation.

As well as its diagnostic uses, it offers a range of therapeutic options and is the best method for imaging during biopsy of small intrahepatic lesions. It is pertinent that as ultrasonic machines have become more user-friendly, scanning technique and the awareness of more subtle changes make it more operator-dependent. The degree of confidence with which positive or negative findings are noted is an important factor.

As with most radiological procedures, adequate clinical information will allow better tailoring of the investigation along with appropriate interpetation, particularly where findings are not pathognomonic.

REFERENCES

1. Ackroyd, N., Gill, R., Griffiths, K. *et al.* (1986) Duplex scanning of the portal vein and portosystemic shunts. *Surgery*, **99**, 591.
2. Barbara, L., Sama, C., Labate, A.M. *et al.* (1987) A population study on the prevalence of gallstone disease: The Sirmione study. *Hepatology*, **7**, 913–917.
3. Bolondi, L., Mazziotti, A., Arienti, V. *et al.* (1984) Ultrasonographic study of portal venous system in portal hypertension and after portosystemic shunt operations. *Surgery*, **95**, 261.
4. Bressler, E.L., Rubin, J.M. & McCracken, S. (1987) Sonographic parallel channel sign: a reappraisal. *Radiology*, **164**, 343–346.
5. Bruneton, J.N., Ladree, D., Carmella, E. *et al.* (1982) Ultrasonographic study of calcified hepatic metastases. *Gastrointestinal Radiology*, **7**, 61.
6. Carlsen, E.N. & Filly, R.A. (1976) Newer sonographic anatomy of the upper abdomen: 1. The portal and hepatic venous anatomy. *Journal of Clinical Ultrasound*, **4**, 85–90.
7. Carr, D., Duncan, J.G., Railton, R. & Smith, C.B. (1976) Liver volume determination by ultrasound: a feasibility study. *British Journal of Radiology*, **49**, 776–778.
8. Choi, B.I., Lee, J.H., Han, M.C., Kim, S.H., Yi, J.G. & Kim, C. (1989) Hilar cholangiocarcinoma: Comparative study with sonography and CT. *Radiology*, **172**, 689–692.
9. Dewbury, K.C. (1980) The visualisation of normal biliary ducts with ultrasound. *British Journal of Radiology*, **53**, 774–780.
10. Dewbury, K.C. & Clarke, B. (1979) The accuracy of ultrasound in the detection of cirrhosis of the liver. *British Journal of Radiology*, **52**, 945–948.
11. Dewbury, K.C., Joseph, A.E.A., Millward-Sadler, G. H. & Birch, S.J. (1980) Ultrasound in the diagnosis of early liver abscess. *British Journal of Radiology*, **53**, 1160.
12. Fowler, R.C. & Reid, W.A. (1988) Ultrasound diagnosis of adenomyomatosis of the gallbladder: Ultrasonic and pathological correlation. *Clinical Radiology*, **39**, 402–406.
13. Gaines, P.A. & Sampson, M.A. (1989) The prevalence and characterization of simple hepatic cysts by ultrasound examination. *British Journal of Radiology*, **62**, 355–357.
14. Garra, B.S., Insana, M.F., Shawker, T.H. & Russel, M.A. (1987) Quantitative estimation of liver attenuation and echogenicity: Normal state versus diffuse liver disease. *Radiology*, **162**, 61–67.
15. Gazelle, G.S. & Haaga, J.R. (1989) Guided percutaneous biopsy of intraabdominal lesions. *American Journal of Roentgenology*, 153, 929–935.
16. Gibney, R., Hendin, A.P. & Cooperberg, P.L. (1987) Sonographically detected hepatic hemangiomas. *American Journal of Roentgenology*, **149**, 953–957.
17. Giorgio, A., Amoroso, P., Fico, P., Lettieri, G., Finelli, L., Stephano, G., Pesce, G., Scala, V., Pierri, P. & Pierri, G. (1986) Ultrasound evaluation of uncomplicated and complicated acute viral

hepatitis. *Journal of Clinical Ultrasound,* **14,** 675–679.

18. Hales, M.R., Allan, J.S. & Hall, E.M. (1959) Injection corrosion studies of normal and cirrhotic livers. *American Journal of Radiology,* **35,** 909.

19. Health and Policy Committee, American College of Physicians. (1988) How to study the gallbladder. *Annals of Internal Medicine,* **109,** 752–754.

20. Hess, C.F., Schmiedl, U., Koelbel, G., Knecht, R. & Kurtz, B. (1989) Diagnosis of liver cirrhosis with US: Receiver-operating characteristic analysis of multidimensional caudate lobe indexes. *Radiology,* **171,** 349–351.

21. Joseph, A.E.A., Dewbury, K.C. & McGuire, P.G. (1979) Ultrasound in the detection of chronic liver disease. *British Journal of Radiology,* **52,** 184–188.

22. Joseph, A.E.A., Dewbury, K.C., Millward-Sadler, G.H. & Clarke, C.W. (1979) Correlation of histopathological and ultrasound appearances of liver metastases. *British Journal of Radiology,* **52,** 518.

23. Kane, R.A. & Katz, S.G. (1982) The spectrum of sonographic findings in portal hypertension. A subject review and new observations. *Radiology,* **142,** 453.

24. Karstrup, S. (1988) Ultrasound diagnosis of cholangiocarcinoma at the confluence of the hepatic ducts. *British Journal of Radiology,* **61,** 987–990.

25. Kuligowska, E., Connors, S.K. & Shapiro, J.H. (1982) Liver abscess: Sonography in diagnosis and treatment. *American Journal of Roentgenology,* **138,** 253.

26. Lee, S.P., Maher, K. & Nicholls, J.F. (1988) Origin and fate of biliary sludge. *Gastroenterology,* **94,** 170–176.

27. van Leeuwen, M.S. (1990) Doppler ultrasound in the evaluation of portal hypertension. In Taylor, K.J.W. & Strandness, D.E. (eds) *Duplex Doppler Ultrasound,* p. 72. New York: Churchill Livingstone.

28. Di Lelio, A., Cestari, C., Lomazzi, A. & Beretta, L. (1989) Cirrhosis: Diagnosis with sonographic study of the liver surface. *Radiology,* **172,** 389–392.

29. Malini, S. & Sabel, J. (1977) Ultrasonography in obstructive jaundice. *Radiology,* **123,** 429–433.

30. Marton, K.I. & Doubilet, P. (1988) How to image the gallbladder in suspected cholecystitis. *Annals of Internal Medicine,* **109,** 722–799.

31. Meire, H.B. (1977) Upper abdominal vascular anatomy demonstrated by grey scale ultrasound. *Ultrasound in Medicine,* **3A,** 357–361.

32. Moriyasu, F., Nishida, O., Ban, N. *et al.* (1987) Ultrasonic Doppler duplex study of hemodynamic changes from portosystemic shunt operations. *Annals of Surgery,* **205,** 151.

33. Nesbit, G.M., Johnson, C.D., James, E.M., MacCarty, R.L., Nagorney, D.M. & Bender, C.E. (1988) Cholangiocarcinoma: diagnosis and evaluation of resectability by CT and sonography as procedures complementary to cholangiography. *American Journal of Roentgenology,* **151,** 933–938.

34. Ohnishi, K., Okuda, K., Ohtsuki, T. *et al.* (1984) Formation of hilar collaterals or cavernous transformation after portal vein obstruction by hepatocellular carcinoma. *Gastroenterology,* **87,** 1150.

35. Powell-Jackson, P.R., Karani, J., Ede, R.J., Meire, H. & Williams, R. (1986) Ultrasound scanning and 99m Tc sulphur colloid scintigraphy in diagnosis of Budd–Chiari syndrome. *Gut,* **27,** 1502–1506.

36. Raby, N., Karani, J., Powell-Jackson, P., Meire, H. & Williams, R. (1988) Assessment of portal vein patency: Comparison of arterial portography and ultrasound scanning. *Clinical Radiology,* **39,** 381–385.

37. Raby, N. & Meire, H.B. (1988) Duplex Doppler ultrasound in the diagnosis of cavernous transformation of the portal vein. *British Journal of Radiology,* **61,** 586.

38. Raghavendra, B.N., Subtramanyam, B.R., Balthazar, E.J., Horrii, S., Megibow, A.J. & Hilton, S. (1983) Sonography of adenomyomatosis of the gallbladder: Radiologic–pathologic correlation. *Radiology,* **146,** 747–752.

39. Raghavendka, B.N., Feiner, H.D., Subramanyam, B.R. *et al.* (1981) Acute cholecystitis: Sonographic–pathologic analysis. *American Journal of Roentgenology,* **137,** 327.

40. Robledo, R., Prieto, M.L., Perez, M., Camunez, F. & Echenagusia, A. (1988) Carcinoma of the hepaticopancreatic ampullar region: Role of ultrasound. *Radiology,* **166,** 409–412.

41. Rogers, J.V., Mack, L.A., Freeny, P.C. *et al.* (1981) Hepatic focal nodular hyperplasia: Angiography, CT, sonography and scintigraphy. *American Journal of Roentgenology,* **137,** 983.

42. Romano, A.J., vanSonnenberg, E., Casola, G., Gosink, B.B., Withers, C.E., McCutchan, J.A. & Leopold, G.R. (1988) Gallbladder and bile duct abnormalities in AIDS: Sonographic findings in eight patients. *American Journal of Roentgenology,* **150,** 123–127.

43. Rome Group for the Epidemiology and Prevalence of Cholelithiasis (GREPCO). (1984) Prevalence of gallstone disease in an Italian adult female population. *American Journal of Epidemiology,* **119,** 796–805.

44. Rome Group for the Epidemiology and Prevention of Cholilithiasis (GREPCO). (1988) The epidemiology of gallstone disease in Rome, Italy. Part 1. Prevalence data in men. *Hepatology,* **8,** 904–906.

45. Ros, P.R., Buck, J.L., Goodman, Z.D., Ros, A.M.V. & Olmsted, W.W. (1988) Intrahepatic cholangiocarcinoma: Radiologic–pathologic correlation. *Radiology,* **167,** 689–693.

46. Sanders, A. & Sanders, R. (1977) Complementary use of B-scan ultrasound and radionuclide imaging techniques. *Journal of Nuclear Medicine,* **18,** 205–219.

47. Sassoon, C., Douillet, P., Cronfait, A.M. *et al.* (1980) Ultrasonographic diagnosis of portal cavernoma in children. A study of 12 cases. *British Journal of Radiology,* **53,** 1047.

48. Sato, S., Ohnishi, K., Sugita, S. & Okuda, K. (1987) Splenic artery and superior mesenteric artery blood flow: nonsurgical Doppler US measurement in healthy subjects and patients with chronic liver disease. *Radiology,* **164,** 347.

49. Saverymuttu, S.H., Joseph, A.E.A. & Maxwell, J.D. (1986) Ultrasound scanning in the detection of hepatic fibrosis and steatosis. *British Medical Journal,* **292,** 13–15.

50. Sheu, J-C., Sung, J-L., Chen, D-S., Yu, J-Y., Wang, T-H., Su, C-T. & Tsang, Y-M. (1984) Ultrasonography of small hepatic tumours using high-resolution linear array real-time instruments. *Radiology,* **150,** 797–802.

51. Stanley, P., Gates, G.F., Eto, R. & Miller, S.W. (1977) Hepatic cavernous hemangiomas and hemangioendotheliomas in infancy. *American Journal of Roentgenology,* **129,** 317–321.

52. Taboury, J., Porcel, A., Tubiana, J-M. & Monnier, J-P. (1983) Cavernous hemangiomas of the liver studied by ultrasound. *Radiology,* **149,** 781–785.

53. Viscomi, G.N., Gonzalez, R. & Taylor, K.J.W. (1981) Histopathological correlation of ultrasound appearances of liver metastases. *Journal of Clinical Gastroenterology,* **3,** 395.

54. Wedmann, B., Borsch, G., Coenen, C. & Paassen, A. (1988) Effect of cholecystectomy on common bile duct diameters: A longitudinal prospective ultrasonographic study. *Journal of Clinical Ultrasound,* **16,** 619–624.

55. Wegener, M., Borsch, G., Schneider, J., Wedmann, B., Winter, R. & Zacharias, J. (1987) Gallbladder wall thickening: A frequent finding in nonbiliary disorders—A prospective ultrasonographic study. *Journal of Clinical Ultrasound,* **15,** 307–312.

56. Weiner, S.N., Koenigsberg, M., Morehouse, H. & Hoffman, J. (1984) Sonography and computed tomography in the diagnosis of carcinoma of the gallbladder. *American Journal of Roentgenology,* **142,** 735.

57. Woodcock, J.P., Gosling, R.G. & Fitzgerald, D.E. (1972) A new non-invasive technique for assessment of superficial femoral artery obstruction. *British Journal of Surgery,* **59,** 226.

58. Wooten, W.B., Green, B. & Goldstein, H.M. (1978) Ultrasonography of necrotic hepatic metastases. *Radiology,* **128,** 447–450.

59. Yoshida, T., Matsue, H., Okazaki, N. & Yoshino, M. (1987) Ultrasonographic differentiation of hepatocellular carcinoma from metastatic liver cancer. *Journal of Clinical Ultrasound,* **15,** 431–437.

60. Yeung, E.Y.C., McCarthy, P., Gompertz, R.H., Benjamin, I.S., Gibson, R.N. & Dawson, P. (1988) The ultrasonographic appearances of hilar cholangiocarcinoma (Klatskin tumours). *British Journal of Radiology,* **61,** 991–995.

CHAPTER 23

Computed Tomography

Richard M. Blaquière

INTRODUCTION

Computed tomography (CT) is a technique involving irradiation of a cross section of tissue by an external X-ray source which rotates around the subject. The X-ray photons which pass through the tissue from any one projection are counted by a bank of detectors, thus building up a profile of the density of the irradiated tissue. The detectors and X-ray tube are linked together in most machines to form the gantry and on modern CT equipment the gantry rotates the full 360° around the abdomen in about 5 seconds or less. The profiles from all the projections are summed and the densities of the different areas are calculated by computer. These densities are termed attenuation values and are measured in Hounsfield Units (HU) in honour of Sir Godfrey Hounsfield who developed the technique. Water has a value of 0 HU and air −1000 HU, while that of liver is between 40 HU and 80 HU.

The digital 'image' produced by the computer can be translated into a visual image by ascribing shades of grey to the various numerical values and displaying the result on a monitor. Changing the range of values over which the grey scale extends—the window width—enables interrogation of the image. The size of the matrix over which the image is displayed determines the size of each picture element or pixel and this is related to the ability of the system to detect both anatomical changes and changes in density. Matrices usually vary between

256×256 to 512×512 pixels although some manufacturers are now enlarging the matrix further. The image produced can be photographed and this hard copy is usually made on film similar to that for conventional radiographs.

TECHNIQUE

The width of the cross section used can be varied and while a standard 8 mm or 10 mm slice is usually employed in examining the liver, occasionally a narrower 4 mm or 5 mm slice is of value. Many sections will be needed to examine a large organ such as the liver and the interval between sections varies between 10 mm and 20 mm depending on whether a dedicated examination is being performed or whether a survey of the whole abdomen is required.

The attenuation value of abnormal liver parenchyma is frequently very similar to that of normal liver. Intravenous (IV) iodinated contrast medium, similar to that used for angiography and intravenous urography, is usually handled differently by normal compared to abnormal liver and this can result in improved detection of abnormal areas. The technique used to give IV contrast is important because the change in density it produces—the enhancement—will vary according to the time that the scan is made after the injection commences. IV contrast rapidly diffuses from the intravascular compartment to the interstitium but the rate at which this occurs is often different in diseased areas. If CT sections are repeated through the same abnormal level a few seconds apart, these temporal changes can be assessed. This is termed dynamic CT and provides an estimate of the vascularity of a lesion.

The rapid leakage of contrast into the interstitium means that the differential enhancement of normal versus abnormal tissue may be lost during the time it takes for the whole of the liver to be examined. This can result in the masking of some abnormalities[17] and has led to the development of various methods of contrast enhancement. Different centres have developed their own methods but the majority give either a bolus of 50 ml of contrast injected by hand followed by a rapid drip infusion of a further 50–100 ml or an infusion of between 100 ml and 150 ml.[105] Frequently the examination is complemented by a preliminary pre-contrast series of slices. Prompted by the need for highly accurate assessment of multifocal primary and multiple secondary tumours prior to hepatic resection, new methods of contrast administration have been explored. This has coincided with technical improvements in CT equipment which allow rapid scanning of sequential slices of the liver during intravenous or intra-arterial contrast injection. This has confusingly also been called dynamic CT but is more correctly, if more cumbersomely, termed sequential or incremental dynamic CT. The techniques have been comprehensively described[36] but can be summarized as follows. For intravenous

administration a pump delivers 50 ml of contrast at a rate of about 5 ml/s and a scanning sequence commences about 45 seconds after this. Contiguous 8 mm or 10 mm slices are made to encompass most of the liver over the next few minutes while further contrast is injected at a rate of 1 ml/s. CT arterial portography is usually performed following hepatic angiography and involves the catheter being left in either the superior mesenteric or, occasionally, hepatic artery and the patient being transferred to an adjacent CT scanner. A similar pump injection and rapid sequence of images are made. Some workers have found that additional CT images delayed for 4–6 hours after IV contrast further improve the detection of tumours.[10]

Contrast agents other than iodinated water-soluble media are also being evaluated. Ethiodized Oil Emulsion 13 (EOE13) is an emulsified form of an iodinated ester of poppy-seed oil which following intravenous injection increases the density of normal hepatic parenchyma. This makes the detection of tumours simpler but, despite the early promise of the technique,[96–98] the agent has not been released for general use. Perfluorooctylbromide, another emulsion, also shows great promise[16,69] but is not yet widely available.

When Lipiodol, which is the iodinated poppy seed oil used in lymphography, is injected into the hepatic artery following angiography it is cleared from the normal liver but persists in hepatocellular carcinoma. CT performed a few days following this detects small tumours which may be missed by conventional CT.[104]

Oral contrast in the form of dilute iodinated water-soluble medium is usually given to opacify the gastrointestinal tract in abdominal CT. Even when a dedicated liver examination is being performed, oral contrast should usually be given to opacify adjacent loops of bowel such as the duodenum and hepatic flexure. This helps to prevent such structures, which can be of the same attenuation as liver parenchyma, from being mistaken for abnormal masses and can also help to show whether they are involved by direct tumour invasion. Usually patients are examined supine but occasionally lateral decubitus examinations are used if artefact from the adjacent bowel is obscuring the liver.

ANATOMY

Computed tomography of the liver provides a series of axial cross-sectional slices and does not have the capability enjoyed by ultrasound and magnetic resonance imaging of direct scanning in other planes. Within these constraints it provides an excellent demonstration of the morphology of the liver.[76]

The liver consists of three lobes, the right, left and caudate, separated by interlobar fissures. The right lobe is the largest with convex superior and right-hand surfaces and a concave inferior surface. The latter is indented posteriorly by the contents of the right renal fossa. The

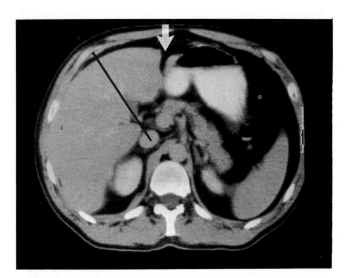

Figure 23.1 Normal liver. The line defines the plane of the interlobal fissure. Note that this is different from the fissure for the ligamentum teres (arrow).

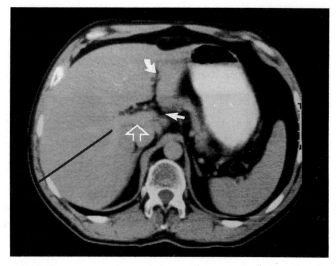

Figure 23.2 The porta hepatis. The enhanced portal vein (open arrow) lies posterior to sections of the hepatic artery shown as two rounded densities. The fissures for the ligamentum venosum (straight arrow) and the ligamentum teres (curved arrow) lie anteriorly. The position of the right intersegmental fissure is deduced by drawing a line, as shown, between the branches of the right portal vein.

left lobe varies in size from a large structure extending to the left lateral wall of the abdomen to a small thin sliver of tissue anterior to the stomach. Rarely it is absent.[9] The right and left lobes are divided into two main segments.

The gallbladder, shown as an oval or rounded structure of near fluid density, lies within a fossa on the inferomedial aspect of the right lobe, lateral to the medial segment of the left lobe. The position of the inferior portion of the gallbladder is variable.

The right and left lobes of the liver are separated by the obliquely orientated interlobar fissure. This is not clearly visible on CT but its position is deduced by drawing a line between the sulcus occupied by the inferior vena cava (IVC) and the superior portion of the gallbladder fossa then continuing this line through the liver parenchyma to the right abdominal side wall (Figure 23.1). The left hepatic lobe is divided into lateral and medial segments by the fissure for the ligamentum teres, or left intersegmental fissure. (In 'classical' anatomy the lateral segment was termed the left lobe while the medial segment was the quadrate lobe.) The left intersegmental fissure contains fat and is readily recognized as a vertical cleft in most patients. It is continuous at its posterior end with the more coronally orientated fissure for the ligamentum venosum (Figure 23.2). The caudate lobe lies posteriorly within the liver and is distinct from the other two lobes. It is bounded anteriorly by the fissure for the ligamentum venosum, which separates it from the posterior aspect of the left lobe. Posterior to the caudate lies the inferior vena cava. The right intersegmental fissure divides the right hepatic lobe into anterior and posterior segments. It is not visualized on CT but lies in a position defined by a line bisecting the anterior and posterior branches of the right portal vein.

The hepatic vessels are best shown on contrast-enhanced

CT (Figure 23.14), although they can be seen as low-density structures coursing within the liver parenchyma on non-enhanced studies. The portal vein passes anterior to the IVC and posterior to both the main hepatic artery and the common bile duct to reach the porta hepatis. The latter structure lies between the posterior end of the left intersegmental fissure and the caudal end of the gallbladder fossa and is also continuous superomedially with the fissure for the ligamentum venosum. The portal vein divides into right and left branches, which enter the liver parenchyma and divide in turn into segmental branches. These form a triad with branches of the hepatic artery and biliary tree running within the parenchyma of the hepatic segments. In contrast, the hepatic veins run in fissures between the hepatic segments. The major hepatic veins are three in number—the right, middle and left. They are most easily seen as they converge on and drain into the IVC at the posterosuperior border of the liver. Since the veins run in the intersegmental fissures they provide important landmarks in the definition of the lobes. This is of increasing importance in the assessment of patients prior to hepatic tumour resection, where CT provides an invaluable adjunct to angiography.[77,83]

The intrahepatic portions of the biliary tree are not normally seen on CT and their visualization implies duct dilatation. The common hepatic and common bile ducts are frequently demonstrated, particularly when narrow contrast-enhanced slices have been obtained. The common hepatic duct is shown as a rounded low-attenuation structure 3–5 mm in diameter lying anterior to the portal vein within the porta hepatis, while the common bile duct can often be traced on serial sections along its course to the duodenum. Within the liver the bile ducts may lie either anterior or posterior to the portal veins.[15]

HEPATIC MASSES

In the strict sense there are no absolute CT criteria which will distinguish benign from malignant tumours, but in a large proportion of patients the CT appearances when taken in conjunction with the clinical, biochemical and other radiological findings will differentiate the two.

MALIGNANT TUMOURS

Hepatocellular carcinoma (HCC)

The CT appearances of HCC are variable but usually these are large focal masses of a similar density to normal liver. They show patchy irregular enhancement with a bolus of intravenous contrast (Figure 23.3) but on more delayed examinations they may become isodense. They are often solitary and can distort the liver contour. Calcification may be present while fatty change is rarely seen.[103] The changes of underlying chronic liver disease such as cirrhosis or haemochromatosis can provide a clue to the correct diagnosis. HCC tends to invade the portal vein and tumour thrombus appears as a low-density area within the vessel. Vascular pooling and rapid filling of hepatic veins indicating arterio-venous shunting may be seen with dynamic CT.[49]

Fibrolamellar carcinoma which occurs in younger patients without previous liver disease frequently shows surface lobulation and is more likely to have calcification and a central scar than the usual form of HCC.[11]

CT is invaluable in the assessment of patients prior to

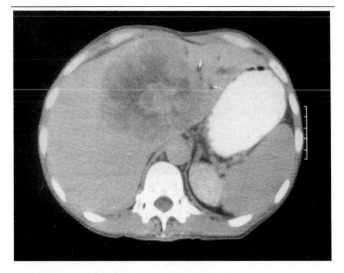

Figure 23.3 Hepatoma. A typical solitary large mass with irregular enhancement, signs of central necrosis, and a faint fleck of calcification. Note the biliary duct dilatation distally (arrows) caused by tumour obstruction.

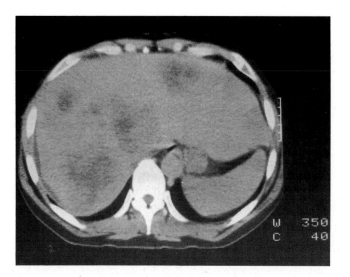

Figure 23.4 Liver metastases. Multiple irregular poorly defined defects of lower attenuation than normal liver.

tumour resection. Both CT arterial portography and Lipiodol-enhanced CT have been used to assess the number of sites of disease. The accuracy of both techniques is greater than that of conventional CT.[24,79] The experience of Lipiodol CT has been mainly in the Far East and the reported use in the United Kingdom has been less encouraging. It may be that this technique is of less value in non-Asian populations.[87]

Metastatic tumours

Metastases are overall the commonest liver malignancy seen and display a variety of CT patterns. The most frequent appearance is of multiple lesions of varying size and of lower density than the adjacent liver parenchyma (Figure 23.4). The margins are often irregular or nodular and there may be a centre of lower density than the periphery due to tumour necrosis. Calcification within a metastasis suggests a primary mucin-secreting tumour such as colonic or ovarian carcinoma, although other metastatic tumours occasionally calcify. The abnormal low density around the calcium usually enables these metastases to be distinguished from non-malignant causes of calcification (Figure 23.5).

Occasionally metastases can appear very similar to cysts having thin walls and an attenuation close to that of water.[6] Scalloped lesions on the surface of the liver due to deposits on or deep to the liver capsule are seen most commonly in patients who have transcoelomic spread of tumour, e.g. metastatic ovarian cancer (Figure 23.6). Some vascular metastases become isodense with normal liver parenchyma when IV contrast is given slowly and may be missed when precontrast images are not made.[13]

Focal masses of low attenuation due to fatty infiltration are occasionally confused with metastases.[102] Conversely, diffuse fatty infiltration can decrease the overall density of the liver, making metastases appear of higher attenuation.

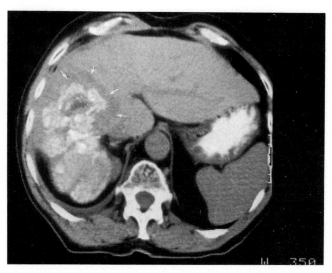

Figure 23.5 Dense tumour calcification in metastases from a primary colonic adenocarcinoma. Note the abnormal low-density tissue (arrows) around the calcified areas.

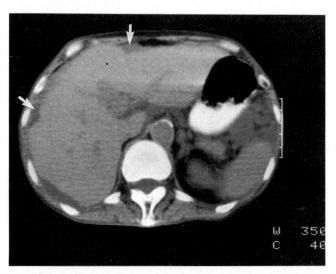

Figure 23.6 Low-attenuation defects on the surface of the liver (arrows) due to metastases from an ovarian carcinoma.

Usually, close attention to technique and to the density of adjacent organs can resolve these difficulties. In cases of doubt, comparison should always be made with the ultrasound and radioisotope findings.[45,54] If, despite these measures, a firm conclusion cannot be reached, CT or ultrasound-guided biopsy will provide the answer.

For many years there has been much discussion of the ideal CT technique for detecting liver metastases. Not only has the need for precontrast scans been questioned but also the volume of contrast, method of administration, speed of injection, and timing of the scan.[1,10,17,67,85,86] This dialogue is reflected in the differing methods used by experienced radiologists.[105] CT has been in clinical use throughout this period and has gained acceptance as the most sensitive radiological technique in the examination

of the liver, although recently its pre-eminence has been threatened by magnetic resonance imaging. It therefore seems likely that all the standard methods of CT examination of the liver are reasonably accurate. Equally, it is becoming clear that the most sensitive methods of examination are those which involve dynamic incremental CT with a powered injector either via the superior mesenteric artery or less invasively via a peripheral vein. Patients being considered for resection of hepatic metastases should ideally have intra-arterial incremental dynamic CT.[36,47,68,79] Both Lipiodol CT and emulsified-oil enhancement have great potential[59,68] but their role is not yet defined.

Other malignant liver tumours

Hepatoblastoma is generally a tumour of childhood. CT is useful firstly to confirm the hepatic origin of the tumour and secondly to demonstrate accurately the extent prior to treatment. CT appearances are usually of a well-defined mass of lower density than normal liver which shows little enhancement with IV contrast. Either calcification, nodularity or a heterogeneous centre are seen in the majority.[29]

Angiosarcoma, which has been linked to occupational exposure to vinyl chloride and other agents as well as thorotrast, has a characteristic enhancement pattern with intravenous contrast which may suggest the diagnosis.[35,61] The recently described entity of epithelioid haemangio-endothelioma can appear on CT either as multiple nodules or as large diffuse masses.[40]

BENIGN TUMOURS

Cavernous haemangioma is a common tumour seen most frequently in women and is often an incidental radiological finding. Fortunately it is one of the few tumours where there are characteristic radiological findings and a confident pathological diagnosis can be made in the majority of patients even when there is a known non-hepatic primary tumour.[39] On pre-contrast CT, haemangiomas are well-defined single or multiple homogeneous areas of lower density than the normal liver. Central areas of low density may be seen particularly in larger tumours and occasionally there is calcification. With a bolus of IV contrast and a dynamic CT technique the characteristic enhancement pattern is shown. Initially the periphery of the lesion becomes dense, sometimes in a nodular fashion, and there is then progressive centripetal enhancement encroaching upon the low-density centre (Figure 23.7). The majority of haemangiomas become isodense with the adjacent liver on delayed CT scans but this may take up to 90 minutes. However, the central low-attenuation clefts seen on the precontrast scans can persist.[90] These probably reflect areas of fibrosis or

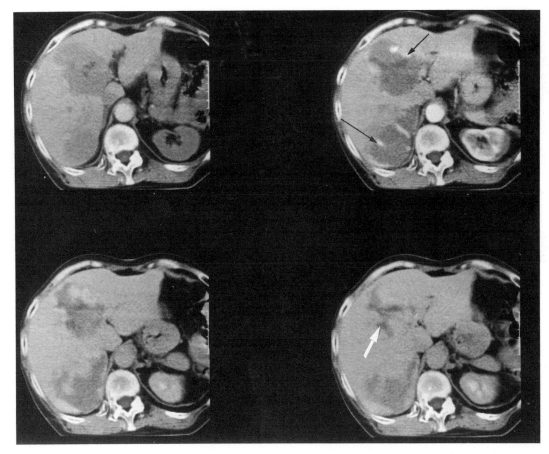

Figure 23.7 Cavernous haemangioma. Serial scans made before, during and after a bolus of IV contrast show the typical enhancement pattern of this tumour. Initially (top left) two low-attenuation hepatic defects are present. Dense peripheral vessels (arrows) opacify early in the contrast phase (top right) and then the densities become more diffuse while the margins of the haemangiomas lose their sharp peripheral definition (bottom left). Five minutes after the injection of contrast (bottom right) most of the haemangiomas are isodense with the adjacent normal liver but central non-enhanced clefts persist (arrow).

necrosis.[12] It is important that strict criteria are rigidly applied since other tumours may show similar peripheral enhancement.[38] In small haemangiomas (less than 2–3 cm) the 'peripheral' early enhancement can involve almost all the tumour, giving an impression of a hyperdense mass.

Although needle biopsy of haemangiomas has been associated with severe haemorrhage the risks have been overstated.[28,92] Nevertheless, biopsy should be reserved for that small group of patients in whom the radiological findings are equivocal and in whom a histological diagnosis is crucial.

Hepatic adenoma and focal nodular hyperplasia (FNH) have certain characteristics in common but differentiation is important since management can differ. In common with most other hepatic tumours, adenomas are usually of lower density than normal liver on pre-contrast CT. Areas of high density centrally due to recent haemorrhage are strongly suggestive of an adenoma.[64] Areas of old haemorrhage are shown by central hypodense zones. A low-density fatty capsule around an adenoma has been reported.[2] With dynamic contrast CT there is some enhancement but the pattern is non-specific.

FNH is usually slightly less dense than normal liver on pre-contrast images but can be isodense and then only detectable by the change in the contour of the liver. A central stellate low-density scar may be present but there should be no evidence of haemorrhage (Figure 23.8). Dynamic CT reveals enhancement which is often vivid and vessels within the central hypodense area strongly suggest the correct diagnosis. On its own CT will only differentiate adenoma from FNH when the appearances are typical. When it is combined with radionuclide imag-

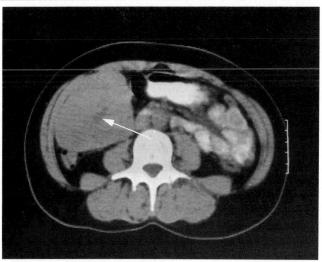

Figure 23.8 Hepatic adenoma shown as a mass projecting from the inferior surface of the liver and containing a central low density 'scar' (arrow).

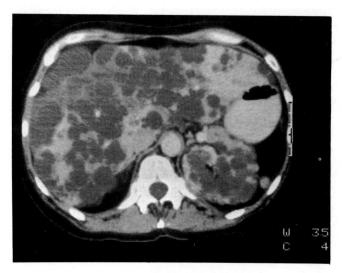

Figure 23.9 Polycystic liver. Innumerable well-defined lesions of water density are scattered throughout the liver. Note the similarity to the cysts involving the left kidney.

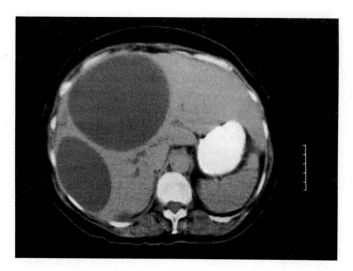

Figure 23.10 Hepatic haematomas of iatrogenic origin mimicking large simple cysts.

ing, ultrasound and angiography a confident diagnosis can be made in the majority of patients.[100]

Nodular regenerative hyperplasia leading to low-attenuation non-enhancing nodules or masses on CT can be mistaken for focal nodular hyperplasia, hepatic adenoma or even metastases.[30]

Rare benign liver tumours: Mesenchymal hamartomas of the liver present on CT as large well-defined non-enhancing cyst-like lesions containing smaller daughter cysts or septa.[52,94] Infantile haemangioendothelioma is seen in the same age group as hepatoblastoma but has a different appearance. While there may be tiny foci of calcium there is marked enhancement, either diffusely or peripherally with IV contrast, similar to that seen in cavernous haemangioma.[60] Hepatic lymphangioma also has a cyst-like appearance and the reported case showed peripheral calcification.[6]

HEPATIC CYSTS

Hepatic cysts are sharply defined round or oval thin-walled lesions of homogeneous fluid density (0–20 HU) which show no enhancement with intravenous contrast. They may be solitary or multiple and can be associated with polycystic renal disease (Figure 23.9). They are a common incidental finding and usually the appearances are characteristic. Small cysts may have an erroneously high-density reading and appear to enhance due to partial volume averaging.[18] (This phenomenon occurs when the slice thickness is greater than the thickness of the lesion so that the density of the lesion is computed with the adjacent tissue contained within the slice, giving an average density).

Lesions which can mimic simple cysts include cystic

primary and secondary tumours, abscesses, hydatid disease, old haematomas and pseudocysts following pancreatitis[6,34] (Figure 23.10). Careful scrutiny of the abnormality and rigorous application of the criteria for the diagnosis of a simple cyst will usually differentiate these other pathologies. Ultrasound is invaluable when the diagnosis is in doubt and if necessary biopsy can be performed.

INFECTION

Intra- and perihepatic pyogenic abscesses are well shown by CT. They appear as low-density lesions with attenuation values between those of cysts and solid tumours, i.e. 20–30 HU. Thus there is an overlap between low-density abscesses and cysts and between high-density abscesses and tumours.[44] Although gas within the abnormality increases the likelihood of an abscess being present, this is less commonly found than in abscesses elsewhere in the body. With intravenous contrast a rim of enhancement appears which is often thick and irregular (Figure 23.11) but this pattern can also be seen in necrotic tumours. Dynamic CT produces the more specific 'double target' sign of enhancement around the low-density centre, surrounded in turn by a less dense ring.[65]

Multiple pyogenic abscesses less than 2 cm in diameter—microabscesses—are uncommon. When they do occur they tend to aggregate as a cluster in an appearance suggesting early coalescence,[51] a feature not seen in fungal microabscesses.

Amoebic liver abscesses have appearances similar to pyogenic abscesses but extrahepatic extension, which is most frequently through the diaphragm, is more common

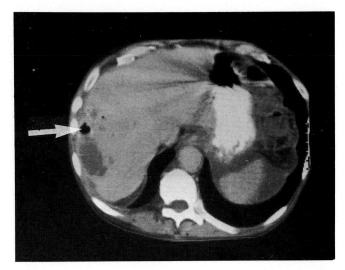

Figure 23.11 Liver abscesses shown as peripheral low-density areas containing gas (arrow) and with marginal enhancement.

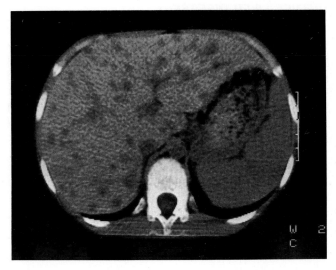

Figure 23.13 Fungal microabscesses appearing as multiple low-density foci in a child immunosuppressed following chemotherapy for leukaemia.

and has been reported in up to 78% of patients.[88] This feature helps to confirm the diagnosis (Figure 23.12).

Fungal infections of the liver usually occur in immuno-compromised patients and are difficult to diagnose. Ultrasound and CT have important complementary roles.[19] The appearance of multiple small rounded low-density lesions on CT in predisposed patients is strongly suggestive of infection by fungi such as *Candida* or *Aspergillus* (Figure 23.13). Despite effective treatment, focal CT abnormalities can persist due to fibrotic nodules.[91] Similar

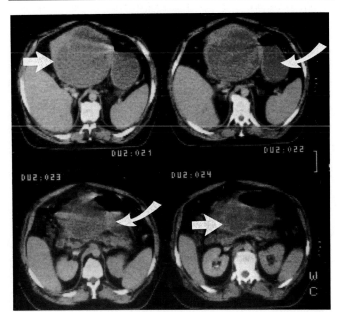

Figure 23.12 Amoebic abscess. A series of scans show a low-density mass (arrows) arising in the left lobe of the liver and extending inferiorly beyond the liver to involve the stomach (curved arrows).

lesions due to extramedullary haemopoiesis have been reported in a patient with acute lymphocytic leukaemia.[55]

In hydatid disease the CT appearance varies according to the parasite, either *Echinococcus granulosus* or *multi-locularis*. *E. granulosus* produces single or multiple well-defined cysts of fluid or low soft-tissue density. A definable wall of raised density is found, is sometimes calcified, and may enhance.[8,26] When daughter cysts consisting of similar smaller lesions within the main cyst are present, the diagnosis is virtually certain. CT may be of some value in assessing response to medical therapy if definitive surgical treatment is not performed.[74] *E. multilocularis* has a completely different CT appearance, being of low soft-tissue density rather than cystic, and with ill-defined margins. Clusters of microcalcification are present in 50% of patients.[31] Such lesions are easily confused with necrotic tumours.

Schistosoma japonica involving the liver causes an unusual and characteristic change on CT. Bands or septa of calcification within the liver parenchyma are found corresponding to the portal fibrosis seen pathologically. Capsular calcification also occurs and where this meets the septal calcification a depression in the hepatic contour is visible. This leads to an appearance resembling a tortoise shell.[4]

Schistosoma mansoni inhabits the superior mesenteric vein, unlike *S. japonica* which favours the colonic and rectal veins and the CT appearances of liver involvement also differ. The periportal fibrosis produced is shown as linear or nodular areas of low attenuation which enhance with intravenous contrast but do not calcify. There could be confusion of such lesions with metastases but careful examination will reveal branching of the abnormal areas in schistosomiasis.[33]

DIFFUSE LIVER DISEASE

Compared to the assessment of focal liver lesions, CT is of limited value in most diffuse liver diseases. Thus patients with viral hepatitis, early cirrhosis and many with infiltration by lymphoma will show no abnormality other than hepatomegaly. Changes secondary to chronic liver disease such as ascites, varices, splenomegaly and portal vein thrombosis are demonstrable by CT and provide important indicators to the presence of occult liver disease. Equally the finding of lymphadenopathy in chronic active hepatitis[43] and primary biliary cirrhosis[82] can lead to a mistaken diagnosis of malignancy. There are a number of diffuse liver diseases which lead to alterations in hepatic density or contour and which can be demonstrated by CT.

Fatty change

This condition causes a decrease in the density of the affected areas. Estimates of decrease in density are made by reference to the spleen, which measures about 7 HU less than normal liver. Gross fatty change will result in marked diminution of density to values close to or less than that of water (Figure 23.14). This causes a characteristic reversal of the normal appearance wherein the normal density hepatic vessels stand out from the less-dense liver parenchyma. CT can be used to quantify the severity of fatty change and when the cause is treatable the changes may resolve.[81]

Fatty change can be diffuse or focal. Focal sparing which may be a result of local alteration in portal blood flow[3] can cause confusion with metastatic disease.[102] Close correlation with radionuclide and ultrasound examinations

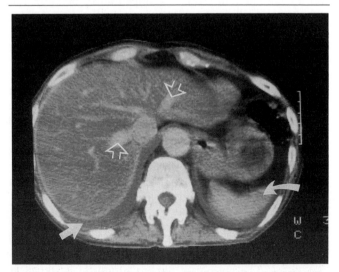

Figure 23.14 Diffuse fatty infiltration of the liver. Despite the administration of IV contrast the liver density is only slightly greater than the adjacent pleural effusion (arrow) and is far less than the enhanced spleen (curved arrow). Note also how the hepatic veins (hollow arrows) stand out from the low-density liver parenchyma.

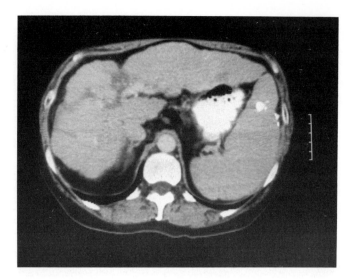

Figure 23.15 Advanced cirrhosis causing contraction of the right lobe of the liver and diffuse nodularity of the surface.

helps to avoid misdiagnosis[45,54] but if doubts still persist radiologically guided biopsy will provide the answer.

Cirrhosis

In early cirrhosis there is frequently no specific CT abnormality although fatty change may be visible. With more advanced disease the hepatic contour becomes nodular due to fibrosis and regeneration nodules (Figure 23.15). The liver shrinks, particularly the right lobe, but the caudate lobe is often spared and may show compensatory hypertrophy. The changes due to portal hypertension may be more obvious than the liver disease.

Deposition diseases

Abnormal hepatic deposition of a number of substances will result in an alteration of the density of the liver parenchyma. Iron deposition in haemochromatosis can lead to a dramatic increase in attenuation values and CT has been proposed as an alternative to liver biopsy in patients with an unexplained raised serum ferritin.[50] A generalized increase in liver density on CT can be due to amiodarone,[84] glycogen storage diseases, gold therapy[62] and probably Wilson's disease.

Congestive heart failure

In some patients with heart failure the liver shows an abnormal pattern of IV contrast enhancement. The most striking change is lobular or patchy areas of increased density separated by linear areas of poor or delayed enhancement (Figure 23.16). The latter may converge on the hepatic veins or lie peripherally. In addition there is usually irregular perivascular enhancement and frequently an overall delay in parenchymal enhancement; on later images the heterogeneous mottled enhancement fades to

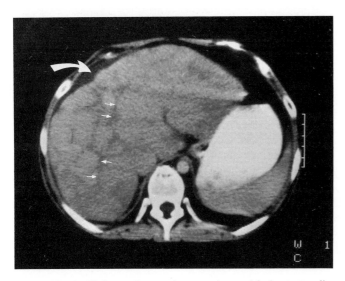

Figure 23.16 Enhanced scan in a patient with long-standing heart failure due to congenital heart disease (note the very small aorta), showing lobulated areas separated by low-attenuation strands (small arrows). The subcapsular low-density area is due to haemorrhage from an earlier liver biopsy (curved arrow).

a more normal homogeneous pattern.[75] Enlargement of the inferior vena cava, reflux of contrast into the hepatic veins and perivascular lymphoedema may also be present.[48,57] It is uncertain why these changes only occur in a minority of patients with congestive heart failure, but it is postulated that they correlate with the degree of hepatic congestion. Their recognition is important so as to avoid confusion with malignant liver disease or Budd–Chiari syndrome, which can look remarkably similar.

Hepatic infarcts

These are rarely diagnosed. Initially they appear on CT as poorly defined non-enhancing low-density areas. With time these become more discrete or merge with other lesions. The abnormalities are generally rounded and lie centrally more often than peripherally but they cannot be differentiated with certainty from abscesses or tumours using CT alone.[58]

Budd–Chiari syndrome (see Chapter 48)

This uncommon syndrome caused by obstruction to hepatic venous drainage has a number of aetiologies including congenital webs, neoplasia and hypercoagulopathies. The CT appearances can vary between the acute and subacute or chronic stages. The diagnosis can be confirmed by finding filling defects in the hepatic veins and inferior vena cava due to thrombi. In the acute stage these may be of raised density.[73] Failure to visualize the hepatic veins is a common finding in chronic disease. There may also be evidence of portal vein and even splenic or mesenteric vein thrombosis.[99] Striking changes in the liver

parenchyma may occur. Acutely the liver is enlarged and of diminished density and there is ascites. With IV contrast there is patchy enhancement around the porta but poor peripheral enhancement.[66] Chronically there are areas of liver atrophy with compensatory hypertrophy of nonaffected areas, notably the caudate lobe. With IV enhancement areas of decreased density at the sites of atrophy have been shown to correspond to areas of local reversal of portal venous flow. They contrast with sites of patchy increased density where the portal flow is in the correct direction. The appearance should not be confused with congestive heart failure, which does not cause hepatic vein thrombosis.

HEPATIC TRAUMA (see Chapter 55)

On CT, subcapsular haematomas are shown as well-defined lenticular low-density areas just deep to the liver capsule, whereas intrahepatic haematomas are rounded collections within the liver itself (Figures 23.16 and 23.17). Acute haemorrhage is of raised density but with time this density decreases to high fluid levels. Hepatic lacerations and fractures appear as irregular linear clefts often extending to the liver surface.

CT enables one to assess other structures such as the spleen, pancreas, kidneys and the volume of free intraperitoneal blood. This makes CT a useful tool in assessing patients who have suffered severe abdominal trauma. Since surgery is required in those patients who are unstable haemodynamically, CT is most valuable in the stable patient with hepatic injuries. The majority of such patients will be treated conservatively and serial CT is used to monitor the resolution of lacerations and haematomas.[37,72] CT is also useful in assessing the changes in those patients who do undergo surgery.[46]

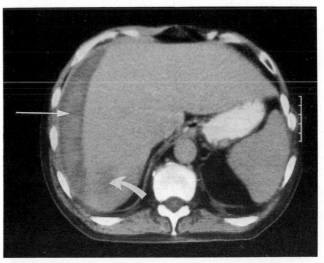

Figure 23.17 A subcapsular haematoma containing areas of raised density due to recent haemorrhage (arrow). An intrahepatic haematoma is represented by the ill-defined low-density area (curved arrow).

BILIARY TRACT DISEASES

Although ultrasound is the corner stone of noninvasive radiological investigation of the biliary tract, CT provides invaluable additional information in a number of conditions and in those patients where ultrasound encounters technical difficulties or is equivocal.

Biliary obstruction

The normal extrahepatic biliary tree may be visible but the normal intrahepatic ducts should not be seen on CT. The presence of intrahepatic branching linear or rounded structures close to water density which enlarge as they approach the porta hepatis implies biliary duct dilatation (Figure 23.18). Care must be taken not to confuse perivascular lymphoedema, which can be due to heart failure, malignant lymphadenopathy or previous lymphatic trauma, with duct dilatation.[57] Extrahepatic biliary dilatation is assumed when the duct measures more than 9 mm, values between 7 and 9 mm being considered equivocal. While intraheptic duct dilatation usually equates with obstruction, this is not necessarily the case with the extrahepatic ducts which, it is assumed, can remain dilated following the passage of a calculus. Biliary duct obstruction may be associated with lobar hepatic atrophy.

By following the course of the dilated ducts the level of the obstruction can be defined. The manner in which the ducts narrow indicates the cause: abrupt tapering of a markedly dilated duct in association with a mass implies tumour; gradual tapering of a moderately dilated common duct implies pancreatitis; abrupt tapering of a moderately dilated system with an intraluminal defect is seen in calculus disease. Bile duct stones may be either high-density calcified lesions or lower-density opacities which are visualized because they are surrounded by bile of near

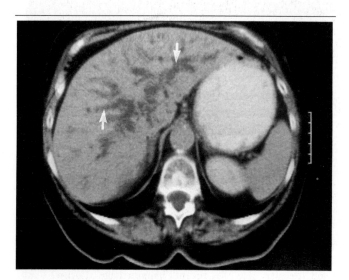

Figure 23.18 Dilated intrahepatic ducts (arrows) converging upon the porta hepatis in a patient with obstructive jaundice.

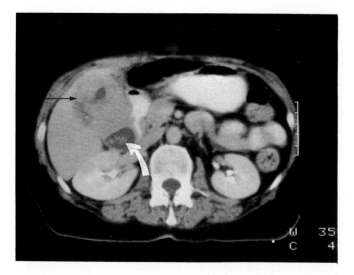

Figure 23.19 Carcinoma (arrow) arising from the wall of the gallbladder and invading the liver. Note the gallstones (curved arrow).

water density, producing the appearance of a target. There is overlap in the appearances of obstruction due to calculi, tumour and inflammation, but using strict criteria for the diagnosis of choledocholithiasis accuracies of 88% have been reported.[7]

The ability of CT to demonstrate not only obstructing masses but also local metastatic adenopathy leads to a high accuracy (92%) in the prediction of malignancy causing suprapancreatic biliary obstruction.[89] This can be invaluable in deciding between surgical resection and palliative drainage procedures.

Gallbladder disease

The CT appearance of gallstones varies according to the amount of calcium they contain. The majority are either densely calcified or have a rim of calcification and are easily detected, but low-density stones are more difficult to identify. Nevertheless, the overall accuracy of gallstone detection by modern CT scanners approaches 90%.[5] Care must be taken to avoid misinterpreting thickening of the gallbladder wall as a large calculus.[70]

In acute cholecystitis a thickened enhancing gallbladder wall is seen and fluid is often present in the gallbladder bed, but it should be remembered that the normal gallbladder wall will show some enhancement.[101] Mural thickening is shown in chronic cholecystitis, while calcification occurs in porcelain gallbladder and mural gas is seen in emphysematous cholecystitis. CT has a high reported accuracy in acute acalculous cholecystitis.[71]

Gallbladder carcinoma is usually shown as an irregular ill-defined enhancing mass in the gallbladder fossa associated with thickening of the gallbladder wall. There may only be irregular mural thickening or an intraluminal mass and the appearances can be complicated since the majority of patients will have chronic gallbladder disease (Figure 23.19). Local invasion, nodal and liver metastases are frequent findings well shown by CT,[32] and have an important bearing on subsequent management.

Biliary duct disease

Cholangiography remains the standard by which all other radiological tests are measured in this group of diseases but CT has an increasingly important role.

Cholangiocarcinoma has three major radiological manifestations—(1) An infiltrating mural tumour often hilar in position which may show raised attenuation on CT but which is often difficult to detect. (2) An exophytic mass often intrahepatic in position and of low attenuation with poor enhancement on CT. (3) An intraluminal polypoid lesion most commonly found in the extrahepatic biliary tree and more readily detected by ultrasound.[22,80] Virtually all patients will show evidence of duct dilatation. CT is good at showing the local spread of disease[32] and therefore in assessing resectability, although sclerosing cholangitis in association with cholangiocarcinoma makes assessment more difficult.

Sclerosing cholangitis causes areas of duct stenosis and dilatation, mural nodularity and wall thickening, all of which can be shown by CT, which in addition may demonstrate an abnormal mural enhancement pattern.[95] Complicating cholangiocarcinoma can also be diagnosed.

Clonorchiasis caused by the Chinese liver fluke *Clonorchis sinensis* transmitted by snails can cause moderate dilatation of the intrahepatic bile ducts, without dilatation of the extrahepatic biliary tree. No more specific findings are seen on CT but when hepatobiliary malignancy is also present there may be more marked dilatation in addition to the signs of the tumour mass.[21] In a series of patients who had peripheral cholangiocarcinoma in addition to clonorchiasis there was an unusual tumour appearance. In addition to the poorly enhancing low-attenuation masses there were stippled areas of high density which corresponded to areas of mucin within the tumour on pathological specimens.[25]

Recurrent pyogenic cholangitis is another disease commoner in the Far East. Duct dilatation, calculi and segmental atrophy are common and during acute attacks, abscesses, bilomas, and abnormal mural or segmental enhancement can be shown. CT is useful in demonstrating the extent of the disease and for guiding further management.[20]

Biliary cystadenoma and cystadenocarcinoma are uncommon tumours usually found in middle-aged women. They are mainly intrahepatic, large (5–7 cm) multilocular lesions of fluid density. Septa, which may enhance, are usually visible on CT in both entities but nodularity

or solid masses as well as coarse calcification suggest cystadenocarcinoma[23,56] (Figure 23.20).

Multiple biliary hamartomas (von Meyenberg complexes) which appear as multiple low-attenuation areas can be confused with hepatic cysts, metastases or micro-abscesses.[27]

Choledochal cyst, a congenital dilatation of the common bile duct leads to extrahepatic duct dilatation and in some patients to intrahepatic dilatation of the main central portions of the ducts without the peripheral tapering seen in patients with biliary obstruction. A further clue to the correct diagnosis is the abrupt change in calibre between the normal and abnormal segments of the duct. The presence of an additional solid mass suggests cholangiocarcinoma, which is a recognized association.

Caroli's disease, another congenital bile duct abnormality, is characterized by multiple low-density tubular structures due to dilated bile ducts which communicate with more rounded areas of focal duct dilatation. In some forms of the disease hepatic fibrosis and cirrhosis predominate.

CT GUIDED BIOPSY AND DRAINAGE (see Chapter 19)

Detailed consideration of the technical aspects is beyond the scope of this text and only a brief review of the application of the technique is presented. It is self-evident that guidance of a biopsy needle to a focal liver lesion using either ultrasound or CT is likely to have a greater accuracy than a blind biopsy and experience has confirmed this. The accuracy for such biopsies now ranges between

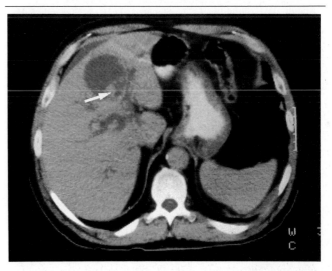

Figure 23.20 Biliary cystadenocarcinoma shown as an intra-hepatic low-attenuation lesion containing mural nodules (arrow). The biliary duct dilatation was a result of tumour extension into the porta hepatis.

83% and 100%.[42] The use of a cutting needle rather than a fine needle increases slightly the risk of complications (1.4% versus 0.83% respectively) but also increases the diagnostic yield.[63] In addition to guiding the needle, CT and ultrasound can ensure that important structures such as the gallbladder, colon and pleural space are not traversed. Furthermore, it appears that the risk of complications in patients with relative contraindications to biopsy, such as ascites, is low when the biopsy needle is guided radiologically.[78] If possible, biopsy of highly vascular malignancies or cavernous haemangiomas should be avoided but not all haemangiomas fulfil the diagnostic criteria and in these circumstances careful fine-needle biopsy can be performed.[28,92]

An extension of the biopsy technique enables the percutaneous drainage of pyogenic abscesses both within and around the liver. Such procedures are successful in between 76% and 87% of patients, success being judged as drainage of the abscess without the need for surgery.[41, 53] Amoebic abscesses are usually treated medically but in patients with complications percutaneous drainage can be used.[93] Percutaneous aspiration and drainage of hydatid cysts is considered to be contraindicated because of the risk of anaphylaxis, but biopsy may be performed inadvertently and it appears that the risk of this complication is low.[14]

REFERENCES

1. Alpern, M.B., Lawson, T.L., Foley, W.D. *et al.* (1986) Focal hepatic masses and fatty infiltration detected by enhanced dynamic CT. *Radiology,* **158**, 45–49.
2. Angres, G., Carter, J.B. & Velasco, J.M. (1980) Unusual ring in liver cell adenoma. *American Journal of Roentgenology,* **135**, 172–174.
3. Arai, K., Matsui, O., Takashima, T. *et al.* (1988) Focal spared areas in fatty liver caused by regional decreased portal flow. *American Journal of Roentgenology,* **151**, 300–302.
4. Araki, T., Hayakawa, K., Okada, J. *et al.* (1985) Hepatic schistosomiasis japonica identified by CT. *Radiology,* **157**, 757–760.
5. Barakos, J.A., Ralls, P.W., Lapin, S.A. *et al.* (1987) Cholelithiasis: evaluation with CT. *Radiology,* **162**, 415–418.
6. Barnes, P.A., Thomas, J.L. & Bernardino, M.E. (1981) Pitfalls in the diagnosis of hepatic cysts by computed tomography. *Radiology,* **141**, 129–133.
7. Baron, R.L. (1987) Common bile duct stones: Reassessment of criteria for CT diagnosis. *Radiology,* **162**, 419–424.
8. Beggs, I. (1983) The radiological appearances of hydatid disease of the liver. *Clinical Radiology,* **34**, 555–563.
9. Belton, R.L. & VanZandt, T.F. (1983) Congenital absence of the left lobe of the liver: A radiologic diagnosis. *Radiology,* **147**, 184.
10. Bernardino, M.E., Erwin, B.C., Steinberg, H.V. *et al.* (1986) Delayed hepatic CT scanning: Increased confidence and improved detection of hepatic metastases. *Radiology,* **159**, 71–74.
11. Brandt, D.J., Johnson, C.D., Stephens, D.H. & Weiland, L.H. (1988) Imaging of fibrolamellar hepatocellular carcinoma. *American Journal of Roentgenology,* **151**, 295–299.
12. Bree, R.L., Schwab, R.E. & Neiman, H.L. (1983) Solitary echogenic spot in the liver: Is it diagnostic of a hemangioma? *American Journal of Roentgenology,* **140**, 41–45.
13. Bressler, E.L., Alpern, M.B., Glazer, G.M. *et al.* (1987) Hypervascular hepatic metastases: CT evaluation. *Radiology,* **162**, 49–51.
14. Bret, P.M., Fond, A., Bretagnolle, M. *et al.* (1988) Percutaneous aspiration and drainage of hydatid cysts in the liver. *Radiology,* **168**, 617–620.
15. Bret, P.M., de Stempel, J.V., Atri, M. *et al.* (1988) Intrahepatic bile duct and portal vein anatomy revisited. *Radiology,* **169**, 405–407.
16. Bruneton, J.N., Falewee, M.N., Francois, E. *et al.* (1989). Liver, spleen, and vessels: Preliminary clinical results of CT with perfluorooctylbromide. *Radiology,* **170**, 179–183.
17. Burgener, F.A. & Hamlin, D.J. (1983) Contrast enhancement of hepatic tumors in CT: Comparison between bolus and infusion techniques. *American Journal of Roentgenology,* **140**, 291–295.
18. Burgener, F.A. & Hamlin, D.J. (1983) Contrast enhancement of focal hepatic lesions in CT: Effect of size and histology. *American Journal of Roentgenology,* **140**, 297–301.
19. Callen, P.W., Filly, R.A. & Marcus, F.S. (1980) Ultrasonography and computed tomography in the evaluation of hepatic microabscesses in the immunosuppressed patient. *Radiology,* **136**, 433–434.
20. Chan, F.L., Man, S.W., Leong, L.L.Y. & Fan, S.T. (1989) Evaluation of recurrent pyogenic cholangitis with CT: Analysis of 50 patients. *Radiology,* **170**, 165–169.
21. Choi, B.I., Kim, H.J., Han, M.C. *et al.* (1989) CT findings of clonorchiasis. *American Journal of Roentgenology,* **152**, 281–284.
22. Choi, B.I., Lee, J.H., Han, M.C. *et al.* (1989) Hilar cholangiocarcinoma: Comparative study with sonography and CT. *Radiology,* **172**, 689–692.
23. Choi, B.I., Lim, J.H., Han, M.C. *et al.* (1989) Biliary cystadenoma and cystadenocarcinoma: CT and sonographic findings. *Radiology,* **171**, 57–61.
24. Choi, B.I., Park, J.H., Kim, B.H. *et al.* (1989) Small hepatocellular carcinoma: Detection with sonography, computed tomography (CT), angiography and Lipiodol–CT. *British Journal of Radiology,* **62**, 897–903.
25. Choi, B.I., Park, J.H., Kim, Y.I. *et al.* (1988) Peripheral cholangiocarcinoma and clonorchiasis: CT findings. *Radiology,* **169**, 149–153.
26. Choliz, J.D., Olaverri, F.J.L., Casas, T.F. & Zubieta, S.O. (1982) Computed tomography in hepatic echinococcosis. *American Journal of Roentgenology,* **139**, 699–702.
27. Cooke, J.C. & Cooke, D.A.P. (1987) The appearances of multiple biliary hamartomas of the liver (von Meyenberg complexes) on computed tomography. *Clinical Radiology,* **38**, 101–102.
28. Cronan, J.J., Esparza, A.R., Dorfman, G.S. *et al.* (1988) Cavernous hemangioma of the liver: Role of percutaneous biopsy. *Radiology,* **166**, 135–138.
29. Dachman, A.M., Pakter, R.L., Ros, P.R. *et al.* (1987) Hepatoblastoma: Radiologic–pathologic correlation in 50 cases. *Radiology,* **164**, 15–19.
30. Dachman, A.H., Ros, P.R., Goodman, Z.D. *et al.* (1987) Nodular regenerative hyperplasia of the liver: Clinical and radiologic observations. *American Journal of Roentgenology,* **148**, 717–722.
31. Didier, D., Weiler, S., Rohmer, P. *et al.* (1985) Hepatic alveolar echinococcosis: Correlative US and CT study. *Radiology,* **154**, 179–186.
32. Engels, J.T., Balfe, D.M. & Lee, J.K.T. (1989) Biliary carcinoma: CT evaluation of extrahepatic spread. *Radiology,* **172**, 35–40.
33. Fataar, S., Bassiony, H., Satyanath, S. *et al.* (1985) CT of hepatic schistosomiasis mansoni. *American Journal of Roentgenology,* **145**, 63–66.
34. Federle, M.P., Filly, R.A. & Moss, A.A. (1981) Cystic hepatic neoplasms: Complementary roles of CT and sonography. *American Journal of Roentgenology,* **136**, 345–348.
35. Fitzgerald, E.J. & Griffiths, T.M. (1987) Computed tomography of vinyl-chloride-induced angiosarcoma of liver. *British Journal of Radiology,* **60**, 593–595.
36. Foley, W.D. (1989) Dynamic hepatic CT. *Radiology,* **170**, 617–622.
37. Foley, W.D., Cates, J.D., Kellman, G.M. *et al.* (1987) Treatment of blunt hepatic injuries: Role of CT. *Radiology,* **164**, 635–638.
38. Freeny, P.C. & Marks, W.M. (1986) Hepatic hemangioma: Dynamic bolus CT. *American Journal of Roentgenology,* **147**, 711–719.
39. Freeny, P.C. & Marks, W.M. (1986) Patterns of contrast enhance-

ment of benign and malignant hepatic neoplasms during bolus dynamic and delayed CT. *Radiology,* **160**, 613–618.

40. Furui, S., Itai, Y., Ohtomo, K. *et al.* (1989) Hepatic epithelioid hemangioendothelioma: Report of five cases. *Radiology,* **171**, 63–68.

41. van Gansbeke, D., Matos, C., Gelin, M. *et al.* (1989) Percutaneous drainage of subphrenic abscesses. *British Journal of Radiology,* **62**, 127–133.

42. Gazelle, G.S. & Haaga, J.R. (1989) Guided percutaneous biopsy of intraabdominal lesions. *American Journal of Roentgenology,* **153**, 929–935.

43. Gore, R.M., Vogelzang, R.L. & Nemcek, A.A. (1988) Lymphadenopathy in chronic active hepatitis: CT observations. *American Journal of Roentgenology,* **151**, 75–78.

44. Halvorsen, R.A., Korobkin, M., Foster, W.L. *et al.* (1984) The variable CT appearance of hepatic abscesses. *American Journal of Roentgenology,* **142**, 941–946.

45. Halvorsen, R.A., Korobkin, M., Ram, P.C. & Thompson, W.M. (1982) CT appearance of focal fatty infiltration of the liver. *American Journal of Roentgenology,* **139**, 277–281.

46. Haney, P.J., Whitley, N.O., Brotman, S. *et al.* (1982) Liver injury and complications in the postoperative trauma patient: CT evaluation. *American Journal of Roentgenology,* **139**, 271–275.

47. Heiken, J.P., Weyman, P.J., Lee, J.K.T. *et al.* (1989) Detection of focal hepatic masses: Prospective evaluation with CT, delayed CT, CT during arterial portography, and MR imaging. *Radiology,* **171**, 47–51.

48. Holley, H.C., Koslin, D.B., Berland, L.L. & Stanley, R.J. (1989) Inhomogeneous enhancement of liver parenchyma secondary to passive congestion: Contrast-enhanced CT. *Radiology,* **170**, 795–800.

49. Hosoki, T., Chatani, M. & Mori, S. (1982) Dynamic computed tomography of hepatocellular carcinoma. *American Journal of Roentgenology,* **139**, 1099–1106.

50. Howard, J.M., Ghent, C.N., Carey, L.S. *et al.* (1983) Diagnostic efficacy of hepatic computed tomography in the detection of body iron overload. *Gastroenterology,* **84**, 209–215.

51. Jeffrey, R.B., Tolentino, C.S., Chang, F.C. & Federle, M.P. (1988) CT of small pyogenic hepatic abscesses: The cluster sign. *American Journal of Roentgenology,* **151**, 487–489.

52. Jennings, C.M., Merrill, C.R. & Slater, D.N. (1987) Case report: The computed tomographic appearances of benign hepatic hamartoma. *Clinical Radiology,* **38**, 103–104.

53. Johnson, R.D., Mueller, P.R., Ferrucci, J.T. *et al.* (1985) Percutaneous drainage of pyogenic liver abscesses. *American Journal of Roentgenology,* **144**, 463–467.

54. Kissin, C.M., Bellamy, E.A., Cosgrove, D.O. *et al.* (1986) Focal sparing in fatty infiltration of the liver. *British Journal of Radiology,* **59**, 25–28.

55. Kopecky, K.K., Moriarty, A.T., Antony, A.C. & Baker, M.K. (1986) Extramedullary hematopoiesis in acute lymphocytic leukemia masquerading as hepatic, renal, and splenic microabscesses. *American Journal of Roentgenology,* **147**, 846–847.

56. Korobkin, M., Stephens, D.H., Lee, J.K.T. *et al.* (1989) Biliary cystadenoma and cystadenocarcinoma: CT and sonographic findings. *American Journal of Roentgenology,* **153**, 507–511.

57. Koslin, D.B., Stanley, R.J., Berland, L.L. *et al.* (1988) Hepatic perivascular lymphedema: CT appearance. *American Journal of Roentgenology,* **150**, 111–113.

58. Lev-Toaff, A.S., Friedman, A.C., Cohen, L.M. *et al.* (1987) Hepatic infarcts: New observations by CT and sonography. *American Journal of Roentgenology,* **149**, 87–90.

59. Lewis, E., AufderHeide, J.F., Bernardino, M.E. *et al.* (1982) CT detection of hepatic metastases with ethiodized oil emulsion 13. *Journal of Computer Assisted Tomography,* **6**(6), 1108–1114.

60. Lucaya, J., Enriquez, G., Amat, L. & Gonzalez-Rivero, M.A. (1985) Computed tomography of infantile hepatic hemangioendothelioma. *American Journal of Roentgenology,* **144**, 821–826.

61. Mahony, B., Jeffrey, R.B. & Federle, M.P. (1982) Spontaneous rupture of hepatic and splenic angiosarcoma demonstrated by CT. *American Journal of Roentgenology,* **138**, 965–966.

62. de Maria, M., De Simone, G., Laconi, A. *et al.* (1986) Gold storage in the liver: Appearance on CT scans. *Radiology,* **159**, 355–356.

63. Martino, C.R., Haaga, J.R., Bryan, P.J. *et al.* (1984) CT-guided liver biopsies: Eight years' experience. *Radiology,* **152**, 755–757.

64. Mathieu, D., Bruneton, J.N., Drouillard, J. *et al.* (1986) Hepatic adenomas and focal nodular hyperplasia: Dynamic CT study. *Radiology,* **160**, 53–58.

65. Mathieu, D., Vasile, N., Fagniez, P.L. *et al.* (1985) Dynamic CT features of hepatic abscesses. *Radiology,* **154**, 749–752.

66. Mathieu, D., Vasile, N., Menu, Y. *et al.* (1987) Budd–Chiari syndrome: Dynamic CT. *Radiology,* **165**, 409–413.

67. Matsui, O., Kadoya, M., Suzuki, M. *et al.* (1983) Work in progress: Dynamic sequential computed tomography during arterial portography in the detection of hepatic neoplasms. *Radiology,* **146**, 721–727.

68. Matsui, O., Takashima, T., Kadoya, M. *et al.* (1987) Liver metastases from colorectal cancers: Detection with CT during arterial portography. *Radiology,* **165**, 65–69.

69. Mattrey, R. (1989) Perfluorooctylbromide: A new contrast agent for CT, sonography, and MR imaging. *American Journal of Roentgenology,* **152**, 247–252.

70. Middleton, W.D., Thorsen, M.K., Lawson, T.L. & Foley, W.D. (1987) False-positive CT diagnosis of gallstones due to thickening of the gallbladder wall. *American Journal of Roentgenology,* **149**, 941–944.

71. Mirvis, S.E., Vainright, J.R., Nelson, A.W. *et al.* (1986) The diagnosis of acute acalculous cholecystitis: A comparison of sonography, scintigraphy, and CT. *American Journal of Roentgenology,* **147**, 1171–1175.

72. Mirvis, S.E., Whitley, N.O., Vainwright, J.R. & Gens, D.R. (1989) Blunt hepatic trauma in adults: CT-based classification and correlation with prognosis and treatment. *Radiology,* **171**, 27–32.

73. Mori, H., Maeda, H., Fukuda, T. *et al.* (1989) Acute thrombosis of the inferior vena cava and hepatic veins in patients with Budd–Chiari syndrome: CT demonstration. *American Journal of Roentgenology,* **153**, 987–991.

74. Morris, D.L., Skene-Smith, H., Haynes, A. & Burrows, F.G.O. (1984) Abdominal hydatid disease: Computed tomographic and ultrasound changes during albendazole therapy. *Clinical Radiology,* **35**, 297–300.

75. Moulton, J.S., Miller, B.L., Dodd, G.D. & Vu, D.N. (1988) Passive hepatic congestion in heart failure: CT abnormalities. *American Journal of Roentgenology,* **151**, 939–942.

76. Mukai, J.K., Stack, C.M., Turner, D.A. *et al.* (1987) Imaging of surgically relevant hepatic vascular and segmental anatomy. Part 1. Normal anatomy. *American Journal of Roentgenology,* **149**, 287–292.

77. Mukai, J.K., Stack, C.M., Turner, D.A. *et al.* (1987) Imaging of surgically relevant hepatic vascular and segmental anatomy. Part 2. Extent and resectability of hepatic neoplasms. *American Journal of Roentgenology,* **149**, 293–297.

78. Murphy, F.B., Barefield, K.P., Steinberg, H.V. & Bernardino, M.E. (1988) CT- or sonography-guided biopsy of the liver in the presence of ascites: frequency of complications. *American Journal of Roentgenology,* **151**, 485–486.

79. Nelson, R.C., Chezmar, J.L., Sugarbaker, P.H. & Bernardino, M.E. (1989) Hepatic tumours: Comparison of CT during arterial portography, delayed CT, and MR imaging for preoperative evaluation. *Radiology,* **172**, 27–34.

80. Nesbit, G.M., Johnson, C.D., James, E.M. *et al.* (1988) Cholangiocarcinomas: Diagnosis and evaluation of resectability by CT and sonography as procedures complementary to cholangiography. *American Journal of Roentgenology,* **151**, 933–938.

81. Nomura, F., Ohnishi, K., Ochiai, T. & Okuda, K. (1987) Obesity-related nonalcoholic fatty liver: CT features and follow-up studies after low-calorie diet. *Radiology,* **162**, 845–847.

82. Outwater, E., Kaplan, M.M. & Bankoff, M.S. (1989) Lymphadenopathy in primary biliary cirrhosis: CT observations. *Radiology,* **171**, 731–733.

83. Pagani, J.J. (1983) Intrahepatic vascular territories shown by computed tomography (CT). *Radiology,* **147**, 173–178.

84. Patrick, D., White, F.E. & Adams, P.C. (1984) Long-term amiodarone therapy: A cause of increased hepatic attenuation on CT. *British Journal of Radiology,* **57**, 573–576.

85. Paushter, D.M., Zeman, R.K., Scheibler, M.L. *et al.* (1989) CT evaluation of suspected hepatic metastases: Comparison of techniques for IV contrast enhancement. *American Journal of Roentgenology,* **152**, 267–271.

86. Platt, J.F. & Glazer, G.M. (1988) IV contrast material for abdominal

CT: Comparison of three methods of administration. *American Journal of Roentgenology*, **151**, 275–277.

87. Raby, N., Karani, J., Michell, M. *et al.* (1989) Lipiodol enhanced CT scanning in assessment of hepatocellular carcinoma. *Clinical Radiology*, **40**, 480–485.

88. Radin, D.R., Ralls, P.W., Colletti, P.M. & Halls, J.M. (1988) CT of amebic liver abscess. *American Journal of Roentgenology*, **150**, 1297–1301.

89. Reiman, T.H., Balfe, D.M. & Weyman, P.J. (1987) Suprapancreatic biliary obstruction: CT evaluation. *Radiology, 163*, 49–56.

90. Scatarige, J.C., Kenny, J.M., Fishman, E.K. *et al.* (1987) CT of giant cavernous hemangioma. *American Journal of Roentgenology*, **149**, 83–85.

91. Shirkhoda, A., Lopez-Berestein, G., Holbert, J.M. & Luna, M.A. (1986) Hepatosplenic fungal infection: CT and pathologic evaluation after treatment with liposomal amphotericin B. *Radiology*, **159**, 349–353.

92. Solbiati, L., Livraghi, T., Pra, L.D. *et al.* (1985) Fine-needle biopsy of hepatic hemangioma with sonographic guidance. *American Journal of Roentgenology*, **144**, 471–474.

93. van Sonnenberg, E., Mueller, P.R., Schiffman, H.R. *et al.* (1985) Intrahepatic amebic abscesses: Indications for and results of percutaneous catheter drainage. *Radiology*, **156**, 631–635.

94. Stanley, P., Hall, T.R., Woolley, M.W. *et al.* (1986) Mesenchymal hamartomas of the liver in childhood: Sonographic and CT findings. *American Journal of Roentgenology*, **147**, 1035–1039.

95. Teefey, S.A., Baron, R.L., Rohrmann, C.A. *et al.* (1988) Sclerosing cholangitis: CT findings. *Radiology*, **169**, 635–639.

96. Thomas, J.L., Bernardino, M.E., Vermess, M. *et al.* (1982) EOE-13 in the detection of hepatosplenic lymphoma. *Radiology, 145*, 629–634.

97. Vermess, M., Doppman, J.L., Sugarbaker, P.H. *et al.* (1982) Computed tomography of the liver and spleen with intravenous lipoid contrast material: Review of 60 examinations. *American Journal of Roentgenology*, **138**, 1063–1071.

98. Vermess, M., Lau, D.H.M., Adams, M.D. *et al.* (1982) Biodistribution study of ethiodized oil emulsion 13 for computed tomography of the liver and spleen. *Journal of Computer Assisted Tomography*, **6**(6), 1115–1119.

99. Vogelzang, R.L., Anschuetz, S.L. & Gore, R.M. (1987) Budd–Chiari syndrome: CT observations. *Radiology*, **163**, 329–333.

100. Welch, T.J., Sheedy, P.F., Johnson, C.M. *et al.* (1985) Focal nodular hyperplasia and hepatic adenoma: Comparison of angiography, CT, US, and scintigraphy. *Radiology*, **156**, 593–595.

101. Whitehouse, R.W. & Martin, D.F. (1986) Contrast-enhanced computed tomography of the normal and abnormal gallbladder. *British Journal of Radiology*, **59**, 1083–1085.

102. Yates, C.K. & Streight, R.A. (1986) Focal fatty infiltration of the liver simulating metastatic disease. *Radiology*, **159**, 83–84.

103. Yoshikawa, J., Matsui, O., Takashima, T. *et al.* (1988) Fatty metamorphosis in hepatocellular carcinoma: Radiologic features in 10 cases. *American Journal of Roentgenology*, **151**, 717–720.

104. Yumoto, Y., Jinno, K., Tokuyama, K. *et al.* (1985) Hepatocellular carcinoma detected by iodized oil. *Radiology*, **154**, 19–24.

105. Zeman, R.K., Clements, L., Silverman, P.M. *et al.* (1988) CT of the liver: A survey of prevailing methods for administration of contrast material. *American Journal of Roentgenology*, **150**, 107–109.

CHAPTER 24

Magnetic Resonance Imaging

Jay P. Heiken

Magnetic resonance imaging (MRI) is based on the phenomenon of nuclear magnetic resonance. The principles were first described in 1946[2,50] but it was not until 1972 that the first two-dimensional proton MR image was generated from a water sample[31] and not until the late 1970s that images of human beings were obtained. As a result of rapid technological advances in this field, MRI became clinically useful by the early 1980s and is now an important diagnostic imaging technique with important applications throughout the body. This chapter reviews some basic concepts of MRI and its current applications in the diagnosis and characterization of hepatic and biliary disorders. Since the role of MRI in evaluating biliary disease is currently quite limited, the majority of the discussion will focus on MRI of the liver.

GENERAL PRINCIPLES OF MAGNETIC RESONANCE IMAGING

As a consequence of their spin, atomic nuclei with an odd number of protons or neutrons have an associated magnetic field, analogous to that of a bar magnet with a north and south pole. In the absence of an externally applied magnetic field, the nuclear magnetic dipoles are randomly oriented. However, when a static external magnetic field is applied, a small percentage of the dipoles align with the magnetic field, producing a net magnetization vector in the direction of the applied field. Although a number of biologically important nuclei can be studied with magnetic resonance techniques, the proton (i.e. the nucleus of the hydrogen atom) is most easy because of its abundance and strong magnetic properties.

Thus, nearly all MR imaging currently in clinical use is based on imaging of protons.

At equilibrium, the net magnetization vector of the aggregate of protons to be imaged lies along the axis of the externally applied static magnetic field. Magnetic resonance signals can be obtained from the protons if they are tipped out of the axis of the static magnetic field. This is done by applying a series of radiofrequency (RF) pulses along an axis perpendicular to the external magnetic field. When each RF pulse is discontinued, the magnetization gradually returns to its equilibrium alignment along the axis of the external magnetic field by a process called relaxation. The process of relaxation is characterized by two time constants, T1 and T2 which are intrinsic properties of each tissue. The changing magnetization produced by the application of the RF pulses induces a voltage in a receiver coil. This voltage can be amplified and detected as a radiofrequency signal from the protons.

In order to produce MR images that contain spatial information, it is necessary to identify the location of the protons producing the MR signals. Spatial encoding is achieved by superimposing three magnetic field gradients on the static magnetic field. These gradients cause a linear variation in the strength of the magnetic field along the spatial coordinates and impose on the protons being imaged characteristics that allow them to be localized to a specific point within the imaged volume.

BASICS OF IMAGE INTERPRETATION

The amplitude of an MR signal is a function of four main parameters; proton density, T1, T2, and flow. By using specific sequences of RF pulses, images that emphasize the contributions of each of these parameters can be produced. Knowledge of a few general principles is helpful in image interpretation. The higher the proton density of a tissue being imaged, the greater the signal that is produced and consequently the brighter the tissue will appear on MR images. Conversely, tissues with low proton density produce low signal intensity and appear dark on MR images. On T1-weighted images, tissues that have a short T1 (e.g. fat) are high in signal intensity (bright) and those with a long T1 (e.g. muscle) are low in signal intensity (dark). On T2-weighted images, tissues with a short T2 (e.g. muscle) have low signal intensity (are dark) and those with a long T2 (e.g. bile or urine) have high signal intensity (are bright). Tissues with intermediate T1 and T2 are medium in signal intensity (grey) on both T1- and T2-weighted images.

The normal liver has an intermediate proton density, T1 and T2 and therefore gives a medium signal intensity on proton-density weighted, T1-weighted and T2-weighted images (see Figure 24.1). The normal T1 and T2 of the liver can be altered by disease or by administration of paramagnetic contrast agents. The proton density of the liver undergoes very little alteration. Most focal hepatic masses (e.g. cysts, benign and malignant neoplasms, abscesses) have prolonged T1 and T2 relaxation compared

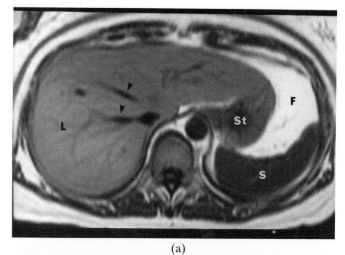

(a)

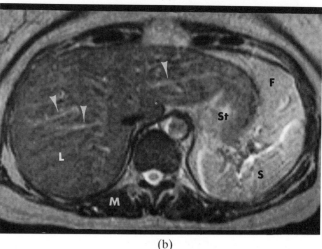

(b)

Figure 24.1 Normal liver. (a) T1-weighted spin echo MR image shows homogeneous intermediate hepatic parenchymal signal intensity (L) that is higher (brighter) than that of the spleen (S), but lower (darker) than that of fat (F). Flowing blood within the hepatic vessels (arrowheads) produces no signal, allowing the vessels to be delineated without the use of intravenous contrast material. St=stomach. (b) T2-weighted spin echo MR image shows homogeneous hepatic parenchymal signal intensity (L) that is somewhat lower (darker) than in (a). Note that the signal intensity of the liver is higher (brighter) than that of muscle (M), but lower (darker) than that of fat (F). On T2-weighted images the hepatic vessels (arrowheads) often appear bright. St=stomach; S=spleen.

with normal liver parenchyma.[12,42] Therefore, these abnormalities appear lower in signal intensity than normal liver on T1-weighted images and higher in signal intensity on T2-weighted images (see Figure 24.2). The MRI appearance of specific focal and diffuse abnormalities of the liver are discussed in more detail below.

TECHNIQUES

Currently the standard technique for MR imaging of the liver is a method called spin-echo. With this technique, each pulse sequence requires approximately 3 to 13

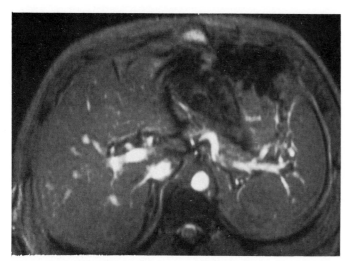

Figure 24.2 Gradient echo image. With gradient echo imaging (a rapid scanning technique), the vessels containing normally flowing blood appear bright.

minutes to image the entire liver. One limitation of this method is that the relatively long imaging time allows artefacts from respiratory motion to degrade the images. A number of motion-suppression techniques have been employed to minimize respiratory artefacts with varying degrees of success. Rapid scanning techniques that allow acquisition of images during a single breath hold are promising in that they not only eliminate respiratory motion artefacts but also decrease overall imaging time. An additional advantage of rapid imaging is that it makes possible the performance of dynamic contrast-enhanced examinations. Nevertheless, at present, spin-echo techniques remain the mainstay of hepatic MR imaging.

Although non-contrast-enhanced MR imaging provides excellent discrimination between normal and abnormal hepatic parenchyma, hepatic signal intensity differences can be increased with the use of intravenous contrast agents. The agent that produces the greatest increase in tissue contrast between normal parenchyma and focal hepatic masses is superparamagnetic iron oxide (ferrite), a compound that is taken up selectively by the reticulo-endothelial system of the liver, spleen, lymph nodes and bone marrow.[61] The crystalline compound acquires a large magnetic moment when placed in a magnetic field, resulting in local magnetic field inhomogeneities that markedly shorten the T2 relaxation of the adjacent normal liver cells. This results in a profound loss of signal from the normal liver tissue. Since the contrast agent is not taken up by tumour cells, hepatic masses stand out on T2-weighted images as foci of higher signal intensity within the very low signal intensity liver. At present, superparamagnetic iron oxide is still an experimental drug and is not yet approved for clinical use. The only intravenous MR contrast agent currently available for clinical use is gadolinium-diethylenetriamine pentaacetic acid (Gd-DTPA). In contrast to iron oxide compounds, Gd-DTPA increases the signal intensity difference between normal and abnormal liver primarily by shortening the T1 relaxation of the tissues in which it is taken up. The biodistribution, excretion and half-life of Gd-DTPA are very similar to those of the iodinated intravenous contrast agents used for excretory urography and computed tomography.[22,60] The main limitation of Gd-DTPA-enhanced imaging of the liver is that it requires rapid imaging of the liver (within the first 2–3 minutes after injection) in order to provide improved detection of focal hepatic lesions. If the liver is imaged more than 3 minutes after the injection of Gd-DTPA, focal lesions may become more difficult to detect. Thus, use of Gd-DTPA as a hepatic contrast agent requires that it be used in conjunction with a rapid imaging technique (see the section on 'Metastases' below).

LIVER

NORMAL LIVER

The anatomy of the liver is well depicted on MR images. The normal liver parenchyma is intermediate in signal intensity (grey) on T1-weighted and proton density-weighted images and slightly lower in signal intensity (darker grey) on T2-weighted images (Figure 24.1). On all pulse sequences the normal hepatic parenchyma is homogeneous. The hepatic and portal veins are easily visualized without the need for intravenous contrast material. Blood vessels appear very low in signal intensity (black) on spin-echo images due to flow-related signal loss (Figure 24.1(a)). On T2-weighted images, slowly flowing venous blood may have high signal intensity owing to a phenomenon called even echo rephasing[78] (Figure 24.1(b)). On gradient echo images (a fast scanning technique) the vessels routinely appear very high in signal intensity (white) (Figure 24.2). Although transaxial images generally show the hepatic vessels adequately, coronal or sagittal images are sometimes helpful to delineate the main portal vein, hepatic veins or inferior vena cava.

FOCAL DISEASE

Metastases

Metastases are generally hypointense on T1-weighted images and hyperintense on T2-weighted images compared with normal hepatic parenchyma (Figure 24.3). They are often heterogeneous in signal intensity, with indistinct margins. Approximately one-quarter of metastases have a central area of hyperintensity ('target' sign) on T2-weighted images, which probably corresponds to central necrosis.[83] A smaller percentage of lesions show a peripheral rim of high signal intensity ('halo' sign), corresponding to changes in the adjacent hepatic parenchyma.

There have been varying opinions of the value of

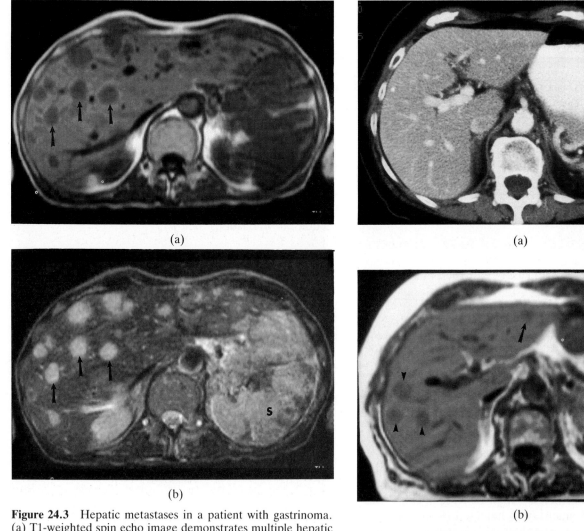

(a)

(b)

Figure 24.3 Hepatic metastases in a patient with gastrinoma. (a) T1-weighted spin echo image demonstrates multiple hepatic masses (arrows) that are lower in signal intensity than the normal liver parenchyma. (b) On the T2-weighted spin echo image the hepatic masses (arrows) are higher in signal intensity than the normal liver. Note that on both T1- and T2-weighted images the metastases have a signal intensity similar to that of the spleen (S).

MRI when compared with contrast enhanced computed tomography (CT). In three studies MRI was found to be superior for the detection of hepatic metastases.[52,73,85] A fourth study showed MRI and CT to be equivalent,[6] whereas an earlier study reported CT to be more useful than MRI.[19] Two recent studies compared MRI with various intravenous and intra-arterial CT methods for the detection of focal hepatic masses in patients being considered for possible hepatic resection.[24,43] Both found MRI to be more sensitive than dynamic intravenous contrast-enhanced CT, but less sensitive than CT arterial portography, an invasive technique reserved for operative candidates. The weight of evidence therefore suggests that MRI is slightly superior to CT in the detection of hepatic metastases (Figure 24.4).

(a)

(b)

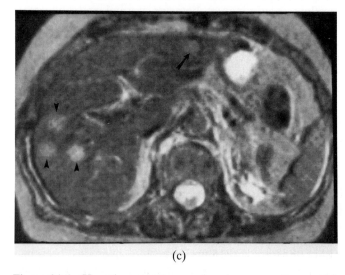

(c)

Figure 24.4 Hepatic metastases of unknown primary. (a) Dynamic-contrast enhanced CT scan shows no definite abnormalities. (b and c) T1-weighted (b) and T2-weighted (c) spin echo MR images show three definite metastases in the right lobe (arrowheads) and one in the left lobe (arrow).

This slight superiority of MRI in the detection of focal hepatic masses may be attributed to several factors:

1. The intrinsic tissue contrast obtainable with MRI is greater than with CT, which depends solely on differences in X-ray attenuation for lesion detection.
2. Fatty change in the liver can obscure focal masses on CT, but does not interfere with the detection of focal masses on MRI. As a significant percentage of patients with cancer have some degree of hepatic fatty change, this is an important advantage of MRI.
3. Peripheral enhancement of metastases on dynamic contrast-enhanced CT examinations can obscure small lesions but this does not occur with non-contrast-enhanced MRI examinations.

Tissue contrast between metastases and normal liver parenchyma can be increased with the administration of intravenous MRI contrast agents. Gd-DTPA, a paramagnetic agent, shortens both T1 and T2 relaxation, but the predominant effect is on T1. Within the first 2–3 minutes after injection of Gd-DTPA, tumour-to-liver contrast is increased, with the normal liver parenchyma increasing in signal intensity due to the T1-shortening effect of Gd-DTPA (Figure 24.5). Since Gd-DTPA quickly enters the extravascular interstitial space, it rapidly enters the tumour, increasing tumour signal intensity and decreasing the tumour-to-liver contrast. Peak tumour-to-liver contrast occurs approximately 1 minute after injection of Gd-DTPA.[22,40] By 4–6 minutes after injection, tumour-to-liver contrast is reduced to pre-contrast levels or below. In order to take advantage of the hepatic contrast-enhancing effect of Gd-DTPA for the detection of hepatic metastases, it is necessary to use rapid scanning techniques such as gradient echo or rapid acquisition spin echo (RASE) imaging.[22,40]

An advantage of using iron oxide particles for hepatic contrast enhancement is that rapid MR imaging techniques are not necessary. Conventional spin echo techniques can be used to obtain images 30 minutes to several hours after injection of the drug.[80] Animal and clinical studies using superparamagnetic iron oxide (ferrite) as a contrast agent have shown increased sensitivity for the detection of hepatic metastases with a decreased threshold size for lesion detectability.[72,76] In these studies, lesions of 2–3 mm could be detected. In another clinical study, iron oxide-enhanced images did not show significantly more metastases than the T2-weighted images.[36] As mentioned, superparamagnetic iron oxide has not yet been approved for clinical use.

Hepatocellular carcinoma

The MRI appearance of hepatocellular carcinoma (HCC) correlates closely with its gross pathological features. Characteristic findings, although not always present, include a pseudocapsule, central scar, intramural septa, daughter nodules and tumour thrombus in portal or hepatic veins.[30] On T1-weighted images the majority

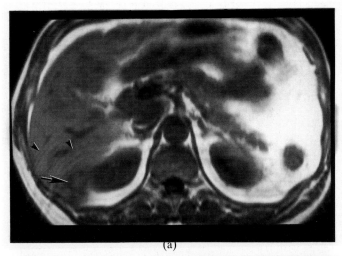

(a)

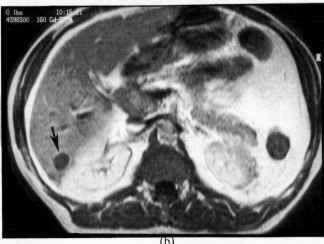

(b)

Figure 24.5 Hepatic metastasis from melanoma. (a) T1-weighted spin echo image shows an ill-defined area of heterogeneous low signal intensity in the right lobe posteriorly (arrow). The alternating high and low signal intensity parallel lines overlying the right lobe (arrowheads) represent 'ghost' artefacts from respiratory motion. (b) Dynamic Gd-DTPA-enhanced MR image using the rapid acquisition spin echo (RASE) technique shows improved delineation of the metastasis (arrow). Note that the improved tumour-to-liver contrast is due to an increase in the signal intensity of the normal hepatic parenchyma.

of HCCs are hypointense compared with normal liver parenchyma (Figure 24.6(a)). Itoh et al.[30] found that nearly half (47%) of HCCs demonstrated by MRI were either hyperintense or isointense on T1-weighted images. This feature helps in differentiating HCC from hepatic metastases, which are nearly always hypointense on T1-weighted images. The relatively high signal intensity on such images has been shown to correlate with fatty change in tumour cells.[58] Nearly all HCCs are hyperintense on T2-weighted images (Figure 24.6(b)).

A pseudocapsule composed of thick, fibrous tissue can be identified in 24–42% of HCCs,[13,30,58] particularly in the smaller tumours. On T1-weighted images, the pseudocapsule appears as a low signal intensity rim (Figure

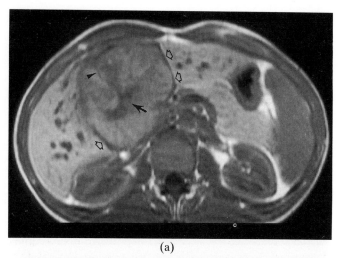

(a)

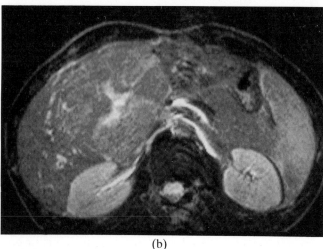

(b)

Figure 24.6 Hepatocellular carcinoma. (a) T1-weighted spin echo image shows a large encapsulated hepatic mass with a central low-signal intensity scar (arrow). The mass is heterogeneous in signal intensity and slightly hypointense compared with normal hepatic parenchyma. The low signal intensity fibrous capsule (open arrows) is well seen. A portion of an internal septum (arrowhead) is also identified. (b) On the T2-weighted spin echo image, the mass is minimally hyperintense compared with normal liver parenchyma and the central scar is now bright. The capsule and septum are not well seen.

24.6(a)). In about one-half of patients the pseudocapsule can also be demonstrated on T2-weighted images as a double-layered peripheral band. An inner, low-intensity band corresponds to fibrous tissue (the pseudocapsule) and an outer high-intensity band represents a zone of compressed small vessels or newly formed bile ducts.[30] A pseudocapsule is not specific for HCC but can also be seen with some adenomas.[58]

Internal features of HCC can include the presence of a central scar or intratumoural septa. A central scar, if present, is low in signal intensity on T1-weighted images but may be either low or high in signal intensity on T2-weighted images (Figure 24.6). Intratumoural septa are thinner than either scars or pseudocapsules and are low in signal intensity on both T1- and T2-weighted images (Figure 24.6). They often divide the mass into compartments of variable signal intensity. The presence of intratumoural septa or a central scar is not specific for HCC but may also be seen with hepatocellular adenoma, focal nodular hyperplasia or giant cavernous haemangioma.[57]

Vascular invasion is much more characteristic of HCC than of other malignant hepatic neoplasms and was identified in 6 of 21 patients in one series.[58] On MRI, tumour thrombus appears as intermediate or high signal intensity material within the portal or hepatic veins on T1- or T2-weighted images respectively. Tumour thrombus can be distinguished from flowing blood within the uninvolved vessels without the use of intravenous contrast material.

Daughter nodules (also called 'satellite lesions') are separate, usually smaller masses that are distinct from the main tumour. They are not specific for HCC.

Dynamic contrast-enhanced MR imaging of most HCCs using gradient echo or rapid spin-echo imaging after intravenous administration of Gd-DTPA shows peak contrast enhancement between 10 seconds and 2 minutes after injection of contrast material. The degree of contrast enhancement is generally slight to moderate, and delayed enhancement is usually minimal.[48,84] A peripheral halo of delayed enhancement, corresponding to fibrous capsular structures, can be identified in 43–55% of patients.[48,84] These enhancement features are useful in differentiating HCC from benign cavernous haemangioma, since haemangioma generally shows early peripheral enhancement with complete high signal intensity fill-in on delayed images.[84] On non-contrast-enhanced images, HCC can be differentiated from benign cavernous haemangioma in 82–95% of cases.[47,49]

Overall, MRI and CT are equivalent in the detection of HCC,[30] but MRI is superior to CT in characterizing these masses, particularly in showing a pseudocapsule and in demonstrating evidence of fatty change.[30,58]

Cavernous haemangioma

MRI has been shown to be useful in distinguishing cavernous haemangiomas from malignant hepatic neoplasms. This differentiation is based on the very long T2 relaxation of cavernous haemangioma compared with other hepatic masses. Consequently, cavernous haemangiomas are higher in signal intensity on T2-weighted images than other hepatic neoplasms (Figure 24.7). Other features characteristic but not diagnostic of cavernous haemangioma include a sharp margin and internal homogeneity,[7,18,28,35,68] although haemangiomas greater than 4 cm in diameter can be heterogeneous in signal intensity from various combinations of haemorrhage, thrombosis, fibrosis, hyalinization, and cystic degeneration.[8,53] Using quantitative characteristics alone (i.e. T2 values or lesion-to-liver signal

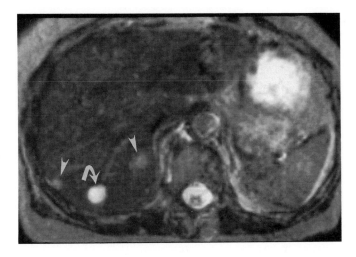

Figure 24.7 Cavernous haemangioma in a patient with hepatic metastases. T2-weighted spin echo image shows a small cavernous haemangioma (curved arrow) which is well circumscribed, homogeneous and very high in signal intensity. Note that the haemangioma is significantly brighter than the less well defined metastases (arrowheads).

intensity ratios), cavernous haemangiomas can be distinguished from malignant hepatic masses (metastases or hepatocellular carcinoma) with an accuracy of 81–92%.[28,41,44,47,49,68] When morphological characteristics are also considered, this differentiation can be made in 90–94% of cases.[41,68] However, vascular metastases such as those from pheochromocytoma, carcinoid and pancreatic islet cell tumours are occasionally difficult to distinguish from cavernous haemangioma because of their marked hyperintensity on T2-weighted images.[34,56] In such instances, dynamic Gd-DTPA enhanced MR imaging may be helpful in making this differentiation. Cavernous haemangiomas typically show early peripheral enhancement with complete hyperintense fill-in on delayed images (Figure 24.8). The peak contrast enhancement of cavernous haemangiomas is generally 2 minutes or later after injection, whereas malignant hepatic neoplasms characteristically show earlier, less intense peak enhancement and hypo- to isointensity compared to liver parenchyma on delayed images.[21,48,84] Contrast-enhanced imaging also distinguishes cavernous haemangiomas from hepatic cysts, which do not increase in signal intensity after injection of Gd-DTPA.

Focal nodular hyperplasia

Focal nodular hyperplasia generally has a signal intensity similar to that of normal liver parenchyma on both T1- and T2-weighted MR images.[39,58,63] A central scar, when present, is generally hypointense on T1-weighted images and hyperintense on T2-weighted images owing to the presence of prominent vascular channels within the fibrous tissue.

Hepatic adenoma

Hepatic adenoma is isointense or slightly hypointense compared with normal liver parenchyma on T1-weighted images and hyperintense on T2-weighted images.[58] On occasion, an adenoma may contain a central vascular scar or a capsule similar to those seen in focal nodular hyperplasia or hepatocellular carcinoma.[57]

Abscess

MRI is useful in both the diagnosis of hepatic abscess and evaluation of its response to treatment. The most widely studied is amoebic liver abscess.[15,51] Before treatment, amoebic abscesses appear as well-circumscribed round or oval masses that are heterogeneously low in signal intensity on T1-weighted images. On T2-weighted images, the abscess cavities demonstrate heterogeneous high signal intensity with a peripheral zone of surrounding high signal intensity corresponding to oedema within the adjacent hepatic parenchyma.[15] After treatment, the abscess cavities tend to become more homogeneously hypo- or hyperintense on T1-weighted or T2-weighted images, respectively, corresponding to central liquefactive necrosis. In addition, post-treatment images show multiple concentric rings of high and low signal intensity.[15,51] On T2-weighted images the central liquefied abscess is surrounded by a high signal intensity band of inflamed granulation tissue and more peripherally by a low-intensity band of collagen. A more peripheral band of high signal intensity, representing locally oedematous hepatic parenchyma, resolves rapidly after successful medical treatment has been initiated.[15] These ring features can also be seen with bacterial liver abscesses[77] and are indistinct prior to therapy. Contrast-enhanced MR imaging using either Gd-DTPA or ferrite particles has been shown to increase the conspicuousness of experimentally induced abscesses in rats and to help define the evolution of the abscess capsule.[64,79]

Hydatid disease

On MRI, hydatid cysts often have a distinctive appearance consisting of a relatively thick (up to 5 mm) low signal intensity peripheral rim, seen best on T2-weighted images in which the hyperintense cyst fluid is sharply demarcated from the intermediate signal intensity hepatic parenchyma.[9,26] On T1-weighted images the cyst fluid is hypointense. Occasionally, multiple internal loculations representing daughter cysts can be identified.[9] Hydatid cysts can usually be differentiated from hepatic abscesses by the presence of a well-defined capsule and lack of surrounding hepatic oedema prior to treatment.

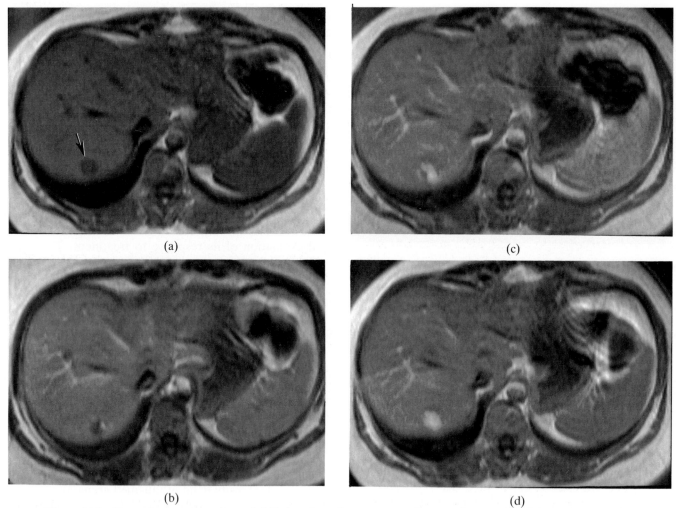

(a)

(b)

(c)

(d)

Figure 24.8 Dynamic contrast-enhanced MR imaging of a cavernous haemangioma using Gd-DTPA and rapid acquisition spin echo (RASE) imaging. (a) Pre-contrast image shows a well-defined hypointense hepatic mass (arrow). (b,c,d) Images obtained 1, 2 and 5 minutes, respectively, after intravenous injection of Gd-DTPA demonstrate gradual centripetal enhancement of the mass with complete enhancement on the 5-minute image (d).

DIFFUSE DISEASE

Iron overload

Spin-echo MRI techniques are very sensitive for detecting clinically significant hepatic iron overload. MRI shows dramatic reductions in the hepatic signal intensity in patients with idiopathic, transfusional or dietary haemosiderosis or haemochromatosis[3,59,67,71] (Figure 24.9). This signal alteration is due to the paramagnetic effect of the ferric ions (Fe^{3+}), which causes shortening of the T1- and T2-relaxation of nearby protons.[67,71] The T2 shortening is the predominant effect and accounts for the reduction in hepatic signal intensity on both T1- and T2-weighted images. Attempts at quantifying liver iron with MRI have been unsuccessful owing to the low hepatic signal intensities in patients with iron overload, the broad range of liver T1- and T2-values observed in normal volunteers, and the fluctuation of values measured in individuals on serial examinations.[4,5,25] These fluctuations are large

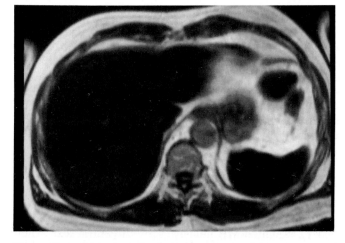

Figure 24.9 Hepatic and splenic iron overload due to repeated blood transfusions. The signal intensity of the liver and spleen are abnormally low on a T1-weighted image.

relative to the expected changes due to hepatic iron deposition. Thus, at present, MRI is not a reliable method for quantifying hepatic iron deposition or for monitoring the treatment of patients with hepatic iron overload.

Fatty change

MRI using conventional spin-echo techniques is generally insensitive in the detection of fatty change of the liver,[12,67,69] although areas of marked fatty change may show increased signal intensity on T1-weighted images[81] (Figure 24.10). Proton chemical shift imaging techniques (proton spectroscopic imaging; phase contrast imaging) have shown improved sensitivity for detecting fatty liver.[23,32,55] These techniques exploit the difference in resonance frequency between protons in fatty acid molecules and protons in water molecules, allowing separation of the fat and water signals. On opposed-phase images in which the fat signal is subtracted from the water signal, fatty liver has lower than normal signal intensity, usually equal to or less than that of muscle[32] (Figure 24.10(c)). Quantitation of the lipid signal fraction can be used to separate fatty liver from normal liver and to corroborate the visual impression of fatty change.[23]

A problem frequently encountered with hepatic computed tomography is difficulty differentiating between focal fatty change and neoplasm. Although chemical shift MRI can differentiate these two entities directly, conventional spin-echo sequences are also capable of making this distinction. Tumour is generally hypointense compared to normal liver parenchyma on T1-weighted images and hyperintense on T2-weighted images, whereas focal fatty change is isointense on T2-weighted images and either isointense or hyperintense on T1-weighted images. Thus, MRI is capable of making a definitive distinction between focal fatty change and hepatic neoplasm.[62]

Cirrhosis

MRI is capable of demonstrating the characteristic morphological features of cirrhosis such as nodularity of the hepatic contour and prominence of the caudate and/or left lobes. Cirrhosis does not significantly alter the T1 and T2 relaxation of liver tissue,[1,12,20,69] and therefore MRI does not have a significant advantage over CT in imaging patients with this disorder. MRI can help to differentiate regenerating nodules from malignant hepatic neoplasms. On T2-weighted images, regenerating nodules appear as foci of low signal intensity,[27,37,46] whereas most malignant neoplasms are hyperintense on such images. The secondary extrahepatic findings of cirrhosis such as portosystemic collaterals, ascites, and splenomegaly are also well-depicted on MRI. In addition, MRI is useful in demonstrating patency of the portal vein or of surgically created portosystemic shunts.[75]

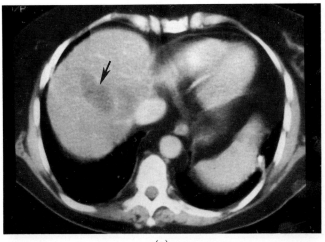

(a)

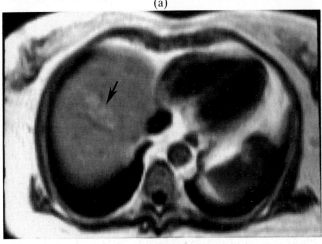

(b)

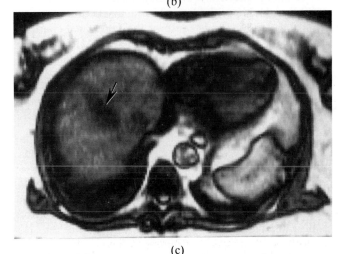

(c)

Figure 24.10 Focal fatty change of the liver. (a) Dynamic contrast-enhanced CT scan shows an ovoid area of low density in the liver (arrow). (b) T1-weighted spin echo image at the same level as (a) shows the abnormal area to be slightly higher in signal intensity (arrow) than the normal hepatic parenchyma. (c) Opposed-phase chemical-shift MR image at the same level as (a) and (b) shows the area of abnormality (arrow) to be hypointense compared with normal liver parenchyma, confirming that the abnormality represents focal fatty change (see text).

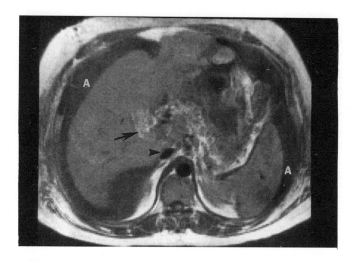

Figure 24.11 Portal vein thrombosis in a patient with portal hypertension. On this T1-weighted spin echo image the portal vein (arrow) contains intermediate signal intensity, rather than the normal vascular signal void as seen in the inferior vena cava (arrowhead). A=ascites.

Hepatitis

Both experimental animal data and preliminary clinical data have demonstrated prolongation of the hepatic T1 and T2 relaxation in hepatitis, with increased signal intensity on T2-weighted MR images.[67,69] Thus, MRI is capable of distinguishing hepatitis from cirrhosis in which no significant alteration in T1 or T2 occurs. In addition, superparamagnetic iron oxide-enhanced MR imaging in patients with hepatitis has shown markedly reduced response to iron oxide because of the functional changes in the hepatic parenchyma.[16] Nevertheless, MRI thus far has not proved to be clinically useful in the evaluation of patients with hepatitis.

Portal vein thrombosis

Magnetic resonance imaging can demonstrate portal vein thrombosis without any administration of intravenous contrast material.[33,45] Because normally flowing blood produces little or no signal on MR images, blood vessels with normal flow appear as regions of signal void. When portal vein thrombosis is present, a significant amount of signal is detected within the portal vein (Figure 24.11). In patients with portal hypertension, distinction between portal vein thrombosis and sluggish flow within the portal vein may be difficult.[82] A helpful sign of intrahepatic portal vein occlusion is segmental hepatic signal intensity difference compared with the remainder of the liver parenchyma. This finding consists of homogeneous higher signal intensity of the affected segment on T2-weighted images and, in some cases, lower signal intensity on T1-weighted images.[29] Another frequent feature of portal vein thrombosis on MRI is the demonstration of periportal collaterals, appearing as multiple small foci of signal void

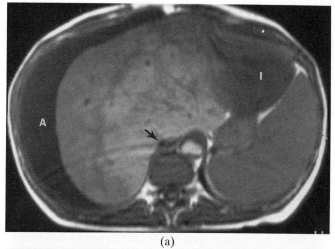

(a)

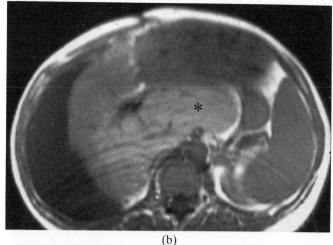

(b)

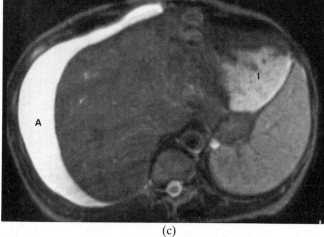

(c)

Figure 24.12 Budd–Chiari syndrome. (a) T1-weighted spin echo image shows heterogeneous hepatic parenchymal signal intensity due to venous congestion. The hepatic veins are not visible and the inferior vena cava (arrow) is compressed. The wedge-shaped zone of low signal intensity in the lateral segment of the left lobe represents an area of infarction (I). Ascites (A) and splenomegaly are also present. (b) A more caudal T1-weighted spin echo image shows enlargement of the caudate lobe (∗). (c) On a T2-weighted image the ascites and infarction are high in signal intensity.

within or surrounding the expected location of the portal vein.[54]

MRI techniques have also been shown to be capable of measuring portal blood flow.[14,74] Since assessment of portal haemodynamics is important in determining treatment in some patients with portal hypertension, MRI can non-invasively provide valuable information in these patients.

Budd–Chiari syndrome

MRI, like other cross-sectional imaging techniques, demonstrates the characteristic morphological features of Budd–Chiari syndrome, including hepatomegaly and marked reduction in calibre or lack of visible hepatic veins and/or intrahepatic inferior vena cava[17,70] (Figure 24.12). The caudate lobe may be enlarged owing to sparing of its venous outflow, which drains directly into the inferior vena cava separate from the hepatic veins. In patients with acute Budd–Chiari syndrome, the caudate lobe may have lower water content and shorter T2 relaxation values than the remaining, congested liver.[66] The hepatic parenchyma is often heterogeneous on both T1- and T2-weighted images owing to the hepatic venous congestion (Figure 24.12). 'Comma-shaped' signal void foci representing intrahepatic collateral vessels have also been described.[70] Ascites is almost invariably present.

BILIARY TRACT

Experience with MRI for evaluation of the biliary system has been limited. Image degradation from motion-related blurring and ghosting has thus far hampered the use of MRI in this area.[65] With motion-suppression techniques and new fast scanning methods, these limitations are currently being overcome.

The normal extrahepatic bile ducts can be identified in the majority of patients, particularly on T1-weighted images. The common bile duct appears as a low signal intensity structure on T1-weighted images and is high in signal intensity on T2-weighted images. In a study of MR imaging of the dilated biliary tract, the dilated intra- and extrahepatic ducts were identified in all 18 patients evaluated.[10] In some cases, dilated intrahepatic bile ducts may be difficult to differentiate from portal veins on conventional spin echo images. In such cases, gradient echo and contrast-enhanced fast scanning techniques may be useful in resolving the ambiguity. Periportal abnormal

signal intensity, consisting of ring-like or linear areas surrounding the intrahepatic portal veins, has been found to be a reliable indicator of bile duct disease.[38] The periportal abnormal intensity, which is low on T1-weighted and high on T2-weighted images, corresponds histologically to oedema, inflammatory cell infiltration, and proliferation of bile ductules in the portal tracts. In a study of a large number of patients this finding was present in all those with biliary diseases, including cholangitis, cholangiocarcinoma and obstructive jaundice.[38] The finding was absent in patients without biliary disease and in those with biliary dilatation without obstructive jaundice or cholangitis. In another study in which nine patients with cholangiocarcinoma were examined by MRI and CT, the investigators concluded that the information obtained with MRI was equal to that obtained with CT.[11]

Despite the optimistic reports of the ability of MRI to detect and evaluate bile duct abnormalities, CT and ultrasound remain the non-invasive imaging procedures of choice for evaluating suspected biliary diseases. Elucidation of the role of MRI in biliary tract imaging will require further investigation.

SUMMARY

The role of MRI in hepatic and biliary imaging is still evolving. MRI has already proved valuable in the detection and characterization of focal hepatic masses, assessment of certain diffuse hepatic parenchymal disorders, and evaluation of hepatic and portal venous blood flow. Further technological advances including improved motion-suppression techniques, rapid scanning methods and the use of intravenous contrast agents offer exciting prospects for the continued expansion of the role of MRI in hepatobiliary imaging. In addition, MR spectroscopy, a technique which is still in its infancy, may become a valuable adjunct to hepatic MR imaging.

The exciting current and potential applications of MRI notwithstanding, enthusiasm for MR imaging of the liver must be counterbalanced with considerations of cost, availability and the relative merits of other non-invasive imaging techniques such as computed tomography and ultrasound both for evaluation of the liver and for detection of extrahepatic disease. Despite rapid advances in hepatic MRI, computed tomography and ultrasound remain the imaging procedures of choice for evaluation of the biliary tract. The role of MRI in hepatic and biliary imaging will continue to evolve for some time.

REFERENCES

1. Bernardino, M.E., Small, W., Goldstein, J. *et al.* (1983) Multiple NMR T2 relaxation values in human liver tissue. *American Journal of Roentgenology*, **141**, 1203–1208.
2. Bloch, F. (1946) Nuclear induction. *Physical Reviews*, **70**, 460–474.
3. Brasch, R.C., Wesbey, G.E., Gooding, G.A. & Koerper, M.A. (1984) Magnetic resonance imaging of transfusional hemosiderosis complicating thalassemia major. *Radiology*, **150**, 767–771.
4. Brown, D.W., Henkelman, R.M., Poon, P.Y. & Fisher, M.M. (1985) Nuclear magnetic resonance study of iron overload in liver tissue. *Magnetic Resonance Imaging*, **3**, 275–282.
5. Chezmar, J.L., Nelson, R.C., Malko, J.A. & Bernardino, M.E. (1990) Hepatic iron overload: diagnosis and quantification by noninvasive imaging. *Gastrointestinal Radiology*, **15**, 27–31.
6. Chezmar, J.L., Rumancik, W.M., Megibow, A.J. *et al.* (1988) Liver

and abdominal screening in patients with cancer: CT vs MR imaging. *Radiology*, **168**, 43–47.

7. Choi, B.I., Han, M.C. & Kim, C.-W. (1990) Small hepatocellular carcinoma versus small cavernous hemangioma: differentiation with MR imaging at 2.0 T. *Radiology*, **176**, 103–106.

8. Choi, B.I., Han, M.C., Park, J.H. *et al.* (1989) Giant cavernous hemangioma of the liver: CT and MR imaging in 10 cases. *American Journal of Roentgenology*, **152**, 1221–1226.

9. Davolio Marani, S.A., Cavossi, G.C., Nicoli, F.A. *et al.* (1990) Hydatid disease: MR imaging study. *Radiology*, **175**, 701–706.

10. Dooms, G.C., Fisher, M.R., Higgins, C.B. *et al.* (1986) MR imaging of the dilated biliary tract. *Radiology*, **158**, 337–341.

11. Dooms, G.C., Kerland, R.K. Jr., Hricak, H. *et al.* (1986) Cholangiocarcinoma: imaging by MR. *Radiology*, **159**, 89–94.

12. Doyle, F.H., Pennock, J.M., Banks, L.M. *et al.* (1982) Nuclear magnetic resonance imaging of the liver: initial experience. *American Journal of Roentgenology*, **138**, 193–200.

13. Ebara, M., Ohto, M., Watanabe, Y. *et al.* (1986) Diagnosis of small hepatocellular carcinoma: correlation of MR imaging and tumor histologic studies. *Radiology*, **159**, 371–377.

14. Edelman, R.R., Zhao, B., Liu, C. *et al.* (1989) MR angiography and dynamic flow evaluation of the portal venous system. *American Journal of Roentgenology*, **153**, 755–760.

15. Elizondo, G., Weissleder, R., Stark, D.D. *et al.* (1987) Amebic liver abscess: diagnosis and treatment evaluation with MR imaging. *Radiology*, **165**, 795–800.

16. Elizondo,G., Weissleder, R., Stark, D.D. *et al.* (1990) Hepatic cirrhosis and hepatitis: MR imaging enhanced with superparamagnetic iron oxide. *Radiology*, **174**, 797–801.

17. Friedman, A.C., Ramchandani, P., Black, M. *et al.* (1986) Magnetic resonance imaging diagnosis of Budd–Chiari syndrome. *Gastroenterology*, **91**, 1289–1295.

18. Glazer, G.M., Aisen, A.M., Francis, I.R. *et al.* (1985) Hepatic cavernous hemangioma: magnetic resonance imaging. *Radiology*, **155**, 417–420.

19. Glazer, G.M., Aisen, A.M., Francis, I.R. *et al.* (1986) Evaluation of focal hepatic masses: a comparative study of MRI and CT. *Gastrointestinal Radiology*, **11**, 263–268.

20. Goldberg, H.I., Moss, A., Stark, D.D. *et al.* (1984) Hepatic cirrhosis: magnetic resonance imaging. *Radiology*, **153**, 737–739.

21. Hamm, B., Fischer, E. & Taupitz, M. (1990) Differentiation of hepatic hemangiomas from metastases by dynamic contrast–enhanced MR imaging. *Journal of Computer Assisted Tomography*, **14**, 205–216.

22. Hamm, B., Wolf, K.-J. & Felix, R. (1987) Conventional and rapid MR imaging of the liver with Gd-DTPA. *Radiology*, **164**, 313–320.

23. Heiken, J.P., Lee, J.K.T. & Dixon, W.T. (1985) Fatty infiltration of the liver: evaluation by proton spectroscopic imaging. *Radiology*, **157**, 707–710.

24. Heiken, J.P., Weyman, P.J., Lee, J.K.T. *et al.* (1989) Detection of focal hepatic masses: prospective evaluation with CT, delayed CT, CT during arterial portography, and MR imaging. *Radiology*, **171**, 47–51.

25. Hernandez, R.J., Sarnaik, S.A., Lande, I. *et al.* (1988) MR evaluation of liver iron overload. *Journal of Computer Assisted Tomography*, **12**, 91–94.

26. Hoff, F.L., Aisen, A.M., Walden, M.E. & Glazer, G.M. (1987) MR imaging in hydatid disease of the liver. *Gastrointestinal Radiology*, **12**, 39–42.

27. Itai, Y., Ohnishi, S., Ohtomo, K. *et al.* (1987) Regenerating nodules of liver cirrhosis: MR imaging. *Radiology*, **165**, 419–423.

28. Itai, Y., Ohtomo, K., Furui, S. *et al.* (1985) Noninvasive diagnosis of small cavernous hemangioma of the liver: advantage of MRI. *American Journal of Roentgenology*, **145**, 1195–1199.

29. Itai, Y., Ohtomo, K., Kokubo, T. *et al.* (1988) Segmental intensity differences in the liver on MR images: a sign of intrahepatic portal flow stoppage. *Radiology*, **167**, 17–19.

30. Itoh, K., Nishimura, K., Togashi, K. *et al.* (1987) Hepatocellular carcinoma: MR imaging. *Radiology*, **164**, 21–25.

31. Lauterbur, P.C. (1973) Image formation by induced local interactions: examples employing nuclear magnetic resonance. *Nature*, **242**, 190–191.

32. Lee, J.K.T., Dixon, W.T., Ling, D. *et al.* (1984) Fatty infiltration

of the liver: demonstration by proton spectroscopic imaging: preliminary observations. *Radiology*, **153**, 195–201.

33. Levy, H.M. & Newhouse, J.H. (1988) MR imaging of portal vein thrombosis. *American Journal of Roentgenology*, **151**, 283–286.

34. Li, K.C., Glazer, G.M., Quint, L.E. *et al.* (1988) Distinction of hepatic cavernous hemangioma from hepatic metastases with MR imaging. *Radiology*, **169**, 409–415.

35. Lombardo, D.M., Baker, M.E., Spritzer, C.E. *et al.* (1990) Hepatic hemangiomas vs metastases: MR differentiation at 1.5 T. *American Journal of Roentgenology*, **155**, 55–59.

36. Marchal, G., Vanhecke, P., Damaerel, P. *et al.* (1989) Detection of liver metastases with superparamagnetic iron oxide in 15 patients: results of MR imaging at 1.5 T. *American Journal of Roentgenology*, **152**, 771–775.

37. Matsui, O., Kadoya, M., Kameyama, T. *et al.* (1989) Adenomatous hyperplastic nodules in the cirrhotic liver: differentiation from hepatocellular carcinoma with MR imaging. *Radiology*, **173**, 123–126.

38. Matsui, O., Kadoya, M., Takashima, T. *et al.* (1989) Intrahepatic periportal abnormal intensity on MR images: an indication of various hepatobiliary diseases. *Radiology*, **171**, 335–338.

39. Mattison, G.R., Glazer, G.M., Quint, L.E. *et al.* (1987) MR imaging of hepatic focal nodular hyperplasia: characterization and distinction from primary malignant hepatic tumors. *American Journal of Roentgenology*, **148**, 711–715.

40. Mirowitz, S.A., Lee, J.K.T., Gutierrez, E. *et al.* (1991) Dynamic gadolinium–DTPA enhanced rapid acquisition spin echo (RASE) MR imaging of the liver. *Radiology* **179**, 371–376.

41. Mirowitz, S.A., Lee, J.K.T. & Heiken, J.P. (1990) Cavernous hemangioma of the liver: assessment of MR tissue specificity with a simplified T2 index. *Journal of Computer Assisted Tomography*, **14**, 223–228.

42. Moss, A.A., Goldberg, H.I., Stark, D.D. *et al.* (1984) Hepatic tumors: magnetic resonance and CT appearance. *Radiology*, **150**, 141–147.

43. Nelson, R.C., Chezmar, J.L., Sugarbaker, P.H. & Bernardino, M.E. (1989) Hepatic tumors: comparison of CT during arterial portography, delayed CT, and MR imaging for preoperative evaluation. *Radiology*, **172**, 27–34.

44. Ohtomo, K., Itai, Y., Furui, S. *et al.* (1985) Hepatic tumors: differentiation by transverse relaxation time (T2) of magnetic resonance imaging. *Radiology*, **155**, 421–423.

45. Ohtomo, K., Itai, Y., Furui, S. *et al.* (1985) MR imaging of portal vein thrombus in hepatocellular carcinoma. *Journal of Computer Assisted Tomography*, **9**, 328–329.

46. Ohtomo, K., Itai, Y., Ohtomo, Y. *et al.* (1990) Regenerating nodules of liver cirrhosis: MR imaging with pathologic correlation. *American Journal of Roentgenology*, **154**, 505–507.

47. Ohtomo, K., Itai, Y., Yoshida, H. *et al.* (1989) MR differentiation of hepatocellular carcinoma from cavernous hemangioma: complementary roles of FLASH and T2 values. *American Journal of Roentgenology*, **152**, 505–507.

48. Ohtomo, K., Itai, Y., Yoshikawa, K. *et al.* (1987) Hepatic tumors: dynamic MR imaging. *Radiology*, **163**, 27–31.

49. Ohtomo, K., Itai, Y., Yoshikawa, K. *et al.* (1988) Hepatocellular carcinoma and cavernous hemangioma: differentiation with MR imaging: efficacy of T2 values at 0.35 and 1.5 T. *Radiology*, **168**, 621–623.

50. Purcell, E.M., Torvey, H.C. & Pound, R.V. (1946) Resonance absorption by nuclear magnetic moment in a solid. *Physical Reviews*, **69**, 37–38.

51. Ralls, P.W., Henley, D.S., Colletti, P.M. *et al.* (1987) Amebic liver abscess: MR imaging. *Radiology*, **165**, 801–804.

52. Reinig, J.W., Dwyer, A.J., Miller, D.L. *et al.* (1987) Liver metastasis detection: comparative sensitivities of MR imaging and CT scanning. *Radiology*, **162**, 43–47.

53. Ros, P.R., Lubbers, P.P., Olmsted, W.W. & Morillo, G. (1987) Hemangioma of the liver: heterogeneous appearance on T2-weighted images. *American Journal of Roentgenology*, **149**, 1167–1170.

54. Ros, P.R., Viamonte, M. Jr., Koka, K. *et al.* (1986) Demonstration of cavernomatous transformation of the portal vein by magnetic resonance imaging. *Gastrointestinal Radiology*, **11**, 90–92.

55. Rosen, B.R., Carter, E.A., Pykett, I.L. *et al.* (1985) Proton

chemical shift imaging: an evaluation of its clinical potential using an in vivo fatty liver model. *Radiology*, **154**, 469–472.

56. Rummeny, E., Saini, S., Wittenberg, J. *et al.* (1989) MR imaging of liver neoplasms. *American Journal of Roentgenology*, **152**, 493–499.

57. Rummeny, E., Weissleder, R., Sironi, S. *et al.* (1989) Central scars in primary liver tumors: MR features, specificity, and pathologic correlation. *Radiology*, **171**, 323–326.

58. Rummeny, E., Weissleder, R., Stark, D.D. *et al.* (1989) Primary liver tumors: diagnosis by MR imaging. *American Journal of Roentgenology*, **152**, 63–72.

59. Runge, V.M., Clanton, J.A., Smith, F.W. *et al.* (1983) Nuclear magnetic resonance of iron and copper disease states. *American Journal of Roentgenology*, **141**, 943–948.

60. Saini, S., Stark, D.D., Brady, T.J. *et al.* (1986) Dynamic spin-echo MRI of liver cancer using gadolinium-DTPA: animal investigation. *American Journal of Roentgenology*, **147**, 357–362.

61. Saini, S., Stark, D.D., Hahn, P.F. *et al.* (1987) Ferrite particles: a superparamagnetic MR contrast agent for the reticuloendothelial system. *Radiology*, **162**, 211–216.

62. Schertz, L.D., Lee, J.K.T., Heiken, J.P. *et al.* (1989) Proton spectroscopic imaging (Dixon method) of the liver: clinical utility. *Radiology*, **173**, 401–405.

63. Schiebler, M.L., Kressel, H.Y., Saul, S.H. *et al.* (1987) MR imaging of focal nodular hyperplasia of the liver. *Journal of Computer Assisted Tomography*, **11**, 651–654.

64. Schmiedl, U., Poajanen, H., Arakawa, M. *et al.* (1988) MR imaging of liver abscesses; application of Gd-DTPA. *Magnetic Resonance Imaging*, **6**, 9–16.

65. Spritzer, C., Kressel, H.Y., Mitchell, D. & Axel, L. (1987) MR imaging of normal extrahepatic bile ducts. *Journal of Computer Assisted Tomography*, **11**, 248–252.

66. Stark, D.D. (1988). Liver. In Stark, D.D. & Bradley, W.G. (eds) *Magnetic Resonance Imaging*, pp.934–1059. St. Louis: C.V. Mosby.

67. Stark, D.D., Bass, N.M., Moss, A.A. *et al.* (1983) Nuclear magnetic resonance imaging of experimentally induced liver disease. *Radiology*, **148**, 743–751.

68. Stark, D.D., Felder, R.C., Wittenberg, J. *et al.* (1985) Magnetic resonance imaging of cavernous hemangioma of the liver: tissue-specific characterization. *American Journal of Roentgenology*, **145**, 213–222.

69. Stark, D.D., Goldberg, H.I., Moss, A.A. & Bass, N.M. (1984) Chronic liver disease: evaluation by magnetic resonance. *Radiology*, **150**, 149–151.

70. Stark, D.D., Hahn, P.F., Trey, C. *et al.* (1986) MRI of the Budd–Chiari syndrome. *American Journal of Roentgenology*, **146**, 1141–1148.

71. Stark, D.D., Moseley, M.E., Bacon, B.R. *et al.* (1985) Magnetic resonance imaging and spectroscopy of hepatic iron overload. *Radiology*, **154**, 137–142.

72. Stark, D.D., Weissleder, R., Elizondo, G. *et al.* (1988) Superparamagnetic iron oxide: clinical application as a contrast agent for MR imaging of the liver. *Radiology*, **168**, 297–301.

73. Stark, D.D., Wittenberg, J., Butch, R.J. & Ferrucci, J.T. Jr. (1987) Hepatic metastases: randomized, controlled comparison of detection with MR imaging and CT. *Radiology*, **165**, 399–406.

74. Tamada, T., Moriyasu, F., Ono, S. *et al.* (1989) Portal blood flow: measurement with MR imaging. *Radiology*, **173**, 639–644.

75. Torres, W.E., Gaylord, G.M., Whitmire, L. *et al.* (1987) The correlation between MR and angiography in portal hypertension. *American Journal of Roentgenology*, **148**, 1109–1112.

76. Tsang, Y.-M., Stark, D.D., Chen, M.C.-M. *et al.* (1988) Hepatic micrometastases in the rat: ferrite-enhanced MR imaging. *Radiology*, **167**, 21–24.

77. Vassiliades, V.C.G. & Bernardino, M.E. (1990) Magnetic resonance imaging of the liver. *Topics in Magnetic Resonance Imaging*, **2**, 1–16.

78. Waluch, V. & Bradley, W.G. Jr. (1984) NMR even echo rephasing in slow laminar flow. *Journal of Computer Assisted Tomography*, **8**, 594–598.

79. Weissleder, R., Saini, S., Stark, D.D. *et al.* (1988) Pyogenic liver abscess: contrast-enhanced MR imaging in rats. *American Journal of Roentgenology*, **150**, 115–120.

80. Weissleder, R., Stark, D.D., Engelstad, B.L. *et al.* (1989) Superparamagnetic iron oxide: pharmacokinetics and toxicity. *American Journal of Roentgenology*, **152**, 167–173.

81. Wenker, J.C., Baker, M.K., Ellis, J.H. & Glant, M.D. (1984) Focal fatty infiltration of the liver: demonstration by magnetic resonance imaging. *American Journal of Roentgenology*, **143**, 573–574.

82. Williams, D.M., Cho, K.J., Aisen, A.M. & Eckhauser, F.E. (1985) Portal hypertension evaluated by MR imaging. *Radiology*, **157**, 703–706.

83. Wittenberg, J., Stark, D.D., Forman, B.H. *et al.* (1988) Differentiation of hepatic metastases from hepatic hemangiomas and cysts by using MR imaging. *American Journal of Roentgenology*, **151**, 79–84.

84. Yoshida, H., Itai, Y., Ohtomo, K. *et al.* (1989) Small hepatocellular carcinoma and cavernous hemangioma: differentiation with dynamic FLASH MR imaging with Gd-DTPA. *Radiology*, **171**, 339–342.

85. Zeman, R.K., Dritschilo, A., Silverman, P.M. *et al.* (1989) Dynamic CT vs 0.5 T MR imaging in the detection of surgically proven hepatic metastases. *Journal of Computer Assisted Tomography*, **13**, 637–644.

CHAPTER 25

Angiography

Robert Dick

At present there are fewer patients requiring angiography for liver and biliary tract diseases than a decade ago. This is because the newer imaging techniques such as duplex Doppler sonography and magnetic resonance imaging (MRI) do not involve ionizing radiation or patient discomfort. Though an invasive investigation, angiography provides, in properly selected patients, diagnostic information which outweighs the risks of irradiation and of the contrast medium used. Angiography is certain to retain its place in diagnosis, and the introduction of non-ionic contrast media (Omnipaque, Niopam) has made the procedure safer. It is increasingly used in an 'interventional' or 'therapeutic' role.[8]

As with computed tomography (CT), angiography provides an anatomical or pathological display yet has the advantage of providing the additional haemodynamic information so important in liver disease. In the investigation of the biliary tract, especially that of the patient with obstructive jaundice, angiography is much less essential in diagnosis than cholangiography and ultrasonography[27] as most biliary tract tumours are avascular. It may nevertheless provide important information if radical surgery is being planned.

Each patient requires an individual rather than an 'algorithmic' type of approach. It is essential that clinicians, radiologists and physicists establish the correct order of investigations. For example, in a patient with acute or continuing gastrointestinal bleeding, angiography is the prime investigation, whereas in suspected cystic liver disease, ultrasonography is pre-eminent. Wherever possible, non-invasive tests should be performed before invasive ones.

In some patients, ultrasonography, radioisotope scanning, CT and angiography will give cumulative information. One or more of these investigations should almost always provide an accurate pre-operative diagnosis of the pathology in patients undergoing an elective laparotomy for liver and biliary disease.

EQUIPMENT, TECHNIQUE AND RISKS

Sophisticated equipment is necessary to achieve the best angiograms. Basic requirements are a high-output generator, X-ray tubes with standard and small (0.3 mm) focal spot for routine and magnification radiography respectively, biplane fluoroscopy, videotape recording, electrically operated flow rate injector, rapid film changers and automatic film processing. Digital vascular subtraction angiography (DSA) is a further desirable refinement and the cost of a modern angiographic unit exceeds £300 000.

Angiography requires meticulous care of the patient both during and after the procedure. By using guided catheters and deflector assemblies operators with reasonable dexterity can become proficient at main trunk and branch catheterization in both the arterial and venous systems. It is important to avoid long examinations and to use the smallest-diameter catheter possible (Fr 5), with as few catheter changes as necessary. The aim is selective catheterization of vessels to give maximum opacification of the territories supplied by the coeliac and superior mesenteric arteries, and of the portal and hepatic venous systems, but keeping the total dose of contrast injected below 1 gram of iodine per kilogram of body weight. Provided that bleeding tendencies are corrected and the risk of further hepatic and/or renal insufficiency is minimized, complications are rare. Non-ionic contrast media are both better tolerated and less toxic than ionic ones and, as they do not cause pain, procedures can be performed under local anaesthesia. If DSA is used, then even small vascular abnormalities can be seen using very small volumes of contrast media (see Figure 25.29); alternatively, contrast injected into veins of the arm or leg may give large-organ information on delayed frames, making arterial catheterization unnecessary. Some clinicians prefer the standard angiogram format to DSA studies.

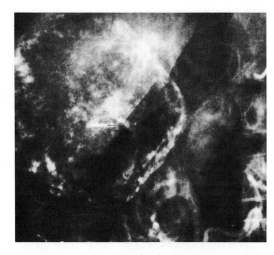

Figure 25.2 Palpable liver mass, 60-year-old male. Discrete blush at 20 s typical of haemangioma. Operative proof. Cure.

LIVER AND BILIARY TUMOURS

Many liver neoplasms have characteristic arteriographic features that differ widely from the normal hepatic arterial pattern (Figure 25.1). If the neoplasm is vascular, it is often possible to distinguish haemangioma, liver-cell adenoma and primary hepatocellular carcinoma (HCC). Haemangioma develops a 'mimosa' blush which persists beyond 12 seconds, and the tumour may be circumscribed (Figure 25.2). Liver cell adenomas (Figure 25.3), HCC and the rare angiosarcoma are usually highly vascular.

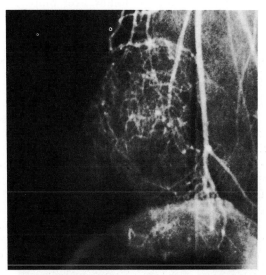

Figure 25.3 Selective hepatic arteriogram. Defined vascular tumour in lower right lobe. Liver cell adenoma. Female on contraceptive pill.

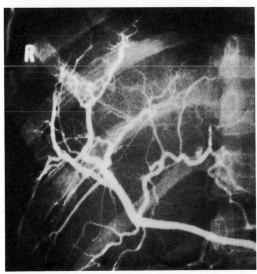

Figure 25.1 Hepatic arteriogram. Normal arterial/arteriolar pattern.

The diagnosis of HCC by angiography is usually straightforward, and is the best method for indicating operability, as angiographic extent correlates well with the surgical findings in 80% of cases.[21] HCC has a bizarre vascularity with dilated tumour arterioles and irregular veins (Figure 25.4). Extrahepatic or intrahepatic arteriovenous shunting may occur.[24] Such early portal venous filling may rarely

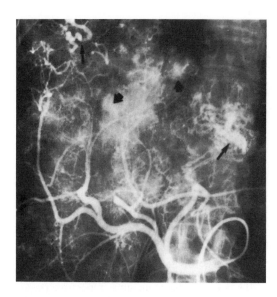

Figure 25.4 Superselective hepatic arteriogram. Diffuse malignant circulation. Tumour stains (short fat arrows) and abnormal veins (long thin arrows). Biopsy = primary liver cell cancer.

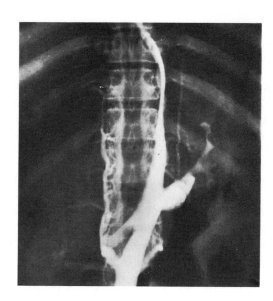

Figure 25.6 Inferior venacavogram. Hepatic cava displaced and invaded by liver cancer right lobe. Vertebral venous plexus fills.

be a feature of cirrhosis or follow liver biopsy, but if widespread is virtually diagnostic of HCC (Figure 25.5). It sometimes occurs locally in regenerative nodules and other neoplasms.[29] Angiograms may show the tumour spreading to hepatic veins, inferior vena cava (Figure 25.6) or extrahepatic structures (Figure 25.7), as well

as the presence of associated cirrhosis (Figure 25.8). Demonstration of an uninvolved lobe, makes consideration of hemihepatectomy worthwhile (Figure 25.9a and b). In inoperable malignancy, an arterial catheter may be left in the hepatic artery, permitting cytotoxic drug perfusion. The possibility of embolizing large tumour

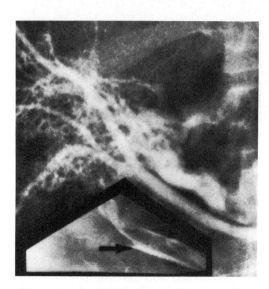

Figure 25.5 Selective hepatic arteriogram. Tumour circulation in liver hilum with shunt to portal vein containing tumour thrombus. Primary liver cancer. Embolized (inset).

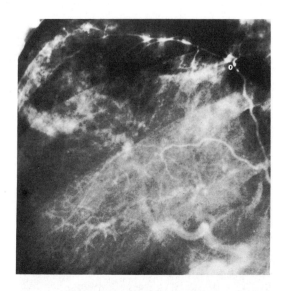

Figure 25.7 Coeliac arteriogram. Peripheral necrotic primary liver cancer. Phrenic artery supply superiorly suggests tumour involves hemidiaphragm (inoperable).

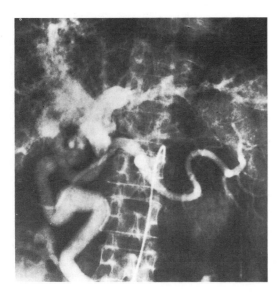

Figure 25.8 Selective coeliac arteriogram. Primary liver cancer in right lobe of liver; massive portal venous shunt. (Large umbilical vein.) Splenomegaly. Courtesy of Dr D. Irving.

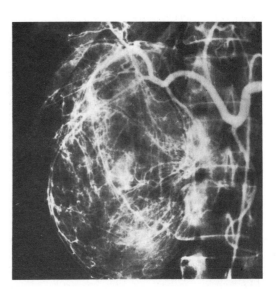

Figure 25.10 Common hepatic arteriogram. Highly vascular tumour right lobe. Carcinoid origin suggested by study. Ileal primary at operation.

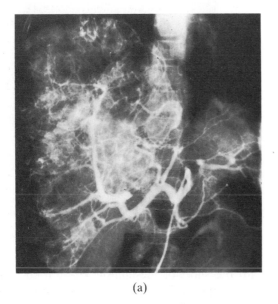

(a)

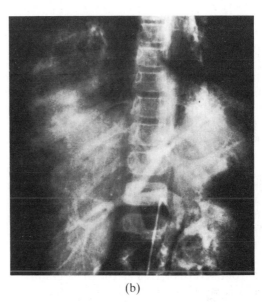

(b)

Figure 25.9 (a) Coeliac arteriogram. Female aged 7 years. Very vascular tumour right lobe. Normal left lobe. Biopsy = multifocal primary liver cell cancer. (b) Superior mesenteric arteriogram. Venous phase. Tumour displaces portal vein branches. Normal left lobe veins. Extended right hemihepatectomy performed. (Portal vein may contribute to blood supply of liver cell adenoma and carcinoma.)

fistulas at the time of arteriography should be considered.

Metastases are much commoner than any other liver neoplasms. They may be highly vascular, especially those of endocrine origin (Figure 25.10). Some are poorly opacified but may have a diagnostic dense peripheral ring of contrast (Figure 25.11). Other metastases, such as the mucoid-secreting colonic variety are totally avascular. If minimal neovascularity is suspected it can be highlighted with the use of pharmacoangiography (Figure 25.12a and b), namely the introduction of intra-arterial drugs prior to injection of contrast. Vasoconstrictors (adrenaline 20 μg), or alternatively, vasodilators (prostaglandins, sodium nitroprusside) have been advocated for injection into the hepatic artery to enhance tumour circulation and

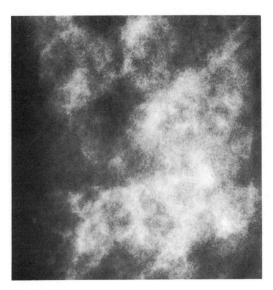

Figure 25.11 Superselective hepatic arteriogram. Capillary phase. Multiple round defects with vascular periphery = metastases. Malignant gastrinomas.

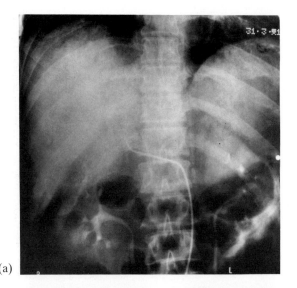

(a)

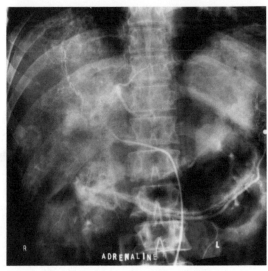

(b)

Figure 25.12 (a) Selective hepatic arteriogram in patient with suspected large-bowl metastases. No tumours visible. (b) Study repeated injecting 15 μg adrenaline prior to a reduced amount of contrast. 'Ringed' metastases clearly shown.

are without added risk to the patient.[10] An adequate volume of contrast agent is the most important factor in opacifying normal or abnormal tissues.

Arteriography is disappointing in the diagnosis of the occasional avascular HCC and of avascular metastases. Very small (1–2 cm) avascular intrahepatic lesions sometimes cause filling defects on a well-filled portal venogram long before they are detected arteriographically.[23] Hepatic lymphoma is always hypovascular and arteriovenous shunting is absent.[7]

Cholangiocarcinomas are usually avascular tumours, causing invasion and fixity of nearby arteries and veins. Dilated bile ducts causing lucencies in the hepatogram phase are distinguished from metastases by their linear shape. The size of the gallbladder can be assessed (Figure 25.13) and the venous phase of the coeliac arteriogram provides important information about the calibre and patency of the splenic, portal and intrahepatic veins. Nevertheless, unless resection is contemplated, angiography is not routinely indicated if cholangiography or ultrasonography have shown the site and probable nature of the biliary pathology.

PORTAL HYPERTENSION

Management of the patient merits an integrated approach, the team consisting of a physician, a surgeon and a radiologist.[4] Timing, of both investigations and treatment, is important.[11] Many patients will require angiography. This should be performed promptly to allow maximum time to plan management. Early in the course of a bleed a slow infusion of Pitressin (vasopressin) (0.1 unit/min)

into the superior mesenteric artery used to be given to lower portal venous pressure and stop variceal bleeding. However, not only did bleeding commonly restart when the drug was discontinued, but Pitressin experimentally is as effective if given by the more simple intravenous route.[13]

Angiography remains the best imaging technique to demonstrate the precise portal venous anatomy, including the number and direction of venous collaterals. Vital haemodynamic information, including flow rates and pressures, is concurrently obtained. The normal portal venous pressure does not exceed 11 mmHg. A pressure in the portal vein of 30 mmHg in a patient with a normal wedge pressure indicates a presinusoidal cause of portal hypertension. Thus, a diagnosis may be made even before angiography has commenced.

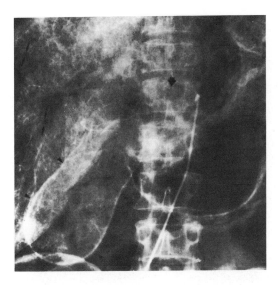

Figure 25.13 Selective coeliac arteriogram. Late hepatogram/portal venous phase. 60-year-old male, carcinoma pancreatic head. Tumour pressure on portal vein (large arrow). Enlarged gallbladder (arrow heads). Multiple small negative defects in liver due to dilated bile ducts (small arrows).

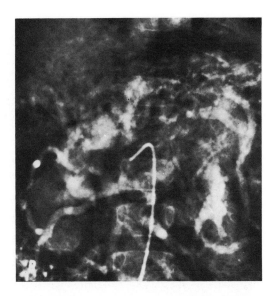

Figure 25.15 Superior mesenteric arteriogram, venous phase. Thrombosed portal vein. Many periportal and gastric collaterals. Past umbilical sepsis.

High-dose arterioportography is advantageous in outlining both the arterial and venous systems at the same examination (Figures 25.14 and 25.15), though duplex Doppler studies may be used as an alternative noninvasive approach.[22]

During angiography, dense variceal filling is not always achieved despite the addition of vasodilators such as bradykinin or prostaglandins,[14] and in some patients elective left gastric pharmacoarteriography should follow.[15] Arteriography in portal hypertension may show associated non-variceal causes of bleeding, namely arteriovenous fistulas, haemangiomas (Figure 25.16), and gastric or duodenal ulcers. In the poor-risk patient the vessel feeding a bleeding ulcer ought to be embolized at once.[2]

Doppler[22] will unquestionably replace much invasive angiography. From the indices time-averaged mean velocity and pulsatility, both the portal vein blood flow and direction may be calculated, though there may be difficulties in interpretation (Figure 25.17).

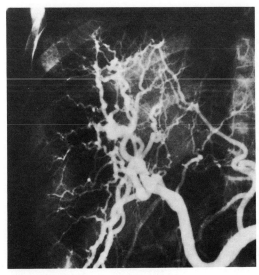

Figure 25.14 Selective hepatic arteriogram. Corkscrewing of arteries and arterioles. Advanced cirrhosis. (Compare with Figure 25.2.)

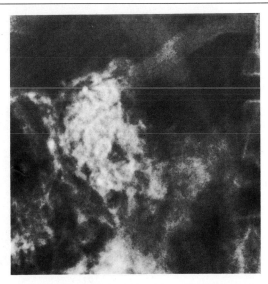

Figure 25.16 Patient with cirrhosis/portal hypertension. Superior mesenteric arteriogram. Capillary haemangioma in duodenal wall (found at endoscopy).

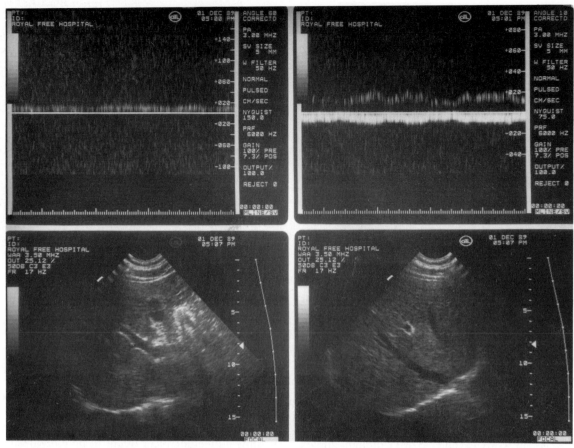

Figure 25.17 Duplex Doppler sonogram demonstrating normal portal and hepatic veins and their accompanying flow tracings.

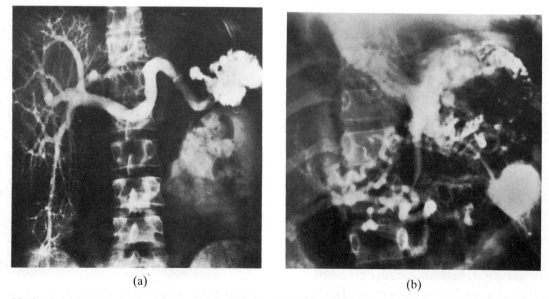

(a)   (b)

Figure 25.18 Splenic portograms. (a) Normal study. Note Riedel's lobe. (b) Child with past portal pyaemia. Splenic and portal vein thrombosis. Oesophageal, gastric and renocaval collaterals.

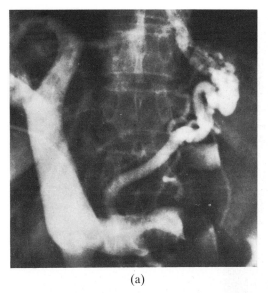

(a)

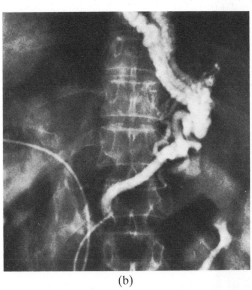

(b)

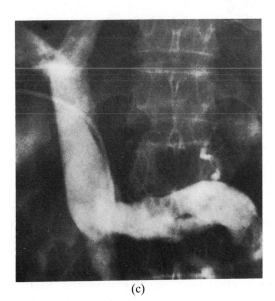

(c)

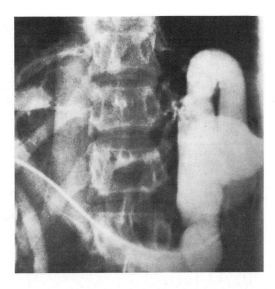

Figure 25.20 Transhepatic portogram. Large retroperitoneal shunt to left renal vein and inferior vena cava.

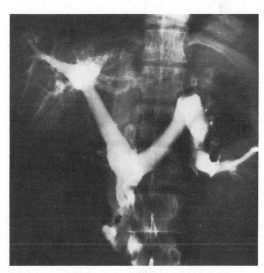

Figure 25.21 Splenic portogram showing patent mesocaval shunt (arrowed). Flow preserved to small cirrhotic liver.

Currently the best method of displaying collaterals, including those in unusual sites, is the direct injection of contrast into the portal venous system; dynamic enhanced CT can also give much information. Splenic pulp injection is quick, and even in inexperienced hands injection of contrast into the splenic pulp using a standard No. 1 green needle, is technically straightforward and free of serious

Figure 25.19 (a) Transhepatic portogram. Left gastric, superior and inferior mesenteric collaterals. (b) Selective left gastric venogram. Gastric and oesophageal varices. (c) Final portogram shows left gastric vein occluded. A thin, short gastric vein remains to be obliterated.

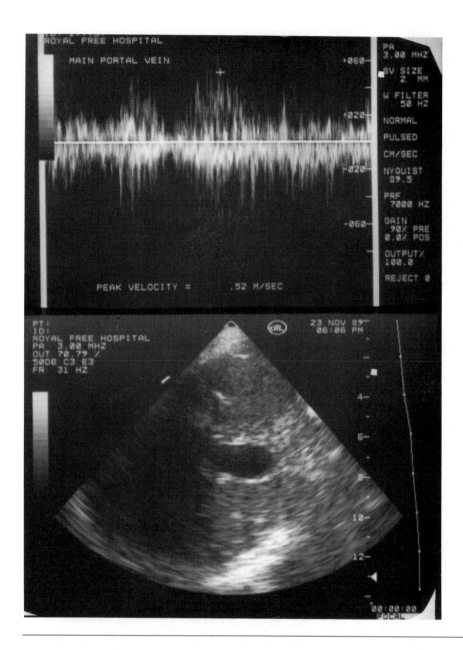

ROYAL FREE HOSPITAL
MAIN PORTAL VEIN

Figure 25.22 Duplex Doppler study in transplanted liver demonstrating grossly dilated portal vein with turbulent flow shown on tracing.

complications if undertaken with care.[9] It is less often performed than previously, though is of value in diagnosis with digital subtraction angiography. The pattern of collateral venous filling depends upon the site of obstruction, the appearance deviating markedly from normal (Figure 25.18). Percutaneous transhepatic portography[16] is possible provided that the portal vein is patent. It gives superb venograms and has the advantage of allowing subsequent selective catheterization and thus thrombosis of gastrooesophageal collaterals (Figure 25.19a, b and c). Access to the portal vein via the umbilical vein has not been universally adopted.

With a good-quality portal venogram, a choice between sclerotherapy and a decompressing surgical shunt can be made for the individual patient. Successful sclerosis of varices by either the oesophagoscope or the transhepatic approach stops acute bleeding instantly and dramatically.

Several centres have now treated large numbers of acutely bleeding patients by transhepatic variceal sclerosis.[17,19,25] The average results of groups cited show a portal vein catheterization rate of 92% and initial variceal sclerosis of 66%. The technique is challenging and initially time-consuming. Useful retroperitoneal shunting veins must be carefully distinguished from large gastric collaterals (Figure 25.20). Thrombin, Gelfoam and Sotradecol combinations and the monomer isobucrylate are four of the commoner agents used. The perfect occluding agent ought to be both easy to handle and cause a guaranteed permanent occlusion. Absolute alcohol is promising in this respect, but whatever agent is used, follow-up studies for up to 2 years indicate recanalization of some veins in over 50% of patients. Thus, the popularity of the technique is waning and following successful sclerotherapy the patient with fair liver function ought, within 4 months,

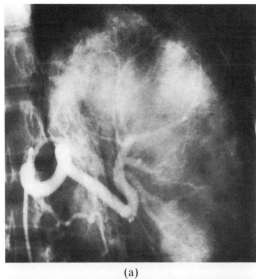

(a)

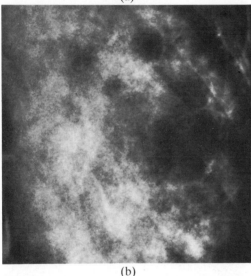

(b)

Figure 25.23 (a) Selective splenic arteriogram. Multiple defects in enlarged spleen were due to sarcoid granuloma. Note lymphogram. (b) Selective left hepatic arteriogram. Multiple abscess cavities in left lobe, confirmed by retrograde cholangiogram.

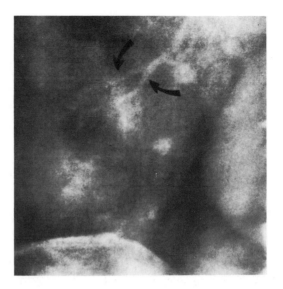

Figure 25.24 Budd–Chiari syndrome. Arteriogram-hepatogram phase. Slow sinusoidal clearance. Note portal vein radicles (arrows).

be shown prior to any type of splenorenal shunt. It cannot be assumed that the anatomy, as demonstrated on a study made weeks or months previously, will remain unaltered. Timely use of ultrasound will make some repeat angiograms unnecessary. Following shunt surgery, patency may be proved by sonography, arteriography, venacavography or, should the spleen remain, splenic pulp injection (Figure 25.21). If the approach is via the venous system (either portal or systemic), pressures may be recorded and should show a significant fall from preoperative readings.

to have elective shunt surgery to decompress the portal system or have oesophageal sclerotherapy. Unfortunately, many patients offered for initial and later repeat sclerotherapy are surgically rejected end-stage cirrhotics with gross ascites and coagulopathy. Serious complications of the procedure are rare in those centres with experience and no subsequent pulmonary emboli have been diagnosed clinically or radiologically.

Hepatic venography and associated manometry are used in portal hypertension both in the diagnostic work-up and sometimes in assessing the response to treatment with drugs such as propranolol[5] (see Chapter 48).

In the preparation of a patient for definitive shunt surgery, angiography should demonstrate the patency of the vessels to be used for the intended portosystemic shunt. The presence and position of the left kidney must

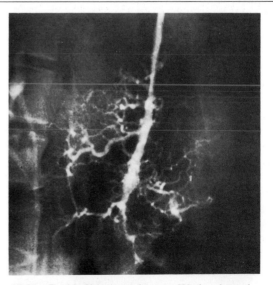

Figure 25.25 Budd–Chiari syndrome. Wedge hepatic venogram, lateral view. Intrahepatic spider's web venous pattern is diagnostic.

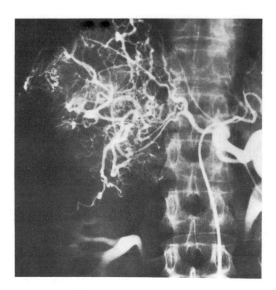

Figure 25.26 Selective coeliac arteriogram. Blood supply of vascular tumour in right hypochondrium is by inferior phrenic arteries, not hepatic. Lesion distorts upper right kidney. Adrenal adenoma.

DUPLEX DOPPLER SONOGRAPHY

This technique has an important role in the assessment of blood flow patterns in portal hypertension[22] and provides useful information concerning blood supply to hepatic tumours as well as in the evaluation of patients for liver transplantation (Figure 25.22). Once it becomes more readily available, this non-invasive technique, preferably with a colour facility, will often replace angiography in the above two groups of patients.

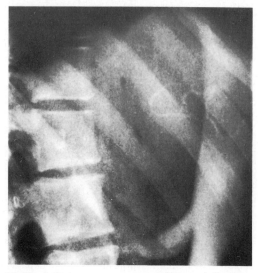

Figure 25.27 Inferior venacavogram. Forward displacement of upper cava due to retroperitoneal tumour.

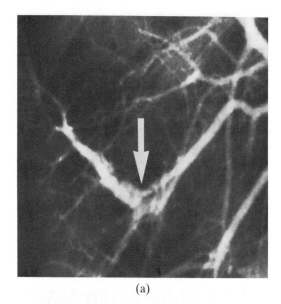

(a)

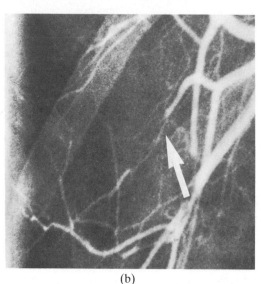

(b)

Figure 25.28 (a) Selective hepatic arteriogram. Patient has traumatic hepatic arterioportal venous shunt (arrows) and haemobilia. (b) Shunt has closed (arrow) following Gelfoam embolization. Immediate cessation of blood loss.

FURTHER APPLICATIONS OF ANGIOGRAPHY

Although they are not indications for angiography, granulomas in liver or spleen appear as well-defined avascular defects, whereas abscesses show the minimal vascularity of a shaggy wall surrounding a necrotic centre (Figure 25.23). Small areas of increased vascularity (pseudotumours) are sometimes seen in the liver of a patient with the Budd–Chiari syndrome.[12] Slowly fading adjacent portal vein radicles may confirm the radiologist's suspicion (Figure 25.24). Other patients with occluded hepatic veins will show a diagnostic plexiform web pattern on wedged hepatic venography (Figure 25.25). These have been

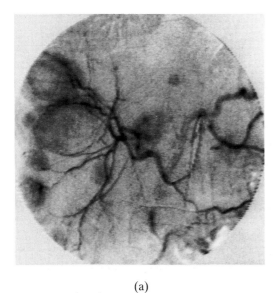

(a)

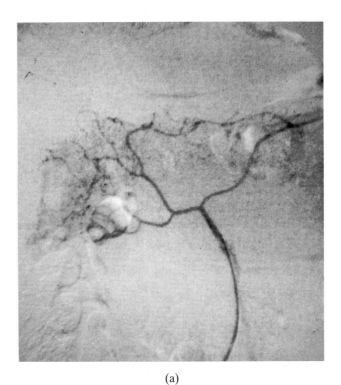

(a)

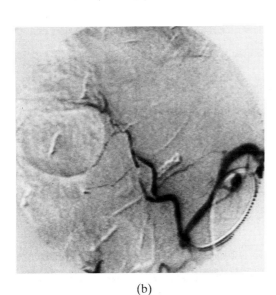

(b)

Figure 25.29 Digital subtraction angiogram (DVSA). 10 ml contrast medium injected into hepatic artery. Multiple vascular metastases. (b) Repeat DVSA following embolization with 5 ml absolute alcohol. Metastases ablated. Symptoms relieved. Courtesy of Dr D. Irving.

proved to be due to venovenous connections between hepatic veins.[18]

In the assessment for liver transplantation, angiography on the recipient is invariably required. This includes coeliac and superior mesenteric arteriography and inferior venacavography, the patency of the portal vein being the single most important factor required.

ANGIOGRAPHIC PITFALLS

Both regenerative nodules and focal nodular hyperplasia may be highly vascular with hepatic arterioportal venous

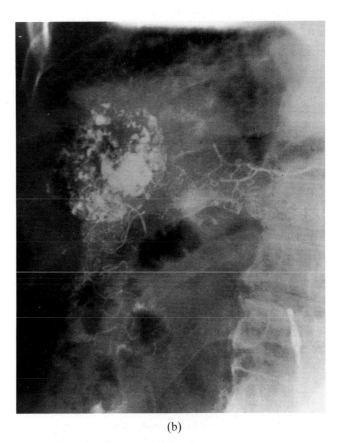

(b)

Figure 25.30 (a) DVSA in patient with high alphafetoprotein. DVSA shows small cirrhotic liver without definite tumour. (b) Radiograph immediately after injection of 10 ml Lipiodol into hepatic arterial catheter. There is immediate uptake in a tumour high in the right lobe.

shunting, and resemble liver cell cancer.[29] The radioisotope scan can prove the presence of a nodule because of increased rather than decreased isotope uptake by the vascular area.[24] Some retroperitoneal tumours may mimic vascular liver masses closely unless their major vascular supply is carefully studied (Figure 25.26). Inferior venacavography is usually decisive (Figure 25.27).

THERAPEUTIC ARTERIAL EMBOLIZATION (INTERVENTIONAL ANGIOGRAPHY)

Many different interventional radiological procedures are available.[28] Embolization should be considered in appropriate patients at the time of angiography. Those with sites of active bleeding, highly vascular neoplasms and arteriovenous fistulas (some iatrogenic in origin) should benefit from timely successful embolization (Figure 25.28a and b).[20] In HCC, symptoms such as abdominal pain may be alleviated by embolization even though life is not prolonged.[6] Symptoms from massive hormone release by endocrine metastases may be relieved or even ablated (Figure 25.29a and b).[1]

Much interest has recently developed in the selective hepatic arterial injection of Lipiodol followed by CT as part of the preoperative assessment of patients with hepatocellular and metastatic cancers[3] (see also Chapter 23). Even small tumours undetectable by conventional angiography take up Lipiodol strongly (Figure 25.30). An extension of this technique is the addition of cytotoxic agents such as Epirubicin to the Lipiodol.[26] Lipiodol labelled with iodine-131 is currently being assessed for the treatment of inoperable cholangiocarcinoma.[19]

REFERENCES

1. Allison, D.J. (1980) Therapeutic embolisation in malignant endocrine tumours. In Veiga-Pines, J.A. (ed.) *Interventional Radiology*, pp. 202–205. Amsterdam: Excerpta Medica.
2. Allison, D.J. (1984) Interventional radiology. *European College of Angiography Meeting*. Helsingor, Denmark.
3. Bruneton, J.N., Kerboul, P., Grimaldi, C. *et al.* (1988) Hepatic interarterial lipiodol: technique, semiologic patterns, and value for hepatic tumours. *Gastrointestinal Radiology*, **13**, 45–51.
4. Burroughs, A.K., Bass, N.M., Osborne, D. *et al.* (1983) Randomised controlled study of transhepatic obliteration of varices and oesophageal stapling transection in uncontrolled variceal haemorrhage. *Liver*, **3**, 122–128.
5. Burroughs, A.K., Jenkins, W.J., Sherlock, S. *et al.* (1983) Controlled trial of propranolol for the prevention of recurrent variceal haemorrhage in patients with cirrhosis. *New England Journal of Medicine*, **309**, 1539–1542.
6. Chuang, V.P. & Wallace, S. (1981) Hepatic artery embolisation in the treatment of hepatic neoplasms. *Radiology*, **111**, 51–58.
7. Chuang, V.P., Bree, R.L. & Bookstein, J.J. (1974) Angiographic features of focal lymphoma of the liver. *Radiology*, **111**, 53–55.
8. Dick, R. (1982) Interventional radiology of the portal venous system. *Annals de Radiologie*, **7**, 441–448.
9. Dilawari, J.B., Chawla, J.K., Raju, J.S. *et al.* (1987) Safety of splenoportovenography as an outpatient procedure. *Lancet*, **2**, 101.
10. Goldstein, H.M., Thaggard, A., Wallace, S. *et al.* (1976) Priscoline-augmented hepatic angiography. *Radiology*, **119**, 275–279.
11. Hayes, P.C., Shepherd, A.N. & Bouchier, I.A.D. (1983) Medical treatment of portal hypertension and oesophageal varices. *British Medical Journal*, **287**, 733–736.
12. Hungerford, G.D., Lunzer, M.R., Dick, R. *et al.* (1976) Pseudometastases in the liver; a presentation of the Budd–Chiari syndrome. *Radiology*, **120**, 627–628.
13. Kauffman, S.L., Harrington, D.P., Barth, K.H. *et al.* (1977) Control of variceal bleeding by superior mesenteric artery vasopressin infusion. *American Journal of Roentgenology*, **128**, 567–570.
14. Legge, D.A. (1977) The use of prostaglandin F2 alpha in selective visceral angiography. *British Journal of Radiology*, **50**, 251–255.
15. Lunderquist, A. (1974) Pharmacoangiography of the left gastric artery in oesophageal varices. *Acta Radiologica; Diagnosis*, **15**, 157–160.
16. Lunderquist, A. & Vang, J. (1974) Transhepatic catheterisation and obliteration of the coronary vein in patients with portal hypertension and oesophageal varices. *New England Journal of Medicine*, **291**, 646–649.
17. Lunderquist, A., Simert, G., Tylen, U. & Vang, J. (1977) Follow-up of patients with portal hypertension and oesophageal varices treated with percutaneous obliteration of gastric coronary vein. *Radiology*, **122**, 59–63.
18. Maguire, R. & Doppman, J.L. (1977) Angiographic abnormalities in partial Budd–Chiari syndrome. *Radiology*, **122**, 629–635.
19. Novell, J.R., Hilson, A., Young, J. *et al.* (1989) Uptake of 131 I Lipiodol by intrahepatic cholangiocarcinoma. *Journal of Hepatology*, **9** (suppl. 1), 5199.
20. O'Halpin, D., Legge, D. & MacErlean, D.P. (1984) Therapeutic arterial embolisation; report of five years experience. *Clinical Radiology*, **35**, 85–93.
21. Okudo, K., Obata, H., Jinouchi, S. *et al.* (1977) Angiographic assessment of gross anatomy of hepatocellular carcinoma; comparison of coeliac angiograms and liver pathology in 100 cases. *Radiology*, **123**, 21–29.
22. Partriquin, H., LaFortune, M., Burns, P.N. *et al.* (1987) Duplex Doppler examination in portal hypertension-technique and anatomy. *American Journal of Radiology*, **149**, 71–76.
23. Pinte, F., Amiel, M., Bourgoin, J. *et al.* (1972) Microangiographie des tumeurs malignes du foie. *Annales de Radiologie*, **15**, 437–443.
24. Reuter, S.R., Redman, H.C. & Siders, D.B. (1970) The spectrum of angiographic findings in hepatoma. *Radiology*, **94**, 89–94.
25. Smith-Laing, G., Camillo, M.E., Dick, R. & Sherlock, S. (1981) Role of percutaneous transhepatic obliteration of varices in the management of haemorrhage from gastro-oesophageal varices. *Gastroenterology*, **80**, 1031–1036.
26. Takayasu, K., Shima, Y., Muramatsu, Y. *et al.* (1987) Hepatocellular carcinoma; treatment with intra-arterial iodized oil with and without chemotherapeutic agents. *Radiology*, **163**, 345–351.
27. Viamonte, M., Jr & Schiff, D. (1977) Diagnostic approach to hepatic malignant neoplasms. *Journal of the American Medical Association*, **238**, 2191–2193.
28. Wilkins, R.A., Nunnerley, H.B., Allison, D.J. *et al.* (1989) The expansion of interventional radiology. Report of a survey conducted by the Royal College of Radiologists. *Clinical Radiology*, **40**, 457–462.
29. Winograd, J. & Palubinskas, A.J. (1977) Arterial-portal venous shunting in cavernous haemangioma of the liver. *Radiology*, **122**, 331–332.

CHAPTER 26

Endoscopic Examination and Therapy in Biliary Tract Disease

H. Neuhaus & M. Classen

Endoscopic cannulation of the papilla of Vater was first reported by McCune *et al.*[150] in 1968. Its more widespread introduction followed the development of new fibre-optic duodenoscopes in 1970. The rapid development of endoscopic–radiological diagnostic and therapeutic procedures in the pancreatic and biliary system resulted in a deluge of mainly enthusiastic reports.[28,45,151,240]

For the first time direct access to the papilla of Vater was possible—the key point of a functional system comprising the duodenum, biliary tract, liver and pancreas. By means of retrograde cannulation the pancreatic ducts and biliary tract were visualized independently of hepatic function, and extrahepatic obstruction was exactly assessed radiologically. In addition, this technique has enabled manometric examination of the two ducts and permitted the collection of pure pancreatic juice and bile for cytological, serological and biochemical examination. With the development of electropapillotomy (EPT) stone extraction from the common bile duct became possible, and 16 years after its introduction EPT has become a generally accepted and routine therapeutic measure. Almost ten years ago complementary techniques for intraductal destruction of stones, drainage of bile, balloon dilatation of stenoses and local irradiation of malignancies were invented. The latest developments of biliary endoscopy are peroral or percutaneous cholangioscopy, biliary endosonography, intraductal laser therapy and implantation of self-expanding metallic stents.

ENDOSCOPIC RETROGRADE CHOLANGIOPANCREATOGRAPHY (ERCP) IN DIAGNOSIS

TECHNICAL ASPECTS

Indications and contraindications

Because of their close topographical and functional relationship, the biliary tract and the pancreatic duct system are visualized under the same procedure of ERCP. This provides an excellent diagnostic method for distinguishing medical and surgical jaundice. Since, even in the absence of jaundice, intravenous cholangiograms often fail to provide diagnostic information, ERCP is indicated for all patients suspected of biliary tract disease. Furthermore, ERCP is indicated on suspicion of pancreatic disease. It permits definitive documentation of chronic pancreatitis, demonstrating ductal abnormalities such as strictures and stones, and thus providing a basis for endoscopic or surgical intervention. Although in patients with obscure epigastric pain a normal pancreatogram cannot exclude relapsing pancreatitis, advanced chronic pancreatitis can be excluded. Pancreatic cancer can be diagnosed by ERCP at the stage at which it usually presents for specialist investigation.

Like other endoscopic examinations, ERCP is contraindicated in severe cardiorespiratory insufficiency or after recent myocardial infarction. In patients with recurrent pancreatitis or continuing pain and hyperamylasaemia, ultrasonographic examination is obligatory prior to ERCP. If pseudocysts can be demonstrated, pancreatography is rarely indicated and should be performed with caution. It may be desirable to test for hepatitis B surface antigen and HIV antibodies in selected patients prior to ERCP. Provided that endoscopes are correctly disinfected, the risk of transmitting viral hepatitis or other infections (e.g. AIDS) is extremely low.[5,23,255] To date only one case of hepatitis B transmission by ERCP has been reported.[149] Previous allergic reactions experienced after intravenous or oral administration of iodine-containing contrast material are not a contraindication to ERCP.

Complications

Respiratory and circulatory reactions to the premedication, aspiration of gastric juice, and perforation of the alimentary tract with the endoscope occur rarely, although it is not easy to determine the risks from the available literature.[65,138,195] Diminution of arterial oxygen saturation following the procedure is common. Complications due to endoscopic manipulation or perforation of the pancreatic or common bile ducts with a plastic catheter are rare.[65,138,180]

Sepsis and pancreatitis are the two main hazards. They occur most frequently after filling an abnormal and poorly draining duct system. In the majority of patients a transient rise in serum amylase and lipase in the absence of pancreatic symptoms is observed after pancreatography, especially if pancreatic parenchymal opacification is present.[228] In 33% of cases an increase of serum amylase is observed even after selective retrograde cholangiography, and in 75% after pancreatography.[126]

Acute pancreatitis following retrograde pancreatography mainly results from excessive and repeated injection of the contrast material; this risk can be diminished by careful fluoroscopic monitoring of the injection by means of a powerful television image-intensifier system. The results of many workers indicate that the risk of severe

pancreatitis is 0.4 – 1.3%.[10,159,192] The role of other factors that may increase the risk of pancreatitis is less clear. Rambow et al. suggested that the routine use of pethidine is deleterious.[191] Only one of six randomized studies comparing low- and high-osmolarity contrast agents showed a reduction in the frequency of clinical pancreatitis in the low-osmolarity contrast group.[36] The use of the newer, more expensive osmolarity medium is recommended in high-risk patients with a history of post-ERCP pancreatitis or spontaneous severe pancreatitis.

Sepsis is the principal cause of mortality following ERCP. It occurs almost exclusively in patients with poor drainage of the pancreatic and biliary system.[127] In pancreatic lesions such as malignant stenosis and pseudocysts, sepsis presumably results from the introduction of infection by the procedure. Patients with biliary stasis invariably have infected bile, and cholangitis and septicaemia may occur as a result of dissemination of bacteria already present if adequate endoscopic drainage is not provided.[89,127] A sudden pressure increase in the biliary tree can cause bacteraemia by cholangiovenous reflux.[94,100]

Instruments

The equipment for duodenoscopy with cannulation of the papilla of Vater consists of a polydirectional, flexible, small-sized endoscope with a high-quality, lateral-viewing optical system and a channel large enough for the passage of tubes, Dormia baskets, biopsy forceps and various other instruments for biliary therapy. These requirements are met by the majority of endoscope manufacturers. Standard forward-viewing endoscopes are suitable only in patients with a Bilroth II partial gastrectomy, when the papilla is approached from below via the afferent loop. The recently developed technology of electronic endoscopes is expected to have a major role in gastrointestinal endoscopy in the 1990s because of presumed improvement in image quality, enhanced teaching abilities, permanent image storage, reproduction and retrieval, and the potential for enhanced imaging by signal processing.[118,226]

Graduated catheters of polyvinylchloride or Teflon, with an outer diameter of 1.5–1.7 mm, are used for the cannulation. Metal tip inserts may facilitate cannulation of the minor papilla or of a smooth or indurated major papilla.

Premedication

Prior to the examination the fasting patient receives an individually 'titrated' dose of a sedating agent whenever necessary under continuous cardiopulmonary monitoring.[62] The mouth and the throat can be swabbed or sprayed with a suitable local anaesthetic. Because of the altered pharmacodynamics of drugs in patients with liver disease, the dosage of sedative must be tailored to avoid respiratory depression or hepatic precoma in susceptible patients. The presence of duodenal ileus is helpful in locating the papilla; intermittent intravenous injection of hyoscine-N-butyl bromide (Buscopan) (20–40 mg) or glucagon (0.5 mg) is effective in achieving this.

Cannulation technique

The patient is examined in the prone position on the x-ray table. The duodenoscope is first introduced into the antrum of the stomach; to avoid strong peristalsis, little air should be insufflated. After locating the pylorus, the tip of the instrument is advanced as near as possible to it by a slight dorsal flexion. The tip is then squared off ventrally in the direction of the lesser curvature and is simultaneously pushed forward until it enters the duodenal bulb with a slight jerk. By turning the instrument through 180°, further introduction is performed with slight air insufflation. The lumen of the descending part of the duodenum then becomes visible.

For cannulation, the endoscope should be straightened. This position can be achieved by hooking the tip of the instrument in the second part of the duodenum and then withdrawing it with a lens facing the patient's left side. Further withdrawal brings the lens up the medial wall of the duodenum to the longitudinal fold and the papilla. The control of the distal tip is thus enhanced and less of the shaft is exposed to radiation. The longitudinal fold is the guide to the papilla, which is located proximally, partly directly on it and partly adjacent to it. The orifice is located in the centre of the papillary area; it is either slit-like or rounded and of variable size. The minor papilla, the end of the duct of Santorini, is located 2 cm above the major papilla towards the posterior wall. The positioning of the catheter tip is crucial for successful cannulation. The tip of the instrument is adjusted so that the extended catheter lies at a right angle with the papillary orifice. After cannulation of the papillary orifice, diluted contrast medium is injected under careful fluoroscopic monitoring. Usually the pancreatic duct is visualized first; cholangiography may then be achieved by placing the catheter tip a short distance inside the papillary orifice and then angling it upwards in a craniodorsal direction.

The technique of cannulation of the papilla is difficult to learn and requires good manual skill by the endoscopist. Both the cannulation success rate and the complication rate depend largely on the skill and experience of the operator. A survey demonstrated that in expert hands there was a 15% failure rate for cannulation and a 3.5% complication rate. In less experienced hands the failure rate was 62% and the complication rate was 15%. With a perfect examination technique the pancreatic duct is visualized in 92% of cases and the common bile duct in 86%.[27] Failure may be due to lack of cooperation by the patient or to abnormal anatomy, as in pyloric or duodenal stenosis, following Billroth II partial gastrectomy, in inflammatory or neoplastic stenosis of the papilla or in the presence of juxtapapillary duodenal diverticula where the papilla is hidden in the diverticulum.

Cholangiographic technique

After cannulation of the papilla, contrast medium should be injected until there is adequate filling of the intrahepatic ducts and the gallbladder. However, in the presence of bile duct stenosis, injection of contrast should be kept to a minimum consistent with making a diagnosis to reduce the risk of producing acute suppurative cholangitis if subsequent drainage is unlikely to be obtained.[127] There is no evidence that routine systemic antibiotic prophylaxis or incorporation of an antibiotic into the injected contrast material is beneficial, but antibiotics should be administered immediately after the procedure if contrast medium has entered poorly drained ducts.[206] Prophylactic antibiotic therapy is indicated if 'high-risk' factors – e.g. duct dilatation noted at ultrasound – are present.

Changing the position of the patient is often more effective than increasing the volume of contrast material. Cystic duct obstruction can be diagnosed if the gallbladder fails to fill after suitable positioning and adequate filling of the intrahepatic tree with contrast has occurred. Filling of the biliary tree commonly provides high-quality retrograde cholangiograms that are easy to interpret. Difficulties in interpretation may result from layering or streaming effects caused by incomplete mixing of contrast material and bile. Air bubbles that are injected together with the contrast material may be confused with common bile duct stones. If this is suspected, rotation of the patient on the body axis with radiographs taken in different positions and projections may prove helpful. After endoscopic sphincterotomy it is sometimes necessary to block the distal common bile duct with a balloon catheter in order to prevent air bubbles and immediate discharge of the contrast medium.

DIAGNOSTIC FINDINGS _____

The papilla of Vater

At endoscopy, hemispherical, papillary and flat-form variants of the papilla are found. Above it the intraduodenal part of the common bile duct penetrates the duodenal wall into the lumen and, together with the major duodenal fold, covers the papilla like a roof. The commonest site for the occurrence of duodenal diverticula is the concave side of the duodenal loop, mainly in the papillary region. Diverticula vary from the size of a pea to that of a tennis ball and occur singly or in groups.[92] The papilla is often located in the border or in the cavity of a diverticulum. Endoscopically the orifice of the diverticulum can be easily recognized by the radial mucosal folds. When manipulating the endoscope near diverticula, the endoscopist must consider the risk of perforation of the thin wall. According to Hoffman and Weiss[93] there is a significant relationship between juxtapapillary duodenal diverticula and gallstones: 74% of patients with duodenal diverticula who were examined also suffered from gallstones. Similar results were found by Kennedy and Thompson.[117] The rate for those patients who had already undergone cholecystectomy was 59%.[117] A decreased pressure of the sphincter of Oddi may lead to bacterial contamination of the biliary tract and development of pigment stones.[144]

A juxta-ampullary carcinoma arising from the distal common bile duct, the head of the pancreas, the duodenum or the papilla of Vater itself can be diagnosed at duodenoscopy.[20,202]

Ulcerated tumours in the area of the papilla are almost exclusively malignant; the histological and cytological proof of malignancy is easily obtained by biopsy and brush cytology.[54,66] The diagnosis of non-ulcerated tumours is difficult. The endoscopic appearance of a coarsely enlarged papilla with a smooth, villous or nodular surface can resemble a carcinoma of the papilla, papillitis or adenomyomatosis of the papilla (Figures 26.1 and 26.2). The results of histological examination may prove falsely negative because only the upper epithelial layers are seized by the biopsy forceps. For reliable histological diagnosis it is necessary in these cases to split the papilla with the electropapillotome and to cut away a larger piece of tissue with the diathermy loop. Furthermore, an enlarged and swollen papilla may be caused by impaction of a gallstone within the papilla. A discharge of pus from the papillary orifice may indicate suppurative cholangitis, while the discharge of blood may indicate a tumour located higher in the biliary tree. A reddened, dilated and irregularly shaped orifice in the presence of upper abdominal pain and transient jaundice may indicate the recent passage of a gallstone through the papilla.

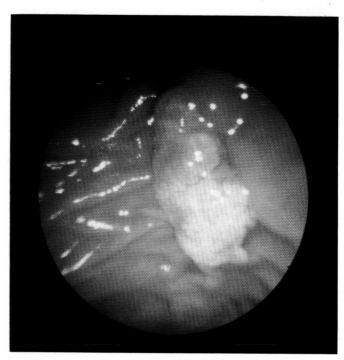

Figure 26.2 Duodenoscopy showing a villous adenoma of the papilla of Vater.

The pancreatic duct system

The course of the main pancreatic duct (MPD) is subject to considerable variation, the ascending type being the most frequent variant.[111,201] (Figure 26.3). The average diameter of the duct is 4 mm in the area of the head, 3 mm in the body and 2 mm in the tail of the pancreas. The normal contour of the wall is smooth. Injection of increasing volumes of contrast material results in opacification of the duct branches (primary, secondary and tertiary), the fine pancreatic ducts and, finally, the acini. Because greater degrees of opacification are

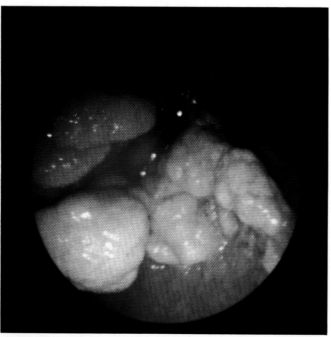

Figure 26.1 Duodenoscopy showing an ampullary carcinoma.

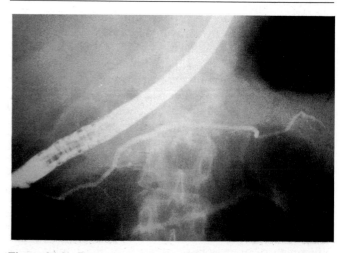

Figure 26.3 Pancreatography via the minor papilla in pancreas divisum. Opacification of the normal main duct and its primary and secondary duct branches.

associated with an increased incidence of pancreatitis, only the main pancreatic duct, the primary and the secondary duct branches should be filled.

Inflammatory pancreatic processes are seen in the pancreatogram as deformations of the duct system or pseudocysts.[112,194,201,211,264] These cysts connect with the duct system in about 60% of cases (Figure 26.4). Filling defects in the area of the duct branches, complete obstruction of the MPD and displacement or narrowing of the common bile duct are indirect signs of pseudocysts.[210] In chronic pancreatitis the earliest changes are minor variations in the calibre of the fine branches. In advanced chronic pancreatitis, marked enlargement and variation in calibre of the MPD and its branches, strictures, obstructions, calculi or coarse acinar opacification are seen in the pancreatogram (Figures 26.5 and 26.6). Using these morphological duct changes, the diagnostic sensitivity of ERCP for chronic pancreatitis ranges between 71% and 93% and the specificity between 89% and 100%.[44]

The Cambridge classification[203] of ERCP in chronic pancreatitis (Table 26.1) should make computerization and comparison of the findings of different observers possible. The radiological differentiation between chronic pancreatitis and carcinoma is difficult and these conditions may coexist.[201,236]

Pancreatic cancer, arising almost exclusively from duct tissue, is seen most commonly on the pancreatogram as complete duct obstruction or stenosis with distal dilatation (Figures 26.7 and 26.8). Rarely, it may appear as a tapering stricture, ectasia or coarse acinar opacification.[20,70,112,236] Special problems arise with cancer involving the head of the pancreas when the pancreatic duct is blocked close to the papilla and pancreatography fails,[236] or when,

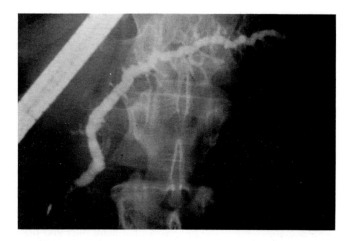

Figure 26.5 Pancreatography in chronic pancreatitis. Enlargement and variation in the calibre of the main pancreatic duct and its branches.

in spite of the tumour, the pancreatogram appears normal. In these cases retrograde cholangiography will sometimes demonstrate a lesion.[139,224] If the pancreatic duct is not blocked by the carcinoma and pancreatography is successful, the diagnostic accuracy of ERCP (92.7%) is much higher than that of computed tomography (58.5%) and ultrasonography (54.4%).[176] A computer program based on 13 ERCP criteria achieved a prospective diagnostic accuracy of 92% in patients with pancreatic head carcinoma.[177]

The first case of a microcystic adenoma communicating with the pancreatic duct and demonstrated by ERCP was recently published.[38] A patient with recurrent pancreatitis caused by a villous adenoma of the duct of Wirsung was reported by Warshaw et al.[252] Kaufman et al. published five cases of pancreatic islet cell tumours with special findings at ERCP, which were different from those of adenocarcinomas.[113] Nevertheless, most cases with such

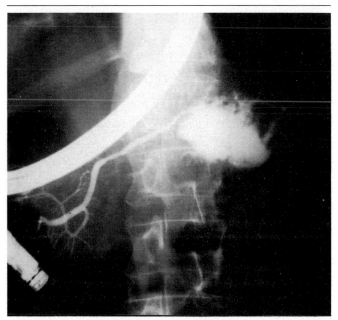

Figure 26.4 Pancreatography with opacification of a pseudocyst after acute pancreatitis.

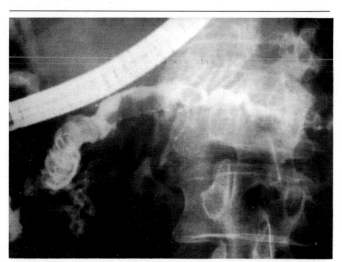

Figure 26.6 Pancreatography in chronic pancreatitis. Prepapillary stenosis and dilatation of the main duct with several intraluminal concrements.

Table 26.1 Grading of chronic pancreatitis by imaging methods

	Endoscopic retrograde pancreatography	Ultrasound or computed tomography
1 Normal	Quality study visualizing whole gland without abnormal features	
2 Equivocal	Less than three abnormal branches	One sign only: Main duct enlarged (<4 mm) Gland enlarged (up to 2 × normal) Cavities (<10 mm) Irregular ducts Focal acute pancreatitis Parenchymal heterogeneity Duct wall echoes increased Irregular head/body contour
3 Mild	More than three abnormal branches ⎫	Two or more signs (as above)
4 Moderate	Abnormal main duct and branches ⎭	
5 Marked	As above with one or more of: Large cavities (>10 mm) Gross gland enlargement (>2 × normal) Intraduct filling defects or calculi Duct obstruction, stricture or gross irregularity Contiguous organ invasion	

From Sarner and Cotton (1984),[203] with kind permission of the authors and the editor of *Gut*.

tumours have a normal pancreatogram and usually the better method for diagnosis and staging is endoscopic ultrasonography. Mistakes in the interpretation of pancreatograms result from injection of insufficient contrast material, the introduction of air bubbles, or faulty positioning causing inadequate filling with contrast material, giving the appearance of complete duct obstruction.

Radiographically it is difficult to distinguish cancer and chronic pancreatitis and additional information is usually required. Positive results have been obtained in 50–80% of cases by cytological examination of pure pancreatic juice aspirated from the intubated main pancreatic duct following secretin stimulation.[85,123] Unfortunately, the results are poor in early cancer, in exocrine pancreatic insufficiency and in tumours located in the body or the tail.[54] Brush cytology from the pancreatic and common bile ducts has also been recommended[66,183,253] (Figure 26.7). In an attempt to provide better diagnosis the measurement of CEA, CA-19-9 and other tumour markers in serum and pure pancreatic juice have been investigated, but none of the antigens described so far has been tumour or pancreas organ-specific.[154]

The biliary tract

The common bile duct in pancreatic disease
Both chronic pancreatitis and cancer are located predominantly in the head of the pancreas. Common bile duct strictures occur in 10–27% of patients with chronic pancreatitis, but infrequently cause significant obstruction.[142, 209] Kalvaria *et al.* investigated the natural history of common bile duct stenosis in chronic alcohol-induced pancreatitis. None of 10 asymptomatic patients and only

29% of 21 patients who predominantly suffered pain had to undergo an operation within 4 years. Even 50% of those who had developed jaundice could be treated conservatively.[110] Knowledge of biliary tract involvement is of great importance in considering pancreatic surgery for patients with chronic pancreatitis. In 75% of patients with cancer of the head of the pancreas, a tight stenosis of the common bile duct with obstruction was observed. Tubular waist-like or thread-like stenoses of the distal common bile duct 3–5 cm in size with distal dilatation are seen on the cholangiogram. It must be stressed that, in patients with cancer of the head of the pancreas when the pancreatic ducts either appear normal or fail to opacify, partial stenosis of the common bile duct is often the abnormality that leads to detection of the pancreatic disease.[139,177]

Bile duct stones
Radiographs of the biliary tree containing gallstones are familiar to clinicians and radiologists and most findings are easy to interpret. Calculi usually float up the duct during injection of contrast and only rarely produce complete obstruction. With impaction of a stone in the papilla of Vater the papilla appears swollen, and on tapping it with the probe it feels hard. In such cases, as well as with impaction of a stone in the lower common bile duct, cannulation of the papilla and injection of contrast may not be possible. Large stones occluding the lumen appear radiologically as convex obstructions in the bile duct or as ring-like lesions. Very small gallstones may easily be overlooked if the volume of contrast medium injected is excessive (Figure 26.9). In such cases detection may be facilitated by late radiographs in the outflow phase

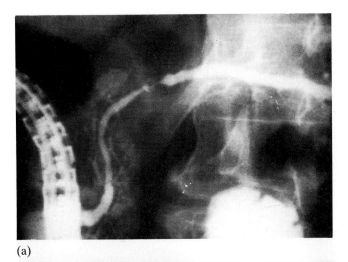

(a)

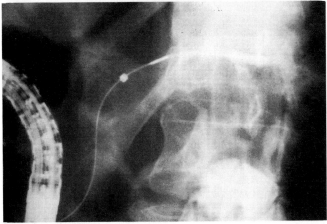

(b)

Figure 26.7 (a) Pancreatography in carcinoma of the pancreatic body. Circumscriptive narrowing of the main duct with prestenotic dilatation. (b) Retrograde catheterization of the stenosis for brush cytology.

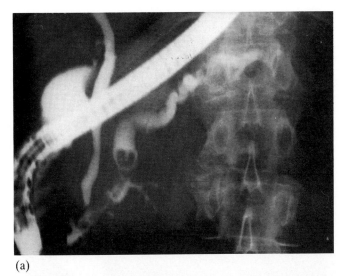

(a)

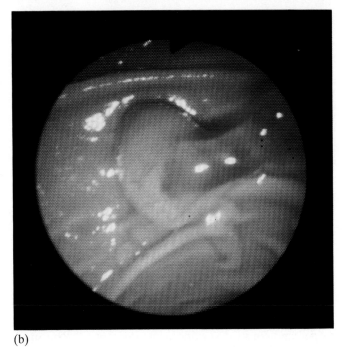

(b)

Figure 26.8 (a) Colloid carcinoma of the pancreas. Filling defect of the main duct due to conglomeration of mucus. (b) Glutinous mucus protruding the papillary orifice.

or by the use of diluted contrast solution. Despite these problems Schölmerich *et al.* found ERCP to be the best method for detection of a biliary origin for acute pancreatitis. The diagnosis of biliary pancreatitis could not be made with a sufficient degree of certainty using laboratory tests, ultrasound or computed tomography.[208] In patients with common bile duct stones, a fine indentation of the distal wall contour of the bile duct seems to indicate secondary cholangitis. Considering the risk of infection by cholangiography in partial duct obstruction, endoscopic papillotomy should, if indicated, follow immediately.

Postoperative syndromes

Choledochoduodenal fistulas are commonly situated on or around the longitudinal fold of the duodenum and are usually caused by the spontaneous passage of gallstones. Ikeda and Okada[102] describe two types of choledochoduodenal fistula. Type I is usually present on the longitudinal fold just proximal to the papilla. It is small and arises from the intramural portion of the common bile duct.

Type II is found in the duodenal mucosa, adjacent to the longitudinal fold. It is large and arises from the extramural portion of the common bile duct. Type II fistulas are probably caused by stones which are too big to enter the narrow intramural portion of the common bile duct. The diagnosis of choledochoduodenal fistula is made by direct observation of the fistula orifice with outflow of bile or contrast medium injected through the papilla. Successful cholangiography performed through the papilla, in addition to visualization of the fistula orifice, confirms the diagnosis.

Formerly the most frequently employed form of biliary–digestive anastomosis was external supraduodenal

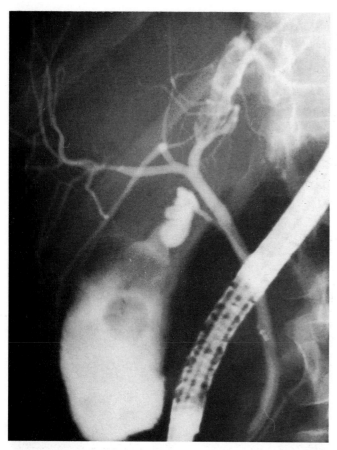

Figure 26.9 Retrograde cholangiography in a patient with gallbladder stones and Caroli's disease. Circumscriptive ductal dilatation and small concretions in the left liver.

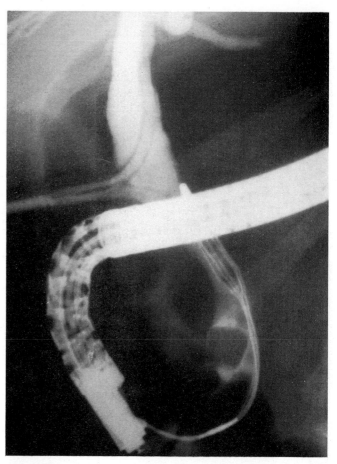

Figure 26.10 Cholangiography in a patient with a T-tube in situ after cholecystectomy and common bile duct exploration. Retrograde extraction of retained stones with a dormia basket after endoscopic papillotomy.

choledochoduodenostomy, where the common bile duct is anastomosed to the anterior wall of the bulb or to the postbulbar duodenum. The anastomosis can be located and cannulated by means of both lateral-viewing duodenoscopes and forward-viewing panendoscopes.[58] The most frequent findings in patients with postoperative complaints are shrinkage of the anastomosis and retention of gallstones or food particles, particularly in the common duct stump below the anastomosis.[58] The stenosed anastomosis can be enlarged by incision using the papillotome of Demling and Classen. Retained gallstones and food remnants in the common duct stump can be extracted with a Dormia basket after endoscopic papillotomy (Figure 26.10). Retrograde cholangiography is difficult to perform following choledochojejunostomy. Gostout reported three patients with Roux-en-Y hepaticojejunostomy, who underwent a successful ERC with the use of a paediatric colonoscope.[77] Following cholecystectomy and bile duct exploration, overlooked or newly formed bile duct stones, stenosis of the papilla of Vater, bile duct strictures and cystic duct remnants can be observed. Strictures of the biliary ductal system may occur after portacaval shunt, partial gastrectomy and liver surgery.

Cholangiocarcinoma
A prospective study carried out in 22 patients with operatively and histologically confirmed carcinoma of the bile ducts demonstrated the high accuracy of ERCP (79%). In comparison sonography (39%), CT (42%) and angiography (55%) were less reliable.[35] Seifert *et al.*[210] distinguish three types of bile duct tumours by means of retrograde cholangiography: (a) stenosis of the duct system with dilatation of the upper duct system and its branches; (b) complete obstruction of common bile duct; and (c) complete obstruction of one of the hepatic ducts without filling of its branches. Spot films demonstrate the irregular contour and sometimes an exophytic border of the constriction.[224] The localization of the cholangiocarcinoma is equally frequent in the areas of the right and left and common hepatic ducts as well as in the triple junction of the common hepatic, cystic and common bile ducts (Figure 26.11). Advanced sclerosing cholangitis may simulate these morphological findings. Carcinomas in the area of the distal common bile duct and the diffuse spreading types are rarely observed. Isolated stenosis found in the bile ducts free of gallstones and in the absence of a

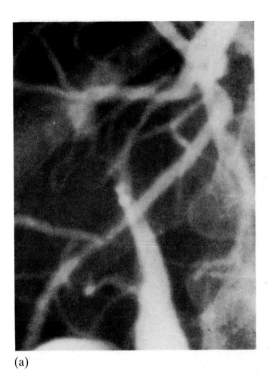

(a)

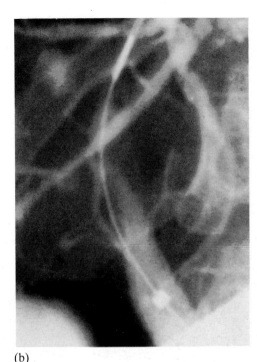

(b)

Figure 26.11
(a) Retrograde cholangiography in cholangiocarcinoma involving the right and left and common hepatic duct. (b) Retrograde catheterization of the left hepatic duct with a brush catheter for cytologic examinations.

history of previous surgery to the ducts are indicative of carcinoma. Differentiation from tumours arising in surrounding tissues, namely the head of the pancreas and the gallbladder, from postoperative strictures, and from inflammatory stenosis is usually possible (Figures 26.12 and 26.13). Establishing a tissue diagnosis of cholangiocarcinoma is difficult but may be safely achieved by a fluoroscopically guided transpapillary biopsy and brush cytology (Figure 26.11).[66,198] Increased sensitivity can be expected from cholangioscopically guided biopsies via the peroral or percutaneous route.[175,243]

Cholecystitis and cholangitis
The role of endoscopic procedures in diagnosis and therapy of biliary infections depends largely on the aetiology and the localization of the inflammation together with the severity of the disease.

Cholecystitis In addition to the clinical picture, ultrasonography is the most important investigation in the diagnosis of acute cholecystitis. Typical criteria include the presence of gallstones, a non-visualized gallbladder, and wall thickening of the inflamed organ. In difficult cases ERCP is able to reveal cystic duct obstruction, which is considered to be a causative factor in the inflammation.[227]

Acute cholangitis Acute cholangitis is generally caused by biliary infection and obstruction, while the mere bacterial contamination of bile does not usually lead to inflammation. Choledocholithiasis and benign biliary strictures represent the most common causes of acute obstructive cholangitis.[179,187] Concomitant biliary pan-

creatitis has been reported.[161] Malignant stenosis rarely induces spontaneous infection. Acute cholangitis is infrequently observed in patients with papillary stenosis, congenital biliary disorders, parasites and sclerosing cholangitis.

Invasive diagnostic or therapeutic approaches to the biliary system may cause iatrogenic cholangitis. The incidence rises significantly in patients with biliary obstruction. Post-ERCP cholangitis is particularly associated with malignant stenosis and when there is fever before the procedure. *Escherichia coli*, *Klebsiella* and streptococci are the predominant pathogens in non-iatrogenic cholangitis, whereas the presence of *Pseudomonas* species in bile and blood cultures indicates contamination of the endoscopic equipment.[32,90] As with ERCP, PTC and associated measures such as percutaneous drainage and cholangioscopy, can cause severe cholangitis, particularly in patients with multiple and proximal biliary tract strictures. Formation of a biliovenous fistula is frequently accompanied by septic complications. In cases of biliary obstruction with intraductal hypertension and simultaneous bile infection, the incidence of bacteraemia rises dramatically, often followed by Gram-negative septicaemia, liver abscess and pylephlebitis. The prognosis of the disease can be improved with timely diagnosis by means of ERCP or PTC and adequate therapy.[78,127,128,131]

Sclerosing cholangitis Continuous biliary obstruction can cause significant bile duct fibrosis due to subclinical inflammation. Aetiological factors like choledocholithiasis, benign strictures, obstructive tumours and congenital disorders can best be differentiated by ERCP. In contrast to these secondary forms of inflammation, the cause of

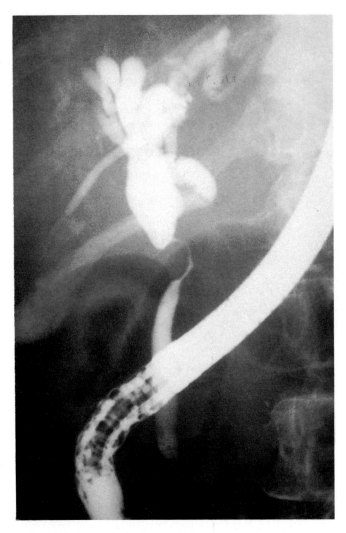

Figure 26.12 Arched stenosis of the common hepatic duct due to periductal metastases in a patient with breast cancer.

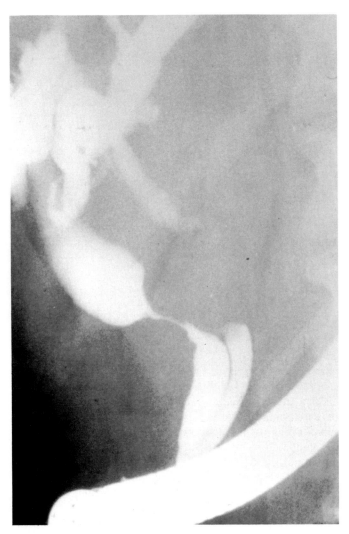

Figure 26.13 Retrograde cholangiography in gallbladder carcinoma. Complete obstruction of the cystic duct and corresponding stenosis of the common bile duct.

primary sclerosing cholangitis is still unclear (see Chapter 37). Chronically progressive inflammation of the biliary tree is associated with ulcerative colitis in 20–40% of the patients.[109] Diagnosis has been significantly improved by ERCP and correspondingly an increasing number of asymptomatic cases can be detected. The differentiation between primary and secondary sclerosing cholangitis is important because of distinct therapeutic measures. The diagnosis of the primary disease requires exclusion of a causal biliary obstruction such as choledocholithiasis.

ERCP, sometimes complemented by PTC, is the most sensitive diagnostic procedure. The spectrum of the radiographic appearances of primary sclerosing cholangitis is broad. In most cases, both intra- and extrahepatic ducts are involved. The intrahepatic changes are normally characterized by irregular stenoses obliterating peripheral ducts and leaving only the more central ducts filled with contrast medium (Figure 26.14). Extrahepatic involvement commonly shows well-defined segments of narrowing.[6,53,143] Diffuse alterations of the entire bile duct

system are not exceptional, but the gallbladder is typically not involved. Localized short stenoses, in contrast, favour the diagnosis of cholangiocarcinoma rather than sclerosing cholangitis. Their presence requires further diagnostic measures such as endoscopic biopsy or brush cytology. Peroral or percutaneous cholangioscopy achieves direct visualization of the findings and facilitates target biopsy.[175]

Recurrent pyogenic cholangitis Recurrent pyogenic cholangitis, predominantly observed in Asia, is clinically characterized by attacks of fever, abdominal pain and jaundice. Bile duct obstruction and recurrent cholangitis are caused by ductal stones secondary to primary bacterial infection. Owing to their diagnostic sensitivity, ERC or PTC in case of failure, should be performed in patients with suspected recurrent pyogenic cholangitis. Typical findings are different diameters of intrahepatic ducts that taper down abruptly, strictures with proximal dilatation of the biliary tree, multiple intra- and extrahepatic calculi

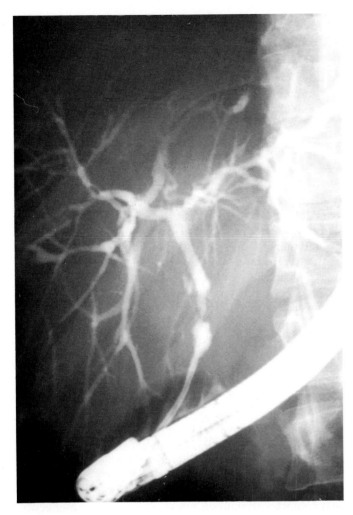

Figure 26.14 Retrograde cholangiography in a patient with ulcerative colitis and primary sclerosing cholangitis, mainly involving the intrahepatic bile ducts with irregular stenoses and peripheral obliterations.

as well as liver abscesses and fistulae. Diseases like clonorchiasis, ascariasis, hepatocellular carcinoma and cholangiocarcinoma may imitate the radiographic appearance of recurrent pyogenic cholangitis.[17]

Common bile duct cysts
Cystic dilatation of the common bile duct is very rarely observed. It may be suspected in patients presenting with intermittent jaundice, upper abdominal pain and an upper abdominal mass. Conventional cholangiography is usually unsuccessful. Since any volume of contrast material may be instilled into the dilated common bile duct by retrograde cholangiography, the diagnosis of even large cysts is possible without difficulty.[178]

Alterations of the intrahepatic bile ducts
Retrograde cholangiography should always attempt to fill the biliary system beyond the bifurcation in order to demonstrate abnormalities of the intrahepatic ducts. Primary alterations of the intrahepatic ducts, such as cystic

ectasia in Caroli's syndrome, intrahepatic gallstones or primary sclerosing cholangitis are infrequent findings but can be readily demonstrated by retrograde cholangiography (Figures 26.9 and 26.15). Secondary alterations of the intrahepatic bile ducts, as in cirrhosis or in metastatic liver disease, are observed more often. Ayoola et al.[6] describe the characteristic changes in cirrhosis as 'pruning' of intrahepatic ducts, with the presence of segments of ductular stenosis, tortuosity, ductular displacement and an absence of dilatation. The stenosis and displacement are due to compression by regenerative nodules; 'pruning' may reflect a severe degree of portal fibrosis. While small metastatic tumour nodules may easily give findings similar to cirrhosis, progressive metastatic liver disease is distinguishable by the presence of irregular dilatation, abrupt obstruction of branches and marked ductular displacement giving rise to 'mass effects'. These findings are probably due to compression of ducts by tumour nodules. In 7 out of 23 patients with primary biliary cirrhosis, irregularities in calibre and a tortuous course of small intrahepatic ducts have been described;[241] it is supposed that these changes are probably related to the distorted hepatic

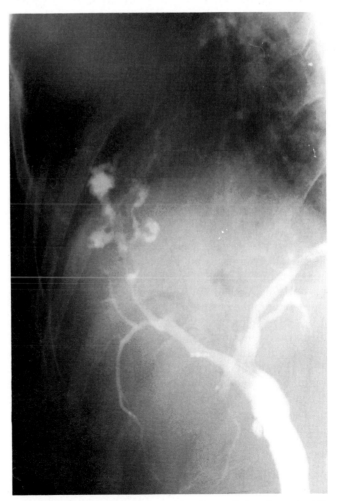

Figure 26.15 Circumscriptive dilatation of intrahepatic bile ducts in Caroli's disease.

architecture of cirrhosis and they may be interpreted as signs that cirrhosis has supervened.

The biliary tree in papillary stenosis

Duodenoscopic assessment of papillary abnormalities in papillitis, adenomyomatosis and ampullary carcinoma has already been mentioned. In such cases deep cannulation of the papilla may be difficult if not impossible, although visualization of the biliary tree can generally be achieved. Common findings in papillary stenosis are dilatation of the extra- and intrahepatic bile ducts as well as the absence of motility of the sphincter of Oddi with consequent delay in emptying of the duct. It must be stressed that the retrogradely filled duct may appear to be larger than when visualized by intravenous cholangiography. Spot films of the papillary region may demonstrate abnormalities of the distal common bile duct such as a thread-like stenosis of the ampullary segment or gross dilatation and irregularity of the contour of the wall. Using fluoroscopy or, preferably, radiocinematography it can be seen that the discharge of the contrast medium is delayed; also, papillary movement is not detectable. In borderline cases the duodenobiliary pressure gradient should, if possible, be measured by manometry to substantiate the diagnosis (see below).

SUPPLEMENTARY PROCEDURES

Choledochal manometry

Microsensor catheters[244] and perfused Teflon catheter systems[2,4,81,158] are available to measure the duodeno-biliary pressure gradient. Microsensor catheters do not readily fit the normal channel of the duodenoscope, so that the sensitive tip is easily damaged. Most centres therefore use a triple-lumen catheter system with side-holes.

Technique Duodenoscopy and cannulation of the papilla are performed in the usual way. Pressure recording is carried out using a triple-lumen catheter with an outer diameter of 1.7 mm. The three manometric channels are perfused with 0.9% saline using a low-compliance pneumohydraulic perfusion system at a reservoir pressure of 7.5 lb/in^2. Pressure changes are monitored by means of external transducers and a 6–8 channel chart recorder. The results are given in mmHg. The duodenobiliary pressure gradient is calculated from the difference between common bile duct and duodenal pressures. Simultaneous recording of ECG and respiration is carried out on separate channels throughout the procedure.

With the introduction of this methodology it has been possible to measure the motor activity of the sphincter of Oddi, including the amplitude and frequency of the sphincter contraction waves as well as their direction of propagation.[4,250]

According to endoscopic manometry studies, the basal pressure of the sphincter of Oddi is about 16 mmHg greater than in the duodenum and approximately 4 mmHg higher than in the common bile duct. Superimposed on the basal sphincter of Oddi pressure is a phasic activity which occurs at a frequency of 3–7 min^{-1}, and reaches contraction amplitudes of 50–120 mmHg.[1] After endoscopic papillotomy the pressure gradient is significantly lower than normal but sphincter activity is still present in about 20% of the patients.[79]

Delayed emptying of contrast medium, a dilated common bile duct or lack of bile duct motility are not reliable criteria for judgement of sphincter of Oddi function. Manometry of the sphincter of Oddi—complementary to scintigraphic techniques—allows patients with a normal sphincter of Oddi to be distinguished from those with dysmotility of the sphincter. 'Dysmotility' is caused either by dyskinesia (nitroglycerin sensitive) or by stenosis (nitroglycerin insensitive).[237] Several studies have shown that endoscopic papillotomy (EPT) is successful in the treatment of sphincter of Oddi-dysfunction. A randomized prospective study of EPT versus sham papillotomy in patients thought to have dysfunction of the sphincter of Oddi showed improvement in pain scores in 17 of 18 cases with elevated sphincter pressure. In contrast, there was improvement in only 3 of 12 patients with dysfunction verified by manometry who underwent the sham procedure.[74]

Toouli et al.[245] reported that patients with common bile duct stones have a higher proportion of retrograde sphincter contractions than normal. This finding gave rise to the hypothesis that this type of sphincter dyskinesia might be a pathogenetic mechanism for the formation of bile duct stones. The possibility has also been suggested that sphincter dyskinesia might also be the consequence of stones. Other groups have not been able to confirm a higher rate of retrograde contractions of the sphincter of Oddi in patients with bile duct stones.[40] Paradoxical motor reactions of the sphincter of Oddi to hormonal stimuli have also been reported. For example, some patients with presumptive sphincter of Oddi dysfunction, show abnormal hypermotility after intravenous injection of cholecystokinin.[1]

Endoscopic manometry of the sphincter of Oddi can be helpful in patients with idiopathic recurrent pancreatitis. Venu et al. found sphincter dysfunction manifested by an elevated basal sphincter pressure of 40 mmHg or more in 17 of 44 patients with unexplained pancreatitis. After endoscopic or surgical sphincterotomy, 16 of the 17 patients remained symptom-free for a mean period of 3 years.[251]

Sphincter of Oddi manometry is not without risk and can induce a predominantly mild pancreatitis.[14] Aspirating triple-lumen catheters seem to reduce the incidence of iatrogenic complications.[215]

Cholangioscopy

A new field of direct visualization of the biliary tract was opened by the development of small-calibre fibre-optic

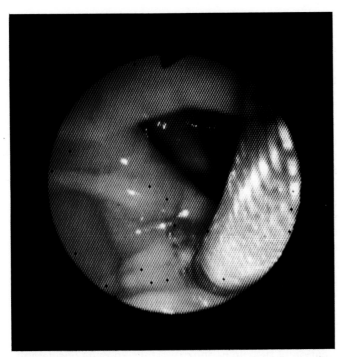

Figure 26.16 Duodenoscopy showing transpapillary insertion of the 'babyscope' into the common bile duct. The light at the tip of the instrument is transilluminating a duodenal diverticulum.

instruments.[174,243] In addition to the diagnostic importance, instrumentation channels of cholangioscopes allow insertion of various forceps and probes for non-surgical interventions in the treatment of cholelithiasis and biliary tumours. The different endoscopic approaches comprise peroral cholangioscopy using the mother–babyscope system, percutaneous transhepatic cholangioscopy and percutaneous or transperitoneal cholecystoscopy.

Technique

Peroral cholangioscopy and cholecystoscopy A long side-viewing duodenoscope (the 'motherscope') is used for the localization of the papilla. After endoscopic papillotomy a thin endoscope ('babyscope') with a maximal outside diameter of 4.5 mm is passed through the instrumentation channel and via the papilla into the common bile duct (Figure 26.16). The babyscope has its own channel of 1.7 mm internal diameter, which facilitates insertion of the cholangioscope over a guide wire as well as various diagnostic and therapeutic interventions. The babyscope, which can be actively angulated in two directions, is fragile and the procedure requires two skilful endoscopists. Peroral direct cholangioscopy using straight or oblique viewing cholangioscopes is even more difficult and seems appropriate only in selected patients with an easily accessible papilla.[247]

Transpapillary endoscopic access to the gallbladder is limited because of the valves in the cystic duct that prevent regurgitation from the common bile duct. Peroral cholecystoscopy by means of the mother–babyscope sys-

tem has been performed in selected patients with dilated cystic ducts and failed in cases with spiral-shaped ducts. The success rate might be improved if it becomes possible to dilate the cystic duct when necessary.[69] The development of a 'grandchild' endoscope that can be inserted through the channel of the babyscope into the gallbladder seems to be feasible.[120] Highly flexible miniscopes of 0.5 mm external diameter can be inserted through catheters into the bile ducts and the gallbladder for direct visualization. The diagnostic value is limited because these sophisticated devices are not steerable and have no instrument channel.[63]

Percutaneous cholangioscopy Percutaneous cholangioscopy is performed according to techniques described by Takada, Yamakawa and Nimura.[174,242,258] Following PTC, a drainage catheter is inserted into the bile ducts through the anterior abdominal wall or right lateral chest wall. The cutaneobiliary fistula or an already existing surgically introduced drainage channel are sequentially dilated every second day by replacing PTC catheters with progressively increasing diameters. At the earliest 7–8 days after initial creation of the fistula, cholangioscopy can be carried out through the sinus tract of a 14–18 French gauge (FG) catheter (Figure 26.17). Cholangioscopes already available have an external diameter of 4.9 mm and a channel size of 2.2 mm. Prototypes with a diameter of 4.1 mm and 1.7 mm, respectively, facilitate cholangioscopy via the sinus tract of a 14 FG catheter.[120] The short working length and manoeuvreability of these endoscopes makes manipulations within the biliary tree easier compared with the peroral approach. Further reduction in the cholangioscope's external diameter will be a main target for future development. To date, the thinnest endoscope with angulation but without an instrument channel is 2.2 mm in external diameter.[120]

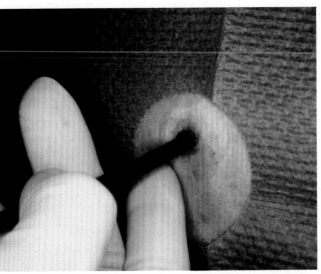

Figure 26.17 Insertion of a cholangioscope into the previously established cutaneobiliary fistula.

Percutaneous cholecystoscopy (a) *Transhepatic approach.* Similarly to the procedure in percutaneous cholangioscopy, a drainage catheter is placed through the 7th or 8th intercostal space into the gallbladder under ultrasonographic or fluoroscopic control. The sinus tract can be dilated immediately after percutaneous cholecystostomy with 10–16 FG dilators. In contrast to the sequential procedure, general anaesthesia is usually required. Percutaneous cholecystoscopy can be carried out one week after creation of the fistula using cholangioscopes as described above.[104] Percutaneous transhepatic cholecystoscopy is an excellent method for precise diagnosis of polypoid lesions of the gallbladder and has therapeutic applications including polypectomy and stone removal. However, the procedure is invasive and should only be performed by experienced physicians in selected cases.[101, 104]

(b) *Transperitoneal approach.* The transperitoneal access to the gallbladder carries the substantial risk of intraperitoneal leakage of bile. A single-stage method including removal of gallstones has been adapted from percutaneous nephrolithotomy and is performed under general or epidural anaesthesia.[16,26] A percutaneous catheter must be left in the gallbladder to establish a track for about 10 days. An exciting development has been the advent of laparoscopic cholecystotomy. This technique allows access to the gallbladder with small-calibre endoscopes under direct visual control. Closure of the gallbladder incision is achieved by means of metal clips and subsequent sealing with fibrin glue.[68]

Associated methods

Depending on the channel size, most cholangioscopes including the babyscope are suitable for performance of target biopsy, brush cytology, laser, electrocoagulation and stone extraction with basket.[167] Lithotripsy can be carried out mechanically and by electrohydraulic or laser lithotripsy under direct visual control.[259]

Indications and diagnostic results

Performance of diagnostic non-surgical cholangioscopy achieves visual and histological differentiation of benign and malignant strictures and polyps as well as other small and multiple lesions mostly detected by ERC or PTC.[141, 175] Cholangioscopic polypectomy might be helpful in the diagnosis of polyps with borderline malignancy.

The intraluminal extent of cancer can be precisely defined so that preoperative tumour staging may be improved.[175] Peroral cholangioscopy is less invasive than the percutaneous approach and carries the risk only of endoscopic sphincterotomy. Tumours located in or proximal to the mid common bile duct can be accessed more easily with a babyscope than neoplasms in the distal biliary tract. According to recently published studies and our own results, successful peroral visualization of biliary stenoses and protruded lesions was obtained in 72/85 patients (Table 26.2). Biopsy studies were effective in 80% of malignant and benign stenoses.[260]

Percutaneous cholangioscopy via the transhepatic route should be used only if the peroral approach fails (Figure 26.18). The risk of the procedure results mainly from the creation of the cutaneobiliary fistula, so that considerable experience in PTC techniques is required.[141] In contrast to the peroral approach, percutaneous cholangioscopy is also appropriate for lesions in the distal common bile duct (Figure 26.19). According to studies of Nimura *et al.*,[175] Chen *et al.*[15a] and our own results, biliary stenoses can be visualized reliably after correct establishment of a sinus tract. Cholangioscopically guided biopsies attained a sensitivity rate of 81% in a total of 217 patients with malignant stenoses (Table 26.3). The results depend on the tumour type, number of biopsies and experience of the endoscopist (Figure 26.20).

To date, percutaneous cholecystoscopy has been performed mainly for non-surgical treatment of gallbladder stones. In one study transhepatic cholecystoscopy was carried out for diagnostic reasons in 72 patients with gallbladder disease (21 carcinoma, 18 with polyps and 33 with cholecystitis). An accurate endoscopic and histological diagnosis was made for all patients and no severe

Table 26.2 Diagnostic peroral cholangioscopy

Author	Indications					
	Malignant stenosis		Benign stenosis		Protruded lesions	
	Patients	Success[a]	Patients	Success[a]	Patients	Success[a]
Riemann[193a]	20	15	7	5	–	–
Yasuda[260]	16	16	8	7	8	7
Authors' group	9	7	11	10	6	5
Total	45	38	26	22	14	12

[a] Endoscopic visualization, guided cholangiography of obstructed segments, biopsy.

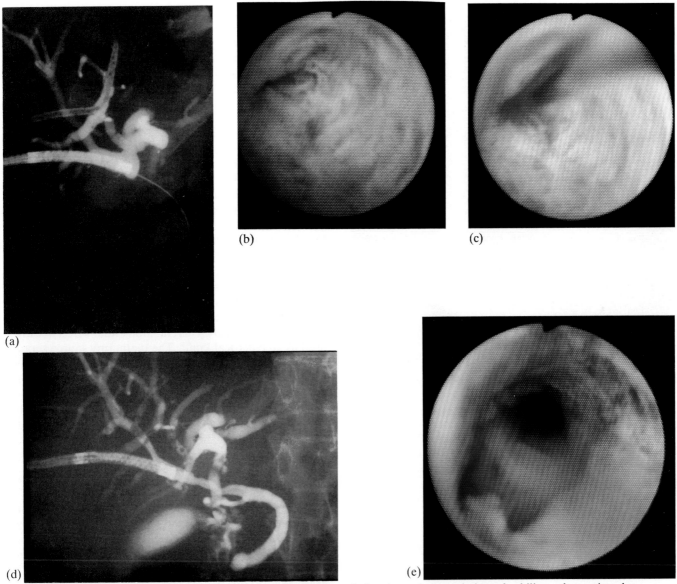

Figure 26.18 (a) Fluoroscopic control of a percutaneous cholangioscopic cannulation of a biliary obstruction due to infiltrative cholangiocarcinoma. (b) Cholangioscopy showing thread-like stenosis of the common bile duct. (c) Cholangioscopic guided cannulation of the obstruction with a guidewire for subsequent dilatation procedures. (d) Cholangioscopic cholangiography demonstrating reopening of the obstruction after dilatation and diathermy. (e) Cholangioscopy showing patency of the common hepatic duct.

complications were observed.[104] However, the clinical value of this time-consuming procedure is limited because most of these patients are candidates for surgery.

CHOLANGIOGRAPHY—WHICH IS THE TECHNIQUE OF CHOICE?

Comparative studies of conventional and retrograde cholangiography have demonstrated the limited diagnostic yield of conventional intravenous methods of opacification.[80] Diagnostic ERCP is therefore preferred by many physicians in patients strongly suspected of having biliary tract disease without clear findings on ultrasonography and computed tomography. In addition, ERCP

has diagnostic utility in so far as it serves as a preliminary manoeuvre for endoscopic therapy such as removal of bile duct stones or placement of drainage catheters. If retrograde opacification of the bile ducts is unsuccessful, PTC using the Chiba needle is indicated.[181] The advantages of the Chiba method using a flexible needle with an outer diameter of 0.7 mm are convincing: it is simple and inexpensive, complications are few, and even non-obstructed ducts may be opacified in most cases. Comparisons between this PTC technique and ERCP have demonstrated that they are complementary rather than competitive procedures.[52,59,60,95] Both procedures have their advantages and disadvantages and each clinician must select the procedure which he regards as most suitable

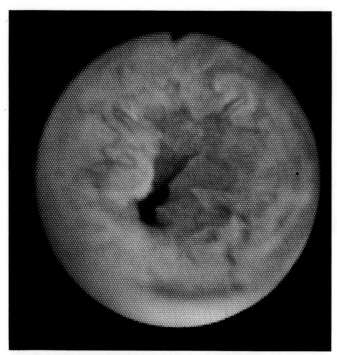

Figure 26.19 Percutaneous cholangioscopic prograde visualization of a normal papilla.

with regard to the facilities and resources available as well as his own personal experience. If complete common bile duct obstruction is demonstrated by ERCP, subsequent performance of PTC is required to locate with reliability the proximal demarcation of the obstructing process, which is important in planning the surgical procedure or measures for biliary drainage.

ENDOSCOPIC THERAPY

Endoscopic papillotomy

Since first reported in 1974 by Kaway and Classen, endoscopic papillotomy (EPT) and its adjunctive techniques as well as the array of indications have developed rapidly.[18,114] Enthusiasm on the one hand and scepticism on the other have been replaced by critical statements based on careful evaluations of management strategies. The worldwide application of EPT in more than 100 000 patients demonstrates acceptance by gastroenterologists and surgeons.[19,28,33,72,115,130,140,164,263] However, various aspects of this procedure, such as the selection of patients, are still under discussion.

Instruments

The same instruments as for diagnostic ERCP are used for EPT. In patients with previous partial gastrectomy, forward-viewing panendoscopes can be used. Several papillotomes have been developed such as the bridged

pulsed papillotome by the Japanese and the arched tracted papillotome by Demling and Classen. Additional recently developed instruments comprise papillotomes with a long, strengthened guiding tip or with a guide wire that may facilitate cannulation of the common bile duct in difficult cases. Precut sphincterotomy using papillotomes with a knife at the tip or a short wire leading to it is recommended if opacification of the biliary tree or insertion of the papillotome are precluded.[47,222] Further instruments such as rotatable or shark-fin shaped papillotomes might be dispensable even in patients after Bilroth II gastrectomy. In these cases the incision of the papilla of Vater is less difficult than adequate endoscopic access to it.

The great majority of procedures carried out to date have been performed with the papillotome developed by Demling and Classen. This papillotome comprises a plastic catheter containing a wire snare. The wire passes out of the lumen of the catheter 3 cm short of the tip and is reintroduced through the wall into the lumen 5 mm from the tip. The wire is drawn taut by application of tension on the proximal end of the catheter. By passing a high-frequency diathermy current along the wire, it can be used as an electrical knife. The diathermy source supplies a current for cutting and/or coagulation. Most endoscopists prefer to use a mixture of cutting and coagulation. Stones are removed from the common bile duct by means of Dormia basket catheters or modified Fogarty catheters that can be passed down the instrument channel of the duodenoscope into the bile duct.

Technique

Premedication, duodenoscopy and filling of the common bile duct with contrast are the same as in diagnostic ERC. The Demling–Classen papillotome is then advanced selectively into the common bile duct under radiological and endoscopic control.[19] After applying tension to the wire and intermittently passing a mixed cutting and coagulation current, the roof of the papilla is slit in the direction between 11 and 12 o'clock for a length of approximately 1.5 cm. The sudden emptying of contrast medium tinged with bile and the successful achieving of an endoscopic view into the lumen of the bile duct indicate that the newly created opening is adequate. The procedure takes 15–30 minutes. When the introduction of the papillotome into the bile duct is impossible, a minicut is performed. With the tip of the catheter of the papillotome fixed in the papillary orifice, a subpapillary mucosal cut is performed by upward movement of the wire. This precutting then permits the deep introduction of the papillotome into the common bile duct and following retraction of the papillotome allows a classical EPT to be performed. Alternatively the papillary roof is incised with the needle knife, which often facilitates selective introduction of the papillotome into the common bile duct.[47,222] This procedure is rarely necessary and potentially dangerous but few data are available.[30]

Table 26.3 Diagnostic percutaneous cholangioscopy

Indication	Nimura[175]		Chen[15a]		Authors' group	
	EV	CB	EV	CB	EV	CB
Malignant tumours	195	151/176	11	6/11	45	18/30
Cholangiocarcinoma	65	55/57	4	4/4	25	11/18
Gallbladder carcinoma	35	27/32	–	–	7	3/3
Hepatocellular carcinoma	22	19/21	–	–	1	0/1
Periductal metastases	–	–	2	0/2	8	1/5
Pancreatic carcinoma	57	38/53	3	0/3	4	3/3
Papillary carcinoma	16	12/13	2	2/2	–	–
Benign stenosis	43		4		18	

EV: endoscopic visualization; number of patients.
CB: correct biopsy.

Results

In most series success rates between 90% and 98% for endoscopic papillotomy in the treatment of bile duct stones are reported by referral centres.[28,56,106,130,248] In approximately 85% of patients the stones disappear spontaneously or can be extracted from the common bile duct by means of balloon catheters or the Dormia basket (Table 26.4; Figures 26.21 and 26.22).

Transhepatic guidewire assistance may improve the results, but a recently published study showed an appreciable complication rate, though not all the complications relate to the access alone.[46,216] These additional techniques of EPT are not standardized and risks can be difficult to estimate. The indication for an individual procedure should therefore be clearly defined.

Complications

As with every invasive therapy, EPT is not without risk of serious complications. The incidence of complications depends on the experience of the investigator. In major reviews[200,212] the complication rates vary between 5% and 8.7% and the EPT-related mortality is approximately 1%[12,21,76,248] (Table 26.5). In our experience, acute pancreatitis and retroperitoneal perforation are rare. By contrast, septic cholangitis is a serious hazard and results from stagnation of bile flow caused by common duct obstruction and simultaneous ascending infection facilitated by papillotomy. Several studies have shown that the complication rate of EPT increases significantly if the common bile duct is not cleared of stones at the initial attempt.[164] A nasobiliary drain is able to achieve a temporary biliary decompression in these cases.[217]

Besides cholangitis, bleeding is a relatively frequent and serious complication of EPT. The risk of bleeding seems to correlate with the length of the incision and with the size of the stones to be removed. Anatomical studies of the arterial blood supply to the papilla of Vater and the distal common bile duct by Spängler[231] stressed the importance of the retroduodenal artery, an anastomotic vessel between the gastroduodenal and the superior mes-

enteric artery. This vessel crosses the terminal common bile duct from the dorsal aspect. From this crossing, branches ramify to lead on to the ventral and dorsal aspects of the common bile duct to the papilla. Arterial bleeding after EPT may originate from the retroduodenal artery itself, from one of its branches in the area of the distal common bile duct, or from another branch which supplies the duodenal wall above the papilla of Vater. Endoscopic suprapapillary Doppler ultrasound can be performed before EPT and frequently indicates arterial and venous signals. The risk of bleeding, however, cannot be eliminated even if an incision is not performed in the direction of a Doppler signal.[169]

Indications

To date, gastroenterologists and surgeons have agreed that EPT is the treatment of choice for common bile duct stones in patients with previous cholecystectomy.[108] Eighty to ninety per cent of bile duct stones can be cleared successfully after sphincterotomy. In patients with the gallbladder in situ, a routine pre-cholecystectomy endoscopic clearance of the bile duct cannot be recommended, if one considers the results of a prospective randomized study of preoperative EPT versus surgery alone for common bile duct stones, which showed no benefit for the combined procedure.[160] According to multivariate analysis of endoscopic and surgical management of bile duct stones, the results of EPT are similar to the surgical approach and the risk of performing both procedures seems to be additive.[155,165] These findings are not surprising in view of the high surgical success rates and low mortality rates of less than 1% in fit patients under the age of 60.[28] Additional risks of a routine preoperative EPT would impair the surgical outcome. In the elderly and patients at risk, however, the combined endoscopic and surgical approach may lower the overall risk owing to simplification and shortening of the surgical procedure. Heinemann *et al.* performed ERCP and stone extraction 2–4 days before cholecystectomy in 728 patients. With this strategy the complication rate was reduced from

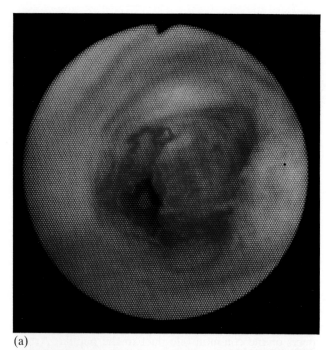

(a)

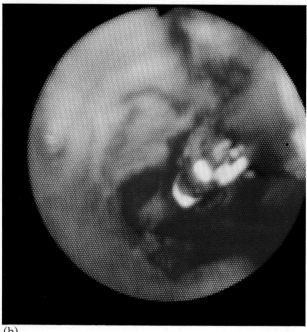

(b)

Figure 26.20 (a) Percutaneous cholangioscopy showing a polypoid cholangiocarcinoma obstructing the right hepatic duct. (b) Cholangioscopic targeted biopsy.

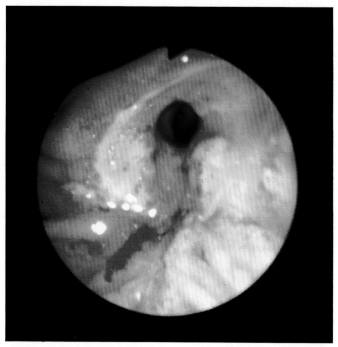

Figure 26.21 Duodenoscopy showing the papilla and the distal part of the common bile duct after previous large endoscopic sphincterotomy.

shown that the long-term complication rate due to the remaining gallbladder is approximately 10% after EPT, which compares favourably with an overall risk for laparotomy in elderly and frail patients (Table 26.6). Evaluation of criteria for the selection of patients who are predisposed to develop gallbladder complications would be of the greatest importance. Initial cholangitis, obstruction of the cyst duct and absence of gallstones were reported as predictors of later gallbladder problems, but these findings have unfortunately not been substantiated in large groups of patients.[37,256] Various techniques of cholecystolithiasis such as extracorporeal shockwave lithotripsy (ESWL), direct litholysis via percutaneous or retrograde gallbladder catheterization, as well as laparoscopic cholecystectomy or cholecystotomy, offer new alternative measures and may avoid long-term complications after endoscopic bile duct clearance. However, these procedures have not yet been performed in larger series of high-risk patients with previous EPT.

Acute suppurative cholangitis, presenting clinically as Charcot's triad of symptoms, with chills and fever, upper abdominal pain and jaundice, is associated with a high operative morbidity and mortality. EPT and drainage procedures are established alternatives to surgical drainage for cholangitis.[17,132,137] Leese *et al.* reported that early EPT in 43 patients with acute cholangitis was associated with a significantly lower 30-day mortality than early surgery in 28 cases despite the fact that the patients undergoing endoscopy had more medical risk factors.[132] Leung reported on 105 patients with acute suppurative cholangitis who did not respond to conservative manage-

21.8% to 2.1%, the residual stone rate was reduced from 2.2% to 0.5%, and the mortality fell from 3.8% to 1%.[88] Two recently published trials on preoperative EPT showed comparable results and indicate that the period of hospitalization is shorter in patients who undergo cholecystectomy after EPT than in those treated with cholecystectomy and choledochotomy.[189,257]

The need for cholecystectomy after endoscopic clearance of the bile duct is controversial. Various studies have

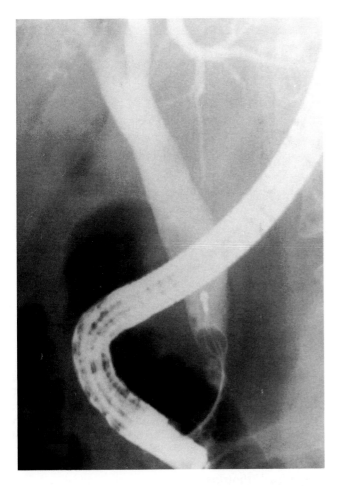

Figure 26.22 Retrograde extraction of a recurrent common bile duct stone with a Dormia basket in a patient with previous cholecystectomy and endoscopic papillotomy.

ment. Endoscopic insertion of a nasobiliary catheter with or without previous EPT was successful in 102 patients. The overall mortality of 4.7% is lower than that reported in comparable surgical studies.[137] In view of these results and the safety of the endoscopic approach, the superiority of emergency endoscopic drainage over urgent surgery is

Table 26.4 Results of endoscopic papillotomies for the removal of stones from the common bile duct

Results	Authors' patients Number (%)	Collective statistic[200] 1974–1986 Number (%)
Spontaneous stone discharge or stone extraction without lithotripsy	902 (87.1%)	12 387 (84 %)
Incomplete success or failure	134 (12.9%)	1563 (10.6%)
No information		796 (5.4%)
Total	1036 (100%)	14 746 (100%)

Table 26.5 Complications of endoscopic papillotomy

	Complication rate (%)		Mortality (%)
	Sahel[200] (n = 18 422)	Seifert[213] (n = 19 218)	Sahel[200] (n = 18 422)
Bleeding	2.56	2.11	0.18
Cholangitis	1.94	0.90	0.40
Acute pancreatitis	1.37	1.09	0.18
Cholecystitis[a]	1.03	n.d.	0.08
Perforation	0.97	0.56	0.11
Impaction of Dormia basket	0.41	–	0.02
Other complications	–	0.79	–
Total	7.63[a]	5.44	0.93[200] 0.84[213]

[a] In relation to 6205 patients with gallbladder in situ.
n.d. = no data.

obvious and the necessity for a randomized study is questionable.

Retained postoperative common bile duct stones with T-tube in situ have traditionally been treated via the T-tube tract by means of instrumentation or dissolution therapy (see Chapter 58). EPT and subsequent endoscopic stone removal have been recommended alternatively as a quick and comparably safe approach[9,225] (Figure 26.10). Patients with an endoscopically–manometrically verified increased sphincter of Oddi pressure due to sphincter dysfunction benefit significantly from EPT.[71,74]

In contrast to a previous restrictive attitude towards ERCP and EPT in acute pancreatitis, various retrospective studies have recently shown that the endoscopic procedure does not aggravate the course of the disease.[50,51,57,116,133,145,163,195,196,199,218] Meanwhile, ERCP is recommended as the diagnostic method of choice for establishing the aetiology in individual cases.[208] In cases of proven ampullary obstruction due to bile duct stones, EPT can readily achieve biliary decompression even in old and fragile patients. In the first controlled trial, patients with predicted severe attacks of acute pancreatitis have significantly benefited from ERCP and EPT compared with conservatively treated patients.[162] The importance of

Table 26.6 Endoscopic management of bile stones without cholecystectomy (collected data)[29,37,48,56,83,103,147,220]

Number of patients	2256
Mean age (years)	74.4
Bile duct clearance	80–93% (mean 90.8%)
Early complications	4–20% (mean 8.6%)
30-day mortality	0–11% (mean 1.2%)
Need for cholecystectomy after EPT	2–7% (mean 2.2%)
follow-up period (n = 847; mean 31 months)	5–18% (mean 8.6%)

Table 26.7 Indications for endoscopic papillotomy (EPT)

EPT of the bile duct orifice
   Common bile duct stones
     after previous cholecystectomy
     with concomitant acute cholangitis or pancreatitis prior to cholecystectomy
     in poor-risk patients with gallbladder in situ
   Acute biliary pancreatitis
   Benign stenosis of manometrically proven dysfunction of the papilla of Vater
   Benign bile duct stricture prior to endoscopic dilatation or stent insertion
   Malignant biliary obstruction for decompression prior to surgery or palliative endoscopic stent implantation
   Extraction of foreign body or parasites from the bile duct
   Insertion of the babyscope into the common bile duct for cholangioscopy
   Insertion of catheters into the biliary tract for various reasons (e.g. retrograde cannulation of the gallbladder, treatment of
     cholangitis, biliary fistula or abscess, intracorporeal lithotripsy)

EPT of the Wirsung duct orifice
   Chronic pancreatitis due to papillary stenosis
   Pancreatic duct stones
   Pancreatic duct strictures prior to endoscopic dilatation or stent placement
   Pancreatic cyst or abscess prior to transpapillary insertion of catheters for drainage
   Insertion of miniscopes for pancreatoscopy

endoscopy in predicted mild cases of acute pancreatitis is less clear.

The development of a variety of adjunctive techniques for biliary and pancreatic duct procedures has led to a considerable expansion of the indications for EPT (Table 26.7).

Only few convincing data exist on the long-term deleterious sequelae of EPT, e.g. bacteriobilia, intrahepatic reflux and unrestricted biliary emptying. Prospective evaluation of sphincter of Oddi function indicated a significant elimination of the sphincter basal pressure after EPT. This effect remained unchanged for at least 2 years, although the amplitude of sphincter of Oddi phasic contraction increased within that period.[73,79] Re-stenosis after EPT is rare and mainly develops in cases with primary ampullary stenosis. Other long-term complications comprise cholecystitis, cholangitis and residual or recurrent bile duct stones. Depending on the patient populations, the rates of further biliary symptoms after EPT vary between 5% and 13%.[87,125,212,213] The comparison of these results with surgical data is difficult owing to different selection criteria.

Management of difficult bile duct stones

In the non-surgical management of bile duct stones EPT can be impossible owing to an inaccessible papilla in patients with anatomical abnormalities of the duodenum or prior gastroduodenal or biliary surgery. If EPT is successful, removal of bile duct stones fails in about 10% of cases from impaction or the large size of the calculi. Difficulties increase with stones above 15 mm in diameter, although every experienced endoscopist will have encountered spontaneous passage of stones larger than 25 mm after EPT. Since big stones may be fragile, an attempt at endoscopic removal is always justified. In case of failure,

the objective of various technically different measures is to reduce the size of the calculi, so that the fragments can be removed without the need for surgical intervention with its attendant risks. If this attempt fails and stones are thought likely to occlude the bile duct, or are already blocking it, the obstacle must be by-passed by a catheter or stent.

Mechanical lithotripsy

The simplest endoscopic adjunct for large stones is a mechanical lithotriptor or 'crushing basket' introduced by Demling *et al.* in 1982.[41] It consists of a wire basket with three or four arms, which is introduced into the bile duct through the instrumentation channel of the duodenoscope. Once the stone is grasped, the mechanically very strong, heavy-duty wires are drawn tight over a winding peg with a milled nut and cut the stone into fragments (Figure 26.23). Similar models with considerable improvements have been introduced by different working groups.[207] A modification by Frimberger *et al.*[67] allows lithotripsy in cases with stone impaction during an attempt to extract the stone with a standard Dormia basket. When the stone is impacted, the endoscope and the Teflon sheath of the Dormia basket are removed and thereafter replaced by a metal spiral sheath, which is passed over the basket wire towards the stone. The success rate of mechanical lithotripsy depends on the selection of patients and seems to correlate negatively with the size of the stone. The main problem is the lack of space within the common bile duct to open the basket around the stone. Conventional baskets are frequently too small and too weak for large stones. Recently developed larger baskets with breaking strengths up to 125 kg have increased the success rate.[207]

In larger trials of mechanical lithotripsy, common bile duct clearance is obtained in 77% up to 94% of patients

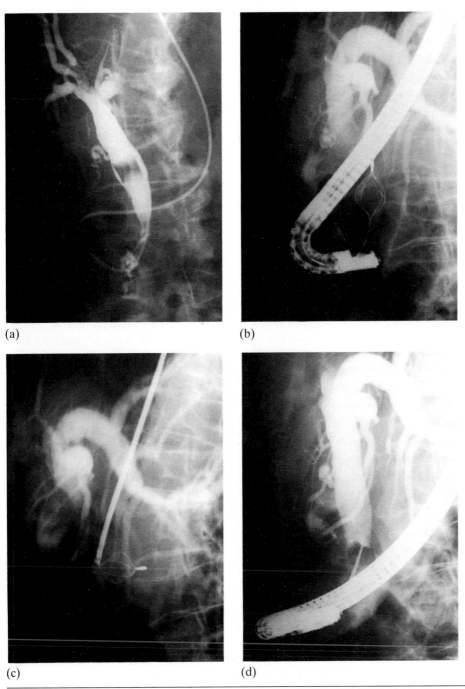

(a)

(b)

(c)

(d)

Figure 26.23 (a) Impacted large common bile duct stone; nasobiliary catheter in situ for establishment of biliary drainage. (b) Endoscopic grasping of the stone with a Dormia basket. (c) After removal of the endoscope the wires of the basket are drawn through a metal sheath by means of a winding peg, leading to stone disintegration. (d) Endoscopic extraction of the stone fragments with a balloon catheter.

with stones not amenable to standard procedures (Table 26.8). Lower success rates may be due to an unfavourable selection of cases with extremely difficult giant calculi.[24] Severe complications are rare and mainly due to EPT. Mechanical lithotripsy is a safe and inexpensive procedure, and should therefore be performed before application of more invasive techniques.

Cholangioscopic electrohydraulic lithotripsy

Since 1975 EHL has been applied for bile duct stones via the percutaneous transhepatic or the transpapillary approach.[119] The technology is simple. A spark discharge from a bipolar co-axial electrode induces shockwaves in a fluid medium. The energy can be absorbed by an abrupt increase in acoustic impedance or resistance such as represented by the stone. Absorption of shockwave energy within the stone leads to a build-up of pressure gradients and formation of brute forces that eventually cause fragmentation. The system includes the generator, which allows the adjustment of the frequency as well as the intensity of the shockwave generation, and the probe with a minimal diameter of 0.8 mm for the transmission of the energy to the surface of the stones. Intracorporeal electrohydraulic lithotripsy is safe provided that the probe

Table 26.8 Results of mechanical lithotripsy

Author	Year	Number of patients (*n*)	Stone diameter (mm)	Success rate (%)
Hagenmüller, Classen[82]	1982	12	24–40	25
Staritz[238]	1983	8	6–28	100
Riemann, Demling[193]	1985	84	22–41	82
Runge[197]	1985	106	10–52	93
Bethge, Hintze[8]	1987	34	8–39	77
Higuchi[91]	1987	30	No data	83
Schneider[207]	1988	209	4–80	88
Siegel[223]	1990	93	No data	94

Table 26.10 Complications of diagnostic and therapeutic percutaneous transhepatic drainage and cholangioscopy; authors' results (1988–1990)

Number of patients	92
Number of cholangioscopies	125
Cholangitis	8
Septicaemia	4
Haemobilia	4
Subcapsular liver haematoma	3
Acute pancreatitis	3
Pneumothorax	1
Procedure-related mortality	1.1%

tip is 1 mm or more away from the duct. When the probe is placed in direct contact with the bile duct wall, the spark energy vaporizes the wall, resulting in perforation at even the lowest power setting.[84] The exact site of spark discharge should therefore be controlled under direct vision during cholangioscopy. Fluoroscopy does not seem to be safe enough, since haemorrhage and perforation of the common bile duct have been observed.[146]

Several groups have worked on the percutaneous biliary approach to direct the EHL probe to the stone (Table 26.9). Direct vision lithotripsy is easy to perform when the patient has a previously dilated T-tube tract large enough to allow passage of a standard choledochoscope. This gives excellent visualization, good tip control and a channel large enough to permit continuous irrigation. When there is no T-tube tract and the papilla is inaccessible, e.g. in patients with previous gastroduodenal or biliary surgery, a cutaneobiliary fistula can be established by sequential dilatation of a percutaneous transhepatic cholangiographic drainage (PTCD) tract. Cholangioscopy

via this sinus tract offers an effective alternative to surgery in patients with difficult bile duct stones not amenable to transampullary manoeuvres. However, the creation of the fistula and the endoscopic procedure may induce severe complications in 10–29% of cases and should be limited to patients in whom all other non-surgical measures have failed[15,106,141] (Table 26.10).

Owing to excellent direct fistula control, complications related to electrohydraulic lithotripsy are rare (Table 26.9). The success rates vary between 83% and 100% depending on the selection of patients in terms of intrahepatic calculi, bile duct strictures and angulations.

When the papilla of Vater is endoscopically accessible, peroral cholangioscopy with a 'mother and baby' dual system provides access to stones in the common bile duct for electrohydraulic lithotripsy during a single ERCP procedure (Figure 26.24). In contrast to the percutaneous access, good targeting of the stones is sometimes difficult to achieve, and sludge and fragments may impair visual control. Two skilled endoscopists are required for the procedure, which has particular limitations in patients with a huge total stone burden and calculi close to the papilla. A few patients have been treated successfully without complications in several centres (Table 26.9). Further improvement of the fragile endoscope system is required.

Table 26.9 Cholangioscopic electrohydraulic lithotripsy

Author	Number of patients	Approach[a]	Procedure-related complications		Bile duct clearance (%)
			Bleeding	Other	
Mo[156]	10	PTCS	1	–	100
Picus[186]	10	T-tube (4)	–	–	100
		PTCS (6)	–	–	100
Chen[15]	10	PTCS	2	1	100
Yoshimoto[261]	40	T-tube (9) PTCS (31)	4	3	95
Liguory[141]	24	PTCS	1	–	83
Yasuda[260]	17	PTCS	–	–	94
	11	POCS	–	–	82
Ponchon[190]	6	POCS	–	–	83
Leung[134]	5	POCS	–	–	100
Neuhaus et al.[170]	8	PTCS	–	–	100
	12	POCS	–	–	63

[a] PTCS: percutaneous transhepatic cholangioscopy. POCS: peroral cholangioscopy (mother–babyscope technique).

Intracorporeal laser lithotripsy

Some attempts to destroy gallstones using different lasers have been made in animals and in man (Table 26.11). The standard continuous-wave neodymium-YAG laser destroys stones by thermal stress and may produce injury to the surrounding tissues.[182] In contrast to this thermal effect, short-pulsed lasers induce shockwave formation. Owing to the thermal relaxation time between single pulses, laser lithotripsy generates less heat and the risk of bile duct damage should be low. Ell *et al.* reported their initial experience in nine patients using a flashlamp-pulsed Nd-YAG laser with a pulse frequency of 1–20 Hz and a pulse duration of 0.1 to 10 ms. Fragmentation was effective in eight patients, and duct clearance was achieved in six without severe complications. The ever shorter

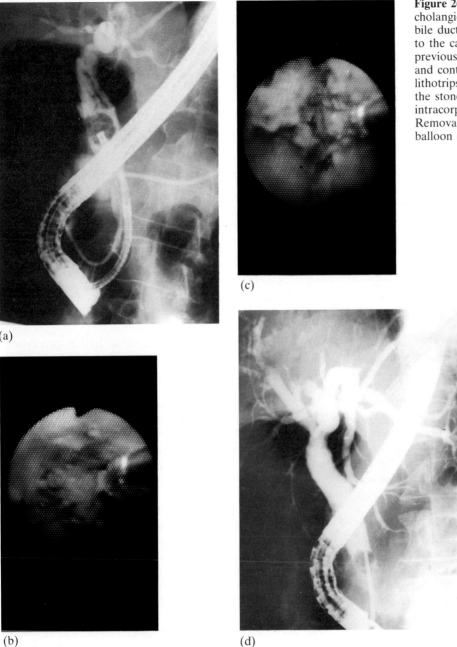

(a)

(b)

(c)

(d)

Figure 26.24 (a) Peroral cholangioscopic cholangiography showing an impacted common bile duct stone. Advancement of the 'babyscope' to the calculus. A nasobiliary catheter was previously inserted for biliary decompression and continuous irrigation with saline during lithotripsy. (b) An 800-μm probe is advanced to the stone. (c) Cholangioscopic controlled intracorporeal electrohydraulic lithotripsy. (d) Removal of the stone fragments with the balloon catheter after successful lithotripsy.

pulse length (1 μs) of a flashlamp-excited dye laser (Candela Laser Corporation, Wayland, MA, USA) produces a higher peak power at a given pulse energy and thus improves the fragmentation efficacy without thermal effects.[121,157]

Pulsed dye laser lithotripsy under peroral or percutaneous cholangioscopic control has achieved safe disintegration of difficult bile duct stones into very small particles provided that the flexible laser fibre with a diameter of 200 or 320 μm can be adequately guided to the stone surface[31,172] (Figure 26.25). Owing to the low risk of bile duct injury, fluoroscopic controlled laser lithotripsy with laser balloons, baskets or special probes seems to be safe enough and would greatly simplify the procedure, which may be employed without sphincterotomy. However, further trials are needed for comparison with simple and cheap alternative methods of lithotripsy.

Extracorporeal shockwave lithotripsy

Since the introduction of extracorporeal shock-wave lithotripsy (ESWL) of bile duct stones,[204] several hundred patients have been successfully treated in various centres (Table 26.12). Bodily immersion of the patient in a tank of degassed water and general anaesthesia during the procedure are no longer necessary. Second-generation devices allow direct coupling of the shockwave head to

Table 26.11 Biliary laser lithotripsy

Author	Number of patients	Type of laser	Approach[a]	Bile duct clearance
Orii[182]	2	CW Nd-YAG	T-tube cholangioscopy (1) PTCS (1)	2
Ell[55]	9	Pulsed Nd-YAG	Transpapillary, x-ray controlled (7) POCS (2)	6
Cotton[31]	25	Pulsed dye laser	T-tube cholangioscopy (5) T-tube x-ray controlled (1) POCS (12) Transpapillary x-ray controlled (7)	20
Neuhaus et al.[172]	14	Pulsed dye laser	POCS (7) PTCS (7)	12

[a] PTCS: percutaneous transhepatic cholangioscopy. POCS: peroral cholangioscopy (mother–babyscope technique).

the patient's skin and treatment under sedation plus analgesia.[239,249] Positioning of the bile duct and monitoring of stone disintegration are achieved by cholangiography by means of a previously inserted nasobiliary catheter and a two-dimensional x-ray system of the lithotripter for fluoroscopic targeting.

Between one and five lithotripsy sessions are required for each patient to obtain stone fragmentation appropriate for spontaneous passage or subsequent endoscopic removal (Figures 26.26 and 26.27). Complete bile duct clearance is achieved in 61–90% of patients with difficult stones (Table 26.12). The differences in the number of procedures and the overall success rates reflect varying levels of aggressive endoscopic management and experience in application of extracorporeal shockwaves. In addition, the energy level of shockwave generation, targeting facilities of the lithotripter and management of the patient's pain during the procedure may have an important impact on the overall results. Reported adverse effects such as pain, skin haematoma and haematuria are mostly mild and there were no life-threatening complications. Considering the high-risk population, the 30-day mortality of 0.9% in the largest series compared favourably with that of open surgery.[205]

In patients with difficult bile duct stones, ESWL is therefore an effective and safe alternative to surgery, but may be time consuming when several ERCP and lithotripsy sessions are required.

Intracorporeal or extracorporeal lithotripsy?
If standard ERCP fails in patients with bile duct stones due to giant or impacted calculi, the cheap, simple and effective performance of mechanical lithotripsy is the method of choice (Figure 26.28). If this measure fails, intracorporeal electrohydraulic or laser lithotripsy under peroral cholangioscopic control may achieve appropriate

stone disintegration within the same ERCP procedure, particularly when access to the papilla is easy, the stone mass is small and the endoscopists are experienced in this field. Otherwise, ESWL offers the more promising alternative. If both procedures have failed or transpapillary manoeuvres are impossible owing to an inaccessible papilla or large stones above a biliary stricture, percutaneous transhepatic cholangioscopy including intracorporeal lithotripsy offers an alternative to surgery in high-risk patients.

Chemical stone dissolution via a bile duct catheter
Dissolution of difficult bile duct stones can be attempted by infusion of various agents via nasobiliary drain or percutaneous transhepatic catheter. Modern solvents for cholesterol stones are mono-octanoin (Capmul), a mono-octanoin preparation detergent (GMOC) and methyl-tert-butyl ether (MTBE). Dissolution of calcium-containing stones is best achieved by a 1% EDTA/bile acid solution. The average duration of therapy is 7 days. The results of various dissolution trials in a large number of patients are, however, disappointing.[184] In 33 patients infusion of MTBE via a nasobiliary catheter contributed to success in only 12 cases. Side-effects such as drowsiness, elevation of liver enzymes and nausea in 26 patients indicate that the use of MTBE for bile duct stones should be restricted, given the availability of alternative, safer and more effective non-surgical measures.[166] Thus the 'chemical revolution' has not yet taken place in choledocholithiasis.

Temporary or permanent biliary drainage for ductal stones
Giant bile duct stones or fragments after insufficient lithotripsy can become impacted through endoscopic manipulations, and obstructive jaundice may result. If bacterial cholangitis is already present, a nasobiliary tube

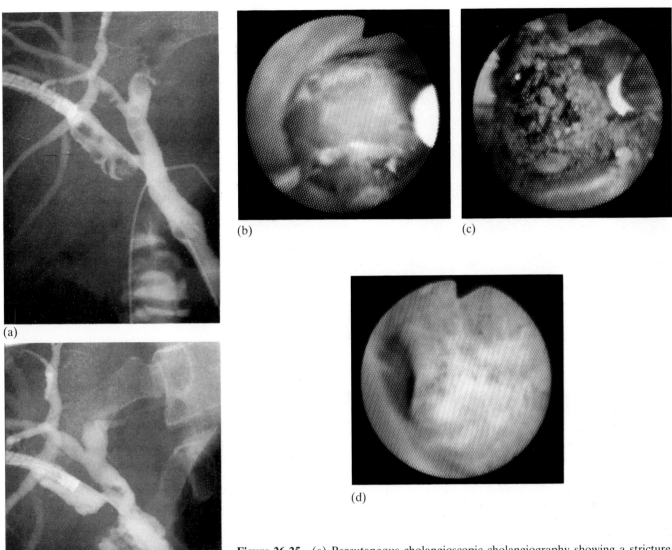

(a)

(b)

(c)

(d)

(e)

Figure 26.25 (a) Percutaneous cholangioscopic cholangiography showing a stricture of the right hepatic duct with proximal dilatation and calculi after previous cholecystectomy and common bile duct exploration. (b) Cholangioscopic visualization of the intrahepatic stones. A 200-μm flexible fibre is pressed to the surface of a calculus for pulsed dye laser lithotripsy. (c) Cholangioscopic controlled stone disintegration. (d) Complete disappearance of stones and fragments; visualization of the dilated postoperative stricture with typical whitish tracks of fibrosis. (e) Cholangioscopic cholangiography demonstrating stone clearance of the intrahepatic biliary tree.

Table 26.12 ESWL for bile duct stones

Author	Number of patients	Complications (%)	Bile duct clearance (%)
Sauerbruch[205]	113	36	86
Bland[11]	42	36	74
Lee[129]	70	7	61
Staritz[239]	33	0	76
Vandermeeren et al.[249]	90	30	90

for the collection of bile to culture bacteria and to monitor the efficacy of antibiotic treatment should first be introduced. Subsequently, an endoscopic endoprosthesis can be implanted as a temporary or long-term measure. The prosthesis is advantageous to the patient as it causes no bile loss and no discomfort. Almost 100% of attempts are successful.

Stent placement as a long-term palliative measure is used as a last resort when no advanced technique of lithotripsy is possible or available in high-risk patients. A recently published study comprising 127 patients with bile duct stones showed successful drain or stent implantation in 98%. Two cases of cholangitis after placement of

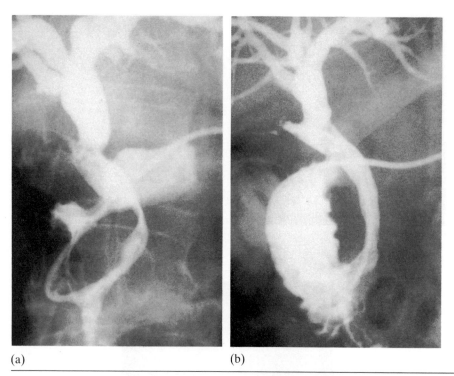

(a)   (b)

Figure 26.26 (a) Cholangiography via a nasobiliary catheter, showing a giant impacted stone in the distal common bile duct. (b) Cholangiographic control after a single treatment with extracorporeal shockwaves demonstrating complete spontaneous disappearance of fragments after successful lithotripsy.

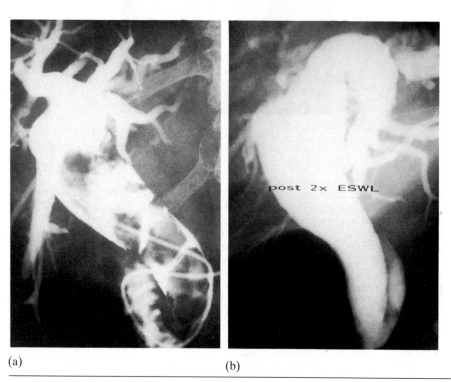

(a)   (b)

Figure 26.27 (a) Cholangiography via a nasobiliary catheter showing multiple impacted large common bile duct stones after previous cholecystectomy. (b) Retrograde cholangiography demonstrating stone clearance of the biliary tree after two sessions of extracorporeal shockwave lithotripsy and endoscopic removal of the fragments.

temporary stents were observed. The 30-day mortality was 3%. Forty-two patients with permanent stents and unfit for further surgical or endoscopic attempts at duct clearance were followed for a mean period of 16 months. Cholangitis developed in four cases and was successfully managed by stent change. These results demonstrate the benefit of nasobiliary catheters for temporary drainage and long-term stenting for biliary decompression in poor-

risk patients not amenable to further endoscopic or surgical procedures.[13]

Endoscopic treatment of gallbladder stones
An interesting alternative to the percutaneous transhepatic contact dissolution of non-calcified gallbladder stones is the peroral transpapillary approach. Success rates of retrograde gallbladder cannulation with or without

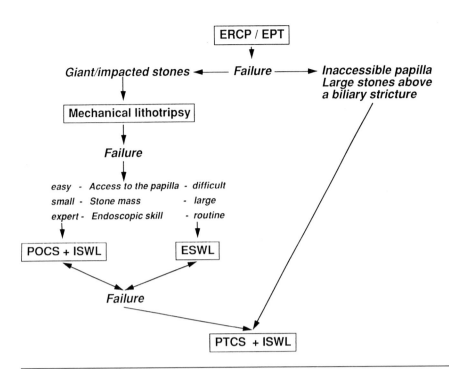

Figure 26.28 Non-surgical treatment of bile duct stones. POCS = peroral cholangioscopy; PTCS = percutaneous transhepatic cholangioscopy; ISWL = intracorporeal shockwave lithotripsy; ESWL = extracorporeal shockwave lithotripsy; EPT = endoscopic papillotomy.

previous EPT vary between 82% and 90% in experienced centres.[64,148,230] Most endoscopists prefer a hydrophilic polymer-coated steerable guidewire (Terumo/Meditech, Meditech Inc., Watertown, MA, USA) called Glidewire, for difficult catheterization of the cystic duct[148,230] (Figure 26.29). Up to 10% of cases have procedure-related complications such as acute pancreatitis.[230] Compared with the percutaneous approach, more (up to 80 ml) MTBE can be instilled into the gallbladder via a naso-vesicular catheter that occludes the cystic duct and prevents spillage of the dissolution agent into the common bile duct. On the other hand, replacement of the catheter for improvement of contact with stones during the dissolution period is much easier via the percutaneous route. The reported dissolution treatment period for the endoscopic technique varies considerably between 2.5 hours and 36 days. Depending on the selection of patients and application of adjunctive techniques like ESWL, complete stone clearance can be achieved in approximately 60% of the patients in whom placement of a nasocystic catheter was successful.[64,230] Studies comparing the percutaneous and the retrograde transpapillary dissolution technique with or without additional ESWL are urgently required.

In contrast to dissolution methods, the direct endoscopic approach to the gallbladder achieves removal of the stones irrespective of their composition. Several technical options are available. Transhepatic cholecystoscopy requires establishment of a stable cutaneovesical fistula and is therefore time consuming.[101,104] Percutaneous transperitoneal cholecystotomy has to be followed by a placement of a Foley catheter over a period of 7–10 days[16] (Figure 26.30). Laparoscopic cholecystotomy may eliminate disadvantages of a 'semiblind' cholecystotomy. Practically every gallbladder can be examined during laparoscopy and can be approached with the appropriate claw instrument.

Frimberger developed a complete set of instruments for this method. A small incision in the fundic region that permits a good overall view can be tailored through the channel of the laparoscope. A sheath is then introduced into the gallbladder, allowing the passage of fibre-endoscope, lithotriptor, and irrigator. After complete removal of stones and fragments, metal clips and fibrin glue seal off the incision again[68] (Figure 26.31). This procedure is even less invasive than the recently developed technique of laparoscopic cholecystectomy and may be carried out without general anaesthesia.[49,185] However, the main drawback of all non-surgical methods that leave the gallbladder in situ is, of course, the risk of gallstone recurrence.

Endoscopic bile drainage

Various endoscopic or percutaneous techniques have been developed to complete or substitute for surgical treatment of biliary strictures and leaks. The advantages and limitations of endoscopic drainage can be discussed on the basis of the experience gained with several hundreds of patients worldwide.

Technique

The guided endoscopic insertion of probes for dilatation or drainage into the common bile duct is greatly facilitated by endoscopic papillotomy. The cut performed usually is small (6–10 mm) and carries little risk of complication.

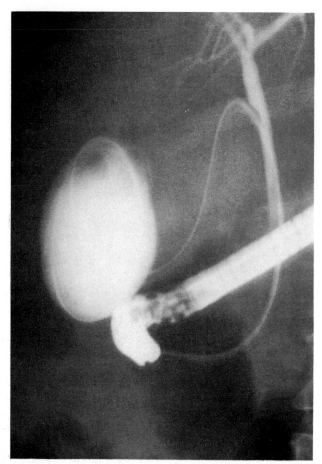

Figure 26.29 Retrograde endoscopic insertion of a nasovesicular catheter over a 'Glidewire' for dissolution of non-calcified gallbladder stones.

Dilatation of benign or malignant biliary strictures

With tapered or balloon catheters this can facilitate the subsequent insertion of drainage probes. Dilatation alone does not seem to be of long-term benefit.[254] Balloon catheters used are a modification of angioplasty catheters. The endoscopic devices are 5 to 8 Fr in diameter and 180 cm in length. The distended balloon measures 2–4 cm in length, with a diameter of 4–10 mm.

Following ERCP and EPT a guidewire is introduced so that its tip comes to rest proximal to the stricture. Dilatation with appropriately sized tapered catheters facilitates the subsequent insertion of the balloon catheter over the guidewire and placement across the stricture. The balloon is then filled with 30–60% radiopaque dye under fluoroscopic control and fully distended to exert a pressure of 4–6 atmospheres (Figure 26.32). Pressure settings, duration of inflation and the number of dilatation procedures required are not as yet standardized.

External bilionasal drainage

For temporary biliary decompression and drainage a 250-cm long polyethylene tube with an outer diameter of 1.7 or 2.2 mm is recommended. This specially preformed catheter adapts to the anatomy of the duodenum and bile ducts and thus decreases the risk of displacement from the bile duct. The drainage catheter is introduced into the bile duct through the instrumentation channel of a duodenoscope. A Seldinger wire facilitates passage through the stenosis. The tip of the drainage catheter with its lateral openings is placed above the stenosis to ensure the flow of congested bile. The other end of the catheter is led through the nose, fixed to the cheek and connected to a plastic bag.

Internal bilioduodenal drainage

Internal drainage of the occluded bile duct is accomplished by the insertion of an endoprosthesis using 8–16-cm long probes made of polyethylene or polyurethane. The 'pig-tail' keeps the tip of the probe well above the stenosis in the bile, and a second 'pig-tail' prevents injury to the duodenal wall. Instead of pig-tail catheters a straight probe with lateral valves can also be used (Amsterdam type). Nowadays, endoprostheses with an outer diameter of 3.4 mm (10 French) or 3.8 mm (11.5 French) should be employed since they achieve better drainage and are occluded less rapidly. An endoscope with an instrument channel measuring 3.7 mm or 4.2 mm, respectively, in diameter is necessary for their insertion. The length of the endoprosthesis is individually tailored according to the anatomy of the bile duct. After endoscopic insertion of a Seldinger wire, the prosthesis is passed with a pushing probe beyond the stenosis. The introduction of the endoprosthesis is controlled both endoscopically and radiologically. The duodenal end of the endoprosthesis should protrude by about 1–2 cm from the papilla of Vater into the duodenal lumen.

Endoscopic insertion and percutaneous transhepatic implantation of endoprostheses are complementary techniques, both having specific advantages. The percutaneous method is technically easier, less expensive, but more invasive. The endoscopic route takes advantage of a more physiological route of access and allows readily an exchange of blocked prostheses.

A combined percutaneous and endoscopic technique is recommended for strictures not amenable to standard endoscopic procedures.[46] A percutaneous transhepatic guidewire is passed through the biliary stricture into the duodenum. The duodenal end of the guidewire is grasped with a basket or a snare passed down a duodenoscope. The radiologist pushes the wire down the transhepatic route, as the endoscopist withdraws the basket tightly closed around the other end of the wire. Endoscopic sphincterotomy and stent insertion is then performed over the guidewire, so that the size of the liver puncture can be minimized. Blockage of endoprostheses is the main problem of endoscopic or percutaneous biliary drainage and therapeutic advances are expected from self-expanding or balloon-expandable metal stents owing to their large lumen and small surface area.

The most common self-expandable stent (Wallstent, Medinvent SA, Lausanne, Switzerland) is made of surgical-grade stainless-steel alloy filaments braided in a tubular fashion. For implantation the diameter of the flexible

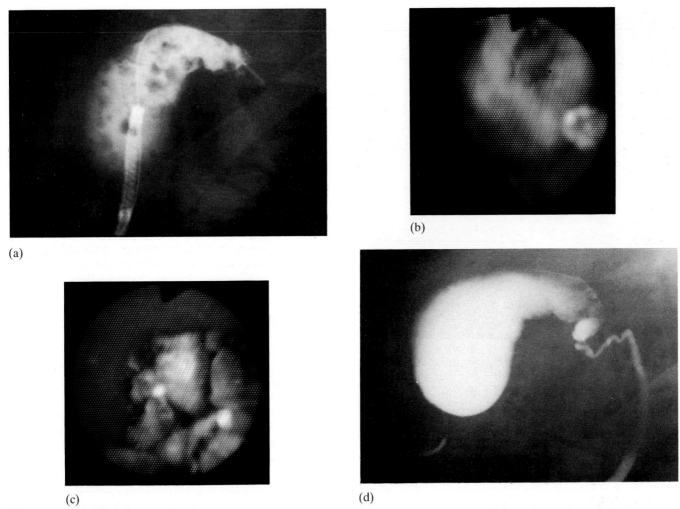

(a)

(b)

(c)

(d)

Figure 26.30 (a) Fluoroscopic control of cholecystoscopy via a percutaneous transhepatic track established by a previously inserted Foley catheter. (b) Cholecystoscopic visualization of a calcified gallbladder calculus. Beginning stone fragmentation by pulsed dye laser lithotripsy showing the outer calcium layers. (c) Complete stone disintegration after laser lithotripsy; 320-μm fibre with a helium aiming beam at 3 o'clock. (d) Cholecystogram demonstrating stone clearance of the gallbladder after percutaneous removal of the fragments with a basket.

prosthesis can be substantially reduced by elongation. The system for insertion and release comprises a 7 or 9 French coaxial catheter with an invaginated rolling membrane, under which the constrained stent is mounted. When the membrane is inflated with contrast medium, the friction between the invaginated membrane and the stent is reduced so that the stent can be slowly released by withdrawing the rolling membrane. During the implantation procedure the position of the prosthesis can be controlled fluoroscopically and endoscopically. The released stent opens by its own expansive force to a diameter up to 30 French. It remains permanently in situ: removal is not possible by endoscopic or percutaneous interventional procedures.

Indications

Absolute therapeutic indications for endoscopic biliary drainage are septic cholangitis, prevention of bile duct obstruction following incomplete transpapillary removal of stones, and inoperable malignant stenoses. A relative therapeutic indication is the preoperative decompression of an obstructed bile duct in order to improve the general condition of the patient. In patients with a benign common bile duct stricture, a conventional endoprosthesis can be positioned across the previously dilated stricture for 1–3 months to promote re-epithelialization of the traumatized duct lumen without restricturing. Endoscopic management can also be indicated in patients with postoperative biliary leaks[39,136] (Figure 26.33).

Diagnostic indications for bilionasal drainage include bacteriological and cytological investigation and possibly also the study of lithogenicity of pure bile.

Contraindications are life-threatening acute cardiopulmonary disease, the acute abdomen, and severe coagulation defects.

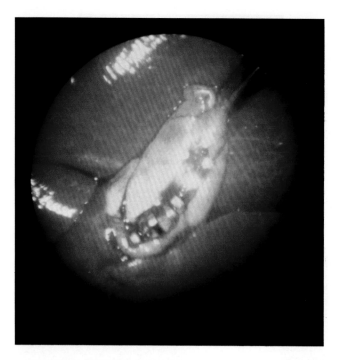

Figure 26.31 Closure of a laparoscopic gallbladder incision with metal clips after stone removal.

Results

Temporary bilionasal drainage According to our survey,[82] bilionasal drainage is most frequently used to prevent stone impaction after EPT (47%) compared with

1% for the management of an already impacted stone, 8.5% for temporary by-pass of malignant bile duct stenosis, 9% for rinsing and chemical dissolution of bile duct stones, and 33% for other diagnostic purposes, mainly bacteriological investigations (Table 26.13). In one patient bile was drained because of jaundice due to chronic pancreatitis.

Insertion of a bilionasal catheter was successful in 95% of cases. In the remaining 5% the papilla of Vater could not be reached endoscopically because of duodenal stenosis, previous Bilroth II gastric resection or hepaticojejunostomy, or intubation failed because of complete bile duct obstruction by tumour. After successful drainage, the serum bilirubin nearly always falls to normal levels unless additional critical disorders, such as severe cholangitis or metastatic disease, are present. Suppurative cholangitis with septicaemia represents an especially important indication for bilionasal drainage, which offers a safe and effective alternative to emergency surgery.[132,137]

Preoperative drainage The question is still unsettled whether preoperative drainage of disturbed bile flow will lower postoperative morbidity and mortality in patients with obstructive jaundice. Biliary decompression prior to laparotomy is theoretically attractive, because jaundice is a prominent surgical risk factor having definitive associations with poor wound healing, bleeding complications and immune dysfunction. In three controlled trials, jaundiced patients with biliary tract obstruction were randomly allocated to surgery either with or without preoperative external biliary drainage.[86,153,188] All studies failed to

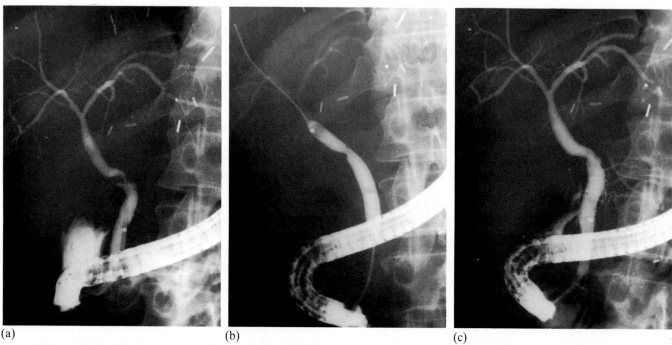

(a) (b) (c)

Figure 26.32 (a) Retrograde cholangiography showing a thread-like stricture of a biliary anastomosis after liver transplantation. (b) Hydrostatic dilatation of the stricture with an endoscopically inserted balloon catheter filled with diluted contrast medium. (c) Retrograde cholangiographic control showing successful dilatation of the stenosis immediately after the procedure.

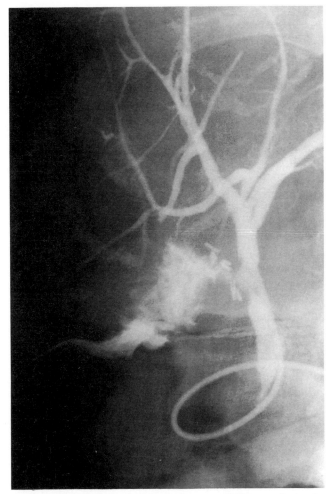

Figure 26.33 Biliary drainage via a nasobiliary catheter in a patient with leakage at the cystic stump after laparoscopic cholecystectomy.

Table 26.13 Indications for endoscopic bilionasal drainage in 609 patients

Indication	Number of patients
Prevention of stone impaction after endoscopic sphincterotomy	288
Diagnostic indication	205
Access for chemical litholysis	57
Malignant bile duct stenosis	52
Overt stone impaction	6
Decompression of bile duct in chronic pancreatitis	1
Total	609

From Hagenmüller and Classen (1982),[82] with kind permission of the publisher, Grune and Stratton.

followed in 18 by temporary stent placement. No early complication was observed. A follow-up study (mean, 4 years) disclosed no recurrence of symptoms or elevated enzymes indicative of recurrent strictures in 18 patients, improvement but minimal clinical symptoms in 4 and an unchanged clinical grade in 1.[75] Berkelhammer *et al.* treated 29 patients with postoperative biliary strictures by endoscopically inserted temporary endoprostheses without routine adjunctive balloon dilatation. Twenty-three of 25 patients with successful stent insertion have had a mean follow-up of 19 months after stent removal; 48%

demonstrate reduction of operative risk with the use of preoperative biliary decompression over an average of 2 weeks. Further trials are warranted to show whether the results can be improved by the less-invasive endoscopic procedure, which provides a physiological internal drainage. In addition, increased drainage time of up to 6 weeks is probably required to improve hepatic function significantly.[122]

Endoscopic treatment of benign strictures Huibregtse *et al.* reported their results in 21 patients in whom endoprostheses were inserted for biliary drainage for benign postoperative strictures. The prostheses had been removed in only 6 patients, with a mean follow-up period of 9 months for these 6 patients. Clinical follow-up for at least 6 months showed that 16 patients had no recurrence of clinical symptoms, 3 patients had one episode of cholangitis and 2 patients had recurrent symptoms.[96] In a recently published trial by Geenen *et al.* on 18 patients with postoperative and 7 with non-operative bile duct strictures, 23 cases had successful balloon dilatation,

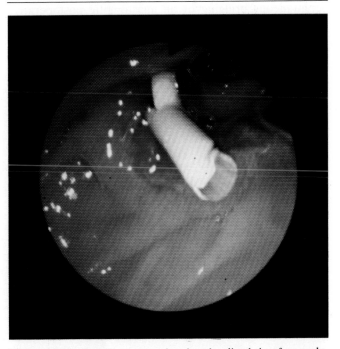

Figure 26.34 Duodenoscopy showing the distal tip of an endoscopically inserted 11.5 French gauge biliary endoprosthesis protruding from the papillary orifice after endoscopic papillotomy. The barb of the prosthesis at 12 o'clock prevents upstream migration of the stent.

had an excellent and 26% a good response.[7] Endoscopic treatment seems also to be effective in selected patients with severe sclerosing cholangitis.[107]

These results indicate that endoscopic biliary endoprosthesis with or without previous balloon dilatation can be used successfully for treatment of benign bile duct strictures. However, much longer follow-up studies are warranted to compare the efficacy with that of surgical procedures.

Percutaneous dilatation of benign strictures is complementary to endoscopy, especially in patients with intrahepatic stenoses. Percutaneous procedures are more invasive and difficult to repeat when compared with endoscopic measures. Various types of self-expanding or expandable metal stents have been implanted via the percutaneous or the endoscopic route in a limited number of patients with benign biliary strictures.[25,105,173] Gianturco expandable metallic stents achieved immediate relief of jaundice and cholangitis in 11 patients with postoperative benign strictures. In a follow-up period of 6–21 months, 9 of the 11 patients had no recurrence of symptoms.[105] Coons reported excellent results with modified Gianturco stents in 8 patients with postoperative strictures and 7 with sclerosing cholangitis.[25] We observed biliary reobstruction due to hyperplastic tissue overgrowth above a Wallstent in 2 of 5 patients with stents for benign strictures. In one case percutaneous cholangioscopy and brush cytology revealed epithelialization of the wire mesh 21 weeks after stent implantation, which promises a trouble-free, long lifespan.[173] The maximal length of follow-up in our patients has been 23 months after percutaneous bridging of an anastomotic postoperative stricture. The irreversibility of metal stent placement means that patients with benign stenoses must be carefully

selected. The procedure seems to be justified when reobstruction occurs in high-risk patients after surgical intervention or balloon dilatation of the stricture.

Palliative endoscopic management of malignant stenoses

The most common indication for internal biliary drainage is malignant biliary obstruction. Endoscopic papillotomy facilitates the initial insertion as well as later replacement of an endoprosthesis (Figure 26.34). Skilled endoscopists have success rates of about 90% in patients with lesions of the papilla or common bile duct.[45,235,246] Complete biliary drainage with subsequent loss of jaundice is more difficult to achieve in patients with hilar tumours, especially those involving the bifurcation (types II and III).[42,235,246] Sufficient palliation is usually obtained by drainage of one liver lobe as long as the drained segments account for more than 20–30% of functional liver volume[45] (Figure 26.35).

Cholangitis and septicaemia are the major early procedure-related complications and occur in 4–10% of cases after drainage of distal biliary tract stenoses.[45,219,246]

The incidence of early cholangitis increases to 20–40% after endoscopic treatment of hilar malignant strictures.[42,45] Placement of multiple stents in patients with hilar tumours causing type II and III strictures reduced the procedure-related mortality and incidence of cholangitis in a retrospective study.[42]

The success rate of endoscopic stent placement reached 97%, when a guidewire was inserted by the percutaneous transhepatic route after failure to cannulate endoscopically.[42] In a recently published trial, however, the combined percutaneous and endoscopic procedure resulted in a total morbidity of 62% and 30-day mortality of 27%.[46]

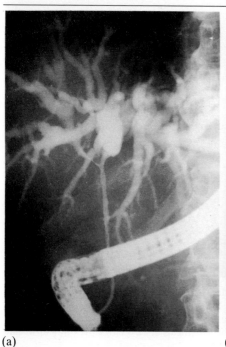 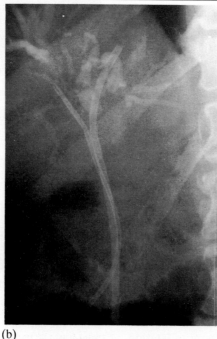

(a) (b)

Figure 26.35 (a) Retrograde cholangiogram showing malignant stenoses of the hepatic bifurcation (Klatskin tumour). (b) Bilateral biliary drainage by two endoscopically inserted plastic endoprostheses (diameter 11.5 French gauge stent in the left hepatic duct and 7 French gauge stent in the right hepatic duct).

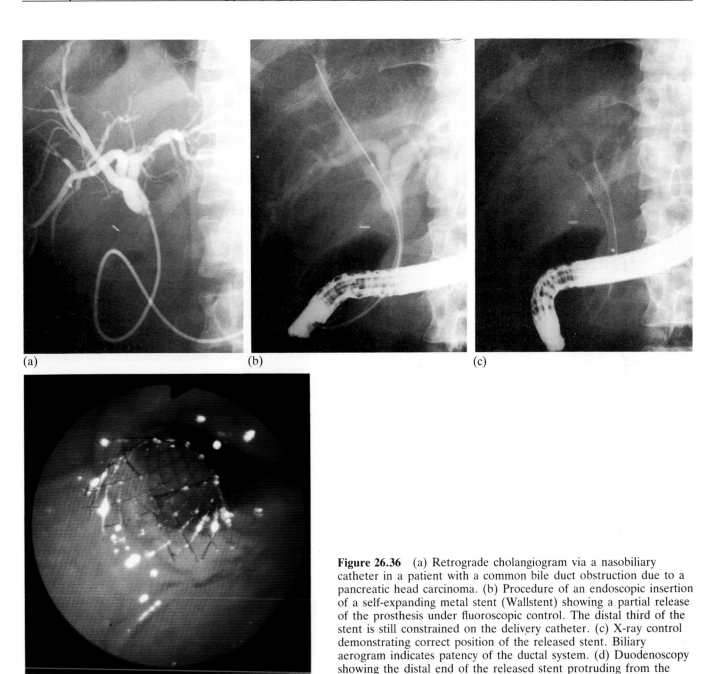

(a)   (b)   (c)

(d)

Figure 26.36 (a) Retrograde cholangiogram via a nasobiliary catheter in a patient with a common bile duct obstruction due to a pancreatic head carcinoma. (b) Procedure of an endoscopic insertion of a self-expanding metal stent (Wallstent) showing a partial release of the prosthesis under fluoroscopic control. The distal third of the stent is still constrained on the delivery catheter. (c) X-ray control demonstrating correct position of the released stent. Biliary aerogram indicates patency of the ductal system. (d) Duodenoscopy showing the distal end of the released stent protruding from the ampulla.

The risk of additional drainage has therefore to be balanced against the risk of complications to undrained segments in bilateral malignant hilar strictures.

Compared with cholangitis, other early procedure-related complications like bleeding, duodenal perforation, stent blockage, pancreatitis or cholecystitis occur rarely. The main drawback of percutaneous or endoscopic stents is blockage after a few months, which frequently leads to septic cholangitis and requires change of the prosthesis. In the majority of cases, reobstruction is the result of slow drainage and bacterial adherence to the stent surface, which is rapidly followed by deposition of glyco-proteins.[135,233] The main determinant of the time to stent blockage seems to be the stent diameter. Long-term patency of French gauge 7 and 8 stents is less than half that of straight 10 FG stents, which showed a mean survival time of 32 weeks in a study of Speer *et al.*[234] Siegel reported similar results for conventional 12 French plastic prostheses.[221] Huibregtse observed an occlusion rate of 21% after a median time of 154 days (range 8–419 days) with polyethylene prostheses.[97] A partial inhibition of stent occlusion by therapy with doxycycline and probably also by aspirin was seen in a placebo-controlled study.[229]

Attempts to prevent blockage of endoprostheses by modifying their shape or composition have so far failed.

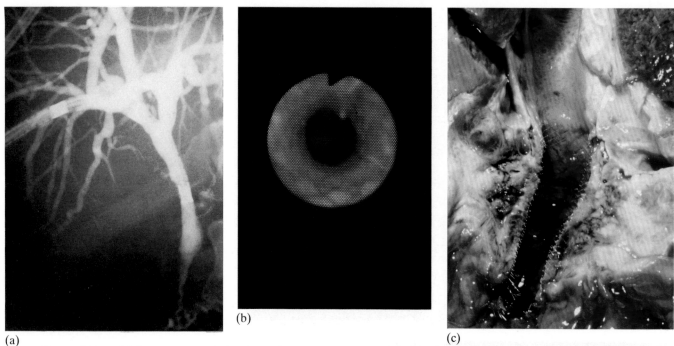

(a)   (c)

(b)

Figure 26.37 (a) Percutaneous cholangioscopic cholangiography showing a distal common bile duct stenosis due to periductal metastases of gastric cancer after previous subtotal gastrectomy. (b) Cholangioscopy of the stenosis after percutaneous implantation of a self-expanding metal stent (Wallstent). (c) Opened common bile duct with a stent in situ surrounded by tumour tissue 90 days after implantation. The diameter of the patent ductal lumen is 8–10 mm.

Self-expanding metal stents, initially developed for use in the urethra and the vascular tree, offer several theoretical advantages over currently available plastic devices.[43,98,168] The large diameter of up to 30 French, the material, and the small surface area suggest a decreased probability of bacterial infection. Fixation of the stent within the duct wall makes dislodgement unlikely. Percutaneously

implanted Gianturco stents achieved divergent clinical results. After initial success, biliary reobstruction occurred in about 10% of 16 patients with malignant biliary obstruction after 6 months.[25] Recurrent jaundice was seen in 8 of 16 cases with malignant strictures treated with Gianturco stents in a European clinical trial.[105] A larger European multicenter study enrolled 103 patients with

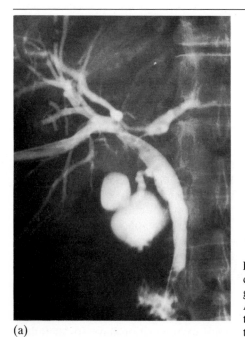

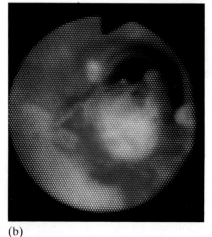

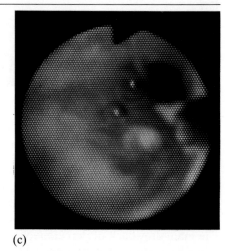

(b)   (c)

(a)

Figure 26.38 (a) Percutaneous cholangiogram showing stenosis of the left hepatic duct at the hilum. (b) Percutaneous cholangioscopy demonstrating a polypoid growing hilar cholangiocarcinoma with obstruction of the left hepatic duct. Advancement of a 800-μm Nd-YAG laser fibre with a helium aiming beam through the instrumentation channel of the cholangioscope. (c) Cholangioscopic intraluminal tumour debulking by laser.

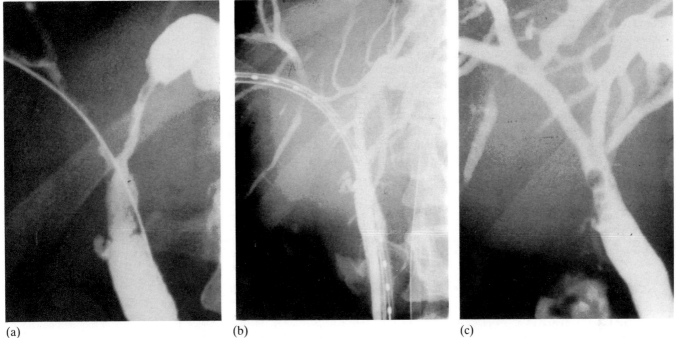

(a) (b) (c)

Figure 26.39 (a) Percutaneous cholangiogram revealing stenoses of both hepatic ducts due to cholangiocarcinoma. (b) Cholangiogram via two transhepatically inserted drainage catheters. Advancement of a probe with radiopaque markers through the right hepatic duct for subsequent precise positioning of the iridium wire. (c) Patency of the hilar ducts 2 months after dilatation and bilateral intraluminal radiotherapy.

malignant biliary stenoses who received an endoscopically placed self-expanding Wallstent. Correct placement of stents was achieved in 97.1% of the patients. Early cholangitis following stent insertion was not seen. Most patients had rapid relief of jaundice. The stent occlusion rate of 5% after a mean period of 175 days (range 40–261) is substantially less than the reported rates for polyethylene stents.[99] In our institute 61 patients with malignant biliary obstruction were treated with percutaneously or endoscopically inserted Wallstents (Figures 26.36 and 26.37). Using guidewire positioning through the stricture, placement of the stent through the tumour was successful in all patients. We observed no early cholangitis, but one case of temporary mild pancreatitis. According to actuarial life-table analysis the probability of stent patency was 81% after 6 months.[171,173]

These preliminary results indicate that stent occlusion by biliary sludge is extremely rare, but biliary reobstruction may occur owing to tumour overgrowth above or below the stent, or tumour ingrowth through the wire mesh of the stent. Since recanalization of the blocked prosthesis can be easily achieved by implantation of a second stent or diathermic cleaning of tumour ingrowth, the irreversibility of stent placement is clinically not relevant in malignant stenoses.[34] Metal stents are, however, much more expensive than plastic prostheses. Randomized controlled trials are warranted to show the cost–benefit ratio and the superiority of metal stents over conventional devices.

Percutaneous implantation of conventional or metal prostheses should be restricted to complex hilar and intrahepatic strictures or difficult extrahepatic stenoses that cannot be managed adequately via the transpapillary route. According to a randomized trial comparing percutaneous and endoscopic procedures for stent insertion, transpapillary placement had a statistically significant higher success rate and a lower complication rate.[232] The results of this trial cannot be extrapolated to other centres, where expertise and case material may be different, but the advantage of the endoscopic approach to percutaneous stenting is accepted by most radiologists and gastroenterologists, at least for lesions of the distal biliary tract.[152] Two randomized studies comparing the endoscopic and surgical palliative management of malignant biliary stenoses failed to show statistically significant differences between endoscopic stenting and surgical by-pass.[3,214]

Interpretation of these trials is difficult owing to small numbers of patients and exclusion of elderly and high-risk cases, in whom randomization is not justified because endoscopic treatment is the preferred option. A larger prospective randomized trial on endoscopic stenting versus bypass surgery for primary low-malignant biliary obstruction in 204 patients was recently completed.[229a] Endoscopic stent placement and surgical by-pass showed a similar drainage success and long-term survival. The incidence of major complications for endoscopy and surgery were 11% and 27% respectively and the corresponding procedure-related 30-day mortality rates were 5% and 18%. These differences were statistically significant. Although initial hospital stay after randomization was shorter in the stented group, more were subsequently readmitted for management of stent blockage and duodenal obstruction. Larger stents may further enhance the superiority of endoscopy over surgery but this should not be extrapolated to fitter patients with small tumours, who should undergo surgery in the hope of resection.

Adjuvant endoscopic biliary tumour therapy comprises lasers, electrocoagulation and internal irradiation[22,61,167,262] (Figures 26.38 and 26.39). Unfortunately, there have yet been no randomized trials to demonstrate that these techniques are superior to simple stent placement. Preliminary results of local biliary tumour debulking by laser under cholangioscopic control indicate that stent placement after successful recanalization appears to be superfluous.[124] A combination of intraductal radiation causing local tumour debulking and ductal fibrosis with implantation of self-expanding metal stents offers theoretically an interesting complementary strategy, which needs to be evaluated in controlled trials.[167,262]

REFERENCES

1. Allescher, H.D. (1989) Papilla of Vater: Structure and function. *Endoscopy*, **21**, 324–329.
2. Allescher, H.D., Neuhaus, H., Hagenmüller, F. & Classen, M. (1990) Effect of *N*-buthylscopolamin on sphincter of Oddi motility in patients during routine ERCP—a manometric study. *Endoscopy*, **22**, 160–163.
3. Andersen, J.R., Sorensen, S.M., Kruse, A. *et al.* (1989) Randomised trial of endoscopic endoprothesis versus operative bypass in malignant obstructive jaundice. *Gut*, **30**, 1132–1135.
4. Arndorfer, R.C., Stef, J.J., Dodds, W.J. *et al.* (1977) Improved infusion system for intraluminal esophageal manometry. *Gastroenterology*, **73**, 23–27.
5. Axon, A.T.R. (1988) Infection and disinfection: special review. *Annual of Gastrointestinal Endoscopy*, **1988**, 181–192.
6. Ayoola, E.A., Vennes, J.A., Silvis, J.E. *et al.* (1976) Endoscopic retrograde intrahepatic cholangiography in liver diseases. *Gastrointestinal Endoscopy*, **22**, 156–159.
7. Berkelhammer, C., Kostan, P. & Haber, G.B. (1989) Endoscopic biliary prothesis as treatment for benign postoperative bile duct strictures. *Gastrointestinal Endoscopy*, **35**, 95–101.
8. Bethge, N. & Hintze, R.E. (1987) Endoskopische Lithotripsie von Gallengangsteinen. *Zeitschrift für Gastroenterologie*, **25**, 119–123.
9. Bickerstaff, K.I., Berry, A.R., Chapman, R.W. & Britton, J. (1988) Early postoperative endoscopic sphincterotomy for retained biliary stones. *Annals of the Royal College of Surgeons England*, **70**, 350–351.
10. Bilbao, M.K., Dotter, C.T., Lee, T.G. & Katon, R.M. (1976) Complications of endoscopic retrograde cholangiopancreaticography (ERCP). A study of 1000 cases. *Gastroenterology*, **70**, 314–320.
11. Bland, K.I. *et al.* (1989) Extracorporeal shock-wave lithotripsy of bile duct calculi. An interim report of the Dornier U.S. Bile Duct Lithotripsy Prospective Study. *Annals of Surgery*, **209**, 743–753.
12. Byrne, P., Leung, J.W. & Cotton, P.B. (1984) Retroperitoneal perforation during endoscopic sphincterotomy. *Radiology*, **150**, 383–384.
13. Cairns, S.R., Dias, L., Cotton, P.B. *et al.* (1989) Additional endoscopic procedures instead of urgent surgery for retained common bile duct stones. *Gut*, **30**, 535–540.
14. Cattau, E.L., Johnson, D.A., Benjamin, S.B. *et al.* (1988) Sphincter of Oddi manometry: a survey of methodology, complications and clinical application. *Gastrointestinal Endoscopy*, **34**, 185 (abstract).
15. Chen, M.F. & Jan, Y.Y. (1990) Percutaneous transhepatic cholangioscopic lithotripsy. *British Journal of Surgery*, **77**, 530–532.
15a. Chen, M.F., Jan, Y.Y. & Lee, T.Y. (1987) Percutaneous transhepatic cholangioscopy. *British Journal of Surgery*, **74**, 728.
16. Chiverton, S.G., Inglis, J.A., Hudd, C. *et al.* (1990) Percutaneous cholecystolithotomy: the first 60 patients. *British Medical Journal*, **300**, 1310–1312.
17. Choi, T.K. & Wong, J. (1986) Endoscopic retrograde cholangiopancreatography and endoscopic papillotomy in recurrent pyogenic cholangitis. *Clinics in Gastroenterology*, **15**, 393–415.
18. Classen, M. & Demling, L. (1974) Endoskopische Sphinkterotomie der Papilla Vateri und Steinextraktion aus dem Ductus Choledochus. *Deutsche Medizinische Wochenschrift*, **99**, 496–497.
19. Classen, M. & Safrany, L. (1975) Endoscopic papillotomy and removal of gallstones. *British Medical Journal*, **iv**, 371–374.
20. Classen, M., Anacker, H., Stadelmann, O. *et al.* (1975) The diagnosis of tumours of the papilla of Vater and of the pancreas by ERCP. In Anacker, H. (ed.) *Efficiency and Limits of Radiologic Examination of the Pancreas*, pp. 203–209. Stuttgart: Thieme.
21. Classen, M. (1987) Endoscopic papillotomy. In Sivak, M.V. (ed.) *Gastroenterologic Endoscopy*, pp. 631–651. Philadelphia, London, Toronto: W.B. Saunders.
22. Classen, M., Hagenmüller, F., Gossner, W. *et al.* (1987) Laser treatment of bile duct cancer via percutaneous choledochoscopy. *Endoscopy*, **19**, 74–75.
23. Classen, M. & Dancygier, H. (1988) Risk of transmitting HIV by endoscopes. *Endoscopy*, **20**, 128.
24. Classen, M., Hagenmüller, F., Knyrim, K. & Frimberger, E. (1988) Giant bile duct stones—non-surgical treatment. *Endoscopy*, **20**, 21–26.
25. Coons, H.G. (1989) Self-expanding stainless steel biliary stents. *Radiology*, **170**, 979–983.
26. Cope, C., Burke, D.R. & Meranze, S.G. (1990) Percutaneous extraction of gallstones in 20 patients. *Radiology*, **176**, 19–24.
27. Cotton, P.B. (1977) Progress report: ERCP. *Gut*, **18**, 316–341.
28. Cotton, P.B. (1984) Endoscopic management of bile duct stones (apples and oranges). *Gut*, **25**, 587–597.
29. Cotton, P.B. (1986) Year follow up after sphincterotomy for stones in patients with gallbladders. *Gastrointestinal Endoscopy*, **32**, 157–158.
30. Cotton, P.B. (1989) Precut papillotomy—a risky technique for experts only. *Gastrointestinal Endoscopy*, **35**(6), 578–579.
31. Cotton, P.B., Kozarek, R.A., Schapiro, R.H. *et al.* (1990) Endoscopic laser lithotripsy of large bile duct stones. *Gastroenterology*, **99**, 1128–1133.
32. Coyan, E.M.J., Falkiner, F.R., Mulvihill, T.E. *et al.* (1984) Pseudomonas aeruginosa-infection following endoscopic retrograde cholangio-pancreatography. *Journal of Hospital Infection*, **5**, 371–376.
33. Cremer, M., Gulbis, A., Toussaint, J. *et al.* (1977) Technique of endoscopic papillotomy. In Delmont, J. (ed.) *The Sphincter of Oddi*, pp. 219–227. Basel: Karger.
34. Cremer, M., Deviere, J., Sugai, B. & Baize, M. (1990) Expandable biliary metal stents for malignancies: endoscopic insertion and diathermic cleaning for tumour ingrowth. *Gastrointestinal Endoscopy*, **36**, 451–457.
35. Crone-Muenzebrock, W., Rowedder, A., Meyer-Panwitt, U. & Kremer, B. (1989) A comparison of the efficacy of sonography, computed tomography, ERCP and angiography in the diagnosis of primary bile duct carcinoma. *Roentgen Fortschritte*, **151**(5), 523–526.
36. Cuncliff, W.J., Cobden, I., Lavelle, M.I. *et al.* (1987) A randomised prospective study comparing two contrast media in ERCP. *Endoscopy*, **19**, 201–202.
37. Davidson, B.R., Neoptolemos, J.P. and Carr-Locke, D.L. (1988) Endoscopic sphincterotomy for common bile duct calculi in patients with gall bladder in situ considered unfit for surgery. *Gut*, **29**, 114–120.
38. Delcenserie, R., Dupas, J.L., Jol, J.P. *et al.* (1988) Microcystic adenoma of the pancreas demonstrated by endoscopic retrograde pancreatography. *Gastrointestinal Endoscopy*, **34**(1), 52–54.
39. Del Olmo, I., Merono, E., Moreira, V.F. *et al.* (1988) Successful

treatment of postoperative external biliary fistulas by endoscopic sphincterotomy. *Gastrointestinal Endoscopy*, **34**, 307–309.

40. De Masi, E., Corazziari, E., Habib, F. *et al.* (1984) Manometric study of the sphincter of Oddi in patients with and without common bile duct stones. *Gut*, **25**, 275–278.

41. Demling, L. & Riemann, J.F. (1982) Mechanischer Lithotriptor. *Deutsche Medizinische Wochenschrift*, **107**, 555.

42. Deviere, J., Baize, M., de Toeuf, J. & Cremer, M. (1988) Long term follow-up of patients with hilar malignant stricture treated by endoscopic internal drainage. *Gastrointestinal Endoscopy*, **34**, 95–101.

43. Dick, R., Gillams, A., Dooley, J.S. *et al.* (1988) Self expandable stainless steel braided endoprosthesis for biliary strictures. *Radiology*, **169**(P), 25 (abstract).

44. Di Magno, E.P. (1986) Ultrasound, computed tomography and endoscopic retrograde pancreatography in the diagnosis of chronic pancreatitis, a comparative evaluation. In Malfertheimer, P. & Ditschuneit, H. (eds.) *Diagnostic Procedures in Pancreatic Disease*, pp. 185–191. Berlin, Heidelberg, New York: Springer.

45. Dowsett, J.F., Vaira, D., Polydorou, A. (1988) Interventional endoscopy in the pancreatobiliary tree. *American Journal of Gastroenterology*, **83**(12), 1328–1336.

46. Dowsett, J.F., Vaira, D., Hatfield, A.R.W. *et al.* (1989) Endoscopic biliary therapy using the combined percutaneous and endoscopic technique. *Gastroenterology*, **96**, 1180–1186.

47. Dowsett, J.F., Polydorou, A.A., Vaira, D. *et al.* (1990) Needle knife papillotomy: how safe and how effective? *Gut*, **31**, 905–908.

48. Dresemann, G., Kautz, G. & Bünte, H. (1988) Langzeitergebnisse nach endoskopischer Sphinkterotomie bei Patienten mit Gallenblase in situ. *Deutsche Medizinische Wochenschrift*, **113**, 500–505.

49. Dubois, F., Berthelot, G. & Levrad, H. (1989) Cholecystektomie par coelioscopie. *La Presse Medicale*, **18**, 980–982.

50. Dupas, J.L., Delcenserie, R. & July, J.P. (1986) Early endoscopic sphincterotomy. An alternative to early surgery in gallstone pancreatitis. *Digestive Diseases and Sciences*, **31**(S), 1199 (abstract).

51. Eimiller, A., Neuhaus, H., Schmid, F. *et al.* (1987) Ergebnisse der Notfallpapillotomie bei akuter Pankreatitis unterschiedlicher Genese. *Zeitschrift für Gastroenterologie*, **25**, 450 (abstract).

52. Elias, E., Summerfield, J.A., Dick, K. & Sherlock, S. (1974) Endoscopic retrograde cholangio-pancreatography in the diagnosis of jaundice associated with ulcerative colitis. *Gastroenterology*, **67**, 907–911.

53. Elias, E., Hamlyn, A.N., Jain, S. *et al.* (1976) A randomized trial of percutaneous transhepatic cholangiography with the Chiba needle versus endoscopic retrograde cholangiography for bile duct visualization in jaundice. *Gastroenterology*, **71**, 439–443.

54. Endo, Y., Morii, T., Tamura, A. & Okuda, S. (1974) Cytodiagnosis of pancreatic malignant tumours by aspiration, under direct vision, using a duodenal fiberoscope. *Gastroenterology*, **67**, 944–951.

55. Ell, C., Lux, G., Hochberger, J. *et al.* (1988) Laserlithotripsy of common bile duct stones. *Gut*, **29**, 746–751.

56. Escorrou, J., Cordova, J.A., Lazorthes, F. *et al.* (1984) Early and late complications after endoscopic sphincterotomy for biliary lithiasis with and without the gallbladder in situ. *Gut*, **25**, 598–602.

57. Escourrou, J., Liguory, C., Boyer, J. *et al.* (1987) Emergency endoscopic sphincterotomy in acute biliary pancreatitis: Results of a multicentre study. *Gastroenterology*, **92**, 1385 (abstract).

58. Farkas, I., Déak, J., Pàlfi, I. & Preisich, P. (1976) Endoscopic retrograde cholangiography in biliodigestive anastomosis. *Endoscopy*, **8**, 127–132.

59. Fischer, M.G., Wolff, W.J., Geffen, A. *et al.* (1974) Antegrade and retrograde visualization of the biliary tree. *American Journal of Gastroenterology*, **61**, 129–132.

60. Fischer, M.G., Wolff, W.J., Geffen, A. & Ozotkay, S. (1975) Combined use of percutaneous transhepatic cholangiography (PTC) and endoscopic ampullary cholangiography in diagnosis of difficult jaundice cases. *American Journal of Gastroenterology*, **63**, 369–380.

61. Fleischer, D., Cattau, E. Jr., Sinofky, E. *et al.* (1989) Development of a laser balloon for the treatment of gastrointestinal obstruction. *Endoscopy*, **21**, 80–85.

62. Fleischer, D. (1990) Monitoring for conscious sedation: perspective of the gastointestinal endoscopist. *Gastrointestinal Endoscopy*, **36**, 19–22.

63. Förster, E.C., Schneider, M.U., Matek, W. & Domschke, W. (1989) Transpapillary cholecystoscopy. *Endoscopy*, **21**, 381–383.

64. Förster, E.C., Matek, W. & Domschke, W. (1990) Endoscopic retrograde cannulation of the gallbladder: direct dissolution of gallstones. *Gastrointestinal Endoscopy*, **36**, 444–450.

65. Forster, A., Gardaz, J.P., Suter, P.M. & Gemperle, M. (1980) Respiratory depression by midazolam and diazepam. *Anesthesiology*, **53**, 494–497.

66. Foutch, P.G., Harlan, J.R., Kerr, D. & Sanowski, R.A. (1989) Wire-guided brush cytology: a new endoscopic method for diagnosis of bile duct cancer. *Gastrointestinal Endoscopy*, **35**(3), 243–247.

67. Frimberger, E., Kuhner, W., Weingart, J. *et al.* (1982) Eine neue Methode der elektrohydraulischen Cholelithotripsie (Lithokasie). *Deutsche Medizinische Wochenschrift*, **107**, 213–215.

68. Frimberger, E. (1989) Operative laparoscopy: cholecystotomy. *Endoscopy*, **21**, 367–372.

69. Fuijta, R., Hirata, N. & Fuijta, Y. (1989) Peroral cholecystoscopy. *Endoscopy*, **21**, 378–380.

70. Fukomoto, K., Nakajima, M., Murakami, K. & Kawai, K. (1974) Diagnosis of pancreatic cancer by endoscopic pancreato-cholangiography. *American Journal of Gastroenterology*, **62**, 210–223.

71. Fullarton, G.M., Hilditch, T., Campbell, A. & Murray, W.R. (1990) Clinical and scintigraphic assessment of the role of endoscopic sphincterotomy in the treatment of sphincter of Oddi dysfunction. *Gut*, **31**, 231–235.

72. Geenen, J. (1978) Endoscopic papillotomy in the United States. In Demling, L. & Classen, M. (eds.) *International Workshop on Endoscopic Papillotomy, Munich, 1976.* Stuttgart: Thieme.

73. Geenen, J.E., Toouli, J., Hogan, W.J. *et al.* (1984) Endoscopic sphincterotomy: follow-up evaluation of effects on the sphincter of Oddi. *Gastroenterology*, **87**, 754–758.

74. Geenen, J.E., Hogan, W.J., Dodds, W.J. *et al.* (1989) The efficacy of endoscopic sphincterotomy after cholecystectomy in patients with sphincter-Oddi-dysfunction. *New England Journal of Medicine*, **320**, 82–87.

75. Geenen, D.J., Geenen, J.E., Hogan, W.J. *et al.* (1989) Endoscopic therapy for benign bile duct strictures. *Gastrointestinal Endoscopy*, **35**(5), 367–371.

76. Goodall, R.J. (1985) Bleeding after endoscopic sphincterotomy. *Annals of the Royal College of Surgeons England*, **22**, 644–646.

77. Gostout, C.J. & Bender, C.E. (1988) Cholangiography, sphincterotomy, and common duct stone removal via Roux-en-Y limb enteroscopy. *Gastroenterology*, **95**, 156–63.

78. Gould, R.J., Vogelzang, R.L., Neimann, H.L. *et al.* (1985) Percutaneous biliary drainage as an initial therapy in sepsis of the bile tract. *Surgery, Gynecology and Obstetrics*, **160**, 523–527.

79. Gregg, J.A. & Carr-Locke, D.L. (1984) Endoscopic pancreatic and biliary manometry in pancreatic, biliary and papillary disease, and after endoscopic sphincterotomy and surgical sphincteroplasty. *Gut*, **25**, 1247–1254.

80. Gundel, H., von Fritsch, E. & Koch, H. (1975) Die Bedeutung der endoskopisch-radiologischen Cholangiographie bei Cholestase und Postcholecystektomie-Syndrom. *Deutsche Medizinische Wochenschrift*, **100**, 1877–1881.

81. Hagenmüller, F., Ossenberg, F.W. & Classen, M. (1977) Duodenoscopic manometry. In Delmont, J. (ed.) *The Sphincter of Oddi*, pp. 72–76. Basel: Karger.

82. Hagenmüller, F. & Classen, M. (1982) Therapeutic endoscopic and percutaneous procedures. In Popper, H. & Schaffner, F. (eds.) *Progress in Liver Diseases*, vol. VII, pp. 299–317. New York: Grune and Stratton.

83. Hansell, D.T., Millar, M.A., Murray, W.R. *et al.* (1989) Endoscopic sphincterotomy for bile duct stones in patients with intact gallbladders. *British Journal of Surgery*, **76**, 856–858.

84. Harrison, J., Morris, D.L., Haynes, J. *et al.* (1987) Electrohydraulic lithotripsy of gallstones—in vitro and animal studies. *Gut*, **28**, 267–271.

85. Hatfield, A.R.W., Smithies, A., Wilkins, R. & Levi, A.J. (1976) Assessment of endoscopic retrograde cholangio-pancreatography (ERCP) and pure pancreatic juice cytology in patients with pancreatic disease. *Gut*, **17**, 14–21.

86. Hatfield, A.R.W., Tobias, R., Terblanche, J. *et al.* (1982)

Preoperative external biliary drainage in obstructive jaundice. A prospective controlled trial. *Lancet*, October 23, 896–899.

87. Hawes, E.R., Cotton, P.B. & Vallon, A.G. (1990) Follow-up 6 to 11 years after duodenoscopic sphincterotomy for stones in patients with prior cholecystectomy. *Gastroenterology*, **98**, 1008–1012.

88. Heinermann, P.M., Boeckl, O. & Pimpl, W. (1989) Selective EPT and preoperative stone removal in bile duct surgery. *Annals of Surgery*, **209**, 267–272.

89. Helm, E.B. & Stille, W. (1984) Infective complications. In Classen, M., Geenen, J. & Kawai, K. (eds.) *Nonsurgical Biliary Drainage*, pp. 60–62. Heidelberg: Springer.

90. Helm, E.B., Bauernfeind, A., Frech, K. & Hagenmüller, F. (1984) Pseudomonas Septikämie nach endoskopischen Eingriffen am Gallengangsystem. *Deutsche Medizinische Wochenschrift*, **109**, 697–701.

91. Higuchi, T. & Kon, Y. (1987) Endoscopic mechanical lithotripsy for the treatment of common bile duct stones. *Endoscopy*, **19**, 216–217.

92. Hintze, R.E. & Bethge, N. (1989) Endoskopische Diagnostik und Therapie bei Patienten mit Duodenaldivertikeln nahe der Papilla Vateri. In *Divertikel des Dünn- und Dickdarms*, pp. 90–100. Wien, Berlin: Ueberreuter Wissenschaft.

93. Hoffmann, L. & Weiss, W. (1977) Clinical importance of juxta-papillary duodenal diverticula. *Acta Endoscopiea*, **13**, 26–34.

94. Huang, T., Bassk, J.A. & Williams, R.D. (1969) The significance of biliary pressure in cholangitis. *Archives of Surgery*, **98**, 629–632.

95. Huchzermeyer, H., Luska, G., Otto, P. & Seifert, I. (1975) The value of the combination of antegrade and retrograde cholangiography in the diagnosis of bile duct obstructions. *Endoscopy*, **7**, 126–133.

96. Huibregtse, K., Katon, R.M. & Tytgat, G.N.J. (1986) Endoscopic treatment of postoperative biliary strictures. *Endoscopy*, **18**, 133–137.

97. Huibregtse, K. (1988) *Endoscopic Biliary and Pancreatic Drainage*. Stuttgart, New York: Georg Thieme Verlag.

98. Huibregtse, K., Cheng, J., Coene, P.P.L.O. *et al.* (1989) Endoscopic placement of expandable metal stents for biliary strictures—a preliminary report on experience with 33 patients. *Endoscopy*, **21**, 280–282.

99. Huibregtse, K., Carr-Locke, D., Cremer, M. *et al.* (1990) Experience with an endoscopically inserted, expandable biliary metal stent (Wallstent). *Gastroenterology* (abstract), **98**, 287.

100. Hultborn, A., Jacobsson, B. & Rosengren, B. (1982) Cholangio-venous reflux during cholangiography. *Acta Chirurgica Scandinavica*, **123**, 111.

101. Ichikawa, K., Nakazawa, S., Naitoh, Y. *et al.* (1988) Clinical evaluation of percutaneous transhepatic cholecystoscopy. *Gastroenterologic Endoscopy*, **30**, 915–925.

102. Ikeda, S. & Okada, Y. (1975) Classification of choledoch-duodenal fiberscopy and its etiological significance. *Gastroenterology*, **69**, 130–137.

103. Ingoldby, C.J.H., El-saadi, J., Hall, R.I. & Denyer, M.E. (1989) Late results of endoscopic sphincterotomy for bile duct stones in elderly patients with gallbladder in situ. *Gut*, **30**, 1129–1131.

104. Inui, K., Nakazawa, S., Yoshino, J. *et al.* (1989) Percutaneous cholecystoscopy. *Endoscopy*, **21**, 361–364.

105. Irving, J.D., Adam, A., Dick, R. *et al.* (1989) Gianturco expandable metallic biliary stents: result of an European clinical trial. *Radiology*, **172**, 321–326.

106. Jeng, K.S., Chiangi, H.J. & Shih, S.C. (1989) Limitations of percutaneous transhepatic cholangioscopy in the removal of complicated biliary calculi. *World Journal of Surgery*, **13**, 603–610.

107. Johnson, G.K., Geenen, J.E., Venu, R.P. & Hogan, W.J. (1987) Endoscopic treatment of biliary duct strictures in sclerosing cholangitis: follow-up assessment of a new therapeutic approach. *Gastrointestinal Endoscopy*, **33**, 9–12.

108. Johnson, A.G. & Hosking, S.W. (1987) Appraisal of the management of bile duct stones. *British Journal of Medicine*, **74**, 555–560.

109. Jorge, A., Findor, J., Esley, C. & Bruch, E. (1988) Primary sclerosing cholangitis. *Zeitschrift für Gastroenterologie*, **26**, 322–330.

110. Kalvaria, I., Bornmann, P.C., Marks, I.N. *et al.* (1989) The spectrum and natural history of common bile duct stenosis in chronic alcohol-induced pancreatitis. *Annals of Surgery*, **210**, 608–613.

111. Kasugai, T., Kuno, N., Kobayashi, S. & Hattori, K. (1972) Endoscopic pancreatocholangiography. I. The normal pancreato-cholangiogram. *Gastroenterology*, **63**, 217–226.

112. Kasugai, T., Kuno, N., Kizu, M. *et al.* (1972) Endoscopic pancreatocholangiography. II. The pathological pancreato-cholangiogram. *Gastroenterology*, **63**, 227–234.

113. Kaufmann, A.R., Sivak Jr., M.V. & Ferguson, D.R. (1988) Endoscopic retrograde cholangiopancreaticography in pancreatic islet cell tumors. *Gastrointestinal Endoscopy*, **34**, 47–51.

114. Kawai, K., Akasaka, Y., Hashimoto, Y. *et al.* (1973) Preliminary report on endoscopical papillotomy. *Journal of Kyoto Prefectural Medical University*, **82**, 353–355.

115. Kawai, K., Akasaka, Y., Murakami, K. *et al.* (1974) Endoscopic sphincterotomy of the ampulla of Vater. *Gastrointestinal Endoscopy*, **20**, 138–151.

116. Kautz, G. & Bünte, H. (1986) ERCP und endoskopische Sphinkterotomie bei akuter Pankreatitis. *Verhandlungen der Deutschen Gesellschaft für Innere Medizin*, **92**, 371–381.

117. Kennedy, R.H. & Thompson, M.H. (1988) Are duodenal diverticula associated with choledocholithiasis? *Gut*, **29**, 1003–1006.

118. Knyrim, K., Seidlitz, H., Vakil, N. *et al.* (1989) Optical performance of electronic imaging systems for the colon. *Gastroenterology*, **96**, 776–782.

119. Koch, H., Stolte, M. & Walz, V. (1977) Endoscopic lithotripsy in the common bile duct. *Endoscopy*, **9**, 95.

120. Komiya, O. (1989) Technical potential and limitation of cholangio-scopes. *Endoscopy*, **21**, 338–340.

121. Kopecky, K.K., Hawes, R.H., Bogan, M.L. *et al.* (1990) Percutaneous pulsed-dye laser lithotripsy of gallbladder stones in swine. *Investigative Radiology*, **25**, 627–630.

122. Koyama, K., Takagi, Y., Ito, K. & Sato, T. (1981) Experimental and clinical studies on the effect of biliary drainage in obstructive jaundice. *American Journal of Surgery*, **142**, 293–299.

123. Kozu, T. (1973) Duodenoscopic collection of intraductal pure pancreatic juice and its application to cytodiagnostis. In Demling, L. & Classen, M. (eds.) *Endoscopy of the Small Intestine with Retrograde Pancreatocholangiography*, pp. 70–73. Stuttgart: Thieme.

124. Kubota, Y., Sek, T., Yamaguchi, T. *et al.* (1990) Palliative recanalization treatment of malignant biliary obstruction by choledochoscopic Nd-YAG-laser irradiation. In *Abstracts of the World Congress of Gastroenterology, Sydney 1990*, p. 787. Abingdon: The Medicine Groupe (UK) Ltd.

125. Kullmann, E., Borch, K. & Liedberg, G. (1989) Long-term follow-up after endoscopic management of retained and recurrent common bile duct stones. *Acta Chirurgica Scandinavica*, **155**, 395–399.

126. LaFerla, G., Gordon, S., Archibald, M. & Murray, W.R. (1986) Hyperamylsaemia and acute pancreatitis following endoscopic retrograde cholangiopancreaticography. *Pancreas*, **1**, 160–163.

127. Lai, C.S., Lo, C.M., Choi, T.K. *et al.* (1989) Urgent biliary decompression after endoscopic retrograde cholangiopancreaticography. *American Journal of Surgery*, **157**, 121–125.

128. Lai, E.L.S. (1990) Management of severe acute cholangitis. *British Journal of Surgery*, **77**, 604–605.

129. Lee, S.H., Fache, J.S. & Burhenne, H.J. (1990) The value of extracorporeal shock-wave lithotripsy in the management of bile duct stones. *American Journal of Roentgenology*, **155**(4), 775–779.

130. Leese, T., Neoptolemos, J.P. & Carr-Locke, D.L. (1985) Successes, failures, early complications and their management following endoscopic sphincterotomy results in 394 consecutive patients from a single centre. *British Journal of Surgery*, **72**, 215–219.

131. Leese, T., Neoptolemos, J.P., Baker, A.R. & Carr-Locke, D.L. (1986) Management of acute cholangitis and the impact of endoscopic sphincterotomy. *British Journal of Surgery*, **73**, 988–992.

132. Leese, T., Neoptolemos, J.P., Baker, A.R. & Carr-Locke, D.L. (1986) Management of acute cholangitis and the impact of endoscopic sphincterotomy. *British Journal of Surgery*, **73**, 988–992.

133. Leung, J.W.L. & Chung, S.C.S. (1987) The role of early ERCP and sphincterotomy in the management of acute biliary pancreatitis. *Gastroenterology*, **92**, 1503.

134. Leung, J.W.L. & Chung, S.C.S. (1989) Electrohydraulic lithotripsy with peroral cholangioscopy. *British Medical Journal*, **299**, 595–598.

135. Leung, J.W.C., Ling, T.K.W., Kung, J.L.S. & Vallance-Owen, J. (1988) The role of bacteria in the blockage of biliary stents. *Gastrointestinal Endoscopy*, **34**, 19–22.

136. Leung, J.W.C., Sung, J.Y., Li, M.K.W. & Metrewel, C. (1988) Biliary stenting as treatment for a spontaneous bile leak. *American Journal of Gastroenterology*, **83**, 1431–1432.

137. Leung, J.W.C., Chung, S.C.S., Sung, J.J.Y. *et al.* (1989) Urgent endoscopic drainage for acute suppurative cholangitis. *Lancet*, **II**, 1307–1309.

138. Liebermann, D.A., Wuerker, C.K. and Katon, R.M. (1985) Cardiopulmonary risk of esophagogastroduodenoscopy: role of endoscope diameter and systemic sedation. *Gastroenterology*, **88**, 468–72.

139. Liguory, C., Gouero, H., Chavy, A. *et al.* (1974) Endoscopic retrograde cholangiopancreatography. *British Journal of Surgery*, **61**, 359–362.

140. Liguory, C., Coffin, J.C., Holler, A. & Chavy, A. (1975) Traitment de la lithiase de la voie biliaire principale par voie endoscopique. *Presse Médicale*, **4**, 20.

141. Liguory, C.L., Lefebvre, J.F., Bonnel, D. *et al.* (1989) Indications for cholangioscopy. *Endoscopy*, **21**, 341–343.

142. Littenberg, G., Afsoudakis, A. & Kaplowitz, N. (1979) Common bile duct stenosis from pancreatitis: a clinical and pathologic spectrum. *Medicine*, **58**, 385–411.

143. Li-Yeng, C. & Goldberg, H.I. (1984) Sclerosing cholangitis: broad spectrum of radiographic features. *Gastrointestinal Radiology*, **9**, 39–47.

144. Lotveit, T., Skar, V. & Osnes, M. (1988) Juxtapapillary duodenal diverticula. *Endoscopy*, **20**, 175–178.

145. Lux, G., Riemann, J.F. & Demling, L. (1984) Biliäre Pankreatitis—Diagnostische und therapeutische Möglichkeiten durch ERCP und endoskopische Papillotomie. *Zeitschrift für Gastroenterologie*, **22**, 346–356.

146. Manegold, B.C., Mennicken, G. & Jung, M. (1982) Endoscopic electrohydraulic disintegration of common bile duct concrements. In *World Congress of Gastroenterology Stockholm, 1982*, Abstract 573.

147. Martin, D.F. & Tweedle, D.E.F. (1987) Endoscopic management of common duct stones without cholecystectomy. *British Journal of Surgery*, **74**, 209–211.

148. McCarthy, J.H., Miller, G.L. & Laurence, B.H. (1990) Cannulation of the biliary tree, cystic duct and gallbladder using a hydrophobic polymer coated steerable guide wire. *Gastrointestinal Endoscopy*, **36**, 386–389.

149. McClelland, D.B.L., Burrell, C.J., Tonkin, R.W. & Heading, R.C. (1978) Hepatitis B absence of transmission by gastrointestinal endoscopy. *British Medical Journal*, **i**: 23–24.

150. McCune, W.S., Shorb, P.E. & Moscovitz, H. (1968) Endoscopic cannulation of the ampulla of Vater: a preliminary report. *Annals of Surgery*, **167**, 752–756.

151. McCune, W.S. (1990) ERCP—the first twenty years. *Gastrointestinal Endoscopy*, **34**, 277–278.

152. McLean, G.K. & Burke, D.R. (1989) Role of endoprostheses in the management of malignant biliary obstruction. *Radiology*, **170**, 961–967.

153. McPherson, G.A.D., Benjamin, J.S., Hodgson, H.J.F. *et al.* (1984) Pre-operative percutaneous transhepatic biliary drainage: the results of a controlled trial. *British Journal of Surgery*, **71**, 371–375.

154. Metzgar, R.S. & Asch, H.K. (1988) Antigens of human pancreatic adenocarcinomas: their role in diagnosis and therapy. December 7–8, 1987, Rockville, MD Conference report. *Pancreas*, **3**, 352.

155. Miller, B.M., Kozarek, R.A., Ryan, J.A. *et al.* (1987) Surgical versus endoscopic management of common bile duct stones. *Annals of Surgery*, **207**, 135–141.

156. Mo, L.R., Hwang, M.H., Yueh, S.K. *et al.* (1988) Percutaneous transhepatic choledochoscopic electrohydraulic lithotripsy (PTCS-EHL) of common bile duct stones. *Gastrointestinal Endoscopy*, **34**, 122–125.

157. Murray, A., Basu, R., Fairclough, P.D. & Wood, R.F.M. (1989) Gallstone lithotripsy with the pulsed dye laser: in vitro studies. *British Journal of Surgery*, **76**, 457–460.

158. Nebel, O.T. (1975) Manometric evaluation of the papilla of Vater. *Gastrointestinal Endoscopy*, **21**, 126–128.

159. Nebel, O.T., Silvis, S.E., Rogers, G. *et al.* (1975) Complications associated with endoscopic retrograde cholangio-pancreatography. Results of the 1974 A.S.G.E. survey. *Gastrointestinal Endoscopy*, **22**, 34–36.

160. Neoptolemos, J.P., Carr-Locke, D.L. & Fossard, D.P. (1987) Prospective randomized study of preoperative endoscopic sphincterotomy versus surgery alone for common bile duct stones. *British Medical Journal*, **294**, 470.

161. Neoptolemos, J.P., Carr-Locke, D.L., Leese, T. & James, D. (1987) Acute cholangitis in association with acute pancreatitis: incidence, clinical features and outcome in relation to ERCP and endoscopic sphincterotomy. *British Journal of Surgery*, **74**, 1103–1106.

162. Neoptolemos, J.P., Carr-Locke, D.L., London, N.J. *et al.* (1988) Controlled trial of urgent endoscopic retrograde cholangiopancreatography and endoscopic sphincterotomy versus conservative treatment for acute pancreatitis due to gallstones. *Lancet*, **2**, 979–983.

163. Neoptolemos, J.P., London, N., Slater, N.D. *et al.* (1986) A prospective study of ERCP and endoscopic sphincterotomy in the diagnosis and treatment of gallstone acute pancreatitis. *Archives of Surgery*, **121**, 697–702.

164. Neoptolemos, J.P., Davidson, B.R., Shaw, D.E. *et al.* (1987) Study of common bile duct exploration and endoscopic sphincterotomy in a consecutive series of 438 patients. *British Journal of Surgery*, **74**, 916–921.

165. Neoptolemos, J.P., Shaw, D.E. & Carr-Locke, D.L. (1989) A multivariate analysis of preoperative risk factors in patients with common bile duct stones—implications for treatment. *Annals of Surgery*, **209**, 157–161.

166. Neoptolemos, J.P., Hall, C., O'Connor, H.J. *et al.* (1990) Methyl-tert-butyl-ether for treating bile duct stones: the British experience. *British Journal of Medicine*, **77**, 32–35.

167. Neuhaus, H. (1989) Endoscopic tumour therapy. *Endoscopy*, **21**, 357–360.

168. Neuhaus, H., Hagenmüller, F. & Classen, M. (1989) Self-expanding biliary stents. Preliminary clinical experience. *Endoscopy*, **21**, 225–228.

169. Neuhaus, H., Hagenmüller, F., Lauer, R. & Classen, M. (1991) A prospective randomized trial of the influence of suprapapillary Doppler ultrasound on endoscopic papillotomy. *Gastrointestinal Endoscopy* (abstract), **37**, 253.

170. Neuhaus, H., Hagenmüller, F. & Classen, M. (1990) Intracorporeal lithotripsy of bile duct stones under cholangioscopic control. In: *Abstracts of the World Congress of Gastroenterology, Sydney 1990*, p. 1061. Abingdon: The Medicine Groupe (UK), Ltd.

171. Neuhaus, H., Hagenmüller, F., Griebel, M. & Classen, M. (1991) Self expanding metal stents versus conventional plastic endoprosthesis for malignant biliary obstruction. *Gastrointestinal Endoscopy* (abstract), **37**, 254.

172. Neuhaus, H., Hoffmann, W., Hogrefe, A. & Classen, M. (1991) Cholangioscope dye laser lithotripsy in the non-surgical treatment of difficult bile duct stones. *Gastrointestinal Endoscopy*, **37**, 254.

173. Neuhaus, H., Hagenmüller, F., Griebel, M. & Classen, M. (1991) Percutaneous cholangioscopic or transpapillary insertion of self-expanding biliary metal stents. *Gastrointestinal Endoscopy*, **37**, 31–37.

174. Nimura, Y., Hayakawa, N., Toyoda, S. *et al.* (1981) Percutaneous transhepatic cholangioscopy. *Stomach & Intestine*, **16**, 681.

175. Nimura, Y., Kamiya, J., Hayakawa, N. & Shionoya, S. (1989) Cholangioscopic differentiation of biliary strictures and polyps. *Endoscopy*, **21**, 351–356.

176. Nix, G., Schmitz, P., Wilson, J. *et al.* (1984) Carcinoma of the head of the pancreas. Therapeutic implications of endoscopic retrograde cholangiopancreatography findings. *Gastroenterology*, **87**, 37–43.

177. Nix, G.A.J.J., van Overbeeke, I.C., Wilson, J.H.P. & Ten Kate, F.J.W. (1988) ERCP diagnosis of tumours in the region of the head of the pancreas. *Digestive Diseases and Sciences*, **33**, 577–586.

178. Nüesch, H.J., Hahnloser, P., Fumagalli, J. *et al.* (1973) Endoskopische retrograde Cholangiographie: Methode der Wahl zur Diagnose der Choledochuszyste. *Deutsche Medizinische Wochenschrift*, **98**, 2069–2070.

179. O'Connor, M.J., Summer, H.W. & Schwartz, M.L. (1982) The

clinical and pathological correlations in mechanical biliary obstruction and acute cholangitis. *Annals of Surgery*, **195**, 419–423.

180. O'Connor, K.W. & Jones, S. (1990) Oxygen desaturation is common and clinically underappreciated during elective endoscopic procedure. *Gastrointestinal Endoscopy*, **36**, 82–84.

181. Okuda, K., Tanikawa, K., Emura, T. *et al.* (1974) Non-surgical percutaneous trans-hepatic cholangiography—diagnostic significance in medical problems of the liver. *American Journal of Digestive Diseases*, **19**, 21–36.

182. Orii, K., Nakahasa, A., Takase, Y. *et al.* (1981) Choledocholithotomy by YAG laser with a choledochofiberscope: case reports of two patients. *Surgery*, **90**, 120–122.

183. Osnes, M., Serck-Hanssen, A. & Myren, J. (1975) Endoscopic retrograde brush cytology (ERBC) of the biliary and pancreatic ducts. *Scandinavian Journal of Gastroenterology*, **10**, 829–831.

184. Palmer, K.R. & Hofmann, A.F. (1986) Intraductal mono-octonoin for the direct dissolution of bile duct stones: experience in 343 patients. *Gut*, **27**, 196–202.

185. Perissat, J., Collet, D.R. & Belliard, R. (1989) Gallstones: laparoscopic treatment—intracorporeal lithotripsy, followed by cholecystotomy or cholecystectomy. A personal technique. *Endoscopy*, **21**, 373–374.

186. Picus, D., Weyman, P.J. & Marx, M.V. (1989) Role of percutaneous intracorporeal electrohydraulic lithotripsy in the treatment of biliary tract calculi. *Radiology*, **170**, 989–993.

187. Pitt, H.A. & Longmire, W.P. (1980) Suppurative cholangitis. In Hardy, J.D. (ed.) *Critical Surgical Illness*, p. 380. Philadelphia: Saunders.

188. Pitt, H.A., Gomes, A.S., Lois, J.F. *et al.* (1985) Does preoperative biliary drainage reduce operative risk or increase hospital cost? *Annals of Surgery*, **201**, 545–552.

189. Ponchon, T., Bory, R., Chavaillon, A. & Fouillet, P. (1989) Biliary lithiasis: combined endoscopic and surgical treatment. *Endoscopy*, **21**, 15–18.

190. Ponchon, T., Chavaillon, A., Ayela, P. & Lambert, R. (1989) Retrograde biliary ultrathin endoscopy enhances biopsy of stenoses and lithotripsy. *Gastrointestinal Endoscopy*, **35**, 292–297.

191. Rambow, A., Staritz, M. & Meyer zum Büschenfelde, K.-H. (1988) Contrast media for ERCP. *Endoscopy*, **20**, 126–127.

192. Riemann, J.F. (1985) Aktuelle gastroenterologische Diagnostik. In Blum, A.L., Siewert, J.R., Ottenjahn, R. & Lehr, L. (eds.), pp. 385–403. Berlin, Heidelberg, New York: Springer.

193. Riemann, J.F., Seuberth, K. and Demling, L. (1985) Mechanical lithotripsy in common bile duct stones. *Gastrointestinal Endoscopy*, **31**, 207–210.

193a. Riemann, J.F., Kohler, B., Harloff, M. & Weber, J. (1989) Die transpapilläre Cholangioskopie. *Deutsche Medizinische Wochenschrift*, **114**, 1775–1779.

194. Robbins, A.H., Messian, R.A., Widrich, W.C. *et al.* (1974) Endoscopic pancreatography. An analysis of the radiologic findings in pancreatitis. *Radiology*, **113**, 293–296.

195. Ross, W.A. (1990) Premedication for upper gastrointestinal endoscopy. *Gastrointestinal Endoscopy*, **35**, 120–126.

196. Rosseland, A.R. and Solhaug, J.H. (1984) Early or delayed endoscopic papillotomy (EPT) in gallstone pancreatitis. *Annals of Surgery*, **199**, 165–167.

197. Runge, D., Gebhardt, J., Burmeister, W. & Wurbs, D. (1981) Mechanische Lithotripsie von Gallengangsteinen. *Deutsche Medizinische Wochenschrift*, **110**, 1981.

198. Rustgi, A.K., Kelsey, P.B., Guelrud, M. *et al.* (1988) Malignant tumours of the bile ducts: diagnosis by biopsy during endoscopic cannulation. *Gastrointestinal Endoscopy*, **35**, 248–251.

199. Safrany, L., Neuhaus, B. & Krause, S. (1980) Endoskopische Papillotomie bei akuter biliärer Pankreatitis. *Deutsche Medizinische Wochenschrift*, **105**, 115–119.

200. Sahel, J. (1987) Komplikationen nach endoskopischer Papillotomie—Ergebnisse einer internationalen Umfrage. *Leber Magen Darm*, **6**, 364–370.

201. Salmon, P.R. (1975) Endoscopic retrograde choledochopancreatography in the diagnosis of pancreatic disease. *Gut*, **16**, 658–663.

202. Salmon, P.R., Rey, J.F., Baddeley, H. *et al.* (1977) ERCP in the diagnosis and management of periampullary carcinoma. In Delmont, J. (ed.) *The Sphincter of Oddi*, pp. 111–114. Basel: Karger.

203. Sarner, M. & Cotton, P.B. (1984) Classification of pancreatitis. *Gut*, **25**, 756–759.

204. Sauerbruch, T., Delius, M., Paumgartner, G. *et al.* (1986) Fragmentation of gallstones by extracorporeal shockwaves. *New England Journal of Medicine*, **314**, 818–822.

205. Sauerbruch, T., Stern, M. and the Study Group for Shock-wave Lithotripsy of Bile Duct Stones (1989) Fragmentation of bile duct stones by extracorporeal shock waves. A new approach to biliary calculi after failure of routine endoscopic measures. *Gastroenterology*, **96**, 146–152.

206. Sauter, G., Grabein, B., Huber, G. *et al.* (1990) Antibiotic prophylaxis of infectious complications with endoscopic retrograde cholangiopancreatography. A randomized controlled study. *Endoscopy*, **22**, 164–167.

207. Schneider, M.U., Matek, W., Bauer R. & Domschke, W. (1988) Mechanical lithotripsy of bile duct stones in 209 patients—effect of technical advances. *Endoscopy*, **20**, 248–253.

208. Schölmerich, J., Gross, V., Johannesson, T. *et al.* (1989) Detection of biliary origin of acute pancreatitis. *Digestive Diseases and Sciences*, **34**(6), 830–833.

209. Scott, J., Summerfield, J.A., Elias, E. *et al.* (1977) Chronic pancreatitis: a cause of cholestasis. *Gut*, **18**, 196–201.

210. Seifert, E., Safrany, L., Stender, H. St. *et al.* (1974) Identification of bile duct tumours by means of endoscopic retrograde pancreatocholangiography (ERCP). *Endoscopy*, **6**, 156–162.

211. Seifert, E., Stender, H., Safrany, L. *et al.* (1974) X-ray findings of pancreatic cysts diagnosed by endoscopic pancreatocholangiography. *Endoscopy*, **6**, 77–83.

212. Seifert, E., Schulte, F. & Chalybäus, C. (1989) Quo vadis endoskopische Sphinkterotomie? *Zeitschrift für Gastroenterologie*, **27**, 77–82.

213. Seifert, E. (1988) Long-term follow-up after endoscopic sphincterotomy (EST). *Endoscopy*, **20**, 232–235.

214. Shepherd, H.A., Royle, G., Ross, A.P. *et al.* (1988) Endoscopic biliary prosthesis in the palliation of malignant obstruction of the distal common bile duct: a randomized trial. *British Journal of Surgery*, **75**, 1166–1168.

215. Sherman, S., Troiano, F.P., Hawes, R.H. & Lehman, G.A. (1990) Sphincter of Oddi manometry: decreased risk of clinical pancreatitis with use of a modified aspirating catheter. *Gastrointestinal Endoscopy*, **36**, 462–466.

216. Shorvon, P.J., Cotton, P.B. & Mason, R.R. (1985) Percutaneous transhepatic assistance for duodenoscopic sphincterotomy. *Gut*, **26**, 1373–76.

217. Siegel, J.H. (1980) Precut papillotomy: A method to improve success of ERCP and papillotomy. *Endoscopy*, **12**, 130–133.

218. Siegel, J.H., Tone, P. & Menikheim, D. (1986) Gallstone pancreatitis: Pathogenesis and clinical forms—the emerging role of endoscopic management. *American Journal of Gastroenterology*, **81**, 774–778.

219. Siegel, J.H. & Snady, H. (1986) The significance of endoscopically placed prostheses in the management of malignant biliary obstruction due to carcinoma in the pancreas: results of nonoperative decompression in 277 patients. *American Journal of Gastroenterology*, **81**, 634–641.

220. Siegel, J.H., Safrany, L., Ben-Zvi, J.S. *et al.* (1987) Duodenoscopic sphincterotomy in patients with gallbladder in situ: Report of a series of 1272 patients. *American Journal of Gastroenterology*, **83**, 1255–1258.

221. Siegel, J.H., Pullano, W., Kodsi, B. *et al.* (1988) Optimal palliation of malignant bile duct obstruction: experience with endoscopic 12 French prostheses. *Endoscopy*, **20**, 137–141.

222. Siegel, J.H., Ben-Zvi, J.S. & Pullano, W. (1989) The needle knife: a valuable tool in diagnostic and therapeutic ERCP. *Gastrointestinal Endoscopy*, **35**(6), 499–503.

223. Siegel, J.H., Ben-Zvi, J.S. & Pullano, W.E. (1990) Mechanical lithotripsy of common bile duct stones. *Gastrointestinal Endoscopy*, **36**, 351–356.

224. Silvis, S.E., Rohrmann, C.A. & Vennes, J.A. (1976) Diagnostic accuracy of endoscopic retrograde cholangiopancreatography in hepatic, biliary and pancreatic malignancy. *Annals of Internal Medicine*, **84**, 438–440.

225. Simpson, C.J., Gray, G.R. & Gillespie, G. (1985) Early endoscopic

sphincterotomy for retained common bile duct stones. *Journal of the Royal College of Surgeons of Edinburgh*, **30**, 288–289.

226. Sivak, M.V. Jr. & Fleisher, D.E. (1983) Colonoscopy with a video endoscope: Preliminary experience with a new type of endoscope (abstract). *Gastrointestinal Endoscopy*, **29**, 187.

227. Sjodahl, R., Tagesson, C. & Watterfors, J. (1978) On the pathogenesis of acute cholecystitis. *Surgery, Gynecology and Obstetrics*, **146**, 199.

228. Skude, W., Wehlin, L., Maruyama, T. & Ariyama, J. (1976) Hyperamylasaemia after duodenoscopy and retrograde cholangio-pancreatography. *Gut*, **17**, 127–132.

229. Smit, J.M., Out, M.M.J., Groen, A.K. *et al.* (1989) A placebo-controlled study on the efficacy of aspirin and doxycyclin in preventing clogging of biliary endoprostheses. *Gastrointestinal Endoscopy*, **35**, 485–489.

229a. Smith, A.C., Dowsett, J.F. & Russell, R.C.G. (1990) Endoscopic stenting versus bypass surgery for primary low malignant biliary obstruction. A prospective randomized trial in 204 patients. In *Abstracts of the World Congresses of Gastroenterology, Sydney 1990*, p. 1174. Abingdon: The Medicine Group (UK).

230. Soehendra, N., Schulz, H., Nam, V.C. *et al.* (1990) ESWL and gallstone dissolution with MTBE via naso-vesicular catheter. *Endoscopy*, **22**, 176–179.

231. Spängler, H.P. (1968) Die Blutversorgung der Papilla Vateri und des papillennahen Choledochusabschnitts. *Anatomischer Anzeiger*, **122**, 371–376.

232. Speer, A.G., Cotton, P.B., Russell, R.C.G. *et al.* (1987) Randomised trial of endoscopic versus percutaneous stent insertion in malignant obstructive jaundice. *Lancet*, **ii**, 57–62.

233. Speer, A.G., Cotton, P.B., Rode, J. *et al.* (1988) Biliary stent blockage with bacterial biofilm. *Annals of Internal Medicine*, **108**, 546–553.

234. Speer, A.G., Cotton, P.B. and MacRae, K.D. (1988) Endoscopic management of malignant biliary obstruction: stents of 10 French gauge are preferable to stents of 8 French gauge. *Gastrointestinal Endoscopy*, **34**, 412–417.

235. Speer, A.G. & Cotton, P.B. (1989) Endoscopic stents for biliary obstruction due to malignancy. In Jacobson, I.M. (ed.) *ERCP, Techniques and Therapeutic Applications*. New York: Elsevier.

236. Stadelmann, O., Safrany, L., Loffler, A. *et al.* (1974) Endoscopic retrograde cholangio-pancreatography in the diagnosis of pancreatic cancer. Experience with 54 cases. *Endoscopy*, **6**, 84–93.

237. Steinberg, W.A. (1988) Sphincter Oddi dysfunction: a clinical controversy. *Gastroenterology*, **95**, 1409–1415.

238. Staritz, M., Ewe, K. & Meyer zum Büschenfelde, K.H. (1983) Mechanical gallstone lithotripsy in the common bile duct: in vitro and in vivo experience. *Endoscopy*, **15**, 316–318.

239. Staritz, M., Rambow, A., Grosse, A. *et al.* (1990) Electromagnetically generated extracorporeal shockwaves for fragmentation of extra- and intrahepatic bile duct stones: indications, success and problems during a 15 month clinical experience. *Gut*, **31**, 222–225.

240. Summerfield, J.A. (1988) Biliary obstruction is best managed by endoscopist. *Gut*, **29**, 741–745.

241. Summerfield, J.A., Elias, E., Hungerford, G.D. *et al.* (1976) The biliary system in primary biliary cirrhosis: a study by endoscopic retrograde cholangiopancreatography. *Gastroenterology*, **70**, 240–243.

242. Takada, T., Suzuki, S., Nakamura, K. *et al.* (1974) Studies on percutaneous biliary tract endoscopy. *Gastroenterologic Endoscopy*, **16**, 106.

243. Takekoshi, T. & Tatagi, K. (1975) Retrograde pancreatocholangioscopy. *Gastroenterologic Endoscopy*, **8**, 172.

244. Tanaka, M. & Ikeda, S. (1988) Sphincter of Oddi Manometry: comparison of microtransducer and perfusion methods. *Endoscopy*, **20**, 184–188.

245. Toouli, J., Geenen, J., Hogen, W.J. *et al.* (1982) Sphincter of Oddi motor activity: a comparison between patients with common bile duct stones and controls. *Gastroenterology*, **82**, 111–117.

246. Tytgat, G.N.J., Bartelsman, J.F.W.M., Den Hartog Jager, F.C.A. *et al.* (1986) Upper intestinal and biliary tract endoprothesis. *Digestive Diseases and Sciences*, **31** (supplement), 57S–76S.

247. Urukami, Y. (1980) Peroral cholangiopancreatoscopy (PDCS) and peroral direct cholangioscopy (PDSCS). *Endoscopy*, **12**, 30.

248. Vaira, D., D'Anna, L., Ainley, C. *et al.* (1989) Endoscopic sphincterotomy in 1000 consecutive patients. *Lancet*, **ii**, 431–434.

249. Vandermeeren, A., Delhaye, M., Gabbrielle, A. & Cremer, M. (1990) In *Abstracts of the World Congress of Gastroenterology, Sydney 1990*, p. 944. Abingdon: The Medicine Groupe (UK), Ltd.

250. Vondrasek, P., Eberhardt, G. & Classen, M. (1974) Endoskopische Halbleiter-Manometrie. *Innere Medizin*, **3**, 188–192.

251. Venu, R.P., Geenen, J.E., Hogan, W. *et al.* (1989) Idiopathic recurrent pancreatitis: an approach to diagnosis and treatment. *Digestive Diseases and Sciences*, **34**, 56–60.

252. Warshaw, A.L., Berr, J. & Gang, D.L. (1987) Villous adenoma of the duct of Wirsung. *Digestive Diseases and Sciences*, **32**(11), 1311–1313.

253. Weidenhiller, S., Flügel, H. & Rösch, W. (1975) Abrasive cytology of the pancreatic and biliary duct in man. *Endoscopy*, **7**, 72–74.

254. Williams, S.J., Avanitidis, D., Ng, M. *et al.* (1990) The role of endoscopic biliary intervention in the management of benign biliary strictures. In: *Abstracts of the World Congress of Gastroenterology, Sydney 1990*, p. 1172. Abingdon: The Medicine Groupe (UK), Ltd.

255. Working Party of the British Society of Gastroenterology (1988) Cleaning and disinfection of equipment for gastrointestinal flexible endoscopy: interim recommendations of a Working Party of the British Society of Gastroenterology. *Gut*, **29**, 1134–1151.

256. Worthley, C.S. & Toouli, J. (1988) Gallbladder non-filling. An indication for cholecystectomy after endoscopic sphincterotomy. *British Journal of Surgery*, **75**, 796–798.

257. Worthley, C.S., Watts, J.McK. & Toouli, J. (1989) Common bile duct exploration or endoscopic sphincterotomy for choledocholithiasis. *Australian and New Zealand Journal of Surgeons*, **59**, 209–216.

258. Yamakawa, T., Mieno, K., Noguchi, T. & Shikata, J. (1976) An improved choledochofiberscope and non-surgical removal of retained biliary tract calculi under direct visual control. *Gastrointestinal Endoscopy*, **22**, 160.

259. Yamakawa, T. (1989) Percutaneous cholangioscopy for management of retained biliary tract stones and intrahepatic stones. *Endoscopy*, **21**, 333–337.

260. Yasuda, K., Nakajima, M., Cho, E. *et al.* (1989) Comparison of peroral and percutaneous cholangioscopy. *Endoscopy*, **21**, 347–350.

261. Yoshimoto, H., Ikeda, S., Tanaka, M. *et al.* (1989) Choledochoscopic electrohydraulic lithotripsy and lithotomy for stones in the common bile duct, intrahepatic ducts and gallbladder. *Annals of Surgery*, **210**, 576–582.

262. Yoshimura, H., Sakaguchi, H., Yoshioka, T. *et al.* (1989) Afterloading intracavitary irradiation and expanding stents for malignant biliary obstruction. *Radiation Medicine*, **7**, 36–41.

263. Zimmon, D.S., Falkenstein, D.B. & Kessler, R.E. (1975) Endoscopic papillotomy for choledocholithiasis. *New England Journal of Medicine*, **293**, 1181–1182.

264. Zimmon, D.S., Falkenstein, D.B., Abraham, R.M. *et al.* (1974) Endoscopic retrograde cholangio-pancreatography (ERCP) in the diagnosis of pancreatic inflammatory disease. *Radiology*, **113**, 287–297.

CHAPTER 27

Peritoneoscopy

Telfer B. Reynolds & Russell E. Cowan

Peritoneoscopy and laparoscopy are synonymous terms, though the latter tends to be used more often when the indication is gynaecological. They are defined similarly in medical dictionaries.[8]

HISTORY

The advanced state of development of peritoneoscopy today owes much to the imagination and ingenuity of the originators of this technique. Ott, a gynaecologist, first examined the abdominal cavity in 1901 using a head mirror and speculum and Kelling in the same year first used optical instruments to perform what he called 'coelioscopy' in the dog by inflating the abdominal cavity with air and examining the contents with a cystoscope. Kelling's technique was published in 1902[24] but its use in humans was not described until 1910 when Jacobaeus[19] published his experience with inspection of the human pleural and peritoneal cavities, again with a cystoscope. One month later, Kelling[25] reported his experience with peritoneoscopy in two patients. Two years later Jacobaeus[20] reported on 45 peritoneoscopic examinations of humans but this was followed by a 10-year interval without further progress until Korbsch[26] rediscovered the technique and developed instruments and methods. Interest in the procedure then flourished, with reports from many peritoneoscopists throughout the world. None contributed more to the technique than Kalk,[22] who designed the instrument that formed the basis of today's peritoneoscopes.

Ruddock[36,37] designed a peritoneoscope with a built-in biopsy facility. He also published his large experience with the procedure. Advances in recent years have stemmed from the introduction of fibreoptics to medical technology, whereby glass-fibre bundles are used to transmit light from the light source down the shaft of the instrument thus providing 'cold light' illumination of the abdominal cavity.[17]

There are many excellent reviews of peritoneoscopic experience in the literature, including those by Caroli and Ricordeau,[5] Barry, Brown and Read,[2] and Hall, Donaldson and Brennan.[14] A colour atlas of peritoneoscopic photographs has been published by Wittman.[46] Developments in the technique and equipment are continuing.

INDICATIONS

With proliferation and refinement of modern imaging techniques and the increasing use of imaging-directed percutaneous biopsy, there has been a substantial decrease in utilization of peritoneoscopy.[10] When considering the indications, it is important to know which organs and how much of them can be seen through the peritoneoscope. In general, one can see the anterior surface of the abdominal viscera as when the abdominal wall is removed at autopsy. This includes the entire anterior surface of the left lobe of the liver, the medial two-thirds of the anterior surface of the right lobe of the liver, the leading edges and the inferior portion of the posterior surfaces of both lobes of the liver, the anterior surface of the gallbladder, the anterior surface of the stomach, parts of the small bowel, colon, mesentery and omentum, and the peritoneum covering the diaphragm, the anterior abdominal wall and the falciform ligament. Not easily seen are the posterior and lateral surfaces of the right lobe of the liver, the duodenum, the cystic and common bile ducts and the retroperitoneal organs such as the kidneys and pancreas. By lifting the left lobe of the liver, Meyer-Burg[29] was able to visualize and biopsy the pancreas in a number of patients who were not obese. Other retroperitoneal structures have also been visualized and biopsied.[30,38] The spleen is visible only if enlarged. The dome of the right lobe of the liver is seen with difficulty. The pelvic organs (bladder, uterus, fallopian tubes and ovaries) are visible, particularly if the patient is placed in the Trendelenberg position and a hand or uterine sound in the vagina is used to manipulate the uterus. Visualization at peritoneoscopy can be increased by using an examining table that tilts in all directions and by inserting a blunt probe into the peritoneal cavity through a separate abdominal puncture.

Assessment of liver disease

A major indication for peritoneoscopy is inspection of the liver surface and evaluation of the size and shape of the organ. When combined with liver biopsy this allows the best assessment of the type and severity of chronic liver disease. Cirrhosis is diagnosed if the surface is

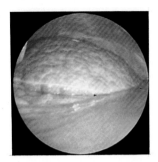

Figure 27.1 Left lobe of liver in a patient with non-alcoholic cirrhosis. The nodules range from 3 to 6 mm in diameter.

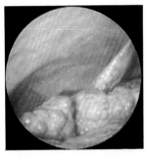

Figure 27.2 Close up view of falciform ligament and medial portions of both left and right liver lobes in a patient with advanced alcoholic cirrhosis. The surface is irregular and lobulated with small regenerative nodules 1 to 2 mm in diameter. The two larger nodules on the left are about 4 mm in diameter.

nodular (Figures 27.1 and 27.2). Small nodules, less than 3 mm in diameter, are most consistent with an alcoholic aetiology, while larger, well-developed nodules suggest non-alcoholic cirrhosis. A liver that is paler than normal with an irregular, granular or coarse sandpaper surface and a thickened leading edge suggests either alcoholic fibrosis or chronic active hepatitis (Figure 27.3). An enlarged liver with a rounded leading edge and a smooth surface is consistent with either a fatty liver or acute alcoholic hepatitis. There is nothing distinctive about the appearance of the liver in acute hepatitis unless the disease is unusually severe with submassive necrosis, when there are often islands of normal-appearing liver surrounded by paler, retracted areas of collapsed parenchyma.

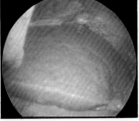

Figure 27.3 Left lobe of the liver in a patient with alcoholic liver disease and extensive fibrosis on microscopic examination. The liver surface is paler than normal and irregular but without well-defined nodules.

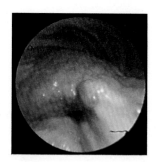

Figure 27.4 In the background is the right lobe of the cirrhotic liver. In the foreground is a tortuous blue collateral vein, 4 to 5 mm in diameter, leading towards the base of the falciform ligament (out of view, to the right).

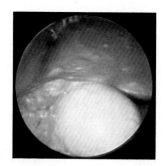

Figure 27.5 Gallbladder and right lobe of liver in a patient with metastatic carcinoma from the pancreas. Numerous small white tumour deposits are evident on the liver surface. These were not seen on ^{99m}Tc sulphur colloid liver scan. The gallbladder is markedly distended and projects 6 to 7 cm below the right lobe margin.

Portal hypertension is recognized at peritoneoscopy by the presence of portal collateral veins. Occasionally a large vein is seen in the falciform ligament (Figure 27.4); more often numerous tiny vessels are present which appear red in colour although they are venules. Tortuous veins are often seen on the undersurface of the diaphragm or on the lateral or anterior walls of the abdominal cavity. The abdominal wall veins are often visible by transillumination in the darkened procedure room. If there are adhesions in the abdomen in patients with portal hypertension, they frequently contain large collateral veins carrying blood from the mesentery or bowel to the abdominal wall.

For recording the progression of liver disease, an accurate, objective description of the liver surface is essential. Nodule size can be estimated relatively accurately if the operator knows the magnification produced by his instrument at a specified distance. A photograph is invaluable for recording the appearance of the liver.

Liver biopsy under direct vision can be performed either through the peritoneoscope or through a separate puncture site. Currently, we prefer to use the Tru-Cut needle and a separate puncture because it gives better specimens with less fragmentation. Direct-vision biopsy is probably little safer than 'blind' biopsy with respect to bleeding except that the operator may have earlier knowledge that bleeding is occurring. Pressure on the liver surface adjacent to a bleeding biopsy site exerted by a probe inserted through the peritoneoscope may be of some value in controlling bleeding. Some advise injection of topical thrombin solution into the biopsy wound or electrocautery via the biopsy needle.[44] We have had no experience with either of the latter two methods. Ruddock[36,37] obtained forceps biopsies of the leading edge of the liver; these are susceptible to artefacts more often because of compression of the specimen.

Evaluation of focal lesions in the liver

Focal lesions detected by hepatic imaging and located within the field of vision of the peritoneoscope can be examined, photographed and biopsied. Metastatic cancer

is usually pale in colour, often has a central umbilication and is easily recognizable (Figure 27.5). Hepatocellular cancer can usually be differentiated from surrounding cirrhotic nodules by its colour, friability and irregularity (Figure 27.6). In some patients, however, the tumour nodules so closely resemble the regenerative nodules of cirrhosis that biopsy is necessary for diagnosis. Less common lesions such as congenital cysts, haemangiomas, hydatid cysts, benign solid tumours and cystadenomas all require experience for ready recognition. When tumour masses appear cystic or highly vascular, the safety of biopsy can be evaluated by first using a fine needle for aspiration.

Because ultrasonic or CT-guided fine-needle biopsy is minimally invasive, has little risk[27,45] and, providing expert cytologic interpretation is available, is highly reliable, it has largely replaced peritoneoscopy for evaluation of focal lesions. However, direct comparisons of the two methods show them to be of approximately equal sensitivity and specificity,[3,9] and frequently complementary.[9] An advantage of peritoneoscopy in suspected metastatic disease is that there may be easily recognizable lesions on the liver surface that are too small to be detected by ultrasound or CT scan. Another advantage in hepato-

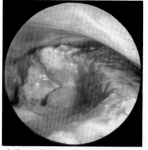

Figure 27.6 Right lobe of liver in a patient with cirrhosis due to hepatitis B. On the lower border of the right lobe just above the gallbladder there are two large, pale, irregular, friable masses of hepatocellular carcinoma. There is blood on the omentum at the bottom of the picture resulting from an aspiration biopsy of the tumour.

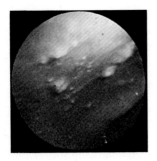

Figure 27.7 Nodules of metastatic carcinoma 1 to 2 mm in diameter on the parietal peritoneum of a patient with ascites caused by metastatic carcinoma.

cellular cancer is that the severity of associated chronic liver disease can be evaluated, which can be important in deciding the feasibility of tumour resection.[21]

Differential diagnosis of ascites

Chronic liver disease causing ascites is usually easily diagnosed at peritoneoscopy. Since much of the peritoneal surface is available for inspection, some of the other causes of ascites can also be identified. In carcinomatous ascites there may be many small neoplastic nodules scattered on the parietal and visceral peritoneum or fewer, larger lesions on the bowel, mesentery or peritoneum (Figure 27.7). In tuberculous or coccidioidal peritonitis there are numerous 0.5–2.0 mm yellow or white tubercles on both the visceral and parietal peritoneum (Figure 27.8). Usually the entire peritoneum is involved; occasionally the disease is limited to the upper or lower abdomen. Biopsy of lesions on the intestinal surface is potentially hazardous but forceps biopsy of a nodule on the peritoneum or mesentery is easy and safe. Peritoneoscopy has been shown to be an effective method of obtaining an early diagnosis in patients with suspected tuberculous peritonitis.[11,47]

In sexually active women with high-protein ascitic fluid, the finding of peritoneal inflammation and/or adhesions in the pelvis or right upper quadrant suggests the possibility of chlamydial peritonitis.[13] Additional diagnostic tests are culture of the fluid for *Chlamydozoa trachomatis*,

immunofluorescent antibody and response to doxycycline treatment.

Staging of lymphoma

Some oncology groups have used peritoneoscopy to look at the liver surface for lymphomatous involvement, to obtain multiple liver biopsies and even to biopsy the spleen.[6,41] Lymph nodes in the posterior abdomen cannot be seen or biopsied at peritoneoscopy because of their location, but Meyer-Burg and Ziegler[30] have used peritoneoscopy for the inspection and biopsy of the supra-gastric lymph nodes in the staging of lymphoma. There is insufficient published experience to judge the safety of splenic biopsy during peritoneoscopy.

CONTRAINDICATIONS

Most contraindications are relative rather than absolute.

Obesity

A thick abdominal wall makes it more difficult to obtain satisfactory anaesthesia of the parietal peritoneum and to penetrate the abdominal wall safely with the peritoneoscopic trocar. Mobility of the peritoneoscope within the abdominal cavity is reduced because the thick abdominal wall tends to hold the instrument in a vertical position. A fatty greater omentum often makes it difficult to view the liver satisfactorily.

Surgical scars

Adhesions frequently form under surgical scars. After cholecystectomy, adhesions often form a curtain in the right upper quadrant, preventing visualization of the right lobe of the liver. Similarly, visualization of the left lobe of the liver may be prevented by adhesions under gastric surgery scars. When portal hypertension is present, adhesions often contain large collateral veins which, if traumatized by the peritoneoscopic trocar or air needle, can bleed seriously. The peritoneoscope should not be inserted, therefore, into the abdomen close to a scar. If a patient has had generalized peritonitis there may be adhesions throughout the abdomen which impair visualization, limit distensibility of the abdomen and constitute a hazard to insertion of the peritoneoscope since loops of bowel can be adherent to the abdominal wall.

Gross coagulation defects

Unless a liver biopsy is performed or an adhesion is torn, the abdominal puncture is the only potential site of bleeding at peritoneoscopy. Since small blood vessels at the puncture site can be clamped and ligated, there is less reason to fear excess bleeding in patients with coagulation defects than there is during percutaneous liver biopsy.

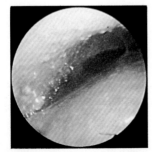

Figure 27.8 Parietal peritoneum and surface of the right lobe of the liver in a patient with tuberculous peritonitis. There are numerous small white tubercles on the peritoneum and a few on the liver surface.

However, patients with grossly abnormal prothrombin times tend to be fragile in many respects, so peritoneoscopy should be performed in such patients only when there is a very strong indication. Trauma to a vein on the peritoneal surface of the abdomen at the puncture site can be overlooked at peritoneoscopy since bleeding will be into the abdominal cavity rather than into the wound and may be temporarily prevented by the tamponade effect of the trocar during the procedure, only to start after removal of the instrument.

Uncooperative patients

Since peritoneoscopy is usually performed without general anaesthesia, some degree of patient cooperation is required. With adequate premedication most apprehensive patients are able to cooperate satisfactorily.

Tense ascites

Visualization at peritoneoscopy is unsatisfactory through ascitic fluid. When marked ascites is present, therefore, it is necessary to remove much of the fluid and replace it with air. In our experience this is not dangerous and does not result in hypovolaemia. Drainage of ascitic fluid from the incision may occur and may persist for several days after the procedure unless the operator is able to suture the hole in the peritoneum. Ascitic fluid extravasation into the tissues of the abdominal wall or into the loose tissues around the male genitalia may also occur if the peritoneal rent is left open while the skin incision is tightly closed.

INSTRUMENTS

Peritoneoscope

Instruments have improved steadily since the introduction of fibre-optic light transmission for endoscopy in 1961.[17] Several excellent instruments are now available, including those made by Storz, Wolff, American Cystoscope Makers, Olympus and Machida. There are both forward oblique and direct-vision telescopes and many contain an operating channel for insertion of a long biopsy needle or probe. Most instruments are insulated to allow safe conduction of an electric current for coagulation. There are slender peritoneoscopes with a diameter as small as 3.4 mm,[12] that are easier to insert through the abdominal wall; however, they provide less illumination in the abdomen. All makes of peritoneoscopes have photographic capabilities which operate either by using a flash bulb at the distal end of the instrument or by using an electronic flash that is conducted from outside the body down the fibre-optic light bundle. Both flexible and ultrasonically equipped peritoneoscopic telescopes are in the process of development.[34,39] Modern instruments are constructed in such a way that they tolerate gas sterilization without loss of optical quality.

Air insufflation needle

For air insufflation most operators, including ourselves, prefer the Veress needle, which has a blunt retractable cannula inside a sharp-pointed needle. The inner cannula springs forward with a clicking sound and projects beyond the point of the needle when the abdominal cavity is entered.

Accessories

Numerous accessories are available, including sterilizable ovens for prewarming telescopes to body temperature. This prevents fogging of the lens after insertion of the telescope into the peritoneal cavity. A suitable alternative is an inexpensive electrical heating pad placed under the tray containing the sterile peritoneoscope. A drop of sterile antifog liquid (UltraStop made by Sigma Chemic, Vienna) placed on the lens immediately prior to insertion of the telescope into the abdomen is also helpful in preventing fogging. There are automatic gas insufflators that give a regulated flow of air or carbon dioxide and provide continuous monitoring of intra-abdominal gas pressure. We prefer hand insufflation with a sterile sphygmomanometer bulb. A variety of biopsy needles is available for insertion through the operating channel of the peritoneoscope or through a separate puncture site. In addition, there are punch-biopsy forceps suitable for biopsying peritoneal nodules.

PREPARATION OF INSTRUMENTS

Care and cleaning of the instruments is best accomplished by a nurse or technician who is familiar with the procedure of peritoneoscopy. Thorough cleaning of the various parts of the instrument after each use is essential. Ethylene oxide gas sterilization clearly provides the greatest possible safety relative to transmission of hepatitis and human immunodeficiency viruses. In this regard, 'wet' sterilization by soaking in activated glutaraldehyde solution poses uncertain risks, although we know of no reported case of transmission of hepatitis or HIV with wet-sterilized endoscopes and activated glutaraldehyde is a known viricidal agent effective against the hepatitis B virus.

TECHNIQUE

Techniques for performance of peritoneoscopy vary considerably and this suggests that the procedure has a large margin of safety with several different ways to achieve the same result. We describe below the method that we have used, with minor modifications, during the past 30 years.

Premedication

We prefer a moderately sedated patient who is not anxious but who is awake enough to respond to commands. Since many patients have severe liver disease and some are habitual drug users, the effect of a given dose of premedication varies markedly. Currently we are using intravenous pethidine (meperidine *USP*) 50–100 mg, followed by intravenous midazolam 2–5 mg, given in the peritoneoscopy room immediately before the procedure. If there is anxiety or pain during the procedure, then additional amounts of either of these medications can be given. Pethidine effect can be reversed by naloxone if indicated. Some workers give atropine routinely as premedication to prevent vagal reactions that occasionally occur in anxious patients. Most peritoneoscopists do not use general anaesthesia for medical peritoneoscopy since it adds risk and expense and the degree of pain and discomfort seldom warrant it. However, Michel and Raynaud[31] have written of the advantages of general anaesthesia of short duration using propanidid. For gynaecological peritoneoscopy, general anaesthesia is usually employed because of pain from tubal manipulation and fulguration.

Location

A procedure room that can also be used for other endoscopy and minor surgery is ideal for peritoneoscopy. There should be an anteroom for changing clothes and a sink for hand scrubbing. The room should contain resuscitation equipment and storage space for the peritoneoscope and attachments. It should be easily darkened and there should be an automatically adjustable table. The use of a surgical suite is unnecessary and, in most hospitals, impractical.

PERFORMANCE OF PERITONEOSCOPY _____

Our patients have a monitor for heart rate and rhythm and an intravenous drip of 5% glucose in water with a port for administration of medications. The operator prepares for the procedure with hand and forearm scrubbing and wears a sterile gown and gloves. The patient's abdomen is prepared and draped in a manner that prevents his visualization of the procedure (Figure 27.9). Selection of entry site for the insufflation needle and the peritoneoscopic trocar is important since insertion of these instruments carries the greatest potential risks for serious injury during the procedure. Many experienced peritoneoscopists use separate entry sites for the air needle and the peritoneoscope but it is probably safer and equally satisfactory to use a single entry site. In choosing a location it is important to avoid: (a) the epigastric vessels which run in the lateral borders of the rectus muscles; (b) the falciform ligament, which may contain large collateral

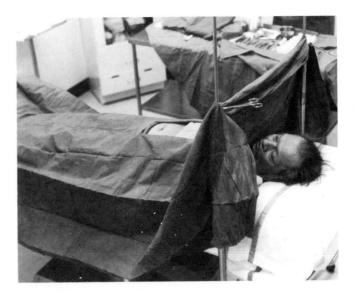

Figure 27.9 Method of draping of the patient for peritoneoscopy.

veins; (c) any collateral veins that are visible on the abdominal wall; and (d) abdominal scars, since these may overlie vascularized adhesions. Obviously, it would be unwise to choose an entry site overlying an abdominal mass or an enlarged liver or spleen. We choose most often a point 2–4 cm below the umbilicus near the midline (Figure 27.10). Should the patient's size or shape indicate that this location will be too far from the liver for optimum visualization, we enter above the umbilicus to the left of the midline to avoid the falciform ligament.

Anaesthesia of the skin and subcutaneous tissue is produced with 1% lignocaine (lidocaine) solution keeping the total dose less than 250 mg. An attempt should be made to anaesthetize the parietal peritoneum. An incision long enough to accommodate the peritoneoscopic trocar is made through the skin and subcutaneous fascia. The Veress needle is then pushed through the abdominal wall, using one hand to exert pressure and the other to keep the needle from abruptly lurching forward when it pierces the parietal peritoneum. When the abdomen is scaphoid it helps to ask the patient to push the umbilicus forward toward the ceiling during insertion of the needle. When the needle tip is in the peritoneal cavity it should move freely and, unless the abdominal wall is thick, it should lie flat (Figure 27.11). Air or carbon dioxide gas is then introduced with a sphygmomanometer bulb or with an automatic insufflation device. If the air or gas does not enter the abdomen with ease, then the needle point may still be located in the tissues of the abdominal wall. If there is any doubt about this one should listen for escaping gas when the needle hulb is open. If there is no return of gas after 100–200 ml have been insufflated, then the needle should be removed and another attempt made to enter the peritoneal cavity. In theory, carbon dioxide gas is safer than air since deaths have occurred during peritoneoscopy from air embolism due to pumping of air into the liver or into a dilated collateral vein.[16,43,46] However, carbon dioxide is somewhat irritating to the peritoneum, is more expensive, and may cause hypercarbia and arrhythmia under certain circumstances.[1,18,28,32,40]

After insufflation of enough air or carbon dioxide to distend the abdomen moderately, the needle is removed (or left in place if a different site is used for peritoneoscope insertion). With air in the abdomen it is easier to ensure anaesthesia of the parietal peritoneum if there is doubt that this was satisfactorily achieved initially. Next, the peritoneoscopy trocar is pushed through the abdominal wall. This requires considerable pressure and it is essential to control the instrument with one hand while pushing with the other in order to avoid moving suddenly several centimetres into the abdominal cavity when the resistance from the abdominal wall is overcome. Better control is achieved when the arms are near full extension and the table is low (Figure 27.12). After penetrating the abdominal wall, the trocar is removed immediately. The trocar sheath should then move easily into the peritoneal cavity with little resistance. If resistance is more than minimal, it is possible that the end of the sheath is still in the abdominal wall with only the tip of the trocar having pierced the peritoneum. If the sheath is freely movable, the peritoneoscopic telescope is next introduced under direct vision with the room darkened. Air or gas is pumped in through the instrument as needed to maintain a satisfactory pneumoperitoneum. The easiest landmark to look for initially is the falciform ligament. Touching the parietal peritoneum, including that over the falciform ligament, causes pain, whereas touching the bowel, omentum or liver does not. After initial inspection of the peritoneal cavity, visualization can be increased by tilting the table in different directions. Occasionally it is helpful to insert a blunt probe through a second entry site to lift the lower edge of the liver or to move omentum away from a suspected mass. We routinely look at as much of the liver surface as possible, the fundus of the gallbladder, the falciform ligament, the parietal peritoneum and the anterior surface of the stomach and bowel. We attempt to see the spleen when the table is tilted to the right and we scan the pelvis in females. We describe the liver surface as objectively as possible and ordinarily take a colour photograph for a permanent record. If a liver biopsy is indicated it can be performed through the operating channel of the peritoneoscope or through a separate puncture site near the area to be biopsied.

If there is much ascites, it must be aspirated to allow visualization, since the fluid prevents adequate light transmission. Most peritoneoscopes have blunt-ended aspiration trocars for removal of ascitic fluid by gentle suction or by siphon drainage. When there is only a small amount of ascites, it is usually possible to see the liver satisfactorily without removing the fluid providing the head of the table is elevated.

At the end of the procedure the peritoneoscope is withdrawn and the air is allowed to escape through the

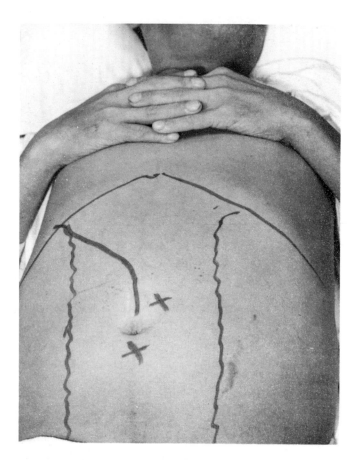

Figure 27.10 Potential entry sites (×) on the abdomen for the air needle and the peritoneoscope. The costal margins and the falciform ligament, represented by the curved line, are outlined in ink. The wavy lines indicate the outer borders of the rectus muscles where the epigastric vessels are located.

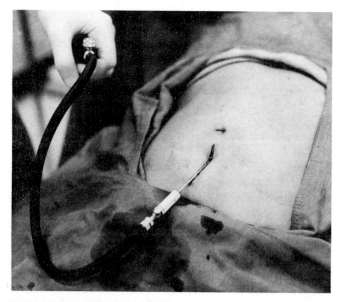

Figure 27.11 When the air needle has penetrated the peritoneum it should lie flat, as pictured, unless the abdominal wall is unusually thick.

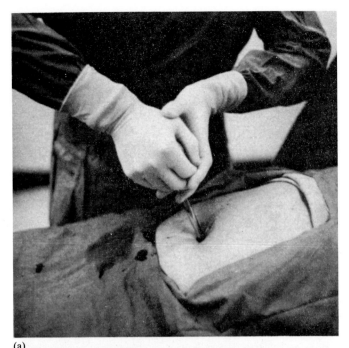

(a)

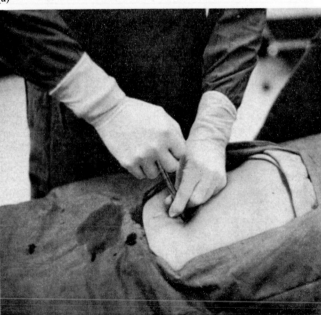

(b)

Figure 27.12 (a) Insertion of the trocar, with force, in this manner, provides potential for injury of abdominal viscera because of poor control over the depth of insertion. (b) By holding the trocar with one hand while pushing with the other, with the table low and the arms extended, the operator has better control over the depth of insertion.

trocar sheath before the latter is finally removed. The wound is closed superficially with interrupted silk sutures. In patients with ascites an attempt should be made to suture the rent in the peritoneum, being careful not to injure the intestine.

Vital signs are recorded immediately before and after the procedure and for 2 or 3 hours postoperatively.

COMPLICATIONS

Peritoneoscopy has a relatively low risk for an invasive procedure. Vilardell, Seres and Marti-Vincente[42] reported a complication rate of 1.2% in 1455 examinations. Bruehl[4] reviewed 63 845 peritoneoscopies performed by 67 physicians and found the complication rate to be 2.5% with a mortality rate of 0.029%. About three-quarters of the procedures included liver biopsy. From a questionnaire sent to physicians in France, Debray and Paolaggi[7] calculated an incidence of relatively serious complications of 0.5% in 35 597 peritoneoscopies, with a mortality of 0.09%. Similar rates of serious complications from reviews of smaller series were reported by Walker, Cooke and Playfair,[44] Handley and Nurick[15] and Barry, Brown and Read.[2] O'Kieffe and Boyce[35] had an overall incidence of complications of 6%, most of them minor. A higher rate of serious complications (2.3%) and mortality (0.49%) was reported by Kane and Krejs in a prospective evaluation of 603 procedures performed by 17 gastroenterologists in Dallas.[23]

Potential major complications are: (a) injection of air into the liver or an abdominal vein, causing air embolism; (b) bleeding into the abdominal cavity from the puncture site in the abdominal wall; (c) bowel perforation (when the bowel is adherent to the anterior abdominal wall); (d) puncture of an ovarian cyst mistaken for ascites; (e) serious bleeding from a liver biopsy; (f) tearing of an adhesion containing a large blood vessel; and (g) injury to abdominal viscera (other than bowel adherent to the abdomen) from the insufflation needle or peritoneoscopic trocar. Many different minor complications have been reported, including subcutaneous emphysema, omental emphysema, leaking of ascites from the wound, leakage of ascites into the anterior abdominal wall and genitalia, and vagal reaction with hypotension and bradycardia. A single case of pneumopericardium complicating peritoneoscopy and associated with surgical emphysema of the neck is an unexplained but minor complication that has been reported.[33]

PERSONAL EXPERIENCE

Over a 30-year period we had 12 major complications in approximately 2400 procedures (0.5%) including all except the last two of the possibilities mentioned above. There were six fatalities; one patient died suddenly, presumably from air embolism; three died as a consequence of bleeding from a traumatized abdominal wall collateral vein; and two patients with hepatocellular cancer and advanced liver disease bled persistently from the liver biopsy site and died 2 and 3 days, respectively, post-peritoneoscopy. Both were considered terminally ill and unsuitable for a surgical attempt to stop the bleeding. Non-fatal major complications were bleeding from an abdominal wall collateral vein that was ligated at laparotomy in two patients, bowel perforation in two patients with tuberculous peritonitis and ovarian cyst perforation in two patients. We know of only one patient who developed an incisional hernia following peritoneoscopy. We have not recognized any instances of deep wound infection or peritonitis.

Clearly, our most serious complication was trauma to large portal collateral veins underlying the trocar entry site. This will be an unavoidable though rare complication if the procedure is performed in patients with portal hypertension. Large collateral veins probably could be detected by preoperative ultrasonic scanning of the planned entry site, but this seems impractical for routine application. In only one of our five patients with this complication did we notice the bleeding during the procedure; presumably the trocar sheath compressed the vein.

In three of the remaining four patients there was excessive bleeding from the incision after removing the trocar as well as deterioration in vital signs. The bag of a Foley catheter inflated after passing it through the incision can be used to compress the bleeding site as a temporary measure. However, surgical intervention under general anaesthesia has been the best solution to this problem in our patients.

We reviewed 300 consecutive peritoneoscopic examinations performed in our liver unit over a $3\frac{1}{2}$-year period to examine the indications, completeness, accuracy and safety of this procedure in our hands. Most of the peritoneoscopies were done by resident staff or Hepatology Fellows under the supervision of one of the authors.

Indications for the procedure in these 300 cases are listed in Table 27.1. This shows that the most common indication was assessment of the type and severity of liver disease, achieved mainly by observation of the surface, leading edge and colour of the liver. Experience with

Table 27.1 Indications for peritoneoscopy in 300 consecutive examinations.[a]

Indications	Number of cases
Assessment of type and severity of liver disease	145
Suspected hepatic malignancy	77
Hepatocellular carcinoma	49
Hepatic metastases	28
Investigation of ascites	43
High protein ascites	20
Suspected tuberculous peritonitis	15
Suspected peritoneal malignancy	5
TB peritonitis versus peritoneal malignancy	2
Miscellaneous	29

[a]The total number of cases exceeds 300 since in some patients there were multiple indications.

Table 27.2 Assessment of accuracy of peritoneoscopic diagnosis by histological confirmation in 165 patients.

Peritoneoscopic diagnosis	Number of cases confirmed	Number of cases not confirmed
Alcoholic liver disease	66	6
Non-alcoholic chronic liver disease ± cirrhosis (chronic active hepatitis, cryptogenic cirrhosis)	23	6
Hepatocellular neoplasia (carcinoma, adenoma)	11	5
Hepatic metastases	20	2
Submassive hepatic necrosis with collapse	4	1
Tuberculous peritonitis	2	2
Peritoneal malignancy	4	1
Others	8	4
Total	138 (84%)	27 (16%)

this procedure has enabled us to recognize reliably the appearance of the liver surface with different types of liver disease. This is especially so with alcoholic liver disease, which forms a major part of our practice. In some patients the indications were multiple; for example, the assessment of alcoholic liver disease and the search for hepatocellular carcinoma suggested by a filling defect on liver scan or the presence of alpha-fetoprotein in the serum. Seventy-seven examinations were performed for suspected primary or secondary hepatic malignancy, including 34 in whom malignancy was suggested by filling defects on liver scan. In 30 (39%) of these examinations, hepatic malignancy was seen with certainty at peritoneoscopy and these included five of the 34 in whom malignancy had been suggested only by liver scan. In another ten patients, hepatic malignancy was detected only by histological examination of liver biopsy tissue taken at peritoneoscopy.

In 43 patients the indication was ascites of uncertain aetiology; 20 had ascites with a high protein content (> 30 g/l). In 27 (63%) of these 43 examinations liver disease was the only abnormality found, while non-hepatic disease was discovered or confirmed in another 8 (19%). In two of the remaining eight cases, adenocarcinoma cells were seen in the ascitic fluid, although no evidence of malignancy was seen at peritoneoscopy, and in another patient the clinical diagnosis of ascites was not confirmed at peritoneoscopy.

Miscellaneous indications for peritoneoscopy included undiagnosed jaundice, hepatomegaly of uncertain cause, the evaluation of abdominal masses and, in three patients with liver disease, the examination of pelvic masses.

In 267 patients (89%) complete examination of the abdominal cavity was possible. The examination was

Table 27.3 Assessment of the value of peritoneoscopy by comparing clinical diagnosis with peritoneoscopic diagnosis (and histological findings when available) in 300 patients.

Clinical diagnosis before peritoneoscopy	Total number	Number confirmed	Number not confirmed
Alcoholic liver disease	148	131	17
Chronic active hepatitis ± cirrhosis	32	21	11
Chronic non-alcoholic liver disease (type unspecified)	23	16	7
Chronic liver disease ± suspected hepatocellular carcinoma	49	13	36
Suspected hepatic metastases	28	17	11
Peritoneamalignancy	7	3	4
Tuberculous peritonitis	17	2	15
Miscellaneous	29	23	6
Total	333	226 (68%)	107 (32%)

incomplete in 25 (8%) because adhesions obscured a part of the abdominal cavity, usually the whole or part of the liver. In eight patients (3%) the procedure was a total failure in that the abdominal cavity was not entered. The gallbladder was seen in 196 examinations (67%) of the remaining 292 patients examined, but was not seen in 73 (25%), despite full examination of the right upper quadrant, because of ascites or a large right hepatic lobe. In another 10 patients (3.5%) visualization of the gallbladder was obscured by adhesions in the right upper quadrant. One patient had undergone a cholecystectomy while in 12 the gallbladder was not mentioned in the peritoneoscopic report. The spleen was seen in only 50 examinations (17%), whereas it was not visible in 205 cases (70%) despite suitable positioning of the patient. Two patients had undergone splenectomy.

Portal hypertension, diagnosed by the presence of portal collateral circulation, was noted in 134 patients (46%), 120 of whom had ascites before or at the time of the procedure. In 20 cases (7%) there was no comment on the presence of increased vascularity but in the remainder, 138 cases, portal hypertension was not diagnosed at peritoneoscopy.

Liver biopsy was performed during only two of the first 65 examinations reviewed and both were by the percutaneous route. This low biopsy rate was due to the lack at that time of a peritoneoscope with an operating channel and it was felt that percutaneous biopsies were best performed as a separate procedure. Since then an instrument with a biopsy channel has been available and also percutaneous biopsies under direct vision have been performed with greater frequency. Thus, the liver was biopsied during 108 (46%) of the remaining 235 examinations and the amount of tissue obtained was sufficient to permit a histological diagnosis in 98 (91%). In six patients, nodules on the peritoneum were biopsied for suspected tuberculous peritonitis or malignant seeding.

The accuracy of peritoneoscopy as a diagnostic pro-

cedure was assessed by comparing the examination findings with the histological diagnosis. This was possible in 164 (55%) of the 300 examinations reviewed and Table 27.2 shows that a high level of accuracy was achieved in recognizing the various macroscopic appearances of alcoholic liver disease, non-alcoholic chronic liver disease and hepatic metastases. The two cases of incorrectly diagnosed tuberculous peritonitis turned out to have malignant nodules on the peritoneum, whereas the one incorrectly diagnosed peritoneal malignancy had tuberculous peritonitis.

The value of the procedure has been assessed by comparing the clinical diagnosis (based on historical information, laboratory data and physical findings) with the peritoneoscopy findings, together with histological information when available (Table 27.3). The total number of confirmed and unconfirmed clinical diagnoses exceeds 300 since some cases had two possible diagnoses before peritoneoscopy and usually only one was correct. In addition to the clinical diagnoses listed in Table 27.3, 20 patients with transudative ascites of unknown cause and 9 with undiagnosed jaundice and hepatomegaly were examined.

A major concern with any diagnostic procedure is its safety. Table 27.4 lists the complications encountered and their frequency in the 235 patients in whom records could be readily obtained for review for postoperative problems. There were no serious complications, though in two patients with cirrhosis the amount of bleeding from the biopsy site initially appeared alarming. Bleeding stopped spontaneously in both cases under direct vision and no blood replacement was required. Incomplete entry into the peritoneal cavity has been considered a complication since it caused the procedure to be abandoned, but in none of these eight cases did any problem follow from the attempt. Leakage of ascites from the wound occurred in 11 patients but ceased quickly with treatment of the ascites and did not interfere with wound healing.

Table 27.4 Complications occurring with 235 peritoneoscopy examinations.

Complications	Number of patients
Incomplete entry into abdominal cavity	8
Bleeding from entry site	1
Subcutaneous emphysema	5
Vagal attack during procedure	2
Emesis during procedure	2
Ascites leak	11
Pain after procedure	15
Hypotension after procedure	2
Fever	3

Subcutaneous emphysema, usually of the abdominal wall but of the mediastinum as well in one case, spontaneously cleared in a few days and caused no more than aesthetic distress. Pain, usually diffusely abdominal and frequently accompanied by bilateral shoulder tip pain, occurred in 15 patients within the first 24 hours of the procedure but never constituted a worrying problem. The shoulder pain is thought to be due to diaphragmatic irritation from retained air. In three patients there was a transient fever, which did not require treatment, within 24 hours of the procedure. The overall incidence of minor complications was 21% (49 in 235 examinations). This is reduced to 10% (24 in 235 examinations) if the eight cases of incomplete entry and those complications that can occur with any surgical procedure—postoperative pain and hypotension in the early postoperative period—are excluded.

REFERENCES

1. Baratz, R.A. & Karis, J.H. (1969) Blood gas studies during laparoscopy under general anesthesia. *Anesthesiology*, **30**, 463–464.
2. Barry, R.E., Brown, P. & Read, A.E. (1978) Physician's use of laparoscopy. *British Medical Journal*, **2**, 1276–1278.
3. Brady, P.G., Goldschmid, S., Chappel, G., Stone, F. & Boyd, W.P. (1987) A comparison of biopsy techniques in suspected focal liver disease. *Gastrointestinal Endoscopy*, **33**, 289–292.
4. Bruehl, W. (1966) Zwischenfalle und Komplikationen bei der Laparoskopie und gezielten Leberpunktion. *Deutsche Medizinische Wochenschrift*, **91**, 2297–2299.
5. Caroli, J. & Ricordeau, P. (1962) Value of peritoneoscopy and peritoneoscopic photography in color and of scintillography in the diagnosis of liver diseases. *Progress in Liver Disease*, **1**, 296–389.
6. Coupland, G.A.E., Townend, D.M. & Martin, C.J. (1981) Peritoneoscopy—use in assessment of intra-abdominal malignancy. *Surgery*, **89**, 645–649.
7. Debray, C.H. & Paolaggi, J.-A. (1976) Accidents de la laparoscopie. *Annales de Medicine Interne*, **127**, 689–692.
8. *Dorland's Illustrated Medical Dictionary* (1974) Philadelphia: W.B. Saunders.
9. Fornari, F., Rapaccini, G.L. & Cavanna, L. (1988) Diagnosis of hepatic lesions: ultrasonically guided fine-needle biopsy or laparoscopy? *Gastrointestinal Endoscopy*, **34**, 231–234.
10. Gandolfi, L., Rossi, A., Leo, P. *et al.* (1985) Indications for laparoscopy before and after the introduction of ultrasonography. *Gastrointestinal Endoscopy*, **31**, 1–3.
11. Geake, T.M., Spitaels, J.M., Moshal, M.G. & Simjee, A.E. (1981) Peritoneoscopy in the diagnosis of tuberculous peritonitis. *Gastrointestinal Endoscopy*, **27**, 66–68.
12. Gips, C.H. (1981) A new slender laparoscope. *Netherlands Journal of Medicine*, **24**, 199–200.
13. Haight, J.B. & Ockner, S. (1988) Chlamydia trachomatis perihepatitis with ascites. *American Journal of Gastroenterology*, **83**, 323–325.
14. Hall, T.J., Donaldson, D.R. & Brennan, T.G. (1980) The value of laparoscopy under local anaesthesia in 230 medical and surgical patients. *British Journal of Surgery*, **67**, 751–753.
15. Handley, R.S. & Nurick, A. W. (1956) Peritoneoscopy: evaluation and report of 136 cases. *British Medical Journal*, **2**, 1211–1214.
16. Hartlieb, J. (1955) Luftembolie bei der Laparoskopie. *Deutsche Medizinische Wochenschrift*, **80**, 1532–1533.
17. Hirschowitz, B.I. (1961) Endoscopic examination of the stomach and duodenal cap with the fiberscope. *Lancet*, **1**, 1074–1078.
18. Hodgson, C., McClelland, R.M.A. & Newton, J.R. (1970) Some effects of the peritoneal insufflation of carbon dioxide at laparoscopy. *Anaesthesia*, **25**, 382–390.
19. Jacobaeus, H.C. (1910) Uber die Moglichkeit, die Zystoskopie bei Untersuchungen seroser Hohlungen anzuwenden. *Munchener Medizinische Wochenschrift*, **57**, 2090–2092.

20. Jacobaeus, H.C. (1912) Uber Laparo- und Thorako-skopie. *Beitrage zue Klinik der Tuberkulose und Spezifischen Tuberkuloseforschung*, **25**, 183–254.
21. Jeffers, L., Spieglman, G., Reddy, R. *et al.* (1988) Laparoscopically directed fine needle aspiration for the diagnosis of hepatocellular cancer: a safe and accurate technique. *Gastrointestinal Endoscopy*, **34**, 235–237.
22. Kalk, H. (1929) Erfahrungen mit der Laparoskopie (zugleich mit Beischreibung eines neuen Intrumentes). *Zeitschrift fur Klinische Medizin*, **111**, 303–348.
23. Kane, M.J. & Krejs, G. (1984) Complications of diagnostic laparoscopy in Dallas: a seven year prospective study. *Gastrointestinal Endoscopy*, **30**, 237–240.
24. Kelling, G. (1902) Uber Oesophagoscopie, Gastroskopie and Colioskopie. *Munchener Medizinische Wochenschrift*, **49**, 21–24.
25. Kelling, G. (1910) Uber die Moglichkeit, die Zystoskopie bei Untersuchungen seroser Hohlungen anzuwenden. Bemerkung zu dem Artikel von Jacobaeus. *Munchener Medizinische Wochenschrift*, **57**, 2358.
26. Korbsch, R. (1921) Die Laparoskopie nach Jacobaeus. *Berliner Klinische Wochenschrift*, **58**, 696.
27. Livraghi, T., Damascelli, B., Lombardi, C. & Spagnoli, I. (1983) Risk in fine needle abdominal biopsy. *Journal of Clinical Ultrasound*, **11**, 77–81.
28. Magno,R., Medegard, A., Bengtsson, R. & Tronstad, S.-E. (1979) Acid-base balance during laparoscopy. *Acta Obstetricia et Gynecologica Scandinavica*, **58**, 81–85.
29. Meyer-Burg, J. (1972) The inspection, palpation and biopsy of the pancreas by peritoneoscopy. *Endoscopy*, **4**, 99–101.
30. Meyer-Burg, J. & Ziegler, U. (1978) The intra-abdominal inspection and biopsy of lymph nodes during peritoneoscopy. *Endoscopy*, **10**, 41–43.
31. Michel, H. & Raynaud, A. (1977) Interet de la laparoscopie sous anesthesie generale. *Endoscopie Digestive*, **2**, 135–136.
32. Motew, M., Ivanovich, A.D., Bieniarz, J. *et al.* (1973) Cardiovascular effects and acid-base and blood gas changes during laparoscopy. *American Journal of Obstetrics and Gynecology*, **115**, 1002–1012.
33. Nicholson, R.D. & Berman, N.D. (1979) Pneumopericardium following laparoscopy. *Chest*, **76**, 605–607.
34. Ohta, Y., Fujiwara, K., Sato, Y. *et al.* (1983) New ultrasonic laparoscope for diagnosis of intra-abdominal diseases. *Gastrointestinal Endoscopy*, **29**, 289–293.
35. O'Kieffe, D.A. & Boyce, H.W., Jr. (1972) Peritoneoscopy: has this procedure come of age? *Medical Annals of the District of Columbia*, **41**, 437–440.
36. Ruddock, J.C. (1934) Peritoneoscopy. *Western Journal of Surgery*, **42**, 392–405.

37. Ruddock, J.C. (1937) Peritoneoscopy. *Surgery, Gynecology and Obstetrics,* **65**, 623–639.

38. Salky, B.A., Bauer, J.J., Gelernt, I.M. & Kreel, I. (1988) The use of laparoscopy in retroperitoneal pathology. *Gastrointestinal Endoscopy,* **34**, 227–230.

39. Sanowski, R.A. & Bellapravalu, S. (1986) Initial experience with a flexible fiberoptic laparoscope. *Gastrointestinal Endoscopy,* **32**, 409–412.

40. Scott, D.B. & Julian, D.G. (1972) Observations on cardiac arrhythmias during laparoscopy. *British Medical Journal,* **1**, 411–413.

41. Veronisi, U., Spinelli, P., Bonadonna, G. *et al.* (1976) Laparoscopy and laparotomy in staging Hodgkin's and non-Hodgkin's lymphoma. *American Journal of Roentgenology,* **127**, 501–503.

42. Vilardell, F., Seres, I. & Marti-Vincente, A. (1968) Complications of peritoneoscopy. A survey of 1455 examinations. *Gastrointestinal Endoscopy,* **14**, 178–180.

43. Wadhwa, R.K., McKenzie, R., Wadhwa, S.R. *et al.* (1978) Gas embolism during laparoscopy. *Anesthesiology,* **48**, 74–76.

44. Walker, R.M., Cooke, A.M. & Playfair, P.L. (1943) Peritoneoscopy. *Proceedings of the Royal Society of Medicine,* **36**, 445–450.

45. Whitmore, L.F., Galambos, J.T., Phillips, V.M. *et al.* (1985) Image guided percutaneous hepatic biopsy: diagnostic accuracy and safety. *Journal of Clinical Gastroenterology,* **7**, 511–514.

46. Whittman, I. (1966) *Peritoneoscopy*, vols I & II. Budapest: Akdemiai Kiado.

47. Wolfe, J.H.N., Behn, A.R. & Jackson, B.T. (1979) Tuberculous peritonitis and role of diagnostic laparoscopy. *Lancet,* **1**, 852–853.

CHAPTER 28

Investigation of the Jaundiced Patient

Stephen Karran, K.C. Dewbury & Ralph Wright

The main problems of diagnosis in the jaundiced patient are:

1. To distinguish between intra- and extrahepatic cholestasis.
2. To identify the site of extrahepatic obstruction.
3. To recognize unusual causes of hepatocellular or haemolytic jaundice that require special management or treatment.
4. To distinguish between acute and chronic hepatocellular disease.

A careful and thorough history and physical examination remain of overriding importance in establishing the diagnosis. Nevertheless, there have been important technical advances that over the past few years have had a profound effect on the rapidity and accuracy of diagnosis in the jaundiced patient. These include serological tests for hepatitis A, hepatitis B, hepatitis C and autoimmune liver disease and radiological and scanning techniques, which not only help to distinguish intrahepatic from extrahepatic

cholestasis but which also localize accurately the site of extrahepatic obstruction. In addition, there have been useful advances in techniques for histological staining of liver biopsy material to identify viral markers and to diagnose certain forms of chronic liver disease such as Wilson's disease, primary biliary cirrhosis and α-1-antitrypsin deficiency.

By contrast, while biochemical tests of liver function may indicate the severity of hepatic damage, they remain disappointing in distinguishing between intra- and extrahepatic cholestasis. Furthermore, certain investigations, such as the standard barium meal, which once were regarded as first-line investigations in the jaundiced patient, are now seldom performed.

The identification of haemolysis as the cause of jaundice is usually not difficult on clinical examination and when simple laboratory investigations are used. The precise cause of the haemolysis may be more difficult to elucidate. In addition, determining the extent to which haemolysis contributes to the jaundice may be problematical when

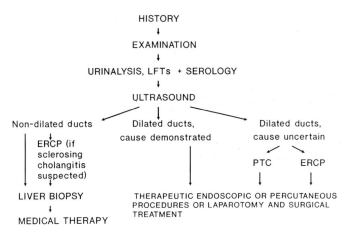

HISTORY
↓
EXAMINATION
↓
URINALYSIS, LFTs + SEROLOGY
↓
ULTRASOUND

Non-dilated ducts   Dilated ducts,   Dilated ducts,
↓   cause demonstrated   cause uncertain
ERCP (if
sclerosing   PTC   ERCP
cholangitis
suspected)   ↓   ↓   ↓
↓
LIVER BIOPSY   THERAPEUTIC ENDOSCOPIC OR PERCUTANEOUS
↓   PROCEDURES OR LAPAROTOMY AND SURGICAL
MEDICAL THERAPY   TREATMENT

Figure 28.1 Proposed schema for the investigation of the jaundiced patient.

it coexists with hepatocellular disease or extrahepatic obstruction. The extent to which breakdown of old red cells from transfused blood contributes to jaundice, particularly in the postoperative period, may also be difficult to determine. When jaundice is mild, and not associated with other symptoms, low-grade haemolysis must be distinguished from Gilbert's syndrome, the commonest form of persistent unconjugated hyperbilirubinaemia. In the neonatal period, haemolytic disease of the newborn has to be distinguished from physiological jaundice, biliary atresia and neonatal hepatitis.

In the absence of features of cholestasis, the diagnosis of hepatocellular jaundice is seldom a problem, although it may be more difficult to identify its cause. The availability of serological markers for viral hepatitis A, B and C, Epstein–Barr virus, cytomegalovirus and leptospiral infection have greatly facilitated precise diagnosis (see Chapter 30). The diagnosis of drug-induced jaundice is based largely on the clinical history with limited help from liver biopsy. The identification of chronic liver disease as a cause of jaundice is usually straightforward once the appropriate clinical, biochemical and other investigations have been undertaken (see Chapters 31 and 32). More difficulty may be encountered if the hepatocellular jaundice is part of an unusual systemic disease (see Chapter 37) or due to a tumour (see Chapters 39 and 60), an infection (see Chapter 38) or a parasite (see Chapter 61). Such cases are less likely to be diagnosed if the disorder is unusual in the particular patient's environment.

The identification of extrahepatic obstruction due to gallstones, tumour or stricture is usually straightforward, but diagnostic difficulty may occur when the extrahepatic obstruction results from conditions such as sclerosing cholangitis, intrahepatic bile duct carcinoma (see Chapters 15, 37, 39, 59 and 60) or parasites (see Chapter 61), or when more than one pathology coexist.

Precise diagnosis is particularly difficult when the situation is complex, for example in the postoperative period (see Chapter 52), in the neonate (see Chapters 44 and 45) and when there has been previous biliary tract surgery

(see Chapter 59). It should be emphasized, however, that in any jaundiced patient in whom the diagnosis is difficult an unusual presentation of a common cause of jaundice such as hepatitis, drugs, gallstones or tumour is still more likely to be found than a rare condition.

In the majority of patients with jaundice, a careful history and clinical examination, together with simple laboratory tests, will provide either the definitive diagnosis or a guide to the underlying pathology. If more elaborate investigations are required, these should be pursued rapidly so that any necessary operative intervention may be undertaken without delay. A hard core of difficult problems requiring extensive investigation remains. With careful organization, it should be possible in most cases to achieve a definitive diagnosis within 3–4 days. It is therefore essential to have a well-established plan of investigation. One such simplified scheme is illustrated in Figure 28.1 (see also Chapters 15 and 59). Diagnostic laparotomy should no longer be necessary in specialist centres.

HISTORY

The important points to establish about the jaundice from the history are:

1. Is it cholestatic?
2. Is it painful and, if so, what is the character of the pain?
3. Is it drug-induced or infective?

A patient with cholestatic jaundice will typically have dark urine, pale stools and pruritis. In some patients none of these features may be present, yet either intrahepatic cholestasis may be demonstrated histologically or an obvious cause of extrahepatic obstruction such as a tumour or a stone may be identified, with or without the biochemical changes of cholestasis. If the history suggests cholestasis, it is particularly important to determine whether the patient has been taking drugs. Analgesics, tranquillizers, psychotropic drugs and the contraceptive pill are so commonly used that the patient may not regard these as significant. In the very young and in the elderly it is important to obtain a history from the relatives and the general practitioner about drug intake.

A history of contact with hepatitis, of travel abroad, of eating raw shellfish or of having used parenteral drugs may suggest viral hepatitis. Such patients often have anorexia, distaste for cigarettes, lassitude, joint pains and urticaria, but many of these symptoms, particularly distaste for cigarettes, occur with other forms of jaundice, including drug-induced and obstructive jaundice. Fluctuation of the depth of discoloration is suggestive of intermittent obstruction as a result of temporary retention of a calculus at the ampulla of Vater or, rarely, a carcinoma at this site, but it can also occur with intrahepatic cholestasis and, when mild, with Gilbert's syndrome.

Pruritus is an important symptom and, although usually steadily progressive, it may fluctuate in both intrahepatic and extrahepatic cholestasis.

A history of biliary 'colic', shoulder tip pain or attacks of acute cholecystitis is strong evidence that the obstructive jaundice is due to calculous disease, although calculi may coexist with neoplastic obstructive lesions or with cirrhosis. Pain of a different nature may indicate more sinister pathology. Pain in the back, for example, is suggestive of pancreatic neoplasm, although penetrating duodenal ulceration may also be responsible. Acute pain referred to the back is suggestive of pancreatitis or gallstones but can also occur with the crises due to rapid haemolysis.

Painless jaundice associated with weight loss is strongly suggestive of neoplasm, particularly carcinoma of the head of the pancreas.

Bruising may be prominent with decompensated hepatocellular jaundice due to hypoprothrombinaemia or the low platelet count associated with hypersplenism, but it can also occur in obstructive jaundice as a result of malabsorption of vitamin K.

It is important to obtain a history of foreign travel, not only because such patients are liable to develop viral hepatitis, but because they may also be exposed to unusual diseases such as malaria and other parasitic infections that can cause hepatocellular or obstructive jaundice. Even in patients who have not been abroad, the diagnosis may be missed because a parasitic infection such as *Fasciola hepatica*, a rare cause of jaundice in the United Kingdom,[3] has not been considered.

The occupational history is also important because this may indicate exposure to a particular infection or to hepatotoxins, while the social and occupational history may suggest alcohol or drug abuse. Some causes of jaundice, such as Wilson's disease and Gilbert's syndrome, are familial. In cholelithiasis there is also sometimes a strong family history. A history of putative autoimmune disease in the patient or family suggests chronic active hepatitis or primary biliary cirrhosis.

PHYSICAL EXAMINATION

A careful examination may provide evidence of the severity of the underlying pathology and its aetiology. Hepatocellular dysfunction may be clearly shown by the presence of cutaneous stigmas such as spider naevi, palmar erythema, Dupuytren's contracture, leuconychia and finger clubbing. Dilated cutaneous collateral veins and a palpable spleen may indicate portal hypertension. Ascites can occur in decompensated cirrhosis but also with disseminated neoplasms. The aetiology may be indicated by its systemic manifestations or by a specific feature. Thus, in alcoholic liver disease there may be other signs of alcoholism, such as peripheral neuropathy, and in drug hypersensitivity reactions there may be other evidence of hypersensitivity, such as a skin rash. Kayser–Fleischer rings suggest Wilson's disease, and xanthomas and xan-

thelasmas are associated with primary biliary cirrhosis. Tattoo marks or scarred antecubital veins may provide the clue to hepatitis B infection.

In the assessment of hepatic size, careful palpation and percussion should start in the iliac fossa. If this procedure is not scrupulously followed, the lower edge of a grossly enlarged organ may be missed, particularly in the obese. The upper border of the liver is defined by percussion; dullness over the liver normally extends upwards as far as the fifth intercostal space. Careful assessment of the

Table 28.1 Laboratory investigations in the jaundiced patient.

Haematological tests
  Full blood count
  Erythrocyte sedimentation rate
  Reticulocyte count
  Haptoglobin levels
  Coombs' test

Liver function tests
  Conjugated and unconjugated bilirubin levels
  Aspartate aminotransferase (AST)
  Alanine aminotransferase (ALT)
  γ-Glutamyl transferase
  Alkaline phosphatase

Proteins
  Albumin
  Globulin
  Prothrombin time (INR)

Immunological and serological tests
  Mitochondrial antibodies
  Smooth muscle and antinuclear antibody
  LKM antibodies
  Immunoglobulins: IgG, IgM, IgA
  Hepatitis B surface antigen (HB_sAg)
  Antibody to Hepatitis C
  IgM antibody to hepatitis A
  Cytomegalovirus antibody
  Epstein–Barr virus antibody (Monospot test)
  Leptospiral agglutinins
  Fasciola complement fixation test
  Amoebic complement fixation test
  Hydatid complement fixation test
  Wassermann reaction and other serological tests for syphilis

α-1-Antitrypsin levels

α-Fetoprotein levels

Serum amylase

Plasma caeruloplasmin levels

Iron and iron binding capacity, Serum Ferritin levels

Spot blood alcohol

Urine
  Urobilin
  Bilirubin
  Haemosiderin
Stools
  Ova
  Parasites

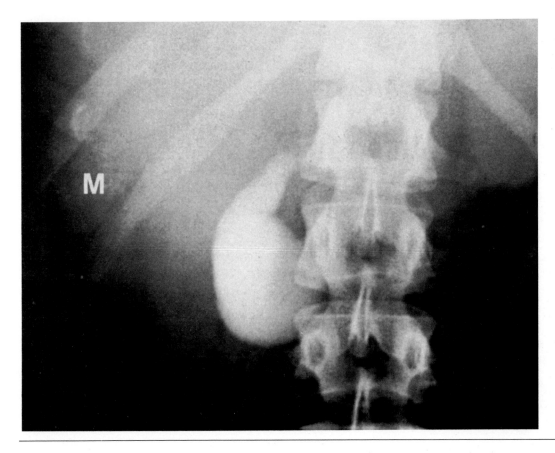

Figure 28.2
Cholecystogram showing calcification in metastases (M) arising from a 'silent' adenocarcinoma of the sigmoid colon in a 35-year-old woman presenting with vague pain in the right hypochondrium.

consistency of the liver is likewise important. Hard irregular areas, for example, strongly suggest neoplastic involvement. A bruit favours portal hypertension or a neoplasm. Splenomegaly can be detected by palpation commencing in the right iliac fossa and progressing upwards and to the left. In difficult cases, rotation of the patient 45° to the right allows the spleen to fall on the clinician's right hand. The left hand should support the rib cage and relax the skin and abdominal musculature by drawing these down and to the right. Percussion may be useful and, in the presence of ascites, the liver and spleen may be ballottable.

The finding of a palpable gallbladder in the presence of obstructive jaundice suggests malignant obstruction to the biliary tree (Courvoisier's law). This obstruction must obviously be below the junction of the cystic and common hepatic ducts, and carcinoma of the head of the pancreas and ampullary lesions are common causes. It is essential, however, to appreciate that the presence of a palpable gallbladder under these circumstances does *not exclude* calculous disease as the cause of the jaundice. Similarly, failure to palpate the gallbladder does not exclude malignancy, either because the biliary tree is involved above the entrance of the cystic duct or because the gallbladder itself may be infiltrated, preventing dilatation. A palpable gallbladder simply implies raised intravesical pressure, which in most cases is due to neoplastic obstruction of the lower ductal system (see Chapter 58).

LABORATORY INVESTIGATIONS

The haematological, biochemical and serological investigations that may be necessary in the diagnosis of the jaundiced patient are listed in Table 28.1 and have been dealt with in Chapters 8, 14, 15 and 18. Unconjugated hyperbilirubinaemia suggests haemolysis, Gilbert's syndrome or one of the rarer causes such as the Crigler-Najjar syndrome. Haemolysis may be associated with anaemia, spherocytosis, reticulocytosis, reduced red cell survival and a positive Coombs' test. In Gilbert's syndrome, the bilirubin is less than 103 μmol/1 (6 mg/dl) and is usually of the order of 50 μmol/1 (3 mg/dl). The plasma unconjugated bilirubin concentrations shows a two- to threefold increase after fasting or after the intravenous administration of 50 mg of nicotinic acid (See Chapter 14).

Standard liver function tests serve only as a general guide in helping to distinguish hepatocellular from obstructive jaundice; these are discussed in Chapters 15 and 18. Marked elevation of the aspartate aminotransferase (AST) suggests hepatocellular necrosis, and alkaline phosphatase levels above 600 international units suggest extrahepatic obstruction, but the latter can also occur with intrahepatic cholestasis and primary biliary cirrhosis. Low albumin and high globulin levels suggest chronic hepatocellular damage, particularly in association with a prolonged

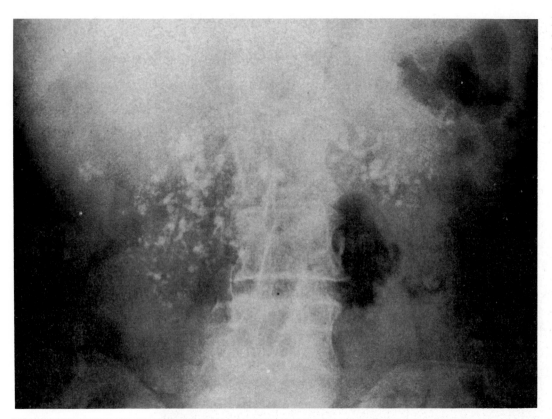

Figure 28.3 Diffuse calcification seen in a case of chronic pancreatitis.

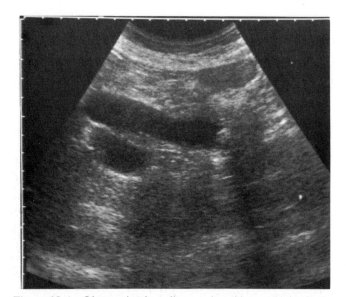

Figure 28.4 Obstructive jaundice produced by a calculus in the dilated common bile duct.

prothrombin time that fails to convert with parenteral vitamin K. Hepatitis B markers suggest acute or chronic hepatitis B infection and IgM antibody to hepatitis A indicates acute hepatitis A infection; IgG antibody to hepatitis C indicates hepatitis C infection (see Chapter 30). Strongly positive antinuclear or smooth muscle antibodies suggest chronic active hepatitis (see Chapter 31) and positive mitochondrial antibodies suggest primary biliary cirrhosis (see Chapter 33). Low α-1-antitrypsin levels favour the chronic liver disease associated with this deficiency (see Chapter 43) and low caeruloplasmin levels favour Wilson's disease (see Chapter 35).

Clearly, the number of tests and the order in which they are performed depend on clinical pointers. Laboratory investigations in the jaundiced infant pose special problems and are discussed in Chapters 44 and 45.

RADIOLOGICAL INVESTIGATIONS

Plain abdominal and chest x-rays

Plain x-rays of the abdomen and chest are simple and quick to perform and may give valuable information. Calcification may be seen in 10–20% of biliary calculi, occasionally in the gallbladder itself, in hepatic metastases (Figure 28.2) and also in chronic pancreatitis (Figure 28.3). Gas may be seen in the biliary tree, portal venous system or in a subphrenic abscess. On the chest film, a primary neoplasm, secondary deposits or pleural effusions may be seen.

Ultrasound

This technique is now established as the prime investigation in the diagnosis of the jaundiced patient (see Chapter 22). It is non-invasive, quick to perform and

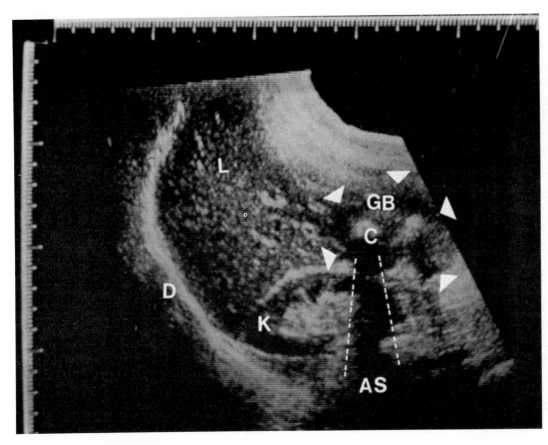

Figure 28.5
Longitudinal scan
through the right lobe of
the liver (L) showing a
thickened gallbladder
(GB, outline indicated
by arrowheads)
containing gallstones and
with distal acoustic
shadowing (AS). The
gallbladder was found to
contain a carcinoma.
C = calculus;
D = diaphragm;
K = right kidney.

accurately separates extrahepatic obstruction from other causes of jaundice by the demonstration of dilated biliary radicles.[2, 8] In experienced hands, the accuracy in detecting ductal dilation is more than 95%. Rarely, diagnostic errors may occur in early acute obstruction because the ducts have not yet become dilated. Ultrasonography is therefore particularly valuable as a screening procedure.

Patients may be separated into three main groups: those without dilated ducts, those with dilated ducts but in whom a definitive cause for the dilation is not shown, and those with dilated ducts in whom the cause of the obstruction is demonstrated (Figure 28.4). A scheme for further investigation is suggested in Figure 28.1. In extrahepatic obstruction, ultrasound imaging will establish the level of the block in approximately 80% of cases.[2, 6] In over 40% of patients, not only the level but also the cause of the obstruction will be demonstrated by ultrasound imaging.[2] Difficulties in achieving a definitive diagnosis arise principally with small lesions at the lower end of the common bile duct, which is often obscured by gas in the duodenum and the colon, or when more than one lesion coexists, such as gallstones and a carcinoma of the gallbladder (Figure 28.5).

When no dilation of the biliary radicles is demonstrated the liver may have a normal echo pattern and liver biopsy may be required, but in a significant proportion of patients a specific echo pattern is shown. This is most commonly either the bright, tightly packed echo pattern seen in many cases of cirrhosis or chronic active hepatitis, or, alternatively, the pattern characteristic of diffuse hepatic metastases (Figure 28.6). Further details of this technique are given in Chapter 22.

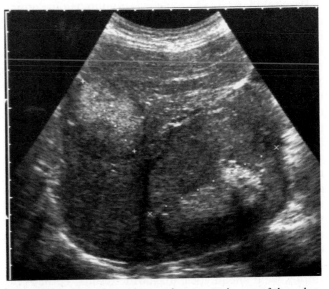

Figure 28.6 Hepatic metastases from a carcinoma of the colon.

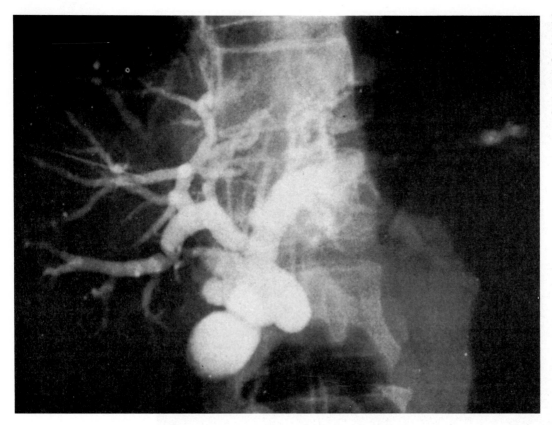

Figure 28.7(a)
Percutaneous
transhepatic
cholangiogram (PTC)
using the Chiba needle.
Dilated ductal system
produced by a carcinoma
of the pancreas.

Radioisotope imaging (see Chapter 21)

Technetium-99*m* sulphur colloid imaging is of limited value in the investigation of the jaundiced patient but may confirm the presence of hepatic metastases or suggest an obstructive aetiology when low activity is seen in the porta hepatis. [131]I rose bengal imaging has also been shown to have prognostic value.

Hepatobiliary agents, such as pyridoxylidine gluta-mate (PGA) and 2,6-dimethylphenylcarbamoylmethyl iminodiacetic acid (HIDA) outline the biliary ducts and common bile duct even in the presence of moderately raised bilirubin levels (103–120 μmol/1 [6–7 mg/dl]). When the common bile duct is patent, activity is seen in the duct after 60 minutes. In the presence of total obstruction, no activity is seen in the duct. In the presence of partial obstruction or jaundice of hepatocel-lular origin the appearance of activity in the gut is delayed. Ultrasound examination may prove helpful in distinguishing these two situations. The precise signifi-cance of delayed appearance of activity in the gut is uncertain. Poor hepatocellular function is associated with impaired excretion and a marked reduction in activity in the gut. This may be confused with partial obstruction. Although in biliary atresia no gut activity is present, there is no good evidence that HIDA studies yield unequivocal diagnostic results. Perhaps the greatest advantage of radioisotope imaging of the biliary tree is that it may be used to quantitate bile flow, permitting an assessment of biliary physiology in post-cholecystectomy syndrome and other post-operative conditions.[9]

Intravenous cholangiography

In this investigation an iodine-containing contrast med-ium, iodipamide (Biligrafin) or ioglycamate (Biligram) is infused over a period of 30 minutes for optimal results. The contrast medium is bound to protein in the plasma and excreted by the liver cells. Bile ducts are outlined and these are optimally demonstrated by tomography. Gallbladder opacification will be demonstrated if the cystic duct is patent. The probability of duct opacification using intravenous cholangiography diminishes rapidly with bilirubin levels above 50 μmol/1 (3 mg/dl).

Intravenous cholangiography nowadays plays only a small part in the investigation of the jaundiced patient. Not only is it unsuccessful in the majority of jaundiced patients, but even when successful the diagnostic yield is low.[1] Comparative studies have shown it to be less accurate than endoscopic retrograde choledochopancrea-tography (ERCP) in the diagnosis of patients undergoing surgery for biliary calculi[7] (see Chapter 26). Intravenous cholangiography has now been largely superseded by ERCP or PTC (see below).

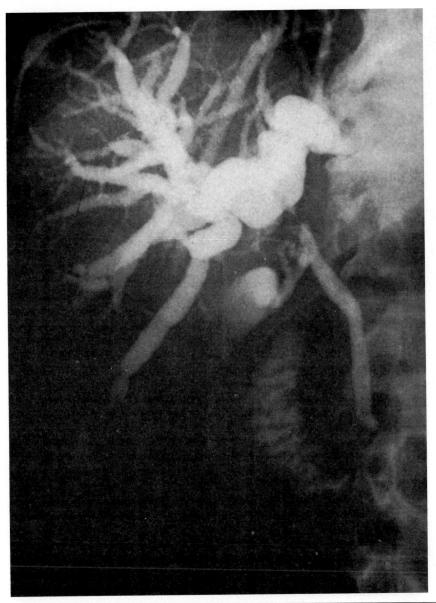

Figure 28.7(b) Percutaneous transhepatic cholangiogram (PTC) using the Chiba needle. Localized stenosis of the common hepatic duct produced by a cholangiocarcinoma causing obstructive jaundice.

Endoscopic retrograde cholangiopancreatography (ERCP)

ERCP has now become an important technique in the investigation of the jaundiced patient. It has several advantages, including visualization of the sphincter of Oddi and definition of both the biliary and pancreatic duct systems. Biopsy of ampullary lesions may also be undertaken if necessary. The lower end of the bile duct is better visualized by ERCP and this should be undertaken if ultrasound has not conclusively demonstrated the cause of obstructive jaundice. In some centres, percutaneous transhepatic cholangiography (PTC) is preferred. The choice between ERCP and PTC is often dependent on the availability of local expertise. A major advance has been the ability to undertake endoscopic therapeutic procedures. These include: sphincterotomy, balloon dilatation of biliary strictures, retrieval of common duct stones, and insertion of biliary endoprostheses for the management of malignant obstructive jaundice (see Chapter 26).

Percutaneous transhepatic cholangiography (PTC)

Percutaneous transhepatic cholangiography (PTC) with the fine-calibre (23-gauge, outer diameter 0.7 mm) thin-walled Chiba needle is another technique for direct opacification of the biliary duct in the jaundiced patient (Figure 28.7a and b). It is safer and more successful than conventional transhepatic cholangiography.

A lateral approach is used with injection of contrast during withdrawal of the needle. The procedure is carried out under fluoroscopic control to identify entry into a bile duct. Aspiration of bile, though desirable, may not be successful and is not essential. Over-filling of the ducts

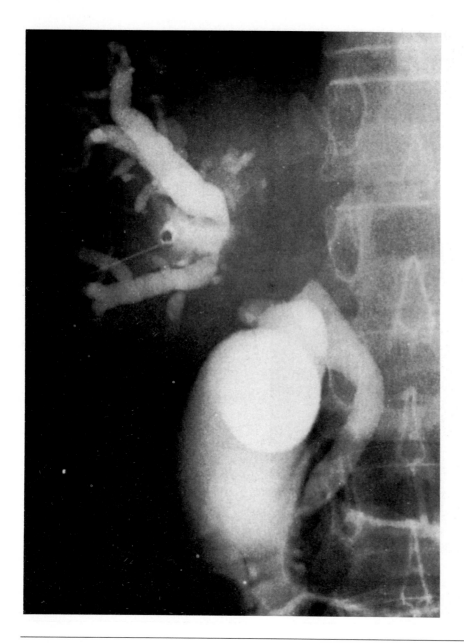

Figure 28.8 A localized ductal carcinoma demonstrated by a combination of ERCP and PTC.

should be avoided. If a surgical lesion of the biliary ducts is demonstrated, immediate laparotomy is not essential but prophylactic antibiotics should be administered while awaiting surgery (see Chapter 58).

Ferrucci and Wittenburg[5] reported successful opacification of the bile ducts in 99% of patients with dilated bile ducts and 82% of normal calibre or sclerosed ducts.

In obstruction of the common bile duct the increased viscosity of stagnant bile may cause poor distal flow of contrast medium and prevent adequate mixing of the injected contrast and bile. This may result in false proximal localization of the site of obstruction; delayed and erect films will reduce this error.

When duct dilatation is present, fine-needle puncture more consistently produces successful intrahepatic cholangiograms than does ERCP.[4] Occasionally, the combined use of PTC and ERCP may be the only way to produce a definitive answer (Figure 28.8). Therapeutic manoeuvres may also be undertaken using a percutaneous transhepatic approach including: balloon dilatation of strictures or the sphincter of Oddi, stone removal and insertion of biliary endoprostheses.

Computed tomography (CT) (see Chapter 23)

This non-invasive investigation yields information similar to that obtained with ultrasound. It does not suffer failures due to gas in the bowel. In diagnosing the cause of obstructive jaundice, CT scanning is probably best reserved for problems that cannot be resolved by ultrasound, or by more direct imaging of the biliary tree by ERCP or PTC. In patients with an established diagnosis of obstructive jaundice due to malignancy—usually already delineated by other techniques—CT scanning provides useful additional information about the anatomical location, nature, extent and suitability for either resection or palliative management by endoscopic or percutaneous biliary endoprosthesis.

OTHER DIAGNOSTIC TECHNIQUES

Gastroscopy, sigmoidoscopy, barium studies and angiography may all provide important information in particular patients. These, however, play a secondary role in the specific investigation of jaundice.

Finally, it may be necessary to obtain a diagnosis more directly, either by percutaneous liver biopsy or at laparoscopy or laparotomy.

Liver biopsy

In the absence of dilated ducts, a liver biopsy is often required and should be performed with the usual precautions. The liver biopsy histology will determine the presence, severity and often the aetiology of acute or chronic liver disease and will help to differentiate the various causes of cholestasis (see Chapter 19).

Laparoscopy

For selected patients this investigation may provide valuable information. When used in combination with ERCP, laparoscopy is particularly accurate; it can be combined with liver biopsy under direct vision. The technique is described in detail in Chapter 27.

Laparotomy

Diagnostic laparotomy should be avoidable in nearly all cases now that other techniques are available. Where such facilities are not readily available, direct visualization and inspection at operation may still be needed. Because it carries a significant morbidity and a definite mortality, particularly in those patients with underlying hepatocellular damage, every effort should be made to reach an accurate diagnosis without recourse to laparotomy.

REFERENCES

1. Blumgart, L.H., Salmon, P.R. & Cotton, P.B. (1974) Endoscopy and retrograde choledochopancreatography in the diagnosis of the patient with jaundice. *Surgery, Gynecology and Obstetrics*, **138**, 565–570.
2. Dewbury, K.C., Joseph, A.E.A., Hayes, S. & Murray, C. (1979) Ultrasound in the evaluation and diagnosis of jaundice. *British Journal of Radiology*, **52**, 276–280.
3. Editorial (1978) Liver fluke in Britain. *British Medical Journal*, **1**, 1091.
4. Elias, E., Hamlyn, A.N., Jain, S. *et al.* (1976) A randomized trial of percutaneous transhepatic cholangiography with the Chiba needle versus endoscopic retrograde cholangiography for bile duct visualization in jaundice. *Gastroenterology*, **71**, 439–443.
5. Ferrucci, J.T. & Wittenburg, J. (1977) Refinements in Chiba needle transhepatic cholangiography. *American Journal of Roentgenology*, **129**, 11–16.
6. Malini, S. & Sabel, J. (1977) Ultrasonography in obstructive jaundice. *Radiology*, **123**, 429–433.
7. Osnes, M., Larsen, S., Lowe, P. *et al.* (1978) Comparison of endoscopic retrograde and intravenous cholangiography in diagnosis of biliary calculi. *Lancet*, **2**, 230.
8. Taylor, K.J. & Rosenfield, A.T. (1977) Greyscale ultrasonography in the differential diagnosis of jaundice *Archives of Surgery*, **112**, 820–825.
9. Lancet Editorial (Anon) (1991) Nuclear Medicine and the hepatobiliary tract. *Lancet*, **337**, 706.

CHAPTER 29

Acute Liver Failure

R.E. Kirsch, M.D. Voigt, S.C. Robson, R.J. Hift, R. Hickman, D. Kahn, S.J. Saunders & J. Terblanche

Acute liver failure has been the subject of a number of recent reviews.[29,133,181,268,269] In this chapter important aspects of diagnosis and management will be presented and related to new observations and hypotheses.

Definitions

Acute liver failure has been defined as a potentially reversible condition, the consequence of severe liver injury, with onset of encephalopathy within 8 weeks of the appearance of first symptoms and in the absence of pre-existing liver disease.[245] This definition has traditionally been used synonymously with the term 'fulminant hepatic failure' (FHF). However, Bernuau *et al.*[25] have suggested that FHF should denote only the development of hepatic encephalopathy within 2 weeks of the onset of jaundice and that 'subfulminant liver failure' should be used to describe the development of encephalopathy 2 weeks to 3 months after the onset of jaundice. The latter has also been termed 'subacute hepatic necrosis'[234] or 'late-onset fulminant hepatic failure'.[99] Bernuau *et al.*[25] also suggested that patients presenting with abnormal hepatic synthetic function, including a greater than 50% decrease in coagulation factors without the development of hepatic encephalopathy, be termed 'severe acute liver failure'. This may progress to FHF with the development of encephalopathy.

Aetiology

Viral, drug-induced and toxic hepatitis account for roughly 90% of all cases of fulminant and subfulminant liver failure.[25,99,164,214,270] The incidence of acute liver failure due to the different forms of viral hepatitis varies geographically and with time (see Chapter 30).

Infection with hepatitis B virus, either alone or in conjunction with hepatitis D virus (delta agent), is the main cause of acute liver failure due to viral infection in Clichy (65%),[25] Athens (75%)[189] and in several centres in the USA (60%).[2] In contrast, these viruses appear to account for only 25% of the cases of acute liver failure resulting from viral infection reported by Gimson in London.[100] Coinfection with hepatitis B virus and the delta agent appears to increase the risk of FHF but does not seem to worsen the prognosis.[105,223]

The incidence of acute liver failure secondary to hepatitis B should be influenced by screening of blood components, the availability of hyperimmune globulin and the advent of effective vaccines for this agent.[65]

The hepatitis A virus accounts for 1.5% of patients with FHF due to viral infection in Athens,[189] 2–4% in the USA,[2] 6% in New Delhi[131] and Clichy[24] and 31% in London.[100] The risk of FHF in patients with hepatitis A infection is very low and ranges from 0.01% to 0.1%.[25] FHF usually develops early in the course and the prognosis may be better than FHF due to other viral causes.[25,100]

Acute liver failure attributed to sporadic non-A, non-B infection ranges from 23% of patients with viral hepatitis in Clichy,[24] 24% Athens,[189] 27% in Denmark[158] to 44% in London.[100] Subfulminant hepatic failure is frequent and an overall mortality of up to 90% has been observed.[25,100] Hepatitis E virus (HEV), (epidemic non-A, non-B hepatitis) infection is the main cause of FHF in pregnant women in Third World countries.[138] Hepatitis C (post-transfusional non-A, non-B hepatitis) is usually mild, but severe hepatitis can occur and probably accounts for a small proportion of cases of fulminant liver failure (see Chapter 30).[289]

There are few convincingly documented reported cases of fulminant or subfulminant hepatitis due to herpes simplex virus, varicella zoster, cytomegalovirus or Epstein–Barr virus.[25,129,158] Encephalopathy in reported cases may relate directly to viral invasion of the central nervous system or to extrahepatic manifestations of disseminated viral infection.

Many drugs may cause acute liver failure (see Chapter 46).[287] The risk of fulminant or subfulminant hepatic failure in patients with drug-induced hepatitis appears to be far greater than in acute viral hepatitis.[25,192] Continued administration of the offending drug appears to be associated with a higher risk of FHF.[231,287] Although several studies have suggested that drug-induced FHF occurs more frequently in patients over 40 years of age, our own experience, based largely on reactions to antituberculosis and anticonvulsant agents, suggests a bimodal age distribution with peaks in both the third and seventh decades.[192]

Toxic hepatic necrosis most commonly due to paracetamol overdose, is the most important cause of acute liver failure in the United Kingdom.[60,260] Concomitant use of enzyme-inducing drugs and/or chronic alcohol ingestion may aggravate paracetamol-induced liver injury. FHF may also be due to ingestion of *Amanita phalloides*[25,81] or may follow exposure to industrial solvents such as chlorinated hydrocarbons.[287] In the Third World, acute liver failure may be associated with the ingestion of food containing aflatoxins[176] and the use of roots, herbs[258] and dichromates by traditional healers.

Other causes of fulminant and subfulminant hepatic failure include ischaemic liver cell necrosis. This may occur as a result of diminished hepatic blood flow associated with low cardiac output states.[13,50,177] Hypovolaemic or septicaemic shock and hepatic artery thrombosis may precipitate massive liver necrosis.[58] FHF may also occur in association with hepatic venous outflow obstruction as in the Budd–Chiari syndrome[152] and veno-occlusive disease of the liver.

Microvesicular steatosis associated with pregnancy, Reye's syndrome and drugs (tetracyclines, valproate) may also be associated with FHF.[59,204,286]

FHF may develop early after liver transplantation as a result of primary graft non-function, hepatic artery thrombosis or acute rejection.[229] FHF may also occur in patients in whom 80% or more of functional normal hepatic parenchyma is removed surgically.[30]

Rarely, acute liver failure may occur in massive malignant infiltration of the liver,[112] jejunal bypass,[18] and hyperthermia.[136]

CLINICAL PRESENTATION

Acute liver failure may develop at any time during the course of hepatitis: encephalopathy may rarely even precede the development of jaundice.[275] In established cases, the major features of FHF include jaundice, encephalopathy, a haemorrhagic diathesis and various metabolic disturbances. Any one of these features may dominate the clinical picture and each may occur in apparent isolation. An important clinical feature of FHF is that the liver is often small and impalpable at presentation. Alternatively, a clinically enlarged liver usually decreases in size as FHF develops. The early stages of fulminant liver failure may therefore mimic several medical conditions, including encephalitis, septicaemia and a variety of metabolic disturbances and intoxications. Later the condition may be dominated by cardiovascular, pulmonary, renal and cerebral dysfunction. Each may mark the onset of multiple organ failure and contribute to morbidity and the high mortality associated with acute liver failure.[27,47]

The early diagnosis of acute liver failure and recognition of associated extrahepatic complications is essential if therapeutic interventions are to succeed.

HEPATIC ENCEPHALOPATHY

Changes in the mental state of patients with acute liver disease usually herald the onset of fulminant hepatic failure. Early recognition is important as this allows rapid institution of appropriate support and transfer, while the patient is stable, to centres with special expertise and, if possible, with established liver transplant programmes.

As Plum and his associates[69,194] have pointed out, the syndrome of hepatic encephalopathy consists of:

1. Personality changes and impaired mental function.
2. Prominent motor abnormalities (asterixis, tremor, paratonia, hyperventilation, hyperactive stretch reflexes and even decerebrate posturing).
3. Alteration of consciousness.
4. Characteristic neuro-ophthalmological changes, including intact pupils and brisk ocular responses.
5. A constellation of laboratory abnormalities.

Most clinicians regard the staging of the depressed level of consciousness as being the most important indicator of the severity of liver failure and consequently of prognosis. Table 29.1 shows one such classification commonly used. In the Fulminant Hepatic Failure Surveillance Study, Trey et al.[247] reported that 17.6% of 284 patients in stage 4 coma survived as did 48% of 13 patients with stage 3 and 66% of 21 patients with stage 2. Most series have shown a mortality of 80–90% of patients who have been in stage 4 for more than a few hours.[22,247] Plum and Hindfelt[194] have emphasized that the broad categories of drowsiness,

stupor or coma are too inclusive for the observer to be able to quantify accurately the day-to-day changes in the severity of encephalopathy. They have pointed out that electroencephalographic and biochemical changes may not closely parallel the clinical course. Guidelines have been developed[41,194] (Table 29.2) to improve the bedside assessment of encephalopathy.

Except in paracetamol toxicity, early onset of encephalopathy, i.e. within the first week of jaundice, appears to be associated with a better prognosis.[182] Other causes of altered mental state must be considered since these may require specific intervention in their own right.

Clinical features

Early diagnosis of encephalopathy requires recognition of subtle signs including personality changes, mental slowing, aggression or flattening of affect.[97,103,235,236] Other signs include restlessness, delirium, motor hyperactivity with facial grimacing, myoclonus, paratonic rigidity (gegenhalten) and seizures.[3] Occasionally these may precede all other manifestations of liver disease.[275] Foetor hepaticus is common but not invariable.[52] Asterixis, the involuntary intermittent relaxation of sustained motor activity, is less specific than fetor hepaticus and is not useful in detecting the early stages of encephalopathy. Tendon reflexes are initially normal, become brisk during stages 2 and 3 when they may be associated with bilateral extensor plantar responses, and are lost during stage 4.[194] Pupillary, oculocephalic and oculovestibular responses are preserved until complications, such as cerebral oedema with brainstem herniation, supervene.

Psychometric and neurophysiological features

Number connection,[53] block design,[224] and digital symbol tests[104] are useful in diagnosing early hepatic encephalopathy. Visual,[45,148,278] and somatosensory evoked

Table 29.1 Stages in the onset and development of hepatic coma.

Grade or stage	Mental state	Tremor	Electroencephalographic changes
Stage 1: prodrome (too often diagnosed in retrospect)	Euphoria, occasionally depression; fluctuant, mild confusion; slowness of mentation and affect; untidy, slurred speech; disordered sleep rhythm	Slight	Usually absent
Stage 2: impending coma	Accentuation of stage 1: drowsiness; inappropriate behaviour; inability to maintain sphincter control	Present (easily elicited)	Abnormal, generalized slowing
Stage 3: stupor	Patient sleeps most of the time but is rousable; speech is incoherent; confusion is marked	Usually present (if patient can cooperate)	Always abnormal
Stage 4: deep coma	Patient may or may not respond to painful stimuli	Usually absent	Always abnormal

Reprinted from Trey *et al.* (1966)[246] (adapted from Adams and Foley[3]), by permission of the *New England Journal of Medicine*.

Table 29.2 A clinical coma profile for bedside use.

Verbal response
  None
  Incomprehensible sounds
  Confused
  Normal

Pupils
  Non-reactive
  Sluggish
  Brisk

Eye opening
  None
  To noxious stimuli only
  To verbal stimuli
  Spontaneous

Oculocephalic-oculovestibular responses
  No reaction
  Partial or dysconjugate
  Full
  Normal

Best motor response
  None
  Abnormal extensor
  Abnormal flexor
  Withdrawal or localizes
  Obeys commands

Respiration
  Nil, on ventilator
  Irregular
  Regular, >22/minute
  Regular, <22/minute

From Plum and Hindfelt (1976),[194] with kind permission of the authors and the publisher, American Elsevier Publishing.

responses[45,237] have been found to be sensitive in detecting early stages of encephalopathy. The standard EEG does not reliably distinguish hepatic encephalopathy from other causes of impaired consciousness.[83,220]

Biochemical tests

Raised blood ammonia levels support the diagnosis of hepatic encephalopathy. However, normal values do not exclude this diagnosis.[54,227] Indeed, in most patients clinical features of encephalopathy precede a rise in the blood ammonia concentration.[54] Measurement of CSF glutamine concentration may also be a useful adjunct to the diagnosis of hepatic encephalopathy but raised levels are not specific for liver disease.[121,265]

The pathophysiology of encephalopathy in fulminant hepatic failure differs in many respects from that seen in chronic portal–systemic shunting.[54] There are numerous superadded metabolic and infective insults,[271] the priming effect of chronic hyperammonaemia is absent[199] and cerebral oedema, which seldom occurs in chronic liver disease, is common.[184]

CEREBRAL OEDEMA _____

Cerebral oedema is thought to be a major cause of death in acute liver failure[21] and to result in significant morbidity in survivors.[179] Ware *et al.*[262] were the first to document the high incidence of cerebral oedema in FHF. More recently cerebral oedema was found in 13 of 16 autopsies, 6 of which showed signs of brainstem coning.[219] The prevalence of cerebral oedema is highest in fulminant hepatic failure, intermediate in subacute hepatic failure, [99] and low in chronic disease. Cerebral oedema is said to occur more frequently in patients with hepatitis B and non-A non-B than hepatitis A but these findings may reflect differences in disease severity.[75]

Pathophysiology

There is still uncertainty as to the mechanism of cerebral oedema in FHF. In general, cerebral oedema may be vasogenic or cytotoxic. In vasogenic oedema, disruption of the blood–brain barrier leads to extravasation of protein-rich fluid. In cytotoxic oedema, the blood–brain barrier is intact but neuroglial cells lose their capacity to maintain solute and water homeostasis and intracellular swelling occurs. Evidence for vasogenic oedema is based on the finding that several animal models of fulminant hepatic failure exhibit increased blood–brain barrier permeability.[120,149,277] However, in some models this increased permeability is not global[141] while in others the blood–brain barrier appears to be intact.[143,150,241]

A cytotoxic mechanism is supported by electron-microscopic studies showing intracellular astrocyte swelling[240] and by the response to mannitol, which requires a largely intact blood–brain barrier in order to be effective.[39] The putative mechanisms for cytotoxic cerebral oedema include a decrease in the activity of the Na^+–K^+ ATPase pump, which is important in neuroglial cellular osmoregulation.[140,233] Serum of patients with fulminant hepatic failure has been shown to inhibit Na^+–K^+ ATPase.[217] Mercaptans,[198] short-chain fatty acids,[57] bile acids, phenolic acids and endotoxin,[216] all of which are known to accumulate in fulminant hepatic failure, have also been shown to inhibit this enzyme. However Na^+–K^+ ATPase activity was not decreased in an experimental, galactosamine-induced, rabbit model of FHF.[82] In other studies where Na^+–K^+ ATPase inhibition was present, inhibition appeared to correlate more closely with encephalopathy[73, 74,217] than with cerebral oedema. This has led some to question whether Na^+–K^+ ATPase inhibition is involved in the pathogenesis of the cerebral oedema associated with acute liver failure.[75]

On balance there is enough evidence to suggest that both vasogenic and cytotoxic mechanisms contribute to the cerebral oedema seen in FHF.[239]

In some models of FHF, raised intracranial pressure may occur in the absence of cerebral oedema.[36] This increase in intracranial pressure has been attributed to vascular engorgement.[64,75] Some workers have demonstrated increased cerebral blood flow in fulminant hepatic failure in man[75] and in experimental animals.[64] Others have found cerebral blood flow to be decreased.[9,228] Thus, it is currently difficult to assess the role that vascular engorgement plays in the pathogenesis of raised intracranial pressure.

Clinical features

Clinical features are related to the intracranial pressure (ICP) and usually occur when pressure exceeds 30 mmHg (normal less than 12 mmHg).[109] Arterial hypertension is a useful indicator of increased ICP.[75] Signs include increased tone, decerebrate posturing, opisthotonos and trismus. There is a tendency to hyperventilation which increases progressively until brainstem coning and respiratory arrest occur. Pupils initially respond sluggishly to light but subsequently dilate and become unresponsive. Oculocephalic and oculovestibular responses are lost with severe raised ICP, which often indicates that brainstem coning has occurred.[109] While loss of pupillary[75] and oculocephalic[111] responses are usually indicative of a poor prognosis, patients with these features have been known to recover. Loss of the oculovestibular response, however, usually indicates irreversible brainstem damage.[111] Papilloedema is rarely seen, even in those patients dying of raised ICP. Several factors may aggravate the effects of acute liver failure on the brain. These include hypoxia, hypercapnoea,[222] hyponatraemia,[119] pyrexia[49] and hypotension.

Continuous arterial monitoring has been recommended as a means of identifying those patients who may be developing clinical features of raised intracranial pressure.[75] Whether ICP should be monitored directly depends on how the attending physician will respond to the information. Indeed, with careful clinical evaluation, experienced staff are able to detect most episodes of sustained intracranial hypertension.[109] This requires intensive monitoring, including examining pupillary responses every 5 minutes, which in practice will be difficult to sustain. Thus, where therapy with mannitol[39] or even thiopentone[90] is contemplated, direct monitoring may be prudent.

HAEMORRHAGE

Bleeding is a common complication of acute liver failure.[96] In Cape Town more than 50% of adults and 70% of children had a major defect of coagulation with life-threatening haemorrhage.[214] The usual sites of bleeding are the nasopharynx, oesophagus, stomach, duodenum, retroperitoneal space and bronchial tree.

Platelets

Gazzard et al. found a platelet count of less than 100×10^9/litre in 46 of 67 patients with acute liver failure.[96] Impaired release of new platelets from the bone marrow and abnormalities of platelet aggregation and adhesion have been described in FHF.[184] The latter have been ascribed to disturbances in arachidonic acid

metabolism, alterations in plasma lipids, and increased levels of von Willebrandt factor, and to the effects of disseminated intravascular coagulation and fibrinolysis.

Coagulation factors

The liver is the major site of synthesis of most coagulation factors. Plasma concentrations fall rapidly in acute liver failure, the rate of disappearance correlating inversely with the half-life of the individual factor. Factors V and VII have the shortest half-lives and therefore fall most rapidly. Prothrombin has a half-life of 2.8–4.4 days, and thus the prothrombin index will not fall immediately.[184]

Fibrinogen levels are commonly decreased in liver failure. This is accounted for by decreased synthesis and accelerated breakdown.[184] Plasma concentrations of fibrin and fibrinogen degradation products are commonly elevated in FHF.[46]

Factor XIII levels are greatly decreased, and this may contribute to poor clot stabilization in liver failure.[178] Factor VIII is exceptional in that the concentration of both its components, the procoagulant protein and the von Willebrandt factor, increase in acute liver failure. The clinical significance of this is unclear but it may reflect endothelial damage.[51]

Procoagulants as well as coagulation inhibitors are disturbed in liver disease. The vitamin K-dependent zymogens, proteins C and S are synthesized by the liver. Antithrombin III and α-2 macroglobulin are also synthesized by the liver and both are profoundly reduced in FHF.[169] Since antithrombin III is an essential cofactor for heparin, the effect of heparin in acute liver failure may be unpredictable.[250]

Fibrinolysis and disseminated intravascular coagulation (DIC)

The role of DIC is not clearly defined in ALF. Elevated levels of some of the fibrin(ogen) degradation products (FDP) are encountered.[184] Fibrin strands have been demonstrated in the vasculature, and consumptive thrombocytopenia is common. Thus, there is evidence to suggest that patients with FHF have a low-grade DIC.

Diagnosis and monitoring

The clotting status may be monitored by assessment of the prothrombin time, partial thromboplastin time, fibrinogen levels, FDPs and platelet count. The prothrombin time is usually regarded as a sensitive indicator of progress and prognosis.[250]

RESPIRATORY COMPLICATIONS

Deranged ventilation and gas exchange are frequent in FHF. This may be due to raised intracranial pressure, metabolic disturbances or local pulmonary abnormalities. Hyperventilation commonly heralds the onset of cerebral oedema, and its severity parallels the depth of coma. This terminates with brainstem coning.

Initially the sensitivity of peripheral chemoreceptors to hypoxia is increased, but this is not maintained when hypoxia is prolonged. Thus, any respiratory complication could lead to a vicious cycle in which the resultant hypoxia would, via hypoxic depression of respiratory drive, lead to a further decrease in P_aO_2. Hypoxaemia most commonly results from pneumonia, gastric aspiration, non-cardiogenic pulmonary oedema, or atelectasis, and less frequently from ventilation–perfusion mismatch, possibly with accompanying perfusion–diffusion defects, pulmonary haemorrhage or respiratory muscle weakness secondary to hypophosphataemia.

Obtunded patients with fulminant hepatic failure frequently vomit and gastric aspiration may result.[181] This may be prevented by nasogastric drainage, treatment of the hepatic encephalopathy and meticulous care of the airways. The latter is particularly important when transporting these patients. As many as 50% of patients with FHF had bacterial pathogens cultured from their sputum, while 20% had radiographic features consistent with bacterial pneumonia.[209,263]

Non-cardiogenic pulmonary oedema occurs in approximately one-third of patients with FHF and is especially frequent in patients with paracetamol overdose who have accompanying metabolic acidosis.[243] Although the pathogenesis is unclear, the finding of a high incidence of both pulmonary and cerebral oedema in patients with fulminant hepatic failure raises the possibility of a central or neurogenic mechanism.[243]

An alternative explanation is that the same factors result in oedema at both sites. Indeed, it has been suggested that patients with fulminant hepatic failure may have abnormal capillary permeability similar to that seen in the adult respiratory distress syndrome.[260] Regardless of the mechanism, the respiratory complications of fulminant hepatic failure require early diagnosis if therapeutic intervention is to succeed.

HYPOGLYCAEMIA

The frequency and importance of hypoglycaemia in patients with acute liver failure has been emphasized.[164,211] In our series, 40% of adults and 44% of children in coma were hypoglycaemic at some time. Several of these patients required very large amounts of oral and intravenous glucose and even then hypoglycaemia was controlled with difficulty.[211] It has been suggested that hypoglycaemia is due to inefficient degradation of insulin by the damaged liver.[101] However, using euglycaemic and hyperglycaemic clamp techniques,[12] Vilstrup *et al.*[255] found that five patients in acute liver failure, with grade 3–4 coma, had tenfold increases in plasma insulin and C-peptide concentration. Insulin sensitivity was decreased to about 15% of the expected value. Calculated metabolic clearance of insulin was normal. In addition, initial glucagon concentrations were increased fiftyfold and were not suppressed by glucose and insulin. Thus, the hyperinsulinaemia of acute liver failure appears to be related to increased secretion rather than to decreased clearance of insulin.

RENAL COMPLICATIONS

Renal insufficiency, which may progress to frank renal failure, is common in acute liver failure. Prerenal uraemia, acute tubular necrosis (ATN), the hepatorenal syndrome (HRS) or combinations of these account for the vast majority of cases. All three conditions present with a decreased clearance of urea and creatinine. Plasma concentrations of both may be misleading. Urea levels may be low owing to decreased production or be increased after gastrointestinal haemorrhage. Similarly, some methods for measuring creatinine concentration may yield falsely low results in the presence of high plasma bilirubin concentrations.[108] In their analysis of 48 patients with fulminant hepatic failure, Wilkinson *et al.* found that 38 had evidence of renal impairment; 4 had prerenal uraemia, 16 ATN and 12 functional renal failure; 6 patients could not be classified.[267]

1 *Prerenal uraemia.* A decreased effective plasma volume is common in acute liver failure. This may be due to dehydration or may reflect a shift of fluid from the intravascular space. Dehydration is often seen in patients with severe nausea, with drowsiness due to impending encephalopathy or after inappropriate sedation. Vomiting, diarrhoea or haemorrhage may also contribute to hypovolaemia.

2 *Acute tubular necrosis.* Patients with acute liver failure are prone to ATN. Hypotension is common;[244] obstructive jaundice has been shown to potentiate anoxic renal damage;[62] and aminoglycosides have been demonstrated to act synergistically with endotoxin in promoting renal tubular dysfunction.[248,276] Finally, several of the causes of acute liver failure also result in renal injury. This would include leptospirosis, paracetamol and carbon tetrachloride poisoning.

3 *Hepatorenal syndrome* (HRS), or functional renal failure is well described in acute liver failure from whatever cause. Ritt *et al.*[206] documented HRS in 8 of 31 and Wilkinson *et al.*[267] in 12 of 48 patients with acute liver failure. HRS appears to be largely functional in origin. The kidneys of patients with HRS regain function when transplanted into recipients with normal livers. Similarly, renal function returns after liver transplantation.[126,144] Renal angiography shows a strikingly abnormal pattern suggestive of severe intrarenal vasoconstriction which is not seen when angiography is repeated shortly after death.[78]

Diagnosis

There is no single test that reliably identifies the cause of renal dysfunction associated with acute liver failure. Epstein *et al.*[79] suggest the simultaneous use of urine sodium concentration, urine-to-plasma creatinine ratio, plasma and urine osmolality and examination of urine sediment. Acute tubular necrosis is characterized by a high urinary sodium concentration (>30 mmol/l), a urine-to-plasma creatinine ratio of less than 20 : 1, a urine osmolality equal to that of plasma and the presence of casts and cellular debris in the sediment. It is often difficult to distinguish prerenal uraemia from HRS. Both have low urine sodium concentrations (<10 mmol/l), urine osmolality at least 100 mosm greater than that of plasma and an unremarkable urine sediment. The urine-to-plasma creatinine ratio is said to be more than 30 : 1 in HRS and less than 30 : 1 in prerenal uraemia. In practice, however, this difference is not reliable and the onus rests on the clinician to exclude prerenal uraemia, which is potentially reversible. Hypovolaemia and even dehydration are notoriously difficult to diagnose in liver disease. Clinical features, central venous pressure (CVP) and even pulmonary capillary wedge pressure (PCWP), may all be misleading. In our experience, the most reliable method of excluding hypovolaemia is to infuse colloid and crystalloids until the plasma space is replete. This is judged by careful observation of the lungs for incipient pulmonary oedema, and of the CVP or PCWP for a sudden rise suggesting that the capacitance of the vasculature has been exceeded. Such a manoeuvre may be vital since renal dysfunction of whatever cause will be aggravated by hypovolaemia. Conversely, overhydration may precipitate cerebral oedema or non-cardiogenic pulmonary oedema.

INFECTION AND IMMUNITY

Bacteriologically proven infections occur in up to 80% of patients with acute liver failure.[209] About 20% of these are associated with bacteraemia or septicaemia.[209] The organisms most frequently isolated are Gram-negative bacilli and Gram-positive cocci.[17,94,171,271] The high frequency of sepsis and endotoxaemia may contribute to multiorgan failure.[28]

The diagnosis of acute bacterial infection in acute liver failure is difficult because confusion, fever, hypotension and leucocytosis may occur in the absence of bacteriologically confirmed sepsis. Common sites of infection include the lungs, urinary tract and cannulae.[209] Blood, sputum, and urine cultures combined with appropriate radiological examinations are vital for early detection of infection.

Fungal infection may occur as a result of the invasion of tissues by *Candida* or *Aspergillus* species with subsequent dissemination. These occur in approximately one third of patients with ALF, usually after 5 days in hospital, and in patients with established renal failure. Suggestive features of fungal infection include deteriorating coma after initial improvement, high white cell count, and a fever unresponsive to antibiotics.[209a]

While immobility, aspiration of blood or secretions and invasive diagnostic or therapeutic procedures are relatively common causes for infection, they do not explain the high incidence of infection found in patients with acute liver failure as compared to other patients in the same intensive care units. Indeed, fatal infections may occur after recovery of consciousness and improvement of hepatic function. Pulmonary abscesses, candida peritonitis and other infections have all resulted in death of apparently convalescing patients.[96,260]

The high incidence of infection in acute liver failure has led several investigators to examine various aspects of immunity in these patients. Complement deficiency, due to activation by circulating endotoxins and reduced hepatic synthesis, is present even in the early stages of acute liver failure.[44,273] Severe deficiencies of complement have been noted in patients with FHF and may result in defective opsonization and serum chemoattractant activity.[272] Patients with fulminant hepatic failure have low levels of fibronectin (plasma opsonizing protein), which may further contribute to defective bacterial clearance and phagocytosis.[122]

Inhibitors of normal chemotactic factors have been detected but may be of secondary importance. Serum factors inhibiting phagocytosis of bacteria have been described.[213] Transfusion of fresh, frozen plasma and replacement of fibronectin in patients with fulminant hepatic failure may improve opsonic function of the patient's serum *in vitro*. This, however, does not appear to augment clearance of opsonized particles *in vivo* nor are there any documented effects on neutrophil function.[122,273]

Neutrophil adherence and locomotion *in vitro* are abnormal in the majority of patients irrespective of the aetiology of acute liver failure.[11,274] Defective Na^+–K^+ ATPase activity in leucocytes may cause these abnormalities, as Na^+–K^+ fluxes are important in cell locomotion.[6] Alternative explanations involve defective expression or blockade of leucocyte integrin receptors by fibronectin or the fibrin(ogen) fragments which result as a consequence of disseminated intravascular coagulation.[208]

Although earlier studies suggested that phagocytic activity of Kupffer cells were preserved in FHF, more recent reports have detailed defective clearance of opsonized particles suggesting damage to these mononuclear phagocytes *in vivo*.[122,173]

High levels of tumour necrosis factor (TNF) and interleukin-1 (IL-1) are released *in vitro* by monocytes/macrophages from patients with acute liver failure.[174] The release of these cytokines, as a result of sepsis and endotoxaemia, may in turn mediate the multiple damage seen in acute liver failure.[28]

BIOCHEMICAL CHANGES

The serum aminotransferases are always elevated early in FHF, frequently to high levels. However, these levels are not useful in predicting which patients with acute liver disease will develop fulminant hepatic failure. Serum bilirubin usually rises soon after the onset of FHF and is mainly conjugated in type. Patients who recover often pass through a phase of marked cholestatic jaundice with very high levels of conjugated bilirubin. Those who die at this stage show large regeneration nodules, with intense cholestasis in hepatocytes. The mechanism is not understood. There is a striking elevation of plasma ligandin levels and the measurement of this cytosolic protein in the plasma may prove to be a good index of liver cell necrosis.[21,186]

Rising α-fetoprotein levels in the plasma may indicate the onset of regeneration.[7,31,32] α-Fetoprotein is synthesized by fetal liver cells[102] and is well established as a serum marker of heptocellular carcinoma.[197] If a sensitive radioimmunoassay is employed in its detection, α-fetoprotein can be found in minute amounts in normal adults.[210] It has been detected in the serum of mice after partial hepatectomy[137,196] and in patients recovering from acute hepatitis,[5,7] suggesting that it accompanies hepatic regeneration.

Karvountzis and Redeker[132] found raised α-fetoprotein levels in 57% of patients with coma complicating fulminant viral hepatitis and in 80% of those who survived. Furthermore, where serial titres were measured, the levels were found to be increasing at the end of the period of coma. In contrast, α-fetoprotein was detected in only 37% of those patients who died, despite the fact that some survived up to 10 days. In those patients in whom α-fetoprotein was detected before death, there was quantitatively more evidence of regeneration at necropsy than in those in whom α-fetoprotein was not detected. The presence of α-fetoprotein was therefore thought to be a favourable prognostic sign and its absence in fulminant hepatitis to be of ominous significance.

Murray-Lyon et al.[172] found that 11 out of 23 survivors of fulminant hepatic failure had raised α-fetoprotein levels compared with 4 out of the 41 fatal cases. The rise in α-fetoprotein levels was found early after the development of grade 4 coma and they felt that it constituted an encouraging prognostic sign at a time when the liver function tests and EEG were unhelpful. This was not the view of Bloomer et al.,[32] who studied serial α-fetoprotein levels in 12 patients with massive hepatic necrosis due to viral hepatitis, ischaemic necrosis and halothane hepatitis. They noted that α-fetoprotein levels were significantly elevated after the eighth day of illness in nine patients, all of whom were shown subsequently at biopsy or necropsy to have histological evidence of hepatic regeneration. Since only one of these nine patients survived, they stated that a rising serum α-fetoprotein level does not necessarily imply ultimate recovery and that it therefore cannot be used to assess prognosis.[32]

HYPONATRAEMIA

Hyponatraemia is common in acute liver failure. Wilkinson et al. found significant hyponatraemia in 48% of their patients with FHF and grade III–IV encephalopathy.[267] Hyponatraemia in acute liver failure is thought to be due to increased total body water rather than to total body sodium depletion. Indeed, total body sodium may be increased.[76] The occasional patient may, however, be sodium deficient. This may be iatrogenic and occur as a

result of lactulose-induced diarrhoea or renal sodium loss. The use of bromocriptine[157] and vasopressin may aggravate hyponatraemia.

Hyponatraemia is most often seen in patients with encephalopathy and renal impairment and these may mask signs of the low plasma sodium concentration. Hyponatraemia produces progressive cerebral oedema and later a compensatory decrease in brain solute concentration. This would aggravate the cerebral oedema and raised intracranial pressure of hepatic encephalopathy.[14]

HYPERNATRAEMIA

Hypernatraemia was present in 11 of the 48 patients described by Wilkinson et al.[267] All 11 died. High plasma sodium concentrations may follow administration of hypertonic saline, bicarbonate or plasma. It is also seen where there has been net loss of water over solute owing to lactulose-induced diarrhoea or to an osmotic diuresis following infusions of dextrose, fructose or mannitol.[267] These patients are often too ill to offset their rising osmolality by increasing oral water intake.[264]

ACID–BASE HOMEOSTASIS

Alkalosis was noted in 49 of 65 observations in 28 patients with fulminant hepatic failure.[202] In contrast, acidosis was present in only 4 of these 28 patients, 3 of whom had ingested toxic amounts of paracetamol.

Alkalosis was most commonly associated with a low P_aCO_2. The mechanism is uncertain. Hyperventilation may be secondary to pulmonary shunting or stimulation of the respiratory centre by hyperammonaemia.[187] Metabolic alkalosis is less common and is often associated with chloride depletion or hypokalaemia.

Lactic acidosis is uncommon in fulminant hepatic failure despite the pivotal role of the liver in lactate metabolism. It is usually encountered where there is shock or septicaemia.[187] When it is present, the prognosis is poor.

HYPOPHOSPHATAEMIA

Dawson et al.[61] found hypophosphataemia in 12 of 13 patients with acute liver failure, most of whom had ingested paracetamol. In one-third, plasma inorganic phosphate levels were less than 0.3 mmol/l. The symptoms of hypophosphataemia, which include irritability, muscle weakness, dysarthria, confusion and coma, have led these authors to postulate a relationship between phosphate depletion and encephalopathy. A subsequent review suggests that current data are insufficient to support this suggestion.[142]

HYPOKALAEMIA, HYPOCALCAEMIA AND HYPOMAGNESAEMIA

While 23 of 38 patients with acute liver failure were found to have hypokalaemia,[267] the incidence of hypocalcaemia and hypomagnesaemia is uncertain, although both have been described.[190] Until such data are available it would seem prudent to measure, and where appropriate to correct, the plasma concentration of these cations in patients with acute liver failure.

MANAGEMENT

INTENSIVE CARE

Intensive care of patients with fulminant liver failure, with careful monitoring of vital functions, is imperative and may be responsible for any improvement in prognosis in recent years. The development of cardiovascular, pulmonary, renal and cerebral complications is common and may mark the onset of multiple organ failure. The early recognition and prompt treatment of these and other complications may influence prognosis.

Principles of management of these complications are similar to those utilized in high-output, low-resistance shock states encountered in septicaemic patients. Early and appropriate treatment of sepsis is imperative.

Correction of bleeding diathesis

As the haemostatic defects in acute liver failure are complex and multifactorial, the response to standard supportive measures is often unpredictable.

Fresh frozen plasma, cryoprecipitate and vitamin K supplementation, where applicable, remain the mainstays of treatment of bleeding in liver disease.[135] Prothrombin and factor IX concentrates are no longer used because of the risk of hepatitis[15] and thromboembolism.[96] Newer measures include the infusion of antithrombin III concentrates (see Chapter 8). These are especially effective in patients with DIC in association with fulminant hepatitis[34] or acute fatty liver of pregnancy.[146] Unfortunately, large amounts of these expensive concentrates are required and there is an associated risk of hepatitis transmission.[135]

Heparin, which may improve coagulation parameters in DIC, increases the risk of haemorrhage and has been shown to have an adverse influence in patients with FHF.[95,98,136,184] Epsilon-aminocaproic acid,[253] exchange tranfusion[93] and plasmapheresis[16] are no longer advocated.

Active bleeding or surgical and invasive procedures (insertion of central venous or arterial catheters) require platelet transfusion, where indicated, and administration of FFP.[184] It is our impression that Haemocel® (gelatin derivatives) may impair thrombocyte function _in vivo_ and promote mucosal and surgical bleeding.

Respiratory support

Oxygen therapy, and intermittent positive pressure ventilation with or without positive end expiratory pressure, should be administered as indicated. Early ventilation, in the absence of specific indications, and prolonged hyperventilation, to prevent cerebral oedema, are of no advantage to patients with FHF.[71] Physiotherapy may aggravate cerebral oedema and should be used only where absolutely necessary.[75]

Maintainence of blood sugar

Hypoglycaemia should be anticipated in every patient with acute liver failure, and regular monitoring of blood glucose concentration is essential. Hypoglycaemia should be corrected parenterally. Total parenteral nutrition has, however, on occasion resulted in hyperglycaemia, presumably due to the insulin insensitivity demonstrated by Vilstrup _et al._[255] Since the hyperglycaemia may not respond to insulin therapy, careful monitoring of glucose levels should be continued in patients receiving total parenteral nutrition.

Management of renal complications

The first step must be to correct hypovolaemia. Thereafter, rigorous attention to the balance between intake and output and careful estimation of the effective intravascular and extravascular volumes are vital. The latter will influence the decision to administer plasma, albumin or crystalloid. As a general rule the use of sodium-containing fluid should be limited, since many patients demonstrate avid sodium retention. Diuretics may induce hypovolaemia, do not improve renal function, and should be used with extreme caution. It is essential to exclude agents known to cause renal damage. Substitution of third-generation cephalosporins for aminoglycosides should be considered. Infections should be vigorously treated.

Dialysis

Dialysis where indicated may be used in the treatment of ATN. There is no evidence that dialysis influences the course of HRS.[79]

Pharmacological maintenance of renal perfusion

Decreased cardiac output,[26] enhanced peripheral vasodilatation,[79] increased activity of renin–angiotensin,[38] kallikrein–kinin,[288] atrial natriuretic peptide,[79] the sympathetic system[205] and alterations in renal prostaglandins[33] have all been incriminated in the pathogenesis of HRS. However, there are as yet no convincing data to support the use of agents designed to counteract their effects.

Correction of electrolyte and acid-base imbalance

The treatment of hyponatraemia is complicated by uncertainty about the relationship between salt administration and the development of central pontine myelinolysis. A number of factors have been associated with an adverse outcome. These include overcorrection and a delay in initiating treatment.[14] Early diagnosis allows treatment to be instituted at a stage where fluid restriction may suffice. When given, sodium replacement should aim to increase plasma sodium concentration at no more than 1–2 mmol/l per hour. The use of hypertonic saline is hazardous and should be reserved for patients with plasma sodium concentrations of 120 mmol/l or less. Demeclocycline should not be used since its use in patients with liver failure appears to be associated with a high incidence of renal deterioration.[188] Urea has been used in chronic liver disease[63] but there are no data on its use in acute liver failure.

Treatment of hypernatraemia depends on its cause. Rapid correction is dangerous since it may cause brain oedema, convulsions and anatomical disruption of brain fibres.[14] Correction using hypotonic fluid should aim to decrease plasma sodium concentration by 1–2 mosmol/l per hour.[14]

Metabolic alkalosis is diminished by repletion of chloride. Overadministration of sodium must be avoided. Acetazolamide and ammonium chloride are contraindicated.[187]

Therapy of lactic acidosis depends on the correction of hypoxia, hypotension, renal failure and shock. The use of bicarbonate in this condition is controversial.[175]

MANAGEMENT OF ENCEPHALOPATHY (see Chapter 47) _____

The ultimate goal in the treatment of hepatic encephalopathy is to improve hepatocellular function. The severity of hepatic encephalopathy is one of the most important prognostic indicators, but it is unclear whether this is because the grade of encephalopathy merely reflects the severity of the underlying liver disease, or whether it contributes independently to a worse prognosis. Prevention or lessening of stupor and coma certainly facilitates the nursing of patients and helps to prevent complications such as aspiration pneumonia. Thus, vigorous management of precomatose patients with encephalopathy is worthwhile.

Rational treatment of hepatic encephalopathy depends on an understanding of its pathophysiology. In the presence of liver failure, potentially neuroactive nitrogenous compounds are absorbed from the intestine, while deranged muscle metabolism alters nitrogen and amino-acid fluxes, which may affect cerebral neurotransmission. The pathophysiological mechanisms by which these compounds lead to neural inhibition in the brain, and hence to hepatic encephalopathy, are increasingly being understood. This is reviewed in detail in Chapter 47. Those theories that provide a rational basis for the use of various suggested therapeutic regimens will be briefly discussed below.

Ammonia intoxication

There is broad agreement that ammonia plays a role in the pathogenesis of hepatic encephalopathy. Nevertheless, ammonia alone is insufficient to account for all the features observed and its precise role and the mechanisms involved remain to be clarified.[40]

Ammonia is an important neurotoxin.[52,54] In patients dying from fulminant hepatic failure, raised glutamine concentration in brain biopsies[201] suggest the presence of increased brain ammonia concentrations.[265] Decreased liver clearance of ammonia as well as hypokalaemia and alkalosis, may contribute to increases in brain ammonia concentration.[52,225]

There are, however, major flaws in the ammonia hypothesis. Ten per cent of patients with hepatic encephalopathy have normal ammonia concentrations.[242] Conversely, patients with raised arterial ammonia concentrations are not consistently found to be encephalopathic. Finally, acute increases of ammonia induce seizures rather than coma in experimental animals.

Despite these reservations, reducing ammonia concentration remains the cornerstone of treatment of hepatic encephalopathy. Ammonia synthesis in the bowel may be decreased by dietary protein restriction. Administration of lactulose or lactitol, orally or per rectum, may be beneficial. These agents acidify the stool,[251] induce mild diarrhoea and stimulate bacterial utilization of nitrogen[256, 266] and short-chain fatty acids,[167] all of which reduce absorption of nitrogenous compounds. Lactulose or lactitol should be given in amounts sufficient to produce two to four loose stools per day. Excessive use may result in fluid and electrolyte imbalance and should be avoided. Although gut sterilization will reduce ammonia formation, the routine use of non-absorbable antibiotics, e.g. neomycin, is not recommended, largely because of the danger of oto- and nephrotoxicity and to a lesser extent because of their theoretical ability to increase endotoxin formation.[75] Agents such as sodium benzoate, arginine, citrulline, ornithine and glutamic acid, which increase incorporation of ammonia into the urea cycle, have been used in chronic hepatic encephalopathy, but not in patients with acute liver failure.[161,283] Alpha-keto acids, which use nitrogen during their conversion to the corresponding amino acid, theoretically should be useful but to date appear to be of limited use in the treatment of encephalopathy.[80,116,259]

Thus, dietary protein restriction and lactulose remain the mainstay of treatment. This should be coupled to the correction of hypokalaemia, fluid balance, pH, and hypoxaemia. Provision of adequate calories and branched-chain amino acids or α-keto acids may improve protein metabolism[139] but do not appear to influence hepatic encephalopathy.[80]

Multifactorial synergistic abnormalities

Ammonia, mercaptans (including the thio-alcohols, methanethiol, dimethylsulphide, dimethyldisulphide), short-chain fatty acids and phenols, when given individually, to experimental animals, have little comagenic effect. However, when given simultaneously, these substances produce a significant depression of consciousness.[280–282] Ammonia, mercaptans and phenols may also suppress hepatic regenerative capacity,[284] thus interfering with recovery.

The implications for therapy include reduced absorption of these compounds from the gut by catharsis and the maintenance of a stable metabolic state in the patient.

False neurotransmitters and amino acid imbalance

Many abnormalities in neurotransmitter metabolism occur in the brain in hepatic encephalopathy. These include decreased noradrenaline,[67] increased serotonin,[19] increased octopamine[67,84] and other amines, as well as marked changes in the concentrations of many amino acids.[19,84,87] The aromatic amine precursors phenylalanine, tyrosine, tryptophan and methionine are increased in the plasma[4,125,159,201] and this suggested that the concentration of their metabolites in body fluids would also be increased. Indeed, raised concentrations of 5-hydroxyindoleacetic acid, the degradation product of 5-hydroxytryptamine (derived from tryptophan), and of homovanillic acid, the degradation product of dopamine (derived from tyrosine), have been found in the cerebrospinal fluid of patients with acute hepatic encephalopathy. Octopamine (derived from tyrosine via tyramine) has also been identified as a false neurotransmitter which is present in increased amounts.[141] The importance of these compounds in the pathogenesis of encephalopathy has yet to be determined. Infusion of extremely high doses of octopamine into the cerebroventricular system of rats does not affect their level of consciousness.[279] In keeping with these observations, initial reports that L-dopa caused striking neurological improvement in three patients with fulminant hepatic failure[191] have not been substantiated in acute or chronic liver disease by controlled trials.[162,254]

The concentration of the branched-chain amino acids—valine, leucine and isoleucine—is depressed in patients with chronic liver disease[123,124] and in animals with experimental encephalopathy.[4,125] Because of their shared transport mechanisms across the blood–brain barrier, the low concentration of branched-chain amino acids have been implicated as one of the causes of the increased brain tryptophan in these patients.[84] However, a clear distinction must be drawn between acute and chronic encephalopathy in this respect, because in fulminant hepatic failure in man the branched-chain amino acids are normal,[86,201] while in the rat they may be elevated.[156] In the study of Record et al.,[201] amino acid concentrations were measured in plasma, whole blood, cerebrospinal fluid and brain tissue in 45 patients with stage 3 or 4 coma due to fulminant hepatic failure. The concentrations of 15 of the 19 amino acids measured were significantly increased in blood and the increases were greater for the amino acids concerned with neurotransmitter metabolism. There was no correlation between the plasma concentrations of these amino acids and changes in the grade of hepatic coma. Plasma concentrations of the branched-chain amino acids were normal, except in those patients who subsequently recovered, in whom the levels were slightly decreased. Phenylalanine, tyrosine and methionine were among the 15 out of 18 amino acids which were significantly increased in cerebrospinal fluid, and among the 15 out of 21 amino acids which were significantly increased in the brain. The increase in tryptophan was associated with significant

elevation in the brain 5-hydroxyindoleacetic acid concentration, suggesting an increase in the 5-hydroxytryptamine turnover in hepatic coma. Brain-to-plasma ratios of most amino acids in patients with hepatic coma were similar to those in control subjects. This suggests that plasma concentration is a major factor controlling the cerebral concentration of branched-chain amino acids. Since cerebrospinal fluid and brain concentrations were increased when plasma concentrations were normal, an increase in brain uptake seems the likely explanation.[201]

Herlin et al.[115] have shown by studies of [^{14}C]insulin uptake into the brain that the blood–brain barrier appears to be intact up to 18 hours after hepatectomy in the rat. This group have also suggested that infused branched-chain amino acids protect the blood–brain barrier from the effects of hepatic failure.[114] We have not been able to confirm this finding in our pig model: CSF amino acid concentrations are just as abnormal in pigs receiving infusions of branched-chain amino acid as in those not.[10] Ammonia alone, despite rapidly increasing brain glutamine levels, does not cause increased uptake of [^{14}C]tryptophan into the brain until after 22 hours of continuous infusion.[154] Recently we have found that prostaglandin $F_{2\alpha}$ prevents the expected rise in the levels of all amino acids except glutamine in the CSF in our pig hepatic failure model. Since the levels of branched-chain and aromatic amino acids and methionine remain normal, this is an effect of potential importance in the management of hepatic encephalopathy.[10] Prostaglandins are known to exist in high concentrations in the brain[232] and to exert some control over cerebral blood flow,[77] neurotransmitter release[118] and intracellular cytoprotection.[226] Their mechanisms in preventing an elevation of CSF amino acids is as yet unclear.

Record and coworkers[201] have taken needle biopsies from the frontal cortex of the brain within an hour of death from 13 patients who later had full autopsy examinations, and from 7 patients dying without evidence of liver disease. These authors point out that some amino acids are found at a significantly higher concentration in brain obtained at autopsy than in tissue frozen immediately after removal during brain surgery. However, good correlation between their patients and the controls led them to believe that this did not introduce a major error into their study. They suggest that the relatively normal concentration of branched-chain amino acids in their patients may be due to the oxidation of these amino acids by extrahepatic tissues, mainly striated muscle,[165] in those patients who survive.[201]

The elevation of amino acids in the plasma may arise from necrotic liver cells or from muscle. The poor nutrition of these patients could result in an increased catabolism of proteins, with release of amino acids (mainly alanine and glutamine) from voluntary muscle for gluconeogenesis. The raised levels of methionine, phenylalanine and tyrosine, however, suggests that these are of hepatic origin. Further evidence for the hepatic origin is that although plasma and tissue amino acids are elevated in dogs after hepatectomy,[89,160,249] the plasma methionine levels fall to very low levels.[160] Thus, it seems likely that the origin of the amino acids in fulminant hepatic failure is both from the liver and from increased catabolism in voluntary muscle.

Our own studies in rats with acute hepatic coma following two-stage hepatic devascularization revealed profound changes in plasma and whole-brain amino acids and putative neurotransmitters. Brain ammonia, glutamine and GABA were increased. Aspartate was decreased, while glutamate was unchanged. An increase in brain tryptophan was accompanied by a similar increase in plasma unbound tryptophan but decreased total plasma tryptophan. These changes occurred in the presence of high plasma levels of the other amino acids, including branched-chain amino acids. Plasma insulin was unchanged, while glucagon levels rose, resulting in a decreased insulin-to-glucagon ratio. These results suggest that, while unbound tryptophan may influence brain tryptophan levels, altered plasma concentrations of neutral amino acids that compete with tryptophan for transport into the brain do not contribute to the increase in brain tryptophan observed during acute hepatic coma.[155] In a separate study we were able to demonstrate an increase in tryptophan transport into the brain of rats subjected to hepatic devascularization. Tryptophan influx occurred mainly via a non-saturable high-capacity system that was not affected by branched-chain amino acids.[155]

In the patients described by Record *et al.*,[201] the brain tryptophan-to-plasma tryptophan ratio was also slightly increased. This suggests that there may be an increased uptake of tryptophan into the brain in hepatic coma. Despite the apparent lack of correlation between the branched-chain amino acids and tryptophan transport, infusions of amino-acid mixtures containing high concentrations of branched-chain amino acids have improved encephalopathy in dogs with portacaval shunts[85] and in man with encephalopathy due to cirrhosis.[86] Maddrey *et al.*[153] have shown that the administration of the α-keto acid analogues of the branched-chain amino acids may have a similar beneficial effect on hepatic encephalopathy. Duffy and Plum[69] suggest that the branched-chain amino acids transaminate with α-ketoglutarate in astrocytes, thereby promoting the synthesis of glutamate. This increase in glutamate would stimulate incorporation of ammonia into glutamine and would restore the transport of reduced equivalents from cytoplasm into mitochondria (the malate aspartate shuttle), a process dependent on an adequate amount of glutamate. Despite these suggestions, we have not been able to confirm any beneficial effect in terms of survival or change in cerebrospinal fluid amino-acid concentrations with branched-chain amino-acid infusions in our pig model. Metanalysis of clinical trials employing branched-chain amino acid (BCAA) therapy in acute and chronic hepatic encephalopathy,[8,80,113] indicates that they are of questionable benefit, at best, in improving coma, although they do improve amino acid profiles[257] and provide nutritional support[139,185] that is at least as

good as a standard protein diet. In addition, no increased benefit has been demonstrated from giving BCAAs in an experimental model of fulminant hepatic failure.[10] Similarly, in practice the α-keto-analogues, despite theoretical advantages, have not lived up to their promise.

Gamma-aminobutyric acid (GABA)

Much attention has been devoted to the role of GABA and the GABA–benzodiazepine receptor complex in the pathogenesis of acute hepatic encephalopathy.[20,215] GABA is recognized as the most important mammalian inhibitory neurotransmitter.[55] Its synthesis from glutamic acid in GABAergic neurons is catalysed by glutamic acid decarboxylase. It is stored in axon vesicles and released into the synapse, during the action potential, by the effect of calcium ions. The binding of GABA to GABA receptors, which are associated with chloride channels, leads either to hyperpolarization or to depolarization of the post-synaptic neurone. Both actions have an inhibitory effect on the central nervous system. GABA released into the synaptic cleft is removed by glial cells and inactivated by GABA-transaminase. Benzodiazepines (BZP) and barbiturates allosterically enhance chloride conductance induced by GABA.

Several lines of evidence[107] support the involvement of the GABA–BZP complex in hepatic encephalopathy.[130] These include a resemblance between coma induced by GABA agonists and hepatic encephalopathy, the enhanced pharmacodynamic effect of BZP in patients with liver disease, and the suggestion that encephalopathy may be reversed by benzodiazepine-receptor antagonists.[106]

The implications for therapy are that the GABA-mimetic agents, especially benzodiazepines and barbiturates, should be avoided in patients with FHF. It is also possible that BZP receptor antagonists such as flumazenil may be useful in the treatment of hepatic encephalopathy. Improvement has been reported in 9 of 14 patients on such therapy,[130] although a recent abstract suggests that flumazenil was of no significant benefit in a controlled trial.[252]

CEREBRAL OEDEMA _____

Effective treatment of cerebral oedema is vital if the prognosis of patients with grade 3–4 encephalopathy is to be improved.

General

In the initial stages, raised intracranial pressure occurs paroxysmally, and may be precipitated by tactile or auditory stimuli. Patients should be nursed in a quiet environment and tactile stimulation should be minimized. Ideally patients should be positioned with their heads raised at 30–45° since this reduces intracranial hydrostatic pressure (ICP). Fluid balance should be managed with the aid of central venous or Swan–Ganz catheters, since raised central venous pressure is associated with raised ICP.[56] Hyponatraemia aggravates cerebral oedema and where possible should be prevented.[119] Similarly, serum osmolality and blood gases should be monitored and maintained within normal limits.

Careful monitoring of blood pressure is vital. In the presence of raised intracranial pressure, hypotension causes a marked reduction in cerebral blood flow and thus needs to be corrected. Hypertension may occur as a compensatory response to raised intracranial pressure and should not be treated with hypotensive agents. Treatment for raised intracranial pressure should be instituted if systolic blood pressure rises above 150 mmHg. Williams' group advocate early institution of specific management for cerebral oedema.[181] This includes the use of osmotic and non-osmotic diuretics, hyperventilation, steroids, prostaglandins and barbiturates. Each of these modalities is discussed below. In addition, recent experimental work has suggested a possible role for hypothermia in relieving cerebral oedema and for branched-chain amino acids in decreasing blood–brain barrier permeability.

Diuretics

Mannitol therapy has been shown to be effective in treating raised intracranial pressure[109] and improving survival in both man[39] and experimental animals.[285] It is the first line of treatment for raised intracranial pressure and is given by rapid bolus infusion, repeated hourly, if necessary. If patients with normal renal function do not have a diuresis, plasma osmolality should be measured and, if below 320 mosm, mannitol should be repeated. Following mannitol, ultrafiltration may be used to remove fluid in oliguric patients. A volume of fluid three to four times that of the mannitol should be removed 15–30 minutes after its administration. Failure to remove sufficient fluid raises intracranial pressure by increasing intravascular volume. Sustained hyperosmolality may further damage the blood–brain barrier.[193]

In a prospective, randomized controlled trial of 44 patients with fulminant hepatic failure, mannitol 1 g/kg was effective in reducing intracranial pressure and improving survival (47.1 vs 5.9%) when compared to control patients or to patients receiving dexamethasone.[39] However, 9 of the 17 patients who received mannitol developed renal failure after the start of therapy. Haemofiltration was not being used and all of these patients died. More recently, Ede et al.[71] obtained a 38% survival rate using lower doses of mannitol combined where necessary with ultrafiltration. In view of the dose-dependent nephrotoxicity of mannitol a dose of 0.3–0.5 g/kg is currently recommended.[181]

Non-osmotic diuretics may be used in addition to mannitol although there have been no controlled studies of these agents in the cerebral oedema of FHF. In other situations, however, cytotoxic oedema[128] and cerebral oedema due to cryogenic brain injury[48] have been improved by furosemide. Theoretically, loop diuretics should be useful since they reduce cerebrospinal fluid secretion by the choroid plexus and increase free water clearance, thus countering the negative free water clearance induced by mannitol.[195]

Barbiturates

In FHF and renal failure, cerebral oedema unresponsive to mannitol therapy has a mortality in excess of 90%. In a recent uncontrolled study, 13 patients with fulminant hepatic failure, oliguric renal failure, intracranial hypertension and grade 4 encephalopathy in whom all other measures had failed were treated with infusion of thiopental. This resulted in a significant reduction of intracranial pressure and improved survival.[90] However, this therapy is dangerous and should not be used routinely until supported by adequately controlled studies.

Hyperventilation

Hypocapnoea induced by hyperventilation reduces cerebral blood flow and consequently intracranial pressure.[145] Short-term hyperventilation may reduce intracranial pressure by up to 20 mmHg.[72] A randomized controlled study of 55 patients with grade 3 or 4 coma showed that prolonged hyperventilation failed to reduce the number of episodes of raised intracranial pressure, the amount of mannitol required, or the mortality.[71]

Corticosteroids

In 1952, Ducci and Katz[68] reported a 66% survival rate, which consisted of two survivors out of three patients. Their analysis of an extended series 10 years later showed a 39% survival rate (9 out of 23 patients).[134] All those who recovered were seen during the first half of the study. This trend for the best results to be obtained during the early part of a series, which has not subsequently been borne out in a larger number of patients, is often seen after the introduction of all additional new forms of therapy. Benhamou et al.[22] reviewed 334 patients, including 60 of their own, of whom 190 were treated with corticosteroids, and found no increased survival in the treated group. Similarly, the European Association for the Study of the Liver found no benefit from the use of corticosteroids.[70] The demonstration that intracranial hypertension could be attenuated in a pig hepatic devascularization model of fulminant hepatic failure by the early administration of corticosteroids[110] led to a randomized, controlled clinical trial to assess whether steroids could prevent cerebral oedema.[39] Dexamethasone, 32 mg immediately, 8 mg four times daily given as soon as stage 3 encephalopathy was reached, did not reduce the occurrence of intracranial hypertension or improve survival. Similarly, Ware et al.[261] were unable to demonstrate any difference between a corticosteroid-treated group and control group in patients with severe viral hepatitis. We do not use corticosteroids in the treatment of our patients.

PROSTAGLANDINS

Prostaglandins have been shown to be effective hepatic cytoprotective agents in animal models[166] and to exert some control over cerebral blood flow,[77] neurotransmitter release[118] and intracellular cytoprotection.[226] Cerebral oedema was improved but hepatocyte damage was aggravated by PGE_2 infusions in a rat model of FHF.[66] In contrast, prostaglandin E_2 blocked the development of fulminant hepatitis in a murine model of FHF.[1] However, in preliminary clinical studies, PGE_1 infusion has resulted in improved liver function and survival in FHF particularly in patients with stage 4 coma. Randomized, double-blind controlled trials are in progress.[1,221]

LIVER TRANSPLANTATION
(see Chapters 56 and 57)

The availability and improved results of liver transplantation have encouraged consideration of this option in selected patients with FHF.[29,35,127,151,180,230] The criteria for transplantation and for the timing of this procedure have yet to be defined. Better prognostic markers are urgently needed[182] to aid these decisions. Patients who are transplanted early may have survived without surgery. On the other hand, transplantation in the presence of stage 4 coma, sepsis, severe hepatorenal syndrome or gastrointestinal haemorrhage is associated with a poor prognosis.[29,127,151,180,229,230] Rapidly progressing encephalopathy, cerebral oedema, severe disturbances of coagulation and/or a shrinking liver indicate that transplantation is necessary. Ideally, patients with FHF should be referred to centres which offer transplantation at an early stage when their clinical condition is likely to be relatively stable. Patients with fulminant hepatic failure should be placed on the urgent transplantation list immediately and their clinical status should be assessed each time a potential donor becomes available.

Pretransplant evaluation should be limited but must include an ultrasonographic assessment of portal vein patency. The height and weight of the recipient are required for a good donor–recipient match. If matching is not possible, anatomic reduction of the donor organ may be required. ABO matching is desirable but not essential.[30]

FHF may be one of the few indications for heterotopic liver transplantation. In this procedure the host liver is left *in situ* and the graft is placed in a non-anatomic position. Recovery of the native liver would in theory allow the eventual removal of the grafted organ. However, heterotopic liver transplantation is associated with technical problems and in practice orthotopic transplantation remains the procedure of choice.[229]

The transplantation procedure is technically less difficult than in chronic liver disease since there are no venous collaterals. However, the operation must be performed as expertly and rapidly as possible, in order to minimize blood loss and resultant haemodynamic instability, which may further damage an already compromised brain. Venovenous bypass should be used in all cases, as it has greatly improved the outcome of transplantation in FHF.[218] It maintains intraoperative haemodynamic stability, decreases intraoperative blood loss and minimizes postoperative renal dysfunction (see Chapter 57).

Liver transplantation in FHF presents a major challenge to the anaesthetist. Maintainance of haemodynamic stability and correction of coagulopathy, acid–base and electrolyte imbalances are vital. Renal dysfunction with decreased or absent urine output adds to the complexity of the procedure. The morbidity and mortality of liver transplantation in FHF are comparable to those of liver transplantation for more conventional indications.[30,35,126,229] Successful transplantation is followed by a return of consciousness within the first few days in the majority of patients.[30] The early period following liver transplantation can be extremely critical, with many complex problems. However, the postoperative management and immunosuppression are similar to those used for any other liver transplant recipient.

The aetiology of FHF is important since it influences therapy and prognosis after transplantation. Hepatitis viruses may infect the transplanted liver. This is particularly important in HBV FHF, where the incidence of graft infection may be as high as 30–50%.[35,126,230] The use of immune serum globulins containing hepatitis B antibodies and of hepatitis B vaccines has failed to prevent hepatitis after transplantation.[35,127,207] The inability to predict graft infection or its severity and the encouraging outcome of patients after transplantation for virus-induced FHF suggest that transplantation should not be excluded because of the risk of graft infection.[127,229]

Transplantation for fulminant hepatic failure due to Wilson's disease is especially worthwhile since the procedure not only saves the patient but also cures the metabolic disorder.[200]

It is unlikely that liver transplantation will become the treatment of choice for patients with fulminant hepatic failure. The capacity of the liver to regenerate in response to injury is well established. Unfortunately, the factors which initiate and control the regenerative response have not yet been elucidated. The apparent lack of adequate regeneration seen in some patients with FHF may be due to a defect in control of the regenerative process or to hepatocellular injury beyond a critical level. Factors which control or modify the regenerative response could in the future be used as a therapeutic modality in patients with hepatic failure. Alternatively, artificial support devices could be used to maintain patients until regeneration occurs.

Key issues in liver transplantation for fulminant hepatic failure include the need for better prognostic markers, the need for objective criteria to determine the optimum timing of the transplant, definition of the relative risks in viral hepatitis, and responsible allocation of donor organs.

EXCHANGE TRANSFUSION, PLASMAPHERESIS, EXTRACORPOREAL LIVER PERFUSION AND CROSS-CIRCULATION

Over the past 20 years several techniques have been designed to support patients with FHF while liver regeneration proceeds. Despite early enthusiasm, exchange transfusion,[203,246] cross-circulation,[214] extracorporeal liver perfusion[88] and plasmapheresis[92,147] have at best been modestly successful in improving encephalopathy and none has improved survival.

CHARCOAL HAEMOPERFUSION

Charcoal haemoperfusion, first reported in 1972,[43] has recently been assessed in a large controlled study of patients with FHF.[183] There was no improvement in survival. In a recent review of charcoal haemoperfusion in FHF, Berk commented that 'use of devices of uncertain capability to correct defects of uncertain character was not likely to be clinically effective'.[23] This state of affairs is likely to persist until the exact pathogenesis of hepatic failure has been elucidated.

HEPATOCYTE TRANSPLANTATION

Hepatocyte transplantation has recently been the subject of two reviews.[37,168] Bumgardner et al. have discussed the most practical source of cells, the procedures necessary for the highest rate of engraftment, the hepatotrophic factors required for promoting engraftment, function and regeneration, and the prevention of rejection.[37] While hepatocyte transplantation has been able to reverse metabolic defects in experimental animals, the use of this procedure in FHF remains a theoretical possibility.

EXPERIMENTAL MODELS OF FHF

A number of experimental models of fulminant hepatic failure have been developed in order to try to elucidate the precise pathophysiology of acute liver disease.[170,238] The most recent of these uses three doses of acetaminophen in the dog. Untreated this resulted in a consistent (90%) mortality rate within 72 hours.[91] A pig model with a similar reproducible survival period has been developed by our group[117] using a combination of hepatic arterial ischaemia followed by injection of carbon tetrachloride into the portal venous system. Both these models satisfy the criteria suggested by Miller et al.[163] and by Terblanche[212,238] and their availability may offer more opportunities to investigate some of the many problems in the management of this complex disorder.

CONCLUSIONS

The clinical syndrome of fulminant hepatic failure is easily recognized but its treatment still poses many problems. The final assessment of any new form of therapy for which increased survival rates are claimed must include prospective controlled trials, as has been emphasized by Chalmers.[42] Such trials can be carried out only in centres where sufficient numbers of patients are seen to make them possible. Thus far, all forms of 'special' treatment assessed in this way have been found wanting, and current management in Cape Town revolves around adequate intensive care and management of specific complications.

REFERENCES

1. Abecassis, M., Falk, J.A., Makowka, L. *et al.* (1987) 16,16-Dimethyl prostaglandin E₂ prevents the development of fulminant hepatitis and blocks the induction of monocyte/macrophage procoagulant activity after murine hepatitis virus strain 3 infection. *Journal of Clinical Investigation,* **80,** 881–889.
2. Acute Hepatic Failure Study Group (1979) Etiology and prognosis in fulminant hepatitis. *Gastroenterology,* **77,** A33 (abstract).
3. Adams, R.D. & Foley, J.M. (1953) The neurological disorder associated with liver disease. In Merritt, H.H. & Hare, C.C. (eds) *Metabolic and Toxic Diseases of the Nervous System,* pp. 198–237. Baltimore: Williams & Wilkins.
4. Aguirre, A., Yoshimura, N., Westman, T. & Fischer, J.E. (1974) Plasma amino acids in dogs with two experimental forms of liver damage. *Journal of Surgical Research,* **16,** 339–345.
5. Akeyama, T., Koyama, T. & Kameda, T. (1972) Alpha-fetoprotein in acute hepatitis. *New England Journal of Medicine,* **287,** 989.
6. Alam, A.N., Wilkinson, S.P., Poston, L. *et al.* (1977) Intracellular electrolyte abnormalities in fulminant hepatic failure. *Gastroenterology,* **72,** 914–917.
7. Alexander, M., Kirsch, R.E., Purves, L. & Saunders, S.J. (1977) Alpha foetoprotein in liver disease: Groote Schuur Hospital experience, 1975–1976. *South African Medical Journal,* **53,** 433–435.
8. Alexander, W.F., Spindel, E., Harty, R.F., & Cerda, J.J. (1989) The usefulness of branched-chain amino acids in patients with acute or chronic hepatic encephalopathy. *American Journal of Gastroenterology,* **84,** 91–96.
9. Almdal, T., Schroeder, T. & Ranek, L. (1989) Cerebral blood flow and liver function in patients with encephalopathy due to acute and chronic liver diseases. *Scandinavian Journal of Gastroenterology,* **24,** 299–303.
10. Alp, M.H. & Hickman, R. (1987) The effect of prostaglandins, branched-chain amino acids and other drugs on the outcome of experimental acute porcine hepatic failure. *Journal of Hepatology,* **4,** 99–107.
11. Altin, M., Rajkouvic, I.A., Hughes R.D. & Williams, R. (1983) Neutrophil adherence in chronic liver disease and fulminant hepatic failure. *Gut,* **24,** 746–750.
12. Andreas, R., Swerdolff, R., Prozefsky, T. & Coleman, D. (1966) Manual feedback technique for the control of blood glucose concentration. In Skeggs, L.T. Jr. (ed.) *Automation in Analytical Chemistry,* pp. 486–489. White Plains, New York: Mediad.
13. Arcidi, J.M. Jr, Moore, G.W. & Hutchins, G.M. (1981) Hepatic morphology in cardiac dysfunction. A clinicopathological study of 1000 subjects at autopsy. *American Journal of Pathology,* **104,** 159–166.
14. Ariett, A. & Papadakis, M.A. (1988) Hyponatraemia and hypernatraemia in liver disease. In Epstein, M. (ed.) *The Kidney in Liver Disease,* pp. 73–86. Baltimore: Williams & Wilkins.
15. Aronson, D.L. (1979) Factor IX complex. *Seminars in Thrombosis and Haemostatis,* **6,** 28–31.
16. Baele, G., Vermeire, P., Demenlenaere, L. & Barber, F. (1973)

Elevation of factor VIII in acute liver necrosis. *Digestion*, **8**, 360–367.

17. Bailey, R.J., Woolf, I.L., Cullens, H. & Williams, R. (1976) Metabolic inhibition of polymorphonuclear leucocytes in fulminant hepatic failure. *Lancet*, **1**, 1162–1163.

18. Baker, A.L., Elson, C., Jaspan, J. & Boyer, J.L. (1979) Liver failure with steatonecrosis after jejunoileal bypass. *Archives of Internal Medicine*, **139**, 289–292.

19. Baldessarini, R.J. & Fischer, J.E. (1973) Serotonin metabolism in rat brain after surgical diversion of portal venous circulation. *Nature; New Biology*, **245**, 25–27.

20. Baraldi, M. & Zeneroli, M.L. (1982) Experimental hepatic encephalopathy: Changes in binding of gamma-amino butyric acid. *Science*, **216**, 427–429.

21. Bass, N.M., Kirsch, R.E., Tuff, S.A. & Saunders, S.J. (1976) Plasma ligandin: A sensitive index of experimental hepatic necrosis. *Gastroenterology*, **71**, A2/895.

22. Benhamou, J.P., Rueff, R.L. & Sicot, C. (1969) Severe hepatic failure: A critical study of current therapy. In Orlandi, F. & Jezequel, A.M. (eds) *Liver and Drugs*, pp. 213–228. London: Academic Press.

23. Berk, P.D. & Goldberg, J.D. (1988) Charcoal hemoperfusion. Plus cà change, plus c'est la mème chose. *Gastroenterology*, **94**, 1228–1230.

24. Bernuau, J., Goudeau, A., Poynard, T. *et al.* (1983) Hepatitis A virus infection: An uncommon cause of fulminant hepatitis with a high survival rate. *Hepatology*, **3**, 821 (abstract).

25. Bernuau, J., Rueff, B. & Benhamou, J.-P. (1986) Fulminant and subfulminant liver failure: Definitions and causes. *Seminars in Liver Disease* **6**(2), 97–106.

26. Better, O.S. & Schrier, R.W. (1983) Disturbed volume homeostasis in patients with cirrhosis of the liver. *Kidney International*, **23**, 303–311.

27. Bihari, D. (1985) Acute liver failure. *Clinics in Anaesthesiology*, **3**, 973–997.

28. Bihari, D.J., Gimson, A.E.S. & Williams, R. (1986) Cardiovascular pulmonary and renal complications of fulminant hepatic failure. *Seminars in Liver Disease*, **6**, 119–128.

29. Bismuth, H., Houssin, D. & Mazmanian, G. (1983) Postoperative liver insufficiency: Prevention and Management. *World Journal of Surgery*, **7**, 505–510.

30. Bismuth, H., Samuel, D., Gugenheim, J. *et al.* (1987) Emergency liver transplantation for fulminant hepatitis. *Annals of Internal Medicine*, **107**, 337–341.

31. Bloomer, J.R., Waldmann, T.A., McIntire, K.R. & Klatskin, G. (1975) Relationship of serum alpha-fetoprotein to the severity and duration of illness in patients with viral hepatitis. *Gastroenterology*, **68**, 342–350.

32. Bloomer, J.R., Waldmann, T.A., McIntire, K.R. & Klatskin, G. (1977) Serum alpha-fetoprotein in patients with massive hepatic necrosis. *Gastroenterology*, **72**, 479–482.

33. Boyer, T.D. & Reynolds, T.B. (1976) The effect of indomethacin on renal blood flow and creatinine clearance in patients with cirrhosis. *Gastroenterology*, **70**, 121A.

34. Braude, S., Arias, J., Hughes, R.D. *et al.* (1981) Antithrombin III infusion during fulminant hepatic failure. *Thrombosis and Haemostasis*, **46**, 369 (abstract).

35. Brems, J.J., Hiatt, J.R., Ramming, K.P. *et al.* (1987) Fulminant hepatic failure: The role of liver transplantation as primary therapy. *American Journal of Surgery*, **154**, 137–141.

36. Brunner, G., Windus, G. & Schmidt, F.W. (1984) Intra cranial pressure and brain oedema in experimental hyper ammonemia. In Kleinberger, G. & Ferenci, P. (eds) *Advances in Hepatic Encephalopathy and Urea Cycle Disease*, pp. 325–330. Basel: Karger.

37. Bumgardner, G.L., Fasola, C. & Sutherland, D.E.R. (1988) Prospects for hepatocyte transplantation. *Hepatology*, **8**, 1158–1161.

38. Cade, R., Wagemaker, H., Vogel, S. *et al.* (1987) Hepatorenal syndrome: Studies of the effect of vascular volume and intraperitoneal pressure on renal and hepatic function. *American Journal of Medicine*, **82**, 427–438.

39. Canalese, J., Gimson, A.E.S., Davis, C. *et al.* (1982) Controlled trial of dexamethasone and mannitol for the cerebral oedema of fulminant hepatic failure. *Gut*, **23**, 625–629.

40. Capocaccia, L., Ferenci, P., Fischer, J.E. & Opolon, P. (1989) Mechanisms of hepatic encephalopathy: Certainties and uncertainties. *Gastroenterology International*, **2**(3), 131–140.

41. Caronna, J.J., Leigh, J., Shaw, D. *et al.* (1975) The outcome of medical coma prediction by bedside assessment of physical signs. *Transactions of the American Neurological Association*, **100**, 25–29.

42. Chalmers, T.C. (1976) A shortage of reliable data. *New England Journal of Medicine*, **294**, 721–722.

43. Chang, T.M.S. (1972) Haemoperfusion over microencapsulated adsorbent in a patient with hepatic coma. *Lancet*, **2**, 1371–1372.

44. Charlesworth, J.A., Lawrence, S., Worsdall, P.A. *et al.* (1977) Acute hepatitis: Significance of changes in complement components. *Clinical and Experimental Immunology*, **28**, 496–501.

45. Chu, N.S. & Yang, S.S. (1988) Portalsystemic encephalopathy: Alterations in somatosensory and brain stem auditory evoked potentials. *Journal of the Neurological Sciences*, **84**, 41–50.

46. Clark, R.D., Gazzard, G.B., Lewis, M.L. *et al.* (1975) Fibrinogen metabolism in acute hepatitis and active chronic hepatitis. *British Journal of Haematology*, **30**, 95–102.

47. Clarke, G.M. (1985) Multiple system organ failure. *Clinics in Anaesthesiology*, **3**, 1027–1057.

48. Clasen, R.A., Pandolfi, S. & Casey, D. (1974) Furosemide and pentobarbital in cryogenic cerebral injury and edema. *Neurology (Minn)*, **24**, 642–648.

49. Clasen, R.A., Pandolfi, S., Laing, I. & Casey, D. (1974) Experimental study of relation of fever to cerebral oedema. *Journal of Neurosurgery*, **41**, 478–481.

50. Cohen, J.A. & Kaplan, M.M. (1978) Left sided heart failure presenting as hepatitis. *Gastroenterology*, **74**, 583–587.

51. Colman, R.W. (1989) The role of plasma proteases in septic shock. *New England Journal of Medicine*, **320**, 1207–1208.

52. Conn, H.O. & Atterbury, C.E. (1987) Cirrhosis. In Schiff, L. & Schiff, E.R. (eds) *Diseases of the Liver*, pp. 725–864. Philadelphia: Lippincott.

53. Conn, H.O. (1977) The trailmaking and number connection tests in assessing mental state in portal–systemic encephalopathy. *American Journal of Digestive Diseases*, **22**, 541–550.

54. Cooper, A.J.L. & Plum, F. (1987) Cerebral ammonia. *Physiology Reviews*, **67**, 440–519.

55. Cooper, J.R., Bloom, F.E. & Roth, R.H. (1982) *The Biochemical Basis of Neuropharmacology*, 4th edn. New York: Oxford University Press.

56. Cuypers, J., Matakis, F. & Potolicchio, S.J. (1976) Effect of central venous pressure on brain tissue pressure and volume. *Journal of Neurosurgery*, **45**, 89–94.

57. Dahl, D.R. (1968) Short chain fatty acid inhibition of rat brain Na^+,K^+ adenosine triphosphatase. *Journal of Neurochemistry*, **15**, 815–820.

58. Dammann, H.G., Hagemann, J., Runge, M. & Kloppel, G. (1982) In vivo diagnosis of massive hepatic infarction by computed tomography. *Digestive Diseases and Sciences*, **27**, 73–79.

59. Davies, M.H., Wilkinson, S.P., Hanid, M.A. *et al.* (1980) Acute liver disease with encephalopathy and renal failure in late pregnancy and the early puerperium. A study of fourteen cases. *British Journal of Obstetrics and Gynaecology*, **87**, 1005–1014.

60. Davis, M. (1986) Protective agents for acetaminophen overdose. *Seminars in Liver Disease*, **6**(2), 138–147.

61. Dawson, D.J., Babbs, C., Warnes, T.W. & Neary, R.H. (1987) Hypophosphataemia in acute liver failure. *British Medical Journal*, **295**, 1312–1313.

62. Dawson, J.L. (1964) Jaundice and anoxic renal damage: Protective effect of mannitol. *British Medical Journal*, **1**, 810–811.

63. Decaux, G., Mols, P., Cauchi, P. & Delwiche, F. (1985) Use of urea for treatment of water retention in hyponatraemic cirrhosis with ascites resistant to diuretics. *British Medical Journal*, **290**, 1782–1783.

64. Dempsey, R.J., & Kindt, G.W. (1982) Experimental acute hepatic encephalopathy: Relationship of pathological cerebral vasodilation to increased intracranial pressure. *Neurosurgery*, **10**, 737–741.

65. Dienstag, J.L. (1989) Passive-active immunoprophylaxis after percutaneous exposure to hepatitis B virus. *Hepatology*, **10**(3), 385–387.

66. Dixit, V. & Chang, T.M.S. (1987) Effects of prostaglandin E_2 on brain edema and liver histopathology in a galactosamine-induced fulminant hepatic failure rat model. *Biomaterials, Artificial Cells and Artificial Organs*, **15**, 559–573.

67. Dodsworth, J.M., James, J.H., Cummings, M.C. & Fischer, J.E. (1974) Depletion of brain norepinephrine in acute hepatic surgery. *Surgery*, **75**, 811–820.

68. Ducci, H. & Katz, R. (1952) Cortisone, ACTH and antibiotics in fulminant hepatitis. *Gastroenterology*, **21**, 357–374.

69. Duffy, T.E. & Plum, F. (1982) Hepatic encephalopathy. In Arias, I., Popper, H., Schachter, D. & Shafritz, D.A. (eds) *The Liver; Biology and Pathobiology*, pp. 693–713. New York: Raven Press.

70. EASL (1979) Randomized trial of steroid therapy in acute liver failure. Report from the European Association for the Study of the Liver. *Gut*, **20**, 620–623.

71. Ede, R.J., Gimson, A.E.S., Bihari, D. & Williams, R. (1986) Controlled hyperventilation in the prevention of cerebral oedema in fulminant hepatic failure. *Journal of Hepatology*, **2**, 43–51.

72. Ede, R.J., Gimson, A.E.S., Canalese, J. & Williams, R. (1982) Cerebral oedema and monitoring of intracranial pressure. *Gastroenterologia Japonica*, **17**, 163–176.

73. Ede, R.J., Gove, C.D. & Williams, R. (1984) Reduced Na^+,K^+-ATPase activity during acute hepatic failure in the rat: A possible cause for encephalopathy and cerebral oedema. *Clinical Science*, **66**, 62p.

74. Ede, R.J., Gove, C.D., Hughes, R.D. *et al.* (1987) Reduced brain Na^+,K^+-ATPase activity in rats with galactosamine-induced hepatic failure: Relationship to encephalopathy and cerebral oedema. *Clinical Science*, **72**, 365–371.

75. Ede, R.J. & Williams, R. (1986) Hepatic encephalopathy and cerebral oedema. *Seminars in Liver Disease*, **6**, 107–118.

76. Edelman, I.S., Leibman, J., O-Meara, M.P. & Birkenfeld, L.W. (1958) Interrelationships between serum sodium concentration, serum osmolarity and total exchangeable sodium, total exchangeable potassium and total body water. *Journal of Clinical Investigation*, **37**, 1236–1256.

77. Ellis, E.F., Kontos, N.A. & Oates, J.A. (1980) The prostaglandin, thromboxane system and coronary and cerebral arterial smooth muscle tone. In Scriabine, J., Keffer, A. & Kuehlf, A. (eds) *Prostaglandins in Cardiovascular and Renal Function*, pp. 209. Jamaica: Spectrum Publications.

78. Epstein, M., Berk, P.D., Hollenberg, N.K. *et al.* (1970) Renal failure in the patient with cirrhosis. The role of active vasoconstriction. *American Journal of Medicine*, **49**, 175–185.

79. Epstein, M. (1988) Hepatorenal syndrome. In Epstein, M. (ed.) *The Kidney in Liver Disease*, pp. 89–118. Baltimore: Willliams & Wilkins.

80. Eriksson, L.S. & Conn, H.O. (1989) Branched-chain amino acids in the management of hepatic encephalopathy: an analysis of variants. *Hepatology*, **10**, 228–246.

81. Faulstich, H. (1979) New aspects of amanita poisoning. *Klinische Wochenschrift*, **57**, 1143–1152.

82. Ferenci, P., Pappas, S.C., Munson, P.J. *et al.* (1984) Changes in the status of neurotransmitter receptors in a rabbit model of hepatic encephalopathy. *Hepatology*, **4**, 186–191.

83. Fisch, B.J. & Klass, D.W. (1988) The diagnostic specificity of triphasic wave patterns. *Electroencephalography and Clinical Neurophysiology*, **70**, 1–8.

84. Fischer, J.E. & Baldessarini, R.J. (1971) False neurotransmitters and hepatic failure. *Lancet*, **2**, 75–80.

85. Fischer, J.E., Funovics, J.M., Aquirra, J.H. *et al.* (1965) The role of plasma amino acids in hepatic encephalopathy. *Surgery*, **78**, 276–290.

86. Fischer, J.E., Rosen, H.M., Ebeid, A.M. *et al.* (1976) The effect of normalization of plasma amino acids on hepatic encephalopathy in man. *Surgery*, **80**, 77–91.

87. Fischer, J.E. (1974) Occurrence of false neurotransmitters. In Williams, R. & Murray-Lyon, I.M. (eds) *Artificial Liver Support*, pp. 31–50. Tunbridge Wells: Pitman Medical.

88. Fischer, M., Botterman, P., von Sommoggy, S. *et al.* (1981) Functional capacity of extracorporeal baboon liver perfusions. In Brunner, G. & Schmidt, F.W. (eds) *Artificial Liver Support*, pp. 280–286. Berlin: Springer-Verlag.

89. Flock, E.B., Lock, M.A., Grundley, J.G. *et al.* (1953) Changes in free amino acids in brain after total hepatectomy. *Journal of Biological Chemistry*, **200**, 529–536.

90. Forbes, A., Alexander, G.J.M., O'Grady, J.G. *et al.* (1989) Thiopental infusion in the treatment of intracranial hypertension complicating fulminant hepatic failure. *Hepatology*, **10**, 306–310.

91. Francavilla, A., Makowka, L., Polimeno, L. *et al.* (1989) A dog model of acetominophen-induced fulminant hepatic failure. *Gastroenterology*, **96**, 470–478.

92. Freeman, J.G., Matthewson, K. & Record, C.O. (1989) Plasmapheresis in acute liver failure. *International Journal of Artificial Organs*, **9**, 433–438.

93. Gallus, A.S., Mucas, C.R. & Hirsh, J. (1972) Coagulation studies in patients with acute infectious hepatitis. *British Journal of Haematology*, **22**, 761–771.

94. Gassner, A., Kleinberger, G., Pichler, M. *et al.* (1981) Infektinem Bei Coma Hepaticum. *Leber, Magen, Darm.*, **11**, 21–24.

95. Gazzard, B.G., Lewis, M.L., Ash, M.I. *et al.* (1974) Coagulation factor concentrate in the treatment of the haemorrhagic diathesis of fulminant liver failure. *Gut*, **15**, 993–998.

96. Gazzard, B.G., Portman, B., Murray-Lyon, I.M. & Williams, R. (1975) Causes of death in fulminant hepatic failure and relationship to quantitative histological assessment of parenchymal damage. *Quarterly Journal of Medicine*, **176**, 615–626.

97. Gazzard, B.G., Price, H. & Dawson, A.M. (1986) Detection of hepatic encephalopathy. *Postgraduate Medical Journal*, **62**(725), 163–166.

98. Gazzard, B.G., Rake, M.O., Flute, P.T. & Williams, R. (1975) Bleeding in relation to the coagulation defect of fulminant hepatic failure. In Williams, R., Murray-Lyon, I.M. (eds) *Artificial Liver Support*. London: Pitman Medical.

99. Gimson, A.E.S., O'Grady, J., Ede, R.J. *et al.* (1986) Late-onset fulminant hepatic failure: Clinical, serological and histological features. *Hepatology*, **6**, 288–294.

100. Gimson, A.E.S., White, Y.S., Eddleston, A.L.W.F. & Williams, R. (1983) Clinical and prognostic differences in fulminant hepatitis type A, B and non-A, non-B. *Gut*, **24**, 1194–1198.

101. Gitler, R.E. (1962) Spontaneous hypoglycaemia. *New York Journal of Medicine*, **62**, 236–250.

102. Gitlin, D. & Boesman, M. (1967) Sites of serum alphafetoprotein synthesis in the human and in the rat. *Journal of Clinical Investigation*, **46**, 1010–1016.

103. Gitlin, N. (1988) Sub-clinical portal–systemic encephalopathy. *American Journal of Gastroenterology*, **83**(1), 8–11.

104. Gitlin, N., Lewis, D.C. & Hinkley, L. (1986) The diagnosis and prevalence of subclinical hepatic encephalopathy in apparently healthy, ambulant, non-shunted patients with cirrhosis. *Journal of Hepatology*, **3**, 75–82.

105. Govindarajan, S., Chin, K.P., Redeker, A.G. & Peters, R.L. (1984) Fulminant B viral hepatitis: Role of delta agent. *Gastroenterology*, **86**, 1417–1420.

106. Grimm, G., Katzenschlager, R., Lenz, K. *et al.* (1988) Improvement of hepatic encephalopathy treated with flumazenil. *Lancet*, **2**, 1392–1394.

107. Haefely, W., Polc, P., Pieri, L. *et al.* (1983) Neuropharmacology of benzodiazepines: Synaptic mechanisms and neural basis of action. In Costa, E. (ed.) *The Benzodiapines: From Molecular Biology to Clinical Practice*, pp. 21–66. New York: Raven Press.

108. Halstead, A.C. & Nanji, A.A. (1982) Artefactual lowering of serum creatinine in the presence of hyperbilirubinaemia—a method-dependent artefact. *Journal of the American Medical Association*, **251**, 38–39.

109. Hanid, M.A., Davies, M., Mellon, P.J. *et al.* (1980) Clinical monitoring of intracranial pressure in fulminant hepatic failure. *Gut*, **21**, 866–869.

110. Hanid, M.A., MacKenzie, R.L., Jenner, R.E. *et al.* (1979) Intracranial pressure in pigs with surgically induced acute liver failure. *Gastroenterology*, **76**, 123–131.

111. Hanid, M.A., Silk, D.B. & Williams, R. (1978) Prognostic value of the oculovestibular reflex in fulminant hepatic failure. *British Medical Journal*, **1**, 1029–1033.

112. Harrison, H.B., Middleton, H.M., Crosby, J.H. & Dasher, N. (1981) Fulminant hepatic failure: An unusual presentation of metastatic liver disease. *Gastroenterology*, **80**, 820–825.

113. Henderson, J., Millikan, W.J. & Warren, W.D. (1982) Manipulation of the amino acid profiles in cirrhosis with hepatic aid or FO80 fails to reverse encephalopathy. *Hepatology*, **2**, 706.

114. Herlin, P.M., James, J.H., Nachbauer, C.A. & Fischer, J.E.

(1983) Effect of total hepatectomy and administration of branched-chain amino acid on regional norepinephrine dopamine and amino acids in rat brain. *Annals of Surgery*, 198, 172–177.

115. Herlin, P.M., James, J.H., Nauchbaver, C. & Fischer, J.E. (1981) The blood-brain barrier is intact eighteen hours after total hepatectomy. *Hepatology*, 1, 515 (abstract).

116. Herlong, H.F., Maddrey, W. C. & Mackenzie, W. (1980) The use of ornithine salts of branched chain amino acids in portal systemic encephalopathy. *Annals of Internal Medicine*, 93, 545–550.

117. Hickman, R. & Alp, M.H. (1986) A predictable pathophysiological model of porcine hepatic failure. *European Journal of Surgical Research*, 18, 283–292.

118. Hillier, K., Roberts, P.J. & Wollard, P. (1976) Catecholamine stimulated prostaglandin synthesis in rat brain synaptosomes. *British Journal of Pharmacology*, 58, 426P–430P.

119. Holliday, M.A., Kalayci, M.N. & Harrah, J. (1968) Factors that limit brain volume changes in response to acute and sustained hyper- and hyponatraemia. *Journal of Clinical Investigation*, 47, 1916–1928.

120. Horowitz, M.E., Schafer, D.F., Molnar, P. *et al.* (1983) Increased blood–brain barrier transfer in a rabbit model of acute liver failure. *Gastroenterology*, 84, 1003–1011.

121. Hourani, B.T., Halin, E.M. & Reynolds, T.B. (1971) Cerebro-spinal fluid glutamine as a measure of hepatic encephalopathy. *Archives of Internal Medicine*, 127, 1033–1036.

122. Hughes, R.D., Imawari, M., Bihari, D. *et al.* (1986) Fibronectin replacement in patients with fulminant hepatic failure. *European Journal of Clinical Investigation*, 16(5), 352–356.

123. Iber, F.L., Rosen, H., Levenson, S.M. & Chalmers, T.C. (1957) The plasma amino acids in patients with liver failure. *Journal of Laboratory and Clinical Medicine*, 50, 417–425.

124. Iob, V., Coon, W.W. & Sloan, M. (1966) Altered concentrations of free amino acids from the plasma of patients with cirrhosis of the liver. *Journal of Surgical Research*, 6, 233–239.

125. Iob, V., Mattson, W.J. Jr, Sloan, M. *et al.* (1970) Alterations in plasma free amino acids in dogs with hepatic insufficency. *Surgery, Gynecology and Obstetrics*, 130, 794–801.

126. Iwatsuki, S., Popovtzer, M.M., Corman, J.L. *et al.* (1973) Recovery from hepatorenal syndrome after orthotopic liver transplantation. *New England Journal of Medicine*, 289, 1155–1159.

127. Iwatsuki, S., Stieber, A.C., Marsh, J.W. *et al.* (1989) Liver transplantation for fulminant hepatic failure. *Transplantation Proceedings*, 21, 2431–2434.

128. James, H.E., Bruce, D.A. & Welsh, F. (1978) Cytotoxic edema produced by 6-amino-nicotinamide and its response to therapy. *Neurosurgery*, 3, 196–200.

129. Jenkins, P.J. & Williams, R. (1980) Fulminant viral hepatitis. *Clinical Gastroenterology*, 9, 171–189.

130. Jones, E.A., Skolnick, P., Gammal, S.H. *et al.* (1989) The gamma-aminobutyric acid A (GABA$_A$) receptor complex and hepatic encephalopathy. Some recent advances. *Annals of Internal Medicine*, 110, 532–546.

131. Joshi, Y.K., Gandhi, B.M. & Tandon, B.N. (1983) Spectrum of hepatitis A virus infection in India. *Hepatology*, 3, 160 (abstract).

132. Karvountzis, G. & Redeker, A.G. (1974) Relation of alpha-fetoprotein in acute hepatitis to severity and prognosis. *Annals of Internal Medicine*, 80, 156–160.

133. Katelaris, P.H. & Jones, D.B. (1989) Fulminant hepatic failure. *Medical Clinics of North America*, 73(4), 953–970.

134. Katz, R., Velasco, M., Klinger, J. & Allesandri, H. (1962) Corticosteroids in the treatment of acute hepatitis in coma. *Gastroenterology*, 42, 258–265.

135. Kelly, D.A. & Summerfield, J.A. (1987) Hemostasis in liver disease. *Seminars in Liver Disease*, 7(3), 182–191.

136. Kew, M., Behrson, H., Seftel, H. & Kent, G. (1970) Liver damage in heatstroke. *American Journal of Medicine*, 49, 192–202.

137. Kew, M.C., Purves, L.P., Branch, W.R. & Behrson, I. (1973) Alphafetoprotein during hepatocellular regeneration. In Saunders, S.J. & Terblanche, J. (eds) *Liver*, pp. 320–321. London: Pitman Medical.

138. Khuroo, M.S., Teli, M.R., Skidmore, S. *et al.* (1981) Incidence and severity of viral hepatitis in pregnancy. *American Journal of Medicine*, 70, 252–255.

139. Kirsch, R.E., Frith, L. & Saunders, S.J. (1976) Stimulation of albumin synthesis by keto analogues of amino acids. *Biochimica et Biophysica Acta*, 442, 437–441.

140. Klatzo, I. (1978) Cerebral oedema and ischemia. *Recent Advances in Neuropathology*, 1, 27–39.

141. Knell, A.J., Davison, A.R., Williams, R. *et al.* (1974) Dopamine and serotonin metabolism in hepatic encephalopathy. *British Medical Journal*, 1, 549–551.

142. Knochel, J.P. (1989) Does hypophosphataemia play a role in acute liver failure? *Hepatology*, 9, 504–505.

143. Knudsen, G.M., Poulsen, H.E. & Paulson, O.B. (1988) Blood–brain permeability in galactosamine-induced hepatic encephalopathy. *Journal of Hepatology*, 6(2), 187–192.

144. Koppel, M.H., Coburn, J.W., Mims, M.M. *et al.* (1969) Transplantation of cadaveric kidneys from patients with hepatorenal syndrome. Evidence for the functional nature of renal failure in advanced liver disease. *New England Journal of Medicine*, 280, 1367–1371.

145. Lassen, N.A. & Christensen, M.S. (1976) Physiology of cerebral blood flow. *British Journal of Anaesthesiology*, 48, 719–734.

146. Laursen, B., Mortensen, J.Z., Frost, L. & Hansen, K.B. (1981) Disseminated intravascular coagulation in hepatic failure treated with antithrombin III. *Thrombosis Research*, 22, 701–740.

147. Kepore, M.J. & Martel, A.J. (1967) Plasmapheresis in hepatic coma. *Lancet*, 2, 771–772.

148. Levy, L.J., Bolton, R.P. & Losowsky, M.S. (1987) The use of visual evoked potential (VEP) in delineating a state of subclinical encephalopathy. A comparison with the number-connection test. *Journal of Hepatology*, 5, 211–217.

149. Livingstone, A.S., Potvin, M., Goresky, C.A. *et al.* (1977) Changes in the blood–brain barrier in hepatic coma after hepatectomy in the rat. *Gastroenterology*, 73, 697–702.

150. Lo, W.D., Ennis, S.R., Goldstein, G.W. *et al.* (1987) The effects of galactosamine-induced hepatic failure upon blood–brain barrier permeability. *Hepatology*, 7, 452–456.

151. Lorber, M.I. (1988) Emergency liver transplantation in fulminant hepatitis. *Hepatology*, 8, 431–432.

152. Maddrey, W.C. (1984) Hepatic vein thrombosis (Budd–Chiari Syndrome). *Hepatology*, 4(1), 445–465.

153. Maddrey, W.C., Weber, F.L., Coulter, A.W. *et al.* (1976) The effects of keto analogues of essential amino acids on portal systemic encephalopathy. *Gastroenterology*, 71, 190–195.

154. Mans, A.M., Biebuyck, J.F. & Hawkins, A.A. (1983) Ammonia selectively stimulates neutral amino acid transport across the blood–brain barrier. *American Journal of Physiology*, 245, C72–C76.

155. Mans, A.M., Biebucyk, J.F., Saunders, S.J. & Kirsch, R.E. (1979) Tryptophan transport across the blood–brain barrier during hepatic failure. *Journal of Neurochemistry*, 33, 409–418.

156. Mans, A.M., Saunders, S.J., Kirsch, R.E. & Biebuyck, J.F. (1979) Correlation of plasma and brain amino acid and putative neurotransmitter alterations during acute hepatic coma in the rat. *Journal of Neurochemistry*, 32, 285–292.

157. Marshall, A.W., Jakobovits, A.W. & Morgan, M.Y. (1982) Bromocriptine-associated hyponatraemia in cirrhosis. *British Medical Journal*, 285, 1534–1535.

158. Mathiesen, L.R., Skinoj, P., Nielson, J.O. *et al.* (1980) Hepatitis A, B and non-A, non-B in fulminant hepatitis. *Gut*, 21, 72–77.

159. Mattson, W.J. Jr, Iob, V., Sloan, M. *et al.* (1970) Alteration of individual free amino acids in brain during acute hepatic coma. *Surgery, Gynecology and Obstetrics*, 130, 263–266.

160. McMenamy, R.H., Vang, J. & Trapanas, T. (1965) Amino acid and alphaketoacid concentration in plasma and blood of the liverless dog. *American Journal of Physiology*, 29, 1046–1052.

161. Mendenhall, C.L., Rouster, S., Marshall, L. & Weesner, R. (1986) A new therapy for portal systemic encephalopathy. *Journal of Gastroenterology*, 81, 540–543.

162. Michel, H., Solere, M., Granier, P. *et al.* (1980) Treatment of cirrhotic hepatic encephalopathy with L-dopa. A controlled trial. *Gastroenterology*, 79, 207–211.

163. Miller, D.J., Hickman, R., Fratter, R. *et al.* (1976) An animal model of fulminant hepatic failure: A feasibility study. *Gastroenterology*, 71, 109–113.

164. Miller, D.J., Saunders, S.J., Hickman, R. & Terblanche, J. (1975) Acute hepatic necrosis: A review of causes and management of

fulminant hepatic failure. In Read, A. (ed.) *Gastroenterology*, pp. 64–90. London: Butterworth.

165. Miller, L.L. (1962) The role of the liver and non-hepatic tissue in the regulation of free amino acid levels in the blood. In Holden, J.T. (ed.) *Amino Acid Pools*, pp. 716–717. Amsterdam: Elsevier.

166. Mizoguchi, Y., Hiroko, T., Miyajima, K. *et al.* (1987) The protective effects of prostaglandin E1 in an experimental massive hepatic cell necrosis model. *Hepatology*, 7, 1184–1188.

167. Mortensen, P.B., Rasmussen, H.S. & Holfug, K. (1988) Lactulose detoxifies in vitro short-chain fatty acid production in colonic contents induced by blood: Implications for hepatic coma. *Gastroenterology*, 94, 750–754.

168. Moscioni, A.D., Chowdhur, J.R., Barbour, R. *et al.* (1989) Human liver cell transplantation. *Gastroenterology*, 96, 1546–1551.

169. Mosvold, J., Abildgaard, U., Jenssen, H. & Anderson, R. (1982) Low antithrombin III in acute hepatic failure at term. *Scandinavian Journal of Haematology*, 29, 48–50.

170. Mullen, K.D., Schafer, D.F., Maynard T.F. *et al.* (1986) Galactosamine-induced fulminant hepatic failure in the rat may be an unsuitable model for acute hepatic encephalopathy: a comparison with the rabbit model. *Gastroenterology*, 90, 1750.

171. Mummery, R.V., Bradley, J.M. & Jeffries, D.J. (1971) Microbiological monitoring of patients with hepatic failure with particular reference to extracorporal porcine liver perfusion. *Lancet*, 2, 60–64.

172. Murray-Lyon, I.M., Orr, A.H., Gazzard, B. *et al.* (1976) Prognostic value of serum alpha-fetoprotein in fulminant hepatic failure including patients treated by charcoal haemoperfusion. *Gut*, 17, 576–580.

173. Murray-Lyon, I.M., Davidson, A.R., Rake, M.O. *et al.* (1973) Hepatic scintiscanning in fulminant hepatic failure. *British Journal of Radiology*, 46, 30–36.

174. Muto, Y., Nouri-Aria, K.T., Meager, A. *et al.* (1988) Enhanced tumour necrosis factor and interleukin-1 in fulminant hepatic failure. *Lancet*, 2, 72–74.

175. Narins, R.G. & Cohen, J. J. (1987) Bicarbonate therapy for organic acidosis: The case for its continued use. *Annals of Internal Medicine*, 106, 615–618.

176. Ngindu, A., Johnson, B.K., Kenya, P.R. *et al.* (1982) Outbreak of acute hepatitis caused by aflatoxin poisoning in Kenya. *Lancet*, 1, 1346–1348.

177. Nouel, O., Henrion, J., Bernuau, J. *et al.* (1980) Fulminant hepatic failure due to transient circulatory failure in patients with chronic heart disease. *Digestive Diseases and Sciences*, 25, 49–52.

178. Nussbaum, M. & Morse, B.S. (1964) Plasma fibrin stabilising factor activity in various diseases. *Blood*, 23, 669–678.

179. O'Brien, C.J., Wise, R.J., O'Grady, A.G. & Williams, R. (1987) Neurological sequelae in patients recovered from fulminant hepatic failure. *Gut*, 28, 93–95.

180. O'Grady, J.G. & Williams, R. (1988) Present position of liver transplantation and its impact on hepatological practice. *Gut*, 29, 566–570.

181. O'Grady, J.G. & Williams, R. (1989) Acute liver failure. *Ballière's Clinical Gastroenterology*, 3(1), 75–89.

182. O'Grady, J.G., Alexander, G.J.M., Hayler, K.M. & Williams, R. (1988) Early indicators of prognosis in acute liver failure and their application to selection of patients for orthotopic liver transplantation. *Gastroenterology*, 94, A578.

183. O'Grady, J.G., Gimson, A.E.S., O'Brien, C.J. *et al.* (1988) Controlled trials of charcoal hemoperfusion and prognostic factors in fulminant hepatic failure. *Gastroenterology*, 94, 1186–1192.

184. O'Grady, J.G., Langley, P.G., Isola, L.M. *et al.* (1986) Coagulopathy of fulminant hepatic failure. *Seminars in Liver Disease*, 6, 159–163.

185. O'Keefe, S.J., Ogden, J. & Dicker, J. (1987) Enteral and parenteral branched chain amino acid-supplemented nutritional support in patients with encephalopathy due to alcoholic liver disease. *Journal of Parenteral and Enteral Nutrition*, 11, 447–453.

186. Ohmi, N. & Arias, I. (1981) Ligandinaemia in primary liver cell cancer in rat and man. *Hepatology*, 1, 316.

187. Oster, J.R. & Perez, G.O. (1988) Acid-base homeostasis and pathophysiology in liver disease. In Epstein, M. (ed.) *The Kidney in Liver Disease*, pp. 119–131. Baltimore: Williams & Wilkins.

188. Oster, J.R., Epstein, M. & Vlarso, H.B. (1976) Deterioration of renal function with demeclocycline administration. *Current Therapeutic Research*, 20, 794–801.

189. Papaevangelou, G., Tassopoulos, N., Roumeliotou-Karayannis, A. & Richardson, C. (1984) Etiology of fulminant viral hepatitis in Greece. *Hepatology*, 4, 369–372.

190. Parbhoo, S.P., James, I.M., Ajdukiewicz, A. *et al.* (1971) Extracorporeal pig liver perfusion in the treatment of hepatic coma due to fulminant hepatitis. *Lancet*, 1, 659–665.

191. Parkes, J.D., Sharpestone, P. & Williams, R. (1970) Levodopa in hepatic coma. *Lancet*, 2, 1341–1343.

192. Parrish, A.G., Robson, S.C., Trey, C. & Kirsch, R.E. (1990) Retrospective survey of drug-induced liver disease at Groote Schuur Hospital, Cape Town – 1983–1987. *South African Medical Journal*, 77, 199–202.

193. Paulson, O.B. & Hertz, M.M. (1978) Blood–brain barrier permeability during short lasting intravascular hyperosmolarity. *European Journal of Clinical Investigation*, 8, 391–396.

194. Plum, F. & Hindfelt, B. (1976) The neurological complications of liver disease. In Vinken, B.J., Bruyn, G.W. & Klawans, H.L. (eds) *Handbook of Clinical Neurology*, vol. 27: *Metabolic and Deficiency Diseases in the Nervous System*, pp. 349–377. New York: American Elsevier Publishing.

195. Pollay, M., Fullenwider, C., Roberts, A. & Stevens, A. (1983) Effect of mannitol and furosemide on blood–brain osmotic gradient and intracranial pressure. *Journal of Neurosurgery*, 59, 945–950.

196. Purves, L.P., Branch, W.R. & Behrson, I. (1973) Alphafetoprotein during hepatocellular regeneration. In Saunders, S.J. & Terblanche, J. (eds) *Liver*, pp. 320–321. London: Pitman Medical.

197. Purves, L.R., & Geddes, E.W. (1972) A more sensitive test for alpha-fetoprotein. *Lancet*, 1, 47–48.

198. Quarforth, G., Ahmed, K. & Zieve, L. (1976) Action of methanethiol of membrane Na^+, K^+ ATPase of rat brain. *Biochemical Pharmacology*, 25, 1039–1044.

199. Raabe, W. & Onstad, G. (1985) Porta-caval shunting changes neuronal sensitivity to ammonia. *Journal of Neurological Science*, 71, 307–314.

200. Rakela, J., Kurtz, S.B., McCarthy, J.T. *et al.* (1986) Fulminant Wilsons disease treated with post dilution hemofiltration and orthotopic liver transplantation. *Gastroenterology*, 90, 2004.

201. Record, C.O., Buxton, C.E., Chase, R.A. *et al.* (1976) Plasma and brain amino acids in fulminant hepatic failure and their relationship to hepatic encephalopathy. *Finnish Journal of Clinical Investigation*, 6, 387–394.

202. Record, C.O., Iles, R.A., Cohen, R.D. *et al.* (1975) Acid-base and metabolic disturbances in fulminating hepatic failure. *Gut*, 16, 144–149.

203. Redeker, A.G. & Yamahiro, H.S. (1973) Controlled trial of exchange transfusion therapy in fulminant hepatitis. *Lancet*, 1, 3–6.

204. Reye, R.D.K., Morgan, G. & Baral, J. (1963) Encephalopathy and fatty degeneration of the viscera: a disease entity in childhood. *Lancet*, 2, 249–252.

205. Ring-Larsen, H., Hesse, B., Henriksen, J.H. & Christensen, N.J. (1982) Sympathetic nervous activity and renal and systemic hemodynamics in cirrhosis: plasma norepinephrine concentration, hepatic extraction and renin release. *Hepatology*, 2, 304–310.

206. Ritt, D.J., Whelan, G., Werner, D.J. *et al.* (1969) Acute hepatic necrosis with stupor or coma. *Medicine*, 48, 151–172.

207. Rizzetto, M., Macagno, S., Chaiberge, E. *et al.* (1987) Liver transplantation in hepatitis delta virus infection. *Lancet*, 2, 469–471.

208. Robson, S.C. (1989) Immune dysfunction in patients with extrahepatic portal venous obstruction. PhD Thesis, University of Cape Town.

209. Rolando, N., Harvey, F., Brahm, J. *et al.* (1990) Prospective study of bacterial infection in acute liver failure: an analysis of fifty patients. *Hepatology*, 11, 49–53.

209a.Rolando, N., Harvey, F., Brahm, J. *et al.* (1991) Fungal infection: a common, unrecognised complication of acute liver failure. *Journal of Hepatology*, 12, 1–9.

210. Ruoshlahti, E. & Seppala, M. (1972) Alpha-fetoprotein in normal human serum. *Nature*, 235, 161–162.

211. Samson, R.I., Trey, C., Timme, A.J. & Saunders, S.J. (1967) Fulminant hepatitis with recurrent hypoglycaemia and haemorrhage. *Gastroenterology*, 54, 291–300.

212. Saunders, S.J. & Terblanche, J. (1975) Animal experience with support systems: Are there appropriate animal models of fulminant hepatic necrosis? In Williams, R. & Murray-Lyon, I.M., (eds) pp. 163–172. London: Pitman Medical.

213. Saunders, S.J., Dowdle, E.B.D., Fiskerstrand, C. *et al.* (1978) Serum factor affecting neutrophil function during acute viral hepatitis. *Gut*, **19**, 930–934.

214. Saunders, S.J., Hickman, R., MacDonald, R. & Terblanche, J. (1972) The treatment of acute liver failure. In Popper, H. & Schaffner, F.F. (eds) *Progess in Liver Disease*, vol. IV, pp. 333–344. New York: Grune & Stratton.

215. Schafer, D.F. & Jones, E.A. (1982) Hepatic encephalopathy and the gamma-aminobutyric acid neurotransmitter system. *Lancet*, **2**, 18–19.

216. Seda, H.W.M., Gove, C.D., Hughes, R.D. & Williams, R. (1984) Inhibition of partially purified rat brain Na^+,K^+-dependent ATPase by bile acid, phenolic acid and endotoxin. *Clinical Science*, **66**, 415–420.

217. Seda, H.W.M., Hughes, R.D., Gove, C.D. & Williams, R. (1984) Inhibition of rat brain Na^+,K^+ATPase activity by serum from patients with fulminant hepatic failure. *Hepatology*, **4**, 74–79.

218. Shaw, B.W., Martin, D.J., Marquez, J.M. *et al.* (1984) Venous bypass in clinical liver transplantation. *Annals of Surgery*, **200**, 524–534.

219. Silk, D.B.A., Hanid, M.A., Trewby, P.N. *et al.* (1977) Treatment of fulminant hepatic failure by polyacronitrile membrane haemodialysis. *Lancet*, **2**, 1–3.

220. Simsarian, J.P. & Harner, R.N. (1972) Diagnosis of metabolic encephalopathy: Significance of triphasic wave patterns in the electroencephalogram. *Neurology*, **22**, 456–465.

221. Sinclair, S.B., Greig, P.D., Blendis, L.M. *et al.* (1989) Biochemical and chemical response of fulminant viral hepatitis due to administration of prostaglandin E (preliminary report). *Journal of Clinical Investigation*, **84**, 1063–1069.

222. Sinhoj, E. & Paulson, O.B. (1969) Carbon dioxide and cerebral circulatory control. *Archives of Neurology*, **20**, 249–252.

223. Smedile, A., Farci, P., Verme, G., Caredda, F. *et al.* (1982) Influence of delta infection on severity of hepatitis B. *Lancet*, **2**, 945–947.

224. Sood, G.K., Sarin, S.K., Mahaptra, J. & Broor, S.L. (1989) Comparative efficacy of psychometric tests in detection of subclinical hepatic encephalopathy in nonalcoholic cirrhotics: Search for a rational approach. *American Journal of Gastroenterology*, **84**, 156–159.

225. Stabenau, J.R. *et al.* (1959) The role of pH gradient in the distribution of ammonia between blood and cerebrospinal fluid, brain and muscle. *Journal of Clinical Investigation*, **38**, 373–383.

226. Stachura, J., Tarnawski, A., Ivery, K.J. *et al.* (1981) Prostaglandin protection of carbon tetrachloride induced liver cell necrosis in the rat. *Gastroenterology*, **81**, 211–217.

227. Stahl, J. (1963) Studies of the blood ammonia in liver disease. Its diagnostic, prognostic and therapeutic significance. *Annals of Internal Medicine*, **58**, 1–24.

228. Stanley, N.N. & Cherniack, N.S. (1976) Effect of liver failure on the cerebral circulatory and metabolic responses to hypoxia in man and the goat. *Clinical Science and Molecular Medicine*, **50**, 15–23.

229. Starzl, T.E., Demetris, A.J. & van Thiel, D. (1989) Liver transplantation. *New England Journal of Medicine*, **321**, 1014–1021, 1092–1099.

230. Stieber, A.C., Ambrosino, G, Van Thiel, D. *et al.* (1988) Orthotopic liver transplantation for fulminant subacute hepatic failure. *Clinics in Gastroenterology*, **17**, 157–165.

231. Stricker, B.H.C. & Spoelstra, P. (1985) *Drug Induced Hepatic Injury*. Amsterdam: Elsevier.

232. Sun, F.F., Chapman, J.P. & McGuire, J.C. (1977) Metabolism of prostaglandin endoperoxides in animal tissues. *Prostaglandins*, **14**, 1055–1074.

233. Sweadner, K. (1970) Two molecular forms of sodium potassium ATPase in brain. *Journal of Biological Chemistry*, **254**, 6060–6067.

234. Tandon, B.N., Joshi, Y.K., Krishnamurthy, L. *et al.* (1982) Subacute hepatic failure: Is it a distinct entity? *Journal of Clinical Gastroenterology*, **4**, 343–346.

235. Tarter, R.E., Arria, A.M., Carra, J. & Van Thiel, D.H. (1987) Memory impairments concomitant with nonalcoholic cirrhosis. *International Journal of Neuroscience*, **32**(3–4), 853–859.

236. Tarter, R.E., Hegedus, A.M., Van Thiel, D.H. & Schade, R.R. (1985) Portal–systemic encephalopathy: Neuropsychiatric manifestations. *International Journal of Psychiatric Medicine*, **15**, 265–275.

237. Tarter, R.E., Sclabassi, R.J., Sandford, S.L. *et al.* (1987) Relationship between hepatic injury status and event related potentials. *Clinical Electroencephalography*, **18**(1), 15–19.

238. Terblanche, J. & Hickman, R. (1991) Animal models of fulminant hepatic failure. *Digestive Diseases and Science*, **36**, 770–774.

239. Traber, P.G., Dal Canto, M., Ganger, D.R. & Blei, A.T. (1989) Effect of body temperature on brain edema and encephalopathy in the rat after devascularization. *Gastroenterology*, **96**, 885–891.

240. Traber, P.G., Dal Canto, M., Ganger, D.R. & Blei, A.T. (1987) Electron microscopy evaluation of brain edema in rabbits with galactosamine-induced fulminant hepatic failure ultrastructure and integrity of the blood–brain barrier. *Hepatology*, **7**, 1272–1277.

241. Traber, P.G., Ganger, D.R. & Blei, A.T. (1986) Brain edema in rabbits with galactosamine-induced fulminant hepatitis. Regional differences and effects in intracranial pressure. *Gastroenterology*, **91**, 1347–1356.

242. Traeger, H.S., Gabuzdas, J., Ballow, A.N. & Davidson, C.S. (1954) Blood ammonia concentration in liver disease and liver coma. *Metabolism*, **3**, 99–109.

243. Trewby, P., Warren, R., Conti, S. *et al.* (1978) The incidence and pathophysiology of pulmonary oedema in fulminant hepatic failure. *Gastroenterology*, **74**, 859–865.

244. Trewby, P.N. & Williams, R. (1977) Pathophysiology of hypotension in patients with fulminant hepatic failure. *Gut*, **18**, 1021–1026.

245. Trey, C. & Davidson, C.S. (1970) The management of fulminant hepatic failure. In Popper, H. & Schaffner, F.F. (eds) *Progress in Liver Disease*, vol. III, pp. 282–298. New York: Grune & Stratton.

246. Trey, C., Burns, D.G. & Saunders, S.J. (1966) Treatment of hepatic coma by exchange blood transfusions. *New England Journal of Medicine*, **274**, 473–481.

247. Trey, C., Lipworth, L., Chalmers, T.C. *et al.* (1968) Fulminant hepatic failure. Presumable contribution of halothane. *New England Journal of Medicine*, **279**, 798–801.

248. Tune, B.M. & Hsu, C.Y. (1985) Augmentation of antibiotic nephrotoxicity by endotoxemia in the rabbit. *Journal of Pharmacology and Experimental Therapy*, **234**, 425–430.

249. Tyce, G.H., Flock, E.V., Owen, C.A. *et al.* (1967) Five hydroxyindole metabolism in the brain after hepatectomy. *Biochemical Pharmacology*, **16**, 979–992.

250. Tygstrup, N. & Ranek, L. (1981) Fulminant hepatic failure. *Clinical Gastroenterology*, **10**, 191–208.

251. Uribe, M., Campello, O., Vargas, F. *et al.* (1987) Acidifying enemas (lactitol and lactose) vs nonacidifying enemas (tap water) to treat acute portal-systemic encephalopathy: A double blind randomized clinical trial. *Hepatology*, **7**, 639–643.

252. Van der Rijt, C.C.D., Schalm, S.W., Meulstee, J. & Stijnen, T. (1989) Flumazenil therapy for hepatic encephalopathy: A double-blind cross-over study. *Hepatology*, **10**, 590 (abstract).

253. Verstraete, M., Vermylen, J. & Collen, D. (1974) Intravascular coagulation in liver disease. *Annual Review of Medicine*, **25**, 447–455.

254. Vij, J.C. & Tandon, B.N. (1978) Controlled trial of levodopa in fulminant hepatitis. *Indian Journal of Medical Research*, **69**, 624–628.

255. Vilstrup, H., Iversen, J. & Tygstrup, N. (1985) Glucoregulation in acute liver failure. *European Journal of Clinical Investigation*, **16**, 193–197.

256. Vince, A., Killingley, M. & Wong, O.M. (1978) Effect of lactulose on ammonia production in a fecal incubation system. *Gastroenterology*, **74**, 544–549.

257. Wahren, J., Denis, J., Desurmont, P. *et al.* (1983) Is intravenous administration of branched-chain amino acids effective in the treatment of hepatic encephalopathy? A multicentre study. *Hepatology*, **3**, 475–480.

258. Wainwright, J. & Schonland, M.M. (1977) Toxic hepatitis in black patients in Natal. *South African Medical Journal*, **51**, 571–573.

259. Walker, S., Gotz, R., Czygan, P. *et al.* (1982) Oral keto analogues of branched amino acids in hyperammonemia in patients with

cirrhosis of the liver: A double blind crossover study. *Digestion,* **24,** 105–111.

260. Ward, M.E., Trewby, P.M., Williams, R. & Strunin, L. (1977) Acute liver failure—experience in a special unit. *Anaesthesia,* **32,** 228–239.
261. Ware, A.J., Cuthbert, J.A., Shorey, J. *et al.* (1981) A prospective trial of steroid therapy in severe viral hepatitis. The prognostic significance of bridging necrosis. *Gastroenterology,* **80,** 219–224.
262. Ware, A.J., D'Agostino, A.M. & Combes, B. (1971) Cerebral oedema: A major complication of massive hepatic necrosis. *Gastroenterology,* **61,** 877–884.
263. Warren, R., Trewby, P., Laws, J. & Williams, R. (1978) Pulmonary complications in fulminant hepatic failure: Analysis of serial radiographs from 100 consecutive patients. *Clinical Radiology,* **29,** 363–369.
264. Warren, S.E., Mitas, J.A. & Swerdin, A.H.R. (1980) Hypernatraemia in hepatic failure. *Journal of the American Medical Association,* **243,** 1257–1260.
265. Watanabe, A., Takei, N., Higashi, T. *et al.* (1984) Glutamic acid and glutamine levels in serum and cerebrospinal fluid in hepatic encephalopathy. *Biochemical Medicine,* **32,** 225–231.
266. Weber, F.L. (1979). The effect of lactulose on urea metabolism and nitrogen excretion in cirrhotic patients. *Gastroenterology,* **77,** 518–523.
267. Wilkinson, S.P., Blendis, L.M. & Williams, R. (1974) Frequency and type of renal and electrolyte disorders in fulminant hepatic failure. *British Medical Journal,* **1,** 186–189.
268. Williams, R. (1986) *Liver Failure.* Edinburgh: Churchill Livingstone.
269. Williams, R. (ed.) (1986) Fulminant hepatic failure. *Seminars in Liver Disease,* **6,** 1–184.
270. Williams, R. (1976) Hepatic failure and development of artificial liver support system. In Popper, H. & Schaffner, F. (eds) *Progress in Liver Disease,* vol. V, pp. 418–435. New York: Grune & Stratton.
271. Wyke, R.J., Canalese, J.C., Gimson, A.E.S. & Williams, R. (1982) Bacteraemia in patients with fulminant hepatic failure. *Liver,* **2,** 45–52.
272. Wyke, R.J., Rajkouvic, I.A., Eddlestone, A.L.W.F. & Williams, R. (1980) Defective opsonization and complement deficiency in serum from patients with fulminant hepatic failure. *Gut,* **21,** 643–649.
273. Wyke, R.J., Rajkouvic, I.A., Silk, D.B.A. & Williams, R. (1978) Impaired bacterial opsonization due to complement deficiency in patients with fulminant hepatic failure. *Gut,* **19,** 984.
274. Wyke, R.J., Yousif-Kadaru, A.G.M., Rajkouvic, I.A. *et al.* (1982) Serum stimulatory activity and leucocyte movement in patients with fulminant hepatic failure. *Clinical and Experimental Immunology,* **50,** 442–449.
275. Zacharski, L.R., Litin, E.M., Mulder, D.W. & Cain, J.C. (1970) Acute, fatal hepatic failure presenting with psychiatric symptoms. *American Journal of Psychiatry,* **127,** 382–386.
276. Zager, R.A. & Prior, R.B. (1986) Gentamycin and gram-negative bacteremia: A synergism for the development of experimental nephrotoxic acute renal failure. *Journal of Clinical Investigation,* **78,** 196–204.
277. Zaki, A.E.O., Wardle, E.N., Canalese, R.J. *et al.* (1983) Potential toxins of acute liver failure and their effects on blood brain barrier permeability. *Experientia,* **39,** 988–991.
278. Zeneroli, M.L., Pinelli, G., Gollini, G. *et al.* (1984) Visual evoked potential: A diagnostic tool for the assessment of hepatic encephalopathy. *Gut,* **25,** 291–299.
279. Zieve, L. (1981) The mechanism of hepatic coma. *Hepatology,* **1,** 360–365.
280. Zieve, L., Doizaki, W.M. & Lyftogt, C. (1984) Brain methanethiol and ammonia concentration in experimental hepatic coma and coma induced by various combinations of these substances. *Journal of Laboratory and Clinical Medicine,* **104,** 655–664.
281. Zieve, L., Doizaki, W.M. & Zieve, J. (1974) Synergism between mercaptans and ammonia or fatty acids in the production of coma: A possible role for mercaptans in the pathogenesis of hepatic coma. *Journal of Laboratory and Clinical Medicine,* **83,** 16–28.
282. Zieve, L., Lyftogt, C. & Draves, K. (1983) Toxicity of fatty acid and ammonia: Interactions with hypoglycemia and Krebs cycle inhibition. *Journal of Laboratory and Clinical Medicine,* **101,** 930–939.
283. Zieve, L., Lyftogt, C. & Raphael, D. (1986) Ammonia toxicity: Comparative protective effects of various arginine and ornithine derivatives, aspartate, benzoate, and carbomyl glutamate. *Metabolism and Brain Disease,* **1,** 25–35.
284. Zieve, L., Shakleton, M., Lyftogt, C. & Draves, K. (1985) Ammonia, octonoate and mercaptan depress regeneration of the normal rat liver after partial hepatectomy. *Hepatology,* **5,** 28–31.
285. Zimmerli, W., Grubinger, C., Tholen, H. *et al.* (1981) Mannitol treatment of cerebral oedema in rats with galactosamine induced severe hepatitis. *Experientia,* **37,** 1323–1325.
286. Zimmerman, H.J. & Ishak, K.G. (1982) Valproate-induced hepatic injury: Analyses of 23 fatal cases. *Hepatology,* **2,** 591–597.
287. Zimmerman, H.J. (1978) *Hepatotoxicity: The Adverse Effects of Drugs and Other Chemicals on the Liver.* New York: Appleton-Century-Crofts.
288. Zipser, R.D. & Liftschitz, M.D. (1988) Prostaglandins and related compounds. In Epstein, M. (ed.) *The Kidney and Liver Disease,* pp. 393–410. Baltimore: Williams & Wilkins.
289. Zuckerman, A.J. (1989) The elusive hepatitis C virus. *British Medical Journal,* **299,** 871–873.

CHAPTER 30

Acute Viral Hepatitis

Joel E. Lavine, F. Geoffrey Bull, G. H. Millward-Sadler & Michael J.P. Arthur

INTRODUCTION

Jaundice is mentioned in the Babylonian Talmud and the writings of Hippocrates, but the first suggestion that it might be infectious in nature came from Pope Zacharias in the eighth century AD; he advised that patients with jaundice should be separated to prevent spread of the contagion.[211] Although Herlitz in Gottingen and Sydenham in London had described epidemics of jaundice, and numerous outbreaks had occurred in the armed forces during the seventeenth, eighteenth and nineteenth centuries, the view was held by Eppinger as late as 1908 that all jaundice was obstructive in origin and due to catarrh in the large bile ducts.[327] McDonald[728] should be credited with first predicting that infective jaundice was produced by an agent smaller than a bacterium, and he postulated that it was due to a virus.

Lürman[688] reported the first recognizable outbreak of serum hepatitis following vaccination of dockers in Bremen with a batch of contaminated vaccine, and during World War II a series of outbreaks after the use of measles and yellow fever vaccine established beyond doubt that hepatitis could be spread by the parenteral route.

As a result of transmission experiments in human volunteers in the 1940s, two types of hepatitis were recognized:[689–691,859,1219] virus hepatitis type A, which occurred sporadically or in small epidemics and could be transmitted both parenterally and by the faecal–oral route; and hepatitis type B, which was originally thought to be transmitted by inoculation only, and could progress to the carrier state. These studies were extended by Krugman and associates at the Willowbrook State School in the late 1950s and 1960s.[607] However, despite early claims, neither of the viruses was visualized or grown in tissue culture.

In 1965, Blumberg, Alter and Visnich,[105] when studying the Ag-system of serum protein allotypes using a simple immunodiffusion technique, discovered a new precipitin line in the serum of an Australian aborigine. This antigen was unrelated to the Ag system, and was termed 'the Australia antigen'. They subsequently showed that the antigen was present at high frequency in patients with leukaemia, as well as in children with Down's syndrome who were living in large institutions but not in those who had not been institutionalized, suggesting an environmental factor. They noted that the presence of the antigen correlated with elevation of the serum transaminase levels and anicteric hepatitis on biopsy. This, and the chance development of hepatitis in a laboratory worker who became Australia antigen positive, led to the conclusion that the Australia antigen was associated with hepatitis.[106] Similar and apparently independent conclusions were reached by Prince[913] in New York and Okochi and Murakami[829] in Japan.

Since then, advances have been rapid. The Australia antigen has been characterized and its specific association with hepatitis B established. In 1977, Rizzetto and colleagues in studies of antigen–antibody systems in hepatitis B, described the delta agent.[953] This was subsequently characterized as an incomplete RNA virus—termed hepatitis D—which is dependent on hepatitis B surface antigen for its transmission. This virus may either co-infect with or super-infect hepatitis B and is now recognized as a significant cause of both fulminant hepatitis and progressive chronic liver disease.

The development of specific serological tests for hepatitis types A and B led to the recognition that there were post-transfusion, sporadic community-acquired, and epidemic-waterborne forms of hepatitis which could not be attributed to either of these viruses and the term non-A non-B (NANB) hepatitis was adopted, often prefixed with the epidemiological subtype. By definition this terminology excluded hepatitis D, or other viruses which may affect the liver, e.g. Ebstein–Barr virus or cytomegalovirus. A major breakthrough in this field occurred in 1988 when Houghton and colleagues from the Chiron corporation were able, using molecular techniques, to clone and identify the major agent responsible for post-transfusion NANB-hepatitis,[203] which they designated as hepatitis C. It should be emphasized that this followed on from exhaustive serial transmission studies in primates,[118–120,123] leading to well characterized highly infectious chimp sera from which they were able to make their original cDNA library. Serological tests for hepatitis C have subsequently become widely available and this virus is now also recognized as a cause of sporadic community acquired viral hepatitis. As screening of blood donors for antibodies to hepatitis C becomes widely adopted, a significant fall in the incidence of post-transfusion hepatitis is anticipated. Through the 1980s, there have also been detailed studies of epidemic-waterborne, enterically transmitted NANB hepatitis that have recently culminated in the molecular cloning and characterization of a fifth hepatotropic virus, now designated as hepatitis E.[946]

This chapter will review each of these five hepatotropic viruses and their specific clinical features in detail, but first, general features common to all causes of acute viral hepatitis are described. Later sections concentrate on other, rarer causes of acute viral hepatitis.

GENERAL FEATURES OF ACUTE VIRAL HEPATITIS

CLINICAL FEATURES

Many cases of viral hepatitis are not associated with significant clinical symptoms and often pass unrecognized. There may be no symptoms at all with minimal liver damage, or anicteric infection with non-specific symptoms but with hepatocellular necrosis and biochemical abnormalities. The non-specific symptoms are those seen in the prodromal phase but stop short of frank icterus.

Icteric attacks can range in severity from mild to fulminant and fatal. Anicteric infection with hepatitis B, C and D may progress to chronic liver disease, but this does not occur with hepatitis A or E. In an individual case it may be difficult to distinguish between the five different forms of viral hepatitis by clinical features alone. Comparative clinical features of infection with hepatitis A, B, C, D and E are summarized in Table 30.1.

Acute icteric hepatitis

The prodromal symptoms of hepatitis vary in severity and duration and some patients present only with overt jaundice. The duration of the pre-icteric symptoms ranges from a few days to 2 weeks and they are mainly gastrointestinal. Anorexia, nausea, malaise, weight loss, distaste for cigarettes, dark urine and pale stools, with or without pruritus, are prominent early symptoms. A decreased olfactory acuity appears to be a factor in the anorexia and improves as the illness subsides.[457]

The appearance of jaundice is usually associated with improvement in symptoms; although anorexia, nausea and lassitude may persist, the temperature settles, the pulse becomes slow and hepatic pain is prominent.

Extrahepatic manifestations of acute viral hepatitis occur and include arthralgia and arthritis, urticaria and angioneurotic oedema,[401,1089] vasculitic and renal lesions,[434,731] Henoch–Schönlein purpura,[394] CSF abnormalities and Guillain–Barré syndrome,[811] myocarditis and cardiomyopathies,[77,1053,1055] pancreatitis,[4,1138] and pleural effusion.[844] These are covered in further detail in the relevant clinical sections for each specific hepatotropic virus. Haematological changes may also occur (see below and Chapter 8).

In most icteric cases, the liver is enlarged and tender but the spleen is palpable in only about 20% of patients. Lymphadenopathy may be present but is usually insignificant, and occasionally there is bruising and purpura.

Lightening of the urine and a return of the stools to normal colour are early signs of recovery. Appetite improves with a gain in weight, but fatigue and lassitude may persist, often for prolonged periods.

Atypical clinical forms of hepatitis

Cholestatic viral hepatitis

Although cholestatic symptoms are a feature in most cases of icteric hepatitis, in some they dominate the clinical picture. Such cases often present acutely with deep jaundice, pronounced pruritis, dark urine and pale stools. In particular, when prodromal symptoms are insignificant, viral hepatitis may be difficult to distinguish from extrahepatic cholestasis and drug-induced cholestasis. In some cases, the symptoms of cholestasis persist for long periods, but this impression may be due to case selection.[302] Recovery is complete and progression to chronic liver disease is unusual.

The liver is usually not much enlarged and seldom tender, and the biochemical features may be indistinguishable from extrahepatic obstruction.

Fulminant hepatitis

In a small proportion of patients, the onset is acute and the illness is rapidly fatal within a period of 1–4 weeks. Usually the patient becomes deeply jaundiced within a few days, with restlessness, hallucinations, drowsiness, vomiting and convulsions. Rarely the onset may be so abrupt that coma and death may supervene in the absence of marked jaundice. The clinical signs are those of acute fulminant hepatic failure (see Chapter 29), with asterixis, constructional apraxia, progressive deterioration in the level of consciousness, fetor hepaticus, gastrointestinal haemorrhage from acute gastric erosions, bruising and purpura, and often renal failure. The liver may decrease in size, which is an ominous sign, as is the development of ascites and oedema.

The serum transaminases, after being very high in the early stages, may fall rapidly to low levels, with prolongation of the prothrombin time and a decrease in the serum albumin levels. In contrast to the normal or low count in typical acute viral hepatitis, there is a leucocytosis and occasionally thrombocytopenia associated with intravascular coagulation (see Chapter 8).

The aetiologic virus in cases of fulminant hepatitis may vary with geographic location. In many parts of the world the severe cases are due to hepatitis B, often in conjunction with hepatitis D infection. Hepatitis E is a significant cause of fulminant hepatitis in developing countries,[933] particularly in pregnant women in the third trimester. In the United Kingdom, viral hepatitis accounts for approximately one-third of all cases of fulminant liver failure and of these, 16% are due to hepatitis A, 29% to hepatitis B often with hepatitis D, and 53% to presumed non-A, non-B viruses.[1256]

Subacute hepatitis

Occasional patients have a severe acute attack and this pursues a more prolonged downhill course with progressive ascites and liver failure, over a period of a few months and terminating in death.[940] Even more exceptionally there may be an apparent period of clinical recovery but with persisting abnormality of liver function before progressive clinical deterioration. Such cases may be difficult to distinguish from chronic active hepatitis of unknown aetiology starting acutely, particularly if immunological markers are absent. These patients are often women. Pathologically, such cases often show bridging hepatic necrosis that is sometimes submassive. Portal hypertension with ascites may develop in such cases owing to collapse of sinusoids and reduction of the intrahepatic vascular space.[1195]

Relapsing hepatitis

Following an apparently complete clinical recovery from typical acute viral hepatitis, one or more relapses may occur, with darkening of the urine, a return of symptoms, particularly nausea and anorexia, and the development of jaundice. This clinicopathological syndrome has been referred to as chronic lobular hepatitis.[904] Occasionally, the liver function tests return to normal between the acute attacks and then relapse, when it may be difficult to exclude the possibility that a different virus is the cause of the second attack. Since there is no cross-immunity, recurrent attacks of viral hepatitis may be due to A, B, C or E, or to superinfection with hepatitis D. There have been several reports of acute hepatitis A in patients with chronic HBV infection.[227,1294] It is more usual, despite clinical recovery, for liver function tests to remain abnormal before the next clinical relapse, but there is again a grey area merging with chronic persistent hepatitis (see Chapter 31).

Two attacks of hepatitis are most likely to occur in drug addicts, haemophiliacs and children in institutions for the mentally retarded. A true relapse of hepatitis is sometimes temporally related to increased physical activity or alcohol abuse. In some series, an increased relapse rate has been reported in patients following treatment with corticosteriods.

Chronic sequelae of acute viral hepatitis

Although the overwhelming majority of patients with viral hepatitis recover completely, a proportion progress to chronic liver disease, particularly after infection with hepatitis B, C or D (see Chapter 31). In some patients there is persistence of symptoms of lethargy, malaise, anorexia and dislike of alcohol and fatty foods, which may last for months. Emotional instability and depression may be striking features. The liver may be palpable and tender and liver function tests may or may not be abnormal. There may be post-hepatitic hyperbilirubinaemia. Liver biopsy may be normal or show features of a resolving hepatitis. These symptoms are often referred to as the post-hepatitis syndrome.[713]

BIOCHEMICAL AND IMMUNOLOGICAL DISTURBANCES

Virtually all the functions of the liver described in Chapter 18 are deranged in acute viral hepatitis. The magnitude of derangement will depend on the severity of hepatocellular necrosis and the degree of cholestasis. Biochemical tests of liver function therefore provide a guide to the diagnosis of acute viral hepatitis and to the assessment of its severity, but have strict limitations and must be interpreted in the light of clinical findings and other investigative procedures in the jaundiced patient (see Chapter 28).

In the typical acute attack of viral hepatitis, serum aspartate aminotransferase (AST) levels become elevated early in the pre-symptomatic period of the disease and may be high in patients who never become icteric. Alanine aminotransferase (ALT) levels are also elevated. By the time clinically overt jaundice develops, the peak levels of aminotransferases have been achieved and they are usually falling. They are of some value in the differential diagnosis of jaundice, as figures in excess of 500 iu/l are seen only in acute hepatitis from any cause and shock or severe heart failure but are rare in extrahepatic obstructive jaundice and in chronic liver disease unless severely decompensated.

Serum bilirubin levels are very variable and are dependent not only on hepatocellular damage but on the degree of cholestasis and the presence of associated haemolysis. Although in general the severity of hepatitis is related to the level of bilirubin, there are striking exceptions, and fulminant hepatitis can occur with relatively little elevation of the bilirubin.

Bilirubinuria may appear before the serum bilirubin level is elevated. Urobilinogen disappears owing to cholestasis at the height of the jaundice in the late icteric phase, and its reappearance may indicate commencing recovery but is of little practical diagnostic value. Similarly, depending on the degree of cholestasis, stools become pale and the reappearance of stercobilin indicates clinical recovery.

Serum alkaline phosphatase levels are usually slightly increased (less than twice normal) in acute viral hepatitis. A level greater than twice the upper limit of normal has been taken as that distinguishing obstructive from hepatocellular jaundice. This level can be misleading as some patients with cholestatic hepatitis may also show levels greater than twice normal and are thus difficult to distinguish from patients with extrahepatic obstruction.

Changes in the plasma lipids and lipoproteins occur in acute viral hepatitis (see Chapter 4), but are not of practical value as tests of liver function.

The serum proteins may provide an important guide to the severity of the hepatitis. Serum albumin levels reflect the ability of the liver to synthesize this protein and are usually normal in an acute attack of hepatitis. Low levels indicate either fulminating severe hepatic damage or chronic liver disease. Serum globulin levels are altered in acute viral hepatitis, with elevation of the IgM levels in HBsAg-negative hepatitis, and of the IgG levels in both hepatitis A and B.[867] Serum complement levels may be low initially, but later rise to normal. The significance of these changes in terms of immune complex formation is doubtful because of the possibility of decreased synthesis by the damaged liver, with subsequent overproduction in response to low levels.[598] Cryoglobulinaemia may be a striking feature.[680]

Apart from the specific immune response to antigens associated with hepatitis A, B, C, D or E, non-specific immune responses occur in viral hepatitis. There is elevation of antibody titres to gut-associated bacteria such as *E. coli*[1175] and to a variety of unidentified viruses and bacteriophage particles present in stools,[19] suggesting a non-specific response to gut-associated antigens, possibly resulting from failure of Kupffer cells in the diseased liver to sequester absorbed antigens (see Chapter 9).

Antibodies to a component of smooth muscle have been demonstrated in a high proportion of patients with viral hepatitis.[336,808,1272] This antibody, which is also detected in other viral infections, such as infectious mononucleosis, may react with a component of the liver cell membrane resembling smooth muscle actomyosin.[470] Antibodies to a liver-specific lipoprotein occur transiently in the serum in a high proportion of patients with viral hepatitis.[533]

HAEMATOLOGICAL CHANGES

These are described in detail in Chapter 8. Many proteins important in the coagulation process, are synthesized in the liver and may provide a sensitive index of hepatocellular dysfunction. As a result of malabsorption of vitamin K, the prothrombin time can be prolonged in cholestasis, whether of extrahepatic or intrahepatic origin, but is readily corrected by giving vitamin K parenterally. A prolonged prothrombin time that vitamin K fails to correct is an indication of severe hepatocellular dysfunction.

As with many viral infections, there may be a leucopenia and, in particular, a lymphopenia with atypical lymphocytes resembling those seen in infectious mononucleosis. Later, there is a relative lymphocytosis, a macrocytosis with a reduced red cell survival[581] and low serum haptoglobulin levels,[1063] but marked haemolysis, which may be associated with a positive Coombs' test, is rare. Throm-

bocytopenia, agranulocytosis, pancytopenia[433,575] and transient red cell aplasia have also been reported.[1019]

The erythrocyte sedimentation rate is usually high in the pre-icteric phase of acute viral hepatitis[1192] but falls to normal with the appearance of jaundice and thereafter fluctuates until recovery. Serum vitamin B_{12} levels are raised in acute viral hepatitis, presumably due to release from damaged hepatocytes;[929] serum iron levels may also be elevated.[975] Serum alpha-fetoprotein levels are high and correlate with the severity of the acute hepatitis.[102, 569] The levels rise during the course of the illness as the serum transaminase levels return towards normal, thus favouring the possibility that alpha-fetoprotein is synthesized during hepatocellular regeneration.

DIFFERENTIAL DIAGNOSIS

The main differences between hepatitis A, B, C, D and E are summarized in Table 30.1. They are usually not sufficient to enable a clear clinical distinction to be made, particularly between hepatitis A, B and C. In Western countries, hepatitis D usually occurs in patients with an obvious parenteral source, e.g. parenteral drug abuse, and hepatitis E is confined to patients who have recently returned from abroad. A firm diagnosis is based on the demonstration of the viruses or their serological markers. The serological tests performed to distinguish between the different specific forms of acute viral hepatitis will vary between different laboratories. Those commonly performed are summarized in Table 30.2.

Icteric viral hepatitis may be difficult to distinguish from other causes of jaundice, particularly those that present clinically with symptoms of hepatocellular failure or cholestasis. The approach to the diagnosis of the jaundiced patient is discussed in Chapter 28. Diagnosis may be particularly difficult in infancy, in the elderly, in pregnancy (Chapter 42) and during the postoperative period (Chapter 52). In these situations the patient may be unable to give a good history, may have received many drugs or blood transfusions, and investigations may have to be limited on clinical grounds. In hepatocellular jaundice, the main distinction has usually to be made from drug-induced jaundice (see Chapter 46), infectious mononucleosis (see Chapter 41), leptospirosis and other bacterial infections of the liver (see Chapter 38), and other viral infections where hepatic involvement is a prominent feature (see below). In addition to the clinical features and serological tests, liver biopsy histology provides the most useful information.

The specialized techniques for the investigation of patients presenting with cholestasis, such as ultrasound and CT scanning (see Chapters 22 and 23), percutaneous cholangiography with the 'skinny' needle (see Chapter 26) and endoscopic retrograde cannulation of the biliary tree (see Chapter 26), have greatly increased the accuracy and speed of diagnosis in such patients.

Anicteric infections or a typical acute attack presenting in the pre-icteric phase are difficult to diagnose clinically.

Table 30.1 Comparative features of hepatitis A, B, C, D and E

	A	B	C	D	E
Incubation (days)	15–49	60–180	14–160 (superinfection)	21–42	21–63
Spread	Epidemic/sporadic	Sporadic/rarely epidemic	Sporadic	Sporadic/rarely epidemic	Epidemic/sporadic
Faecal–oral	Very common	Doubtful	Doubtful	No	Very common
Parenteral	Rare	Common	Common	Common	Not known
Sexual	No	Common	Probable	Rare	No
Perinatal	No	Common	Probable	Rare	No
Clinical					
Onset	Acute	Insidious/acute	Insidious/acute	Insidious/acute	Acute
Fulminant	Rare	Uncommon, increases with HDV infection	Uncommon, often late onset	Uncommon, more frequent with superinfection	Uncommon, more frequent in pregnancy
Chronic	No	Common	Common	Common	No
Abnormal LFTs	Short-lived	Prolonged	Usually prolonged	Prolonged	Short-lived
Viraemia	Transient	Transient and chronic	Transient and chronic	Transient and chronic	Transient
Virus	27-nm RNA	42-nm DNA	50–60-nm RNA	36-nm RNA	32–34-nm RNA
Classification	Picornavirus	Hepadnavirus	Flavivirus	Unique, unclassified	Calicivirus
Genome size	7.48 kb	3.2 kb	~10 kb	1.7 kb	7.6 kb
Immunization					
Passive	Effective	Variable, effective if given early post-exposure	Possible protective effect	Protective against coinfection with HBV, *not* superinfection	Not known
Active	Early clinical studies encouraging	Effective	Not available (1992)	Use HBV vaccine No HDV vaccine available	Not available (1992)

Table 30.2 Serological tests commonly performed in the clinical evaluation of acute viral hepatitis

Hepatitis	First-line tests	Second-line tests
A	IgM anti-HAV	–
B	HBsAg HBeAg	IgM anti-HBc DNA polymerase activity HBV-DNA (serum)
C	Anti-HCV (C-100-3 EIA)	HCV-RNA (serum) by PCR second-generation anti-HCV tests C-100-3 C-33-C } by immunoblot assay C-22
D	Anti-HDV	HDV-RNA (serum)
E	Anti-HEV Available 1992	Immunoelectron microscopy of stools HEV-RNA in stools

The chief cause of concern is the liability of such cases to spread the infection to health-care personnel and patients, and the danger to the patient himself of inadvertent surgery when presenting with gastrointestinal symptoms.

Distinction between acute viral hepatitis and a relapse or decompensation of chronic liver disease is based on clinical, biochemical and histological features.

GENERAL PATHOLOGY OF ACUTE VIRAL HEPATITIS

The standard histological changes of acute hepatitis are similar for hepatitis A, B, C, D and E, both grossly and microscopically, and individual cases cannot be separated other than by techniques for demonstrating the virus.[1124]

Macroscopic changes

The clinically enlarged and tender liver is seen at laparoscopy to be a swollen and reddened organ[170] (see Chapter 27). With more severe degrees of jaundice the liver may also be slightly green, but this is always less marked in hepatitis than in large bile duct obstruction for a given level of serum bilirubin.[271]

Microscopic changes

These have been extensively described.[93,96,515,758,869,875,903] There is cell death and degeneration with a mesenchymal reaction, hepatocyte regeneration and sometimes repair. The sinusoids are dilated where loss of hepatocytes has occurred but elsewhere are narrowed by enlarged hepatocytes showing ballooning degeneration and by twinning of cell plates from regeneration. The inflammatory reaction further complicates the histological features by obscuring and filling the sinusoids. This combination of changes results in considerable disorganization of the microanatomical architecture of the acinus. It is usually maximal around the terminal hepatic vein, though not confined to that zone (Figure 30.1).

Cell damage

This is present throughout the acinus but is most striking in the perivenular area and shows considerable variation between cases. In mild and anicteric forms of viral hepatitis the damage may be minimal and virtually confined to the perivenular zone. This damage to hepatocytes can be identified as ballooning degeneration and acidophil degeneration. Hepatocytes showing ballooning degeneration are swollen to twice normal or more (Figure 30.2). The nucleus may be normal in appearance, but degenerative changes ranging from pyknosis to nuclear inclusions have also been described.[991] The nucleus is surrounded by a cuff of granular cytoplasm with fine strands of cytoplasm radiating from this cuff to the plasma membrane. There is no staining between the strands which gives the cell a peripheral pallor. The plasma

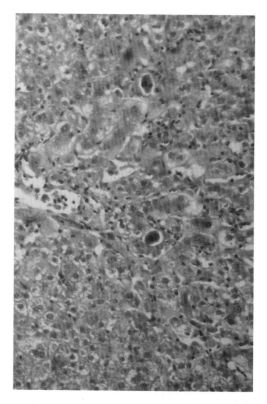

Figure 30.1 Patient with acute hepatitis B. The terminal hepatic vein is on the centre left margin. The parenchyma around the terminal hepatic vein is disorganized from cell damage and loss and the cell plate pattern is difficult to define.

membrane is often sharply defined, but focal defects may be seen along its length. Electron-microscopically there is a striking dilatation of the endoplasmic reticulum, swelling of mitochondria and a loss of ribosomes and glycogen. Fine granules of bile and lipofuscin may be

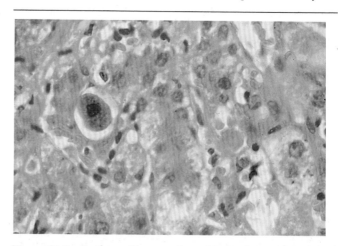

Figure 30.2 Patient with acute hepatitis B. Generalized swelling of hepatocytes has encroached on the sinusoidal space, which can best be identified by the small nuclei of the sinusoidal and inflammatory cells. Ballooned hepatocytes are particularly prominent at bottom right. A hepatocyte showing acidophil degeneration has rounded contours, a deeply eosinophilic cytoplasm and a shrunken hyperchromatic nucleus.

identified within the cytoplasm. These changes have been attributed to bile retention, but where bile is absent cholate stasis has been postulated (Chapter 15).[904] Bile stasis rarely reflects morphologically the degree of bilirubinaemia.

Bile can be visualized as granules within hepatocytes, mostly perivenular and also as thrombi within and often distending the bile canaliculi. Some bile is also present in Kupffer cells. While the bile in the canaliculi is conjugated, that present in Kupffer cells is unconjugated, a discrepancy attributed to subsequent deconjugation in the Kupffer cell by lysomal β-glucuronidase.[270] Kupffer cells are also involved in the catabolism of effete red cells and therefore any unconjugated bilirubin present could represent failure of release into the blood.[98]

Ballooning degeneration affects a large proportion of the hepatocytes in the parenchyma and, although it is a reversible cell degeneration, lysis may occur. Conversely, acidophil degeneration is irreversible and represents cell death (Figure 30.2). Affected hepatocytes are scattered singly throughout the parenchyma, are small and have uniformly acidophilic, deeply staining cytoplasm. The cell outline may be angulated at points of residual contact with other hepatocytes but often is rounded and then completely separated by a clear space from its neighbours. Within this condensed cell body the nucleus, if still present, shows either pyknosis or karyorrhexis. Electron microscopically the cells are relatively electron-dense with the residual organelles compacted together. The membranes of the endoplasmic reticulum are without a lumen, glycogen and ribosomes are absent and surface microvilli are sparse or absent.

Apart from the active hepatocellular degeneration there is also usually evidence from collapse of the reticulin architecture of preceding loss of hepatocytes (Figure 30.3). This passive collapse may be local and minor or may be more significant, representing confluent loss of hepatocytes. In the early stages reticulin fibres remain slightly apart and regeneration can reconstitute the cell plate. None the less, this passive collapse of the fibre scaffold may form a template in which abnormal connective-tissue septa may be formed. As well as hepatocellular damage, there may be bile duct damage in a small proportion of cases. The damage is usually segmental along the bile duct, may not extend round the whole circumference and when present in a biopsy does not affect all bile ducts.[909,1005] A variable degree of bile duct proliferation may be present. It has been suggested that bile duct damage is associated with chronicity[909] and with non-A, non-B hepatitis.[651,1005]

Mesenchymal reaction

Portal tracts contain an inflammatory infiltrate predominantly mononuclear and mostly lymphocytic, but with an admixture of plasma cells, macrophages and some neutrophil and eosinophil leucocytes (Figure 30.4). There is an overflow of mononuclear cells into periportal sinusoids. The lytic necrosis of hepatocytes in the limiting plate can blur the margins of the portal tract which with clusters of mononuclear cells in this area produces features that overlap with piecemeal necrosis (Figure 30.4).[60]

Within the sinusoids there is an infiltrate of lymphocytes with occasional plasma cells. The significance of plasma cells is disputed but they are present in greatest numbers during the acute phase of liver cell damage and are less

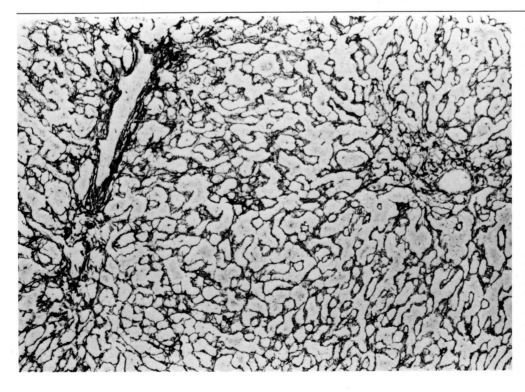

Figure 30.3 Reticulin preparation with portal tract to the right and terminal hepatic venule to the left. Condensed reticulin can be particularly seen around the efferent vein and results from loss of hepatocytes. (Reticulin.)

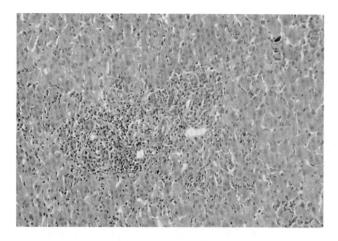

Figure 30.4 Portal tract heavily infiltrated by mononuclear cells. The infiltrate spills out into periportal sinusoids so that the limiting plate is ill-defined.

frequent with resolution.[93,515] Kupffer cells also show focal proliferation, particularly in areas where cell death has been prominent. On occasions they can be found surrounding an acidophil body.[515] These macrophages are also hypertrophied with bulky cytoplasm laden with phagocytosed debris, bile, lipofuscin, ceroid pigment and sometimes haemosiderin (Figure 30.5). The concurrence of both ceroid and haemosiderin pigments within focally hyperplastic macrophages is particularly suggestive of drug- or viral-induced hepatitis. It has been suggested that this focal hyperplasia, combined with hypertrophy, may impede the sinusoidal blood flow and that the consequent hypoxia in the adjacent hepatocytes further contributes to the cell damage.[990] The pigment-laden macrophages slowly disappear with resolution and persist longest in the portal tracts.

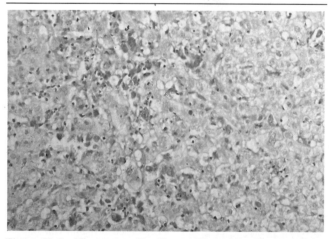

Figure 30.5 Numerous Kupffer cells in the sinusoids are swollen and laden with phagocytosed fragments of cell death identified as a granular red ceroid pigment after diastase-PAS staining.

Regeneration

Regenerative activity starts within 48 hours of hepatocellular damage (see Chapter 11). Mitotic activity is not often observed in liver biopsies but the consequences of regeneration can be seen. These are (a) small foci of twinning of cell plates; (b) increased numbers of hepatocytes with two or more nuclei; and (c) increased variation in size and staining of hepatocyte nuclei.

Evolution of changes

Strict chronological or clinical correlations are not usually possible, but early, middle and late stages can be identified. An overall concept of the morphological evolution has been presented.[93] The features of early viral hepatitis are not well documented, but focal liver cell necrosis, many mitoses in hepatocytes, a mononuclear infiltrate in portal tracts and hyperplasia of sinusoidal cells have been described.[271] In chimpanzees experimentally infected with hepatitis B virus a lymphocytic infiltration of sinusoids and portal tracts with hyperplasia of Kupffer cells precedes the parenchymal degenerative changes.[65] Parenchymal degeneration persists for varying periods, up to several months in some instances, but eventually the active parenchymal degeneration and the cholestasis subside. In the stage of resolution the emphasis is on evidence of previous cell death with prominent regeneration. There may be a residual lymphocyte infiltrate in portal tracts but more characteristic are the clusters of ceroid-laden macrophages within sinusoids. These ceroid-laden macrophages persist and may still be present in the portal tracts 4–6 months after the onset of jaundice.

Differential diagnosis

Features that are most characteristic of a particular viral infection are detailed later under that virus. The major differential diagnosis is from a drug-induced hepatitis.

Differentiation between a viral and a drug-induced hepatitis is difficult and frequently impossible on morphological criteria. Guidelines have been published[94] and drug-induced liver disease is considered in Chapter 46. A pattern of hepatocellular damage resembling viral hepatitis has been described with heat stroke.[94,440] The clinical history with the associated neurological complications and evidence of rhabdomyolysis should clearly identify such cases.

Morphological variants

Cholestatic hepatitis

In cholestatic hepatitis the parenchymal changes of viral hepatitis are present but are less pronounced, although canalicular cholestasis is severe.[1069] Within portal tracts, there is proliferation of bile ductules around the edges and these ductules may be distended and filled with bile. There is an increased proportion of neutrophils within the inflammatory infiltrate in the portal tracts and these neutrophils usually surround the proliferating bile ductules. Consequently, large bile duct obstruction may be mimicked. This variant was clearly described in association with an outbreak of viral hepatitis in New Delhi.[428,1262] The cholestasis may persist for many months but there is no indication that this morphological variant of hepatitis predisposes to chronic liver disease.

Drug addiction hepatitis
Intravenous drug addiction is frequently associated with a viral hepatitis. The morphological features are dependent upon the particular virus transmitted. Particulate matter such as talc may be mixed with the drug. Classically this produces granulomatous lung disease and right heart endocarditis, but rarely sufficient may enter the systemic circulation to reach the liver and produce a granulomatous reaction around the foreign material in portal tracts.[1302] Polarized light will clearly identify doubly-refractile material such as talc.

Relapsing hepatitis (chronic lobular hepatitis)
Chronic lobular hepatitis[902] may be regarded as prolonged or unresolved acute hepatitis lasting for more than 6 months. The condition is more fully considered in Chapter 31.

Massive hepatic necrosis
Massive hepatocellular damage results in fulminant liver failure. Biopsies are rarely performed in the acute stages, so that most information is derived from autopsy studies such as the classical observation of Lucké,[684,685] and more recently confirmed by studies on livers removed from patients with acute hepatic failure treated by liver transplantation. Different patterns of gross pathology have been described which represent the rate of massive necrosis along a timescale rather than variations on a disease process.

In the earliest stages, up to one week, the liver is approximately normal in size and weight, or only slightly smaller. The majority of dead hepatocytes have not disintegrated and the stroma is still separated by this residual effete parenchyma. At a slightly later stage, hepatocytes are lost, predominantly around the efferent veins, and dilated sinusoids are passively filled with blood. The overall result is a soft liver with a wrinkled capsule and a congested cut surface.

Submassive hepatic necrosis
Longer survival allows more complete disintegration of hepatocytes with corresponding collapse of the architecture. Bile retention is prominent in hepatocytes, canaliculi and Kupffer cells and there is a pronounced mononuclear infiltrate in portal tracts. Cell death is not uniform throughout the liver; some areas appear to be totally effaced while other areas of liver show lesser degrees of damage. Large areas of collapsed stroma contain ductular structures. There is controversy whether they are prolifer-

ating bile ductules or metaplastic hepatocytes. Following the confluent loss of hepatocytes, portal tracts may be approximated to each other. The consequence of this more complete cell loss is a small and limp liver that is heavily bile-stained and has a very wrinkled capsule. The differences are later further accentuated by hepatocellular regeneration so that over a period of 2–3 months the liver macroscopically may show bulging regenerative masses of parenchyma separated by large areas of collapse. This pattern is interpreted by some as cirrhosis and by others as submassive hepatic necrosis.[315] As the pattern is one of progressive hepatocellular death exceeding regeneration, of relentless clinical deterioration and of increasing liver failure with a relatively well-defined and short timescale, the latter terminology seems most appropriate.

Prognostic morphological features
A vast majority of patients with viral hepatitis improve without sequelae and only a small proportion progress to chronic liver disease.[74] Numerous attempts have been made to identify clinical, serological and morphological features which may affect prognosis and predict those patients at risk. Clinically, those patients who develop cirrhosis are older and include more females than the average.[100] The risk of chronic liver disease is also related to the specific virus infection. Chronicity is more common in association with the hepatitis B, C and D viruses than with the hepatitis A and E viruses. Morphological features that have been associated with an adverse prognosis include confluent necrosis, piecemeal necrosis, an impaired regenerative response, bile duct damage and an excessive proportion of plasma cells.

Bridging hepatic necrosis
This term, suggested by Conn,[225] has replaced subacute hepatic necrosis and should be confined to the appearance of confluent necrosis linking portal tracts with terminal hepatic veins (Figure 30.6). It should not be used to described the confluent necrosis that links these venules to each other or links portal tracts together. In their series, Boyer and Klatskin[115] describe complications in half of the patients with liver biopsies defined by them as showing bridging hepatic necrosis. Many of these patients develop cirrhosis. Similar results, but with a lower instance of complications, have been reported by others.[1235] Not all examples progress and there are well-documented instances of complete recovery of normal liver structure and function in patients whose biopsies showed bridging hepatic necrosis.[1082,1152] A prospective study on bridging hepatic necrosis failed to demonstrate any effect of bridging hepatic necrosis on outcome, even in the non-treated group.[1236] Others have suggested that persistence of bridging hepatic necrosis after the sixteenth week is usually associated with chronicity. The conflicting results reported by Ware and his colleagues[1235,1236] can be explained on this basis. Their prospective study only accepted patients whose acute illness at presentation was

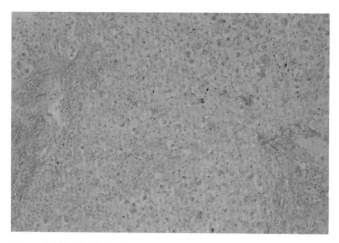

Figure 30.6 Bridging hepatic necrosis. Loss of hepatocytes has resulted in collapse of the cell plates with formation of a bridge of collagen (blue) between portal tract (left) and terminal hepatic vein (right). (MSB trichrome.)

less than 1 month on admission and the average duration of their patients' illnesses was 6–7 weeks from admission to the trial. Consequently they were probably examining liver biopsies during the earlier stages of the evolution of the disease.

Such findings have implied that it is the failure to resolve bridging hepatic necrosis that is the significant factor leading to chronicity and that this presumably occurs by inadequate regenerative activity. This would be consistent with the suggestion that relative lack of regenerative capacity was a major contribution to massive hepatic necrosis secondary to viral infection.[869]

Bridging hepatic necrosis could predispose to chronic liver disease in several ways. It could provide a septum formed by the passive collapse of reticulin fibres along which active fibrogenesis can produce a bridge of mature collagen between tract and efferent veins. Blood vessels form within this collagen bridge, bypass the parenchyma, and thus produce a vascular shunt. It has been suggested also that the presence of such a pattern of necrosis simply facilitates the progression of a chronic hepatitis so that the architecture is more quickly disrupted.[96] Alternatively it may be a morphological representation of cell death in excess of regeneration.[315,869] These three pathogenetic mechanisms are not mutually exclusive and the identification of bridging hepatic necrosis in a liver biopsy should be regarded as an adverse prognostic feature.

Impaired regeneration

Viral hepatitis is frequently much more severe in patients over 40 years of age[115,315,558,712] while survivors are almost invariably under the age of 30 years.[558] This relative influence of age has been attributed to increasing impairment of hepatocellular regeneration with age.[315,869,870] This has some morphological correlations. Extensive simultaneous death of hepatocytes can produce fulminating acute hepatic failure before regeneration has had time

to develop. For lesser degrees of cell death, the rate of regeneration may be crucial; it is therefore interesting to note that the average age of patients dying with submassive hepatic necrosis is 68 years.[315] It is logical speculation that when cell death and regeneration are approximately balanced, the effects of such architectural distortion as bridging hepatic necrosis could be much more significant and therefore contribute to the development of cirrhosis.

A major problem in confirming this concept is the accurate histological identification of regenerative capacity in the individual patient. Apart from the number of mitoses and the twinning of cell plates, the *lack* of architectural disarray in the presence of confluent hepatocellular damage may be ominous.[869] This lack reflects the absence of regeneration within the typical histological pattern of acute viral hepatitis.

Piecemeal necrosis (see Chapter 31)

Considerable difficulty arises in distinguishing piecemeal necrosis from the overspill of inflammatory cells into periportal areas that is seen in non-complicated acute viral hepatitis. This is particularly true in hepatitis A infections.[1144] Features of active fibrogenesis, rosette formation of hepatocytes, an intimate relationship between lymphocytes and hepatocytes, and a periportal and portal reaction that is out of proportion to the perivenular changes suggest piecemeal necrosis. Also, it is rare for hepatocytes to be isolated within fibrous tissue by simple spillover from portal tracts.

Despite the emphasis on chronicity, piecemeal necrosis may occasionally occur in acute viral hepatitis and then it has been suggested that chronicity is a likely outcome.[96,293] The rate at which piecemeal necrosis then produces architectural distortion by fibrosis is influenced by the presence of bridging hepatic necrosis.[96]

It is unlikely that the piecemeal necrosis is present in all cases of acute viral hepatitis progressing to chronic liver disease, nor does the presence of piecemeal necrosis indicate inevitable chronic liver disease.[96,293,338] In a survey of 17 biopsies showing chronic active hepatitis from patients with acute viral hepatitis, only 3 patients progressed to chronic liver disease.[338] If hepatitis A is excluded, then piecemeal necrosis seems to be a reliable indicator: chronic liver disease developed in 95% of patients with hepatitis B and 89% of patients with non-A, non-B hepatitis associated with piecemeal necrosis.[1207]

Plasma cells are a component of the infiltrate in piecemeal necrosis and are present in small numbers in uncomplicated hepatitis. They are particularly prominent in biopsies showing piecemeal necrosis or bridging hepatic necrosis and have been implicated as an adverse prognostic feature when present in large numbers in a biopsy.[98,293,516]

Bile duct damage

Damage to bile ducts was described in acute hepatitis by Poulsen and Christoffersen,[909] who also reported that these cases progressed to chronic liver disease (Figure

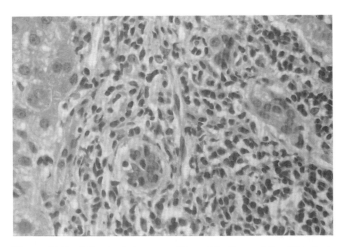

Figure 30.7 Bile duct damage: the epithelium of the bile ducts in this inflamed portal tract has lost polarity and mononuclear inflammatory cells have breached the bile duct basement membranes.

30.7). Piecemeal necrosis was a prominent feature in the majority of their cases. Bile duct damage has also been described in acute cholestatic viral hepatitis and in this morphological environment is not associated with chronicity. Bile duct lesions may be a prominent feature of one form of non-A, non-B hepatitis,[1005] possibly hepatitis C, whereas acute cholestatic viral hepatitis may have an association with hepatitis E. This suggests that bile duct damage may be a feature of particular viral infections rather than a pathological process resulting in secondary chronic complications.

TREATMENT OF THE ACUTE ATTACK _____

In the absence of specific antiviral agents effective against the viruses in the acute phase of hepatitis, treatment has traditionally consisted mainly of bed-rest and dietary advice, although each is controversial.

During the acute attack, patients often have marked malaise, lassitude, anorexia and nausea, and therefore require bed-rest and dietary restriction, particularly of fatty foods. They should be adequately hydrated with correction of electrolyte disturbances and be given a high calorie intake. In the severe or fulminant case, a treatment regimen for fulminant hepatic failure should be instituted (see Chapter 29).

Whether early ambulation predisposes to relapse and chronicity is doubtful. Studies during World War II suggesting that early ambulation increased the frequency of relapse were not confirmed, provided the patients had some bed-rest during the day,[179,804] although there is some suggestion that strenuous physical activity early in the illness might have an untoward effect.[603] While they are acutely ill, patients should be confined to bed, with gradual convalescence if symptoms improve. Return to bed-rest is appropriate if symptoms recur or liver function tests deteriorate sharply. Patients should be advised to reduce their intake of fatty food if it produces nausea, and it is conventional to advise abstention from alcohol for 6 months, although the evidence that either influences the outcome of the illness or progression to chronicity is marginal. In a randomized controlled study of continued alcohol consumption compared to abstention during convalescence from acute viral hepatitis, no adverse effects on recovery or prognosis were observed from moderate alcohol consumption (mean 26 g ethanol/day).[1172]

Details of treatments specific to individual types of viral hepatitis are discussed further in the relevant clinical sections, but some are worthy of general consideration. Corticosteroids have been used in the treatment of acute viral hepatitis, with some improvement in the patient's feeling of well-being and in liver function tests. However, early studies showed that the duration of the illness was unaffected, and unless treatment was continued into convalescence relapse was likely to occur.[330] Because of their side-effects, corticosteroids are therefore seldom recommended in uncomplicated cases of acute viral hepatitis. Their use in prolonged cholestasis and the fulminant form of the disease has been advocated in the past,[1031] but several studies have reported that corticosteroid treatment may be harmful and may be associated with prominent side-effects.[103,422,786]

Nevertheless, there are some patients with autoimmune chronic active hepatitis who present acutely,[37] and have the histological pattern of piecemeal necrosis, in whom corticosteroids may be effective. If this histology or immunological features such as hyperglobulinaemia with autoantibodies exist, then corticosteroids are indicated.

Treatment with drugs such as levamisole, acyclovir, interferons and other antiviral agents has been undertaken more frequently in chronic rather than acute hepatitis and is discussed further in Chapter 31.

The naturally occurring flavenoid, (+)-cyanidanol-3, widely studied as a protective agent against various hepatotoxic agents, has been evaluated clinically in acute viral hepatitis. It is thought to act as a free radical scavenger and has antioxidant properties inhibiting lipid peroxidation by hepatotoxic chemicals.[630] Some controlled clinical studies[104,1007] in acute viral hepatitis have shown a marginally increased rapidity of resolution of biochemical tests of liver function or clearance of HBsAg, but others have shown no differences from controls and the benefit, if any, is negligible.[226,630]

In patients with severe viral hepatitis and fulminant liver failure, liver transplantation should be considered. The indications for, and timing of, liver transplantation in fulminant liver failure are discussed in Chapter 56. Survival rates as high as 71% have been reported for patients with fulminant hepatic failure undergoing liver transplantation,[82] but there are significant problems with recurrent infection in the grafted liver with hepatitis B, D and C. These are discussed further in the relevant clinical sections for each virus.

General preventative measures in acute viral hepatitis

There is considerable variation in attitudes regarding the policy for isolation of sporadic cases of acute hepatitis. In Western society, mild cases are usually managed at home, but if severe are admitted either to an isolation unit in infectious disease hospitals or to a side-room in a general hospital.

There is little evidence that isolation in the home will reduce the spread of infection to other family members, since it is likely that they will already have been exposed during the incubation period. Simple measures in the home regarding disposal of urine and stools, handwashing and the use of separate eating utensils are usually advised. The value of passive immunization of contacts is discussed later.

Patients are usually admitted to hospital only if the jaundice persists for more than 2–3 weeks or if they are acutely ill, but if repeated sporadic cases occur in a closed community such as a school, isolation of mild cases may be attempted to contain the spread.

In hospital, the patient with acute hepatitis should be isolated in a single cubicle wherever possible. Adequate facilities should be available for the disposal of urine, faeces, soiled linen, syringes and needles, not only to prevent spread in the hospital ward but to prevent infection of ancillary and laboratory staff. Medical attendants should consider using special gowns, gloves and eye protection, particularly when handling patients' blood or if undertaking invasive procedures such as endoscopy. Measures specific to preventing spread of hepatitis A, B, C, D and E are described in the relevant sections, as are passive and active immunization against the specific forms of viral hepatitis (where available).

Table 30.3 Properties of hepatitis A virus

- Unique member of family Picornaviridae with single serotype
- "Full" and "empty" non-enveloped particles
- Isolated from faeces, serum, bile and liver
- Buoyant density of 1.42–1.27 g/ml
- Three of four capsid polypeptides with M_r 30–33 kD, 21–27 kD, 23 kD and ?2.5 kD
- Non-structural proteins:
  (a) VPg linked to 5′ end of genome
  (b) RNA-dependent RNA polymerase
  (c) Protease
- Viral genome (+) strand RNA of 7.48 kb with 3′ poly(A) tract and non-coding sequence at 5′ terminus
- Inactivated by formaldehyde at 37°C for 72 h, chlorine and ultraviolet irradiation
- Resistant to inactivation by ether, heating at 60°C, acid, and storage in the cold

COURSE AND PROGNOSIS

The course and prognosis of acute viral hepatitis are variable, and in part dependent on the specific aetiological agent. Further details are given later in the relevant specific clinical sections.

HEPATITIS A

PROPERTIES OF HEPATITIS A VIRUS (see Table 30.3)

The first definitive identification of the virus of HAV was reported in 1973 by Feinstone, Kapakian and Purcell[343] using immune electron microscopy. They visualized 27-nm particles in acute-phase stool specimens in two of four subjects inoculated with the MS-1 strain of hepatitis A virus. Faecal shedding of these particles was greatest during the prodromal phase and for 5 days before the onset of jaundice, when aminotransferase levels were at their peak. The virus remained detectable in stools for up to 2 weeks during the late acute or early convalescent phase.[237,284] Antibody, as detected by clumping of these particles, could be demonstrated in sera obtained during well-documented hepatitis A epidemics, experimentally acquired MS-1, and Joliot Prison infections, but not in pre-inoculation specimens nor in individuals with acute non-bacterial gastroenteritis.[921]

Morphology and protein structure

Electron microscopy of immune-precipitated HAV particles reveals that they are 27–32 nm in diameter and have cubic symmetry (Figure 30.8). "Full" particles unpenetrated by stain and "empty" particles can be identified and are indistinguishable antigenically. There are three major particles of varying buoyant density ranging from 1.27 to 1.42 g/ml (major density of 1.34, sedimentation coefficient of 158 S). Further characterization has demonstrated three major polypeptides of molecular weight 30–33 kD, 24–25 kD and 21–27 kD, thus resembling the VP1, VP2 and VP3 proteins composing the capsid of enteroviruses.[236,429,472,1049] A fourth structural protein is predicted by analogy to other picornaviruses but has not been positively demonstrated in HAV.

Physical and chemical studies on the stability of HAV show that it is relatively resistant to inactivation by ether; acid at pH 3.0 for 3 h at 25°C; heating at 60°C for 1 h; or to storage at −20°C for years. The virus may be inactivated by autoclaving at 121°C for 20 min, formalin 3% for 5 min at 5°C; halogens; or by sodium hypochlorite 5 mg/l at 20°C for 10 min.[917]

Relationships with Picornaviridae

Hepatitis A virus is classified in the Picornaviridae, a family of small (22-nm) non-enveloped spherical viruses. There are four genera, of which two, the enteroviruses

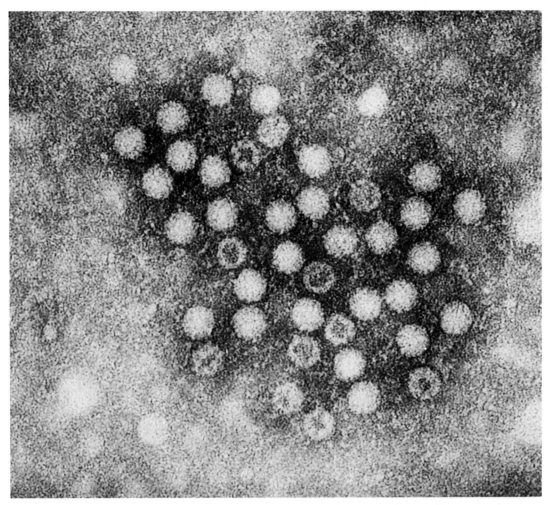

Figure 30.8 Hepatitis A virus, showing both full and empty particles. The particles measure 26–28 nm in diameter. Magnification, × 300 000. (Electron micrograph from a series by Anthea Thornton and A.J. Zuckerman, London School of Hygiene and Tropical Medicine.)

and rhinoviruses, include many human pathogens. All have a similar size, structure and replicative strategy dependent on a single-stranded RNA genome. Homology is particularly evident between HAV and the enterovirus genus, of which human poliovirus 1 is the prototype, although there are also differences which are considered sufficient grounds for placing it in a separate genus.[472]

Picornaviridae infect by attaching to receptors on susceptible cells, typically hepatocytes in the case of HAV. After penetration, the single-stranded RNA, MW 2.5×10^6 daltons, is rapidly uncoated and serves directly as a messenger RNA for the synthesis of a large viral polyprotein. This is cleaved into specific viral proteins which include three structural proteins from which the viral capsomeres are formed. There are probably 60 such capsomeres arranged with characteristic cubic symmetry in an icosahedral structure, the viral procapsid. Replication of the viral RNA and its enclosure in this protein shell to form the nucleocapsid occurs in the cytoplasm. The virus is finally exteriorized from the cell from vacuoles or rupture of the cell membrane, although HAV is not usually cytopathic. Similar replicative strategies have been documented for the other positive single-stranded RNA

viruses, which include not only picornaviridae but flaviviridae, togaviridae, coronaviridae and caliciviridae.

Genome structure

The genomes of a number of wild-type, attenuated, cell-culture-adapted, and neutralization-resistant mutants of HAV have been reverse-transcribed into cDNA, cloned and partially or fully sequenced[213,214,527,672,800,858,1158,1213] (Figure 30.9). Examination of the primary sequence reveals a genome length of 7470–7478 base pairs, depending on the strain. This is similar to human poliovirus RNA. Sequences from HAV isolated from disparate geographical areas are highly similar. A 734-bp non-coding region precedes the single open reading frame (ORF), which extends to base number 7415. The ORF is followed by a short 62-bp 3′ non-coding region terminated by a variable-length polyadenylated tract.

The highly conserved non-coding region has a number of features in common with the picornaviridae, including a stem-and-loop structure and a tract of high (95%) pyrimidine content. Although the functions of this region are unknown, it may be involved in stimulation of

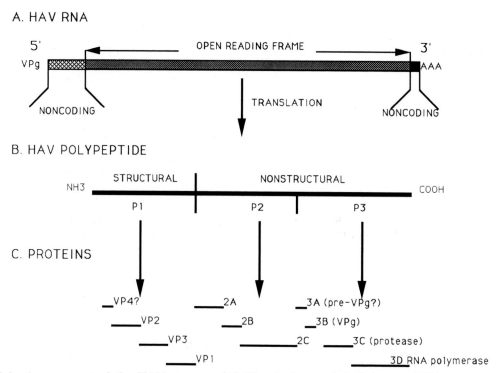

Figure 30.9 Arrangement of the HAV genome. (A) The single-stranded, (+)-sense RNA genome contains a covalently linked protein (VPg) attached to the 5'-terminus. A 5'-non-coding sequence of 734 nucleotides precedes the single open reading frame which extends to nucleotide 7415. The ORF is followed by a short 62-bp 3'-non-coding sequence which is highly variant between HAV strains. A poly (A+) tract (AAA) of variable length is linked to the 3' terminus. (B) The translated HAV-RNA produces a single polypeptide with a structural amino-terminal end (P1) and a non-structural carboxy-terminal end (P2 and P3). (C) Post-translational proteolytic processing of the polypeptide precursor produces a variety of structural and non-structural proteins. Structural products VP1, 2, 3 and perhaps 4 compose the viral capsid. The non-structural proteins derived from P2 and P3 are indicated, with proposed functions of some products shown. Proteins 2A, 2B and 3A demonstrate distinct differences from other picornaviruses, and their functions are unknown. Sizes of non-coding and coding RNA and structural and non-structural polypeptides are approximately proportioned. See text for references and further detail.

viral protein synthesis[472] and may also influence viral adaptation in cell culture.[216]

In vitro translation of the viral linear RNA to protein demonstrates that HAV has a (+) strand genome. The single ORF encodes a precursor polypeptide which undergoes post-translational processing by a viral protease,[263] a hallmark of picornaviruses. The polypeptide is divided into various domains which are destined to be structural (P1) or non-structural (P2 and P3) proteins (Figure 30.9). Structural proteins compose the viral capsid, produced from VP1, VP2 and VP3 and the putative fourth protein, VP4. Protein products from the non-structural regions are derived as depicted in Figure 30.9 and by analogy to picornaviruses are likely to include a protease and an RNA-dependent RNA polymerase. Recent evidence indicates that the 3C sequence encodes for a protease which cleaves the P2–P3 junction of HAV[534] (see Figure 30.9). The function of the 3' non-coding region is unknown, and the primary nucleotide sequence in this region is highly variable. Further, a peptide (VPg) is bound to the 5' end of the RNA,[1244] and an RNA-dependent RNA polymerase encoded by the virus is associated with the genome.[924]

For further information, several excellent reviews have recently been written on the biophysical and molecular biological features of the hepatitis A virus.[215,237,429,472, 1050,1160]

Antigenic composition and determinants

HAV has a single serotype by virtue of a single immuno-dominant epitope. The antigenic integrity of this epitope appears to be conformation-dependent as it is detected on intact virions but not on isolated individual structural proteins.[472,655] Antibodies prepared in rabbits to intact HAV bind to isolated HAV structural proteins and will neutralize infectivity in cell culture; conversely, antibodies raised to isolated structural proteins and synthetic peptides representing VP1 epitopes do not recognize the intact virus and are incapable of neutralizing infectivity.[371] Convalescent HAV antibodies and rabbit anti-HAV will bind to fusion proteins produced in *E. coli* by transformation with plasmids containing the amino-terminal portion of Trp E fused with the VP1 cDNA sequence[541] and to a portion of VP1 produced by an expression vector.[841]

Multiple related immunogenic sites have been identified

by mapping with monoclonal antibodies produced to intact HAV. Of 16 stable hybridomas produced, the antibodies from 9 were able to compete with polyclonal anti-HAV from serum. The competitive monoclonal antibodies recognize disrupted HAV proteins in immunoblot analysis and at least one class of antibodies bound to a determinant on VP1.[497] Other studies have shown that three conformation-dependent epitopes (two of which overlap) combine to form a single immunodominant site on the virion.[655,1086] Several HAV mutants have been selected which escape neutralization by specific monoclonal antibodies. One mutant has a mis-sense mutation in VP3 replacing an aspartic acid residue with a histidine or alanine residue, another replaces a residue at position 102 of VP1. This indicates that VP3 and VP1 are important regions for binding neutralizing antibodies as with other picornaviruses such as polio and human rhinovirus.[883]

LABORATORY DETECTION OF HAV INFECTION

A range of techniques is available for detection of HAV or HAV antigen in body fluids and stools, and for antibodies to HAV in serum. The virus may be demonstrated in stools and body fluids by electron microscopy. However, this technique is time consuming and relatively insensitive. The viral RNA may be demonstrated with more sensitivity by molecular hybridization to radio-labelled cDNA probes[837,1159] or single-stranded RNA probes.[535] However, since most viral shedding precedes overt liver abnormalities, evidence of infection with HAV in the routine clinical setting is based on detection of specific antibodies to HAV by RIA or EIA. Serum IgG antibodies indicate previous exposure and immunity to HAV, while a rising titre is indicative of a recent infection.[928]

Following infection, IgM antibodies to HAV appear in the serum within a few weeks, usually preceding clinical presentation, and may remain detectable for several months, sometimes up to a year[653] (Figure 30.10). In a prospective study of IgM anti-HAV in 59 patients, marked

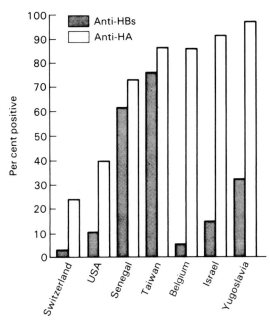

Figure 30.11 Relationships between prevalences of anti-HA and anti-HBs in young adults by country. (From Szmuness et al.[1119] with kind permission of the authors and the editor of the American Journal of Epidemiology.)

variability in the duration of its persistence was observed, ranging from 30 to 420 days, though most were seronegative by 120 days.[554a] A non-specific increase in polyclonal IgM is also common. Diagnosis of acute infection is therefore now usually based on detection of IgM to HAV in serum either by RIA[653,968] or EIA.[304,777] In these methods, antibodies to human IgM are coated to a solid phase, typically the wells of a plastic microtitre plate, and used to capture IgM in the serum under test. The presence of specific IgM to HAV is established by further incubation with HAV antigen, either radiolabelled or conjugated to a suitable enzyme. In the latter instance the activity of enzyme bound via HAV antigen to specific IgM on the solid phase is determined visually or spectrophotometrically following incubation with substrate. These tests are sensitive, specific and sufficiently reliable to allow diagnosis of acute infection to be confirmed with a single serum sample. Recently, detection of IgM anti-HAV in saliva has been demonstrated to be a satisfactory alternative to serum for the diagnosis of acute hepatitis A infection.[852]

EPIDEMIOLOGY OF HEPATITIS A

This has been fully reviewed by Dienstag et al.,[289] Purcell et al.[922] and Vyas et al.[1222] Hepatitis A has a worldwide distribution, but the true geographical incidence cannot be determined with accuracy. Studies of the prevalence of anti-HAV in blood donors show that it varies from 29% (in Switzerland) to 90% (in Israel and Yugoslavia), and indicate considerable geographical variation[1119] (Figure 30.11). Furthermore, only 5–10% of 18–19-year-

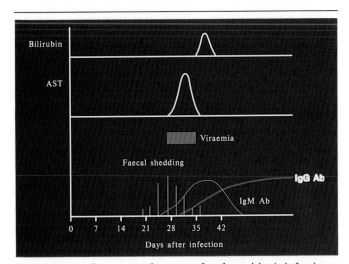

Figure 30.10 Sequence of events after hepatitis A infection.

olds in the USA and Switzerland have antibody, compared with over 90% in Israel and Yugoslavia. In a study of blood donors in West Scotland and children admitted to a Glasgow hospital, the prevalence of anti-HAV was 16% at age 5, 30% at age 15, and 78% at age >40 years.[612] Nevertheless, in most communities the majority of cases occur in childhood. A seasonal incidence, with a peak in late autumn, is usually observed, but is reported to be disappearing in the USA.[141]

In most temperate countries, especially in relatively closed communities such as Greenland, hepatitis A occurs in epidemics every 5–25 years.[1061,1062] In England, Wales and Ireland, there appears to be a 7-year cycle, with peaks of incidence reported in 1982 and 1989.[892] Hepatitis A is hyperendemic in tropical countries, particularly in the developing countries where infection occurs at an early age owing to poor hygiene. In the USA the prevalence of anti-HAV is higher in the lower socioeconomic groups, who are affected at an earlier age.[289,1267]

Improved socioeconomic conditions in Israel have been associated with a decrease in the incidence of hepatitis A in 1–4-year-olds, but the overall incidence has increased, largely owing to a doubling of the incidence in the 5–9-year-old age group.[420] Later exposure to the virus with an increase in clinical, rather than subclinical, infection was suggested as a possible explanation for this paradoxical rise in incidence of hepatitis A. Another factor related to both ethnic and socioeconomic group that appears to be a risk factor for hepatitis A infection is sibship size. In a multiple logistic regression analysis, sibship size emerged as the most important variable to correlate with positive serology for HAV in a study of 522 males aged 25–44 in Israel.[419]

Methods of spread

Documentation of the methods of spread of hepatitis A has been based on transmission experiments and studies of both sporadic and epidemic outbreaks in susceptible communities.[289]

Voegt showed that hepatitis with a short incubation period could be transmitted by duodenal juice.[1219] The importance of the faecal–oral route as a mode of transmission was firmly substantiated by the transmission experiments of MacCallum and Bradley,[689] Krugman and associates[607] and others.[690,691] The periods of infectivity ranged from 14 to 21 days before the onset of jaundice to the seventh or eighth day after jaundice, but were consistently negative thereafter, despite persistence of abnormal liver function tests. Based on these studies, the incubation period, that is the interval to the onset of first symptoms, ranged from 15 to 49 days. Clinical observations produce comparable figures; studies in general practice estimated an incubation period of 26–35 days[882] and point-source outbreaks similarly indicated an incubation period of 4–6 weeks.[189,286,1223]

These observations have been confirmed and extended by the direct examination of the shedding of hepatitis A

in stools, using immune electron microscopy, and by measuring specific antibody to hepatitis A in serum in transmission experiments or in sporadic outbreaks of hepatitis A in man, as well as in experimental infection of chimpanzees (see Figure 30.10). Dienstag et al.[284] studied the pattern of faecal shedding of HA Ag detected by immune electron microscopy in Joliot Prison volunteers inoculated with the MS-1 strain of HAV. Stool shedding of particles was observed 28–41 days after inoculation at the time of onset of prodromal symptoms, and peak elevation of the serum transaminase. In one study in chimpanzees, faecal shedding of HAV was noted 15–51 days after intravenous or oral inoculation of infected stools, and correlated with the peak transaminase elevation and histological necrosis in the liver.[285] Anti-HAV in serum developed 22–47 days after inoculation. Similar results were reported in four other chimpanzees.[1155] Purcell et al.[922] have determined the infectivity titre of HAV in various clinical specimens from patients acutely infected with the virus by inoculating susceptible chimpanzees and marmosets. There was a direct relationship between the challenge dose and the severity of the resultant hepatitis, with an inverse relationship between the infecting dose of HAV and the incubation period. The highest tires of HAV were detected in acute-phase stool samples. Acute-phase serum and saliva were much less infectious; the serum specimens all contained IgM anti-HAV which may have partly neutralized the virus. Urine and semen samples were not infectious for HAV.

Spread of infection most commonly occurs sporadically by the faecal–oral route as a result of direct contact. On occasions, in a susceptible community, explosive epidemics can occur. For example, in an epidemic in Greenland 93% of those affected were aged between 1 and 25 years, suggesting widespread immunity in the adult population, probably resulting from a similar epidemic documented in 1947–1948.[1062] Epidemics have also been traced to point-source contamination of food[189,444,682] or water supplies[1223] and there has been serological confirmation of an outbreak of hepatitis A due to ingestion of incompletely cooked mussels contaminated by sewage.[287] In the south of England a statistically significant association between hepatitis A and the consumption of cockles, but not other seafoods, has been reported in a case-controlled study.[830] A massive epidemic of hepatitis A in Shangai in 1988 affecting 292 301 people has been attributed to eating infected hairy clams from the Qidong beach area.[496] Hepatitis A occured in 11.92% of those who had consumed hairy clams compared to 0.52% of controls. Clam consumption preceded clinical symptoms by a mean period of 30 days and the risk of hepatitis A correlated with the number of clams consumed and with eating raw or lightly cooked clams. The source of infection was confirmed by a combination of immunological, immune electron-microscopic and molecular hybridization techniques. These demonstrated HAV in extracts of pooled alimentary gland and branchia from 1000 hairy clams both in those obtained from markets in Shangai and those from Qidong. The hairy clams were heavily contaminated, each containing 2–8 $TCID_{50}$ HAV, explaining the observation that approximately 12% of cases of hepatitis A in this epidemic had eaten just one clam. In a case control study in Japan, consumption of raw oysters was a significant risk factor for hepatitis A infection, and this was put forward as an explanation for the observed seasonal peak of cases in March each year.[465] In Livorno, Italy, consumption of raw mussels and clams was identified as the most likely source of an observed doubling of the annual incidence of hepatitis A infection in 1984. Following the introduction of comprehensive control measures in 1985, the annual incidence fell dramatically from 46 to 2.3 per 100 000 population.[741] In contrast, shellfish was thought to be a significant factor in only 56 of 25 451 reported cases of hepatitis A infection in a 9 year period in England, Wales and Ireland.[892]

Other foods have also been implicated in the spread of hepatitis A infection. Approximately 1000 food-handlers with hepatitis A were reported to the US Center for Disease Control (CDC) between 1975 and 1980, accounting for approximately 7% of reported cases per year.[167] In recent food-borne hepatitis A outbreaks, case control studies have suggested that vehicles of transmission include salads; foods routinely handled after cooking e.g. hamburger buns, and mixed bar drinks.[682,769] Customers who microwave their food before consumption appear to be protected from risk of developing hepatitis A.[769]

For members of a Westernized society, another significant risk factor for development of hepatitis A is travel to endemic areas. In the series of 25 451 reported cases in England, Wales and Ireland, 15% reported recent travel abroad, of whom 82% had visited high-prevalence areas, particularly the Indian subcontinent.[892] Of 233 French volunteer field workers in west and central Africa, seroconversion for IgG to HAV was documented in 48.1%.[637]

There is also evidence to indicate that HAV may be transmitted by the parenteral route. Transient viraemia during the late incubation period and early icteric phase of hepatitis A has been documented repeatedly by transmission experiments or by the inadvertent transfusion of infected blood.[1037] The prevalence of anti-HAV is greater amongst Norwegian drug addicts, occurring in 43% compared to 5% of an age-matched general population.[474] Moreover, the prevalence of anti-HAV correlated with the presence of markers for hepatitis B infection, suggesting possible parenteral transmission of HAV in this group.

Although circumstantial evidence suggests that transmission by urine can occur, this mode of spread is infrequent and has not been documented directly. Similarly, there have been occasional reports of spread attributable to infected nasopharyngeal secretions, including a large food-borne outbreak.[660]

Homosexual spread is unusual except under special circumstances of promiscuity involving frequent oral–anal contact, for example as occurs amongst communities in San Francisco.[233] A high incidence of hepatitis A has also been reported amongst male homosexuals in Holland.[241]

SPECIFIC CLINICAL FEATURES OF HEPATITIS A ___

The typical sequence of events after HAV infection is summarized in Figure 30.10. The incubation period ranges from 15 to 49 days, but during the prodromal phase faecal shedding occurs and is associated with transient viraemia. In a typical case the peak of transaminasaemia is heralded by intense nausea, anorexia and vomiting, which precedes the onset of jaundice. HAV is not usually detectable in the stools or serum once jaundice is clinically overt. Hepatitis A infection can present in a variety of atypical forms (see section on general clinical features of viral hepatitis) but two features are noteworthy:

1. Anicteric cases are common, based on the frequent finding of anti-HAV in subjects who have never been jaundiced and cannot recall an episode of hepatitis.[1120, 1125] The ratio of subclinical to clinical infections may be as high as 1:10 to 1:20 in some communities.
2. Some cases develop a marked and often prolonged intrahepatic cholestatic phase of their illness,[405] particularly the elderly. This may initially be difficult to distinguish clinically from extrahepatic bile duct obstruction.

Extrahepatic manifestations are much less common in HAV than in HBV infection.[1089] Those specifically reported in serologically proven HAV infection include arthritis and cutaneous vasculitis associated with cryoglobulinaemia and vascular deposits of IgM and complement;[250,506] toxic epidermal necrolysis;[1250] bradycardia and hypotension;[406] fatal myocarditis;[299] and renal failure in the absence of severe liver damage.[1184] Rarer complications include optic neuritis, transverse myelitis, and polyneuritis.[496]

Haematological manifestations may also occur (see section on general clinical features of viral hepatitis and Chapter 8). Thrombocytopenia, aplastic anaemia, and red-cell aplasia are all reported in serologically proven hepatitis A.[296,496,714]

There are no specific biochemical features of HAV infection, which cannot therefore be distinguished from other forms of viral hepatitis by standard liver function tests alone. When studied serially, the rise in aspartate aminotransferase (AST) is more rapid and less prolonged in HAV infection than in HBV.[607] In acute viral hepatitis, an elevated IgM level is relatively specific to HAV infection,[867,1301] but the need for such tests has been obviated by the development of specific serological tests for each of the viruses.

SPECIFIC PATHOLOGICAL FEATURES OF HEPATITIS A ___

The general features of an acute hepatitis are present but cholestasis is more pronounced and the periportal inflammation and hepatocellular damage are more prominent than in either hepatitis B or non-A, non-B hepatitis.[610,1015,1144] Bile thrombi and cholestatic liver cell rosettes can be particularly prominent, while immunocyto-chemically, cytokeratins appear in hepatocytes showing ductular transformation. Abnormal bile duct epithelium resembling the bile duct lesions in septicaemia may also be found.[1015]

Specific demonstration of HAV in the liver

After the identification of the virus of hepatitis A by immunoelectron microscopy in stools,[286,288,343] a similar and antigenically identical 27-nm particle was demonstrated in the hepatocyte cytoplasm.[1011] Immunofluorescent studies of experimentally infected chimpanzees also showed cytoplasmic localization and failed to demonstrate any nuclear antigen.[717] Positive reactions were obtained before any clinical, biochemical or morphological evidence of hepatitis. Initially, many hepatocytes showed faint fluorescence and this progressed to intense fluorescence in a few hepatocytes. Occasionally staining can be obtained after biochemical resolution of the hepatitis.

The virus has been grown in human hepatoma cell cultures,[262] and other culture systems.[263] The virus yield is low but sufficient to support the concept that HAV is a member of the family of picornaviridae viruses, although it has an unusually long period of replication.[263]

The virus and viral antigens have also been demonstrated within infected tissue culture cells using monoclonal antibodies to the hepatitis A virus and an immunogold pre-embedding technique.[245] Numerous antigenic sites were labelled within the cytoplasm of the infected cell. In cells showing cytopathic change multivesicular bodies were heavily labelled, whereas in cells not showing cytopathic changes cytoplasmic myelin figures were labelled and vesicles containing virus-like particles were also observed. In sequential studies infected cells showing cytopathic change showed early formation of long helical polyribosomes followed by hypertrophy and cysternal dilatation and degranulation of the rough endoplasmic reticulum. Large myelin-like structures and annulate lamellae appeared at a later stage as did the 24–27-nm virus-like particles within cytoplasmic vesicles.[1162]

HAV has also been demonstrated in the resected liver and follow-up biopsies of the transplanted liver in two patients using immunocytochemical and in-situ hybridization techniques. There was strong granular staining of the cytoplasm of many hepatocytes, using a monoclonal antibody to HAV. Probing for HAV-specific genomic sequences using a cDNA probe to the 3' end of the genome showed a predominantly nuclear/perinuclear pattern.[332]

PATHOGENESIS OF HEPATITIS A

Although a cytopathic effect of the hepatitis A virus can be demonstrated in tissue culture,[245,1162] the appearance of clinical evidence of liver disease with the immune response to the virus suggests a major role for cellular and/or humoral immunity in the pathogenesis of the liver disease. When human T lymphocytes in the liver biopsies of two patients with acute HAV infection were isolated,

42% and 53% respectively of the subsequent CD8[+] clones were HAV-specific when tested against HAV-infected skin fibroblasts.[1196] Similarly, in a marmoset model of hepatitis A infection, close interaction was identified between hepatocytes and lymphocytes by electron microscopy.[507] Although immune complexes have been demonstrated in the serum during experimental hepatitis A infection in chimpanzees,[700,701] they appear before the onset of liver disease and are usually formed by complexes of IgM with hepatitis A virus capsid polypeptides and RNA.[701] Immunocytochemically, IgM is present as granular deposits in the sinusoidal cells and HAV antigens have also been located in the Kupffer cell cytoplasm.[1016] It is believed that the immune complexes are a reflection of the viraemic phase of the disease[700] but it has also been suggested that the presence of the virus in Kupffer cells leads to their functional impairment and consequently the clinical and biochemical manifestations of disease.[1016]

PROGNOSIS AND CLINICAL OUTCOME IN HEPATITIS A

Hepatitis A is usually a benign, self-limiting disease, with the majority of patients making a full recovery with normal liver function tests within 2 months. A small number may develop the post-hepatitis syndrome with malaise, lassitude and depression. In a follow-up study of 1212 patients infected with HAV in the Shanghai epidemic, clinical recovery with normal liver function occured in 63.4% at 2 months, 20.4% at 3 months, 8.6% at 4 months, 4.8% at 5 months and 1.5% at 6 months.[496] The disease persisted beyond 6 months in 1.3% of cases. Progressive chronic liver disease is thought never to occur, but a biphasic relapsing illness associated with recurrent faecal shedding of HAV has been reported from Argentina.[1057,1136] There are also sporadic case reports of persistently abnormal liver function tests for up to 4 years[727] associated with liver fibrosis and persistence of IgM anti-HAV antibodies.[229,727]

Two factors are associated with increased severity of HAV infection: age greater than 50 years[616,793] and previous infection with HBV,[847] particularly in those with chronic active hepatitis B or cirrhosis.[496] If HAV infection occurs during pregnancy the prognosis for mother and fetus is good, with no reported increase in severity of hepatitis, or maternal or perinatal death rate.[496]

Fulminant liver failure is rare in HAV infection, and the mortality rate is estimated to be 0.14% in hospitalized cases.[654] In the Shanghai epidemic, fatal fulminant hepatitis A occurred in 8.55/10 000 cases.[496] In European tertiary referral centres for fulminant liver failure, HAV infection is responsible for 46/943 (4.9%) of cases in the King's College Hospital series[1256] and 4% of 502 cases in the Hôpital Beaujon series in France.[82]

TREATMENT OF HEPATITIS A

In the uncomplicated case of acute hepatitis A no specific therapy is of proven benefit, but attention to the general measures outlined earlier is recommended. Patients with the severe cholestatic form of viral hepatitis A may derive some symptomatic benefit from a short course of prednisolone (30 mg/day) to improve pruritus and general well-being, and to reduce the serum bilirubin,[307,405] but prolonged treatment with corticosteroids is not advocated.

The antioxidant compound (+)-cyanidanol-3 has been subjected to a controlled trial in the management of acute HAV infection but no benefit was observed above placebo.[879] In studies of HAV infection in the human hepatoma cell line PLC/PRF/5, four antiviral agents have emerged as being potential chemotherapeutic agents. These were ribavirin, amantadine, pyrazofurin and glycyrrhizin,[242] but they have not been evaluated in clinical HAV infection.

PREVENTION OF HEPATITIS A

This has recently been reviewed in detail by Iwarson.[522]

Immunoprophylaxis

In 1945 several field trials clearly established that human normal immune serum globulin (HNIG) could prevent hepatitis A infection if given before or within 1–2 weeks of exposure.[379,442] Administration of HNIG between 2 and 3 weeks after exposure to HAV is not effective in preventing clinical manifestations of the disease.[418] Preparations of HNIG from various sources in different parts of the world have been shown to be effective in either preventing or attenuating infection.[116,230,895] This is presumed to be due to the presence of high-titre anti-HAV in normal serum pools as a result of the frequency of infection in childhood. HNIG prepared, for example, from plasma pools in the USA and UK appears to be effective in preventing hepatitis A acquired abroad.

By attenuating the infection with HNIG, rather than preventing it completely, so-called passive–active immunity may theoretically result in natural lifelong immunity. Under such circumstances, the immunized individual excretes the virus at some stage, and it has been feared that such undetected ambulant cases might be a hazard to contacts, but this does not appear to be clinically significant.

Since HNIG is readily available and is effective in protecting 80–90% of contacts if administered before or within 1–2 weeks of exposure, its widespread use has been advocated. Recommendations for the use of HNIG are based on epidemiological data identifying groups at risk. The following recommendations are based on those of the Advisory Committee on Immunization Practices,[8] the WHO Expert Committee on Viral Hepatitis,[1267] and the Joint Committee on Vaccination and Immunization of the Department of Health (UK).

Close household contacts should all be given HNIG unless there is a clear history of hepatitis A infection in the past. Secondary attack rates are highest for children, but although they are low in adults the disease is often severe and therefore HNIG is recommended for them as well. School and work contacts should not be given HNIG routinely unless repeated cases are occurring, suggesting a common-source outbreak.

In prisons or in institutions for the mentally retarded, periodic outbreaks of hepatitis may occur and these may be contained by the administration of HNIG to patients and staff. Hospital and laboratory personnel should not be given routine prophylactic HNIG, but reliance on prevention of spread should be based on stringent precautions in dealing with infected material.

There is good evidence that travel abroad in tropical areas or developing countries where hepatitis A is common is associated with an increased risk of infection. It is therefore recommended that HNIG should be given in a dose of 0.02–0.12 ml/kg body weight intramuscularly and repeated at 6 months if there is continuing risk of exposure by residence abroad in such countries.

Individuals who handle non-human primates, particularly chimpanzees, are liable to develop hepatitis A, and HNIG in doses of 0.5 ml/kg body weight administered 4-monthly is advisable.

Current recommendations include the suggestion that individuals requesting HNIG should first be tested for anti-HAV antibodies to assess the need for prophylaxis, particularly if repeated HNIG administration is likely. This may obviate the need for HNIG in 13–60% of cases, depending on age and past medical history.[851,1146]

In the United Kingdom there have been concerns expressed about the falling titre of anti-HAV in blood donors and in HNIG preparations,[460] leading to the suggestion that the new inactivated hepatitis A vaccines (see below) could be used to immunize plasmapheresis donors as a method of preparing anti-HAV for clinical use in the future.[522]

Active immunization

Although hepatitis A is usually a relatively mild infection acquired in childhood, there is evidence that the age of infection in Western communitites is increasing. Since attacks may be more severe in the older age group, it can be argued that active immunization in childhood would be advantageous.

Hepatitis A vaccines are under commercial development and are likely to become available for clinical use in the near future.[522] Three different approaches have been adopted in attempts to produce a vaccine to HAV: a live attenuated virus vaccine, an inactivated virus vaccine; and the development of recombinant polypeptide vaccines.

Serial passage of HAV in cell cultures has made it possible to produce attenuated variants with reduced infectivity but retained antigenicity. In marmosets and chimpanzees these provide immunity without development of clinically significant infection.[557,918] Attenuated live vaccines have been used in human volunteers with some success. Mao *et al.* report use of an attenuated live H_2 strain of HAV in 12 volunteers, none of whom developed abnormalities of liver function and all of

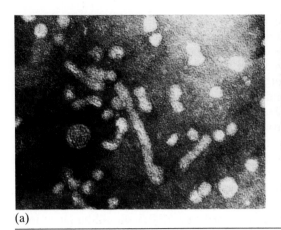
(a)

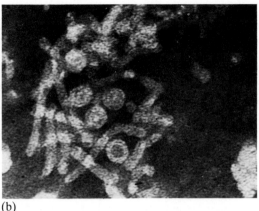
(b)

Figure 30.12 Hepatitis B surface antigen in serum. (a) Numerous small spherical particles (19 to 20 nm) predominate. (b) Long filamentous particles (40 to 45 nm) are seen. Dane particles are present in both (a) and (b), but are most frequent in (b), where an 'empty' Dane particle can also be identified.

whom seroconverted to become anti-HAV positive with neutralizing antibodies.[698] Using 10^7 TCID$_{50}$ of the F1 variant of HAV strain CR326F as an attenuated live virus vaccine, Midthun et al.,[749] report antibody to HAV in 100% of recipients, with neutralizing antibody present at 3 and 6 months after vaccination but no adverse effects on liver function. One potential advantage of live attenuated vaccines is their potential oral use for development of mucosal immunity, but the relevance of this has been questioned in HAV infection.[1087] A potential disadvantage is reversion to a virulent strain and this has encouraged the development of inactivated virus vaccines. These are prepared by various different techniques but are

Table 30.4 Properties of hepatitis B virus

Virion
- 42-nm spherical particles with lipid-rich outer envelope containing various surface antigens encoded by the virus
- Central hexagonal core 27 nm in diameter
- Up to 10^8 particles/ml serum

Core
- 27-nm hexagonal structure containing the viral genome and reverse transcriptase, encapsidated by core antigen
- Buoyant density in CsCl of 1.33 g/ml
- DNA genome formed by reverse transcription of RNA
- Genome relaxed, circular, partially double-stranded 3.2 kb with covalently-bound protein on 5' end of minus strand and RNA oligonucleotide on 5' end of plus strand
- Four open reading frames: pre-S and S, C, P and X
- Major proteins: HBcAg (M_r 22 kD). Viral polymerase encoding reverse transcriptase, terminal protein primer for DNA synthesis, and genome encapsidation function

Small particles and filaments
- 22-nm spheres and rods up to several hundred nanometres in length
- Buoyant density in CsCl of 1.17–1.21 g/ml
- In great excess of virions in serum, up to 500 mg/l
- Major polypeptides composed of glycosylated and non-glycosylated surface antigen

usually grown in cell culture (e.g. fibroblast) and then inactivated by exposure to formalin. In one study, such a vaccine coupled to aluminium hydroxide as an adjuvant induced anti-HAV antibodies in 100% of human volunteer recipients after three doses given at 1-month intervals.[353] Significant anti-HAV titres persisted in all recipients at 12 months.[354] Similar results were obtained in eight human volunteers injected with an inactivated hepatitis A vaccine prepared at the Walter Reed Army Institute.[1058] Commercial preparations of inactivated HAV vaccines are currently in clinical trial and should be available for clinical use in the near future.[522]

The future of HAV vaccination lies in the production of recombinant polypeptides for use as immunogens. The strategy is to insert the genetic sequences for the capsid proteins VP$_0$, VP$_1$ or VP$_3$ into expression vectors that can then generate the polypeptide/protein. Recombinant VP$_0$, VP$_1$ and VP$_3$ proteins have been used to immunize animals, which show a stable neutralizing antibody response when exposed to subimmunogenic doses of HAV.[372,541,910] The potential advantage of this technology is the eventual large-scale production of a highly purified, safe, effective and potentially inexpensive product.

HEPATITIS B

PROPERTIES OF HEPATITIS B VIRUS (see Table 30.4)

Human hepatitis B virus (HBV) is a prototype member in the family of Hepadnaviridae (for *hepa*totropic *DNA* *vir*uses). This family of viruses has numerous unique and remarkable aspects of structure and propagation which may inform rational approaches for antiviral strategies. Electron microscopy of HBV particles in serum reveals a number of forms: 43-nm double-shelled 'Dane particles' with 22–25-nm electron-dense inner cores; 20-nm spheres in 10^3-fold to 10^6-fold excess over the 'Dane particles'; and 20-nm diameter filaments of variable length (Figure 30.12).[251,965] Rods and spheres may reach concentrations of 10^{13}

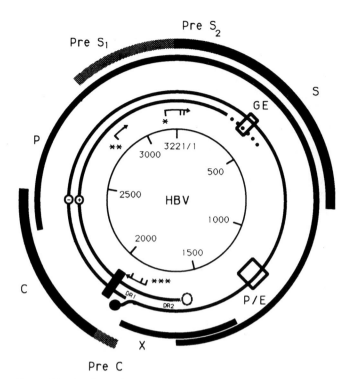

Figure 30.13 Organization of the HBV (strain adw2) genome. The position of the four ORFs (S, C, P and X) relative to their position in the viral genome is indicated. The internal calibration circle designates nucleotide number, ranging from 1 to 3221, beginning and ending at the unique EcoRI restriction site. Positions of transcript initiation are shown next to asterisks; the start sites for the 3.5-kb and 2.1-kb messages have three asterisks and one asterisk, respectively, while the start site for the 2.4-kb message has two asterisks. Positions of important *cis*-acting regulatory elements are also depicted, including the transcription termination element (TATAAA) (dark rectangle bisecting area of double-stranded DNA), the genomic promoter/enhancer element (P/E), the glucocorticoid-responsive enhancer (GE), and the direct repeat elements (DR1 and DR2). Positions of the terminal protein primer attached to the 5′ end of (−) strand DNA (dark circle) and the RNA oligonucleotide attached to the 5′ end of (+) strand DNA (stippled hollow circle) are included.

particles/ml. They are composed of lipid, protein and carbohydrate, sedimenting at 1.18 g/ml in caesium chloride. Along with host-derived lipid, these particles contain 24-kD hepatitis B surface antigen (HBsAg) in fantastic abundance at concentrations of 50–300 μg/ml serum. These subviral, non-infectious lipoprotein particles may serve as 'dummy particles' to bind neutralizing antibodies, a potential purpose for this enormous synthetic effort. Dane particles are the actual virions, containing nucleic acid as well as lipid, carbohydrate and protein. Removal of the viral envelope, containing HBsAg, with non-ionic detergent, unveils an inner core or nucleocapsid, whose chief structural component is a 21-kD hepatitis core antigen (HBcAg). The nucleocapsid also contains nucleic acid and a virus-derived polymerase, which incorporates

deoxyribonucleotide triphosphates into DNA without addition of exogenous template or primer.[964]

Genome structure

Disruption of the nucleocapsid with sodium dodecyl sulphate reveals the novel hepadnaviral genome, composed of relaxed circular DNA. Only 3.2 kb in size, the HBV genome is the smallest known for a non-defective animal virus (Figure 30.13). Two remarkable structural asymmetries exist within the genome: first, the 5′ end of the (−) strand is covalently bound to a protein,[383] while the 5′ end of the (+) strand is bound to an RNA oligonucleotide;[1254] and second, the two strands of DNA are of unequal size. The partially double-stranded DNA has a unit-length (−) strand (designated '(−)' because it is complementary to the virion mRNAs) and a shorter (+) strand. The (+) strand has a fixed 5′ end, but the 3′ end is variably terminated, not only between isolates but between each virus within an isolate. The (+) strand ranges from 15 to 60% of unit-length. The endogenous polymerase reaction alluded to above, in which deoxyribonucleotides mixed with virion cores are incorporated into DNA without addition of exogenous template, primer or polymerase, proceeds by elongation of the 3′ end of (+) strand DNA to repair the single-stranded gap region.[964,966,1103] The relaxed circular conformation is maintained by a 224-base-pair cohesive terminus at the 5′ end of the (+) strand; denaturation of the genome leads to formation of linear single strands of DNA.[987]

Genome organization

Molecular cloning and sequencing of numerous HBV isolates of various subtypes[187,587,834,1074,1193,1194] has revealed unprecedented parsimony in genetic arrangement. The compact 3.2-kb genome is achieved by overlapping structural open reading frames (ORFs), and *cis*-acting regulatory elements with structural ORFs, in over half of the genome. Every nucleotide in the genome encodes at least one structural element, and no intervening sequences are present. Owing to the overlapping functional arrangement, the mutation rate of the genome is very low, approximately 2×10^4 base substitutions per site per year. This rate is 1 to 2 orders of magnitude lower than for other DNA viruses during replication.[393] Examination of the nucleotide sequence reveals four ORFs, all encoded by (−) strand DNA. The four ORFs are designated S (surface antigen), C (core antigen), P (polymerase) and X (a transactivator). As evident in Figure 30.13, the P ORF overlaps all other ORFs, either partially (as with C and X) or wholly (as with S). The 5′ portion of pre-C overlaps with the 3′ terminus of X. Additionally, the C and S ORFs encode more than one protein product by virtue of numerous translation initiation codons in-frame within the same ORF. Thus, pre-S₁, pre-S₂ and S contain common nucleotide and amino acid sequences within all of S; pre-S₁ and pre-S₂ contain common amino acid sequences within all of pre-S_2; while pre-S_1 has a unique sequence of 119 amino acids at the NH_3 terminus. All three terminate at the 3′ end with the same translational stop codon. Similarly, pre-C contains all the nucleotide sequences in C, along with unique sequences at the 5′ end. The conserved regulatory sequences interspersed with the overlapping structural elements are also depicted in Figure 30.13. These include the 11-base-pair repeats DR1 and DR2, involved in the initiation of DNA replication, the TATAAA signal responsible for transcriptional cleavage and polyadenylation, and transcriptional enhancer elements which augment expression from the viral promoters.

Replication of HBV

The unique mechanism by which HBV propagates is a distinguishing feature of the hepadnaviral family. Although the virus particle contains DNA, the genome amplifies and replicates via an RNA intermediate, requiring utilization of a virally-encoded reverse transcriptase.[1105] To facilitate understanding of the complicated viral life cycle, a schematic is presented in Figure 30.14a. An overview of the major steps is as follows. *Step 1*: The mature virion containing partially double-stranded

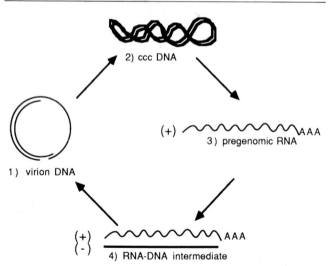

Figure 30.14a Overview of the hepatitis B viral life-cycle. (1) The intact virion containing partially double-stranded circular DNA enters a host cell and uncoats. The viral DNA undergoes a number of processing events (see text) to form covalently-closed circular (ccc) DNA. (2) The cccDNA, found exclusively in the nucleus, is the template for transcription of all viral messages including the pre-genomic RNA. (3) Pre-genomic RNA, so designated because it serves as the template for reverse transcription, is encapsidated with the virally-encoded reverse transcriptase. AAA designates a polyadenylation tract. (4) Sequestered within viral capsids, the pre-genomic RNA serves as the template for (−) strand DNA synthesis. Plus strand synthesis then proceeds using (−) strand DNA as template, forming a partially double-stranded DNA which is found in budded and now mature propagated virions. (Adapted from Ref. 366.)

DNA attaches, enters and uncoats in a permissive host cell. *Step 2*: The virion DNA matures into covalently closed circular DNA. *Step 3*: Genomic RNA is transcribed from the covalently closed circular DNA template. This genomic RNA is sequestered by an encapsidation reaction, serving as the template for Step 4. *Step 4*: Genomic RNA is reverse-transcribed to form (−) strand DNA. The (−) strand DNA then is replicated to form (+) strand DNA, bringing the cycle back to Step 1.[366,1106,1254]

Uptake of HBV

Little is known about the means of entry of HBV into host cells. Since the envelope proteins pre-S_1, pre-S_2 and S reside on the virion surface and are available for interaction with cellular membranes, they are considered leading candidates for mediating viral attachment to cells. However, the prime suspect is pre-S_1 protein, based on the consideration that Dane particles, containing one-third pre-S_1 in the envelope, obviously bind to cellular membranes, while abundant subviral particles which lack pre-S_1 protein do not. Indeed, experimental evidence confirms that only recombinant synthetic hepatitis B surface antigen particles containing some pre-S_1 protein could bind to human liver plasma membranes. This attachment was saturable and could be prevented by monoclonal antibodies specific for pre-S_1 protein.[896] Other studies using naturally obtained virions and 20-nm particles confirmed that virions attached to liver plasma membranes while subviral particles did not, and that the viral attachment was inhibited by monoclonal antibodies recognizing a sequential epitope between amino acids 27 and 49 of the pre-S_1 domain.[897]

Topographic analyses of pre-S_1 protein in viral envelope using monoclonal antibodies and protease digestion demonstrate that the amino-terminal portion of pre-S_1 is located on the virion surface.[623,872] Recent experiments by Kuroki and Ganem with duck hepatitis B virus have identified a candidate receptor for the virus on the plasma membrane of duck hepatocytes. This 180-kD protein binds specifically to a pre-S affinity column and demonstrates species and tissue specificity. The protein appears to be glycosylated, as it binds to a lectin column; binding can be prevented if the cells are treated first with tunicamycin (Kuroki and Ganem, personal communication).

No information is available on the fate of virions once attachment to host cells occurs, and the mechanism of entry, viral uncoating, and processing and transport of the genome to the nucleus remain to be elucidated.

Production of covalently closed circular DNA

Covalently closed circular (ccc) DNA is the first novel nucleic acid to appear in infections, preceding the appearance of viral RNA.[1106] This form is located exclusively in the nucleus and is requisite for persistence of viral infection. Many steps are necessary for conversion of partially double-stranded DNA to ccc DNA. These include: (1) completion of the single-stranded gap by extension of the 3′ end of (+) strand DNA to form a completely double-stranded DNA; (2) removal of the covalently bound protein from the 5′ end of the (−) DNA strand and removal of the RNA oligonucleotide from the 5′ end of the (+) DNA strand; (3) removal of the terminal redundancy from the (−) DNA strand; and (4) ligation of the 5′ and 3′ ends of each strand to form the cccDNA. The machinery and mechanisms by which this processing is achieved have not been explored.

Experiments by Tuttleman *et al.*[1188] using bromodeoxyuridine labelling revealed that the persistent cccDNA form replicates by reverse transcription of open circular forms, not by semiconservative replication of cccDNA. This indicated that reinfection of cells is required to perpetuate the cccDNA species, although the question remained whether virions have to exit the cell and then re-enter via the plasma membrane, or whether an intracellular pathway exists for reinfection. Utilizing the drug suramin, which blocks cellular entry of virus, Wu *et al.*[1281] have demonstrated that persistence of infection and continued formation of cccDNA primarily involve intracellular pathways which recycle encapsidated and reverse-transcribed viral genomes to the cell nucleus.

Synthesis of pregenomic RNA
Covalently closed circular DNA serves as the template for viral transcription, probably utilizing cellular RNA polymerase II. Two major classes of transcripts are synthesized (*vide infra*), only one of which, the 3.5-kb species, encodes all of the viral genetic information. This larger species is designated the pregenomic species because of its ultimate destination to and replication in viral cores.

Fine structure mapping of the 3.5-kb species in ground squirrel hepatitis virus actually reveals three species, varying by 31 nucleotides at the 5′ end. The larger two contain the AUG start codon for the precore gene product, but the smallest of the 3.5-kb transcripts initiates between the precore and core translation start sites. Only the smallest 3.5-kb transcript is found in viral cores, indicating stringent specificity in encapsidation of pregenome.[322] Site-directed mutagenesis of the precore AUG results in packaging of all three 3.5-kb transcripts (H. Schaller, personal communication). This suggests that the larger 3.5-kb transcripts are not packaged, owing to phenomena related to precore translation or secretory processing.

The pregenomic RNA is larger than the unit-length cccDNA because of a terminal redundancy, which contains a polyadenylation signal. This variant polyadenylation signal, TATAAA, must be ignored on the first pass of transcription and recognized and used on the second pass. The mechanism of this differential signal use has been investigated in ground squirrel hepatitis virus, and it appears that multiple DNA sequences upstream of the variant polyadenylation signal increase the efficiency of its use. The upstream sequences are not included in the 5′ end of the pregenomic RNA, as transcription initiation begins between the helper signal and the TATAAA

polyadenylation signal, but are present only at the 3′ end of the RNA.[978] (Figure 30.13).

Requirements for recognition and packaging of the pregenomic RNA into viral cores are being investigated. Stringent size requirements are likely to exist, and the primary sequence signal for packaging pregenomic RNA has been identified within an 85-nucleotide stem–loop structure at the 5′ end of the pregenomic RNA.[545] Aside from the obvious requirement for core antigen and RNA for encapsidation, translation of the P ORF is also required.[466] This ensures that every encapsidated RNA is capable of undergoing reverse transcription. Encapsidation of genomes defective for the polymerase gene product is inefficient, even when normal polymerase is provided in *trans*.[466]

Minus-strand DNA synthesis
Viral DNA synthesis occurs solely within nucleocapsids. Once pregenomic RNA is sequestered within nucleocapsids, (−) strand DNA synthesis commences with utilization of a protein primer.[778] Precipitation of protein primer–DNA complex with monoclonal antibodies specific for the amino terminal of the P ORF reveals that the protein primer is derived from the virus.[113]

Mapping of the 5′ end of (−) strand DNA after proteolytic digestion of the bound protein reveals that the DNA initiates within a DR1 element residing within a region of terminal redundancy[665,779,1025] (Figure 30.14b). Because DNA synthesis could originate in either the 5′ or 3′ DR1 element, Seeger and Maragos designed an expression vector for the production of infectious virus and found that initiation of reverse transcription began within the 3′ copy of DR1.[1026] Once initiated, DNA synthesis proceeds to the 5′ end of pregenomic RNA.

Plus-strand DNA synthesis
The RNA template in the (−) strand DNA/RNA intermediate is hydrolysed as (−) strand DNA synthesis proceeds. This hydrolysis is mediated by the RNase H activity encoded within the P ORF gene product.[930] Minus-strand DNA is then free to serve as the template for (+) strand DNA synthesis. The initiation site for (+) strand DNA has been mapped to the 3′ end of DR2[1025] (Figure 30.14b). The RNA oligonucleotide attached to the 5′ end of (+) DNA[664] is the primer for the synthesis of this strand; the RNA oligonucleotide is derived from the 5′ end of the original RNA pregenome, which was hydrolysed by RNase H to leave a capped oligonucleotide terminating at the 3′ end of the upstream DR1.[665,1025] The mechanism by which the RNA oligonucleotide undergoes transposition and binding to the DR2 site of (−) strand DNA is unknown. Initiation of (+) strand DNA synthesis is followed by progressive extension to the 5′ end of (−) strand DNA. At this point, in order to elongate further the (+) strand, the template containing the redundancy (*r*) at the 5′ end of (−) strand DNA must be substituted with the *r* at the 3′ end of (−) strand DNA, which generates an open circular molecule (Figure

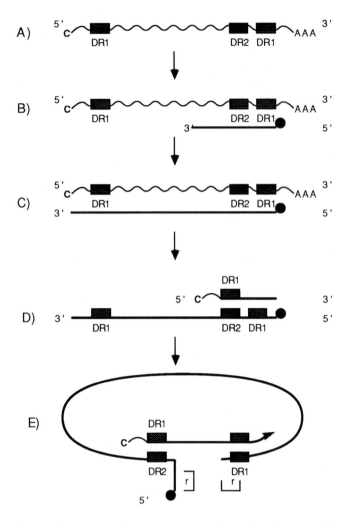

Figure 30.14b Replicative strategy of hepatitis B virus. (A) The capped polyadenylated pregenomic RNA containing direct repeat elements 1 and 2 (DR1 and DR2) serves as the template for reverse transcription. (B) Minus strand DNA synthesis initiates within the 3' DR1 element of pre-genomic RNA. (C) Minus strand DNA elongates to the 5' end of the RNA template. (D) Plus strand DNA synthesis begins when a capped RNA oligonucleotide, terminating with a DR1 element, is transposed to the DR2 site of (−) strand DNA. This oligonucleotide is probably formed by partial hydrolysis of pre-genomic RNA by RNase H. Plus strand DNA elongation proceeds until the 5' end of (−) strand DNA is reached. (E) Further elongation of (+) strand DNA requires switching the 5' end of the (−) DNA template for the 3' end of the (−) DNA template. This can occur because of the terminal redundancy present at the 5' and 3' ends of (−) strand DNA. The C represents the cap on RNA, r represents the terminal redundancy. The solid circle denotes a terminal protein primer covalently attached to (−) strand DNA, the stippled boxes represent direct repeat elements. Wavy lines denote RNA, solid lines denote DNA.

30.14b). From here, (+) strand synthesis could continue until reaching the 5' end of (−) strand DNA again, but, for reasons not known, (+) strand synthesis variably terminates as (+) strand DNA approaches 15–60% the total length of its template.

Viral transcription

All HBV transcripts are produced from (−) strand DNA and are capped, polyadenylated and terminated at a common 3' position. There are two major families of transcripts: the genomic 3.5-kb species and the subgenomic 2.4-kb and 2.1-kb species. The genomic RNAs serve two functions, as template for reverse transcription, and as messenger RNA for production of core antigen and polymerase. Subgenomic RNA is not encapsidated and serves as mRNA for pre-S_1, pre-S_2 and S (and perhaps X) proteins (Figure 30.13).

Fine structure mapping of the 3.5-kb and 2.1-kb species reveals that each is composed of multiple related transcripts varying at the 5' terminus (Figure 30.13). The 3.5-kb species has three transcripts differing by 31 nucleotides; only the smallest, which lacks the precore AUG, is encapsidated as the replicative template. The larger two of the 3.5-kb transcripts contain the precore AUG and therefore probably produce HBeAg as well as HBcAg and polymerase.[322] The 2.1-kb species also has three 5' variant transcripts, of which only the longest contains the pre-S_2 AUG. This transcript probably encodes the pre-S_2 protein, while the shorter two encode S.[176,1085] The 2.4-kb species appears to be a single transcript with the 5' end originating 38 nucleotides upstream of the translation initiation codon for pre-S_1.[1254] This transcript appears to encode pre-S_1. No other mRNAs are produced in abundance, although a low-abundance 0.7-kb mRNA is probably responsible for encoding the X protein.[1113] Alternatively spliced transcripts in low abundance have also been identified in transfected hepatoma cells and in naturally infected livers. These spliced transcripts have been characterized and genetically analysed. Although HBV mutants unable to produce spliced transcripts are replication-competent in vitro, it is not yet known what role they may play in natural infections.[1277]

Transcriptional regulatory elements

Regulatory elements required for RNA polymerase binding and initiation of HBV ORF transcription have been identified upstream of the major viral transcripts and the X ORF. These promoter elements lack a consensus TATAA element within 100 nucleotides of the 3.5-kb and 2.1-kb transcripts, which is the usual eukaryotic sequence utilized to properly initiate transcription approximately 30 nucleotides downstream.[322] Variations from this consensus sequence may explain the multiplicity of initiation sites demonstrated with HBV. Using putative HBV promoter elements linked to reporter genes, investigators identified a critical 84-bp region upstream of the genomic RNA start site[1284] and a 200-bp region immediately preceding the 2.1-kb transcript[934] as viral promoters. When HBV promoters were linked to a reporter chloramphenicol acetyltransferase gene, then transfected into a human hepatoma cell line, the relative promoter strengths were precore >X>pre-S_2>pre-S_1.[40]

Two orientation-independent, *cis*-acting enhancer

elements have been identified in HBV. The first, residing in a 100–200-base-pair region 600 base pairs upstream of the genomic RNA start site, enhances both the genomic RNA and X promoters.[476,1035] This enhancer appears to work best in liver cells,[525,1035] augmenting expression 3-fold to 20-fold[476] or 20-fold to 100-fold[40] in liver cells, compared to only 2-fold to 5-fold in non-liver cells. A second enhancer, apparently lacking species or tissue specificity, mediates the effect of steroids by binding to a glucocorticoid-receptor complex. This 30-base-pair glucocorticoid-responsive enhancer is located 340 base pairs upstream from the HBV EcoRI site, within the S ORF. Its activity is more modest, perhaps augmenting expression 3-fold to 5-fold.[1185]

The HBV genomic enhancer must bind a number of cellular transactivation factors in order to mediate its effect. These factors are, to varying degrees, tissue- and species-specific in distribution and confer, in part, the tissue tropism and species specificity characteristic of hepadnaviral infection. Transactivating factors E, TGT3, EP and NF-I all bind to the 83-base-pair-long HBV DNA enhancer fragment.[83,840] The positive factor E is responsive to phorbol ester, while EP is the factor identical to EF-C, which binds the polyoma virus enhancer.[840]

In addition to binding cellular transactivators, the HBV genome appears to produce a powerful pleiotropic transactivator from the X ORF. This product may alter the viral disease course, activating cellular genes, augmenting viral gene expression, diminishing the host immune response or modifying cellular proto-oncogene expression, predisposing to hepatocellular carcinoma. The transactivator role of X was proposed based on genome sequence comparisons between HTLV and HBV.[755] X has since been shown to activate both pol II and pol III promoters[47] up to 20-fold to 40-fold. A variety of heterologous viral promoter and enhancer combinations are demonstrably activated by the X gene product; notably, the LTR elements from HIV,[1029] HTLV-1, RSV and the HSV-thymidine kinase gene[1078,1189] and the SV40 enhancer and early promoter. The X gene product also positively transactivates the homologous HBV core enhancer/promoter element in permissive cells.[217] Recent studies by Seto *et al.* demonstrate that X acts through the AP-1 and AP-2 sites and that X has a transcription activation domain.[1030]

Tissue specificity

The remarkable species specificity and tissue tropism of HBV appears to result from (1) the interaction of the viral envelope protein(s) with a limited number of cell types containing the viral receptor, and (2) the specificity of host cell transactivation factors with the viral genomic promoter/enhancer element. Studies by Kuroki and Ganem (personal communication) demonstrate that the pre-S protein of duck hepatitis B virus binds to a specific 180-kD membrane-bound candidate receptor protein which has limited tissue distribution in host animals. Replication appears limited to animals which exhibit this

membrane-bound protein. Further factors restrict HBV replication once DNA enters a host cell, as replicative intermediates are found only in productively infected cells in vivo, in primary hepatocytes infected in vitro,[819] and in transfected hepatoma cells such as HepG2.[1108] It appears that the restricted production of genomic RNA to these cell populations is limited by the presence of liver-specific proteins binding to sequence-specific areas on HBV, notably to 17- and 12-base-pair-long palindromes in the HBV enhancer and promoter domains, respectively.[476,556] The production of 2.1-kb mRNA is not as restricted as 3.5-kb mRNA. This transcript can be found in multiple cell types from different species and tissues,[366] although some preferential liver and kidney expression is found in some transgenic mice containing the HBV genome with the S promoter.[148] This transcript also demonstrates developmental and male sex hormone regulation in transgenic mice, as expression of 2.1-kb transcripts could be diminished by castration of male mice, then restored by provision of testosterone to these animals.[266,337]

Extrahepatic forms of HBV and other mammalian hepadnaviruses have been observed in tissues such as peripheral blood leucocytes, pancreas, kidney and spleen.[366,640,967] Generally, the copy number in these tissues is far lower than in liver tissue. However, Korba *et al.*[592] demonstrated that replication of woodchuck hepatitis virus in peripheral blood leucocytes can be stimulated in vitro by a lipopolysaccharide mitogen. This finding suggests that extracellular factors may provide signals which stimulate viral replication in extrahepatic tissues under certain conditions which have yet to be elucidated.

Viral proteins

The P ORF product

Isolation and characterization of the P ORF gene product has not been achieved. Sequence homology in the P ORF to other gene sequences encoding reverse transcriptase in retroid elements (such as retroviruses and calimoviruses) led to suspicion that the P ORF encoded a polymerase.[1165]

Genomic analysis of the P ORF has revealed four domains. The amino terminal domain probably encodes the protein primer for (−) strand DNA synthesis. This is followed downstream by a spacer region, which is followed by a domain encoding RNA- and DNA-directed DNA polymerase function. Site-directed mutagenesis of conserved sites in this region results in the production of nucleocapsids containing only single-stranded RNA. The last domain, at the 3′ end of the P ORF, encodes RNase H activity, required for hydrolysis of RNA in the RNA–DNA replication intermediate. The multifunctional gene product appears to be expressed as a single translational unit.[930] The P ORF gene product appears also to play an essential role in packaging of genomic RNA, independent of its role in reverse transcription.[466]

The P ORF can theoretically encode a protein of

90 kD. Activity gel analysis of virion proteins run on SDS–polyacrylamide gel electrophoresis and then renatured reveals two polymerase activities migrating at 90 and 70 kD. These activities can be immunoprecipitated with antibodies to peptides prepared from the P ORF.[68,69] The translation of P appears to arise by de-novo initiation at the internal P ORF AUG in 3.5-kb transcripts, not by formation of core–pol fusion proteins, followed by post-translational proteolytic processing, as found in retroviruses.[183,1003]

The X ORF product

The X ORF gene product has not been isolated from virions. From the nucleic acid sequence, the gene product is predictably 17 kD in size. In vitro transcription and translation of cloned X-region HBV DNA demonstrates a 17-kD product.[591] Purified X protein cloned in _E. coli_ is 16.5 kD.[1280] Screening of chronic viral carrier sera reveals the occasional presence of antibodies directed to a synthetic X product.[591,747] At present, the only known function for X is that of a generalized transactivator (_vide supra_). Production of X appears to be essential for viral replication, as frameshift mutants in a region past the P ORF–X ORF overlap fail to propagate in vivo.[366] Strong evidence suggests that the X gene product is a serine/threonine protein kinase, and that this kinase activity is required for the transactivating function. The kinase activity is present in intact virions. Although the X gene product cannot bind to DNA substrates directly, apparently it is responsible for phosphorylating other transactivators which do bind to the HBV enhancer and other heterologous viral promoter elements.[1280] The transactivating activity of X antigen resides within amino acids 32 to 148, and the N- and C-terminal residues are dispensable for this activity.[951]

C ORF products

The major structural component of the viral capsid is hepatitis B core antigen (HBcAg). This antigen is only present in serum as an internal component of Dane particles; immunoprecipitation of HBcAg can only be achieved after removal of the viral envelope with non-ionic detergent.[964] HBcAg derived from viral cores in serum appears to be a single species on gel electrophoresis. This 21-kD protein has 183–185 amino acids, of which the carboxy-terminal 34 amino acids are rich in arginine. The basic carboxy-terminal end confers non-specific DNA binding activity to this protein,[871] although RNA binding activity has not been demonstrated. Within hepatocytes, HBcAg from native cores appears heterogeneous on gel electrophoresis. Heterogeneity is removed by treatment of the cores with alkaline phosphatase, indicating that HBcAg is a phosphoprotein while within the cell.[919] Since HBcAg becomes dephosphorylated in the course of viral export, phosphorylation may play a role in viral maturation.

Another antigen found in the serum of HBV-infected patients is hepatitis Be antigen (HBeAg). This soluble 16-kD antigen, antigenically and physically different from HBsAg and HBcAg, is now known to be produced from the same ORF as HBcAg (Figure 30.13). The C ORF has two in-frame translation initiation codons, separated by a short distance, which can encode 29 amino acids. HBeAg appears to be synthesized beginning with the first AUG, while HBcAg is synthesized beginning with the second. The 29-amino-acid leader sequence appears to be a signal sequence responsible for altering the intracellular pathway and subsequent processing between HBeAg and HBcAg. The signal sequence ultimately directs the precore protein to the endoplasmic reticulum, Golgi and cellular membrane, and to a secretory pathway leading to its presence in serum, whereas the core protein accumulates as particles in cytoplasm and, to some extent, in nuclei.[1002] In the course of precore processing, 19 amino-terminal acids are cleaved, along with 34 carboxy-terminal amino acids.[843] As a portion of the C ORF resembles an aspartyl protease coding domain,[756] it appeared that conversion of HBcAg to HBeAg might involve self-cleavage; however, site-directed mutagenesis of the putative protease domain did not alter HBcAg or HBeAg processing.[531,801]

The production of precore protein does not appear to be necessary for viral infection or replication. Introduction of frameshift mutations in vitro in the precore region still results in productive infection,[181,1001] and spontaneous termination codons may arise in this region in the course of normal human infections. These variant strains appear to occur in individuals with HBsAg-positive viraemia who are also positive for anti-HBe.[825,1168]

S ORF products

The envelope of virions is composed of approximately equimolar ratios of pre-S_1, pre-S_2 and S proteins. All three proteins are required for virion assembly and infection.[1190] These proteins share common antigenic determinants, as they share the 226 amino acids which compose S. The S protein has both non-glycosylated and glycosylated forms, designated $p24^S$ and $gp27^S$ respectively. Middle S, or pre-S_2 protein, has a unique amino terminus of 55 amino acids preceding the common S sequence. Pre-S_2 also has non-glycosylated and glycosylated forms, designated $p33^S$ and $gp36^S$ respectively. Last, large S protein, or pre-S_1, has 174 unique amino acids at the amino terminus preceding S, with 119 unique amino acids preceding pre-S_2. The non-glycosylated and glycosylated forms of pre-S_1 are termed $p39^S$ and $gp42^S$ respectively.[450,504]

The pivotal role of the immune response to surface antigens in the resolution or persistence of HBV infection has led to intensive interest in the structural and immunogenic properties of these molecules. The epitopes unique to pre-S_1 and pre-S_2 appear to be on the surface of the virion, as monoclonal antibodies to these epitopes can bind to intact virions,[988] and the unique epitopes can be removed by limited proteolysis, leaving only the S determinants.[450] Antibodies to all three proteins usually appear during the course of natural infection, any of which are protective and neutralizing. In some individuals, antibodies to pre-S are produced without production of detectable antibody to S. The genetic basis for variation in immune response has been pursued in inbred mice. Responses to pre-S and S are controlled by distinct H-2 genes.[751] Some epitopes of pre-S and S are recognized by B cells in different mouse strains, while other pre-S and S epitopes are recognized by T cells.[753] Some mice non-responders to S develop antibodies to S when immunized with pre-S$_2$, indicating that T helper cells directed to pre-S$_2$ provide help to B cells directed to S.[752] Although these experiments with mice may not be wholly applicable to humans, the results indicate that inclusion of the highly immunogenic pre-S$_2$ in recombinant vaccines may be useful for those individuals who do not respond to S alone.[1178]

Viral mutants

Chronic carriers of HBV may exhibit emergence and gradual takeover of wild-type HBV by mutant forms. On occasion, the emergence of these forms may be accompanied by serological conversion in the patient from HBeAg to anti-HBe positivity. The advent of polymerase chain reaction (PCR) technology has facilitated detailed analysis of the mutants in HBsAg-positive, anti-HBe positive individuals. Santantonio *et al.* found that 41 of 42 carriers with this serological pattern contained mutations in the precore region which prevented HBeAg expression: 33 were infected predominantly or exclusively with variants containing a stop codon; two had a mixture of wild-type and a precore stop codon mutant virus; and three had precore variants with mutations of the precore translation initiation codon.[986] Some patients with precore stop variants may be more prone to suffer fulminant hepatitis than those with wild-type virus. In a recent survey, 9 of 10 patients with HBV and fulminant hepatitis had a preponderance of the variant recovered from serum, while 0 of 8 patients with acute hepatitis demonstrated this change.[597] Another study demonstrated a source outbreak of fulminant hepatitis stemming from an anti-HBe positive carrier in which all five fulminant cases were found to have a common viral variant containing two mutations in the precore region.[661] Other mutations in the presurface/surface, X and C regions were present, which may also or alternatively impact on the clinical response in these infections. (See also Prevention of Hepatitis B—escape mutants of hepatitis B virus.)

Systems for studying hepadnaviruses

Animal hepadnaviruses

An outbreak of primary hepatocellular carcinoma associated with chronic hepatitis in captive Eastern woodchucks (*Marmota monax*) at the Philadelphia zoo led to the discovery of woodchuck hepatitis virus (WHV), a viral homologue of HBV.[1104] This fortunate discovery was

followed quickly by the discovery of other hepatitis B viruses, that of ground squirrel hepatitis virus (GSHV) affecting Beechey ground squirrels (*Spermophilus beecheyi*),[704] duck hepatitis B virus (DHBV) affecting Pekin ducks (*Anas domesticus*),[715] and heron hepatitis virus (HHV) which affects herons.[1083] Each virus has been characterized, cloned and sequenced, allowing detailed comparisons.[249,364,365,588,696,716,1024,1046] The family of hepadnaviridae has many similarities: (1) a narrow host range and relative hepatotropism; (2) a life cycle characterized by reverse transcription of an RNA intermediate; (3) production of copious defective subviral particles containing surface antigens; (4) a partially double-stranded 3.3-kb DNA genome with a relaxed circular conformation; and (5) a compact genome with overlapping open reading frames for core antigen, surface antigen and polymerase. Within the family of hepadnaviridae there appears to be a subdivision into mammalian hepadnaviruses (HBV, GSHV, WHV) and avian hepadnavirus (DHBV, HHV). These two groups differ in that mammalian hepadnaviruses (1) exhibit greater nucleotide sequence homology with each other compared to the avian viruses, (2) have four open reading frames (S, C, P and X) while the avian virus (without X) has three, (3) demonstrate antigenic cross-reactivity which does not extend to the avian viruses, and (4) vary in their virion ultrastructure from the avian hepadnaviruses.[967]

Non-HBV members of hepadnaviridae fortuitously provide models for studying viral-associated pathogenesis (Table 30.5). Mammalian hepadnaviruses can all cause chronic active hepatitis of varying degrees and are associated with hepatocellular carcinoma (HCC). Infection of woodchucks with WHV provokes a particularly virulent hepatitis which can cause HCC in 25% of animals by the time they average 52 months old.[850] Infection of ground squirrels with GSHV results in a less severe degree of hepatic inflammation, with a diminished incidence of HCC occurring in these animals, usually in later life.[705] A significant incidence of HCC has never been demonstrated in domesticated DHBV-infected Pekin ducks bred in the United States.

In-vitro systems

Both immortalized hepatoma cells in culture and primary hepatocytes are available to study the hepadnaviral life cycle. Primary hepatocytes prepared by collagenase perfusion of newborn duckling[1187] or fetal human liver[819] are permissive for infection and replication of DHBV or HBV respectively in the first few days after culture. Transformed human hepatoma cells, such as HepG2 or Huh7, transfected with naked DNA, are permissive for viral replication.[5,1108,1283] HepG2 cells transfected with HBV DNA produce virions in media which are infectious to chimpanzees,[1109] confirming the replication competence of this system. However, immortalized hepatoma cells cannot be infected, presumably because they lack viral receptor.

The availability of these in-vitro systems and animal

Table 30.5 Comparison of hepadnaviruses

| Virus | Host | Size (kb) | ORFs | Pathological consequences | | |
				Healthy carrier	Chronic hepatitis[a]	Hepatocellular carcinoma[a]
HBV	Humans	3.2	4	Yes	++	++
WHV	Eastern woodchucks	3.3	4	Yes	+++	+++
GSHV	Beechey ground squirrels	3.3	4	Yes	+	++
DHBV	Pekin duck	3.0	3(no X)	Yes	0	0 (in USA)

+ = rare; ++ = occasional; +++ = frequent.

models has provided unprecedented opportunity to study viral biology and pathogenesis. Cloned hepadnaviral genomes may be genetically manipulated and reintroduced into isolated cells or animals to address fundamental questions in the viral life cycle. Many of the studies following have utilized such approaches.

LABORATORY DETECTION OF HEPATITIS B INFECTION

Techniques for the laboratory detection of hepatitis B infection have recently been reviewed.[484] Those commercially available include tests for HBsAg, HBeAg, HBV-DNA (by hybridization methodology), anti-HBs, anti-HBe, anti-HBc and IgM anti-HBc. These tests provide information for clinical use, but for research purposes other tests are available, including HBV-DNA by polymerase chain reaction (PCR), pre-S_1 and pre-S_2 antigens and their respective antibodies, and tests for HBV-DNA polymerase activity. Each of these tests and their clinical significance is reviewed below. The sequence of serological changes is discussed further later (see Specific Clinical Features of Hepatitis B).

Hepatitis B surface antigen and antibody

Earlier tests for HBsAg and anti-HBs, which included the original immunodiffusion technique, complement fixation and counterimmunoelectrophoresis, have now been replaced with third generation tests which are both highly sensitive and specific. These include various forms of radioimmunoassay (RIA), haemagglutination assays and enzyme immunoassays (EIA). Their merits have been reviewed[62,490,920] but, because of their relative simplicity and similar sensitivity to RIA,[1261] EIAs have become the most widely used tests for detecting HBsAg and anti-HBs.

Detection of HBsAg in the serum is indicative of active infection with hepatitis B, but the absolute level of surface antigenaemia carries no clinical significance and is not related to the degree of infectivity.[484] For example, high levels of HBsAg may be seen in otherwise healthy carriers of HBV.[482] In an individual patient a decreasing titre of HBsAg is indicative of a resolving infection[363] and is probably an earlier prognostic marker than changes in

HBeAg status. Serum samples must be at least 10–14 days apart if a significant change is to be observed.

Even techniques as sensitive as RIA and EIA for detection of HBsAg are not infallible, and occasional cases occur that are negative for HBsAg by standard RIAs or EIAs but positive for other serological tests such as DNA polymerase activity, anti-HBc or HBV-DNA. The development of monoclonal antibody reagents to detect HBsAg[1227] has improved sensitivity and such tests are now commercially available as one-step monoclonal EIAs. False negative results have also been reported with these assays, probably owing to a mutation in the 'a' epitope of HBsAg.[949]

Anti-Hbs is generally found only after clearance of HBsAg from serum and usually persists long term. A 'window' may occur between loss of HBsAg and development of anti-HBs. Occasionally in chronic carriers both HBsAg and anti-HBs may coexist.[1040] Naturally acquired anti-HBs has been seen as conferring immunity against HBV, but the protective value of low titres is not established.[600] Anti-HBs also occurs after active vaccination and is normally successful in conferring immunity (see Prevention of Hepatitis B).

Subtyping of hepatitis B surface antigen and antibody

The commonest technique used for subtyping is a counterimmunoelectrophoretic method employing cross-absorbed monovalent reagents. Other techniques include passive haemagglutination and reverse passive haemagglutination. With all these methods, high-titre specific antisera are required. Subtyping can also be carried out by a double-label radioimmunoassay.[157] Subtyping may be of particular value in sero-epidemiological studies (see Epidemiology of Hepatitis B).

Pre-S antigens and antibodies

Tests for pre-S antigens and antibodies are currently considered to be research tools, but it has been suggested that their detection may have some clinical relevance. Methods are not standardized and variable sensitivity may explain some of the discrepant results which have been reported.

Using sensitive assays, pre-S_1 and pre-S_2 antigens have been reported in the sera of 95% of cases of acute hepatitis B,[265] and in general their presence correlates with positivity for HBV-DNA and markers of viral replication.[192,614] Pre-S$_1$ and pre-S$_2$ antigens have however, also been reported in the sera of patients who are HBV–DNA-negative with no markers of active viral replication.[265,1205] Pre-S antigens appear early in acute HBV infection[127] but early disappearance is common and may indicate subsequent clinical resolution.[265] Persistence of pre-S antigens has been associated with chronic HBV infection[192,265,614] and pre-S$_2$ antigen persistence is associated with poor outcome in fulminant hepatitis B.[128]

Anti-pre-S antibodies develop early in the clinical course of acute HBV infection,[452] usually at a stage when HBsAg is detectable and before development of anti-HBs. It has been suggested that the intensity of the anti-pre-S$_2$ antibody response is closely correlated with subsequent resolution of HBV infection,[1183] and failure to develop anti-pre-S$_2$ antibodies has been associated with a poor prognosis in fulminant hepatitis B.[128] Early claims that anti-pre-S antibodies may play a role in elimination of the virus[1150] have not been substantiated and it is now clear that they may persist in high titre in chronic HBV infection.[144,454] The anti-pre-S antibody response is biphasic, with a second peak detectable in the convalescent phase.[144] Long-term persistence of anti-pre-S antibodies in serum may occur as described for, but independent of, anti-HBs.[452]

At present it is not clear that tests for pre-S$_1$ and pre-S$_2$ antigens and their respective antibodies provide information that is of greater value than that obtained from tests that are routinely available in clinical practice.

Hepatitis B core antigen and antibody

Hepatitis B core antigen is readily detectable in liver in HBV infection (see section on specific pathology of HBV infection) but is not usually detectable in serum unless specific manipulations are undertaken to reveal HBcAg contained within intact virions. In a recent study employing high-molarity treatment of serum, HBcAg levels measured by RIA correlated well with serum HBV-DNA in chronic HBV infection.[191] In acute HBV infection, HBcAg positivity persisted despite HBV-DNA clearance and correlated with maximum liver damage, leading to the suggestion that this may have occurred due to release of HBcAg from HBV-infected hepatocytes undergoing lysis.[191]

Anti-HBc is usually measured by commercially available EIAs. It develops early in acute HBV infection and persists long term. Anti-HBc may be present in acute infection in the absence of HBsAg[514] and also persists as a marker of previous infection after HBsAg clearance, making it a valuable tool in sero-epidemiological surveys of HBV infection.[484] Anti-HBc does not develop after hepatitis B vaccination and it may therefore be used to distinguish HBV infection from previous vaccination.[484]

IgM anti-HBc is usually measured by commercially available RIAs or EIAs. A knowledge of the sensitivity of the method employed is important for subsequent interpretation of results. IgM anti-HBc develops early and is present in high titre in acute hepatitis B, but may also persist in low titre for prolonged periods in chronic HBV infection.[58,188,1056] Modern tests are therefore designed to detect IgM anti-HBc above a pre-defined level and are usually indicative of recent HBV infection. The duration of detection of IgM anti-HBc using such tests is variable, ranging from 2 to 134 weeks after acute HBV infection.[188,671] IgM anti-HBc is particularly useful in distinguishing recent and current HBV infection from remote previous infection and is also useful in diagnosing HBV infection when HBsAg is negative, e.g. in some cases of fulminant hepatitis B or in the recovery phase of acute hepatitis B after clearance of HBsAg and before appearance of anti-HBs.

Titres of IgM anti-HBc may rise with spontaneous reactivation of HBV infection associated with reappearance of HBV-DNA and DNA polymerase activity in the serum, i.e. markers of active viral replication.[1056] The nature of this response has recently been investigated in more detail in acute icteric hepatitis superimposed on chronic HBsAg carriage. IgM anti-HBc was separated by rate zonal centrifugation into 19 S and 7–8 S forms; the 19 S form was observed in reactivation of chronic hepatitis B and was associated with a severe clinical course (mortality 5/9 cases), whereas the 7–8 S form was observed more frequently in HDV superinfection (see Hepatitis D) and was associated with a more benign clinical course (mortality 1/9 cases).[1142]

'e' Antigen and antibody

Detection of HBeAg in the serum is of particular value in the clinical evaluation of the patient with HBV infection because of its association with viral replication, active liver damage and infectivity.[484] The 'e' antigen is derived from the nucleocapsid gene of HBV[842] and is a fragment of the virus core, probably formed by autocleavage of the core protein[756] (see section on properties of HBV-C ORF products). It is found only in HBsAg-positive sera and is usually measured by commercially available RIAs or EIAs, as is HB 'e' antibody.

HBeAg is found in the serum early in acute HBV infection but disappears in association with the appearance of 'e' antibody in resolving infection.[481] Persistence of HBeAg is associated with continuing infectivity, viral replication and liver damage, with subsequent development of chronic liver disease. In a Caucasian population, patients who are HBeAg positive usually have detectable HBV-DNA in the serum, but other ethnic groups may exhibit discordance; e.g. 87% of an HBeAg-positive Asian population were reported to be HBV-DNA-negative.[1017] It is important to note that patients with chronic liver disease due to HBV are not universally HBeAg positive; some cases of chronic active hepatitis may be negative for HBeAg and positive for HBe antibody.[432] These patients are usually HBV-DNA positive together with other markers of viral replication. This clinical and serological picture may also be seen with the 'e' negative mutant of HBV in which there is an adenine–thymidine mutation which creates a stop codon in the pre-core gene and prevents 'e' antigen synthesis (see section on properties of HBV+HBV mutants). A negative HBeAg result does not therefore equate to a zero risk of infectivity, although in general the risk of infectivity is lower than in HBeAg-positive sera.

Recent studies have separated HBeAg into small and large molecular forms by agarose gel electrophoresis, with preliminary results suggesting that large HBeAg correlates with severity of chronic liver disease.[621]

HBV-DNA and DNA polymerase activity

HBV-DNA can be detected in serum using either hybridization techniques or the polymerase chain reaction. In the hybridization methods, cloned radiolabelled HBV-DNA of high specific activity is used as a probe which is hybridized either with extracted viral nucleic acids[107,131,549] or with nucleic acids retained on a nitrocellulose filter after spotting of serum samples.[807,1018] These methods will detect in the order of 10–500 pg/ml (approximately 10^6 genome equivalents) of HBV-DNA[484] and are now commercially available. A recently described modification of the spot-hybridization technique using a digoxigenin-labelled probe reports detection of 1–3 pg/ml of HBV-DNA.[802]

In acute viral hepatitis, HBV-DNA is not found during the incubation period but becomes detectable, after HBsAg is present in serum, at the onset of clinical symptoms.[432,1264,1299] HBV-DNA is cleared from the serum rapidly in acute self-limited HBV infection, usually disappearing before HBeAg and invariably before biochemical resolution of the hepatitis. HBV-DNA usually remains detectable in patients with persisting HBeAg and in patients with chronic HBV-related liver disease. The presence of HBV-DNA in serum (measured by dot hybridization) implies active viral replication, ongoing liver disease and infectivity.[432,481,484]

The polymerase chain reaction method of detecting HBV-DNA is extremely sensitive and is currently used predominantly as a research tool. This assay and its modifications are reported to detect as few as 1 to 3 virus genomes in serum samples.[1288,1299] With this extraordinary level of sensitivity, this assay must be performed under carefully controlled conditions in order to avoid false positive results. Notwithstanding these reservations, it appears that HBV-DNA (measured by PCR) is detectable in the majority of HBsAg-positive sera. HBV-DNA (by PCR) was detected in 95–100% of those who were both HBsAg and HBeAg positive and in 41–78% of those who were HBsAg positive but negative for HBeAg.[52,846] In the latter group, patients with abnormal transaminases were more likely to be positive for HBV-DNA by PCR.[52] Positive results for HBV-DNA by PCR have also been reported in 4–11% of HBsAg-negative blood donors in Taiwan and in 13% of those with anti-HBs antibodies.[846,

[1230] Transfusion of blood positive for HBV-DNA by PCR but negative for other HBV markers was reported to cause an apparent non-A, non-B hepatitis in 1 of 9 cases, with no reported cases of HBV transmission.[1230] In contrast, transmission of HBV to chimpanzees has been reported following experimental inoculation of human blood that was negative for other serological markers of HBV but positive for HBV-DNA by PCR.[1153]

In clinical practice, detection of HBV-DNA by hybridization methods is more valuable that the PCR technique because it is indicative of a high level of viral replication and more likely to be associated with ongoing liver damage. Patients who are negative for HBV-DNA by dot hybridization but positive by PCR are a low infective risk in daily life but should obviously be excluded from blood donation wherever possible.

HBV-DNA polymerase activity is another research tool which has been used as a measure of active viral replication. It is an endogenous DNA polymerase of the hepatitis B virus and is encoded by the P-ORF (see Properties of Hepatitis B Virus). DNA polymerase activity is released into the serum but its value as a marker of viral replication has largely been superseded by direct measurements of HBV-DNA. Antibodies to DNA polymerase are also described, but they are not currently thought to be of clinical value.[182,345]

EPIDEMIOLOGY OF HEPATITIS B

Hepatitis B infection has a worldwide distribution with marked geographical variation in prevalence. Current estimates suggest that 300–400 million people worldwide have chronic HBV infection, and that acute and chronic hepatitis B lead to 250 000 deaths per annum.[702] The prevalence of serological markers of HBV infection in different parts of the world is summarized in Table 30.6. Recent examples of populations with a high reported prevalence rate for HBsAg positivity include 31% in Kiribati (formerly the Gilbert Islands);[1157] 20% in Tonga;[1226] 19.9% in Cameroon;[198] 16.7% in Saudi Arabia;[318] 11.4% in Eastern Kenya;[500] 10.8% in Ethiopia;[565] 9.9% in Black South African mineworkers;[308] and 8.3% in Singapore.[878] Within areas with an intermediate or low reported prevalence of HBsAg positivity (see Table 30.6), some communities have much higher rates of HBsAg carriage; for example, the aboriginal populations of Australia and New Zealand, ranging from 5% to 19%,[158,473,759] and the Inuit eskimo populations of Canada with 3.9% to 6.9%.[50,636]

The prevalence of HBV infection in the community will depend on a wide range of factors, including social customs such as tribal scarification, parenteral drug abuse, sexual promiscuity, homosexuality, exposure to insect-borne vectors and population density. Additional factors facilitate development of chronicity and the carrier state, including male sex, vertical transmission and immunodeficiency. Each of these factors is discussed in further detail later (see Methods of Spread). Thus, in different

Table 30.6 Geographic distribution of HBV infection

Prevalence	HBsAg+ve (%)	Any serological marker of HBV infection (%)	Region/country
High	8–15	>60	Southeast Asia, China, Phillipines, Indonesia, Middle East, Africa, Pacific Islands, Arctic (Eskimo), Amazon Basin
Intermediate	2–7	20–60	East and Southern Europe, USSR, Central Asia, Japan, Israel, South America (northern)
Low	<2	<20	North America, Western Europe, Australia, New Zealand, South America (southern)

Adapted from ref. 702 with permission.

populations there will be striking differences in the age of acquiring infection, and in whether it is predominantly rural or urban. In Western communities it is predominantly urban, whereas in developing countries it is common in the more primitive rural communities.

Subtyping has provided information not only about spread within a community but also about spread from one community to another. Figure 30.15 illustrates the geographical distribution of HBsAg subtypes predominant in particular communities. In a Canadian study of 63 symptom-free blood donors, some of whom had immigrated from abroad in childhood, the subtype correlated with that predominating in their country of birth rather than in their country of domicile.[340] Similarly, retrospective typing of an epidemic in Sweden in 1953 showed it to be predominantly ad, which is the usual subtype in Sweden, whereas another epidemic in 1972 was ay, suggesting that it had been introduced from abroad.[519] In a study of acute HBV infection in Japan, 31 of 137 cases were found to have travelled abroad at some time during the incubation period. In the majority, the HBV subtype matched that known to be prevalent in the country they had visited rather than that found in Japan, indicating that their HBV infection had been imported.[1041]

Reliable data on the *incidence* of acute HBV infection are less readily available, largely because most developing countries do not compile this information and in Western countries under-reporting of cases is a significant problem.[30] This notwithstanding, figures for the USA and England, Wales and Ireland reveal some interesting trends. The reported incidence of HBV infection in the USA rose from 7.0 to 11.5 per 100 000 population from 1979 to 1985 (60% increase), but fell again to 9.4/100 000 in 1989.[702] In England, Wales and Ireland the number of reported cases rose from an average of about 1000 cases per annum between 1975 and 1979 to a peak of almost 2000 cases in 1984, with a subsequent sustained fall from 1985 to a total of 644 reported cases in 1988 (see Figure 30.16); the latter figure is equivalent to an annual incidence of 6/100 000 population.[889,891] The reasons for this decline in the UK series are multifactorial but probably include (i) less parenteral spread of HBV infection by drug abusers because of a reduction in use of shared needles and syringes and a change to other routes of drug administration, and (ii) decreased homosexual and heterosexual transmission of HBV infection, consequent upon alterations in sexual habits and practices with widespread awareness of HIV infection.[891] In the USA,

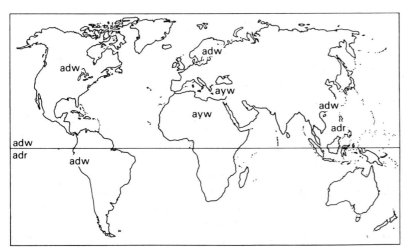

Figure 30.15 Geographical distribution of HBsAg subtypes.

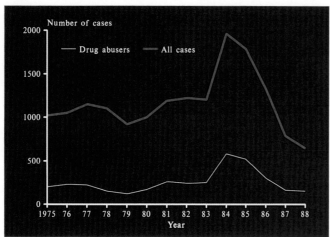

Figure 30.16 Annual reported incidence of acute hepatitis B in England, Ireland and Wales. (Reproduced with permission from Polakoff *et al.*[891]) This contrasts with recent trends in the USA (see text).

Table 30.7 Methods of spread of HBV—Western countries

	USA (% of reported cases)	England, Wales and Ireland (% of reported cases)
Heterosexual activity	26[a]	6.7
Drug abuse	23	24.2
Homosexual activity	8	7.5
Health-care employment	3	3.1
Household and other contacts	2	3.7[b]
Transfusions and dialysis	1	1.4
Travel abroad	ND[c]	8.4[b]
Tattooing	ND	2.3
Surgery, dentistry or injection	ND	3.0
Institutionalized/mental handicap	ND	0.6
Unknown	37	39.1

[a]Heterosexual activity in the US series included sexual contact with acute cases, carriers and multiple partners. Information on multiple partners was not available in the England, Wales and Ireland series.
[b]Some of the household contacts and acquisition abroad may have been sexual but this was not specified.
[c]Data adapted from refs 702 and 891.
ND = no data. Results reflect reported associations not proven routes of infection.

homosexual transmission of HBV infection is also decreasing, but heterosexual spread and transmission by parenteral drug abuse continued to rise between 1985 and 1989.[702]

Methods of spread

Methods of spread of HBV infection vary according to geographic region. In developing countries with a high prevalence of HBV infection, vertical transmission from mother to infant at or soon after birth (perinatal transmission) or horizontal transmission in infancy or early childhood are the most important methods of spread. On a worldwide basis, perinatal and early-childhood transmission thus account for the gross majority of HBV infections and these are described in greater detail below.

In Western countries the majority of infections are acquired in adolescence and adulthood. Transmission occurs by a variety of routes, but parenteral and sexual spread (both homosexual and heterosexual) appear to be the most important. Table 30.7 summarizes recent data concerning mode of transmission for reported cases of acute HBV infection in the USA and in England, Wales and Ireland. Methods of spread of HBV infection that are more relevant to Westernized societies are described later, including discussion of specific problems such as HBV in haemodialysis units, medical personnel and institutes for the mentally handicapped.

Perinatal transmission of hepatitis B

Perinatal transmission of HBV from carrier mothers to infants is rare in Western communities[269,1014] but is common in developing regions.[71,72,721,1091] The risk of perinatal transmission is closely related to both the HBeAg status of the mother[269,824] and to maternal serum HBV-DNA levels (hybridization method).[644] The risk of developing HBV infection is 70–90% for infants born to

HBeAg-positive mothers and 10–40% for infants born to HBeAg-negative mothers.[644,1093,1282] Infants born to mothers with very high levels of serum HBV-DNA (>80 pg/ml) are at high risk of HBV infection[644] and 10–15% may acquire infection despite both passive and active vaccination at birth.[512,646] This has led to the suggestion that patients with high levels of serum HBV-DNA may benefit from delivery by caesarean section[646] (see below).

Transmission from mother to infant usually occurs at the time of birth or shortly thereafter by inapparent inoculation of the infant with infected blood or liquor,[269] and HBsAg and HBeAg are only rarely detected in cord blood. In a series of 51 high-risk Senegalese neonates born to mothers who were chronic carriers of HBsAg, none had IgM anti-HBc in cord blood, suggesting that none had been primarily infected in utero.[407,633] Nine infants were positive for HBsAg and HBeAg in cord blood, but this was thought to be due to contamination by maternal blood. Further evidence for transmission during the birth process is provided by the observation that infants of HBsAg-positive, HBeAg-positive mothers who were delivered by caesarean section were much less likely to become infected (<10%) and to have HBV-DNA in their serum (0/30) than infants delivered vaginally (24.9% infected, HBV-DNA found in 13/67).[645] In contrast, it has been suggested that intrauterine HBV infection may rarely occur by transplacental transfer of maternal blood during threatened abortion or threatened pre-term labour.[666]

Although perinatal transmission is relatively uncommon in Western communities, it is a significant problem within high-risk subpopulations. One example is the children born to the immigrant Southeast Asian community in the USA.[360] Screening of high-risk groups for HBsAg in the prenatal period has been advocated in Western countries, but such a policy will not prevent all cases of perinatal HBV transmission.[543,734] It has been suggested that consideration should be given to screening all pregnant women for HBsAg.[615,866]

Perinatal infection rarely leads to serious liver disease during the first few years of life, although acute viral hepatitis progressing to cirrhosis can occur.[1273] If the mother has acute hepatitis B infection during the second, and particularly during the third, trimester the infant frequently becomes infected with elevated transaminases.[1013,1014,1273] More commonly, perinatal transmission leads to chronic infection with variable degrees of liver disease (see Chapter 31); more than 90% of infected infants born to HBeAg-positive mothers and 40–70% of infected infants born to HBsAg-positive, HBeAg-negative mothers will remain chronically infected.[1091–1093,1282]

Horizontal transmission of hepatitis B
In areas with a high prevalence of HBV, neonates who escape perinatal transmission remain at high risk of acquiring the disease in early childhood by horizontal transmission. This may occur both within families, particularly from mothers or sibs[559,678] or from other HBV-infected members of the community. In Asian children born to HBsAg-positive mothers but not infected at birth, 60% of those born to HBeAg-positive and 40% born to HBeAg-negative mothers will become infected with HBV by the age of 5 years.[70]

The relative importance of perinatal (vertical) transmission compared to horizontal transmission in early childhood varies from one community to another, even within a single geographical location. In a study of two adjacent villages in Africa, perinatal transmission was the commonest mode of infection in one village, but horizontal transmission was more common in the other.[1252] In some countries, e.g. Namibia,[114] Ethiopia[1180] and Egypt,[499] horizontal transmission of HBV appears to be more important than perinatal transmission. This is important to recognize, because such populations should be targeted for early immunization, which is effective in preventing chronic HBV infection acquired by horizontal transmission.[1253]

Horizontal transmission of HBV within families also occurs in areas with a low prevalence of hepatitis B infection. For example, studies in Spain,[908] Sweden[669] and Australia[1257] have reported the presence of HBV markers in 30–45% of household contacts of chronic HBsAg carriers. The risk was highest for contacts of HBeAg-positive carriers[908,1257] and for those in contact with more than one chronic HBV carrier, markers were present in 75.9% of cases.[908] In the Australian study, family contacts of Asian patients were more likely to be positive for HBV markers than contacts of Caucasian patients and it was estimated that the risk of non-sexual

and non-vertical transmission of HBV in Asian families was 18%.[1257]

This pattern of horizontal transmission to children is reported in other Western societies, where subpopulations with a high prevalence of HBV infection are at particular risk. For example, in the USA, horizontal childhood transmission of HBV infection is most commonly observed in Alaskan Eskimos, Pacific Islanders, and infants of first-generation immigrants from regions of the world with a high prevalence of HBV infection.[702] Horizontal transmission of HBV infection has also been reported within day-care centres and nurseries.[252,445,812]

The mode of horizontal transmission of HBV in childhood is uncertain. The possibility that it is transmitted within families by routes other than those involving overt or inapparent inoculation of serum must be considered. HBsAg has been detected in the stools of patients with acute hepatitis B,[425,821,1176] and has also been detected in urine[101] and saliva.[1234]

In the early Willowbrook transmission experiments, it was shown that administration of the MS-2 serum pool by mouth could produce long-incubation-period hepatitis.[607] It has also been suggested that HBV2, a variant of HBV described in Spain, has an improved ability for spread by the oral route.[312] Despite these observations, there is no clear indication that oral spread is involved in transmission of HBV within families. Transmission by contact with saliva or by open wounds have been suggested as alternative methods of familial spread,[252] but it is not clear that this is important on a worldwide basis. Although HBsAg may be detected in breast milk,[269] transmission by this route is thought to be unlikely and conventional advice suggests that there is no absolute contraindication to carrier mothers breast-feeding their infants. More recent studies using PCR have, however, demonstrated HBV-DNA in maternal colostrum.[770]

Sexual transmission of hepatitis B
Sexual transmission of HBV is increasingly recognized as an important method of spread, particularly in communities with a low prevalence of HBV infection. In these circumstances, perinatal and childhood transmission are rare and HBV infection tends to occur in adolescence and early adulthood.[702]

Hepatitis B may be acquired by either homosexual or heterosexual contact (see Table 30.7). HBsAg is present in many body fluids other than blood, including semen[448,673] and saliva.[1234] Transmission of HBV may occur during either vaginal or anal intercourse, but salivary spread may also be important.[1216] The practice of safe sex and use of condoms decreases the risk of HBV transmission, but only synthetic condoms are impermeable to hepatitis B virions, whereas natural condoms are not.[765]

Homosexual transmission is common in Western societies, accounting for 7.5–8% of reported cases of HBV infection in recent series (see Table 30.7). In the USA this represents a dramatic reduction compared with the 20% of cases reported from 1980 to 1985.[32] This is thought to reflect a change in sexual practices within the homosexual community related to prevention of spread of HIV infection.

Markers of HBV infection are common in homosexual men[532,1117] and many are HBeAg positive, implying a high degree of infectivity.[1052] This is reflected in the observation that there is a 70% risk of acquiring HBV infection after 5 years of homosexual activity, and that this is associated with receptive anal intercourse and promiscuity.[294,609,1009] In a series of 48 HBsAg-positive homosexual men presenting at a sexually transmitted disease clinic, 29% had acute hepatitis, 48% had chronic persistent hepatitis, 17% had chronic active hepatitis and 6% had cirrhosis.[791]

Heterosexual activity, particularly with multiple partners, is increasing in importance as a risk factor for HBV infection in the USA[32] (see Table 30.7). Sexual partners of intravenous drug abusers, prostitutes, and their clients are at particularly high risk, but risk of HBV infection is not confined to these groups. Risk increases with duration of heterosexual activity, sexual promiscuity, history of other sexually transmitted diseases and positive serology for syphilis.[29,31,735,974] Sexual transmission may occur when the primary case has acute hepatitis B[589] but may also occur from asymptomatic chronic HBsAg carriers, particularly if the index case is HBeAg positive or serum HBV-DNA positive.[1140] Heterosexual transmission may occur between spouses and in cases of acute HBV infection this may account for a significant proportion of all spread to household contacts.[589] In chronic carriers, transmission of HBV from female to male spouse appears to be more efficient than from male to female, with HBV seropositivity reported in 100% of husbands of HBeAg-positive wives in a Chinese population.[586]

Transmission of HBV has also been reported after artificial insemination[92] and screening of semen donors for HBsAg is now recommended.

Parenteral transmission of hepatitis B

Parenteral transmission of HBV occurs following exposure to infected blood or blood products during parenteral drug abuse, medical transfusion or other procedures involving contaminated needles or instruments, e.g. tribal scarification, tattooing or acupuncture.

Parenteral drug abuse is an important method of spread of HBV, particularly in developed countries (see also Hepatitis D and Hepatitis C). Transmission of HBV can be eliminated in parenteral drug abusers by provision of disposable syringes and needles, assuming that they are not subsequently shared. Schemes to provide disposable materials are controversial and this mode of spread of HBV infection continues to be a major problem. In the USA, HBV infection attributable to parenteral drug abuse has continued to increase since 1985 and now accounts for 23% of reported cases[702] (see Table 30.7). In England, Wales and Ireland, parenteral drug abuse accounts for a similar percentage (24.2%) of cases of HBV infection,

but the absolute number of cases fell dramatically in 1988 to only 20% of that reported in 1985[891] (see Table 30.7). The reasons for this are unclear, but a change to alternative routes of drug abuse, decreased recruitment to parenteral drug abuse, and a reduction in needle/syringe sharing, have all been suggested. Regional variations occur within the UK and one series from Manchester has reported that 51% of 283 cases of acute HBV infection could be attributed to parenteral drug abuse.[649] Cyclical outbreaks of HBV infection due to parenteral drug abuse have occurred in Sweden since 1969, when more than 50% of reported cases were attributed to this cause.[206] From 1976 to 1985 the number of cases of HBV infection in Sweden have declined, but parenteral drug abuse continues to be the most important risk factor, accounting for between 20% and 52% of cases.[206]

Risk of infection with HBV is associated with duration of drug abuse, with one US study demonstrating markers of previous HBV infection in 95% of cases after 5 years of parenteral drug abuse.[993] In this study, those that remained free of HBV infection tended to be less than 25 years old, with an infrequent drug habit (less than once per month) and to have been abusing drugs for less than 2 years. These are obviously an important group to target in vaccination programmes.

In areas with a high prevalence of HBV infection, parenteral drug abuse remains a significant risk factor for HBV infection. In a study of 390 parenteral drug abusers in Taiwan, the rate of HBsAg carriage, at 22.1%, was similar to that of the general population, but the prevalence of markers of previous HBV infection was significantly higher at 99.2%.[207]

Spread of HBV by transfusion of blood or blood products has become less important in countries which have introduced routine screening of all donors for HBsAg (and other markers of HBV infection). This method of spread now accounts for less than 1% of cases of HBV infection in the USA and England, Ireland and Wales[702, 891] and for 2–3% of cases annually in Sweden.[206]

Before the recognition of Australia antigen (HBsAg) and the introduction of routine screening, transmission of HBV by transfusion of blood or blood products was a significant problem. Much of the early data do not distinguish between hepatitis B or C, but nevertheless these studies are instructive. It was recognized that hepatitis could be transmitted by the transfusion of blood or blood products during World War II.[75] The attack rate varied from less than 1% to over 10%, depending on the number of donors contributing to the pool of dried human plasma[719] and, in the case of transfusion of whole blood, bore a linear relationship to the number of units transfused for up to six units per patient.[784] Reported attack rates following blood transfusion varied in different countries, and were dependent on factors such as the source of donor blood and the duration of follow-up. In the USA, an incidence as high as 18% was reported,[436] whereas in the United Kingdom it was less than 1%.[737] A cooperative study in the USA defined a risk which ranged from 0 to

8.6 per 100 patients and confirmed a high risk with transfused blood obtained from commercial donors and a correlation with the volume of blood transfused.[414]

Hepatitis also occurred after the administration of other blood derivatives such as commercially prepared plasma fractions. Such preparations were shown to be contaminated with HBsAg.[85,477,478,1010,1304] These included clotting factor concentrates, cryoprecipitates and fibrinogen, including radioiodinated fibrinogen used in the diagnosis of deep vein thrombosis.[515] The clotting factor concentrates which were most likely to transmit hepatitis were factors II, VII, VIII, IX and X.[212,828,1080] This had serious consequences, particularly in haemophiliacs, who developed chronic liver disease after repeated treatment with factor VIII or IX concentrates.[1080] It is now clear that hepatitis C is also implicated in post-transfusion hepatitis and in the chronic liver disease of haemophiliacs (see Hepatitis C and Chapters 8 and 38).

Use of serum- or plasma-derived proteins in other products may also lead to transmission of HBV. A major epidemic of HBV infection occurred in 1942 following use of yellow-fever vaccine that had been stabilized with human serum. Approximately 50 000 US army personnel injected with this vaccine developed icteric hepatitis and estimates suggest that 330 000 were infected in total. Follow-up studies performed on 597 of these veterans in 1985 demonstrated that 97% of those who received the implicated vaccine and became jaundiced were positive for anti-HBs compared to 76% who received implicated vaccine but remained well and 13% of those who received a different vaccine.[1022] Only one subject remained HBsAg positive in 1985.

The introduction of routine screening of donors for HBsAg has not completely eradicated HBV transmission following transfusion of blood or blood products.[1023] HBV may be transmitted by subjects who are HBsAg negative but anti-HBc positive,[352,479] presumably due to low levels of circulating virus. In French blood donors, HBV-DNA was found in the serum in 5 of 247 donors who were negative for all other markers of HBV infection and who had normal transaminases.[301] Circulating HBV-DNA (in either the presence or absence of anti-HBc) may therefore explain the small numbers of cases of HBV transmission by blood or blood products that continue to occur. There have also been reports of HBV transmission by heat-treated factor VIII concentrate that was negative for HBsAg and for HBV-DNA by dot hybridization.[117] This indicates that heat treatment is not effective at eradicating HBV and suggests that blood products with levels of HBV-DNA too low to be detected by the dot hybridization technique may transmit HBV infection (see section on laboratory detection of HBV-DNA by PCR).

There are other forms of parenteral spread of hepatitis B infection which include tattooing, acupuncture and tribal scarification. These each have the potential for sharing of non-sterile needles or instruments, and hence for HBV transmission. The association between tattooing and hepatitis B has been suspected since the 1950s. Studies have demonstrated spread of HBV infection from both contaminated needles and tattooing dye.[788] In Australian naval personnel there is a correlation between the prevalence of HBV markers and a history of tattooing, particularly if performed in Asia.[861] This contrasts with a study of Norwegian merchant seamen, in whom the prevalence of HBV markers was associated with a history of frequent casual sexual contacts in foreign countries, but not with tattooing.[1047]

HBV infection may also occur after acupuncture. In one large outbreak reported from Rhode Island, USA, 35 from a total of 366 patients treated at one acupuncture clinic developed HBV infection.[567] The risk of developing HBV was related to the number of acupuncture needles in the treatment course; patients receiving less than 150 needles had an attack rate of 9%, compared to 33% for patients who received 450 needles or more.

Conventional medical treatment may also lead to transmission of HBV infection. In a medical centre in Haifa, Israel, an outbreak of hepatitis B infection was attributed to use of a common multiple-dose vial of heparin and normal saline flush solution, thought to have been contaminated by the blood of a known HBsAg-positive patient.[836] Transmission of HBV in Egypt has also been attributed to parenteral antischistosomal therapy.[498]

Hepatitis B may also result from the accidental inoculation of minute quantities of blood when toothbrushes, razors and hair scissors are used communally. The sporadic hepatitis seen in Swedish trail runners, well documented epidemiologically, is now known to be usually due to hepatitis B, probably resulting from contaminated scrubbing brushes used for cleaning the legs after running.[86]

Scarification is presumed to be an important method of spread of HBV transmission in primitive communities, but the extent to which it contributes to the high frequency of HBV carriers is not certain. In the horizontal transmission of HBV infection observed in institutionalized Black children in South Africa, the prevalence of HBV markers was significantly correlated with a history of scarification.[2]

More controversial is the role of insect vectors, which might be an important factor accounting for the high prevalence of hepatitis B in tropical communities. HBsAg has been detected in mosquitoes[914] and bedbugs.[809] There is no evidence that the virus replicates in these insects, but HBsAg has been shown to persist for several weeks in bedbugs after they have been fed HBV artificially. HBsAg was detected in 25 of 29 pools of blood-fed mosquitoes caught at an institution for Black children in South Africa,[2] and this was suggested as a possible factor in the observed high level of horizontal HBV transmission.

Other methods of spread of hepatitis B that are of specific interest include transmission within haemodialysis units, transmission from patients to health-care personnel (and vice versa) and transmission within institutions. Each will be discussed in further detail.

Transmission of hepatitis B in haemodialysis units

The dangers of viral hepatitis in association with haemodialysis were not appreciated in the early 1960s, when this technique was first introduced, until several outbreaks were reported, including some deaths among members of staff.[708]

Once routine testing for HBsAg became established, it was clear that infection was widespread within many dialysis units, that staff were more severely affected than patients (who usually had a mild illness or were asymptomatic), and that there was a high secondary attack rate in the relatives of patients undergoing haemodialysis.[180,681,887,1186] For example, in a survey of 583 patients and 451 medical personnel in 15 haemodialysis centres in the USA, HBsAg was detected in 16.8% of patients and 2.4% of staff, and anti-HBs in 34% of patients and 31.3% of staff respectively. Sixty-one per cent of family contacts of dialysis patients with a history of hepatitis B infection patients had one or other of these markers.[1116] These studies suggest that, although haemodialysis patients may not have overt liver disease, they are likely to transmit more severe infection to contacts, including family members, than do other carriers of HBsAg such as blood donors.

The higher infectivity of haemodialysis patients compared with other HBsAg carriers has been confirmed serologically. In one study almost all the HBsAg-positive haemodialysis patients had HBeAg and DNA polymerase activity in their serum whereas none of the other carriers had them.[162] A high incidence of HBeAg in dialysis patients has been confirmed by Miller and coworkers.[754]

Although hepatitis B is often introduced into dialysis units by patients who have had previous blood transfusions, cross-infection within units is the chief means of perpetuating hepatitis B.[888] Spread to staff occurs in a variety of ways as a result of contact with patients' blood, usually by inapparent inoculation. There is some evidence that airborne spread may also occur.[17] Nursing staff in haemodialysis units are at particularly high risk of acquiring HBV infection. In one study of new HBV infections in staff in a haemodialysis unit in Southern Israel, 7 out of 9 cases occurred in nursing staff.[361] The methods of spread of hepatitis in dialysis units and to the household contacts have been thoroughly reviewed.[708,1266]

Some cases of dialysis-associated hepatitis do not have HBV markers or evidence of hepatitis A.[1118] It is now recognized that many of these cases may be due to hepatitis C (see Epidemiology of Hepatitis C).

The outcome of the liver disease in patients who have HBsAg in their circulation before or after renal transplantation has been variable. In one report, there was a fivefold increase in deaths from hepatic failure in HBsAg-positive patients compared with those who were negative,[884] although this had not been found in previous studies.[1101] Immunosuppression after renal transplantation leads to reactivation of HBV replication as determined by serial measurements of serum HBV-DNA in graft recipients[259] and this may contribute to the poor prognosis in this group.

There are strong indications for the immunization of patients who are likely to undergo haemodialysis or renal transplantation, as well as for medical and nursing personnel and ancillary staff who may be involved in their clinical care.[426,631]

Transmission of hepatitis B to medical personnel

Health-care employment is recorded as a potential factor in approximately 3% of reported cases of HBV infection per annum in the USA and England, Wales and Ireland[702,891] (see Table 30.7). Most studies indicate an increased risk of HBV infection in health-care workers but this is in part dependent on the nature of their employment and their degree of exposure to patients' blood or contaminated secretions.

In Rochester, Minnesota, a population-based study of the incidence of acute hepatitis B demonstrated a fivefold increase in medical employees.[839] Recent evidence suggests that the incidence of acute hepatitis B is decreasing in health-care workers in the USA, probably due to hepatitis B immunization.[32]

In general, studies of HBV markers in health-care personnel also show an increased prevalence compared to the general population. In one American survey, dentists and physicians had a threefold to fivefold greater prevalence of HBV markers than volunteer blood donors. Similar findings are reported from other centres; in Toronto HBV markers were found in up to 10% of health-care personnel,[577] whereas in Hamburg 2.2% were carriers of HBsAg.[528] In hospital workers in Senegal 17.8% were positive for HBsAg and 79.2% had anti-HBc in their serum, indicating previous infection.[971] The prevalence of HBV markers was related to duration of service in the hospital and peaked in those who had been employed for 2–3 years. The overall prevalence of HBV markers is much lower in medical staff in the UK (1.1–6%).[1070]

Studies have demonstrated that laboratory personnel, particularly those handling patients' blood, have an increased risk of developing hepatitis B or markers of HBV infection.[424,857] The risk of developing HBV infection may be up to fivefold greater in hospital staff who are frequently exposed to blood or blood products compared to those who are not.[577] However, in an analysis of HBV in health care workers admitted to one liver unit,[156] including a high proportion who developed severe liver disease, specific inoculation injuries were not the usual mode of transmission.

Dentists and dental technicians are another group at high risk of developing hepatitis B[997] and up to 26% in some surveys have serum markers of current or previous HBV infection.[945,998,1072] In the USA the HBsAg carrier rate in dentists (0.9%) is greater than that observed in volunteer blood donors (0.1–0.2%),[785] but in Denmark the carrier rate in dentists is no higher than in the general population.[11] Extensive contamination with HBsAg has been described in dental surgeries,[880] probably owing to dissemination of aerosols and microdroplets containing HBV-contaminated saliva and blood. The prevalence of HBV markers in dentists is significantly associated with age and numbers of years in practice, but not with numbers of patients seen, nor numbers of high-risk patients treated.[945] Use of gloves and other protective measures, e.g. eye shields, does not appear significantly to reduce the risk of HBV infection in dental surgeons.[945, 997]

Health-care workers in institutions for the mentally retarded are also at increased risk of acquiring HBV, with one study demonstrating seroconversion in 13 employees during 539 person-years of occupational exposure.[677] The increased risk of HBV infection in haemodialysis staff is described above.

Transmission of hepatitis B from medical personnel to patients

Transmission of HBV from medical personnel to patients is rare and, as determined by serum markers of infectivity, the overall risk to patients of acquiring HBV infection from their medical attendants is very low. In a survey of 36 000 medical staff in Austria, only 210 were found to be HBsAg positive and of these HBV-DNA (by dot hybridization) was found in only 15.[468,469]

Nevertheless, transmission of HBV to patients is recorded, particularly from dentists, haemodialysis unit staff, and gynaecologists. In dentists the rate of HBsAg carriage is little higher than that of other health-care workers, but the nature of their contact is such as to facilitate spread and examples of outbreaks of hepatitis B attributable to HBsAg-positive dentists have been reported in the USA.[950]

Outbreaks of hepatitis B attributable to gynaecological surgery have also been reported.[6,634,1246] Following three cases of acute HBV infection after gynaecological surgery in the UK, the surgeon was found to be HBsAg and HBeAg positive.[1246] Analysis of sera in 247 patients operated on by this surgeon demonstrated markers of HBV infection in 9%. Hysterectomy (10/42) and caesarian section (10/51) carried the greatest risk of infection.

The medicolegal aspects of transmission of HBV from medical staff to patients, and in particular the action which should be taken if doctors or other medical personnel are found to be carriers of HBsAg, have been reviewed.[631] It was concluded that only those involved in haemodialysis or intensive-care units should be screened; if found positive, they should be directed to alternative areas of medical employment. In the UK, the department of health recommends that for surgeons, gynaecologists and other staff, transfer to low-risk medical occupations should occur only if they are identified as the definite source of a transmitted outbreak of hepatitis B in their patients. This policy has been criticized and pre-employment testing has been suggested.[1073]

Transmission of hepatitis B in institutions

It has been recognized for many years that there is a high prevalence of viral hepatitis in institutions for the mentally retarded.

Several important facts about the epidemiology of hepatitis B have emerged from the examination of patients and staff in such institutions. Although there is variation in the prevalence of HBV markers between institutions, it is usually much higher than in the general population. The frequency of HBV markers increases with the duration of stay in the institution and is greater in patients than in staff, although the latter also have an increased incidence (Figure 30.17). The HBsAg carrier rate in Down's syndrome is considerably greater than that for other mentally retarded patients.[106,579,1112,1115] This is probably due to a defective antibody response and to impaired cell-mediated immunity resulting in a more prolonged carrier state, since all patients are equally exposed.[1112,1115] The patients in mental institutions often develop anicteric infections; for example, none of 26 children who developed HBV markers after admission to one institution were clinically jaundiced.[1115]

Mentally handicapped carriers, particularly those with Down's syndrome, are more likely to have HBeAg and less likely to have anti-HBe than other carriers. Of 26 mentally handicapped HBsAg carriers, 12 had HBeAg (Figure 30.17) and none had anti-HBe, whereas only one of 50 blood donors or antenatal carriers who were HBsAg positive had HBeAg.[578] Mentally handicapped carriers also have a high prevalence of HBV-DNA in the serum. In one study, 24% of a total of 493 mentally handicapped males had HBV-DNA in their serum, with the highest prevalence of HBV-DNA observed in those with Down's syndrome.[1204] The high frequency of HBV markers is probably due to recurrent exposure by the non-parenteral route, the HBeAg-positive HBV-DNA-positive carriers acting as a potent reservoir of infection.

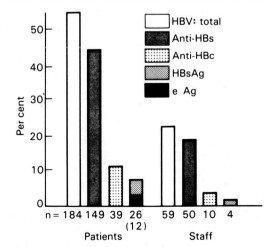

Figure 30.17 HBV markers in patients and staff in an institute for the mentally retarded. (From Kingham _et al._[579] with kind permission of the authors and the editor of the _British Medical Journal._)

Outbreaks of hepatitis B have also been described in other institutions, such as a tuberculosis unit.[351] In this outbreak, 11 out of 37 HBsAg-positive patients were jaundiced, a high proportion became carriers and spread occurred to domestic and medical staff as well as to household contacts, particularly spouses.

SPECIFIC CLINICAL FEATURES OF HEPATITIS B ___

The incubation period for hepatitis B ranges from 60 to 180 days, with a mean of 90 days.[1305] The explanation for this wide range is unclear. The size of the inoculum may be a factor but it is not a crucial one as there is considerable variation in the incubation period whether HBV is spread by transfusion of large volumes of blood or by the inoculation of small quantities, for example by needlestick or personal contact. More relevant may be the concentration of intact virions and anti-HBs in a particular inoculum. Nevertheless, transmission experiments performed in the 1950s demonstrated that dilution of serum (known to transmit icteric hepatitis) before inoculation prolonged the incubation period.[64]

The sequence of events and serological changes in acute HBV infection are summarized in Figure 30.18a and contrasts with that observed in chronic HBV infection (Figure 30.18b). Specific details of individual serological tests are described earlier (see Laboratory Detection of HBV Infection).

In acute hepatitis B infection, HBsAg, HBeAg and HBV-DNA (by dot hybridization) become detectable in the serum about 6 weeks after the primary infection and several weeks before biochemical evidence of liver damage or onset of clinical symptoms. Thus, viral replication precedes the onset of clinical hepatitis. They remain positive during the prodromal phase and early acute illness, although HBeAg may be cleared before clinical presentation in some cases. With the onset of clinical symptoms, anti-HBc and IgM anti-HBc also become detectable and remain so into the convalescent phase of the illness. In a typical resolving case of acute hepatitis B infection, HBeAg and HBV-DNA (by dot hybridization) are cleared from the serum, often when the patient is still symptomatic. HBV-DNA may remain detectable by PCR at this stage. With clearance of HBeAg, anti-HBe usually becomes detectable, but there may be a 'window' before this occurs and, owing to the relatively low sensitivity of the commercially available EIAs, anti-HBe may remain undetectable in some cases despite clearance of HBeAg. Eventually, HBsAg and HBV-DNA (by PCR) are cleared from the serum and this is associated with a fall in titre of IgM anti-HBc.

Anti-HBs is the last marker to appear in the serum and is only detectable as antibody excess once HBsAg has disappeared from the serum, although complex formation with antigen may occur much earlier and the anti-HBs response may be an important factor in eliminating HBsAg from the serum. There may therefore be a period when neither HBsAg nor anti-HBs is detectable in serum

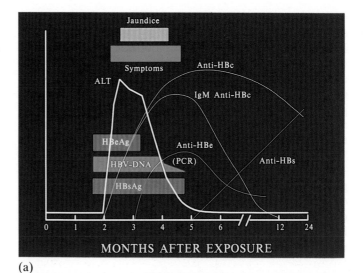

(a)

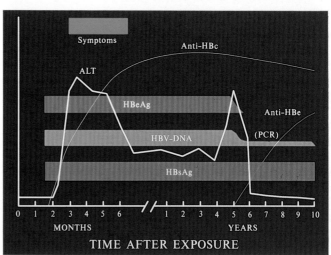

(b)

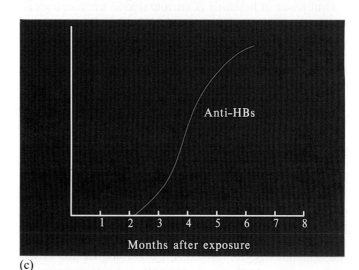

(c)

Figure 30.18 Sequence of events after HBV infection. (a) Classic acute hepatitis B infection. (b) Acute infection followed by chronic hepatitis B. (c) Primary antibody response to hepatitis B (HBsAg) vaccine. (Reproduced with kind permission of Hoofnagle[484] and Thieme Medical Publishers Inc.)

and the only serological indicators of recent HBV infection are IgM anti-HBc and IgG anti-HBc. The titre of anti-HBc gradually falls during convalescence in the uncomplicated acute case but normally persists long-term at low titre, together with anti-HBs.

The serological changes of chronic HBV infection are summarized in Figure 30.18b and described in Chapter 31. The serological response to vaccination against hepatitis B (with HBsAg) is summarized in Figure 30.18c and consists of development of anti-HBs only, with no other HBV markers (see Prevention of Hepatitis B).

The serological features of two clinically important HBV syndromes are worthy of further consideration. In chronic carriers of HBsAg with little or no evidence of ongoing liver damage, acute icteric hepatitis may be superimposed. This may be related to infection with other viruses (see Hepatitis D and C) but may also be related to spontaneous reactivation of hepatitis B.[1056,1167] The latter is associated with active viral replication, and is accompanied by detection of HBV-DNA in the serum and rising titres of IgM anti-HBc. Thus, on serological data alone, it may be difficult to distinguish spontaneous reactivation from acute infection with HBV.

In fulminant hepatitis due to acute HBV infection, the serological features may be atypical. HBsAg may not be detectable in up to 20% of cases[389,849] and HBV-DNA is absent in up to 90% of cases of fulminant HBV infection.[82] In these circumstances the diagnosis of fulminant hepatitis B can be confirmed by detection of IgM anti-HBc.

The clinical presentation of acute hepatitis B is as described earlier (see General Features of Acute Viral Hepatitis). The entire clinical spectrum may be observed ranging from asymptomatic cases to anicteric infection, typical acute icteric viral hepatitis, cholestatic hepatitis, or rarely severe fulminant hepatitis with liver failure.

Extrahepatic manifestations are relatively prominent in HBV infection and may occur in acute as well as chronic infection. Those which are clearly associated with acute hepatitis B infection include *a serum sickness-like syndrome* with arthralgia and arthritis, urticaria, and angioneurotic oedema related to immune complex deposition.[22,401] Rashes and arthropathy have been reported in up to 25% of cases of acute HBV infection.[1089] Joint symptoms usually precede the onset of jaundice, but may persist throughout the illness and occasionally continue after resolution of the clinical hepatitis.

A necrotizing vasculitis indistinguishable from *polyarteritis nodosa* occurs in HBV infection[398,1028] and is thought to be related to immune complex deposition.[398,399,1173] Although reported most frequently in association with chronic hepatitis B, vasculitis and polyarteritis nodosa are also reported in acute HBV infection.[731] Polyarteritis nodosa may also occur in anicteric cases[51] or in the recovery phase of acute HBV infection.[375] The clinical features of this syndrome are diverse and may include abdominal pain, neurological involvement, myalgia, hypertension, renal disease, skin involvement (Figure 30.19), cardiac involvement, arthritis and Raynaud's syn-

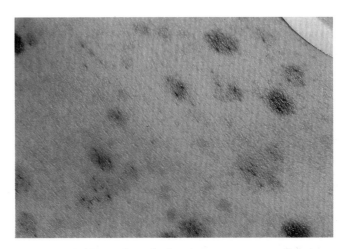

Figure 30.19 Purpuric rash due to cutaneous vasculitis in an HBsAg-positive patient with polyarteris nodosa.

drome.[731] The authors have recently seen a case of spontaneous reactivation of hepatitis B associated with polyarteritis manifesting with a peripheral neuropathy, gut infarction leading to perforation, neuropsychiatric symptoms, proteinuria and diffuse cutaneous vasculitis (Figure 30.19), culminating in liver failure due to hepatic arterial involvement and infarction of the liver.

Hepatitis B-associated glomerulonephritis is related to deposition of immune complexes in the glomerular basement membrane.[628,1209] It is normally associated with chronic HBV infection and the pathological features are of a membranous or membranoproliferative glomerulonephritis. Morphological changes resembling glomerulonephritis have also been reported in acute hepatitis B.[317]

Neurological manifestations reported in association with acute hepatitis B include *seizures*,[137,253] and *Guillain–Barré syndrome* (GBS).[88,811,1126] Tabor has reviewed eight reported cases of GBS (age range 21–76 years) in patients with acute HBV infection.[1126] Neurological symptoms developed 3–9 weeks after the onset of acute hepatitis, and in 3 of 4 patients in whom lumbar puncture was performed HBsAg was detected in the CSF. All eight patients recovered from GBS after 2–6 months, usually at the time of recovery from the acute hepatitis.

Mononeuritis usually occurs in association with HBV-related polyarteritis nodosa (see above), but has also been reported as isolated neurological manifestation in acute hepatitis B.[862]

Other rare extrahepatic manifestations associated with acute hepatitis B include *pleural effusions*,[210,1123] and *acute pericarditis*.[7] In these cases, HBsAg was detected in pleural or pericardial fluid.

Papular acrodermatitis of childhood (Gianotti's syndrome)[386] is an erythematous papular skin eruption, usually confined to the face, buttocks and limbs, that is associated with inguinal or axillary lymphadenopathy and occurs in acute hepatitis B infection. The skin rash usually precedes the onset of hepatitis, which may be anicteric. The rash usually resolves within 15–20 days of its onset.

Haematological manifestations of acute HBV infection are described in further detail in Chapter 8. The most serious is *aplastic anaemia*, which may be fatal.[736]

The *biochemical abnormalities* observed in acute hepatitis B infection are similar to those seen in any other cause of viral hepatitis and are described earlier (see General Features of Viral Hepatitis). In comparison with hepatitis A infection, the rise in transaminases in acute hepatitis B tends to be more gradual and more prolonged.[607] In some studies of hepatitis B, a prolonged clinical course has been associated with lower bilirubin levels during the acute attack.[810,1038]

SPECIFIC PATHOLOGICAL FEATURES OF HEPATITIS B

Specific demonstration of hepatitis B virus in the liver

The component parts of hepatitis B virus can be demonstrated in the liver by a variety of techniques. These range from simple light and electron microscopic visualization through immunocytochemical localization to in situ hybridization. These are all mostly easily demonstrated in chronic hepatitis B. Ground glass hepatocytes are not a feature of acute hepatitis B infection.

Hepatitis B surface antigen

In both acute and chronic hepatitis B virus infection of hepatocytes, HBsAg is only present in the cytoplasm and is particularly concentrated around the hepatocyte membrane.[10,314,972] There is no nuclear localization.[65,314,427,972] Sequential biopsies of self-limited acute hepatitis B in chimpanzees have demonstrated transient cytoplasmic fluorescence with accentuation of staining of the hepatocyte membrane.[65,479] Similarly, in man positive cytoplasmic fluorescence was found in the early stages of acute viral hepatitis[10] and it has been suggested that persistent cytoplasmic localization suggests transition to chronic liver disease.[427,935,952]

Various histochemical techniques identify HBsAg in hepatocyte cytoplasm[1042] but none is positive in acute hepatitis B.[268] A positive result should either suggest an acute exacerbation of chronic hepatitis B or a viral superinfection in a chronic hepatitis B carrier.[758] In areas endemic for hepatitis B, immunocytochemical identification of cytoplasmic HBsAg can be useful in identifying true acute hepatitis B. Correlation of tissue HBsAg with serological tests or HBV and HAV markers demonstrated that many cases diagnosed clinically as acute hepatitis B were examples of superinfection or reactivation of unrecognized hepatitis B carriers.[1102]

Electron microscopy has consistently failed to demonstrate HBsAg in hepatocytes in fulminant or non-complicated acute hepatitis B.[722]

Pre-S polypeptides

Pre-S_1 and pre-S_2 polypeptides are thought to have a role in the binding of the virus to hepatocyte cell membrane receptors. Both pre-S_1 and pre-S_2 can be detected immunocytochemically within the hepatocyte.[431] There is no apparent correlation between the presence of pre-S_1 or pre-S_2 with the degree of liver damage. Both polypeptides could be demonstrated in liver whether showing chronic active hepatitis or a carrier state. It has been suggested that pre-S_1[1149] and pre-S_2[143] are related to viral replication. This seems unlikely as both polypeptides can be demonstrated in biopsies from e-antigen-positive or e-antibody-positive patients.[431]

It is possible that pre-S proteins may be another antigenic target for cytotoxic T cells.[495] Membranous expression of both pre-S_1 and pre-S_2 polypeptides was identified in over 50% of 80 livers with a strong correlation with core antigen. Membranous expression of both S_1 and S_2 proteins was particularly localized to areas of inflammatory activity and liver cell necrosis.

Hepatitis B core antigen

The core antigen is found predominantly in the nucleus of the hepatocyte in both acute and chronic hepatitis B infection. Immunocytochemical and ultrastructural studies show that in acute hepatitis many biopsies are negative.[427,838] Even in positive cases, only occasional cells can be demonstrated by electron microscopy to contain intranuclear particles and these are scanty in number.[818] In sequential liver biopsies in experimentally infected chimpanzees, core antigen can be demonstrated in the nucleus of hepatocytes during the incubation period and up to the time of maximal elevation of the serum transaminases:[480] this is a stage when liver biopsies are unlikely to be obtained in man.

Confirmatory evidence has come from studies on hepatitis B virus DNA-transfected HepG2 tissue-culture cells. Three patterns of core antigen expression were identified: (a) cells with nuclear core antigen, (b) cells with cytoplasmic core antigen, and (c) cells with both nuclear and cytoplasmic core antigen. Hepatitis B virus DNA was only expressed in the culture medium from cells expressing cytoplasmic core antigens.[970] In the tissue-culture model, core particles can be identified budding into the cysterna of the endoplasmic reticulum.

The morphology of core particles is identical in acute and chronic hepatitis. They have been most extensively studied in chronic infections, where they are much more numerous. They are small (21–25 nm diameter) and round, with a slightly angular periphery. They may have an electron-dense core but this is not always seen (see Chapter 31).

Hepatitis B e antigen

There is no visible morphological structure to the e antigen demonstrable in routine light- or electron-microscopically examined tissue. No satisfactory demonstration of e antigen in the liver has been made in acute hepatitis B by immunocytochemical methods.

Hepatitis B viral DNA

Hepatitis B viral DNA has mostly been studied in chronic hepatitis B infections[411,412,748] or inferred from related hepadnavirus infections in experimental animal systems such as the Pekin duck.[536,1106] Particularly from the experimental studies, replication was associated with prominent viral DNA in the hepatocyte cytoplasm (see Replication of HBV).

Immune response

Immunoglobulin, particularly IgG, and complement have been immunocytochemically demonstrated in the liver.[44,952] Immunoglobulin when present is almost invariably in the nucleus and could represent immune complexes with core antigen which may fix complement.[382] Morphological demonstration of complement in acute viral hepatitis may indicate an adverse prognosis. Of 47 patients with acute hepatitis B infection, complement was demonstrated in 10 patients. All progressed to chronic liver disease, although this was of varying severity. Of the 37 remaining patients only 3 developed chronic liver disease.[952] There is a humoral component to the immune response in acute hepatitis B: anti-LSP antibodies are first detected at the onset of liver injury when there is no evidence of cellular immunity to the same antigenic complex.[1210]

Cellular immune responses have mostly been studied in chronic hepatitis B (see Chapter 31). Immunocytochemical studies in acute hepatitis B shows CD-4$^+$ lymphocytes in portal areas with CD-8$^+$ mononuclear cells infiltrating the parenchyma and in contact with damaged hepatocytes. The appearances supported the concept of cytotoxic liver cell damage.[796] Increased expression of β_2-microglobulin is also seen on hepatocytes in acute hepatitis B.[797] This expression was maximal in the perivenular zone, particularly in association with bridging hepatic necrosis, and is thought to reflect an increased display of HLA-A, B and C antigens, thus increasing the susceptibility of hepatocytes to T cell-mediated immune response.

PATHOGENESIS OF HEPATITIS B _____

The pathogenesis of the tissue damage in acute HBV infection will be determined by the ability of HBV to gain access to the hepatocyte and by the consequences of HBV expression in the hepatocyte.

Access of HBV

The method by which the virus gains access and the explanation of its limited host range and hepatic specificity are still unclear. The suggestion that polymerized human albumin facilitates entry of the virus into the cell is controversial.[1275] HBsAg only reacts with artificially polymerized albumin and not with native albumin, and binding sites for polymerized serum albumin and native albumin on the hepatocyte membrane are distinct. The latter appear to be non-specific and binding is only weak. Also, similar receptors have not been demonstrated in other species affected by hepadnaviruses for the appropriate polyalbumin. A number of factors may modulate access of HBV to the liver cell; as well as antibodies to polyalbumin these include antibodies to other antigens, such as the pre-S$_1$ and pre-S$_2$ antigens on the Dane particle,[1291] and anti-idiotype antibodies. There may be modification of the immune attack on the cell and the continuing access of the virus to the cell may vary according to the relative states of free and integrated HBV-DNA within the hepatocyte.

Consequence of HBV within the hepatocyte

The hepatocellular damage associated with HBV infection could be due to either of two causes that are not mutually exclusive. The virus may exert a direct cytopathic effect upon the hepatocyte or the hepatocyte may be damaged by an immune response to viral antigens that are expressed on the surface membrane of the cell.

Cytopathic effect

The ability of the hepatitis B virus to infect hepatocytes while producing vast quantities of HBsAg in asymptomatic carriers with minimal evidence of liver disease indicated that the virus was not necessarily cytopathic. In addition, cell lines expressing HBsAg do not show functional or growth impairment. Initially therefore, a direct cytopathic effect of the virus was discounted and the possibility of a cytopathic effect in other circumstances was ignored. Hoofnagle *et al.*[481] were the first to propose a direct cytopathic effect, which was soon demonstrated when large quantities of cytoplasmic HBV-DNA were found in damaged hepatocytes in the absence of an adjacent inflammatory infiltrate.[149] If tissue culture cell lines are modified to express hepatitis B core antigen then cytopathic effects can be observed,[1287] so that cytopathic change may be more related to the viral production of DNA or core antigen rather than of the surface antigen.

Immune response

The abnormal immune response which undoubtedly occurs could be mediated in several different ways (Figure 30.20). Varying sizes of immune complexes have been observed in a small number of patients with HBsAg-positive liver disease suggesting that the hepatic damage might be mediated by immune complex injury.[16] There is no doubt that circulating immune complexes of HBsAg

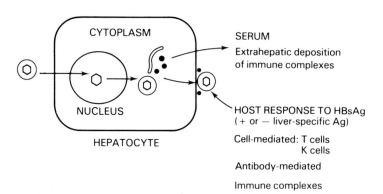

Figure 30.20 Diagram to illustrate immunopathological mechanisms in hepatitis infection. (After Wright.[1274])

can be observed in the serum, particularly in acute viral hepatitis, but there is little direct evidence of immune complex damage in the liver when measured by immunofluorescent techniques,[314] as can be observed in extrahepatic sites. On the other hand, an enhanced anti-HBs response has been observed in patients with fulminant hepatitis B[1265] and it has been suggested that this results in an intense ischaemic necrosis of hepatocytes due to an Arthus reaction. The patients with fulminant hepatitis B had lower HBsAg and HBV-DNA concentrations in the serum, higher IgM anti-HBc titres and were unlikely to have HBeAg. More recent studies have failed to show such clear-cut differences between fulminant and uncomplicated acute HBV infection.[91,333]

There is more convincing evidence that cell-mediated immune reactions to HBsAg may be important in determining the outcome of infection and possibly the pathogenesis of the hepatic injuries. Clinical evidence favours a defective cellular immune response to the virus because (a) defective cell-mediated immunity such as in patients with Down's syndrome, chronic renal failure or lepromatous leprosy favours the carrier state; (b) hepatic failure may develop after stopping cytotoxic therapy; and (c) drugs which modify the immune response, such as levamisole, transfer factor and interferon, may induce liver cell necrosis. It has been suggested that defective T cell function with impaired cell-mediated immunity to HBsAg may determine whether the infection is self-limited or persists with varying degrees of liver damage.[303] This possibility has been studied extensively in both acute and chronic liver disease, but the results have been contradictory, partly because of the inadequacy of in vitro techniques for assessing T cell function and cell-mediated immunity, and partly because impure antigens have been used.

A cell-mediated immune reaction to HBsAg has been reported early in the acute phase of viral hepatitis,[1212] whereas chronic carriers fail to show evidence of cell-mediated immunity to HBsAg. Such results suggest that a specific cell-mediated immune reaction to HBsAg is necessary to eliminate the infection and prevent the carrier state. They do not provide convincing evidence of an abnormal, cell-mediated immune reaction to HBsAg in the pathogenesis of the hepatocellular necrosis.[438]

Crucial to the understanding of the mechanisms of cell damage and acute and chronic HBV infection are the serial studies of intrahepatic and serological factors modifying viral replication and the immune response. Since the opportunity to obtain serial liver biopsies in patients during the incubation period and early acute stages of HBV infection is very limited, most correlations have occurred in patients with chronic HBV infection. In acute hepatitis and in the early phase of chronic active hepatitis, hepatocytes in different parts of the same liver will be undergoing cell damage, be refractory to viral infection and be regenerating simultaneously, so that clear-cut distinctions between these various processes is difficult. It has been postulated that T cell cytotoxicity directed against the core antigen is responsible for hepatocyte damage in acute and chronic hepatitis B[780] (Figure 30.21). In 28 patients with chronic HBV infection, only hepatocytes expressing HBcAg on their surface were susceptible, whereas HBsAg-positive hepatocytes were unaffected:[803] cytotoxicity could be blocked by monoclonal anti-HBc

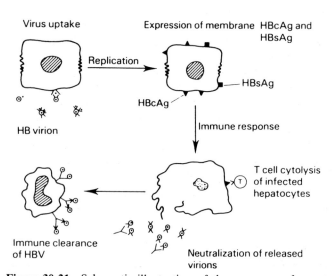

Figure 30.21 Schematic illustration of the sequence of events in acute HBV infection, from virus uptake through replication and liver cell damage to recovery. (From Mondelli and Eddleston,[780] with kind permission of the authors and the editor of _Seminars in Liver Disease._)

but not by monoclonal anti-HBs. This is consistent with those earlier studies which demonstrated that IgG eluted from liver cell membranes in chronic hepatitis B is core-antigen-specific. T-cell cytotoxicity is greater than non-T-cell cytotoxicity; the latter non-T-cell cytoxicity is blocked by liver specific antigens (LSP). Using a specific T-lymphocyte migration inhibition assay, a specific sensitization to core but not to surface antigen or LSP has been demonstrated.[1211]

In acute viral hepatitis, both surface and core antigens are expressed on the hepatocyte membrane. Viral infection stimulates expression of interferon-α and major histocompatibility complex class I glycoproteins and this expression coincides with elevation of the serum transaminases. It has been proposed that these class I molecules, together with the HBV antigens exposed on the hepatocyte membrane, target hepatocytes for cytotoxic attack by cytotoxic T lymphocytes.[599,1154] Interferon-α activates the 2–5A oligoadenylate synthetase/endonuclease system and other enzymes that inhibit viral synthesis, preventing reinfection of hepatocytes.[449,1154] Another factor may be the development of neutralizing antibodies to the envelope of the virus.

The explanation for the development of chronic infection is not clear. Any explanation of the development of the carrier state has to take into account the predisposition of immunosuppressed patients to develop the carrier state with little liver damage, and the much greater likelihood of chronic liver disease developing after perinatal infection and in males. The high frequency of the development of chronicity and the rarity of fulminant hepatitis may relate to modulation of the infant's immune response to maternal nucleocapsid e and core antigens and their respective antibodies.[1154] Impaired production of interferon-α has been demonstrated in patients with chronic active hepatitis, but there is no evidence that pre-existing deficiency of interferon is important in the development of chronic liver disease.[449] In this context it is of interest that cells transfected with the HBV genome have a defective response to interferon.[833]

The demonstration of membrane expression of core and e nucleocapsid antigens as well as envelope antigens (pre-S₁, pre-S₂ and S proteins) by specific monoclonal antibodies has enhanced the study of their possible role in hepatocellular necrosis.[283,347–349,1211] Transfection of rat fibroblasts[385] with hepatitis B surface and core antigen genes will enable the construction of HBV virions in cells and their production and release on the liver cell surface to be studied[970] and hopefully will clarify the pathogenetic mechanisms.

PROGNOSIS AND CLINICAL OUTCOME IN HEPATITIS B

Many cases of acute hepatitis B infection run a subclinical or anicteric course and do not come to clinical attention. This is particularly true in developing countries, where hepatitis B infection is usually acquired in the perinatal period or in early childhood and, in the majority, is not associated with a clinically significant illness. As discussed earlier, acquisition of HBV infection by perinatal or early childhood transmission is associated with a high rate of development of the chronic carrier state (see Chapter 31) with the attendant risk of hepatocellular carcinoma in the 2nd to 4th decade (see Chapter 39). In contrast, children who develop a typical acute icteric hepatitic illness with HBV infection rarely, if ever, progress to develop chronic liver disease.[548]

In a typical case of acute icteric hepatitis B infection acquired in adolescence or adulthood, the clinical course tends to be more prolonged than for hepatitis A, there is a greater risk of developing fulminant hepatitis, and there is also the potential for chronicity. In the majority of cases (>90%), however, the disease is self-limiting with spontaneous complete recovery. The traditional view[810,939] that 5–10% of patients with acute hepatitis B retain markers of active viral replication and progress to develop chronic liver disease has been challenged, with recent data suggesting that progression may occur in as few as 0.2–3%.[111,1139] In these more recent studies, recognition of cases of acute icteric hepatitis due to spontaneous reactivation of chronic HBV infection, or to hepatitis D superinfection, may account for the apparent decrease in the proportion of acute cases that progress to chronic liver disease. Earlier studies may therefore have overestimated the risk of developing chronic liver disease after acute hepatitis B infection. An indication of the risk of progressing to chronic liver disease is obtained from liver histology. The presence of bridging necrosis (from portal tracts to terminal hepatic veins) is strongly associated with development of chronicity.[115]

Fulminant hepatitis with onset of liver failure and hepatic encephalopathy (see Chapter 29) is a rare sequela of acute hepatitis B infection, occurring in less than 1% of cases.[111,939] In tertiary referral centres for fulminant liver failure in Europe, acute hepatitis B infection accounts for a significant proportion of cases, with 9% of a total of 943 cases reported in the King's College Hospital series, and 32% of a total of 502 cases reported from the Hopital Beaujon, France.[82,1256] Co-infection and superinfection with hepatitis D are further important causes of fulminant liver failure in patients with HBV infection and these will be discussed later (see Hepatitis D).

TREATMENT OF ACUTE HEPATITIS B

In the uncomplicated cases of acute hepatitis B, attention to general measures, as described earlier (see General Features of Acute Viral Hepatitis) and reviewed by Dusheiko,[307] is recommended, but no specific therapy is in regular use.

Several treatments have been tested in controlled trials for treatment of uncomplicated acute hepatitis B. Reduced ALT and AST levels have been reported after treatment with (+)-cyanidanol-3 in acute hepatitis B, but with no significant improvement in rate of clearance of HBsAg or subsequent development of the chronic carrier state.[879] The proven benefit of interferons in chronic hepatitis B has led to their use in acute HBV infection. In a randomized controlled trial of interferon-α in the management of uncomplicated hepatitis B in Greece, no benefit was observed from a regime of 3–10 million units t.i.d. for 3 weeks.[1141] The role of interferons in the management of chronic hepatitis B is described in Chapter 31.

In fulminant hepatitis B, the usual therapeutic measures for treatment of liver failure are undertaken (see Chapter 29). Corticosteroids have been used but they have no beneficial effect on either morbidity or mortality.[307] Similarly, interferons have been tried in the treatment of fulminant hepatitis B, but without any beneficial effect.[750, 984]

The only successful treatment for fulminant hepatitis B infection is liver transplantation,[82] with an improvement in survival from approximately 25% to 60–70% at 1 year. Unfortunately, recurrent HBV infection in the liver graft is a significant problem despite attempts to prevent it with passive immunization, combined active and passive immunization or interferon-α therapy.[1163]

PREVENTION OF HEPATITIS B _____

Prevention of HBV infection is now possible following the development of safe, effective vaccines. Currently their use in developing countries is limited by expense and difficulties with appropriate delivery. In Western countries, strategies for the use of HBV vaccines are still evolving. They have been used predominantly in high-risk groups and, as will be discussed later, this strategy may not be the most appropriate. Until there is widespread immunization against HBV, there remains the need to employ *routine preventative measures* and the occasional requirement for *post-exposure prophylaxis*. These subjects will be discussed, followed by a review of *active immunization* against HBV infection.

Routine preventative measures against HBV infection

Simple measures are discussed earlier (see General Preventative Measures in Acute Viral Hepatitis), but several important points should be made with respect to HBV infection.

In developing countries, spread of HBV occurs predominantly in the perinatal period or during early childhood and the preventative measures outlined below are not likely to have a significant impact on HBV transmission. In areas with a low prevalence of HBV infection, simple measures may help prevent the common methods of spread. For example, the use of condoms or practice of 'safe sex' may help prevent the spread of HBV infection in the promiscuous homosexual or heterosexual communities. Screening of blood donors for HBsAg is clearly mandatory and has been effective[23,400,416,1023] in preventing all but the rare case when other markers of

HBV, or HBV-DNA, are present in donor blood in the absence of detectable HBsAg.[352,479,1153]

Other forms of parenteral spread of HBV infection are also potentially preventable, although sharing of needles and syringes by parenteral drug abusers is common despite their knowledge of the risks involved. Adequate sterilization or the use of disposable needles or instruments prevents spread by acupuncture, tattooing or scarification.

Prevention of spread of HBV infection within hospitals is a matter for considerable concern. The extent to which blood, faeces, urine and other biological fluids from patients with hepatitis or HBsAg carriers should be identified and specially handled by laboratory staff is controversial. In the United Kingdom, such material is identified and labelled as being a 'hepatitis risk', and sent to the laboratory in sealed containers and dealt with separately.

The whole question of the management of patients with acute hepatitis or of the chronic HBsAg carrier in a general hospital and the precautions which should be taken to prevent spread should be viewed in relation to the following facts:

1 Many cases of acute hepatitis are no longer infectious at the time of admission to hospital with deep jaundice.
2 Spread from acute cases is most likely to occur if they are admitted to hospital during the incubation period or pre-icteric phase and therefore will not be identified as a hepatitis risk. Furthermore, a high proportion of HBsAg carriers seen as patients in a general hospital will not be identified. For example, in one survey of consecutive admissions to a general hospital, 84% of the patients found to be HBsAg positive had not been identified and the test had not been specifically requested.[857] Such patients will therefore be nursed and their blood or other body fluids handled in the laboratory without special precautions.
3 The majority of HBsAg carriers in a general hospital will be HBeAg negative and may have anti-e and will therefore be less likely to spread hepatitis B. This does not apply to carriers in dialysis units, those with Down's syndrome or immunosuppressed patients.
4 As discussed earlier, although some surveys have reported a high incidence of HBV markers in hospital personnel, including dentists, the frequency with which they develop clinically overt hepatitis compared with the general population may not be of the same magnitude.

In the authors' view, in a community with a low HBsAg carrier rate, simple precautions (see General Preventative Measures in Acute Viral Hepatitis) should be taken in those with acute hepatitis and if possible they should be accommodated in a side-room. HBsAg carriers requiring dental extraction, endoscopy or surgery should be left to the end of the operating session and the theatre and instruments must be sterilized after use. Dentists and endoscopists should be encouraged to wear gloves under these circumstances. Laboratory personnel and postmortem attendants should take simple practical precautions when handling *all* specimens. These include avoidance of mouth-pipetting, eating, smoking and drinking in the laboratory, or the use of equipment or containers that allow spillage of blood. There should be special facilities for handwashing, and clean protective clothing should be worn, including gloves if practicable, particularly if abrasions are present on the hands. Should spillage of potentially contaminated material occur, the work area should be cleaned with hypochlorite, formaldehyde or glutaraldehyde solution as appropriate.

The whole subject is fully reviewed by Cossart,[234] and methods advocated for the control of hepatitis in laboratories have been proposed by the WHO Expert Committee on Viral Hepatitis.[1266,1267] We would, however, agree with the view of the WHO Expert Committee on Viral Hepatitis that 'there is no evidence that the identification of patients who are HBsAg positive so that their specimens can be specially labelled or handled would lead to any greater reduction of the occupational risk of hepatitis B than would result from the meticulous attention to procedures for the safe handling of all clinical specimens.'[1267]

Post-exposure prophylaxis against HBV infection

Known exposure to HBV infection may occur in individuals who have not previously received, or have not responded, to active HBV vaccination. In Western societies the most frequent clinical situations in which this occurs are after needlestick and other forms of parenteral exposure or after sexual exposure; whereas in developing countries, birth to an HBsAg-positive mother is more relevant. In each of these circumstances post-exposure prophylaxis is appropriate and usually consists of a combination of both passive immunoprophylaxis and active immunization.[260,384,1308]

Passive immunoprophylaxis is imparted by administration of hepatitis B immune globulin (HBIG), which is prepared from pooled plasma that contains a high titre of anti-HBs. The recommended dose of HBIG (200 iu/ml of anti-HBs) for adults is 0.05–0.07 ml/kg body weight, given as early as possible post-exposure. HBIG should preferably be given within 48 hours, but a first dose should not be given more than 7 days post-exposure. In some regimes a second dose is recommended after an interval of 30 days.[264]

The mode of action of HBIG in preventing HBV transmission is uncertain. The titre of anti-HBs in serum after HBIG administration is not predictive of protective potency[384] and it has been suggested that HBIG may attenuate rather than prevent HBV transmission, leading to passive–active immunization.[292]

HBIG, if given alone, is only partially effective in preventing clinically significant post-exposure HBV infection. In the controlled study of Krugman and Giles,[608] HBIG given within 4 hours of experimental innoculation of the MS-2 serum pool failed to prevent development of

HBV infection in 4 of 10 innoculated children. In clinical practice, where the degree of exposure to HBV is less clearly defined, HBIG is more effective but does not prevent HBV transmission in all. A study conducted in England and Wales between 1975 and 1987, demonstrated that 53 (0.6%) of 9370 post-exposure HBIG recipients developed acute hepatitis B.[893] The highest rate of 3.7% occurred in those who had been sexually exposed (*n*=564), which compares with reported rates of 0.9% after accidental innoculation (*n*=2056), 0.2% after exposure through skin abrasions or minor contact via mucous membranes (*n*=5747), and no reported cases in 1003 recipients who did not meet the recognized criteria for HBIG administration.

There is some evidence to suggest that HBIG may only delay the onset of HBV infection. Earlier studies of HBIG administered to hospital staff and patients found a decreased rate of HBV infection at 8 months, but by 12 months the rate of HBV infection was similar to that of the untreated group.[415,1020] In a study of post-exposure prophylaxis in haemodialysis unit staff, HBIG given alone was less effective than HBIG plus active vaccination, with HBV infection occurring in 11/33 compared to 1/24 cases respectively.[771] The co-administration of anti-HBs (in HBIG) does not interfere with the subsequent response to active vaccination, providing they are injected at different sites. It has been suggested that administration of anti-HBs may even enhance the subsequent response to HBsAg vaccines,[766] but others have been unable to confirm this observation.[652]

For the prevention of perinatal transmission of HBV, the recommended dose of HBIG is 0.13 ml/kg body weight given as a single dose immediately after delivery or as soon as possible thereafter, preferably within 12 hours. Several studies from different parts of the world have shown that HBIG given within 48 hours of birth will reduce the likelihood of perinatal transmission,[63,71,590,799,941] but infection may occur as passive immunity wanes at 6–9 months unless the infant is actively immunized. Comparative information is available for infants born to high-risk (HBsAg-positive, HBeAg-positive) mothers in the UK. In the period from 1982–1985 such infants received HBIG alone, whereas combined HBIG and active immunization was routinely administered after 1985. At 1 year of age, 11 of 124 infants who received four doses of HBIG and 4 of 20 infants who received three doses were positive for HBsAg. This compares with HBsAg positivity in only 1 of 54 infants who received HBIG followed by later active immunization and 4 of 102 that received combined HBIG and active immunization at birth (2 of these 4 did not complete a full course of active immunization).[890] In other studies, HBIG in combination with either serum-derived[194] or yeast-derived[1096] vaccines has been shown to prevent perinatal HBV transmission in 90–95% of infants born to HBsAg-positive mothers (see Active Immunization Against HBV infection).

One recently highlighted potential pitfall of HBIG

administration is that some preparations also contain anti-HIV antibodies, which are thus passively transferred to recipients. This has been reported to lead to a false diagnosis of HIV infection in HBIG recipients in infancy.[9] In contrast, serological studies in adults have demonstrated no detectable passive transfer of HIV antibodies, even when they were known to be present in the original HBIG preparation.[876]

Interest in passive immunoprophylaxis has been rekindled by the desire to prevent re-infection of grafts in patients undergoing liver transplantation for fulminant or chronic HBV infection. Future developments may see more attention paid to HBIG or monoclonal antibody preparations directed against either the pre-S_1 or pre-S_2 epitopes of HBV.[384] Anti-pre-S_1 and anti-pre-S_2 are neutralizing antibodies that, theoretically at least, offer the best option for preventing HBV reinfection of liver grafts.

The relative failure of passive immunization for post-exposure prophylaxis has led to the suggestion that this may be better replaced by accelerated active vaccination programmes,[521,1218,1225] in which doses are given at 0, 2 and 6 weeks after exposure. These accelerated regimes appear to be effective but are not at present in widespread use (see below).

Active immunization against HBV infection

Vaccines for use in the prevention of HBV infection have been available for clinical use since the mid 1980s. Those that are commercially available include *plasma-derived vaccines* and *recombinant vaccines*, both of which are preparations of purified HBsAg. Experience with these vaccines indicates that they are highly efficacious in preventing HBV infection. Other novel developments in this field have included *polypeptide subunit vaccines, hybrid vaccinia virus vaccines and other hybrid virus or particle HBV vaccines*. Active vaccination against hepatitis B has recently been reviewed.[384,1308]

The mode of action of HBV vaccines is not well understood. It is presumed that HBsAg induces development of anti-HBs and that the latter is protective, but induction of T-cell-dependent immunity may also be important. The induction of antibodies against pre-S_1 and pre-S_2 by plasma-derived vaccines has been emphasized,[384] but this contrasts with the response to the widely used recombinant vaccines which induce anti-HBs only, yet offer good protection against HBV infection.

Recommended vaccination schedules

It is currently recommended that both plasma-derived and recombinant HBV vaccines are administered by intramuscular injection in the deltoid muscle for adults and the lateral aspect of the thigh for children. Gluteal injection is not recommended as it often leads to an inadequate response. The standard regime is 3 doses of vaccine (20 µg in adults and 10 µg in children) at 0, 1 month and 6 months. Alternative timing, doses or routes

of vaccine administration have also been reported to give a satisfactory anti-HBs response (see below).

Indications and strategies for use of hepatitis B vaccines

Indications for the use of hepatitis B vaccines have been summarized in a number of publications.[520,1269–1271,1307, 1308] At present, Zuckerman's recommendations are applicable for clinical use in Great Britain and other Western countries. In brief, vaccination is proposed for the following.

1. Health-care personnel who are exposed to blood or blood products, who are staff of residential institutions for the mentally handicapped, staff involved in haemodialysis or the treatment of haemophilia, dentists, and ancillary staff exposed to such increased-risk patients.
2. Medical personnel exposed to HBV by an accidental needlestick injury, in which case HBIG plus immediate active immunization at a contralateral site should be instituted.
3. Patients about to enter a residential institution for the mentally retarded, patients on maintenance haemodialysis or those requiring frequent blood transfusion or transfusion of blood products, and immunosuppressed patients or patients requiring frequent renal dialysis.
4. Patients in whom sexual spread is likely, for example amongst spouses, promiscuous homosexuals and prostitutes. It is also appropriate to vaccinate other family members who have close daily contact with patients who are HBsAg positive. Parenteral drug abusers and their sexual contacts should also be vaccinated.
5. Infants of mothers who are carriers of HBV, particularly those who are e-antigen-positive, in which case a combination of HBIG and vaccination may be the treatment of choice.
6. Much more controversial would be the need to immunize people who frequently travel abroad to endemic areas, the staff of custodial institutions such as prisons, ambulance and rescue staff, and selected police and military personnel.

A similar strategy of vaccinating high-risk groups has been employed in the USA since hepatitis B vaccines became available for clinical use, but the overall incidence of hepatitis B has increased from ~200 000 to ~300 000 cases per annum throughout this period (see Epidemiology of Hepatitis B). This has led to the suggestion that universal vaccination of children (and possibly adolescents) should be considered in the USA.[553] Although studies performed in societies with sophisticated health-care systems have demonstrated that vaccination of high-risk groups is cost-effective,[42,136,627] it is not clear that a universal vaccination strategy can be justified on grounds of cost–benefit alone.

In regions of the world with an intermediate or high prevalence of HBV infection, current recommendations are for a universal vaccination strategy.[264,1306] The Center for Disease Control, Atlanta, and the World Health Organization now recommend that hepatitis B vaccine be administered together with the expanded programme on immunization (EPI).[396,720] When given together with EPI, hepatitis B vaccines are satisfactorily immunogenic.[881,1181] Successful application of this strategy is both fiscally and logistically difficult in underdeveloped countries, but there remains the potential, at least, for eradication of hepatitis B.

Specific vaccines for prevention of hepatitis B

Plasma derived vaccines Over the past decade, a number of plasma-derived vaccines have been developed in the USA, Europe and Japan and these have undergone clinical trials. In most instances the 22-nm particles have been used, but the methods used to purify and inactivate the virus have varied. In the preparation marketed by Merck Sharp & Dohme, small particles are concentrated from the plasma of hepatitis B carriers by ammonium sulphate precipitation, isopycnic banding and rate-zonal sedimentation. The antigen is then digested with pepsin and exposed to 8 mol/l urea solution to facilitate the removal of liver and blood plasma components. After a further purification step of gel filtration, it is treated with formalin and adsorbed onto an alum adjuvant.[464,1121] All protein in the final product is HBsAg and is free of human albumin and other extraneous proteins and pyrogens; each batch is safety-tested in chimpanzees. This preparative procedure will destroy all known infective agents, including the human immunodeficiency virus (HIV). Because this vaccine was originally prepared from donations from New York homosexuals, the possibility that it transmitted HIV infection caused considerable concern, but no example of such transmission has been reported. Vaccines prepared from adw or ayw subtypes are equally safe and immunogenic.[848]

After vaccination, 85–95% or more of healthy individuals develop detectable anti-HBs, but a lower response is reported in Africa, with only 67% of adults aged 21–70 years developing antibodies.[1127] After successful vaccination, anti-HBs titres fall with time and by 4 years are below 10 iu/l in 34% of vaccinees.[537] The duration of persistence of anti-HBs is related to the peak titre after the third dose of vaccine, such that all adult vaccinees with peak titres greater than 10 000 iu/l had titres that remained above 10 iu/l at 6 years post-vaccination.[537] Similar results were obtained in infants born to HBeAg-positive mothers; all vaccinees with titres greater than 1000 iu/l had titres that remained above 10 iu/l at 4 years.[675]

Three other vaccines produced from HBsAg-positive plasma have been produced and subjected to extensive clinical trials, one from the Pasteur Institute,[246] one from the Central Laboratory of the Netherlands Red Cross Blood Transfusion Service[272] and another from the Green Cross Corporation in Osaka.[638] The Pasteur vaccine was prepared by lipoprotein elimination, precipitation of immune complexes, concentration and treatment of the purified HBsAg with formalin. Three injections of 5 μg of vaccine with aluminium hydroxide as adjuvant are given at monthly intervals. The Netherlands Red Cross vaccine was prepared by two cycles of heat-inactivation and was given in three or four monthly injections of 3 μg, depending on the trial subjects being studied (see below). The Green Cross Corporation method of preparing vaccine is similar but includes a formaldehyde treatment step.

For plasma-derived HBV vaccines a WHO Report[1270] has stressed the importance of the need for the establishment of international reference preparations. These should be adequately inactivated and prepared and should be safety-tested in chimpanzees and human volunteers.

Many controlled clinical trials have now been conducted using the plasma-derived subviral particle vaccines mentioned above. Subjects include homosexual men, medical staff, dialysis patients and newborn infants. In a controlled, randomized, double-blind clinical trial in 1083 homosexual men from New York, Szmuness and associates[1121] showed that the attack rate of hepatitis B was 3.2% in vaccine recipients compared with 25.6% in placebo recipients. The vaccine is virtually totally protective when given pre-exposure and partially effective when given post-exposure. This was confirmed by a study in male homosexuals using the Netherlands Red Cross vaccine[240] in which anti-HBs was detected in 89–95% of vaccinated individuals. Similar results were obtained in subsequent trials using the Merck vaccine, the Pasteur Institute vaccine and the Netherlands Red Cross vaccine in medical staff.[246,272,1122] In some societies, use of the vaccine has had a dramatic effect on the incidence of HBV infection. For example, in Alaska, a comprehensive programme of screening all Alaskan natives for HBsAg and the strategy of vaccinating all susceptible persons and neonates have led to a marked reduction in the annual incidence of acute hepatitis B in that community from 215 to 14 cases per 100 000 population.[730]

Of major importance worldwide is the prevention of the perinatal transmission of HBV, which has wide implications in relation to the development of chronic liver disease and hepatocellular carcinoma. As indicated earlier, the administration of HBIG within 24–48 h of birth will reduce the frequency of the carrier state in newborn infants, but they remain susceptible after the first year of life. Two major randomized controlled trials from Taiwan involving 17 500 women[71,72] and from Hong Kong involving 9072 women[1263] have shown clearly that combined HBIG and active immunization protects over 90% of infants of HBeAg-positive mothers. Almost all of the infants would otherwise have become infected with HBV and 70% would have become chronic carriers. This and other smaller studies provide firm guidelines for the prevention of perinatally transmitted hepatitis B.[632] The infants of HBsAg-positive mothers, particularly those who are HBeAg positive, should be given HBIG at birth and actively immunized even if born by caesarean section.

Babies of HBeAg-negative mothers should be immunized in endemic areas, and the babies of 'high-risk' mothers in non-endemic areas should also be offered immunization.

The economic and logistical problems of trying to use this method of prevention in the Third World are considerable,[45,1269] but it is likely to prove the most effective way of reducing chronic liver disease and hepatocellular carcinoma worldwide. This is currently under careful evaluation in the Gambia.[1148]

Trials of hepatitis B vaccines in haemodialysis patients have given variable results. In three early trials of plasma-derived vaccines, two appeared to show its efficacy in a substantial number of patients studied.[247,272] In one contrary report using the Merck vaccine,[1095] the population studied showed both a low antibody response rate to hepatitis B vaccine and a low viral attack rate. This large placebo-controlled study of 1311 patients receiving haemodialysis in the USA showed that only 50% of vaccine recipients responded adequately, and that the incidence of HBV infection was virtually identical in the vaccine and placebo recipients. A point of concern was that some individuals who appeared to develop an anti-HBs response were not protected, and it has been suggested[633] that the antibody response to HBsAg may not always be fully protective against HBV infection. More recent studies have confirmed a poor response rate (47% develop anti-HBs) in haemodialysis patients receiving plasma-derived vaccines[855,1090] according to standard regimens. In contrast, further multiple doses of plasma-derived vaccine have been reported to give a 92% seroconversion rate in haemodialysis patients.[1206] A poor response to plasma-derived vaccines has also been reported in Down's syndrome and other forms of mental retardation;[48,451] in the elderly;[267] in alcoholics—particularly in those with liver disease;[743] in type I (insulin-dependent) diabetics;[911] and in HIV-positive homosexual men[169,221,679] and HIV-positive haemophiliacs.[697,835]

A small proportion of normal subjects also fail to respond to hepatitis B vaccines, and the cellular and genetic basis for this have been investigated. Abnormalities of both B and T cell function are described,[201,316] and there is an association between non-response and homozygosity for the extended or fixed major histocompatibility complex (MHC) haplotype [HLA-B8, SC01, DR3].[21] The presence of this MHC haplotype on both chromosomes appears to be associated with the absence of a dominant immune response gene in the MHC.

In those that fail to respond to a standard regimen of plasma-derived vaccine, a small proportion (18%) will respond to a fourth dose, but the majority fail to develop a sustained antibody response to either the plasma-derived or recombinant vaccines.[538,1243] There are reports of non-responders developing HBV infection.[112] Various adjuvant therapies have been used in an attempt to enhance the immune response to hepatitis B vaccines; oral administration of taurine enhances the response rate in normal volunteers[517,622] and thymopentin[298] interferon-

γ[926] and interleukin-2[746] have all been reported to improve the response in patients with renal disease.

Recombinant vaccines   An important advance in the prevention of hepatitis B has been the application of recombinant DNA technology to produce new vaccines. On a global scale this is the most important application of molecular biology to date in preventing human disease. Potentially such vaccines could be produced in large quantities and at low cost, making large-scale worldwide vaccination a technical possibility.

The HBV genome encoding HBsAg has been incorporated into a variety of expression vectors, including yeasts (_Saccharomyces cerevisae_), _E.coli_ and mammalian cell lines. Preparations of yeast-derived recombinant vaccines are currently widely available for clinical use. These are safe, immunogenic and effective in preventing hepatitis B infection. In the UK and many other countries they are currently used in preference to the plasma-derived vaccines, largely because of the perception that there is an improved safety record.

These vaccines are prepared by fermentation of the yeasts containing part of the HBV genome, followed by lysis and extraction of the HBsAg particles. The preparation from SmithKline Beecham is further purified by precipitation steps, ion-exchange and gel permeation chromatography and caesium chloride ultracentrifugation.[873] The purified non-glycosylated HBsAg particles are spherical and resemble the 22-nm particles found in serum in human infection.[99,873] Structural characterization by mass spectrometry has confirmed that these particles have the primary structure of HBsAg.[456]

When they are injected as a vaccine into humans, the antibody response to yeast-derived vaccines is similar to that observed with the plasma-derived vaccines. Antibodies (anti-HBs) are directed against the 'a' determinant of HBsAg, with monoclonal studies indicating that there is a response to the RFHBs epitope, which is known to be protective.[441,1237] With the standard regimen of three doses of 10–20 μg of recombinant yeast-derived vaccine, 97–100% of normal healthy young adults develop anti-HBs.[87,155,408,994] Although the level of anti-HBs achieved is initially higher with plasma-derived compared to recombinant yeast-derived vaccines,[248,547] after an interval of 11 months there is little difference in antibody levels.[547] Protective levels of anti-HBs (>10 iu/ml) were observed in 97% of recipients of the early batches of the Merck Sharp & Dohme preparation of recombinant yeast-derived vaccine at 1 year, and in 68% at 2 years of follow-up,[155] which compares favourably with plasma-derived vaccines. Other studies of recombinant yeast-derived vaccines have reported protective levels of anti-HBs persisting in 78% of vaccinees at 3 years and in 68% at 4 years.[540]

Recombinant yeast-derived vaccines are also effective in neonates and children, producing protective levels (>10 iu/ml) in 100% in some reports.[739,976] As for plasma-derived vaccines, infants born to HBsAg-positive mothers have a low seroconversion rate (84%) with recombinant yeast-derived vaccines.[739] A relatively poor response is also observed in parenteral drug abusers (76%),[977] haemodialysis patients (55%)[139,140] and HIV-positive homosexuals.[639]

Recombinant yeast-derived vaccines appear to be as efficacious as the plasma-derived vaccines in preventing HBV infection, with low rates of HBV infection reported in high-risk groups.[39] In a study of 183 homosexuals, only 2 developed serological evidence of HBV infection, without clinically overt hepatitis, over a follow-up period of 7 months.[916] Protective efficacy has also been demonstrated for institutionalized patients with mental handicap[1197] and for infants born to HBsAg-positive, HBeAg-positive mothers.[901] In the latter study, only 2 (3.6%) of 55 vaccinated infants developed HBV infection over a follow-up period of 13 months.

Alternative timing, doses or routes of vaccine administration

Short dose intervals of 0, 2 and 6 weeks give rise to protective antibody levels more rapidly than the standard regimen but the peak titre is lower.[1225] In the more conventional regimen, an increased interval between the second and third dose (i.e. 0, 2 and 12 months) promotes an even higher peak titre and is theoretically valuable in prolonging the duration of acquired immunity.[539]

There has been considerable interest in low-dose intramuscular or intradermal use of the plasma-derived HBV vaccines, principally to reduce the cost of, and thereby extend, vaccination programmes in developing countries. Low-dose intramuscular regimens using three doses of 2 μg of plasma-derived vaccine have been reported to give rise to protective levels of antibody in 90% of normal adult volunteers[453] and 91.2% of 650 healthy children aged 2–12 years.[760] A follow-up study of these children at 1 year demonstrated that 89% still had detectable anti-HBs, although one vaccinee developed clinical hepatitis B.[761] Low-dose intramuscular regimens have also been advocated for vaccination of neonates,[643,789,1292] but this is controversial and considered inadvisable for infants born to high-risk (HBsAg-positive, HBeAg-positive) mothers.[511,641]

Intradermal injection of low doses (2 μg) of plasma-derived HBV vaccines have also been reported to give rise to satisfactory levels of anti-HBs in adult volunteers[209,451,576] and in children,[776] that persist in the majority for at least 2 years.[513,576] Intradermal administration of recombinant vaccine (1 μg) has been reported to give an inferior anti-HBs response compared with intradermal plasma-derived vaccine (2 μg).[142,624] The intradermal route is technically more difficult and poor technique may lead to subcutaneous injection, which is relatively ineffective at stimulating an adequate anti-HBs response.[1224] As low-dose intramuscular administration seems equally effective, there seems little justification for use of the intradermal technique.

The duration of immunity after HBV vaccination is unknown, but is related to the titre of anti-HBs. If this falls below 10 iu/l there may be a risk of infection, and this has led to the suggestion that booster doses of vaccine should be given in these circumstances[36,815,1259] or at 5–6-year intervals in infants.[1293] Although this approach has been criticized,[387] there is evidence from a study performed in Senegalese infants that protective efficacy falls in the 5th and 6th year post-vaccination from 100% to 67%.[239]

Complications of hepatitis B vaccines

The majority of complications of hepatitis B vaccination are relatively minor and consist largely of pain and swelling at the site of injection. There are isolated case reports of erythema nodosum after use of both plasma-derived and recombinant yeast-derived vaccines.[295,404] Type I hypersensitivity to the minute quantity (<10 pg/ml) of yeast proteins in the recombinant vaccines, manifesting as pain and swelling of the entire arm, has also been reported.[133] Uveitis has been observed after use of plasma-derived vaccine.[362]

In a post-marketing surveillance study of spontaneously reported neurological adverse events after vaccination with plasma-derived vaccine (Heptavax-B, MSD), a total of 41 possible adverse events were reported from an estimated total of 850 000 vaccinations.[1036] These consisted of Bell's palsy (10 cases), Guillain–Barré syndrome (9 cases), convulsions (5 cases), lumbar radiculopathy (5 cases), optic neuritis (5 cases), transverse myelitis (4 cases) and brachial plexus neuropathy (3 cases). Of these, the only one found to be present more often than expected (by some of the analyses) was Guillain–Barré syndrome, and it was concluded that there was no significant epidemiological association between the vaccine and adverse neurological events.

New developments in hepatitis B vaccines

The various alternative approaches to vaccination against hepatitis B have recently been reviewed.[384,1308] New vaccines are required to improve efficacy, to reduce costs, and to simplify the method of delivery, making them more applicable for use in developing countries. Several different candidate vaccines have been developed.

Polypeptide subunit vaccines are synthetic peptides that correspond to components of the primary sequence of HBsAg or the pre-S proteins. They have the advantage that they can be prepared in pure form and are theoretically safer than other vaccines. Many different peptides have been synthesized and used as antigens in this context. In general they tend to be poorly immunogenic in comparison with plasma-derived or recombinant HBsAg particles, but their immunogenicity is improved if they are presented in micellar form.[13,138,300,1307,1308] Those that have been investigated include peptides that correspond to a 25-kD non-glycosylated and 30-kD glycosylated form of polypeptide I of HBsAg (designated p25 and gp30 respectively).[1308] In micellar form, synthetic peptides corresponding to HBsAg have been demonstrated to be immunogenic in young adults.[471] A synthetic peptide containing the entire 55 amino acids of the pre-S$_2$ region has also been found to be immunogenic in chimpanzees and to protect against intravenous challenge with live HBV.[321] These vaccines are not yet available for clinical use.

Hybrid vaccines are prepared by insertion of components of the HBV genome into other live viruses to produce chimeric forms. Genomic sequences of HBsAg have been inserted into vaccinia virus to produce stable hybrids that are capable of producing significant levels of HBsAg.[1071] Rabbits vaccinated with the purified hybrid virus developed immunity to HBV, as did three chimpanzees. This vaccine has several potential advantages, including low cost, long storage life and ease of administration, e.g. by skin scratch technique. Unfortunately, the potential for altered virulence of the vaccinia virus after genetic recombinations is unknown and this has not yet been developed as a vaccine for human use.

Another approach has been to produce hybrids of HBV genomic sequences in live recombinant adenoviruses, which would thus be suitable for oral administration. In a chimpanzee model, live human adenoviruses type 4 (ad4) and type 7 (ad7) containing the HBsAg genome, given sequentially by mouth, produced significant circulating levels of anti-HBs in two animals.[683] When challenged with live HBV, one chimpanzee was protected and the other developed a modified disease course. This is a promising development with important potential for human disease.

Hepatitis B core antigen has also been used to produce hybrids with synthetic viral peptides. This has been successful in improving immunogenicity for a number of different viral polypeptides,[208] including pre-S and S sequences of HBV.[1084] With these constructs, antibody responses against both HBcAg and the additional epitopes (S or pre-S) are observed, suggesting that this approach has considerable potential.

New recombinant vaccines are also under development. Considerable attention has been paid to developing vaccines derived from yeasts, *E.coli* or mammalian cells that express additional components of the HBV genome. A recombinant vaccine that contains the sequences for S and pre-S$_2$ has been prepared from mammalian cells,[1177] and used as an immunogen in human volunteers. This recombinant vaccine elicited a good anti-HBs response, but there was also an early high-titre production of anti-pre S$_2$. A yeast-derived recombinant vaccine that contains S, pre-S$_1$ and pre-S$_2$ domains has also been demonstrated to elicit an antibody response to all three components in rabbits. Vaccines that contain pre-S$_1$ and pre-S$_2$ sequences may potentially be more efficacious in preventing HBV infection, but this remains to be proved.

Recombinant methods have also been used to express core antigen (HBcAg) in *E.coli* for use as a hepatitis B vaccine. The particles produced are 21 nm in diameter and identical in appearance to those observed in HBV-infected liver.[1285] Such *E.coli*-derived core particles are immunogenic in chimpanzees, particularly after treatment

with sodium dodecyl sulphate to reveal 'e' antigen.[794] Challenge experiments with live HBV performed in two chimps demonstrated complete protection in one and modified disease in the other. Studies of this vaccine in humans are anticipated.

Escape mutants of hepatitis B virus

In addition to the 'e' antigen-negative mutants of hepatitis B virus described earlier, recent evidence indicates that replicating, pathogenic, forms of HBV may occur in which there are mutations affecting the 'a' determinant of HBsAg. These have recently been reviewed.[561,1308] These mutants of HBV first came to light in Italy, when immunized infants of HBsAg-positive mothers, all of whom had a satisfactory anti-HBs response to vaccine, later developed evidence of HBV infection, with HBsAg in the serum.[1295] In further studies, an HBV isolate from one of these cases was sequenced, with the finding that a point mutation from guanosine to adenosine had occurred at nucleotide position 587.[168] This results in a glycine to arginine substitution at position 145 of the 'a' determinant of the HBsAg, which alters the epitope sufficiently to render the vaccine-generated anti-HBs antibodies ineffective at neutralizing the mutant virus. An identical mutant has also been described in a liver transplant case treated with monoclonal anti-HBs to prevent graft reinfection. The patient became HBsAg positive again, but this antigen was not recognized by the monoclonal anti-HBs, and sequencing data confirmed a point mutation at nucleotide position 587.[732]

To date, the emergence of such escape mutants is not widespread in subjects vaccinated against hepatitis B, but these observations have led to the suggestion that future hepatitis B vaccines may need to include mutant virus sequences in their design.

HEPATITIS D

INTRODUCTION

Astute observations by Rizzetto and his colleagues in Italy in 1977 led to their discovery of delta agent hepatitis. While examining liver biopsy specimens for hepatitis B core antigen immunofluorescence in nuclei, these researchers found that some nuclei exhibited immunofluorescence even though no hepatitis B core particles were evident by electron microscopy. The new antigen, designated delta, was found only in liver cell nuclei of HBsAg-positive patients, but not in all. Furthermore, expression of HBcAg and delta antigen were mutually exclusive. Patients expressing the delta antigen were found to have a higher prevalence and severity of liver disease than those who did not.[953] These findings, along with their later finding that the delta agent was a defective infectious agent enveloped by the surface antigens of

HBV, led to the rapid characterization of the molecular biology of this defective virus and fuller understanding of why some cases of hepatitis B virus are more fulminant than others.

PROPERTIES OF HEPATITIS D VIRUS (see Table 30.8) _____

Classification

The delta agent was designated hepatitis delta virus (later hepatitis D virus or HDV) once it became clear that this agent was a distinct entity.[960] Hepatitis D virus is the smallest animal virus known and is the only defective RNA virus infecting animal cells. Owing to its unique structure and life cycle, this virus is unclassified and unrelated to any other known animal virus. The virus most resembles small pathogenic defective RNA viruses of plants, composed of viroids, satellite viruses and satellite RNAs.[595,1231] Viroids are unencapsidated, self-replicating molecules, while plant satellite RNA viruses are helper-dependent for replication and require helper virus protein for encapsidation. Satellite viruses are helper-dependent as well, but they are encapsidated by satellite protein which is encoded by the genomic RNA.[129] Hepatitis D virus resembles all of the subviral RNA agents in differing ways: (1) HDV requires helper function (as do satellite RNAs) from hepatitis B virus; (2) HDV resembles viroids and satellite RNAs in the mechanism of replication by 'rolling circle', the extensive intramolecular base pairing giving rise to an unbranched rod-like genome, and in the conserved regions required for self-ligation and cleavage; and (3) HDV resembles satellite viruses in encoding a protein required for encapsidation.

Table 30.8 Properties of hepatitis D virus
_____

- Unclassified satellite virus of hepatitis B virus
- 36-nm particles with indistinct internal structure enveloped by HBV surface proteins
- Replication restricted to liver
- Buoyant density of 1.24–1.25 g/ml
- Viral genome composed of single-stranded covalently closed circular 1.7-kb RNA
- Single known gene product (delta antigen) required for encapsidation and replication
- RNA genome undergoes autocatalytic cleavage and ligation
- Can be propagated in primary tissue culture or in woodchuck and chimpanzee animal models

HDV structure

Morphology

Visualization of HDV in liver or serum by electron microscopy reveals 36-nm particles with an indistinct internal structure. Delta RNA and antigen are detectable within the particles, but a defined core structure, as seen with HBV, is not apparent.[956] This size corresponds with that found by filtration, as HDV filtered through a polycarbonate membrane is retained by a 30-nm filter.[447] Sedimentation velocity is intermediate between that of Dane particles (HBV virions) and 22-nm HBsAg-containing particles, while the buoyant density determined in caesium chloride is 1.24–1.25 g/ml.[956]

Composition

Hepatitis D virus is composed of a single-stranded RNA genome associated with two forms of HDAg encapsidated by envelope derived from pre-surface and surface antigens of hepatitis B virus. The resistance of HDV-RNA to exogenous RNase and the release of HDAg after treatment of the virion with non-ionic detergents demonstrates that HDV-RNA and HDAg are internal components within an HBsAg coat.

The encapsidated genome, visualized by electron microscopy under denaturing conditions, is a covalently closed circular molecule and therefore not polyadenylated.[596] Under non-denaturing conditions, the genome is a closed, circular, unbranched rod structure.[196] The single strand of RNA is of plus (sense) polarity, determined by strand-specific hybridization to single-stranded DNA probes. Three complete viral sequences have been published, obtained by sequencing overlapping cDNA clones.[618,694,1231] These three isolates are 90% similar and 1679–1683 bases in length. Computer-generated analyses of lowest free energy configurations reveal the unbranched rod structure to be due to extensive intramolecular base pairing, as 70% of the genome is complementary.[1231] Two domains in the genome, encompassing 295 base pairs, are highly conserved in every isolate and span a UV-sensitive cross-linking site.[130] These viroid-like domains are probably involved in replication and engage in autocatalytic cleavage and ligation.[619,1032,1279]

Primary sequencing of genomic and antigenomic RNA reveals five long (>300 nucleotides) open reading frames (ORF). Translation of each ORF in bacteria reveals only one protein product recognized by antisera from infected patients—the hepatitis D antigen from ORF5.[1239]

Hepatitis D antigen in infected animals is present in two forms at 24 and 27 kD.[109] However, ORF5 cDNA translated in vitro by rabbit reticulocyte lysates or in transfected COS cells produces only a single variety, ranging from 24 to 26 kD.[184,1239] Predictions from primary sequence data reveal HDAg proteins of either 195 amino acids[618] or 214 amino acids.[694,1231] The reason for this sequence discrepancy and HDAg heterogeneity has become more clear; specific base transitions occur owing to RNA replication-associated mutagenesis. One extremely frequent site for mis-sense mutation during genome replication is in the termination codon at amino acid position 195, which extends the polypeptide to the next termination signal at position 214.[687] Replication of the genomes encoding the short 24-kD and long 27-kD HDAg have been studied by viral cDNA transfection in vitro. Only the short form of HDAg supported HDV genome replication, whereas the long form acted as a potent dominant-negative repressor of replication. These results may have important implications in natural infections, where the generation of long-form genomes may lead to self-limiting infection.[185,395]

Antibodies to HDAg are non-neutralizing. Human IgG monoclonal antibodies have been produced by Epstein–Barr virus transformation of peripheral leucocytes. The single epitope recognized by the two monoclonal antibodies was also recognized by polyclonal antibodies. The monoclonal antibodies recognized both denatured and native HDAg, indicating that the epitope is linear and related to the HDAg primary sequence.[886]

The envelope of HDV contains surface antigens derived from HBV. However, the composition of the envelope varies from that found in HBV and more resembles the composition of HBsAg in 22-nm HBsAg particles found in isolated HBV infections. Using the nomenclature detailed earlier on the molecular biology of HBV, HDV envelope contains 95% p24 and gp27^s, 5% p33^s and gp36^s (glycosylated pre-S$_2$ proteins) and 1% p39 and gp42^s (pre-S$_1$, non-glycosylated and glycosylated proteins).[109]

Virion life cycle

The mechanism by which HDV attaches to and enters host cells is unknown. Since HDV resides in an envelope contributed by HBV, presumably the viral receptor is common. Most likely the pre-S$_1$ protein in the envelope of HDV is the ligand binding the virus to receptor.

The helper role of HBV appears limited to supplying envelope in order to allow HDV to bind and reinfect cells. No helper functions are required for HDV replication intracellularly, as complete HDV cDNA clones transfected into cultured human hepatoma cells replicate normally.[620]

Replication

The genome of HDV in serum particles is unit-length, single-stranded RNA of plus polarity. However, replicating HDV-RNA in liver exhibits a variety of forms. Genomic (+) strands are in excess of antigenomic strands in a ratio of 20 : 1 or 30 : 1. Genomic RNA is predominantly single-stranded, whereas antigenomic RNA is generally found in double-stranded molecules, hybridized to genomic RNA. No DNA intermediates are detectable.[413] This arrangement has analogy to plant viroids, where replication occurs via a rolling-circle mechanism. In this replication strategy, the genomic-length, circular (+)

strand is used as the template for successive rounds of minus-strand synthesis, which is multimeric and linear. The multimeric linear minus strand then serves as the template for plus-strand synthesis, generating linear duplexed complementary RNA strands.[129] Host cell-derived, RNA-dependent RNA polymerase is required. The autocatalytic splicing and ligating properties of isolated HDV RNA are probably responsible for the production of unit-length circular genomes from the multimeric linear precursor.[619,1032,1033,1278,1279]

Essential aspects of HDV replication and transcription of HDAg are mediated by HDV-RNA autocatalysis. A highly conserved viroid-like region within HDV can undergo self-cleavage and ligation; this activity is pH-independent but divalent cation-dependent. An area as small as 117 nucleotides around the cleavage site is adequate, with the cleavage leaving a phosphodiester bond. The 5′ fragment has a terminal uridyl 2′, 3′ cyclic monophosphate residue, while the 3′ fragment gives a 5′ hydroxyl group. Apposition of complementary RNA in the area of the cleavage site is required for ribozyme activity.[619,1032,1033,1278,1279]

Hepatitis DAg has an undefined but essential role in HDV replication. Trimers of complete viral cDNA carrying a frameshift mutation in the HDAg open reading frame exhibited 40-fold diminished levels of replicative forms when transfected into human hepatoma cells. The normal level of replication can be restored by cotransfection of the wild-type HDAg open reading frame, indicating that HDAg can act in *trans*.[620] Hepatitis DAg is probably translated from a cytoplasmic, polyadenylated antigenomic mRNA which is 800 base pairs in length. This recently characterized mRNA species is 500 times less abundant than full-length genomic RNA. The 5′ terminus and the 3′ site at which the poly(A) is added has been characterized.[493]

Apparently, HDAg has RNA-binding activity which is specific for HDV-RNA. Under conditions of high salt and an excess amount of unrelated RNA, both genomic and antigenomic HDV-RNA bound to HDAg, several different regions of genomic and antigenomic RNA could compete for HDAg binding, indicating the binding of antigen is probably specific for a secondary folded structure unique to HDV RNA. The middle third of HDAg was sufficient for binding HDV RNA.[186,668]

HDV infection appears to be directly cytopathic. An interesting hypothesis on the molecular pathobiology of this infection has recently been advanced. Extensive complementarity exists between two regions of human 7SL RNA (a structure involved in the translocation of secretory and membrane-associated proteins) and antigenomic HDV RNA. Spanning two 48 and 44 HDV nucleotide domains, there are regions of 73% and 77% base complementarity respectively. Thus, the replicative intermediate of HDV may injure cells by annealing to host RNA, interfering with cellular protein sorting.[806]

Experimental systems for study of HDV

The host range of HDV infection is limited to those animals allowing replication of hepadnaviruses. Chimpanzees can be inoculated to allow superinfection or co-infection.[108,923] Chronic HDV infection may occur, although less frequently than in humans. Fulminant hepatitis is also less frequent than in human infection.[900] Cloned HDV cDNA may be studied by direct inoculation of multimeric nucleic acid into the chimpanzee liver.[1110]

HDV can replicate in woodchucks as well. Human serum infected with HDV results in an infection with serological patterns similar to chimp or human infection. The viruses from woodchucks or chimps have similar biophysical properties, but the HDV acquires the WHV envelope after initial infection.[899] HDV replicates in non-neoplastic liver tissue of woodchucks, as well as in hepatocellular carcinoma tissue. No replication is evident in any extrahepatic tissues including spleen, kidney or peripheral leucocytes.[805] No attempts have been made to propagate this virus in ground squirrels.

There are no immortalized tissue-culture systems which support hepadnaviral or HDV infection, presumably because de-differentiated hepatoma cells lack the viral receptor. However, WHV-infected primary woodchuck hepatocytes prepared by collagenase perfusion are viable for many months in culture and can support propagation of woodchuck-passaged HDV, although only a small fraction of hepatocyte nuclei are infected.[202,1143]

LABORATORY DETECTION OF HDV INFECTION

Routine laboratory tests for detection of HDV infection include commercially available RIAs and EIAs for total and IgM anti-HDV antibodies and for delta antigen in serum. Delta antigen may also be demonstrated by immunohistochemistry in liver biopsy specimens. Delta antigen and *HDV-RNA* in serum may be detected by immunoblotting or dot hybridization techniques respectively, but these are currently used predominantly as research tools.

The interrelationship between HBV and HDV serology in differentiating the diagnosis of HBV/HDV co-infection from HDV superinfection of chronic HBV infection is described later (see Specific Clinical Features of Hepatitis D Infection).

Total anti-HDV antibodies become positive late in the clinical course of HDV infection and are usually negative in the acute phase of the disease.[41,151,981] Acute and convalescent sera are therefore required in order to interpret results if this test alone is used to diagnose HDV infection. If acute-phase sera are not available, a sample taken 30 days after the onset of symptoms is diagnostic of HDV infection in 92% of cases.[981] In patients who experience acute self-limited co-infection with both HDV and HBV, total anti-HDV titres are usually low and remain detectable in serum for an average of 9 months

(5.5 months after clearance of HBsAg).[164] A persistent high titre of total anti-HDV is highly suggestive of chronic HDV-related liver disease occurring in a patient with chronic HBV infection who has become superinfected with HDV.[256]

IgM anti-HDV antibodies are detected earlier in the course of HDV infection[1066] and are of considerable clinical value, with positive results found in 77–93% of acute cases.[41,153] The commercially available tests do not differentiate between HDV/HBV co-infection and superinfection with HDV; in one report IgM anti-HDV was present in 27/36 cases of co-infection and 14/17 cases of superinfection.[153] In patients with self-limiting co-infections, the IgM response is usually short-lived, but in chronic HDV infection the IgM anti-HDV response is variable, ranging from completely negative in some patients to fluctuating or persistently high titres in others.[256] Two different forms of IgM anti-HDV antibodies have recently been described; a 19 S pentameric form and a 7–8 S monomeric form, which can be separated in the laboratory by rate-zonal centrifugation. The higher molecular weight (19 S) form is detected predominantly in acute HDV infection, whereas the 7 S form is found most frequently in association with chronic HDV infection.[530] Moreover, in cases of acute HDV infection that progressed to become chronic, a sequential change from 19 S to 7–8 S forms was observed. The different molecular weight forms of IgM anti-HDV do not differentiate co-infection from superinfection.

Delta antigen becomes detectable (by RIA or EIA) in serum in the late incubation period of acute HDV infection[1034] and may persist into the symptomatic stage in approximately 20% of cases.[41] Using a sensitive technique for detection of delta antigen (Deltassay), positive results have been reported in up to 83% of cases of acute HDV infection, with 37/42 positive in cases of HBV/HDV co-infection and 12/17 positive in cases of HDV superinfection.[153] In chronic HDV infection, delta antigen is often undetectable in serum by conventional EIA or RIA techniques, but immunoblotting reveals positive results in the majority of cases.[89]

Delta antigen can also be detected in liver biopsy material and this is an important method of confirming the diagnosis of hepatitis D (see Specific Pathological Features of Hepatitis D).

HDV-RNA in serum can be detected by dot hybridization, using either cDNA or single-stranded (antisense) RNA probes for HDV. In acute HDV infection, serum HDV-RNA is detected in 61–90% of cases during the symptomatic phase of the illness, but becomes negative after clinical recovery.[1068,1303] In chronic HDV infection, serum HDV-RNA is detected in 58–75% of cases,[1068,1303] and in some remains detectable in multiple samples over a period of several years.[1068] In chronic HDV infection, positive results for HDV-RNA are usually accompanied by positive results for IgM anti-HDV in serum and positive immunohistochemistry for delta antigen at liver biopsy.[1068]

EPIDEMIOLOGY OF HEPATITIS D

Geographical distribution

The original descriptions of delta virus found a high incidence in southern Italy, but hepatitis D infection has now been found throughout the world.[1039] In addition to southern Italy, other high-incidence areas include parts of eastern Europe and western Asia,[1039,1137] Venezuela,[430,905,1170] Columbia,[145,146] the Amazon Basin,[84,1039] and some Pacific Islands.[1079]

Although delta infection is only found in association with HBV infection, not all high-HBV-prevalence areas have a high incidence of infection with the delta agent. In the Far East, superinfection with delta is an uncommon event. Earlier studies from Taiwan indicated that only 5% of patients with chronic HBV liver diseases have delta antibody in their serum,[193] but in a more recent study using a combination of tests for both total and IgM anti-HDV and delta antigen, the reported prevalence of HDV superinfection among patients with chronic hepatitis was much higher at 25%.[1179]

Despite its worldwide distribution, there is considerable local geographical variation with, for instance, a far higher incidence in southern compared with northern Italy.[334] Geographical variations in the prevalence of anti-HDV are also reported in Japan, with 9.8% positive in the eastern suburban area of Kure compared with 2.7% in other areas.[1133]

Studies in the UK have included retrospective immunofluorescent analysis of liver biopsies stored from 1973. Positive staining of liver nuclei using an anti-delta antibody was found in the biopsies from 7 out of 15 drug addicts.[1214] By contrast, studies in Sweden indicated that delta agent infection did not exist prior to 1973 but had been increasing progressively in incidence amongst HBsAg-positive drug addicts since then.[439]

More recent studies have shown a relatively low prevalence (2.6%) of markers for HDV in hepatitis B carriers in the UK,[566] although in one UK series containing a significant number of parenteral drug abusers and haemophiliacs a much higher prevalence was found (13%).[1247]

In addition to Italy, other parts of Western Europe have a relatively high prevalence of markers for HDV infection; for example, in Spain the overall prevalence of HDV markers was 19.4% in all HBsAg carriers tested. Within this study, however, the prevalence among parenteral drug abusers was 68% whereas the prevalence amongst HBsAg carriers with no clear-cut risk factor for HDV infection was much lower at 7.3%.[175] Thus the prevalence of HDV markers within a community is related not only to geographical variations but also to social factors which increase the risk of transmission of HDV. It is also evident that the prevalence of HDV markers is much higher in those with chronic liver disease (6.7–100%) than in asymptomatic HBsAg carriers (0–24%) irrespective of geographical location.[84,154,339,1171] This is undoubt-

edly related to increased risk of progression of chronic liver disease in HDV superinfection of chronic HBV infection (see Specific Clinical Features, Prognosis and Outcome of Hepatitis D Infection).

Methods of spread

HDV is transmitted by many of the same mechanisms as HBV. Consequently, for a particular community, the mode of transmission will be particularly influenced by the composition of the population at risk. In areas of low HBV endemicity, superinfection with HDV is confined largely to haemophiliacs and to parenteral drug abusers. Thus between one-third and two-thirds of HBsAg-positive parenteral drug abusers may have markers of HDV infection, with prevalence rates recorded at 31% in Ireland, 64% in Italy, 64–68% in Spain, 67% in New York, and 91% in Taiwan.[154,175,494,816,931] The spread of HDV by needlestick transmission in a population of drug addicts in Sweden has been documented: starting with the initial patients in 1973, 72% of all known drug addicts had been infected by HDV by 1981. In this time only four non-drug-addict patients showed evidence of HDV infection.[439] Co-infection with both HBV and HDV is also a significant problem in parenteral drug abusers, occurring in 10.5% in a series from west Scotland.[726] In a severe outbreak of acute hepatitis in parenteral drug abusers in the USA, approximately 50% were found to be co-infected with HBV and HDV.[658] In this study, markers of HDV infection were detected in 33% of sexual contacts of parenteral drug abusers infected with HBV and HDV, indicating that HDV can also be sexually transmitted. In contrast, HDV infection is rare in homosexual men.[657,1242,1247]

Reports from the early 1980s indicate that as many as half in some series of patients with haemophilia in the USA and Italy had evidence of HDV infection.[958] The risk was related to the infusion of commercially available factor VIII concentrates and was not as great if clotting factor concentrates were made from single plasma donations. More recent reports still indicate a high prevalence of HDV markers in haemophiliacs (~33%)[154,175] in some countries, but modern screening methods for HBsAg and viral inactivation procedures for clotting factor concentrates have substantially reduced the risk of transmission of HDV by this route.

The risk of post-blood-transfusion delta hepatitis varies with the sensitivity of the techniques used to screen out hepatitis B virus-positive blood donations. With the use of radioimmunoassay to screen all donations in the USA and UK, the incidence should be negligible. The risk theoretically remains with less sensitive techniques because of the known propensity for HBsAg and HBcAg to decrease in blood and liver in association with active HDV infection.[955] Screening of blood donations for HDV markers is not considered necessary, as the rare case in which these may be positive in the absence of HBsAg is likely to reflect past HDV infection.[961] Awareness of the risks of hepatitis B infection may account for the relative paucity of reports of HDV infections in haemodialysis units, but in one unit an episode involving five patients using the same HBsAg-positive dialysis equipment has been recorded.[703]

There are areas where HDV infection has a high prevalence and appears to be endemic. In these areas different modes of transmission apply. In an outbreak of HDV infection among the native Indian population of Venezuela, transmission of infection correlated with poor sanitary conditions and may also have occurred via similar routes to those implicated in hepatitis B virus transmission, e.g. via sexual intercourse and by contamination of open skin wounds.[430,905]

Infection is probably also maintained by horizontal transmission from patients with combined chronic HBV and HDV infection. In a similar outbreak in the Santa Marta region of Columbia, infection occurred most frequently in children under the age of 15 years, suggesting that HDV infection was horizontally transmitted.[146] Clustering of HDV infection in families has been found,[1067] but there is little evidence for vertical transmission.[1296] Very few hepatitis B virus carrier mothers have markers of HDV infection and, even in those who do, perinatal transmission of HDV only occurs in conjunction with active neonatal HBV infection. This is usually a complication in those mothers who are HBeAg positive. Neonatal HDV infection is an infrequent occurrence, therefore, because most mothers harbouring HDV are anti-HBe antibody positive and because the combination of HBeAg positivity and HDV infection results in more severe liver disease, with a decrease in fecundity.

SPECIFIC CLINICAL FEATURES, OUTCOME AND PROGNOSIS OF HEPATITIS D INFECTION _____

Infection with HDV usually produces clinical liver disease, but the specific outcome is largely determined by the hepatitis B virus status in the patient. HDV may co-infect with HBV, or it may superinfect in a patient who already has chronic HBV infection (Figure 30.22). Latent HDV infection may also occur rarely in the apparent absence of HBV infection (in liver transplant recipients—see below).

Hepatitis D co-infection with HBV may be distinguished from superinfection by the presence or absence of IgM anti-HBc antibodies.

Co-infection with HBV and HDV is characterized by the presence of HDV markers and IgM anti-HBc antibodies in the serum, whereas patients with HDV superinfection have HDV markers but are IgM anti-HBc antibody negative.

Co-infection with HBV/HDV usually presents clinically with acute viral hepatitis, often characterized by a biphasic rise in transaminases, a feature that is rarely observed in acute hepatitis B alone (see Figure 30.22a).[670] Such co-infection results in a higher frequency of fulminant hepatitis than when there is infection with HBV alone,

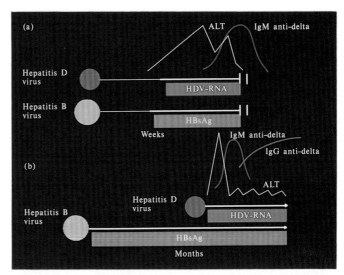

Figure 30.22 (a) Sequence of events in acute hepatitis with simultaneous coinfection by both the hepatitis B virus and the delta agent. The serum aminotransferase levels frequently show a biphasic pattern with IgM antibody to the delta agent appearing with the second peak in ALT levels. Clearance of the HBV infection automatically terminates the delta infection, although IgM antibody persists in decreasing titres for some weeks. (b) Sequence of events in chronic HBV infection with delta superinfection. There is a sharp rise in some serum aminotransferase levels (dotted lines) followed by increasing titres of IgM anti-delta antibody. The raised aminotransferases return towards their baseline value but may show fluctuating small peaks with persistent delta infection. IgG antibody then appears in increasing titre replacing IgM. (Adapted with permission from Rizzetto.[960] © 1983 American Association for the Study of Liver Diseases.)

[409,605,1065] but progression to chronic liver disease is rare.[152,1064] In patients co-infected with HBV/HDV, fulminant hepatitis develops in 2–7.5% of cases.[152,853] The majority of patients co-infected with HBV and HDV make a spontaneous clinical recovery, with no long-term sequelae. In one series the mortality rate for HDV/HBV co-infection was 0 compared to 25% in chronic HBsAg-positive patients superinfected with HDV.[1171]

Superinfection with HDV can lead to different patterns of liver disease in patients with chronic HBV infection. Acute fulminant hepatitis can result and, unless the patient is screened for IgM antibody to HBcAg (which is negative in such cases), the association with HDV infection may be missed. The presentation will then be of a patient with acute HBsAg-positive fulminant hepatitis.[165,334,409,430,865]

Approximately one-third of patients with fulminant hepatitis B as characterized by the presence of IgM anti-HBc antibody also have HDV markers in their serum, compared with only 4% of patients with non-fulminant acute hepatitis B.[409] In a tertiary referral centre for fulminant hepatic failure at the Hôpital Beaujon, Paris, HDV infection accounted for 13% of a series of 502 adult cases, with an overall mortality of 79.5% in the HDV group.[82]

Most HBsAg carriers superinfected with HDV develop an acute hepatitis followed by chronic progressive liver damage;[223,244,932,954,959,979] thus the asymptomatic carrier may convert to chronic persistent hepatitis (CPH) or chronic active hepatitis (CAH), patients with CPH may show an episode of increased parenchymal damage or convert to CAH, and patients with CAH may show exacerbation of their disease activity. In some studies progression to chronic liver disease is reported in 78–90% of cases of HDV superinfection in patients with chronic HBV infection, with the majority developing chronic active hepatitis or cirrhosis.[152,853] In contrast, other studies have reported a slower and less aggressive outcome, with chronic active hepatitis developing in 46% of cases.[667] There appears to be correlation with the HBeAg status of the patient. Those chronic HBV carriers who are HBeAg positive are most likely to develop a severe fulminating illness when superinfected with HDV, whereas chronic HBsAg carriers who are anti-HBe antibody positive usually develop chronic HDV-related liver disease. This information must be interpreted with some caution, because recent evidence indicates that HDV superinfection can inhibit HBV replication and increase the rate of seroconversion from HBeAg positive to HBeAg negative, with appearance of anti-HBe antibody.[501,604,663] This does not occur in HBV/HDV coinfection,[380] and in some cases of HDV superinfection continuing HBV replication has been documented.[335] Rarely, HDV superinfection may lead to a self-limited infection with subsequent clearance of both HDV and HBV.[959]

Despite the almost invariable association with HBV, there is a negative correlation between HDV and hepatocellular carcinoma.[193,243,570]

Recent evidence suggests that *latent HDV infection* may rarely occur in the absence of HBV markers in patients who have undergone liver transplantation for combined HBV/HDV infection.[962] In these patients, a latent asymptomatic recurrence of HDV infection occurs in the grafted liver, with reactivation and clinical hepatitis precipitated only by the subsequent return of HBV infection to the graft.

SPECIFIC PATHOLOGICAL FEATURES OF HEPATITIS D

Although hepatitis D virus RNA is associated with the 35–37-nm subset hepatitis B surface antigen particles, no inner structure can be identified even after the surface antigen has been removed using detergents. Immunocytochemically, delta antigen can be identified in hepatocyte nuclei.[159,953,1100,1156] Small amounts of delta antigen can also be found in the hepatocyte cytoplasm. There is no corresponding morphological structure to this immunocytochemical pattern; immunoelectron-microscopy shows positive staining of dense, round, 20–30-nm structures with soft, indistinct edges in the nuclei.[159] These round bodies lack standard morphological viral substructures.

They are also found in HBsAg-negative cases of chronic hepatitis and some cases of hepatitis B core antigen-positive livers that lack delta agent.[159] Similar structures have also been described in the nuclei of chimpanzees infected with the hepatitis A virus.[992] Possible delta–antidelta immune complexes can sometimes be identified in hepatocyte nuclei by the presence of immunoglobulin and complement.[957]

Immunological demonstration of hepatitis D has identified that infection is always associated with significant liver pathology. The minimal lesion observed is chronic persistent hepatitis, but severe liver disease progressing rapidly to cirrhosis or to fulminant liver failure is more common.[244,410,662,905,960,1100] There are no special features which separate HDV superinfection from a severe chronic active hepatitis B infection[1215] or fulminant liver failure from any cause,[410] but there are features which are more consistently present which should further suggest hepatitis D infection. Many cases have increased numbers of hepatocytes showing granular acidophil degeneration of the cytoplasm.[905,906,1215] It is uncommon for this acidophil degeneration to be associated with an inflammatory reaction, and it is suggested that the virus is directly cytopathic to the hepatocyte.

A more specific variation in the features of HDV infection occurs in northern South America. Liver biopsies show an intense microvesicular fatty change as well as numerous hepatocytes showing acidophil degeneration.[84,145,906] An occasional case has been described outside the Amazon Basin.[650,905]

Sanded nuclei are more typical of chronic hepatitis B virus infection[95,782] but have also been described in delta-positive, core-negative hepatocyte nuclei.[782]

Hepatitis delta virus has been transmitted to chimpanzees.[956] In the chimpanzee chronic hepatitis B carrier, infection results in a marked deterioration of liver function tests, with evidence of active hepatocellular damage and the formation of acidophil bodies in the liver biopsies. On electron microscopy, cytoplasmic tubular structures indistinguishable from those found in other non-A, non-B hepatitides are found.[550] Woodchucks can also be superinfected with HDV provided that the woodchuck hepatitis virus surface antigen is present.[898] Again the virus forms 35–37-nm particles in the blood, composed of a core of RNA coated by the woodchuck hepatitis virus surface antigen.

TREATMENT AND PREVENTION OF ACUTE HEPATITIS D

There is no active treatment for delta infection once established. Steroids are of no known benefit. Interferon-α has been used in the treatment of chronic HDV-related liver disease with some short-term benefit (see Chapter 31), but this drug is not appropriate for the treatment of acute hepatitis D.

As HDV can only replicate in the presence of HBV,

vaccination with a hepatitis B vaccine will automatically protect against infection with HDV. A recombinant HDV vaccine comprised of 64 amino acids containing a major immunogenic epitope from the N-terminal sequence of delta antigen has been developed and used in woodchucks. Despite a significant anti-HDV response, the vaccine did not protect animals from experimental HDV superinfection.[555]

HEPATITIS C

PROPERTIES OF HEPATITIS C VIRUS (see Table 30.9) _____

Relationship to parenterally transmitted NANB hepatitis

With the development of reliable serological tests for HAV, HBV and other hepatotropic viruses such as CMV and EBV, it was apparent that there was a residue of post-transfusion hepatitis for which other, as yet unidentified, infectious agents were likely to be responsible.[344,584,915] In this form of post-transfusion hepatitis clinical symptoms are very variable, asymptomatic cases are common and abnormalities of liver function tests are often transient. However, chronic progressive liver disease is a common sequel. This hepatitis is defined by exclusion as parenterally transmitted non-A, non-B hepatitis (PT-NANBH).

Surrogate markers, notably elevated ALT value in combination with antibodies to hepatitis B core antigen, are of some value in excluding blood which transmits PT-NANB hepatitis,[1094] but this method lacks sensitivity and specificity.

Transmission studies showed that NANB hepatitis could be transferred by inoculation to chimpanzees from patients with PT-NANBH, and that at least one infectious agent

Table 30.9 Properties of hepatitis C virus

_____

- Predominant cause of parenterally transmitted non-A, non-B hepatitis
- Distantly related to flavivirus and pestivirus families and some RNA plant virus supergroups
- 50–60 nm enveloped single-stranded positive-polarity RNA virus
- Approximate 10-kb genome with single open reading frame
- Numerous structural and non-structural protein products derived from single polyprotein precursor
- Single non-structural epitope identified with non-neutralizing antibody
- No homology to other hepatitis viruses
- Very low titres in sera

was involved.[1043] Infectivity, which was associated with the formation of characteristic tubular ultrastructures in hepatocytes,[1289] was abolished by passage through 80-nm filters[446] or treatment with organic solvents,[119] implicating a small, enveloped virus.[120] However, as extensive efforts to isolate the putative infectious agent(s) using conventional virological and immunological techniques were unsuccessful,[25,290,291] it was inferred that levels of virus and viral antigens in serum were probably very low, perhaps only 10^2 to 10^4 viral particles per millilitre of blood in chronic NANB infection.[121,1240]

The breakthrough in defining the aetiological agent came from the work of Houghton and colleagues at the Chiron Corporation, Emeryville, California, USA. They succeeded in cloning the genome of a small, positively stranded RNA virus which had not previously been described.[203] They demonstrated a clear association between serum antibodies in patients with well-documented NANBH and recombinant proteins of this virus, now designated HCV. This, and the reports that followed, confirmed that HCV was responsible for most PT-NANBH and a substantial proportion of NANBH that was community-acquired.[27,204,617,772,787]

Initial cloning studies of HCV

The novel approach adopted by the Chiron group to define the PT-NANB agent employed a strategy which did not require isolation of the agent.[203,487] They reasoned that the failure of conventional approaches was probably due to low titres of virus or viral antigens in plasma. On the other hand, following prolonged immunological challenge during chronic infection or convalescence from NANBH, detectable levels of specific antibodies to the agent might be produced. They therefore opted to clone the agent from total nucleic acids in infected plasma, amplify the encoded polypeptides in an expression vector and assess the antigenicity of these peptides by their exclusive reactivity to sera from patients with NANBH. Their scheme for isolating the cDNA of the putative infectious agent is outlined below and in Figure 30.23.

A high-titre plasma was obtained from chimpanzees with chronic NANBH acquired after inoculation with the agent contaminating a human factor VIII concentrate implicated in the transmission of NANBH.[118] The plasma was centrifuged sufficiently to pellet all viruses and the concentrate was treated so that DNA or RNA from viral genomes would be released. After denaturing to ensure single-stranded forms, cDNA was prepared using reverse transcriptase with random oligonucleotide primers.

Next, a lambda gt11 cDNA library was constructed in *E. coli* to express sequences of the viral genome encoding peptides. After screening approximately 10^6 recombinant phage colonies for reactivity with convalescent serum from a patient infected with NANBH, one particular cDNA clone, 5.1.1, was isolated which reacted strongly with the patient's serum and that of other patients with NANBH. A panel of sera from patients with a variety

High-titre, HCV-infected chimpanzee serum
↓
Ultracentrifugation to pellet virus
↓
Recovery and denaturation of nucleic acids in pellet
↓
Random priming of template and reverse transcription to synthesized cDNA
↓
Construction of λgt11 cDNA expression library
↓
Differential immunoscreening of library to isolate clone unique to infected sera
↓
Enzyme-linked immunoassay using antibodies to fusion protein expressed from unique clone

Figure 30.23 Scheme for isolation of HCV cDNA and development of assay for anti-HCV.[203,617]

of other liver disorders was unreactive, indicating the specificity of the reagent.[203]

A larger overlapping cDNA clone, C100, incorporating the 5.1.1 clone, was then engineered from the same library. This hybridized with RNA of up to 10^4 nucleotides (consistent with the genome of a small virus) found in low abundance in the liver and plasma of chimpanzees infected with the NANB agent, but not with RNA from uninfected human and chimpanzee livers.[203]

The C100 peptide is a sequence of 363 amino acids located in the non-structural, NS4, region of HCV (Figure

30.24).[204] In view of its diagnostic potential as an HCV-specific antigen, the C100 clone was fused to the human gene for superoxide dismutase to promote efficient expression of the recombinant protein in *E. coli* and yeast. The product from yeast, C100–3, was purified for use as antigen in an EIA for HCV.[617] This assay, now available commercially, has been widely applied in seroepidemiological investigations of NANBH in blood donors, haemophiliacs and community-acquired infections.[27,328,571,695,787]

Further cDNA clones, overlapping with both termini of C100, were similarly produced by 'walking' the genome with repeated PCR reactions and the sequence for three-quarters of its length towards the 3′ terminus, encoding the non-structural proteins, was reported.[487]

The use of strand-specific probes prepared from the cDNA showed that the genome was a single, positively stranded RNA with a single, large ORF. The expected translational product would be a polyprotein of about 3000 amino acids.[203,204] This showed partial homologies in organization and sequence with other viruses, including a non-structural protein, NS3, of flaviviruses and pestiviruses.[757] These archetypal studies have now been extended by the Chiron group and others to complete the genomic sequence of the prototypic strain, HCV₁ as well as Japanese isolates.[205,488,563,826,1129] This has established the main features of genomic organization, including the location of the structural nucleocapsid and envelope peptides, perhaps the most pertinent to the development of diagnostics and vaccines.

The tentative relationship between HCV and the flaviviruses and pestiviruses[204,563,757] has been strengthened,

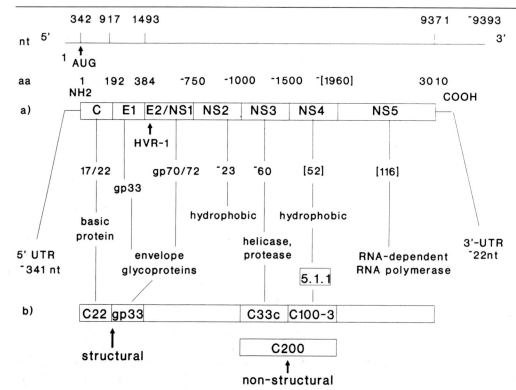

Figure 30.24 Organization of the ORF of HCV-1. (a) The ORF of the polyprotein of HCV-1 is represented by the open box. Approximate boundaries of specific protein coding domains are indicated by vertical lines. Initiating nucleotide (nt) and amino acid (aa) positions are numbered above. Protein nomenclature adopts that used with flaviviruses and pestiviruses: C, nucleocapsid; E1 and E2, envelope; NS (1–5), non-structural. Some putative functions are indicated. The sizes of glycosylated (gp) and non-glycosylated proteins (p) either observed experimentally or deduced (in square brackets) are expressed in kilodaltons. (b) The nomenclature and location of some cloned antigenic proteins used in EIA for antibodies to HCV.

although unique features of HCV provide grounds for placing HCV into a third genus of the Flaviviridae family.[437] Sequence studies of other HCV isolates have demonstrated variability of parts of the genome, while some parts are highly conserved.[323–325,611,820,826,1130,1131] These studies are detailed in the following sections.

Genomic structure of HCV

The identification of HCV by molecular cloning[617] enabled its genomic RNA sequence to be determined.[205,487,488,563,826,1129] Comparison of the nucleotide and its predicted encoded amino acid sequence with databank sequences revealed homologies with other viruses and identified sequences associated with specific functions. By analogy, this suggested how the functions and location of HCV proteins might be assigned. Further, since current methods of viral classification are based on genomic structure and organization,[54] the molecular cloning approach has inevitably focused attention on the phylogenetic relationships between HCV and other viruses. Thus, despite minimal morphological data and the current inability to propagate HCV in tissue culture, the basic layout of the genome and location of its structural and non-structural proteins has been inferred.[204,205,563,826,1129]

The first available sequence data for HCV covered three-quarters of the genome towards the 3' terminus encoding the non-structural viral proteins.[203,487] It showed small homologies with other viruses, including the non-structural proteins of flaviviruses and pestiviruses as well as plant virus supergroups.[757] These homologies were colinear in the case of flaviviruses and pestiviruses. Notably, the canonical sequence Gly-Asp-Asp characteristic of RNA-dependent RNA polymerases was positioned towards the 3' terminus, as in Dengue virus, a flavivirus.[174] The hydrophobicity profile of the non-structural amino acid sequence resembles that of flaviviruses.[204]

In common with many animal viruses, the genomic RNA was positively stranded[203] but unlike the alphavirus families togavirus and rubivirus,[1251] with its only member, rubella, there is a single large ORF coding for protein, which was soon shown to extend almost to the 5' terminus.[204,205,826] This genomic arrangement is a hallmark of flaviviruses[1251] and the closely related pestiviruses.[205,218–220]

The organization of the flavivirus genome and its translational products is well described for the prototypic member, yellow fever virus,[947] and the closely related agents of Dengue[435,948] and West Nile fevers.[1249] Comparable information is available for the related pestivirus group which includes bovine diarrhoeal virus and hog cholera virus.[218–220]

The complete or nearly complete nucleotide sequence from the 5' terminus to the previously disclosed sequence[487] covering the non-structural region of the genome has now been determined for HCV isolated from human and chimpanzee carriers.[205,488,563,826,1129]

The untranslated regions (UTR)

The genome begins with a short UTR[826,1130] now believed to be 341 nucleotides (nt) in length.[437] This is followed by a single ORF for protein encompassing almost the entire genome. In the prototypic strain, HCV-1, this is 9033 nt,[205] equivalent to a translational product of 3011 amino acids or 3010 in two Japanese isolates.[563,1129] This ORF represents most of the genome since the following 3'-UTR is short, about 27 nt,[437] or 54/55 nt.[563,1129]

Sequencing of the 5'-UTR showed that it was 99% conserved, even in HCV isolates comparing humans and chimpanzees.[826] This was also implied by the high sensitivity with which PCR primers based on the 5'-UTR sequence detected HCV genomes from a wide range of geographical locations.[368,554,826]

A more detailed analysis of the 5' (and 3') terminal UTRs is now available.[437] The 5'-UTR shows remarkable sequence homology to bovine diarrhoeal virus and hog cholera virus but not to other viruses, including flaviviruses where the 5'-UTR is considerably shorter.[826] There are four blocks of sequence, 18–37 nt, with greater than 70% homology and numerous small tracts of identity throughout the region. There were a number of small ORFs, a feature of pestiviruses which is not found in most flaviviruses, and overall sequence identity to the pestivirus 5'-UTR was almost 50%. The extreme 5' terminus of 22 nt is capable of forming a stable hairpin structure by intramolecular base-pairing. It is not known whether this is capped. The strict maintenance of the nucleotide sequence among diverse HCV isolates, and close similarity to the 5'-UTR of pestiviruses, suggests that it is a highly evolved structure with an essential regulatory role in viral replication.

Following the stop codon at the 3' terminus of the ORF of HCV-1, there is a short RNA sequence of 27 nt which is polyadenylated. Several other polyadenylated RNA species terminating further upstream from this tract were also demonstrated. They have not been detected in two Japanese isolates which contain larger 3'-UTR regions of 54 and 55 nt respectively[563,1129] and the significance of these subgenomic RNA molecules remains unknown.

Protein coding sequence

The protein coding sequence of HCV-1 starts with the AUG codon at nucleotide 342 and continues to the close of the ORF at nucleotide 9375, equivalent to a polyprotein of 3011 amino acids; 3010 in two Japanese isolates.[563,1129]

The first upstream region, equivalent to about 120 amino acids, was over 90% conserved between the two HCV strains obtained from human and chimpanzee carriers.[826] Traits of basic amino acids were frequent, consistent with the role of a structural nucleocapsid protein in close physical association with the viral nucleic acid.[563,826,1130] On the other hand, downstream from nucleotides 1205–2014, conservation diminished to about 75%. There are fifteen potential sites for glycosylation from nucleotides 929 to 2276 and there is evidence of many point mutations between the HCV strains. These are properties which would be expected for a protein on the exterior of the virus, possibly located on protruding spikes, and subject to selection pressure by immune mechanisms while in the mammalian host.[563,826]

In vitro translation of the pestivirus and flavivirus genomes and processing by microsomal membrane fractions has shown that the polyprotein is translated from one initiation point at the amino terminus of the core protein. Proteins are glycosylated, although not all potential sites may be used, and cleaved to produce the mature viral proteins. Cleavage may occur at signal sequences characteristically associated with hydrophobic stretches preceding the structural proteins. Other sequences are probably involved in the correct insertion of glycoproteins in the lipid bilayer.[947,948]

With flaviviruses and pestiviruses, in-vitro transcription/translation of the genomes has enabled the translational products to be identified, suggested mechanisms for their processing and established the relationship with the genomic sequence.

This approach, using in-vitro transcription/translation, has now been extended to HCV, with RNA transcripts prepared from cDNA encoding the amino-terminal one-third of the genome. These were translated and processed using a rabbit reticulocyte lysate in the presence of a microsomal membrane fraction.[462] Other similar expression systems are actively being investigated.[489]

Four major membrane-associated proteins were detected. Comparison of the products of various deletion mutants with the predicted amino acid sequences enabled these peptides to be ordered as NH_2-p22-gp35-gp70-p19-COOH. The p22, of 191 amino acid residues, was the non-glycosylated basic peptide corresponding to the core peptide, which by analogy to flaviviruses would be cleaved close to its COOH terminus. The p19 has a similar size and location to the NS2A region of flaviviruses. The gp70 and gp35 are both heavily glycosylated and unlike p22 and p19 were transported into the microsomal membrane. The location of gp70 suggests that it is equivalent to the NS1 region of flaviviruses. Here the protein, although glycosylated, is not structural but is expressed on the surface of infected cells.[163,1000] In pestiviruses the equivalent protein is gp35/55, where it probably represents the second structural envelope protein. In HCV it is therefore referred to as E2/NS1. The other putative envelope protein, E1, would be derived from gp35. Coupled with the hydrophobicity profile, the E1 and E2/NS1 regions located between core and NS2A show a greater resemblance to the envelope region of pestiviruses rather than of flaviviruses. The functions of the non-structural proteins of these viruses are fairly speculative.

The largest, NS5, contains a canonical sequence towards its 3′ terminus which is characteristic of viral RNA polymerases. The NS3 may have proteolytic activity and its hydrophobicity profile suggests that it could bridge the Golgi membrane to function in the processing and assembly of the virus. A second domain, probably encoding a helicase function, involved with viral RNA replication,

is also present. The NS2 and NS4 are highly hydrophobic although not particularly well-conserved. In flaviviruses and pestiviruses each region encodes two proteins, e.g. NS2A and NS2B, but functions have not been ascribed to them.

Classification of HCV

The tenuous relationship between HCV and flaviviruses suggested on the basis of the original cloning data has now been substantiated.[204,563,757] Flaviviruses, previously classified in the family Togaviridae, are now regarded as a genus of the family Flaviviridae[1251] and pestiviruses have been suggested as a second genus.[220] These viruses share major features in genomic organization with HCV, including the positioning of the structural proteins from the 5′ terminus, with the relatively well-defined capsid preceding the putative envelope sequence.[218–220]

Homologies are also evident between the non-structural protein domains in number, size and location of signature sequences characteristically associated with particular functions. The similarities in hydrophobicity profiles of the polyproteins of the three viral types are particularly striking,[205] although the HCV genome of 9391 nt is somewhat shorter than either flavivirus (~10.3 kb) or pestivirus (12–13 kb) genomes.[218–220] Yet there are only small tracts of nucleotide sequence identity in the ORF, suggesting the distinctiveness of the HCV genome.

However, the 5′-UTRs of HCV and pestiviruses are remarkably similar even at the nucleotide level, with major homologies, and quite unlike the corresponding region of flaviviruses.[437]

In summary, current data indicate that HCV is somewhat intermediate in properties between flaviviruses and pestiviruses and until further information is available, particularly on the transcriptional strategy of HCV, it has been suggested that HCV might be considered as a third genus of the Flaviviridae.[204,205,437]

Subtypes and variants of HCV

The RNA viruses, lacking a proof-reading facility for the viral RNA polymerase, express a very high mutation rate, perhaps in the order of one error per 10^4 nucleotides synthesized.[505,594] Thus, assuming ongoing viral replication and host surveillance during chronic infection with HCV, genetic drift with the emergence of new viral strains is expected, perhaps accompanied by shifts in virulence and pathogenicity. The first evidence for this came with the detection of nucleotide heterogeneity in HCV isolates from Japanese patients, where only 80% homology with the NS5 region of HCV_1 was evident.[562,611] Similar observations with regard to the NS3/NS4 domains were soon reported.[1131]

In general, estimates of the variability in the sequences of non-structural genes are high, irrespective of whether the data were obtained from cloned genomes or by direct sequencing of HCV isolates by reverse transcription and

PCR. However, deletions, insertions and reading frame shifts have not been detected and, owing to degeneracy in the amino acid code, not all the nucleotide substitutions necessarily produce amino acid substitution. Thus, some localities in the non-structural protein may be highly conserved to maintain functional activity. The NS2 region is probably the most variable, although overall hydrophobicity seems to be highly conserved.

Some parts of the nucleotide sequence are remarkably well conserved. In particular the conservation of the short 5'-UTR sequences and, to a lesser extent, the putative core region immediately downstream indicates that mutations in these regions are generally detrimental to viral replication.[826]

In contrast, the putative envelope genes E1 and E2/NS1 are highly variable, a variability which is not uniformly distributed but localized upstream of E2/NS1 as hypervariable regions (HVR).[463,1241] The first, HVR1, of about 30 nt between nucleotides 1514–1541 (amino acid residues 391–400) is present in isolates in the United States related to HCV1,[820] and in both the HJ and BK Japanese isolates, both of which have been completely sequenced.[563,1129] The Japanese strains also have at least one other region, HVR2, further downstream between nucleotides 1763–1781.[462,463]

Evidence for the differential evolution of the HCV genome has come from isolates taken 13 years apart from an American patient chronically infected with HCV. In particular, it showed a 39-nt domain overlapping with HVR1 which differed in 28.2% of nucleotides, with a high percentage of these changes leading to amino acid substitutions. This compared to only 0.7% of nucleotides in the highly conserved 5'-UTR.[820,1241] This hypervariability would give the product of the E2/NS1 region, the glycosylated peptide gp70,[462,489] a propensity for antigenic variation consistent with location on the exterior of the virus,[826] and the additional HVR2 in Japanese isolates may imply that rather more of this protein is exposed on the viral exterior than in the HCV1 strain. Together these observations show that the E2/NS1 region is evolving rapidly even in a single chronically infected individual. However, most potential glycosylation sites and all of the 30 cysteine residues are conserved.[820]

The heterogeneity of the HCV genome suggests that distinct subtypes of HCV may predominate in different geographical locations and evidence for this is now accumulating. Thus, in one study of 19 HCV-RNA-positive plasmas in Japan, using primers to the NS5 region in the PCR method, two sequence patterns, K_1 and K_2, were detected to which 13 and 6 of the strains could be assigned. The prototypical strain was distinct and did not seem to be represented in this Japanese series[324,325] although it is frequently detected in Japanese haemophiliacs.[461]

Distinct strains of HCV have also been detected in Edinburgh, Scotland. Here phylogenetic analysis of the NS3 region of HCV carriers showed that NS3 sequences were highly conserved, in a group of intravenous drug users, consistent with infections from a single source.

However, amongst haemophiliacs there was a different sequence type. This was also highly conserved despite the likelihood that these patients had been infected with a factor VIII preparation containing donations from a wide geographical range. The reason is unclear, but these subjects were co-infected with HIV and probably immunologically compromised.[1051] Houghton and colleagues, in a recent review of HCV heterogeneity have suggested a classification for the 15 described variants into three distinct subgroups (I, II and III) according to their nucleotide and amino acid homologies.[489]

During chronic infection there is clearly an opportunity for co-infection with either an *in situ* evolved variant or one acquired through secondary infection. However, thus far no relationship between such variants and pathogenicity, virulence, or viral persistence has been described.

LABORATORY DETECTION OF HCV INFECTION ____

The immediate practical application of the cloning of HCV has been the development of specific serological tests to detect HCV infection. Antibody assays based on recombinant peptide antigens have become generally available in EIA format from commercial sources with the first generation of tests using the non-structural antigen encoded by the 5.1.1[617] and the larger overlapping C100 clones. In second-generation tests, increased sensitivity and specificity have been achieved by addition of structural antigens to the panel.[199,486,564,792,827,1203]

The HCV genome has been detected directly in low abundance in serum and in liver by reverse transcription of the RNA in vitro followed by exponential, but specific, amplification of the cDNA using adaptations[367,554,1240] of the recently devised PCR technique.[823,980] The essential specific oligonucleotide primers were based initially on the non-structural cDNA sequence,[487] but sensitivity is clearly improved with more conserved sequences from the structural and, particularly, 5'-UTR of the genome.[369,826]

Together these assays detecting either HCV-RNA or antibodies to HCV have provided a wealth of complementary seroepidemiological data on HCV infection and have shown that 90% of PT-NANBH and much of the sporadic community-acquired NANBH, hitherto defined by exclusion or surrogate markers,[1094] can be attributed unequivocally to HCV (see Epidemiology of Hepatitis C). Transfusion centres in many countries have recently introduced the C100–3 EIA for detection of HCV, but there is valid concern about the relatively low sensitivity of this assay.[729,783] The improvements obtained by including recombinant or synthetic structural antigens from the nucleocapsid region are likely to overcome these reservations in the near future.[486,792,827]

Anti-C100–3 EIA

Antibodies to HCV as measured by the anti-C100–3 EIA are associated with hepatitis C infection and the presence of HCV-RNA in three recognized patterns (Figure 30.25):

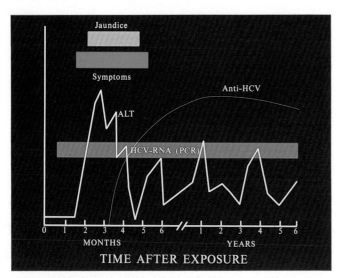

Figure 30.25 Typical sequence of events in a case of acute hepatitis C that progresses to chronic infection with liver disease. (Reproduced with kind permission of Hoofnagle[484] and Thieme Medical Publishers.)

1. An acute resolving hepatitis paralleled by transient rapid elevation of ALT and HCV-RNA. Antibodies to C100–3 develop in about one-third of cases, with seroconversion commonly occurring in 3–6 months.
2. A chronic hepatitis with elevated ALT, persistence of viral RNA and anti-C100–3. (There is evidence that the virus may persist at least 13 years.)[820]
3. A chronic hepatitis with fluctuating levels of ALT. Viral RNA and anti-C100–3 cannot always be detected in serum.[328,560]

In all these situations, anti-C100–3 may not be detected for weeks or months after initiation of infection by inoculation of HCV-positive material,[27,328] demonstration of HCV-RNA by PCR,[367,368,826,1240] or onset of abnormal liver function;[329] and even when it is present, antibody titres are low (1/10 to 1/100). Thus, this test is not the most sensitive index of HCV infection.[560]

The first commercially available C-100–3 EIA (Ortho) has also been unduly prone to low specificity. Particularly implicated were frozen sera and sera with elevated levels of immunoglobulins, autoantibodies or immune complexes. False positive results have been encountered in patients with liver disease irrespective of aetiology, rheumatoid disease[1151] and some healthy individuals, notably Africans with relatively high levels of immunoglobulins.[417,729] A non-specific association of immunoglobulin with the solid-phase antigen is likely to be responsible, although antibodies to the superoxide dismutase component have also been suggested.[503] However, it is likely that such problems can be alleviated to a considerable extent by technical improvements in the test.

Assays for IgM antibodies to C-100–3 have been developed, but do not seem to confer any diagnostic advantage in acute hepatitis C. In patients with acute resolving hepatitis C, IgM antibodies disappear within 6 months but persist in patients who go on to develop chronic hepatitis C infection.[926]

As well as the relatively late IgG antibody response to the C100–3 epitope,[27,328,617] there must also be some question as to whether all strains of HCV express the sequence encoding the relevant 5.1.1 epitope. As the non-structural region is poorly conserved, the sequence of the prototypic HCV strain may be less common in Japan, with obvious implications for the sensitivity of the C100–3 assay in these situations.[325,1131]

Recombinant immunoblot assays (RIBA)

At present a confirmatory test based on specific neutralization is not yet available commercially, but so called supplementary tests are produced (RIBA and RIBA-2; Ortho Diagnostics Systems).[310] The first of these (RIBA) uses discrete bands of the *E. coli* 5.1.1 and yeast C100–3 recombinant clones along with appropriate controls on a nitrocellulose strip. Although responses to both antigens do not always occur, the assay appears to be specific and of comparable sensitivity to the EIA for C100–3.[329,894,1059,1060]

This assay has now been largely superseded by the four antigen RIBA-2 supplementary test, which has additional antigens, designated as C33c and C22–3 (Fig 30.24) derived from the non-structural and core regions respectively, of the virus. Initial reports with this assay suggest that a positive result is indicative of infectivity and risk of transmission of PT-NANBH.[1203] It is also evident that some blood donors implicated in PT-NANBH are negative by EIA or RIBA-2 for anti C-100–3 but positive for antibodies against C33c and C22.[311]

A similar dot-blot assay using C-100, core (putative capsid) and C33c recombinant polypeptides as antigens (Matrix HCV: Abbott) has been described and also appears to be a good supplementary assay for detection of HCV infection.[763]

Assays employing structural antigens

Synthetic peptides derived from the published nucleocapsid sequence[826] have now been used to develop further EIAs for the detection of HCV infection.[486,827] Epitopes on these structural peptides are immunogenic and the antibody response to them can be detected before the anti-C100–3 response.[199,827] Moreover, these assays demonstrate an increased sensitivity of HCV detection in acute and chronic NANB hepatitis compared with the C100–3 EIA, particularly those employing a combination of peptides from both structural and non-structural regions.

The product of the core gene, p22, has also been produced in a baculovirus expression system and used as antigen in an EIA.[199] Of 58 NANB hepatitis patients, 49 were positive for p22 antibody, 42 for anti C100–3 antibody, and 39 had both antibodies. In post-transfusion patients, p22 antibody was detected in 13/23 at 1–3 months post-transfusion; 4/13 had anti-C100–3 at this stage. However, in five patients neither antibody was detected at 30 months after transfusion and in two others only anti-C100–3 was detected.

An EIA employing three different synthetic peptides as HCV antigens has recently been introduced (HCV C-200 C-22 EIA; United Biomedical, New York). In comparison with the C-100–3 EIA, preliminary data suggest that the HCV C-200 C22 EIA is both more specific and more sensitive for detection of HCV infection and may be a useful alternative to RIBA-2 as a confirmatory assay.[67]

Infection with HCV is also associated with antibody production to GOR47–1, an epitope encoded by a single-copy gene of the host.[767] These antibodies are present in the acute phase of HCV infection before anti-C100–3 is detected. The recent report that the epitope cross-reacts with an epitope on the viral core suggests that assays based on this epitope will have similar sensitivity to the second-generation assays.[768] It has also been suggested that this may represent a link between HCV infection and autoimmune liver disease.[768]

Polymerase chain reaction

The PCR technique has been developed into a highly sensitive and specific procedure to detect HCV infection using primers to the most conserved regions of the genome, the 5′-UTR[368] and the following capsid peptide sequences.[826] It is the only method for direct detection of the viral genome in serum or tissue samples and this can be positive many months before anti-C100–3 is detected. However, the test protocol is relatively complicated and labour-intensive, taking 2–3 days to perform. A high throughput of samples increases the risk of non-specific reactions, particularly by contamination with specific cDNA produced.[626] The RNA extraction steps before reverse transcription are also rather cumbersome.[827] It is therefore likely that PCR procedure will remain in the domain of the reference laboratory for the forseeable future.

Use of a second stage of amplification using primer pairs internal to those used in the first stage ('nested' primers) increases sensitivity markedly and maintains specificity, while avoiding the use of radiolabelled nucleotides and autoradiography.[790] This was first applied to HCV using primers deduced from the non-structural sequence of HCV-1.[367,554] It is now known that primers to the 5′-UTR generally provide more sensitivity since this region is highly conserved among HCV isolates.[368]

EPIDEMIOLOGY OF HEPATITIS C

Following the introduction of assays for the detection of antibodies to hepatitis C, the seroepidemiology of this infection and modes of transmission have been re-defined. Earlier studies of parenterally transmitted and sporadic

community-acquired non-A, non-B hepatitis (PT-NANBH and CA-NANBH respectively) had provided information about the epidemiology of these conditions, but this was largely inferred from clinical observations. Testing for anti-HCV has not only served to confirm many of these earlier observations but has also provided a more comprehensive knowledge of the modes of transmission and prevalence of this infection. It is now apparent that hepatitis C infection is responsible for most, if not all, cases of PT-NANBH worldwide, and a large proportion of cases of CA-NANBH in developed countries.

The information presented in this section concentrates on data derived from studies which have used serological tests for antibodies directed against HCV. These became available in 1989 and the majority of epidemiological and transmission studies reported since then have used the EIA for anti-C100–3. This assay has significant limitations in the detection of HCV infection, which have been summarized by Alter[34] (see Laboratory Detection of HCV Infection). These include problems leading to an underestimate of HCV infection: for example, failure to detect HCV infection in 25–40% of blood donors implicated in PT-NANBH; failure to detect HCV infection in some individuals who test positive for antibodies to other recombinant HCV antigens or are positive for HCV-RNA by PCR; and a tendency for titres of anti-C100–3 antibodies to decrease both with time after infection and increasing age. Other problems may lead to an overestimate of HCV infection, for example false positive results in patients with raised immunoglobulins.

Notwithstanding these difficulties, the anti-C100–3 assay has provided valuable information about the seroepidemiology and transmission of HCV infection, as described below. A more precise and comprehensive picture will undoubtedly emerge over the next few years as second-generation tests for anti-HCV and assays for HCV-RNA become more widely applied.

Geographical distribution, prevalence and incidence of HCV infection

Hepatitis C infection is distributed throughout the world, with some minor geographical variations in the prevalence of HCV markers. This information is derived largely from testing for anti-C100–3 in volunteer blood donors and is summarized in Table 30.10.

The most notable feature is that in comparison with HBV infection there is relative geographical consistency in the prevalence of HCV infection. Regional variations are documented within some countries, for example, the prevalence of HCV infection in southern Italy is approximately twice that observed in northern Italy[1054] (further examples are evident in Table 30.10). Within one geographical area, the prevalence of HCV markers varies according to the type of population under investigation. In one study of blood donors in Chicago, USA, a striking difference in the prevalence of HCV markers was found

Table 30.10 Geographical distribution and prevalence of anti-HCV

Region	Type of study	No. of subjects studied	Prevalence of anti-HCV (%)	Reference
Europe				
UK, London	Blood donors	1 100	0.55	367
UK, north east	Blood donors	1 120	0.18	134
France (various)	Blood donors	25 137	0.68	526
Germany, north	Blood donors	2 114	0.24	613
Germany, central and south	Blood donors	1 009	0.79	613
Italy, north	Blood donors	8 068	0.68	1054
Italy, south	Blood donors	3 049	1.38	1054
Spain	Healthy pregnant women	241	1.2	328
USA				
Wisconsin	Blood donors	15 881	0.54	744
Greater New York	Volunteer blood donors	446	0.9–1.4	1097
Chicago	Volunteer blood donors	6 118	0.8	255
	Paid blood donors	3 718	10.49	255
Far East				
Taiwan	Blood donors	420	0.95	195
Taiwan	Healthy subjects	1 419	0.28	648
	Paid blood donors	500	0.8	648
	Healthy pregnant women	793	0.4	648
Africa				
South Africa	Urban black blood donors	498	1.2	319
	Asian blood donors	500	0.8	319
	White blood donors	500	0.6	319

between volunteer and paid blood donors (0.54% and 10.49% respectively). In most countries, there are well-defined risk groups with a high prevalence of HCV markers, and these tend to be overrepresented in the paid blood donor population. The high risk groups identified in studies of HCV prevalence are summarized for several different countries in Table 30.11, and methods of spread in these groups are discussed in further detail below.

There are few longitudinal studies of the incidence of documented HCV infection from around the world,

largely because the assay for anti-HCV has only recently become widely available. The most detailed information comes from the CDC survey of NANBH in four sentinel counties in the USA.[33] The incidence of NANBH was unchanged over a 7-year surveillance period at 7.1 cases per 100 000 population, but the pattern of risk factors changed, with a decline in the proportion of post-transfusion cases from 17% to 6% of the total and a marked rise in cases attributed to drug abuse from 21% to 42%. Analysis of stored sera revealed that anti-HCV was found

Table 30.11 Prevalence of anti-HCV in high-risk groups

Patient group	Spain (%)	UK (%)	Taiwan (%)
PT-NANBH	85	–[a]	24–86.5
Chronic liver disease and previous transfusion	62	–	–
Haemophiliacs	70	–	90
Parenteral drug abusers	70	80.6	81
Haemodialysis patients	20	1	–
Homosexual men	8	26 (HIV+ve)	–
		4 (HIV−ve)	
Sexual partners of drug addicts	6	–	–
Mental handicap	–	6	–

Data in this table are derived from ref. 328 (Spain), ref. 783 (UK), ref. 195 and ref. 647 (Taiwan).
[a]Dash indicates no data quoted in the selected references.

in 48% of the total number of cases of NANBH after 6 weeks and in 68% after 6 months of follow-up.

Methods of spread

Hepatitis C was initially identified as the agent responsible for a large proportion of cases of post-transfusion NANBH, indicating that *parenteral spread* was a clinically important mode of transmission of this virus. Serological surveys of patients with CA-NANBH have revealed a group who are anti-HCV positive but in whom there is no obvious parenteral source of infection, suggesting that this virus may also be transmitted by *non-parenteral routes*. In the USA, hepatitis C is responsible for the majority of all cases of NANBH, with a parenteral source of infection or other identifiable risk factor present in 60% of cases,[33] suggesting that non-parenteral spread may be important in the remaining 40%. In countries with a low incidence of post-transfusion NANBH and relatively low levels of intravenous drug abuse, non-parenteral spread may be more important in the epidemiology of hepatitis C infection.

Parenteral spread of hepatitis C

Hepatitis C is the principal cause of PT-NANBH and is thus common in groups of patients who have received multiple transfusions of blood or blood products, including coagulation factors prepared from human plasma. Hepatitis C is also prevalent among parenteral drug abusers and may be transmitted by any other parenteral exposure.

Transfusion-associated hepatitis C

Before the introduction of screening of blood donors for risk of NANB virus transmission, the risk of PT-NANBH was reported at between 7% and 17% (average ~10%) in the USA[1,585] with similar figures reported in Canada,[341] Spain[459] and Italy.[224] In the UK,[222,737] the Netherlands[942] and Australia,[235] in studies which included patients receiving multiple transfusions, PT-NANBH was less common, occuring in 1–3% of cases. More recently, a much lower incidence was reported in London, UK, with only 1/387 recipients (0.26%) of more than three units of blood developing biochemical evidence of PT-NANBH.[228] Throughout the 1980s the incidence of PT-NANBH has declined in the USA to an estimated 3–4% of all transfusions.[381] Exclusion of high risk donors and introduction of surrogate tests such as measurement of ALT and anti-HBc in donor blood have probably all contributed to this decline.

The development of serological assays for detection of anti-HCV has unequivocally demonstrated that the majority of post-transfusion NANBH is caused by hepatitis C. In blood transfusion recipients from many different parts of the world, anti-HCV antibodies have been reported in 9–25% of cases of acute resolving NANBH and 60–100% of cases of chronic NANBH (see Table 30.12). Seroconversion to anti-HCV positivity (as measured by the C-100–3 EIA) occurs late in the majority of

Table 30.12 Detection of anti-HCV in patients with post-transfusion NANB hepatitis

Country	Type of PT-NANBH	Percentage of patients anti-HCV+ve	Reference
USA	1. Chronic	71	617
	2. Acute resolving	60	27
	Chronic	100	27
Japan	Acute resolving	15	617
	Chronic	78	617
Italy	Chronic	84	617
Netherlands	Acute resolving	25	1201
	Chronic	60	1201
Germany	Acute resolving	20	969
	Chronic	79	969
Spain	Chronic	84	329
Taiwan	1. Chronic	86.5	647
	2. Chronic	58.5	1228
Canada	Acute resolving	9	342
	Chronic	61	342

cases, with a mean delay of 22 weeks after transfusion and 15 weeks after the onset of symptoms. This may account for the lower anti-HCV positivity rate in acute post-transfusion NANBH. In addition, follow-up studies of anti-HCV antibodies in patients with acute resolving hepatitis have shown that they tend to disappear with time.[27] In studies of chronic post-transfusion NANBH in which there has been both a prolonged follow-up and regular serum sampling, more than 85% of cases are anti-HCV positive (by the C100–3 EIA)[27,329] and these antibodies have been reported to persist for up to 7 years.[31] With testing for antibodies to other HCV antigens and for HCV-RNA in serum, it has been suggested that hepatitis C may account for over 90% and possibly 100% of cases of chronic post-transfusion NANBH,[381] but this has yet to be established.

The clear role for hepatitis C in post-transfusion NANBH has led to the introduction of screening for anti-HCV (by the C100–3 EIA) in blood donors in many countries. This will not eradicate transfusion-associated hepatitis C, as some implicated donations are negative for anti-HCV in this assay but positive for antibodies to other hepatitis C antigens.[311] Until improved tests for the detection of HCV infection are widely available for screening of blood donors, it is inevitable that transfusion-associated hepatitis C will continue to occur. It is estimated that the introduction of screening of blood donors for anti-HCV (by C100–3 reactivity) will reduce the incidence of transfusion-associated hepatitis C by a further 50–70%, compared with the level of protection provided by surrogate tests alone.[381]

The risk of transmitting hepatitis C by transfusion of anti-HCV-positive donor blood has been determined by retrospective analysis of stored aliquots of transfused sera;

reports of transmission of HCV infection have varied from 17% (1/6) in the UK,[367] to 46% (16/35) in the Netherlands,[1202] and 88% (14/16) in the USA.[329] Some of this variation may be explained by the relatively small numbers of anti-HCV-positive transfusions in each study. Supplementary tests (see Laboratory Detection of HCV Infection) such as the RIBA-2[1203] or detection of HCV-RNA in serum by nested PCR[367] may help to predict infectivity of sera positive for anti-HCV by the C100–3 EIA and are therefore helpful in subsequent assessment and counselling of anti-HCV-positive blood donors.

Coagulation factors and other blood products may also transmit HCV infection, which is therefore particularly prominent in haemophiliacs and patients with other inherited coagulation defects. Chronic liver disease is a common problem in haemophiliacs receiving regular clotting factor concentrates, with many having persistently elevated transaminases and at least 20% of these having chronic active hepatitis or cirrhosis at liver biopsy.[12,443] With the ability to test for and detect anti-HCV, it is now clear that hepatitis C is a major cause of chronic liver disease in haemophilia.[695] The reported prevalence of anti-HCV antibodies in haemophiliacs ranges from 59% to 85%.[132,328,686,695,814,885,1008] The prevalence of anti-HCV antibodies increases with severity and duration of haemophilia[1008] and is related to use of commercial factor VIII concentrates that antedated viral inactivation procedures.[686,885] Haemophiliacs at presentation or those who have received only heat-treated or solvent-detergent treated concentrates are seronegative for anti-HCV antibodies.[686,814,854,885] The presence of HCV-RNA in different batches and sources of clotting factor concentrates has been investigated using nested PCR.[369] These authors found HCV-RNA in a wide variety of clotting factor concentrates, particularly those prepared from paid donors that had not been heat-treated. Preparations from volunteer donors that had been heated to 80°C for 72 h were negative for HCV-RNA, but HCV-RNA could be detected in preparations that had been heated at 60°C for 20–32 h, including some that had also been treated with heptane as a solvent. These studies emphasize the risk of HCV infection in haemophiliacs if appropriate measures are not taken to inactivate HCV in clotting factor concentrates prepared from human donors.

PT-NANB hepatitis is also reported after prolonged use of intravenous immunoglobulin preparations in patients with agammaglobulinaemia.[659,1255] Many intravenous immunoglobulin preparations contain anti-HCV antibodies[863,925] and it is possible that these preparations may also transmit HCV, albeit rarely.[925] Careful evaluation of these products for HCV-RNA is warranted.

Parenteral drug abuse

It has long been recognized that parenteral drug abusers are at high risk of developing acute or chronic PT-NANB hepatitis, in addition to hepatitis B and D. Parenteral drug abuse was identified as a risk factor in 42% of cases of NANB hepatitis in a US series[33] and as the major factor in a recent Swedish series of NANB hepatitis.[606] The prevalence of anti-HCV antibodies in parenteral drug abusers ranges from 48% to 74%,[328,392,1051,1199] and is related to duration of drug abuse. In an Australian study, 66% were anti-HCV positive within 2 years of starting regular parenteral drug abuse, rising to 100% after 8 years[78] HCV-RNA has been detected in the plasma of 7/13 anti-HCV-positive parenteral drug abusers, indicating the high risk of transmission from shared needles.[1051]

Other forms of parenteral spread

A high prevalence of anti-HCV antibodies has been reported in haemodialysis patients, ranging from 0–37% in Germany,[1004] 18.7% in Japan,[1134] and 17.3–24% in Italy.[388,781] Many of these patients had also been transfused, but seropositive cases occurred in each of these haemodialysis centres in patients who had not received blood transfusions. The prevalence of anti-HCV antibodies correlated with the duration of treatment by haemodialysis[781,1004] and was associated with raised transaminases, indicative of liver injury.[781]

Transmission of hepatitis C has also been recorded in medical personnel after needlestick injury. In one case report, a surgeon developed hepatitis C with eventual seroconversion after a needlestick injury contaminated with blood from a parenteral drug abuser.[1191] In another, a nurse received a needlestick injury from a patient who was in the incubation phase of transfusion-associated hepatitis C. When tested 4 weeks after the needlestick incident, the patient was anti-HCV negative (and remained so for the next 2 years) but HCV-RNA positive. The nurse became HCV-RNA positive 13 weeks after the original incident at the onset of acute hepatitis, and seroconverted to anti-HCV positive 3 weeks later.

An outbreak of hepatitis C has also been reported from a plasmapheresis centre, in which 25/171 donors (15%) developed clinically overt hepatitis.[1300] Of these, 12 were tested for anti-HCV and all had seroconverted to anti-HCV positive by 18 months. The source of hepatitis C infection was traced to re-use of a buffer-dispensing needle and tubing which was connected to the centrifuge bottle to resuspend the pelleted cells after each donation.

Non-parenteral spread of hepatitis C

Hepatitis C may occur in individuals with no obvious parenteral route of infection. Several alternative routes of transmission have been implicated, including *sexual transmission, perinatal transmission and horizontal transmission* within families and households. In some patients with hepatitis C, neither parenteral spread nor any of these other factors can be identified, and these are termed *sporadic community-acquired* cases.

Sexual transmission of hepatitis C The role of sexual transmission in HCV infection is controversial. In a case control study, NANB hepatitis was significantly associated with a history of multiple heterosexual partners or a history of sexual or household contact with a subject who had previously had hepatitis.[31] The risk of acquiring NANB hepatitis was increased 11-fold for those with a history of multiple sexual partners, and 6-fold for those with a history of sexual/household contact with a partner with previous hepatitis. This study indicated that sexual transmission could be implicated in as many as 11% of cases of NANB hepatitis. The same group have reported a high prevalence of anti-HCV antibodies in heterosexuals with multiple partners (16%) and in those with a history of sexual/household contact with a partner with previous hepatitis (14%).[35]

In contrast, other studies have found little evidence of sexual transmission of HCV. The sexual partners of anti-HCV-positive haemophiliacs were all reported to be seronegative for anti-HCV.[1012] Similarly, anti-HCV antibodies have not been reported in the sexual partners of patients with transfusion-associated hepatitis C.[328,331] In one study of the sexual partners of anti-HCV-positive parenteral drug abusers, anti-HCV was found in only 1/19 cases.[328] Another study reports anti-HCV antibodies in 11% of sexual contacts of drug abusers, but there was a strong correlation with coexistent infection with either HIV or HBV.[1169] In summary, there is some evidence for heterosexual transmission of HCV, but it appears to be a relatively infrequent event.

Homosexual transmission of HCV also seems to be rare, but the prevalence of anti-HCV antibodies in homosexuals, although low, is higher than for the general population, ranging from 4% to 16%.[328,740,783,1169] In most studies there is a correlation between infection with HIV and the presence of anti-HCV antibodies.

Perinatal transmission of hepatitis C Perinatal transmission of hepatitis C is a possible route by which the worldwide pool of HCV infection could be maintained. Initial studies failed to demonstrate any significant degree of seroconversion to anti-HCV positivity in infants born to anti-HCV-positive mothers.[943,1098,1245] One exception to this was infants born to mothers who were positive for both anti-HCV and anti-HIV, of whom 44% seroconverted to anti-HCV positive between age 6 months and 1 year.[391]

Failure to detect anti-HCV antibodies in infants born to anti-HCV-positive mothers does not completely exclude the possibility of HCV transmission. More recently this subject has been investigated using assays for HCV-RNA and other molecular techniques to sequence HCV isolates in different family members. These studies have demonstrated that 8/10 infants born to anti-HCV-positive mothers had HCV-RNA detectable in their serum, that this persisted continuously from birth for follow-up periods of 2–19 months, and that anti-HCV was negative in all the HCV-RNA-positive infants after age 9 months.[1147] Persisting HCV-RNA positivity was observed for infants born to anti-HCV-positive mothers both with and without

concurrent HIV infection. As liver damage was minimal in these infants, it was suggested that acquisition of hepatitis C at birth may lead to an HCV carrier state. Supportive data for this have been obtained from Japan, where one family has been described in which the grandmother, mother and daughter are all HCV-RNA positive.[509] Moreover, sequencing data from a region of the HCV genome that encodes for the viral envelope protein—a hypervariable region that usually shows 16% nucleotide sequence variation within Japan—demonstrated that this sequence was identical in mother and daughter and almost identical in the grandmother.

These studies demonstrate conclusively that HCV may be acquired by perinatal transmission. Although the global importance of this remains to be established, it is potentially an important turning point in the epidemiology of HCV infection.

Horizontal and familial transmission of hepatitis C Perinatal and sexual transmission may play a role in the clustering of HCV within families, but it is also possible that horizontal transmission may occur from one family member to another. Seropositivity for anti-HCV has been reported in 8–34% of relatives of anti-HCV-positive index cases.[161,502,551,582] The method of spread of HCV within families is uncertain, but inapparent parenteral spread is one possibility.

Hepatitis C infection is also common within some long term institutions for mentally retarded children, with a prevalence of 11.1% recorded in one centre[1221] and 6% in another.[783] Again the method of spread is uncertain, but inapparent parenteral transmission is a likely candidate.

HCV-RNA has been documented in the saliva of patients with chronic hepatitis,[1128,1229] and this is one possible route of transmission within families or institutions. HCV in saliva is infective, as determined by reported transmission of hepatitis C following a human bite.[309]

Sporadic community acquired hepatitis C In a large proportion of cases of NANB hepatitis, the route of transmission of infection is not apparent and the patient does not belong to any of the recognized high-risk groups. In the USA, approximately 40% of cases of NANB hepatitis are in this group.[33] Current evidence indicates that the gross majority of these cases of NANB hepatitis are caused by hepatitis C, with seroconversion to anti-HCV positivity reported in 30% in acute NANBH,[783] rising to 60–80% in chronic NANBH.[33,381,617] Inapparent parenteral transmission or non-parenteral transmission by unrecognized routes must explain the spread of HCV in these cases, but as yet this is poorly understood. Although HCV is a flavivirus and is closely related to other arthropod-borne viruses, there is no evidence that it is transmitted by insect vectors to man.

SPECIFIC CLINICAL FEATURES OF HEPATITIS C

The typical sequence of events after hepatitis C infection is summarized in Figure 30.25. Many studies of the clinical features of PT-NANBH antedate the development of serological tests for anti-HCV, but features reported in these earlier studies are presumed to be indicative of the clinical features of HCV infection, as the majority of cases of PT-NANBH are now known to be due to hepatitis C.

The incubation period for PT-NANBH is usually between 6 and 12 weeks but ranges from 2 to 26 weeks.[290] The incubation period for PT-NANBH acquired from treatment with clotting factor concentrates is towards the shorter end of this spectrum (4 weeks)[55,492] and this may be related to the high concentration of HCV in these preparations.

There are no specific clinical features which distinguish hepatitis C from other forms of viral hepatitis, and a wide spectrum of clinical presentation may be observed.[24] In PT-NANBH, a high proportion of cases are asymptomatic and many are detected only by careful analysis of serial liver function tests. In the majority, the clinical hepatitis is mild in the acute phase and only 25% of cases become jaundiced. Severe fulminant hepatitis may rarely occur, as may late-onset hepatic failure, both of which carry a poor prognosis (see Prognosis and Outcome of Hepatitis C).

Fluctuations in the serum transaminases are a characteristic feature of hepatitis C. These may be very striking, with a relapsing 10–15-fold variation from week to week.

The clinical course and features of sporadic community-acquired hepatitis C are less clearly defined. Many mild cases are presumably treated in the community and only those who remain unwell require further assessment or hospitalization. At that stage they are a selected group and tend to have a severe and often protracted clinical course. Progression to chronic liver disease is discussed later (see Prognosis and Outcome of Hepatitis C).

Extrahepatic manifestations are less common with hepatitis C infection than in hepatitis B, but several are described. In acute hepatitis C infection, there are isolated case reports of urticaria[944] and erythema nodosum.[297] Transient arthritis has been reported in the prodromal phase of acute NANB hepatitis.[290,864] Other reported extrahepatic manifestations of hepatitis C infection include cryoglobulinaemia, cutaneous vasculitis,[306] and bone marrow aplasia[59,171,278,1297] (see Chapter 8).

SPECIFIC PATHOLOGICAL FEATURES OF HEPATITIS C

The identification of hepatitis C virus is now clarifying the field of non-A, non-B virus hepatitis. It is also helping to confirm the pathological changes which previously had been attributed to parenterally transmitted non-A, non-B virus hepatitis. As yet, specific morphological identification of the virus has not been made either in tissue or in blood.

Apart from fatty change, which is more common in HDV and non-A, non-B hepatitis,[55,56,279] three main features can be identified. These are cytopathic changes, sinusoidal and portal infiltrates, and bile duct damage. It has been suggested that these different patterns represent stages of evolution rather than different forms of hepatitis.[279]

Cytopathic change[276,279,651,1220] consists of an intense granular eosinophilia of scattered single hepatocytes. This has been recorded as being present in up to 100% of biopsies showing non-A, non-B hepatitis.[651] There is rarely a Kupffer cell reaction around the degenerate hepatocytes and it is thought they represent cytopathic damage by the virus. Appearances are virtually identical to those produced by hepatitis D. Microvesicular fatty change can be seen in many of the other hepatocytes.

Sinusoidal infiltrates (Figure 30.26) usually consist of lymphocytes with macrophages and are disproportionate to the degree of apparent parenchymal damage. These features have been particularly found in association with intravenous drug addiction[1248] and intravenous factor VIII administration.[55] Semiquantitative and morphometric analysis of the pathology of chronic non-A, non-B hepatitis suggested that the sinusoidal infiltrates and the acidophil bodies were the most characteristic histological sign of non-A, non-B hepatitis.[1220] Equally characteristic, particularly once chronic hepatitis develops, are the lymphoid aggregates which focally expand the portal tracts.[651,996]

Bile duct damage (Figure 30.7) with lymphocytes infiltrating the bile duct epithelium is particularly prominent in non-A, non-B hepatitis.[995] It was originally noted as an adverse prognostic feature in liver biopsies showing acute hepatitis[909] when 14 cases of acute non-B hepatitis progressed to chronic liver disease and three of these to cirrhosis. As bile duct damage can be present in cholestatic hepatitis without evidence of chronic liver disease, the adverse nature of this feature would seem more related

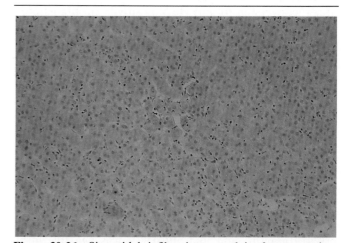

Figure 30.26 Sinusoidal infiltrations: nuclei of mononuclear cells in sinusoids form a prominent feature. Acidophil bodies, ballooning degeneration and collapse of cell plates are relatively minor features.

to the virus likely to cause chronic infection. Although only present in 30% of a series of 40 liver biopsies from patients with non-A, non-B hepatitis,[651] this lesion may be underestimated because of its focal nature.

There have been many attempts to identify the virus by electron microscopy. Changes are frequently found in hepatocyte nuclei from patients with non-A, non-B hepatitis. Electron-dense particles which can range in size from 15 to 30 nm have been described (Table 30.13). Unfortunately, these are not specific, having been identified also in hepatitis D infection[159,160,550] as well as a variety of other virus hepatitides and non-virus-related liver diseases.[275]

Cytoplasmic changes have also been described.[273,274,1248] These are similar to changes described in the chimpanzee which appear to represent specific forms of cytoplasmic damage induced by these viral infections and not by the virus itself.[989]

Ultrastructurally there is a marked lymphocytic interaction with hepatocytes and sinusoidal endothelial cells. Damaged hepatocytes showed loss of microvilli, with lymphocytes in close contact with the plasma membrane.[508] Immunocytochemical studies confirmed the central role of cytotoxic T cells within the space of Disse, but also demonstrated a higher proportion of NK lymphocytes in acute than in chronic non-A, non-B hepatitis.[281]

Experimental pathology

Ultrastructurally, particles ranging between 15 and 30 nm in size with a median size of 25–27 nm have been consistently found in the nuclei of chimpanzee hepatocytes during the course of non-A, non-B hepatitis.[147,273,523,1043] Although consistently present in non-A, non-B hepatitis, they can also be found in hepatitis B infections and also occasionally in chimpanzees with no known viral infection.[275] Cytoplasmic changes also commonly and consistently occur in chimpanzee hepatocytes during the course of non-A, non-B hepatitis. Four types of inclusion

have been identified.[874] The first are sponge-like inclusions with a dense reticulomatrix within which are some profiles of smooth endoplasmic reticulum. The second type of inclusion is formed from focal segments of smooth endoplasmic reticulum where two curved lengths of membrane are opposed and thickened and the small gap between them is filled with a matrix of moderate electron density. The third and most common change is a cylindrical complex formed by a parallel arrangement of double membranes, approximately 25 nm in diameter, with each double membrane filled by a moderately dense matrix.[147,523,874,1043] The fourth change is usually present in association with these cylindrical complexes and is formed from arrays of microtubular aggregates. Since these changes are not necessarily specific for non-A, non-B hepatitis and can be found in chimpanzees superinfected with hepatitis D,[160,550] it is possible that they represent hepatocellular degeneration rather than a specific viral pathology.[989] An experimental study of the sequential changes occurring in chimpanzees infected with hepatitis C virus suggests that these inclusions represent a host response to the expression of interferon.[1044] The protein of these microtubular aggregates has been isolated and partially sequenced. It is a single protein with a molecular weight of 44 kD. This p44 protein was not found in uninfected chimpanzees and the partial amino acid sequence so far has no homology to any known proteins.[475]

PROGNOSIS AND OUTCOME OF HEPATITIS C

Information about prognosis and outcome is largely derived from studies of PT-NANBH, but it is assumed that the majority of these cases were due to hepatitis C. In patients with PT-NANBH, approximately 50% have an acute resolving hepatitis and 50% develop chronic hepatitis, of whom approximately 20% develop cirrhosis.[90,593] For patients documented to be seropositive for anti-HCV, a higher proportion (80%) have been reported to develop chronic liver disease.[813] In one study that compared outcome for chronic PT-NANBH with that

Table 30.13 Ultrastructural liver changes recorded in human non-A, non-B hepatitis

Author/reference	No. of patients	Nuclear particles	Size (nm)	Cytoplasmic alteration	Type
Bamber et al.[57]	12	8	20–35	0	–
Busachi et al.[150]	8	5 (2)	15–27 (+31–46)	7	Lamellae
De Vos et al.[273]	1	1	Not stated	1	Tubules
De Vos et al.[274]	2	Not stated	–	2	Tubules
De Vos et al.[275]	31	28	20–29	0	–
Dienes et al.[279]	22	6	Not stated	0	–
Dienes et al.[280]	1	1	20–27	0	–
Gmelin et al.[397]	1	1	25–30	–	–
Spichtin et al.[1081]	18	17	20–29	0	Laminar bodies
Weller et al.[1248]	8	2	27–30	2	
Total	106	71		14	

for chronic CA-NANBH, anti-HCV seropositivity was documented in 75% of patients in each group and patient follow-up ranged from 3 to 20 years.[485] In the chronic PT-NANBH group ($n=24$), 29% improved with normalization of liver function tests (after 5 years), 55% had chronic persistent hepatitis and 16% had chronic active hepatitis with cirrhosis. In patients with chronic CA-NANBH ($n=62$), 2% showed remission, 43% had stable chronic persistent hepatitis and 55% progressed to chronic active hepatitis or cirrhosis. In this study, progression to cirrhosis and development of complications took many years in both forms of chronic hepatitis C infection. One exception to this is patients who are co-infected with both HCV and HIV, in whom a rapid progression to cirrhosis within 3 years of the onset of hepatitis has been reported.[709] The relationship between HCV and hepatocellular carcinoma is described in Chapters 31 and 39.

Severe fulminant hepatitis is a rare complication of acute hepatitis C infection. In the King's College Hospital series, presumed NANB hepatitis was the commonest viral cause of fulminant hepatic failure, accounting for 158/338 viral cases from a total of 943 cases from all causes.[1256] Hepatic failure in NANBH often occurs between 6 weeks and 6 months after the onset of first symptoms, and this has been termed late-onset hepatic failure. In a UK series, 90% of cases of late-onset hepatic failure were due to NANBH.[390] The proportion of these cases of fulminant or late-onset hepatic failure which are due to hepatitis C infection is unclear. Most of these patients are anti-HCV negative, but this may simply reflect the fact that seroconversion to anti-HCV positivity tends to occur late in the disease. Measurement of HCV-RNA or antibodies to other HCV antigens in such patients may improve our understanding of the role of HCV in fulminant or late-onset hepatic failure.

TREATMENT AND PREVENTION OF HEPATITIS C

There are no specific treatments of proven benefit in the acute phase of either PT-NANBH, CA-NANBH or serologically proven hepatitis C infection. Interferons have been used for the treatment of chronic hepatitis C with some benefit and this is reviewed in Chapter 31. Recent studies have suggested that treatment with natural interferon-β may decrease HCV-RNA in the acute phase of hepatitis C and prevent progression to chronic hepatitis,[831] but numbers were small and these preliminary results await confirmation. Cyanidanol-3 has been reported to improve transaminase levels significantly in acute NANB hepatitis,[879] but treatment with this compound has not gained widespread acceptance.

In severe fulminant hepatitis C, liver transplantation may be the only effective treatment. Results are similar to those obtained with other causes of fulminant liver failure, with an approximate 60% 1-year survival rate after liver transplantation. Recurrence of HCV infection in liver grafts is reported to be problematic in some studies, but not in others. Some studies have reported

frequent loss of anti-HCV after liver transplant,[423,937] whereas others report persisting anti-HCV antibodies in the majority.[710] In each of these studies, recurrent hepatitis in the liver graft was unusual and often not related to anti-HCV status. Further light has recently been shed on this by studies of pre- and post-transplant HCV-RNA status in patients with chronic hepatitis C undergoing liver transplantation in San Francisco, USA. Of 23 patients who were serum HCV-RNA positive before transplantation, 15 (65%) remained HCV-RNA positive post-transplantation and 73% of these had histological hepatitis.[1276] In the majority histological features were mild, but one death occurred due to liver failure in a patient with chronic active hepatitis C in the liver graft, over a follow-up period of 12.5 months.

At present there are no vaccines available for the prevention of hepatitis C. The molecular cloning of HCV led to the expectation that vaccines would follow, but recent evidence concerning the heterogeneity of this virus suggests that development of effective vaccines will pose some difficulties. However, recent advances in the development of vaccines to related flaviviruses and pestiviruses give some cause for optimism.[489]

Before the introduction of blood donor screening for anti-HCV, studies in patients undergoing cardiac surgery investigated the role of immune serum globulin (ISG) in the prevention of PT-NANBH. In those given ISG there was a significant reduction in the incidence of PT-NANBH.[14,983] The need for ISG prophylaxis in patients receiving multiple transfusions has been partially negated by the introduction of blood donor screening for anti-HCV. This appears to be effective in preventing a significant proportion of, but not all, transfusion-associated hepatitis C. In a recent report from Japan which compared PT-NANBH in the period before introduction of anti-HCV screening with the period immediately after, a pronounced effect was observed.[529] In patients receiving 1–10-unit transfusions, the incidence of PT-NANBH fell from 4.9% to 1.9%, and for those receiving 11–20-unit transfusions it fell from 16.3% to 3.3% of cases. Failure to prevent some cases of transfusion-associated hepatitis reflects recruitment of HCV-infected donors who did not exhibit anti-HCV as determined by the C100–3 EIA.

HEPATITIS E

PROPERTIES OF HEPATITIS E VIRUS
(Table 30.14)

An epidemiologically distinct form of non-A, non-B viral hepatitis, principally transmitted by the faecal–oral route, has been recognized globally in regions where sanitation is poor and the populace is malnourished.[121] This form of hepatitis has been entitled water-borne hepatitis, epidemic hepatitis or enterically-transmitted non-A, non-B hepatitis (ET-NANBH). Convalescent sera obtained from patients in one outbreak aggregated virus-like particles in stool

Table 30.14 Properties of hepatitis E virus

- Major cause of enterically transmitted epidemic non-A, non-B hepatitis
- Non-enveloped 32–34-nm virus probably in the calicivirus family
- Genome single plus-strand 7.6 kb RNA which is polyadenylated
- No homology to other hepatitis viruses

specimens from a temporally and geographically distinct outbreak, providing evidence for a common aetiological agent. The virus appeared by electron microscopy as 27–34-nm particles and sedimented at 183 S.[123]

Further characterization of the virus has been facilitated by passage in cynomologous macaques, initially inoculated with human faecal material.[123] After serial faecal–oral passage of virus in the animal, macaque faecal material was inoculated intravenously into another macaque, from which infectious gallbladder bile was obtained to facilitate molecular cloning of the virus.[946]

A cDNA library was cloned in the bacteriophage vector λgt10 after isolation of RNA present in bile from both infected and uninfected macaques. Of six cloned inserts, one yielded a 1.3-kb cDNA which detected a uniquely hybridizing band present in infected but not uninfected macaque bile. These sequences were not present in genomic DNA from infected or uninfected macaque liver, nor in that from normal human liver, indicating that the cDNA was derived from RNA not present endogenously in mammalian genomes. To demonstrate convincingly that this virus was the pathogen common to most, if not all, outbreaks of enterically transmitted non-A, non-B hepatitis, RNA isolated from faecal specimens obtained from outbreaks in Mexico, Tashkent, USSR, Borneo, Somalia and Pakistan all hybridized positively with the cDNA probe.[946]

Further characterization of this virus, now designated hepatitis E (HEV), indicates that the viral genome is positive-sense, single-stranded RNA which is polyadenylated. The 7.6-kb RNA encodes a consensus-sequence for RNA-directed RNA polymerase, but no other similarities to known viral or non-viral sequences are apparent. Based on size, sedimentation, lack of a viral envelope and characteristics of the viral genome, it appears that HEV belongs to the calicivirus family.[946]

Expression of recombinant proteins from cloned HEV will facilitate the development of diagnostic assays and may provide the ability to develop vaccines against this widespread virus.

LABORATORY DETECTION OF HEV INFECTION

At present there are no routine assays for HEV infection and the diagnosis is usually made clinically on the basis of epidemiological likelihood of exposure to HEV and absence of serum markers for HAV, HBV and HCV.

Attempts to develop RIAs and EIAs for HEV have, until recently, been unsuccessful. Techniques such as immunoelectron microscopy (IEM) have previously been used to identify virus-like particles (VLPs) in stools or to identify sera that contain antibodies with the ability to aggregate VLPs in known HEV-infected stool samples.[125] The observation that a fluorescein (FITC)-labelled IgG fraction (prepared from an IEM-positive convalescent serum in a case of HEV infection) reacts with HEV antigen in the liver of infected cynos monkeys,[601] led to the development of a fluorescent antibody (FA) blocking assay.[602] In this assay, the ability of unknown sera to block the fluorescent interaction between FITC-IgG and HEV antigen in cynos liver is presumed to signify the presence of anti-HEV antibodies.

More recently the molecular cloning of HEV (see Properties of Hepatitis E Virus) has facilitated direct detection of genomic sequences of HEV in stool specimens.[946] Antibodies to HEV have now been successfully detected in acute and convalescent sera with an EIA which uses recombinant HEV antigens.[1309] This promising development may soon lead to a commercially available assay.

EPIDEMIOLOGY OF HEPATITIS E

Massive epidemics of waterborne viral hepatitis were first reported from India in the mid-1950s.[1217] Although originally assumed to be due to hepatitis A, a retrospective analysis of sera taken and stored at the time of the outbreak revealed no evidence of acute infection with either HAV or HBV.[1262] These data gave the first clear indication that an enterically transmitted non-A non-B hepatitis (ET-NANBH) virus was responsible for this form of epidemic hepatitis. Many similar outbreaks were subsequently reported, predominantly from India, southeast Asia, and the USSR (see Table 30.15). Epidemic waterborne spread, associated with poor standards of hygiene and faecal contamination of drinking water, was a feature of many of these outbreaks.

Analysis of stool specimens from an outbreak of ET-

Table 30.15 Geographical distribution of epidemic HEV infection

Country/region	Year	No. of cases	Reference
Delhi, India	1955	29 300	1217
Kirgiz, USSR	1955	10 800	1027
Katmandhu, Nepal	1973	>10 000	552
Burma	1976	20 000	795
			125
Algeria	1980	780	79
Ethiopian refugees			
Sudan	1985	>2 000	177
Somalia	1985	>3 000	177
Huitzila, Mexico	1986	90	178
Kunpur, North India	1991	79 000	936

NANBH in Nepal by IEM using convalescent sera led to the description of 27–30-nm and 32–34-nm virus-like particles.[552] Furthermore, transmission experiments in tamarins demonstrated that infected animals developed antibodies capable of aggregating these particles by IEM.[552] Similar VLPs were subsequently identified in stool samples from Burmese, Tashkent USSR and Mexican outbreaks.[123,124,795] Of major importance was the observation that acute and convalescent sera from many geographically diverse epidemics of ET-NANBH (as listed in Table 30.15) reacted specifically with these VLPs.[124] The presence of anti-HEV antibodies was subsequently confirmed, using the fluorescent antibody blocking assay (see Laboratory Detection of HEV Infection), in 77–100% of sera from cases of ET-NANBH from Asia, Africa and North America.[602] Within India, retrospective analyses of samples from 10 separate epidemics of ET-NANBH, spanning 35 years, have demonstrated evidence of HEV infection in 9 of them.[933] These studies provide evidence that geographically and chronologically distant epidemics of ET-NANBH are due to an aetiological agent now designated as HEV.

These observations have recently been confirmed using molecular techniques to identify genomic sequences of HEV in stool specimens from five geographically distinct epidemics of ET-NANBH[946] (see Properties of Hepatitis E Virus). HEV genome has also been identified in 16 stool specimens from the recent massive epidemic of ET-NANBH involving 79 000 cases in Kanpur, an industrial city in northern India, between January and April 1991.[936] The discovery and characterization of HEV, and epidemiological features of HEV infection have recently been reviewed.[126]

Although HEV infection is reported predominantly in epidemic form, it is also endemic in many developing countries. For example, sporadic acute cases occur commonly in India.[573,1135] Immigrants from these regions may also import HEV infection to the Western world, as described for Pakistani immigrants to the USA.[257] Travellers to endemic regions are also at risk of developing HEV infection.[355]

CLINICAL FEATURES AND OUTCOME OF HEV INFECTION

The incubation period for hepatitis E ranges from 3 to 9 weeks with an average of 6 weeks.[933] In large epidemics the attack rate is highest in adolescents and young adults (2.9%), with a lower rate in children under the age of 14 years (1.4%) and in those over the age of 40 years (2.0%). This is strikingly different from HAV, which predominantly infects young children, but the explanation for this is unknown.

In the majority of patients, HEV causes an acute self-limiting hepatitis, from which the majority make a complete recovery. The usual clinical features are those of any viral hepatitis and include dark urine (92%), jaundice (87%), nausea (84%), abdominal pain (75%),

fever (54%) and pruritus (55%).[693] Severe hepatitis with fulminant hepatic failure (FHF) is reported in 0.5–3% of cases,[572,933] but a characteristic and as yet unexplained feature of HEV infection is the development of FHF in approximately 20% of women infected in the third trimester of pregnancy.[572,933] Hepatitis E infection has not been reported to cause chronic liver disease.

SPECIFIC PATHOLOGICAL FEATURES OF HEPATITIS E

The outbreak of epidemic hepatitis in New Delhi in 1956 was associated with the pattern of cholestatic viral hepatitis which has been described previously. Subsequent demonstration that this epidemic was not due to infection with either the A or B viruses, and the epidemiological characteristics of the outbreak suggest that it was due to the hepatitis E virus.[1262] A similar cholestatic hepatitis in which large ballooned hepatocytes with clear cytoplasm were prominent has also been described in an epidemic waterborne hepatitis in which there was no evidence of either A or B virus infection.[1232] Viral particles are not normally present in the liver of patients with acute hepatitis. None the less, in a study of a patient with fulminant hepatitis and IgM antibody to HEV, virus-like particles were detected in small bile ductules and sinusoidal lining cells.[46]

Hepatitis E virus has been experimentally transmitted to cynomologus macaques and tamarins. Virus-like particles of 27–37 nm have been recovered from the animals and successfully transmitted into further animals. These transmissions were associated with a self-limiting acute hepatitis.[123,1076] Virus particles of appropriate size were also found in the cytoplasm of the damaged hepatocytes.[1076]

TREATMENT AND PREVENTION OF HEPATITIS E

There are no specific treatments for HEV infection and management is confined to general supportive measures. Prevention of HEV infection is by improving standards of hygiene, with particular attention to preventing faecal contamination of drinking water. At present there are no vaccines available to prevent HEV infection.

OTHER VIRUSES

Although recent work has clearly identified two additional hepatitis viruses, hepatitis C and hepatitis E, among the non-A, non-B hepatitides, there still remains the theoretical possibility of more viral agents (hepatitis F?). The current evidence suggests that any such candidate will not be numerically important as a cause of transmitted hepatitis. Identification will of course be dependent initially on a process of careful exclusion of other known causes.

Many other viruses affect the liver and it is impossible

to be comprehensive. These viruses range from yellow fever, where acidophil degeneration of hepatocytes was first described,[238] to the haemorrhagic fever viruses of Lassa fever and Ebola haemorrhagic fever. For these many viruses hepatitis is either produced as part of a systemic illness or as a consequence of an opportunistic infection in an immunosuppressed host. Viruses contributing to neonatal hepatitis are also discussed in Chapter 44.

Flaviviruses

Yellow fever
Yellow fever results from infection with an RNA flavivirus transmitted by mosquitoes. Replication of the virus occurs in both vector and host. The virus is endemic in jungle primates of both Africa and Central and South America, and the cycle is between primate and mosquito. Man is involved when incidentally exposed to jungle (or sylvan) yellow fever. An urban variety of yellow fever exists in which the cycle is between man and mosquito and other primates are incidentally involved. The virus is identical for these varieties but the mosquito vectors differ. In the Americas the mosquito *Aedes aegypti* transmits urban yellow fever and *Haemogogus* species complete the jungle cycle. In Africa several species of aedine mosquitoes can transmit both urban and jungle yellow fever.[232] Outbreaks may occur in other countries, as demonstrated by the epidemic of yellow fever that occurred in Swansea in 1865.[738]

Most infections are clinically inapparent, although they are usually more severe in older age groups. Outbreaks appear to vary in virulence and the incidence of complications.[544,963] Five reasons have been suggested for this.[231] These are the immune status of the population, the difficulty of diagnosis of isolated cases, lack of means for investigation, variations in ecological conditions that influence the circulation of the virus in the wild and in man-to-man transmission, and negligence.

The most common presenting complaints are fever, headaches, nausea and vomiting, with jaundice in more severe cases. Abdominal, chest and/or joint pains may be present. Leucopenia is initially present followed by a leucocytosis. Central nervous system involvement, renal failure and evidence of a bleeding diathesis appear to be adverse prognostic features.[544]

The changes in the liver have been documented by biopsy in man[359,568] and experimentally in monkeys.[1161] These confirm the prominent acidophil degeneration of hepatocytes in the mid-zone (Figure 30.27) as described in the autopsy studies performed by Councilman.[238] Even in severe cases there is sparing of a rim of perivenular and periportal hepatocytes.[568] In addition, fatty change and ballooning degeneration of other hepatocytes may be seen; these occur early in the course of the disease.[359] Experimentally, the earliest feature is acidophil necrosis of Kupffer cells 24 hours after inoculation. Yellow fever virus is immunocytochemically present in these cells.

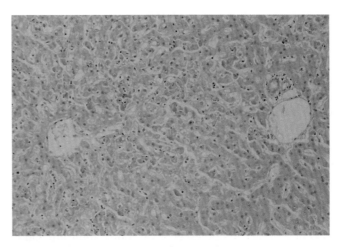

Figure 30.27 Yellow fever. Extensive midzonal hepatocellular damage extending into the perivenular zone. Acidophil bodies are numerous but the inflammatory infiltrate is relatively slight in both sinusoids and portal tracts.

Hepatocellular damage does not occur until the third day post-inoculation but then rapidly increases.[1161] Immuno-electron microscopy demonstrates virus-specific antigens incorporated into cytoplasmic membranes as well as on the envelopes of extracellular virions in tissue culture cells infected with the yellow fever virus.[378] There is no evidence of chronic liver disease resulting from yellow fever that cannot be explained by concomitant infection with hepatitis B virus.

Treatment is non-specific; supportive measures are required such as correction of electrolyte imbalance and control of renal failure when necessary. Prophylaxis is obviously more desirable; approximately 90% of any population vaccinated with the stabilized yellow fever 17D vaccine develop haemagglutination inhibition antibodies.[982,1260]

Other flaviviruses
Two closely related flaviviruses, dengue and Nile valley fever virus are occasionally associated with liver disease. Dengue has indistinguishable liver lesions and a virus can be isolated from the liver in patients who die of the disease.[973] West-Nile virus has also been isolated from four patients with hepatitis[718]

Adenoviruses
Historically, adenoviruses were frequently isolated from patients with hepatitis during the search for the infective agents of hepatitis A and B. Adenoviruses are both ubiquitous and relatively easily isolated by laboratory techniques. They are also known to be excreted in the faeces intermittently over many years so that reactivation of such viruses during an episode of hepatitis is possible. It has been shown that antibody titres to adenovirus will rise during the course of other infections such as viral and mycoplasmal pneumonias.[356] Adenovirus infections of

the liver are associated with focal areas of coagulative necrosis of hepatocytes. Hepatocytes surrounding these necrotic foci usually contain large intranuclear inclusions of adenovirus which can be confirmed both by electron microscopy and by immunocytochemistry. Such examples of adenovirus hepatitis are usually associated with congenital or acquired severe immunodeficiency.[822,1208]

Herpes viruses

Infectious mononucleosis

Infectious mononucleosis is now well established as an infection with the Epstein–Barr virus (EBV); there is an extensive literature with several reviews.[49,197,629] Typically infection occurs in adolescence or young adult life and is characterized by fever, malaise, sore throat and lymphadenopathy. Clinically, hepatitis with hepatomegaly occurs in up to 15% of cases but abnormal elevation of serum aminotransferases is almost universal.[305,377] Rarely there may be profound hyperbilirubinaemia[692] and exudative ascites.[699] During investigation of a child presenting with high fever and subsequently demonstrated to have Epstein–Barr virus infection, ultrasound revealed a distended gallbladder with increased wall thickness up to 0.6 cm.[1077] The clinical presentation may closely mimic infectious hepatitis and then be wrongly diagnosed, but the serological reactions are usually characteristic and diagnostic.[467,674]

The features on liver biopsy have to be distinguished from a malignant lymphomatous infiltrate (see Chapter 41).[674] Hepatocellular damage is not usually pronounced, but regenerative, particularly mitotic, activity may be disproportionately increased. Extensive hepatocellular necrosis can occur,[15] but death from hepatic failure is extremely rare, as is progression to chronicity.[61] One case report of cirrhosis in a 27-year-old woman with chronic Epstein–Barr virus infection was also complicated by chronic infection with chlamydia and hepatitis A virus.[43]

Hepatitis due to infection with or reactivation of the Epstein–Barr virus has now become a complication of liver transplantation (see Chapter 56).[635,706]

Cytomegalovirus

This DNA virus is identical on electron microscopy to the herpes viruses with which it is usually grouped. Several antigenic subtypes exist.[402]

Infection with this virus is very common and most cases are asymptomatic, although overwhelming infection can occur. It can be transmitted transplacentally to the fetus[1114] and in or around the neonatal period. The peak incidence of infection is in young adult life. Infection may present as a febrile systemic illness, a hepatitis, an atypical mononucleosis syndrome usually with hepatitis, or as a Guillain–Barré syndrome.[1006] It can be associated with ascites.[845] Infection is commonly followed by a prolonged excretion of the virus, which is often intermittent and occurs in the presence of high serum antibody titres.[402] Patients on immunosuppressive therapy are particularly

prone to infection as are those undergoing cardiac surgery.[1075] In normal individuals the pathological features are identical to those of viral hepatitis, with hepatocytes showing acidophil degeneration and a mixed inflammatory infiltrate in the portal tracts and parenchyma.[1164] A granulomatous hepatitis has also been described,[110,1145] sometimes similar to those found in *Coxiella burnetii* infections.[676] Cytomegalovirus inclusions can be demonstrated in hepatocytes and vascular endothelium in approximately 20% of cases[458] (Figure 30.28). Cytomegalovirus hepatitis in immunocompromised hosts seems to be characterized by the consistent presence of viral inclusions within hepatocytes and by the paucity of an inflammatory reaction. Cytomegalovirus infection occurring in patients with chronic hepatitis B surface antigenpositive liver disease resulted in acute hepatic failure.[1198]

The diagnosis of the cytomegalovirus hepatitis as distinct from other forms of viral hepatitis is difficult. It has been suggested that after liver transplantation, weekly quantitative monitoring of cytomegalovirus antigenaemia should be undertaken, as it is a sensitive early marker of active CMV infection.[1200]

Herpes simplex

This DNA virus causes disseminated infection with hepatitis in neonatal life and it can also present as a fulminant hepatitis.[81] Both strains of herpes simplex virus (HSV-1 and HSV-2) have been isolated from cases of generalized disease.[798] In adults, clinical hepatitis is usually part of a disseminated infection, usually in immunosuppressed individuals and particularly after organ transplantation,[625] or as a result of concurrent illness such as Hodgkin's disease or ulcerative colitis.[1045] None the less, primary infection in previously healthy individuals[733] and in pregnant women[860] has been recorded. Even in adults with genital herpes and no evidence of systemic illness, mild elevation of serum aminotransferases may be found in

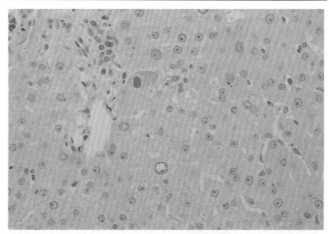

Figure 30.28 Cytomegalovirus. A mild cholestatic hepatitis in a middle aged male was associated with the presence of large eosinophilic intranuclear inclusions, in this instance in a periportal hepatocyte. Many identical inclusions were present in duodenal and gastric biopsies.

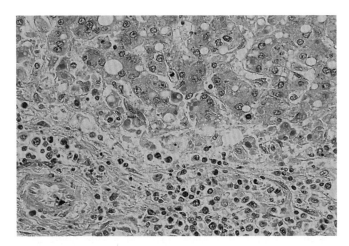

Figure 30.29 Herpes simplex. Perivenular hepatocytes show focal coagulative necrosis and disruption of the cell plate. Numerous large dense eosinophilic viral inclusion bodies are present within hepatocytes.

approximately 10–20% of patients. These levels return to normal with resolution of the genital lesions.[764]

The clinical features of systemic infection are fever, a severe disseminated intravascular coagulation syndrome with leukopenia, thrombocytopenia and prolonged prothrombin and partial thromboplastin times as well as evidence of involvement of multiple organs such as encephalitis, myocarditis or hepatitis.[625] The primary focal lesion may be oral, frequently with severe buccal and pharyngeal ulceration, but oesophageal and primary geni-

tal infection have been recorded.[326,1290] When associated with pregnancy there is the additional risk of disseminated herpes infection in the fetus.

In the liver there are small punctate haemorrhagic foci of necrosis with a variable, usually mononuclear reaction. Hepatocytes around the necrotic focus usually contain typical intranuclear inclusion bodies (Figure 30.29).[642]

Treatment with cytosine arabinoside has now been superseded by acyclovir, which can be administered intravenously.

Herpes zoster/varicella

This is unusual in adults but may be severe in immunosuppressed individuals.[546,856] The characteristics of the skin rash, with isolation of the virus from the vesicles, should establish the diagnosis in doubtful cases. Pneumonitis is the most severe complication. In the liver, small foci of necrosis 1–3 mm in diameter are found.[190] New inclusions are readily demonstrable in the epidermal cells of the skin vesicles but their presence in hepatocytes is not so consistent. A rare example of post-necrotic cirrhosis following varicella hepatitis in a transplant patient has been recorded.[20] Acyclovir may be beneficial in treating varicella in immunocompromised individuals.[546]

Enteroviruses

This group of viruses is one genus of the family of picornaviruses and includes polio virus, coxsackie virus A and B and echoviruses. The 27-nm hepatitis A virus is morphologically similar to the enteroviruses and is classi-

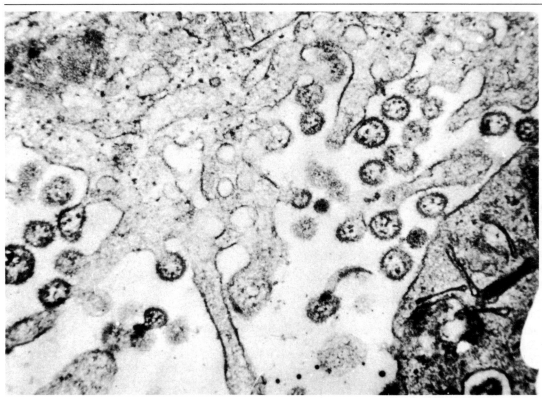

Figure 30.30 Lassa fever. Lassa virus budding out from cell surface. The virus particles contain granules characteristic of the family Arenaviridae and these have been shown to be host ribosomes. Vero cell culture, × 98 000. (Courtesy of Dr A. Baskerville, Microbiological Research Establishment, Porton Down, UK.)

Coxsackie viruses

Coxsackie group B viruses classically cause epidemic myalgia but have been associated with a wide variety of syndromes in adults[76,346] and have been implicated in the pathogenesis of some cardiomyopathies and may cause severe myocarditis.[938] Hepatic involvement is documented only rarely, despite the widespread organ involvement found in most adult infections. A clinically significant hepatitis has been recorded but is associated with a myocarditis.[421,938,1107] The liver shows a non-specific portal tract inflammatory infiltrate with micro-abscesses containing neutrophils in the parenchyma. Virus-like particles are present in the hepatocyte cytoplasm on electron microscopy.[421] Fulminating liver disease is produced in neonates.[775,907] The more severe nature of the disease in neonates is probably related to their poorly developed immune competence; with AIDS and liver transplantation, fulminant hepatic failure in the adult due to coxsackie B viruses may become of greater significance.

Coxsackie group A viruses usually cause herpangina, upper respiratory tract infection or aseptic meningitis. There is no good evidence for liver disease due to coxsackie group A viruses.

Echoviruses

These can cause severe hepatic necrosis in neonates[491,774] but involvement in adults is rarely recorded. Abnormal liver function tests have been found in one of two adult siblings presenting with pneumonitis and aseptic meningitis[999]

Arenaviruses

These are a group of morphologically indistinguishable but markedly pleomorphic viruses that have both common and specific antigenic characteristics[97,172]

Lassa fever

First identified in 1969, this disease attained publicity because of its infectivity and high mortality rate of between one-third and two-thirds of cases.[357] Since then outbreaks have continued to occur in various parts of West Africa, but serological studies indicate generalized infection within this area.[724] A prospective study in Sierra Leone demonstrated that Lassa fever was responsible for between 10% and 16% of all adult medical admissions and for approximately 30% of all adult deaths in the hospitals studied, suggesting that the disease was endemic in this area.[725] The virus is a negative-stranded RNA arenavirus (Figure 30.30) transmitted to man from a rodent host, *Mastomys natalensis*, which forms the reservoir for human infection. Clinical infection is characterized by fever with generalized organ involvement; pneumonia, myocarditis, encepha-

lopathy, nephropathy and myositis and a haemorrhagic diathesis can all occur. The severity of the haemorrhagic diathesis seems to be a marker of cases with a high mortality. In a study of 213 cases of Lassa fever, 17 (11%) had abnormal bleeding; of these, 6 patients died.[358] Lassa fever in the last trimester of pregnancy also seems to have a particularly severe outcome, but evacuation of the uterus can significantly improve the mother's chance of survival.[912] Death is usually from sudden cardiovascular collapse.[172] Barrier nursing of these patients is successful in preventing transmission to hospital staff.[350,455]

In the liver, focal necroses and diffuse hepatocellular damage can be seen, with perivenular accentuation of the damage. Acidophil bodies have been described as a prominent feature.[313] There is a vigorous macrophage response to cellular damage but lymphocytic infiltration is scanty.[723] Virus particles have been demonstrated in the space of Disse and in the bile canaliculus by electron microscopy.[1258]

Treatment should involve barrier nursing and general supportive measures in the intensive-care unit. Systemically administered ribavirin is a viricidal agent effective for Lassa fever.[258]

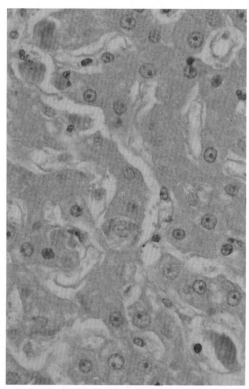

Figure 30.31 Ebola virus. Marked eosinophil degeneration of individual hepatocytes is present. In one hepatocyte (centre) an eosinophil cytoplasmic inclusion is forming to the left of the nucleus. (Day 6; courtesy of Dr A. Baskerville, Microbiological Research Establishment, Porton Down, UK.)

Argentinian and Bolivian haemorrhagic fevers

Both these fevers are due to arenaviruses and both are associated with a hepatitis similar to that described for Lassa fever.[200,320]

Filoviridae

Marburg virus

In 1967, personnel working with African green monkeys in Marburg, Frankfurt and Belgrade became seriously ill.[711,1099] Five of the 27 patients died. The early symptoms were high fever, conjunctivitis and an enanthema, followed by an exanthem with hepatitis, diarrhoea, renal abnormalities and bleeding tendency. Encephalitis or myocarditis was sometimes clinically present. Leucopenia was characteristically present from the first day of illness and could change to a leucocytosis. There was an atypical lymphocytosis and a profound thrombocytopenia.[374] The virus has subsequently been shown to be present in Central Africa[403] and to be more common in savanna zones than in rain forests.[1166] The physicochemical properties of the virus have been defined, as has its relationship to the Ebola virus.[574] The virus has an elongated tubular form 70–80 nm in diameter in which there is a core 35–40 nm in diameter with a hollow centre. The tubules may be branched and spikes may be present on the surface. An enlarged head or torus can be identified on some tubules. Many tubules appear to be formed from incomplete outer coat.[18,580,868]

The main changes in the liver are necroses starting off as acidophil degeneration of hepatocytes. Mild fatty change may be present. Scanty lymphocytic and histiocytic inflammatory cell infiltrate is present and hyperplastic Kupffer cells around the necroses are laden with ceroid pigment.[73] Long-term complications of the hepatitis have not been described.

Ebola virus

Two simultaneous outbreaks of a severe viral haemorrhagic fever occurred in the Sudan and in Zaire in 1976.[510,1268] The mortality was approximately 70% in over 500 cases. A population survey demonstrated antibody titres to Ebola virus in 12.4% of Central African populations from six countries,[403] suggesting that the disease is endemic, possibly with a monkey reservoir. The virus has been accidentally imported into the United States in a colony of cynomolgus monkeys.[524]

Clinically, patients present with a sudden onset of high fever, chills, headache, myalgia, anorexia, nausea, abdominal pain, sore throat and profound prostration. On around the fifth day of the acute phase an exanthematous rash on the trunk precedes haemorrhagic manifestations, particularly from mucosal surfaces. Haemorrhagic complications usually have a fatal outcome within a week.[135,1111] Transmission of infection requires very close contact with the patient and there is no evidence of droplet transmission. An outbreak can be contained by strict isolation, use of protective clothing and careful handling and disposal of body fluids and excretions.

The virus is very similar to Marburg virus.[574] The liver

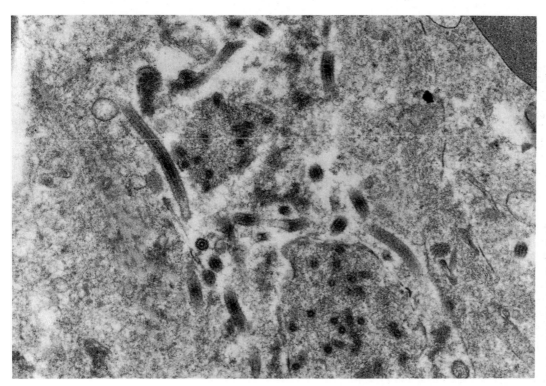

Figure 30.32 Ebola virus: the viral particles are long tubular structures of extraordinary length cut through in various tangential planes in the hepatocyte cytoplasm. Note the central core to the particles. EM × 44 000. Courtesy of Dr A. Baskerville.

shows numerous foci of necrosis (Figure 30.31) and viral particles can be seen within the hepatocyte cytoplasm and bile canaliculi (Figure 30.32). The virus also replicates in endothelial cytoplasm[66] and its presence can be confirmed using immunological techniques.[376]

Treatment is supportive; no specific viricidal agent or vaccination programme is currently available.

Paramyxoviruses

Measles

Elevated aminotransferase levels with hepatomegaly have been recorded during the course of measles in two adults.[1048] A review of 65 adults with measles found liver involvement in 52 patients and clinical jaundice in 5. The hepatitis was associated with a more severe illness, including a higher occurrence of secondary bacterial infections, but resolved completely with no evidence of chronic liver disease.[373] Liver biopsy features were non-specific and no viral particles were found by electron microscopy in three young adults investigated for hepatitis with associated measles.[773] Multinucleate hepatocytes and a severe hepatitis with cholangitis were identified in a child suffering from a common variable immunodeficiency syndrome during the course of a severe systemic intercurrent illness attributed to measles.[173]

Other paramyxoviruses

Paramyxovirus-like particles have been found in the cytoplasm of hepatocytes from patients with severe hepatitis. The other characteristic feature was the syncytial change in the hepatocytes, with up to 30 nuclei present in some cells. Patient's ages ranged from 5 months to 41 years.[877] The nature of these particles and their relationship to other paramyxoviruses remains to be established.

Miscellaneous

Rubella

A 24-year-old woman with rubella had raised serum aminotransferases during the course of her infection.[1298] Liver biopsy in a 24-year-old man with rubella and raised serum transaminases showed an acute hepatitis; cytotoxic T-cells were the dominant component of the inflammatory infiltrate.[832]

Parvoviruses

A hepatitis has been identified in fetuses with transplacentally transmitted maternal parvovirus infection. The affected fetus was commonly stillborn with hydrops fetalis.[38,745]

REFERENCES

1. Aach, R.D., Szmuness, W., Mosley, J.W. *et al.* (1981) Serum alanine aminotransferase of donors in relation to the risk of non-A, non-B hepatitis in recipients. The Transfusion-Transmitted Viruses Study. *New England Journal of Medicine,* **304,** 989–994.
2. Abdool Karim, S.S., Coovadia, H.M., Windsor, I.M. *et al.* (1988) The prevalence and transmission of hepatitis B virus infection in urban, rural and institutionalized black children of Natal/KwaZulu, South Africa. *International Journal of Epidemiology,* **17,** 168–173.
3. Aceti, A., Taliani, G., De Bac, C. & Sebastiani, A. (1990) Anti-HCV false positivity in malaria. *Lancet,* **336,** 1442–1443.
4. Achord, J.L. (1968) Acute pancreatitis with infectious hepatitis. *Journal of the American Medical Association,* **205,** 837–840.
5. Acs, G., Sells, M.A., Purcell, R.H. *et al.* (1987) Hepatitis B virus produced by transfected Hep G2 cells causes hepatitis in chimpanzees. *Proceedings of the National Academy of Sciences of the USA,* **84,** 4641–4644.
6. A District Control of Infection Officer (1987) Acute hepatitis B following gynaecological surgery. *Journal of Hospital Infection,* **9,** 34–38.
7. Adler, R., Takahashi, M. & Wright, H.T. (1978) Acute pericarditis associated with hepatitis B infection. *Pediatrics,* **61,** 716–719.
8. Advisory Committee on Immunization Practices (1978) *Immune Globulins for Protection against Viral Hepatitis.* Atlanta: Center for Disease Control.
9. Albersheim, S.G., Smyth, J.A., Solimano, A. & Cook, D. (1988) Passively acquired human immunodeficiency virus seropositivity in a neonate after hepatitis B immunoglobulin. *Journal of Pediatrics,* **112,** 915–916.
10. Alberti, A., Realdi, G., Tremolada, F. & Spina, G.P. (1976) Liver cell surface localization of hepatitis B antigen and of immunoglobulins in acute and chronic hepatitis and in liver cirrhosis. *Clinical and Experimental Immunology,* **25,** 396–402.
11. Aldershvile, J., Brock, A., Dietrichson, O. *et al.* (1978) Hepatitis B virus infections among Danish dentists. *Journal of Infectious Diseases,* **137,** 63–66.
12. Aledort, L.M., Levine, P.H., Hilgartner, M. *et al.* (1985) A study of liver biopsies and liver disease among hemophiliacs. *Blood,* **66,** 367–372.
13. Alexander, H. & Lerner, R.A. (1984) Chemically synthesized peptide analogues of the hepatitis surface antigen. In Chisari F.V. (ed.) *Advances in Hepatitis Research,* Ch 24, pp 223–229. New York: Masson Publishing.
14. Al-Khaja, N., Roberts, D.G., Belboul, A. *et al.* (1991) Gamma globulin prophylaxis to reduce post-transfusion non-A, non-B hepatitis after cardiac surgery with cardiopulmonary bypass. *Scandinavian Journal of Thoracic and Cardiovascular Surgery,* **25,** 7–12.
15. Allen, U.R. & Bass, B.H. (1963) Fatal hepatic necrosis in glandular fever. *Journal of Clinical Pathology,* **16,** 339–341.
16. Almeida, J.D. & Waterson, A.P. (1969) Immune complexes in hepatitis. *Lancet,* **2** 983–986.
17. Almeida, J.D., Chisholm, G.D., Kulatilake, A.K. *et al.* (1971) Possible airborne spread of serum hepatitis virus within a haemodialysis unit. *Lancet,* **2,** 849–850.
18. Almeida, J.D., Waterson, A.P. & Simpson, D.I.H. (1971) Morphology and morphogenesis of the Marburg agent. In Martini, G.A. & Siegert, R. (eds) *Marburg Virus Disease.* Proceedings of a Symposium, pp. 84–97. Berlin, New York: Springer-Verlag.
19. Almeida, J.D., Gay, F.W. & Wreghitt, T.G. (1974) Pitfalls in the study of hepatitis A. *Lancet,* **2,** 748–751.
20. Alonso, E.M., Fox, A.S., Franklin, W.A. & Whitington, P.F. (1990) Post necrotic cirrhosis following varicella hepatitis in a liver transplant patient. *Transplantation,* **49,** 650–653.
21. Alper, C.A., Kruskall, M.S., Marcus-Bagley, D. *et al.* (1989) Genetic prediction of nonresponse to hepatitis B vaccine. *New England Journal of Medicine,* **321,** 708–712.
22. Alpert, E., Isselbacher, K.J. & Scheur, P.H. (1971) The pathogenesis of arthritis associated with viral hepatitis. *New England Journal of Medicine,* **285,** 185–189.
23. Alter, H.J., Holland, P.V., Purcell, R.H. *et al.* (1972) Post transfusion hepatitis after exclusion of commercial and hepatitis-B antigen positive donors. *Annals of Internal Medicine,* **77,** 691–699.

24. Alter, H.J. & Dienstag, J.L. (1984) The evolving spectrum of non-A, non-B hepatitis. In Chisari, F.V. (ed.) *Advances in Hepatitis Research*, pp. 281–292. New York: Masson Publishing.

25. Alter, H.J. (1985) Post transfusion hepatitis: clinical features, risk and donor testing. In Zuckerman, A.J. (ed.) *Infection, Immunity and Blood Transfusion*, pp. 47–61. New York: Alan R. Liss.

26. Alter, H.J. (1988) Transfusion-associated non-A, non-B hepatitis: the first decade. In Zuckerman, A.J. (ed.), *Viral Hepatitis and Liver Disease*, pp 537–542. London: Liss.

27. Alter, H.J., Purcell, R.H., Shih, J.W. *et al.* (1989) Detection of antibody to hepatitis C virus in prospectively followed transfusion recipients with acute and chronic non-A, non-B hepatitis. *New England Journal of Medicine*, **321**, 1494–1500.

28. Alter, M.J., Gerety, R.J., Smallwood, L.A. *et al.* (1982) Sporadic non-A, non-B hepatitis: frequency and epidemiology in an urban US population. *Journal of Infectious Diseases*, **145**, 886–893.

29. Alter, M.J., Ahtone, J., Weisfuse, I. *et al.* (1986) Hepatitis B virus transmission between heterosexuals. *Journal of the American Medical Association*, **256**, 1307–1310.

30. Alter, M.J., Mares, A., Hadler, S.C. & Maynard, J.E. (1987) The effect of underreporting on the apparent incidence and epidemiology of acute viral hepatitis. *American Journal of Epidemiology*, **125**, 133–139.

31. Alter, M.J., Coleman, P.J., Alexander, W.J. *et al.* (1989) Importance of heterosexual activity in the transmission of hepatitis B and non-A, non-B hepatitis in the United States. *Journal of the American Medical Association*, **262**, 1201–1205.

32. Alter, M.J., Hadler, S.C., Margolis, H.S. *et al.* (1990) The changing epidemiology of hepatitis B in the United States. Need for alternative vaccination strategies. *Journal of the American Medical Association*, **263**, 1218–1222.

33. Alter, M.J., Hadler, S.C., Judson, F.N. *et al.* (1990) Risk factors for acute non-A, non-B hepatitis in the United States and association with hepatitis C virus infection. *Journal of the American Medical Association*, **264**, 2231–2235.

34. Alter, M.J. (1991) Inapparent transmission of hepatitis C: Footprints in the sand. *Hepatology*, **14**, 389–391.

35. Alter, M.J., Horsburgh, C.R., Mayer, K.H. & Seage, G.R. (1991) Association of hepatitis C virus antibody with high risk behaviours in the United States. In Hillinger, F.B., Lemon, S.M. & Margolis, H.S. (eds) *Viral Hepatitis and Liver Disease*. Baltimore: Williams & Wilkins.

36. Ambrosch, F., Frisch-Niggemeyer, W., Kremsner, P. *et al.* (1987) Persistence of vaccine-induced antibodies to hepatitis B surface antigen and the need for booster vaccination in adult subjects. *Postgraduate Medical Journal*, **63**, 129–135.

37. Amontree, J.S., Stuart, T.D. & Bredfeldt, J.E. (1989) Autoimmune chronic active hepatitis masquerading as acute hepatitis. *Journal of Clinical Gastroenterology*, **11**, 303–307.

38. Anand, A., Gray, E.S., Brown, T. *et al.* (1987) Human parvovirus infection in pregnancy and hydrops foetalis. *New England Journal of Medicine*, **316**, 183–186.

39. Andre, F.E. (1989) Summary of safety and efficacy data on a yeast-derived hepatitis B vaccine. *American Journal of Medicine*, **87**, 14S-20S.

40. Antonucci, T.K., & Rutter, W.J. (1989) Hepatitis B virus (HBV) promoters are regulated by the HBV enhancer in a tissue-specific manner. *Journal of Virology*, **63**, 579–583.

41. Aragona, M., Macano, S., Caredda, F. *et al.* (1987) Serological response to the hepatitis delta virus in hepatitis D. *Lancet*, **1**, 478–480.

42. Arevalo, J.A. & Washington, A.E. (1988) Cost-effectiveness of prenatal screening and immunization for hepatitis B virus. *Journal of the American Medical Association*, **259**, 365–369.

43. Ariad, S., Yanai, I. & Sobel, R. (1989) Chronic infection with Epstein–Barr virus, chlamydia and hepatitis A virus, terminating in cirrhosis and nasopharyngeal carcinoma. *Israeli Journal of Medical Science*, **25**, 328–331.

44. Arnold, W., Meyer zum Büschenfelde, K.H., Hess, G. & Knolle, J. (1975) Intranuclear IgG in hepatocytes of patients with hepatitis-B-core-antigen (HBcAg) in liver tissue. *Digestion*, **12**, 277.

45. Arthur, M.J.P., Hall, A.J. & Wright, R. (1984) Hepatitis B, hepatocellular carcinoma, and strategies for prevention. *Lancet*, **1**, 607–610.

46. Asher, L.V., Innis, B.L., Shrestha, M.P. *et al.* (1990) Virus-like particles in the liver of a patient with fulminant hepatitis and antibodied hepatitis E virus. *Journal of Medical Virology*, **31**, 229–233.

47. Aufiero, B. & Schneider, R.J. (1990) The hepatitis B virus X-gene product *trans*-activates both RNA polymerase II and III promoters. *EMBO Journal*, **9**, 497–504.

48. Avanzani, M.A., Söderström, T., Wahl, M. *et al.* (1988) IgG subclass deficiency in patients with Down's syndrome and aberrant hepatitis B vaccine response. *Scandinavian Journal of Immunology*, **28**, 465–470.

49. Axelrod, P. & Feinstone, A.J. (1990) Infectious mononucleosis in old adults. *American Family Physician*, **42**, 1599–1606.

50. Baikie, M., Ratnam, S., Bryant, D.G. *et al.* (1989) Epidemiologic features of hepatitis B virus infection in northern Labrador. *Canadian Medical Association Journal*, **141**, 791–795.

51. Baker, A.L., Kaplan, M.M., Benz, W.C. *et al.* (1972) Polyarteritis associated with Australia antigen-positive hepatitis. *Gastroenterology*, **62**, 105–110.

52. Baker, B.L., Di Bisceglie, A.M., Kaneko, S. *et al.* (1991) Determination of hepatitis B virus DNA in serum using the polymerase chain reaction: Clinical significance and correlation with serological and biochemical markers. *Hepatology*, **13**, 632–636.

53. Balayan, M.S., Andjaparidze, A.G., Savinskaya, S.S. *et al.* (1983) Evidence for a virus in non-A, non-B hepatitis transmitted via the fecal-oral route. *Intervirology*, **20**, 23–31.

54. Baltimore, D. (1971) Expression of animal virus genomes. *Bacteriology Review*, **35**, 235–241.

55. Bamber, M., Murray, A., Arborgh, B.A.M. *et al.* (1981) Short incubation non-A, non-B hepatitis transmitted by factor VIII concentrates in patients with congenital coagulation disorders. *Gut*, **22**, 854–859.

56. Bamber, M., Murray, A.K., Weller, I.V.D.,*et al.* (1981) Clinical and histological features of a group of patients with sporadic non-A, non-B hepatitis. *Journal of Clinical Pathology*, **34**, 1175–1180.

57. Bamber, M., Murray, A.K., Lewin, J. *et al.* (1981) Ultrastructural features in chronic non-A, non-B (NANB) hepatitis: a controlled blind study. *Journal of Medical Virology*, **8**, 267–275.

58. Bänninger, P., Altorfer, J., Frösner, G.G. *et al.* (1983) Prevalence and significance of anti-HBc IgM (radioimmunoassay) in acute and chronic hepatitis B and in blood donors. *Hepatology*, **3**, 337–342.

59. Bannister, P., Miloszewski, K., Barnard, D. & Losowsky, M.S. (1983) Fatal marrow aplasia associated with non-A, non-B hepatitis. *British Medical Journal*, **286**, 1314–1315.

60. Baptista, A., Bianchi, L., De Groote, J. *et al.* (1988) Review: The diagnostic significance of periportal hepatic necrosis and inflammation. *Histopathology*, **12**, 569–580.

61. Bar, R.S., Adlard, J. & Thomas, F.B. (1975) Lymphopenic infectious mononucleosis. *Archives of Internal Medicine*, **135**, 334–337.

62. Barbara, J.A.J., Howell, D.R., Cleghorn, T.E. *et al.* (1977) A comparison of different methods of screening blood donations for HBsAg. *Vox Sanguinis*, **32**, 4–9.

63. Barbara, J.A.J., Howell, D.R., Contreras, M. *et al.* (1984) Indications for hepatitis B immunoglobulin for neonates of HBsAg carrier mothers. *British Medical Journal*, **289**, 880.

64. Barker, L.F. & Murray, R. (1972) Relationship of virus dose to incubation time of clinical hepatitis and time of appearance of hepatitis-associated antigen. *American Journal of the Medical Sciences*, **263**, 27–33.

65. Barker, L.F., Chisari, F., McGrath, P.P. *et al.* (1973) Transmission of type B viral hepatitis to chimpanzees. *Journal of Infectious Diseases*, **127**, 648–662.

66. Baskerville, A., Fisher-Hoch, S.P., Neild, G.H. & Dowsett, A.B. (1985) Ultrastructural pathology of experimental ebola haemorrhagic fever virus infection. *Journal of Pathology*, **147**, 199–209.

67. Bassetti, D., Cutrupi, V., Dallago, B. & Alfonsi, P. (1991) Second generation RIBA to confirm diagnosis of HCV infection (correspondence). *Lancet*, **337**, 912–913.

68. Bavand, M.R. & Laub, O. (1988) Two proteins with reverse transcriptase activities associated with hepatitis B virus-like particles. *Journal of Virology*, **62**, 626–628.

69. Bavand, M., Feitelson, M, and Laub, O. (1989) The hepatitis B

virus-associated reverse transcriptase is encoded by the viral *pol* gene. *Journal of Virology*, **63**, 1019–1021.

70. Beasley, R.P.& Huang, L.Y. (1983) Postnatal infectivity of hepatitis B surface antigen-carrier mothers. *Journal of Infectious Diseases*, **147**, 185–190.

71. Beasley, R.P., Hwang, L.-Y., Lee, G.C.-Y. *et al.* (1983) Prevention of perinatally transmitted hepatitis B virus infections with hepatitis B immune globulin and hepatitis B vaccine. *Lancet*, **2**, 1099–1102.

72. Beasley, R.P., Hwang, L.-U., Stevens, C.E. *et al.* (1983) Efficacy of hepatitis B immunoglobulin for prevention of perinatal transmission of the hepatitis B virus carrier state: final report of a randomized double-blind placebo-controlled trial. *Hepatology*, **3**, 135–141.

73. Bechtelsheimer, H., Korb, G. & Gedigk, P. (1972) The morphology and pathogenesis of 'Marburg' virus hepatitis. *Human Pathology*, **3**, 255–264.

74. Beebe, G.W. & Simon, A.H. (1970) Cirrhosis of the liver following viral hepatitis; a 20-year mortality follow-up. *American Journal of Epidemiology*, **62**, 279–286.

75. Beeson, P.B. (1943) Jaundice occurring one to four months after transfusion of blood or plasma. *Journal of the American Medical Association*, **121**, 1332–1334.

76. Begovac, J., Puntaric, V., Borcic, D. *et al.* (1988) Mononucleosis-like syndrome associated with a multisystem coxsackie virus type B3 infection in adolescents. *European Journal of Paediatrics*, **147**, 426–427.

77. Bell, H. (1971) Cardiac manifestations of viral hepatitis. *Journal of the American Medical Association*, **218**, 387–391.

78. Bell, J., Batey, R.G., Farrell, G.C. *et al.* (1990) Hepatitis C virus in intravenous drug users. *Medical Journal of Australia*, **153**, 274–276.

79. Bellabes, H., Bernatallah, A. & Bourguermouh, A. (1984) Non-A/non-B epidemic viral hepatitis in Algeria: Strong evidence for its water spread. In Vyas, G.N., Dienstag, J.L. & Hoofnagle, J.H. (eds) *Viral Hepatitis and Liver Disease,* p. 637. New York: Grune & Stratton.

80. Bellobuono, A., Mozzi, F., Petrini, G. *et al.* (1990) Infectivity of blood that is immunoblot intermediate reactive on hepatitis C virus antibody testing. *Lancet*, **336**, 309.

81. Benador, N., Mannhardt, W., Schranz, D. *et al.* (1990) Three cases of neonatal herpes simplex virus infection presenting as fulminant hepatitis. *European Journal of Paediatrics*, **149**, 555–559.

82. Benhamou, J.-P. (1991) Fulminant and subfulminant liver failure: Definition and causes. In Williams, R. & Hughes, R.D. (eds) *Acute Liver Failure*, pp. 6–10. London: Miter Press Limited.

83. Ben-Levy, R., Faktor, O., Berger, I. & Shaul, Y. (1989) Cellular factors that interact with the hepatitis B virus enhancer. *Molecular and Cellular Biology*, **9**, 1804–1809.

84. Bensabath, G., Hadler, S.C., Soares, M.C. *et al.* (1987) Hepatitis delta virus infection and Labrea hepatitis. Prevalence and role in fulminant hepatitis in the Amazon Basin. *Journal of the American Medical Association*, **258**, 479–483.

85. Berg, J.V.R., Berntsen, K.O., Björling, H. *et al.* (1974) Recovery of hepatitis B antibody from human plasma products separated by a modified Cohn fractionation. *Vox Sanguinis*, **27**, 302–309.

86. Berg, R., Ringerts, O. & Espmark, A. (1971) Australia antigen in hepatitis amongst Swedish trail finders. *Acta Pathologica et Microbiologica Scandinavica, Section B, Microbiology*, **79**, 423–427.

87. Bergamini, F. & Zanetti, A. (1987) Immunogenicity of yeast-derived hepatitis B vaccines in young adults. *Postgraduate Medical Journal*, **63**, 137–138.

88. Berger, J.R., Ayyar, D.R. & Sheremata, W.A. (1981) Guillain–Barré syndrome complicating acute hepatitis B. *Archives of Neurology*, **38**, 366–368.

89. Bergmann, K.F. & Gerin, J.L. (1986) Antigens of hepatitis delta virus in the liver and serum of humans and animals. *Journal of Infectious Diseases*, **514**, 702–705.

90. Berman, M., Alter, H.J., Ishak, K.G. *et al.* (1979) The chronic sequelae of non-A, non-B hepatitis. *Annals of Internal Medicine*, **91**, 1–6.

91. Bernuau, J., Goudeau, A., Poynard, T. *et al.* (1986) Multivariate analysis of prognostic factors of fulminant hepatitis B. *Hepatology*, 6, 97–106.

92. Berry, W.R., Gottesfeld, R.L., Alter, H.J. & Vierling, J.M. (1987) Transmission of hepatitis B virus by artificial insemination. *Journal of the American Medical Association*, **257**, 1079–1081.

93. Bianchi, L., De Groote, J., Desmet, V.J. *et al.* (1971) Morphological criteria in viral hepatitis. Review by an International Group. *Lancet*, **1**, 333–337.

94. Bianchi, L., De Groote, J., Desmet, V.J. *et al.* (1974) Guidelines for diagnosis of therapeutic drug induced liver injury in liver biopsies. Review by an international group. Lancet, **1**, 854–857.

95. Bianchi, L. & Gudat, F. (1976) Sandered nuclei in hepatitis B. Eosinophilic inclusions in liver cell nuclei due to excess in hepatitis B core antigen formation. *Laboratory Investigation,* **35**, 1–5.

96. Bianchi, L., De Groote, J., Desmet, V.J. *et al.* (1977) Acute and chronic hepatitis revisited. *Lancet*, **2**, 914–919.

97. Bishop, D.H. (1989) Infection and coding strategies of arenaviruses, phleboviruses, and nairoviruses. *Review of Infectious Diseases*, **11** (Suppl.4), S722-S729.

98. Bissell, D.M., Hammaker, L. & Schmid, R. (1972) Hemaglobin and erythrocyte catabolism in rat liver: the separate roles of parenchymal and sinusoidal cells. *Blood*, **40**, 812–822.

99. Bitter, G.A., Egan, K.M., Burnette, W.N. *et al.* (1988) Hepatitis B vaccine produced in yeast. *Journal of Medical Virology*, **25**, 123–140.

100. Bjorneboe, M. (1974) Viral hepatitis and cirrhosis. *Clinics in Gastroenterology*, **3**, 409–418.

101. Blainey, J.D., Earle, A., Flewett, T.H. & Williams, L.K.L. (1971) Is the urine infective in serum hepatitis? *Lancet*, **1**, 797.

102. Bloomer, J.R., Waldmann, T.A., McIntyre, K.R. & Klatskin, G. (1975) Relationship of serum alpha-fetoprotein to the severity and duration of illness in patients with viral hepatitis. *Gastroenterology*, **68**, 342–350.

103. Blum, A.L., Stutz, R. & Haemmerli, U.P. (1969) A fortuitously controlled study of steroid therapy in acute viral hepatitis. *American Journal of Medicine*, **47**, 82–92.

104. Blum, A.L., Berthet, P., Doelle, W. *et al.* (1977) Treatment of acute viral hepatitis with (+)-cyanidanol-3. *Lancet*, **2**, 1153–1155.

105. Blumberg, B.S., Alter, H.J. & Visnich, S. (1965) A 'new' antigen in leukemia sera. *Journal of the American Medical Association*, **191**, 541–546.

106. Blumberg, B.S., Gerstley, B.J.S., Hungerford, D.A. *et al.* (1967) A serum antigen (Australia antigen) in Downs's syndrome, leukaemia and hepatitis. *Annals of Internal Medicine*, **66**, 924–931.

107. Bonino, F., Hoyer, B., Nelson, J. *et al.* (1981) Hepatitis B virus DNA in the sera of HBs antigen carriers: a marker of active hepatitis B virus replication in liver. *Hepatology*, **1**, 386–391.

108. Bonino, F., Hoyer, B., Shih, J. *et al.* (1984) Delta hepatitis agent: structural and antigenic properties of the delta-associated particles. *Infection and Immunity*, **43**, 1000–1005.

109. Bonino, F., Heermann, K.H., Rizzetto, M., & Gerlich, W.H. (1986) Hepatitis delta virus: protein composition of delta antigen and its hepatitis B virus-derived envelope. *Journal of Virology*, **58**, 945–950.

110. Bonkowsky, H.L., Lee, R.V. & Klatskin, G. (1975) Acute granulomatous hepatitis. Occurrence in cytomegalovirus mononucleosis. *Journal of the American Medical Association*, **233**, 1284–1288.

111. Bortolotti, F., Bertaggia, A., Crivellaro, C. *et al.* (1986) Chronic evolution of acute hepatitis type B: prevalence and predictive markers. *Infection*, **14**, 64–67.

112. Bortolotti, F., Crivellaro, C., Pornaro, E. & Realdi, G. (1988) Hepatitis B in a nonresponder to hepatitis B vaccine. *Infection*, **16**, 119–120.

113. Bosh, V., Bartenschlager, R., Radziwill, G. *et al.* (1988) The duck hepatitis B virus P-gene codes for protein strongly associated with the 5′ end of the viral DNA minus strand. *Virology*, **166**, 475–485.

114. Botha, J.F., Ritchie, M.J.J., Dushieko, G.M. *et al.* (1984) Hepatitis B virus carrier state in black children in Ovamboland: role of perinatal and horizontal infection. *Lancet*, **1**, 1210–1212.

115. Boyer, J.L. & Klatskin, G. (1970) Pattern of necrosis in acute viral hepatitis. *New England Journal of Medicine, 283*, 1063–1071.

116. Brachott, D., Lifschitz, I., Mosley, J.W. *et al.* (1975) Potency of fragmented IgG; two studies of postexposure prophylaxis in type

A hepatitis. *Journal of Laboratory and Clinical Medicine*, **85**, 281–286.

117. Brackman, H.-H. & Egli, H. (1988) Acute hepatitis B infection after treatment with heat-inactivated factor VIII concentrate. *Lancet*, **2**, 967.

118. Bradley, D.W., Cook, E.H., Maynard, J.E. *et al.* (1979) Experimental infection of chimpanzees with antihemophilic factor (factor VIII) materials; recovery of virus-like particles associated with non-A, non-B hepatitis. *Journal of Medical Virology*, **3**, 253–269.

119. Bradley, D.W., Maynard, J.E., Popper, H. *et al.* (1983) Post transfusion non-A, non-B hepatitis: Physicochemical properties of two distinct agents. *Journal of Infectious Diseases*, **148**, 254–265.

120. Bradley, D.W., McCaustland, K.A., Cook, E.H. *et al.* (1985) Post transfusion non-A, non-B hepatitis in chimpanzees: Physicochemical evidence that the tubule-forming agent is a small, enveloped virus. *Gastroenterology*, **88**, 773–779.

121. Bradley, D.W.& Maynard, J.E. (1986) Etiology and natural history of post-transfusion and enterically-transmitted non-A, non-B hepatitis. *Seminars in Liver Disease*, **6**, 56–66.

122. Bradley, D.W., Krawczynski, K., Humphrey, C.D.& McCaustland, K.A. (1987) Biochemically silent posttransfusion non-A, non-B hepatitis interferes with superinfection by hepatitis A virus. *Intervirology*, **27**, 86–90.

123. Bradley, D.W., Krawczynski, K., Cook, E.H., Jr. *et al.* (1987) Enterically transmitted non-A, non-B hepatitis: serial passage of disease in cynomologous macaques and tamarins and recovery of disease-associated 27- to 34-nm viruslike particles. *Proceedings of the National Academy of Sciences of the USA*, **84**, 6277–6281.

124. Bradley, D.W., Andjaparidze, A., Cook, E.H. *et al.* (1988) Aetiological agent of enterically transmitted non-A, non-B hepatitis. *Journal of General Virology*, **69**, 731–738.

125. Bradley, D.W. (1990) Isolation and characterization of hepatitis E virus (HEV). In Bianchi, L., Gerok, W., Maier, K.-P. & Dienhardt, F. (eds) *Infectious Diseases of the Liver*, pp. 317–331. Dordrecht: Kluwer.

126. Bradley, D.W., Krawczynski, K., Beach, M.J. & Purdy M.A. (1991) Non-A, non-B hepatitis: Toward the discovery of hepatitis C and E viruses. *Seminars in Liver Disease*, **11**, 128–146.

127. Brahm, J., Vento, S., Rondanelli, E.G. *et al.* (1988) Sequential studies of pre-S2 antigenemia and anti-pre-S2 antibodies in relation to viral replication in acute hepatitis B followed from the early incubation phase. *Journal of Medical Virology*, **24**, 205–209.

128. Brahm, J., Fagan, E.A., Budkowska, A. *et al.* (1991) Prognostic significance of pre-S2 antigen and antibody in fulminant hepatitis B. *Journal of Hepatology*, **13**, 49–55.

129. Branch, A.D. and Robertson H.D. (1984) A replication cycle for viroids and small infectious RNAs. *Science*, **223**, 450–455.

130. Branch, A.D., Benenfeld, B.J., Baroudy, B.M. *et al.* (1989) An ultraviolet-sensitive RNA structural element in a viroid-like domain of the hepatitis delta virus. *Science*, **243**, 649–652.

131. Brechot, C., Hadchouel, M., Scotto, J. *et al.* (1981) Detection of hepatitis B virus DNA in liver and serum: a direct appraisal of the chronic carrier state. *Lancet*, **2**, 765–768.

132. Brettler, D.B., Alter, H.J., Dienstag, J.L. *et al.* (1990) Prevalence of hepatitis C virus antibody in a cohort of hemophilia patients. *Blood*, **76**, 254–256.

133. Brightman, C.A.J., Scadding, G.K., Dumbreck, L.A. *et al.* (1989) Yeast-derived hepatitis B vaccine and yeast sensitivity. *Lancet*, **1**, 903.

134. Brind, A.M., Codd, A.A., Cohen, B.J. *et al.* (1990) Low prevalence of antibody to hepatitis C virus in North East England. *Journal of Medical Virology*, **32**, 243–248.

135. British Medical Journal. (1977) Ebola virus infection (editorial). *British Medical Journal*, **2**, 539–540.

136. Brook, M.G., Lever, A.M.L., Kelly, D. *et al.* (1989) Antenatal screening for hepatitis B is medically and economically effective in the prevention of vertical transmission: Three years experience in a London hospital. *Quarterly Journal of Medicine*, **71**, 313–317.

137. Brooks, B R. (1977) Viral hepatitis type B presenting with seizure. *Journal of the American Medical Association*, **237**, 472–473.

138. Brown, S.E., Howard, C.R., Zuckerman, A.J. & Steward, M.W. (1984) Affinity of antibody responses in man to hepatitis B vaccine determined with synthetic peptides. *Lancet*, **2**, 184–187.

139. Bruguera, M., Cremades, M., Mayor, A. *et al.* (1987) Immunogen-

icity of a recombinant hepatitis B vaccine in haemodialysis patients. *Postgraduate Medical Journal*, **63**, 155–158.

140. Bruguera, M., Cremades, M., Rodicio, J.L. *et al.* (1989) Immunogenicity of a yeast- derived hepatitis B vaccine in hemodialysis patients. *American Journal of Medicine*, **87**, 30S-32S.

141. Bryan, J.A. & Gregg, M.B. (1975) Viral hepatitis in the US 1970–73: an analysis of morbidity trends and the impact of HBsAg testing on surveillance and epidemiology. *American Journal of the Medical Sciences*, **270**, 271–282.

142. Bryan, J.P., Sjogren, M., Iqbal, M. *et al.* (1990) Comparative trial of low-dose, intradermal, recombinant- and plasma-derived hepatitis B vaccines. *Journal of Infectious Diseases*, **162**, 789–793.

143. Budkowska, A., Dubrenil, P. & Pillot, J. (1988) Prognostic value of pre-S2 epitopes of hepatitis B virus and anti-pre-S2 response evaluated by monoclonal assays. In Zuckerman, A.J. (ed.) *Viral Hepatitis and Liver Disease*, pp. 287–289. London: Alan R Liss.

144. Budkowska, A., Dubrenil, P., Maillard, P. *et al.* (1990) A biphasic pattern of anti-pre-S responses in acute hepatitis B virus infection. *Hepatology*, **12**, 1271–1277.

145. Buitrago, B., Popper, H., Hadler, S.C. *et al.* (1986a) Specific histologic features of Santa Marta hepatitis: A severe form of hepatitis δ-virus infection in Northern South America. *Hepatology*, **6**, 1285–1291.

146. Buitrago, B., Hadler, S.C., Popper, H. *et al.* (1986b) Epidemiologic aspects of Santa Marta hepatitis over a 40-year period. *Hepatology*, **6**, 1292–1296.

147. Burk, K.H., Cabral, G.A., Dreesman, G.R. *et al.* (1981) Ultrastructural changes and virus-like particles localised in liver hepatocytes of chimpanzees infected with non-A, non-B hepatitis. *Journal of Medical Virology*, **7**, 1–19.

148. Burk, R.D., DeLoia, J.A., Elawady, M.K. & Gearhart, J.D. (1988) Tissue preferential expression of the hepatitis B virus (HBV) surface antigen gene in two lines of HBV transgenic mice. *Journal of Virology*, **62**, 649–654.

149. Burrell, C.J., Gowans, E.J., Jibert, A.R. *et al.* (1982) Hepatitis B virus DNA detection by in situ cyto-hybridisation: Implications for viral replication strategy and pathogenesis of chronic hepatitis. *Hepatology*, **2**, 85S-91S.

150. Busachi, C.A., Realdi, G., Alberti, A. *et al.* (1981) Ultrastructural changes in the liver of patients with chronic non-A, non-B hepatitis. *Journal of Medical Virology*, **7**, 205–212.

151. Buti, M., Esteban, R., Jardi, R. *et al.* (1986) Serological diagnosis of acute delta hepatitis. *Journal of Medical Virology*, **18**, 81–85.

152. Buti, M., Esteban, R., Jardi, R. *et al.* (1987) Clinical and serological outcome of acute delta infection. *Journal of Hepatology*, **5**, 59–64.

153. Buti, M., Esteban, R., Jardi, R. *et al.* (1987) Serological markers for delta hepatitis. *Lancet*, **1**, 815.

154. Buti, M., Esteban, R., Jardi, R. *et al.* (1988) Epidemiology of delta infection in Spain. *Journal of Medical Virology*, **26**, 327–332.

155. Butterly, L., Watkins, E. & Dienstag, J.L. (1989) Recombinant-yeast-derived hepatitis B vaccine in healthy adults: safety and two-year immunogenicity of early investigative lots of vaccine. *Journal of Medical Virology*, **27**(2), 155–159.

156. Callender, M.E., White, Y.S. & Williams, R. (1982) Hepatitis B virus infection in medical and health care personnel. *British Medical Journal*, **284**, 324–326.

157. Cameron, C.H. & Dane, D.S. (1974) Radioimmunoassay and saturation analysis. *British Medical Bulletin*, **30**, 90–92.

158. Campbell, D.H., Sargent, J.W. & Plant, A.J. (1989) The prevalence of markers of infection with hepatitis B virus in a mixed-race Australian community. *Medical Journal of Australia*, **150**, 489–492.

159. Canese, M.G., Rizzetto, M., Arico, S. *et al.* (1979) An ultrastructural and immunohistochemical study on the delta antigen associated with the hepatitis B virus. *Journal of Pathology*, **128**, 169–175.

160. Canese, M.G., Rizzetto, M., Novara, R. *et al.* (1984) Experimental infection of chimpanzees with the HBsAg-associated delta agent: an ultrastructural study. *Journal of Medical Virology*, **13**, 63–72.

161. Caporaso, N., Morisco, F., Romano, M. *et al.* (1990) Familial clustering of hepatitis C virus infection and chronic liver disease. *Italian Journal of Gastroenterology*, **22**, 281–282.

162. Cappel, R., De Cuyper, F. & van Beers, D. (1977) e Antigen and antibody, DNA polymerase and inhibitors of DNA polymerase in

acute and chronic hepatitis. *Journal of Infectious Diseases,* **136,** 617–622.

163. Cardiff, R.D. & Lund, J.K. (1976) Distribution of dengue-2 antigens by electron immunocytochemistry. *Infect Immun.,* **13,** 1699–1709.

164. Caredda, F., Antinori, S., Pastecchia, C. & Moroni, M. (1987) HBV/HDV coinfection. *Lancet,* **2,** 455.

165. Caredda, F., Antinori, S., Pastecchia, C. *et al.* (1988) A possible misdiagnosis in patients presenting with acute HBsAg-negative hepatitis: the role of hepatitis delta virus. *Infection,* **16,** 358–359.

166. Cariani, E., Zonaro, A., Primi, D. *et al.* (1991) Detection of HCV RNA and antibodies to HCV after needlestick injury. *Lancet,* **337,** 850.

167. Carl, M., Francis, D.P. & Maynard, J.E. (1983) Food-borne hepatitis A: recommendations for control. *Journal of Infectious Diseases,* **148,** 1133–1135.

168. Carman, W.F., Zanetti, A.R., Karayiannis, P. *et al.* (1990) Vaccine-induced escape mutant of hepatitis B virus. *Lancet,* **336,** 325–329.

169. Carne, C.A., Weller, I.V.D., Waite, J. *et al.* (1987) Impaired responsiveness of homosexual men with HIV antibodies to plasma derived hepatitis B vaccine. *British Medical Journal,* **294,** 866–868.

170. Caroli, J. & Ricordeau, P. (1961) Value of peritoneoscopy and peritoneoscopic photography in color and of scintillography in the diagnosis of liver disease. In Popper, H. & Schaffner, F. (eds) *Progress in Liver Diseases,* Vol. 1, pp. 296–314. New York: Grune & Stratton.

171. Carquel, A., Vigano, P., Davoli, C. *et al.* (1983) Sporadic acute non-A, non-B hepatitis complicated by aplastic anemia. *American Journal of Gastroenterology,* **78,** 245–247.

172. Casals, J. (1976) Arenaviruses. In Evans, A.S. (ed.) *Viral Infections in Humans,* pp. 103–125. New York: Plenum Press.

173. Case Records of the Massachussetts General Hospital (1988) Weekly clinicopathological exercises. *New England Journal of Medicine,* **319,** 495–509.

174. Castle, E. & Wengler, G. (1987) Nucleotide sequence of the 5'-terminal untranslated part of the genome of the flavivirus West Nile virus. *Archives of Virology,* **92,** 309–313.

175. Castro, A., Pedreira, J. and Sanchez, P. (1989) Hepatitis delta infection in North-west Spain. *Lancet,* **1,** 665.

176. Cattaneo, R., Will, H., Hernandez, N. & Schaller, H. (1983) Signals regulating hepatitis B surface antigen transcription. *Nature,* **305,** 336–338.

177. Centers for Disease Control (1987) Enterically transmitted non-A, non-B hepatitis — East Africa. *Morbidity and Mortality Weekly Report,* **36,** 241–244.

178. Centers for Disease Control (1987) Enterically transmitted non-A, non-B hepatitis — Mexico. *Morbidity and Mortality Weekly Report,* **36,** 597–602.

179. Chalmers, T.C., Eckhardt, R.D., Reynolds, W.E. *et al.* (1955) The treatment of acute infectious hepatitis. Controlled studies of the effects of diet, rest and physical reconditioning on the acute course of the disease and on the incidence of relapses and residual abnormalities. *Journal of Clinical Investigation,* **34,** 1163–1235.

180. Chalmers, T.C. (1973) Hemodialysis-associated hepatitis. *Journal of the American Medical Association,* **225,** 412–414.

181. Chang, C., Enders, G., Sprengel, R. *et al.* (1987) Expression of the precore region of an avian hepatitis B virus is not required for viral replication. *Journal of Virology,* **61,** 3322–3325.

182. Chang, L.-J., Dienstag, J., Ganen, D. & Varmus, H. (1989) Detection of antibodies against hepatitis B virus polymerase antigen in hepatitis B virus-infected patients. *Hepatology,* **10,** 332–335.

183. Chang, L.J., Pryciak, P., Ganem, D. & Varmus, H.E. (1989) Biosynthesis of the reverse transcriptase of hepatitis B viruses involves *de novo* translational initiation, not ribosomal frameshifting. *Nature,* **337,** 364–368.

184. Chang, M.F., Baker, S.C., Soe, L.H. *et al.* (1988) Human hepatitis delta antigen is a nuclear phosphoprotein with RNA-binding activity. *Journal of Virology,* **62,** 2403–2410.

185. Chao, M., Hsieh, S.Y. & Taylor, J. (1990) Role of two forms of hepatitis delta virus antigen: evidence for a mechanism of self-limiting genome replication. *Journal of Virology,* **64,** 5066–5069.

186. Chao, M., Hsieh, S.Y. & Taylor, J. (1991) The antigen of hepatitis delta virus: Examination of *in vitro* RNA-binding specificity. *Journal of Virology,* **65,** 4057–4062.

187. Charney, P., Pourcel, C., Louise, A. *et al.* (1979) Cloning in *Escherichia coli* and physical structure of hepatitis B virion DNA. *Proceedings of the National Academy of Sciences of the USA,* **76,** 2222–2226.

188. Chau, K.H., Hargie, M.P., Decker, R.H. *et al.* (1983) Serodiagnosis of recent hepatitis B infection by IgM class anti-HBc. *Hepatology,* **3,** 142–149.

189. Chaudhuri, A.K.R., Cassie, G. & Silver, M. (1975) Outbreak of food-borne type A hepatitis in Greater Glasgow. *Lancet,* **2,** 223–225.

190. Cheatham, W.J., Weller, T.H., Dolan, T.F. & Dower, J.C. (1956) Varicella: report of two fatal cases with necropsy, virus isolation and serologic studies. *American Journal of Pathology,* **32,** 1015–1035.

191. Chemello, L., Pontisso, P., Schiavon, E. *et al.* (1988) Hepatitis B core antigen in serum during acute hepatitis B. *Journal of Medical Virology,* **24,** 361–367.

192. Chemin, I., Baginski, I., Petit, M.A. *et al.* (1991) Correlation between HBV DNA detection by polymerase chain reaction and pre-S1 antigenemia in symptomatic and asymptomatic hepatitis B virus infections. *Journal of Medical Virology,* **33,** 51–57.

193. Chen, D.-S., Lai, M.-Y. & Sung, J.-L. (1984) Delta agent infection in patients with chronic liver diseases and hepatocellular carcinoma — an infrequent finding in Taiwan. *Hepatology,* **4,** 502–503.

194. Chen, D.-S., Hsu, N.H.-M., Sung, J.-L. *et al.* (1987) A mass vaccination program in Taiwan against hepatitis B virus infection in infants of hepatitis B surface antigen-carrier mothers. *Journal of the American Medical Association,* **257,** 2597–2603.

195. Chen, D.-S., Kuo, G.C., Sung, J.-L. *et al.* (1990) Hepatitis C virus infection in an area hyperendemic for hepatitis B and chronic liver disease: The Taiwan experience. *Journal of Infectious Diseases,* **162,** 817–822.

196. Chen, P-J, Kalpana, G., Goldberg, J. *et al.* (1986) The structure and replication of the genome of the hepatitis delta virus. *Proceedings of the National Academy of Sciences of the USA,* **83,** 8774–8778.

197. Chetham, M.F & Roberts, K.B. (1991) Infectious mononucleosis in adolescence. *Paediatric Annual,* **20,** 206–213.

198. Chiaramonte, M., Stroffolini, T., Ngatchu, T. *et al.* (1991) Hepatitis B virus infection in Cameroon: A seroepidemiological survey in city school children. *Journal of Medical Virology,* **33,** 95–99.

199. Chiba, J., Ohba, H., Matsuura, Y. *et al.* (1991) Serodiagnosis of hepatitis C virus (HCV) infection with an HCV core protein molecularly expressed by a recombinant baculovirus. *Proceedings of the National Academy of Sciences of the USA,* **88,** 14641–14645.

200. Child, P.L., MacKenzie, R.B., Valverde, L.R. & Johnson, K.M. (1967) Bolivian haemorrhagic fever: a pathologic description. *Archives of Pathology,* **83,** 434–445.

201. Chiou, S.-S., Yamauchi, K., Nakanishi, T. & Obata, H. (1988) Nature of immunological non-responsiveness to hepatitis B vaccine in healthy individuals. *Immunology,* **64,** 545–550.

202. Choi, S.S., Rasshofer, R. & Roggendorf, M. (1988) Propagation of woodchuck hepatitis delta virus in primary woodchuck hepatocytes. *Virology,* **167,** 451–457.

203. Choo, Q.L., Kuo, G., Weiner, A.J. *et al.* (1989) Isolation of a cDNA clone derived from a blood-borne non-A, non-B viral hepatitis genome. *Science,* **244,** 359–362.

204. Choo, Q-L., Weiner, A.J., Bradley, D.W. *et al.* (1990) Hepatitis C virus: The major causative agent of viral non-A, non-B hepatitis. *British Medical Bulletin,* **46,** 423–441.

205. Choo, Q.-L., Richman, K.H., Itan, J.H. *et al.* (1991) Genetic organisation and diversity of the hepatitis C virus. *Proceedings of the National Academy of Sciences of the USA,* **88,** 2451–2455.

206. Christenson, B. (1987) Epidemiology of hepatitis B in Sweden. *Journal of Infection,* **15,** 269–277.

207. Chung, D.-C., Ko, Y.-C., Chen, C.-J. *et al.* (1989) Seroepidemiology of hepatitis B virus, hepatitis D virus, and human immunodeficiency virus infections among parenteral drug abusers in Southern Taiwan. *Journal of Medical Virology,* **28,** 215–218.

208. Clarke, B.E., Newton, S.E., Carroll, A.R. *et al.* (1987) Improved immunogenicity of a peptide epitope after fusion to hepatitis B core protein. *Nature,* **330,** 381–384.

209. Clarke, J.A., Hollinger, F.B., Lewis, E. *et al.* (1989) Intradermal inoculation with Heptavax-B. *Journal of the American Medical Association*, **262**, 2567–2571.

210. Cocchi, P. & Silenzi, M. (1976) Pleural effusion in HBsAg-positive hepatitis. *Journal of Pediatrics,* **89**, 329–330.

211. Cockayne, E.A. (1912) Catarrhal jaundice, sporadic and epidemic and its relation to acute yellow atrophy of the liver. *Quarterly Journal of Medicine*, **6**, 1.

212. Cohen, B.J. & Richmond, J.G. (1982) Electron microscopy of hepatitis core antigen synthesized in *E. coli*. *Nature*, **296**, 677–678.

213. Cohen, J.I., Ticehurst, J.R., Purcell, R.H. *et al.* (1987) Complete nucleotide sequence of wild-type hepatitis A virus: comparison with different strains of hepatitis A virus and other picornaviruses. *Journal of Virology*, **61**, 50–59.

214. Cohen, J.I., Rosenblum, B., Ticehurst, J.R. *et al.* (1987) Complete nucleotide sequence of an attenuated hepatitis A virus: comparison with wild-type virus. *Proceedings of the National Academy of Sciences of the USA,* **84**, 2497–2501.

215. Cohen, J.I. (1989) Hepatitis A virus: insights from molecular biology. *Hepatology*, **10**, 889–895.

216. Cohen, J.I., Rosenblum, B., Feinstone, S.M. *et al.* (1989) Attenuation and cell culture adaptation of hepatitis A virus (HAV): a genetic analysis with HAV cDNA. *Journal of Virology,* **63**, 5364–5370.

217. Colgrove, R., Simon, G. & Ganem, D. (1989) Transcriptional activation of homologous and heterologous genes by the hepatitis B virus X gene product in cells permissive for viral replication. *Journal of Virology*, **63**, 4019–4026.

218. Collett, M.S., Larson, R., Gold, C., *et al.* (1988A) Molecular cloning and nucleotide sequence of the pestivirus bovine viral diarrhea virus. *Virology*, **165**, 191–199.

219. Collett, M.S., Larson, R., Belzer, S.K. & Retzel, E. (1988B) Proteins encoded by bovine viral diarrhea virus: The genomic organisation of a pestivirus. *Virology*, **165**, 200–208.

220. Collett, M.S., Anderson, D.K. & Retzel, E. (1988C) Comparisons of the pestivirus boving viral diarrhoea virus with members of the flaviviridae. *Journal of General Virology*, **69**, 2637–2643.

221. Collier, A.C., Corey, L., Murphy, V.L. & Handsfield, H.H. (1988) Antibody to human immunodeficiency virus (HIV) and suboptimal response to hepatitis B vaccination. *Annals of Internal Medicine,* **109**, 101–105.

222. Collins, J.D., Bassendine, M.F., Codd, A.A. *et al.* (1983) Prospective study of post-transfusion hepatitis after cardiac surgery in a British centre. *British Medical Journal*, **287**, 1422–1424.

223. Colombo, M., Cambieri, R., Rumi, M.G. *et al.* (1983) Long-term delta superinfection in hepatitis B surface antigen carriers and its relationship to the course of chronic hepatitis. *Gastroenterology*, **85**, 235–239.

224. Colombo, M., Oldani, S., Donato, M.F. *et al.* (1987) A multicenter prospective study of postransfusion hepatitis in Milan. *Hepatology*, **7**, 709–712.

225. Conn, H.O. (1976) Chronic hepatitis: reducing an iatrogenic enigma to a workable puzzle. *Gastroenterology*, **70**, 1182–1184.

226. Conn, H.O. (1983) Cyanidanol: will a hepatotrophic drug from Europe go West? *Hepatology*, **3**, 121–123.

227. Conteas, C., Henry, K., Rakela, J. & Weliky, B. (1983) Acute type A hepatitis in three patients with chronic HBV infection. *Digestive Diseases and Sciences*, **28**, 684–686.

228. Contreras, M., Barbara, J.A.J., Anderson, C.C. *et al.* (1991) Low incidence of non-A, non-B post-transfusion hepatitis in London confirmed by hepatitis C virus serology. *Lancet*, **337**, 753–757.

229. Cook, D.J., Riddell, R.H., Chernesky, M.A. & Salena, B.J. (1989) Relapsing hepatitis A infection with immunological sequelae. *Canadian Journal of Gastroenterology*, **3**, 145–148.

230. Co-operative Study (1971) Prophylactic gamma globulin for prevention of endemic hepatitis. Effects of US gamma globulin upon the incidence of viral hepatitis and other infectious diseases in US soldiers abroad. *Archives of Internal Medicine*, **128**, 723–738.

231. Cordellier, R. (1990) Yellow fever in Western Africa, 1973–87. Observed facts – studies realised, campaign, prevention and forecast. *World Health Statistical Quarterly*, **43**, 52–67.

232. Cordellier, R. (1991) The epidemiology of yellow fever in Western Africa. *Bulletin of the World Health Organisation*, **69**, 73–84.

233. Corey, L. & Holmes, K.K. (1980) Sexual transmission of hepatitis A in homosexual men: incidence and mechanism. *New England Journal of Medicine*, **302**, 435–438.

234. Cossart, Y.E. (1977) *Virus Hepatitis and its Control*. London: Baillière Tindall.

235. Cossart, Y.E., Kirsch, S. & Ismay, S.L. (1982) Post-transfusion hepatitis in Australia. *Lancet*, **1**, 208–213.

236. Coulepis, A.G., Locarnini, S.A., Westaway, E.G. *et al.* (1982) Biophysical and biochemical characterization of hepatitis A virus. *Intervirology*, **18**, 107–127.

237. Coulepis, A.G., Anderson, B.N. & Gust, I.D. (1987) Hepatitis A. *Advances in Virus Research*, **32**, 129–169.

238. Councilman, W.T. (1890) Pathologic histology of yellow fever. In Sternberg, G.M. (ed.) *Report on Etiology and Prevention of Yellow Fever*, pp. 151–159. U.S. Marine Hospital Service, Public Health Report Bulletin 1.

239. Coursaget, P., Yvonnet, B., Chotard, J. *et al.* (1986) Seven-year study of hepatitis B vaccine efficacy in infants from an endemic area (Senegal). *Lancet*, **2**, 1143–1145.

240. Coutinho, R.A., Lelie, N., Lent, P.A.-Van *et al.* (1983) Efficacy of a heat inactivated hepatitis B vaccine in male homosexuals: outcome of a placebo-controlled double blind trial. *British Medical Journal*, **286**, 1305–1308.

241. Coutinho, R.A., Lent, P.A.-Van, Lelie, N. *et al.* (1983) Prevalence and incidence of hepatitis A among male homosexuals. *British Medical Journal*, **287**, 1743–1745.

242. Crance, J.M., Biziagos, E., Passagot, J. *et al.* (1990) Inhibition of hepatitis A virus replication in vitro by antiviral compounds. *Journal of Medical Virology*, **31**, 155–160.

243. Craxi, A., Raimondo, G., Giannuoh, G. *et al.* (1983) Delta agent and hepatocellular carcinoma. In Rizzetto, M., Verme, G. & Bonino, F. (eds) *Viral Hepatitis and Delta Infection*. New York: Alan R Liss.

244. Craxi, A., Raimondo, G., Longo, G. *et al.* (1984) Delta agent infection in acute hepatitis and chronic HBsAg carriers with and without liver disease. *Gut*, **25**, 1288–1290.

245. Cromeans, T., Humphrey, C., Sobsey, M. & Fields, H. (1989) Use of immunogold pre-embedding technique to detect hepatitis A viral antigenic infected cells. *American Journal of Anatomy*, **185**, 314–320.

246. Crosnier, J., Jungers, P., Courouce, A.-M. *et al.* (1981a) Randomized placebo-controlled trial of hepatitis B surface antigen vaccine in French haemodialysis unit. I. Medical staff. *Lancet*, **1**, 455–459.

247. Crosnier, J., Jungers, P. & Courouce, A.M. (1981b) Randomized placebo-controlled trial of hepatitis B surface antigen vaccine in French haemodialysis unit. II. Haemodialysis patients. *Lancet*, **1**, 777–780.

248. Crovari, P., Crovari, P.C., Petrilli, R.C. *et al.* (1987) Immunogenicity of a yeast-derived hepatitis B vaccine (Engerix-B) in healthy young adults. *Postgraduate Medical Journal*, **63**, 161–164.

249. Cummings, I.W., Bronne, J.K., Salsar, W.A. *et al.* (1980) Isolation, characterization and comparison of recombinant DNAs derived from genomes of human hepatitis B virus and woodchuck hepatitis virus. *Proceedings of the National Academy of Sciences of the USA*, **77**, 1842–1846.

250. Dan, M. & Yaniv, R. (1990) Cholestatic hepatitis, cutaneous vasculitis, and vascular depostis of immunoglobulin M and complement associated with hepatitis A virus infection. *American Journal of Medicine*, **89**, 103–104.

251. Dane, D.S., Cameron, C.H. & Briggs, M. (1970) Virus-like particles in serum of patients with Australia antigen associated hepatitis. *Lancet*, **2**, 695–698.

252. Davis, L.G., Weber, D.J. & Lemon, S.M. (1989) Horizontal transmission of hepatitis B virus. *Lancet*, **1**, 889–892.

253. Davison, A.M., Williams, I.R., Mawdsley, C. & Robson, J.S. (1972) Neuropathy associated with hepatitis in patients maintained on haemodialysis. *British Medical Journal*, **1**, 409–411.

254. Dawson, D.G., Spivey, G.H., Korelitz, J.J. & Schmidt, R.T. (1987) Hepatitis B: risk to expatriates in South East Asia. *British Medical Journal*, **294**, 547.

255. Dawson, G.J., Lesniewski, R.R., Stewart, J.L. *et al.* (1991) Detection of antibodies to hepatitis C virus in US blood donors. *Journal of Clinical Microbiology*, **29**, 551–556.

256. De Cock, K.M., Govindarajan, S. & Redeker, A.G. (1987)

Serological response to hepatitis delta virus in hepatitis D. *Lancet*, **1**, 1438.

257. De Cock, K.M., Bradley, D.W., Sandford, N.L. *et al.* (1987) Epidemic non-A, non-B hepatitis in patients from Pakistan. *Annals of Internal Medicine*, **106**, 227–230.

258. Deeter, R.G. & Khanderia, U. (1986) Recent advances in antiviral therapy. *Clinical Pharmacology*, **5**, 961–976.

259. Degos, F., Lugassy, C., Degott, C. *et al.* (1988) Hepatitis B virus and hepatitis B-related viral infection in renal transplant recipients. *Gastroenterology*, **94**, 151–156.

260. De Groote, J.J. (1987) Therapeutic measures after hepatitis B virus infection: Postexposure prophylaxis. *Postgraduate Medical Journal*, **63**, 33–39.

261. Deinhardt, F. (1976) Hepatitis in primates. *Advances in Virus Research*, **20**, 113–157.

262. Deinhardt, F., Scheid, R., Gauss-Müller, V. *et al.* (1981) Propagation of human hepatitis A virus in cell lines of primary hepatocellular carcinomas. In Maupas, P. & Melnick, J. (eds) *Hepatitis B Virus and Primary Hepatocellular Carcinoma*, pp 109–113. Basel: S. Karger.

263. Deinhardt, F. & von der Helm, K. (1984) Cloning and expression of hepatitis A virus DNA in prokaryotic cells. In Chisari, F.V. (ed.) *Advances in Hepatitis Research*, pp. 263–267. New York: Masson Publishing.

264. Deinhardt, F.D. & Zuckerman, A.J. (1985) Immunisation against hepatitis B: report on a WHO meeting on viral hepatitis in Europe. *Journal of Medical Virology*, **17**, 209–217.

265. Delfini, C., Colloca, S., Taliani, G. *et al.* (1989) Clearance of hepatitis B virus DNA and pre-S surface antigens in patients with markers of acute viral replication. *Journal of Medical Virology*, **28**, 169–175.

266. DeLoia, J.A., Burk, R.D. & Gearhart, J.D. (1989) Developmental regulation of hepatitis B surface antigen expression in two lines of hepatitis B virus transgenic mice. *Journal of Virology*, **63**, 4069–4073.

267. Denis, F., Mounicer, M., Hessel, L. *et al.* (1984) Hepatitis B vaccination in the elderly. *Journal of Infectious Diseases*, **149**, 1019.

268. Deodhar, K.P., Tapp, E. & Scheuer, P.J. (1975) Orcein staining of hepatitis B antigen in paraffin sections of liver biopsies. *Journal of Clinical Pathology*, **28**, 66–70.

269. Derso, A., Boxall, E.H., Tarlow, M.J. & Flewett, T.H. (1978) Transmission of HBsAg from mother to infant in four ethnic groups. *British Medical Journal*, **1**, 949–952.

270. Desmet, V.J., Bullens, A.M. & De Groote, J. (1970) A clinical and histochemical study of cholestasis. *Gut*, **2**, 516–523.

271. Desmet, V.J. & De Groote, J. (1974) Histological diagnosis of viral hepatitis. *Clinics in Gastroenterology*, **3**, 337–354.

272. Desmyter, J., Colaert, J., de Groote, G. *et al.* (1983) Efficacy of heat-inactivated hepatitis B vaccine in haemodialysis patients and staff. Double blind placebo-controlled trial. *Lancet*, **2**, 1322–1332.

273. De Vos, R., De Wolf-Peeters, C., Fevery, J. & Desmet, V.J. (1981) Non-A non-B hepatitis in man: further evidence in favour of hepatitis-B like particles. *Liver*, **1**, 298–300.

274. De Vos, R., De Wolf-Peeters, C., Vanstapel, M.J. *et al.* (1982) New ultrastructural marker in hepatocytes in non-A, non-B viral hepatitis. *Liver*, **2**, 35–44.

275. De Vos, R., Vanstapel, M.J., Desmyter, J. *et al.* (1983) Are nuclear particles specific for non-A, non-B hepatitis? *Hepatology*, **3**, 532–544.

276. De Wolf-Peeters, C., De Vos, R., Desmet, V.J. & Fevery, J. (1981) A light microscopic marker of non-A, non-B viral hepatitis. *Journal of Clinical Pathology*, **34**, 814.

277. De Wolf-Peeters, C., De Vos, R., Desmet, V. *et al.* (1981) Human non-A, non-B hepatitis: ultrastructural alterations in hepatocytes. *Liver*, **1**, 50–55.

278. Dhingra, K., Michels, S.D., Winton, E.F. & Gordon, D.S. (1988) Transient bone marrow aplasia associated with non-A, non-B hepatitis. *American Journal of Hematology*, **29**, 168–171.

279. Dienes, H.P., Popper, H., Arnold, W. & Lobeck, H. (1982) Histological observations in human hepatitis non-A, non-B. *Hepatology*, **2**, 562–571.

280. Dienes, H.P., Grun, M., Hess, G. & John, H.D. (1983) Simultaneous infection with non-A, non-B and B viruses in a patient exhibiting different histologic patterns of acute hepatitis. *Liver*, **3**, 385–391.

281. Dienes, H.P., Hutteroth, T., Hess, G. & Meuer, S.C. (1987) Immunoelectron microscopic observations on the inflammatory infiltrates and HLA antigens in hepatitis B and non-A, non-B. *Hepatology*, **7**, 1317–1325.

282. Dienes, H.P., Purcell, R.H., Popper, H. & Ponzetto, A. (1990) The significance of infections with two types of viral hepatitis demonstrated by histologic features in chimpanzees. *Journal of Hepatology*, **10**, 77–84.

283. Dienes, H.P., Gerlich, W.H., Worsdorfer, M. *et al.* (1990) Hepatic expression patterns of the large and middle hepatitis B virus surface proteins in viremic and nonviremic chronic hepatitis B. *Gastroenterology*, **98**, 1017–1023.

284. Dienstag, J.L., Feinstone, S.M., Kapikian, A.Z. *et al.* (1975) Faecal shedding of hepatitis-A antigen. *Lancet*, **1**, 765–767.

285. Dienstag, J.L., Feinstone, S.M., Purcell, R.H. *et al.* (1975) Experimental infection of chimpanzees with hepatitis A virus. *Journal of Infectious Diseases*, **132**, 532–545.

286. Dienstag, J.L., Routenberg, J.A., Purcell, R.H. *et al.* (1975) Foodhandler-associated outbreak of hepatitis type A. An immune electron microscopic study. *Annals of Internal Medicine*, **83**, 647–650.

287. Dienstag, J.L., Gust, I.D., Lucas, C.R. *et al.* (1976) Mussel-associated viral hepatitis type A: serological confirmation. *Lancet*, **1**, 561–563.

288. Dienstag, J.L., Feinstone, S.M., Purcell, R.H. *et al.* (1977) Non-A, non-B post-transfusion hepatitis. *Lancet*, **1**, 560–562.

289. Dienstag, J.L., Szmuness, W., Stevens, C.E. & Purcell, R.H. (1978) Hepatitis A virus infection: new insights from seroepidemiologic studies. *Journal of Infectious Diseases*, **137**, 328–340.

290. Dienstag, J.L. (1983) Non-A, non-B hepatitis. I. Recognition, epidemiology, and clinical features. *Gastroenterology*, **85**, 439–462.

291. Dienstag, J.L. (1983) Non-A, non-B hepatitis. II. Experimental transmission, putative virus agents and markers, and prevention. *Gastroenterology*, **85**, 743–768.

292. Dienstag, J.L. (1989) Passive-active immunoprophylaxis after percutaneous exposure to hepatitis B virus. *Hepatology*, **10**, 385–387.

293. Dietrichson, O., Juhl, E., Christoffersen, P. *et al.* (1975) Acute viral hepatitis; factors possibly predicting chronic liver disease. *Acta Pathologica et Microbiologica Scandinavica. Section A: Pathology*, **83**, 183–188.

294. Dietzman, D.E., Harnisch, J.P., Ray, C.G. *et al.* (1977) Hepatitis B surface antigen (HBsAg) and antibody to HBsAg: Prevalence in homosexual and heterosexual men. *Journal of the American Medical Association*, **238**, 2625–2626.

295. DiGiusto, C.A. & Bernhard, J.D. (1986) Erythema nodosum provoked by hepatitis B vaccine. *Lancet*, **2**, 1042.

296. Doménech, P., Palomeque, A., Martinez-Gutiérrez A. *et al.* (1986) Severe aplastic anaemia following hepatitis A. *Acta Haematologica*, **76**, 227–229.

297. Domingo, P., Ris, J., Martinez, E. & Casas, F. (1990) Erythema nodosum and hepatitis C. *Lancet*, **336**, 1377.

298. Donati, D. & Gastaldi, L. (1988) Controlled trial of thymopentin in hemodialysis patients who fail to respond to hepatitis B vaccination. *Nephron*, **50**, 133–136.

299. Doorduyn, P.K. & Stuiver, P.C. (1989) Acute hepatic failure in hepatitis A. *Lancet*, **1**, 675.

300. Dreesman, G.R. (1984) Polypeptide and synthetic peptide vaccines for hepatitis B virus. In Chisari, F.V. (ed.) *Advances in Hepatitis Research*, Ch 23, pp. 216–222. New York: Masson Publishing.

301. Driss, F., Boboc, B., Zarski, J.P. *et al.* (1989) An epidemiological and clinica study of transaminase levels and hepatitis B antibodies in 1100 blood donors. *Vox Sanguinis*, **57**, 43–48.

302. Dublin, I.N., Sullivan, B.H., LeGolvan, P.C. & Murphy, L.C. (1960) The cholestatic form of viral hepatitis. Experiences with viral hepatitis at Brooke Army Hospital during the years 1951–1953. *American Journal of Medicine*, **29**, 55–72.

303. Dudley, F.J., Fox, R.A. & Sherlock, S. (1972) Cellular immunity and hepatitis-associated, Australia antigen liver disease. *Lancet*, **1**, 723–726.

304. Duermeyer, W. & van der Veen, J. (1978) Specific detection of IgM antibodies by ELISA applied in hepatitis A. *Lancet*, **2**, 684–685.

305. Dunnet, W.N. (1963) Infectious mononucleosis. *British Medical Journal*, **1**, 1187–1191.

306. Durand, J.M., Lefevre, P., Harle, J.R., *et al.* (1991) Cutaneous vasculitis and cryoglobulinaemia type II associated with hepatitis C virus infection. *Lancet*, **337**, 499–500.

307. Dusheiko, G.M. (1989) Review article: the management of hepatitis A, B, D and non-A non-B. *Alimentary Pharmacology & Therapeutics*, **3**, 1–20.

308. Dusheiko, G.M., Brink, B.A., Conradie, J.D. *et al.* (1989) Regional prevalence of hepatitis B, delta, and human immunodeficiency virus infection in southern Africa: a large population survey. *American Journal of Epidemiology*, **129**, 138–145.

309. Dusheiko, G.M., Smith, M. & Scheuer, P.J. (1990) Hepatitis C virus transmitted by human bite. *Lancet*, **336**, 503–504.

310. Ebeling, F., Nankkarinen, R. & Leikola, J. (1990) Recombinant immunoblot assay for hepatitis C virus antibody as predictor of infectivity. *Lancet*, **335**, 982–983.

311. Ebeling, F., Naukkarinen, R., Myllylä, G. & Leikola, J. (1991) Second generation RIBA to confirm diagnosis of HCV infection (correspondence). *Lancet*, **337**, 912–913.

312. Echevarría, J.M., León, P., Domingo, C.J. *et al.* (1991) Characterization of HBV2-like infections in Spain. *Journal of Medical Virology*, **33**, 240–247.

313. Edington, G.M. & White, H.A. (1972) The pathology of Lassa fever. *Transactions of the Royal Society of Tropical Medicine and Hygiene*, **66**, 381–389.

314. Edgington, T.S. & Ritt, D.J. (1971) Intrahepatic expression of serum hepatitis virus-associated antigens. *Journal of Experimental Medicine*, **134**, 871–885.

315. Edmondson, H. & Peters, R.L. (1977) Liver. In Anderson, W.A.D. & Kissane, J.M. (eds) *Pathology*, pp. 1321–1438. St Louis: C V Mosby.

316. Egea, E., Iglesias, A., Salazar, M. *et al.* (1991) The cellular basis for lack of antibody response to hepatitis B vaccine in humans. *Journal of Experimental Medicine*, **173**, 531–538.

317. Eknoyan, G., Gyorkey, F., Dichoso, C. *et al.* (1972) Renal morphological and immunological changes associated with acute viral hepatitis. *Kidney International*, **1**, 413.

318. El-Hazmi, M.A.F. (1989) Hepatitis B virus in Saudi Arabia. *Journal of Tropical Medicine and Hygiene*, **92**, 56–61.

319. Ellis, L.A., Brown, D., Conradie, J.D. *et al.* (1990) Prevalence of hepatitis C in South Africa: Detection of anti-HCV in recent and stored serum. *Journal of Medical Virology*, **32**, 249–251.

320. Elsner, B., Schwarz, E., Mando, O.G. *et al.* (1973) Pathology of 12 fatal cases of Argentine haemorrhagic fever. *American Journal of Tropical Medicine and Hygiene*, **22**, 229–236.

321. Emini, E.A., Larson, V., Eichberg, J. *et al.* (1989) Protective effect of a synthetic peptide comprising the complete preS2 region of the hepatitis B virus surface protein. *Journal of Medical Virology*, **28**, 7–12.

322. Enders, O., Ganem, D. & Varmus, H. (1985) Mapping the major transcripts of ground-squirrel hepatitis virus: the presumptive template for reverse transcriptase is terminally redundant. *Cell*, **42**, 297–308.

323. Enomoto, N., Takada, N., Takase, S. *et al.* (1990a) Nucleotide sequences and subtypes of hepatitis C virus genomes. *Gastroenterologia Japonica*, **25**, 404.

324. Enomoto, N., Takada, N., Takase, S. *et al.* (1990b) Nucleotide sequences and subtypes of hepatitis C virus genomes. *Gastroenterologia Japonica*, **25**, 405.

325. Enomoto, N., Takada, A., Nakao, T. & Date, T. (1990) There are two major types of hepatitis C virus in Japan. *Biochemical and Biophysical Research Communications*, **170**, 1021–1025.

326. Epon, L., Kosinski, K. & Hirsch, M.S. (1976) Hepatitis in an adult caused by herpes simplex virus type I. *Gastroenterology*, **71**, 500–504.

327. Eppinger, H. (1908) Die pathogene des Ikterus. *Ergebnisse der Inneren Medizin und Kinderheikunde*, **1**, 107.

328. Esteban, J.I., Esteban, R., Viladomiu, L. *et al.* (1989) Hepatitis C virus antibodies among risk groups in Spain. *Lancet*, **2**, 294–297.

329. Esteban, J.I., Gonzalez, A., Hernandez, J.M. *et al.* (1990) Evaluation of antibodies to hepatitis C virus in a study of transfusion-associated hepatitis. *New England Journal of Medicine*, **323**, 1107–1112.

330. Evans, A.S., Sprinz, H. & Nelson, R.S. (1953) Adrenal hormone therapy in viral hepatitis. I. The effect of ACTH and cortisone in severe and fulminant cases. *Annals of Internal Medicine*, **38**, 1115, 1134, 1148.

331. Everhart, J.E., Di Bisceglie, A.M., Murray, L.M. *et al.* (1990) Risk for non-A, non-B (type C) hepatitis through sexual or household contact with chronic carriers. *Annals of Internal Medicine*, **112**, 544–545.

332. Fagan, E., Yousef, G., Brahm, J. *et al.* (1990) Persistence of hepatitis A virus in fulminant hepatitis and after liver transplantation. *Journal of Medical Virology*, **30**, 131–136.

333. Fagan, E.A. & Williams, R. (1990) Fulminant viral hepatitis. *British Medical Bulletin*, **46**, 462–480.

334. Farci, P., Smedile, A., Lavarini, C. *et al.* (1983) Delta hepatitis in inapparent carriers of hepatitis B surface antigen. A disease simulating acute hepatitis B progressive to chronicity. *Gastroenterology*, **85**, 669–673.

335. Farci, P., Karayiannis, P., Lai, M.E. *et al.* (1988) Acute and chronic hepatitis delta virus infection: Direct or indirect effect on hepatitis B virus replication? *Journal of Medical Virology*, **26**, 279–288.

336. Farrow, L.J., Holborow, E.J., Johnson, G.D. *et al.* (1970) Autoantibodies and the hepatitis-associated antigen in acute infective hepatitis. *British Medical Journal*, **2**, 693–695.

337. Farza, H., Salmon, A., Hadchouel, M. *et al.* (1987) Hepatitis B surface antigen gene expression is regulated by sex steroids and glucocorticoids in transgenic mice. *Proceedings of the National Academy of Sciences of the USA*, **84**, 1187–1191.

338. Fauerholdt, L., Asnaes, S., Ranek, L. *et al.* (1977) Significance of suspected chronic aggressive hepatitis in acute hepatitis. *Gastroenterology*, **73**, 543–548.

339. Fay, O., Tanno, H., Gatti, H. *et al.* (1987) Anti-delta antibody in various HBsAg positive Argentine populations. *Journal of Medical Virology*, **22**, 257–262.

340. Feinman, S.V., Berris, B.K., Sinclair, J.C. *et al.* (1973) Relation of hepatitis B antigen subtypes in symptom-free carriers to geographical origin and liver abnormalities. *Lancet*, **2**, 867.

341. Feinman, S.V., Berris, B. & Borarski, S. (1988) Postransfusion hepatitis in Toronto, Canada. *Gastroenterology*, **95**, 464–469.

342. Feinman, S.V., Berris, B. & Herst, R. (1991) Anti-HCV in post-transfusion hepatitis: deductions from a prospective study. *Journal of Hepatology*, **12**, 377–381.

343. Feinstone, S.M., Kapikian, A.Z. & Purcell, R.H. (1973) Hepatitis A: detection by immune electron microscopy of virus-like antigen associated with acute illness. *Science*, **182**, 1026–1028.

344. Feinstone, S.M., Kapikian, A.Z., Purcell, R.H. *et al.* (1975) Transfusion-associated hepatitis not due to viral hepatitis type A or B. *New England Journal of Medicine*, **292**, 767–770.

345. Feitelson, M.A., Millman, I., Duncan, G.D. & Blumberg, B.S. (1988) Presence of antibodies to the polymerase gene product(s) of hepatitis B and woodchuck hepatitis virus in natural and experimental infections. *Journal of Medical Virology*, **24**, 121–136.

346. Feldman, R.G., Bryant, J., Ives, K.N. & Hill, N.C. (1987) A novel presentation of coxsackie B2 virus infection during pregnancy. *Journal of Infection*, **15**, 73–76.

347. Ferrari, C., Penna, A., Giuberti, T. *et al.* (1987) Intrahepatic nucleocapsid antigen specific T cells in chronic active hepatitis. *Journal of Immunology*, **139**, 539–544.

348. Ferrari, C., Chisari, F.V., Rubera, E. *et al.* (1988a) Functional modulation of hepatitis B core antigen specific T lymphocytes by an autoreactive T cell clone. *Journal of Immunology*, **141**, 1155–1160.

349. Ferrari, C., Penna, A., DegliAntoni, A. & Fiaccadori, F. (1988b) Cellular immune response to hepatitis B virus antigens. An overview. *Journal of Hepatology*, **7**, 21–33.

350. Fisher-Hoch, S.P., Price, M.E., Craven, R.B. *et al.* (1985) Safe intensive-care management of a severe case of Lassa fever with simple barrier nursing techniques. *Lancet*, **2**, 1227–1229.

351. Fitzgerald, G.R., Grimes, H., Reynolds, M. *et al.* (1975) Hepatitis-associated-antigen-positive hepatitis in a tuberculosis unit. *Gut*, **16**, 421–428.

352. Flanagan, P., Nuttall, P. & James, V. (1989) Post-transfusion hepatitis in Trent Regional Health Authority, 1988. *British Medical Journal*, **299**, 656–657.

353. Flehmig, B., Heinricy, U. & Pfisterer, M. (1989a) Immunogenicity of a killed hepatitis A vaccine in seronegative volunteers. _Lancet_, **1**, 1039–1041.

354. Flehmig, B. & Heinricy, U. (1989b) Hepatitis A vaccine — response to correspondence. _Lancet_, **2**, 114.

355. Fortier, D., Treadwell, T.L. & Koff, R.S. (1989) Enterically transmitted non-A, non-B hepatitis: Importation from Mexico to Massachusetts. _New England Journal of Medicine_, **320**, 1281–1282.

356. Foy, H.M., Cooney, M.K., McMahan, R. & Grayston, J.T. (1973) Viral and mycoplasmal pneumonia in a prepaid medical care group during an 8 year period. _American Journal of Epidemiology_, **97**, 93–102.

357. Frame, J.D., Baldwin, J.M., Jr, Gocke, D.J. & Troup, J.M. (1970) Lassa fever, a new virus disease of man from West Africa. I. Clinical description and pathological findings. _American Journal of Tropical Medicine and Hygiene_, **19**, 670–676.

358. Frame, J.D. (1989) Clinical features of Lassa fever in Liberia. _Review of Infectious Diseases_, **11** (Suppl. 4), S783–S789.

359. Francis, T.I., Moore, D.L., Edington, G.M. & Smith, J.A. (1972) A clinicopathological study of human yellow fever. _Bulletin of the World Health Organisation_, **46**, 659–667.

360. Franks, A.L., Berg, C.J., Kane, A.M. et al. (1989) Hepatitis B virus infection among children born in the United States to Southeast Asian refugees. _New England Journal of Medicine_, **321**, 1301–1305.

361. Fraser, G.M., Fraser, D., Chazan, R., et al. (1987) Hepatitis B infections in a chronic hemodialysis unit in a country where hepatitis B is endemic: A prospective study. _American Journal of Epidemiology_, **126**, 500–505.

362. Fried, M., Conen, D., Conzelmann, M. & Steinemann, E. (1987) Uveitis after hepatitis B vaccination. _Lancet_, **2**, 631–632.

363. Frösner, G.G., Shomerus, K.H., Wiedman, K.H. et al. (1982) Diagnostic significance of quantitative determination of hepatitis B surface antigen in acute and chronic hepatitis B infection. _European Journal of Clinical Microbiology_, **1**, 52–58.

364. Galibert, F., Chen, T.N., & Mandart, E. (1982) Nucleotide sequence of a cloned woodchuck hepatitis virus genome: comparison with the hepatitis B virus sequence. _Journal of Virology_, **41**, 51–65.

365. Ganem, D., Greenbaum, L. & Varmus, H.E. (1982) Virion DNA of ground squirrel hepatitis virus: structural analysis and molecular cloning. _Journal of Virology_, **44**, 374–383.

366. Ganem, D. & Varmus, H.E. (1987) The molecular biology of the hepatitis B viruses. _Annual Review of Biochemistry_, **56**, 651–693.

367. Garson, J.A., Tedder, R.S., Briggs, M. et al. (1990) Detection of hepatitis C viral sequences in blood donations by "nested" polymerase chain reaction and prediction of infectivity. _Lancet_, **335**, 1419–1422.

368. Garson, J.A., Ring, C., Tuke, P. & Tedder, R.A. (1990) Enhanced detection by PCR of hepatitis C virus RNA. _Lancet_, **336**, 878–879.

369. Garson, J.A., Tuke, P.W., Makris, M. et al. (1990) Demonstration of viraemia patterns in haemophiliacs treated with hepatitis-C-virus contaminated factor VIII concentrates. _Lancet_, **336**, 1022–1025.

370. Garson, J.A., Preston, F.E., Makris, M. et al. (1990) Detection by PCR of hepatitis C virus in factor VIII concentrates. _Lancet_, **335**, 1473.

371. Gauss-Muller, V. & Deinhardt, F. (1988) Immunoreactivity of human and rabbit antisera to hepatitis A virus. _Journal of Medical Virology_, **24**, 219–228.

372. Gauss-Müller, V., Mingquan, Z., von der Helm, K. & Deinhardt, F. (1990) Recombinant proteins VP1 and VP3 of hepatitis A virus prime for neutralizing response. _Journal of Medical Virology_, **31**, 277–283.

373. Gavish, D., Kleinmann, Y., Morag, A. & Chajek-Shaul, T. (1983) Hepatitis and jaundice associated with measles in young adults. An analysis of 65 cases. _Archives of Internal Medicine_, **143**, 674–677.

374. Gear, J.H. (1989) Clinical aspects of African viral haemorrhagic fevers. _Review of Infectious Diseases_, **11** (Suppl. 4), S777–S782.

375. Gehr, M.K., Chopra, S., Chung, T.J. & Hamburger, R.J. (1982) Polyarteritis nodosa after HBsAg hepatitis in a patient undergoing hemodialysis. _Archives of Internal Medicine_, **142**, 1554–1556.

376. Geisbert, T.W. & Jahrling, P.B. (1990) Use of immunoelectron microscopy to show ebola virus during the 1989 United States epizootic. _Journal of Clinical Pathology_, **43**, 813–816.

377. Gelb, D., West, M. & Zimmerman, H.J. (1962) Serum enzymes in disease: IX. Analysis of factors responsible for elevated values in infectious mononucleosis. _American Journal of Medicine_, **33**, 249–261.

378. Gelderblom, H.R., Kocks, C., L'Age-Stehr, J. & Reupke, H. (1985) Comparative immunoelectron microscopy with monoclonal antibodies on the yellow fever virus-infected cells: Pre-embedding labelling vs immunocryoultramycrotomy. _Journal of Virological Methods_, **10**, 225–239.

379. Gellis, S.S., Stokes, J., Brother, G.M. et al. (1945) The use of human immune serum globulin (γ globulin) in infectious (epidemic) hepatitis in the Mediterranean theater of operations. _Journal of the American Medical Association_, **128**, 1062–1063.

380. Genesca, J., Jardi, R., Buti, M. et al. (1987) Hepatitis B virus replication in acute hepatitis B, acute hepatitis B virus-hepatitis delta virus coinfection and acute hepatitis delta superinfection. _Hepatology_, **7**, 569–572.

381. Genesca, J., Esteban, J.I. & Alter, H.J. (1991) Blood-borne non-A, non-B hepatitis: Hepatitis C. _Seminars in Liver Disease_, **11**, 147–164.

382. Gerber, M.A., Sarno, E. & Vernace, S.J. (1976) Immune complexes in hepatocytic nuclei of HB Ag-positive chronic hepatitis. _New England Journal of Medicine_, **294**, 922–925.

383. Gerlich, W. & Robinson, W.S. (1980) Hepatitis B virus contains protein attached to the 5' terminus of its complete DNA strand. _Cell_, **21**, 801.

384. Gerlich, W.H., Deepen, R., Heermann, K.-H. et al. (1990) Prospects in immune prophylaxis of hepatitis B. In Bianchi, L., Gerok, W., Maier, K.-P. & Deinhardt, F. (eds) _Infectious Diseases of the Liver_, pp. 297–303. Dordrecht: Kluwer.

385. Gholson, C.F., Siddiqui, A. & Vierling, J.N. (1990) Cell surface expression of hepatitis B surface and core antigens in transfected rat fibroblast cell lines. _Gastroenterology_, **98**, 968–975.

386. Gianotti, F. (1973) Papular acrodermatitis of childhood. An Australia antigen disease. _Archives of Diseases of Children_, **48**, 794–799.

387. Gilks, W.R., Hall, A.J. & Day, N.E. (1989) Timing of booster doses of hepatitis B vaccine. _Lancet_, **2**, 1273–1275.

388. Gilli, P., Moretti, M., Soffritti, S. & Menini, C. (1990) Anti-HCV positive patients in dialysis units? _Lancet_, **336**, 243–244.

389. Gimson, A.E., Tedder, R.S., White, Y.S. et al. (1983) Serological markers in fulminant hepatitis B. _Gut_, **24**, 615–617.

390. Gimson, A.E., O'Grady, J., Ede, R.J. et al. (1986) Late onset hepatic failure: Clinical, serological and histological features. _Hepatology_, **6**, 288–294.

391. Giovannini, M., Tagger, A., Ribero, M.L. et al. (1900) Maternal-infant transmission of hepatitis C virus and HIV infections: a possible interaction. _Lancet_, **335**, 1166.

392. Girardi, E., Zaccarelli, M., Tossini, G. et al. (1990) Hepatitis C virus infection in intravenous drug users: Prevalence and risk factors. _Scandinavian Journal of Infectious Diseases_, **22**, 751–752.

393. Girones, R. & Miller, R.H. (1989) Mutation rate of the hapadnavirus genome. _Virology_, **170**, 595–597.

394. Gitlin, N. (1973) Extrahepatic manifestations of long incubation hepatitis (MS-2 hepatitis): an association with Henoch-Schönlein syndrome. Liver. _Proceedings of the International Liver Conference, Cape Town_, pp. 47–48. London: Pitman Medical.

395. Glenn, J.S. & White, J.M. (1991) Trans-dominant inhibition of human hepatitis delta virus genome replication. _Journal of Virology_, **65**, 2357–2361.

396. Global Advisory Group of the Expanded Programme on Immunisation (1988) _Weekly Epidemiology Record_, **63**, 9–12.

397. Gmelin, K., Kommerell, B., Waldherr, R. & Ehrlich, B.V. (1980) Intranuclear virus-like particles in a case of sporadic non-A, non-B hepatitis. _Journal of Medical Virology_, **5**, 317–322.

398. Gocke, D.J., Hsu, K., Morgan, C., Bombardieri, S. et al. (1970) Association between polyarteritis and Australia antigen. _Lancet_, **2**, 1149–1153.

399. Gocke, D.J., Hsu, K., Morgan, C. et al. (1971) Vasculitis in association with Australia antigen. _Journal of Experimental Medicine_, **134**, 330–336.

400. Gocke, D.J. (1972) A prospective study of post-transfusion hepa-titis. The role of Australia antigen. *Journal of the American Medical Association*, **219**, 1165–1170.

401. Gocke, D.J. (1975) Extrahepatic manifestations of viral hepatitis. *American Journal of Medical Sciences*, **270**, 49–52.

402. Gold, E. & Nankervis, G.A. (1976) Cytomegalovirus. In Evans, A.S. (ed.) *Viral Infections of Humans*, pp. 143–161. New York: Plenum Press.

403. Gonzalez, J.P., Josse, R., Johnson, E.D. *et al.* (1989) Antibody prevalence against haemorrhagic fever viruses in randomized representative Central African populations. *Research in Virology*, **140**, 319–331.

404. Goolsby, P.L. (1989) Erythema nodosum after Recombivax HB hepatitis B vaccine. *New England Journal of Medicine*, **321**, 1198–1199.

405. Gordon, S.C., Reddy, K.R., Schiff, L. & Schiff, E.R. (1984) Prolonged intrahepatic cholestasis secondary to acute hepatitis A. *Annals of Internal Medicine*, **101**, 635–637.

406. Gordon, S.C., Patel, A.S., Veneri, R.J. *et al.* (1989) Case report: Acute type A hepatitis presenting with hypotension, bradycardia, and sinus arrest. *Journal of Medical Virology*, **28**, 219–222.

407. Goudeau, A., Yvonnet, B., Lasage, G. *et al.* (1983) Lack of anti-HBc IgM in neonates with HBsAg carrier mothers argues against transplacental transmission of hepatitis B virus infection. *Lancet*, **1**, 1103–1104.

408. Goudeau, A., Denis, F., Mounier, M. *et al.* (1987) Comparative multicentre study of the immunogenicity of different hepatitis B vaccines in healthy volunteers. *Postgraduate Medical Journal*, **63**, 125–128.

409. Govindarajan, S., Chin, K.P., Redeker, A.G. & Peters, R.L. (1984) Fulminant B viral hepatitis: role of delta agent. *Gastroenterology*, **86**, 1417–1420.

410. Govindarajan, S., De Cock, K.M. & Peters, R.L. (1985) Morphologic and immunohistochemical features of fulminant delta hepatitis. *Human Pathology*, **16**, 262–267.

411. Gowans, E.J., Burrell, C.J., Jilbert, A.R. *et al.* (1981) Detection of hepatitis B virus DNA sequences in infected hepatocytes by in situ hybridization. *Journal of Medical Virology*, **8**, 67–78.

412. Gowans, E.J., Burrell, C.J., Jilbert, A.R. *et al.* (1983) Patterns of single and double stranded hepatitis B virus DNA and viral antigens accumulated in infected liver cells. *Journal of General Virology*, **64**, 1229–1239.

413. Gowans, E.J., Baroudy, B.M, Negro, F. *et al.* (1988) Evidence for replication of hepatitis delta virus RNA in hepatocyte nuclei after in vivo infection. *Virology*, **167**, 274–278.

414. Grady, G.F. & Bennett, A.J.E. (1972) National transfusion hepatitis study. Risk of post-transfusion hepatitis in the United States. *Journal of the American Medical Association*, **220**, 692–701.

415. Grady, G.F. & Lee, V.A. (1975) Hepatitis B immune globulin-prevention of hepatitis from accidental exposure among medical workers. *New England Journal of Medicine*, **293**, 1067–1070.

416. Grady, G.F. (1978) Transfusions and hepatitis: update in 1978. *New England Journal of Medicine*, **298**, 1413–1415.

417. Gray, J.J., Wreghitt, T.G., Friend, P.J. *et al.* (1990) Differentiation between specific and non-specific hepatitis C antibodies in chronic liver disease. *Lancet*, **335**, 609–610.

418. Green, M.S. & Dotan, K. (1988) Efficacy of immune serum globulin in an outbreak of hepatitis A virus infection in adults. *Journal of Infection*, **17**, 265–270.

419. Green, M.S. & Zaaide, Y. (1989) Sibship size as a risk factor for hepatitis A infection. *American Journal of Epidemiology*, **129**, 800–805.

420. Green, M.S., Block, C & Slater, P.E. (1989) Rise in the incidence of viral hepatitis in Israel despite improved socioeconomic conditions. *Reviews of Infectious Diseases*, **11**, 464–469.

421. Gregor, G.R., Geller, S.A., Walker, G.F. & Campomanes, B.A. (1975) Coxsackie hepatitis in an adult with ultrastructural demonstration of the virus. *Mount Sinai Journal of Medicine*, **12**, 575–580.

422. Gregory, P.B., Knauer, C.M., Kempson, R.L. & Miller, R. (1976) Steroid therapy in severe viral hepatitis. A double blind, randomized trial of methylprednisolone versus placebo. *New England Journal of Medicine*, **294**(13), 681–687.

423. Grendele, M., Gridelli, B., Colledan, M. *et al.* (1989) Hepatitis C virus infection and liver transplantation. *Lancet*, **2**, 1221–1222.

424. Grist, N.R. (1976) Hepatitis in clinical laboratories, 1973–74. *Journal of Clinical Pathology*, **29**, 480–483.

425. Grob, P.J. & Jemelka, H.I. (1972) Faecal SH-antigen in acute hepatitis. *American Journal of Diseases of Children*, **123**, 400–401.

426. Grob, P. (1982) Hepatitis B vaccination of renal transplant and haemodialysis patients. *Scandinavian Journal of Infectious Diseases. Supplementum*, **38**, 28–32.

427. Gudat, F., Bianchi, L., Sonnabend, W. *et al.* (1975) Pattern of core and surface expression in liver tissue reflects state of specific immune response in hepatitis B. *Laboratory Investigation*, **32**, 1–9.

428. Gupta, D.N. & Smetana, H.F. (1957) The histopathology of viral heaptitis seen in the Delhi epidemic (1955–56). *Indian Journal of Medical Research, Supplement*, **45**, 101.

429. Gust, I.D. & Feinstone, S.M. (1988) *Hepatitis A*. Boca Raton, Fla: CRC Press.

430. Hadler, S.C., de Monzon, M., Ponzetto, A. *et al.* (1984) An epidemic of severe hepatitis due to delta virus infection in Yucpa Indians in Venezuela. *Annals of Internal Medicine*, **100**, 339–344.

431. Hadzic, N., Alberti, A., Portmann, B. & Vergani, D. (1991) Detection of hepatitis B virus pre-S1 and pre-S2 determinants in paraffin wax embedded liver tissue: Importance of reagents used. *Journal of Clinical Pathology*, **44**, 554–557.

432. Hadziyannis, S.J., Lieberman, H.M., Karvountzis, G.G. & Shafritz, D.A. (1983) Analysis of liver disease, nuclear HBcAg, viral replication, and hepatitis B virus DNA in liver and serum of HBeAg vs anti-HBe positive carriers of hepatitis B virus. *Hepatology*, **3**, 656–662.

433. Hagler, L., Pastore, R.A. & Bergin, J.J. (1975) Aplastic anemia following viral hepatitis: report of two fatal cases and literature review. *Medicine*, **54**(2), 139–164.

434. Hague, R.V. (1975) Acute glomerulonephritis complicating Australia antigen-negative viral hepatitis. *Scandinavian Journal of Infectious Diseases*, **7**, 277–279.

435. Hahn, Y.S., Galler, R., Hunkapiller, T. *et al.* (1988) Nucleotide sequence of dengue 2 RNA and comparison of the encoded proteins with those of other flaviviruses. *Virology*, **162**, 167–180.

436. Hampers, C.L., Prager, D. & Senior, J.R. (1964) Post-transfusion anicteric hepatitis. *New England Journal of Medicine*, **271**, 747–754.

437. Han, J.H., Shyamala, V., Richman, K.H. *et al.* (1991) Characterisation of the terminal regions of hepatitis C viral RNA: Identification of conserved sequences in the 5′ untranslated region and poly (A) tails at the 3′ end. *Proceedings of the National Academy of Sciences in the USA*, **88**, 1711–1715.

438. Hanson, R.G., Hoofnagle, J.H., Minuk, G.Y. *et al.* (1984) Cell-mediated immunity to hepatitis B surface antigen in man. *Clinical and Experimental Immunology*, **57**, 257–264.

439. Hansson, B.G., Moestrup, T., Widell, A. *et al.* (1982) Infection with delta agent in Sweden: introduction of a new hepatitis agent. *Journal of Infectious Diseases*, **146**, 472–478.

440. Hassanein, T., Perper, J.A., Tepperman, L. *et al.* (1991) Liver failure occurring as a component of exertional heatstroke. *Gastroenterology*, **100**, 1442–1447.

441. Hauser, P., Voet, P., Simoen, E. *et al.* (1987) Immunological properties of recombinant HBsAg produced in yeast. *Postgraduate Medical Journal*, **63**, 83–91.

442. Havens, W.P. & Paul, J.R. (1945) Prevention of infectious hepatitis with γ globulin. *Journal of the American Medical Association*, **129**, 270–272.

443. Hay, C.R.M., Preston, F.E., Triger, D.R. & Underwood, J.C.E. (1985) Progressive liver disease in haemophilia: an understated problem? *Lancet*, **1**, 1495–1498.

444. Hayashi, H., Yagi, A., Ichimiya, H. *et al.* (1988) An outbreak of foodborne hepatitis A in a factory: A possible shift in age of patients in Japan. *International Journal of Epidemiology*, **17**, 870–873.

445. Hayashi, J., Kashiwagi, S., Nomura, H. *et al.* (1987) Hepatitis B virus transmission in nursery schools. *American Journal of Epidemiology*, **125**, 492–498.

446. He, L-F, Alling, D., Popkin, T. *et al.* (1987) Determining the size of non-A, non-B hepatitis virus by filtration. *Journal of Infectious Diseases*, **156**, 636–640.

447. He, L.F., Ford, E., Purcell, R.H. *et al.* (1989) The size of the hepatitis delta agent. *Journal of Medical Virology*, **27**, 31–33.

448. Heathcote, J., Cameron, C.H. & Dane, D.S. (1974) Hepatitis B antigen in saliva and semen. *Lancet*, **1**, 71–73.

449. Heathcote, J., Kim, Y.-I., Yim, C.K. *et al.* (1989) Interferon-associated lymphocyte 2′, 5′-oligoadenylate synthetase in acute and chronic viral hepatitis. *Hepatology*, **9**, 105–109.

450. Heermann, K.H., Goldmann, U., Schwartz, W. *et al.* (1984) Large surface proteins of hepatitis B virus containing the pre-S sequence. *Journal of Virology*, **52**, 396–402.

451. Heijtink, R.A., de Jong, P., Schalm, S.W. & Masurel, N. (1984) Hepatitis B vaccination in Down's syndrome and other mentally retarded patients. *Hepatology*, **4**, 611–614.

452. Heijtink, R.A., de Wilde, G.A., van Hattum, J. & Schalm, S.W. (1989a) Long-term immune reactivity to pre-S(2)-antigen after acute hepatitis B infection. *Journal of Medical Virology*, **27**, 95–99.

453. Heijtink, R.A., Knol, R.M. & Schalm, S.W. (1989b) Low-dose (2μg) hepatitis B vaccination in medical students: comparable immunogenicity for intramuscular and intradermal routes. *Journal of Medical Virology*, **27**, 151–154.

454. Hellström, U.B. & Sylvan, S.P.E. (1987) The immune response against pre-S2-encoded peptides and human serum albumin during hepatitis B virus infection. *Postgraduate Medical Journal*, **63**, 165–168.

455. Helmick, C.G., Webb, P.A., Scribner, C.L. *et al.* (1986) No evidence for increased risk of Lassa fever infection in hospital staff. *Lancet*, **2**, 1202–1205.

456. Hemling, M.E., Carr, S.A., Capiau, C. & Petre, J. (1988) Structural characterization of recombinant hepatitis B surface antigen protein by mass spectrometry. *Biochemistry*, **27**, 699–705.

457. Henkin, R.I. & Smith, F.R. (1971) Hyposmia in acute viral hepatitis. *Lancet*, **1**, 823–826.

458. Henson, D.E., Grimley, P.M. & Strano, A.J. (1974) Post natal cytomegalovirus hepatitis. *Human Pathology*, **5**, 93–103.

459. Hernandez, J.M., Piqueras, J., Carreras, A. & Triginer, J. (1983) Posttransfusion hepatitis in Spain. A prospective study. *Vox Sanguinis*, **44**, 231–237.

460. Higgins, G., Wreghitt, T.G., Gray, J.J. *et al.* (1990) Hepatitis A virus antibody in East Anglian blood donors. *Lancet*, **336**, 1330.

461. Hijikata, M., Kato, N., Mori, S. *et al.* (1990) Frequent detection of hepatitis C virus US strain in Japanese hemophiliacs. *Japanese Journal of Cancer Research*, **81**, 1195–1197.

462. Hijikata, M., Kato, N., Ootsuyama, Y. *et al.* (1991) Gene mapping of the putative structural region of hepatitis C virus genome by in vitro processing analysis. *Proceedings of the National Academy of Sciences of the USA*, **88**, 5547–5551.

463. Hijikata, M., Kato, N., Ootsuyama, Y. *et al.* (1991) Hypervariable regions in the putative glycoprotein of hepatitis C virus. *Biochemical and Biophysical Research Communications*, **175**, 220–228.

464. Hilleman, M., Buynak, K.E., McAleer, W. & McLean, A. (1981) Human hepatitis B vaccine. In *Proceedings of the European Symposium on Hepatitis B*, pp. 120–139. Hoddesdon: Merck Sharp and Dohme.

465. Hino, K. (1987) Epidemiological and experimental study of acute hepatitis type A with special reference to seasonal occurrence. *Acta Hepatologica Japonica*, **28**, 853–862.

466. Hirsch, R.C., Lavine, J.E., Chang, L-J. *et al.* (1990) Polymerase gene products of hepatitis B viruses are required for genomic RNA packaging as well as for reverse transcription. *Nature*, **344**, 552–555.

467. Hoagland, R.J. (1967) *Infectious Mononucleosis*. New York: Grune & Stratton.

468. Hoffmann, H., Tuma, W., Heinz, F.X. *et al.* (1987) Patient's risk of hepatitis B infection from medical staff. *Lancet*, **1**, 169–170.

469. Hoffmann, H., Tuma, W., Heinz, F.X., *et al.* (1988) Infectivity of medical staff for hepatitis B. *Infection*, **16**, 171–174.

470. Holborrow, E.J. (1972) Immunological aspects of viral hepatitis. *British Medical Bulletin*, **28**, 142–144.

471. Hollinger, F.B., Troisi, C., Heiberg, D., *et al.* (1986) Response to hepatitis B polypeptide vaccine in micelle form in a young adult population. *Journal of Medical Virology*, **19**, 229–240.

472. Hollinger, F.B. & Ticehurst, J. (1990) Hepatitis A virus. In Fields, B.N., Knipe, D.M. *et al.* (eds) *Virology*, 2nd Edn. pp. 637–666. New York: Raven Press.

473. Holman, C.D.J., Bucens, M.R., Quadros, C.F. & Reid, P.M. (1987) Occurrence and distribution of hepatitis B infection in the aboriginal population of Western Australia. *Australian and New Zealand Journal of Medicine*, **17**, 518–525.

474. Holter, E. & Siebke, J.-Chr. (1988) Hepatitis A in young Norwegian drug addicts and prison inmates. *Infection*, **16**, 91–94.

475. Honda, Y., Condo, J., Maeda, P. *et al.* (1990) Isolation and purification of a non-A, non-B hepatitis-associated microtubular aggregates protein. *Journal of General Virology*, **71**, 1999–2004.

476. Honigswachs, J., Faktor, O., Dikstein, R. *et al.* (1989) Liver-specific expression of hepatitis B virus is determined by the combined action of the core gene promoter and the enhancer. *Journal of Virology*, **63**, 919–924.

477. Hoofnagle, J.H. & Barker, L.F. (1976) Hepatitis B virus and albumin products. *Proceedings of Workshop on Albumin*. WH400 W927, pp. 305–314. Maryland: Bethesda NIH.

478. Hoofnagle, J.H., Gerety, R.J., Thiel, J. & Barker, L.F. (1976) The prevalence of hepatitis B surface antigen in commercially prepared plasma products. *Journal of Laboratory and Clinical Medicine*, **88**(1), 102–113.

479. Hoofnagle, J.H., Seeff, L.B., Bales, Z.B. *et al.* (1978) Type B hepatitis after transfusion with blood containing antibody to hepatitis B core antigen. *New England Journal of* Medicine, **298**, 1379–1383.

480. Hoofnagle, J.H., Michalak, T., Nowoslawski, A. *et al.* (1978) Immunofluorescence microscopy in experimentally induced type B hepatitis in the chimpanzee. *Gastroenterology*, **74**, 182–187.

481. Hoofnagle, J.H., Dusheiko, G.M., Seeff, L.B. *et al.* (1981) Seroconversion from hepatitis B e antigen to antibody in chronic type B hepatitis. *Annals of Internal Medicine*, **94**, 744–748.

482. Hoofnagle, J.H., Shafritz, D.A. & Popper, H. (1987) Chronic type B hepatitis and the "healthy" HBsAg carrier state. *Hepatology*, **7**, 758–763.

483. Hoofnagle, J.H. & Di Bisceglie, A.M. (1991) Serologic diagnosis of acute and chronic viral hepatitis. *Hepatology*, **11**, 73–83.

484. Hoofnagle, J.H. & Di Bisceglie, A.M. (1991) Serologic diagnosis of acute and chronic viral hepatitis. *Seminars in Liver Disease*, **11**, 73–83.

485. Hopf, U., Möller, B., Küther, D. *et al.* (1990) Long-term follow-up of posttransfusion and sporadic chronic hepatitis non-A, non-B and frequency of circulating antibodies to hepatitis C virus (HCV). *Journal of Hepatology*, **10**, 69–76.

486. Hosein, B., Fang, C.T., Popovsky, M.A., *et al.* (1991) Improved serodiagnosis of hepatitis C virus infection with synthetic peptide antigen from capsid protein. *Proceedings of the National Academy of Sciences of the USA*, **88**, 3647–3651.

487. Houghton, M., Choo, Q-L, & Kuo, G. (1989) European Patent Application 88,310,922.5 and Publ. 318,216.

488. Houghton, M., Choo, Q.-L. & Kuo, G. (1990) European Patent Application 90,302,806 and Publ. 388,232.

489. Houghton, M., Weiner, A., Han, J. *et al.* (1991) Molecular biology of the hepatitis C viruses: Implications for diagnosis, development and control of viral disease. *Hepatology*, **14**, 381–388.

490. Howard, C.R. & Burrell, C.J. (1976) Structure and nature of hepatitis B antigen. *Progress in Medical Virology*, **22**, 36–103.

491. Ho Yen, D.O., Hardy, R. McClure, J. *et al.* (1989) Fatal outcome of echovirus 7 infection. *Scandinavian Journal of Infectious Diseases*, **21**, 459–461.

492. Hruby, M.A. & Scharf, V. (1978) Transfusion-related short-incubation hepatitis in hemophilia patients. *Journal of the American Medical Association* **240**, 1355–1357.

493. Hsieh, S.Y., Chao, M., Coates, L. & Taylor, J. (1990) Hepatitis delta virus genome replication: a polyadenylated mRNA for delta antigen. *Journal of Virology*, **64**, 3192–3198.

494. Hsu, H.-M., Wang, Y.-F., Lo, S.-H. *et al.* (1990) Hepatitis D virus infection among intravenous drug abusers in Taiwan: Analysis of risk factors and liver function tests. *Journal of Medical Virology*, **31**, 76–81.

495. Hu, K.Q., Hao, L.J., Zhang, Y.Y. & Wang, Y.K. (1989) Intrahepatic expression of pre-S proteins of the hepatitis B virus and its possible relation to liver cell necrosis. *American Journal of Gastroenterology*, **84**, 1538–1542.

496. Hu, M., Kang, L. & Yao, G. (1990) An outbreak of Hepatitis A in Shanghai. In Bianchi, L., Gerok, W., Maier, K.P. & Deinhardt,

F. (eds) *Infectious Diseases of the Liver*, pp. 361–372. London: Kluwer.

497. Hughes, J.V., Stanton, L.W., Tomassini, J.E. *et al.* (1984) Neutralizing monoclonal antibodies to hepatitis A virus: partial localization of a neutralizing antigenic site. *Journal of Virology*, **52**, 465–473.

498. Hyams, K.C., Mansour, M.M., Massoud, A. & Dunn, M.A. (1987) Parenteral antischistosomal therapy: A potential risk factor for hepatitis B infection. *Journal of Medical Virology*, **23**, 109–114.

499. Hyams, K.C., Osman, N.M., Khaled, E.M. *et al.* (1988) Maternal-infant transmission of hepatitis B in Egypt. *Journal of Medical Virology*, **24**, 191–197.

500. Hyams, K.C., Okoth, F.A., Tukei, P.M. *et al.* (1989) Epidemiology of hepatitis B in Eastern Kenya. *Journal of Medical Virology*, **28**, 106–109.

501. Ichimura, H., Tamura, I., Tsubakio, T. *et al.* (1988) Influence of hepatitis delta virus superinfection on the clearance of hepatitis B virus (HBV) markers in HBV carriers in Japan. *Journal of Medical Virology*, **26**, 49–55.

502. Idéo, G., Bellati, G., Pedraglio, E. *et al.* (1990) Intrafamilial transmission of hepatitis C virus. *Lancet*, **335**, 353.

503. Ikeda, Y., Toda, G., Hashimoto, N. & Kurokawa, K. (1990) Antibody to superoxide dismutase, autoimmune hepatitis, and antibody tests for hepatitis C virus. *Lancet*, **335**, 1345–1346.

504. Imamura, T., Araki, M., Miyanohara, A. *et al.* (1987) Expression of hepatitis B virus middle and large surface antigen genes in *Saccharomyces cerevisiae*. *Journal of Virology*, **61**, 3543–3549.

505. Imazeki, F., Omata, M. & Ohto, M. (1990) Heterogeneity and evolution rates of delta virus RNA sequences. *Journal of Virology*, **64**, 5594–5599.

506. Inman, R.D., Hodge, M., Johnston, M.E.A. *et al.* (1986) Arthritis, vasculitis, and cryoglobulinemia associated with relapsing hepatitis A virus infection. *Annals of Internal Medicine*, **105**, 700–703.

507. Inoue, O. (1985) Morphological studies on the mechanism of hepatocellular injury during acute phase of infection in marmosets inoculated with hepatitis A virus. *Acta Pathologica Japonica*, **35**, 1319–1331.

508. Inoue, O., Itakura, H., Toriyama, K. *et al.* (1987) Ultrastructural study of lymphocyte interaction with hepatocytes and endothelial cells in acute non-A, non-B hepatitis. *Acta Pathologica Japonica*, **37**, 207–212.

509. Inoue, Y., Miyamura, T., Unayama, T. *et al.* (1991) Maternal transfer of HCV. *Nature*, **353**, 609.

510. International Commission (1978) Ebola haemorrhagic fever in Zaire, 1976. Dysentery, malaria, filariasis, measles, amoebiasis, pneumonia, tuberculosis and goitre. *Bulletin of the World Health Organization*, **56**, 271–293.

511. Ip, H.M., Wong, V.C.W., Leli, P.N. & Reesink, H.W. (1987) Should the dose of hepatitis B vaccine be reduced in newborn babies? *Lancet*, **2**, 1218–1219.

512. Ip, H.M., Lelie, P.N., Wang, V.C. *et al.* (1989) Prevention of hepatitis B virus carrier state in infants according to maternal serum levels of HBV DNA. *Lancet*, **1**, 406–410.

513. Irving, W.L., Parsons, A.J., Kurtz, J.B. & Juel-Jensen, B.E. (1987) Intradermal hepatitis B vaccine. *Lancet*, **2**, 561.

514. Irwin, G.R., Allen, R.G., Segal, H.G. *et al.* (1977) Serodiagnosis of hepatitis B virus infection by antibody to core antigen. *Journal of Infectious Diseases*, **136**, 31–36.

515. Ishak, K.G. (1973) Viral hepatitis: the morphologic spectrum. In Gall, E.A. & Mostofi, F.K. (eds) *The Liver* (International Academy of Pathology Monograph), pp. 218–268. Baltimore: Williams & Wilkins.

516. Ishak, K.G. (1976) Light microscopic morphology of viral hepatitis. *American Journal of Clinical Pathology*, **65**, 787–827.

517. Ishizaka, S., Kuriyama, S., Kikuchi, E., *et al.* (1990) A novel oral adjuvant for hepatitis B virus (HBV) vaccines. *Journal of Hepatology*, **11**, 326–329.

518. Itoh, Y., Iwakiri, S., Kitajima, K. *et al.* (1986) Lack of detectable reverse transcriptase activity in human and chimpanzee sera with a high infectivity for non-A, non-B hepatitis. *Journal of General Virology*, **67**, 777–779.

519. Iwarson, S., Magnius, L., Lindholm, A. & Lundin, P. (1973) Subtypes of hepatitis B antigen in blood donors and post-transfusion hepatitis: clinical and epidemiological aspects. *British Medical Journal*, **1**, 84–87.

520. Iwarson, S. (ed.) (1982) Vaccination against hepatitis B. *Scandinavian Journal of Infectious Diseases. Supplementum*, **36**, 79–81.

521. Iwarson, S. (1989) Post-exposure prophylaxis for hepatitis B: active or passive? *Lancet*, **2**, 146–148.

522. Iwarson, S. (1990) Hepatitis A virus immunisation. *Lancet*, **336**, 1590.

523. Jackson, D., Tabor, E. & Gerety, R.J. (1979) Acute non-A, non-B hepatitis: specific ultrastructural alterations in endoplasmic reticulum of infected hepatocytes. *Lancet*, **2**, 1249–1250.

524. Jahrling, P.B., Geisbert, T.W., Dalgard, D.W. *et al.* (1990) Preliminary report: Isolation of ebola virus from monkeys imported to USA. *Lancet*, **335**, 502–505.

525. Jameel, S. & Siddiqui, A. (1986) The human hepatitis B virus enhancer requires *trans*-acting cellular factors for activity. *Molecular and Cellular Biology*, **6**, 710–715.

526. Janot, C., Couroucé, A.M. & Maniez, M. (1989) Antibodies to hepatitis C virus in French blood donors. *Lancet*, **2**, 796–797.

527. Jansen, R.W., Newbold, J.E. & Lemon, S.M. (1988) Complete nucleotide sequence of a cell culture-adapted variant of hepatitis A virus: comparison with wild-type virus with restricted capacity for in vitro replication. *Virology*, **163**, 299–307.

528. Janzen, J., Tripatzis, I., Wagner, U. *et al.* (1978) Epidemiology of hepatitis B surface antigen (HBsAg) and antibody to HBsAg in hospital personnel. *Journal of Infectious Diseases*, **137**, 261–265.

529. Japanese Red Cross Non-A, Non-B Hepatitis Research Group. (1991) Effect of screening for hepatitis C virus antibody and hepatitis B virus core antibody of incidence of post-transfusion hepatitis. *Lancet*, **338**, 1040–1041.

530. Jardi, R., Buti, M., Rodriguez-Frias, F. *et al.* (1991) Clinical significance of two forms of IgM antibody to hepatitis delta virus. *Hepatology*, **14**, 25–28.

531. Jean-Jean, O., Salhi, S., Carlier, D. *et al.* (1989) Biosynthesis of hepatitis B virus e antigen: Directed mutagenesis of the putative aspartyl protease site. *Journal of Virology*, **63**, 5497–5500.

532. Jeffries, M.D.J., James, W.H., Jeffries, F.J.G. *et al.* (1973) Australia antigen (hepatitis-associated) in patients attending a venereal disease clinic. *British Medical Journal*, **2**, 455–456.

533. Jensen, D.M., McFarlane, I.G., Portmann, B.S. *et al.* (1978) Detection of antibodies directed against a liver-specific membrane lipoprotein in patients with acute and chronic active hepatitis. *New England Journal of Medicine*, **299**, 1–7.

534. Jia, X.-Y., Ehrenfeld, E. & Summers, D.F. (1991) Proteolytic activity of hepatitis A virus 3C protein. *Journal of Virology*, **65**, 2595–2600.

535. Jiang, X., Estes, M.K. & Metcalf, T.G. (1987) Detection of hepatitis A virus by hybridization with single-stranded RNA probes. *Applied and Environmental Microbiology*, **53**, 2487–2495.

536. Jilbert, A.R., Freiman, J.S., Burrell, C.J. *et al.* (1988) Virus-liver cell interactions in duck hepatitis B virus infection. A study of virus dissemination within the liver. *Gastroenterology*, **95**, 1375–1382.

537. Jilg, W., Schmidt, M. & Deinhardt, F. (1988) Persistence of specific antibodies after hepatitis B vaccination. *Journal of Hepatology*, **6**, 201–207.

538. Jilg, W., Schmidt, M. & Deinhardt, F. (1988) Immune response to hepatitis B revaccination. *Journal of Medical Virology*, **24**, 377–384.

539. Jilg, W., Schmidt, M. & Deinhardt, F. (1989) Vaccination against hepatitis B: Comparison of three different vaccination schedules. *Journal of Infectious Diseases*, **160**, 766–769.

540. Jilg, W., Schmidt, M. & Deinhardt, F. (1989) Four-year experience with a recombinant hepatitis B vaccine. *Infection*, **17**, 70–76.

541. Johnston, J.M., Harmon, S.A., Binn, L.N. *et al.* (1988) Antigenic and immunogenic properties of a hepatitis A virus capsid protein expressed in *Escherichia coli*. *Journal of Infectious Diseases*, **157**, 1203–1211.

542. Joint Committee on Vaccination and Immunisation. (1990) Immunoprophylaxis of Hepatitis A. In Salisbury, D. & Miller, C. (eds) *Immunisation against Infectious Disease*, pp. 96–97. London: HMSO.

543. Jonas, M.M., Schiff, E.R., O'Sullivan, M.J. *et al.* (1987) Failure of centers for disease control criteria to identify hepatitis B infection

in a large municipal obstetrical population. *Annals of Internal Medicine*, **107**, 335–337.

544. Jones, E.M.M. & Wilson, D.C. (1972) Clinical features of yellow fever cases at Vom Christian Hospital during the 1969 epidemic on the Jos Plateau, Nigeria. *Bulletin of the World Health Organization*, **46**, 653–657.

545. Junker-Niepmann, M., Bartenschlager, R. & Schaller H. (1990) A short cis-acting sequence is required for hepatitis B virus pregenome encapsidation and sufficient for packaging of foreign RNA. *EMBO J*, **9**, 3389–3396.

546. Jura, E., Chadwick, E.G., Josephs, S.H. *et al.* (1989) Varicella-zoster virus infections in children infected with human immunodeficiency virus. *Paediatric Infectious Diseases Journal*, **8**, 586–590.

547. Just, M., Berger, R. & Just, V. (1987) Reactogenicity and immunogenicity of a recombinant hepatitis B vaccine compared with a plasma-derived vaccine in young adults. *Postgraduate Medical Journal*, **63**, 121–123.

548. Kaganov, B.S., Nisevich, N.I., Uchaikin, V.F. *et al.* (1990) Acute viral hepatitis B in children: lack of chronicity. *Lancet*, **336**, 374–375.

549. Kam, W., Rall, L.B., Smuckler, E.A. *et al.* (1982) Hepatitis B viral DNA in liver and serum of asymptomatic carrier. *Proceedings of the National Academy of Sciences of the USA*, **79**, 7522–7526.

550. Kamimura, T., Ponzetto, A., Bonino, F. *et al.* (1983) Cytoplasmic tubular structures in liver of HBsAg carrier chimpanzees infected with delta agent and comparison with cytoplasmic structures in non-A, non-B hepatitis. *Hepatology*, **3**, 631–637.

551. Kamitsukasa, H., Harada, H., Yakura, M. *et al.* (1989) Intrafamilial transmission of hepatitis C virus. *Lancet*, **2**, 987.

552. Kane, M.A., Bradley, D.W., Shrestha, S.M. *et al.* (1984) Epidemic non-A, non-B hepatitis in Nepal: Recovery of a possible etiologic agent and transmission studies in marmosets. *Journal of the American Medical Association* 252, 3140–3145.

553. Kane, M.A., Alter, M.J., Hadler, S.C. & Margolis, H.S. (1989) Hepatitis B infection in the United States. Recent trends and future strategies for control. *American Journal of Medicine, 87*, 11S-13S.

554. Kaneko, S., Unoura, M., Kobayashi, K. *et al.* (1990) Detection of serum hepatitis C virus RNA. *Lancet*, **335**, 976.

554a. Kao, H.W., Asheavi, M. & Redeker, A.G. (1984) The persistence of Hepatitis A IgM antibody after acute hepatitis A. *Hepatology*, **4**, 933–936.

555. Karayiannis, P., Saldanha, J., Monjardino, J. *et al.* (1990) Immunization of woodchucks with recombinant hepatitis delta antigen does not protect against hepatitis delta virus infection. *Hepatology*, **12**, 1125–1128.

556. Karpen, S., Banerjee, R., Zelent, A. *et al.* (1988) Identification of protein-binding sites in the hepatitis B virus enhancer and core promoter domains. *Molecular and Cellular Biology*, **8**, 5159–5165.

557. Karron, R.A., Daemer, R., Ticehurst, J. *et al.* (1988) Studies of prototype live hepatitis A virus vaccines in primate models. *Journal of Infectious Diseases*, **157**, 338–345.

558. Karvountzis, G.G., Redeker, A.G. & Peters, R.L. (1975) Long term follow-up studies of patients surviving fulminant viral hepatitis. *Gastroenterology*, **67**, 870–877.

559. Kashiwagi, S., Hayashi, J., Nomura, H. *et al.* (1988) Changing pattern of intrafamilial transmission of hepatitis B virus in Okinawa, Japan. *American Journal of Epidemiology*, **127**, 783–787.

560. Katayama, T., Saito, I., Katayama, T. *et al.* (1990) Blood screening for non-A, non-B hepatitis by hepatitis C virus antibody assay. *Transfusion*, **301**, 374–376.

561. Katkov, W.N. & Dienstag, J.L. (1991) Prevention and therapy of viral hepatitis. *Seminars in Liver Disease*, **11**, 165–174.

562. Kato, N., Ohkoshi, S. & Shomotohno, K. (1989) Japanese isolates of the non-A, non-B hepatitis viral genome show sequence variations from the original isolate in the USA. *Proceedings of the Japanese Academy*, **65B**, 219–223.

563. Kato, N., Hijikata, M., Ootsuyama, Y. *et al.* (1990) Molecular cloning of the human hepatitis C virus genome from Japanese patients with non-A, non-B hepatitis. *Proceedings of the National Academy of Sciences in the USA, 87*, 9524–9528.

564. Kato, N., Hijikata, M., Ootsuyama, Y. *et al.* (1990) A structural protein encoded by the 5' region of the hepatitis C virus genome

565. Kefene, H., Rapicetta, M., Rossi, G.B. *et al.* (1988) Ethiopian National Hepatitis B Study. *Journal of Medical Virology*, **24**, 75–83.

566. Kelly, V., Kensit, J. & Barrett, A. (1989) Hepatitis D (delta) infection in South-east London. *Lancet*, **1**, 45.

567. Kent, G.P., Brondum, J., Keenlyside, R.A. *et al.* (1988) A large outbreak of acupuncture-associated hepatitis B. *American Journal of Epidemiology*, **127**, 591–598.

568. Kerr, J.A. (1973) Liver pathology in yellow fever. *Transactions of the Royal Society of Tropical Medicine and Hygiene*, **67**, 882.

569. Kew, M.C., Purves, L.R. & Bershon, I. (1973) Serum alpha-fetoprotein levels in acute viral hepatitis. *Gut*, **14**, 939–942.

570. Kew, M.C., Dusheiko, G.M., Hadziyannis, S.J. & Patterson, A. (1984) Does delta infection play a part in the pathogenesis of hepatitis B virus related hepatocellular carcinoma? *British Medical Journal*, **288**, 1727.

571. Kew, M.C., Houghton, M., Choo, Q.-L. & Kuo, G. (1990) Hepatitis C virus antibodies in Southern African blacks with hepatocellular carcinoma. *Lancet*, **335**, 873–874.

572. Khuroo, M.S., Teli, M.R., Skidmore, S. *et al.* (1981) Incidence and severity of viral hepatitis in pregnancy. *American Journal of Medicine*, **70**, 252–255.

573. Khuroo, M.S., Deurmeyer, W., Zargar, S.A. *et al.* (1983) Acute sporadic NANB hepatitis in India. *American Journal of Epidemiology*, **118**, 360–364.

574. Kiley, M.P., Cox, N.J., Elliott, L.H. *et al.* (1988) Physicochemical properties of Marburg virus: Evidence for three distinct virus strains and their relationship to the ebola virus. *Journal of General Virology*, **69**, 1957–1967.

575. Kindmark, C.-O., Sjolin, J., Nordlinder, H. *et al.* (1984) Aplastic anaemia in a case of hepatitis B with a high titer of hepatitis B antigen. *Acta Medica Scandinavica*, **215**, 89–92.

576. King, J.W., Taylor, E.M., Crow, S.D. *et al.* (1990) Comparison of the immunogenicity of hepatitis B vaccine administered intradermally and intramuscularly. *Reviews of Infectious Diseases*, **12**, 1035–1043.

577. King, S.M., Jarvis, D.A., Shaw, J. *et al.* (1987) Prevalence of hepatitis B surface antigen and antibody (hepatitis B virus markers) in personnel at a children's hospital. *American Journal of Epidemiology*, **126**, 480–483.

578. Kingham, J.G.C. & Wright, R. (1978) Unpublished observations.

579. Kingham, J.G.C., McGuire, M.J., Paine, D.H.D. & Wright, R. (1978) Hepatitis B in a hospital for the mentally subnormal in Southern England. *British Medical Journal*, **2**, 594–596.

580. Kissling, R.E., Robinson, R.Q., Murphy, F.A. & Whitfield, S. (1968) Green monkey agent of disease. *Science*, **161**, 1364.

581. Kivel, R.M. (1961) Hematologic aspects of acute viral hepatitis. *American Journal of Digestive Diseases*, **6**, 1017–1031.

582. Kiyosawa, K., Sodeyama, T., Tanaka, E. *et al.* (1991) Intrafamilial transmission of hepatitis C virus in Japan. *Journal of Medical Virology*, **33**, 114–116.

583. Kniskern, P.J., Hagopian, A., Burke, P. *et al.* (1988) A candidate vaccine for hepatitis B containing the complete viral surface protein. *Hepatology*, **8**, 82–87.

584. Knodell, R.G., Conrad, M.E., Dienstag, J.L. & Bell, C.J. (1975) Etiological spectrum of post-transfusion hepatitis. *Gastroenterology*, **69**, 1278–1285.

585. Knodell, R.G., Conrad, M.E., Dienstag, J.L. *et al.* (1978) Etiological spectrum of post- transfusion hepatitis. *Gastroenterology*, **72**, 111–121.

586. Ko, Y.-C., Yen, Y.-Y., Yeh, S.-M. & Lan, S.-J. (1989) Female to male transmission of hepatitis B virus between Chinese spouses. *Journal of Medical Virology*, **27**, 142–144.

587. Kobayashi, M. & Koike, K. (1984) Complete nucleotide sequence of hepatitis B virus DNA of subtype adr and its conserved gene organization. *Gene*, **30**, 227–232.

588. Kodama, K., Ogasawara, N., Yoshikawa, H. & Murakami, S. (1985) Nucleotide sequence of a cloned woodchuck hepatitis virus genome: Evolutional relationship between hepdnaviruses. *Journal of Virology*, **56**, 978–986.

589. Koff, R.S., Slavin, M.M., Connelly, L.J.D. & Rosen, D.R. (1977)

Contagiousness of acute hepatitis B. Secondary attack rates in household contacts. *Gastroenterology*, **72**, 297–300.

590. Kohler, P.F., Dubois, R.S., Merrill, D.A. & Bowes, W.A. (1974) Prevention of chronic neonatal hepatitis B virus infection with antibody to the hepatitis B surface antigen. *New England Journal of Medicine*, **291**, 1378–1380.

591. Koike, K., Akatsuka, T. & Miyamura, T. (1988) Characterization of hepatitis B virus X gene: *In vitro* translation of mRNA from COS-1 cells transfected with the X gene. *Virology*, **163**, 233–235.

592. Korba, B.E., Cote, P.J. & Gerin, J.L. (1988) Mitogen-induced replication of woodchuck hepatitis virus in cultured peripheral blood lymphocytes. *Science*, **241**, 1213–1216.

593. Koretz, R.L., Stone, O. & Gitnick, G.L. (1980) The long-term course of non-A, non-B post-transfusion hepatitis. *Gastroenterology*, **79**, 893–898.

594. Kornberg, A. (1980) *DNA Replication*. San Francisco: Freeman.

595. Kos, A., Dijkema, R., Arnberg, A.C. *et al.* (1986) The hepatitis delta virus possesses a circular RNA. *Nature*, **323**, 558–560.

596. Kos, A., de Reus, A., Dubbeld, M. *et al.* (1987) Biological and molecular characterization of the hepatitis delta virus. *Progress in Clinical and Biological Research*, **234**, 83–87.

597. Kosaka, Y., Takase, K., Kojima, M. *et al.* (1991) Fulminant hepatitis B: Induction by hepatitis B virus mutants defective in the precore region and incapable of encoding e antigen. *Gastroenterology*, **100**, 1087–1094.

598. Kosmidis, J.C. & Leader-Williams, L.K. (1972) Complement levels in acute infectious hepatitis and serum hepatitis. *Clinical and Experimental Immunology*, **11**, 31–35.

599. Kourinski, M. & Claveri, J.P. (1989) MHC-antigen interaction: What does the T-cell see? *Advances in Immunology*, **45**, 107.

600. Koziol, D.E., Alter, H.J., Kirchner, J.P. *et al.* (1976) The development of HBsAg-positive hepatitis despite the previous existence of antibody to HBsAg. *Journal of Immunology*, **117**, 2260–2262.

601. Krawczynski, K. & Bradley, D.W. (1989) Enterically transmitted non-A, non-B hepatitis: Identification of virus-associated antigen in experimentally infected cynomolgus macaques. *Journal of Infectious Diseases*, **159**, 1042–1049.

602. Krawczynski, K., Bradley, D.W., Ajdukiewicz, A. *et al.* (In press) Virus associated antigen and antibody of epidemic non-A, non-B hepatitis: Serology of outbreaks and sporadic cases. In Shikata, T. (ed.) *Proceedings of International Symposium of Non-A, Non-B Hepatitis and Blood-Borne Infectious Diseases, Tokyo 1989*. Amsterdam: Elsevier.

603. Krikler, D.M. & Zilberg, B. (1966) Activity and hepatitis. *Lancet*, **2**, 1046–1047.

604. Krogsgaard, K., Kryger, P., Aldershvile, J. *et al.* (1987) δ-Infection and suppression of hepatitis B virus replication in chronic HBsAg carriers. *Hepatology*, **7**, 42–45.

605. Krogsgaard, K., Mathiesen, L.R., Aldershvile, J. *et al.* (1988) Delta infection and hepatitis B virus replication in Danish patients with fulminant hepatitis B. *Scandinavian Journal of Infectious Diseases*, **20**, 127–133.

606. Krogsgaard, K., Wantzin, P., Mathiesen L.R. *et al.* (1990) Early appearance of antibodies to hepatitis C virus in community acquired acute non-A, non-B hepatitis is associated with progression to chronic liver disease. *Scandinavian Journal of Infectious Diseases*, **22**, 399–402.

607. Krugman, S., Giles, J.P. & Hammond, J. (1967) Infectious hepatitis: evidence for two distinctive clinical, epidemiological and immunological types of infection. *Journal of the American Medical Association*, **200**, 365–373.

608. Krugman, S. & Giles, J.P. (1973) Viral hepatitis, type B (MS-2 strain); further observations on natural history and prevention. *New England Journal of Medicine*, **288**, 755–760.

609. Kryger, P., Pedersen, N.S., Mathieson, L. *et al.* (1982) Increased risk of infection with hepatitis A and B viruses in men with a history of syphilis: Relation to sexual contacts. *Journal of Infectious Diseases*, **145**, 23–26.

610. Kryger, P. & Christoffersen, P. (1983) Liver histopathology of the hepatitis A virus infection: a comparison with hepatitis type B and non-A, non-B. *Journal of Clinical Pathology*, **36**, 650–654.

611. Kubo, Y., Takeuchi, K., Boonmar, S. *et al.* (1989) A cDNA fragment of hepatitis C virus isolated from an implicated donor of post-transfusion non-A, non-B hepatitis in Japan. *Nucleic Acid Research*, **17**, 10367–10372.

612. Kudesia, G. & Follett, E.A.C. (1988) Hepatitis A in Scotland – is it a continuing problem? *Scottish Medical Journal*, **33**, 231–233.

613. Kühnl, P., Seidl, S., Stangel, W. *et al.* (1989) Antibody to hepatitis C virus in German blood donors. *Lancet*, **2**, 324.

614. Kuijpers, L., Koens, M., Murray-Lyon, I. *et al.* (1989) Pre-S proteins in hepatitis B. *Journal of Medical Virology*, **28**, 47–51.

615. Kumar, M.L., Dawson, N.V., McCullough, A.J. *et al.* (1987) Should all pregnant women be screened for hepatitis B? *Annals of Internal Medicine*, **107**, 273–277.

616. Kumashiro, R., Sata, M., Suzuki, H. *et al.* (1988) Clinical study of acute hepatitis type A in patients older than fifty years. *Acta Hepatologica Japonica*, **29**, 457–462.

617. Kuo, G., Choo, Q-L, Alter, H.J. *et al.* (1989) An assay for circulating antibodies to a major etiologic virus of human non-A, non-B hepatitis. *Science*, **244**, 362–364.

618. Kuo, M.Y., Goldberg, J., Coates, L. *et al.* (1988a) Molecular cloning of hepatitis delta virus RNA from an infected woodchuck liver: sequence, structure, and applications. *Journal of Virology*, **62**, 1855–1861.

619. Kuo, M.Y., Sharmeen, L., Dinter-Gottlieb, G., & Taylor, J. (1988b) Characterization of self-cleaving RNA sequences on the genome and antigenome of human hepatitis delta virus. *Journal of Virology*, **62**, 4438–4444.

620. Kuo, M.Y., Chao, M., & Taylor, J. (1989) Initiation of replication of the human hepatitis delta virus genome from cloned DNA: role of delta antigen. *Journal of Virology*, **63**, 1945–1950.

621. Kurai, K., Iino, S., Kurokawa, K. *et al.* (1991) Large molecular form of serum HBeAg in chronic hepatitis B virus infection: relation to liver cell damage. *Hepatology*, **13**, 1057–1060.

622. Kuriyama, S., Tsujii, T., Ishizaka, S. *et al.* (1988) Enhancing effects of oral adjuvants on anti-HBs responses induced by hepatitis B vaccine. *Clinical and Experimental Immunology*, **72**, 383–389.

623. Kuroki, K., Floreani, M., Mimms, L.T. & Ganem, D. (1990) Epitope mapping of the preS1 domain of the hepatitis B virus large surface protein. *Virology*, **176**, 620–624.

624. Kurtz, J.B., Alder, M.J., Mayon-White, R.T. *et al.* (1989) Plasma-derived versus recombinant hepatitis B vaccines. *Lancet*, **1**, 451.

625. Kusne, S., Schwartz, M., Breinig, M.K. *et al.* (1991) Herpes simplex virus hepatitis after solid organ transplantation in adults. *Journal of Infectious Diseases*, **163**, 1001–1007.

626. Kwok, S. & Higuchi, R. (1989) Avoiding false positives with PCR. *Nature*, **339**, 237–238.

627. Lahaye, D., Strauss, P., Baleux, C. & van Ganse, W. (1987) Cost-benefit analysis of hepatitis-B vaccination. *Lancet*, **2**, 441–442.

628. Lai, K.N., Lai, F.M-M. & Tam, J.S. (1989) Comparison of polyclonal and monoclonal antibodies in determination of glomerular deposits of hepatitis B virus antigens in hepatitis B virus-associated glomerulonephritides. *American Journal of Clinical Pathology*, **92**, 159–165.

629. Lambore, S., McSherry, J. & Kraus, A.S. (1991) Acute and chronic symptoms of mononucleosis. *Journal of Family Practitioner*, **33**, 33–37.

630. Lancet (1982) (+)-Cyanidanol-3 (editorial). *Lancet*, **1**, 549.

631. Lancet (1983) The hepatitis B carrier in hospital (editorial). *Lancet*, **2**, 1285–1286.

632. Lancet (1984) Prevention of perinatally transmitted hepatitis B infection (editorial). *Lancet*, **1**, 939–941.

633. Lancet (1984) Hepatitis B vaccine and haemodialysis (editorial). *Lancet*, **2**, 962–963.

634. Lancet — Collaborative Study, Central Public Health Laboratory, London (1980) Acute hepatitis B associated with gynaecological surgery. *Lancet*, **1**, 1–6.

635. Langnas, A.N., Castaldo, P., Markin, R.S. *et al.* (1991) The spectrum of Epstein–Barr virus infection with hepatitis following liver transplantation. *Transplantation Proceedings*, **23**, 1513–1514.

636. Larke, R.P.B., Froese, G.J., Devine, R.D.O. & Petruk, M. (1987) Extension of the epidemiology of hepatitis B in circumpolar regions through a comprehensive serologic study in the Northwest Territories of Canada. *Journal of Medical Virology*, **22**, 269–276.

637. Larouze, B., Gaudebout, C., Mercier, E. *et al.* (1987) Infection with hepatitis A and B viruses in French volunteers working in tropical Africa. *American Journal of Epidemiology*, **126**, 31–37.

638. Lau, J.Y.N., Lai, C.L., Wu, P.C. & Lin, H.J. (1989) Comparison of two plasma-derived hepatitis B vaccines: Long-term report of a prospective, randomized trial. *Journal of Gastroenterology and Hepatology*, **4**, 331–337.

639. Laukamm-Josten, U., von Laer, G., Feldmeier, H. *et al.* (1987) Active immunization against hepatitis B: Immunogenicity of a recombinant DNA vaccine in females, heterosexual and homosexual males. *Postgraduate Medical Journal*, **63**, 143–146.

640. Lavine, J.E., Lake, J.R., Ascher, N.L. *et al.* (1991) Persistent hepatitis B virus following interferon-α therapy and liver transplantation. *Gastroenterology*, **100**, 263–267.

641. Lee, C.-Y., Hwang, L.-Y. & Beasley, R.P. (1989) Low-dose hepatitis B vaccine. *Lancet*, **2**, 860–861.

642. Lee, J.C. & Fortuny, I.E. (1972) Adult herpes simplex hepatitis. *Human Pathology*, **3**, 277–281.

643. Lee, K.-S., Lee, H., Moon, S.J. *et al.* (1987) Hepatitis B vaccination of newborn infants: Clinical study of new vaccine formulation and dose regimen. *Hepatology*, **7**, 941–945.

644. Lee, S.-D., Lo, K.-J., Wu, J.-C. *et al.* (1986) Prevention of maternal-infant hepatitis B transmission by immunization: The role of serum hepatitis B virus DNA. *Hepatology*, **6**, 369–373.

645. Lee, S.-D., Lo, K.-J., Tsai, Y.-T. *et al.* (1988) Role of caesarean section in prevention of mother-infant transmission of hepatitis B virus. *Lancet*, **2**, 833–834.

646. Lee, S.-D., Lo, K.-J., Tsai, Y.-T. & Wu, J.-C. (1989) Maternal hepatitis B virus DNA in mother-infant transmission. *Lancet*, **2**, 719.

647. Lee, S.-D., Tsai, Y.-T., Hwang, S.-J. *et al.* (1991) A prospective study of post- transfusion non-A, non-B (type C) hepatitis following cardiovascular surgery in Taiwan. *Journal of Medical Virology*, **33**, 188–192.

648. Lee, S.-D., Chan, C.-Y., Wang, Y.-J. *et al.* (1991) Seroepidemiology of hepatitis C virus infection in Taiwan. *Hepatology*, **13**, 830–833.

649. Leen, C.L.S., Davison, S.M., Flegg, P.J. & Mandal, B.K. (1989) Seven years experience of acute hepatitis B in a regional department of infectious diseases and tropical medicine. *Journal of Infection*, **18**, 257–263.

650. Lefkowitch, J.H., Goldstein, H., Yatto, R. & Gerber, M.A. (1987) Cytopathic liver injury in acute delta virus hepatitis. *Gastroenterology*, **92**, 1262–1266.

651. Lefkowitch, J.H. & Apfelbaum, T.F. (1989) Non-A, non-B hepatitis: Characterisation of liver biopsy pathology. *Journal of Clinical Gastroenterology*, **11**, 225–232.

652. Lelie, P.N., van Amelsfoort, P.J.A.J., de Groot, C.S.M. *et al.* (1989) Lack of immune potentiation by complexing HBdAg in a heat-inactivated hepatitis B vaccine with antibody in hepatitis B immunoglobulin. *Hepatology*, **10**, 36–38.

653. Lemon, S.M., Brown, C.D., Brooks, D.S. *et al.* (1980) Specific immunoglobulin M response to hepatitis A virus determined by solid-phase radioimmunoassay. *Infection and Immunity*, **28**, 927–936.

654. Lemon, S.M. (1985) Type A viral hepatitis: new developments in an old disease. *New England Journal of Medicine*, **313**, 1059–1067.

655. Lemon, S.M. & Ping, L-H. (1989) Antigenic structure of hepatitis A virus. In Semler, B.L. & Ehrenfeld, E. (eds) *Molecular Aspects of Picornavirus Infection and Detection*, pp. 193–208. Washington, D.C.: American Society for Microbiology.

656. León, A., Cantón, R., Elía, M. & Mateos, M. (1991) Second-generation RIBA to confirm diagnosis of HCV infection. *Lancet*, **337**, 912–913.

657. León, P., López, J.A., Contreras, G. & Echevarría, J.M. (1988) Antibodies to hepatitis delta virus in intravenous drug addicts and male homosexuals in Spain. *European Journal of Clinical Microbiology and Infectious Diseases*, **7**, 533–535.

658. Lettau, L.A., McCarthy, J.G., Smith, M.H. *et al.* (1987) Outbreak of severe hepatitis due to delta and hepatitis B viruses in parenteral drug abusers and their contacts. *New England Journal of Medicine*, **317**, 1256–1262.

659. Lever, A.M.L., Webster, A.D.B., Brown, D. & Thomas, H.C. (1984) Non A, non B hepatitis occurring in agammaglobulinaemic patients after intravenous immunoglobulin. *Lancet*, **2**, 1062–1064.

660. Levy, B.S., Fontaine, R.E., Smith, C.A. *et al.* (1975) A large food-borne outbreak of hepatitis A. Possible transmission via oropharyngeal secretions. *Journal of the American Medical Association*, **234**, 289–294.

661. Liang, T.J., Hasegawa, K., Rimon, N. *et al.* (1991) A hepatitis B virus mutant associated with an epidemic of fulminant hepatitis. *New England Journal of Medicine*, **324**, 1705–1709.

662. Liaw, Y.-F., Chen, T.-J., Chu, C.-M. & Liu, H.-H. (1990) Acute hepatitis delta virus superinfection in patients with liver cirrhosis. *Journal of Hepatology*, **10**, 41–45.

663. Liaw, Y.-F., Dong, J.-T., Chiu, K.-W. *et al.* (1991) Why most patients with hepatitis delta virus infection are seronegative for hepatitis B e antigen. *Journal of Hepatology*, **12**, 106–109.

664. Lien, J-M., Aldrich, C.E. & Mason, W.S. (1986) Evidence that a capped oligoribonucleotide is the primer for duck hepatitis B virus plus-strand DNA synthesis. *Journal of Virology*, **57**, 229–236.

665. Lien, J-M., Petcu, D.J., Aldrich, C.E. & Mason, W.S. (1987) Initiation and termination of duck hepatitis B virus DNA synthesis during virus maturation. *Journal of Virology*, **61**, 3832–3840.

666. Lin, H.-H., Lee, T.-Y., Chen, D.-S. *et al.* (1987) Transplacental leakage of HBeAg-positive maternal blood as the most likely route in causing intrauterine infection with hepatitis B virus. *Journal of Pediatrics*, **111**, 877–881.

667. Lin, H.-H., Liaw, Y.-F., Chen, T.-J. *et al.* (1989) Natural course of patients with chronic type B hepatitis following acute hepatitis delta virus superinfection. *Liver*, **9**, 129–134.

668. Lin, J.H., Chang, M.F., Baker, S.C. *et al.* (1990) Characterization of hepatitis delta antigen: specific binding to hepatitis delta virus RNA. *Journal of Virology*, **64**, 4051–4058.

669. Lindberg, J. & Lindholm, A. (1988) HBsAg-positive Swedish blood donors: Natural history and origin of infection. *Scandinavian Journal of Infectious Diseases*, **20**, 377–382.

670. Lindh, G., Mattsson, L., von Sydow, M. & Weiland, O. (1990) Acute hepatitis B and hepatitis D co-infection in the Stockholm region in the 1970s and 1980s — A comparison. *Infection*, **18**, 357–360.

671. Lindsay, K.L., Nizze, J.A., Koretz, R. & Gitnick, G. (1986) Diagnostic usefulness of testing for anti-HBc IgM in acute hepatitis B. *Hepatology*, **6**, 1325–1328.

672. Linemeyer, D.L., Menke, J.G., Martin-Gallardo, A. *et al.* (1985) Molecular cloning and partial sequencing of hepatitis A viral cDNA. *Journal of Virology*, **54**, 247–255.

673. Linneman, C.C. & Goldberg, S. (1974) Hepatitis-B antigen in saliva and semen. *Lancet*, **1**, 320.

674. Lloyd-Still, J.D., Scott, J.P. & Crussi, F. (1985) The spectrum of Epstein-Barr virus hepatitis in children. *Paediatric Pathology*, **5**, 337–351.

675. Lo, K.-J., Lee, S.-D., Tsai, Y.-T. *et al.* (1988) Long-term immunogenicity and efficacy of hepatitis B vaccine in infants born to HBeAg-positive HBsAg-carrier mothers. *Hepatology*, **8**, 1647–1650.

676. Lobdell, D.H. (1987) "Ring" granulomas in cytomegalovirus hepatitis. *Archives of Pathology and Laboratory Medicine*, **111**, 881–882.

677. Lohiya, G., Lohiya, S., Caires, S. & Nizibian, R. (1986) Occupational risk of hepatitis B from institutionalized mentally retarded HBsAg carriers: A prospective study. *Journal of Infectious Diseases*, **154**, 990–995.

678. Lok, A.S.-F., Lai, C.-L., Wu, P.-C. *et al.* (1987) Hepatitis B virus infection in Chinese families in Hong Kong. *American Journal of Epidemiology*, **126**, 492–499.

679. Loke, R.H.T., Murray-Lyon, I.M., Coleman, J.C. *et al.* Diminished response to recombinant hepatitis B vaccine in homosexual men with HIV antibody: An indicator of poor prognosis. *Journal of Medical Virology*, **31**, 109–111.

680. London, T.W. (1977) Hepatitis B virus and antigen–antibody complex diseases. *New England Journal of Medicine*, **296**, 1528–1529.

681. London, W.T., Difiglia, M., Sutnick, A.I. & Blumberg, B.S. (1969) An epidemic of hepatitis in a chronic haemodialysis unit. Australia antigen and differences in host response. *New England Journal of Medicine*, **281**, 571–578.

682. Lowry, P.W., Levine, R., Stroup, F. *et al.* (1989) Hepatitis A outbreak on a floating restaurant in Florida, 1986. *American Journal of Epidemiology*, **129**, 155–164.

683. Lubeck, M.D., Davis, A.R., Chengalvala, M. *et al.* (1989)

Immunogenicity and efficacy testing in chimpanzees of an oral hepatitis B vaccine based on live recombinant adenovirus. *Proceedings of the National Academy of Sciences of the USA*, **86**, 6763–6767.

684. Lucké, B. (1944) The pathology of fatal epidemic hepatitis. *American Journal of Pathology*, **20**, 471–593.

685. Lucké, B. & Mallory, T. (1946) The fulminant form of epidemic hepatitis. *American Journal of Pathology*, **22**, 867–945.

686. Ludlam, C.A., Chapman, D., Cohen, B. & Litton, P.A. (1989) Antibodies to hepatitis C virus in haemophilia. *Lancet*, **2**, 560–561.

687. Luo, G., Chao, M., Hsieh, S-Y. *et al.* (1990) A specific base transition occurs on replicating hepatitis delta virus RNA. *Journal of Virology*, **64**, 1021–1027.

688. Lürman (1885) Eine Icterusepidemie. *Berliner Klinische Wochenschrift*, **22**, 20.

689. MacCallum, F.O. & Bradley, W.H. (1944) Transmission of infective hepatitis to human volunteers. *Lancet*, **2**, 228.

690. MacCallum, F.O. (1972) Historical perspectives. *Canadian Medical Association Journal*, **106**, 423–426.

691. MacCallum, F.O. (1972) Early studies of viral hepatitis. *British Medical Bulletin*, **28**, 105–108.

692. Mahoney, D.J. Jr., Fernbach, D.J., Starke, J.R. & Reid, B.S. (1987) Profound hyperbilirubinaemia: An unusual presentation of childhood infectious mononucleosis. *Paediatric Infectious Diseases Journal*, **6**, 73–74.

693. Maier, K.-P. (1990) Non-A, non-B hepatitis: infections by the enteral and parenteral route. In Bianchi, L., Gerok, W., Maier, K.-P. & Deinhardt, F. (eds) *Infectious Diseases of the Liver*, pp. 309–316. Dordrecht: Kluwer.

694. Makino, S., Chang, M.F., Shieh, C.K. *et al.* (1987) Molecular cloning and sequencing of a human hepatitis delta virus RNA. *Nature*, **329**, 343–346.

695. Makris, M., Preston, F.E., Triger, D.R. *et al.* (1990) Hepatitis C antibody and chronic liver disease in haemophilia. *Lancet*, **335**, 1117–1119.

696. Mandart, E., Kay, A. & Galibert, F. (1984) Nucleotide sequence of a cloned duck hepatitis B virus genome: comparison with woodchuck and human hepatitis B virus sequences. *Journal of Virology*, **49**, 782–792.

697. Mannucci, P.M., Zanetti, A.R., Gringeri, A. *et al.* (1989) Long-term immunogenicity of a plasma-derived hepatitis B vaccine in HIV seropositive and HIV seronegative hemophiliacs. *Archives of Internal Medicine*, **149**, 1333–1337.

698. Mao, J.S., Dong, D.X., Zhang, H.Y. *et al.* (1989) Primary study of attenuated live hepatitis A vaccine (H2 strain) in humans. *Journal of Infectious Diseases*, **159**, 621–624.

699. Marano, A.R., Lanse, S.B., Garsten, J.J. *et al.* (1986) Exudative ascites complicating infectious mononucleosis. *American Journal of Gastroenterology*, **81**, 808–811.

700. Margolis, H.S., Nainan, O.V., Krawczynski, K. *et al.* (1988) Appearance of immune complexes during experimental hepatitis A infection in chimpanzees. *Journal of Medical Virology*, **26**, 315–326.

701. Margolis, H.S. & Nainan, O.V. (1990) Identification of virus components in circulating immune complexes isolated during hepatitis A virus infection. *Hepatology*, **11**, 31–37.

702. Margolis, H.S., Alter, M.J. & Hadler, S.C. (1991) Hepatitis B: Evolving epidemiology and implications for control. *Seminars in Liver Disease*, **11**, 84–92.

703. Marinucci, G., Valeri, L., Di Giacomo, C. *et al.* (1983) Spread of delta (δ) infection in a group of haemodialysis carriers of HBsAg. In Rizzetto, M., Verme, G. & Bonino, F. (eds) *Viral Hepatitis and Delta Infection*. New York: Allan R Liss.

704. Marion, P.L., Oshiro, L., Regnery, D.C. *et al.* (1980) A virus in Beechey ground squirrels that is related to hepatitis B virus of man. *Proceedings of the National Academy of Sciences of the USA*, **77**, 2941–2945.

705. Marion, P.L., Van Davelaar, M.J., Knight, S.S. *et al.* (1983) Hepatocellular carcinoma in ground squirrels persistently infected with ground squirrel hepatitis virus. *Proceedings of the National Academy of Sciences of the USA*, **83**, 4543–4546.

706. Markin, R.S., Wood, R.P, Shaw, B.W. Jr. *et al.* (1990) Immunohistologic identification of Epstein-Barr virus induced hepatitis reactivation after OKT-3 therapy following orthotopic liver transplant. *American Journal of Gastroenterology*, **85**, 1014–1018.

707. Markoff, L. (1989) In vitro processing of dengue virus structural proteins: cleavage of the pre-membrane protein. *Journal of Virology*, **63**(8), 3345–3352.

708. Marmion, B.P. & Tonkin, R.W. (1972) Control of hepatitis in dialysis units. *British Medical Bulletin*, **28**, 169–179.

709. Martin, P., Di Bisceglie, A.M., Kassianides, C. *et al.* (1989) Rapidly progressive non-A, non-B hepatitis in patients with human immunodeficiency virus infection. *Gastroenterology*, **97**, 1559–1561.

710. Martin, P., Muñoz, S.J., Di Bisceglie, A.M. *et al.* (1991) Recurrence of hepatitis C virus infection after orthotopic liver transplantation. *Hepatology*, **13**, 719–721.

711. Martini, G.A., Knauff, H.G., Schmidt, H.A. *et al.* (1968) A hitherto unknown infectious disease contracted from monkeys. 'Marburg-virus' disease. *German Medical Monthly*, **13**, 457–470.

712. Martini, G.A. & Baltzer, G. (1972) Complications of viral hepatitis. *Canadian Medical Association Journal*, **106**, 508–512.

713. Martini, G.A. & Strohmeyer, G. (1974) Post hepatitis syndromes. *Clinics in Gastroenterology*, **3**, 377–390.

714. Mashiko, N. (1988) Mechanisms of thrombocytopenia in acute hepatitis A. *Acta Hepatologica Japonica*, **29**, 711–718.

715. Mason, W.S., Seal, G. & Summers, J. (1980) Virus of Pekin ducks with structural and biological relatedness to human hepatitis B virus. *Journal of Virology*, **36**, 829–836.

716. Mason, W.S., Aldrich, G., Summers, J. & Taylor, J.M. (1982) Asymmetric replication of duck hepatitis B virus DNA in liver cells: free minus-strand DNA. *Proceedings of the National Academy of Sciences of the USA*, **79**, 3997–4001.

717. Mathieson, L.R., Feinstone, S.M., Purcell, R.H. & Wagner, J.A. (1977) Detection of hepatitis A antigen by immunofluorescence. *Infection and Immunity*, **18**, 524–530.

718. Mathiot, C.C., Zalez, J.P. & Georges, A.J. (1988) Current problems of arbo viruses in Central Africa. *Bulletin de la Societé de Pathologie Exotique Filiales*, **81**, 396–401.

719. Maycock, W. d'A. (1965) Control of serum hepatitis. *Report on a European Symposium Convened by the WHO, Prague, 1964*, p. 82. Copenhagen: World Health Organisation.

720. Maynard, J.E., Kane, M.A. & Hadler, S.C. (1989) Global control of hepatitis B through vaccination: Role of hepatitis B vaccine in the expanded programme on immunization. *Reviews of Infectious Diseases*, **11**, S574–S578.

721. Mazzur, S. & Watson, T.M. (1974) Excess males among siblings of Australia antigen carriers. *Nature*, **250**, 60–61.

722. McCaul, T.F., Fagan, E.A., Tovey, G. *et al.* (1986) Fulminant hepatitis. An ultrastructural study. *Journal of Hepatology*, **2**, 276–290.

723. McCormick, J.B., Walker, D.H., King, I.J. *et al.* (1986) Lassa virus hepatitis: A study of fatal Lassa fever in humans. *American Journal of Tropical Medicine and Hygiene*, **35**, 401–407.

724. McCormick, J.B., Webb, P.A., Krebbs, J.W. *et al.* (1987) A prospective study of the epidemiology and ecology of Lassa fever. *Journal of Infectious Diseases*, **155**, 437–444.

725. McCormick, J.B., King, I.J., Webb, P.A. *et al.* (1987) A case-controlled study of the clinical diagnosis and course Lassa fever. *Journal of Infectious Diseases*, **155**, 445–455.

726. McCruden, E.A.B. & Follett, E.A.C. (1990) Evidence of past delta co-infection with acute hepatitis B in intravenous drug abusers in the west of Scotland. *Journal of Infection*, **21**, 151–155.

727. McDonald, G.S.A., Courtney, M.G., Shattock, A.G. & Weir, D.G. (1989) Prolonged IgM antibodies and histopathological evidence of chronicity in hepatitis A. *Liver*, **9**, 223–228.

728. McDonald, S. (1908) Acute yellow atrophy. *Edinburgh Medical Journal*, **15**, 208.

729. McFarlane, I.G., Smith, H.M., Johnson, P.J. *et al.* (1990) Hepatitis C virus antibodies in chronic active hepatitis: pathogenetic factor or false-positive result? *Lancet*, **335**, 754–757.

730. McMahon, B.J., Rhoades, E.R., Heyward, W.L. *et al.* (1987) A comprehensive programme to reduce the incidence of hepatitis B virus infection and its sequelae in Alaskan natives. *Lancet*, **2**, 1134–1136.

731. McMahon, B.J., Heyward, W.L., Templin, D.W. *et al.* (1989) Hepatitis B-associated polyarteritis nodosa in Alaskan eskimos: clinical and epidemiologic features and long-term follow-up. *Hepatology*, **9**, 97–101.

732. McMahon, G., McCarthy, L.A., Dottavio, D. *et al.* (1991) Surface

antigen and polymerase gene variation in hepatitis B virus isolates from a mononclonal antibody treated liver transplant patient. In Hollinger, F.B., Lemon, S.M. & Margolis, H.S. (eds) *Viral Hepatitis and Liver Disease*. Baltimore: Williams & Wilkins.

733. McMinn, P.C., Lim, I.S., McKenzie, P.E. *et al.* (1989) Disseminated herpes simplex virus infection in an apparently immunocompetent woman. *Medical Journal of Australia*, **151**, 588–590.

734. McQuillan, G.M., Townsend, T.R., Johannes, C.B. *et al.* (1987) Prevention of perinatal transmission of hepatitis B virus: The sensitivity, specificity, and predictive value of the recommended screening questions to detect high-risk women in an obstetric population. *American Journal of Epidemiology*, **126**, 484–491.

735. McQuillan, G.M., Townsend, T.R., Fields, H.A. *et al.* (1989) The seroepidemology of hepatitis B virus in the United States, 1976–80. *American Journal of Medicine*, **87**(Suppl. 3A), 5–10.

736. McSweeney, P.A., Carter, J.M., Green, G.J. & Romeril, K.R. (1988) Fatal aplastic anemia associated with hepatitis B viral infection. *American Journal of Medicine*, **85**, 255–256.

737. Medical Research Council Working Party on Post-transfusion Hepatitis. (1974) Post- transfusion hepatitis in a London hospital: results of a two-year prospective study. *Journal of Hygiene*, **73**, 173–188.

738. Meers, P.D. (1986) Yellow fever in Swansea, 1865. *Journal of Hygiene, London*, **97**, 185–191.

739. Meheus, A., Alisjahbana, A., Vranckx, R. *et al.* (1987) Immunogenicity of a recombinant DNA hepatitis B vaccine in neonates. *Postgraduate Medical Journal*, **63**, 139–141.

740. Melbye, M., Biggar, R.J., Wantzin, P. *et al.* (1990) Sexual transmission of hepatitis C virus: cohort study (1981–9) among European homosexual men. *British Medical Journal*, **301**, 210–212.

741. Mele, A., Rastelli, M.G., Gill, O.N. *et al.* (1989) Recurrent epidemic hepatitis A associated with consumption of raw shellfish, probably controlled through public health measures. *American Journal of Epidemiology*, **130**, 540–546.

742. Melnick, J.L. (1982) Classification of hepatitis A virus as enterovirus type 72 and hepatitis B virus as hepatoma virus type I. *Intervirology*, **18**, 105–106.

743. Mendenhall, C., Roselle, G.A., Lybecker, L.A. *et al.* (1988) Hepatitis B vaccination. Response of alcoholics with and without liver injury. *Digestive Diseases and Sciences*, **33**, 263–269.

744. Menitove, J.E., Richards, W.A. & Destree, M. (1990) Early US experience with anti-HCV kit in blood donors. *Lancet*, **336**, 244–245.

745. Metzman, R., Anand, A., DeGiulio, P.A. & Kniseley, A.S. (1989) Hepatic disease associated with intrauterine parvovirus B19 infection in a newborn premature infant. *Journal of Paediatric Gastroenterology and Nutrition*, **9**, 112–114.

746. Meuer, S.C., Dumann, H., Meyer zum Büschenfelde, K.-H. & Köhler, H. (1989) Low-dose interleukin-2 induces systemic immune responses against HBsAg in immunodeficient nonresponders to hepatitis B vaccination. *Lancet*, **1**, 15–17.

747. Meyers, M.L., Trepo, L.V., Nath, N. *et al.* (1986) Hepatitis B virus polypeptide X expression in *Escherichia coli* and identification of specific antibodies in sera from hepatitis B virus infected humans. *Journal of Virology*, **57**, 101–109.

748. Michitaka, K., Horiike, N., Nadano, S. *et al.* (1988) Change of hepatitis B virus DNA distribution associated with the progression of chronic hepatitis. *Liver*, **8**, 247–253.

749. Midthun, K., Ellerbeck, E., Gershman, K. *et al.* (1991) Safety and immunogenicity of a live attenuated hepatitis A virus vaccine in seronegative volunteers. *Journal of Infectious Diseases*, **163**, 735–739.

750. Milazzo, S., Galli, M., Fassio, P.G. *et al.* (1985) Attempted treatment of fulminant viral hepatitis with human fibroblast interferon. *Infection*, **13**, 130–133.

751. Milich, D. & Chisari, F. (1982) Genetic regulation of the immune response to hepatitis B surface antigen (HBsAg). *Journal of Immunology*, **129**, 320–325.

752. Milich, D., McNamara, M., McLachlan, A. *et al.* (1985) Distinct H-2-linked regulation of T-cell responses to the pre-S and S regions of the same hepatitis B surface antigen polypeptide allows circumvention of nonresponsiveness to the S region. *Proceedings of the National Academy of Sciences of the USA*, **82**, 8168–8172.

753. Milich, D., Thornton, G., Neurath, A. *et al.* (1985) Enhanced

immunogenicity of the pre-S region of hepatitis B surface antigen. *Science*, **228**, 1195–1198.

754. Miller, D.J., Williams, A.E., Le Bouvier, G.L. *et al.* (1978) Hepatitis B in hemodialysis patients: significance of HBeAg. *Gastroenterology*, **74**, 1208–1213.

755. Miller, R.H. & Robinson, W.S. (1984) Hepatitis B viral DNA forms in nuclear and cytoplasmic fractions of infected human liver. *Virology*, **137**, 309–399.

756. Miller, R.H. (1987) Proteolytic self-cleavage of hepatitis B virus core may generate serum e antigen. *Science*, **236**, 722–725.

757. Miller, R.H. & Purcell, R.H. (1990) Hepatitis C virus shares amino acid sequence similarity with pestiviruses and flaviviruses as well as members of two plant virus supergroups. *Proceedings of the National Academy of Sciences of the USA*, **87**, 2057–2061.

758. Millward-Sadler, G.H. (1976) Pathological aspects of virus hepatitis. In Truelove, S.C. & Ritchie, J. (eds) *Topics in Gastroenterology*, pp. 29–54. Oxford: Blackwell Scientific.

759. Milne, A., Allwood, G.K., Moyes, C.D. *et al.* (1987) A seroepidemiological study of the prevalence of hepatitis B infections in a hyperendemic New Zealand community. *International Journal of Epidemiology*, **16**, 84–90.

760. Milne, A., Dimitrakakis, M., Allwood, G. *et al.* (1987) Immunogenicity of low doses of hepatitis B vaccine in children: A study in 650 New Zealand children. *Journal of Medical Virology*, **23**, 401–405.

761. Milne, A., Dimitrakakis, M., Campbell, C. *et al.* (1987b) Low-dose vaccination against hepatitis B in children: One-year follow-up. *Journal of Medical Virology*, **22**, 387–392.

762. Milne, A., Brawner, T.A., Dumbill, P.C. *et al.* (1989) Comparison of the immunogenicity of reduced doses of two recombinant DNA hepatitis B vaccines in New Zealand children. *Journal of Medical Virology*, **27**, 264–267.

763. Mimms, L., Vallari, D., Ducharme, L. *et al.* (1990) Specificity of anti-HCV ELISA assessed by reactivity to three immunodominant HCV regions. *Lancet*, **336**, 1590–1591.

764. Minuk, G.Y. & Nicolle, L.E. (1986) Genital herpes and hepatitis in healthy young adults. *Journal of Medical Virology*, **19**, 269–275.

765. Minuk, G.Y., Bohme, C.E., Bowen, T.J. *et al.* (1987) Efficacy of commercial condoms in the prevention of hepatitis B virus infection. *Gastroenterology*, **93**, 710–714.

766. Minuk, G.Y., Bohme, C.E. & Bowen, T.J. (1989) Passive and active immunization against hepatitis B virus infection: Optimal scheduling in healthy young adults. *Clinical and Investigative Medicine*, **12**, 175–180.

767. Mishiro, S., Hoshi, Y., Takeda, K. *et al.* (1990) Non-A, non-B hepatitis specific antibodies directed at host-derived epitope: implication for an autoimmune process. *Lancet*, **336**, 1400–1403.

768. Mishiro, S., Takeda, K., Hoshi, Y. *et al.* (1991) An autoantibody cross-reactive to hepatitis C virus core and a host nuclear antigen. *Autoimmunity*, **10**, 269–273.

769. Mishu, R., Hadler, S.C., Boaz, V.A. *et al.* (1990) Foodborne hepatitis A: Evidence that microwaving reduces risk? *Journal of Infectious Diseases*, **162**, 655–658.

770. Mitsuda, T., Yokota, S., Mori, T. *et al.* (1989) Demonstration of mother-to-infant transmission of hepatitis B virus by means of polymerase chain reaction. *Lancet*, **2**, 886–888.

771. Mitsui, T., Iwano, K., Suzuki, S. *et al.* (1989) Combined hepatitis B immune globulin and vaccine for postexposure prophylaxis of accidental hepatitis B virus infection in hemodialysis staff members: Comparison with immune globulin without vaccine in historical controls. *Hepatology*, **10**, 324–327.

772. Miyamura, T., Saito, I., Katayama, T. *et al.* (1990) Detection of antibody against antigen expressed by molecularly cloned hepatitis C virus cDNA: application to diagnosis and blood screening for posttransfusion hepatitis. *Proceedings of the National Academy of Sciences of the USA*, **87**, 983–987.

773. Modai, D., Pik, A., Marmor, Z. *et al.* (1986) Liver dysfunction in measles, liver biopsy findings. *Digestive Diseases and Sciences*, **31**, 333.

774. Modlin, J.F. (1986) Perinatal echovirus infection: insights from a literature review of 61 cases of serious infection and 16 outbreaks in nurseries. *Review of Infectious Diseases*, **8**, 918–926.

775. Modlin, J.F. (1988) Perinatal echovirus and type B coxsackie virus infections. *Clinics in Perinatology*, **15**, 233–246.

776. Mok, Q., Underhill, G., Wonke, B. *et al.* (1989) Intradermal hepatitis B vaccine in thalassaemia and sickle cell disease. *Archives of Disease in Childhood,* **64**, 535–540.

777. Moller, A.M. & Mathiesen, L.R. (1979) Detection of immunoglobulin M antibodies to hepatitis A virus by enzyme-linked immunosorbent assay. *Journal of Clinical Microbiology,* **10**, 628–632.

778. Molnar-Kimber, K.L., Summers, J., Taylor, J. & Mason, W.S. (1983) Protein covalently bound to minus-strand DNA intermediates of duck hepatitis B virus. *Journal of Virology,* **45**, 165–172.

779. Molnar-Kimber, K.L., Summers, J. & Mason, W.S. (1984) Mapping of the cohesive overlap of duck hepatitis B virus DNA and of the site of initiation of reverse transcription. *Journal of Virology,* **51**, 181–191.

780. Mondelli, M. & Eddleston, A.L.W.F. (1984) Mechanisms of liver cell injury in acute and chronic hepatitis B. *Seminars in Liver Disease,* **4**, 47–58.

781. Mondelli, M.U., Cristina, G., Filice G. *et al.* (1990) Anti-HCV positive patients in dialysis units? *Lancet,* **336**, 243–244.

782. Moreno, A., Ramon-y-Cajal, S., Marazuela, M. *et al.* (1989) Sandered nuclei in delta patients. *Liver,* **9**, 367–371.

783. Mortimer, P.P., Cohen, B.J., Litton, P.A. *et al.* (1989) Hepatitis C virus antibody. *Lancet,* **2**, 798.

784. Mosley, J.W. (1965) The surveillance of transfusion-associated viral hepatitis. *Journal of the American Medical Association,* **193**, 1007–1010.

785. Mosley, J.W., Edwards, V.M., Casey, G. *et al.* (1975) Hepatitis B virus infection in dentists. *New England Journal of Medicine,* **293**, 729–734.

786. Mosley, J.W., Combes, B., Volwiler, W. & Zimmerman, H.J. (1976) Corticosteroids in fulminant hepatitis. *New England Journal of Medicine,* **295**(16), 898–899.

787. Mosley, J.W., Aach, R.D., Hollinger, B. *et al.* (1990) Non-A, non-B hepatitis and antibody to hepatitis C virus. *Journal of the American Medical Association,* **263**, 77–78.

788. Mowatt, N.A.G., Albert-Recht, F., Brunt, P.W. & Walker, W. (1973) Outbreak of serum hepatitis associated with tattooing. *Lancet,* **1**, 33–34.

789. Moyes, C.D., Milne, A., Dimitrakakis, M. *et al.* (1987) Very- low-dose hepatitis B vaccine in newborn infants: An economic option for control in endemic areas. *Lancet,* **1**, 29–31.

790. Mullis, K.B. & Faloona, F.A. (1987) Specific synthesis of DNA in vitro via a polymerase catalysed chain reaction. *Methods in Enzymology,* **155**, 335–350.

791. Munck, L.K., Petersen, C.S., Bech, K. *et al.* (1988) Hepatitis B in symptomless Danish homosexual men. *Genitourinary Medicine,* **64**, 39–42.

792. Muraiso, K., Hijikata, M., Ohkoshi, S. *et al.* (1990) A structural protein of hepatitis C virus expressed in *E. coli* facilitates accurate detection of hepatitis C virus. *Biochemical and Biophysical Research Communications,* **172**, 511–516.

793. Muraoka, H. (1990) Clinical and epidemiological study on factors of serious development of viral hepatitis type A. *Japanese Journal of Gastroenterology,* **87**, 1383–1391.

794. Murray, K., Bruce, S.A., Wingfield, P. *et al.* (1987) Protective immunisation against hepatitis B with an internal antigen of the virus. *Journal of Medical Virology,* **23**, 101–107.

795. Myint, H., Soe, M.M., Khin, T. *et al.* (1985) A clinical and epidemiological study of an epidemic of non-A, non-B hepatitis in Rangoon. *American Journal of Tropical Medicine and Hygiene,* **34**, 1183–1189.

796. Nagafuchi, S., Kashiwagi, S., Tsuji, Y. *et al.* (1989) Delayed-type hypersensitivity skin reaction to HBsAg and immunohistopathologic study of liver in patients with acute type B viral hepatitis. *Microbiology-Immunology,* **33**, 539–548.

797. Nagafuchi, Y. & Scheuer, P.J. (1986) Expression of beta 2-microglobulin on hepatocytes in acute and chronic type B hepatitis. *Hepatology,* **6**, 20–23.

798. Nahmias, A.J. & Josey, W.E. (1976) Epidemiology of herpes simplex viruses 1 and 2. In Evans, A.S. (ed.) *Viral Infections in Humans,* pp. 253–271. New York: Plenum Press.

799. Nair, P.V., Weissman, J.Y., Tong, M.J. *et al.* (1984) Efficacy of hepatitis B immune globulin in prevention of perinatal transmission of the hepatitis B virus. *Gastroenterology,* **87**, 293–298.

800. Najarian, R., Caput, D., Gee, W. *et al.* (1985) Primary structure and gene organization of human hepatitis A virus. *Proceedings of the National Academy of Sciences of the USA,* **82**, 2627–2631.

801. Nassal, M., Galle, P.R. & Schaller, H. (1989) Proteaselike sequence in hepatitis B virus core antigen is not required for e antigen generation and may not be part of an aspartic acid-type protease. *Journal of Virology,* **63**, 2598–2604.

802. Naoumov, N.V., Lau, J.Y.N., Daniels, H.M. *et al.* (1991) Detection of HBV-DNA using a digoxigenin-labelled probe. *Journal of Hepatology,* **12**, 382–385.

803. Naumov, N.V., Mondelli, M., Alexander, G.J.M. *et al.* (1984) Relationship between expression of HBV antigens in isolated hepatocytes and autologous lymphocyte cytotoxicity in patients with chronic HBV infection. *Hepatology,* **4**, 63–68.

804. Nefzger, M.D. & Chalmers, T.C. (1963) The treatment of acute infectious hepatitis. Ten year follow-up study of the effects of diet. *American Journal of Medicine,* **35**, 299–309.

805. Negro, F., Korba, B.E., Forzani, B. *et al.* (1989) Hepatitis delta virus (HDV) and woodchuck hepatitis virus (WHV) nucleic acids in tissues of HDV-infected chronic WHV carrier woodchucks. *Journal of Virology,* **63**, 1612–1618.

806. Negro, F., Gerin, J.L., Purcell, R.H. & Miller, R.H. (1989) Basis of hepatitis delta virus disease? *Nature,* **341**, 111.

807. Neurath, A.R., Strick, N., Barker, L. & Krugman, S. (1982) Radioimmunoassays of hidden viral antigens. *Proceedings of the National Academy of Sciences of the USA,* **79**, 4415–4419.

808. Newble, D.I., Holmes, K.T., Wangel, A.G. & Forbes, I.J. (1975) Immune reactions in acute viral hepatitis. *Clinical and Experimental Immunology,* **20**, 17–28.

809. Newkirk, M.M., Downe, A.E.R. & Simon, J.B. (1975) Fate of ingested hepatitis B antigen in blood sucking insects. *Gastroenterology,* **69**, 982–987.

810. Nielsen, J.O., Dietrichson, O.& Juhl, E. (1974) Incidence and meaning of the 'e' determinant among hepatitis-B-antigen positive patients with acute and chronic liver diseases. *Lancet,* **2**, 913–915.

811. Niermeijer, P. & Gips, C.H. (1975) Guillain-Barré syndrome in acute HBsAg positive hepatitis. *British Medical Journal,* **2**, 732–733.

812. Nigro, G. & Taliani, G. (1989) Nursery-acquired asymptomatic B hepatitis. *Lancet,* **1**, 1451–1452.

813. Nishioka, K., Watanabe, J., Furuta, S. *et al.* (1991) Antibody to the hepatitis C virus in acute hepatitis and chronic liver diseases in Japan. *Liver,* **11**, 65–70.

814. Noel, L., Guerois, C., Maisonneuve, P. *et al* (1989) Antibodies to hepatitis C virus in haemophilia. *Lancet,* **2**, 560–561.

815. Nommensen, F.E., Go, S.T. & MacLaren, D.M. (1989) Half-life of Hbs antibody after hepatitis B vaccination: An aid to timing of booster vaccination. *Lancet,* **2**, 847–849.

816. Novick, D.M., Facri, P., Croxson, T.S. *et al.* (1988) Hepatitis D virus and human immunodeficiency virus antibodies in parenteral drug abusers who are hepatitis B surface antigen positive. *Journal of Infectious Diseases,* **158**, 795–803.

817. Nowak, T., Färber, P.M. & Wengler, G. (1989) Analyses of the terminal sequences of West Nile virus structural proteins and of the in vitro translation of those proteins allow the proposal of a complete scheme of the proteolytic cleavages modeled in their synthesis. *Virology,* **169**, 365–376.

818. Nowoslawski, A., Brzosko, W.J., Madalinski, K. & Krawczynski, K. (1970) Cellular localisation of Australia antigen in the liver of patients with lymphoproliferative disorders. *Lancet,* **1**, 494–498.

819. Ochiya, T., Tsurimoto, T., Ueda, K. *et al.* (1989) An *in vitro* system for infection with hepatitis B virus that uses primary human fetal hepatocytes. *Proceedings of the National Academy of Sciences of the USA,* **86**, 1875–1879.

820. Ogata, N., Alter, H.J., Miller, R.H. & Purcell, R.H. (1991) Nucleotide sequence and mutation rate of the H strain of hepatitis C virus. *Proceedings of the National Academy of Sciences of the USA,* **88**, 3392–3396.

821. Ogra, P.L. (1973) Immunologic aspects of hepatitis-associated antigen and antibody in human body fluids. *Journal of Immunology,* **110**, 1197–1205.

822. Ohbu, M., Sasaki, K., Okudara, M. *et al.* (1987) Adenovirus hepatitis in a patient with severe combined immunodeficiency. *Acta Pathologica Japonica,* **37**, 655–664.

823. Ohkoshi, S., Kato, N., Kinoshita, T. *et al.* (1990) Detection of

hepatitis C virus RNA in sera and liver tissues of non-A, non-B patients using the polymerase chain reaction. *Japanese Journal of Cancer Research*, **81**, 862–865.

824. Okada, K., Kamiyama, I., Inomata, M. *et al.* (1976) e Antigen and anti-e in the serum of asymptomatic carrier mothers as indicators of positive and negative transmission of hepatitis B virus to their infants. *New England Journal of Medicine*, **294**, 746–749.

825. Okamoto, H., Yotsumoto, S., Akahane, Y. *et al.* (1990) Hepatitis B viruses with precore region defects prevail in persistently infected hosts along with seroconversion to the antibody against e antigen. *Journal of Virology*, **64**, 1298–1303.

826. Okamoto, H., Okada, S., Sugiyama, Y. *et al.* (1990A) The 5'-terminal sequence of the hepatitis C virus genome. *Japanese Journal of Experimental Medicine*, **60**, 167–177.

827. Okamoto, H., Okada, S., Sugiyama, Y. *et al.* (1990B) Detection of hepatitis C virus RNA by a two-stage polymerase chain reaction with two pairs of primers deduced from the 5'-noncoding region. *Japanese Journal of Experimental Medicine*, **60**, 215–222.

828. Oken, M.M., Hootkin, L. & DeJager, R.L. (1972) Hepatitis after Koyne administration. *American Journal of Digestive Diseases*, **17**, 271–274.

829. Okochi, K. & Murakami, S. (1968) Observations on Australia antigen in Japanese. *Vox Sanguinis*, **15**, 374–385.

830. O'Mahoney, M.C., Gooch, C.D., Smyth, D.A. *et al.* (1983) Epidemic hepatitis A from cockles. *Lancet*, **1**, 518–520.

831. Omata, M., Yokosuka, O., Takano, S. *et al.* (1991) Resolution of acute hepatitis C after therapy with natural beta interferon. *Lancet*, **338**, 914–915.

832. Onji, M., Kumon, I., Kanaoka, M. *et al.* (1988) Intrahepatic lymphocyte subpopulations in acute hepatitis in an adult with rubella. *American Journal of Gastroenterology*, **83**, 320–322.

833. Onji, M., Lever, A.M.L., Saito, I. & Thomas, H.C. (1989) Defective response to interferons and cells transfected with the hepatitis B virus genome. *Hepatology*, **9**, 92–96.

834. Ono, Y., Onda, H., Sasada, R. *et al.* (1983) The complete nucleotide sequences of the cloned hepatitis B virus DNA: subtype adr and adw. *Nucleic Acids Research*, **11**, 1747–1757.

835. Oon, L.L.E., King, A., Higgins, J.A., *et al.* (1991) Protective antibodies to hepatitis B virus in haemophiliacs. *Journal of Medical Virology*, **33**, 19–25.

836. Oren, I., Hershow, R.C., Ben-Porath, E. *et al.* (1989) A common-source outbreak of fulminant hepatitis B in a hospital. *Annals of Internal Medicine*, **110**, 691–698.

837. Oren, R., Shouval, D. & Tur-Kaspa, R. (1989) Detection of hepatitis A virus RNA in serum from patients with acute hepatitis. *Journal of Medical Virology*, **28**, 261–263.

838. Orr, W. (1974) The detection of hepatitis B antigen in hepatic parenchyma by the fluorescent antibody technique. *American Journal of Clinical Pathology*, **64**, 257–262.

839. Osmon, D.R., Melton III, J., Keys, T.F. *et al.* (1987) Viral hepatitis. A population-based study in Rochester, Minn, 1971–1980. *Archives of Internal Medicine*, **147**, 1235–1240.

840. Ostapchuk, P., Scheirle, G. & Hearing, P. (1989) Binding of nuclear factor EF-C to a functional domain of the hepatitis B virus enhancer region. *Molecular and Cellular Biology*, **9**, 2787–2797.

841. Ostermayr, R., von der Helm, K., Gauss-Muller, V. *et al.* (1987) Expression of hepatitis A virus cDNA in *Escherichia coli*: antigenic VP1 recombinant protein. *Journal of Virology*, **61**, 3645–3647.

842. Ou, J., Laub, O. & Rutter, W. (1986) Hepatitis B virus gene function: The precore region targets the core antigen to cellular membranes and causes the secretion of the e antigen. *Proceedings of the National Academy of Sciences of the USA*, **83**, 1578–1582.

843. Ou, J-H., Yeh, C-T. & Yen, T.S.B. (1989) Transport of hepatitis B virus precore protein into the nucleus after cleavage of its signal peptide. *Journal of Virology*, **63**, 5238–5243.

844. Owen, R.L. & Shapiro, H. (1974) Pleural effusion, rash, and anergy in icteric hepatitis. *New England Journal of Medicine*, **291**, 963–965.

845. Ozsoylu, S., Kocak, N. & Yuce, A. (1989) Ascites related to cytomegalovirus infection. *European Journal of Paediatrics*, **149**, 142–143.

846. Pao, C.C., Yao, D.-S., Lin, C.-Y. *et al.* (1991) Serum hepatitis B virus DNA in hepatitis B virus seropositive and seronegative

patients with normal liver function. *American Journal of Clinical Pathology*, **95**, 591–596.

847. Papachristou, A.A., Dumas, A.S. & Katsouyannopoulos, V.C. (1991) Dissociation of alanine aminotransferase values in acute hepatitis A patients with and without past experience to the hepatitis B virus. *Epidemiology and Infection*, **106**, 397–402.

848. Papaevangelou, G.J., Vissoulis, C.G., Roumeliotou-Karayannis, A.J. *et al.* (1982) Comparison of safety and immunogenicity of ADW and AYW hepatitis B vaccines. *Journal of Medical Virology*, **9**, 231–236.

849. Papaevangelou, G., Tassopoulos, N., Roumeliotou-Karayannis, A. & Richardson, C. (1984) Etiology of fulminant viral hepatitis in Greece. *Hepatology*, **4**, 369–372.

850. Paronetto, F. & Tennant, B.C. (1990) Woodchuck hepatitis virus infection: A model of human hepatic diseases and hepatocellular carcinoma. In Popper, H. & Schaffner, F. (eds) *Progess in Liver Diseases*, Vol. IX., pp. 463–484. Philadelphia: W.B. Saunders.

851. Parry, J.V., Farrington, C.P., Perry, K.R. *et al.* (1988) Rational programme for screening travellers for antibodies to hepatitis A virus. *Lancet*, **1**, 1447–1449.

852. Parry, J.V., Perry, K.R., Panday, S. & Mortimer, P.P. (1989) Diagnosis of hepatitis A and B by testing saliva. *Journal of Medical Virology*, **28**, 255–260.

853. Pasetti, G., Calzetti, C., Degli Antoni, A. *et al.* (1988) Clinical features of hepatitis delta virus infection in a Northern Italian area. *Infection*, **16**, 345–348.

854. Pasi, K.J., Evans, J.A., Skidmore, S.J. & Hill, F.G.H. (1990) Prevention of hepatitis C virus infection in haemophiliacs. *Lancet*, **335**, 1473–1474.

855. Pasko, M.T., Bartholomew, W.R., Beam, T.R. Jr. *et al.* (1988) Long-term evaluation of the hepatitis B vaccine (Heptavax-B) in hemodialysis patients. *American Journal of Kidney Diseases*, **11**, 326–331.

856. Patti, M.E., Selvaggi, K.J. & Kroboth, F.J. (1990) Varicella hepatitis in the immunocompromised adult: a case report and a review of the literature. *American Journal of Medicine*, **88**, 77–80.

857. Pattison, C.P., Maynard, J.E. & Berquist, K.R. (1975) Epidemiology of hepatitis B in hospital personnel. *American Journal of Epidemiology*, **101**, 59–64.

858. Paul, A.V., Tada, H., von der Helm, K. *et al.* (1987) The entire nucleotide sequence of the genome of human hepatitis A virus (isolate MBB). *Virus Research*, **88**, 153–171.

859. Paul, J.R., Havens, W.P., Sabin, A.B. & Philip, C.B. (1945) Transmission experiments in serum jaundice and infectious hepatitis. *Journal of the American Medical Association*, **128**, 911–915.

860. Pauranik, A., Jain, S. & Maheshwari, M.C. (1987) Herpes simplex virus type 2 encephalitis in peripartum period preceded by hepatitis. *Japanese Journal of Medicine*, **26**, 84–87.

861. Pavli, P., Bayliss, G.J.A., Dent, O.F. & Lunz, M.R. (1989) The prevalence of serological markers for hepatitis B virus infection in Australian naval personnel. *Medical Journal of Australia*, **151**, 71–75.

862. Pelletier, G., Elghozi, D., Trepo, C. *et al.* (1985) Mononeuritis in acute viral hepatitis. *Digestion*, **32**, 53–56.

863. Pérez-Trallero, E., Cilla, G., Iturriza, M., *et al.* (1990) Commercial immunoglobulins and HCV. *Lancet*, **336**, 1590.

864. Perrillo, R.P., Pohl, D.A., Roodman, S.T. & Tsai, C.C. (1981) Acute non-A, non-B hepatitis with serum sickness-like syndrome and aplastic anemia. *Journal of the American Medical Association*, **245**, 494–496.

865. Perrillo, R.P., Chau, K.H., Overby, L.R. & Decker, R.H. (1983) Anti-hepatitis B core immunoglobulin M in the serologic evaluation of hepatitis B virus infection and simultaneous infection with type B, delta agent, and non-A, non-B viruses. *Gastroenterology*, **85**, 163–167.

866. Pesce, A.F., Crewe, E.B. & Cunningham, A.L. (1989) Should all pregnant women be screened for hepatitis B surface antigen? *Medical Journal of Australia*, **150**, 19–21.

867. Peters, C.J. & Johnson, K.M. (1972) Serum immunoglobulin levels in Australia antigen positive and Australia antigen negative hepatitis. *Clinical and Experimental Immunology*, **11**, 381–391.

868. Peters, D., Muller, G. & Slenczka, W. (1971) Morphology, development, and classification of the Marburg virus. In Martini,

G. A. & Siegert, R. (eds) *Marburg Virus Disease*. Proceedings of a Symposium, pp. 68–823. New York: Springer-Verlag.

869. Peters, R.L. (1975) Viral hepatitis: a pathologic spectrum. *American Journal of the Medical Sciences*, **270**, 17–31.

870. Peters, R.L., Omata, M., Aschavai, O. & Liew, C.T. (1978) Protracted viral hepatitis with impaired regeneration. In Vyas, G.N., Cohen, S.N. & Schmid, R. (eds) *Viral Hepatitis*, pp. 79–84. Philadelphia: Franklin Institute Press.

871. Petit, M.A., & Pilot, J. (1985) HBC and HBE antigenicity and DNA binding activity of major core protein P-22 in hepatitis B virus core particles isolated from the cytoplasm of human liver cells. *Journal of Virology*, **53**, 543–551.

872. Petit, M.A., Capel, F., Riottot, M.M. *et al.* (1987) Antigenic mapping of the surface proteins of infectious hepatitis B virus particles. *Journal of General Virology*, **68**, 2759–2767.

873. Pêtre, J., Van Wijnendaele, F., De Neys, B. *et al.* (1987) Development of a hepatitis B vaccine from transformed yeast cells. *Postgraduate Medical Journal*, **63**, 73–81.

874. Pfeiffer, U., Thomssen, R., Legler, K. *et al.* (1980) Experimental non-A non-B hepatitis: four types of cytoplasmic alteration in hepatocytes of infected chimpanzees. *Virchows Archiv. B. Cell Pathology*, **33**, 233–243.

875. Phillips, M.J. & Poucell, S. (1981) Modern aspects of the morphology of viral hepatitis. *Human Pathology*, **12**, 1060–1084.

876. Phillips, M. & Cummins, L.M. (1988) Absence of seroconversion following treatment with hepatitis B immune globulin containing antibody to human immunodeficiency virus. *Hepatology*, **8**, 497–498.

877. Phillips, M.J., Blendis, L.M., Poucell, S. *et al.* (1991) Syncytial giant-cell hepatitis. Sporadic hepatitis with distinctive pathological features, a severe clinical course and paramyxoviral features. *New England Journal of Medicine*, **324**, 455–460.

878. Phoon, W.O., Fong, N.P., Lee, J. & Leong, H.K. (1987) A study on the prevalence of hepatitis B surface antigen among Chinese adult males in Singapore. *International Journal of Epidemiology*, **16**, 74–78.

879. Piazza, M., Guadagnino, V., Picciotto, L. *et al.* (1983) Effect of (+)-Cyanidanol-3 in acute HAV, HBV, and non-A, non-B viral hepatitis. *Hepatology*, **3**, 45–49.

880. Piazza, M., Guadagnino, V., Picciotto, L. *et al.* (1987) Contamination by hepatitis B surface antigen in dental surgeries. *British Medical Journal*, **295**, 473–474.

881. Piazza, M., Da Villa, G., Picciotto, L. *et al.* (1988) Mass vaccination against hepatitis B in infants in Italy. *Lancet*, **2**, 1132.

882. Pickles, W.N. (1930) Epidemic catarrhal jaundice: outbreak in Yorkshire. *British Medical Journal*, **1**, 1944.

883. Ping, L.H., Jansen, R.W., Stapleton, J.T. *et al.* (1988) Identification of an immunodominant antigenic site involving the capsid protein VP3 of hepatitis A virus. *Proceedings of the National Academy of Sciences of the USA*, **85**, 8281–8285.

884. Pirson, Y., Alexandre, G.P. & Ypersele, C. (1977) Long-term effect of HBs antigenemia on patient survival after renal transplantation. *New England Journal of Medicine*, **296**(4), 194–196.

885. Pistello, M., Ceccherini-Nelli, L., Cecconi, N. *et al.* (1991) Hepatitis C virus seroprevalence in Italian haemophiliacs injected with virus-inactivated concentrates: Five year follow-up and correlation with antibodies to other viruses. *Journal of Medical Virology*, **33**, 43–46.

886. Pohl, C., Baroudy, B.M., Bergmann, K.F. *et al.* (1987) A human monoclonal antibody that recognizes viral polypeptides and in vitro translation products of the genome of the hepatitis D virus. *Journal of Infectious Diseases*, **156**, 622–629.

887. Polakoff, S., Cossart, Y.E. & Tillett, H.E. (1972) Hepatitis in dialysis units in the UK. *British Medical Journal*, **2**, 94.

888. Polakoff, S. (1976) Hepatitis B in retreat from dialysis units in the United Kingdom in 1973. *British Medical Journal*, **1**, 1579.

889. Polakoff, S. (1987) Decrease in acute hepatitis B incidence in England and Wales in 1985–86. *Lancet*, **1**, 380.

890. Polakoff, S. & Vandervelde, E.M. (1988) Immunisation of neonates at high risk of hepatitis B in England and Wales: national surveillance. *British Medical Journal*, **297**, 249–253.

891. Polakoff, S. (1989) Acute viral hepatitis B: Laboratory reports 1985–8. *Communicable Diseases Report*, **29**, 3–6.

892. Polakoff, S. (1990) Reports of clinical hepatitis A from Public Health and hospital microbiology laboratories to the PHLS Communicable Disease Surveillance Centre during the period 1980–1988. *Journal of Infection*, **21**, 111–117.

893. Polakoff, S. (1990) Public Health Laboratory Service surveillance of prophylaxis by specific hepatitis B immunoglobulin in England and Wales during the period 1975–1987. *Journal of Infection*, **21**, 213–220.

894. Polesky, H.F. & Hanson, M.R. (1989) Transfusion-associated hepatitis C virus (non-A, non-B) infection. *Archives of Pathology and Laboratory Medicine*, **113**, 232–235.

895. Pollock, T.M., & Reid, D. (1969) Immunoglobulin for the prevention of infective heaptitis in persons working overseas. *Lancet*, **1**, 281.

896. Pontisso, P., Petit, M-A., Bankowski, M.J. & Peeples, M.E. (1989) Human liver plasma membranes contain receptors for the hepatitis B virus pre-S1 region and, via polymerized human serum albumin, for the pre-S2 region. *Journal of Virology*, **63**, 1981–1988.

897. Pontisso, P., Ruvoletto, M-G., Gerlich, W.H. *et al.* (1989) Identification of an attachment site for human liver plasma membranes on hepatitis B virus particles. *Virology*, **173**, 522–530.

898. Ponzetto, A., Purcell, R.H. & Gerin, J.L. (1983) Experimental transmission of the delta agent to the eastern woodchuck (Marmota monax). *Progress in Clinical and Biological Research*, **143**, 107–112.

899. Ponzetto, A., Cote, P.J., Popper, H. *et al.* (1984) Transmission of the hepatitis B-associated delta agent to the eastern woodchuck. *Proceedings of the National Academy of Sciences of the USA*, **81**, 2208–2212.

900. Ponzetto, A., Negro, F., Popper, H. *et al.* (1988) Serial passage of hepatitis delta virus (HDV) in chronic hepatitis B virus (HBV) carrier chimpanzees. *Hepatology*, **8**, 1655–1661.

901. Poovorawan, Y., Sanpavat, S., Pongpunlert, W. *et al.* (1989) Protective efficacy of a recombinant DNA hepatitis B vaccine in neonates of HBe antigen-positive mothers. *Journal of the American Medical Association*, **261**, 3278–3281.

902. Popper, H. & Schaffner, F. (1971) The vocabulary of chronic hepatitis. *New England Journal of Medicine*, **284**, 1154–1156.

903. Popper, H. (1972) The pathology of viral hepatitis. *Canadian Medical Association Journal*, **106**, 447–452.

904. Popper, H. & Schaffner, F. (1976) Chronic hepatitis: taxonomic, etiologic and therapeutic problems. In Popper, H. & Schaffner, F. (eds) *Progress in Liver Diseases*, Vol. 5, pp. 531–558. New York: Grune & Stratton.

905. Popper, H., Thung, S.N., Gerber, M.A. *et al.* (1983) Histologic studies of severe delta agent infection in Venezuelan Indians. *Hepatology*, **3**, 906–912.

906. Popper, H., Buitrago, B., Hadler, S.C. *et al.* (1987) Pathology of hepatitis delta infection in the Amazon Basin. *Progress in Clinical and Biological Research*, **234**, 121–128.

907. Porres, E.R., Verthammer, J., Moss, N. *et al.* (1985) Fatal coxsackie virus B4 infection in a neonate. *South Medical Journal*, **78**, 1254–1256.

908. Porres, J.C., Carreño, V., Bartolomé, J. *et al.* (1989) A dynamic study of the intrafamilial spread of hepatitis B virus infection: Relation with the viral replication. *Journal of Medical Virology*, **28**, 237–242.

909. Poulsen, H. & Christoffersen, P. (1969) Abnormal bile duct epithelium in liver biopsies with histological signs of viral hepatitis. *Acta Pathologica et Microbiologica Scandinavica*, **76**, 383–390.

910. Powdrill, T.F. & Johnston, J.M. (1991) Immunologic priming with recombinant hepatitis A virus capsid proteins produced in *Escheria coli*. *Journal of Virology*, **65**, 2686–2690.

911. Pozzilli, P., Arduini, P., Visalli, N. *et al.* (1987) Reduced protection against hepatitis B virus following vaccination in patients with type 1 (insulin-dependent) diabetes. *Diabetologia*, **30**, 817–819.

912. Price, M.E., Fisher-Hoch, S.P., Craven, R.B. & McCormick, J.B. (1988) A prospective study of maternal and foetal outcome in acute Lassa fever infection during pregnancy. *British Medical Journal*, **297**, 584–587.

913. Prince, A.M. (1968) An antigen detected in the blood during the incubation period of serum hepatitis. *Proceedings of the National Academy of Sciences of the USA*, **60**, 814–821.

914. Prince, A.M., Metselaar, D., Kafuko, G.W. *et al.* (1972) Hepatitis B antigen in wild-caught mosquitoes in Africa. *Lancet*, **2**, 247–250.

915. Prince, A.M., Brotman, B., Grady, G.F. *et al.* (1974) Long-incubation post-transfusion hepatitis without serological evidence of exposure to hepatitis-B virus. *Lancet*, **2**, 241–246.

916. Prinsen, H., Goilav, C., Safary, A. *et al.* (1987) Immunogenicity and tolerance of a yeast-derived hepatitis B vaccine in homosexual men. *Postgraduate Medical Journal*, **63**, 147–150.

917. Provost, P.J., Wolanski, B.S., Miller, W.J. *et al.* (1975) Physical, chemical and morphologic dimensions of human hepatitis A virus strain CR326. *Proceedings of the Society for Experimental Biology and Medicine*, **148**, 532–539.

918. Provost, P.J., Conti, P.A., Giesa, P.A. *et al.* (1983) Studies in chimpanzees of liver, attenuated hepatitis A vaccine candidates. *Proceedings of the Society for Experimental Biology and Medicine*, **172**, 357–363.

919. Pugh, J., Zweidler, A. & Summers, J. (1989) Characterization of the major duck hepatitis B virus core particle protein. *Journal of Virology*, **63**, 1371–1376.

920. Purcell, R.H. (1975) Current status of diagnostic tests for viral hepatitis. In Mathieu, A. & Kahan, B.D. (eds) *Immunologic Aspects Anaesthetic and Surgical Practices*, pp. 205–226. New York: Grune & Stratton.

921. Purcell, R.H., Dienstag, J.L., Feinstone, S.M. & Kapikian, A.Z. (1975) Relationship of hepatitis A antigen to viral hepatitis. *American Journal of Medical Science*, **270**, 61–71.

922. Purcell, R.H., Feinstone, S.M., Ticehurst, J.R. *et al.* (1984) Hepatitis B virus. In Vyas, G.N., Dienstag, J.L. & Hoofnagle, J. (eds) *Viral Hepatitis and Liver Disease*, pp. 9–22. New York: Grune & Stratton.

923. Purcell, R.H., Satterfield, W.C., Bergmann, K.F. *et al.* (1987) Experimental hepatitis delta infection in the chimpanzee. In Rizzetto, M., Gerin, J.L. & Purcell, R.H. (eds) *The Hepatitis Delta Virus and Its Infection*, pp. 27–36. New York: Alan R. Liss, Inc.

924. Putnam, J.R. & Phillips, B.A. (1981) Picornaviral structure and assembly. *Microbiology Review*, **45**, 287–315.

925. Quinti, I., Paganelli, R., Scala, E. *et al.* (1990) Hepatitis C virus antibodies in gammaglobulin. *Lancet*, **336**, 1377.

926. Quiroga, J.A., Castillo, I., Porres, J.C. *et al.* (1990) Recombinant γ-interferon as adjuvant to hepatitis B vaccine in hemodialysis patients. *Hepatology*, **12**, 661–663.

927. Quiroga, J.A., Campillo, M.L., Catillo, I. *et al.* (1991) IgM antibody to hepatitis C virus in acute and chronic hepatitis C. *Hepatology*, **14**, 38–43.

928. Rabinowitz, M., Hallak, A., Grunberg, J. *et al.* (1987) A modified, solid phase radioimmunoassay for the differential diagnosis of acute and convalescent phases of hepatitis A infection. *American Journal of Clinical Pathology*, **88**, 738–742.

929. Rachmilewitz, M., Moshkowitz, B., Rachmilewitz, B. *et al.* (1972) Serum vitamin B12 binding proteins in viral hepatitis. *European Journal of Clinical Investigation*, **2**, 239–242.

930. Radziwill, G., Tucker, W. & Schaller, H. (1990) Mutational analysis of the hepatitis B virus P gene product: Domain structure and RNase H activity. *Journal of Virology*, **64**, 613–620.

931. Raimondo, G., Smedile, A., Gallo, L. *et al.* (1982) Multicentre study of prevalence of HBV-associated delta infection and liver disease in drug addicts. *Lancet*, **1**, 249–251.

932. Raimondo, G., Longo, G. & Squadrito, G. (1983) Exacerbation of chronic liver disease due to hepatitis B surface antigen after delta infection. *British Medical Journal*, **286**, 845.

933. Ramalingaswami, V. & Purcell, R.H. (1988) Waterborne non-A non-B hepatitis. *Lancet*, **1**, 571–573.

934. Raney, A.K., Milich, D.R. & McLachlan, A. (1989) Characterization of hepatitis B virus major surface antigen gene transcriptional regulatory elements in differentiated hepatoma cell lines. *Journal of Virology*, **63**, 3919–3925.

935. Ray, M.B., Desmet, V.J., Fevery, J. *et al.* (1976) Distribution patterns of hepatitis B surface antigen (HBsAg) in the liver of hepatitis B patients. *Journal of Clinical Pathology*, **29**, 94–100.

936. Ray, R., Aggarwal, R., Salunke, P.N. *et al.* (1991) Hepatitis E virus genome in stools of hepatitis patients during large epidemic in north India. *Lancet*, **338**, 783–784.

937. Read, A.E., Donegan, E., Lake, J. *et al.* (1991) Hepatitis C in patients undergoing liver transplantation. *Annals of Internal Medicine*, **114**, 282–284.

938. Read, R.B., Ede, R.J., Morgan-Capner, P. *et al.* (1985) Myocarditis and fulminant hepatic failure from coxsackie virus B infection. *Postgraduate Medical Journal*, **61**, 749–752.

939. Redeker, A.G. (1975) Viral hepatitis: clinical aspects. *American Journal of the Medical Sciences*, **270**, 9–16.

940. Redeker, A.G. (1978) Advances in clinical aspects of acute and chronic liver disease of viral origin. In Vyas, G.N., Cohen, S.N. & Schmid, R. (eds) *Viral Hepatitis*, pp. 425–429. Philadelphia: Franklin Institute Press.

941. Reesink, H.W., Reerink-Brongers, E., Lafaber-Schut, B.J.T. *et al.* (1979) Prevention of chronic HBsAg carrier state in infants of HBsAg-positive mothers by hepatitis B immunoglobulin. *Lancet*, **2**, 436–437.

942. Reesink, H.W., Leentvaar-Knypers, A., Van der Poel, C.L. *et al.* (1988) Non-A, non-B postransfusion hepatitis in open heart surgery patients in the Netherlands: Preliminary results of a prospective study. In Zuckerman, A.J. (ed.) *Viral Hepatitis and Liver Disease*, pp. 558–560. New York: Alan R. Liss.

943. Reesink, H.W., Wong, V.C.W., Ip, H.M.H. *et al.* (1990) Mother-to-infant transmission and hepatitis C virus. *Lancet*, **335**, 1216–1217.

944. Reichel, M. & Mauro, T.M. (1990) Urticaria and hepatitis C. *Lancet*, **336**, 822–823.

945. Reingold, A.L., Kane, M.A. & Hightower, A.W. (1988) Failure of gloves and other protective devices to prevent transmission of hepatitis B virus to oral surgeons. *Journal of the American Medical Association* **259**, 2558–2560.

946. Reyes, G.R., Purdy, M.A., Kim, J.P. *et al.* (1990) Isolation of a cDNA from the virus responsible for enterically transmitted non-A, non-B hepatitis. *Science*, **247**, 1335–1339.

947. Rice, C.M., Lencehs, E.M., Eddy, S.R. *et al.* (1985) Nucleotide sequence of yellow fever virus: implications for flavivirus gene expression and evolution. *Science*, **229**, 726–733.

948. Rice, C.M., Strauss, E.G. & Strauss, J.H. (1986) Structure of the flavivirus genome. In Schlesinger, S. & Schlesinger, M.J. (eds) *The Togaviridae and Flaviviridae*, pp. 279–326. New York: Plenum Press.

949. Rice, S.J. (1988) False negativity with one-step monoclonal assay for hepatitis B surface antigen. *Lancet*, **1**, 1786.

950. Rimland, D., Parkin, W.E., Miller, P.H.G.B. & Schrack, W.D. (1977) Hepatitis B outbreak traced to an oral surgeon. *New England Journal of Medicine*, **296**(17), 953–958.

951. Ritter, S.E., Whitten, T.M., Wuets, A.T. & Schloemer, R.H. (1991) An internal domain of the hepatitis B virus X antigen is necessary for transactivating activity. *Virology*, **182**, 841–845.

952. Rizzetto, M., Bonino, F., Diana, S. & Verme, G. (1976) Prognostic significance of in-vitro complement fixation in liver biopsy specimens from patients with acute viral hepatitis type B. *Lancet*, **2**, 436–438.

953. Rizzetto, M., Canese, M.G., Aricó, J. *et al.* (1977) Immunofluorescence detection of a new antigen-antibody system (delta-antidelta) associated to the hepatitis B virus in the liver and in the serum of HBsAg carriers. *Gut*, **18**, 996–1003.

954. Rizzetto, M., Shih, J.W.K., Gocke, D.J. *et al.* (1979) Incidence and significance of antibodies to delta antigen in HBV infection. *Lancet*, **2**, 986–990.

955. Rizzetto, M., Canese, M.G., Gerin, J.L. *et al.* (1980) Transmission of hepatitis B virus-associated delta antigen to chimpanzees. *Journal of Infectious Diseases*, **141**, 590–602.

956. Rizzetto, M., Hoyer, B., Canese, M.G. *et al.* (1980) Delta agent: association of delta antigen with hepatitis B surface antigen and RNA in serum of delta-infected chimpanzees. *Proceedings of the National Academy of Sciences of the USA*, **77**, 6124–6128.

957. Rizzetto, M., Canese, M.G., Purcell, R.H. *et al.* (1981) Experimental HBV in delta infections of chimpanzees: occurrence and significance of intrahepatic immune complexes of hepatitis B core antigen and delta antigen. *Hepatology*, **1**, 567–579.

958. Rizzetto, M., Morello, C., Mannucci, P.M. *et al.* (1982) Delta infection and liver disease in haemophilic carriers of the hepatitis B surface antigen. *Journal of Infectious Diseases*, **145**, 18–22.

959. Rizzetto, M., Verme, G., Recchia, S. *et al.* (1983) Chronic hepatitis in carriers of hepatitis B surface antigen, with intrahepatic expression of the delta antigen. An active and progressive disease unresponsive to immunosuppressive treatment. *Annals of Internal Medicine*, **98**, 437–441.

960. Rizzetto, M., Bonino, F., Verme, G. *et al.* (1983) Nomenclature: a proposal to designate the delta agent as hepatitis D virus. In Rizzetto, M., Gerin, J.L. & Purcell, R.H. (eds) *The Hepatitis Delta Virus and its Infections.* New York: Alan R. Liss.

960a. Rizzetto, M. (1983) Delta agent. *Hepatology*, 3, 729–737.

961. Rizzetto, M., Ponzetto, A. & Marinucci, G. (1988) Transfusion-related delta hepatitis. *Transfusion Medicine Reviews*, 2, 224–228.

962. Rizzetto, M. (1990) Hepatitis delta: the virus and the disease. *Journal of Hepatology*, 11, S145–S148.

963. Robbins, F.C., Mahmoud, A.A.F. & Warren, K.S. (1977) Algorithms in the diagnosis and management of exotic diseases. XIX. Major tropical viral infections: smallpox, yellow fever and Lassa fever. *Journal of Infectious Diseases*, 135, 341–346.

964. Robinson, W.S. & Greenman, R.L. (1974) DNA polymerase in the core of the human hepatitis B virus candidate. *Journal of Virology*, 13, 1231–1236.

965. Robinson, W.S. & Lutwick, L.J. (1976) The virus of hepatitis, type B. *New England Journal of Medicine*, 295, 1168–1175.

966. Robinson, W.S. (1977) The genome of hepatitis B virus. *Annual Review of Microbiology*, 31, 357–377.

967. Robinson, W.S. (1990) Hepadnaviridae and their replication. In Fields, B.N. & Knipe, D.M. (eds) *Virology*, pp. 2137–2170. New York: Raven Press.

968. Roggendorf, M., Frosner, G.G., Deinhardt, F. & Sheid, R. (1980) Comparison of solid-phase test systems for demonstrating antibodies against hepatitis A virus (anti-HAV) of the IgM class. *Journal of Medical Virology*, 5, 47–62.

969. Roggendorf, M., Deinhardt, F., Rasshofer, R. *et al.* (1989) Antibodies to hepatitis C virus. *Lancet*, 2, 324–325.

970. Roingeard, P., Lu, S.L., Sureau, C. *et al.* (1990) Immunocytochemical and electron microscopic study of hepatitis B virus antigen and complete particle production in hepatitis B virus DNA transfected HepG2 cells. *Hepatology*, 11, 277–285.

971. Romieu, I., Sow, I., Lu, S. *et al.* (1989) Prevalence of hepatitis B markers among hospital workers in Senegal. *Journal of Medical Virology*, 27, 282–287.

972. Roos, C.M., Feltkampf-Vroom, T.M. & Helder, A.W. (1976) The localisation of hepatitis B antigen and immunoglobulin G in liver tissue: an immunofluorescence, light and electron microscopic study. *Journal of Pathology*, 118, 1–8.

973. Rosen, L., Khin, M.M. & U, T. (1989) Recovery of virus from the liver of children with fatal Dengue: reflections on the pathogenesis of the disease and its possible analogy with that of yellow fever. *Research in Virology*, 140, 351–360.

974. Rosenblum, L.S., Hadler, S.C., Castro, K.G. *et al.* (1990) Heterosexual transmission of hepatitis B virus in Belle Glade, Florida. *Journal of Infectious Diseases*, 161, 407–411.

975. Rumball, J.M., Stone, C.M. & Hasset, C. (1959) The behaviour of serum iron in acute hepatitis. *Gastroenterology*, 36, 219–223.

976. Rumi, M.G., Romeo, R., Bortolini, M. *et al.* (1989) Immunogenicity of a yeast- recombinant hepatitis B vaccine in high-risk children. *Journal of Medical Virology*, 27, 48–51.

977. Rumi, M., Colombo, M., Romeo, R. *et al.* (1991) Suboptimal response to hepatitis B vaccine in drug users. *Archives of Internal Medicine*, 151, 574–578.

978. Russnak, R. & Ganem, D. (1990) Sequences 5' to the polyadenylation signal mediate differential poly(A) site use in hepatitis B viruses. *Genes and Development*, 4, 764–776.

979. Sagnelli, E., Piccinino, F., Pasquale, G. *et al.* (1984) Delta agent infection: An unfavourable event in HBsAg positive chronic hepatitis. *Liver*, 4, 170–176.

980. Saiki, R.K., Gelfand, D.H., Stoffel, S. *et al.* (1988) Primer-directed enzymatic amplification of DNA with a thermostable DNA polymerase. *Science*, 239, 487–491.

981. Salassa, B., Daziano, E., Bonino, F. *et al.* (1991) Serological diagnosis of hepatitis B and delta virus (HBV/HDV) coinfection. *Journal of Hepatology*, 12, 10–13.

982. Saluzzo, J.F., Some, L., Baudon, D. *et al.* (1985) The use of stabilised yellow fever vaccine 17D at the time of the yellow fever epidemic in Burkina Faso. *Bulletin de la Societé de Pathologie Exotique Filiales*, 78, 536–540.

983. Sanches-Quijano, A., Pineda, J.A., Lissen, E. *et al.* (1988) Prevention of post-transfusion non-A, non-B hepatitis by non-specific immunoglobulin in heart surgery patients. *Lancet*, 1, 1245–1249.

984. Sanchez-Tapias, J.M., Mas, A. & Costa, J. (1987) Recombinant alpha 2C interferon therapy in fulminant viral hepatitis. *Journal of Hepatology*, 5, 205–210.

985. Sansonno, D.E., Fiore, G., Pietropaolo, F. *et al.* (1988) Hepatitis A virus and non-A, non-B virus superinfections in HBsAg chronic carriers. *Digestion*, 39, 197–203.

986. Santantonio, T., Jung, M.C., Miska, S. *et al.* (1991) Prevalence and type of pre-C HBV mutants in anti-HBe positive carriers with chronic liver disease in a highly endemic area. *Virology*, 183, 840–844.

987. Sattler, F. & Robinson, W.S. (1979) Hepatitis B viral DNA molecules have cohesive ends. *Journal of Virology*, 32, 226–233.

988. Schaeffer, E., Snyder, R. & Sninsky, J. (1986) Identification and localization of pre-S encoded polypeptides from woodchuck and ground squirrel hepatitis viruses. *Journal of Virology*, 57, 173–182.

989. Schaff, Z., Gerety, R.J., Gremley, P.M. *et al.* (1985) Ultrastructural and cytochemical study of hepatocytes and lymphocytes during experimental non-A, non-B infections in chimpanzees. *Journal of Experimental Pathology*, 2, 25–36.

990. Schaffner, F. (1966) Intralobular changes in hepatocytes and the electron microscopic mesenchymal response in acute viral hepatitis. *Medicine*, 45, 547–552.

991. Schaffner, F. (1970) The structural basis of altered hepatic function in viral hepatitis. *American Journal of Medicine*, 49, 658–668.

992. Schaffner, F., Dienstag, J.L., Purcell, R.H. & Popper, H. (1977) Chimpanzee livers after infection with human hepatitis viruses A and B. Ultrastructural studies. *Archives of Pathology and Laboratory Medicine*, 101, 113–117.

993. Schatz, G., Hadler, S., McCarthey, J. *et al.* (1990) Outreach to needle users and sexual contacts: A multi-year, community-wide hepatitis B/delta hepatitis control program in Worcester, Massachusetts. In Coursaget, P. & Tong, M.J. (eds) *Progress in Hepatitis B Immunization.* London: John Libbey.

994. Scheiermann, N., Gesemann, K.M., Kreuzfelder, E. & Paar, D. (1987) Effects of a recombinant yeast-derived hepatitis B vaccine in healthy adults. *Postgraduate Medical Journal*, 63, 115–119.

995. Scheuer, P.J., Teixeira, M.R., Weller, I.V.D. *et al.* (1979) Pathology of acute hepatitis A, B, and non-A, non-B. *Gastroenterology*, 79, 1124.

996. Scheuer, P.J. (1989) Non-A, non-B hepatitis. *Virchows Archives Series A*, 415, 301–303.

997. Scheutz, F., Melbye, M., Esteban, J.I. *et al.* (1988) Hepatitis B virus infection in Danish dentists. *American Journal of Epidemiology*, 128, 190–196.

998. Schiff, E.R., de Medina, M., Woodman, S. *et al.* (1982) VA cooperative study on hepatitis and dentistry. *Hepatology*, 2, 688.

999. Schleissner, L.A. & Portnoy, L. (1968) Hepatitis and pneumonia associated with echovirus type 9 infection in two adult siblings. *Annals of Internal Medicine*, 68, 1315–1319.

1000. Schlesinger, J.J., Brandriss, M.W., Cropp, C.B. & Monath, T.P. (1986) Protection against yellow fever in monkeys by immunization with yellow fever virus nonstructural protein NS1. *Journal of Virology*, 60, 1153–1155.

1001. Schlict, H.J., Salfeld, J. & Schaller, H. (1987) The duck hepatitis B virus pre-C region encodes a signal sequence which is essential for synthesis and secretion of processed core proteins but not for virus formation. *Journal of Virology*, 61, 3701–3709.

1002. Schlict, H.J. & Schaller, H. (1989) The secretory core protein of human hepatitis B virus is expressed on the cell surface. *Journal of Virology*, 63, 5399–5404.

1003. Schlict, H.J., Radziwill, G. & Schaller, H. (1989) Synthesis and encapsidation of duck hepatitis B virus reverse transcriptase do not require formation of core-polymerase fusion proteins. *Cell*, 56, 85–92.

1004. Schlipköter, U., Roggendorf, M., Ernst, G. *et al.* (1990) Hepatitis C virus antibodies in haemodialysis patients. *Lancet*, 335, 1409.

1005. Schmid, M., Pirovino, M., Altorfer, J. *et al.* (1982) Acute hepatitis non-A, non-B; are there any specific light microscopic features. *Liver*, 2, 61–67.

1006. Schmitz, H. & Enders, G. (1977) Cytomegalovirus as a frequent cause of Guillain–Barré syndrome. *Journal of Medical Virology*, **1**, 21–27.

1007. Schomerus, H., Wideman, K.H., Dolle, W. *et al.* (1984) (+)-Cyanidanol-3 in the treatment of acute viral hepatitis: a randomized controlled trial. *Hepatology*, **4**, 331–335.

1008. Schramm, W., Roggendorf, M., Rommel, F. *et al.* (1989) Prevalence of antibodies to hepatitis C virus (HCV) in haemophiliacs. *Blut*, **59**, 390–392.

1009. Schreeder, M.T., Thompson, S.E., Hadler, S.C. *et al.* (1982) Hepatitis B in homosexual men: Prevalence of infection and factors related to transmission. *Journal of Infectious Diseases*, **146**, 7–15.

1010. Schroeder, D.D. & Mozen, N.M. (1970) Australia antigen: distribution during Cohn ethanol fractionation of human plasma. *Science*, **168**, 1462–1464.

1011. Schulman, A.N., Dienstag, J.L., Jackson, D.R. *et al.* (1976) Hepatitis A antigen particles in the liver, bile, and stool of chimpanzees. *Journal of Infectious Diseases*, **134**(1), 80–84.

1012. Schulman, S. & Grillner, L. (1990) Antibodies against hepatitis C in a population of Swedish haemophiliacs and heterosexual partners. *Scandinavian Journal of Infectious Diseases*, **22**, 393–397.

1013. Schweitzer, I.L. & Spears, R.L. (1970) Hepatitis associated antigen (Australia antigen) in mother and infant. *New England Journal of Medicine*, **283**, 570–572.

1014. Schweitzer, I.L., Mosley, J.W., Edwards, M.A.V.M. & Overby, L.B. (1973) Factors influencing neonatal infection by hepatitis B virus. *Gastroenterology*, **65**, 277–283.

1015. Sciot, R., Van Damme, B. & Desmet, V.J. (1986) Cholestatic features in hepatitis A. *Journal of Hepatology*, **3**, 172–181.

1016. Sciot, R., De Vos, R., De Wolf-Peeters, C. & Desmet, V.J. (1986) Hepatitis A: a Kupffer cell disease? *Journal of Clinical Pathology*, **39**, 1160–1161.

1017. Scott, J.S., Pace, R.A., Sheridan, J.W. & Cooksley, W.G. (1990) Discordance of hepatitis B e antigen and hepatitis B viral deoxyribonucleic acid. *Journal of Medical Virology*, **32**, 225–231.

1018. Scotto, J., Hadchouel, M., Hery, C. *et al.* (1983) Detection of hepatitis B viral DNA in serum by a simple spot hybridization technique: comparisons with results for other viral markers. *Hepatology*, **3**, 279–284.

1019. Sears, D.A., George, J.N. & Gold, M.S. (1975) Transient red blood cell aplasia in association with viral hepatitis. Occurrence four years apart in siblings. *Archives of Internal Medicine*, **135**, 1585–1589.

1020. Seeff, L.B., Zimmerman, H.J., Wright, E.C. *et al.* (1975) Efficacy of hepatitis B immune serum globulin after accidental exposure. Preliminary report of the Veterans Administration Co-operative Study. *Lancet*, **2**, 939–941.

1021. Seeff, L.B., Zimmerman, H.J., Wright, E.C. *et al.* (1977) A randomized, double blind controlled trial of the efficacy of immune serum globulin for the prevention of post-transfusion hepatitis. *Gastroenterology*, **72**, 111–121.

1022. Seeff, L.B., Beebe, G.W., Hoofnagle, J.H. *et al.* (1987) A serologic follow-up of the 1942 epidemic of post-vaccination hepatitis in the United States army. *New England Journal of Medicine*, **316**, 965–970.

1023. Seeff, L.B. (1987) Transfusion-associated hepatitis B: Past and present. *Transfusion Medicine Reviews*, **2**, 204–214.

1024. Seeger, C., Ganem, D. & Varmus, H.S. (1984) The cloned genome of ground squirrel hepatitis virus is infectious in the animal. *Proceedings of the National Academy of Sciences in the USA*, **81**, 5849–5842.

1025. Seeger, C., Ganem, D. & Varmus, H.S. (1986) Biochemical and genetic evidence for the hepatitis B virus replication strategy. *Science*, **232**, 477.

1026. Seeger, C. & Maragos, J. (1990) Identification and characterization of the woodchuck hepatitis virus origin of DNA replication. *Journal of Virology*, **64**, 16–23.

1027. Sergeev, N.W., Paktoris, E.A., Ananev, W.A. *et al.* (1957) General characteristics of Botkin's disease occurring in Kirgiz Republic of USSR in 1955–56. *Soviet Healthcare Kirgizii*, **5**, 16–23.

1028. Sergent, J.S., Lockshin, M.D., Christian, C.L. & Gocke, D.J. (1976) Vasculitis with hepatitis B antigenemia. *Medicine*, **55**, 1–18.

1029. Seto, E., Yen, T.S.B., Peterlin, B.M. & Ou, J-H. (1988) Trans-activation of the human immunodeficiency virus long terminal repeat by the hepatitis B virus X protein. *Proceedings of the National Academy of Sciences of the USA*, **85**, 8286–8290.

1030. Seto, E., Mitchell, P.J. & Yen, T.S.B. (1990) Transactivation by the hepatitis B virus X protein depends on AP-2 and other transcription factors. *Nature*, **344**, 72–74.

1031. Shaldon, S. & Sherlock, S. (1957) Virus hepatitis with features of prolonged bile retention. *British Medical Journal*, **2**, 734–738.

1032. Sharmeen, L., Kuo, M.Y., Dinter-Gottlieb, G. & Taylor, J. (1988) Antigenomic RNA of human hepatitis delta virus can undergo self-cleavage. *Journal of Virology*, **62**, 2674–2679.

1033. Sharmeen, L., Kuo, M.Y. & Taylor, J. (1989) Self-ligating RNA sequences on the antigenome of human hepatitis delta virus. *Journal of Virology*, **63**, 1428–1430.

1034. Shattock, A.G. & Morgan, B.M. (1984) Sensitive enzyme immunoassay for the detection of delta antigen and anti-delta, using serum as the delta antigen source. *Journal of Medical Virology*, **13**, 73–82.

1035. Shaul, Y., Riter, W.J. & Laub, O. (1985) Human hepatitis B viral enhancer element. *EMBO Journal*, **4**, 426–430.

1036. Shaw, F.E., Graham, D.J., Guess, H.A. *et al.* (1988) Postmarketing surveillance for neurologic adverse events reported after hepatitis B vaccination. *American Journal of Epidemiology*, **127**, 337–352.

1037. Sheretz, R.J., Russell, B.A. & Reuman, P.D. (1984) Transmission of hepatitis A by transfusion of blood products. *Archives of Internal Medicine*, **144**, 1579–1580.

1038. Sherlock, S. (1976) Predicting progression of acute type-B hepatitis to chronicity. *Lancet*, **2**, 354–356.

1039. Sheron, N. & Alexander, G.J.M. (1990) Hepatitis C, D and E virus infection. In Farthing, M.J.G. (ed.) *Baillière's Clinical Gastroenterology*, Vol. 4(3), pp. 749–774. London: Baillière Tindall.

1040. Shiels, M.T., Taswell, H.F., Czaja, A.J. *et al.* (1987) Frequency and significance of concurrent hepatitis B surface antigen and antibody in acute and chronic hepatitis B. *Gastroenterology*, **93**, 675–680.

1041. Shiina, S., Fujino, H., Yasuda, H. *et al.* (1988) HBs antigen subtypes among acute hepatitis patients in Japan: Evidence of imported hepatitis. *American Journal of Gastroenterology*, **83**, 727–729.

1042. Shikata, T., Uzawa, T., Yoshiwara, N. *et al.* (1974) Staining methods of Australia antigen in paraffin section: detection of cytoplasmic inclusion bodies. *Japanese Journal of Experimental Medicine*, **44**, 25–36.

1043. Shimuzu, Y.K., Feinstone, S.M., Purcell, R.H. *et al.* (1979) Non-A, non-B hepatitis: Ultrastructural evidence for two antigens in experimentally infected chimpanzees. *Science*, **205**, 197–200.

1044. Shimuzu, Y.K., Weiner, A.J., Rosenblatt, J. *et al.* (1990) Early events in hepatitis C virus infection of chimpanzees. *Proceedings of the National Academy of Sciences of the USA*, **87**, 6441–6444.

1045. Shlien, R.D., Meyers, S., Lee, J.A. *et al.* (1988) Fulminant herpes simplex hepatitis in a patient with ulcerative colitis. *Gut*, **29**, 257–261.

1046. Siddiqui, A., Marion, P.L. & Robinson, W.S. (1981) Ground squirrel hepatitis virus DNA molecular cloning and comparison with hepatitis B virus DNA. *Journal of Virology*, **38**, 393–397.

1047. Siebke, J.C., Wessel, N., Kvandal, P. & Lie, T. (1989) The prevalence of hepatitis A and B in Norwegian merchant seamen. A serological study. *Infection*, **17**, 77–80.

1048. Siegel, D. & Hirschman, S.Z. (1977) Hepatic dysfunction in acute measles infection of adults. *Archives of Internal Medicine*, **137**, 1178–1179.

1049. Siegl, G., Frosner, G.G., Gauss-Muller, V. *et al.* (1981) The physicochemical properties of infectious hepatitis A viruses. *Journal of General Virology*, **57**, 331–341.

1050. Siegl, G. (1988) Virology of hepatitis A. In Zuckerman, A.J. (ed.) *Viral Hepatitis and Liver Disease*, pp. 3–7. New York: Alan R. Liss.

1051. Simmonds, P., Zhang, L.-Q., Watson, H.G. *et al.* (1990) Hepatitis C quantification and sequencing in blood products, haemophiliacs, and drug users. *Lancet*, **336**, 1469–1472.

1052. Simmons, P.D., Islam, M.N., Knott, S. *et al.* (1977) e Antigen among male homosexual patients. *British Medical Journal*, **2**, 1458.

1053. Singh, D.S., Gupta, P.R., Gupta, S.S. *et al.* (1989) Cardiac changes in acute viral hepatitis in Varanasi (India): case reports. *Journal of Tropical Medicine and Hygiene*, **92**, 243–248.

1054. Sirchia, G., Bellobuono, A., Giovanetti, A. & Marconi, M. (1989) Antibodies to hepatitis C virus in Italian blood donors. *Lancet*, **2**, 797.

1055. Sisto, A., Doesburg, N. Van, Deal, C. *et al.* (1989) Decompensated cardiomyopathy mimicking hepatitis in a 13-year-old girl. *Journal of Pediatric Gastroenterology and Nutrition*, **9**, 126–130.

1056. Sjogren, M. & Hoofnagle, J.H. (1985) Immunoglobulin M antibody to hepatitis B core antigen in patients with chronic type B hepatitis. *Gastroenterology*, **89**, 252–258.

1057. Sjogren, M.H., Tanno, H., Ray, O. *et al.* (1987) Hepatitis A virus in stool during clinical relapse. *Annals of Internal Medicine*, **106**, 221–226.

1058. Sjogren, M.H., Binn, L.N., Dubois, D.R. *et al.* (1991) Immunogenicity of an inactivated hepatitis A vaccine. *Annals of Internal Medicine*, **114**, 470–471.

1059. Skidmore, S. (1990) Recombinant immunoblot assay for hepatitis C antibody. *Lancet*, **335**, 1346.

1060. Skidmore, S.J., Pasi, K.J. & Hill, F.G.H. (1990) The use of the anti-hepatitis C virus (HCV) assay in assessing clinical findings in patients receiving blood products. *International Symposium in Viral Hepatitis and Liver Disease, Houston, Texas, USA, April 1990* (Abstract).

1061. Skinhoj, P. (1975) Natural history of viral hepatitis in Greenland. *American Journal of the Medical Sciences*, **270**, 305–307.

1062. Skinhoj, P., Mikkelsen, F. & Hollinger, F.B. (1977) Hepatitis A in Greenland: importance of specific antibody testing in epidemiologic surveillance. *American Journal of Epidemiology*, **105**(2), 140–147.

1063. Skrede, S., Blomhoff, J.P., Elgjo, K. & Gjone, E. (1973) Biochemical tests in evaluation of liver function. *Scandinavian Journal of Gastroenterology*, **8**, 37–45.

1064. Smedile, A., Dentico, P., Zanetti, A. *et al.* (1981) Infection with the HBV associated delta (δ) agent in HBsAg carriers. *Gastroenterology*, **81**, 992–997.

1065. Smedile, A., Farci, R., Verme, G. *et al.* (1982) Influence of delta infection on severity of hepatitis B. *Lancet*, **2**, 945–947.

1066. Smedile, A., Lavarini, C., Crivelli, O. *et al.* (1982) Radioimmunoassay detection of IgM antibodies to the HDV-associated delta antigen: Clinical significance in delta infection. *Journal of Medical Virology*, **9**, 131–138.

1067. Smedile, A., Lavarini, C., Arico, S. *et al.* (1983) Epidemiological patterns of infection with hepatitis B virus-associated delta agent in Italy. *American Journal of Epidemiology*, **117**, 223–229.

1068. Smedile, A., Rizzetto, M., Denniston, K. *et al.* (1986) Type D hepatitis: The clinical significance of hepatitis D virus RNA in serum as detected by a hybridization-based assay. *Hepatology*, **6**, 1297–1302.

1069. Smetana, H.F. (1975) The New Delhi epidemic 1955–1956. In Hartmann, F., Lo Grippo, G.A., Mateer, J.G. & Little, B.J. (eds) *Hepatitis Frontiers*. Boston: Brown & Co.

1070. Smith, C.E.T. (1987) A study of the prevalence of markers of hepatitis B infection in hospital staff. *Journal of Hospital Infection*, **9**, 39–42.

1071. Smith, G.I., Mackett, M. & Moss, B. (1983) Infectious vaccinea virus recombinants that express hepatitis B virus surface antigen. *Nature*, **302**, 402–495.

1072. Smith, H.M., Alexander, G.J.M., Birnbaum, W. & Williams, R. (1987) Does screening high risk dental patients for hepatitis B virus protect dentists? *British Medical Journal*, **295**, 309–310.

1073. Snashall, D. (1989) Transmission of hepatitis B from gynaecologist to patient. *Lancet*, **1**, 505–506.

1074. Sninsky, J.J., Siddiqui, A., Robinson, W.S. & Cohen, S.N. (1979) Cloning and endonuclease mapping of the hepatitis B virus genome. *Nature*, **279**, 346–348.

1075. Snover, D.C., Hutton, S., Balfour, H.H. Jr. & Bloomer, J.R. (1987) Cytomegalovirus infection of the liver in transplant recipients. *Journal of Clinical Gastroenterology*, **9**, 659–665.

1076. Soe, S., Uchida, T., Suzuki, K. *et al.* (1989) Enterically transmitted non-A, non-B hepatitis in cynomologus monkeys: Morphology and probable mechanism of hepatocellular necrosis. *Liver*, **9**, 135–145.

1077. Song, R.Y., Peck, R. & Murray, H.G. (1989) Persistent high fever and gall-bladder wall thickening in a child with primary Epstein–Barr viral infection. *Australian Paediatric Journal*, **25**, 368–369.

1078. Spandau, D.F. & Lee, C-H. (1988) *trans*-activation of viral enhancers by the hepatitis B virus X protein. *Journal of Virology*, **62**, 427–434.

1079. Speed, B.R., Dimitrakakis, M., Thoma, K. & Gust, I.D. (1989) Control of HBV and HDV infection in an isolated Pacific island: 1. Pattern of infection. *Journal of Medical Virology*, **29**, 13–19.

1080. Spero, J.A., Lewis, J.H., van Thiel, D.H. *et al.* (1978) Asymptomatic structural liver disease in hemophilia. *New England Journal of Medicine*, **298**, 1373–1378.

1081. Spichtin, H.-P., Gudat, F., Berthold, H. *et al.* (1984) Nuclear particles of non-A, non-B type in healthy volunteers and patients with hepatitis B. *Hepatology*, **4**, 510–514.

1082. Spitz, R.D., Keren, D.F., Boitnott, J.K. & Maddrey, W.C. (1978) Bridging hepatic necrosis. Aetiology and prognosis. *American Journal of Digestive Diseases*, **23**, 1076–1078.

1083. Sprengel, R., Kaleta, E.F. & Will, H. (1988) Isolation and characterization of a hepatitis B virus endemic in herons. *Journal of Virology*, **62**, 3832–3839.

1084. Stahl, S.J. & Murray, K. (1989) Immunogenicity of peptide fusions to hepatitis B virus core antigen. *Proceedings of the National Academy of Sciences of the USA*, **86**, 6283–6287.

1085. Standring, D.N., Rutter, W.J., Varmus, H.D. & Ganem, D. (1984) Transcription of the hepatitis B surface antigen gene in cultured murine cells initiates within the pre-surface region. *Journal of Virology*, **50**, 563–571.

1086. Stapleton, J.T. & Lemon, S.M. (1987) Neutralization escape mutants define a dominant immunogenic neutralization site on hepatitis A virus. *Journal of Virology*, **61**, 491–498.

1087. Stapleton, J.T., Binn, L.N. & Lemon, S.M. (1991) The role of secretory immunity in hepatitis A virus infection. *Journal of Infectious Diseases*, **163**, 7–11.

1088. Stark, R., Rümenapf, T., Meyers, G. & Thiel, H.J. (1990) Genomic localization of hog cholera virus glycoproteins. *Virology*, **174**, 286–289.

1089. Steigman, A. (1973) Rashes and arthropathy in viral hepatitis. *Mount Sinai Journal of Medicine*, **40**, 752–757.

1090. Steketee, R.W., Ziarnik, M.E. & Davis, J.P. (1988) Seroresponse to hepatitis B vaccine in patients and staff of renal dialysis centers, Wisconsin. *American Journal of Epidemiology*, **127**, 772–782.

1091. Stevens, C.E., Beasley, R.P., Tsui, J. & Lee, W.C. (1975) Vertical transmission of hepatitis B antigen in Taiwan. *New England Journal of Medicine*, **292**, 771–774.

1092. Stevens, C.E., Neurath, R.A., Szmuness, W. *et al.* (1978) Correlations between HBeAg/anti-HBe, HBsAg titer, HBsAg-associated albumin binding sites and infectivity. In Vyas, G.N., Cohen, S.N. & Schmid, R. (eds) *Viral Heptatitis*, pp. 211–215. Philadelphia: Franklin Institute Press.

1093. Stevens, C.E., Neurath, R.A., Beasley, R.P. *et al.* (1979) HBeAg and anti-HBs detection by radioimmunoassay. Correlation with vertical transmission of hepatitis B virus in Taiwan. *Journal of Medical Virology*, **3**, 237–241.

1094. Stevens, C.E., Aach, R.D., Hollinger, F.B. *et al.* (1984) Hepatitis B virus antibody in blood donors and the occurrence of non-A, non-B hepatitis in transfusion recipients. An analysis of the transfusion-transmitted viruses study. *Annals of Internal Medicine*, **101**, 733–738.

1095. Stevens, C.E., Alter, H.J., Taylor, P.E. *et al.* (1984) Dialysis Vaccine Trial Study Group: Immunogenicity and efficacy. *New England Journal of Medicine*, **311**, 496–501.

1096. Stevens, C.E., Taylor, P.E., Tong, M.J. *et al.* (1987) Yeast-recombinant hepatitis B vaccine. *Journal of the American Medical Association*, **257**, 2612–2616.

1097. Stevens, C.E., Taylor, P.E., Pindyck, H. *et al.* (1990) Epidemiology of hepatitis C virus. A preliminary study in volunteer blood donors. *Journal of the American Medical Association*, **263**, 49–53.

1098. Stevens, C.E. (In press) Perinatal and sexual transmission of HCV. In Hollinger, E.B., Lemon, S.M. & Margolis, H.S. (eds)

Viral Hepatitis and Liver Disease. Baltimore: Williams & Wilkins Co.

1099. Stille, W., Böhle, E., Helm, E. *et al.* (1968) An infectious disease transmitted by Cercopithecus aethiops (green monkey disease). *German Medical Monthly*, **13**, 470–478.

1100. Stocklin, E., Gudat, F., Krey, G. *et al.* (1981) Delta antigen in hepatitis B: immunohistology of frozen and paraffin embedded liver biopsies and relation to HBV infection. *Hepatology*, **1**, 238–242.

1101. Strom, T.B. & Merrill, J.P. (1977) Hepatitis B, transfusions and renal transplantation (editorial). *New England Journal of Medicine*, **296**(4), 225–226.

1102. Su, I.J., Kuo, T.T. & Liaw, Y.F. (1985) Hepatocyte hepatitis B surface antigen. Diagnostic evaluation of patients with clinically acute hepatitis B surface antigen-positive hepatitis. *Archives of Pathology and Laboratory Medicine*, **109**, 400–402.

1103. Summers, J.A., O'Connell, A. & Millman, I. (1975) Genome of hepatitis B virus: restriction enzyme cleavage and structure of DNA extracted from Dane particles. *Proceedings of the National Academy of Sciences of the USA*, **72**, 4597–4601.

1104. Summers, J., Smolec, J.M. & Snyder, R. (1978) A virus similar to human hepatitis B virus associated with hepatitis and hepatoma in woodchucks. *Proceedings of the National Academy of Sciences of the USA*, **75**, 4533–4537.

1105. Summers, J. & Mason, W.S. (1982) Replication of the genome of a hepatitis B-like virus by reverse transcription of an RNA intermediate. *Cell*, **29**, 403–415.

1106. Summers, J. (1988) The replication cycle of hepatitis B viruses. *Cancer*, **61**, 1957–1962.

1107. Sun, N.C. & Smith, V.M. (1966) Hepatitis associated with myocarditis. Unusual manifestation of infection with coxsackie virus group B type 3. *New England Journal of Medicine*, **274**, 190–193.

1108. Sureau, C., Romet-Lemonne, J.L., Mullins, J.I. & Essex, M. (1986) Production of hepatitis B virus by a differentiated human hepatoma-cell line after transfection with cloned circular DNA. *Cell*, **47**, 37–47.

1109. Sureau, C., Eichberg, J.W., Hubbard, G.B. *et al.* (1988) A molecularly cloned hepatitis B virus produced in vitro is infectious in a chimpanzee. *Journal of Virology*, **62**, 3064–3067.

1110. Sureau, C., Taylor, J., Chao, M. *et al.* (1989) Cloned hepatitis delta virus cDNA is infectious in the chimpanzee. *Journal of Virology*, **63**, 4292–4297.

1111. Sureau, P.H. (1989) First hand clinical observations of haemorrhagic manifestations in ebola haemorrhagic fever in Zaire. *Review of Infectious Diseases*, **11** (Suppl. 4), S790–S793.

1112. Sutnick, A.I., Bugbee, S.J., London, T.A. *et al.* (1973) Lymphocyte function in normal people with persistent Australia antigen. *Journal of Laboratory and Clinical Medicine*, **82**, 79–85.

1113. Suzuki, T., Masui, N., Kajino, K. *et al.* (1989) Detection and mapping of spliced RNA from a human hepatoma cell line transfected with the hepatitis B virus genome. *Proceedings of the National Academy of Sciences of the USA*, **86**, 8422–8426.

1114. Szeifert, G., Csecsei, K., Toth, Z. & Papp, Z. (1985) Prenatal diagnosis of ascites caused by a cytomegalovirus hepatitis. *Acta Paediatrica Hungarica*, **26**, 311–316.

1115. Szmuness, W., Prince, A.M., Etling, G.F. & Pick, R. (1972) Development and distribution of hemaglutinating antibody against the hepatitis B antigen in institutionalized populations. *Journal of Infectious Diseases*, **126**, 498–506.

1116. Szmuness, W., Prince, A.M., Grady, G.F. *et al.* (1974) Hepatitis B infection. A point-prevalence study in 15 US hemodialysis centers. *Journal of the American Medical Association*, **227**, 901–906.

1117. Szmuness, W., Much, I, Prince, A.M. *et al.* (1975) On the role of sexual behaviour in the spread of hepatitis B infection. *Annals of Internal Medicine*, **83**(4), 489–495.

1118. Szmuness, W., Dienstag, J.L., Purcell, R.H. *et al.* (1977) Hepatitis type A and hemodialysis: a seroepidemiologic study in 15 US centers. *Annals of Internal Medicine*, **87**(1), 8–12.

1119. Szmuness, W., Dienstag, J.L., Purcell, R.H. *et al.* (1977) The prevalence of antibody to hepatitis A antigen in various parts of the world. A pilot study. *American Journal of Epidemiology*, **5**, 392–398.

1120. Szmuness, W., Purcell, R.H., Dienstag, J.L. *et al.* (1977) Antibody to hepatitis A antigen in institutionalized mentally retarded patients. *Journal of the American Medical Association*, **237**, 1702–1705.

1121. Szmuness, W., Stevens, C.E., Zang, E.A. *et al.* (1981) A controlled clinical trial of the efficacy of the hepatitis B vaccine (Heptavax B): a final report. *Hepatology*, **1**, 377–385.

1122. Szmuness, W., Stevens, C.E., Harley, E.J. *et al.* (1982) Hepatitis B vaccine in medical staff of hemodialysis units. Efficacy and subtype cross-protection. *New England Journal of Medicine*, **307**, 1481–1486.

1123. Tabor, E., Russell, R.P., Gerety, R.J., *et al.* (1977) Hepatitis B surface antigen and e antigen in pleural effusion: A case report. *Gastroenterology*, **73**, 1157–1159.

1124. Tabor, E., Gerety, R.J., Drucker, J.A. *et al.* (1978) Transmission of non-A, non-B hepatitis from man to chimpanzee. *Lancet*, **1**, 463–466.

1125. Tabor, E., Jones, R., Gerety, R.J. *et al.* (1979) Asymptomatic viral hepatitis types A and B in an adolescent population. *Pediatrics*, **62**, 1026–1030.

1126. Tabor, E. (1987) Guillain–Barré syndrome and other neurologic syndromes in hepatitis A, B and non-A, non-B. *Journal of Medical Virology*, **21**, 207–216.

1127. Tabor, E., Gerety, R.J., Cairns, J. & Bayley, A.C. (1990) Antibody responses of adults, adolescents, and children to a plasma-derived hepatitis B vaccine in a rural African setting. *Journal of Medical Virology*, **32**, 134–138.

1128. Takamatsu, K., Koyanagi, Y., Okita, K. & Yamamoto, N. (1990) Hepatitis C virus RNA in saliva. *Lancet*, **336**, 1515.

1129. Takamizawa, A., Mori, C., Fuke, I. *et al.* (1991) Structure and organisation of the hepatitis C virus genome isolated from human carriers. *Journal of Virology*, **65**, 1105–1113.

1130. Takeuchi, K., Kubo, Y., Boonmar, S. *et al.* (1990) The putative nucleocapsid and envelope protein genes of hepatitis C virus determined by comparison of the nucleotide sequences of two isolates derived from an experimentally infected chimpanzee and healthy human carriers. *Journal of General Virology*, **71**, 3027–3033.

1131. Takeuchi, K., Boomar, S., Kubo, Y. *et al.* (1990) Hepatitis C viral cDNA clones isolated from a healthy carrier donor implicated in post-transfusion non-A, non-B hepatitis. *Gene*, **91**, 287–291.

1132. Takeuchi, K., Kubo, Y., Boonmar, S. *et al.* (1990) Nucleotide sequence of core and envelope genes of the hepatitis C virus genome derived directly from human healthy carriers. *Nucleic Acids Research*, **18**, 4626.

1133. Tamura, I., Ichimura, H., Itoh, Y. *et al.* (1987) Prevalence of antibody to delta antigen among HBV carriers in Japan. *Journal of Medical Virology*, **22**, 217–221.

1134. Tamura, I., Kobayashi, Y., Koda, T. *et al.* (1990) Hepatitis C virus antibodies in haemodialysis patients. *Lancet*, **335**, 1409.

1135. Tandon, B.N., Gandi, B.M., Joshi, Y.K. *et al.* (1985) Hepatitis virus non-A, non-B: the cause of a major public health problem in India. *Bulletin of the World Health Organisation*, **63**, 931–934.

1136. Tanno, H., Fay, O.H., Rojman, J.A. & Palazzi, J. (1988) Biphasic form of hepatitis A virus infection: a frequent variant in Argentina. *Liver*, **8**, 53–57.

1137. Tapalaga, D., Forzani, B., Hele, C. *et al.* (1986) Prevalence of the hepatitis delta virus in Rumania. *Hepato-Gastroenterology*, **33**, 238–239.

1138. Taranto, D., Carrato, A., Romano, M. *et al.* (1989) Mild pancreatic damage in acute viral hepatitis. *Digestion*, **42**, 93–97.

1139. Tassopoulos, N.C., Papaevangelou, G.J., Sjogren, M.H. *et al.* (1987) Natural history of acute hepatitis B surface antigen-positive hepatitis in Greek adults. *Gastroenterology*, **92**, 1844–1850.

1140. Tassopoulos, N.C., Papaevangelou, G.J., Roumeliotou-Karayannis, A. *et al.* (1987) Detection of hepatitis B virus DNA in asymptomatic hepatitis B surface antigen carriers: relation to sexual transmission. *American Journal of Epidemiology*, **126**, 587–591.

1141. Tassopoulos, N.C., Hadziyannis, S.J. & Wright, G.E. (1989) Recombinant human interferon alpha-2b in the management of acute type B hepatitis. *Hepatology*, **10**, 576.

1142. Tassopoulos, N.C., Sjogren, M.H. & Purcell, R.H. (1990) 19S and 7-8S forms of IgM antibody to hepatitis B core antigen in acute icteric hepatitis superimposed on hepatitis B surface antigen carriage. *Infection*, **18**, 376–380.

1143. Taylor, J., Mason, W., Summers, J. *et al.* (1987) Replication of human hepatitis delta virus in primary cultures of woodchuck hepatocytes. *Journal of Virology*, **61**, 2891–2895.

1144. Teixeira, M.R., Weller, I.V.D., Murray, A. *et al.* (1982) The pathology of hepatitis A in man. *Liver*, **2**, 53–60.

1145. Ten Napel, C.H.H., Houthoff, H.J. & The, T.H. (1984) Cytomegalovirus hepatitis in normal and immune compromised hosts. *Liver*, **4**, 184–194.

1146. Tettmar, R.E., Masterton, R.G. & Strike, P.W. (1987) Hepatitis A immunity in British adults—An assessment of the need for pre-immunisation screening. *Journal of Infection*, **15**, 39–43.

1147. Thaler, M.M., Park, C.-K., Landers, D.V. *et al.* (1991) Vertical transmission of hepatitis C virus. *Lancet*, **338**, 17–18.

1148. The Gambia Hepatitis Study Group (1987) The Gambia Hepatitis Intervention Study. *Cancer Research*, **47**, 5782–5787.

1149. Theilmann, L., Klinkert, M., Gmelin, K. *et al.* (1986) Detection of pre-S1 proteins in serum and liver of HBsAg-positive patients: A new mark of hepatitis B virus infection. *Hepatology*, **6**, 186–190.

1150. Theilmann, L., Klinkert, M.-Q., Gmelin, K. *et al.* (1987) Detection of antibodies against pre-S1 proteins in sera of patients with hepatitis B virus (HBV) infection. *Journal of Hepatology*, **4**, 22–28.

1151. Theilmann, L., Blazek, M., Goeser, T. *et al.* (1990) False-positive anti-HCV tests in rheumatoid arthritis. *Lancet*, **335**, 1346.

1152. Theodore, E. & Niv, Y. (1978) The clinical course of subacute hepatic necrosis. *American Journal of Gastroenterology*, **70**, 600–606.

1153. Thiers, V, Nakajima, E., Kremsdorf, D. *et al.* (1988) Transmission of hepatitis B from hepatitis-B-seronegative subjects. *Lancet*, **2**, 1273–1276.

1154. Thomas, H.C., Jacyna, M., Walters, J. & Main, J. (1988) Virus-host interaction in chronic hepatitis B virus infection. *Seminars in Liver Disease*, **8**, 342–349.

1155. Thornton, A., Tsiquaye, K.N. & Zuckerman, A.J. (1977) Studies on human hepatitis A virus in chimpanzees. *British Journal of Experimental Pathology*, **58**, 352–358.

1156. Thung, S.N. & Gerber, M.A. (1983) Immunohistochemical study of delta antigen in an American metropolitan population. *Liver*, **3**, 392–397.

1157. Tibbs, C.J. (1987) Hepatitis B, tropical ulcers, and immunisation strategy in Kiribati. *British Medical Journal*, **294**, 537–540.

1158. Ticehurst, J.R., Racaniello, V.R., Baroudy, B.M., *et al.* (1983) Molecular cloning and characterization of hepatitis A virus cDNA. *Proceedings of the National Academy of Sciences of the USA*, **80**, 5885–5889.

1159. Ticehurst, J.R., Feinstone, S.M., Chestnut, T. *et al.* (1987) Detection of hepatitis A virus by extraction of viral RNA and molecular hybridization. *Journal of Clinical Microbiology*, **25**, 1822–1829.

1160. Ticehurst, J., Cohen, J.I., Feinstone, S.M. *et al.* (1989) Replication of hepatitis A virus: new ideas from studies with cloned cDNA. In Semler, B.L. & Ehrenfeld, E. (eds) *Molecular Aspects of Picornavirus Infection and Detection*, pp. 27–50. Washington, D.C.: American Society for Microbiology.

1161. Tiggert, W.D., Berge, T.O., Gochenour, W.S. *et al.* (1960) Experimental yellow fever. *Transactions of the New York Academy of Sciences*, **22**, 323–333.

1162. Tinari, A., Ruggeri, F.M., Divizia, M. *et al.* (1989) Morphological changes in HAV-infected Frp/3 cells and immunolocalization of HAAG. *Archives of Virology*, **104**, 209–224.

1163. Todo, S., Demetris, A.J., Van Thiel, D. *et al.* (1991) Orthotopic liver transplantation for patients with hepatitis B virus-related liver disease. *Hepatology*, **13**, 619–626.

1164. Toghill, P.J., Bailey, M.E., Williams, R. *et al.* (1967) Cytomegalovirus hepatitis in the adult. *Lancet*, **1**, 1351–1354.

1165. Toh, H., Hayashida, H. & Miyata, T. (1983) Sequence homology between retroviral reverse transcriptase and putative polymerases of hepatitis B virus and cauliflower mosaic virus. *Nature*, **305**, 827–829.

1166. Tomori, O., Fabiyi, A., Sorungbe, A. *et al.* (1988) Viral haemorrhagic fever antibodies in Nigerian populations. *American Journal of Tropical Medicine and Hygiene*, **38**, 407–410.

1167. Tong, M.J., Sampliner, R.E., Govindarajan, S. & Co, R.L. (1987) Spontaneous reactivation of hepatitis B in Chinese patients with HBsAg-positive chronic active hepatitis. *Hepatology*, **7**, 713–718.

1168. Tong, S., Li, J., Vitvitski, L. & Trépo, C. (1990) Active hepatitis B virus replication in the presence of anti-HBe is associated with viral variants containing an inactive pre-C region. *Virology*, **176**, 596–603.

1169. Tor, J., Llibre, J.M., Carbonell, M. *et al.* (1990) Sexual transmission of hepatitis C virus and its relation with hepatitis B virus and HIV. *British Medical Journal*, **301**, 1130–1133.

1170. Torres, J.R. & Mondolfi, A. (1991) Protracted outbreak of severe delta hepatitis: Experience in an isolated Amerindian population of the upper Orinoco basin. *Reviews of Infectious Diseases*, **13**, 52–55.

1171. Toukan, A.U., Abu-El-Rub, O.A., Abu-Laban, S.A. *et al.* (1987) The epidemiology and clinical outcome of hepatitis D virus (delta) infection in Jordan. *Hepatology*, **7**, 1340–1345.

1172. Tözün, N., Forbes, A., Anderson, M.G. & Murray-Lyon, I.M. (1991) Safety of alcohol after viral hepatitis. *Lancet*, **337**, 1079–1080.

1173. Trepo, C.G., Zuckerman, A.J., Bird, R.C. & Prince, A.M. (1974) The role of circulating hepatitis B antigen/antibody immune complexes in the pathogenesis of vascular and hepatic manifestations in polyarteritis nodosa. *Journal of Clinical Pathology*, **27**, 863–868.

1174. Trewby, P.N. & Williams, R. (1977) Pathophysiology of hypotension in patients with fulminant hepatic failure. *Gut*, **18**, 1021–1026.

1175. Triger, D.R., Alp, M.H. & Wright, R. (1972) Bacterial and dietary antibodies in liver disease. *Lancet*, **1**, 60–63.

1176. Tripatzis, I. (1972) Australia antigen in urine and feces. *American Journal of Diseases of Children*, **123**, 401–404.

1177. Tron, F., Degos, F., Bréchot, C. *et al.* (1989) Randomized dose range study of a recombinant hepatitis B vaccine produced in mammalian cells and containing the S and preS2 sequences. *Journal of Infectious Diseases*, **160**, 199–204.

1178. Trosi, C.L., and Hollinger, F.B. (1990) Hepatitis B vaccines. In Popper, H. & Schaffner, F. (eds) *Progress in Liver Diseases*, Vol. IX, pp. 405–442. Philadelphia: W.B. Saunders.

1179. Tsai, J.-F., Margolis, H.S., Fields, H.A. *et al.* (1990) Hepatitis delta virus superinfection among patients with chronic hepatitis B in Southern Taiwan. *Scandinavian Journal of Infectious Diseases*, **22**, 403–405.

1180. Tsega, E., Tsega, M., Mengesha, B. *et al.* (1988) Transmission of hepatitis B virus infection in Ethiopia with emphasis on the importance of vertical transmission. *International Journal of Epidemiology*, **1**, 874–879.

1181. Tsega, E., Tafesse, B., Nordenfelt, E. *et al.* (1990) Immunogenicity of hepatitis B vaccine simultaneously administered with the expanded programme on immunisation (EPI). *Journal of Medical Virology*, **32**, 232–235.

1182. Tsiquaye, K.N., Harrison, T.J., Portmann, B. *et al.* (1984) Acute hepatitis A infection in hepatitis B chimpanzee carriers. *Hepatology*, **4**, 504–509.

1183. Tsuda, F., Masuko, K., Mitsui, T. *et al.* (1988) Antibody against the translation product of the pre-S2 region of hepatitis B virus and the resolution of infection after accidental needlestick exposure. *American Journal of Gastroenterology*, **83**, 943–947.

1184. Tsuru, T., Ishibashi, H., Matsuishi, E. *et al.* (1990) Acute renal failure associated with acute type A hepatitis with a mild liver damage. *Fukuoka Acta Medica*, **81**, 337–341.

1185. Tur-Kaspa, R., Burk, R., Shaul, Y. *et al.* (1986) Hepatitis B virus DNA contains a glucocorticoid-responsive element. *Proceedings of the National Academy of Sciences in the USA*, **83**, 1627–1631.

1186. Turner, G.C. & Bruce White, G.B. (1969) SH antigen in haemodialysis associated hepatitis. *Lancet*, **2**, 121–124.

1187. Tuttleman, J.S., Pugh, J.C. & Summers, J.W. (1986) In vitro experimental infection of primary duck hepatocyte cultures with duck hepatitis B virus. *Journal of Virology*, **58**, 17–25.

1188. Tuttleman, J.S., Pourcel, C. & Summers, J. (1986) Formation of the pool of covalently closed circular viral DNA in hepadnavirus-infected cells. *Cell*, **47**, 451–460.

1189. Twu, J-S.& Schloemer, R.H. (1987) Transcriptional *trans-*

activating function of hepatitis B. virus. *Journal of Virology*, **61**, 3448–3453.

1190. Ueda, K., Tsurimoto, T. & Matsubara, K. (1991) Three envelope proteins of hepatitis B virus: large S, middle S, and major S proteins needed for the formation of Dane particles. *Journal of Virology*, **65**, 3521–3529.

1191. Vaglia, A., Nicolin, R., Puro, V. *et al.* (1990) Needlestick hepatitis C virus seroconversion in a surgeon. *Lancet*, **336**, 1315–1316.

1192. Vahrman, J. (1971) Viral hepatitis and the E.S.R. *British Medical Journal*, **2**, 466–467.

1193. Valenzuela, P., Gray, P., Quiroga, M. *et al.* (1979) Nucleotide sequence of the gene coding for the major protein of hepatitis B virus surface antigen. *Nature*, **280**, 815–819.

1194. Valenzuela, P., Quiroga, M., Zaldivar, J. *et al.* (1980) The nucleotide sequence of the hepatitis B viral genome and the identification of the major viral genes. In Fields, B.N., Jaenisch, R. & Fox, C.F. (eds) *Animal Virus Genetics*, pp. 57–71. New York: Academic Press.

1195. Valla, D., Flejou, J.-F., Lebrec, D. *et al.* (1989) Portal hypertension and ascites in acute hepatitis: Clinical, hemodynamic and histological correlations. *Hepatology*, **10**, 482–487.

1196. Vallbracht, A., Maier, K., Stierhof, Y.-D. *et al.* (1989) Liver-derived cytotoxic T cells in hepatitis A virus infection. *Journal of Infectious Diseases*, **160**, 209–217.

1197. Van Damme, P., Vranckx, R., Safary, A. *et al.* (1989) Protective efficacy of a recombinant deoxyribonucleic acid hepatitis B vaccine in institutionalized mentally handicapped clients. *American Journal of Medicine*, **87**, 26S–29S.

1198. Vandelli, C., Zannini, A., Piaggi, V. *et al.* (1987) What is the effect of a cytomegalovirus infection when superimposed on HBsAg-positive chronic hepatitis? *Journal of Hepatology*, **4**, 343–348.

1199. van den Hoek, J.A.R., van Haastrecht, H.J.A., Goudsmit, J. *et al.* (1990) Prevalence, incidence, and risk factors of hepatitis C virus infection among drug users in Amsterdam. *Journal of Infectious Diseases*, **162**, 823–826.

1200. van der Berg, A.P., Klompmaker, I.J., Haagsma, E.B. *et al.* (1991) Antigenaemia in the diagnosis and monitoring of active cytomegalovirus infection after liver transplantation. *Journal of Infectious Diseases*, **164**, 265–270.

1201. van der Poel, C.L., Reesink, H.W., Lelie, P.N. *et al.* (1989) Anti-hepatitis C antibodies and non-A, non-B post-transfusion hepatitis in The Netherlands. *Lancet*, **2**, 297–298.

1202. van der Poel, C.L., Reesink, H.W., Schaasberg, W. *et al.* (1990) Infectivity of blood seropositive for hepatitis C virus antibodies. *Lancet*, **335**, 558–560.

1203. van der Poel, C.L., Cuypers, H.T.M., Reesink, H.W. *et al.* (1991) Confirmation of hepatitis C virus infection by new four-antigen recombinant immunoblot assay. *Lancet*, **337**, 317–319.

1204. van Ditzhuijsen, Th.J.M., de Witte-van der Schoot, E., van Loon, A.M. *et al.* (1988) Hepatitis B virus infection in an institution for the mentally retarded. *American Journal of Epidemiology*, **128**, 629–638.

1205. van Ditzhuijsen, T.J.M., Kuijpers, L.P.C., Koens, M.J. *et al.* (1990) Hepatitis B pre-S1 and pre-S2 proteins: Clinical significance and relation to hepatitis B virus DNA. *Journal of Medical Virology*, **32**, 87–91.

1206. van Geelen, J.A., Schalm, S.W., de Visser, E.M. & Heijtink, R.A. (1987) Immune response to hepatitis B vaccine in hemodialysis patients. *Nephron*, **45**, 216–218.

1207. Van Stapel, M.J., van Steenbergen, W., de Wolf-Peeters, C. *et al.* (1983) Prognostic significance of piecemeal necrosis in acute viral hepatitis. *Liver*, **3**, 346–357.

1208. Varki, N.M., Bhuta, S., Drake, T. & Porter, D.D. (1990) Adenovirus hepatitis in two successive liver transplants in a child. *Archives of Pathology and Laboratory Medicine*, **114**, 106–109.

1209. Venkataseshan, V.S., Lieberman, K., Kim, D.U. *et al.* (1990) Hepatitis-B-associated glomerulonephritis: Pathology, pathogenesis, and clinical course. *Medicine*, **69**(4), 200–216.

1210. Vento, F., McFarlane, B.M., Vento, T.G. *et al.* (1988) Serial study of liver-directed autoantibodies and autoreactive T-lymphocytes in acute viral hepatitis B. *Journal of Autoimmunity*, **1**, 299–307.

1211. Vento, S., Heggarty, J.E., Alberti, A. *et al.* (1985) T lymphocyte

sensitization to HBcAg in hepatitis B virus mediated unresponsiveness to HBsAg in hepatitis B virus related to chronic liver disease. *Hepatology*, **5**, 192–197.

1212. Vento, S., Rondanelli, E.G., Ranieri, S. *et al.* (1987) Prospective study of cellular immunity to hepatitis-B-virus antigens from the early incubation phase of acute hepatitis B. *Lancet*, **2**, 119–122.

1213. Venuti, A., Di Russo, C., Del Grosso, N. *et al.* (1985) Isolation and molecular cloning of a fast-growing strain of human hepatitis A virus from its double-stranded replicative form. *Journal of Virology*, **56**, 579–588.

1214. Vergani, D., Mieli-Vergani, G., Hussain, M.J. *et al.* (1983) Delta infection in the UK. *Lancet*, **1**, 305.

1215. Verme, G., Amoroso, P., Lettieri, G. *et al.* (1986) A histological study of hepatitis delta virus liver disease. *Hepatology*, **6**, 1303–1307.

1216. Villarejos, F.V.M., Kirsten, P.H., Visona, K.A. *et al.* (1974) Role of saliva, urine and feces in the transmission of type B hepatitis. *New England Journal of Medicine*, **291**, 1375–1378.

1217. Viswanathan, R. (1957) Infectious hepatitis in Delhi (1955–56): A critical study: Epidemiology. *Indian Journal of Medical Research*, **45**, 1–30.

1218. Vodopija, I., Ljubičič., M., Baklaič, Ž. *et al.* (1989) Post-exposure prophylaxis for hepatitis B. *Lancet*, **2**, 1161–1162.

1219. Voegt, H. (1942) Zur aetiologie der hepatitis epidemica. *Munchener Medizinische Wochenschrift*, **89**, 76–79.

1220. Volma, J., Luders, C.J. & Henning, H. (1985) Semi-quantitative and morphometric investigations on the histopathology of chronic hepatitis non-A, non-B. *Z. Gastroenterology*, **23**, 632–642.

1221. Vranckx, R. & Van Damme, P. (1990) Hepatitis C in institutionalized children. *New England Journal of Medicine*, **323**, 64.

1222. Vyas, G.N., Dienstag, J.L. & Hoofnagle, J.H. (eds) (1984) *Viral Hepatitis and Liver Disease*. New York: Grune & Stratton.

1223. Wacker, W.E.C., Riordan, J.F., Snodgrass, P.J. *et al.* (1972) The Holy Cross hepatitis outbreak: clinical and chemical abnormalities. *Archives of Internal Medicine*, **130**, 357–360.

1224. Wahl, M. & Hermodsson, S. (1987) Intradermal, subcutaneous or intramuscular administration of hepatitis B vaccine: side effects and antibody response. *Scandinavian Journal of Infectious Diseases*, **19**, 617–621.

1225. Wahl, M., Hermodsson, S. & Iwarson, S. (1988) Hepatitis B vaccination with short dose intervals — a possible alternative for post-exposure prophylaxis? *Infection*, **16**, 229–232.

1226. Wainwright, R.B., McMahon, B.J., Bender, T.R. *et al.* (1986) Prevalence of hepatitis B virus infection in Tonga: Identifying high risk groups for immunization with hepatitis B vaccine. *International Journal of Epidemiology*, **15**, 567–571.

1227. Wands, J.R., Marciniak, R.A., Isselbacher, K.J. *et al.* (1982) Demonstration of previously undetected hepatitis B viral determinants in an Australian aboriginal population by monoclonal anti-HBs antibody radioimmunoassay. *Lancet*, **1**, 977–980.

1228. Wang, J.-T., Wang, T.-H., Lin, J.-T. *et al.* (1990) Hepatitis C virus in a prospective study of posttransfusion non-A, non-B hepatitis in Taiwan. *Journal of Medical Virology*, **32**, 83–86.

1229. Wang, J.-T., Wang, T.-H., Lin, J.-T. *et al.* (1991) Hepatitis C virus RNA in saliva of patients with post-transfusion hepatitis C infection. *Lancet*, **337**, 48.

1230. Wang, J.-T., Wang, T.-H., Sheu, J.-C. *et al.* (1991) Detection of hepatitis B virus DNA by polymerase chain reaction in plasma of volunteer blood donors negative for hepatitis B surface antigen. *Journal of Infectious Diseases*, **163**, 397–399.

1231. Wang, K-S, Choo, Q-L, Weiner, A.J. *et al.* (1986) Structure, sequence and expression of the hepatitis delta viral genome. *Nature*, **323**, 508–513.

1232. Wang, X.C., Liu, X.M., Tan, C.Z. *et al.* (1990) Epidemic non-A, non-B hepatitis in Xing Jiang. Clinical and pathologic observations. *Chinese Medical Journal (Engl.)* **103**, 890–898.

1233. Warburton, A.R.E., Wreghitt, T.G., Rampling, A. *et al.* (1991) Hepatitis A outbreak involving bread. *Epidemiology and Infection*, **106**, 199–202.

1234. Ward, R., Borchert, P., Wright, A. & Cline, E. (1972) Hepatitis B antigen in saliva and mouth washings. *Lancet*, **2**, 726–727.

1235. Ware, A.J., Eigenbrodt, E.H. & Combes, B. (1975) Prognostic significance of subacute hepatic necrosis in acute hepatitis. *Gastroenterology*, **68**, 519–524.

1236. Ware, A.J., Cuthbert, J.A., Shorey, J. *et al.* (1981) A prospective trial of steroid therapy in severe viral hepatitis. *Gastroenterology*, **80**, 219–224.

1237. Waters, J.A., O'Rourke, S.M., Richardson, S.C. *et al.* (1987) Qualitative analysis of the humoral immune response to the "a" determinant of HBs antigen after inoculation with plasma-derived or recombinant vaccine. *Journal of Medical Virology*, **21**, 155–160.

1238. Weiland, E., Stark, R., Haas, B. *et al.* (1990) Pestivirus glycoprotein which induces neutralising antibodies form part of a disulfide-linked heterodimer. *Journal of Virology*, **64**, 3563–3569.

1239. Weiner, A.J., Choo, Q.L., Wang, K.S. *et al.* (1988) A single antigenomic open reading frame of the hepatitis delta virus encodes the epitope(s) of both hepatitis delta antigen polypeptides p24 delta and p27 delta. *Journal of Virology*, **62**, 594–599.

1240. Weiner, A.J., Kuo, G., Bradley, D.W. *et al.* (1990) Detection of hepatitis C viral sequences in non-A, non-B hepatitis. *Lancet*, **335**, 1–3.

1241. Weiner, A.J., Brauer, M.J., Rosenblatt, J. *et al.* (1991) Variable and hypervariable domains are found in the regions of HCV corresponding to the flavivirus envelope and NS1 proteins and the pestivirus envelope glycoproteins. *Virology*, **180**, 842–848.

1242. Weisfuse, I.B., Hadler, S.C., Fields, H.A. *et al.* (1989) Delta hepatitis in homosexual men in the United States. *Hepatology*, **9**, 872–874.

1243. Weissman, J.Y., Tsuchiyose, M.M., Tong, M.J. *et al.* (1988) Lack of response to recombinant hepatitis B vaccine in nonresponders to the plasma vaccine. *Journal of the American Medical Association*, **260**, 1734–1738.

1244. Weitz, M., Baroudy, B.M., Maloy, W.L. *et al.* (1986) Detection of a genome-linked protein (VPg) of hepatitis A virus and its comparison with other picornaviral VPgs. *Journal of Virology*, **60**, 124–130.

1245. Wejstal, R., Hermodsson, S., Iwarson, R. & Norkrans, G. (1990) Mother to infant transmission of hepatitis C virus infection. *Journal of Medical Virology*, **30**, 178–180.

1246. Welch, J., Webster, M., Tilzey, A.J. *et al.* (1989) Hepatitis B infections after gynaecological surgery. *Lancet*, **1**, 205–207.

1247. Weller, I.V.D., Karayiannis, P., Lok, A.S.F. *et al.* (1983) Significance of delta agent infection in chronic hepatitis B virus infection: a study in British carriers. *Gut*, **24**, 1061–1063.

1248. Weller, I.V.D., Cohn, D., Sierralta, A. *et al.* (1984) Clinical, biochemical, serological, histological and ultrastructural features of liver disease in drug abusers. *Gut*, **25**, 417–423.

1249. Wengler, G. & Wengler, G. (1981) Terminal sequences of the genome and replicative form RNA of the flavivirus west Nile virus: absence of poly [A] and possible role in RNA replication. *Virology*, **113**, 544–555.

1250. Werblowsky-Constantini, N., Livshin, R., Burstein, M. *et al.* (1989) Toxic epidermal necrolysis associated with acute cholestatic viral hepatitis A. *Journal of Clinical Gastroenterology*, **11**, 691–693.

1251. Westaway, E.G., Brinton, M.A., Gaidamovich, S.Ya. *et al.* (1985) Flaviviridae. *Intervirology*, **24**, 183–192.

1252. Whittle, H.C., Bradley, A.K., McLaughlan, M. *et al.* (1983) Hepatitis B virus infection in two Gambian villages. *Lancet*, **1**, 1203–1206.

1253. Whittle, H.C., Inskip, H., Hall, A.J. *et al.* (1991) Vaccination against hepatitis B and protection against chronic viral carriage in The Gambia. *Lancet*, **337**, 747–750.

1254. Will, H., Reiser, W., Weimer, T. *et al.* (1987) Replication strategy of human hepatitis B virus. *Journal of Virology*, **61**, 904–911.

1255. Williams. P.E., Yap, P.L., Gillon, J. *et al.* (1989) Transmission of non-A, non-B hepatitis by pH4-treated intravenous immunoglobulin. *Vox Sanguinis*, **57**, 15–18.

1256. Williams, R. & Wendon, J. (1991) Clinical syndrome and aetiology of fulminant hepatic failure. In Williams, R. & Hughes, R.D. (eds) *Acute Liver Failure*, pp.1–5. London: Miter Press.

1257. Williams, S.J., Batey, R.G., Craig, P.I., *et al.* (1987) Hepatitis B in Australia: Determinants of intrafamily spread. *Australian and New Zealand Journal of Medicine*, **17**, 220–227.

1258. Winn, W.C., Monath, T.P., Murphy, F.A. & Whitfield, S.G. (1975) Lassa virus hepatitis. Observations on a fatal case from the 1972 Sierra Leone epidemic. *Archives of Pathology*, **99**, 599–604.

1259. Wismans, P.J., van Hattum, J., Mudde, G.C. *et al.* (1989) Is booster injection with hepatitis B vaccine necessary in healthy responders? *Journal of Hepatology*, **8**, 236–240.

1260. Wolga, J., Rodhain, F., Hannoun, C. *et al.* (1986) Evaluation of thermostable yellow fever vaccine from the Pasteur Institute of International Travellers. *Journal of Biological Standardization*, **14**, 289–295.

1261. Wolters, G., Kuijpers, L.P.C., Kacaki, J. & Schuurs, H.W.M. (1977) Enzyme-linked immunosorbent assay for hepatitis B surface antigen. *Journal of Infectious Diseases*, **136**, 311–317.

1262. Wong, D.C., Purcell, R.H., Sreenivasan, M.A. *et al.* (1980) Epidemic and endemic hepatitis in India: evidence for a non-A, non-B hepatitis virus aetiology. *Lancet*, **2**, 876–878.

1263. Wong, V.C.W., Ip, H.M., Reesink, H.W. *et al.* (1984) Prevention of the HBsAg carrier state in newborn infants of mothers who are chronic carriers of HBsAg and HBeAg by administration of hepatitis-B vaccine and hepatitis-B immunoglobulin. *Lancet*, **1**, 921–929.

1264. Wood, J.R., Taswell, H.F., Czaja, A.J. & Rabe, D. (1988) Pattern and duration of HBV DNA seropositivity in acute hepatitis B. *Digestive Diseases and Sciences*, **33**, 477–480.

1265. Woolf, I., El Sheikh, N., Cullens, H. *et al.* (1976) Enhanced production in pathogenesis of fulminant viral hepatitis type B. *British Medical Journal*, **2**, 669–671.

1266. World Health Organisation (1973) Viral hepatitis: report of a WHO Scientific Group, Geneva. Technical Report Series, No. 512.

1267. World Health Organisation (1977) Advances in viral hepatitis: report of the WHO Expert Committee on Viral Hepatitis. Technical Report Series, No. 602.

1268. World Health Organisation International Study Team (1978) Ebola haemorrhagic fever in Sudan, 1976. *Bulletin of the World Health Organisation*, **56**, 247–270.

1269. World Health Organisation (1982) Prevention of liver cancer. Technical Report Series, No. 691.

1270. World Health Organisation Report (1983) Viral hepatitis: the use of normal and specific immunoglobulin. *WHO Weekly Epidemiological Record*, **58**, 237.

1271. World Health Organisation Hepatitis Programme (1983) Hepatitis programme. *Lancet*, **2**, 350.

1272. Wright, R. (1970) Australia antigen and smooth-muscle antibody in acute and chronic hepatitis. *Lancet*, **1**, 521–522.

1273. Wright, R., Perkins, J.R., Bower, B.D. & Jerome, D.W. (1970) Cirrhosis associated with the Australia antigen in an infant who acquired hepatitis from her mother. *British Medical Journal*, **4**, 719–721.

1274. Wright, R. (1977) Immunology of gastrointestinal and liver disease. In Turk, J. (ed.) *Current Topics in Immunology*. London: Edward Arnold.

1275. Wright, T.L. & Ganem, D. (1989) The polyalbumin hypothesis: Where is it in 1989? *Gastroenterology*, **96**, 250–254.

1276. Wright, T.L., Ferrell, L., Donegan, E. *et al.* (1991) Impact of hepatitis C viral (HCV) infection on the allograft following liver transplantation. *Hepatology*, **14**, 51A.

1277. Wu, H.L., Chen, P.J., Tu, S.J. *et al.* (1991) Characterization and genetic analysis of alternatively spliced transcripts of hepatitis B virus in infected human liver tissues and transfected HepG2 cells. *Journal of Virology*, **65**, 1680–1686.

1278. Wu, H.N., Lin, Y.J., Lin, F.P. *et al.* (1989) Human hepatitis delta virus RNA subfragments contain an autocleavage activity. *Proceedings of the National Academy of Sciences of the USA*, **86**, 1831–1835.

1279. Wu, H.N. & Lai, M.M. (1989) Reversible cleavage and ligation of hepatitis delta virus RNA. *Science*, **243**, 652–654.

1280. Wu, J.Y., Zhuo, Z.-Y., Judd, A. *et al.* (1990) The hepatitis B virus-encoded transcriptional trans-activator hbx appears to be a novel protein serine-threonine kinase. *Cell*, **63**, 687–695.

1281. Wu, T.-T., Coates, L., Aldrich, C.E. *et al.* (1990) In hepatocytes infected with duck hepatitis B virus, the template for viral RNA synthesis is amplified by an intracellular pathway. *Virology*, **175**, 255–261.

1282. Xu, Z.Y., Liu, C.B., Francis, D.P. *et al.* (1985) Prevention of perinatal acquisition of hepatitis B virus carriage using vaccine: Preliminary report of a randomized, double-blind placebo-controlled and comparative trial. *Pediatrics*, **76**, 713–718.

1283. Yaginuma, K., Shirakata, Y., Kobayashi, M. *et al.* (1987) Hepatitis B virus (HBV) particles are produced in a cell-culture system by transient expression of transfected HBV DNA. *Proceedings of the National Academy of Sciences of the USA*, **84**, 2678–2682.

1284. Yaginuma, K. & Koike, K. (1989) Identification of a promoter region for 3.6-kilobase mRNA of hepatitis B virus and specific cellular binding protein. *Journal of Virology*, **63**, 2914–2920.

1285. Yamaguchi, M., Hirano, T., Sugahara, K. *et al.* (1988) Electron microscopy of hepatitis B virus core antigen expressing yeast cells by freeze-substitution fixation. *European Journal of Cell Biology*, **47**, 138–143.

1286. Yasuda, A., Kimura-Kuroda, J., Oginoto, M. *et al.* (1990) Induction of protective immunity in animals vaccinated with recombinant vaccinia viruses that express Pre M and E glycoprotein of Japanese encephalitis virus. *Journal of Virology*, **64**, 2788–2795.

1287. Yoakum, G.H., Korba, B.E., Lechner, J.F. *et al.* (1983) High frequency transfection and cytopathology of hepatitis B core antigen gene in human cells. *Science*, **222**, 385.

1288. Yokosuka, O., Omata, M., Tada, M. *et al.* (1989) Supersensitive detection method of HBV DNA using polymerase chain reaction. *Acta Hepatologica Japonica*, **30**, 178–181.

1289. Yoshizawa, H., Itoh, Y., Iwakiri, S. *et al.* (1981) Demonstration of two different types of non-A, non-B hepatitis By reinjection and cross-challenge studies in chimpanzees. *Gastroenterology*, **81**, 107.

1290. Young, E.J., Killam, A.P. & Greene, J.F., Jr. (1976) Disseminated herpes virus infection. Association with primary genital herpes in pregnancy. *Journal of the American Medical Association*, **235**, 2731–2733.

1291. Yuki, N., Hayashi, N., Katayama, K. *et al.* (1990) Quantitative analysis of pre-S1 and pre-S2 in relation to HBsAg expression. *Hepatology*, **11**, 38–43.

1292. Yvonnet, B., Coursaget, P., Lebouleux, D. *et al.* (1987) Low-dose hepatitis B vaccine immunisation in children. *Lancet*, **1**, 169.

1293. Yvonnet, B., Coursaget, P., Chotard, J. *et al.* (1987) Hepatitis B vaccine in infants from an endemic area: Long-term anti-HBs persistence and revaccination. *Journal of Medical* Virology, **22**, 315–321.

1294. Zachoval, R., Roggendorf, M. & Deinhardt, F. (1983) Hepatitis A infection in chronic carriers of hepatitis B virus. *Hepatology*, **3**, 528–531.

1295. Zanetti, A.R., Tanzi, E., Manzillo, G. *et al.* (1988) Hepatitis B variant in Europe. *Lancet*, **2**, 1132–1133.

1296. Zanetti, R.A., Tanzi, E., Ferroni, P. *et al.* (1983) Vertical transmission of the HBV-associated delta agent. In Rizzetto, M., Verme, G. & Bonino, F. (eds) *Viral Hepatitis and Delta Infection*. New York: Alan R Liss.

1297. Zeldis, J.B., Dienstag, J.L. & Gale, R.P. (1983) Aplastic anemia and non-A, non-B hepatitis. *American Journal of Medicine*, **74**, 64–68.

1298. Zeldis, J.B., Miller, J.G. & Dienstag, J.L. (1985) Hepatitis in an adult with rubella. *American Journal of Medicine*, **79**, 515–516.

1299. Zeldis, J.B., Lee, J.H., Mamish, D. *et al.* (1989) Direct method for detecting small quantities of hepatitis B virus DNA in serum and plasma using the polymerase chain reaction. *Journal of Clinical Investigation*, **84**, 1503–1508.

1300. Zhang, W.H., Liu, C.B., Sun, Y.D. *et al.* (1990) Hepatitis C virus causing non-A, non-B hepatitis in plasmapheresis centre. *Lancet*, **336**, 353.

1301. Zhuang, H., Kaldor, J., Locarnini, S.A. & Gust, I.D. (1982) Serum immunoglobulin levels in acute A, B and non-A, non-B hepatitis. *Gastroenterology*, **82**, 549–553.

1302. Zientara, M. & Moore, S. (1970) Fatal talc embolism in a drug addict. *Human Pathology*, **1**, 324–327.

1303. Zignego, A.L., Dubois, F., Samuel, D. *et al.* (1990) Serum hepatitis delta virus RNA in patients with delta hepatitis and in liver graft recipients. *Journal of Hepatology*, **11**, 102–110.

1304. Zuckerman, A.J., Taylor, P.E., Bird, G. & Russell, S.M. (1971) The Australia (hepatitis-associated) antigen in fibrinogen and other fractions of human plasma. *Journal of Clinical Pathology*, **24**, 2–7.

1305. Zuckerman, A.J. (1975) *Human Viral Hepatitis*. Amsterdam and Oxford: North-Holland.

1306. Zuckerman, A.J. (1982) Priorities for immunisation against hepatitis B. *British Medical Journal*, **2**, 686–688.

1307. Zuckerman, A.J. (1984) Alternative hepatitis B vaccines: polypeptide micelle vaccines. In Chisari, F.V. (ed.) *Advances in Hepatitis Research*. Ch. 26, pp. 238–240. New York: Masson Publishing.

1308. Zuckerman, A.J. (1990) Vaccines against hepatitis A and B. In Farthing, M.J.G. (ed.) *Baillière's Clinical Gastroenterology*, Vol. 4(3), pp. 775–788. London: Baillière Tindall.

1309. Goldsmith, R., Yarbough, P.O., Reyes, G.R. *et al.* (1992) Enzyme linked immunosorbent assay for diagnosis of acute sporadic hepatitis E in Egyptian children. *Lancet*, **339**, 328–331.

CHAPTER 31

Chronic Hepatitis

Meron R. Jacyna, G.H. Millward-Sadler & Howard C. Thomas

The phrase 'chronic hepatitis' denotes chronic inflammation of the liver continuing without improvement for 6 months or more.[160] Pathologically, the term specifies a chronic, non-granulomatous, predominantly lymphocytic inflammation of the liver. There are a number of distinct pathological subtypes—for example, chronic active hepatitis and chronic persistent hepatitis—which can be diagnosed histologically. The 'gold standard' for diagnosing chronic hepatitis is liver biopsy. This procedure confirms the diagnosis of chronic hepatitis, excludes other concomitant hepatic diseases (for example, alcoholic liver disease, haemochromatosis, etc.), and, by allowing an estimate of the severity of the hepatitis to be made, can aid in determining the prognosis for the individual patient.

Although there are several different causes of chronic hepatitis, the clinical features are common to all causes and reflect the pathophysiological effects of the final common pathway—which is hepatocellular damage. Similarly, the different pathological subtypes of chronic hepatitis, which reflect the severity of the inflammation at one point in time, can generally be found in any and all causes of chronic hepatitis. Thus, initially we shall consider the general clinical and histological characteristics of chronic hepatitis.

GENERAL ASPECTS OF CHRONIC HEPATITIS

CLINICAL FEATURES

Symptoms

Although the commonest symptom of chronic hepatitis is fatigue, many patients have no symptoms at all and the hepatitis may be detected only incidentally, for example during screening for a life-insurance medical or other routine health check. Symptoms, if they do occur, are usually vague. They include anorexia and general malaise. Pain over the liver is sometimes reported, particularly with exercise, and muscle cramps may also be seen in a proportion of patients. Patients may also present with dyspepsia or epigastric discomfort, although, since this symptom is very commonly found in the general population (36% of the general population experience indigestion every month[201]), its significance in this group of patients is unclear. These symptoms may develop insidiously and patients may have been unwell for many months before seeking medical attention. It has also been our experience that some patients with chronic hepatitis may initially be mistakenly labelled as chronic fatigue syndrome (also called myalgic encephalomyelitis, or post-viral syndrome) and it is only after investigation that the true diagnosis of chronic hepatitis is established.

Certain types of chronic hepatitis may have specific symptoms. For example, amenorrhoea and arthralgia in a young girl with suspected chronic hepatitis may suggest

chronic autoimmune hepatitis. Subjects with chronic viral hepatitis are more likely to have had previous transfusion of blood or blood products, to have had a previous episode of jaundice, to be homosexual, or to be intravenous drug abusers. If information about these features is not volunteered, they should be specifically sought. The history should also include information on recent foreign travel; family history and contact with jaundiced subjects and a detailed drug history is very important.

Signs

Most patients have no physical signs to indicate the underlying hepatic inflammation. In particular tenderness over the liver, which may be seen in acute viral hepatitis, is not generally seen. As the inflammation persists and hepatocellular damage progresses, ultimately cirrhosis and hepatocellular failure develop and the signs of liver failure appear: palmar erythema, spider naevi and other skin telangiectases, jaundice, bruising and prolonged bleeding, splenomegaly, confusion, ascites, peripheral oedema. Generally, the signs of chronic hepatitis are not specific, but there are some features that may suggest the cause for the underlying hepatitis. The Kaiser–Fleischer rings of Wilson's disease are one example. Chronic hepatitis in a young girl with acne, arthropathy and alveolitis is most likely to be due to chronic autoimmune hepatitis. Similarly, chronic hepatitis in a male homosexual, intravenous drug abuser, or tattooed individual is more likely to be due to chronic hepatitis B or delta infections.

HISTOLOGICAL FEATURES

The hallmark of this chronic inflammatory reaction is the lymphocyte. As in any chronic inflammation, there is cellular damage with regeneration and, particularly in more severe cases, repair. It is the regenerative and repair processes that ultimately lead an aggressive chronic hepatitis over a period of time into cirrhosis.

The chronic inflammation and each of its individual components of cell damage, regeneration, inflammation and repair will vary in severity with time. However, histological examination of liver obtained by needle liver biopsy, in spite of the small sample volume obtained (one millionth of the total liver volume) results in a reasonable overall assessment of the degree and severity of hepatic inflammation at the time at which the biopsy was taken. Arbitrary dividing lines have been drawn separating the hepatitis (as assessed histologically) into grades of severity and these are discussed below.

Chronic persistent hepatitis

Chronic persistent hepatitis (CPH) is a histological diagnosis based on the appearance of normal hepatic architecture, with a mononuclear cell infiltrate within the portal tracts. The mononuclear cells are predominantly lymphocytes, although occasional plasma cells and macrophages may also be present. The portal tracts may be slightly expanded by fibrous spurs, but there is no destruction of the limiting plate by piecemeal necrosis; this negative feature separates this condition from chronic active hepatitis (Figure 31.1).

This hallmark of CPH—the lymphocyte, macrophage and plasma cell infiltrate within the portal tract—is sometimes termed 'portal triaditis'. In smaller portal tracts the infiltrate is uniformly distributed, but in larger ones it is focal and peripheral. Occasional cells may spill over into periportal sinusoids but there is no piecemeal necrosis. There may be minimal portal tract fibrosis with an occasional slender fibrous spur extending into the parenchyma. The limiting plates (between the portal tract and hepatocyte columns) are orderly and are only interrupted by a very occasional focal cluster of mononuclear cells. These are sometimes seen around a degenerate hepatocyte.

The importance of CPH is that it does not produce significant architectural distortion, i.e. it does not lead to cirrhosis. However, CPH may later progress to chronic active hepatitis,[2,93] which may readily advance to cirrhosis.[2] With CPH associated with hepatitis B infection, this change to chronic active hepatitis is more likely to occur in patients with persistence of HBV-DNA in the serum.[93]

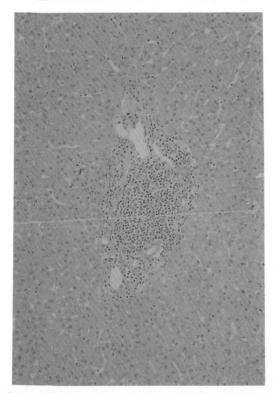

Figure 31.1 Chronic persistent hepatitis: the portal tract is expanded by a mononuclear inflammatory infiltrate but the architecture and cell plate patterns are well preserved. There is no piecemeal necrosis.

On occasion, liver biopsy may demonstrate features of CPH when the diagnosis has been previously established as chronic active hepatitis. Although it is possible that this is the result of biopsy sampling error, it is more usually due to spontaneous remission or successful treatment of a previous chronic active hepatitis. In this case, residual fibrosis from the preceding piecemeal necrosis may be identified. This will have expanded the portal tracts and may have isolated solitary or small groups of hepatocytes around the periphery.

CPH is usually caused by chronic viral infection, although the morphological criteria outlined are not specific and may be found in other conditions not due to persistent virus infection. These include the non-specific reactive changes sometimes seen in the liver in patients with systemic infections such as septicaemia, or systemic illnesses such as malignant disease or inflammatory bowel disease.

Chronic lobular hepatitis

Chronic lobular hepatitis (CLH) is defined as a hepatitis in which architectural preservation is good, piecemeal necrosis is slight or at most moderate, and there is some scattered parenchymal damage (sometimes termed 'spotty necrosis'). This injury to the hepatocytes may be seen as acidophil or ballooning degeneration (Figure 31.2). The morphological features are indistinguishable from those of a typical acute hepatitis and it is only the length of history that establishes the inflammatory process as chronic. As in a resolving acute hepatitis there may be focal collapse of the reticulin architecture distorting the cell plates around the terminal hepatic vein, which indicates previous loss of hepatocytes. Small focal hyperplastic clusters of hypertrophied and ceroid-laden Kupffer cells can be found within the sinusoids. Focal knots of hepatocytes three or four cells across are present and reflect the cellular regeneration following cell loss. CLH may reflect a prolonged unresolved course of acute hepatitis (for example, due to a virus or a drug), or may represent a relapsing hepatitis.

Chronic active hepatitis

The pathology of chronic active hepatitis (CAH) is dominated by the process of piecemeal necrosis. This is defined as the combination of inflammatory cells and fibroblastic activity destroying the parenchyma, and surrounding and isolating small groups of hepatocytes at the interface between parenchyma and collagen. This ultimately leads to architectural distortion, which may vary from mild enlargement of the portal tracts through to frank cirrhosis. CAH is the most serious form of chronic hepatitis, with the worst prognosis. There are several well defined components to the overall histological lesion of CAH.

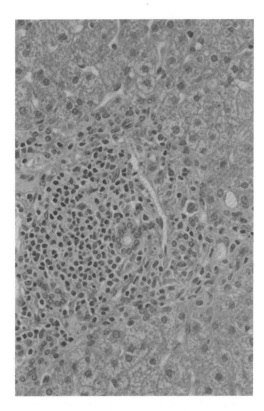

Figure 31.2 The portal tract is expanded by a chronic inflammatory infiltrate which occasionally spills over into periportal sinusoids. Acidophil degeneration of hepatocytes may be seen and an acidophil body is present on the edge of the portal tract on the right.

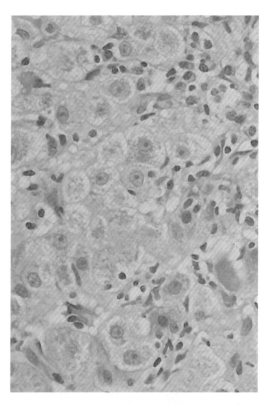

Figure 31.3 Piecemeal necrosis. The edge of an expanded portal tract is just present top right. An inflammatory infiltrate including plasma cells blurs the interface with the hepatocytes which show ballooning and acidophil degenerative changes. H&E.

Mesenchymal reaction

There are three elements to this: (a) an inflammatory infiltrate composed of lymphocytes with a variable number of plasma cells and some macrophages; (b) Kupffer cell hyperplasia; and (c) increased fibroblastic activity (Figure 31.3). The inflammatory cell infiltrate is variable in intensity and is mainly centred on portal tracts and established fibrous bands, but from these it extends into the parenchyma. Extensive sinusoidal infiltrates of lymphocytes and plasma cells are a feature of the most active disease (Figure 31.3). At the edges of portal tracts and fibrous septa with parenchyma, the lymphocytes surround and isolate single or small groups of hepatocytes.

Careful study of this intimate association of hepatocyte with lymphocyte suggests that the lymphocytes come into direct surface contact with hepatocyte plasma membranes and also invaginate directly into the hepatocyte. This contact is associated with the expression of adhesion molecules such as the thrombospondin receptor on the hepatocytes and the corresponding ligands on the inflammatory cells[286–288] and is usually associated with degenerative changes in the hepatocyte cytoplasm.[145] Direct extension by lymphocytes into the cytoplasm of degenerating hepatocytes is also observed. Damage to sinusoidal endothelial cells with cytoplasmic swelling and increase in micropinocytotic vesicles and dense bodies is also

apparent in areas of piecemeal necrosis.[12] Small foci where hepatocytes have been lost or destroyed are marked for a short period by a small collection of lymphocytes with Kupffer cells and occasional plasma cells. Kupffer cells are hyperplastic in focal areas of cell death, but also may be diffusely prominent throughout the sinusoids. There is rarely the hypertrophy with focal proliferation within and obstructing the sinusoids that is a feature of acute viral hepatitis. Similarly, phagocytosis of pigments is not a prominent feature, although small amounts of bile, lipofuscin or ceroid can be demonstrated by specific staining techniques.

The active fibrogenesis which is part of this reaction is responsible for the permanent isolation of single or small groups of hepatocytes. On electron microscopy, new collagen is laid down in the space of Disse, together with the basement membrane and microfibrillary collagens[114] (see Chapter 32).

Piecemeal necrosis

Piecemeal necrosis occurs irregularly throughout the liver and with varying intensity, so that on biopsy some portal tracts may contain a discrete inflammatory infiltrate mimicking chronic persistent hepatitis, whilst adjacent tracts may show a florid piecemeal necrosis. The intensity of the inflammatory infiltrate and the extent to which hepatocytes are isolated is the index of activity of the process (i.e. mild or severe). The lesion also varies in intensity with time, so that biopsies showing very little activity may be found during the natural course of the disease.

The significance of piecemeal necrosis in the pathogenesis and evolution of CAH has been questioned. Although its significance in the transition of acute into chronic hepatitis has been reaffirmed,[21,81,234] other studies have found that acute hepatitis with piecemeal necrosis may not invariably progress to chronicity.[95] Whether or not CAH progresses to cirrhosis relates to the severity of the histological lesion and subdivision into two grades of CAH, mild and severe CAH, may be helpful (discussed below).

Parenchymal degeneration

Descriptions of CAH include mention of continuing acidophil and ballooning degeneration of hepatocytes.[9,190,234] This cell lysis may become confluent and features resembling bridging hepatic necrosis as described in acute viral hepatitis are then found.[9,21,43,56,233] A zone of collapsed reticulin extends from a portal tract or abnormal fibrous spur into the parenchyma towards an efferent vein. Initially, these reticulin fibres may be separated slightly, but in the presence of piecemeal necrosis with its active fibrosis they are rapidly converted to collagen. It has been proposed that these bridges of necrosis permit more rapid spread of piecemeal necrosis throughout the liver so that architectural distortion is thus rapidly consolidated.[21] The presence of such features in a group of chronic hepatitis patients may be associated with a worse prognosis.[43,56,233]

Parenchymal regeneration

One of the prominent features of chronic active hepatitis is the regenerative activity identified by twinning of cell plates, formation of knots of hepatocytes and increased variation in hepatocyte nuclear size and staining. More florid regeneration includes the formation of multinucleate hepatocytes (Figure 31.4). These are usually giant hepatocytes with three or four nuclei, but occasionally syncytial hepatocytes with many nuclei may be found.[223] Regenerating hepatocytes may also form rosettes (Figure 31.5). These are usually adjacent to portal tracts and are small groups of four to eight hepatocytes around a central bile canaliculus which is visible as a lumen. A thin fibrous band surrounds this rosette and isolates it from adjacent parenchyma.

Regenerative activity may be irregular in distribution throughout the biopsy. Active areas, with twinning of plates to form intraparenchymal nodules, may compress the adjacent inactive parenchyma,[213] and the architectural distortion from these regeneration nodules may thus simulate the appearances of cirrhosis.

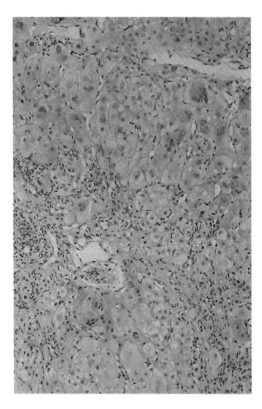

Figure 31.4 Piecemeal necrosis. Many regenerating multinucleated hepatocytes are present. Occasional hepatocytes show acidophil or ballooning degeneration and piecemeal necrosis is prominent in this field. H&E.

Bile ducts

Bile duct lesions have been described in chronic active hepatitis;[47] they differ from those found in acute viral hepatitis[218] and primary biliary cirrhosis and are more often seen in non-A non-B hepatitis.[79] The bile duct lesion in CAH is segmental, affecting both large and small interlobular ducts, and consists of focal hyperplasia of the bile duct epithelium so that the lumen may be narrowed or occluded (Figure 31.6). These hyperplastic epithelial cells may have an abundant clear empty cytoplasm and occasional mitoses may also be identified.

Mild CAH and severe CAH

On the basis of the criteria described above, CAH can be subdivided into two grades of severity; mild CAH and severe CAH. The intensity of the inflammatory infiltrate and the extent to which hepatocytes are isolated are used as measures of the activity. A grading system that assigns numerical scores to different parameters of activity has been proposed and may be of use in quantifying changes in liver biopsies associated with therapeutic procedures.[149] In severe CAH, the fibrous septae extend into the hepatocyte columns and isolate individual groups of cells into rosettes. Bridging necrosis between the portal tracts and terminal hepatic vein is also a prominent feature of severe CAH, which frequently progresses to cirrhosis.[43,56] On the other hand, in mild CAH there is only slight

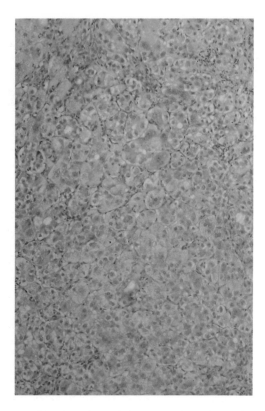

Figure 31.5 Rosettes. Many hepatocytes have formed regenerative rosettes with a small central lumen. These are not confined to, but are particularly frequent in the periportal zone bottom left. H&E.

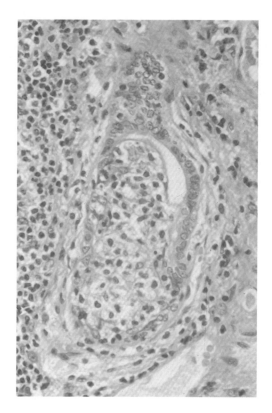

Figure 31.6 Hyperplastic bile duct epithelium with almost complete obliteration of the lumen. Epithelial cells have abundant vacuolated cytoplasm. H&E. From Millward-Sadler (1976) reference 190, with kind permission of the publisher, Blackwell Scientific.

erosion of the limiting plate, with some piecemeal necrosis but no bridging necrosis or rosettes. Studies suggest that mild CAH generally does not progress to cirrhosis.[9,56,71, 233] However, the division of the histological appearance into either mild or severe CAH may not be clear-cut, and of course a mild CAH may later progress to a severe CAH and vice versa.

With severe CAH, cirrhosis may be evident at the time of the initial liver biopsy. This is often the case with the more aggressive type of severe CAH frequently found in autoimmune chronic hepatitis. This is sometimes termed 'active' cirrhosis or, more precisely, chronic active hepatitis with cirrhosis. If the cause of the chronic hepatitis is successfully treated, or a spontaneous remission occurs, then the inflammation resolves but the cirrhosis persists. This is sometimes called 'inactive' (burnt-out) cirrhosis and may be indistinguishable from other causes of cirrhosis for which no active inflammation is seen.

INVESTIGATIONS USED IN DIAGNOSIS

Biochemical serology

The biochemical hallmark of hepatitis is a raised serum transaminase. Two enzymes are commonly measured; aspartate transaminase (AST) and alanine transaminase

(ALT). Generally, both tests supply equivalent information, although there is some evidence that the ALT may be a slightly more sensitive and specific marker of hepatic inflammation.[54] Thus, in most types of hepatitis the ALT is usually higher than the AST. The only exception to this is in acute alcoholic hepatitis, where the AST rises higher than the ALT; this may be a useful pointer towards the diagnosis of alcohol-induced hepatic inflammation.[51]

The commonest cause of an acutely raised serum transaminase is acute viral hepatitis. In this situation, the levels rise to several thousand international units per litre (IU/l) but in a successfully resolving acute hepatitis rapidly return to normal, usually within 3 months. A persistently elevated transaminase level (for 6 months or more) usually indicates continuing hepatic damage from an underlying chronic disorder. There are many possible causes of this; for example, fatty liver due to obesity or diabetes, alcohol abuse, congestive cardiac failure, haemochromatosis, or the various causes of chronic hepatitis to be described shortly. Aspartate transaminase is also present in muscle and other tissues and thus it should be remembered that muscle diseases, in particular myositis, may also cause an elevated serum AST. Alanine transaminase, however, is found only in the liver; thus if myositis is suspected in a patient with a raised AST, simultaneous measurement of

ALT and creatine kinase will help differentiate liver from muscle damage. Elevated serum transaminases are also frequently seen in patients presenting with thyrotoxicosis. Again this can be simply distinguished from chronic hepatitis by measurement of thyroid function tests.

In chronic hepatitis, the transaminase rise is less marked than in acute drug or viral hepatitis. The transaminase levels may be only slightly raised above normal, but are usually between 50 and 250 IU/l and rarely exceed 500 IU/l. The raised ALT or AST may be discovered in patients with obvious signs or symptoms suggesting underlying chronic hepatitis. More commonly the abnormality is noted incidentally via biochemical screening during a routine medical checkup, or by profiling—that is, performing a battery of biochemical tests during the routine investigative 'work-up' of patients. Generally in chronic hepatitis, the higher the serum transaminase level the greater the degree of hepatic damage seen histologically. Thus monitoring of serum transaminases is useful during treatment of chronic hepatitis (e.g., steroids in chronic autoimmune hepatitis, interferon-α in chronic non-A non-B hepatitis), where a falling AST/ALT is a helpful monitor of the beneficial effects of treatment. Again there are exceptions to this rule; in Wilson's disease, for example, there may be a florid chronic active hepatitis with severe fulminant liver failure, but the transaminases and alkaline phosphatase may be inappropriately low.[178,243] Similarly, there are reports that in chronic non-A non-B hepatitis there may be a very poor correlation between the serum biochemistry and the histological severity of the underlying hepatic inflammation.[235]

Patients with chronic hepatitis, particularly chronic active hepatitis, almost invariably have a raised serum transaminase. In chronic persistent hepatitis the transaminases may be only minimally raised, or may fluctuate between normal and slightly raised—this is particularly the case with chronic non-A non-B hepatitis.[80] Thus, in a patient who is suspected as having chronic hepatitis, monitoring of the serum transaminases over several months may be required. Very occasionally, even subjects with chronic active hepatitis or cirrhosis have been reported as having normal liver biochemistry at some time.[70] Fortunately, these are extremely uncommon cases and usually occur because the biochemistry was taken infrequently, or at a time when the hepatitis was in a quiescent phase (i.e. CPH), and later became more active.

Although raised levels of serum transaminases are the hallmark of a chronic hepatitic process, minor elevations of the other hepatic enzymes, such as gamma-glutamyl transpeptidase and alkaline phosphatase, may also be seen, particularly if there is a cholestatic component to the chronic hepatitis.

Other serological investigations

Other blood tests that should be performed in the event of a persistently raised serum transaminase (AST) are:

Hepatitis B surface antigen—if positive, hepatitis e antigen hepatitis e antibody
Antibody to hepatitis C
Anti-nuclear, anti-smooth muscle and antimitochondrial antibodies
Copper and caeruloplasmin (except in the elderly)
Iron and transferrin
α$_1$-Antitrypsin
Alpha-fetoprotein
Creatine phosphokinase
Thyroid function tests
Fasting glucose

Although it may be possible from these serological tests confidently to confirm or exclude certain diagnoses (such as chronic hepatitis due to HBV infection, or deranged LFTs due to thyrotoxicosis, polymyositis, etc.), other diagnoses which may be prompted by abnormal serological tests (such as α$_1$-antitrypsin deficiency, haemochromatosis, diabetic fatty liver, Wilson's disease, chronic autoimmune hepatitis) usually require a liver biopsy for definitive confirmation.

Liver biopsy

Although serological tests may indicate the true diagnosis, a liver biopsy is the most important component of the 'work-up' of a patient with suspected chronic hepatitis. Percutaneous liver biopsy is essential for the initial management of patients with suspected chronic hepatitis and may be repeated during follow-up in order to assess the response to therapy. It is felt by most authorities that a liver biopsy should be performed in any individual with a persistently raised serum transaminase.[131] A liver biopsy confirms (or otherwise) the diagnosis of chronic hepatitis, may allow a firm diagnostic label to be applied (e.g. chronic hepatitis due to Wilson's disease, or chronic hepatitis due to hepatitis B infection), allows assessment of the severity of the inflammation (at the time the liver biopsy was taken), excludes other concomitant hepatic diseases (for example, alcoholic liver disease, haemochromatosis), and aids in attempting to predict the prognosis for the individual patient. As there are now specific treatments available for most types of chronic hepatitis, establishing the correct diagnosis and assessing the severity of the disease is vital, and can only be achieved with certainty with a liver biopsy. The small risk of the procedure (in terms of morbidity and mortality) is heavily outweighed by all these considerations.

SPECIFIC CAUSES OF CHRONIC HEPATITIS

CHRONIC VIRAL HEPATITIS: OVERVIEW

Since the characterization of the non-A non-B hepatitis agents into two types, hepatitis C (predominantly parenterally transmitted) and hepatitis E (enterally spread), there are now known to be at least five viruses (A to E) which principally cause acute hepatitis.[155,156] Of these, it is now accepted that only three (hepatitis B, hepatitis D (delta) and hepatitis C) can progress to chronic hepatitis. There is some evidence that occasionally hepatitis A infection may take a protracted course, particularly in patients who have been immunosuppressed. A recent report describes a patient with hepatitis A infection for 3 years following a course of steroids.[180] However, this is a most uncommon event; a study of 451 patients with hepatitis A infection revealed no evidence of chronicity in any patient.[163] There are no published series of hepatitis A infection progressing to cirrhosis. The periportal inflammation associated with hepatitis A closely mimics piecemeal necrosis and can result in a misdiagnosis unless the findings are correlated with serological markers of hepatitis A infection. Differentiation from piecemeal necrosis can also be made if the inflammatory infiltrate is analysed for the lymphocyte subtypes that are present (see Chapter 30).[237]

CHRONIC HEPATITIS B INFECTION _____

Epidemiology and subjects at risk

The hepatitis B virus (HBV) is a partially double-stranded DNA virus which causes both acute and chronic hepatitis in man. Although the vast majority of infected adult individuals have an acute, self-limiting infection (Figure 31.7), it is the individuals with persistent HBV infection who run the major health risks. On a worldwide basis, more than 250 million people are estimated to suffer from chronic HBV infection, the vast majority of whom live in China and the Far East. Overall, 50% of these chronic carriers can be expected to die prematurely, either as a

result of chronic inflammatory liver disease or secondary to the development of hepatocellular carcinoma.[14] Chronic HBV infection is relatively uncommon in Western Europe and North America, compared with the less-developed Eastern European and Third World states. For example, in the United Kingdom, HBV is not a common cause of chronic hepatitis,[87] whereas HBV is responsible for 25–60% of cases of chronic active hepatitis and/or cirrhosis in Greece,[112] Africa,[8] and Iraq.[26] A similarly high incidence of chronic HBV infection of 10–15% is seen in the Middle East, but the highest rates are observed in Southeast Asia and China. In Taiwan, 70–90% of the population have markers suggesting exposure to the hepatitis B virus at some time in their life.[14,15]

The age at which infection occurs appears to be important in the development of the carrier state. In Southeast Asia and China for example, vertical transmission (mother to baby) is common at, or around, the time of birth. Ninety per cent of babies born to HBV e antigen-positive mothers become infected with HBV and more than 90% of these will develop a chronic carrier state.[15] These infants probably receive a large innoculum of virus from maternal blood before or during birth, and also by close contact with secretions during labour. As will be seen later, this, by far the largest group of chronically infected patients (generally Chinese/eastern Asians), do not respond to antiviral therapy as readily as individuals who acquire their infection in adulthood. In contrast, patients with chronic HBV infection seen in Western Europe and the USA have mostly acquired their infection in adulthood as a result of intravenous drug abuse or sexual activity.[298] Only 1–5% of this group of adults infected with HBV will develop chronic infection, as most will develop an acute HBV infection which is successfully cleared.

Following exposure in adulthood, there is also a greater likelihood (6-fold increase) of male compared to female subjects remaining chronically infected. The reasons for this difference are not known, although it may be speculated that they are hormonal in origin. There is a glucocorticoid-responsive element in the genome of HBV,[277] and other studies have indicated that HBsAg gene expression is regulated by sex steroids and glucocorticoids.[92] In addition, HBs antigen is cleared more slowly in male inbred mice than female mice of the same genotype, suggesting that phagocytic cells in males do not 'see' the viral protein as readily as females.[61]

In addition to age and sex, chronic hepatitis B infection is more likely to develop in individuals who have a defective host (immune) response against the virus. Individuals particularly at risk of HBV infection include multiply transfused patients, haemophiliacs, haemodialysis patients, intravenous drug abusers and those in institutions for the mentally handicapped. Patients with immunodeficiency states are also liable to become chronically infected, and an increased chronic HBV infection rate has been reported in patients with lepromatous leprosy,[20] Down's syndrome,[257] those receiving immunosuppress-

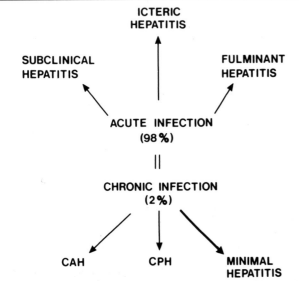

Figure 31.7 Outcome of infection with the hepatitis B virus. Most adult infected individuals spontaneously clear infection, but a small minority will progress to chronic infection.

ive or cytotoxic chemotherapy[125,291] and those with immunodeficiency disorders, such as hypo- or agammaglobulinaemia. The medical and paramedical staff and household contacts involved with such patients will also be at increased risk (see Chapter 30).

The host response to hepatitis B virus infection

Several studies have suggested that HBV is not a cytopathic virus and that the cause of the inflammation seen in chronically infected subjects is not directly due to the virus but is in fact due to the host cell-mediated immune response.[4] The principal observations are:

1. The absence of hepatocellular damage during the early phase of acute hepatitis infection in both clinical and experimental conditions in spite of high levels of virus replication.
2. The discrepancy between the consistent presence of HBsAg in hepatocytes showing an abundance of HBV-DNA,[111] and the observed inverse relationship between the number of HBsAg-positive hepatocytes and active liver cell damage.[113,259]
3. The reduction in hepatic inflammatory activity that accompanies the administration of immunosuppressive drugs, such as prednisolone.[126]

If the host immune response is inadequate, chronic viral persistence may occur, but in an overaggressive reaction the results may be severe hepatitis culminating in fulminant hepatitis. The individual components of this response are discussed below.

Cellular immunity

Elimination of HBV-infected hepatocytes is primarily dependent on the cell-mediated arm of the immune system, which recognizes HBV-infected hepatocytes and destroys them. Studies in patients with chronic HBV infection suggest that the nucleocapsid (HBcore and HBe) antigens are an important target for this cell-mediated cytotoxicity.[88,215] Whereas antibodies are often directed to conformational epitopes—this is true of the HB core epitope[292]—helper and cytotoxic T cells usually recognize epitopes on short linear peptides produced by degradation of viral proteins within the antigen-presenting cells (in the case of helper T cells) and in the infected host cell (in the case of cytotoxic T cells). The cytotoxic T cells recognize the linear viral peptides physically associated with the MHC class I glycoprotein antigens, and the MHC–virus antigen complex is the signal that the T cell responds to, and initiates the death of the infected cell. Uninfected hepatocytes usually express very little MHC class I glycoprotein,[263] but in the early stage of acute HBV infection, after the production of interferon-α by the host, MHC expression on hepatocytes increases and coincidentally transaminase levels rise (Figure 31.8). Interferon also activates several intracellular enzymes, including 2-5 A oligoadenylate synthetase (2-5AOS), endonucleases and a protein kinase, which inhibit viral protein synthesis by either destroying the mRNA or inhibiting translation. These interferon-induced changes would also be expected to produce an antiviral state in uninfected regenerating liver cells, preventing reinfection during the lysis of infected hepatocytes.

Humoral immunity

Virus neutralizing antibodies are directed to epitopes on the envelope of the virus (Figure 31.9). This is composed of three polypeptides each with the same carboxyl terminus and are designated the large, middle and small envelope proteins. The amino-terminal 120-amino-acid region of the large protein, which is not present in the middle and small proteins, is designated pre-S_1. This hydrophilic area is myristilated, and recent data indicate that the region 21–47aa is capable of binding to the

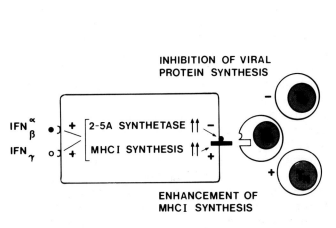

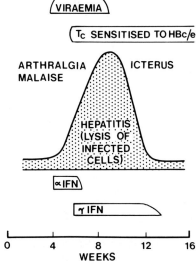

Figure 31.8 Clearance of HBV infected hepatocytes is dependent on an interplay between interferon and the host immune response.

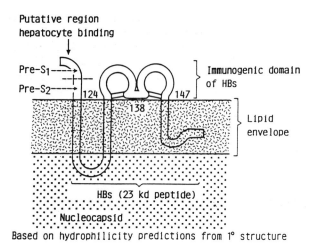

Putative region
hepatocyte binding

Pre-S$_1$
Pre-S$_2$
124 147
138

Immunogenic domain
of HBs

Lipid
envelope

HBs (23 kd peptide)

Nucleocapsid

Based on hydrophilicity predictions from 1° structure

Figure 31.9 Structure of the hepatitis B surface protein, including the pre-S$_1$ and S$_2$ domains.

membrane of the hepatocyte[202] and is therefore probably involved in virus uptake. The antibodies found in convalescent serum bind predominantly to the epitopes of the HBs-gene-encoded region,[169] the carboxyl terminal region that is present in all the envelope proteins. Two hydrophilic regions of this polypeptide, amino acids 124–148, form loops because of intramolecular disulphide bridges, and are the binding region for the majority (more than 80%) of the antigen-binding capacity of convalescent sera. Using monoclonal antibodies binding to these regions, it has been possible to show that antibody to the region 124–136 when administered to chimpanzees will prevent infection. Antibodies to this region, as well as to other epitopes on the S-gene-encoded polypeptide, are present in the serum of patients convalescent from HBV infection and in normal subjects immunized with plasma-derived and recombinant DNA-produced HBs vaccine.[135] Although patients recovered from HBV, or vaccinated with HBs antigen, are protected from further infection, there has been considerable debate on the importance of antibodies to the middle and large pre-S$_2$- and pre-S$_1$-bearing polypeptides. During natural infection, antibodies to pre-S$_1$ and pre-S$_2$ appear before antibodies to the HBs region.[31,136] If, as has been postulated,[202] the pre-S$_1$ region is important for binding of HBV to the hepatocyte during infection, antibodies to this region would be virus-neutralizing, and therefore their presence may be important in preventing entry of HBV particles into uninfected hepatocytes. Interference with the production of anti-envelope antibodies thus may be expected to lead to protracted HBV infection, and this is seen in agammaglobulinaemic patients who, when exposed to HBV, frequently develop chronic infection.

Mechanisms of viral persistence

Successful recovery from HBV infection is dependent on the integrated activities of the patient's interferon and immune systems as described above, and chronic HBV infection arises when the virus exploits primary defects in these defences or neutralizes essential components of the hosts' interferon and immune response. Elimination of HBV-infected hepatocytes is achieved by natural killer and cytotoxic T cells, which recognize and destroy HBV-infected hepatocytes.[265] The humoral (antibody) response to epitopes on the lipid–protein coat which envelopes the virus is of lesser importance and appears to be mainly responsible for protective immunity against reinfection.

It is likely that there are many different reasons why, in some adults and in most neonates, there is a failure of the patient's interferon and/or immune systems to eliminate infected hepatocytes from the liver. For example, in neonates, immaturity of the immune system and transplacental transfer of maternal anti-HBc may be important; in adults, quantitative and qualitative abnormalities in the interferon response may be more crucial.

Infection during the neonatal period

This large group of patients is largely representative of chronic HBV carriers from Southeast Asia and China, who mostly acquire their infection at or around the time of birth and who are by far the largest group of chronic carriers. Prior to birth, HBV e antigen (HBeAg) passes across the placenta from mother to fetus. HBeAg is a low-molecular-weight soluble protein which is part of the nucleocapsid pre-core/core gene (C) product (Figure 31.10). When the full pre-core/core gene is translated (from the first AUG codon), a secretory protein is produced. The pre-core encoded region functions as a signal peptide[206,229] directing this protein to the cell membrane, ultimately to be secreted from the cell. This protein takes up a conformation that displays the HBe epitopes. When translation of the nucleocapsid open-reading frame starts at the second AUG codon, the HBcore protein is produced. This, probably because of the absence of the pre-core encoded signal sequence and the presence of the carboxyterminal nucleophilic sequence, is not secreted and assembles around HBV RNA–DNA complexes to form virus nucleocapsids.

The pre-core region of the genome is not necessary for the production of infectious virus particles.[41] Its continued presence within the small genome of the virus therefore probably confers some biological advantage by altering the virus-to-host relationship. The only known function conferred on the infected cell by the presence of this pre-core region is the ability to secrete soluble HBe antigen (HBeAg),[206,229] and it is likely that secretion of HBeAg into the blood alters the balance between the host and the virus, favourably for the virus. About 5% of patients with chronic HBV hepatitis do not have HBe antigen detectable in the serum, and this group of patients have a more severe and rapidly progressive liver disease.[22,300] The reason for this failure to produce HBe antigen is the presence of a mutation in the pre-core region of the HBV genome, resulting in a novel stop codon which prematurely terminates translation.[37] Other mutations within the

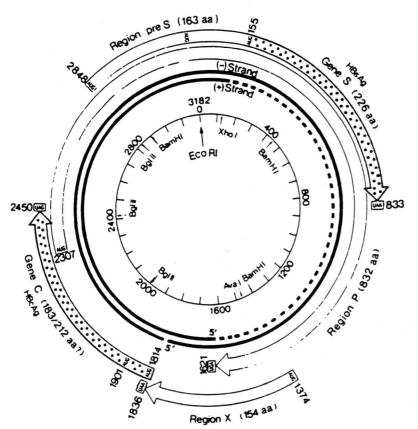

Figure 31.10 Genomic structure of the hepatitis B virus. The pre-core region (region 1836 to 1901) is where initiation of the HB 'e' protein commences.

genomic structure of the hepatitis B virus appear relatively commonly and may confer an advantage to the virus by subtly altering viral protein structures and thus allowing it to evade the host immune system.[60]

It is likely that transmission of HBeAg from mother to fetus is also one of the factors leading to virus chronicity, by preventing elimination of infected hepatocytes in the neonate. Normally, elimination of infected hepatocytes is achieved by natural killer cells and cytotoxic T cells, which recognize infected hepatocytes displaying HBV antigens (particularly peptides derived from the nucleocapsid antigens) on the cell surface in association with MHC class I proteins.[265] In the immunologically immature neonate, circulating HBeAg may reduce the cytotoxic T cell response against infected hepatocytes (possibly by inducing immune tolerance against the nucleocapsid 'target' antigens displayed on the cell surface) and thus reduce the degree of hepatic inflammation, lessening the risk of death to the host and elimination of the virus (both of which are disadvantageous to the virus). In this way a protracted infection is more likely, which is of course advantageous to the virus; a healthy host with persistent infection is much more likely to spread the virus to other individuals than a sick host with severe liver disease.

It has been speculated that a further factor that may lead to the development of chronicity in neonates is the active transport of maternal IgG anti-HBc via placental Fc receptors to the fetus.[3,215] The first host-induced immunological marker of HBV infection is antibody to the core protein (anti-HBc), which appears shortly after the time HBsAg is first detected in the serum.[122] Anti-HBc is not a neutralizing antibody and high titres of anti-HBc in the absence of HBsAg or anti-HBs may indicate the presence of continuing replication of HBV in the liver and infective HBV particles in the sera.[123] Cytotoxic T cells sensitized to nucleocapsid proteins displayed in the hepatocyte membrane recognize and destroy HBV-infected hepatocytes,[88,215] but anti-HBc and anti-HBe block this cytotoxic T-cell killing of HBV-infected hepatocytes.[82,192,215] Usually the epitopes recognized by antibodies and cytotoxic T cells are different, but this inhibition of T-cell-mediated hepatocytolysis by nucleocapsid antibodies suggests that the epitopes recognized are the same, or displayed near to each other on the cell membrane. This blocking effect may be due to simple steric hindrance if the B and cytotoxic T cell epitopes are displayed close to each other on the cell membrane.[215] Thus maternal anti-HBc transfer to the fetus may modulate T-cell-mediated lysis of infected cells,[271] which, together with the immaturity of the neonatal immune system,[200] and by analogy to chronic measles infection of the central nervous system,[101,142,211] may be another mechanism leading to viral persistence (Figure 31.11). Consistent with this hypothesis is the observation that some adult patients progressing from acute to chronic infection produce anti-HBc before those who clear the virus,[168] and injection of monoclonal anti-HBc and anti-HBe along with an infectious inoculum of HBV into

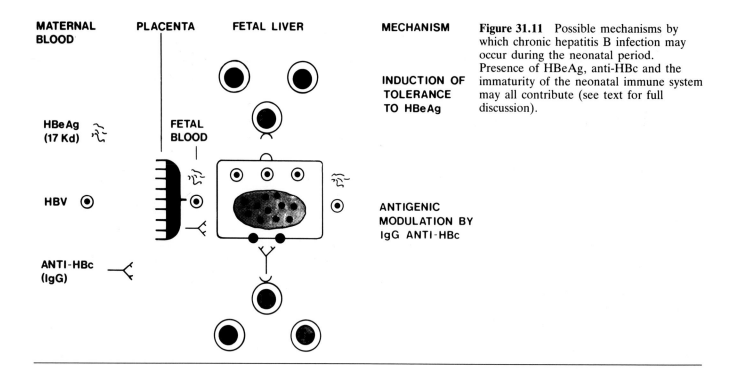

Figure 31.11 Possible mechanisms by which chronic hepatitis B infection may occur during the neonatal period. Presence of HBeAg, anti-HBc and the immaturity of the neonatal immune system may all contribute (see text for full discussion).

chimpanzees results in a protracted infection lasting 12–18 months.[136]

Infection after the neonatal period

The reasons for development of chronicity in this group may differ from those in patients who acquire their infection around the time of birth. There is evidence that abnormalities of the interferon response may contribute significantly to the development of the chronic HBV-infected state. The interferons, and interferon-α in particular, are essential for successful elimination of virus infections; they enhance MHC class I display and induce an intracellular antiviral state which blocks virus replication.[164,254] Thus a deficiency of interferon or interference with the hepatocyte response to interferon may lead to the establishment of a chronic carrier state. Interferon-α production by the host during the early phase of acute HBV infection is believed to be critically important for successful resolution during a typically self-limiting acute HBV infection.[214] Studies of peripheral blood mononuclear cells (PBMC) taken from patients with acute[164] and chronic[1,133,144] HBV infection have revealed that the production of interferon-α is subnormal. It is possible that this reduced production of interferon is directly attributable to HBV infection of the PBMC (in particular the T4 and T8 subsets),[158] and suppression of interferon production in cells, by the core region of the HBV genome, has been shown.[279] However, as reduced interferon production is also seen in lymphocytes taken from patients with a typically resolving acute HBV infection,[164] it is unlikely that an interferon deficiency per se is the cause of most cases of persistent HBV infection. This is further supported by studies showing that interferon-α therapy in chronic hepatitis B only results in clearance of

HBV infection in about a third of treated patients.[139] If persistence of infection was due to deficient interferon production by PBMC in all cases, then it might be expected that much higher seroconversion rates with interferon-α therapy would be seen.

In acute HBV infection, interferon-α is responsible for the initial increase in MHC class I antigen display on hepatocyte membranes and the activation of the 2-5A oligoadenylate synthetase (2-5OAS), endonuclease and protein kinase systems which results in an effective antiviral state within the liver (Figure 31.8). In chronic HBV-infected subjects there is evidence of an abnormal response of HBV-infected hepatocytes to interferon: levels of 2-5OAS are only minimally elevated[132] and MHC class I proteins are present only in very low density on these infected hepatocytes.[132,196] Similarly the PBMCs of patients with chronic hepatitis B infection also display a lack of MHC class I expression and 2-5OAS enzyme activation.[216] It seems likely that this abnormal cellular response to interferon is directly attributable to the virus. In vitro transfection of HBV into cells in tissue culture makes them specifically unresponsive to interferon; they remain susceptible to lysis by Sindbis virus and MHC induction does not occur.[205] MHC class I display is critical for recognition and elimination of HBV-infected hepatocytes by cytotoxic T cells and the decreased MHC expression, in addition to the reduced 2-5OAS activation, increases the likelihood of persistent HBV infection. The mechanism of this virus-induced abnormal interferon response is not clear, but one hypothesis is that it may be due to interference by HBV-DNA polymerase. One study has shown that cells, when transfected with the HBV-DNA polymerase gene, produce polymerase protein and become unresponsive to the effects of interferon-α.[100] Transfection with other HBV genes, however, does not affect the cellular response to interferon. This effect of HBV-DNA polymerase on the interferon response appears to be clinically relevant as determined by the second part of this study, which examined liver biopsies (by immunohistochemistry) taken from patients with chronic HBV infection treated with interferon-α. The interferon-inducible protein, β-2-microglobulin, was detected on 45% of normal hepatocytes, but on only 8% of hepatocytes expressing the polymerase protein.[100]

Serological diagnosis of chronic hepatitis B infection

The serological markers of a hepatitis B infection are sufficiently specific and sensitive that it is possible to diagnose confidently most cases of chronic hepatitis B infection by their use alone. However, as indicated earlier, a liver biopsy is an essential component of management in order to confirm the presence of chronic hepatitis, grade the severity of the histological lesion, exclude other possible concomitant disorders, and allow prognostication.

The first serological marker to appear in HBV infection is HBsAg, which is present in the blood 1–10 weeks after exposure to the virus and 2–8 weeks before the onset of hepatitis.[70] Excess HBsAg can be seen in the serum by electron microscopy as 22-nm particles. These particles possibly confer a biological advantage to the virus, as they may 'divert' antibody to HBsAg (anti-HBs) away from intact whole virus particles, and thus reduce the chances of virus neutralization by these anti-envelope antibodies. HBsAg persists during the acute phase of the illness and is usually cleared late in the convalescent period following the formation of anti-HBs. Failure to clear HBsAg within 6 months indicates a chronic HBsAg carrier state.

HBcAg is only found in the liver and is not detectable free in the sera of infected individuals. A soluble component of the core protein, HBeAg, is detectable in the sera of patients with replicating HBV and appears in the blood within a few days of the appearance of HBsAg.[199] In a typically resolving acute HBV infection, HBeAg is 'cleared' from the serum within 2 weeks,[199] but, similarly to HBsAg, a chronic carrier state with continuing viral replication and hepatic inflammation occurs if HBeAg persists for 6 months or more. At about the same time HBeAg is first detected in the blood, HBV-DNA polymerase activity is also observed. Both HBeAg and HBV-DNA polymerase detection in the sera correlate well with the presence of circulating intact HBV 'Dane' particles, and thus indicate high infectivity of the patient.

HBV-DNA can also be detected in the sera of patients with acute or persisting chronic viral replication, but although this is the most reliable way of determining the presence of HBV infection and of active viral replication (and thus infectivity of an individual), testing for HBV-DNA is not widely available and at present is only used as a research tool.

The first host-induced immunological marker of HBV infection is antibody to the core protein (anti-HBc), which appears at, or shortly after the time that HBsAg and HBeAg are first detected in the blood.[122] Anti-HBc may be either IgM class (usually indicating active viral replication in the acute or chronic phase) or IgG (usually seen during both the acute and chronic phases of infection and also in the convalescent period). It is not a neutralizing antibody and high titres of anti-HBc in the absence of HBsAg or anti-HBs may indicate the presence of continuing replication of HBV in the liver and infective HBV particles in the sera.[123] Anti-HBe appears after anti-HBc and, like anti-HBc, is not a neutralizing antibody. However, several studies have now shown that loss of HBeAg and the development of anti-HBe correlates well with the cessation of easily detectable viral replication in the liver and a biochemical and histological resolution of hepatic inflammation in the majority of infected individuals.[124,221] Anti-HBe may persist for several months or years but, unlike anti-HBc, is gradually lost from the serum. Anti-HBs is a neutralizing, protective antibody which is the last antibody to appear during HBV infection and is usually detected in the late convalescent period. The appearance of anti-HBs usually indicates recovery from infection and the patient is thereafter protected against reinfection.

On the basis of the serological tests described above, chronic HBV infection can be subdivided into one of three types: active HBeAg-positive infection, active HBeAg-negative infection (anti-HBe or 'pre-core mutant' hepatitis), and finally the inactive HBsAg carrier state.

HBsAg-positive, HBeAg-positive, HBV-DNA-positive patients

The presence of HBeAg in the serum always indicates hepatitis B viral replication, and thus HBV-DNA (and DNA-polymerase, the viral enzyme responsible for virus replication) will also be detected in the serum. HBeAg in the serum indicates the presence of circulating intact HBV 'Dane' particles and thus these patients are highly infectious; for example, 90% of babies born to HBeAg-positive mothers become infected with HBV.[15] Subjects with HBeAg-positive HBV infection always have hepatic inflammation of variable severity, ranging from very mild CPH, through to severe CAH with cirrhosis. Subjects may be asymptomatic with no signs of chronic liver disease, or may present with the symptoms and stigmata of frank cirrhosis. The rate of progression of the chronic hepatitis varies from subject to subject; many individuals (particularly those who were infected during the neonatal period) may carry the virus for many years without obvious harm, whilst some people may develop a rapidly progressive CAH over a short period of time. Overall, it is estimated that 50% of this group of patients will die as a direct result of chronic inflammatory liver disease or secondary to the development of hepatocellular carcinoma.[14] As a consequence, antiviral strategies directed at this group of patients are important and are discussed more fully later.

HBsAg-positive, HBeAg-negative, HBV-DNA-positive patients

This group exhibit HBV replication, as evidenced by the detection of HBV-DNA and DNA-polymerase in the serum. HBeAg is not detected in the serum but patients are usually positive for antibodies to HBe (anti-HBe) and thus this infection is sometimes called anti-HBe-positive hepatitis. HBeAg is a protein produced from the pre-core/core region of the HBV genome of the core protein and is not necessary for the production of infectious virus particles.[41] This failure to produce HBe antigen is due to a mutation occurring in the pre-core region of the HBV genome, resulting in a novel stop codon which prematurely terminates translation.[37] Thus, the virus can produce core protein and the other gene products (the surface, DNA-polymerase and X proteins), but not the 'e' protein. About 5% of patients with chronic HBV hepatitis do not have HBe antigen detectable in the serum, and generally this group of patients have a more severe and rapidly progressive liver disease.[22,300] This has led some observers to speculate that the function of HBeAg may be to reduce the inflammatory process by an (as yet) undetermined effect on the cell-mediated immune system. Thus, this 'pre-core' mutant virus appears to cause a more aggressive hepatitis than the non-mutated HBeAg-producing virus and there is some evidence that it may be more frequently involved in producing fulminant hepatitis B infection.[38]

In order to diagnose anti-HBe chronic HBV infection with absolute certainty, it is usually necessary to have firm proof of active hepatitis B viral replication, such as the presence of HBV-DNA and/or DNA-polymerase in the serum. These more specialized tests are not generally available. A study of anti-HBe-positive patients with chronic hepatitis from Taiwan has suggested that one-third of these patients have evidence of continuing HBV replication, and a further one-third have evidence of chronic delta infection.[300] It therefore seems likely that the remaining anti-HBe-positive patients with chronic hepatitis have non-A non-B infection. Thus, if tests for active viral replication are not available, the diagnosis of anti-HBe-positive HBV infection can still be made with a reasonable degree of certainty by excluding chronic delta infection (delta antibodies, and stains for delta antigen in liver biopsy material) and chronic non-A non-B hepatitis (antibody to hepatitis C virus).

HBsAg-positive, HBeAg-negative, HBV-DNA-negative patients

This group of patients have no evidence of viral replication (HBeAg, HBV-DNA and DNA-polymerase all negative) and no evidence of hepatic inflammation, and are thus called 'HBsAg carriers' (to contrast them from HBV-infected individuals with active viral replication and hepatitis). Serum transaminases are usually normal in this group of patients, suggesting no hepatic inflammation,

and a liver biopsy is not indicated in this group of patients in the absence of any biochemical evidence to suggest hepatitis. If performed, a liver biopsy is usually normal and shows no inflammation, although 'ground-glass' hepatocytes (containing HBsAg) may be seen. In the absence of markers of hepatitis B virus replication (HBeAg, HBV-DNA and DNA-polymerase), biochemical and histological evidence of chronic hepatitis in a patient who is positive for HBsAg alone is not due to chronic HBV infection and is usually due to another cause, for example concomitant chronic non-A non-B or delta infections.

The continued expression of HBsAg in the serum in the absence of active HBV replication is probably due to integration of the HBV genome into the host genome. It is now clear that HBV-DNA becomes covalently integrated into the hepatocyte genome at some time during chronic infection.[27,241] The continuous secretion of the viral coat protein (HBsAg) in the absence of active viral replication probably represents this phase, in which the viral DNA has become integrated into the host DNA and some of the viral genes are transcribed and translated as though they were hepatocyte genomic DNA. This integration event may be involved (late in the infection) in the malignant transformation of hepatocytes.[240] The cells containing integrated sequences must evade the immune elimination processes, and probably do so by not expressing HB core and HBe antigens (the putative targets for cytotoxic T cells) on their cell surface.[262] Since the preferred site for integration on the viral genome is in the promoter region of the HBcore gene,[72] this transcription unit is therefore destroyed during the integration process and thus no nucleocapsid antigens are produced. HBsAg however, continues to be expressed in these cells because this gene is intact in the integrated viral sequence.[72] As long as the cell is not recognized by the cytotoxic T cells as being infected, integration of the virus will result in viral persistence. Whether HBV integrates or not is dependent on the duration of infection and is usually found if infection has been present for 2 or more years. Studies of attempts at eliminating HBV infection using interferon therapy have indicated that patients who have had chronic infection for many years, and who have integrated HBV-DNA, are much less likely to clear HBs antigen than patients with a short period of chronicity and in whom integration is not found.[210] In individuals who have 'cleared' replicating virus (HBV-DNA, HBV-DNA polymerase and HBe antigen all negative) and have no evidence of liver disease, reactivation of infection (from integrated HBV) has sometimes been seen when immunosuppressive therapy is given or acquired immune dysfunction occurs.[67,125]

Clinical features of chronic hepatitis B infection

In patients infected in adulthood, males are more commonly affected. The symptoms and signs are not specific for hepatitis B infection and are those of progressive hepatocellular damage. Most patients are asymptomatic but some patients present with symptoms and signs of frank liver failure, such as ascites, variceal haemorrhage or encephalopathy.

Although arthralgia, arthritis and urticaria are well-recognized clinical features of acute viral hepatitis, they may also occur in chronic hepatitis B infection and occasionally a variety of other extrahepatic manifestations may be seen. For example, an association between glomerulonephritis and hepatitis B was described by Combes *et al.*,[53] who demonstrated HBsAg, IgG and complement in the glomerular basement membrane by immunofluorescence. The deposits are nodular and glomeruli show a membranoproliferative or membranous pattern associated with immune complex deposition.[104] This may be a common cause of glomerulonephritis in certain parts of the world, particularly in children.[33] Some patients with chronic hepatitis B may show a hypersensitivity angiitis, similar to polyarteritis nodosa[239] but this may also occur in association with acute infection[185] (see Chapter 30). A very small number of HBsAg-positive patients (with Dane particles in their serum) may present with purpura and arthralgia as essential mixed cryoglobulinaemia,[165] but presentations are uncommon.

Histology and morphology of chronic hepatitis B infection

Patients with chronic HBV hepatitis will show a spectrum of histological appearances as described previously and as seen in other causes of chronic hepatitis, but there are some histological features (such as ground-glass hepatocytes) that are specific to this infection. Patients may have a very minimal hepatic inflammation and fall into the category of mild CPH, or a more severe CAH with cirrhosis. Chronic lobular hepatitis may also be seen. One direct comparative study of HBsAg-positive and negative cases of chronic active hepatitis showed a significantly higher incidence of parenchymal and portal inflammation in the HBsAg-negative group (mostly auto-immune hepatitis), and a more prominent plasma cell component in the infiltrates,[48] but a similar study by Schalm and co-workers failed to find any significant differences between HBsAg-positive and negative patients.[232]

HBsAg carriers

In HBsAg carriers without active viral replication, the liver biopsy architecture is usually normal and inflammation is absent or confined to portal tracts and minimal. Ground-glass hepatocytes may be observed (Figure 31.12). These are cells with an increased volume of cytoplasm in which there is a finely granular or stippled, pale-staining eosinophilic zone.[113] This zone may form the bulk of the cytoplasm, when there is usually a halo separating it from the plasma membrane, or it may form a discrete inclusion, sometimes crescentic in shape and occasionally perinuclear

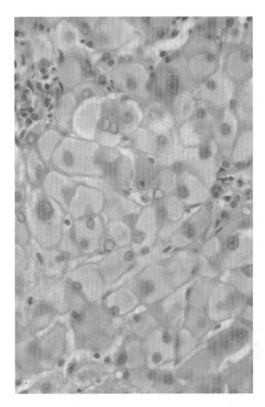

Figure 31.12 Ground glass hepatocytes in chronic hepatitis B infection. Most hepatocytes have a large discrete area of finely stippled, pale, eosinophilic cytoplasm pushing the nucleus to one side and sometimes separated from the plasma membrane by a clear non-staining rim, H&E.

in location. These cells may be widely dispersed throughout the biopsy or may form confluent clusters in any part of the acinus. They are most frequent and readily recognized in asymptomatic carriers, but have also been found in chronic active hepatitis and cirrhosis due to HBV. These cells are also orcein-positive (Figure 31.13), which separates them from the identical appearances that can be produced by drug-induced hyperplasia of the smooth endoplasmic reticulum.[266,297] Orcein (or aldehyde fuchsin) staining reveals HBsAg in the hepatocyte cytoplasm,[73,244] as well as elastic fibres. It is likely that these stains demonstrate sulphonic acid groups formed by the oxidation of disulphide bonds,[244] in which HBsAg is particularly rich.[289] Immunocytochemical techniques also confirm and demonstrate HBsAg in the cytoplasm.[113,190,244] Immunoperoxidase staining for HBsAg is thought to be more sensitive; some orcein-negative hepatocytes can be positively stained by this method.[190] The core antigen, if present, is usually confined to the nucleus with little evidence of cytoplasmic expression.[258] With integration of the HBV-DNA into the genome of the cell, expression of core antigen slowly disappears. Electron microscopic examination of hepatocytes from HBsAg carriers reveals parallel tubular forms, spherical particles and 'owl-eye bodies' within the smooth endoplasmic reticulum.[102,253]

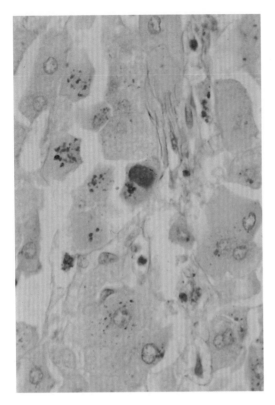

Figure 31.13 Orcein-positive hepatocytes. A large brown inclusion within the cytoplasm of a hepatocyte in the centre of the field represents orcein-positive staining of hepatitis B surface antigen in the cell. Note the difference from the multiple small orcein-positive granules of copper binding protein that are present in many of the other hepatocytes. Orcein.

Interestingly, these are not often seen in patients with chronic active hepatitis.[5]

Chronic HBV infection with active replication

This group of patients always have hepatic inflammation of variable severity ranging from very mild CPH through to severe CAH with cirrhosis, and orcein stains may demonstrate HBsAg in the cytoplasm of hepatocytes. It is also possible to stain for the markers of active viral replication. Correlation of histological features with the different markers of HBV expression has suggested that parenchymal damage and inflammation was significantly correlated with evidence of HBV replication.[209] Hepatitis B core antigen and particles can be demonstrated by immunofluorescent, immunoperoxidase and electron-microscopic techniques.[130,190,259] These core particles are 21–25 nm in size, found mostly in or on the surface of the hepatocyte nucleus, and correspond morphologically to the inner compartment of the Dane particle.[130] They are more frequently observed in immunosuppressed subjects, and during successful elimination of HBV from the liver the amount of demonstrable nuclear HBcAg diminishes.[231] With increasing degrees of inflammation, the expression of nuclear HBcAg becomes much more focal

in distribution,[25,85,258] but there is increased expression of core antigen within the cytoplasm.[129,258,302]

The pattern of e antigen expression has been differentiated from core antigen using monoclonal antibodies in biopsies from HBsAg carriers.[194] The e antigen was more commonly co-expressed in both nucleus and cytoplasm than the core antigen, which was usually confined to the nucleus. Immunoelectron microscopy of the e antigen has confirmed its presence in the nucleus and in the cytoplasm, where it can be located within the cytosol or the endoplasmic reticulum as well as on the plasma membrane.[301] The presence of e antigen in the serum is associated with evidence of HBV replication and therefore correlates with the expression of HBV-DNA and core antigen in the liver.[189,269] Nonetheless, chronic active hepatitis does sometimes occur in patients with antibodies to the e antigen: evidence of continuing viral replication can be seen by the demonstration of core antigen and/or HBV-DNA in these biopsies.[22,189,258] This presumably relates to infection with the core mutant HBV that is unable to secrete e antigen.[37,300]

HBV-DNA can be localized within the infected hepatocyte by molecular probes and autoradiography.[110,187] Generally, these special methods of demonstrating morphological markers of virus replication are only used as research tools. In situ hybridization studies have suggested that the HBV-DNA is more commonly localized to areas of the biopsy that show piecemeal necrosis or bridging hepatic necrosis.[187]

CHRONIC DELTA HEPATITIS INFECTION

Background

The hepatitis delta virus (HDV) is a small RNA virus which can cause either an acute, sometimes fulminant hepatitis or a more slowly progressive chronic hepatitis. HDV is a defective virus and cannot produce its own external envelope; instead it utilizes HBV surface protein (HBsAg) to form its outer coat.[195] It is therefore totally dependent on HBsAg for its propagation and hepatotropism. Replication of HDV, however, is totally independent of HBV replication; thus HDV infection may co-exist in inactive HBsAg carriers who do not have active HBV replication.[246] If infection with HBV and HDV occur at the same time (co-infection), an acute self-limiting infection (which may be fulminant) occurs in the majority of patients and few become chronically infected.[226] However, if HDV superinfection occurs in a patient who already is a chronic HBV carrier (with either active (HBV-DNA positive) or inactive (HBsAg carrier) infection), then a chronic HDV hepatitis results in 70–90% of cases.[226]

The HDV genome is known to produce at least one protein; the delta antigen. This is a phosphorylated polypeptide capable of binding RNA, which accumulates predominantly in the nucleoplasm of the nuclei of infected hepatocytes.[195] Identification of this protein in the nuclei of hepatocytes, or less reliably in the serum, is a useful way of establishing the diagnosis of chronic HDV hepatitis. The function(s) of this protein is as yet unclear.

Clinical features of chronic HDV hepatitis

There are no specific clinical features of chronic HDV hepatitis and the diagnosis of chronic HDV hepatitis should always be considered in any HBsAg-positive patient with chronic hepatitis. However chronic hepatitis in certain clinical scenarios may implicate the delta agent as a cause. These include a rapidly progressive HBsAg-positive chronic active hepatitis with cirrhosis developing very early; anti-HBe chronic HBV infection, particularly if HBV-DNA is negative; known chronic HBV carriers who develop a secondary 'flare-up' or worsening of their hepatitis; and subjects with chronic hepatitis from geographical areas where HDV is known to be prevalent (e.g. southern Italy,[103,248] Brazil,[99] Venezuela[217] and the Middle East[245]).

Serological identification of chronic HDV infection

The serological diagnosis of chronic HDV infection is often difficult. The presence of HDV infection in HBsAg-positive patients can be identified by detection of delta antigen or HDV-RNA in serum, or by demonstration of anti-HDV seroconversion. The most reliable and specific method of detecting HDV infection is molecular hybridization for HDV-RNA,[249] but this method is not readily available in most laboratories involved in screening for HDV infection. Although more freely available, detection of delta antigen in serum by radioimmunoassay (RIA) is not a reliable way of diagnosing HDV infection and studies have shown that only 2–80% of patients with acute HDV infection will have detectable delta antigen present in the serum.[137,242] This antigen disappears from serum within a few days.[248] Thus, absence of circulating delta antigen (by RIA) does not exclude HDV infection. Western blotting for delta antigen in serum may increase the sensitivity of detection,[17] but, like HDV-RNA, is not freely available. At present, the diagnosis of acute HDV infection is best established by the detection of IgM anti-HDV, which persists in the serum for a brief period in low titre during the acute illness.[247] In the event of successful elimination of HBV/HDV infection, anti-HDV disappears from the serum within 6 months in most patients, although a minority may have low titre IgG anti-HDV detectable long after the convalescent period.[203] Previous HDV infection cannot be reliably diagnosed using current serological methods. In chronic HBV/HDV infections however, high titres of both IgM and IgG anti-HDV are present[226] and the diagnosis can be confirmed by demonstrating the presence of delta antigen in liver tissue specimens by immunofluorescence.[246]

Molecular basis of pathogenicity

It is not known at present how HDV contributes to the worsening of the hepatitis seen in patients with chronic HBV infection. Circumstantial evidence suggests that the HDV-RNA genome may interact or interfere with intracellular functions, in an analogous way to the plant viroids with which HDV shares certain similarities.[195] Further circumstantial evidence (results of antiviral therapy with interferon-α) supports the suggestion that HDV may be directly cytopathic to the liver. This is discussed in more detail later in this chapter.

Natural history and prognosis of chronic HDV hepatitis

Several studies have looked at the natural history of HDV infection.[23,63] These have indicated that a rapidly progressive and scarring inflammation resulting in cirrhosis within 12 months may be seen in about 15% of cases. A further 15% have a benign disease with spontaneous remission of the inflammation, and the remaining 70% have a slowly progressive development of cirrhosis. Thus, chronic HDV infection is a more aggressive and destructive inflammation than chronic HBV hepatitis and untreated carries a worse prognosis.

Histology and morphology of chronic HDV hepatitis

Infection with HDV is always associated with significant histological evidence of hepatic injury. Although chronic persistent hepatitis may occur, it is usual to have more severe grades of hepatic inflammation, and severe liver disease progressing rapidly to cirrhosis or liver cell failure is frequently seen.[62,108,217,285] There are no specific features which separate chronic HDV hepatitis from chronic HBV hepatitis. In some instances there is a non-fatty foamy cytoplasmic degeneration of hepatocytes.[109,161] Many cases have increased numbers of hepatocytes showing granular acidophil degeneration of the cytoplasm,[217,285] but similar changes have also been observed in non-A non-B hepatitis. It is uncommon for this acidophil degeneration to be associated with an inflammatory reaction and it further supports the contention that, unlike HBV, HDV is a directly cytopathic agent. None the less, an analysis of the distribution of different lymphocyte subsets composing the inflammatory infiltrate in the various parts of the acinus in patients with chronic active delta hepatitis has shown that there is no difference from a chronic active hepatitis B infection without delta. It has therefore been suggested that T-cell-mediated immunity may still have a role in the pathogenesis of chronic delta hepatitis.[49] The relative importance of this role remains to be elucidated but it has been separately recorded that parenchymal lymphocytic infiltrates were more commonly clustered around hepatocytes morphologically expressing either the delta antigen or cytoplasmic hepatitis B core antigen.[150]

The structure of the delta virus is not well understood.

The outer envelope consists of HBsAg antigen which, when removed, reveals no discernible inner structure. Using an immunofluorescent system however, delta antigen can be detected within the nuclei of infected hepatocytes. IgG, representing delta antigen–anti-delta immune complexes, can also sometimes be identified within the nucleus.[225] Immunoelectron microscopy may reveal positive staining for delta antigen in the nuclei as dense round structures with soft, indistinct edges and a diameter of approximately 20–30 nm.[36,150] However, these bodies do not have any standard morphological viral substructure, nor are they unique to infections with HDV.

CHRONIC HEPATITIS C INFECTION

The cloning and sequencing of the hepatitis C virus (HCV), the agent now known to be responsible for most cases of non-A non-B (NANB) hepatitis,[45] was a major breakthrough for virologists and hepatologists dealing with this disease. Prior to this discovery, the diagnosis of chronic non-A non-B hepatitis was predominantly a diagnosis of exclusion. It was considered in patients with chronic hepatitis and a history of parenteral exposure to blood, blood products or intravenous drug abuse, only when the other known causes of chronic hepatitis had been excluded. However, subsequent to the discovery of HCV and the development of an antibody test (anti-HCV) for the detection of this agent,[152] it is now clear that most cases of chronic NANB hepatitis are due to HCV and also that many cases of so-called 'cryptogenic' chronic hepatitis (chronic hepatitis in an individual with no apparent parenteral exposure, and with no other known cause for chronic hepatitis) are also due to this agent.[176] In spite of this, there are still a small minority of cases of chronic NANB hepatitis which have been caused by exposure of the affected individual to an infectious agent which is not HCV but may represent another, as yet, undiscovered NANB virus.[156] Thus, although the anti-HCV test has considerably advanced our ability to diagnose chronic NANB hepatitis more confidently, there are still occasions when, in spite of a negative anti-HCV test, clinical factors will indicate the diagnosis of chronic NANB/C hepatitis.

Serological diagnosis

The hepatitis C virus (HCV) is an RNA virus that appears to be related to the flaviviridae. Its nature is discussed more fully in Chapter 30. Subsequent to the discovery of this agent,[45] a solid-phase enzyme-linked assay has been developed using an expressed viral polypeptide antigen (C100-3). This assay detects antibodies (anti-HCV) to a non-structural region of the virus.[152] Using this assay, it is now clear that HCV infection is the cause of most cases of chronic NANB hepatitis; reports indicate that 70–80% of patients in the USA, Japan and Italy with parenterally acquired chronic NANB hepatitis have antibodies to this virus.[152] As well as antibodies to the virus, HCV nucleic

acid sequences have also been detected in the livers of anti-HCV-positive patients with chronic NANB hepatitis,[293] indicating continuing viraemia in patients with chronic infection. Many studies have now reported on the incidence of antibodies to HCV (anti-HCV) in normal individuals and various disease states. The incidence in apparently healthy UK blood donors is between 0.5 and 1%,[155] whilst certain population groups, notably haemophiliacs and intravenous drug abusers, have a much higher rate of anti-HCV positivity, varying between 64–78% and 48–70%, respectively.[90,228]

Unfortunately, there appears to be a relatively high incidence of false positive anti-HCV tests, particularly in patients with high serum globulin levels, which are often seen in patients with cirrhosis and autoimmune liver disease in particular.[184] Anti-HCV is also rarely found in the early phase of NANB hepatitis and generally does not become detectable until 20 weeks after infection.[6] Thus, the current (first-generation) anti-HCV test, which only detects antibody to one of the non-structural proteins of HCV, will be unlikely to help in the differential diagnosis of acute viral hepatitis but should prove extremely useful in patients with chronic HCV hepatitis.

Epidemiology and natural history

Chronic HCV infection appears to occur all over the world. It is found in North America (where it is more common than HBV infection) and Western Europe as well as the Middle East and Far East.[155] Preliminary data from several countries have indicated that there may be considerable genomic variability between strains of HCV from different countries.[156] This is now being taken into account in future vaccine design (see Chapter 30).

The morbidity of this disease is high. It is estimated that approximately 40–50% of patients acquiring HCV infection will develop chronic hepatitis, with 15–20% of these subjects progressing to cirrhosis.[80,222] For example, in the United States it has been estimated that at least 6000 patients per annum develop cirrhosis as a direct consequence of chronic NANB hepatitis.[115] Like the delta virus, it appears that HCV is a directly cytopathic agent. Again, the main evidence for this comes from the pattern of response of HCV to interferon therapy.

Histology

A spectrum of histological abnormalities, ranging from mild CPH through to severe CAH with cirrhosis, may be seen in chronic HCV/NANB hepatitis. There are no histological features which are diagnostic: however, there are some features which may suggest the possibility of chronic NANB/HCV infection.[79] These include the presence of follicular lymphoid aggregates, sinusoidal mononuclear cell infiltration[294] focal bile duct damage,[10] microvesicular fatty change and eosinophilic granular hepatocytes with acidophilic bodies (Figure 31.14). Although these histological features are not specific for

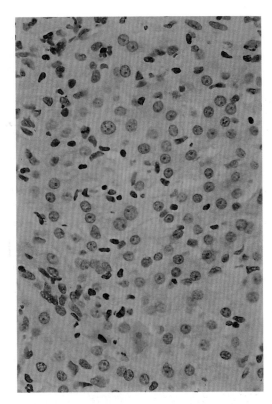

Figure 31.14 Hepatitis non-A non-B/hepatitis C infection. There is some disorganization of the liver cell plate, but the more obvious feature is the mononuclear cell infiltrate in the sinusoids in the relative absence of hepatocyte degeneration or fibrosis. H&E.

NANB/HCV hepatitis, taken together with an appropriate history and absence of markers of HBV and HDV infection they may act as pointers towards this diagnosis. Careful immunoelectron microscopic analysis of the different lymphocyte subsets in the inflammatory infiltrate and of their status with regard to the expression of activation markers failed to show any significant differences from hepatitis B.[78]

The hepatitis C virus has not definitively been morphologically identified at the ultrastructural level, although there are several reports of intranuclear particles[11,34,74] and of cytoplasmic changes.[74,75,294] The intranuclear changes have been seen in other conditions such as delta hepatitis[36] and the cytoplasmic tubules and lamellae appear to be a response to focal damage rather than viral inclusions.

Clinical features of chronic NANB/HCV hepatitis

There are no specific clinical features of chronic NANB/HCV hepatitis and the symptoms and signs are as discussed earlier under the heading general clinical features. Biochemically, however, the disease may be distinguished by marked fluctuations in the height of the serum transaminase levels[80] and on occasion the serum

transaminases may even be normal. This is not usually seen in other types of chronic hepatitis.

Link with other hepatic disease

Several papers have indicated that anti-HCV positivity is not uncommon in patients who also have other liver disorders, for example hepatitis B infection,[94] primary biliary cirrhosis,[90] alcoholic cirrhosis,[32,90] and autoimmune disease.[89] There is also a very strong correlation between anti-HCV positivity and the development of hepatocellular carcinoma.[32,44,52,84,270] Although the data are still scarce, it does suggest that chronic HCV infection may be a co-factor in some patients who are known to have other hepatic disease. However other studies are conflicting on the incidence of anti-HCV in different types of chronic hepatitis[65] and there is some evidence that false positive anti-HCV tests may be common,[184] particularly in cirrhotic patients who have raised levels of immunoglobulins. Until the advent of readily available confirmatory tests for the presence of HCV infection (such as polymerase chain reaction and/or HCV probe hybridization), the true relationship between this virus and other inflammatory hepatic diseases will remain unclear. The relationship of HCV infection to autoimmune chronic hepatitis characterized by liver–kidney–microsomal antibodies is discussed in the next section.

CHRONIC AUTOIMMUNE ('LUPOID') HEPATITIS ___

Clinical features

Waldenstrom first drew attention to chronic liver disease in young women with jaundice, acne, amenorrhoea, hepatosplenomegaly and hyperglobulinaemia.[290] Within the next few years, there were several reports of chronic active liver disease in young women[13,151] and women at the menopause,[39] with features suggesting an immune disturbance. These included a positive LE cell phenomenon,[143] which led to the term 'lupoid' hepatitis[170] and a prominent plasma cell infiltrate in the liver, hence the term 'plasma cell hepatitis'.[107] The histological lesion found in this group of patients is usually chronic active hepatitis, often severe, and the development of cirrhosis is a frequent event if patients are not treated.

Early studies of the clinical features of autoimmune hepatitis were confused by the inability to exclude other causes of chronic hepatitis. After the discovery of HBsAg and the hepatitis B virus, chronic active hepatitis was initially simply classified as HBsAg-positive or negative. Patients who were HBsAg-positive were more likely to be males of an older age group, and nowadays are recognized to represent patients with chronic HBV hepatitis. Patients with HBsAg-negative chronic active hepatitis were more likely to be young women, or women at the menopause, and are now recognized as having autoimmune hepatitis. The general clinical differences

Table 31.1 Clinical and immunological distinctions between HBsAg-positive and HBsAg-negative chronic active hepatitis

	HBsAg-positive	HBsAg-negative
Age	Often elderly	Often young
Sex	Mostly males	Usually females
Multisystem disease	Rare	Common
Antinuclear factor	Rare	Common
Smooth muscle antibody	Rare	Common
Anti-HBc	Common	Rare
Liver-specific antibodies	Rare	Common
Hyperglobulinaemia	Moderate	Marked
HLA-B8 distribution	Normal	Increased
Geographical distribution	Variable	Probably universal
Response to corticosteroids	Unknown	Favourable
Prognosis	Unknown	Usually poor

Data from Wright.[299]

between these two groups of patients is shown in Table 31.1.

Early studies of the clinical features of chronic active hepatitis, including many patients who today would be classified as chronic autoimmune hepatitis, are still relevant today. In the series from the UK reported by Read et al.,[220] 81 patients were described, of whom 49 were female and 49 were under 21 years of age. In 13 patients, other autoimmune phenomena such as thyroid disease, arthralgia, ulcerative colitis or renal disease were the presenting features. Thus, it is likely that autoimmune hepatitis accounts for many of these cases. On physical examination, the patients often looked well but could have mild jaundice, prominent spider naevi and palmar erythema. Cutaneous striae and gynaecomastia occurred in young males. The spleen was palpable in the majority of patients and the liver was usually increased but occasionally reduced in size. Amenorrhoea was a common feature in young women, as were acne and skin rashes, including those resembling lupus erythematosus, purpura and splinter haemorrhages. Additional features were arthralgia, pulmonary infiltration and associated diseases such as thyroiditis, ulcerative colitis and diabetes. Renal abnormalities included albuminuria, the nephrotic syndrome and renal tubular acidosis.

The series from Australia reported by Mistilis et al.[191] was strikingly similar, including age and sex incidence, mode of presentation, a progressive downhill course, the presence of multisystem involvement and an association with putative autoimmune disease. Even in those patients who presented insidiously, jaundice and episodes of deteriorating liver function soon developed during the course of the disease. This was often associated with anorexia, marked fatigue, abdominal pain, the development of new spider naevi, fever, haemorrhagic phenomena and ascites. Death usually occurred from liver failure with or without bleeding varices, but in a few patients the course was so unpredictable that remissions occurred even after hepatic failure. In rare instances chronic autoimmune

hepatitis may present acutely and a diagnosis of an acute viral hepatitis made.[59]

Untreated, the prognosis is not good. In the Australian series, half the deaths occurred in the first few years when the disease was most active, and only 6 patients survived 10 years. This reflects the severity of the hepatitis. This is also seen in the serum transaminases, which are often consistently at 300–500 IU/l, compared to chronic HBV hepatitis where the transaminases are mostly under 200 and usually less than 100 IU/l. In chronic autoimmune hepatitis, hypergammaglobulinaemia of some degree is almost always seen, sometimes to very high values.

Haematological changes include an anaemia which is often normochromic, and leucopenia is also occasionally observed. A positive LE cell phenomenon was found in 10 of the 81 British patients and 9 of the 60 cases examined in the Australian series. The clinical and biochemical features in these two series are summarized in Table 31.2.

Apart from the associated clinical extrahepatic manifestations noted in the series cited above, other reports have noted that multisystem disease is not uncommon in autoimmune hepatitis. Golding and associates[105] found a high frequency of Sjögren's syndrome, renal tubular acidosis and pulmonary diffusion defects, as well as a small number of patients with peripheral neuropathy, ulcerative colitis, thyroid disease and arthropathy. Fibrosing alveolitis,[278] ulcerative colitis,[120] arthropathy, autoimmune haemolytic anaemia,[208] neutropenia[19] and rheumatoid nodules[98] have all been reported, and patients with a primary diagnosis of autoimmune hepatitis may present with symptoms and signs of disease affecting virtually any

Table 31.2 Comparison of two large series of chronic active hepatitis

	Read, Sherlock and Harrison[220]	Mistilis, Skyring and Blackburn[191]
Total number of patients	81	82
Males	32	17
Females	49	65
Age	40<20 yrs	32<20 yrs
Onset:		
Acute jaundice	28%	32%
Insidious jaundice	37%	48%
Anicteric	22%	20%
Splenomegaly	77%	49% (at onset)
Hepatomegaly	72%	75% (at onset)
Spider naevi	Nearly 100%	45% (at onset)
Amenorrhoea	All young women	38% (premenopausal)
Ulcerative colitis	6%	11%
Arthralgia	11%	18%
Varices	2%	42%
Ascites	15%	41%
Bilirubin 50–170 μmol/l (3–10 mg/100 ml)	Most patients	Most patients
Globulin	>50g/l 53%	>35g/l
Albumin	<30g/l 33%	Mean 31g/l
LE cells	16%	15%

other organ system in the body. It has been claimed that the incidence of associated autoimmune diseases is lower in postmenopausal patients when compared with the younger age groups.[159]

Immunological changes

A number of immunological phenomena have been described, including humoral and cell-mediated reactions to liver-specific antigens, but their role in the disease process remains unclear. Although autoimmune models resembling the lesion seen in man have been produced by the injection of liver-specific lipoproteins into rabbits and mice, their relevance to autoimmune hepatitis in man is unclear.[35,148]

Humoral mechanisms

Hyperglobulinaemia is one of the most striking immunological abnormalities in chronic active hepatitis. All three major immunoglobulin classes are involved, although the rise is most pronounced in the IgG levels.[96] The mechanism of the hyperglobulinaemia is probably complex. Evidence of increased C1q, but not C3, catabolism suggested a deficiency of C4 or C2[261] which has now been confirmed.[197] Abnormalities of immune regulation have also been demonstrated.[118] Serum complement levels may be low, but they can be correlated with low serum albumin levels and a prolonged prothrombin time, which suggests that they are due to defective synthesis by the diseased liver rather than to complement utilization in immune complex formation.[97] However, there is some evidence for in vivo inactivation of C3 in chronic active hepatitis, which favours the latter possibility;[260] its binding properties to isolated hepatocytes have been described.[219]

Another striking immunological abnormality is the range of autoantibodies observed.[83] Initial reports were of non-organ-specific autoantibodies, but a liver-specific membrane reactive autoantibody has also been described.[128] Antinuclear antibody,[154] often of the IgG class, occurs in over half the patients and is present at high titre; about 10% of patients have a positive LE cell phenomenon and DNA-binding antibodies, which were originally thought to be specific for systemic lupus erythematosus, may also be seen.[69] Smooth-muscle antibodies were initially described by Johnson et al.[141] These antibodies occur in 40–60% of HBsAg-negative chronic active hepatitis at high titre.[147] Although the highest titres and strongest reactions are usually found in chronic autoimmune hepatitis, smooth-muscle antibodies are also present in other forms of liver disease and in viral infections.[7,119] The broad-reacting high-titre smooth-muscle antibody found in chronic autoimmune hepatitis has been shown to be directed against actin[28,166] and other components of the cytoskeleton.[153]

An antibody reacting with microsomal membranes is found particularly in the sera of young patients with clinically active disease in the absence of other autoantibodies.[250] This antibody is distinct from the mitochondrial antibody that is commonly present in primary biliary cirrhosis but in only a small proportion of patients with chronic autoimmune hepatitis.[83]

Antibodies to liver-specific lipoprotein (LSP) have also been found and studies have suggested that they correlate with the presence of piecemeal necrosis.[140,296] There is evidence that some antibody activity is directed to the asialoglycoprotein receptor.[181] The LSP antibodies may be of practical value in predicting a relapse of chronic autoimmune hepatitis after withdrawal of treatment.[183] Liver-specific antibodies, however, may not be completely specific for the liver.[89,182] On the basis of the presence of autoantibodies, some authorities have subdivided chronic autoimmune hepatitis into two distinct types; a 'classical' type I autoimmune hepatitis, with elevated titres of anti-smooth muscle and anti-nuclear antibodies, and a less common type II autoimmune hepatitis, which is defined by the presence of antibodies to liver and kidney microsomes (anti-LKM).[121] Patients with type II autoimmune hepatitis generally have a more aggressive disease and tend to present much younger, when between 2 and 14 years of age.[121] Both groups respond well to steroids, although type II patients may require higher doses.

Cell-mediated immunity

Patients with chronic autoimmune hepatitis often have impaired cell-mediated immunity as demonstrated by skin-testing, decreased numbers of circulating T cells and impaired lymphocyte transformation responses.[268] Both the number and function of non-specific suppressor cells[118] are diminished in these patients. A defect in antigen-specific suppressor cell functions may be responsible for the development of autoantibodies reacting with liver membrane antigens.[281] Several studies of lymphocyte cytotoxicity in chronic autoimmune hepatitis have been performed[252,284] and the whole subject of cellular immune reactions in autoimmune hepatitis has been reviewed.[186,264] Overall, it was concluded that in autoimmune hepatitis an antibody-dependent cellular immune reaction is the major effector mechanism of liver cell destruction.[188] One study has demonstrated specific helper T-cell clones in patients with autoimmune hepatitis which react with liver-specific lipoprotein and the asialoglycoprotein receptor, both known targets of immune attack in autoimmune hepatitis.[295] These T-cell clones stimulate autologous B lymphocytes to produce autoantibodies directed at these self-antigens.[295] The rapid response of the hepatic inflammation to treatment with immunosuppressive therapy is also supportive of this contention.

Diagnosis

Unfortunately there is no single diagnostic test for chronic autoimmune hepatitis and the diagnosis of autoimmune hepatitis is based on clinical, histological, biochemical and immunological findings, and the exclusion of other known causes for chronic hepatitis. The clinical features which may suggest this diagnosis have already been detailed. In women, overlap may occur between chronic autoimmune hepatitis and primary biliary cirrhosis. As in chronic autoimmune hepatitis, hypergammaglobulinaemia and other immunological phenomena, such as autoantibody formation (in particular antimitochondrial antibody) are frequently seen in primary biliary cirrhosis.[83] Although a liver biopsy usually differentiates between chronic active hepatitis and primary biliary cirrhosis, it may sometimes be difficult definitively to distinguish between these two conditions. A similar problem may occur in distinguishing chronic autoimmune hepatitis from primary sclerosing cholangitis, where autoimmune phenomena such as organ-specific and non-organ-specific antibodies and hypergammaglobulinaemia and an increased incidence of HLA B8 and DR3 also occur. Cholangiographic examination, however, usually demonstrates multifocal strictures involving the intra- and extra-hepatic ducts which are diagnostic of primary sclerosing cholangitis.

Aetiology

Although the evidence of both cell-mediated and humoral immune activation and the rapid response to immunosuppressive therapy indicates that the hepatocellular inflammation is specifically mediated by the immune system, the trigger for this autoimmune assault on the liver is not known. Linkage disequilibrium studies have indicated that in autoimmune hepatitis there is a strong association between HLA-B8 and DR3, and also with specific immunoglobulin allotypes.[172] This suggests a genetically determined HLA-linked aberration in regulation of immune responses, as HLA-DR3 may be linked with a regulator gene for suppressor cells. Thus, there exists the possibility that autoimmune hepatitis represents a defective immune response to hepatocytes, which may be initiated by an environmental 'trigger', possibly an infectious agent.

High-titre antibodies to a variety of bacterial and viral antigens, particularly enterobacteria, measles, rubella and cytomegalovirus,[46,273,275] have been also observed in chronic autoimmune hepatitis, and there is an overall correlation between the presence of antinuclear antibody, smooth muscle antibody and these viral antibody titres, but no cross-reactivity.[274] The measles and rubella virus titres are particularly high. One study has suggested that persistent genomic material from the measles virus can be detected in patients with chronic autoimmune hepatitis,[227] leading to speculation that this virus may trigger the disease.

More recently a number of studies have suggested that HCV infection may play a role in the development of autoimmune hepatitis. A study from Spain on 34 patients with type I autoimmune hepatitis, has revealed that nearly half (15 patients) were anti-HCV positive.[90] Another study has shown that 86% of patients with type II (anti-LKM-positive) autoimmune hepatitis are anti-HCV-positive.[162] Absorption studies excluded the possibility that a common antibody is involved[162] and the authors

have suggested that HCV infection in some way increases or modifies membrane expression of the LKM antigen (a 50-kDa protein, p450dbl, which is found on rat hepatocyte membranes). Other studies from Japan have shown that, during HCV infection, specific cytotoxic T cell clones are found which lyse hepatocytes from patients with chronic NANB hepatitis and autoimmune hepatitis, but not from patients with acute hepatitis A or B infections, or chronic hepatitis B infection.[134]

Unfortunately, antibody tests for the presence of virus infection may not be completely specific and false positive antibody results may occur, particularly in patients whose immune systems are generally activated (as is seen in autoimmune hepatitis) and also in patients with cirrhosis, where immunoglobulin levels are generally raised. Thus, the raised titres of measles and rubella antibodies, and the presence of antibodies to HCV in autoimmune hepatitis may be spurious and relate simply to the hypergammaglobulinaemia. Indeed in the case of antibodies to HCV, it seems highly likely that at least a proportion of patients who are anti-HCV-positive, particularly those with cirrhosis, are not infected with this virus.[184] One study from the United States has shown that the rate of anti-HCV positivity in steroid-treated autoimmune (and cryptogenic) chronic hepatitis is much lower than the rate seen in untreated patients.[65] This suggests that treatment and a reduction in globulin levels may result in a lower rate of anti-HCV positivity. In support for this, a study from Sweden has shown a highly significant fall in the rate of anti-HCV positivity in chronic autoimmune hepatitis (from 33% down to 1%) during steroid treatment.[236]

The latest virus incriminated as a trigger for chronic autoimmune hepatitis is hepatitis A: three relatives of patients with autoimmune chronic hepatitis developed autoimmune hepatitis after subclinical hepatitis A infection.[283] In two of the subjects, specific helper T cells and antibodies to the asialoglycoprotein receptor persisted and increased after acute hepatitis A. The authors recommend that relatives of patients with autoimmune hepatitis should be vaccinated against hepatitis A (when the vaccine becomes available within the next year or two).

Histology

The histology of chronic autoimmune hepatitis is indistinguishable from the general features described earlier. The histological lesion is more likely to be chronic active hepatitis (often severe), which may co-exist with evidence of established cirrhosis at the time of first diagnosis ('active cirrhosis'). More active parenchymal inflammation and an increased number of plasma cells are pointers favouring autoimmune as opposed to chronic viral hepatitis.

DRUG-INDUCED CHRONIC HEPATITIS

Several drugs have been shown to induce a clinical and histological picture of chronic hepatitis[175] (Table 31.3). These include laxatives containing oxyphenisatin,[57]

Table 31.3 Drug-induced chronic active hepatitis (CAH)

Drugs producing an illness clinically and histologically resembling idiopathic CAH
    Oxyphenisatin
    Methyldopa
    Nitrofurantoin
    Dantrolene

Drugs producing an illness histologically resembling CAH
    Isoniazid
    Halothane

Drugs which very rarely have been associated with liver injury compatible with CAH
    Sulphonamides
    Propylthiouracil
    Asprin
    Paracetamol (acetaminophen)
    Chlorpromazine

Data from Maddrey.[175]

methyldopa,[106] nitrofurantoin,[18,255] dantrolene,[40,280] isoniazid[174] and paracetamol (acetaminophen),[24] and several others. The importance of a detailed drug history must again be emphasized in any patient with proven or suspected chronic hepatitis. If there is a failure to normalize serum transaminases upon withdrawal of a drug, then liver biopsy is mandatory to exclude other causes of chronic hepatitis. This may show chronic active hepatitis and may even reveal features of established cirrhosis. It is usually impossible histologically to distinguish between drug-induced chronic hepatitis and that from other causes. If a drug is suspected as the cause for chronic hepatitis, then removal of the drug and close monitoring of serum transaminases during this withdrawal period may enable the diagnosis to be made.

CHRONIC HEPATITIS IN ALCOHOLIC LIVER DISEASE

The effects of excessive alcohol consumption on the liver are varied. Generally, however, the spectrum of lesions extends from mild fatty changes, through acute alcoholic hepatitis (the histological infiltrate for which is the polymorph), to cirrhosis. Chronic active hepatitis is not frequently seen—indeed, the mechanism by which this lesion arises in alcoholic liver disease is poorly understood.[58] Although it is possible that alcohol may rarely produce a chronic hepatitis in a similar fashion to drug-induced chronic hepatitis, it is also possible that the hepatitis is actually caused by another process, for example co-existent chronic NANB/HCV hepatitis. In support of this contention, a recent study from Spain looked at 15 patients with alcoholic cirrhosis and found that 7 (45%) were anti-HCV positive.[90] These results were confirmed in a further study from Spain, which found that 39% of alcoholic cirrhotics were anti-HCV-positive,[32] although this study also revealed that an even higher proportion of patients with alcoholic cirrhosis who also had hepatocel-

lular carcinoma were anti-HCV-positive (77%; 23 of 30 patients). Another study from Italy has examined patients with chronic liver disease associated with alcohol abuse and found that 14 of 40 such patients (35%) were anti-HCV positive.[29] Ten of these 14 anti-HCV-positive patients also had chronic active hepatitis (CAH) on liver biopsy, whereas none of the 26 anti-HCV-negative alcoholic liver disease patients had CAH on biopsy.[29]

There may be one or two interpretations of these data; firstly the possibility that these results are spurious and for some reason (possibly the raised serum globulin levels), patients with alcoholic cirrhosis, especially those patients who also have hepatocellular carcinoma, have a high false positive anti-HCV rate. The second possibility is that these results are genuine and that a subgroup (about one-third) of Italian and Spanish patients with chronic liver disease associated with alcohol abuse will also have co-existing HCV infection, which may cause chronic active hepatitis and thus play a role in the evolution of their liver disease. The implications of this are that co-existing HCV infection may determine the nature and severity of the hepatic lesion in some patients who consume large amounts of alcohol. Further studies in this area are required.

WILSON'S DISEASE

Wilson's disease (see also Chapter 35) can present as a chronic active hepatitis. It may also present as fulminant liver failure. Histological differentiation from the other causes of hepatitis may be difficult. Although demonstration of excess copper in the liver (or its absence) is helpful, the simplest way to establish this diagnosis is through serum estimation of copper and caeruloplasmin. Measurement of the copper content of the liver biopsy specimen is also diagnostic.

α₁-ANTITRYPSIN DEFICIENCY

This condition in both adults and children can pursue a prolonged course with intermittent jaundice, and the histological features may sometimes be indistinguishable from other causes of chronic hepatitis.[117,276] However, a distinction can be made on the basis of the detection of PAS-positive globules in the liver, which can be shown immunologically to be retained α₁-antitrypsin, and the demonstration of the phenotype in the serum. This is discussed more fully in Chapter 43.

CRYPTOGENIC CHRONIC HEPATITIS

Cryptogenic chronic hepatitis should now indicate chronic hepatitis in which autoantibody markers, B and C viral markers, and evidence for other specific aetiologies are absent.[66] Studies from around the world (Europe and the Far East) suggests that 12–26% of patients with chronic hepatitis may fall into this category.[173] It is likely that many (if not all) of these patients are either autoantibody-negative chronic autoimmune hepatitis, or anti-HCV-negative chronic non-A non-B hepatitis. Another NANB virus may be involved in some of these cases. Many patients with cryptogenic chronic hepatitis may improve with steroid treatment,[65] suggesting that an underlying immunological disorder may be responsible for the majority. Other cases may need antiviral therapy. The relevance of this finding to the treatment of cryptogenic chronic hepatitis is discussed later.

TREATMENT OF CHRONIC HEPATITIS

GENERAL PRINCIPLES

Although therapy is available to control most types of chronic hepatitis, it may not be possible completely to 'cure' the patient; for example, chronic autoimmune hepatitis can be controlled by long-term immunosuppressive therapy, but relapses are common if therapy is discontinued. In the case of chronic viral hepatitis, approximately 50–70% of chronic NANB/HCV hepatitis but only 40–50% of chronic HBV patients will respond to interferon.[138,139] Thus, patients with chronic hepatitis need support and regular follow-up over long periods of time.

Patients should have regular monitoring of serum biochemistry and, in the case of viral hepatitis, of virus serology. In patients who have already developed cirrhosis, ultrasonography and estimations of alpha-fetoprotein should be performed at least yearly in order to exclude the development of hepatocellular carcinoma. The diet should be mixed, balanced and low in fat, and it would also seem sensible for patients to avoid large amounts of alcohol. Although patients with chronic hepatitis may feel tired, exercise is often well tolerated[224] and therefore should be encouraged.

Once the particular cause of the chronic hepatitis is established, patients can be treated in the specific ways described below. The indications for treatment should also reflect the severity of the inflammatory process; for example, patients with chronic persistent hepatitis (CPH) are less likely to progress to cirrhosis than patients with chronic active hepatitis,[16] although it must be remembered that reports of patients with CPH who later progressed to chronic active hepatitis and cirrhosis have been published.[2]

SPECIFIC THERAPIES

Chronic viral hepatitis

A variety of different antiviral agents including acyclovir, adenine arabinoside, interleukins and several other drugs have been tried in all three types of chronic viral hepatitis (HBV, HDV and NANB/HCV) with variable success. Although many of these agents have demonstrable antiviral activity, there may be problems with severe side-effects (for example, in the case of adenine arabinoside), or the antiviral effect may not be sufficient to result in a clinically significant response (in the case of acyclovir). The only antiviral agent with proven clinical efficacy, tolerable side-effects and broad range of activity against all three types of chronic viral hepatitis is interferon-α.

Immunosuppressive therapy, for example prednisolone, was initially thought to be beneficial in chronic viral hepatitis and was widely used. This has now been shown to be untrue, and patients with chronic viral hepatitis should not be treated with steroids or any other form of immunosuppressive therapy as they are likely to affect adversely the course of their disease. For example, in the case of chronic hepatitis B infection, controlled trials have now revealed that steroids are hazardous and can result in serious hepatic decompensation.[126] Thus, corticosteroids alone should not be used in chronic hepatitis B infection, unless they are given as a short ('priming') course prior to interferon-α therapy. The rationale for using them in this way is that the abrupt withdrawal of the steroids results in a modest stimulation of the immune system. This may help increase the response rates of interferon-α-treated patients with chronic hepatitis B infection, particularly those who acquired their infection during the neonatal period. In chronic NANB/HCV hepatitis, immunosuppressive therapy may appear to improve the hepatic inflammation as determined by monitoring of the serum transaminases. However, histologically there is very frequently a worsening in the degree of liver damage compared to patients with chronic NANB hepatitis who are not treated with this form of therapy.[235] The same is seen in chronic delta infection and further emphasizes the point that immunosuppressive therapy may be harmful in chronic viral hepatitis from any cause.

At present, the best single-agent therapy for chronic viral hepatitis of any cause is interferon-α. The interferons are naturally synthesized proteins that are produced in response to viral infection and other stimuli.[254] There are three major forms: interferon-α, produced by monocytes and transformed B lymphocytes; interferon-β, originating primarily from fibroblasts; and interferon-γ, made by T lymphoblasts. All three types of interferon have broad antiviral and immunomodulatory properties[212] that theoretically make them ideal therapeutic agents for chronic viral hepatitis, but only interferon-α has been studied extensively.

Chronic hepatitis B infection

Antiviral therapy is only required for patients with active viral replication; HBsAg 'carriers' without liver disease and with no evidence of active viral replication do not require treatment. In patients who are HBeAg-positive, the goal of interferon therapy is permanent disappearance of HBV e antigen from the serum and the development

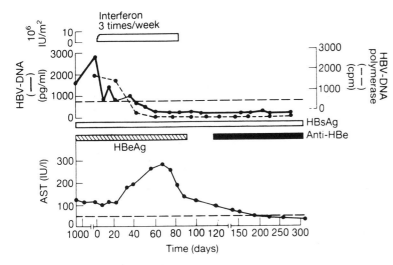

Figure 31.15 Effect of interferon-α, administered thrice weekly, to a patient with chronic hepatitis B infection. Note the rapid, early fall in viral DNA and DNA-polymerase, but the later seroconversion (from HBeAg positive to negative) associated with a delayed biochemical hepatitis. Loss of HBsAg is not important, and rarely occurs unless the patient has been a carrier for less than 4 years.

of antibody to HBe (seroconversion), which is associated with a permanent loss of replicating HBV from the liver and also results in a biochemical and histological remission in the majority of infected individuals.[124,221] In anti-HBe-positive patients, monitoring of the inhibition of viral replication, and thus the success of therapy, is more difficult and requires sequential measurement of HBV-DNA and/or DNA-polymerase.

There are two types of interferon-α commercially available: recombinant and lymphoblastoid interferons-α. Both types of interferon-α must be administered by intramuscular injection (generally 5–10 million units thrice weekly) and both are equally efficacious in chronic hepatitis B. In HBeAg-positive individuals who acquired their infection in adulthood, a 3-month course of thrice-weekly recombinant or lymphoblastoid interferon-α will produce seroconversion rates (loss of HBeAg) in 40–50% of subjects.[30,86,177] A review of the factors that appear to predict a seroconversion response indicates that Chinese chronic carriers (presumably infected from birth) show a very poor response, whereas European and North American carriers (who usually acquire their infection in adulthood) respond best.[139] Attempts to improve the response rates to interferon-α have focused on combination therapies, in particular further stimulation of the immune system by the use of a short 'priming' course of prednisolone prior to the interferon-α therapy.[139,210]

Other factors that are predictive of a seroconversion response to interferon-α therapy are high serum transaminases,[30] marked inflammatory activity on hepatic biopsy,[30] the presence of IgM anti-HBc[42] and low serum HBV-DNA.[210] Impairment of the host immune system, and in particular infection with the HIV virus, reduces the likelihood of a response to interferon-α treatment.[179] Other studies reveal that 3 months of therapy is as effective as and better tolerated than 6 months of therapy,[238] and also that thrice-weekly injections for 3 months are more effective and probably better tolerated than daily injections for 1 month.[167]

The mechanism of action of interferon in chronic hepatitis B infection is unknown, but several changes in the immune system and in the infected hepatocyte are believed to be important. An increase in MHC class I protein display in the hepatocyte occurs within 24 hours of starting therapy.[214] Interferon-α also stimulates the cell-mediated immune system and causes an increase in the CD4/CD8 ratio.[212] Changes in humoral immunity also occur, and patients who respond to therapy either have IgM anti-HBc present before treatment or develop it during the course of therapy.[42] The earliest sign of a response to interferon-α therapy is a fall in serum HBV-DNA and DNA polymerase levels (Figure 31.15), and a low pre-treatment serum HBV-DNA level is the most significant predictor of whether or not the patient will respond to therapy.[210] It is thus clear that, in addition to its immunostimulatory action, the direct effect of the interferon-α on HBV replication is also very important.

The main side-effects of interferon treatment are fever, chills and myalgia, which occur for a few hours after the initial interferon injections are given. These side-effects are generally well tolerated by most patients, although a small minority of patients may find them unacceptable and require interferon dose reductions. Interferon is a naturally produced substance and no major side-effects have yet been reported at doses of less than 10 million units three times a week. Thrombocytopaenia and dementia rarely may occur with higher dosage schedules.

Recent attempts to increase the response rates of chronic HBV patients to interferon-α by the addition of other antiviral agents, such as acyclovir or pre-interferon prednisolone, have been tried. Further stimulation of the immune system by 'priming' with pre-interferon prednisolone therapy has not been shown to be better than interferon therapy alone in adult acquired infection,[210] but preliminary results in neonatally acquired chronic HBV infection appear promising.[139] The few studies in this sphere have been analysed in detail in a recent critical review.[139]

Chronic delta hepatitis infection

There have been very few studies on the use of interferon-α in chronic delta (HDV) infection. Several small studies have indicated that both lymphoblastoid or recombinant interferon-α (high doses, of 5–10 million units thrice weekly) inhibit HDV replication, resulting in a fall in serum HDV-RNA levels and a corresponding improvement in biochemical and histological parameters of inflammation.[127] One controlled trial conducted in Italy[230] showed that 9 of 12 treated patients and none of 12 controls improved while on thrice-weekly recombinant interferon-α therapy given for 12 weeks. The pattern of improvement with interferon-α therapy is different from that seen in patients with chronic HBV infection successfully responding to interferon-α treatment. Unlike the delayed 'sero-conversion hepatitis' seen in chronic HBV infection, in chronic HDV hepatitis there is an immediate fall in serum transaminases, suggesting that it is the direct antiviral effect of interferon on HDV replication which results in the rapid reduction in hepatic inflammation. The benefit is not often permanent; in the trial described above[230] when assessed one year after the interferon had been stopped, all but one patient had relapsed. In this patient, however, there was permanent loss of HDV from the liver. At present the best option with chronic HDV infection is probably long-term interferon therapy in an attempt to suppress disease activity and reduce the high risk of progression to cirrhosis. Cure may only occur when HBs antigen is cleared.[91]

Chronic non-A non-B/HCV hepatitis

Interferons-α have now been studied in chronic NANB hepatitis, and initial uncontrolled studies indicated encouraging results,[267] with aminotransferase levels returning to normal within 2 months of therapy in approximately 80% of patients. Randomized controlled studies have now been performed in several centres, and results confirm the earlier findings of rapid normalization of aminotransferase levels while on low-dose (3–5 million units thrice weekly) interferon in 50–70% of patients.[68,77,138] Unlike the response seen in chronic hepatitis B infection, there is usually a rapid fall in serum aminotransferase levels during therapy (Figure 31.16). In parallel with the biochemical improvement, there is also histological improvement with suppression of hepatocellular degeneration and reduction of inflammation in treated patients.[68,79,204] Non-responders to interferon are more likely to have a more severe liver disease,[76] and higher doses of interferon used for longer periods of time may be more successful in this group of patients. Of course the long-term goal is a permanent 'cure', with normalization of aminotransferase levels and histology even after treatment has been discontinued. Data from these studies have also indicated that sustained remissions may be achieved in up to 50% of patients who respond to interferon therapy and who are treated for 6–12 months continuously. Even if relapse does occur on stopping therapy, continuous low-dose interferon is reasonably well tolerated by patients and

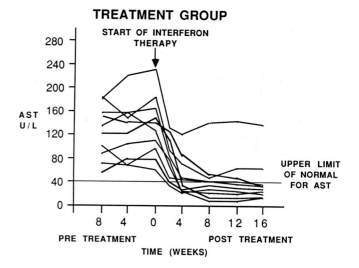

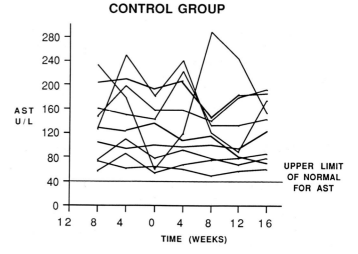

Figure 31.16 Effect of interferon-α on patients with chronic non-A non-B/C hepatitis. Note the rapid fall in serum aminotransferases (unlike in chronic hepatitis B infection). Also note the typical wide fluctuations in serum aminotransferases seen in the untreated control group. Taken from Jacyna 1989 (reference 138), with permission from the publisher.

may be an acceptable inconvenience in view of the high risk of development of cirrhosis.

Chronic autoimmune hepatitis

The mortality of untreated chronic autoimmune hepatitis is high; in most series 50% of patients die within 5 years. Because of the florid histological and immunological features, immunosuppressive therapy was tried and has now become the mainstay of therapy. Early uncontrolled studies reported on the use of corticosteroids[157,207] and azathioprine[171] with promising results and several randomized controlled trials have also been reported. Cook *et al.*, in a trial of 49 patients with autoimmune hepatitis,[55] found a striking reduction in mortality in the treated group (15 mg prednisolone per day) compared with the controls (13% vs 48%). Long-term follow-up of this group of patients has shown that the benefits of prednisolone therapy continue for 10–15 years.[146] Treated patients also developed a significantly higher serum albumin and lower bilirubin and globulin levels.[55] In a large prospective controlled trial from the Mayo clinic,[251] prednisolone therapy, with or without azathioprine, significantly improved life expectancy, histological resolution, and clinical and biochemical amelioration. It has now been convincingly shown that prednisolone is superior to azathioprine,[198] but the side effects at 15 or 20 mg of prednisolone per day are significant and sometimes serious. Although it is common practice to start with higher doses of prednisolone, it would appear that the optimum dose, in terms of maximal histological and clinical remission for the lowest rate of side-effects, is 10 mg prednisolone with 50 mg azathioprine.[256] The response to corticosteroid therapy should be monitored biochemically (serum transaminases) and histologically (repeat liver biopsy). Studies on the relapse rates seen after stopping prednisolone therapy are variable, but are generally quite high—from 50% to 75%.[64,116] Thus, although there is a chance that permanent biochemical and histological improvement may be seen after 1 year of continuous steroid therapy, the likelihood is that immunosuppressive therapy will need to be continued for many years.

Cryptogenic and other types of chronic hepatitis

Many patients with cryptogenic chronic hepatitis may improve with steroid treatment,[64,66] suggesting that an underlying immunological disorder may be responsible for the majority of cases. On this basis, it seems reasonable initially to treat most patients with cryptogenic chronic hepatitis with prednisolone (with or without azathioprine), particularly if there are features that may suggest an underlying autoimmune process, for example raised globulins.[176] Unfortunately, patients with chronic NANB hepatitis mistakenly 'treated' with prednisolone may show an improvement in serum transaminases, but histologically the degree of liver damage proceeds with greater vigour than if the patients were untreated.[235] Thus, a repeat liver biopsy after 6 months therapy is advisable in patients with cryptogenic chronic hepatitis, even if biochemical evidence suggests that the treatment is beneficial. In the case of patients with cryptogenic chronic active hepatitis who actually have autoantibody-negative autoimmune hepatitis but are mistakenly diagnosed as chronic NANB/HCV and treated with interferon-α, there may be a rapid and dramatic deterioration in the serum transaminases.[282] This is readily apparent within 48 hours of treatment and should be easily detected by careful monitoring of the serum transaminases during the early stages of interferon-α therapy. In this situation, changing the treatment to steroids may produce a rapid normalization of biochemistry.

The treatment of Wilson's disease with copper-chelating agents (e.g. penicillamine) and of α₁-antitrypsin deficient chronic hepatitis is discussed in Chapters 35 and 43, as is the role of liver transplantation as definitive treatment for chronic delta and autoimmune hepatitis and α₁-antitrypsin deficiency in Chapters 56 and 57. In the case of suspected drug- or alcohol-induced chronic hepatitis, withdrawal of the offending agent usually produces an amelioration in the degree of hepatic inflammation. If there is no improvement in the hepatic inflammation with withdrawal, then another underlying cause of chronic hepatitis should be suspected (for example, chronic NANB/HCV hepatitis).

REFERENCES

1. Abb, J., Zachoval, R., Eisenberg, J. et al. (1985) Production of interferon alpha and interferon gamma by peripheral blood leucocytes from patients with chronic hepatitis B infection. *Journal of Medical Virology*, **16**, 171–176.
2. Aldershvile, J., Dietrichson, A., Skinhoj, P. et al. (1982) Chronic persistent hepatitis: serological classification and meaning of the hepatitis system. *Hepatology*, **2**, 243–246.
3. Alexander, G.J.M. & Eddleston, A.L.W.F. (1986) Does maternal antibody to core antigen prevent recognition of transplacental transmission of hepatitis B virus? *Lancet*, **1**, 296–297.
4. Alexander, G.J.M. (1990) Immunology of hepatitis B virus infection. *British Medical Bulletin*, **46**, 354–367.
5. Almeida, J.D., Gioannini, P., Scalise, G. et al. (1973) Electron microscope study of a case of Australia antigen positive chronic hepatitis. *Journal of Clinical Pathology*, **26**, 113–119.
6. Alter, H.J., Purcell, R.H., Shih, J. W. et al. (1989) Detection of antibody to hepatitis C virus in prospectively followed transfusion recipients with acute and chronic non-A non-B hepatitis. *New England Journal of Medicine*, **321**, 1494–1500.
7. Andersen, P. (1974) Indirect immunofluorescence studies of smooth muscle antibodies. *Acta Pathologica et Microbiologica Scandinavica*, **82**, 577–584.
8. Anthony, P.P., Vogel, C.L., Sadikali, F. et al. (1972) Hepatitis-associated antigen and antibody in Uganda: correlation of serological testing with histopathology. *British Medical Journal*, **1**, 403–406.
9. Baggenstoss, A.H., Soloway, R.D., Summerskill, W.H.J. et al. (1972) Chronic active liver disease. The range of histologic lesions, their response to treatment and evolution. *Human Pathology*, **3**, 183–184.
10. Bamber, A., Murray, A., Arborgh, B.A.M. et al. (1981) Short incubation non-A, non-B hepatitis transmitted by Factor VIII concentrates in patients with congenital coagulation disorders. *Gut*, **22**, 854–859.
11. Bamber, A., Murray, A., Lewin, J. et al. (1981) Ultrastructural features in chronic non-A, non-B (NANB) hepatitis: a controlled blind study. *Journal of Medical Virology*, **8**, 267–275.
12. Bardadin, K.A. & Desmet, V.J. (1985) Ultrastructural observations on sinusoidal endothelial cells in chronic active hepatitis. *Histopathology*, **9**, 171–181.
13. Bearn, A.G., Kunkel, H.G. & Slater, R.J. (1956) The problem of chronic liver disease in young women. *American Journal of Medicine*, **21**, 3–15.
14. Beasley, R.P., Hwang, L., Lin, C. et al. (1981) Hepatocellular carcinoma and hepatitis B virus; a prospective study of 22,700 men in Taiwan. *Lancet*, **2**, 1129–1132.
15. Beasley, R.P., Hwang, L., Lin, C. et al. (1981) Hepatitis B immune globulin efficacy in the interruption of perinatal transmission of hepatitis B virus carrier state. *Lancet*, **2**, 387–393.
16. Becker, M.D., Scheuer, P., Baptista, A. et al. (1970) Prognosis of chronic persistent hepatitis. *Lancet*, **1**, 53–57.
17. Bergmann, K.F. & Gerin, J.L. (1986) Antigens of hepatitis Delta virus in the liver and serum of humans and animals. *Journal of Infectious Disease*, **514**, 702–705.

18. Black, M., Rabin, L. & Schatz, N. (1980) Nitrofurantoin-induced chronic active hepatitis. *Annals of Internal Medicine, 92*, 62–64.

19. Boxer, L.A., Yokoyama, M. & Wiebe, R.A. (1972) Autoimmune neutropenia associated with chronic active hepatitis. *American Journal of Medicine, 52*, 279–282.

20. Blumberg, B.S., Melartin, L., Lechat, M. *et al.* (1967) Association between lepromatous leprosy and Australia antigen. *Lancet, 2*, 173–176.

21. Bolin, T.D., Davis, A.E. & Liddlelow, A.G. (1973) Liver disease and cell mediated immunity in hepatitis-associated antigen carriers. *Gut, 14*, 365–368.

22. Bonino, F., Rosina, F., Rizetto, M. *et al.* (1986) Chronic hepatitis in HBsAg carriers with serum HBV DNA and anti-HBe. *Gastroenterology, 90*, 1268–1273.

23. Bonino, F., Negro, F., Baldi, M. *et al.* (1987) The natural history of chronic Delta hepatitis, In Rizetto, M., Gerin, J.L. & Purcell R.H. (eds) *Hepatitis Delta Virus and Its Infection*, pp. 145–152. New York: Alan R Liss.

24. Bonkowsky, H.L., Mudge, G.H. & McMurty, R.J. (1978) Chronic hepatic inflammation and fibrosis due to low doses of paracetamol. *Lancet, 1*, 1016–1018.

25. Bortolotti, F., Alberti, A., Cadrobbi, P. *et al.* (1985) Prognostic value of hepatitis B core antigen (HBcAg) expression in the liver of children with chronic hepatitis type B. *Liver, 5*, 40–47.

26. Boxall, E.H., Flewett, T.H., Paton, A. *et al.* (1976) Hepatitis B surface antigen and cirrhosis in Iraq. *Gut, 17*, 119–121.

27. Brechot, C., Scotto, J., Charnay, P. *et al.* (1981) Detection of hepatitis B virus DNA in liver and serum. A direct appraisal of the chronic carrier state. *Lancet, 2*, 765–767.

28. Bretherton, L., Brown, C., Pedersen, J.S. *et al.* (1983) ELISA assay for IgG autoantibody to G-actin: comparison of chronic active hepatitis and acute viral hepatitis. *Clinical and Experimental Immunology, 51*, 611–616.

29. Brillanti, S., Barbara, L., Miglioli, M. *et al.* (1989) Hepatitis C virus: a possible cause of chronic hepatitis in alcoholics. *Lancet, 2*, 1390–1391.

30. Brook, M.G., Chan, G., Yap, I. *et al.* (1989) Randomised controlled trial of treatment with lymphoblastoid alpha-interferon in Europid males with chronic hepatitis B virus infection. *British Medical Journal, 299*, 652–656.

31. Brown, S.E., Howard, C.R., Zuckerman, A.J. *et al.* (1984) Affinity of antibody responses in man to hepatitis B vaccine determined with synthetic peptides. *Lancet, 1*, 184–187.

32. Bruix, J., Barrera, J.M., Calvet, X. *et al.* (1989) Prevalence of antibodies to hepatitis C virus in Spanish patients with hepatocellular carcinoma and cirrhosis. *Lancet, 2*, 1004–1006.

33. Brzosko, W.J., Krawcynski, K., Nazarewicz, T. *et al.* (1974) Glomerulonephritis associated with hepatitis B surface antigen immune complexes in children. *Lancet, 2*, 477–482.

34. Busachi, C.A., Realdi, G., Alberti, A. *et al.* (1981) Ultrastructural changes in the liver of patients with chronic non-A, non-B hepatitis. *Journal of Medical Virology, 7*, 205–212.

35. Butler, R.C. (1984) Studies of experimental chronic active hepatitis in the rabbit. II. Immunological findings. *British Journal of Experimental Pathology, 65*, 509–519.

36. Canese, M.G., Rizetto, M., Arico, S. *et al.* (1979) An ultrastructural and immunohistochemical study of the delta antigen associated with the hepatitis B virus. *Journal of Pathology, 128*, 169–175.

37. Carman, W.F., Jacyna, M.R., Hadziyannis, S. *et al.* (1989) Mutation preventing formation of hepatitis B e antigen in patients with chronic hepatitis B infection. *Lancet, 2*, 588–591.

38. Carman, W.F., Fagan, E., Hadziyannis, S. *et al.* (1991) Association of a precore genomic variant of Hepatitis B virus with fulminant hepatitis B infection. *Hepatology, 14*, 219–222.

39. Cattan, R., Vesin, P. & Bodin, H. (1957) Cirrhoses dysproteinemiques d'origine inconnue chez la femme. *Bulletin de la societé Medicale des Hopitaux de Paris, 73*, 608–616.

40. Chan, C.H. (1990) Dantrolene sodium and hepatic injury. *Neurology, 40*, 1427–1432.

41. Chang, C., Enders, G., Sprengel, R. *et al.* (1987) Expression of the pre-core region of an avian hepatitis B virus is not required for viral replication. *Journal of Virology, 61*, 3322–3325.

42. Chen, G., Karayiannis, P., McGarvey, M.J. *et al.* (1989) Subclasses of antibodies to hepatitis B core antigen in chronic HBV infection;

changes during treatment with alpha-interferon: Changes during treatment with interferon and predictors of response. *Gut, 30*, 1123–1128.

43. Chen, T.J. & Liaw, Y.F. (1988) The prognostic significance of bridging hepatic necrosis in chronic type B hepatitis: a histopathologic study. *Liver, 8*, 10–16.

44. Chiaramonte, M., Farinati, F., Faginoli, S. *et al.* (1990) Antibody to hepatitis C virus in hepatocellular carcinoma. *Lancet, 2*, 301–302.

45. Choo, Q.-L., Kuo, G., Weiner, A. *et al.* (1989) Isolation of a cDNA clone derived from a blood-borne non-A non-B viral hepatitis genome. *Science, 244*, 359–362.

46. Christie, K.E., Endresen, C. & Haukenes, G. (1984) IgM antibodies in sera from patients with chronic active hepatitis with the measles virus matrix protein and nucleo-protein. *Journal of Medical Virology, 14*, 149–157.

47. Christoffersen, P., Dietrichson, O., Faber, V. *et al.* (1972) The occurrence of abnormal bile duct epithelium in chronic aggressive hepatitis. *Acta Pathologica et Microbiologica Scandinavica; Section A, Pathology, 80*, 294–303.

48. Christoffersen, P., Dietrichson, O. & Nielsen, J.O. (1973) Histological changes in two serologically defined groups of chronic hepatitis. *Acta Pathologica et Microbiologica Scandinavica: Section A, Pathology, 81*, 698–702.

49. Chu, C.M. & Liaw, Y.F. (1989) Studies on the composition of the mononuclear cell infiltrates in liver from patients with chronic active delta hepatitis. *Hepatology, 10*, 911–915.

50. Chu, C.M., Karayainnis, P., Fowler, M.J.F. *et al.* (1985) Natural studies of chronic HBV infection in Taiwan: Studies of HBV-DNA in serum. *Hepatology, 5*, 431–434.

51. Cohen, J.A. & Kaplan, M.M. (1979) The SGOT/SGPT ratio—an indicator of alcoholic liver disease. *Digestive Diseases and Sciences, 24*, 835–838.

52. Colombo, M., Kuo, G., Choo, Q.-L. *et al.* (1989) Prevalence of antibodies to hepatitis C virus in Italian patients with hepatocellular carcinoma. *Lancet, 2*, 1006–1008.

53. Combes, B., Stastny, P., Shoery, J. *et al.* (1971) Glomerulonephritis with deposition of Australia antigen–antibody complexes in glomerular basement membrane. *Lancet, 2*, 234–237.

54. Coodley, E.L. (1971) Enzyme diagnosis in hepatic disease. *American Journal of Gastroenterology, 56*, 413–419.

55. Cook, C.G., Mulligan, R. & Sherlock, S. (1971) Controlled prospective trial of corticosteroid therapy in active chronic hepatitis. *Quarterly Journal of Medicine, 40*, 159–185.

56. Cooksley, W.G., Bradbear, R.A., Robinson, W. *et al.* (1986) The prognosis of chronic active hepatitis without cirrhosis in relation to bridging necrosis. *Hepatology, 6*, 345–348.

57. Cooksley, W.G.E., Cowen, A.E. & Powell, L.W. (1973) The incidence of oxyphenisatin ingestion in chronic active hepatitis; a prospective controlled study of 29 patients. *Australian and New Zealand Journal of Medicine, 3*, 124–128.

58. Crapper, R.M., Bathal, P.S., Mackay, I.R. *et al.* (1983) Chronic active hepatitis in alcoholic patients. *Liver, 3*, 327–337.

59. Crapper, R.M., Bhathal, P.S., Mackay, I.R. & Frazer, I.H. (1986) 'Acute' autoimmune hepatitis. *Digestion, 34*, 216–225.

60. Crawford, D.H. (1990) Hepatitis B virus escape mutants. *British Medical Journal, 301*, 1058–1059.

61. Craxi, A., Montano, L., Goodall, A. & Thomas, H.C. (1982) Genetic and sex-linked factors influencing HBs antigen clearance. *Journal of Medical Virology, 9*, 117–123.

62. Craxi, A., Rainmondo, G., Longo, G., *et al.* (1984) Delta agent infection in acute hepatitis and chronic HBsAg carriers with and without liver disease. *Gut, 25*, 1288–1290.

63. Craxi, A., Di Marco, V., Magrin, S. *et al.* (1987) The natural history of chronic type B hepatitis in Southern Italy: effect of HBV replication and of HDV infection. In Rizzetto, M., Gerin, J.L. & Purcell, R.H. (eds) *The Hepatitis Delta Virus and Its Infection*, pp. 153–165. New York: Alan R. Liss.

64. Czaja, A.J., Ludwig, J., Baggenstoss, A.H. *et al.* (1981) Corticosteroid-treated chronic active hepatitis in remission. *New England Journal of Medicine, 304*, 5–9.

65. Czaja, A.J., Taswell, H.F., Rakela, J. *et al.* (1990) Frequency and significance of antibody to hepatitis C virus in severe corticosteroid-treated cryptogenic chronic active hepatitis. *Mayo Clinic Proceedings, 65*, 1303–1313.

66. Czaja, A.J., Hay, J.E. & Rakela, J. (1990) Clinical features and prognostic implications of severe corticosteroid-treated cryptogenic chronic active hepatitis. *Mayo Clinic Proceedings*, **65**, 23–30.
67. Davis, G.L., Hoofnagle, J.H. & Waggoner, J.G. (1984) Spontaneous reactivation of chronic hepatitis B infection. *Gastroenterology*, **86**, 230–235.
68. Davis, G.L., Balart, L., Schiff, E. *et al.* (1989) Treatment of chronic hepatitis C with recombinant alpha-interferon. A multicenter randomized controlled trial. *New England Journal of Medicine*, **321**, 1501–1506.
69. Davis, P. & Read, A.E. (1975) Antibodies to double stranded (native) DNA in chronic active hepatitis. *Gut*, **16**, 413–415.
70. De Francis, R., D'Arminio, A., Vecchi, M. *et al.* (1980) Chronic asymptomatic HBsAg carriers; histological abnormalities and diagnostic and prognostic value of serologic markers of HBV. *Gastroenterology*, **79**, 521–527.
71. De Groote, J., Desmet, V.J., Gedigk, P. *et al.* (1968) A classification of chronic hepatitis. *Lancet*, **2**, 626–628.
72. Dejean, A. (1985) Specific hepatitis B virus integration in hepatocellular carcinoma DNA through a viral 11-base-pair direct repeat. *Proceedings of the National Academy of Sciences of the USA*, **81**, 5350–5358.
73. Deodhar, K.P., Tapp, E. & Scheuer, P.J. (1975) Orcein staining of hepatitis B antigen in paraffin sections of liver biopsies. *Journal of Clinical Pathology*, **28**, 66–70.
74. De Vos, R., De Wolf-Peeters, C., Fevery, J. & Desmet, V.J. (1981) Non-A, non-B hepatitis in man: further evidence in favour of hepatitis-B like particles. *Liver*, **1**, 298–300.
75. De Vos, R., De Wolf-Peeters, C., Vanstapel, M.J. *et al.* (1982) New ultrastructural marker in hepatocytes in non-A, non-B viral hepatitis. *Liver*, **2**, 35–44.
76. Di Bisceglie, A.M., Lisker-Melman, M., Martin, P. *et al.* (1989) Factors predicting the outcome of alpha-interferon therapy for chronic non-A non-B hepatitis. *Gastroenterology*, **96**, A593.
77. Di Bisceglie, A.M., Martin, P., Kassianides, C. *et al.* (1989) Recombinant interferon alpha therapy for chronic hepatitis C. A randomized, double-blind, placebo-controlled controlled trial. *New England Journal of Medicine*, **321**, 1506–1510.
78. Dienes, H.P., Hutteroth, T., Hess, G. & Meuer, S.C. (1987) Immunoelectron microscopic observations on the inflammatory infiltrates and HLA antigens in hepatitis B and non-A, non-B. *Hepatology*, **7**, 1317–1325.
79. Dienes, H.P., Popper, H., Arnold, W. *et al.* (1982) Histologic observations in human hepatitis non-A non-B. *Hepatology*, **2**, 562–571.
80. Dienstag, J. (1983) Non-A Non-B hepatitis. In Thomas, H.C. & McSween, R.N.M. (eds) *Recent Advances in Hepatology*, Vol. 1, pp. 25–55. Edinburgh: Churchill Livingstone.
81. Dietrichson, O., Juhl, E., Christoffersen, P. *et al.* (1975) Acute viral hepatitis; factors possibly predicting liver disease. *Acta Pathologica et Microbiologica Scandinavica; Section A, Pathology*, **83**, 183–188.
82. Doherty, P.C. & Zinkernagel, R.M.A. (1975) Biological role for the major histocompatibility antigen. *Lancet*, **1**, 1405–1409.
83. Doniach, D., Roitt, I.M., Walker, J.G. *et al.* (1966) Tissue antibodies in primary biliary cirrhosis, active chronic lupoid hepatitis, cryptogenic cirrhosis and other liver disease and their clinical implications. *Clinical and Experimental Immunology*, **1**, 237–262.
84. Ducreux, M., Buffet, C., Dussaix, E. *et al.* (1990) Antibody to hepatitis C virus in hepatocellular carcinoma. *Lancet*, **2**, 301.
85. Dusheiko, G. & Paterson, A. (1987) Hepatitis B core and surface antigen expression in HBeAg and HBV DNA positive chronic hepatitis B: correlation with clinical and histological parameters. *Liver*, **7**, 228–232.
86. Dusheiko, G.M., Kassianides, C., Song, E. *et al.* (1988) Loss of hepatitis B surface antigen in three controlled trials of recombinant alpha-interferon for treatment of chronic hepatitis B infection. In Zuckerman, A.J. (ed.) *Viral Hepatitis and Liver Disease*, pp. 844–847. New York: Alan R. Liss.
87. Eddleston, A.L.W.F., Stern, R.B., Reed, W.D. *et al.* (1973) Detection of hepatitis B antigen by radio-immunoassay in chronic liver disease and hepatocellular carcinoma in Great Britain. *Lancet*, **2**, 690–694.
88. Eddleston, A.W.L.F., Mondelli, M., Mieli-Vergani, G. *et al.* (1982) Lymphocyte cytotoxicity to autologous hepatocytes in chronic hepatitis B infection. *Hepatology*, **2**, 122S–127S.
89. Edgington, T.S. (1984) Antihepatocyte antibodies and hepatitis. *Hepatology*, **4**, 346–347.
90. Esteban, J.I., Esteban, R., Viladomiu, L. *et al.* (1989) Hepatitis C virus antibodies among risk groups in Spain. *Lancet*, **2**, 294–297.
91. Farci, P., Karayiannis, P. & Brook, M.G. (1989) Treatment of chronic hepatitis delta virus infection with human lymphoblastoid alpha-interferon. *Quarterly Journal of Medicine*, **73**, 1045–1054.
92. Farza, H., Salman, A., Hadchouel, M. *et al.* (1987) Hepatitis B surface antigen gene expression is regulated by sex steroids and glucocorticoids in transgenic mice. *Proceedings of the National Academy of Sciences of the USA*, **84**, 1187–1191.
93. Fattovich, G., Brollo, L., Alberti, A. *et al.* (1990) Chronic persistent hepatitis type B can be a progressive disease when associated with sustained virus replication. *Journal of Hepatology*, **11**, 29–33.
94. Fattovich, G., Tagger, A., Brollo, L. *et al.* (1989) Liver disease in anti-HBe positive chronic HBsAg carriers and hepatitis C virus. *Lancet*, **2**, 797–780.
95. Fauerholdt, L., Asnaes, S., Ranek, L. *et al.* (1977) Significance of suspected 'chronic aggressive hepatitis' in acute hepatitis. *Gastroenterology*, **73**, 543–548.
96. Feizi, T. (1968) Immunoglobulins in chronic liver disease. *Gut*, **9**, 193–198.
97. Finlayson, N.D.C., Krohn, K., Fauconnet, M.H. *et al.* (1972) Significance of serum complement levels in chronic liver disease. *Gastroenterology*, **63**, 653–659.
98. Fitz, J.G., Petri, M. & Hellmann, D. (1987) Chronic active hepatitis presenting with rheumatoid nodules and arthritis. *Journal of Rheumatology*, **14**, 595–598.
99. Fonseca, J.C.F. & Simonetti, J.P. (1987) Epidemiology of the hepatitis delta virus in Brazil. In Rizzetto, M., Gerin, J.L. & Purcell, R.H. (eds) *The Hepatitis Delta Virus and its Infection*, pp. 507–514. New York: Alan R. Liss.
100. Foster, G.R., Goldin, R.D., Ackrill, A.M. *et al.* (1991) Expression of the terminal protein region of hepatitis B virus inhibits cellular responses to interferon alpha and gamma and double-stranded RNA. *Proceedings of the National Academy of Science of the USA*, **88**, 2888–2892.
101. Fujinam, R.S. & Oldstone, M.B.A. (1981) Alterations in expression of measles virus polypeptides by antibody: molecular events in antibody induced antigenic modulation. *Journal of Immunology*, **125**, 78–85.
102. Gerber, M.A., Hadziyannis, S.J., Vissoulis, C. *et al.* (1974) Hepatitis B antigen; nature and distribution of cytoplasmic antigen in hepatocytes of carriers. *Proceedings of the Society for Experimental Biology and Medicine*, **145**, 863–867.
103. Giusti, G. & Sagnelli, E. (1987) Epidemiology of HDV infection in Southern Italy. In Rizzetto, M., Gerin, J.L. & Purcell, J.H. (eds) *The Hepatitis Delta Virus and its Infection*, pp. 367–377. New York: Alan R. Liss.
104. Gocke, D.J. (1978) Immune complex phenomena associated with hepatitis. In Vyas, G.N., Cohen, S.N. & Schmid, R. (eds) *Viral Hepatitis*, pp. 277–284. Philadelpha: Franklin Institute Press.
105. Golding, P.L., Smith, M. & Williams, R. (1973) Multisystem involvement in chronic liver disease: Studies on the incidence and pathogenesis. *American Journal of Medicine*, **55**, 772–782.
106. Goldstein, G.B., Lam, K.C. & Mistilis, S.P. (1973) Drug-induced active chronic hepatitis. *Digestive Diseases and Sciences*, **18**, 177–184.
107. Good, R.A. (1956) Plasma-cell hepatitis and extreme hypergammaglobulinaemia in adolescent females. *American Journal of Disease of Children*, **92**, 508–509.
108. Govindarajan, S., De Cock, K.M. & Redeker, A.G. (1986) Natural course of delta superinfection in chronic hepatitis B virus-infected patients: histopathologic study with multiple liver biopsies. *Hepatology*, **6**, 640–644.
109. Govindarajan, S., Fields, H.A., Humphrey, C.D. & Margolis, H.S. (1986) Pathologic and ultrastructural changes of acute and chronic delta hepatitis in an experimentally infected chimpanzee. *American Journal of Pathology*, **122**, 315–322.
110. Gowans, E.J., Burrell, C.J., Jilbert, A.R. *et al.* (1981) Detection

of hepatitis B virus DNA sequences in infected hepatocytes by in situ hybridisation. *Journal of Medical Virology*, **8**, 67–78.

111. Gowans, E.J., Burrel, C.J., Jilbert, A.R. *et al.* (1983) Patterns of single and double stranded hepatitis B virus DNA and viral antigens accumulated in infected liver cells. *Journal of General Virology*, **64**, 1229–1239.

112. Hadziyannis, S.J., Merikas, G.E. & Afroudakis, A.P. (1970) Hepatitis-associated antigen in chronic liver disease. *Lancet*, **2**, 100–101.

113. Hadziyannis, S.J., Gerber, M.A., Vissoulis, C. *et al.* (1973) Cytoplasmic hepatitis B antigen in 'ground-glass' hepatocytes of carriers. *Archives of Pathology*, **96**, 327–330.

114. Hahn, E.G. & Schuppan, D. (1983) Collagen metabolism in liver disease. In Bianchi, L., Gerok, S. & Landman, L. *Liver in Metabolic Disease*. Falk Symposium no. 35, pp. 309–323. Lancaster: MTP Press.

115. Halliday, C. & Henahan, J. (1986) Congress report; 1986 World Congress of Gastroenterology. *Gastroenterology in Practice*, **2**, 6–16.

116. Hegarty, J.E., Nouri Aria, K.T.N., Portmann, B. *et al.* (1983) Relapse following treatment withdrawal in patients with autoimmune chronic active hepatitis. *Hepatology*, **3**, 685–689.

117. Hodges, J.R., Millward-Sadler, G.H., Barbatis, C. *et al.* (1981) Heterozygous MZ alpha-1-antitrypsin deficiency in adults with chronic active hepatitis and cryptogenic cirrhosis. *New England Journal of Medicine*, **304**, 557–560.

118. Hodgson, H.J.F., Wands, J.R., Isselbacher, K.J. *et al.* (1978) Alteration in suppressor cell activity in chronic active hepatitis. *Proceedings of the National Academy of Sciences of the USA*, **75**, 1549–1553.

119. Holborow, E.J., Hemsted, E.H. & Mead, S.V. (1973) Smooth muscle antibodies in infectious mononucleosis. *British Medical Journal*, **3**, 323–325.

120. Holdsworth, M.J., Hall, E. & Sherlock, S. (1965) Ulcerative colitis in chronic liver disease. *Quarterly Journal of Medicine*, **34**, 211–217.

121. Homberg, J.-C., Abuaf, N., Bernard, O. *et al.* (1987) Chronic active hepatitis associated with anti-liver-kidney microsome antibody type 1: a second type of autoimmune hepatitis. *Hepatology*, **7**, 1333–1339.

122. Hoofnagle, J.H., Gerety, J.R., Ni, L.Y. *et al.* (1978) Antibody to hepatitis B core antigen; a sensitive indicator of hepatitis B virus replication. *New England Journal of Medicine*, **290**, 1336–1339.

123. Hoofnagle, J.H., Seeff, L.B., Bales, Z.B. *et al.* (1978) Type B hepatitis after transfusion with blood containing antibody to hepatitis B core antigen. *New England Journal of Medicine*, **298**, 1379–1385.

124. Hoofnagle, J.H., Dusheiko, G.M., Seeff, L.B. *et al.* (1981) Seroconversion from hepatitis B e antigen to antibody in chronic hepatitis B infection. *Annals of Internal Medicine*, **94**, 744–748.

125. Hoofnagle, J.H., Dusheiko, G.M., Schafer, D.F. *et al.* (1982) Reactivation of chronic hepatitis B virus infection by cancer chemotherapy. *Annals of Internal Medicine*, **96**, 447–449.

126. Hoofnagle, J.H., Davis, G.L., Pappas, C. *et al.* (1986) A short course of prednisolone in chronic type B hepatitis: report of a randomised, double blind, placebo controlled trial. *Annals of Internal Medicine*, **104**, 12–17.

127. Hoofnagle, J.H., Mullen, K., Peters, M. *et al.* (1987) Treatment of chronic delta hepatitis with recombinant human alpha interferon. In Rizetto, M., Gerin, J.L. & Purcell, R.H. (eds) *Delta Hepatitis Virus and its Infection*, pp. 291–298. New York: Alan R. Liss.

128. Hopf, U., Meyer Zum Buschenfeld, K.H. & Arnold, W. (1976) Detection of a liver membrane autoantibody in HBsAg negative chronic active hepatitis. *New England Journal of Medicine*, **294**, 574–580.

129. Hsu, H.C., Lin, Y.H., Chang, M.H. *et al.* (1988) Pathology of chronic hepatitis B virus infection in children: with special reference to the intrahepatic expression of hepatitis B virus antigens. *Hepatology*, **8**, 378–382.

130. Huang, S.N. (1975) Structural and immunoreactive characteristics of hepatitis B core antigen. *American Journal of the Medical Sciences*, **270**, 131–139.

131. Hultcranz, R., Glaumann, H., Lindberg, G. *et al.* (1986) Liver investigation in 149 asymptomatic patients with moderately elev-

ated activities of serum aminotransferases. *Scandinavian Journal of Gastroenterology*, **21**, 109–113.

132. Ikeda, T., Pignatelli, M., Lever, A.M.L. *et al.* (1986) Relationship of HLA protein display to activation of 2-5A synthetase in HBe antigen or anti-HBe positive chronic HBV infection. *Gut*, **27**, 1498–1501.

133. Ikeda, T., Lever, A.M.L. & Thomas, H.C. (1986) Evidence for a deficiency of interferon production in patients with chronic HBV acquired in adult life. *Hepatology*, **6**, 962–965.

134. Imawari, M., Nomura, M., Kaieda, T. *et al.* (1990) Cytotoxicity of a non-A non-B hepatitis specific T-cell clone, TA-NB-2, on hepatocytes from patients with various liver diseases. In *Proceedings of the First International Symposium on Non-A Non-B Hepatitis, Tokyo* (in press).

135. Ishihara, K., Waters, J., Pignatelli, M. *et al.* (1987) Characterisation of the polymerised and monomeric human serum albumin binding sites on hepatitis B surface antigen. *Journal of Medical Virology*, **21**, 89–95.

136. Iwarson, S., Tabor, E., Thomas, H.C. *et al.* (1985) Neutralisation of hepatitis B virus infectivity by a murine monoclonal antibody: An experimental study in the chimpanzee. *Journal of Medical Virology*, **16**, 89–96.

137. Jacobsen, I.M., Dienstag, J.L., Werner, B.G. *et al.* (1985) Epidemiology and clinical impact of hepatitis D virus (delta) infection. *Hepatology*, **5**, 188.

138. Jacyna, M.R., Brooks, G., Loke, R.H.T. *et al.* (1989) Randomised controlled trial of lymphoblastoid alpha-interferon in chronic non-A non-B hepatitis. *British Medical Journal*, **298**, 80–82.

139. Jacyna, M.R. & Thomas, H.C. (1990) Antiviral therapy: hepatitis B infection. *British Medical Bulletin*, **46**, 368–382.

140. Jensen, D.M., McFarlane, I.G., Portmann, B.S. *et al.* (1978) Detection of antibodies directed against a liver-specific membrane lipoprotein in patients with acute and chronic hepatitis. *New England Journal of Medicine*, **299**, 1–7.

141. Johnson, G.D., Holborow, E.J. & Glynn, L.E. (1965) Antibody to smooth muscle in patients with liver disease. *Lancet*, **2**, 878–879.

142. Joseph, B.S., Cooper, N.R. & Oldstone, M.B.A. (1975) Immunologic injury of cultured cells infected with measles virus: Role of IgG antibody and the alternate pathway of complement. *Journal of Experimental Medicine*, **141**, 761–774.

143. Joske, R.A. & King, W.E. (1955) The LE cell phenomenon in active chronic viral hepatitis. *Lancet*, **2**, 477–479.

144. Kato, Y., Nakagawa, H. & Kobayashi, K. (1982) Interferon production by peripheral lymphocytes in HBsAg positive liver disease. *Hepatology*, **2**, 789–790.

145. Kawanishi, H. (1977) Morphologic association of lymphocytes with hepatocytes in chronic liver disease. *Archives of Pathology and Laboratory Medicine*, **101**, 286–290.

146. Kirk, A.P., Jain, S., Pocock, S. *et al.* (1980) Late results of Royal Free Hospital controlled trial of prednisolone therapy in hepatitis B surface antigen negative chronic active hepatitis. *Gut*, **21**, 78–85.

147. Klatskin, G. (1975) Persistent HB antigenaemia: associated clinical manifestations and hepatic lesions. *American Journal of the Medical Sciences*, **270**, 33–40.

148. Klingenstein, R.J. & Wands, J.R. (1984) The development of animal models in chronic active hepatitis. In Cohen, S. & Soloway, R.D. (eds) *Chronic Active Hepatitis*, pp. 249–259. New York: Churchill Livingstone.

149. Knodell, R.G., Ishak, K.G., Black, W.C. *et al.* (1981) Formulation and application of a numerical scoring system for assessing histological activity in asymptomatic chronic active hepatitis. *Hepatology*, **1**, 431–435.

150. Kojima, T., Callea, F., Desmyter, J. *et al.* (1990) Immuno-light and electron microscopic features of chronic hepatitis D. *Liver*, **10**, 17–27.

151. Kunkel, H.G., Ahrens, E.H., Eisenmenger, W.J. *et al.* (1951) Extreme hypergammaglobulinaemia in young women with liver disease of unknown aetiology. *Journal of Clinical Investigation*, **30**, 654–659.

152. Kuo, G., Choo, Q.-L., Alter, H.J. *et al.* (1989) An assay for circulating antibodies to a major etiologic virus of human non-A non-B hepatitis. *Science*, **244**, 362–366.

153. Kurki, P., Miettinen, A., Salaspuro, M. *et al.* (1983) Cytoskeleton

antibodies in chronic active hepatitis, primary biliary cirrhosis and alcoholic liver disease. *Liver*, **3**, 297–302.

154. Kurki, P., Gripenberg, M., Teppo, A.M. *et al.* (1984) Profiles of anti-nuclear antibodies in chronic active hepatitis, primary biliary cirrhosis and alcoholic liver disease. *Liver*, **4**, 134–138.

155. *Lancet* Editorial (1990) Hepatitis C virus upstanding. *Lancet*, **335**, 1431–1432.

156. *Lancet* Editorial (1990) The A to F of viral hepatitis. *Lancet*, **336**, 1158–1160.

157. Last, P.M. (1957) The treatment of active chronic infectious hepatitis with ACTH and cortisone. *Medical Journal of Australia*, **1**, 672–676.

158. Laure, F., Chatenoud, L., Pasquinelli, C. *et al.* (1987) Frequent lymphocyte infection by hepatitis B virus in haemophiliacs. *British Journal of Haematology*, **65**, 181–185.

159. Lebovics, E., Schaffner, F., Klion, F.M. & Simon, C. (1985) Autoimmune chronic active hepatitis in postmenopausal women. *Digestive Diseases and Sciences*, **30**, 824–828.

160. Leevy, C.M. & Tygstrup, N. (eds) (1976) *Standardisation of Nomenclature, Diagnostic Criteria and Diagnostic Methodology for Diseases of the Liver and Biliary Tree*. Basel: S. Karger.

161. Lefkowitch, J.H., Goldstein, H., Yatto, R. & Gerber, M.A. (1987) Cytopathic liver injury in acute delta virus hepatitis. *Gastroenterology*, **92**, 1262–1266.

162. Lenzi, M., Ballardinin, G., Fusconi, M. *et al.* (1990) Type 2 autoimmune hepatitis and hepatitis C virus infection. *Lancet*, **1**, 258–259.

163. Lesnicar, G. (1988) A prospective study of viral hepatitis A and the question of chronicity. *Hepato-gastroenterology*, **35**, 69–72.

164. Levin, S. & Hahn, T. (1982) Interferon system in acute viral hepatitis. *Lancet*, **1**, 592–594.

165. Levo, Y., Gorevic, P.D., Kassab, H.J. *et al.* (1977) Association between hepatitis B virus and essential mixed cryoglobulinaemia. *New England Journal of Medicine*, **296**, 1501–1504.

166. Lidman, K., Biberfeld, G., Fagraeus, A. *et al.* (1976) Anti-actin specificity of human smooth muscle antibodies in chronic active hepatitis. *Clinical and Experimental Immunology*, **24**, 266–272.

167. Lok, A.S.F., Weller, I.V.D., Karayiannis, P. *et al.* (1984) Thrice weekly lymphoblastoid interferon is effective in inhibiting hepatitis B virus replication. *Liver*, **4**, 45–49.

168. Lok, A.S.F., Karayiannis, P., Jowett, T. *et al.* (1988) Studies of HBV replication during acute hepatitis followed by recovery and acute hepatitis progressing to chronic disease. *Journal of Hepatology*, **51**, 671–679.

169. Machida, A., Kishimoto, S., Ohruma, H. *et al.* (1983) A hepatitis B surface antigen polypeptide (p31) with the receptor for polymerised human as well as chimpanzee albumin. *Gastroenterology*, **85**, 268–274.

170. Mackay, I.R., Taft, L.I. & Cowling, D.C. (1956) Lupoid hepatitis. *Lancet*, **2**, 1323–1326.

171. Mackay, I.R. (1968) Chronic hepatitis; effect of prolonged suppressive treatment and comparison of azathioprine with prednisolone. *Quarterly Journal of Medicine*, **37**, 379–392.

172. Mackay, I.R. (1984) Genetic aspects of immunologically mediated liver disease. *Seminars in Liver Disease*, **4**, 13–202.

173. Mackay, I.R. (1985) Autoimmune diseases of the liver; chronic active hepatitis and primary biliary cirrhosis. In Rose, N.R. & Mackay, I.R. (eds) *The Autoimmune Diseases*, pp. 291–337. Orlando: Academic Press.

174. Maddrey, W.C. & Boitnott, J.K. (1973) Isoniazid hepatitis. *Annals of Internal Medicine*, **79**, 1–12.

175. Maddrey, W.C. (1983) Drug-induced chronic active hepatitis. In Cohen, S. & Soloway, R.D. (eds) *Chronic Active Liver Disease*, pp. 131–146. Edinburgh: Churchill Livingstone.

176. Martin, P. (1990) Hepatitis C: from laboratory to bedside. *Mayo Clinic Proceedings*, **65**, 1372–1376.

177. Mazella, G., Saracco, G., Rizetto, M. *et al.* (1988) Human lymphoblastoid interferon for the treatment of chronic hepatitis B. *American Journal of Medicine*, **85** (suppl. 2A), 141–142.

178. McCollough, A.J., Fleming, C.R., Thistle, J.L. *et al.* (1983) Diagnosis of Wilson's disease presenting as fulminant hepatic failure. *Gastroenterology*, **84**, 161–166.

179. McDonald, J.A., Caruso, L., Karayiannis, P. *et al.* (1987) Diminished responsiveness of male homosexual chronic hepatitis B carriers with HTLV-III antibodies to recombinant alpha-interferon. *Hepatology*, **7**, 719–723.

180. McDonald, G.S.A., Courtney, M.G., Shattock, A.G. *et al.* (1989) IgM antibodies and histopathological evidence of chronicity of hepatitis A. *Liver*, **9**, 223–228.

181. McFarlane, B.M., McSorley, C.G., Vergani, D. *et al.* (1986) Serum antibodies reacting with the hepatic asialoglycoprotein receptor (hepatic lectin) in acute and chronic liver disorders. *Journal of Hepatology*, **3**, 196–208.

182. McFarlane, I.G., Wojcicka, B.M., Williams, R. *et al.* (1980) Antigens of the human liver. *Clinical and Experimental Immunology*, **40**, 1–7.

183. McFarlane, I.G., Hegarty, J.E., McSorley, C.G. *et al.* (1984) Antibodies to liver-specific protein predict outcome of treatment withdrawal in autoimmune chronic active hepatitis. *Lancet*, **2**, 954–956.

184. McFarlane, I.G., Smith, H.M., Johnson, P.J. *et al.* (1990) Hepatitis C virus antibodies in chronic active hepatitis: pathogenetic factor or false positive? *Lancet*, **335**, 754–758.

185. McMahon, B.J., Heyward, W.L., Templin, D.W. *et al.* (1989) Hepatitis B-associated polyarteritis nodosa in Alaskan Eskimos: clinical and epidemiologic features and long-term follow-up. *Hepatology*, **9**, 97–101.

186. Meyer zum Buschenfelde, K.H. & Manns, M. (1984) Mechanisms of autoimmune liver disease. *Seminars in Liver Disease*, **4**, 26–36.

187. Michitaka, K., Horiike, N., Nadano, S. *et al.* (1988) Change of hepatitis B virus DNA distribution associated with the progression of chronic hepatitis. *Liver*, **8**, 247–253.

188. Mieli–Vergani, G., Vergani, D., Jenkins, P.J. *et al.* (1979) Lymphocyte cytotoxicity to autologous hepatocytes in HBsAg-negative chronic active hepatitis. *Clinical and Experimental Immunology*, **38**, 16–21.

189. Milani, S., Ambu, S., Patussi, V. *et al.* (1988) Serum HBV DNA and intrahepatic hepatitis B core antigen (HBcAg) in chronic hepatitis B virus infection: correlation with infectivity and liver histology. *Hepatogastroenterology*, **35**, 306–308.

190. Millward-Sadler, G.H. (1976) Pathological aspects of virus hepatitis. In Truelove, S. & Ritchie, J.A. (eds) *Topics in Gastroenterology*, Vol. 4, pp. 29–54. Oxford: Blackwell Scientific.

191. Mistilis, S.P., Skyring, A.P. & Blackburn, C.R.B. (1968) Natural history of chronic active hepatitis. I. Clinical features, course, diagnostic criteria, morbidity, mortality and survival. *Australasian Annals of Medicine*, **17**, 214–223.

192. Mondelli, M., Mieli–Vergani, G., Alberti, A. *et al.* (1982) Specificity of T lymphocyte cytotoxicity to autologous hepatocytes in chronic hepatitis B virus infection; evidence that T cells are directed against HBV antigen expressed on hepatocytes. *Journal of Immunology*, **129**, 2773–2778.

193. Mondelli, M. & Eddleston, A.L.W.F. (1984) Mechanisms of liver cell injury in acute and chronic hepatitis B virus infection. *Seminars in Liver Disease*, **4**, 47–59.

194. Mondelli, M., Tedder, R.S., Ferns, B. *et al.* (1986) Differential distribution of hepatitis B core and e antigens in hepatocytes: analysis by monoclonal antibodies. *Hepatology*, **6**, 199–204.

195. Monjardino, J.P. & Saldanha, J.A. (1990) Delta hepatitis. *British Medical Bulletin*, **46**, 399–407.

196. Montano, L., Miescher, G.C. *et al.* (1982) Hepatitis B virus and HLA display in the liver during chronic hepatitis B virus infection. *Hepatology*, **2**, 557–561.

197. Munoz, L.E., De Villiers, D., Markham, D. *et al.* (1982) Complement activation in chronic liver disease. *Clinical and Experimental Immunology*, **47**, 548–554.

198. Murray-Lyon, I.A., Stern, R.B. & Williams, R. (1973) Controlled trial of prednisolone and azathioprine in active chronic hepatitis. *Lancet*, **1**, 735–737.

199. Mushahwar, I.K., McGrath, L.C., Drnec, J. *et al.* (1981) Radioimmunoassay for detection of hepatitis e antigen and its antibody: Results of clinical evaluation. *American Journal of Clinical Pathology*, **76**, 692–697.

200. Nash, A.A. (1985) Tolerance and suppression in virus disease. *British Medical Bulletin*, **41**, 41–45.

201. Nebel, O.T., Furnes, M.F., Castell Do. *et al.* (1976) Symptomatic gastroesophageal reflux; incidence and precipitating factors. *American Journal of Digestive Disease*, **21**, 953–956.

202. Neurath, A.R., Kent, S.B.H., Stricer, K. *et al.* (1986) Identification and chemical synthesis of a host receptor binding site on hepatitis B virus. *Cell,* **46**, 429–436.

203. Novick, D.M. (1985) Hepatitis D virus antibody in HBsAg-positive and HBsAg-negative substance abusers with chronic liver disease. *Journal of Medical Virology,* **15**, 351–359.

204. Omata, M., Yoshimi, I., Yokosuka, O. *et al.* (1989) Histological changes of the liver by treatment of chronic non-A non-B hepatitis with recombinant leukocyte interferon alpha. *Digestive Diseases and Sciences,* **34**, 330–337.

205. Onji, M., Lever, A.M.L., Saito, I. *et al.* (1989) Defective response to interferons in cells transfected with the hepatitis B genome. *Hepatology,* **9**, 92–96.

206. Ou, J., Lauk, O. & Rutter, W. (1986) Hepatitis B gene function: The pre-core region targets the core antigen to cellular membranes and causes the secretion of the HBe antigen. *Proceedings of the National Academy of Sciences of the USA,* **83**, 1578–1582.

207. Page, A.R. & Good, R.A. (1960) Plasma-cell hepatitis with special attention to steroid therapy. *American Journal of Diseases of Children,* **99**, 288–314.

208. Panush, R.S., Wilkinson, L.S. & Fagan, R.R. (1973) Chronic active hepatitis associated with eosinophilia and Coombs positive haemolytic anaemia. *Gastroenterology,* **64**, 1015–1019.

209. Paz, M.O., Brenes, F., Karayiannis, P. *et al.* (1986) Chronic hepatitis B virus infection. Viral replication and patterns of inflammatory activity: serological, clinical and histological correlations. *Journal of Hepatology,* **3**, 371–377.

210. Perillo, R.P., Schiff, E.R., Davis, G.L. *et al.* (1990) A randomized, controlled trial of interferon alpha-2b alone and after prednisolone withdrawal for the treatment of chronic hepatitis B. *New England Journal of Medicine,* **323**, 295–301.

211. Perrin, L.H., Joseph, B.S., Cooper, N.R. *et al.* (1976) Mechanisms of injury of virus infected cells by antiviral antibody and complement: Participation of IgG, F(ab) and the alternate complement pathway. *Journal of Experimental Medicine,* **143**, 1027–1041.

212. Peters, M., Davis, G.L., Dooley, J.S. *et al.* (1986) The interferon system in acute and chronic viral hepatitis. In Popper, H. & Schaffner, F. (eds) *Progress in Liver Disease,* Vol. 8, pp. 453–467. New York: Grune and Stratton.

213. Peters, R.L. (1975) Viral hepatitis: a pathologic spectrum. *American Journal of Medicine,* **270**, 17–31.

214. Pignatelli, M., Waters, J., Lever, A.M.L. *et al.* (1986) HLA class I antigens in hepatocyte membrane during recovery from acute hepatitis infection and during interferon therapy of chronic hepatitis B infection. *Hepatology,* **6**, 349–353.

215. Pignatelli, M., Waters, J., Lever, A.M.L. *et al.* (1987) Cytotoxic T-cell responses to the nucleocapsid proteins of HBV in chronic hepatitis. *Journal of Hepatology,* **4**, 15–21.

216. Poitrine, A., Chousterman, S., Chousterman, M. *et al.* (1985) Lack of in vivo activation of the interferon system in HBsAg positive chronic active liver disease. *Hepatology,* **5**, 171–174.

217. Popper, H., Thung, S.N., Gerber, M.A. *et al.* (1983) Histologic studies of severe delta agent infection in Venezuelan Indians. *Hepatology,* **3**, 906–912.

218. Poulsen, H. & Christofferseon, P. (1969) Abnormal bile duct epithelium in liver biopsies with histological signs of viral hepatitis. *Acta Pathologica et Microbiologica Scandinavica,* **76**, 383–390.

219. Ramodori, G., Lenzi, M., Dienes, H.P. *et al.* (1983) Binding properties of mechanical and enzymologically isolated hepatocytes for IgG and C3. *Liver,* **3**, 358–368.

220. Read, A.E., Sherlock, S. & Harrison, C.V. (1963) Active 'juvenile' cirrhosis considered as part of a systemic disease and the effect of corticosteroid therapy. *Gut,* **4**, 378–393.

221. Realdi, G., Alberti, A., Rugge, M. *et al.* (1980) Seroconversion from hepatitis B e antigen to anti-HBe in chronic hepatitis B infection. *Gastroenterology,* **79**, 195–199.

222. Realdi, G., Alberti, A., Rugge, M. *et al.* (1982) Long term follow up of acute and chronic non-A non-B post-transfusion hepatitis; evidence of progression to liver cirrhosis. *Gut,* **23**, 270–275.

223. Richey, J., Rogers, S. & Van Thiel, D.H. (1977) Giant multinucleated hepatocytes in an adult with chronic active hepatitis. *Gastroenterology,* **73**, 570–574.

224. Ritland, S., Petlund, C.F., Knudsen, T. *et al.* (1983) Improvement of physical capacity after long-term training in patients with chronic active hepatitis. *Scandinavian Journal of Gastroenterology,* **18**, 1083–1087.

225. Rizzetto, M., Canese, M.G., Purcell, R.H. *et al.* (1981) Experimental HBV in delta infections of chimpanzees: occurrence and significance of intrahepatic immune complexes of hepatitis B core antigen and delta antigen. *Hepatology,* **1**, 567–579.

226. Rizzetto, M. (1983) The delta agent. *Hepatology,* **3**, 729–734.

227. Robertson, D.A.F., Zhang, S.L., Guy, E.G. *et al.* (1987) Persistent measles virus genome in autoimmune chronic active hepatitis. *Lancet,* **2**, 9–11.

228. Roggendorf, M., Deinhardt, F., Rasshofer, R. *et al.* (1989) Antibodies to hepatitis C virus. *Lancet,* **2**, 324–325.

229. Roosinck, M., Jamcel, S., Loukin, S. *et al.* (1986) Expression of hepatitis B viral core region in mammalian cells. *Molecular and Cell Biology,* **6**, 1393–1400.

230. Rosina, F., Saracco, G., Lattore, V. *et al.* (1987) Alpha 2 recombinant interferon in the treatment of chronic hepatitis delta hepatitis. In Rizzetto, M., Gerin, J.L. & Purcell, R.H. (eds) *Hepatitis Delta Virus and its Infection,* pp. 299–303. New York: Alan R. Liss.

231. Sanchez-Tapias, J.M., Vilar, J.H., Costa, J. *et al.* (1985) Natural history of chronic persistent hepatitis B. Relationship between hepatitis B virus replication and the course of the disease. *Journal of Hepatology,* **1**, 15–27.

232. Schalm, S.W., Summerskill, W.H.J., Gitnick, G.I. *et al.* (1976) Contrasting features and responses to treatment of severe chronic active liver disease with and without hepatitis B surface antigen. *Gut,* **17**, 781–786.

233. Schalm, S.W., Korman, M.G., Summerskill, W.H.J. *et al.* (1977) Severe chronic active hepatitis. Prognostic significance of initial morphological patterns. *American Journal of Digestive Diseases,* **22**, 973–980.

234. Scheuer, P.J. (1977) Chronic hepatitis: a problem for the pathologist. *Histopathology,* **1**, 5–19.

235. Schoeman, M.N., Liddle, C., Bilou, M. *et al.* (1990) Chronic NANB hepatitis: a lack of correlation between biochemical and morphological activity and effects of immunosuppressive therapy on disease progression. *Australian and New Zealand Journal of Medicine,* **20**, 56–62.

236. Schvarcz, R., Von Sydow, M. & Weiland, O. (1990) Autoimmune chronic active hepatitis: changing reactivity for antibodies to hepatitis C virus after immunosuppressive therapy. *Scandinavian Journal of Gastroenterology,* **25**, 1175–1180.

237. Sciot, R., Van den Oord, J.J., De Wolf Peeters, C. & Desmet, V.J. (1986) In situ characterisation of the (peri)portal inflammatory infiltrate in acute hepatitis A. *Liver,* **6**, 331–336.

238. Scully, L.J., Shein, R., Karayiannis, P. *et al.* (1987) Lymphoblastoid interferon therapy of chronic hepatitis B infection; a comparison of 12 vs. 24 weeks of thrice weekly treatment. *Hepatology,* **5**, 51–58.

239. Sergent, J.S., Lockshin, M.D., Christian, C.L. *et al.* (1976) Vasculitis with hepatitis B antigenaemia; long-term observations in nine patients. *Medicine (Baltimore),* **55**, 1–18.

240. Shafritz, D.A. & Kew, M. (1981) Identification of integrated hepatitis B virus sequences in human hepatocellular carcinoma. *Hepatology,* **1**, 1–8.

241. Shafritz, D., Shouval, D., Sherman, H.I. *et al.* (1981) Integration of hepatitis B virus DNA into the genome of liver cells in chronic liver disease and hepatocellular carcinoma. *New England Journal of Medicine,* **305**, 1067–1073.

242. Shattock, A.G., Irwin, F.M., Morgan, B.M. *et al.* (1985) Increased severity and morbidity of acute hepatitis in drug abusers with simultaneously acquired hepatitis B and hepatitis D virus infection. *British Medical Journal,* **290**, 1377.

243. Shaver, W.A., Bhatt, H. & Coombes, B. (1986) Low serum alkaline phosphatase activity in Wilson's disease. *Hepatology,* **6**, 859–863.

244. Shikata, T., Uzawa, T., Yoshiwara, N. *et al.* (1974) Staining methods of Australia antigen in paraffin section; detection of cytoplasmic inclusion bodies. *Japanese Journal of Experimental Medicine,* **44**, 25–36.

245. Shobokshi, O.A. & Serbour, F.E. (1987) Prevalence of delta antigen/antibody in various HBsAg positive patients in Saudi Arabia. In Rizzetto, M., Gerin, J.L. & Purcell, R.H. *The Hepatitis*

Delta Virus and its Infection, pp. 471–475. New York: Alan R. Liss.

246. Smedile, A., Dentico, P., Zanetti, A. *et al.* (1981) Infection with the delta agent in chronic HBsAg carriers. *Gastroenterology*, **81**, 992–997.

247. Smedile, A., Lavarini, C., Crivello, O. *et al.* (1982) Radioimmunoassay detection of IgM antibodies to the HBV-associated delta antigen. *Journal of Medical Virology*, **9**, 131–138.

248. Smedile, A., Lavarini, C., Farci, P. *et al.* (1983) Epidemiologic patterns of infection with the hepatitis B virus-associated delta agent in Italy. *American Journal of Epidemiology*, **117**, 223–229.

249. Smedile, A., Baroudy, B.M., Bergmann, K.F. *et al.* (1987) Clinical significance of HDV-RNA in HDV disease. In Rizzetto, M., Gerin, J.L. & Purcell, R.H. (eds) *Hepatitis Delta Virus and its Infection*, pp. 231–234. New York: Alan R. Liss.

250. Smith, M.G.M., Williams, R., Walker, G. *et al.* (1974) Hepatic disorders associated with liver/kidney microsomal antibodies. *British Medical Journal*, **2**, 80–84.

251. Soloway, R.E., Summerskill, W.H.J., Baggenstoss, A.H. *et al.* (1972) Clinical, biochemical and histological remission of severe chronic active liver disease; a controlled study of treatments and early prognosis. *Gastroenterology*, **63**, 820–833.

252. Stefanini, G.F., Meliconi, R., Miglio, F. *et al.* (1983) Lymphocytotoxicity against autologous hepatocytes and membrane-bound IgG in viral and autoimmune chronic active hepatitis. *Liver*, **3**, 36–45.

253. Stein, O., Fainaru, M. & Stein, Y. (1972) Visualisation of virus-like particles in endoplasmic reticulum of hepatocytes of Australia antigen carriers. *Laboratory Investigation*, **26**, 262–269.

254. Stewart, W.E. (1979) *The Interferon System*, 2nd edn. New York: Springer-Verlag.

255. Stricker, B.H., Blok, A.P., Claas, F.H. *et al.* (1988) Hepatic injury associated with the use of nitrofurans: a clinicopathological study of 52 reported cases. *Hepatology*, **8**, 599–606.

256. Summerskill, W.H.J., Korman, M.G., Ammon, H.V. *et al.* (1975) Prednisone for chronic active liver disease; dose titration, standard dose and combination with azathioprine compared. *Gut*, **16**, 876–883.

257. Sutnick, A.I., London, W.T., Gertsley, B.J.S. *et al.* (1968) Anicteric hepatitis associated with Australia antigen. Occurrence in patients with Downs Syndrome. *Journal of the American Medical Association*, **205**, 670–674.

258. Suzuki, K., Uchida, T. & Shikata, T. (1987) Histopathological analysis of chronic hepatitis B virus (HBV) infection in relation to HBV replication. *Liver*, **7**, 260–270.

259. Tapp, E. & Jones, D.M. (1977) HBcAg and HBcAg in the livers of asymptomatic HB antigen carriers. *Journal of Clinical Pathology*, **30**, 671–677.

260. Teisberg, P. & Gjone, E. (1973) Circulating conversion products of C3 in liver disease; evidence for in vivo activation of the complement system. *Clinical and Experimental Immunology*, **14**, 509–514.

261. Thomas, H.C., Potter, B.J., Elias, E. & Sherlock, S. (1979) Metabolism of the third component of complement in acute type B hepatitis, HB surface antigen positive glomerulonephritis, polyarteritis nodosum, and HB surface antigen positive and negative chronic liver disease. *Gastroenterology*, **76**, 673–685.

262. Thomas, H.C. (1982) Immunological mechanisms in chronic hepatitis B virus infection. *Hepatology*, **2**, 116S.

263. Thomas, H.C., Shipton, U. & Montano, L. (1982) The HLA system: Its relevance to the pathogenesis of liver disease. *Progress in Liver Disease*, **7**, 517–527.

264. Thomas, H.C. & Lok, A.S.F. (1984) The immunopathology of autoimmune and hepatitis B virus-induced chronic hepatitis. *Seminars in Liver Disease*, **4**, 36–46.

265. Thomas, H.C., Jacyna, M.R. & Waters, J. (1988) Virus-host interaction in chronic hepatitis B virus infection. *Seminars in Liver Disease*, **8**, 342–349.

266. Thomsen, P., Poulsen, H. & Petersen, P. (1977) Different types of ground glass hepatocytes in human liver biopsies. Morphology, recurrence and diagnostic significance. *Scandinavian Journal of Gastroenterology*, **11**, 113–119.

267. Thomson, B.J., Doran, M., Lever, A.M.L. *et al.* (1987) Alpha-interferon therapy for non-A non-B hepatitis transmitted by gammaglobulin replacement therapy. *Lancet*, **1**, 539–541.

268. Toh, B.H., Roberts-Thomson, I.C., Matthews, J.D. *et al.* (1975) Depression of cell-mediated immunity in old age and the immunopathic diseases, lupus erythematosus, chronic hepatitis and rheumatoid arthritis. *Clinical and Experimental Immunology*, **14**, 193–202.

269. Tozuka, S., Uchida, T., Suzuki, K. *et al.* (1989) State of hepatitis B virus DNA in hepatocytes of patients with noncarcinomatous liver disease. Its special relationship with necroinflammatory activity and the stage of disease. *Archives of Pathology and Laboratory Medicine*, **113**, 20–25.

270. Tremolada, F., Benvegnu, L., Casarin, C. *et al.* (1990) Antibody to hepatitis C virus in hepatocellular carcinoma. *Lancet*, **2**, 300–301.

271. Trevisan, A., Realdi, G., Alberti, A. *et al.* (1982) Core-antigen specific immunoglobulin G bound to the liver cell membrane in chronic hepatitis B. *Gastroenterology*, **82**, 218–222.

272. Trevisan, A., Gudat, F., Guggenheim, R. *et al.* (1982) Demonstration of albumin receptors on isolated human hepatocytes by light and scanning EM. *Hepatology*, **2**, 832–835.

273. Triger, D.R., Alp, M.H. & Wright, R. (1972) Bacterial antigens and dietary antibodies in liver disease. *Lancet*, **1**, 60–63.

274. Triger, D.R., Kurtz, J.B. & Wright, R. (1974) Viral antibodies in chronic liver disease. *Gut*, **15**, 94–98.

275. Triger, D.R., Kurtz, J.B., MacCallum, F.O. *et al.* (1972) Raised antibody titres to measles and rubella viruses in chronic active hepatitis. *Lancet*, **1**, 665–667.

276. Triger, D.R., Millward-Sadler, G.H., Czaykowski, A.A. *et al.* (1976) Alpha-1-antitrypsin deficiency and liver disease in adults. *Quarterly Journal of Medicine*, **45**, 351–372.

277. Tur-Kaspa, R., Burk, R., Shaul, Y. *et al.* (1986) Hepatitis B virus DNA contains a glucocorticoid-responsive element. *Proceedings of the National Academy of Sciences of the USA*, **83**, 1627–1631.

278. Turner-Warwick, M. (1968) Fibrosing alveolitis and chronic liver disease. *Quarterly Journal of Medicine*, **37**, 133–149.

279. Twu, J.S., Lee, C.H., Lin, P.M. *et al.* (1988) Hepatitis B virus suppresses expression of human beta-interferon. *Proceedings of the National Academy of Sciences of the USA*, **85**, 252–256.

280. Utili, R., Boitnott, J.K. & Zimmerman, H.J. (1977) Dantrolene-associated hepatic injury; incidence and character. *Gastroenterology*, **72**, 610–616.

281. Vento, S., Hegarty, J.E., Bottazzo, G. *et al.* (1984) Antigen-specific suppressor cell function in autoimmune chronic active hepatitis. *Lancet*, **1**, 1200–1203.

282. Vento, S., Di Perri, G., Garofano, T. *et al.* (1989) Hazards of interferon therapy for HBV-negative chronic hepatitis. *Lancet*, **2**, 926.

283. Vento, S., Garofano, T. & Di Perri *et al.* (1991) Identification of hepatitis A virus as a trigger for autoimmune chronic hepatitis type 1 in susceptible individuals. *Lancet*, **337**, 1183–1187.

284. Vergani, G.M. & Eddleston, A.W.L.F. (1981) Autoimmunity to liver membrane antigens in acute and chronic hepatitis. *Clinics in Immunology and Allergy*, **1**, 181–197.

285. Verme, G., Amoroso, P., Lettieri, G. *et al.* (1986) A histological study of hepatitis delta virus liver disease. *Hepatology*, **6**, 1303–1307.

286. Volpes, R., van den Oord, J.J. & Desmet, V.J. (1990) Hepatic expression of intercellular adhesion molecule-1 (ICAM-1) in viral hepatitis B. *Hepatology*, **12**, 148–154.

287. Volpes, R., van den Oord, J.J. & Demset, V.J. (1990) Immunohistochemical study of adhesion molecules in liver inflammation. *Hepatology*, **12**(1), 59–65.

288. Volpes, R., van den Oord, J.J. & Desmet, V.J. (1990) Adhesive molecules in liver disease. Immunohistochemical distribution of thrombospondin receptors in chronic HBV infection. *Journal of Hepatology*, **10**, 297–304.

289. Vyas, G.N., Williams, E.W., Klaus, G.G.B. *et al.* (1972) Hepatitis-associated Australia antigen, protein, peptides and amino acid composition of purified antigen with its use in determining sensitivity of the haemagglutination test. *Journal of Immunology*, **108**, 1114–1116.

290. Waldenstrom J. (1950) *Leber, blutproteine und nahrungsweiss stoffwechs.* Sonderband XV. Tagung. Bad Kissingen, p. 8.

291. Wands, J.R., Davis, T.E., Humphrey, R.L. *et al.* (1975) Serial studies on hepatitis B surface antigen and antibody following bone marrow transplantation for acute leukaemia. *Gastroenterology*, **69**, 879–884.

292. Waters, J.A., Jowett, T.P. & Thomas, H.C. (1986) Identification of dominant epitopes of the nucleocapsid (HBc) of the hepatitis B virus. *Journal of Medical Virology*, **19**, 79–86.

293. Weiner, A.J., Kuo, G., Bradley, D.W. *et al.* (1990) Detection of hepatitis C virus sequences in non-A non-B hepatitis. *Lancet*, **335**, 1–3.

294. Weller, I.V.D., Cohn, D., Sierralta, A. *et al.* (1984) Clinical, biochemical, serological, histological and ultrastructural features of liver disease in drug abusers. *Gut*, **25**, 417–423.

295. Wen, L., Peakman, M., Lobo-Yeo, A. *et al.* (1990) T cell directed hepatocyte damage in autoimmune chronic active hepatitis. *Lancet*, **336**, 1527–1530.

296. Wiedman, K.H., Bartholomew, T.C., Brown, D.J.C. *et al.* (1984) Liver membrane antibodies detected by immunoradiometric assay in acute and chronic virus-induced and autoimmune liver disease. *Hepatology*, **4**, 199–203.

297. Winkler, K., Junge, U. & Creutzfeldt, W. (1977) Ground glass hepatocytes in unselected liver biopsies. Ultrastructure and relationship to hepatitis B antigen. *Scandinavian Journal of Gastroenterology*, **2**, 167–170.

298. Wright, R.A. (1975) Hepatitis B and the HBsAg carrier: An outbreak related to sexual contact. *Journal of the American Medical Assocation*, **232**, 717.

299. Wright, R. (1977) Immunology of gastrointestinal and liver disease. In Turk, J. (ed.) *Current Topics in Immunology*. London: Edward Arnold.

300. Wu, J.C., Lee, S.D., Tsay, S.H. *et al.* (1988) Symptomatic anti-HBe positive chronic hepatitis B in Taiwan with special reference to persistent HBV replication and HDV superinfection. *Journal of Medical Virology*, **25**, 141–148.

301. Yamada, G., Takaguchi, K., Matsueda, K. *et al.* (1990) Immuno-electron microscopic observation of intrahepatic HBeAg in patients with chronic hepatitis B. *Hepatology*, **12**, 133–140.

302. Yoo, J.Y., Howard, R., Waggoner, J.G. & Hoofnagle, J.H. (1987) Peroxidase-anti-peroxidase detection of hepatitis B surface and core antigen in liver biopsy specimens from patients with chronic type B hepatitis. *Journal of Medical Virology*, **23**, 273–281.

Index

Carcinosarcoma, 1106
Cardiac matters, *see* Heart
Carnitine, parenteral nutrition-associated
        deficiency and supplementation, 134
Caroli's disease (congenital dilation of
        intrahepatic duct), 1218
    CT imaging, 565
β-Carotene
    absorption, 113
    in protoporphyria, 405
    sources, 112
Casoni test, 1568, 1569
Catabolism of hormones, 175, *see also*
        Hypercatabolism
Catalase, peroxisomal, ethanol oxidation
        and, 910–11
Catecholamines
    growth/regeneration and, 263–4
    hepatic encephalopathy and, 1270–1
Catheterization
    carbohydrate metabolic studies via, 46
        in liver disease, 50–1
    drainage probe insertion facilitated by,
        622
    for endoscopy, 596, 597
    for portal venography, 590
Caudate lobe, anatomy, 6
Cavernous haemangioma, *see*
        Haemangiomas
Cavernous transformation, Doppler
        ultrasound, 548
CD antigens in T-cell lymphoma, 1142
CD8 cells in liver disease, 236
Cefoperazone, pharmacokinetics, 441, 442
Cefotaxime, pharmacokinetics, 441, 443
Cefoxitin, pharmacokinetics, 443
Ceftazidime, pharmacokinetics, 443
Ceftriaxone, pharmacokinetics, 441
Cell, *see also specific cell types/components
        and* Histology; Ultrastructure
    death, cirrhosis as a feature of, 831–2, 834
    as extracellular matrix sources, 844–5
    regeneration, *see* Regeneration
    in viral hepatitis, 721–3
        access, 721
        damage/degeneration, 686–7, 721, 748
Cell-mediated immunity
    autoimmune hepatitis and, 807
    HBV and, 721, 721–3, 795
    primary sclerosing cholangitis and, 1021–2
Cell plates, parenchymal, 17, 18
    biopsy histology, 485, 486
Central nervous system in Wilson's disease,
        971–4
Centrilobular zone, *see* Perivenular zone
Cephalosporins, pharmacokinetics, 441,
        442–3
Cephalothin, pharmacokinetics, 441, 443
Cephamycins, pharmacokinetics, 441
Cephapirin, pharmacokinetics, 441
Cephazolin, pharmacokinetics, 443
Cerebrospinal fluid in hepatic
        encephalopathy, 1266
Cerebrotendinous xanthomatosis, 301, 305
Cerebrum
    in hepatic encephalopathy, 1265, 1266–8
    oedema, in acute hepatic failure, 10–18,
        661–2, 669–70
Ceroid pigment, staining for, 482, 483, 484
Cestodes (tapeworms), 1541, 1566–71
c-fos, metalloproteinase regulation and, 853
Chemical dissolution, 618, 1481–2, 1483–4
    of bile duct stones, 618, 1483–4
    of gallbladder stones, 1481–2

Chemotactic factors, acute hepatic failure
        and, 664
Chemotherapy
    antimicrobial, *see* Antibiotics *and specific
        (types of) antibiotics*
    cytotoxic, 1127–8, 1130–3
        embolization with, 1130
        infusion, *see* Infusion
        metastatic tumours, 1098, 1127–8
        pancreatic cancer, 1532–3
        primary tumours (in general), 1127,
            1129–30, 1130–2, 1132–3
        toxicity, 1247–9
Chenodeoxycholic acid (CDCA), 292
    in cirrhosis, 308
    metabolism, 295–6
    toxicity, 311
    treatments using, 131, 311
Chest
    pain in, in chronic cholecystitis, 1465
    X-ray, of jaundiced patient, 652
Children, 1189–232, *see also* Infants and
        neonates *and conditions not
        mentioned below*
    biopsies, 479
    cholestasis in, 114, 1195–6, 1196, 1197,
        1386
    cirrhosis
        alpha-1-antitrypsin deficiency and, 1176,
            1179–80, 1182
        genetic counselling, 1182
        Indian, 826, 1201
    liver disorders (in general), 1189–207, *see
        also specific disorders*
        medical aspects, 1189–207
        surgical aspects, 1208–32, 1419
    nutritional assessment in, 138
    papular acrodermatitis, HBV-associated,
        719–20
    radionuclide imaging, 530
    rheumatoid arthritis, 1004
    transplantation in, 1213, 1226, 1419,
        1450–3
    trauma, 1414
Chimpanzees, HDV infection, 736
Chlamydia spp., 1046
Chlorambucil
    in primary biliary cirrhosis, 895
    toxicity, 1248
Chloramphenicol
    adverse effects, 1243
        ultrastructural features, 499
    pharmacokinetics, 441–4
Chlordiazepoxide, pharmacokinetics, 437
Chlormethiazole, pharmacokinetics, 433
Chloroquine in clonorchiasis, 1555
Chlorpromazine
    damage caused by, immunological
        phenomena associated with,
        239–40
    pharmacokinetics, 438
Chlortetracycline, toxicity, 1243
Cholangiocarcinomas, 1099–101, 1520–8
    aetiology, 1099, 1553
    angiography, 586, 1523
    clinical features, 1099
    clonorchiasis and, association, 1553
    CT imaging, 565, 579
    diagnosis, 1521
        endoscopic, 602–3
    extent of, 1522–4
    hilar, 1520–7
    incidence, 1520
    location, 1520

    in middle third of bile duct, 1527–8
    MR imaging, 579
    natural history, 1520
    pathology, 1099–100
    percutaneous transhepatic
        cholangiography, 655, 1521, 1522,
        1523, 1524
    prognosis/course, 1100
    sclerosing cholangitis and
        differentiation, 1510, 1521
        primary, 1023
    treatment, 594, 1101, 1440, 1441, 1524–7
        endoscopic, 628, 629
    ultrasonography, 542–4
Cholangiography, 595–610, 654, 1474–5,
        1494–5
    in biliary atresia, 1211
    endoscopic retrograde, *see* Endoscopic
        retrograde
        cholangio(pancreato)graphy
    intravenous, of jaundiced patient, 654
    operative, 1474–5
    percutaneous transhepatic, 655–6, 1494–5
        of carcinomas, 654, 655, 1521, 1522,
            1523, 1524
        of jaundiced patient, 655–6
    in primary biliary cirrhosis, 889
    in primary sclerosing cholangitis, 1020–1,
        1022
Cholangiojejunostomy, retrograde
        intrahepatic, 1506
Cholangiopancreatography, endoscopic
        retrograde, *see* Endoscopic
        retrograde
        cholangio(pancreato)graphy
Cholangiopathy, infantile obstructive, 374
Cholangioscopic electrohydraulic lithotripsy,
        615–16
Cholangioscopy, 606–8
    percutaneous (transhepatic; PTC), 607,
        609–10, 611
    peroral, 607, 608
Cholangitis, 603–5, 612–13, 1466, 1472, *see
        also* Pericholangitis
    acute, 603
    ascending, 1466
        biliary atresia surgery complicated by,
            1212
    CT imaging, 565
    endoscopy
        diagnostic, 603–5
        therapeutic, 612–13, 1472
    intrahepatic, 374
    management principles, 1472
    pyogenic, *see* Pyogenic cholangitis
    sclerosing, *see* Sclerosing cholangitis
    suppurative, acute, 612–13
Cholecalciferol (vitamin D_3), 114, *see also* 1,
        25-Dihydroxyvitamin D_3; 25-
        Hydroxyvitamin D_3
Cholecystectomy, 1472–7
    bile composition affected by, 278
    gallbladder carcinoma, 1517–18, 1518–19
    jaundice following, 1379
    laparoscopic, 1476–7
    retrograde, 1474
    syndrome following, 1479
Cholecystitis, 544–5, 1460–6
    acalculous, 1461–2
        acute, 1215, 1461
        aetiology, 1461
        in AIDS, 1044
        in parenteral nutrition, 134
    acute/acute-on-chronic, 1215, 1460–3